Stell and Maran's
Textbook of Head and Neck Surgery and Oncology

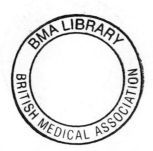

Primum non nocere (first, do no harm).

Hippocrates (*c.*460–377BC)

Every surgeon carries about him a little cemetery, in which from time to time he goes to pray, a cemetery of bitterness and regret, of which he seeks the reason for certain of his failures.

René Leriche (1951)

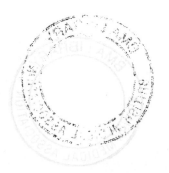

Stell and Maran's Textbook of Head and Neck Surgery and Oncology

Fifth edition

Edited by

John C Watkinson MSc MS FRCS DLO

Consultant Head and Neck and Thyroid Surgeon, Queen Elizabeth Hospital,
University of Birmingham NHS Trust. Formerly Hunterian Professor, Royal College of Surgeons of England, UK

Ralph W Gilbert MD FRCSC

Deputy Chief, Otolaryngology-Head and Neck Surgery, University Health Network; and Professor, Department of
Otolaryngology-Head and Neck Surgery, University of Toronto, Ontario, Canada

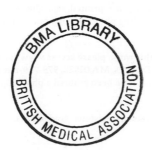

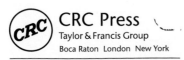

CRC Press
Taylor & Francis Group
Boca Raton London New York

CRC Press is an imprint of the
Taylor & Francis Group, an **informa** business

CRC Press
Taylor & Francis Group
6000 Broken Sound Parkway NW, Suite 300
Boca Raton, FL 33487-2742

© 2000 by Taylor & Francis Group, LLC
CRC Press is an imprint of Taylor & Francis Group, an Informa business

Visit the Taylor & Francis Web site at
http://www.taylorandfrancis.com

and the CRC Press Web site at
http://www.crcpress.com

JCW: I wish to thank my secretary, Angela Roberts, for her help and patience during the writing of this book. To my patients for their understanding, and to Ralph Gilbert for his enduring friendship and unlimited help during all stages of the book's transition. As ever, to my parents and grandparents for their wisdom and understanding and lastly to Esmé, Helen and William since without their ongoing love and support, none of this would have been worthwhile.

RWG: I wish to thank John Watkinson for the vision and ability to pull together this most recent edition of Stell and Maran. I would also like to thank all my mentors who have contributed so greatly to my passion for head and neck surgery and taught me so many of the secrets of this subspecialty. Among these, I would like to especially acknowledge Professor Patrick Gullane, my mentor and friend, without whom I would not be involved in the writing and editing of this book. Finally to my family Anita, Richard and Emily for their love, support and understanding of my passion and commitment to this profession.

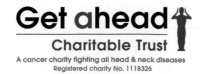

Get ahead

Charitable Trust

A cancer charity fighting all head & neck diseases
Registered charity No. 1118326

A proportion of the royalties from the sales of this book will be donated to the Get A-Head Charitable Trust, which fights head and neck diseases (including cancer) by funding research, promoting education and providing state-of-the-art equipment.

Contents

PART THREE: ENDOCRINE DISEASE

Section editor: John C Watkinson

PART FOUR: MALIGNANT DISEASE

Section A Surgery by primary site
Section editors: Ken MacKenzie and Gerald McGarry

Key to reference annotations

Seminal primary article = ●
Key review paper = ◆
First formal publication of a management guideline = ✳

Contributors

Patrick Addison BSc (Hons) MBChB MD FRCS (Plast)
Consultant Plastic Surgeon, St Johns Hospital and Royal Hospital for Sick Children, Edinburgh, UK

Kim Ah-See MB ChB
Consultant ENT Surgeon, Aberdeen Royal Infirmary, Aberdeen, UK

Shahzada Ahmed BSc(hons) MB ChB DLO FRCS
ENT Department, University Hospitals Birmingham NHS Foundation Trust, Birmingham, UK

Lorraine M Albon FRCP
Consultant in Diabetes, Endocrinology and Acute Medicine, Portsmouth Hospitals NHS Trust, Portsmouth, UK

Jawaher Ansari MBBS MRCP FRCR
Consultant Clinical Oncologist, The Beatson West of Scotland Cancer Centre, Glasgow, UK

Nigel Beasley FRCS
Consultant Head and Neck Surgeon, University Hospitals Nottingham, Queens Medical Centre Campus, Nottingham, UK

Rocco Bellantone MD
Professor of Surgery, Head Division of General and Endocrine Surgery, Dean, Università Cattolica del Sacro Cuore, Rome, Italy

Martin A Birchall MD (Cantab) FRCS FRCS (Oto) FRCS (ORL)
Professor of Laryngology, University College London, Consultant in Otolaryngology, Head and Neck Surgery, The Royal National Throat Nose and Ear Hospital, Royal Free Hampstead NHS Trust, London, UK

Kristien Boelaert MD PhD MRCP
Senior Clinical Lecturer and Consultant Endocrinologist, School of Clinical and Experimental Medicine, College of Medical and Dental Sciences, University of Birmingham, UK

Patrick J Bradley MBA FRCS FRACS(Hon) FRCSLT(Hon)
Honorary Professor and Emeritus Consultant Head and Neck Oncologic Surgeon, Nottingham University Hospitals, Queens Medical Centre Campus, Nottingham, UK

James S Brown MD FRCS FDSRCS
Consultant Oral and Maxillofacial Surgeon, University Hospital Aintree, Liverpool; Honorary Professor in Molecular and Clinical Cancer Medicine University of Liverpool, Liverpool, UK

Andrew K Chan BMedSci MBChB MRCP FRCR
Consultant Clinical Oncologist, University Hospitals Coventry and Warwickshire NHS Trust, Coventry, UK

John M Chaplin MBChB FRACS
Consultant Head and Neck, Endocrine and Reconstructive Surgeon, Department of Otolaryngology Head and Neck Surgery, Auckland City Hospital, Auckland, New Zealand

Nellie Cheah MBBS MRCP FRCR
Consultant Clinical Oncologist, Department of Oncology and Radiotherapy, Penang General Hospital, Penang, Malaysia

Daniel TT Chua MB ChB FRCR FHKAM(Radiology)
Consultant, Department of Clinical Oncology, Hong Kong Sanatorium and Hospital, Hong Kong SAR, China

Jonathan Clark FRACS
Consultant Head and Neck Surgeon, Sydney Head and Neck Institute, Royal Prince Alfred Hospital, Sydney, Australia

Peter Clarke BSc FRCS
ENT Consultant, Charing Cross Hospital, London, UK

Helen Cocks MD MBChB FRCS (ORLHNS)
Consultant Head and Neck Surgeon, Sunderland Royal Hospital, Sunderland, UK

Marc A Cohen MD
Assistant Professor, Otolaryngology/Head and Neck Surgery, Weill Cornell Medical College/New York Presbyterian Hospital, New York, NY, USA

Rogan Corbridge MB BS ARCO FRCS (Eng) FRCS (ORL)
Consultant ENT Surgeon, Royal Berkshire Hospital, Reading, UK

Graham Cox MS BS BDS (Hons) FRCS (Eng) FRCS (ORL)
Consultant ENT Surgeon and Macmillan Head and Neck Surgical Oncologist, Oxford University Hospitals, Oxford, UK

Carmela De Crea MD
Assistant Professor of Surgery, Università Cattolica del Sacro Cuore, Rome, Italy

Andrew Davies MBBS MSc MD FRCP
Consultant in Palliative Medicine, St Luke's Cancer Centre, Royal Surrey County Hospital NHS Foundation Trust, Guildford, UK

Stephen Dover FDSRCS FRCS
Consultant Oral, Maxillofacial and Craniofacial Surgeon Departments of Maxillofacial and Craniofacial Surgery, University Hospital Birmingham NHS Foundation Trust, and Birmingham Children's Hospital NHS Foundation Trust, Birmingham, UK; Honorary Senior Lecturer, University of Birmingham Birmingham, UK

Simone Eerenstein MD PhD
Department of Otolaryngology/Head and Neck Surgery, VU University Medical Centre/Cancer Centre, Amsterdam, The Netherlands

R James A England FRCS (ORL-HNS)
Consultant Otolaryngologist, Thyroid Surgeon, Hull Royal Infirmary, UK

Johannes J Fagan MBChB MMed FCS(ORL)
Professor, Chairman, Division of Otolaryngology, University of Cape Town, Cape Town, South Africa

Debra Fitzgerald
Formerly Clinical Audit Project Manager, Head and Neck Office, University Hospitals Birmingham NHS Foundation Trust, Birmingham, UK

Jayne A Franklyn MD PhD FRCP FMedSci
William Withering Professor of Medicine, Head, School of Clinical and Experimental Medicine, College of Medical and Dental Sciences, University of Birmingham, Birmingham, UK

Ian Ganly MB ChB PhD FRCS FRCS-ORL
Associate Professor, Head and Neck Service, Department of Surgery, Memorial Sloan-Kettering Cancer Center, New York, NY, USA

Ralph W Gilbert MD FRCSC
Deputy Chief, Otolaryngology–Head and Neck Surgery, University Health Network, Professor, Department of Otolaryngology–Head and Neck Surgery, University of Toronto, Ontario, Canada

Neil Gittoes BSc MBChB PhD FRCP
Consultant Encocrinologist and Honorary Senior Lecturer, University Hospitals Birmingham NHS Foundation Trust, UK

John Glaholm MB BS BSc FRCP FRCR
Consultant Clinical Oncologist, The Cancer Centre, University Hospitals Birmingham NHS Foundation Trust, Birmingham, UK

Michael Gleeson MD FRCS FRACS(Hon) FDS (Hon)
Professor of Otolaryngology and Skull Base Surgery, The National Hospital for Neurology and Neurosurgery, London, UK; Guy's, Kings and St Thomas' Hospitals, London, UK

David G Grant MB ChB BSc FRCS (ORL-HNS)
Senior Associate Consultant, Department of Otolaryngology Head and Neck Surgery, Mayo Clinic, Jacksonville, FL, USA

Robert J Grimer FRCS FRCSEd (Orth)
Consultant Orthopaedic Oncologist, Royal Orthopaedic Hospital Birmingham, UK

Patrick J Gullane CM MB FRCSC FACS FRACS(Hon) FRCS(Hon)
Otolaryngologist-in-Chief, University Health Network, Wharton Chair in Head and Neck Surgery, Princess Margaret Hospital, Professor and Chairman, Department of Otolaryngology – Head and Neck Surgery, University of Toronto, Toronto, Ontario, Canada

Gillian L Hall FRCPath FDS
Department of Oral Pathology, Liverpool University Dental Hospital, Liverpool, UK

Kevin J Harrington PhD FRCR FRCP
Reader in Biological Cancer Therapies, The Institute of Cancer Research, London, UK

Barney Harrison MB BS MS FRCS
Consultant Endocrine Surgeon, Royal Hallamshire Hospital, and Honorary Senior Clinical Lecturer, University of Sheffield, Sheffield, UK

Andrew Hartley MRCP FRCR
Consultant Clinical Oncologist, University Hospitals Birmingham NHS Foundation Trust, Birmingham, UK

Michael L Hinni MD
Associate Professor, Department of Otolaryngology Head and Neck Surgery, Mayo Clinic, Phoenix, AZ, USA

Jarrod Homer FRCS MD
Consultant Head and Neck Surgeon and Otolaryngologist, Manchester Royal Infirmary; Honorary Reader, University of Manchester, Manchester, UK

David J Howard FRCS FRCSEd
Emeritus Professor of Head and Neck Oncology, Imperial College London, Emeritus Senior Lecturer, University College London, UK

Richard M Irving MD FRCS (ORL-HNS)
Consultant Skull Base Surgeon, University Hospitals Birmingham NHS Foundation Trust, Birmingham, UK

Petra J Jankowska BSc MRCP FRCR
Beacon Centre, Taunton and Somerset NHS Foundation Trust, Taunton, UK

Jean-Pierre Jeannon FRCS (ORL-HNS)
Consultant Otorhinolaryngologist Head and Neck Surgeon, Department of Otorhinolaryngology, Head and Neck Surgery, Guy's and St Thomas' Hospital, London, UK

Alan Johnson MB ChB ChM FRCS(Edin) FRCS(Glas)
ENT Department, University Hospitals Birmingham NHS Foundation Trust, Birmingham, UK

Rajive M Jose MBBS MS FRCS (PLASTIC SURGERY)
Specialist Registrar, Department of Plastic Surgery, University Hospitals Birmingham NHS Foundation Trust, Birmingham, UK

Rehan Kazi MS DNB FRCS FACS PhD
Team Leader (Outcomes), Royal Marsden Hospital, London, UK

Dae Kim MBChB BDS MRCS FRCS (Orl-HNS) MSc PhD
Consultant Head and Neck and Endocrine Surgeon, Department of Otolaryngology, Queen Alexandra Hospital, Portsmouth, UK

C René Leemans MD PhD
Professor and Chair, Department of Otolaryngology–Head and Neck Surgery, VU University Medical Centre/VUmc Cancer Centre, Amsterdam, The Netherlands

David Lesnik MD
Clinical Fellow in Thyroid and Parathyroid Surgery, Massachusetts Eye and Ear Infirmary, Boston, MA, USA

Celestino Pio Lombardi MD
Assistant Professor of Surgery, Università Cattolica del Sacro Cuore, Rome, Italy

Valerie J Lund CBE MS FRCS FRCSEd
Professor of Rhinology, University College London, Honorary
Consultant ENT Surgeon, Royal Free, University College and
Moorfields Hospitals, London, UK

Kenneth MacKenzie MBChB FRCSEd
Consultant Otorhinolaryngologist and Head and Neck Surgeon
Glasgow Royal Infirmary; Honorary Clinical Senior Lecturer,
University of Glasgow, Glasgow, UK

Prem Mahendra MD FRCP FRCPath
Consultant Haemato-Oncologist, Centre for Clinical
Haematology, University Hospitals Birmingham NHS Foundation
Trust, Birmingham, UK

Richard CW Martin MBChB FRACS MS
Surgical Oncologist/Head and Neck Surgeon, New Zealand
Melanoma Unit, Waitemata District Health Board, Northshore
Hospital and the University of Auckland, Auckland, New Zealand

Thomas PC Martin BA(Hons) FRCS(ORL-HNS)
National Otology Fellow, Addenbrooke's Hospital NHS Trust,
Cambridge, UK

Tim Martin MSc FRCS FRCS (OMFS) FDSRCS
Oral and Maxillofacial Surgeon, University Hospitals Birmingham
NHS Foundation Trust; and Honorary Senior Lecturer, Faculty of
Dentistry and Medicine, University of Birmingham, Birmingham,
UK

Des McGuire RN BPhil Dip HE (MENTAL HEALTH), MBACP
Head and Neck Counsellor, ENT/Maxillofacial Department,
University Hospitals Birmingham NHS Foundation Trust,
Birmingham, UK

Gerald W McGarry MB ChB FRCS (Glas) FRCS (Ed) FRCS (ORL-HNS) MD
Consultant ENT Surgeon, Glasgow Royal Infirmary, Glasgow, UK

Nick P McIvor
Consultant Otolaryngologist, Head and Neck Surgeon, Auckland
District Health Board, New Zealand

Hisham Mehanna PhD BMedSc(hons) MBChB(hons) FRCS FRCS (ORL-HNS)
Honorary Professor of Head and Neck and Thyroid Surgery
Director, Institute of Head and Neck Studies and Education,
University Hospital, Coventry, UK

Ram Moorthy FRCS (ORL-HNS)
Consultant ENT Surgeon, Wexham Park Hospital, Wexham, UK

Laura Moss FRCP FRCR LLM
Consultant Clinical Oncologist, Velindre Hospital, Cardiff, UK

Zoë Neary
Macmillan Head and Neck Clinical Nurse Specialist, Queen
Elizabeth Hospital, University Hospitals Birmingham NHS
Foundation Trust, Birmingham, UK

Peter C Neligan MB FRCS (I) FRCSC, FACS
Professor of Surgery and Director of the Center for
Reconstructive Surgery, University of Washington Medical
Center, Seattle WA, USA

Andrew J Nicol MBChB FCS
Associate Professor, Trauma Surgeon and Head of Trauma Centre,
Groote Schuur Hospital, University of Cape Town, Cape Town,
South Africa

Chris M Nutting MD MRCP FRCR
Consultant Clinical Oncologist, Head and Neck Unit, Royal
Marsden NHS Foundation Trust, London, UK

Tadhg P O'Dwyer DLO FRCS FRCS(I)
Consultant Otolaryngologist Head and Neck Surgeon, Mater
University Hospital, Dublin, Ireland

Julie Olliff BMedSci BMBS FRCP FRCR FBIR
Consultant Radiologist, Imaging, University Hospitals
Birmingham NHS Foundation Trust, Birmingham, UK

Alison Page BSc MBChB MRCP FRCR
Consultant Radiologist, Imaging, University Hospitals
Birmingham NHS Foundation Trust, Birmingham, UK

Vinidh Paleri MS FRCS (ORL-HNS)
Consultant Head and Neck and Thyroid Surgeon, Otolaryngology-
Head and Neck Surgery, Newcastle upon Tyne Hospitals NHS
Trust; Honorary Clinical Senior Lecturer, Northern Institute for
Cancer Research, Newcastle University, Newcastle upon Tyne, UK

Carsten E Palme MB BS FRACS
Consultant Surgeon, Clinical Senior Lecturer, Otolaryngology
Head and Neck Surgery, Westmead Hospital, University of
Sydney, Sydney, Australia

Benedict Panizza MBBS MBA FRACS
Associate Professor, Director, Department of Otolaryngology,
Head and Neck Surgery, Co-Director, Queensland Skull Base Unit,
University of Queensland, Princess Alexandra Hospital, Brisbane,
Australia

Sat Parmar FDSRCS FRCS FRCS (OMFS)
Oral and Maxillofacial Head and Neck Surgeon, University
Hospitals Birmingham NHS Foundation Trust, Birmingham, UK

Snehal G Patel MD FRCS
Associate Professor, Laboratory of Epithelial Cancer Biology, Head
and Neck Service, Department of Surgery, Memorial Sloan
Kettering Cancer Center, New York, NY, USA

Andre Potenza MD
Clinical Fellow in Thyroid and Parathyroid Surgery, Massachusetts
Eye and Ear Infirmary, Boston, MA, USA

Christian Potter MA FRCS (Eng) FRCS (ORL)
Consultant ENT Surgeon, South Devon Healthcare Trust, Torbay
Hospital, Torbay, UK

J Paul M Pracy MBBS FRCS (ORL-HNS)
Consultant Otolaryngologist Head and Neck Surgeon, University
Hospitals Birmingham NHS Foundation Trust, Birmingham, UK

Rabin Pratap Singh BDS MFDS RCS (Eng)
Royal Orthopaedic Hospital, Birmingham, UK

Marco Raffaelli MD
Assistant Professor of Surgery, Università Cattolica del Sacro Cuore, Rome, Italy

Gregory W Randolph MD FACS
Director General and Thyroid Surgical Services, Mass Eye and Ear Infirmary; Member Endocrine Surgical Service, Mass General Hospital; Associate Professor Otolaryngology Head and Neck Surgery, Harvard Medical School, MA, USA

Guy Rees FRCS FRACS
Consultant Otolaryngologist and Head and Neck Surgeon, Royal Adelaide Hospital, Adelaide, Australia

Kate Reid BSc Hons (Speech Sci) MRCSLT
Speech and Language Therapist, University Hospitals Birmingham NHS Foundation Trust, Birmingham, UK

Peter Rhys-Evans MB BS LRCP FRCS DCC(Paris)
Consultant Head and Neck and Thyroid Surgeon, Royal Marsden Hospital, London, UK

Maria Rogers RGN MHS Post-graduate diploma ENB 338, 998, 931
University Hospitals Birmingham NHS Foundation Trust, Birmingham, UK

Simon N Rogers FDSRCS FRCS MD
Consultant Surgeon, Regional Maxillofacial Unit, University Hospital Aintree, Liverpool and Professor in the Evidence-Based Practice Research Centre (EPRC), Faculty of Health, Edge Hill University, Ormskirk, UK

Nicholas J Roland MBChB MD FRCS
Consultant Otolaryngology/Head and Neck Surgeon, Department of Otolaryngology and Head and Neck Surgery, University Hospital Aintree, Liverpool, UK

Nick Rowell MA MD FRCP FRCR
Consultant in Clinical Oncology, Kent Oncology Centre, Maidstone Hospital, Maidstone, UK

Jatin P Shah MD PhD(Hon) FACS FRCS(Hon)
Elliott W Strong Chair in Head and Neck Oncology, Professor of Surgery, Chief, Head and Neck Service, Department of Surgery, Memorial Sloan-Kettering Cancer Center, New York, NY, USA

Ashok R Shaha MD FACS
Jatin P Shah Chair in Head and Neck Surgery and Oncology, Professor of Surgery, Laboratory of Epithelial Cancer Biology, Head and Neck Service, Department of Surgery, Memorial Sloan-Kettering Cancer Center, New York NY, USA

Neil Sharma MRCS DOHNS
Specialty Registrar, Otolaryngology, Head and Neck Surgery, North Western Deanery, Manchester, UK; Clinical Research Fellow, School of Clinical and Experimental Medicine, University of Birmingham, Birmingham, UK

Patrick Sheahan MD FRCSI (ORL-HNS)
Consultant Otolaryngologist, Head and Neck Surgeon, South Infirmary Victoria University Hospital, Cork, Ireland

Taimur Shoaib MB ChB FRCSEd DMI(RCSEd) MD FRCS(Plast)
Consultant Plastic and Reconstructive/Head and Neck Surgeon, Canniesburn Plastic Surgery Unit, Glasgow Royal Infirmary Glasgow, UK

Ricard Simo FRCS (ORL-HNS)
Consultant Otorhinolaryngologist Head and Neck Surgeon Department of Otorhinolaryngology, Head and Neck Surgery, Guy's and St Thomas' Hospital, London, UK

Bhuvanesh Singh MD PhD
Associate Professor, Director, Laboratory of Epithelial Cancer Biology, Head and Neck Service, Memorial Sloan-Kettering Cancer Center, New York, New York, USA

Nick Slevin FRCR FRCP
Consultant in Clinical Oncology, The Christie and Honorary Senior Lecturer, University of Manchester, UK

C Arturo Solares MD
Assistant Professor, Head and Neck Surgery, Neurosurgery, Co-Director, Skull Base Center, Georgia Health and Sciences University, Augusta GA, USA

David S Soutar MBChB FRCS(Ed) FRCS(Glas) ChM
Consultant Plastic Surgeon (retired), Canniesburn Plastic Surgery Unit, Glasgow Royal Infirmary, Glasgow, UK

Mrinal Supriya FRCS ED (OTOL-HNS)
Specialist Registrar, Aberdeen Royal Infirmary, Aberdeen, UK

Conrad V Timon MD FRCS(Oto)
Consultant Otolaryngologist Head and Neck Surgeon, St James' Hospital, Dublin and Professor of Otolaryngology, Trinity College Dublin, Ireland

Iñigo Tolosa BSc (Hons) ClinPsyD PGDiploma
Consultant Clinical Psychologist, Cancer Centre, University Hospitals Birmingham NHS Foundation Trust, Birmingham, UK

Nawaz Walji MB ChB MRCP FRCR
Consultant Clinical Oncologist, University Hospitals Coventry and Warwickshire NHS Trust, Coventry, UK

Adrian T Warfield FRCPath
Consultant Histopathologist and Cytopathologist, University Hospitals Birmingham NHS Foundation Trust, and Honorary Senior Clinical Lecturer, University of Birmingham, UK

John C Watkinson MSc MS FRCS DLO
Consultant Head and Neck and Thyroid Surgeon, Department of Otolaryngology Head and Neck Surgery, University Hospitals Birmingham NHS Foundation Trust, Birmingham, UK

Keith Webster MMedSci FRCS FRCS (OMFS) FDSRCS
Oral and Maxillofacial Surgeon, University Hospitals Birmingham NHS Foundation Trust; and Honorary Senior Lecturer, Faculty of Dentistry and Medicine, University of Birmingham, Birmingham, UK

William Ignace Wei MBBS MS FRCS FRCSE FRACS (Hon) FACS (Hon) FHKAM (Surg) (ORL)
Director, Li Shu Pui ENT, Head and Neck Surgery Centre, Head Department of Surgery, Hong Kong Sanatorium and Hospital, Hong Kong SAR, China

Nicholas White BSc MD FRCS
Consultant Plastic and Craniofacial Surgeon, Department of Plastic Surgery, University Hospitals Birmingham NHS Foundation Trust, Birmingham, UK

Richard Wight MB BS FRCS
Chair, National Comparative Head and Neck Audit (DAHNO), SSCRG Head and Neck National Cancer Intelligence Network, Consultant Head and Neck Surgeon, South Tees Hospitals, NHS Foundation Trust, UK

Janet A Wilson MD FRCSEd FRCSEng FRCSLT (Hon)
Professor of Otolaryngology Head and Neck Surgery, University of Newcastle; Honorary Consultant Otolaryngologist, Freeman Hospital, Newcastle upon Tyne, UK

Julia A Woolgar PhD FRCPath FDS RCS Eng
Senior Lecturer and Consultant Oral Pathologist, Liverpool University Dental Hospital, Liverpool, UK

Steve Worrollo FIMPT
Consultant Maxillofacial Prosthetist, Department of Maxillofacial Prosthetics, University Hospitals Birmingham NHS Foundation Trust, Birmingham, and Birmingham Children's Hospital NHS Foundation Trust, Birmingham, UK

Volkert B Wreesmann MD PhD
Fellow, Laboratory of Epithelial Cancer Biology, Head and Neck Service, Memorial Sloan-Kettering Cancer Center, New York, New York, USA

Lok H Yap MB BCh BAO FRCS FRCS(PLASTIC SURGERY)
Consultant Plastic Surgeon, Department of Plastic Surgery, University Hospitals Birmingham NHS Foundation Trust, Birmingham, UK

Preface

Having been interested in head and neck oncology for nearly 30 years, we are both proud to have been involved in this fifth edition of *Stell and Maran's Textbook of Head and Neck Surgery and Oncology*. Since the last edition was published ten years ago, significant advances have been made in both the diagnosis and treatment of head and neck diseases and cancer. The aim of this book is to update colleagues on recent developments in molecular biology, highlight changes in methods for pathological diagnosis to include the emerging importance of the human papilloma virus, advances in chemoradiation together with technological developments to include minimally invasive surgery, nerve monitoring, the harmonic scalpel and the robot. Side by side, we were keen to include new techniques in reconstruction, as well as covering audit and quality of life.

The main changes in the book from the last edition include division into sections on benign and malignant disease, treatments with both radiotherapy and chemotherapy, as well as an endocrine section and one on reconstruction. Each section has its own editors and within the sections, most chapters are written by at least two authors chosen for their recognized expertise in each specific field. Selected editors, subeditors and chapter authors bring a significant international flavour to this historically well-established British textbook.

The scope of head and neck cancer management ranges from laboratory science to palliative care, and within this is included treatment with surgery (as well as reconstruction), clinical oncology and subsequent rehabilitation with emphasis on quality of life. Subspecialization is now the norm and therefore some might question the continued wisdom of producing a one volume concise text attempting to address this unique discipline. However, we still believe that the way this book is written providing concise approaches with treatment plans and key points for the specific sites within head and neck cancer continues to be as valid today as it was nearly 40 years ago, when the book was first conceived by Professors Philip Stell and Arnold Maran.

We hope that in its current form, the book will continue to be a major resource not only for trainees but established practitioners in otolaryngology, maxillofacial surgery, plastic surgery, as well as endocrine surgery and clinical oncology whose specific work includes a major head and neck practice, but also for those professions allied to medicine, such as speech and language therapy, head and neck oncology and Macmillan nurses, as well as dieticians. The algebraic sum of care includes all these disciplines in one form or another, and the care for patients with these diseases continues to evolve. Best practice we feel is represented in this book, and the *UK Effective Head and Neck Cancer Management Guidelines* (second edition) can be found on the website of the British Association of Otolaryngologists (www.entuk.org).

We gratefully acknowledge all the authors (and in particular the section editors) in this book for their time, effort and expertise in making it such a wonderful source of information for patients with head and neck disease.

Ralph W Gilbert
John C Watkinson
2011

Foreword from Arnold Maran

When this book was first published 40 years ago, the late Philip Stell and I had completed eight head and neck surgery courses. The book was, essentially, 'The Book of the Course'. By dint of including every fact ever known about head and neck cancer surgery we managed to fill 453, A5 pages in the form of 19 chapters. Each of us had completed a Head and Neck Fellowship in the United States and we brought back the right product at the right time. Although throat surgery was labelled as an integral part of ENT, the soft tissue surgical skills of a generation had been dulled by the repeatable success of first, the fenestration and then the stapedectomy operations, the results of which were spectacular.

When Stell and I started trying to make head and neck surgery an integral part of the specialty of otolaryngology, it was not difficult because it was being performed half-heartedly by general surgeons, variably by plastic surgeons and badly by singly qualified oral surgeons. Although our otolaryngological colleagues welcomed the introduction of the subspecialty onto their surgical menu, it was only nurtured as a subspecialty (through cross-referrals) in a few centres. As Professor Stell was wont to say, 'Amateurs teaching amateurs to be amateurs'.

Little wonder then that well-trained oral and maxillofacial surgeons entered the scene bringing in new levels of expertise. If there is anything remaining that gives me a sense of pride, it is the fact that I oiled the collegiate wheels to create a Specialty Fellowship for doubly qualified oral surgeons, a step which caused a quantum leap in standards. They, together with a new generation of oncologists, form part of the multidisciplinary teams around the country that make life so much better for the unfortunate patients on whom we pioneers had little alternative other than the performance of often very mutilating resections. At low points I always remembered what the famous pioneer John Conley once said to me, 'If you don't do the operation, the tumour will!' Those who suffered these gross ministrations might, were they alive, have the satisfaction of knowing that their suffering has made life much better for today's patients who are unfortunate enough to have a head and neck cancer.

I am grateful first to my colleague Professor Janet Wilson for persuading me to resurrect the book for a third edition in 1993 and to Dr Mark Gaze who 'introduced' radiotherapy to the book. But my biggest thanks is to John Watkinson, who carried on the Stell and Maran tradition of head and neck courses with international contributors and who has had enough belief in the need for the book to shepherd it through two subsequent editions. His hard work and focus has culminated in the magnificently illustrated book you are now holding and of which he and his contributors can be justly proud.

I feel certain that were he alive, Philip Stell would echo these sentiments.

Arnold Maran
2011

Foreword from Janet Wilson

The latest edition of this landmark textbook is a great credit to John Watkinson and his team of experts. While losing nothing of the essentials of the craft of head and neck surgery, the book has expanded steadily in terms of scope and insight. The well-chosen introductory chapters set the scene of the twenty-first century head and neck disease knowledge base. This review is then set against key concerns on the overall management strategy and clinical decision-making which underpin every successfully treated head and neck condition. These considerations run through the majority of the book and make it essential reading, not just for surgeons but for all professional groups involved in the challenging yet rewarding management of this complex area.

It was inevitable that as basic science knowledge expanded, patient-focused considerations emerged, and techniques of assessment and reconstructive surgery became ever more complex, that the size of *Stell and Maran* would increase over the years. Nonetheless, the editors have worked extremely hard to ensure that the finished work retains the manageable size which has always made it so appealing both to trainees at the start of their career and to experts seeking a comprehensive update.

Excitingly, the publication of the present edition coincides with what appear to be the first real-world examples of allowing patient-specific biological factors to optimize treatment schedules. Furthermore, at a time when many anticipated a welcome fall in the incidence of squamous cancer due to international efforts to curtail cigarette smoking, in fact the growth of virally induced, particularly oropharyngeal lesions has led to a disease increase. Certain countries are also experiencing a considerable increase in disorders of the thyroid gland – and endocrine disease now comprises an important and substantial section of the book.

As the knowledge has undergone exponential growth over the decades, so the painstaking selection of key material by John Watkinson and his team has become all the more valuable. The reader picking up this beautifully illustrated volume draws on the combined wisdom and surgical expertise of an impressively well-informed international team. The book is a joy to own, a pleasure to read and, above all, a powerful force to advance treatment standards in the huge variety of head and neck conditions.

I regard it as a great pleasure and privilege to have been associated with *Stell and Maran* for over 20 years.

Janet Wilson
2011

Arnold Maran: a personal perspective

'I do not believe, however, that what I've described is the sort of thing that one human being should inflict on another'. This was said to me and others who were attending a course given in New York in 1966 by the outstanding head and neck surgeon of my generation, the suave, urbane Dr John Conley. He was referring to the application of the operation that he had just described to us, the total glossolaryngectomy.

As a young, aspiring head and neck surgeon, I was disappointed to hear this from the master of so many 'big, big operations' for which he was famous; these were the days where the extent and complexity of the surgery performed was also a measure of the man. It was a time when surgeons were still labelled courageous even though it was their patients who were taking all the risks. But even for the great John Conley, exenteration of the entire mouth and throat was a step too far. It took both the late Philip Stell and me another quarter of a century to start sharing the same philosophy and ask ourselves, 'What on earth are we doing to people?'

So why is this new much enhanced edition of our original slim volume now being produced thirty-four years after its birth? Why is there still such a specialty as Head and Neck Surgery? The reason, of course, is that between the first edition of the book in 1972 and now we have not developed an effective alternative. Neither radiotherapy nor chemotherapy have, on their own, been deemed to be the cure of squamous carcinoma apart from certain small tumours. The truth remains that if the surgeon does not operate and the patient is left with no treatment then the tumour will 'do the operation'.

No-one who reads this book believes in their heart that cancer is a surgical disease, but until the 'magic bullet' is discovered the head and neck surgeon has a role. In practising this subspecialty we are unlike other cancer surgeons. They are usually able to leave the patient with only a scar that can be hidden by clothes, even though they may have a catheter and a bag, a cough and a weak voice or an ostomy bag into which their bowels empty near their trouser pocket. Such can, however, on the whole be disguised and physiological and anatomical problems are compatible with attending a dinner party without discomfiting the other guests. We, on the other hand, interfere with very visible anatomy and can affect, in turn, the physiology of speech, swallowing, chewing and breathing in such a way that is impossible to disguise and may attract unwanted attention from onlookers.

Since I started to practise head and neck surgery, however, things have improved enormously because of the cascade of reconstructive procedures; so much so that the specialty is now virtually unrecognizable to that which we practised in the 1960s.

People have been operating on the head and neck for centuries. Anecdotes of the Egyptians, Greeks and Chinese making holes in heads and throats do not, however, form any part of the evolution of our specialty and they should be relegated to the realms of history and archaeology.

Nineteenth-century surgeons sliced off cancers of the face or lip and cauterized the base, because that was the repertoire of almost all of surgery – cutting and cauterizing. Surgeons could do this in the mouth and, for a long time, the larynx, where it was attractive to perform a tracheostomy and excise bits of the larynx opened by a laryngofissure, in between the patient's swallows and coughs. Although survival figures were published, or rather claimed, in order to enhance the reputation of the surgeon, these were the days of eminence-based rather than evidence-based surgery and it is doubtful if there were any survivors other than from superficial verrucous tumours. The cause of death was always infection and/or haemorrhage.

The man who resurrected the specialty was Dr Hayes Martin who was the original Head of Service at the Memorial Hospital, New York. He was armed with the lessons he had learned from war, namely the control of sepsis by wide debridement, penicillin and delayed primary closure. He had learned the basic steps of the new specialty of plastic surgery and used tubed pedicle flaps. He also had access to stored blood and plasma, and was able to keep patients alive after major procedures. His three surgical pillars were total laryngectomy, the combined mandibular and oral cavity resection (COMMANDO) operation and the radical neck dissection (or rather the avoidance of 'nit picking' nodes out of a neck showing signs of metastatic disease). There was virtually no reconstruction. Patients may have been cured of their cancers but many were left with considerable impediments.

Things had improved by the time Stell and I started; we had the Wookey flaps and the forehead flap introduced by the late Ian McGregor. It was a start, but for every Wookey flap that worked, five became unusable over a period of months as they progressively shrank before application. While the forehead flap was robust, it did leave the patient with the uncomfortable task of explaining that it was a surgical procedure rather than an unfortunate accident that had caused his facial deformity.

The early head and neck surgeons of the 1960s and 1970s were able to do far more operations than today because there were fewer of us operating. We developed good judgement as to what was and what was not possible. The problem for the patients, however, is that good judgement comes from experience, and experience is learned from bad judgement. Stell and I learned how to deal with carotid blow-outs before we learned not to make vertical incisions in irradiated necks. We learned that if a patient could not eat then he has to be fed parenterally with enough calories to encourage healing. We learned how to avoid creating raised intracranial pressure after watching patients die of it. We were able to learn slowly by a thing that is no longer fostered during surgical education, at least in the UK – a learning curve.

The single biggest factor that improved head and neck surgery was the discovery of the blood supply to the skin. It is astonishing that we had to wait until the 1970s before an apparently simple thing like the way blood supplies skin was explained. Once it was revealed, however, the cascade of reconstruction began. The deltopectoral flap became the workhorse of reconstruction and things further improved with the advent of the pectoralis myocutaneous flap. We turned a blind eye to its incommodious bulk because of its unfailing reliability. Larger defects were closed with the latissimus dorsi flap, but we still had not solved the problem of replacing the mandible. We used free bone grafts carved to shape and wired into place, although many free bone grafts to the jaw failed and the mechanism by which those who did survive remained uncertain. All that was to end with the advent of the free flap.

The key to this was learning a new technology, namely small vessel anastomosis. Up until now, the learning curve of reconstruction had been incremental, by which I mean that it was not difficult to move from Wookey, to forehead, to deltopectoral and to myocutaneous. However, to learn small vessel anastomosis took time, patience, a steady hand and good eyesight. If the technique was learned, however, the surgeon could not only do better cancer surgery but could also close any hole with tissue that was thin, that survived and that functioned.

The introduction of this new technology did wonders for the surgical civil war that had raged over the 'ownership' of head and neck surgery for the previous fifty years. The only surgeons who could perform the whole repertoire on their own became those who could join blood vessels together – the rest had to call on help or do the fashionable thing and 'work in teams'. There is, of course, nothing to be criticized about team working, in fact it is the tenet of modern surgery and the patient benefits because the tired surgeon makes mistakes and to perform a modern head and neck cancer excision and reconstruction solo is tiring.

The original civil war had been between the general and ENT surgeons in the United States, and between plastic surgery and ENT in the United Kingdom. In both countries, the initial 'winners' were the ENT surgeons who went on to change the name of their specialty to Otolaryngology–Head and Neck Surgery (not one that would have been recommended by a marketing man). I was not alone in deploring this change because a surgeon cannot make his reputation by a name, only by ability.

Maxillofacial surgeons had always had an interest in the specialty, but were handicapped because their leaders had not bitten the bullet and demanded dual qualification. When their specialty association finally made the brave decision in the early 1980s that all oral and maxillofacial consultants should be dually qualified the Royal College of Surgeons of Edinburgh co-operated by making available a specialty fellowship in maxillofacial surgery. The same demand was not made of the maxillofacial surgeons in the United States and there, head and neck surgery became the unchallenged province of the otolaryngologist. However, it then became 'unfashionable', or rather non-remunerative, especially in the United States. The advent of managed health care relegated head and neck surgery to the poor earner category. The patients were mostly from deprived communities, poor, smoking and drinking to excess and incompetent in the area of self-care and help. The rewards for doing emotionally and technically demanding surgery became unattractive for most newly qualified American otolaryngologists and so there is now a dearth of head and neck surgeons, both in academic and private practice. To a newly qualified resident, the gentle art of otology, facial plastic surgery or endoscopic rhinology proved greater attractions.

In the United Kingdom, there is not a dearth of surgeons but a dearth of experience. Cancer of the head and neck in the UK has the same prevalence as cancer of the pancreas, which is considered inoperable unless it is in the tail. But while cancer of the pancreas only occurs in one site, head and neck cancers occur in eight different sites. Some are seen first by the dentists, some by the otolaryngologists, some by the plastic surgeons and some by the generalists. Until recently, this has been the greatest problem both for the practitioners and the patients.

The volume–outcome curve in any form of surgery is unimportant after a hundred or so operations, but it is vital in the first fifty. There are many head and neck surgeons in the UK today who have, in their repertoire, operations in which they are basically 'inexperienced' because the condition is so rare, but they are nonetheless able to offer to operate on patients in spite of the recommendations of the Bristol Inquiry by Professor Kennedy. I therefore welcome the move taken by the Senate of Surgery a few years ago when they decided to sanction training for only a few. The original specialty, whether it is plastics, ENT or maxillofacial, is unimportant because the further specialist training will be tailored to their specific needs.

I have concentrated in this brief review of the history of the subspecialty on the surgical aspects. It is salutary to go back to the writings of Hayes Martin who foresaw the end of the surgical side of the specialty with the 'new' radiotherapy. 'New' technologies that are successful, such as the polio vaccine, antibiotics for specific infections and surgery for the drainage of abscesses are immediate, obvious and beneficial. We are seeing the same false hopes raised by every new 'add-on' to radiotherapy as our predecessors saw in the 1930s and 1940s. The 'magic bullet' will not be radiotherapy or even a variant, but, like surgery, it is for the moment the best we can offer patients.

The newer chemotherapy drugs do seem to show some benefit. In the 1960s and 1970s, when the drugs used for the treatment of mesodermal tumours were applied to squamous carcinomas, there were only two outcomes – ill patients became more ill and hirsute patients became smooth. There were no cures and if one is permitted to quote Dr Conley again, 'If your treatment is worse than the disease then you become the disease'.

So what can readers of this book learn from the past?

- Follow the Oslerian principle of not creating harm.
- In the local situation, work with your colleagues and do not compete, because the only loser will be the patient.
- Audit and believe the results.
- And, finally, be holistic and ask whether what you plan for a particular patient would be what you would do to a relative.

If you do these things you will not make the mistake of not learning from history and you will be a good head and neck 'doctor'.

Arnold Maran
2011

List of abbreviations used

2D	two-dimensional	CCH	C cell hyperplasia
3D CRT	three-dimensional conformal radiotherapy	CCI	Charlson comorbidity index
3D	three-dimensional	CCRT	concomitant cheoradiotherapy
ABG	arterial blood gas	CD	Cowden's disease
ACC	adenoid cystic carcinoma	CDK	cyclin-dependent kinases
ACE	adult comorbidity evaluation	CEA	carcinoembryonic antigen
ACTH	adrenocorticotropic hormone	CFD	colour flow Doppler
ADC	apparent diffusion coefficient	CFDS	colour flow Doppler Sonography
ADH	alcohol dehydrogenase; antidiuretic hormone	CGCL	central giant cell lesion
		CGRP	calcitonin gene-related peptide
ADMH	autosomal dominant mild hyperparathyroidism	CHEP	cricohyoidoepiglottopexy
		CHP	cricohyoidopexy
AF	atrial fibrillation	CJD	Creutzfeldt–Jakob disease
AFAP	attenuated familial adenomatous polyposis	CML	chronic myeloid leukaemia
AFTN	autonomously functioning thyroid nodules	CN	cranial nerve
AIDS	acquired immunodeficiency syndrome	CNS	central nervous system
AJCC	American Joint Committee on Cancer	CNS	clinical nurse specialist
ALDH	acetaldehyde dehydrogenase	COF	conventional ossifying fibroma
ALT	anterolateral thigh	COG	Children's Oncology Group
APUD	amine precursor and uptake decarboxylase	COPD	chronic obstructive pulmonary disease
ARDS	adult respiratory distress syndrome	CRF	corticotrophin-releasing factor
ARF	acute renal failure	CRH	corticotrophin-releasing hormone
ARSAC	Administration of Radioactive Substances Advisory Committee	CRP	C-reactive protein
		CRT	chemoradiotherapy
ART	antiretroviral therapy	CSA	circumflex scapula artery
ASA	American Society of Anesthesiologists	CSCCHN	cutaneous SCC of the head and neck
ASSIDS	Assessment of Intelligibility of Dysarthric Speech	CSF	cerebrospinal fluid
		CSR	calcium-sensing receptor
ATA	American Thyroid Association	CT	calcitonin
ATLS	Advanced Trauma Life Support	CT	computed tomography
ATP	adenosine triphosphate	CTRT	chemoradiation
BAETS	British Association of Endocrine and Thyroid Surgeons	CTV	clinical target volume
		CUP	carcinoma of unknown primary origin
BAHA	bone anchored hearing aid	CV	central venous
BAHNO	British Association of Head and Neck Oncologists	CVP	central venous pressure
		CXR	chest x-ray
BAMMF	buccinator artery myomucosal flap	DAHNO	Data for Head and Neck Oncology
BCC	basal cell carcinoma	DAT	digital audiotape
bFGF	basic fibroblast growth factor	DCIA	deep circumflex iliac artery
BFHH	benign familial hypocalciuric hypercalcaemia	DI	diabetes insipidus
		DIC	disseminated intravascular coagulation
BIPP	bismuth and iodoform paraffin paste	DLBCL	diffuse large cell B-cell lymphoma
BMI	body-mass index	DLT	dose-limiting toxicities
BMP	bone morphogenic proteins	DM	distant metastasis
BRAF	B-Raf	DMSA	dimercaptosuccinic acid
BTA	British Thyroid Association	DNES	diffuse neuroendocrine system
CADCAM	computer-aided design, computer-aided manufacture	DTC	differentiated thyroid carcinoma
		DVH	dose–volume histograms
CAP	College of American Pathologists	DVT	deep vein thrombosis
CBC	complete blood count	DWI	diffusion-weighted imaging

EA	early intracellular antigen	FTUMP	follicular tumour of uncertain malignant potential
EAC	external auditory canal	FVPTC	follicular variant of papillary thyroid carcinoma
EAM	external auditory meatus		
EBRT	external beam radiation therapy	G-CSF	granulocyte colony-stimulating factor
EBSLN	external branch of the superior laryngeal nerve	GBR	guided bone regeneration
		GCS	Glasgow Coma Score
EBV	Epstein–Barr virus	GCT	giant cell tumour
ECD	extracapsular dissection	GDNF	glial cell line-derived neurotrophic factor
ECG	electrocardiogram	GFR	growth factor receptor
ECOG	Eastern Co-operative Oncology Group	GH	growth hormone
ECS	extracapsular spread	GHRH	GH-releasing hormone
EGF	epidermal growth factor	GI	gastrointestinal
EGFR	epidermal growth factor receptor	GORTEC	Groupe d'Oncologie Radiotherapie Tête et Cou
ELS	endoscopic laser surgery		
EMA	epithelial membrane antigen	GTV	gross tumour volume
EMG	electromyogram; electromyography	H&E	haematoxylin and eosin
EMI	elective mucosal irradiation	HA	hydroxyapatite
END	elective neck dissection	HBO	hyperbaric oxygen
ENT	ear, nose and throat	HCTA	helical CT angiography
ENoG	electroneuronography	HDR	high-dose rate
EORTC	European Organisation for Research and Treatment of Cancer	HIF	hypoxia inducible factor
		HIV	human immunodeficiency virus
EPI	electronic portal imaging	HL	Hodgkin's lymphoma
EPSTSSG	European Paediatric Soft Tissue Sarcoma Study Group	HLA	human leukocyte antigen
		HMWCK	high molecular weight cytokeratins
ESR	erythrocyte sedimentation rate	HNC	head and neck cancer
ETA	European Thyroid Association	HNPG	head and neck paragangliomas
ETE	extrathyroidal extension	HNSCC	head and neck squamous cell carcinoma
EUA	examination under anaesthesia	HPT-JT	hyperparathyroidism or hereditary hyperparathyroidism with jaw tumours
FACT	Functional Assessment of Cancer Therapy		
FAMM	facial artery muscular mucosal	HPT	hyperparathyroidism
FAP	familial adenomatous polyposis	HPV	human papilloma virus
FBC	full blood count	HRQOL	health-related quality of life
FD	fibrous dysplasia	HSV	herpes simplex virus
FDG-PET	^{18}F-fluorodeoxyglucose positron emission tomography	HTA	hyalinizing trabecular adenoma
		HTT	hyalinizing trabecular tumours
FEES	flexible endoscopic evaluation of swallowing	IAC	internal auditory canal
		ICA	internal carotid artery
FEESST	flexible endoscopic evaluation of swallowing with sensory testing	ICIDH	International Classification of Impairment Disabilities and Handicaps
FESS	functional endoscopic sinus surgery	ICP	intracranial pressure
FGF	fibroblast growth factor	ICRU	International Commission on Radiation Units and Measurements
FHH	familial hypercalcaemic hypocalciuria; familial hypocalciuric hypercalcaemia		
		ICU	intensive care units
FIHP	familial isolated hyperparathyroidism	ID	inferior dental
FMTC	familial medullary thyroid cancer	IG	image guidance
FNA	fine needle aspiration	IGF	insulin-like growth factors
FNAB	fine needle aspiration biopsy	IGRT	image-guided radiotherapy
FNAC	fine needle aspirate cytology	IHC	immunohistochemistry
FND	functional neck dissection	IJV	internal jugular vein
FSH	follicle-stimulating hormone	ILN	inferior laryngeal nerve
fT3	free T3	IM	internal margin
fT4	free T4	IMAP	internal mammary artery perforator
FTC	follicular thyroid carcinoma	IMRA	immunoradiometric
FTSG	full-thickness skin grafts	IMRT	intensity-modulated radiotherapy
FTT	free tissue transfer		

IONM	intraoperative nerve monitoring	MOFT	multiple oxyphil follicular tumours
IPSS	inferior petrosal sinus sampling	MPNT	malignant peripheral nerve sheath tumour
ISH	*in-situ* hybridization	MPT	maximal phonation time
ISO	International Organization for Standardization	MR	magnetic resonance
ITA	inferior thyroid artery	MRA	magnetic resonance angiography
ITU	intensive treatment unit	MRI	magnetic resonance imaging
JNA	juvenile nasopharyngeal angiofibroma	mRNA	messenger ribonucleic acid
KD	Kikuchi disease	MRND	modified radical neck dissection
KFI	Kaplan–Feinstein index	MRSA	methicillin resistant *Staphylococcus aureus*
KIN	keratinocyte intraepithelial neoplasia	MSI	microsatellite instability
KS	Kaposi's sarcoma	MSK	Memorial Sloan Kettering
KSHV	Kaposi sarcoma-associated virus	MSLT	Melanoma Sentinel Lymph Trial
KTP	potassium titanyl phosphate	MST	maximum stimulation test
KWD	Kawasaki disease	MTC	medullary thyroid carcinoma
LAT	lateral aberrant thyroid	MVD	mean vessel density
LDH	lactate dehydrogenase	NCASP	National Clinical Audit Support Programme
LDR	low-dose rate	NCDB	National Cancer Database
LH	luteinizing hormone	NCDS	National Cancer Dataset
LIN	laryngeal intraepithelial neoplasia	NEC	neuroendocrine carcinoma
LMWH	low molecular weight heparin	NEMS	nanoelectromechanical systems
LND	anterolateral neck dissection	NET	nerve excitability test
LOH	loss of heterozygosity	NET	neuroendocrine tumour
LRC	locoregional control	NF1	neurofibromatosis 1
LRF	locoregional flaps	NFA	non-functioning adenoma
LTBR	lateral temporal bone resection	NG	nasogastric
MAB	monoclonal antibodies	NGF	neural growth factor
MACH-NC	Meta-analysis of Chemotherapy on Head and Neck Cancer	NHL	non-Hodgkin lymphomas
MACS	minimal access cranial suspension	NHS	National Health Service
MALT	mucosa-associated lymphoid tissue	NIC	National Institute of Cancer
MAPK	mitogen activated protein kinase	NICE	National Institute for Health and Clinical Excellence
MARCH	Meta-analysis of Radiotherapy in Carcinomas of the Head and Neck	NIH	National Institutes for Health
MCC	Merkel cell carcinoma	NMSC	melanoma and non-melanoma skin cancer
MCT	medium chain triglyceride	NOS	not otherwise specified
MDADI	MD Anderson Dysphagia Inventory	NOTES	natural orifice transluminal endoscopic surgery
MDCT	multirow detector computed tomography	NPC	nasopharyngeal carcinoma
MDT	multidisciplinary team	NSHPT	neonatal severe HPT
MDTM	multidisciplinary team meeting	NTM	non-tuberculous atypical mycobacterial adenitis
MEMS	microelectromechanical systems		
MEN	multiple endocrine neoplasia	NTTBR	near total temporal bone excision
MFH	malignant fibrous histiocytoma	OAR	organs at risk
MI	myocardial infarction	OD	osseous dysplasias
MIBG	metaiodobenzylguanidine	OGTT	oral glucose tolerance test
MIFC	minimally invasive follicular carcinoma	OIN	oral intraepithelial neoplasia
MIP	minimally invasive parathyroidectomy	ONB	olfactory neuroblastoma
MIRA	Minimally Invasive Robotic Association	OPG	orthopantomogram
MIS	minimally invasive surgery	OPSCC	oropharyngeal squamous cell carcinoma
MIVAT	minimally invasive video-assisted thyroidectomy	OPSE	oropharyngeal swallow efficiency
		ORF	open reading frames
MLC	multileaf collimators	OTT	overall treatment time
MMM	mucosal malignant melanoma	PAS	periodic acid Schiff
MMP	matrix metalloproteinases	PC	parathyroid carcinoma
MND	modified neck dissection	PCNSL	primary central nervous system lymphoma
MNG	multinodular goitre	PCR	polymerase chain reaction
		PDGF	platelet-derived growth factor

PDTC	poorly differentiated thyroid carcinoma		SIGN	Scottish Intercollegiate Guidelines Network
PE	pharyngo-oesophageal		SIN	squamous intraepithelial neoplasia
PE	pulmonary embolism		SIRS	systemic inflammatory response syndrome
PEEP	positive end expiratory pressure		SLE	systemic lupus erythematosus
PEG	percutaneous endoscopic gastroscopy		SLN	superior laryngeal nerve
PET	positron emission tomography		SLT	speech and language therapist
PF	cisplatin, 5-fluorouracil		SM	set-up margin
PGL	persistent generalized lymphadenopathy		SMA	smooth muscle actin
PHTS	PTEN hamartoma tumour syndrome		SMAS	superficial musculoaponeurotic system
PIF	palatal island flap		SNB	sentinel node biopsy
PIF	prolactin inhibitory factor		SND	selective neck dissection
PIN	penile intraepithelial neoplasia		SNUC	sinonasal undifferentiated carcinoma
PL	partial laryngectomy		SOFT	solitary oxyphil follicular tumour
PLAT	paraganglioma-like adenoma of the thyroid		SOHND	supraomohyoid neck dissection
PLND	posterolateral neck dissection		SPA	salivary pleomorphic adenoma
PORT	postoperative radiotherapy		SPECT	single photon emission computed
PPAR	peroxisome proliferation activated receptor			tomography
PSSHN	Performance Status Scale for Head and Neck		SPIO	superparamagnetic iron oxide
pT	primary tumour		SSND	superselective neck dissection
PTAH	phosphotungstic acid haematoxylin		SSRI	selective serotonin reuptake inhibitors
PTC	papillary thyroid carcinoma		STIR	short tau inversion recovery
PTFE	polytetrafluoroethylene		STS	soft tissue sarcomas
PTG	parathyroid glands		STSG	split-thickness skin grafts
PTH	parathyroid hormone		SUS	Secondary Uses Services
PTHrP	parathyroid hormone-related peptide		SVR	secondary voice restoration
PTU	propylthiouracil		TB	tuberculosis
PTV	planning target volume		TCP	tricalcium phosphate
PVC	polyvinylchloride		TDAA	thoracodorsal angular artery
QoL	quality of life		TEP	tracheoesophageal
QRT-PCR	quantitative reverse transcriptase-		TFT	thyroid function tests
	polymerase chain reaction		TG	thyroglobulin
RAI	radioactive iodine		TGFα	transforming growth factor-alpha
RFLP	restriction fragment length polymorphism		TGF-β	transforming growth factor-beta
rhTSH	recombinant human TSH		THORP	titanium hollow osseointegrated
RIS	radiation-induced sarcoma			reconstruction plate
RLN	recurrent laryngeal nerve		THW	thyroid hormone withdrawal
RLNP	recurrent laryngeal nerve palsy		TK	tyrosine kinase
RND	radical neck dissection		TKI	tyrosine kinase inhibitor
RP	rapid prototyping		TLM	transoral laser microsurgery
RT-PCR	reverse transcription-polymerase chain		TMJ	temporomandibular joint
	reaction		TND	therapeutic node dissection
RT	radiation therapy; radiotherapy		TNF	tumour necrosis factor
Rb	retinoblastoma		TNM	tumour, node, metastasis
SAGES	Society of American Gastrointestinal and		TO	tracheo-oesophageal
	Endoscopic Surgeons		TOM	therapy outcome measure
SALT	speech and language therapist		TORS	transoral robotic surgery
SAN	spinal accessory nerve		TPF	docetaxel, cisplatin, 5-fluorouracil
SCC	squamous cell carcinoma		TPF	temporoparietal fascia
SCCHN	squamous cell cancer of the head and neck		TPN	total parenteral nutrition
SCM	sternocleidomastoid muscle		TPO	thyroid peroxidase
SCN	solid cell nests		TR	thyroid hormone receptor
SCPL	supracricoid partial laryngectomy		TRH	thyrotropin releasing hormone
SEER	Surveillance Epidemiology and End Results		TSG	tumour suppressor genes
sEMG	surface electromyography		TSH	thyroid-stimulating hormone
SI	signal intensity		TTF-1	thyroid transcription factor-1
SIADH	syndrome of inappropriate ADH secretion		Tg	thyroglobulin

UADT	upper aerodigestive tract	VCA	viral capsid antigen
UCNT	undifferentiated carcinoma of nasopharyngeal type	VEGF	vascular endothelial growth factor
		VFSS	video fluoroscopy swallowing study
UICC	Union Internationale Contre le Cancer	VHI	Voice Handicap Index
URLNP	unilateral RLNP	VPQ	Voice Performance Questionnaire
US	ultrasound	VoiSS	Voice Symptom Scale
USPIO	ultrasmall superparamagnetic iron oxide	WBC	white blood cell
USS	ultrasound scanning	WBS	whole body scan
UV	ultraviolet	WHO	World Health Organization
UW-QoL	University of Washington Quality of Life	WIFC	widely invasive follicular carcinoma
VA	Veterans Affairs	XIAP	X-linked inhibitor of apoptosis protein
VAPP	Voice Activity and Participation Profile	ZES	Zollinger Ellison syndrome

History of head and neck surgery

RALPH W GILBERT AND JOHN C WATKINSON

Because the newer methods of treatment are good, it does not follow that the old ones were bad: for if our honourable and worshipful ancestors had not recovered from their ailments, you and I would not be here today.

Confucius, 551–478BC

This book, the original concept of the named authors, Philip Stell and Arnold Maran, is a reflection of the modern history of head and neck surgery: continuous innovation through the integration of knowledge, imagination and teamwork of health-care professionals from a variety of disciplines committed to the treatment of head and neck tumours. The pace of change in the treatment of head and neck tumours has accelerated in the last two to three decades with a remarkable transition from predominantly ablative surgery to combined therapies focused on preservation of the form and function of the anatomic structures of the head and neck. This chapter will summarize the history of head and neck surgery, with information gleaned from published summaries of this history and original articles.[1]

Some of the earliest attempts at head and neck surgery can likely be credited to Egyptian physicians who attempted ablative and reconstructive procedures of the oral cavity and lip. The 'Edwin Smith Papyrus', the origins of which are dated at approximately 3000BC, contains some of the first descriptions of surgical management of mandibular and nasal fractures, as well as lip tumours.

Arguably, the first documented efforts of reconstructive head and neck surgery are found in the Sanskrit texts of ancient India written approximately 2600 years ago. During this period of Indian history, reconstructive surgery of the nose and ear was highly valued, as invaders from surrounding territories would often stigmatize their victims by amputating the nose or ear. The early Hindu justice system also imposed harsh penalties on those found guilty of being unfaithful to a spouse by amputating either the genitalia or the nose. It is

therefore logical that the nose, a structure of dignity and unique personal identity, would become a focus of reconstructive head and neck surgery. In his *Sushruta Samhita* (Sushruta's compendium), Sushruta, regarded as the 'father of Indian surgery' described a variety of surgical techniques for reconstruction of head and neck defects. Considerable controversy exists over the time period of his contributions with dates ranging from 600BCE to 1000AD. He contributed to many fields of medicine, but he is said to have laid the foundations for a variety of pedicled and rotation flaps, and was the pioneer of reconstructive nasal surgery having described more than 15 methods of nasal reconstruction, similar to many of the techniques utilized in the nineteenth and twentieth centuries.

Whether Helenistic or Roman physicians were exposed to the Indian techniques through Alexander the Great's expedition to India in the fourth century BCE is of debate. Certainly, Roman and Hellenistic physicians described similar techniques to those described in India. Aulus Cornelius Celsus, considered to be the greatest of the Roman medical authors and surgeons, also described a variety of techniques similar to those practised in India in his medical text of the first century, *De Medecina*, and is credited with one of the first head and neck cancer procedures describing excision of a lip malignancy.[2]

The development of surgery of the head and neck certainly continued in the Middle Ages. However, following the fall of Rome in the fifth century and the diffusion of Barbarians and Christianity throughout the Middle Ages, a significant decline in the advancement of all surgery, in particular reconstruction, occurred. This decline was certainly aided by Pope Innocent III who prohibited surgical procedures of all types. It is interesting to note that physicians of the time considered surgery to be a manual skill and below their intellectual and societal stature. The development of the concept of the barber surgeon appeared and the decline of the role of surgery and surgeons began.

The period of Renaissance in the fourteenth century signalled a rebirth of science, medicine and the world of surgery. In the fifteenth century, the Branca family became prominent in wound reconstruction and the reintroduction of the Indian method of nasal reconstruction.[3] The family apparently zealously protected the techniques they had developed from outside observers and the surgical techniques were passed down through family members. Branca's son Antonius inherited this technique and modified it through the use of a delayed skin flap from the arm. This Italian method, as it became known, was eventually transferred to other families of surgeons.

Descriptions of these various techniques may have contributed to Gasparro Tagliacozzi's interest in nasal reconstruction. Tagliacozzi, incorrectly referred to as the originator of the Italian method, made significant contributions to facial reconstructive surgery. Working in Bologna in the latter half of the sixteenth century, Tagliacozzi described and refined the use of distant pedicled flaps for a variety of head and neck reconstructions.[4]

In the seventeenth century, Pimpernelle first described tongue surgery for malignancy. In the following 200 years, there were very few publications and developments in head and neck surgery.

The modern era was heralded by the development of the achromatic microscope, which allowed pathologists to first view tissues under magnification. In 1835, Mirault[5] and Langenbeck described wedge excision of the tongue with ligation of the lingual artery to control bleeding; a major advance to reduce the bleeding associated with these procedures. Roux, in 1839, first described access procedures to the oral cavity. His technique was the first description of lip splitting incisions combined with mandibular osteotomy. The mid-nineteenth century was dominated by developments in the pathologic description of tumours, including those by the father of modern oncologic pathology, Virchow. In the latter part of the century, the description of various surgical access approaches to the head and neck began to appear.

Gordon Buck from New York was the first to describe the laryngofissure approach to remove laryngeal tumours in 1851. The famous Viennese surgeon, Theodore Bilroth, introduced techniques of bilateral mandibular osteotomy for oral access in 1862 and described the first total laryngectomy in 1873. Interestingly, this operation so widely used today rapidly fell out of favour as the perioperative mortality was extremely high (one in 25 of Bilroth's patients survived one year).

In the latter part of the century, Kocher described the technique of lateral mandibular osteotomy along with the first description of the importance of neck node management in mucosal tumors of the head and neck.[6] In 1885, Henry Butlin published his work on diseases of the tongue.[7] He described premalignant lesions of the tongue and advocated for early diagnosis and treatment. He also described the importance of the lymph nodes of the tail of the parotid as metastatic sites for advanced oral tumours.

The early twentieth century was dominated by developing knowledge of the lymphatics of the head and neck and improvements in surgical technique. Polya in 1902, described the lymphatic drainage of the oral cavity, demonstrating that 50 per cent of the lymphatics traversed the mandibular periosteum leading to an interest in en-bloc resections and the foundations of the original composite resection for oral cancer. In 1906, the American surgeon and father of neck dissection George Crile described his approach to head and neck tumours, becoming the foundation of the present-day radical and functional approaches to neck dissection.[8] Crile was an extremely creative surgeon developing pneumatic suits for patients to maintain their blood pressure during extensive surgical procedures. He also developed a carotid clamp that would allow reductions in carotid flow without complete occlusion. In 1913, Gluck and Sorensen described improved approaches to the creation of tracheostome and repair of the pharynx in laryngectomy. The approaches of Gluck and Soerensen arguably became the foundation of modern laryngopharyngeal ablative and reconstructive surgery.[9]

In the 1930s, surgical techniques continued to evolve along with interest in the use of radiation therapy for the treatment of head and neck tumours. In 1932, GL Semken described radical neck dissection and en-bloc resection of the tongue and the associated lymphatic structures. In 1932, Ward performed and described the first composite resection.

A major innovation for head and neck management was described in 1934 by Hayes Martin and Ellis, that of the use of final needle aspiration cytology as a diagnostic tool; a development which would dramatically alter the treatment of head and neck malignancy and thyroid disease over the next 75 years.[10]

The 1930s and 1940s were dominated by attempts at the treatment of head and neck tumours with radiotherapy. A renaissance of interest in surgical approaches to head and neck diseases occurred in the late 1940s and 1950s as the early and late effects of this primitive form of radiation became evident.

The 1940s and 1950s were dominated by development in surgical technique and an increasing interest in organ-preserving surgical procedures. Gluck and Portmann described the technique of vertical hemilaryngectomy to extirpate small volume laryngeal lesions and reported large series of patients with successful outcomes.[11] In 1951, Alonso from Uruguay, one of the fathers of partial laryngeal surgery, described techniques of vertical and horizontal supraglottic laryngectomy and wrote the following prophetic statement:

> Cancer is a terrible disease, but I do not accept that the surgeon's scalpel may be more destructive than the disease itself. The war against the larynx must stop, since its removal is unnecessary and ineffective in many cases. To take away the disease without excising a healthy glottis to make an effort to preserve the function of the organ, to strive not to return a disabled person to the society: that is my motto.[12]

In 1951, Hayes Martin published his seminal work on head and neck surgery describing his techniques and outcomes for patients over the previous three decades at Memorial Sloan Kettering.[13] In 1952, Conley and Pack extended concepts of vascular surgery to neck tumours, describing approaches to vascular tumours and malignancy involving the carotid.[14]

Management of neck disease evolved in the 1960s and 1970s following the descriptions of selective neck dissection by Soares in South America and Bocca in Italy.[15, 16] The current approaches to neck dissection arose from refinements of approaches popularized by these authors and provided an evidence basis from work done by Shah,[17] Byers,[18] Medina[19] and others.

The 1960s, 1970s and 1980s were dominated academically by giants in the field who literally changed the face of head and neck surgery through their enormous contributions to the evidence basis of head and neck surgery. Through their fellowship training programmes their skills were extended to other countries of the world and provided the academic foundation for the next generation of surgical leaders. A list of individuals of this era would include, but not be limited to, Dr Hayes Martin (USA), Dr John Conley (USA), Philip Stell (UK), Arnold Maran (UK), Joseph Ogura (USA), Dr Douglas Bryce (Canada), Dr M Lederman (UK), Sir Donald Harrison (UK) and Dr Richard Jesse (USA).

The 1980s and 1990s saw the continued development of surgical technique, including major innovation in the techniques of delivering radiotherapy, including 3D conformal radiation and intensity modulated radiotherapy (IMRT).

The major surgical innovations of this era were the increasing interest in minimally invasive surgery of the larynx and endoscopic endonasal and skull base surgery. Jako and colleagues from the United States and Kleinsasser from Germany influenced the developments in minimally invasive surgery of the larynx. The techniques advocated by these creative surgeons have been expanded and popularized by others. Most notable among these was Dr Wolfgang Steiner[20] and his colleagues from Germany, whose systematic approach to the endoscopic laser excision of laryngeal tumours has changed the management approach to early and advanced laryngeal malignancy.

In the early 1980s, Messerklinger, Stammberger[21] and colleagues from Austria introduced the concept of functional endoscopic sinus surgery providing the technical foundation for the developments in minimally invasive nasal surgery. A number of groups around the world, most notably Kassam, Carrau and Snyderman[22] from the United States have extended these concepts and techniques, developing transnasal approaches to the management of skull base tumours.

The last two decades have seen an expanded interest in multimodality therapy combining surgery and radiotherapy or chemotherapy and radiation, with surgery reserved for salvage. This evolution in approach has evolved from surgeons becoming increasingly involved in clinical trials and the interest of surgeons in developing an evidentiary basis for the treatments they offer. Perhaps the most prominent of these trials have been the laryngeal organ preservation trials in the United States[23] and the evolution of clinical trials evaluating the role of chemotherapy, radiation therapy, molecular targeted therapy and surgery in the United States and Europe.

The most important surgical innovations of the past 40–50 years have, however, been in the development of reconstructive approaches to ablative defects of the head and neck. In the 1960s, a number of surgical innovations changed the morbidity of head and neck reconstruction. The increasing use of axial pattern flaps made reconstruction of large oral cavity and neck defects more reliable and less costly to the patient in terms of prolonged hospitalization. Foremost among these were the descriptions of the forehead flap for oral reconstruction popularized by McGregor and McGregor[24] and the deltopectoral flap described in the

United States by Bakamjian and colleagues.[25] In the late 1970s, the description of the pectoralis major myocutaneous flap by Ariyan[26] transformed head and neck oncologic surgery as patients could be offered a single stage reliable reconstruction with minimal donor site morbidity. In addition, the ease of harvest and transfer of the pectoralis major flap made it a technique that any head and neck-trained surgeon could perform, broadening the scope of reconstructive surgery to other disciplines outside plastic surgery.

The late 1960s and early 1970s heralded the era of reconstructive microsurgery. The concept of free tissue transfer had been developed years earlier, but was limited by the quality and availability of microvascular sutures, quality instruments and magnification. Jacobsen and Suarez first described the repair of vessels under 2 mm in 1960. The first free tissue transfer of a composite of skin was performed by Taylor and Daniel in 1973.[27] Subsequent developments in reconstructive microsurgery have resulted in the description of a plethora of free tissue transfers available for head and neck reconstruction championed by a number of extremely gifted reconstructive microsurgeons, including Harii, Buncke, Manktelow and many others.

The more notable among these flaps are: the free forearm flap described by Yang in 1983[28] and popularized for oral cavity and oromandibular reconstruction by Soutar; the free fibular transfer originally described by Taylor in 1977[29] and popularized by Hidalgo and Rekow for mandibular reconstruction in 1995;[30] and the anterolateral thigh flap described by Song et al. in 1984[31] and popularized for head and neck reconstruction by Wei and colleagues in 2002.[32]

The community of specialties performing head and neck oncologic and reconstructive surgery has changed dramatically over the past 40 years. Head and neck oncologic surgery in the 1950s and 1960s was largely the domain of general and plastic surgeons, with the majority of reconstruction performed by plastic surgeons. In the last three decades of the twentieth century, however, major changes in the specialties treating defects of the head and neck had evolved. Increasingly in Europe and North America, otolaryngologists with subspecialty training in head and neck surgery and reconstructive microsurgery began to develop an interest and expertise in head and neck surgery that extended beyond the treatment of laryngeal cancer. At the same time in Europe, maxillofacial surgery began its evolution as a specialty and increasingly maxillofacial surgeons treated and reconstructed congenital, traumatic and oncologic defects of the head and neck.

With regard to thyroid surgery, goitre (guttur, Latin for throat) has been recognized as a discrete condition since earliest recorded times (2000BC). Normal thyroid anatomy was not generally understood until the renaissance when the gland was named glandulam thyroideam (Latin for shield shaped). The first thyroidectomy was performed in 1646, but the ten-year-old patient died and the surgeon was imprisoned. In the 1850s, mortality rates remained high (approximately 40 per cent), but following key advances in anaesthesia, the discovery of antisepsis and the development of the haemostat by Spencer Wells, surgeons such as Billroth and Kocher improved mortality rates from 12.6 per cent in the 1880s to 0.2 per cent in 1898. Kocher was a meticulous surgeon with low complication rates. He described the incision for thyroidectomy, as well as other surgical advances, and became the first surgeon to be awarded the Nobel Prize in 1909.[33]

Kocher trained Halstead who subsequently trained Crile, Mayo and Lahey, who in turn trained Oliver Beahrs. In the UK, James Berry and Cecil Joll further championed advances, as did Sir Thomas Dunhill in Australia who pioneered one-stage near-total thyroidectomy for benign disease. Further advances regarding the anatomy of the recurrent laryngeal nerve, parathyroids (including extracapsular dissection) and the external branch of the superior laryngeal nerve allowed surgeons to further refine their techniques.[34]

Before 1948, the thyroid gland was the domain of the general surgeon, but following the inception of the NHS and development of ENT as a specialty, over the last 50 years head and neck surgery has been shared between otolaryngologists and general and endocrine surgeons. More and more in the United Kingdom, thyroid disease and malignancy is treated in a multidisciplinary setting by a team which includes both endocrinologists as well as surgeons from backgrounds in both general and endocrine surgery, as well as otolaryngology.

THE FUTURE

In the next ten years, further refinements will occur in the selection and application of the myriad of treatment options for head and neck malignancy. Increased characterization of genomic and proteinomic profiles of tumours will allow us to better select patients for these therapies, providing a more individualized approach to head and neck cancer treatment. Surgical innovation with the introduction of more minimally invasive approaches, including robotics, will continue to develop and expand with the goal of reducing the morbidity associated with treatment. In the reconstructive arena, the major innovations are clearly in tissue engineering and transplantation. Tissue engineering may offer the potential to create composite tissue constructs that will replace the current approaches, including free tissue transfer and the associated donor site morbidity. Composite tissue allografts (CTA) or transplantation clearly have the potential to dramatically change the field of reconstructive surgery of the head and neck. Certainly, the recent experience with partial facial transplantation in France has highlighted the opportunities of this technology, as well as the ethical dilemmas associated with the technique.

REFERENCES

1. Conley JJ, Vonfraekel PH. Historical aspects of head and neck surgery. *Annals of Otology, Rhinology, and Laryngology* 1956; **65**: 643–55.
2. Pardon M. Celsus and the Hippocratic Corpus: The originality of a 'plagiarist'. A brief history of wound care medicine in history. *Celsus* (AD 25), plastic surgeon: On the repair of defects of the ears, lips, and nose. *Studies in Ancient Medicine* 2005; **31** (Suppl.): 403–11.
3. Branca A. *Ersatz der Nase aus der Haut des Oberarms*, cited in Hirsch A, Biographisches Lexikon. Berlin: Urban & Schwarzenberg, 1929.
4. Tagliacozzi G. *De curtorum chirugia per insitionem libri duo*. Venice: Gaspar Bindonus Jr, 1597.
5. Mirault G. Memoire sur la ligature de la langue et sur celle de l'artere linguale en particulier; precede d'une observation de cancer de la langue gueri par la ligature de cet organe. *Memoires de l'Academie de Medicine, Paris* 1835; **4**: 35–68.
6. Kocher T. Ueber radialheilulng des krebes. *Zeitschrifte für Chirurgie* 1880; **13**: 134–66.
7. Butlin HT. Excision and dissection of the head. *British Medical Journal* 1894; **1**: 785.
8. Crile G. Excision of cancer of the head and neck with special reference to the plan of dissection based on 132 operations. *Journal of the American Medical Association* 1906; **47**: 1780.
9. Gluck T, Soerensen J. Die Resektion und Extirpation des Larynx, Pharynx und Esophagus. In: Katz L, Preysing H, Blumenfeld F (eds). *Handbuch der Speciellen Chirurgie des Ohres und der Oberen Luftwege*, vol. IV. Wurzburg: Verlag von Curt Kabitsch, 1931.
10. Martin HE, Ellis EB. Aspiration biopsy. *Surgery of Gynecology and Obstetrics* 1934; **59**: 578–89.
11. Portmann G. La laryngectomie totale en trois temps; operation de securite. *Presse Medicine* 1940; **48**: 633.
12. Alonso JM. Conservative surgery of cancer of the larynx. *Transactions of the American Academy of Ophthalmology and Otolaryngology* 1947; **51**: 633–42.
13. Martin HE, Del Valle B, Ehrlich L *et al.* Neck dissection. *Cancer* 1951; **4**: 441.
14. Conley JJ, Pack GT. Surgical procedure for lessening the hazard of carotid bulb excision. *Surgery* 1952; **31**: 845–58.
15. Bocca E. Functional problems connected with bilateral radical neck dissection. *Journal of Laryngology and Otology* 1953; **67**: 567–77.
16. Bocca E. Conservative neck dissection. *Laryngoscope* 1975; **85**: 1511–15.
17. Shah JP, Andersen PE. The impact of patterns of nodal metastasis on modifications of neck dissection. *Annals of Surgical Oncology* 1994; **1**: 521–32.
18. Byers RM. Modified neck dissection. A study of 967 cases from 1970 to 1980. *American Journal of Surgery* 1985; **150**: 414–21.
19. Medina JE, Byers RM. Supraomohyoid neck dissection: rationale, indications, and surgical technique. *Head and Neck* 1989; **11**: 111–22.
20. Steiner W. Experience in endoscopic laser surgery of malignant tumours of the upper aero-digestive tract. *Advances in Otorhinolaryngology* 1988; **39**: 135–44.
21. Stammberger H, Posawetz W. Functional endoscopic sinus surgery. Concept, indications and results of the Messerklinger technique. *European Archives of Otorhinolaryngology* 1990; **247**: 63–76.

22. Snyderman CH, Carrau RL, Kassam AB *et al*. Endoscopic skull base surgery: principles of endonasal oncological surgery. *Journal of Surgical Oncology* 2008; **97**: 658–64.

23. The Department of Veterans Affairs Laryngeal Cancer Study Group. Induction chemotherapy plus radiation compared with surgery plus radiation in patients with advanced laryngeal cancer. *New England Journal of Medicine* 1991; **324**: 1685–90.

24. McGregor IA, McGregor FM. *Cancer of the face and mouth. Pathology and management for surgeons.* Edinburgh: Churchill Livingstone, 1986.

25. Bakamjian V, Littlewood M. Cervical skin flaps for intraoral and pharyngeal repair following cancer surgery. *British Journal of Plastic Surgery* 1964; **17**: 191–210.

26. Ariyan S. The pectoralis major myocutaneous flap. A versatile flap for reconstruction of the head and neck area. *Plastic and Reconstructive Surgery* 1979; **63**: 73–81.

27. Taylor GI, Daniel RK. The free flap: composite tissue transfer by vascular anastomosis. *Australia and New Zealand Journal of Surgery* 1973; **43**: 1–3.

28. Yang GF. [Free grafting of a lateral brachial skin flap]. *Zhonghua Wai Ke Za Zhi* 1983; **21**: 272–4.

29. Taylor GI. Microvascular free bone transfer: a clinical technique. *Orthopedic Clinics of North America* 1977; **8**: 425–47.

30. Hidalgo DA, Rekow A. A review of 60 consecutive fibula free flap mandible reconstructions. *Plastic and Reconstructive Surgery* 1995; **96**: 585–96; discussion 597–602.

31. Song YG, Chen GZ, Song YL. The free thigh flap: a new free flap concept based on the septocutaneous artery. *British Journal of Plastic Surgery* 1984; **37**: 149–59.

32. Wei FC, Jain V, Celik N *et al*. Have we found an ideal soft-tissue flap? An experience with 672 anterolateral thigh flaps. *Plastic and Reconstructive Surgery* 2002; **109**: 2219–26; discussion 2227–30.

33. Slough CM, Johns R, Randolph GW *et al*. History of thyroid and parathyroid surgery. In: Randolph G (ed.). *Surgery of the thyroid and parathyroid glands.* Philadelphia, PA: Saunders, 2003: 3–11.

34. Welbourne RB. *The history of endocrine surgery.* New York: Praegar, 1990.

INTRODUCTION TO HEAD AND NECK SURGERY

Section editor: René Leemans

2

Epidemiology and prevention of head and neck cancer

IAN GANLY AND SNEHAL G PATEL

> To study the phenomenon of disease without books is to sail an uncharted sea, while to study books without patients is not to go to sea at all.
>
> Sir William Osler (1849–1919)

INTRODUCTION

Squamous cell cancer constitutes the most common head and neck malignancy and is related to tobacco and/or alcohol usage. Non-squamous malignancy includes thyroid cancer, salivary gland cancer and sarcomas. These malignancies are not associated with tobacco and/or alcohol usage. According to the National Cancer Institute's Surveillance Epidemiology and End Results (SEER) programmes of the United States, between 1975 and 2001 the incidence for most head and neck cancer sites has globally decreased, except for tongue (up 16 per cent), tonsil (up 12 per cent), nasal cavity and sinuses (up 12 per cent), salivary glands (up 20 per cent) and thyroid (up 52 per cent). Estimated new head and neck cancer cases and deaths for 2007 are shown in **Table 2.1**.

SQUAMOUS MALIGNANT TUMOURS

Squamous cell carcinoma of the head and neck encompasses cancer of the oral cavity, oropharynx, larynx and hypopharynx, nasopharynx, nasal cavity and paranasal sinuses. The main causative factors are tobacco and alcohol usage. In the UK, head and neck cancer represents 5–10 per cent of all tumours making it the eighth most common cancer in males and sixteenth most frequent in females. However, the incidence of head and neck cancer varies with geography with high rates being reported in France, India, South America and Eastern Europe.[1, 2, 3] In most regions, the majority of cancers arise in the larynx. In the Indian subcontinent, head and neck cancer accounts for 45 per cent of all malignancies with oral cancer being the most common type accounting for one-third of all cancers.[4] For nasopharyngeal carcinoma, there are wide geographical differences with very high rates in Southeast Asia. This is due to Epstein–Barr virus and inhalation of carcinogens from cured fish and other aetiological agents.

Men are two to three times more commonly affected than women and the incidence increases with age with 98 per cent of cases occurring in patients over 40 years of age. The two most important factors in the aetiology of head and neck cancer are tobacco and alcohol. There is a synergistic interaction between these two agents which is supermultiplicative for the mouth, additive for the larynx and between additive and multiplicative for the oesophagus.[5] A large case–control study from the United States shows good evidence of a dose–response relationship for both tobacco and alcohol.[6, 7] Other factors are also implicated in the aetiology of head and neck cancer; there is a great deal of statistical evidence supporting agents such as diet, viruses, occupational agents, pollutants, genetic influences, but few case-controlled epidemiological studies have been carried out.

Since the histologic distribution and aetiopathologic considerations for cancers at various sites within the head and neck are distinct, the epidemiology and prevention of these tumours will be discussed in more detail under separate anatomic sites.

Table 2.1   Estimated new cancer cases and deaths in the United States, 2007.

	Estimated cases			Estimated deaths		
	Both sexes	Male	Female	Both sexes	Male	Female
Oral cavity/oropharynx	34 360	24 180	10 180	7550	5180	2370
Tongue	9800	6930	2870	1830	1180	650
Mouth	10 660	6480	4180	1860	1110	750
Other oral cavity	2100	1460	640	1680	1270	410
Oropharynx	11 800	9310	2490	2180	1620	560
Larynx	11 300	8960	2340	3660	2900	760
Thyroid	33 550	8070	25 480	1530	650	880

Cancer of the oral cavity and oropharynx

EPIDEMIOLOGY

It is estimated that in 2007 there will be 22 560 new cases of oral cavity cancer in the United States, 14 870 male and 7690 female. In the UK, it is the 20th most common cancer. The incidence and mortality increase with age with over 85 per cent of cases occurring after the fifth decade. Over the last 30 years, there has been a slight increase in oral cancer mainly attributable to the increase in tongue cancer in young men.[8, 9, 10, 11] When patients newly diagnosed with oral and oropharyngeal cancers are carefully examined, about 15 per cent will have another cancer in nearby areas, such as the larynx, oesophagus or lung. Of those who are cured of oral or oropharyngeal cancer, 10–40 per cent will develop a second cancer of the upper aerodigestive tract at a later time. Lung cancer often also occurs in these patients. For this reason, it is important for patients with oral and oropharyngeal cancer to have follow-up examinations for the rest of their lives and to avoid smoking and drinking, which increase the risk for these second cancers.

Cancer of the oropharynx is the third most common head and neck cancer after larynx and oral cavity. In 2007, it is estimated that there were 11 800 new cases of oropharynx cancer in the United States, 9310 male and 2490 female. In the UK, it has an incidence of 0.8 per 100 000 population per annum. This accounts for 10.9 per cent of all head and neck cancers.[12] Raised incidence rates are observed in the Netherlands, India, France and Italy.[12] There has been a slight increase in tonsil and base of tongue cancer over the last decade and this is largely due to human papilloma virus (HPV) infection of the palatine and lingual tonsils.[13]

AETIOLOGY

Tobacco

Cigarettes

Tobacco is the most important factor and over 90 per cent of patients have a history of smoking. Tobacco contains over 30 known carcinogens, such as polycyclic aromatic hydro-carbons and nitrosamines.[14] There is a synergistic interaction with alcohol due to the increased mucosal absorption of these carcinogens as a result of the increased solubility of the

carcinogens in alcohol compared with aqueous saliva. The use of filtered cigarettes reduces this exposure[15, 16] and stopping smoking reduces the risk of head and neck cancer. The risk of oral cancer is reduced by 30 per cent in those who have discontinued for between one and nine years and by 50 per cent for those over nine years,[17] but it is unlikely that it ever returns to the baseline as compared to the rest of the population.

Pipe and cigar smokers have an increased risk of oral cancer compared to other head and neck subsites.[18] This is thought to be due to the type of tobacco used. There are two major types of tobacco – black or dark (air-cured) tobacco is used in the manufacture of cigars and pipe blends and blond (flue-cured) tobacco is used for cigarettes. Black tobacco cigarette users have a three-fold relative risk of oral cavity and pharyngeal cancer when compared to blond tobacco cigarette users.[19] This is because the extract of black tobacco cigarettes is more carcinogenic than blond tobacco cigarettes.[20]

In the oropharynx, the sites most commonly affected are those in prolonged contact with surface carcinogen. The crypts of the tonsils, the glossotonsillar sulcus and the tongue base are bathed in saliva to a greater extent than the soft palate or post-pharyngeal wall and are thus more common sites in cases where smoking and alcohol are aetiological factors.

Smokeless tobacco

Oral cancer is strongly associated with different forms of smokeless tobacco consumed by chewing. These include bidi, chutta, paan, khaini and toombak. This is particularly common in the Indian subcontinent and accounts for the high incidence of oral cancer in these countries. Oral cancer increases in a dose-dependent fashion with these agents.[21, 22] There is also a strong association between the site of oral cancer and the site where the tobacco is placed. In India and parts of Asia, oral tobacco is mixed with betel leaf, slated lime and areca nut to form a quid called 'paan'. The lime lowers the pH which accelerates the release of alkaloids from both the tobacco and areca nut. Chewing paan correlates with alveolobuccal cancer.[23] Paan is also strongly associated with a premaligant lesion oral submucus fibrosis.[24] Bidi smoking causes cancer of the oral commissure, oral tongue and also the base of the tongue. Reverse smoking (chutta) is associated with cancer of the hard palate and palatine arch in India.[25] Other forms of smokeless tobacco include khaini and toombak. Khaini is a mixture of tobacco and lime that is retained in the inferior gingivobuccal sulcus and leads to cancer in this site.[26] Toombak, the form used in the Sudan, has been extensively studied. It contains very high levels of nitrosamines.[27] Toombak-associated carcinogens have high prevalence of p53 protein aberration.

Marijuana

When marijuana is smoked, a wide range of potential carcinogens are released and absorbed, including polycyclic aromatic hydrocarbons, benzopyrene, phenols, phytosterols, acids and terpenes.[28] A study from Memorial Sloan Kettering Cancer Center reported an overall risk of 2.6 compared to non-users.[29]

Alcohol

Alcohol is believed to act in a synergistic fashion with tobacco in the aetiology of oral and oropharyngeal cancer.[30, 31, 32] However, some case–control and cohort studies have shown an increased risk of cancer even in non-smokers.[33] Over the past few decades, alcohol consumption has been steadily increasing and this matches the increase in oral cancer mortality.[34] There is variation in oral cavity sites with higher risk of buccal cancer than floor of the mouth cancer in non-drinkers and a higher risk of lateral tongue cancer than other tongue cancers in non-drinkers. In the oropharynx, tumours arise more commonly in the glossotonsillar sulci and more posteriorly in the pharyngoepiglottic fold.

The precise mechanism by which alcohol causes cancer is not clearly defined as alcohol itself is not a carcinogen. Possible mechanisms include:

1. Alcohol may act as a solvent increasing the cellular permeability of tobacco carcinogens through the mucosa of the upper aerodigestive tract.[30]
2. The non-alcohol constituents of various alcoholic beverages may have carcinogenic activities.
3. The immediate metabolite of ethanol is acetaldehyde and this may have a locally damaging effect on cells.[35]
4. Chronic alcohol use may upregulate enzymes of the cytochrome P450 system which may result in the activation of procarcinogens into carcinogens.
5. Alcohol can also decrease the activity of DNA repair enzymes resulting in increased chromosomal damage.
6. Alcohol impairs immunity due to a reduction in T cell number, decreased mitogenic activity and macrophage activity.
7. Alcohol is high in calories, which suppresses appetite in heavy drinkers. Metabolism is further damaged by liver disease resulting in nutritional deficiencies and therefore lowered resistance to cancer.

Dental factors

Poor oral hygiene is associated with oral cancer, although no causal relationship has ever been established. This may be due to chronic inflammation of the gingiva.[36] Painful or loose fitting dentures have also been associated with oral and oropharyngeal cancer.[37, 38] This may also be due to chronic inflammation. There is some evidence suggesting mouthwashes containing alcohol may also be important,[39] although it is possible that the cancer risk is due to other factors, for example, patients may use the mouthwash to disguise the smell of tobacco or disguise the smell of alcohol.

Occupational exposure

Wood dust exposure is associated with the risk of oral cancer,[40] as well as pharyngeal and laryngeal cancer.[41] Occupations involving exposure to organic chemicals and coal products are also at increased risk.[41]

Infections

In head and neck cancer, several viruses have been implicated in carcinogenesis, including human papilloma virus (HPV), human immunodeficiency virus (HIV), herpes simplex virus (HSV) and Epstein–Barr virus (EBV).

Human papillomavirus

Human papilloma virus has been extensively studied and there seems to be a definite association between virus and tumour formation.[13, 42] In particular, between 30 and 100 per cent of verrucous carcinomas have HPV.[43] The proportion of cancers with HPV varies with site with a strong association with tonsil cancer.[44, 45] Steinberg[43] reported HPV infection to be highest in tonsil (74 per cent), followed by larynx (30 per cent), tongue (22 per cent), nasopharynx (21 per cent) and floor of the mouth (5 per cent). HPV exists in many different serotypes and specific serotypes are associated with head and neck cancer. For example, benign lesions such as the common wart are associated with 'low risk types' and include HPV 6, 11, 13, 32.[46] High risk types are associated with premalignant lesions and squamous cell carcinoma and include HPV 16, 18, 31, 33, 35, 39.[46, 47] HPV 16 and 18 appear to be the most common types associated with squamous cell carcinoma. HPV 31, 33 and 35 are more commonly associated with cervical cancer and are not found in oral cancer.[48, 49] The E6 and E7 open reading frames (ORFs) of the high risk HPVs are particularly important. They bind to and inactivate tumour suppressor genes p53 and pRb, respectively.[50] This allows uncontrolled cell proliferation which can result in genomic instability and cellular transformation.[51] There is no relationship between clinical stage and HPV status in squamous cell carcinoma of the head and neck. This suggests HPV infection is not a late event in the evolution of head and neck cancer. As mentioned above, the highest incidence of HPV is found in tonsil cancer suggesting that there is a predilection of HPV infection for patients with tonsillar carcinoma.[44, 45] Patients with HPV-positive tonsil cancer tend to be young, non-smokers and non-drinkers. The molecular characteristics are completely different to HPV-negative tonsil cancers, where p53 is often mutated due to carcinogens in tobacco smoke and amplification of cyclin D1. Probably due to the different pathogenetic origin, HPV-positive tonsil cancers have a better prognosis.

Human immunodeficiency virus

A recent study from New York showed HIV infection in 5 per cent of head and neck cancer patients.[52] In patients under 45 years, HIV infection was present in over 20 per cent. Due to the depressed immunity in HIV patients, the head and neck cancers observed were larger and more advanced in the HIV group. In addition, HIV infection is more common in inner city populations and certain socioeconomic groups and this will also contribute to the advanced stage at presentation of these patients.

Herpes simplex virus

Several studies have shown that patients with oral cancer have higher antibodies to herpes simplex virus, but this does not prove a causal relationship.[53] Antibody levels are higher in smokers and even higher in smokers with oral cancer. It is possible that the immunosuppression produced by smoking may lead to HSV chronic carrier state, resulting in raised antibody levels. HSV-type protein has been reported in 42 per cent of patients with oral cancer and 0 per cent in control patients.[54] However, there is little evidence that HSV gene sequences are present in oral cancer cells or any evidence of gene integration. Therefore, there is currently little emphasis on HSV in head and neck cancer.

Epstein–Barr virus

There is no evidence that EBV is associated with oral cancer. However, this virus is strongly associated with nasopharyngeal carcinoma. The association is strongest for WHO types II and III.[55] Eighty-one per cent of Greenland Eskimos have EBV, a population with a high incidence of undifferentiated nasopharyngeal cancer, suggesting that a chronic carrier state exists in endemic populations.

Nutritional factors

Several studies suggest high fruit and vegetable intake is associated with a decreased risk of head and neck cancer. This may be due to increased intake of the antioxidants or free radical scavenging vitamins A, C and E.[56, 57] La Vecchia et al.[58] estimated that up to 15 per cent of oral and pharyngeal cancers in Europe can be attributed to dietary deficiencies. Some studies have shown an increased risk with red meat intake and salted meat.[59, 60]

Inflammatory

Gastro-oesophageal reflux disease

Reflux has been documented in 36–54 per cent of patients,[61, 62] which could suggest reflux to be a risk factor in laryngeal and pharyngeal cancer. However, no direct causal association has been reported.

Precancer

Leukoplakia and erythroplakia are significant factors important in the aetiology of oral cancer. Submucous fibrosis is a well-recognized precancerous condition, resulting in tumours in the orpharynx, particularly on the anterior palatoglossal fold.

Genetic and immunologic predisposition

Although smoking is the main risk factor, not all people who smoke develop head and neck cancer. Therefore, genetic and immunologic factors also play a role. There are several genetic conditions which are associated with increased risk. Li–Fraumeni syndrome, an autosomal dominant condition involving mutation of the *p53* gene, has been associated with head and neck cancer in patients with minimal tobacco exposure.[63] Fanconi's anemia, Bloom syndrome and ataxia-telangiectasia are autosomal recessive disorders associated with increased chromosomal fragility and cancer

susceptibility. There is an increased incidence of head and neck cancer in each of these conditions.[64, 65, 66, 67] There is a genetic susceptibility in the capacity to metabolize carcinogens and repair consequent DNA damage. This involves polymorphisms in *GST* genes,[68, 69, 70] *CYP* genes[71, 72] and the cytochrome P450 system.[73]

Immunologic factors are also important. Patients treated for bone marrow transplants and organ transplants have an increased incidence of skin cancer and oral cavity cancer. This may be due to the long-term use of immunosuppressive drugs.[74]

PREVENTION OF CANCER OF THE ORAL CAVITY AND OROPHARYNX

Screening

Cancers of the oral cavity are generally easily amenable to early detection during routine screening examinations by a doctor or dentist, or by self-examination. Regular dental check ups that include an examination of the entire mouth are important in helping to find oral and oropharyngeal cancers (and precancers) early. Many doctors and dentists recommend that patients look at their mouth in a mirror every month. The American Cancer Society also recommends that doctors examine the mouth and throat as part of a routine cancer-related check-up. On the other hand, tumours of the oropharynx remain relatively asymptomatic and may not be easily accessible to early detection even by an experienced clinician. A high index of suspicion is necessary in adults who present with an otherwise asymptomatic neck mass, especially if there is a history of tobacco and/or alcohol abuse.

Reducing risk factors

Most oral cavity and oropharyngeal cancer can be prevented by avoiding known risk factors. Tobacco and alcohol are the most important risk factors for these cancers. The best approach is never to start smoking and limit the intake of alcoholic beverages. Quitting tobacco and alcohol greatly lowers the risk of developing these cancers, even after many years of use. Exposure to ultraviolet radiation is an important and avoidable risk factor for cancer of the lips, as well as for skin cancer. Exposure to ultraviolet rays can be reduced by avoiding the midday sun, wearing a wide-brimmed hat and using sunscreen. Avoiding sources of oral irritation (such as dentures that do not fit properly) may also decrease the risk for oral cancer. A poor diet has been related to oral cavity and oropharyngeal cancer. The American Cancer Society recommends eating a variety of healthful foods, with an emphasis on plant sources. This includes eating at least five servings of fruit and vegetables every day, as well as servings of whole grain foods from plant sources such as breads, cereals, grain products, rice, pasta or beans. Eating fewer red meats, especially those high in fat or processed is also recommended. A diet rich in antioxidants, such as carotene, vitamins C and E, seems to prevent head and neck squamous cell cancer in heavy smokers and drinkers.[75]

Chemoprevention

At one time, it was thought that because leukoplakia or erythroplakia often preceded the development of oral cancer, surgically removing these areas would prevent cancer from developing. However, recent studies have found that even when these areas are completely removed, people with certain types of erythroplakia and leukoplakia are still at increased risk of developing a cancer in some other area of their mouth. This risk is particularly high if the affected tissue appears abnormal under the microscope (dysplastic) and has an abnormal amount of DNA in its cells (aneuploidy). One reason surgery does not help prevent cancer is that the entire lining of the mouth can be considered 'precancerous'. This is referred to as 'field cancerization'.[76, 77] Chemoprevention may be beneficial in patients with leukoplakia or erythroplakia. For example, isotretinoin (13-*cis*-retinoic acid) is a drug chemically related to vitamin A (a retinoid). When used by patients with oral cavity or oropharyngeal cancer, isotretinoin may reduce the risk of developing a second cancer in the head and neck region. Unfortunately, side effects of this medicine limit its use.[78] Another approach has been to develop oral rinses that contain anticancer compounds. A common class of drugs being tested is the non-steroidal anti-inflammatory drugs.[79] Clinical trials using gene therapy and vaccine therapy are also underway.[80, 81]

Cancer of the larynx and hypopharynx

EPIDEMIOLOGY

The American Cancer Society estimated that 11 300 new cases of laryngeal cancer (8960 in men and 2340 in women) would be diagnosed, and 3660 people (2900 men and 760 women) would die from the disease in the United States in 2007. These numbers are falling by around 2 to 3 per cent a year, mainly because fewer people are smoking. About 60 per cent of larynx cancers start in the glottis, 35 per cent develop in the supraglottic region and the remaining 5 per cent occur in the subglottis.

Cancer of the hypopharynx accounts for 10 per cent of all squamous cell cancers of the upper aerodigestive tract.[82] In the UK, the overall incidence is 1 per 100 000 per annum. There is a high incidence in Northern France of 14.8 per 100 000.[83] Subsites of the hypopharynx include pyriform fossa (70 per cent), postcricoid area (15 per cent) and posterior pharyngeal wall (15 per cent). The pyriform fossa is the most common subsite in North America and France. Postcricoid lesions appear more commonly in Northern Europe. The mean age at presentation is 60 years. Pyriform fossa and post-pharyngeal wall have a male predominance of 5 to 20:1 in North America[84, 85] with 50:1 in France.[86] Postcricoid lesions show a female preponderance 1.5:1.[87, 88, 89]

AETIOLOGY

Tobacco

There is a strong association between laryngeal cancer and cigarette smoking. The relative risk of laryngeal cancer between smokers and non-smokers is 15.5 in men and 12.4 in women.[90] Environmental tobacco smoke also increases the risk of laryngeal cancer.[91]

Alcohol

The combined use of tobacco and alcohol increases the risk of laryngeal cancer by 50 per cent over the estimated risk, if these factors were considered additive.[92, 93, 94] Different alcoholic beverages have different carcinogenic content. Beer contains the carcinogen nitrosodimethylamine, while wines contain the carcinogen tannin. Dark liquors (whisky, rum) have greater organic compounds (esters, acetaldehyde) than light liquors (vodka, gin). The risk of laryngeal and hypopharyngeal cancer is increased with dark alcohol intake. Risk is greater for hypopharyngeal cancer than laryngeal cancer.[95] This variation in the risk of alcohol is shown for different sites in the larynx, i.e. supraglottic cancer patients are more likely than glottic and subglottic patients to be heavy drinkers of alcohol.[96, 97]

Occupational factors

Laryngeal cancer is associated with nickel and mustard gas exposure.[98] There may also be association with asbestos exposure.[99, 100] Machinists and car mechanics are at increased risk.[101, 102] Long-term exposure to sulphuric and hydrochloric acid in battery plant workers have increased risk.[103]

Radiation

Postcricoid carcinoma is associated with previous radiation[87, 104] and sideropenic dysphagia.[87, 88, 89] Between 4 and 6 per cent have a history of Patterson Brown–Kelly or Plummer Vinson syndrome. Radiation is also implicated in posterior pharyngeal wall carcinomas.[105]

Nutritional factors

Several studies associate high fruit and vegetable intake with a decreased risk of head and neck cancer. This may reflect increased intake of the antioxidants or free radical scavenging vitamins A, C and E.[106, 107]

Infection

As in oral cavity and oropharyngeal cancer, human papilloma viruses may also be a factor in some cases of laryngeal and hypopharyngeal cancer.

Immunosuppression

Laryngeal and hypopharyngeal cancers are more common in people who are immunosuppressed due to HIV or due to organ transplantation.

PREVENTION

Reducing risk factors

Most laryngeal and hypopharyngeal cancers can be prevented by avoiding the known risk factors. Tobacco use is the most important cause of cancer in these areas. Because alcohol abuse acts synergistically with tobacco smoke, it is especially important to avoid the combination of drinking and smoking. In the workplace, adequate ventilation and the use of industrial respirators when working with cancer-causing chemicals are important preventive measures. As in all head and neck cancers, malnutrition and vitamin deficiencies are also important and eating a healthy balanced diet is recommended.

Chemoprevention

Chemoprevention is the use of drugs to stop cancer from developing. This may involve preventing precancerous lesions, such as dysplasia from becoming cancerous or preventing cancer from recurring once it has been treated. They may also prevent the development of a second tumour in the head and neck area. Various chemopreventive agents are being tested to see if they can reduce the risk of developing a second primary tumour. Several retinoid analogues (chemicals related to vitamin A) are currently being studied. The drug most commonly studied is isotretinoin (Accutane™).

Cancer of the nasopharynx

EPIDEMIOLOGY

Nasopharyngeal cancer (NPC) is rare with an incidence in the UK of 0.5/100 000. It accounts for 1–2 per cent of all head and neck cancers. In the United States, there are approximately 2000 cases per year. However, in southern China and Hong Kong, the disease is endemic with an incidence rate of 50 per 100 000.[108] It is also common among the Inuits of Alaska. It is also found more often in immigrant groups in the United States, such as recent Chinese immigrants and those from Southeast Asia, such as the Hmong. In the last few years, the rate at which Americans, including Chinese immigrants, have been developing this cancer has been slowly dropping.

There are three subtypes:

1. WHO type 1: keratinizing squamous cell carcinoma
2. WHO type 2: non-keratinizing (differentiated) carcinoma
3. WHO type 3: undifferentiated carcinoma.

In North America, type 1 accounts for 68 per cent of cases.[109] In the Far East, type 2 and 3 account for 95 per cent of cases.[110]

NPC affects a younger age group than other head and neck cancers. In endemic areas, the incidence rises from age 20 to peak in the fourth and fifth decades.[111] All NPCs show a male preponderance of 3:1. In the United States, it is 50 per cent more common in blacks than in whites.

AETIOLOGY

Nasopharyngeal cancer is the result of interaction of genetic and environmental factors.

Genetic factors

The genetic association is with different types of HLA types: in ethnic Chinese, NPC is associated with HLA types A2, B17 and Bw46.[112] HLA B17 carries the same risk as Bw46 and is associated with younger onset disease and poorer prognosis.[113] In addition, family members of people with NPC are more likely to get this cancer.

Environmental factors

The most important environmental factor is infection by EBV. Almost all nasopharyngeal cancer cells contain EBV.

There is a strong association between undifferentiated nasopharynx cancer and positive serology for EBV antigens. Antibody titres to EBV antigens correlate with stage of disease and a fall reflects tumour response to treatment, whereas a rise in antibody levels means progression of disease.[114, 115]

Dietary factors are also important. People who live in areas of Asia, northern Africa and the Arctic region, where NPC is common, typically eat diets very high in salt-cured fish and meat. Studies indicate that foods preserved in this way that are cooked at high temperatures may produce chemicals that can damage DNA. Ho[116] has reported accumulation of carcinogenic nitrosamines in salted fish. In southeast China, the rate of this cancer is dropping as people begin eating a more 'western' diet.

PREVENTION

Reducing risk factors

Most people in the United Kingdom and United States who develop nasopharyngeal cancer have no known risk factors, so their cancers could not have been prevented. Because certain dietary factors have been associated with NPC risk, eliminating them is one way to reduce the number of cases in parts of the world where NPC is common, such as southern China, northern Africa and the Arctic region. Descendants of Southeast Asians who immigrated to the United States and eat a typical 'American diet', for example, have lower risk of developing NPC.

Early detection and screening

In some parts of the world, such as China, where NPC is common, some effort is underway for screening for this cancer. Subjects are first selected if their blood shows evidence of infection with the EBV; these patients are then subsequently given regular examinations. This strategy can also be applied to families where one member has developed NPC. It is not yet known if this intervention will lower the death rate from this cancer. Some cases of NPC can be found early in the course of the disease because they result in symptoms that cause patients to seek medical attention. The symptoms may even seem unrelated to the nasopharynx (e.g. in adults, persistent fullness in one ear). In some other cases, NPC may not cause symptoms until it has reached an advanced stage. Most of the time, however, the cancer spreads to lymph nodes in the neck before any symptoms occur. Over 80 per cent of patients are in an advanced stage when they are diagnosed.

Cancer of the nasal cavity and paranasal sinuses

EPIDEMIOLOGY

Cancers of the nasal cavity and paranasal sinuses are rare. About 2000 people in the United States develop cancer of the nasal cavity and paranasal sinuses each year. Men are about 50 per cent more likely than women to get this cancer. Nearly 80 per cent of the people who get this cancer are between the ages of 45 and 85 years. These cancers also occur much more often in certain areas of the world, such as Japan and South Africa. About 60–70 per cent of cancers of the nasal cavity and paranasal sinuses occur in the maxillary sinus, 20–30 per cent in the nasal cavity, 10–15 per cent in the ethmoid sinuses, and less than 5 per cent in the frontal and sphenoid sinuses.

AETIOLOGY

As in all head and neck cancer, smoking tobacco is a risk factor for nasal cavity cancer. Occupational factors are also important. These include occupational exposure to dusts from wood, textiles and leather, and even perhaps flour. Other substances linked to this type of cancer are glues, formaldehyde, solvents used in furniture and shoe production, nickel and chromium dust, mustard gas, isopropyl ('rubbing') alcohol and radium. HPV infection may also be important; HPV DNA type 16 has been detected in over 50 per cent of non-keratinizing carcinomas.[117]

PREVENTION

Reducing risk factors

The best way to prevent cancer of the nasal cavity and paranasal sinuses is to avoid the known risk factors, such as cigarette smoking. Environmental protective measures include adequate ventilation and the use of respirators can reduce occupational exposure to airborne carcinogens. However, because many people with cancer of the nasal cavity and paranasal sinuses have no known risk factors, there is currently no way to prevent all of these cancers.

Early detection and screening

Small cancers of the nasal cavity and paranasal sinuses usually do not cause any specific symptoms. Many of the symptoms of nasal cavity and paranasal sinus cancers can also be caused by benign conditions, such as infections. For these reasons, many of these cancers are not recognized until they have grown large enough to block the nasal airway or sinuses, or until they have spread to adjacent tissues, regional lymph nodes or even to distant areas of the body. Because cancers of the nasal cavity and paranasal sinuses occur so rarely, routine testing of people without any symptoms is not recommended.

NON-SQUAMOUS MALIGNANT TUMOURS

Carcinoma of the thyroid

EPIDEMIOLOGY

In the year 2007, in the United States, it was estimated that there would be 33 550 new cases of thyroid cancer diagnosed. It is more common in women with a ratio of 3:1 and affects mainly young people with nearly two-thirds of cases in the age group 20–55 years. The most common type is differentiated (80 per cent), which includes papillary (85 per cent) and follicular (15 per cent) cancer. Poorly differentiated

cancer accounts for 10 per cent of cases, anaplastic 5 per cent and medullary thyroid cancer 5 per cent. The incidence of thyroid cancer is increasing and this increase is mostly related to papillary carcinoma diagnosis, without any significant difference in the less frequent histologies. The increase is the result of the incidental detection of early thyroid cancer because of increasing use of imaging, such as computed tomography (CT), magnetic resonance imaging (MRI), ultrasound (US) and positron emission tomography (PET)[118] Between 1988 and 2002, the increased number of thyroid cancers is the result of increased numbers of small nodules (<1 cm in 49 per cent of cases and <2 cm in 87 per cent of cases). The increase is therefore due to subclinical diagnosis rather than a true disease incidence. As a result, the mortality rates for well-differentiated thyroid cancer have remained relatively static and the prognosis is excellent with a five-year survival of all cases of 97 per cent. Medullary thyroid cancer (MTC), which constitutes approximately 5 per cent of all thyroid malignancies, originates from the parafollicular C cells, secretes calcitonin and occurs in both sporadic and hereditary forms.[119, 120]

AETIOLOGY

Diet low in iodine

Thyroid cancer is more common in areas of the world where diets are low in iodine.[121]

Radiation

A history of radiation treatment in childhood is a known risk factor. In the past, radiation was used to treat children with acne, fungal infections of the scalp, an enlarged thymus and tonsillar and adenoidal hypertrophy. Subsequent studies showed that there was an increased incidence of thyroid cancer in these children.[122] In contrast, exposure to radiation in adults carries little risk of thyroid cancer. Children exposed to radioactive fallout from nuclear power plant accidents or nuclear weapons also have an increased incidence of thyroid cancer. For example, children exposed to nuclear fallout from Chernobyl have an eight times incidence of thyroid cancer.[123, 124, 125]

Hereditary conditions

Inherited medical conditions, such as Gardner syndrome, familial polyposis and Cowden disease, have an increased incidence of thyroid cancer. Certain families also have an increased incidence of papillary thyroid cancer. Seventy-five per cent of MTC occur as a sporadic form and 25 per cent as a hereditary form. The hereditary forms can occur in three different settings: as a single component in a hereditary disease (FMTC), in the hereditary syndrome multiple endocrine neoplasia syndrome type A (MEN-2A) associated with parathyroid disease and phaeochromocytoma and finally in the hereditary syndrome MEN-2B associated with phaeochromocytoma and a specific phenotype characterized by mucosal ganglioneuromas, intestinal ganglioneuromatosis and a marfanoid habitus. Both MEN-2 syndromes are autosomal dominant genetic disorders characterized by mutations in the RET proto-oncogene.[126, 127] Patients can now be stratified into high-, intermediate- and low-risk groups according to the type of RET mutation.[128]

PREVENTION

Reducing risk factors

Most people with thyroid cancer have no known risk factors. Therefore, it is not possible to reliably prevent most cases of this disease.

Early detection and screening

Most cases of thyroid cancer can be found early by the detection of a neck lump either by the patient or by their doctor on routine examination. It is unusual for early thyroid cancer to present with any symptoms. In MTC, 80 per cent are familial and 20 per cent sporadic. In the familial forms, mutation of the RET proto-oncogene is present. It is therefore possible to screen family members of patients with MTC for RET mutations. There are several types of mutations which can be classified into low-, intermediate- and high-risk mutations.[128] If present, these patients can then be treated by prophylactic thyroidectomy. The age of thyroidectomy is also influenced by the type of RET mutation; patients with high risk mutations can be offered prophylactic thyroidectomy as early as three years of age.[129]

Salivary gland carcinomas

EPIDEMIOLOGY

There are two main types of salivary glands, the major salivary glands (parotid, submandibular and sublingual glands) and the minor salivary glands. About 80 per cent of all salivary gland tumours are in the parotid gland, 10–15 per cent in the submandibular gland and the rest in the sublingual and minor salivary glands. Most tumours of the parotid gland are benign, whereas 40 per cent of submandibular gland tumours and 80 per cent of minor salivary gland tumours are malignant. There are several different types of malignant tumours of the salivary glands due to the different types of cells which make up normal salivary glands. These include mucoepidermoid carcinoma, adenoid cystic carcinoma, acinic cell carcinoma, polymorphous low-grade adenocarcinoma and rare adenocarcinomas, such as basal cell, clear cell, salivary duct and mucinous adenocarcinoma. Salivary gland carcinomas are not common and occur with an annual rate of 1.2 per 100 000 in the United States. About one-third of patients are under the age of 55 years. The incidence of these cancers is increasing, but the cause for this is unknown. The survival depends on cell type and stage of the cancer. The overall five-year survival rate is 68 per cent for all people with salivary gland cancer.

AETIOLOGY

Exposure to radiation to the head and neck area for other medical reasons, e.g. radiotherapy for squamous cell cancer, increases the risk of salivary gland cancer.[130] Industrial exposure to radioactive substances and also accidental exposure from atomic bomb blasts also increase the risk of salivary gland cancer.[130] Some studies have also suggested that working with certain metals (nickel alloy dust) and minerals (silica dust) may increase the risk for salivary gland cancer. In men, smoking and heavy alcohol consumption was also associated with higher risk, but these factors were not strongly related to salivary gland cancer in women.[131] Hormonal dependence may also be important; early menarche and nulliparity are associated with increased risk, whereas older age at full-term pregnancy and long duration of oral contraceptive use are associated with reduced risk.[132] Female patients with salivary gland tumours are also 0.5 times more likely to develop breast cancer.[133] Diets low in vegetables and high in animal fat may also be an important factor.[134]

PREVENTION

Avoiding certain risk factors, such as radioactive substances, nickel dust and silica dust, may help reduce the risk of developing salivary gland cancer. These cancers can also be found early when the patient or doctor notices a lump within the gland. Checking the salivary gland for lumps should therefore be a routine part of a general medical or dental check-up.

Sarcomas of the head and neck

EPIDEMIOLOGY

Sarcomas of the head and neck constitute less than 1 per cent of head and neck malignancies. They are divided into those arising from soft tissue sarcomas (STS)[135] and those arising from bone (osteosarcoma).[136] Soft tissue sarcomas comprise a heterogeneous group with varied histology and behaviour, and include chondrosarcoma, dermatofibrosarcoma protuberans, Ewing's sarcoma, leiomyosarcoma, liposarcoma, malignant fibrous histiocytoma, malignant peripheral nerve sheath tumour, rhabdomyosarcoma and synovial sarcoma.[135] Rhabdomyosarcoma is rare in adults, but is the most common soft tissue sarcoma in children with over 30 per cent occurring in the head and neck. Dermatofibrosarcoma protuberans is a rare tumour of the dermis that has a high recurrence rate. Malignant fibrous histiocytoma is the most common soft tissue sarcoma in middle and late adulthood. Only 4 per cent of liposarcomas occur in the head and neck with the neck being the most common site. Synovial sarcomas occur in the 20–50 year age group with the majority arising in the parapharyngeal space. The most common site of chondrosarcoma in the head and neck is the larynx, maxilla and skull base. Most occur in the age group of 30–60 years. The most common site in the larynx is the posterior lamina of the cricoid cartilage (75 per cent). Malignant peripheral nerve sheath tumours are extremely rare, but more common in patients with neurofibromatosis type 1 (NF1).

Osteogenic sarcoma is a rare highly malignant tumour with an incidence of one in 100 000 with only 7 per cent occurring in the head and neck region. The majority of these arise in the mandible followed by the maxilla. Head and neck osteosarcoma is most common between the ages of 30 and

40 years in comparison to long bone osteosarcoma which is most common in the teenage years.

AETIOLOGY

Genetic predisposition

Studies have shown that some groups of individuals are at an increased risk of developing soft tissue sarcoma. Among them are genetically predisposed individuals, such as those suffering from neurofibromatosis who are at risk of malignant peripheral nerve sheath tumour (MPNT), people with the Li–Fraumeni syndrome and children with retinoblastoma who are predisposed to osteosarcoma, rhabdomyosarcoma and fibrosarcoma. Other heritable syndromes associated with an increased risk of STS include Gardner's syndrome and nevoid basal cell carcinoma syndrome.

Radiation

Previous exposure to irradiation is another well-documented risk factor[137] for both soft tissue sarcoma and osteogenic sarcoma. Although radiation-induced sarcoma (RIS) is a well-recognized long-term complication of radiation therapy for other sites, the head and neck are less commonly affected. It is difficult to implicate therapeutic irradiation in the causation of head and neck tumours because of the inherent risk of multiple primary tumours in these patients. In addition, patients with certain types of primary tumours, such as retinoblastomas, have an increased sensitivity to radiation therapy, but are at increased risk for the development of sarcoma irrespective of the type of treatment.

Occupational factors

Environmental carcinogens, and chemicals like urethane, ethylene derivatives and polycyclic hydrocarbons, have also been reported to increase the risk of STS at sites other than the head and neck.

Viruses

The role of viruses in the pathogenesis of STS has been investigated, but apart from the association of HIV with Kaposi's sarcoma and the observation that viral oncogenes, such as the *src* in the Rous sarcoma virus, can transform cells in culture, no conclusive proof is available for a viral aetiology. Immunosuppression attributable to either HIV infection or antirejection medication in organ transplant recipients has been reported to have predisposed to leiomyosarcoma of the liver in paediatric patients who had a latent Epstein–Barr virus (EBV) infection.

Trauma

Trauma most often draws attention to a tumour and there is no conclusive evidence to support the association of sarcomas to scar tissue. A possible association between artificial implants and soft tissue sarcomas has been debated for a few years and angiosarcomas have been reported to arise around previously placed vascular grafts.[138]

Other factors

Patients with chronic lymphoedema have an increased incidence of soft tissue sarcoma formation.[139] Patients with Paget's disease of bone, particularly the skull, are predisposed to osteogenic sarcoma.[140, 141]

PREVENTION

Reducing risk factors

Most people with sarcoma have no known risk factors. Therefore, it is not possible to reliably prevent most cases of this disease.

EARLY DETECTION AND SCREENING

Most cases of sarcoma often present late due to the rarity of the disease. Early detection may be possible in patients with a genetic predisposition, such as neurofibromatosis, Gardner's syndrome and children with retinoblastoma.

KEY LEARNING POINTS

Squamous cell cancer of the oral cavity and oropharynx

- The incidence of oral cavity SCC is increasing, particularly in young men.
- There is a high incidence (15 per cent) of second primaries in patients with oral cavity cancer.
- The main causative factors are tobacco and alcohol.
- There is synergistic interaction between tobacco and alcohol.
- There is a strong association with human papilloma virus, particularly in tonsil cancer.
- Leukoplakia, erythroplakia and submucus fibrosis are important precancerous conditions.
- Genetic predisposition syndromes include Li–Fraumeni, Fanconi's, Bloom and ataxia telangiectasia.

Squamous cell cancer of the larynx and hypopharynx

- Cancer of the larynx accounts for 30 per cent of head and neck cancer.
- Sixty per cent of larynx cancers are glottic, 35 per cent supraglottic and 5 per cent subglottic.
- Larynx cancer has male predisposition M:F of 4:1.
- Cancer of the hypopharynx accounts for 10 per cent of head and neck cancer.
- The main subsite is pyriform fossa, then postcricoid, then posterior pharyngeal wall.
- The male predisposition M:F is 20:1 in pyriform fossa and posterior pharyngeal wall cancer.
- There is a female predisposition M:F of 1:1.5 in postcricoid cancer.
- Main causative factors are tobacco and alcohol.
- Synergistic interaction between tobacco and alcohol.

- Heavy alcohol consumption associated with supraglottic larynx cancer and hypopharynx cancer.
- There is an association with human papilloma virus in larynx cancer.
- Radiotherapy and sideropenic anaemia are associated with postcricoid cancer.

Squamous cell cancer of the nasopharynx

- Cancer of the nasopharynx accounts for 1–2 per cent of head and neck cancer.
- There is an increased incidence in Southeast Asia.
- There is a male predisposition M:F of 3:1.
- It is more common in the young with peak age of 40–50 years.
- Eighty per cent of cases present with advanced stage disease.
- There is a genetic predisposition with association with HLA types A2, Bw16, B17.
- There is a strong association with Epstein–Barr virus infection and consumption of salt cured fish.
- Antibody levels to EBV correlate with stage of disease and response to therapy.

Squamous cell cancer of the nasal cavity and paranasal sinuses

- Cancer of the nasal cavity and paranasal sinuses is rare.
- There is a male predisposition with age at presentation of 45–85 years.
- The most common site is maxillary sinus, then nasal cavity, then ethmoid sinus, then sphenoid and frontal sinus.
- The majority of patients present with advanced stage disease.
- Causative factors include tobacco and exposure to wood dust.

Thyroid cancer

- There is a female predisposition of F:M of 3:1.
- It affects mainly young patients with peak age 20–55 years.
- There is increasing incidence due to incidental detection through increased use of imaging.
- It has an association with low iodine diet.
- There is a strong association with previous radiation exposure.
- There is an association with multiple endocrine neoplasia (MEN) syndrome.
- There is an increased incidence in patients with Gardner's syndrome, familial polyposis and Cowden disease.

Salivary gland cancer

- The majority of parotid gland tumours are benign (80 per cent).
- Forty per cent of submandibular and 80 per cent of minor salivary gland tumours are malignant.

- There is heterogeneous histology due to multiple cell types in salivary gland tissue.
- The most common salivary gland cancers are mucoepidermoid, adenoid cystic and acinic cell carcinoma.
- There is an association with previous radiation exposure.

Head and neck sarcoma

- Head and neck sarcoma is uncommon.
- There is an association with previous radiation exposure.
- There is an association with polycyclic hydrocarbon exposure.
- Human immunodeficiency virus is associated with Kaposi's sarcoma.
- Genetic predisposition in neurofibromatosis includes Li–Fraumeni syndrome and Gardner's syndrome.

REFERENCES

1. Johnson NW. Oral cancer: a worldwide problem. *FDI World* 1997; **6**: 19–21.
2. Moore SR, Johnson NW, Pierce AM, Wilson DF. The epidemiology of mouth cancer: a review of global incidence. *Oral Diseases* 2000; **6**: 65–74.
3. Moore SR, Johnson NW, Pierce AM, Wilson DF. The epidemiology of tongue cancer: a review of global incidence. *Oral Diseases* 2000; **6**: 75–84.
4. Sankaranarayanan R. Oral cancer in India: a clinical and epidemiological review. *Oral Surgery, Oral Medicine, and Oral Pathology* 1990; **69**: 325–30.
5. Franceschi S, Talamani R, Barra S et al. Smoking and drinking in relation to cancer of the oral cavity, pharynx, larynx and oesophagus in Northern Italy. *Cancer Research* 1990; **50**: 6502–7.
6. Blot WJ, McLaughlin JK, Winn DM et al. Smoking and drinking in relation to oral and pharyngeal cancer. *Cancer Research* 1988; **48**: 3282–7.
7. Blot WJ. Alcohol and cancer. *Cancer Research* 1992; **52**(Suppl. 7): 2119s–23s.
8. Hindle I, Downer MC, Speight PM. The epidemiology of oral cancer. *British Journal of Oral and Maxillofacial Surgery* 1996; **34**: 471–6.
9. Moller H. Changing incidence of cancer of the tongue, oral cavity, and pharynx in Denmark. *Journal of Oral Pathology and Medicine* 1989; **18**: 224–9.
10. Boyle P, MacFarlane GJ, Scully C. Oral cancer: necessity for prevention strategies. *Lancet* 1993; **342**: 1129.
11. MacFarlane GJ, Boyle P, Scully C. Oral cancer in Scotland: changing incidence and mortality. *British Medical Journal* 1992; **305**: 1121–3.
12. Powell J, Robin PE. Cancer of the head and neck: the present state. In: Rhys Evans PH, Robin PE, Fielding JWL

(eds). *Head and neck cancer.* London: Castle House Publications, 1983.

◆ 13. Fakhry C, Gillison ML. Clinical implications of human papillomavirus in head and neck cancers. *Journal of Clinical Oncology* 2006; **24**: 2606–11.

14. International Agency for Research on Cancer. Tobacco smoking. IARC Monographs on the Evaluation of the Carcinogenic Risk of Chemicals to Humans. Washington DC: IARC, 1986.

● 15. Mashberg A, Boffetta P, Winkelman R, Garfinkel L. Tobacco smoking, alcohol drinking, and cancer of the oral cavity and oropharynx among US veterans. *Cancer* 1993; **72**: 1369–72.

◆ 16. Moulin JJ, Mur JM, Cavelier C. Comparative epidemiology in Europe of cancers related to tobacco (lung, larynx, pharynx, oral cavity). *Bulletin du Cancer* 1985; **72**: 155–8.

17. MacFarlane GJ, Zheng T, Marshall JR *et al.* Alcohol, tobacco, diet and the risk of oral cancer: a pooled analysis of three case-control studies. *European Journal of Cancer. Part B, Oral Oncology* 1995; **31B**: 181–7.

18. Kahn HA. The Dorn study of smoking and mortality among US veterans: report on eight and one half years of observation. *National Cancer Institute Monograph* 1966; **19**: 1–25.

19. De Stefani E, Boffetta P, Oreggia F *et al.* Smoking patterns and cancer of the oral cavity and pharynx: a case-control study in Uruguay. *Oral Oncology* 1998; **34**: 340–6.

20. Munoz N, Correa P, Bock FG. Comparative carcinogenic effect of two types of tobacco. *Cancer* 1968; **21**: 376–89.

21. Ko YC, Huang YL, Lee CH *et al.* Betal quid chewing, cigarette smoking and alcohol consumption related to oral cancer in Taiwan. *Journal of Oral Pathology and Medicine* 1995; **24**: 450–3.

22. Thomas S, Wilson A. A quamtitative evaluation of the role of betal quid in oral carcinogenesis. *European Journal of Cancer. Part B, Oral Oncology* 1993; **29B**: 265–71.

◆ 23. IARC Monographs on the Evaluation of the Carcinogenic Risk of Chemicals to the Human. Tobacco habits other than smoking: betal-quid and areca nut chewing and some related nitrosamines. Lyon: International Agency for Research on Cancer, 1985: 37.

24. Gupta PC, Mehta FS, Daftary DK *et al.* Incidence rates of oral cancer and natural history of oral precancerous lesions in a ten year follow up study of Indian villagers. *Community Dentistry and Oral Epidemiology* 1980; **8**: 283–333.

25. Reddy CRRM. Carcinoma of hard palate in relation to reverse smoking of chuttas. *Journal of the National Cancer Institute* 1974; **53**: 615–61.

● 26. Mehta FS, Gupta PC, Daftary DK *et al.* An epidemiologic study of oral cancer and precancerous conditions among 101 761 villagers in Maharashtra, India. *International Journal of Cancer* 1972; **10**: 134–41.

27. Idris AM, Ahmed HM, Malik MO. Toombak dipping and cancer of the oral cavity in the Sudan: a case-control study. *International Journal of Cancer* 1995; **63**: 477–80.

28. Nahas G, Latour C. The human toxicity of marijuana. *Medical Journal of Australia* 1992; **156**: 495–7.

29. Zhang ZF, Morgenstern H, Spitz MR *et al.* Marijuana use and increased risk of squamous cell carcinoma of the head and neck. *Cancer Epidemiology* 1999; **8**: 1071–8.

◆ 30. McCoy DG, Wynder EL. Etiological and preventive implications in alcohol carcinogenesis. *Cancer Research* 1979; **39**: 2844–50.

◆ 31. Blot WJ, McLaughlin JK, Winn DM *et al.* Smoking and drinking in relation to oral and pharyngeal cancer. *Cancer Research* 1988; **48**: 3282–7.

● 32. Brugere J, Guenel P, Leclerc A, Rodriguez J. Differential effects of tobacco and alcohol in cancer of the larynx, pharynx and mouth. *Cancer* 1986; **57**: 391–5.

33. Kato I, Nomura AM. Alcohol in the aetiology of upper aerodigestive tract cancer. *European Journal of Cancer. Part B, Oral Oncology* 1994; **30B**: 75–81.

34. Hindle I, Downer MC, Speight PM. The association between introral cancer and surrogate markers of smoking and alcohol consumption. *Community Dental Health* 2000; **17**: 107–13.

35. Enwonwu CO, Meeks VI. Bionutrition and oral cancer in humans. *Critical Reviews in Oral Biology and Medicine* 1995; **6**: 5–17.

36. Maier H, Zoller J, Herrmann A *et al.* Dental status and oral hygiene in patients with head and neck cancer. *Otolaryngology and Head and Neck Surgery* 1993; **108**: 655–61.

37. Velly AM, Franco EL, Schlecht N *et al.* Relationship between dental factors and risk of upper aerodigestive tract cancer. *Oral Oncology* 1998; **34**: 284–91.

38. Young TB, Ford CN, Brandenburg JH. An epidemiologic study of oral cancer in a statewide network. *American Journal of Otolaryngology* 1986; **7**: 200–8.

39. Winn DM, Blot WJ, McLaughlin JK *et al.* Mouthwash use and oral conditions in the risk of oral and pharyngeal cancer. *Cancer Research* 1991; **51**: 3044–7.

40. Schildt EB, Eriksson M, Hardell L, Magnuson A. Occupational exposures as risk factors for oral cancer evaluated in a Swedish case-control study. *Oncology Reports* 1999; **6**: 317–20.

◆ 41. Maier H, Dietz A, Gewelke U, Heller WD. Occupational exposure to hazardous substances and risk of cancer in the area of the mouth cavity, oropharynx, hypopharynx and larynx. A case-control study. *Laryngorhinootologie* 1991; **70**: 93–8.

42. Brandsma JL, Abramson AL. Association of papillomavirus with cancers of the head and neck. *Archives of Otolaryngology and Head and Neck Surgery* 1989; **115**: 621–5.

◆ 43. Steinberg BM. Viral etiology of head and neck cancer. In: Harrison LB, Sessions RB, Hong WK (eds). *Head and neck cancer: a multidisciplinary approach*. Philadelphia, PA: Lippincott-Raven, 1999: 35–47.

♦ 44. Snijders PFF, van den Brule AAJC, Meijer CJLM, Walboomers JMM. Papillomaviruses and cancer of the upper digestive and respiratory tracts. *Current Topics in Microbiology and Immunology* 1994; **186**: 177–98.

● 45. Paz IB, Cook N. Human papillomavirus (HPV) in head and neck cancer. An association of HPV16 with squamous cell carcinoma of Waldeyer's tonsillar ring. *Cancer* 1997; **79**: 595–604.

46. Snijders PIF, Scholes AGM, Hart CA. Prevalence of mucosatropic human papillomaviruses in squamous cell carcinomas of the head and neck. *International Journal of Cancer* 1996; **66**: 464–9.

♦ 47. Androphy EJ. Molecular biology of human papilloma virus infection and oncogenesis. *Journal of Investigative Dermatology* 1994; **103**: 248–56.

48. Woods KV, Shillitoe EJ, Spitz MR, Storthz K. Analysis of human papillomavirus DNA in oral squamous cell carcinomas. *Journal of Oral Pathology and Medicine* 1993; **22**: 101–8.

♦ 49. Yeudall WA. Human papillomavirus and oral neoplasia. *European Journal of Cancer. Part B, Oral Oncology* 1992; **28B**: 61–6.

50. Bernard HU, Apt D. Transcriptional control and cell type specificity of HPV gene expression. *Archives of Dermatology* 1994; **130**: 210–15.

51. Sugarman PB, Shillitoe EJ. The high risk human papilloma viruses and oral cancer: evidence for and against a causal relationship. *Oral Diseases* 1997; **3**: 130–47.

● 52. Singh B, Balwally AN, Shaha AR *et al*. Upper aerodigestive tract squamous cell carcinoma. The human immunodeficiency virus connection. *Archives of Otolaryngology and Head and Neck Surgery* 1996; **122**: 639–43.

53. Larsson PA, Edstrom S, Westin T *et al*. Reactivity against herpes simplex virus in patients with head and neck cancer. *International Journal of Cancer* 1991; **49**: 14–18.

54. Kassim KH, Daley TD. Herpes simplex virus type proteins in human oral squamous cell carcinoma. *Oral Surgery, Oral Medicine, Oral Pathology, Oral Radiology, and Endodontics* 1988; **65**: 445–8.

♦ 55. Hording U, Albeck H, Daugaard S. Nasopharyngeal carcinoma: histopathologic types and association with Epstein–Barr virus. *European Journal of Cancer. Part B, Oral Oncology* 1993; **29**: 137–9.

● 56. McLaughlin JK, Gridley G, Block G *et al*. Dietary factors in oral and pharyngeal cancer. *Journal of the National Cancer Institute* 1988; **80**: 1237–43.

57. La Vecchia C, Tavani A. Fruit and vegetables and human cancer. *European Journal of Cancer Prevention* 1998; **7**: 3–8.

58. La Vecchia C, Tavani A, Franceschi S *et al*. Epidemiology and prevention of oral cancer. *Oral Oncology* 1997; **33**: 302–12.

59. Tavani A, Gallus S, La Vecchia C *et al*. Diet and risk of oral and pharyngeal cancer. An Italian case-control study. *European Journal of Cancer Prevention* 2001; **10**: 191–5.

60. De Stefani E, Oreggia F, Ronco A *et al*. Salted meat consumption as a risk factor for cancer of the oral cavity and pharynx: a case-control study from Uruguay. *Cancer Epidemiology, Biomarkers and Prevention* 1994; **3**: 381–5.

61. Biacabe B, Gleich LL, Laccourreye O *et al*. Silent gastroesophageal reflux disease in patients with pharyngolaryngeal cancer: further results. *Head and Neck* 1998; **20**: 510–14.

62. Chen MY, Ott DJ, Casolo BJ *et al*. Correlation of laryngeal and pharyngeal carcinomas and 24 hour pH monitoring of the esophagus and pharynx. *Otolaryngology and Head and Neck Surgery* 1998; **119**: 460–2.

● 63. Li FP, Correa P, Fraumeni JF. Testing for germ line p53 mutations in cancer families. *Cancer Epidemiology, Biomarkers and Prevention* 1991; **1**: 91–4.

● 64. Kutler DI, Auerbach AD, Satagopan J *et al*. High incidence of head and neck squamous cell carcinoma in patients with Fanconi anemia. *Archives of Otolaryngology and Head and Neck Surgery* 2003; **129**: 106–12.

65. Snow DG, Campbell JB, Smallman LA. Fanconi's anemia and post-cricoid carcinoma. *Journal of Laryngology and Otology* 1991; **105**: 125–7.

● 66. Berkower AS, Biller HF. Head and neck cancer associated with Bloom syndrome. *Laryngoscope* 1988; **98**: 746–8.

● 67. Hecht F, Hecht BK. Cancer in ataxia-telangiectasia patients. *Cancer Genetics and Cytogenetics* 1990; **46**: 9–19.

68. Park LY, Muscat JE, Kaur T *et al*. Comparison of GSTM polymorphisms and risk for oral cancer between African Americans and Caucasians. *Pharmacogenetics* 2000; **10**: 123–31.

69. Gronau S, Konig-Greger D, Rettinger C, Riechelmann H. GSTM1 gene polymorphisms in patients with head and neck tumors. *Laryngorhinootologie* 2000; **79**: 341–4.

● 70. Buch SC, Notani PN, Bhisey RA. Polymorphism at GSTM1, GSTM3 and GSTT1 gene loci and susceptibility to oral cancer in an Indian population. *Carcinogenesis* 2002; **23**: 803–7.

71. Sato M, Sato T, Izumo T, Amagasa T. Genetically high susceptibility to oral squamous cell carcinoma in terms of combined genotyping of CYP1A1 and GSTM1 genes. *Oral Oncology* 2000; **236**: 267–71.

72. Sreelekha TT, Ramadas K, Pandey M *et al*. Genetic polymorphisms of CYP1A1, GSTM1 and GSTT1 genes in Indian oral cancer. *Oral Oncology* 2001; **37**: 593–8.

● 73. Bouchardy C, Hirvonen A, Coutelle C *et al*. Role of alcohol dehydrogenase 3 and cytochrome p450E1 genotypes in susceptibility to cancers of the upper aerodigestive tract. *International Journal of Cancer* 2000; **87**: 734–40.

♦ 74. Lisner M, Patterson B, Kandel R *et al*. Cutaneous and mucosal neoplasms in bone marrow transplant recipients. *Cancer* 1990; **65**: 473–6.

75. Suzuki T, Wakai K, Matsuo K et al. Effect of dietary antioxidants and risk of oral, pharyngeal and laryngeal squamous cell carcinoma according to smoking and drinking habits. *Cancer Science* 2006; **97**: 760–7.

76. Slaughter DP, Southwick HW, Smejkal W. Field cancerization in oral stratified squamous epithelium; clinical implications of multicentric origin. *Cancer* 1953; **6**: 963–8.

77. Braakhuis BJ, Tabor MP, Kummer JA et al. A genetic explanation of Slaughter's concept of field cancerization: evidence and clinical implications. *Cancer Research* 2003; **63**: 1727–30.

78. Khuri FR, Lee JJ, Lippman SM et al. Randomised phase III trial of low-dose isotretinoin for prevention of second primary tumors in stage I and II head and neck cancer patients. *Journal of the National Cancer Institute* 2006; **98**: 426.

79. Boyle JO. A randomised study of sulindac in oral premalignant lesions. ClinicalTrials.gov. Available from http://clinicaltrials.gov/ct2/show/NCT00299195.

80. Clayman GL, Lippman SM. Gene therapy in preventing cancer in patients with premalignant carcinoma of the oral cavity and pharynx. ClinicalTrials.gov. Available from http://clinicaltrials.gov/ct2/show/NCT00064103.

81. Strome SE. MAGE-A3/HPV 16 vaccine for squamous cell carcinoma of the head and neck. ClinicalTrials.gov. Available from http://clinicaltrials.gov/ct2/show/NCT00257738.

82. Silver CE. *Surgery for cancer of the larynx and related structures*, 2nd edn. Philadelphia: WB Saunders, 1996.

83. Adenis L, Lefebvre JL, Cambier L. Registre des cancers des voies aerodigestives superieures des departments du Nord et du Pas-de-Calais 1984–1986. *Bulletin du Cancer Paris* 1988; **75**: 745–50.

84. Driscoll WG, Nagorsky MJ, Cantrell RW, Johns ME. Carcinoma of the pyriform sinus: analysis of 102 cases. *Laryngoscope* 1983; **93**: 556–60.

85. Eisbach KJ, Krause CJ. Carcinoma of the pyriform sinus. A comparison of treatment modalities. *Laryngoscope* 1977; **87**: 1904–10.

86. Van den Brouck C, Eschwege F, De La Rochefordiere A et al. Squamous cell carcinoma of the pyriform sinus: a retrospective study of 351 cases treated at the Institut Gustave-Roussy. *Head and Neck Surgery* 1987; **10**: 4–13.

87. Stell PM, Carden EA, Hibbert J, Dalby JE. Post cricoid carcinoma. *Clinical Oncology* 1978; **4**: 215–26.

88. Farrington WT, Weighill JS, Jones PH. Post cricoid carcinoma (10 year retrospective study). *Journal of Laryngology and Otology* 1986; **100**: 79–84.

89. Kajanti M, Mantyla M. Carcinoma of the hypopharynx. *Acta Oncologica* 1990; **29**: 903–7.

90. Raitiola HS, Pukander JS. Etiological factors of laryngeal cancer. *Acta Otolaryngologica Supplement* 1997; **529**: 215–17.

91. Vineis P, Airoldi L, Veglia P et al. Environmental tobacco smoke and risk of respiratory cancer and chronic obstructive pulmonary disease in former smokers and never smokers in the EPIC prospective study. *British Medical Journal* 2005; **330**: 277.

92. Maier H, Dietz A, Gewelke U et al. Tobacco and alcohol associated cancer risk of the upper respiratory and digestive tract. *Laryngorhinootologie* 1990; **69**: 505–11.

93. Olsen J, Sabreo S. Fasting. U. Interaction of alcohol and tobacco as risk factors in cancer of the laryngeal region. *Journal of Epidemiology and Community Health* 1985; **39**: 165–8.

94. Guenel P, Chastang JF, Luce D et al. A study of the interaction of alcohol drinking and tobacco smoking among French cases of laryngeal cancer. *Journal of Epidemiology and Community Health* 1988; **42**: 350–4.

95. Rothman KJ, Cann CI, Fried MP. Carcinogenicity of dark liquor. *American Journal of Public Health* 1989; **79**: 1516–20.

96. Altieri A, Garavello W, Bosetti C et al. Alcohol consumption and risk of laryngeal cancer. *Oral Oncology* 2005; **41**: 956–65.

97. Menvielle G, Luce D, Goldberg P et al. Smoking, alcohol drinking and cancer risk for various sites of the larynx and hypopharynx. A case-control study in France. *European Journal of Cancer Prevention* 2004; **13**: 165–72.

98. Ries LAG. Rates. In: Harras A (ed.) *Cancer: rates and risks*. Washington DC: National Institutes of Health, 1996: 9–55.

99. Hinds MW, Thomas DB, O'Reilly HP. Asbestos, dental X-rays, tobacco, and alcohol in the epidemiology of laryngeal cancer. *Cancer* 1979; **44**: 1114–20.

100. Burch JD, Howe GR, Miller AB et al. Tobacco, alcohol, asbestos and nickel in the etiology of cancer of the larynx: a case-control study. *Journal of the National Cancer Institute* 1981; **67**: 1219–21.

101. Flanders WD, Rothman KJ. Occupational risk for laryngeal cancer. *American Journal of Public Health* 1982; **72**: 369–72.

102. Zagraniski RT, Kelsey JL, Walter SD. Occupational risk factors for laryngeal carcinoma: Connecticut, 1975–1980. *American Journal of Epidemiology* 1986; **124**: 67–76.

103. Coggon D, Pannett B, Wield G. Upper aerodigestive cancer in battery manufacturers and steel workers exposed to mineral acid mists. *Occupational and Environmental Medicine* 1996; **53**: 445–59.

104. Harrison DFN, Thompson AE. Pharyngolaryngoesophagectomy with pharyngogastric anastamosis for cancer of the hypopharynx: review of 101 operations. *Head and Neck Surgery* 1986; **8**: 418–28.

105. Jones AS, Stell PM. Squamous cell carcinoma of the posterior pharyngeal wall. *Clinical Otolaryngology* 1991; **16**: 462–5.

106. Esteve J, Riboli E, Pequignot G et al. Diet and cancers of the larynx and hypopharynx: the IARC multi-center study in southwestern Europe. *Cancer Causes and Control* 1996; **7**: 240–52.

107. La Vecchia C, Negri E, D'Avanzo B *et al*. Dietary indicators of laryngeal cancer risk. *Cancer Research* 1990; **50**: 4497–500.

◆ 108. YuM. *Nasopharyngeal carcinoma: epidemiology and dietary factors*. Lyon: IARC Scientific Publications, 1991: 104.

109. Perez CA. Nasopharynx. In: Perez CA, Brady LW (eds). *Principles and practice of radiation oncology*, 2nd edn. Philadelphia: JB Lippincott, 1991: 617–43.

110. Altun M, Fandi A, Dupuis O *et al*. Undifferentiated nasopharyngeal cancer (UCNT): Current diagnostic and therapeutic aspects. *International Journal of Radiation Oncology, Biology, Physics* 1995; **32**: 859–77.

111. Lin T, Chang H, Chen C *et al*. Risk factors for nasopharyngeal carcinoma. *Anticancer Research* 1986; **6**: 791–6.

112. Chan SH, Day NE, Kunaratnam N, Chia KB. HLA and nasopharyngeal carcinoma in Chinese – a further study. *International Journal of Cancer* 1983; **32**: 171–6.

113. Chan S, Day N, Khor T *et al*. HLA markers in the development and prognosis of NPC in Chinese. In: Grundman E, Krueger GRF, Ablashi DV (eds). *Cancer campaign*. Vol. 5: Nasopharyngeal carcinoma. Stuttgart: Gustav Fischer, 1981: 205–11.

● 114. Henle W, Henle G, Ho JHC *et al*. Antibodies to Epstein Barr virus in nasopharyngeal carcinoma, other head and neck neoplasms and control groups. *Journal of the National Cancer Institute* 1970; **44**: 225–31.

● 115. Henle H, Ho JHC, Henle G *et al*. Antibodies to Epstein. Barr virus related antigens in nasopharyngeal carcinoma: comparison of active cases and long term survivors. *Journal of the National Cancer Institute* 1973; **51**: 361–9.

116. Ho JHC. Stage classification of nasopharyngeal carcinoma: a review. In: de The G, Ito Y (eds). *Nasopharyngeal carcinoma: etiology and control*. Lyon: International Agency for Research on Cancer, 1978: 94–114.

117. El-Mothy SK, Lu DW. Prevalence of high risk human papillomavirus DNA in nonkeratinising (cylindrical cell) carcinoma of the sinonasal tract: a distinct clinicopathologic and molecular disease entity. *American Journal of Surgical Pathology* 2005; **29**: 1367–72.

● 118. Davies L, Welch HG. Increasing incidence of thyroid cancer in the United States, 1973–2002. *Journal of the American Medical Association* 2006; **295**: 2164–7.

● 119. Steiner AL, Goodman AD, Powers SR. Study of a kindred with pheochromocytoma, medullary thyroid carcinoma, hyperparathyroidism and Cushing's disease; multiple endocrine neoplasia type 2. *Medicine* 1968; **47**: 371–409.

● 120. Williams ED, Pollock DJ. Multiple mucosal neuromata with endocrine tumors: a syndrome allied to Von Recklinghausen's disease. *Journal of Pathology and Bacteriology* 1966; **91**: 71–80.

121. Sehestedt T, Knudsen N, Perrild H, Johansen C. Iodine intake and incidence of thyroid cancer in Denmark. *Clinical Endocrinology* 2006; **65**: 229–33.

122. Palmer JA, Mustard RA, Simpson WJ. Irradiation as an etiologic factor in tumours of the thyroid, parathyroid and salivary glands. *Canadian Journal of Surgery* 1980; **23**: 39–42.

◆ 123. Williams ED. Chernobyl and thyroid cancer. *Journal of Surgical Oncology* 2006; **94**: 670–7.

124. Bogdanova TI, Zurnadzhy LY, Greenebaum E *et al*. A cohort study of thyroid cancer and other thyroid diseases after the Chornobyl accident: pathology analysis of thyroid cancer cases in Ukraine detected during the first screening (1998–2000). *Cancer* 2006; **107**: 2559–66.

◆ 125. Hoffman FO, Ruttenber AJ, Greenland S, Carroll RJ. Radiation exposure and thyroid cancer. *Journal of the American Medical Association* 2006; **295**: 1060–2.

● 126. Mulligan LM, Eng C, Attie T *et al*. Diverse phenotypes associated with exon 10 mutations of the RET proto-oncogene. *Human Molecular Genetics* 1994; **12**: 2163–7.

◆ 127. Hansford JR, Mulligan LM. Multiple endocrine neoplasia type 2 and RET: from neoplasia to neurogenesis. *Journal of Medical Genetics* 2000; **37**: 817–27.

◆ 128. Kikumori T, Evans D, Lee JE *et al*. Genetic abnormalities in MEN-2. In: Doherty GM, Skogseid B (eds.) *Surgical endocrinology*. Philadelphia: Lippincott Williams & Wilkins, 2001: 531–40.

129. Butter A, Gagne J, Al-Jazaeri A *et al*. Prophylactic thyroidectomy in pediatric carriers of multiple endocrine neoplasia type 2A or familial medullary thyroid carcinoma: mutation in C620 is associated with Hirschsprung's disease. *Journal of Pediatric Surgery* 2007; **42**: 203–6.

◆ 130. Sun EC, Curtis R, Melbye M *et al*. Salivary gland cancer in the United States. *Cancer Epidemiology Biomarkers and Prevention* 1999; **8**: 1095–100.

131. Horn-Ross PL, Ljung BM, Morrow M. Environmental factors and the risk of salivary gland cancer. *Epidemiology* 1997; **8**: 414–19.

132. Horn-Ross PL, Morrow M, Ljung BM. Menstrual and reproductive factors for salivary gland cancer risk in women. *Epidemiology* 1999; **10**: 528–30.

133. In der Maur CD, Klokman WJ, van Leeuwen FE *et al*. Increased risk of breast cancer development after diagnosis in salivary gland tumour. *European Journal of Cancer* 2005; **41**: 1311–15.

134. Horn-Ross PL, Morrow M, Ljung BM. Diet and the risk of salivary gland cancer. *American Journal of Epidemiology* 1997; **146**: 171–6.

◆ 135. Patel SG, Shaha AR, Shah JP. Soft tissue sarcomas of the head and neck: an update. *American Journal of Otolaryngology* 2001; **22**: 2–18.

● 136. Patel SG, Meyers P, Huvos AG *et al.* Improved outcomes in patients with osteogenic sarcoma of the head and neck. *Cancer* 2002; **95**: 1495–503.

◆ 137. Patel SG, See AC, Williamson PA *et al.* Radiation induced sarcoma of the head and neck. *Head and Neck* 1999; **21**: 346–54.

138. Ben-Izhak O, Vlodavsky E, Ofer A *et al.* Epithelioid angiosarcoma associated with a Dacron vascular graft. *American Journal of Surgical Pathology* 1999; **23**: 1418–22.

139. Eby CS, Brennan MJ, Fine G. Lymphangiosarcoma: a lethal complication of chronic lymphoedema. Report of two cases and review of the literature. *Archives of Surgery* 1967; **94**: 223–30.

◆ 140. Mankin HJ, Hornicek FJ. Paget's sarcoma: a historical and outcome review. *Clinical Orthopaedics and Related Research* 2005; **438**: 97–102.

141. Fuchs B, Pritchard DJ. Etiology of osteosarcoma. *Clinical Orthopaedics and Related Research* 2002; **397**: 40–52.

3

Molecular biology as applied to head and neck oncology

VOLKERT B WREESMANN AND BHUVANESH SINGH

A mighty flame followeth a tiny spark.

Dante Alighieri, *The Divine Comedy*

INTRODUCTION

In 1960, the discovery of the Philadelphia (Ph) chromosome, a reciprocal translocation between chromosomes 9 and 22 [t(9;22)(q34;q11.2)], in chronic myeloid leukaemia (CML), was the first clear evidence suggesting cancer was a genetic disease.[1] The Ph chromosome represents a fusion of the tyrosine kinase proto-oncogene c-Abl (chromosome 9q34) with the serine/threonine kinase gene BCR (chromosome 22q11.2) and directly promotes the development of CML by increasing tyrosine kinase signalling (**Figure 3.1**). Moreover, the clinical importance of genomic aberrations was highlighted by the significant response to c-Abl tyrosine kinase inhibitors in patients with CML containing the Ph translocation. These findings ushered in the genomic era of cancer research which focused on the identification of genetic aberrations that could be targeted for therapeutic benefit. The advent of high throughput genetic screen tools has accelerated discovery, allowing the identification of many genetic abnormalities present in individual cancers. Extrapolation of screening data suggests that cancer cells contain as many as 12 000 individual aberrations.[2, 3] However, no clinical or biological significance could be attached to the vast majority of newly identified genetic abnormalities. Mathematical models suggest that only between five and ten critical aberrations are essential in cancer pathogenesis.[3] The biological mechanisms underlying the striking accumulation of molecular changes and the identification of cancer-causing

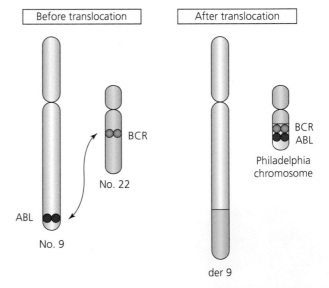

Figure 3.1 Creation of the Philadelphia chromosome through reciprocal exchange of genetic material between chromosomes 9 and 22. Fusion of the c-Abl-containing region of distal chromosome 9 to the BCR-containing region of chromosome 22 results in formation of a chimeric oncogene that causes chronic myeloid leukaemia.

primary events among the large pool of secondary 'passenger mutations' has been an important focus of contemporary cancer research. Although much is known about the molecular basis for head and neck squamous cell carcinoma (HNSCC) pathogenesis, it has not translated into clinical application due to the high level of genetic complexity present in these cancers. In this chapter, we will discuss the genetic basis for HNSCC pathogenesis while highlighting those events that may have therapeutic implications.

GENETIC BASIS FOR CANCER DEVELOPMENT

Normal cells can acquire genetic aberrations due to the inherent infidelity of DNA replication machinery. However, this innate mutagenesis is rarely sufficient to support cancer development on its own, as mutations are random and those that affect cancer-related genes also activate protective measures in cells to block oncogenesis. It is now accepted that cancer pathogenesis requires an environment that promotes the development of genetic aberrations, characterized by increased genetic damage or decreased inherent genetic repair and protective mechanisms.[4] While inherited mutations (germline mutations) in several protective genes have been associated with increased cancer risk, much less is known about normal variations (polymorphisms) in the sequence of individual genes (much like skin colour or blood type) that alter gene function and cancer susceptibility. In addition, mutagenic environmental factors can induce genetic mutations (somatic mutations) in cells, which, once established, can be inheritable and propagated in subsequent cell divisions. Accordingly, cancer results from an imbalance in factors promoting the development and accumulation of genetic events and those that prevent, exclude or repair genetic damage.

CARCINOGENS THAT PROMOTE HNSCC

Tobacco, alcohol, betel nut and sexually transmitted viral pathogens (human papilloma virus (HPV)) have all been associated with an increased risk of HNSCC.[5] Each of these carcinogens promotes progression to HNSCC by contributing to the accumulation of genetic aberrations, the rate and accumulation of which is dependent on a balance between carcinogen dosage and host susceptibility. Tobacco smoke is an aerosol containing vapour and particulate components with more than 4000 chemicals, at least 60 of which have been shown to be carcinogenic. Tobacco carcinogens are broadly grouped into polycyclic aromatic hydrocarbons (i.e. benzo[a]pyrenes), heterocyclic aromatic amines, aromatic amines, aldehydes, asz-arenes (dibenz[a,h]acridine and 7H-dibenzo[c,g]carbazole), N-nitrosamines (N-nitrosodiethylamine), as well as other agents. Many of these compounds are tumorigenic in mice. Once absorbed, most tobacco carcinogens require activation by cellular enzymes (i.e. cytochrome P450 group) to promote tumorigenesis and their effects can be offset by detoxifying enzymes (i.e. *GSTM1*). Dysfunction of these enzymatic pathways has been associated with increased risk for HNSCC.[6]

Chronic alcohol exposure results in increased cancer incidence in animal models, confirming its carcinogenic role.[7] Similar to tobacco, carcinogens in alcohol require its metabolism to an active intermediate (acetaldehyde) by alcohol dehydrogenase (ADH), CYP2E1 (along with reactive oxygen species) or catalase. Acetaldehyde is then inactivated by conversion to acetate by acetaldehyde dehydrogenase (ALDH). Acetaldehyde exerts its carcinogenic effect primarily by direct binding to DNA, but also alters methyl transfer, resulting in genetic hypomethylation, which in turn affects the transcription of multiple genes. In addition, reactive oxygen species are generated during alcohol metabolism, which also have mutagenic effects. Factors promoting accumulation of acetaldehyde, including increased alcohol consumption, increased alcohol metabolism, or decreased conversion to acetate result in increased rates of cancer formation. For example, deficiency of ALDH2, which is common in Asians, increases the risk for esophageal cancer formation up to 16-fold relative to those with normal ALDH2.[8] Alcohol also promoted cytochrome P450 activity which increases activation of procarcinogens (both for tobacco and alcohol). In addition, alcohol can also act as a solvent to facilitate entry of carcinogens into cells, especially in the upper aerodigestive tract.

Recent studies show that the human papilloma virus may be responsible for development of HNSCC.[9] HPV is a retrovirus that primarily infects transitional epithelial tissues. The HPV family contains over 70 different types that can be divided into low- and high-risk categories with respect to their ability to promote cancer development. HPV types 16 and 18 are the most common high-risk types associated with cervical and anogenital cancers, while 6 and 11 are low-risk types that cause non-cancer pathologies (e.g. papillomas and condylomas). Infection with high-risk HPV subtypes has been shown to transform benign human keratinocytes in culture, a phenomenon that is not observed with low-risk HPV types. Early viral proteins, E6 and E7, are essential for transforming effects and are more potent in high-risk HPV types. Their functions are discussed in the following sections. A meta-analysis of published trials, including 5046 HNSCC cancer specimens, shows a 26 per cent prevalence of HPV, with the vast majority being HPV type 16 (HPV-16).[10] The predominant location of HPV-associated tumours is in the oropharynx, with a predilection for non-smokers (up to 50 per cent of cases). Similar to cervical cancers, detection of HPV in HNSCC is associated with sexual history, implicating direct exposure as a cause for infection.[11] In addition, immunosuppression has been suggested to increase the risk for infection and development of HPV-related HNSCC.[12]

INHERITED SUSCEPTIBILITY TO HNSCC

Susceptibility to the carcinogenic effects of tobacco, alcohol and HPV varies widely between individuals, and is dependent on hereditary factors.[13] A significant role for hereditary susceptibility factors in the development of HNSCC is suggested by several observations. For example, observational evidence suggests that a two- to 14-fold increased incidence of HNSCC is present in first-degree relatives of patients with HNSCC.[14, 15] Several studies and meta-analyses suggest that

Table 3.1 Genetic cancer syndromes associated with HNSCC.

Syndrome	Gene	HNSCC	Other cancers
Fanconi	FANC family	> 500-fold higher rate	Haematological
FAMMM	p16	Increased	Melanoma, pancreas
N/A	RNASEL	1.5-fold increased risk	Prostate, cervix, breast
Bloom	BLM (DNA helicase)	Increased	Multiple leukaemias, lymphomas and carcinomas
Xeroderma pigmentosum	XP-A to XP-G	Increased	UV-induced skin cancer
Ataxia telangiectasia	ATM	Increased	Leukaemia, lymphoma
Li–Fraumeni	p53	Increased	Lymphoma, sarcoma

certain inherited genetic polymorphisms can increase HNSCC risk by affecting the function of carcinogen activating enzymes (i.e. cytochrome P450 group or ADH) or detoxifying enzymes (GSTM1 or ALDH).[16] Polymorphisms in prominent cell cycle regulators, such as cyclin D1 (CCND1), p53 and P21 (Waf1/CIP1) have also been associated with susceptibility for HNSCC. A study by Storey and colleagues demonstrates a polymorphism at codon 72 in the *p53* gene, which modifies susceptibility of p53 to HPV-mediated degradation, is associated with an increased risk of HNSCC development.[17, 18] However, the exact role of these polymorphisms in HNSCC pathogenesis has yet to be validated.

In contrast, several inherited mutations are clearly associated with increased risk for HNSCC development.[19] These mutations and the resulting heritable syndromes including Li–Fraumeni syndrome (p53 mutation), Fanconi anaemia (FANCA-A to FANCA-M mutations), Bloom's syndrome (BLM mutation), and dyskeratosis congenita (DKCA mutation) have an increased incidence of squamous cell carcinoma of mucosal membranes.[18, 20, 21, 22, 23, 24] The causative genes involved in these inherited syndromes function in DNA repair and surveillance of genetic stability, which explains a higher rate of cancer development in affected patients (**Table 3.1**). It remains unclear why affected patients feature a predilection for SCC development, but it is of interest that some of the genes (p53, BLM, FANCA-M) can be found inactivated uniquely in the genetic blueprint of HNSCC tumours (but not in their host genomes) occurring in the general population (sporadic HNSCC).[18] The collective data suggest that these genes are likely involved in key pathways, inactivation of which is an early event in the development of HNSCC. However, the infrequent inactivation of these genes in the germline of HNSCC patients suggests they likely represent a minor fraction of hereditary influences in HNSCC development.

SOMATIC GENETIC MUTATIONS IN CANCER

The interplay between the cumulative exposure to carcinogens and host susceptibility factors drives cancer pathogenesis through induction of somatic genomic mutations. Cancer-causing somatic genetic aberrations can be divided into two broad categories: those that affect proto-oncogenes and those that affect tumour suppressor genes (**Figure 3.2**).[25]

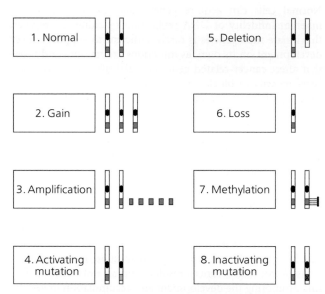

Figure 3.2 Normal pair of (paternally and maternally derived) chromosomes with centromere represented by black dot and both alleles of target gene sequence represented by orange regions (1), and most common genetic alterations that affect the gene sequence to activate it (in the case of the oncogene, 2–4) or inactivate it (in the case of the tumour suppressor gene, 5–8). Note that complete inactivation of tumour suppressor genes requires a combination of two separate inactivational events, each affecting one of two alleles.

Proto-oncogenes are activators of oncogenesis, as they promote cellular growth, neovascularization (angiogenesis), cellular dissociation from the environment and cellular migration. Proto-oncogenes are activated by diverse genetic events including chromosomal gain or amplification that increase gene dosage, activating mutations that result in changes or increases in gene activity, or translocation/rearrangement in chromosomes that produce novel genes (such as the Philadelphia translocation) (**Figure 3.1**). Tumour suppressor genes typically have no direct functional effects on oncogenesis, but normally function to limit the effects of cancer-causing events to the extent that they may induce programmed cell death to assure that detrimental aberrations are not propagated. Their loss allows a permissive environment for cancer pathogenesis, characterized by genetic instability that fosters accumulation of other genetic abnormalities.

Tumour suppressor genes are commonly inactivated through loss of genetic information, inactivating mutations (i.e. missense/nonsense mutations), decreased protein production (i.e. mutation or hypermethylation gene promotor or increased activity of micro-RNAs) or increase in protein turnover (i.e. ubiquitin-based proteasome degradation). Combined, genetic abnormalities confer cells with growth self-sufficiency, insensitivity to antigrowth and cell death signals, limitless replicative potential and an ability to detach from and invade surrounding structures and spread to distant anatomic sites.[26, 27]

GENETIC PROGRESSION MODEL FOR HNSCC

Global genomic screening tools have revealed that HNSCC are characterized by an array of genomic alterations (**Figure 3.3**). Accumulating evidence suggests that genetic aberrations develop in an arbitrary manner, with those providing survival advantages selected for in a Darwinian manner in individual cells.[4, 28] As critical genetic aberrations

accumulate, mucosal keratinocytes progress through distinct histopathological stages from benign squamous hyperplasia to dysplasia, carcinoma *in situ* and finally invasive carcinoma. Individual genomic aberrations accumulate at different stages of the progression axis,[29, 30] but it remains to be determined if they directly contribute to or are required for progression (**Figure 3.4**). The current model of progression to HNSCC suggests deletion of the chromosomal 9p21 region as an early event, given that it is detectable in a significant proportion of hyperplastic lesions of the upper aerodigestive tract. The candidate gene 9p21 region includes p16 and/or p14^{arf}. Another early event in HNSCC progression is deletion of the chromosomal 3p region that is first detectable in benign squamous hyperplasia. The subsequent transformation from hyperplasia to dysplasia appears to be associated with amplification of the 3q26.3 locus and p53 mutation, identifiable in early dysplastic lesions, carcinoma *in situ* and HNSCC. The transformation of dysplasia to malignancy is also associated with 11q13 amplification (activation of cyclin D1), gains of the chromosomal regions 7q11.2 (EGFR activation), 8q23-24 and deletions of 13q21, 14q23, 4p and

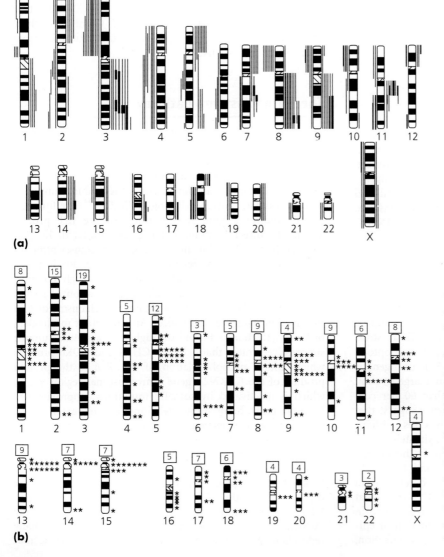

(a)

(b)

Figure 3.3   (a) Ideogram showing common chromosomal alterations identified by comparative genomic hybridization (CGH) in HNSCC. Each vertical line on either side of the ideogram represents an aberration detected in a single tumour. Thin vertical lines indicate losses (left) and gains (right) of the chromosomal region. The chromosomal locations of high-level gene amplification are shown by thick lines (right). (b) Ideogram showing the most common chromosomal breakpoints identified by spectral karyotyping of HNSCC chromosomes. The number of breakpoints in each chromosome that were identified by SKY, but could not be precisely assigned to a chromosomal band, are noted in the box on top of the chromosome.

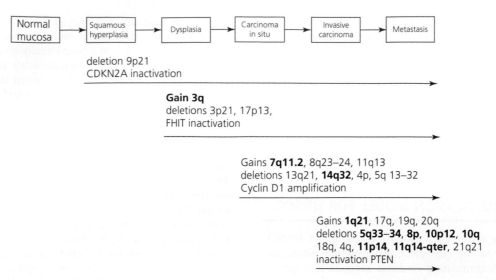

Figure 3.4 Tumour progression model for HNSCC, showing that histologic progression from normal mucosa to invasive carcinoma and ultimately metastasis is associated with a stepwise accumulation of specific genetic alterations (genetic alterations associated with metastatic progression are highlighted in bold).

5q13-32. Subsequent gains of 1q21, 17q, 19q, 20q and deletions of 5q33-34, 8p, 10p12, 10q, 18q, 4q, 11p14, 11q14-qter and 21q21 and PTEN inactivation appear to be associated with initiation of the metastatic process.[31] The gene targets and the functional and clinical significance of most of these aberrations remain to be defined.

COMMON MOLECULAR SIGNALLING PATHWAYS AFFECTED IN HNSCC

In addition to uncharacterized genomic alterations, HNSCC are characterized by multiple alterations in well-characterized biochemical signalling pathways that control oncogenic properties, such as the balance between cell survival and cell death (apoptosis), angiogenesis, invasion and metastasis. The most common signalling pathways affected in HNSCC are described below (**Figure 3.5**).

The p53 pathway

The p53 protein is a transcription factor that plays an essential role in the pathogenesis of human cancers, including HNSCC.[32] The p53 pathway is activated by cellular stress resulting in either cell cycle arrest to allow repair or apoptosis in case of severe event. The importance of p53 in oncogenesis is evident from the fact that it is mutated in a large fraction of human malignancies, including more than 60 per cent of HNSCC. Moreover, several lines of evidence suggest that the p53 pathway may be inactivated in cases without detectable genetic mutations in p53. Approximately 10–15 per cent of HNSCC feature overexpression of the human variant of mouse double minute proteins 2 and 4 (MDM2 and MDM4), which promote proteasome-based degradation of p53 by ubiquitination. Similarly, the p14[ARF] gene that inhibits the association of p53 with MDM2 is inactivated in HNSCC by homozygous deletion, somatic mutation or epigenetic silencing. In addition, in cases with HPV infection,

the E6 viral oncoprotein binds and degrades p53. Aberrations may also be present in other proteins in the p53 pathway including BCL2, p21, BCL-Xl, caspase, BAX and other p53 family members (p73 and p63). Combined, these abnormalities result in p53 pathway inactivation in more than 95 per cent of HNSCC.

The retinoblastoma pathway

The retinoblastoma pathway plays a central part in regulation of cell cycle progression from the G1 phase into the S phase, the commitment step in the cell cycle.[33] Detrimental alterations in components of the Rb pathway are required for cancer development, as shown from their ubiquitous presence in human cancer, including HNSCC.[5, 34] The function of Rb revolves around its inhibition of the E2F protein activity by direct binding. When phosphorylated, Rb dissociates from E2F, allowing it to activate transcription of genes required for progression into S phase. Rb is phosphorylated by cyclin-dependent kinases through complex regulatory networks. Although direct inactivation of pRB is uncommon in HNSCC, several indirect mechanisms of pRB inactivation have been identified. An important mechanism of Rb inactivation is fuelled through p16, a central tumour suppressive protein that activates CDK4 and CDK6 proteins which inhibit phosphorylation of Rb. P16 is the protein product of the CDKN2A gene (chromosomal region 9p21), which is inactivated by somatic mutations (approximately 5–15 per cent), homozygous deletions (approximately 30–60 per cent) and epigenetic silencing by hypermethylation (approximately 10–20 per cent). As a result of these and other events, immunohistochemical analysis demonstrates that p16 absence is present in at least 80 per cent of HNSCC. In addition, the pRB protein is sequestered and tagged for degradation by the E7 protein in HPV-infected tumours. HPV positivity and intrinsic p16 silencing are mutually exclusive events, suggesting that they are functionally redundant. Activation of cyclin D1, a proto-oncogene that

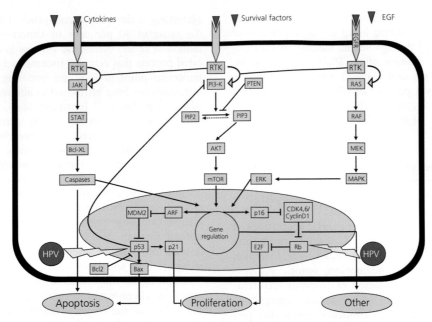

Figure 3.5 Simplification of most common signalling pathways affected in HNSCC. Activational relationships between sequential factors are represented by arrows, whereas inhibition is represented by barred lines. Transmembrane receptor tyrosine kinase (*RTK*) receptors including *EGFR* and several other unidentified receptors are activated by various extracellular ligands (represented by red triangles) and activate cytoplasmic protein cascades, such as RAS-MAPK pathway, PI3-kinase/AKT pathway and JAK-STAT pathway, ultimately resulting in modulation of the intranuclear gene regulation machinery. As a result, the activity of the two most important intranuclear signalling pathways including the p53 pathway and the Rb pathway is modulated, resulting in a shifted balance between cell death (apoptosis) and cell survival (proliferation) signals. In addition, altered gene regulation results in modulation of several other cellular properties including induction of angiogenesis, invasion and metastasis. Human papilloma virus (HPV) is typically present in cytoplasmic vesicles (episomes) and degrades p53 and Rb proteins with the use of its E6 (p53) and E7 (Rb) proteins.

exerts its positive effect on cell cycle progression by promoting phosphorylation of pRB by cdk4, is another important mechanism for inactivation of the Rb pathway in HNSCC. Constitutive activation of cyclin D1 through chromosomal amplification (of locus 11q13) (**Figure 3.2**) can be identified in approximately 30 per cent of HNSCC. The collective data suggest that inactivation of the retinoblastoma pathway is required for HNSCC development.

Epidermal growth factor receptor pathway

The ErbB/HER family of tyrosine kinase receptors, including epidermal growth factor receptor (EGFR/ERBb1), Her2Neu (ERBb2), ErbB3 and ErbB4, are important activators of mitogenic signalling.[34] ERBb tyrosine kinases possess an extracellular N-terminal ligand-binding domain, a transmembrane region and a C-terminal intracellular domain which includes the kinase domain and multiple phosphorylation sites. These receptors are activated by various ligands, including tumour necrosis factor alpha (TNFα) and EGF. Ligand binding induces homodimerization or heterodimerization with other ErbB receptors (receptor crosstalk) and results in receptor activation by autophosphorylation. The activated receptor recruits intracellular signalling complexes which activate mitogenic signalling pathways, such as the RAS/MEK/ERK cascade, the STAT cascade, the PI3K/AKT cascade, and several angiogenic, cell adhesion and cell cycle regulatory pathways.

Overexpression of EGFR and its ligands is well documented in HNSCC and premalignant mucosa and occurs in 40–95 per cent of cases. EGFR overexpression in HNSCC is a result of several factors, including transcriptional induction and genetic amplification. In addition, constitutively active EGFR through point mutation in the kinase domain or deletions in the extracellular domain have been described in HNSCC, but appear to be rare. Overexpression of other ErbB receptors in HNSCC is common, but underlying mechanisms are less well defined.

The PI3-kinase pathway

The PI3-kinase pathway is an important downstream effector of the EGFR and many other membrane-based receptors and is a central player in cancer pathogenesis.[35] In normal cells, activation of upstream signalling factors, such as EGFR, results in the recruitment of PI3K isoforms to the plasma membrane that subsequently generate 3'-phosphorylated phosphoinositides (PI3, 4P, PI3, 4, 5). Phosphoinositol triphosphate (PIP3) activates PDK1, resulting in phosphorylation of AKT. AKT is the active component of the pathway, promoting cellular survival by affecting the function of many proteins by phosphorylation to promote cell survival. The tumour gene phosphatase and tensin homologue gene (PTEN) is an important negative regulator of the PI3K-AKT pathway activity by regulating PIP3 dephosphorylation, which decreases the phosphorylated AKT fraction and promotes G1 arrest.

Constitutive activation of components of the PI3K cascade is common in HNSCC, occurring in up to 70–90 per cent of cases. It may be achieved through several mechanisms including chromosomal amplification of the PIK3CA locus (chromosome 3q26.3; 30/40 per cent of cases), activating mutations in PI3K (approximately 5 per cent of HNSCC), amplification of AKT (20–30 per cent), or somatic mutation, homozygous deletion or methylation of the PTEN locus in HNSCC.[36]

DNA repair pathways and genetic instability

Several lines of evidence suggest genomic instability is a cardinal feature of progression to HNSCC.[13, 37] This is confirmed by progressive accumulation of genetic aberrations as a keratinocyte evolves into an HNSCC. Factors promoting genomic instability may include deficiencies in DNA repair, chromosome cohesion and condensation, mitotic progression, spindle assembly and regulation of chromosomal telomere length. A key method in which genome integrity is disputed in HNSCC is through abnormalities in the p53 pathway, an inherited mutation which can lead to many different cancers, as demonstrated in patients with Li–Fraumeni syndrome.[19] Similarly, studies on telomerase, the enzyme that controls the length of telomeres (repetitive sequences of DNA, located at chromosomal ends) which linearly correlate with cellular lifespan, demonstrate that this pathway is also aberrant in HNSCC.[38, 39] Overall, the precise contribution of individual pathways to genomic instability in HNSCC remains to be defined.

Angiogenesis

Tumours cannot grow to sizes beyond 5–10 mm without access to the circulatory system for oxygen and nutrients and release of their metabolic waste products. As a consequence, neoangiogenesis is required for HNSCC progression.[26, 27, 40] Tumours secrete multiple soluble factors, including vascular endothelial growth factor (VEGF), acidic and basic fibroblast growth factor (FGF1/2), and interleukin 8 (IL-8) to promote vascular ingrowth. In addition, adhesion molecules mediating cell–cell and cell–matrix interactions, such as integrins and cadherins, also contribute to proangiogenic signals. Several studies have linked neoangiogenesis to development and progression of HNSCC.[41] Consistent with this, histopathological studies show increased microvessel density accompanies tumour progression.[42] Upregulation of VEGF family members including VEGF-A, VEGF-B, VEGF-C and VEGF-D, VEGF-E and FGF proteins and downregulation of thrombospondin-1 have been revealed in a high percentage of HNSCC and some of these factors have also been detected in serum of HNSCC patients.[43]

Cellular adhesion, dissociation, invasion, migration and metastasis

In contrast to normal cells, cancer cells have an acquired capability to survive dissociation from their normal environment, invade their environment and metastasize.[26, 27, 44]

Metastasis is the unique end product of this cascade and is the cause of 90 per cent of cancer-related mortality. The induction of the metastatic process is an extremely complicated process that remains incompletely understood. From a molecular point of view, an initiating role in the onset of metastasis has been attributed to aberrant homeostasis of cell adhesion pathways.[44] In recent years, important groups of cell adhesion proteins have been identified, including proteins from the cadherin and integrin superfamily. These membrane-bound receptors are central regulators of cell–cell interactions (cadherins) and cell–matrix interactions (integrins). In normal cells, the interactions of cadherins with the outside environment transmit intracellular antigrowth regulatory signals. Not surprisingly, cancer cells are marked by a significant downregulation of cadherins. In addition, the normal integrin profile present at the cell membrane of normal cells may be altered in cancer cells to switch from recognition of and interaction with the physiologic outside environment to adaptation to novel matrix components and associated alteration of intracellular signalling. In addition to cell adhesion molecules, a second important biochemical mechanism involved in invasion and metastasis includes the increased activity of extracellular protease enzymes aimed at degradation of extracellular material during preparation of escape to and settlement in distant anatomic locations. To fulfil this requirement, protease genes, such as the matrix metalloproteinases (MMPs), are upregulated and inhibitors of protease enzymes, such as the TIMPs, are downregulated in both cancer cells and surrounding stroma cells. Alterations of integrins, cadherins, MMPs and TIMPs are common in HNSCC and correlate with the pathological features and clinical outcome of HNSCC.[45]

CLINICAL UTILITY OF MOLECULAR CHANGES IN HNSCC

Molecular diagnostics

The identification of tumour-specific (somatic) molecular alterations in HNSCC and their earliest neoplastic precursors, coupled with the development of highly sensitive molecular analytic techniques, such as the polymerase chain reaction (PCR), provides several opportunities for improved molecular diagnostics of HNSCC.[46] The improved sensitivity of molecular diagnosis over traditional histopathologic assessment of oral neoplasia is evident from studies showing that premalignant lesions containing 3p14 or 9p21 alterations have a significantly higher likelihood of evolving into HNSCC (37 per cent) compared to premalignant lesions without these changes (6 per cent).[47] These data were confirmed and extended by the observation that premalignant lesions that harbour additional deletions of 4q, 8p, 11q and 17p had an even higher risk of developing into HNSCC.[48] Several studies have demonstrated a correlation between the presence of genetically abnormal cells in histologically benign mucosa within the surgical margins of HNSCC resection specimens and a higher risk for local recurrence.[49] Possibilities for improvement of molecular staging are further suggested by data demonstrating the accuracy of PCR-detected molecular alterations in histologically benign lymph node aspirates and associated reduction of survival.[50] Also, Califano and colleagues[51] demonstrated that histologically benign tissue taken during primary tumour localization examinations of unknown primary HNSCC contained the identical molecular alterations as the lymphatic metastasis. Several studies have demonstrated the possibility of distinguishing primary lung cancer from lung-metastatic HNSCC based on p53 mutation analysis or global expression profiling.[52, 53, 54, 55, 56] Recently, studies have included PCR-based analysis of promotor hypermethylation events and mitochondrial DNA mutations instead of traditional LOH analysis, suggesting that it may improve sensitivity and specificity.[57, 58] Tumour-specific methylation events can be detected in the saliva and serum of patients with HNSCC, foreseeing development of a non-invasive routine screening test for smokers and drinkers.[57, 58] The complement of data foreshadows the introduction of molecular detection of HNSCC in risk groups and molecular staging in HNSCC patients once the findings are validated and analytic techniques optimized.

Molecular staging of HNSCC

As clinical behaviour of individual tumours is directly determined by the complement of its genetic aberrations, molecular factors may be better predictors of clinical outcome than currently used clinicopathological factors. Indeed, several studies suggest that molecular analysis of HNSCC is associated with improved outcome prediction compared to traditional staging (**Table 3.2**).

p53 mutation was identified as an independent predictor of poor outcome after surgery with or without radiation therapy in several trials. In addition, p53 mutation was identified as an independent predictor of chemotherapy alone, and chemoradiation resistance in several HNSCC studies.[59] These studies confirm *in vitro* work which has shown that cell lines with p53 mutation are more sensitive to cisplatin treatment, which may relate to a decreased capacity for DNA repair in affected cells.[60] Nonetheless, the evidence for p53 mutation as an independent predictor of outcome in HNSCC remains based on small studies with heterogeneous study populations and needs appropriate confirmation.[61] Also, the clinical relevance of p53 inactivation by other means

than point mutation and prognostic evaluation of alterations in p53 pathway members (BCL2, p21, MDM2, BCL-Xl, caspases, BAX, p73 and p63) needs further delineation.

Several studies have suggested that alterations in the Rb pathway may also be of prognostic significance in HNSCC. Several studies show independent prognostic significance associated with the presence of cyclin D1 overrepresentation in HNSCC series treated with surgery with or without radiation therapy even after controlling for clinicopathological variables by multivariate analysis.[62]

Human papillomavirus is well known to compromise p53 and Rb pathways (see above under The retinoblastoma pathway) in oropharyngeal cancers is one of the strongest outcome predictors. Overall, HPV-positive tumours have improved outcomes relative to HPV-negative cases.[63] The prognostic value of HPV positivity is well defined in oropharyngeal carcinoma patients treated with chemoradiotherapy.[64] Studies from Worden *et al.*[65] and Kumar *et al.*[66] strongly suggest that oropharyngeal carcinoma patients treated with chemoradiation should be stratified for HPV status in clinical management and trials. Recent work indicates that the genetic composition of HPV-positive and HPV-negative cancers may be different, suggesting putative molecular markers that may be of predictive value.[67] Kumar and colleagues[66] report an association between *p16* and HPV status, suggesting that *p16* may serve as a surrogate marker for HPV infection. Recent work suggests that combining the EGFR expression status with HPV status may improve prognostic analysis of chemoradiotherapy treatment.[68, 69]

Alterations in EGFR and several of its downstream effectors have been associated with prognostic significance in multivariate analyses.[34] These studies suggest that constitutive activity of the EGFR pathway results in aggressive tumour behaviour. Multiple studies have reported EGFR overexpression as an independent predictor of poor outcome after surgery ± radiation therapy.[70] Also, EGFR overexpression is associated with chemotherapy and chemoradiation resistance.[70] These findings are in line with the observed modulation of chemotherapy and radiation therapy resistance of other human tumours by ErbB receptors.[69] This may relate to the proficiency of ErbB receptors to activate a pro-survival state in cancer cells through activation of downstream pathways including the RAS/MEK/ERK cascade, the STAT cascade, the PI3K/AKT cascade, and several angiogenic, cell adhesion and cell cycle regulatory pathways.

Constitutive activation of PI3-kinase through 3q26 amplification is strongly associated with survival after surgery with or without radiation therapy of HNSCC.[71] Also, overexpression of AKT provides an independent survival benefit in patients with HNSCC.[72, 73] A prognostic role for other EGFR-induced survival factors, such as the STATs, the PLC/gamma factors and members of the MEK pathway is currently under investigation. Members of pathways involved in angiogenesis, cellular adhesion, invasion and metastasis, such as the VEGF, MMPs, TIMPs, integrins and cadherins, the expression and activity of which may be influenced by the EGFR pathway, have been the subject of many prognostic studies with promising results.[40] For example, it appears that VEGF expression is an independent predictor of surgical and chemotherapy outcome, suggesting that resistance to these treatments is conferred through the activation of neoangiogenesis.[40]

Table 3.2 Clinical relevance of molecular factors in HNSCC.

Molecular alteration	Prognostic significance	Therapeutic agents
P53 pathway	P53	ONYX-15, adP53
Rb pathway	Cyclin D1	In progress
EGFR pathway	EGFR	Cetuximab, panitumumab gefitinib, erlotinib
PI3K/AKT pathway	PI3 K, AKT	Everolimus, temsirolimus
Human papilloma virus	HPV	Vaccination, immunotherapy
Angiogenesis	VEGF	Bevacizumab
DNA repair	Unclear	PARP inhibitors

In addition to the above-described molecular factors, a significant number of uncharacterized chromosomal aberrations have been associated with poor outcome of HNSCC, including deletions of 3p, 5q11, 6q14, 8p21-23, 9p21, 10q, 11q23, 14q, 17p, 18q, 21q11 and 22q and gains of 3q26 and 11q13, 12q24.[74] Some of these genomic abnormalities (3p, 3q26, 9p21) also represent early events in the HNSCC progression model, suggesting that the clinical course of HNSCC may be determined early in its pathogenesis (**Figure 3.3**). Overall, the prognostic assessment of individual molecular factors has revealed important support for their mechanistic and vital role in HNSCC pathogenesis and the hypothesis that molecular factors can be used as strong prognostic factors. However, a significant degree of outcome variation remains unexplained by the analysis of individual molecular factors. Given the multifactorial nature and genetic complexity of cancer, it is now clearly accepted that the accuracy of molecular staging may be improved significantly by analysis of multiple factors in concert.[75]

A convincing example of the improved predictive power of combined molecular assessment is provided by breast cancer analysis. Using microarray-based global gene expression profiling (**Figure 3.6**), van de Vijver and colleagues identified a 70-gene poor prognosis signature that outperformed clinicopathological factors in the prediction of distant metastasis.[76, 77] The molecular signature was an independent predictor of disease outcome in 295 patients and has been validated in several independent patient groups.[76, 77, 78] The poor prognosis signature consisted of genes regulating cell cycle, invasion, metastasis and angiogenesis, which supports its direct relationship with oncogenesis. Several other groups have reported equivalent findings in breast cancer and other tumour types. At the Netherlands Cancer Institute, a chip with the breast cancer signature has been developed and is currently being tested in clinical practice.

Microarray studies of HNSCC confirm the improved prognostic analysis of large-scale molecular profiling. A microarray study by Chung and colleagues, who investigated the gene expression profile of 60 HNSCC, identified a high risk gene expression profile predictive of lymph node metastasis (80 per cent accuracy).[79, 80] Pramana and colleagues[81] independently confirmed the association of this profile with poor outcome after chemoradiation treatment of HNSCC. Roepman and colleagues identified (in 92 tumours) and independently validated (in 27 tumours) 102 predictor genes that predicted the presence of lymph node metastasis with 86 per cent accuracy compared to 68 per cent accuracy of clinical diagnosis in their cases.[82] In addition, Ganly and colleagues identified and externally validated MDM2 and ERBB2 (Her2Neu) as predictors of regional recurrence after chemoradiation therapy of laryngeal carcinoma, further implicating the importance of p53 and receptor tyrosine kinase signalling in HNSCC.[83] Reproducibility issues associated with RNA-based microarray analysis may be overcome by recently developed improvements in DNA-based microarray analysis, which will further increase the accuracy of molecular prediction. Despite this, the assessment of increasing numbers of predictor variables has unmasked multiple statistical issues. Significant effort has been placed on development of robust analytic approaches that may further solidify the value of molecular prediction in cancers such as HNSCC. In addition, the identification of molecular

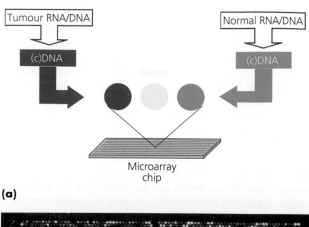

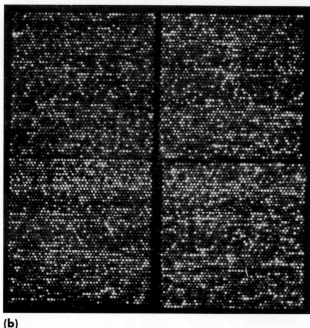

Figure 3.6   (a) Schematic description of microarray analysis. Tumour and normal reference RNA (or DNA) is reversely transcribed into complementary DNA (cDNA) (or directly used in case of DNA) and differentially labelled with a red fluorescent and green fluorescent agent, respectively. Equal amounts of labelled tumour and reference DNA are hybridized onto chips dotted with several thousands of individual gene sequences. With the use of a computer-assisted microscope and spectral analysis, the green-to-red colour ratio for each dot (gene) is calculated, the intensity of which represents overrepresentation (red-to-green ratio >1), underrepresentation (red-to-green ratio <1) or equal representation (red-to-green ratio $=1$) of the sequence in tumour tissue relative to the normal reference tissue. (b) Image of dotted microarray chip after hybridization, showing clear variations of green-to-red ratio ($=$ gene expression level or DNA copy number) between dots.

prognostic factors will be critically dependent on assembly of homogeneous study populations as the molecular profile of HNSCC is known to be influenced by multiple clinicopathologic variables that may obscure survival correlations.

In addition to prognostic analysis of individual or combined molecular markers, HNSCC can be stratified in several different subgroups based on divergent global molecular profiles, some of which are associated with poor clinical outcome. Ginos and colleagues performed microarray analysis of 41 HNSCC and demonstrated categorization into several different expression signatures, one of which was associated with recurrence.[84]

Despite these promising findings, the key question that remains is whether any of the putative predictors can be used to individualize treatment selection. Unfortunately, unlike the example of kinase mutations in other solid tumours, the predictive value of individual or combined molecular markers remains insufficient for routine clinical use in HNSCC. Even more importantly, the inherent genetic differences that predict response to chemotherapy, which may not only serve as treatment selectors, but also as therapeutic targets, remain unidentified.

Molecular therapeutic targets

The unique presence of somatic molecular alterations in cancer cells holds an opportunity for targeted HNSCC treatment.[85] Targeted treatment has a theoretical advantage over the standard treatment, due to the ability to selectively target cancer cells and spare their normal environment. This is exemplified by treatment of chronic leukaemia and gastrointestinal stromal tumours with the respective BCR/Abl and cKIT targeting agent Gleevec.[86] The characteristic molecular pathways of HNSCC, such as those governed by p53, Rb, EGFR and VEGF, are currently targeted with novel agents in preclinical and clinical trials to establish their efficacy. Of these, cetuximab, an anti-EGFR antibody, given concomitantly with radiation has been shown to be superior to radiation alone without adding to high-grade toxicity.[85, 87] Additional anti-EGFR agents are also showing promising results in combination with chemotherapy and/or radiation therapy, including panitumumab and the tyrosine kinase inhibitors (TKI) gefitinib and erlotinib.[85]

Other approaches have also been employed in HNSCC with some success. Bevacizumab, a monoclonal antibody to VEGF, has been tested in phase II studies of HNSCC patients alone or in combination with EGFR inhibitors.[88] Single agent treatment with angiogenesis blockers, such as bevacizumab, demonstrate response rates in the order of 4 per cent, that may increase to 14 per cent when combined with erlotinib.[88] In addition, several general tyrosine kinase inhibitors that inhibit multiple tyrosine kinase pathways simultaneously have been developed (sorafenib, sunitinib and others), and are the subject of clinical trials based on successful preclinical treatment of HNSCC cells. HNSCC with defects in DNA repair pathways are currently targeted by inhibitors of poly(ADP-ribose)polymerase (PARP), a nuclear enzyme that corrects DNA damage in DNA repair-deficient tumour cells recovering from radiation therapy.[89] Reactivation of p53 protein function with genetically modified viral vectors has also undergone clinical trials.[90, 91, 92, 93] ONYX-15 is an E1B-deleted adenovirus that replicates exclusively in p53 mutated cells. The agent, applied through intratumoral injection, yielded a 13 per cent response rate as a single agent and a 63 per cent rate in combination with cisplatin and 5-fluorouracil in patients with HNSCC. A second adenoviral vector, Adp53 which leads to p53 re-expression, showed modest activity in phase II trials, with a 12 per cent response rate in the

unresectable patients and 27 per cent of respectable patients surviving beyond 18 months.[94] Given the complexity of biochemical signalling pathways in human tumours, it is clear that targeted treatment of HNSCC will be most efficacious when multiple signalling pathways are blocked simultaneously, and in conjunction with standard treatment.[95, 96]

CONCLUSION

The past few years have brought significant advancements in our understanding of the biology of HNSCC. As genetic screening technologies continue to improve, we expect further improvement in delineation of the HNSCC genome. It is expected that prognostic markers and biological therapies that are derived from increased knowledge will lead to a significant and expanding role in the treatment of HNSCC in the future.

KEY EVIDENCE

- Cancer is caused by a random accumulation of genetic alterations. Genetic alterations critical for cancer cell survival are selected for in a Darwinian manner, and these critical alterations may be exploited for diagnostic, prognostic and therapeutic benefit.[1, 2, 3, 4, 25, 26, 27, 86]
- Evidence for viability of targeted treatment in HNSCC has been derived from a recent study showing improved survival of conventionally treated HNSCC with addition of cetuximab, a monoclonal antibody to EGFR.[95]

KEY LEARNING POINTS

- Cancer results from an imbalance in factors promoting the development and accumulation of genetic mutations and those that prevent, exclude or repair genetic damage.
- Extrapolation of screening data suggests that cancer cells contain as many as 12 000 individual aberrations, but biological and mathematical models suggest that only between 10 and 60 critical aberrations are essential in cancer pathogenesis.
- Genetic mutations develop in an arbitrary manner, with those providing survival advantages selected for in a Darwinian manner in individual cells.
- Critical molecular alterations for cancer development typically activate genes that promote oncogenesis (proto-oncogens) or inactivate genes that limit oncogenesis.

- Combined, the complement of genetic abnormalities confers cells with growth self-sufficiency, insensitivity to antigrowth and cell death signals, limitless replicative potential and an ability to detach from and invade surrounding structures and spread to distant anatomic sites.
- HNSCC development is increased in the presence of tobacco exposure, alcohol exposure, oncogenic HPV exposure and (non-)syndromal hereditary susceptibility factors including Fanconi anaemia, dyskeratosis congenita, Bloom's syndrome, Li–Fraumeni syndrome and specific polymorphisms in carcinogen-activating enzymes, detoxifying enzymes and cell cycle regulator genes.
- Histological progression of mucosal keratinocytes from benign squamous hyperplasia to dysplasia, carcinoma *in situ* and finally invasive carcinoma is paralleled by a stepwise increase in genomic complexity with accumulation of specific molecular alterations at specific stages along the histologic progression axis.
- Common molecular signalling pathways affected in HNSCC include the p53 pathway, the retinoblastoma pathway, the epidermal growth factor receptor pathway, the PI3-kinase pathway, and several DNA repair and genetic instability pathways, angiogenesis pathways and cellular adhesion, dissociation, invasion, migration and metastasis pathways.
- The unique presence of somatic molecular alterations in cancer cells has been shown to provide an opportunity for improved diagnostics, improved staging and cancer-specific treatment of HNSCC, but further development is needed to establish these unequivocally into clinical practice.

REFERENCES

1. Nowell PC. Discovery of the Philadelphia chromosome: a personal perspective. *Journal of Clinical Investigation* 2007; **117**: 2033–5.
2. Parmigiani G, Boca S, Lin J et al. Design and analysis issues in genome-wide somatic mutation studies of cancer. *Genomics* 2009; **93**: 17–21.
3. Sjoblom T, Jones S, Wood LD et al. The consensus coding sequences of human breast and colorectal cancers. *Science* 2006; **314**: 268–74.
4. Cahill DP, Kinzler KW, Vogelstein B, Lengauer C. Genetic instability and darwinian selection in tumours. *Trends in Cellular Biology* 1999; **9**: M57–60.
5. Singh B. Molecular pathogenesis of head and neck cancers. *Journal of Surgical Oncology* 2008; **97**: 634–9.
6. Ho T, Wei Q, Sturgis EM. Epidemiology of carcinogen metabolism genes and risk of squamous cell carcinoma of the head and neck. *Head and Neck* 2007; **29**: 682–99.
7. Viswanathan H, Wilson J. Alcohol – the neglected risk factor in head and neck cancer. *Clinical Otolaryngology and Allied Sciences* 2004; **29**: 295–300.
8. Morita M, Kumashiro R, Kubo N et al. Alcohol drinking, cigarette smoking, and the development of squamous cell carcinoma of the esophagus: epidemiology, clinical findings, and prevention. *International Journal of Clinical Oncology* 2010; **15**: 126–34.
9. Chung CH, Gillison ML. Human papillomavirus in head and neck cancer: its role in pathogenesis and clinical implications. *Clinical Cancer Research* 2009; **15**: 6758–62.
10. Kreimer AR, Clifford GM, Boyle P, Franceschi S. Human papillomavirus types in head and neck squamous cell carcinomas worldwide: a systematic review. *Cancer Epidemiology, Biomarkers and Prevention* 2005; **14**: 467–75.
11. D'Souza G, Kreimer AR, Viscidi R et al. Case-control study of human papillomavirus and oropharyngeal cancer. *New England Journal of Medicine* 2007; **356**: 1944–56.
12. Gillison ML. Oropharyngeal cancer: a potential consequence of concomitant HPV and HIV infection. *Current Opinion in Oncology* 2009; **21**: 439–44.
13. Sturgis EM, Wei Q. Genetic susceptibility – molecular epidemiology of head and neck cancer. *Current Opinion in Oncology* 2002; **14**: 310–17.
14. Foulkes WD, Brunet JS, Sieh W et al. Familial risks of squamous cell carcinoma of the head and neck: retrospective case-control study. *British Medical Journal* 1996; **313**: 716–21.
15. Mork J, Moller B, Glattre E. Familial risk in head and neck squamous cell carcinoma diagnosed before the age of 45: a population-based study. *Oral Oncology* 1999; **35**: 360–7.
16. Sturgis EM, Wei Q, Spitz MR. Descriptive epidemiology and risk factors for head and neck cancer. *Seminars in Oncology* 2004; **31**: 726–33.
17. Storey A, Thomas M, Kalita A et al. Role of a p53 polymorphism in the development of human papillomavirus-associated cancer. *Nature* 1998; **393**: 229–34.
18. Friedlander PL. Genomic instability in head and neck cancer patients. *Head and Neck* 2001; **23**: 683–91.
19. Prime SS, Thakker NS, Pring M et al. A review of inherited cancer syndromes and their relevance to oral squamous cell carcinoma. *Oral Oncology* 2001; **37**: 1–16.
20. Kutler DI, Singh B, Satagopan J et al. A 20-year perspective on the International Fanconi Anemia Registry (IFAR). *Blood* 2003; **101**: 1249–56.
21. Kutler DI, Auerbach AD, Satagopan J et al. High incidence of head and neck squamous cell carcinoma in patients with Fanconi anemia. *Archives of Otolaryngology – Head and Neck Surgery* 2003; **129**: 106–12.

22. German J. Bloom's syndrome. XX. The first 100 cancers. *Cancer Genetics and Cytogenetics* 1997; **93**: 100–6.

23. Berkower AS, Biller HF. Head and neck cancer associated with Bloom's syndrome. *Laryngoscope* 1988; **98**: 746–8.

24. Alter BP, Giri N, Savage SA, Rosenberg PS. Cancer in dyskeratosis congenita. *Blood* 2009; **113**: 6549–57.

25. Lengauer C, Kinzler KW, Vogelstein B. Genetic instabilities in human cancers. *Nature* 1998; **396**: 643–9.

26. Hahn WC, Weinberg RA. Rules for making human tumor cells. *New England Journal of Medicine* 2002; **347**: 1593–603.

27. Hahn WC, Weinberg RA. Modelling the molecular circuitry of cancer. *Nature Reviews. Cancer* 2002; **2**: 331–41.

28. Gatenby RA, Vincent TL. An evolutionary model of carcinogenesis. *Cancer Research* 2003; **63**: 6212–20.

29. Ha PK, Benoit NE, Yochem R *et al.* A transcriptional progression model for head and neck cancer. *Clinical Cancer Research* 2003; **9**: 3058–64.

30. Califano J, van der Riet P, Westra W *et al.* Genetic progression model for head and neck cancer: implications for field cancerization. *Cancer Research* 1996; **56**: 2488–92.

31. Bockmuhl U, Schluns K, Schmidt S *et al.* Chromosomal alterations during metastasis formation of head and neck squamous cell carcinoma. *Genes Chromosomes Cancer* 2002; **33**: 29–35.

32. Gasco M, Crook T. The p53 network in head and neck cancer. *Oral Oncology* 2003; **39**: 222–31.

33. Du W, Searle JS. The rb pathway and cancer therapeutics. *Current Drug Targets* 2009; **10**: 581–9.

34. Kalyankrishna S, Grandis JR. Epidermal growth factor receptor biology in head and neck cancer. *Journal of Clinical Oncology* 2006; **24**: 2666–72.

35. Bussink J, van der Kogel AJ, Kaanders JH. Activation of the PI3-K/AKT pathway and implications for radioresistance mechanisms in head and neck cancer. *Lancet Oncology* 2008; **9**: 288–96.

36. Pedrero JM, Carracedo DG, Pinto CM *et al.* Frequent genetic and biochemical alterations of the PI 3-K/AKT/PTEN pathway in head and neck squamous cell carcinoma. *International Journal of Cancer* 2005; **114**: 242–8.

37. Minhas KM, Singh B, Jiang WW *et al.* Spindle assembly checkpoint defects and chromosomal instability in head and neck squamous cell carcinoma. *International Journal of Cancer* 2003; **107**: 46–52.

38. Hahn WC, Stewart SA, Brooks MW *et al.* Inhibition of telomerase limits the growth of human cancer cells. *Nature Medicine* 1999; **5**: 1164–70.

39. McCaul JA, Gordon KE, Clark LJ, Parkinson EK. Telomerase inhibition and the future management of head-and-neck cancer. *Lancet Oncology* 2002; **3**: 280–8.

40. Seiwert TY, Cohen EE. Targeting angiogenesis in head and neck cancer. *Seminars in Oncology* 2008; **35**: 274–85.

41. Walsh JE, Lathers DM, Chi AC *et al.* Mechanisms of tumor growth and metastasis in head and neck squamous cell carcinoma. *Current Treatment Options in Oncology* 2007; **8**: 227–38.

42. Lentsch EJ, Goudy S, Sosnowski J *et al.* Microvessel density in head and neck squamous cell carcinoma primary tumors and its correlation with clinical staging parameters. *Laryngoscope* 2006; **116**: 397–400.

43. Riedel F, Gotte K, Schwalb J *et al.* Serum levels of vascular endothelial growth factor in patients with head and neck cancer. *European Archives of Otorhinolaryngology* 2000; **257**: 332–6.

44. Gupta PB, Mani S, Yang J *et al.* The evolving portrait of cancer metastasis. *Cold Spring Harbor Symposia on Quantitative Biology* 2005; **70**: 291–7.

45. Ziober BL, Silverman SS Jr, Kramer RH. Adhesive mechanisms regulating invasion and metastasis in oral cancer. *Critical Reviews in Oral Biology and Medicine* 2001; **12**: 499–510.

46. Hu YC, Sidransky D, Ahrendt SA. Molecular detection approaches for smoking associated tumors. *Oncogene* 2002; **21**: 7289–97.

47. Mao L, Lee JS, Fan YH *et al.* Frequent microsatellite alterations at chromosomes 9p21 and 3p14 in oral premalignant lesions and their value in cancer risk assessment. *Nature Medicine* 1996; **2**: 682–5.

48. Rosin MP, Cheng X, Poh C *et al.* Use of allelic loss to predict malignant risk for low-grade oral epithelial dysplasia. *Clinical Cancer Research* 2000; **6**: 357–62.

49. Bradley PJ, MacLennan K, Brakenhoff RH, Leemans CR. Status of primary tumour surgical margins in squamous head and neck cancer: prognostic implications. *Current Opinion in Otolaryngology and Head and Neck Surgery* 2007; **15**: 74–81.

50. Ferris RL, Xi L, Raja S *et al.* Molecular staging of cervical lymph nodes in squamous cell carcinoma of the head and neck. *Cancer Research* 2005; **65**: 2147–56.

51. Califano J, Westra WH, Koch W *et al.* Unknown primary head and neck squamous cell carcinoma: molecular identification of the site of origin. *Journal of the National Cancer Institute* 1999; **91**: 599–604.

52. Talbot SG, Estilo C, Maghami E *et al.* Gene expression profiling allows distinction between primary and metastatic squamous cell carcinomas in the lung. *Cancer Research* 2005; **65**: 3063–71.

53. Vachani A, Nebozhyn M, Singhal S *et al.* A 10-gene classifier for distinguishing head and neck squamous cell carcinoma and lung squamous cell carcinoma. *Clinical Cancer Research* 2007; **13**: 2905–15.

54. Leong PP, Rezai B, Koch WM *et al.* Distinguishing second primary tumors from lung metastases in patients with head and neck squamous cell carcinoma. *Journal of the National Cancer Institute* 1998; **90**: 972–7.

55. Geurts TW, van Velthuysen ML, Broekman F *et al.* Differential diagnosis of pulmonary carcinoma following

head and neck cancer by genetic analysis. *Clinical Cancer Research* 2009; **15**: 980–5.

56. Geurts TW, Nederlof PM, van den Brekel MW *et al.* Pulmonary squamous cell carcinoma following head and neck squamous cell carcinoma: metastasis or second primary? *Clinical Cancer Research* 2005; **11**: 6608–14.

57. Glazer CA, Chang SS, Ha PK, Califano JA. Applying the molecular biology and epigenetics of head and neck cancer in everyday clinical practice. *Oral Oncology* 2009; **45**: 440–6.

58. Ha PK, Chang SS, Glazer CA *et al.* Molecular techniques and genetic alterations in head and neck cancer. *Oral Oncology* 2009; **45**: 335–9.

59. Lothaire P, de Azambuja E, Dequanter D *et al.* Molecular markers of head and neck squamous cell carcinoma: promising signs in need of prospective evaluation. *Head and Neck* 2006; **28**: 256–69.

60. Mandic R, Schamberger CJ, Muller JF *et al.* Reduced cisplatin sensitivity of head and neck squamous cell carcinoma cell lines correlates with mutations affecting the COOH-terminal nuclear localization signal of p53. *Clinical Cancer Research* 2005; **11**: 6845–52.

61. Tandon S, Tudur-Smith C, Riley RD *et al.* A systematic review of p53 as a prognostic factor of survival in squamous cell carcinoma of the four main anatomical subsites of the head and neck. *Cancer Epidemiology, Biomarkers and Prevention* 2010; **19**: 574–87.

62. Thomas GR, Nadiminti H, Regalado J. Molecular predictors of clinical outcome in patients with head and neck squamous cell carcinoma. *International Jouarnal of Experimental Pathology* 2005; **86**: 347–63.

63. Fakhry C, Westra WH, Li S *et al.* Improved survival of patients with human papillomavirus-positive head and neck squamous cell carcinoma in a prospective clinical trial. *Journal of the National Cancer Institute* 2008; **100**: 261–9.

64. Ang KK, Harris J, Wheeler R *et al.* Human papillomavirus and survival of patients with oropharyngeal cancer. *New England Journal of Medicine* 2010; **363**: 24–35.

65. Worden FP, Moyer J, Lee JS *et al.* Chemoselection as a strategy for organ preservation in patients with T4 laryngeal squamous cell carcinoma with cartilage invasion. *Laryngoscope* 2009; **119**: 1510–17.

66. Kumar B, Cordell KG, Lee JS *et al.* Response to therapy and outcomes in oropharyngeal cancer are associated with biomarkers including human papillomavirus, epidermal growth factor receptor, gender, and smoking. *International Journal of Radiation Oncology, Biology, Physics* 2007; **69**: S109–11.

67. Braakhuis BJ, Snijders PJ, Keune WJ *et al.* Genetic patterns in head and neck cancers that contain or lack transcriptionally active human papillomavirus. *Journal of the National Cancer Institute* 2004; **96**: 998–1006.

68. Hong A, Dobbins T, Lee CS *et al.* Relationships between epidermal growth factor receptor expression and human papillomavirus status as markers of prognosis in oropharyngeal cancer. *European Journal of Cancer* 2010; **46**: 2088–96.

69. Zaczek A, Brandt B, Bielawski KP. The diverse signaling network of EGFR, HER2, HER3 and HER4 tyrosine kinase receptors and the consequences for therapeutic approaches. *Histology and Histopathology* 2005; **20**: 1005–15.

70. Quon H, Liu FF, Cummings BJ. Potential molecular prognostic markers in head and neck squamous cell carcinomas. *Head and Neck* 2001; **23**: 147–59.

71. Singh B, Stoffel A, Gogineni S *et al.* Amplification of the 3q26.3 locus is associated with progression to invasive cancer and is a negative prognostic factor in head and neck squamous cell carcinomas. *American Journal of Pathology* 2002; **161**: 365–71.

72. Fenic I, Steger K, Gruber C *et al.* Analysis of PIK3CA and Akt/protein kinase B in head and neck squamous cell carcinoma. *Oncology Reports* 2007; **18**: 253–9.

73. Gupta AK, McKenna WG, Weber CN *et al.* Local recurrence in head and neck cancer: relationship to radiation resistance and signal transduction. *Clinical Cancer Research* 2002; **8**: 885–92.

74. Wreesmann VB, Singh B. Chromosomal aberrations in squamous cell carcinomas of the upper aerodigestive tract: biologic insights and clinical opportunities. *Journal of Oral Pathology and Medicine* 2005; **34**: 449–59.

75. Wreesmann VB, Shi W, Thaler HT *et al.* Identification of novel prognosticators of outcome in squamous cell carcinoma of the head and neck. *Journal of Clinical Oncology* 2004; **22**: 3965–72.

76. van de Vijver MJ, He YD, van't Veer LJ *et al.* A gene-expression signature as a predictor of survival in breast cancer. *New England Journal of Medicine* 2002; **347**: 1999–2009.

77. van't Veer LJ, Dai H, van de Vijver MJ *et al.* Gene expression profiling predicts clinical outcome of breast cancer. *Nature* 2002; **415**: 530–6.

78. Bogaerts J, Cardoso F, Buyse M *et al.* Gene signature evaluation as a prognostic tool: challenges in the design of the MINDACT trial. *Nature Clinical Practice. Oncology* 2006; **3**: 540–51.

79. Chung CH, Parker JS, Ely K *et al.* Gene expression profiles identify epithelial-to-mesenchymal transition and activation of nuclear factor-kappaB signaling as characteristics of a high-risk head and neck squamous cell carcinoma. *Cancer Research* 2006; **66**: 8210–18.

80. Chung CH, Parker JS, Karaca G *et al.* Molecular classification of head and neck squamous cell carcinomas using patterns of gene expression. *Cancer Cell* 2004; **5**: 489–500.

81. Pramana J, Van den Brekel MW, van Velthuysen ML *et al.* Gene expression profiling to predict outcome after chemoradiation in head and neck cancer. *International Journal of Radiation Oncology, Biology, Physics* 2007; **69**: 1544–52.

82. Roepman P, Wessels LF, Kettelarij N *et al.* An expression profile for diagnosis of lymph node metastases from primary head and neck squamous cell carcinomas. *Nature Genetics* 2005; **37**: 182–6.

83. Ganly I, Talbot S, Carlson D *et al.* Identification of angiogenesis/metastases genes predicting chemoradiotherapy response in patients with laryngopharyngeal carcinoma. *Journal of Clinical Oncology* 2007; **25**: 1369–76.

84. Ginos MA, Page GP, Michalowicz BS *et al.* Identification of a gene expression signature associated with recurrent disease in squamous cell carcinoma of the head and neck. *Cancer Research* 2004; **64**: 55–63.

85. Le Tourneau C, Siu LL. Molecular-targeted therapies in the treatment of squamous cell carcinomas of the head and neck. *Current Opinion in Oncology* 2008; **20**: 256–63.

86. Waller CF. Imatinib mesylate. *Recent Results in Cancer Research* 2010; **184**: 3–20.

87. Bernier J. Cetuximab in the treatment of head and neck cancer. *Expert Review of Anticancer Therapy* 2006; **6**: 1539–52.

88. Rapidis AD, Vermorken JB, Bourhis J. Targeted therapies in head and neck cancer: past, present and future. *Reviews on Recent Clinical Trials* 2008; **3**: 156–66.

89. Khan K, Araki K, Wang D *et al.* Head and neck cancer radiosensitization by the novel poly(ADP-ribose) polymerase inhibitor GPI-15427. *Head and Neck* 2010; **32**: 381–91.

90. Ganly I, Kirn D, Eckhardt G *et al.* A phase I study of Onyx-015, an E1B attenuated adenovirus, administered intratumorally to patients with recurrent head and neck cancer. *Clinical Cancer Research* 2000; **6**: 798–806.

91. Khuri FR, Nemunaitis J, Ganly I *et al.* A controlled trial of intratumoral ONYX-015, a selectively-replicating adenovirus, in combination with cisplatin and 5-fluorouracil in patients with recurrent head and neck cancer. *Nature Medicine* 2000; **6**: 879–85.

92. Nemunaitis J, Ganly I, Khuri F *et al.* Selective replication and oncolysis in p53 mutant tumors with ONYX-015, an E1B-55kD gene-deleted adenovirus, in patients with advanced head and neck cancer: a phase II trial. *Cancer Research* 2000; **60**: 6359–66.

93. Nemunaitis J, Khuri F, Ganly I *et al.* Phase II trial of intratumoral administration of ONYX-015, a replication-selective adenovirus, in patients with refractory head and neck cancer. *Journal of Clinical Oncology* 2001; **19**: 289–98.

94. Nemunaitis J, O'Brien J. Head and neck cancer: gene therapy approaches. Part II: Genes delivered. *Expert Opinion on Biological Therapy* 2002; **2**: 311–24.

95. Thomas SM, Grandis JR. The current state of head and neck cancer gene therapy. *Human Gene Therapy* 2009; **20**: 1565–75.

96. Boehm AL, Sen M, Seethala R *et al.* Combined targeting of epidermal growth factor receptor, signal transducer and activator of transcription-3, and Bcl-X(L) enhances antitumor effects in squamous cell carcinoma of the head and neck. *Molecular Pharmacology* 2008; **73**: 1632–42.

Assessment and staging

NICK ROLAND

Measure twice, cut once.

INTRODUCTION

There is no more an important aspect of head and neck cancer care than the initial evaluation of the patient and the patient's tumour. The practice requires specific expertise and judgement. Regrettably, it is a process which is still occasionally carried out incorrectly and by surgeons who do not have proficiency. The surgeon must 'get it right the first time'. The consequence of not doing so can be disastrous.

In general, the first decision to be made in a patient with a confirmed head and neck cancer is whether or not to treat the patient before deciding what form of management strategy is appropriate. Deciding which patients with head and neck cancer should be treated is often more difficult than in many other fields of surgery, because there are seldom absolute objective signs that demonstrate the patient is beyond treatment.

There are several important points when it comes to making the ultimate decision with regard to treatment planning. These are:

- age of the patient;
- tumour factors (site and extent of the tumour);
- intercurrent disease (comorbidity);
- social circumstances;
- patient's wishes.

Some patients should not be treated, usually because a combination of advanced stage and poor general condition makes the mutilating effects of surgery not worthwhile. It should be noted, however, that although a head and neck tumour may be incurable, there are very few that are unresectable. Virtually every structure in the head and neck to which a tumour may be fixed can be removed in continuity and repaired in some way, shape or form. It is important to remember, therefore, that although the vast majority of patients with head and neck cancer are potentially treatable that not all are curable.

Treatment should not begin until the surgeon and patient have a clear understanding of the goals of treatment. If a patient is unfit for surgery because of advancing age or poor general health, then consideration should be given to whether or not palliative treatment is appropriate by radiotherapy and/or chemotherapy, or whether purely supportive measures will suffice with no active anticancer treatment at all. A final decision on treatment often hinges on a full assessment of the patient including physiological age and general condition.

The aim of this chapter is primarily to describe why and how we appraise a patient and their tumour. The chapter will address the general principles applicable to the topic of evaluation, classification and staging. In addition, the limitations and pitfalls of this process are described.

HISTORY

The clinical features of malignant disease are manifest by the primary tumour, secondary deposits and the general effects of cancer. Taking the history from a patient with a head and neck tumour is no different from taking the history of a patient with any other medical or surgical condition.

1. **Age.** The age of the patient will prove to be an important determinant in treatment planning. This will be due to specific age-related tumour factors and patient comorbidity factors. It may also be complicated by evocative perceptions on the part of the carers and their individual attitudes to age. When a young person develops a head and neck tumour, it often carries a sinister significance. A genetic predisposition or alteration in immune status may have caused their tumour to develop. Elderly people often have impaired functional organ reserve or significant comorbidity. They are less able to be successfully rehabilitated with regard to speech and swallowing than are younger patients after major surgery.
2. **Social circumstance.** Social circumstance is particularly important to consider in context with the patient's environmental and cultural background. Most head and neck procedures violate normal anatomy and physiology, and usually the psyche of the patient. Every patient who has a head and neck operation requires not only physical support, but psychosocial support afterwards. The decision on the appropriate modality of primary treatment should take into consideration factors such as the patient living alone, if they are unable to read and write or if they are an alcoholic.
3. **Risk factors.** Enquiry should be made into the presence of risk factors for the development of cancer of the head and neck, such as the use of tobacco products, alcohol abuse, and environmental exposure to wood dust or heavy metals.
4. **Related symptoms.** Symptoms related to the tumour will give a hint as to the anatomical position. The duration of symptoms may give a clue to the tumour behaviour. Patients who have had symptoms for a protracted period of many months, but with a small confined tumour, will probably have indolent disease. Those patients with a short history of weeks, but with a tumour causing multiple symptoms due to local extent, will have a more aggressive disease. A tumour that is growing very quickly may not be amenable to treatment by any modality and can act as a 'clinical biological indicator', so that any treatment may indeed be worse than the end point of the disease itself. The situation where the operation was a success and the patient a failure is not a desirable end result.

Table 4.1 Eastern Co-operative Oncology Group (ECOG) scale.

Grade	Description
0	Fully active, able to carry on all predisease activities without restriction (Karnofsky 90–100)
1	Restricted in physically strenuous activity, but ambulatory and able to carry out work of a light or sedentary nature, e.g. for example, light housework, office work (Karnofsky 70–80)
2	Ambulatory and capable of self-care, but unable to carry out any work activities. Up and about more than 50% of waking hours (Karnofsky 50–60)
3	Capable of only limited self-care, confined to bed or chair 50% or more of waking hours (Karnofsky 30–40)
4	Completely disabled. Cannot carry out any self-care. Totally confined to bed or chair (Karnofsky 10–20)

5. **Previous medical history.** The patient's previous medical history should be properly documented. It is paramount to assess the patient's risks pertaining to intercurrent diseases and that from their head and neck tumour. Comorbidity will compromise planned operative procedures, chemoradiation and the patient's overall prognosis. Disorders which will potentiate anaesthetic problems, bleeding (anticoagulants, aspirin) and postoperative recovery should be clearly recorded. Tumours that develop in immunocompromised individuals seldom do well by any modality. The patient's general condition should always be classified using one of the methods of measuring performance status such as the Eastern Co-operative Oncology Group (ECOG) scheme[1] or the Karnofsky status (**Table 4.1**).[2]
6. **Patients who have been treated elsewhere.** If one is assessing a patient who has had treatment elsewhere, it is important not to assume anything that has gone on before and to start again, both in the history-taking and in the clinical examination, in order not to get caught out. In patient assessment, a useful aphorism to remember is 'good judgement is usually the result of experience, but experience has usually resulted from previous bad judgement'.

EXAMINATION OF THE PRIMARY SITE

When assessing the primary lesion, its exact position, borders and effect on function should be delineated both by inspection and where posssible by palpation.

A good light source and head lamp should be used to inspect the oral cavity and oropharynx. Palpation of the tongue and tongue base by a gloved finger may reveal a tumour which is not obvious on inspection alone. In addition to primary tumour assessment, it is important to assess the patient's dentition and to seek the advice of a restorative dentist if the oral cavity is to be involved in surgical or radiotherapy treatment.

Fibreoptic endoscopy provides excellent access to the nasal cavity, nasopharynx and larynx for clinical examination. The mucosa of the tongue base can be inspected by asking the patient to protrude the tongue. Vocal cord movement should be assessed on phonation. Vocal fold mucosal wave can be further gauged by stroboscopy. The piriform fossa can be exposed by asking the patient to blow their cheeks out against their closed mouth.

A permanent record of the findings should be made preferably by photographs with written description from the examiner. In the absence of this facility, drawings or a pre-printed set of illustrations should be used. Although one ought to think in terms of T-staging, it is advised that a stage is not conferred until all of the appropriate investigations have been completed.

It is important to have a copy of the current TNM (tumour, node, metastasis) staging system, American Joint Committee on Cancer (AJCC) or Union Internationale Contre le Cancer (UICC)[3, 4] both in clinic and in the operating room to facilitate accurate staging.

EXAMINATION OF THE NECK

Involved lymph nodes rarely produce symptoms until they are quite large. Therefore, the surgeon must depend mainly on physical examination to detect clinically enlarged nodes. Detailed drawings using prepared diagrams complement the written report.

The triangles of the neck and the lymph nodes that they contain are examined in turn (**Figures 4.1** and **4.2**). Having inspected the neck from the front, the clinician stands behind

the patient and flexes his or her head slightly. Palpation then takes place in a systematic manner to include all lymph node groups and cervical anatomy (**Table 4.2**).[4] The position, size and number of nodes should be established. Fixation of the nodes to adjacent anatomical structures or skin should be defined and clearly documented. As with assessment of the primary tumour, think in terms of N-staging, but a stage should not be conferred until all of the appropriate investigations have been completed.

Clothing should be removed until the points of the shoulders can be seen. The index fingers are placed on both mastoid processes and the clinician works down the trapezius muscle until the fingers meet at the clavicle. There are nodes under the trapezius muscle and, because of this, fingers should be inserted under the anterior border of the muscle with the thumb pressing down on the top with the shoulder blades forward. When the clavicle is reached, the posterior triangle (level V) is palpated. Here, the nodes lie between the skin and muscles of the floor of the triangle and therefore can be rolled between these two surfaces. Tension is taken off the sternomastoid muscle by passive, gentle lateral movement of the head to the examined side. The fingers are placed in front of, and medial to, the sternomastoid with the thumb behind it, thus forming a 'C' around the muscle. The examination progresses down the muscle carefully because 80 per cent of the nodes lie under the muscle within the jugular chain (levels II–IV) of the deep cervical lymph nodes. The smallest node which can be easily palpated in the jugular chain is probably 1 cm. The jugulodigastric node is the largest normal node in the neck and can be palpated in many normal people. Most clinically positive nodes occur in the upper jugular chain (levels II and III), but the most superior jugular nodes (level II), including the junctional nodes, are difficult to

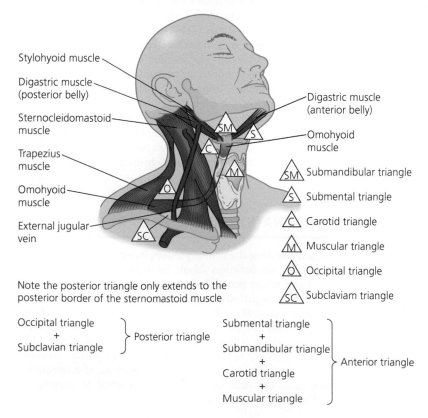

Stylohyoid muscle

Digastric muscle (posterior belly)

Sternocleidomastoid muscle

Trapezius muscle

Omohyoid muscle

External jugular vein

Digastric muscle (anterior belly)

Omohyoid muscle

SM Submandibular triangle

S Submental triangle

C Carotid triangle

M Muscular triangle

O Occipital triangle

SC Subclaviam triangle

Note the posterior triangle only extends to the posterior border of the sternomastoid muscle

Occipital triangle
+
Subclavian triangle   } Posterior triangle

Submental triangle
+
Submandibular triangle
+
Carotid triangle
+
Muscular triangle   } Anterior triangle

Figure 4.1 The triangles of the neck.

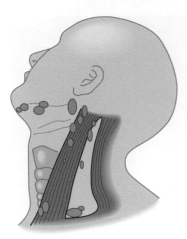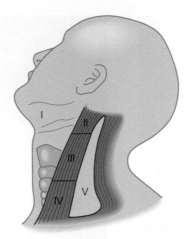

Figure 4.2   Lymph node levels.

Table 4.2   Lymph node levels.

Level	Nomenclature of anatomical site of lymph node
I	Contains the submental and submandibular triangles bounded by the posterior belly of the digastric muscle, the hyoid bone inferiorly and the body of the mandible superiorly
II	Contains the upper jugular lymph nodes and extends from the level of the hyoid bone inferiorly to the skull base superiorly
III	Contains the middle jugular lymph nodes from the hyoid bone superiorly to the cricothyroid membrane inferiorly
IV	Contains the lower jugular lymph nodes from the cricothyroid membrane superiorly to the clavicle inferiorly
V	Contains the posterior triangle lymph nodes bounded by the anterior border of the trapezius posteriorly, the posterior border of the sternocleidomastoid muscle anteriorly and the clavicle inferiorly
VI	Contains the anterior compartment lymph nodes from the hyoid bone superiorly to the suprasternal notch inferiorly. On each side, the medial border of the carotid sheath forms the lateral border
VII	Contains the lymph nodes inferior to the suprasternal notch in the upper mediastinum

palpate, particularly in men, and positive lymph nodes in the lower jugular area (level IV) may be difficult to feel since they are often small, deep and mobile.

Attention should be paid to the suprasternal notch and the space within it (the space of Burns), as clinically positive cricothyroid and pretracheal nodes may be discovered. The trachea is palpated and at this point the size of the thyroid gland is assessed. Then, working upwards, the mobility of the larynx and pharynx on the prevertebral fascia is assessed and, in particular, a note made of any pain on palpation of the trachea which may indicate direct invasion of this structure by direct extension from a postcricoid carcinoma.

The submandibular gland and nodes along with the submental nodes (level I) should now be examined. These are all easier to feel and nodes down to 0.5 cm can usually be palpated. At the posterior border of the submandibular gland, the examination continues upwards over the face to assess the preauricular nodes.

A number of normal structures can be confused with a lymph node in the neck. The lateral tips of the transverse processes of both C_1 and C_2 can simulate lymph nodes, as can the parotid tail, superior horn of the thyroid cartilage and the carotid bulb. Irradiated and obstructed submandibular glands may also simulate lymph node enlargement.

The reliability of the neck examination depends on the experience and ability of the examiner, the gross anatomy of the individual neck and whether or not there has been previous treatment, such as surgery and/or radiotherapy. A fat, thick or a muscular neck can make evaluation difficult, as can a recent incisional biopsy or tracheostomy.

It is important to remember that there is a well-recognized error in tumour palpation in general, with considerable intraobserver and interobserver variation when estimating tumour size. These pitfalls of tumour measurement are particularly common in head and neck cancer. There is considerable error in palpating the neck, with significant variation between experienced observers. The use of calipers or another measuring tool is therefore advised.[5]

FINE NEEDLE ASPIRATION CYTOLOGY

Fine needle aspiration cytology (FNAC) is the mainstay initial investigation for patients who present with cervical lymphadenopathy. With the advent of rapid access neck lump clinics, an FNAC result is obtained easily and in many cases a diagnosis procured immediately. In these clinics, a surgeon and cytopathologist are available for the evaluation and aspiration of neck masses. Ideally, the clinic should also have an ultrasound facility as this will improve the adequacy of aspirates.

An early indication as to the tissue or tumour of origin may thus greatly influence the early management of a patient with head and neck swelling, reducing dramatically both patient anxiety and resource consumption. The early detection of, for example, a colloid goitre, lymphoma or adenocarcinoma will lead to a very different clinical approach from

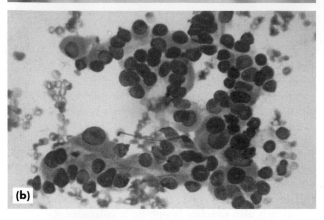

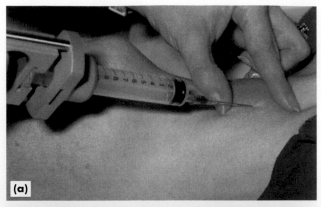

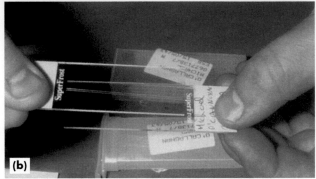

Figure 4.3 Fine-needle aspiration cytology showing (a) squamous cell carcinoma and (b) papillary carcinoma of the thyroid gland.

Figure 4.4 Technique for fine-needle aspiration cytology showing (a) aspiration of a solitary thyroid nodule and (b) smearing.

the detection of a pleomorphic adenoma or a squamous cell carcinoma. In the head and neck, FNAC is of particular value because of the multiplicity of accessible organs and the heterogeneous pathology encountered (**Figure 4.3**).

The necessary equipment should be kept in a small box ready for use and comprises a 20-mL syringe, 21-G needles, microscope slides, slide carriers, fixative spray and skin swabs. Air is expelled from a syringe and a needle attached. The lump is stabilized with the left hand as the needle enters (**Figure 4.4**). Suction is applied, and while this is maintained, several radial passes are made within the substance of the swelling. The suction is released and the needle withdrawn through the skin. The tissue core should thus be retained within the needle itself, rather than transferred to the syringe. The needle is disconnected and 10 mL of air aspirated into the syringe. This is then reconnected to the needle and the specimen expelled on to a slide. A second slide is used to smear the specimen and this process repeated with further slides until the smear is of the right thickness. This can be judged only with experience and feedback from the cytologist. Both fixed and air-dried slides should be sent to the laboratory. The slides should be sprayed at once with alcohol fixative, if Papanicolaou or similar stains are to be used. In addition, they should be air-dried for May–Grünwald–Giemsa to be used. Blood in the specimen will cause a drying artefact, but may not render it useless. If fluid is aspirated, this should be sent in a clean universal container so that a cytospin preparation can be obtained.

In many cases, a preliminary diagnosis is achieved in the clinic. However, in some situations, the aspirate may be inadequate for purpose or interpretation difficult. The submission of inadequate material for diagnosis is simply remedied by repeating the aspirate. Cystic lesions are particularly difficult as cyst content rather than epithelial cells may be aspirated. Ultrasound-guided fine needle biopsy is particularly useful in these cases and in neck masses which are difficult to define by palpation alone.

The ability to apply immunohistochemistry has increased the validity of cytology in many of the disease diagnoses, particularly lymphoma. However, FNAC is no substitute for histology, especially in the determination of nodal architecture in lymphoma, the malignant potential of a follicular thyroid tumour, of extracapsular spread in squamous carcinoma, or in the distinction of a pleomorphic from a monomorphic adenoma. Incisional biopsy of a lymph node is rarely justified as a squamous carcinoma may be implanted into the tissues. Similarly, open biopsy is contraindicated in pleomorphic adenoma or nodal deposits of squamous carcinoma. Although the former practice of Tru-cut needle core biopsies has now been superseded by FNAC, it may be useful in certain instances. In the diagnosis of anaplastic carcinoma, adequate information may be obtained from an outpatient Tru-cut needle core biopsy, if tissue cannot be obtained under general anaesthesia for various reasons.

FNAC is regarded as safe by most authorities. Some report no cell seeding at all, while others have detected spillage of 10^2–10^4 cells, but have also shown that the number of cells required to cause a seeded growth in humans is about twice that observed. There are no reports of seeding of head and neck tumours, including parotid tumours. Care should be applied if a lump seems to be pulsatile or obviously vascular to avoid inadvertent aspiration of a carotid body tumour. Suspicion of such a lesion is largely regarded either as a contraindication or an indication for the use of a finer (23 G) needle.

Several studies have confirmed the excellent diagnostic accuracy of FNAC.[6, 7, 8] To achieve this high degree of diagnostic accuracy, the cytopathologist must be well trained in the interpretation of head and neck aspiration cytology. If the findings of FNAC do not correlate with the clinical picture, the surgeon should pursue other diagnostic investigations. Clinical acumen should prevail. It is said that FNAC is as useful as the combined intelligence of the surgeon and cytologist. Regular constructive liaison between the two is pivotal.

GENERAL EXAMINATION

General health

The patient's general health should be assessed with the usual investigations. All patients undergoing major surgery should have a full blood count, urea and electrolytes, liver function tests along with a chest x-ray, electrocardiogram (ECG) and thyroid function tests. Occult hypothyroidism is not uncommon in the elderly nor in those patients having revision treatment when previous surgery or radiotherapy to the thyroid gland can affect its function. Patients should be assessed for deep vein thrombosis (DVT) prophylaxis. Specialist head and neck imaging is discussed subsequently (Chapter 6, Head and neck pathology), but as patients are at risk of metastases and a second primary within the chest, a computed tomography (CT) scan of the chest should be considered as an alternative to a chest x-ray.

A decision as to whether the patient is fit for surgery and general anaesthetic should be made following discussion with the anaesthetist who shares the final responsibility for the patient's health during any such procedure. The American Society of Anaesthesiologists (ASA) scoring guide estimates a patient's anaesthetic risk based on age, medical comorbidities, anatomical abnormalities and prior anaesthetic experience.[9] The ASA score gives an objective assessment of a patient's ability to tolerate a planned surgical procedure. The anaesthetist may order further investigations deemed appropriate on the basis of the patient's comorbidity.

Nutritional status

Head and neck cancer can cause difficulty in eating and swallowing. In addition, head and neck cancer patients are often heavy smokers and alcohol drinkers who are prone to poor nutrition. Malnutrition can compromise wound healing, immunological function and increase susceptibility to infection. Nutritional status should be assessed with a dietician and preoperative feeding may be required. This may be done orally, intravenously, via a nasogastric tube, feeding gastrostomy or jejunostomy or, more commonly a percutaneous gastrostomy (PEG). The type of feed and route of administration should be a joint decision with the dietician. Consideration should be given when postoperative feeding problems may be predicted (i.e. in oral, oropharyngeal, laryngeal surgery and radiotherapy) to request preoperative PEGs.

Dental assessment

Presurgical dental assessment is very important for head and neck cancer patients, as many have high levels of dental neglect and dental anxiety. In these patients, subsequent dental problems are inevitable without effective dental intervention. Assessment by a maxillofacial prosthodontist/ dental oncologist should take place ideally prior to any definitive treatment. This is especially important for the dentate patient with oral and oropharyngeal tumours and patients requiring maxillectomy with prosthetic obturation. Definitive decisions regarding a cancer patient's dental and periodontal disease management are best made prior to definitive surgery, allowing any necessary dental extractions to be undertaken at the same time as the ablative surgery, which in turn gives adequate time for socket healing prior to the commencement of any postoperative radiotherapy. Advice is also useful for patients planned for access mandibulotomy procedures, where the position of the mandibulotomy cut can be discussed, often with agreed sacrifice of a lower incisor tooth. Patients requiring composite reconstruction following segmental mandibulectomy should also be discussed where the choice of composite reconstruction will affect future oral rehabilitation, possibly with the use of dental implants.

Psychological assessment

Head and neck cancer patients not only suffer the burden of suffering a life-threatening disease, but they are often unable to conceal their affliction which frequently affects basic social functions such as eating and swallowing. Furthermore, treatments of the cancer can result in disfigurement and dysfunction. Pretreatment psychosocial evaluation is therefore extremely important in these patients. Factors to consider include smoking habits, alcohol dependence, coping skills, personality disorders, a history of psychiatric illness and substance abuse. The presence of comorbidities and level of social support are also important. Awareness of these factors and the expertise of a psychologist and patient support groups are vital. Pretreatment counselling allows appropriate medical support for alcohol and nicotine withdrawal and to reduce patient anxiety and uncertainty.

RADIOLOGY

Imaging is integral to the assessment of the patient, providing vital information about the primary tumour, neck nodes and distant metastases. The primary role of radiology is not usually one of diagnosis, but is one of accurate staging of the extent and spread of disease. There is an emphasis on those

essential that the invasion of the tumour into local structures is identified. Appreciation of potential treatment options in this context will increase awareness of the significance of getting this right. A drawing is made of the operative findings or on to a preprinted set of illustrations. Multiple photographs should be taken and also placed in the case file. It is important to think in terms of TNM staging, but to avoid consigning a stage at this time.

PATHOLOGY

It is important to have a relationship with the head and neck pathologist, to discuss cases regularly and to record details in an agreed and systematic manner. Specimens should be pinned out and details relating to the primary and nodal disease recorded accordingly.

Pathological tumour size should be recorded along with tumour thickness, which is important in tumours, such as the oral cavity and melanoma. The margins relating to microscopic resection should be commented on. Multifocality of the tumours should also be recorded, along with the presence or absence of perineural, vascular, lymphatic and bone invasion. Differentiated thyroid tumours should be reported as thyroglobulin positive or negative.

Cervical lymph nodes should be recorded on a diagram relating to the levels involved and the report should include which nodes were sampled, the number of nodes sampled, the number of nodes which contained tumour, their pathological site and whether or not there was extracapsular spread. This report should form part of a minimum data set. The allocation of a pN_0 classification to a neck dissection must satisfy the following criteria. Histological examination of a selective neck dissection specimen will ordinarily include six or more lymph nodes, while histological examination of a radical or modified radical neck dissection will ordinarily include ten or more lymph nodes.[1, 2]

It is important to record the type of growth (histology) along with the pathological TNM stage and overall stage. Histological differentiation of the tumour is a factor included in the UICC and AJC staging systems (**Table 4.3**).[3, 4]

The histological grading of squamous cell carcinoma represents estimation by the pathologist of the expected biologic behaviour of the neoplasm. It has been suggested that such information, in conjunction with other characteristics of the primary tumour, would be useful in the rational approach to therapy.[14] Others have reserved doubts as to the validity of the method because of its subjective nature.[15, 16]

In a systematic review of 3294 patients, it was found that 46 per cent of patients with poorly differentiated tumours

had a nodal metastasis at presentation compared with only 28 per cent differentiated tumours. Distant metastases at presentation were found in 3.4 per cent of poorly differentiated tumours, compared with 1.8 per cent of well-differentiated tumours. Primary and nodal recurrence rates rose for poorly differentiated tumours and survival fell significantly for poorly differentiated tumours.[17] In another retrospective review of over 1000 patients, grade and distant metastases were considered. It was found that patients with well-differentiated tumours are at low risk of metastases and patients with poorly differentiated tumours are at high risk of distant metastases. It was suggested they should be considered for systemic chemotherapy.[18]

Although grading is a common practice, it has not evolved as an important factor in planning therapeutic strategies. It should be used in conjunction with other pathological and stage parameters in providing an overall picture of the tumour's aggressiveness and remains an adjunctive part of the TNM system.[3, 4]

THE MULTIDISCIPLINARY TEAM MEETING

Assessment is not merely a process of a surgeon examining the patient, arranging scans and taking a biopsy of a tumour. It is advisable to obtain as many opinions as possible and not to rush in with a treatment. A multidisciplinary approach should provide each patient with a thorough and well-organized evaluation and treatment plan (Chapter 47, Multidisciplinary team working).

In the United Kingdom, there is legislation through the Improving Outcomes Guidance document that every patient with a diagnosis of head and neck cancer is discussed at a multidisciplinary team meeting (MDTM)[19] The core team should include a head and neck surgeon, oncologist, radiologist, pathologist, clinical nurse specialist, dietitian, speech therapist and psychologist. The meetings should be held on a weekly basis and serve a population of approximately one million patients. There should be facility for discussion of base of skull tumours (neurosurgeons will be present) and thyroid tumours (endocrinology and nuclear medicine physicians present) either within the head and neck multidisciplinary team (MDT) or as a separate meeting.

It is important for each member of the team to have a fundamental knowledge of each other's role and expertise. Awareness of the combined capability and experience available within the MDT is an essential element of the head and neck surgeon's role. However, every member of the MDT should harness this easily accessible facility for their patients.

STAGING OF CANCER

Staging is the process of subdivision of cases of cancer into groups in which the behaviour may be similar. Staging of head and neck cancer is a system designed to express the relative severity, or extent, of the disease. It is meant to facilitate an estimation of prognosis and provide useful information for treatment decisions. Classification by anatomical extent of the disease as determined clinically and

Table 4.3 Grading based on differentiation.

Grade	G, Histopathological grading
GX	Grade of differentiation cannot be assessed
G1	Well differentiated
G2	Moderately differentiated
G3	Poorly differentiated
G4	Undifferentiated

histopathologically (when possible) is the one that the TNM system primarily uses.

The concept is that an orderly progression of disease takes place with enlargement of and invasion by the primary tumour (T) followed by spread to the regional lymph nodes (N) and eventually spread beyond these nodes to distant metastatic sites (M). The stage at diagnosis in the life history of an individual cancer is numerically assigned a TNM classification. These individual TNM classifications are then assembled into four stage groups (stages I–IV), each with similar survival outcomes based on the observation that better survival is anticipated for cancers with less extension.

Aims of the TNM staging system

Cancer is a heterogeneous disease, or rather group of diseases, and the natural history and response to treatment can be both wide and varied. So there are obvious advantages in a staging system for head and neck squamous cell carcinoma (HNSCC). It is important for both clinical and therapeutic research and as an acceptable and reproducible method of staging all sites within the region. It is mandatory to allow any meaningful comparison to be made between different centres, both nationally and internationally. The goals of any cancer staging system are therefore, by definition, far reaching and multiple in nature. The system should act as a dictionary, allowing individual physicians and surgeons to compare and exchange information using language and vocabulary that they can all understand (**Box 4.2**).

It is worth looking at a few of these points in more detail. First and foremost, staging acts as a guide to the appropriate treatment. The question, 'How should a patient with carcinoma of the larynx be treated?' cannot be answered without reference to staging. A patient with a small tumour confined to the true vocal cord which remains mobile can be successfully treated either by surgery or by irradiation with voice preservation, but a patient with an advanced transglottic carcinoma, causing airway obstruction and invading the thyroid cartilage with nodal metastases, usually requires laryngectomy and neck dissection.

Second, the stage of a tumour acts as a guide to prognosis. Accurate prognosis is important, not only to satisfy a patient who wants to know the likelihood of successful treatment, but also to ensure the equivalence of groups in clinical trials. For example, suppose a new form of treatment is being compared with standard practice in the treatment of oropharyngeal carcinoma. If there arises, by chance, a preponderance of more advanced cases in the conventional treatment arm, the survival rate in the experimental arm may be greater, even if in reality there is no difference between the treatments, stage by stage. Prerandomization stratification by stage will prevent this source of error.

Staging also permits more reliable comparison of results between centres by allowing an estimate of case mix. For example, if hospital A publishes better survival figures for laryngeal cancer, it may be assumed that it is a better hospital offering better treatment than other hospitals. Yet, different hospitals serve different populations and consequently the pattern of cancer cases they see may be different. The observed discrepancy may therefore result from the fact that hospital B serves a large population of socially disadvantaged patients who present late with advanced disease. If survival figures are published separately for each stage, it may be found that there is no difference between hospital A and hospital B or even that truly better results from hospital B have been masked by the large proportion of poor prognostic cases treated there.

Finally, staging allows a more reliable examination of reasons behind time trends. For example, the incidence of both malignant melanoma and testicular cancer is increasing in Scotland, yet the proportion of patients dying from these diseases is diminishing. It might be assumed that the improved survival from melanoma has been caused by the development of effective systemic therapy, as is the case for testicular tumours. In fact, examination of the distribution of stages at presentation shows that more cases of melanoma are now being diagnosed early as a result of a public education campaign, but the prognosis of advanced cases has not changed.

TNM staging nomenclature

Over the last decade, the two principal staging classifications for head and neck cancer, those of the AJCC and the UICC, have undergone a convergent evolution and are now, to all intents and purposes, identical.[3, 4]

Details can be found in the current UICC handbook.[3] For each primary site in the head and neck, the factors taken into account in the stage classification are described in the appropriate chapter of the UICC handbook, to which every head and neck surgeon should have access. The following general definitions apply to all sites.

The TNM system for describing the anatomical extent of head and neck cancer is based on the assessment of three components, namely T, the extent of the primary tumour, N, the presence or absence and extent of regional lymph-node metastases and M, the presence or absence of distant metastases. All cases are identified by T, N and M categories, which must be accurately determined and recorded before treatment is commenced. The system is confined to carcinoma for all sites and malignancy must be confirmed by histological examination. Two classifications have been described for each head and neck site:

1. Clinical classification (pretreatment clinical classification, designated cTNM) is evidence acquired before primary treatment. It is based on information available prior to first definitive treatment. The clinical stage is essential to selecting and evaluating primary therapy. The UICC classification suggests that for each site the specific methods of

---

Box 4.2   Benefits of staging

- An aid to planning therapy
- Indication of prognosis
- Comparison of results of treatment
- Facilitate exchange of information between treatment centres

investigation available for TNM classifications should be listed. These include mandatory methods, such as clinical examination and biopsy, which should always be employed to establish the extent of the tumour, and additional methods, such as conventional radiography, along with other special investigations. For cTNM, traditional staging demands that certain prerequisite patient assessment be performed and its use reflects the level of certainty according to the particular diagnostic method used.

2. Pathological classification (postsurgical histopathological classification, designated pTNM). The pTNM classification is based on evidence acquired before treatment, supplemented or modified by additional information acquired either surgically or pathologically. Further information regarding the primary lesion may be recorded under the headings 'G' for histopathological grading, 'L' for lymphatic invasion and 'V' for venous invasion. The presence or absence of residual tumour after treatment may be described by the symbol 'R'. The pathological stage gives information for estimating prognosis and calculating end results.[4]

Within the TNM classification, the oral cavity, pharynx, larynx, maxillary sinus, salivary and thyroid glands are all listed as primary sites, the pharynx being subdivided by convention into the nasopharynx, oropharynx and hypopharynx. The cervical oesophagus is listed as a subsite.

Multiple tumours should be classified independently and in the case of multiple synchronous tumours in one organ, the tumour with the highest T category should be classified and the multiplicity or number of tumours indicated in parentheses.

Each site is described under a TNM heading (mandatory) and a cTNM and pTNM classification (optional). After being assigned various TNM categories, patients are grouped into a number of clinical stages (see **Table 4.6**). Classification is distinguished from staging, which is the grouping of cancers with similar crude survival rates.

The C-factor, or certainty factor, reflects the validity of classification according to the diagnostic methods employed (C1–C5). C1 would be evidence from standard diagnostic means, whereas C5 is evidence from autopsy. Generally speaking, pretherapeutic clinical staging of head and neck cancers should be based on a C2 factor. That would be evidence obtained by special diagnostic means, e.g. radiographic imaging (e.g. CT, MRI or US), endoscopy, biopsy and cytology.[3]

Method of staging

The aim is to define in each patient all of the factors relevant to the natural history and outcome of the relevant disease, thereby enabling a patient with cancer to be grouped with other similar cases. The sex and age of the patient, the duration and severity of symptoms and signs, and the presence and severity of intercurrent disease should all be documented.

CT and MRI are now established as the mainstay investigations in the preoperative work up of patients with head

and neck cancer. Scans to evaluate the primary site should be performed prior to biopsy to avoid the effect of upstaging from the oedema caused by biopsy trauma. There is a natural desire to confer a stage on the tumour at presentation in the clinic and certainly after endoscopy. This should be avoided. It is better to rely on descriptive text to avoid changing the stage as more information becomes available. The clinical (pretreatment) classification (cTNM) based on examination, imaging, endoscopy and biopsy should be clearly documented in the case file only when all of the above information is collated. This will improve the chance that at least a certainty factor of 2 is applied. The UICC book should be available in every theatre and clinic to assist in applying the correct stage. Once the clinical stage is assigned, it should not be changed on the basis of subsequent information. Clinical staging ends if a decision is made not to treat the patient.

Most of the reasons for staging do not immediately appear to benefit the individual patient and so it might be tempting for the busy surgeon to make no attempt at the staging process beyond a brief assessment for the purposes of choosing either treatment A or B, or worse still for them to assign hurriedly a wholly inaccurate stage. Yet, if the biology of cancer is to be more fully understood and if treatments are to be improved, it is imperative that staging should be carried out fully and accurately on every patient.

While assessment of the tumour, nodes and metastases is usually sufficient for the staging purposes, other factors which are sometimes taken into account include the histological differentiation or grade of the tumour, along with the patient's age and sex, for example, in cases of soft-tissue sarcoma and differentiated thyroid carcinoma. For tumours such as lymphoma, which do not follow an orderly progression from primary tumour to nodal involvement and then distant metastases, special staging systems have been devised.

Even for epidermoid cancer, there are a variety of different staging classifications. Although these have similar aims and use similar data, the systems differ in important regards and therefore lead to groupings which may not be directly comparable and may thus preclude a meaningful exchange of data not only between centres but also between countries. The use of 'alternative systems' is therefore discouraged, other than for research purposes, and then only when correlation to TNM staging is available.

PRIMARY TUMOUR (T) STAGING

The extent of primary tumour is indicated by the suffixes 1, 2, 3 or 4, representing progressively more advanced disease. Increase in size is usually the sole criterion for categories 1, 2 and 3, while 4 often indicates direct extension (spread by continuity and contiguity) from outside the primary site, or invasion of underlying bone or cartilage (**Table 4.4**). Other criteria are applied in special circumstances, such as fixation of the vocal cord in laryngeal carcinoma and the degree of extrapharyngeal extension in nasopharyngeal carcinoma. A uniform description of advanced tumours as T4a (resectable) and T4b (unresectable) has been introduced to define the concept of inoperable fixation.[3, 4]

T_0 is used when there is no evidence of a primary tumour, T_{1s} used when the primary is non-invasive or carcinoma *in*

Table 4.4 Primary tumour classification.

Stage	T, Primary tumour
TX	Primary tumour cannot be assessed
T0	No evidence of primary tumour
Tis	Carcinoma *in situ*
T1, T2, T3, T4 (T4a, T4b)	Increasing size and/or local extent of the primary tumour

Table 4.5 Nodal status classification.

N-stage	N, Regional lymph nodes
NX	Regional lymph nodes cannot be assessed
N0	No regional lymph node metastasis
N1	Metastasis in a single ipsilateral lymph node. 3 cm or less in greatest dimension
N2	N2a: Metastasis in a single ipsilateral lymph node, more than 3 cm, but not more than 6 cm in greatest dimension N2b: Metastasis in multiple ipsilateral lymph nodes, none more than 6 cm in greatest dimension N2c: Metastasis in bilateral or contralateral lymph nodes, none more than 6 cm in greatest dimension
N3	Metastasis in a lymph node more than 6 cm in greatest dimension

Table 4.6 Stage grouping.

Stage			
0	Tis	N0	M0
I	T1	N0	M0
II	T2	N0	M0
III	T1, T2	N1	M0
	T3	N0, N1	M0
IVA	T1, T2, T3	N2	M0
	T4a	N0, N1, N2	M0
IVB	Any T	N3	M0
	T4b	Any N	M0
IVC	Any T	Any N	M1

situ and T_x when for some reason the extent of the primary tumour cannot be assessed. A frequent error is in the assignment of stage for a primary of unknown origin. This should be T_0 and not T_x as is sometimes given.

CERVICAL NODE (N) STAGING

The presence of cervical lymph node metastases remains the most significant prognostic indicator of survival and disease recurrence in squamous cell carcinoma of the head and neck.

Lymph nodes are described as ipsilateral, bilateral, contralateral or midline; they may be single or multiple and are measured by size, number and anatomical location (**Table 4.5**). During clinical examination, the actual size of the nodal mass should be measured and allowance made for the intervening soft tissues.[5] It is well recognized that most masses over 3 cm in diameter are not single nodes, but represent confluent nodes or tumour in the soft-tissue compartments of the neck. Midline nodes are considered ipsilateral nodes, except in the thyroid. Direct extension of the primary tumour into lymph nodes is classified as lymph node metastasis.[3, 4]

Imaging for node detection and delineation is advisable if the neck is being scanned as part of the evaluation of the primary tumour, if there is a high chance of occult disease (e.g. supraglottic primary), to assess the extent of nodal disease, to define any deep nodal fixation, or if clinical detection is difficult because of a short fat or previously irradiated neck.

Lymph nodes are subdivided into specific anatomic sites and grouped into seven levels for ease of description (**Table 4.2**). The pattern of lymphatic drainage varies for different anatomic sites. However, the location of the lymph node metastases has prognostic significance. Survival is significantly worse when metastases involve lymph nodes beyond the first echelon of lymphatic drainage.[20] It is particularly poor for lymph nodes in the lower regions of the neck, i.e. level IV and level V (supraclavicular area).

The seventh edition of the UICC booklet alludes to the importance of levels in some sites, but does not present any definitions. The AJCC *Cancer staging manual* gives a much more thorough account. It recommends that each N staging category be recorded to show, in addition to the established parameters, whether the nodes involved are located in the upper (U) or lower (L) regions of the neck, depending on their location above or below the lower border of the thyroid cartilage.[3, 4]

Under the current joint classification, the clinical findings regarding regional cervical lymphadenopathy are defined for each site independent of the primary tumour. The definitions of the N categories for all head and neck sites, except nasopharynx and thyroid, are the same. The natural history and response to treatment of cervical nodal metastases from nasopharynx are different, in terms of their impact on prognosis, so they justify a different N classification. Regional lymph node metastases from well-differentiated thyroid cancer do not significantly affect the ultimate prognosis and therefore also justify a unique system.

METASTASES (M) STAGING

The presence or absence of distant metastases is indicated by M_1 or M_0, respectively. M_1 can be subdivided further to include the anatomical area involved, such as pulmonary (PUL), hepatic (HEP) or brain (BRA).

The role of imaging in confirmation of metastic disease status has already been discussed. While it would be inadvisable to contemplate major surgery before excluding the presence of distant metastases, in practice very few patients with squamous cell carcinoma have disease outside the head and neck at presentation. The converse situation, of a secondary lesion in the head and neck, should be considered when adenocarcinoma occurs in the cervical lymph nodes or salivary glands. A primary lesion particularly in the breast, bowel or chest should then be excluded.

Stage grouping

A tumour with four degrees of T, three degrees of N and two degrees of M will have 24 potential TNM categories. In head and neck cancer, with subdivision of T stage (at least six options) and N stage (six options) there are potentially 48 TNM categories (and more depending on further subdivision of T stage at individual sites). This is clearly too many for easy use. Even in the largest reported patient series, there will be some combinations with too few patients for meaningful comparison. It has therefore been felt necessary to condense these into a convenient number of TNM stage groups (**Table 4.6**). The grouping adopted is designed to ensure, as far as possible, that each group is more or less homogeneous in respect of survival; in addition, that the survival rates of these groups for each cancer site are distinctive. Carcinoma *in situ* is categorized as stage 0; cases with distant metastasis as stage IV. The exception to this grouping is for thyroid and nasopharyngeal carcinoma (Chapter 23, Surgical management of differentiated thyroid cancer and Chapter 30, Pharynx: nasopharynx, respectively).[3, 4]

Advanced tumours (stage IV) have been divided into three categories: stage IVA, advanced resectable disease; stage IVB, advanced unresectable disease; and stage IVC, advanced distant metastatic disease.

A patient with a primary of unknown origin (T_0) will be staged according to the N status, i.e. stage III or IV disease. The importance of carefully excluding a primary site is already discussed and the implications of its position will have an effect on prognosis in this subgroup of patients.[21]

LIMITATIONS OF T STAGING

The TNM system provides head and neck surgeons with a common means of communication that is clinically orientated and based on pretreatment diagnostic studies. No one system is perfect and the criticisms that were aimed at the old classifications focused on the numerous subcategories that contained so few cases per category that statistical conclusions could not be drawn. In addition, there was lack of agreement on anatomical boundaries, the staging of cervical lymphadenopathy and the fact that host tumour responses and histopathological findings were not taken into account. The main limitations are as follows:

- crude system;
- tumour size not consistently related to prognosis;
- debatable anatomical boundaries;
- can be difficult to accurately assess clinical extent;
- inconsistencies;
- omissions.

For the majority of sites in the head and neck, emphasis is placed on tumour size. It is however, well recognized that T stage alone is of limited prognostic significance in many head and neck carcinomas. It is a significant factor in the presence of nodes on presentation. Patients with larger tumours are more likely to have nodes than those with smaller tumours.[22] In carcinoma of the larynx, the poorer prognosis with increased T stage is explained by the increasing propensity to nodal metastases with larger tumours. If nodal metastases are removed as a confounding factor, then T stage per se does not influence prognosis.[23]

Tumours of the larynx are classified according to the number of anatomical surfaces involved, rather than size. This has led to a number of problems. For example, a large 3 cm tumour of the supraglottis may still remain T_1, whereas in the glottis this will almost certainly be a T_3. This mitigates against supraglottic tumours in terms of outcome. In addition, depth of invasion is not measured, but is of prognostic and therapeutic importance. For example, a superficial tumour of the vocal cord mucosa would be T_{1a}. The same tumour may be deeply infiltrating into the vocalis muscle and yet the stage will still remain T_{1a}. These tumours of the same stage would require different resections if laser was chosen as the modality of treatment. A further classification system has been proposed based on the type of cordectomies in this situation.[24]

Tumours of the hypopharynx are classified in terms of both their size and anatomical extent. In the past, the anatomical boundaries of the hypopharynx have been contentious, and it is occasionally difficult to be certain of the exact origin of some of the larger tumours. The dual listing of the aryepiglottic fold in both the supraglottis and hypopharynx (hypopharyngeal aspect of the aryepiglottic fold) sites particularly invokes a problem trying to classify the site of origin in some situations.

In the oral cavity and particularly the oropharynx, the size of the tumour is not always easily measured. There is little difficulty in defining a T_1 or T_4 tumour, but problems can occur when the tumour measures between 1.5 and 3 cm. Furthermore, increasing severity with a T_4 tumour is reflected in deep invasion into muscle, bone or adjacent structures. Bony invasion of the mandible demonstrated radiographically is classified as T_4 disease. However bony erosion is not easily defined. The 2 cm lesion in the anterior floor of the mouth that involves the alveolar ridge and is adherent to the periosteum will not necessarily demonstrate bony erosion on radiographic evaluation. Most surgeons agree that the underlying bone should be included in the surgical resection (either a rim or complete resection) and therefore T_2 and T_4 disease may require essentially the same treatment.

A similar problem is encountered in determining the depth of invasion of lesions into the soft tissue of the floor of the mouth. Superficial invasion of the sublingual area as opposed to invasion of the mylohyoid muscle can be subtle. There is then a reliance on the predictive power of radiographic modalities including CT and MRI. Depth of invasion of lesions of the floor of mouth has been shown to be of prognostic significance and this is similarly difficult to assess by either clinical or radiographic means.[22]

Further confusion relating to prognostic staging of primary disease surrounds the fact that bony involvement of the medial or inferior walls of the maxillary sinus receive only a T_2 classification, but when oral carcinoma involves the antrum (erosion of the inferior wall of the sinus), the classification is T_{4a}. This apparent disparity is explained by the discrepancy in behaviour of the two separate bone involvements and subsequent specific behaviour of these diseases.

There is no mention of the cervical trachea as a subsite within the current lung staging system which is interesting as it was included in previous UICC and AJCC manuals. The reason for its exclusion is that there is currently too little information on outcome to construct a realistic staging system. In addition, there is no mention in either system of a TNM classification for carcinoma of the external auditory meatus or middle ear, although one has been proposed in the past.

LIMITATIONS OF N STAGING

There is approximately a 50 per cent reduction in five-year survival rate with the development of cervical lymph node metastases in patients with squamous cell carcinoma of the head and neck. Although the presence of cervical node metastases is of undoubted importance, there are still some fundamental and basic difficulties in classifying node status.

The main criticisms are as follows:

- observer variability (presence of nodal disease and size measurement);
- no inclusion of immunological status;
- importance of extracapsular spread;
- N2 (bilateral involvement) implies better prognosis than N3 (large nodes greater than 6 cm).

The reliability of clinical examination of nodes is contentious with studies showing that observers disagree on their presence.[25] Furthermore, palpable nodes do not always harbour tumour. During clinical examination, the size of the node should be measured with calipers, and allowance made for the intervening soft tissues. There is considerable observer error in estimating the size of the node by palpation alone without a measuring device.[5] Most masses over the size of 3 cm in diameter are not single nodes, but will represent confluent nodes or tumour in the soft tissue compartments of the neck.

One of the main criticisms over the last decade has been the failure of the TNM system to provide a description of the level of nodal involvement. Various studies have confirmed the importance of this parameter[20] and now it is included in the current classification.[4] Although the AJCC manual gives a detailed description of lymph node levels, the inclusion is merely that a designation of 'U' or 'L' may be used to indicate metastasis above the lower border of the cricoid (U) or below the lower border of the cricoid (L).[4] It is advised that specific lymph node level (as well as U/L category) be documented in the case file and on the database, for ease in future use.

The immunological and pathological status of lymph nodes is not included. This is not so surprising as the evidence for importance of immunology of lymph nodes is conflicting. For example, it has been stated by some authorities that the presence of reticular hyperplasia[26] and evidence of lymphocytic stimulation[27] in lymph nodes is a good prognostic sign, whereas a double-blind retrospective study has shown no correlation between lymph node morphology and survival or metastases.[28]

The presence of extracapsular nodal spread has been shown to be associated with significant decline in survival and high rate of local-regional recurrence.[29] Extracapsular spread is noted in a majority of lymph nodes larger than 3 cm and in a significant number of nodes less than 2 cm.[30] The situation is even worse when there is tumour freely extending through into the soft tissues of the neck.[31] Imaging studies showing amorphous spiculated margins of involved nodes or involvement of internodal fat resulting in loss of normal oval or round nodal shape strongly suggest extracapsular tumour spread. However, despite the obvious importance, extracapsular spread is not an integral part of N status classification.

In addition, inclusion of bilateral or contralateral disease as N2 is confusing since it implies a better prognosis than N3 disease. The word fixation has, at least, been removed from previous nodal classifications since it was open to wide and varied subjective interpretation. However, it is worth noting that the present classification of N3 disease includes nodes which are greater than 6 cm in size which are usually fixed.

LIMITATIONS OF PATHOLOGICAL STAGING

The pathological assessment of the primary tumour (pT) entails a resection of the primary tumour or biopsy adequate to evaluate the highest pT category. The system, even with the aforementioned guidelines, is open to sampling errors and inter- and intraobserver errors. It is advised that pT is derived from the actual measurement of the unfixed tumour in the surgical specimen, as up to 30 per cent shrinkage occurs.

Direct extension of the primary tumour into lymph nodes is classified as a lymphn-node metastasis. Of course, it could be argued that this extension has a completely different biology and perhaps outcome to a tumour that has truly metastasized. Similarly contentious is that a tumour nodule in the connective tissue of a lymph drainage area without histological evidence of residual lymph node is classified in the pN category as a regional lymph node if it has a smooth contour. A tumour with an irregular contour is classified in the pT category, i.e. discontinuous extension.[3]

In contrast to clinical staging, when size is a criterion for pN classification, measurement is made of the metastasis, not of the entire lymph node. Although there is an instruction to identify extracapsular nodal spread, it is still not a quantitative factor in the pN classification.

There have been many suggestions for other pathological factors to be included in the pathological stage.

Numerous attempts have been made to correlate the microscopic appearance of a tumour with its biological behaviour and patient prognosis. Although studies have found a higher incidence of cervical lymph node metastases in poorly differentiated tumours,[17] the single most important pathological feature correlating with cervical node metastases appears to be the tumour–host interface. Tumours with infiltrating margins have a poorer prognosis than those with pushing edges.[32, 33] Vascular and nerve sheath invasion also increases the probability of lymphn-node metastases.[34] These observations prompted multifactorial analysis of the cell population (structure, differentiation, nuclear polymorphism, mitosis) and of the tumour–host relationship (mode of invasion, stage of invasion, vascular invasion, cellular response).[35]

While some studies report a close correlation between histological malignancy scores and the outcome of disease,[35, 36] other investigations have found no significant improvement on conventional grading.[37] Critics of these grading systems have pointed out that they are extremely labour intensive and the criteria used have a subjective element with wide inter- and intraobserver error by the histopathologist.[38] In addition, it is argued that the pooling of statistically significant and less important parameters results in a compromised conclusion of no clinical value.[37] Hence, these systems have not been adopted for regular use in clinical practice nor do they form part of pathological staging.

The challenge seems to be how to incorporate nonanatomic prognostic factors with the TNM system. For example, the use of biomolecular markers and measures of cell kinetics have been suggested as potential prognostic indices for tumour behaviour. Some studies have found that certain markers influence outcome, but the results are not consistent and they too have not found regular use in clinical practice.[39, 40, 41, 42, 43]

LIMITATIONS OF STAGE GROUPING

Despite the obvious value of staging, both in the management of individual patients, and for the grouping of patients in trials and reports of treatment, it does have its limitations. The most insidious of these is that attempts to increase the accuracy of staging leads to greater complexity, and hence paradoxically to more errors and an increased likelihood of non-compliance by the person responsible for staging. Advances in methods of collecting and recording data will hopefully reduce these errors.

There are now seven stages for head and neck cancers arising at mucosal sites (0, I, II, III, IVa, IVb, IVc) and six stages for salivary gland cancers (I, II, III, IVa, IVb, IVc). Differentiated thyroid cancers also have six stages (I, II, III, IVa, IVb, IVc) with undifferentiated (anaplastic) cancers having three as all cases are stage IV (IVa, IVb, IVc). Many authorities have concluded that problems exist with the current staging system.[44, 45, 46, 47] One of the main criticisms is that the size of some groups defined by the combinations of the TNM classifications is small, preventing accurate prediction from previous experience.

Compelling arguments have been advanced suggesting the different ways grouping the same T, N and M categories may result in an improved system.

The TANIS score combines the integers of the T and N to create a new score. Thus, a T1N0 would be a TANIS 1 and T2N2 would be a TANIS 4, etc. First reported by Jones et al.,[47] this is an easy system to use evaluated primarily for cancers of the oral cavity and oropharynx. It treats T and N as equivalent with respect to survival. The advantages of the TANIS score are its ease of application, ability to define a reasonable number of groups, and ability to be applied retrospectively if the TNM score is known. The main disadvantage is that the concept of T and N equivalence does not hold true. Many studies have confirmed the more significant impact of N status over T status. For example, a T2N0 carcinoma does not have the same survival as a T1N1 at any site, though both of these would be TANIS 2.

Others have also tried to improve on the current stage grouping and TANIS system with subtle variations.[48, 49, 50]

They more or less all claim that their system is an improvement on any other. Lydiatt et al.[51] provide a review of these. They observe that one of the main disadvantages is that the systems are not intuitive and would require a chart for most clinicians to stage their patients. Analyses comparing the authors' system to other systems including the UICC/AJCC are flawed, because each one is not independent of the authors' system. Therefore, because the system was created from the database, it would naturally perform well. The true test is whether the results from an independent database would yield similar results.

The five major sites of the head and neck (oral cavity, oropharynx, larynx, hypopharynx and paranasal sinuses) share the same system. Arguably they should be independent of each other. One advantage of an independent system is better groupings within each site. Different systems are in use for the nasopharynx and thyroid, which are considered to be sufficiently different with respect to risk factors, behaviour and treatment. In their rebuttal of these views, the AJCC Task Force maintains the opinion that independent systems would create problems for clinicians and investigators not remembering which group was staged by which system. They are of the view that any new system should be comprehensive and easily applicable to all the major sites.[51]

CONCLUSIONS

The current TNM system relies on morphology of the tumour (anatomical site and extent of disease) with little or no attention given to patient factors. However, the literature does suggest that symptom severity[52] and comorbidity[53] have a significant impact on outcomes. It is therefore recommended that these data be recorded.

Definitions of TNM categories may be altered or expanded for clinical or research purposes as long as the basic definitions are recorded and not changed. Changes in the TNM classification should and will only occur, based on the appropriate collection, presentation and analysis of data, in the forum of the UICC and AJCC.[3, 4]

All of the above inconsistencies make the head and neck a complicated region in which to apply a single concept of classification. However, the end result embraces the orderly description of disease with increasing size and extent and one which lends itself to incorporation into a staging system, so that comparisons of treatment results might be meaningful. The current system, while fallible, is founded on sound principles and represents the combined work and experience of many physicians and surgeons who have spent years treating head and neck cancer. Any shortcomings or criticism of the system must reflect the complexity of the disease rather than any actual deficiencies within the staging classification.

In recent years, the advent of sophisticated imaging technology has made assessment much more accurate. Cases are often demonstrated to be more extensive than is clinically apparent, and are accordingly put into higher stages. **Table 4.7**, shows the results of treatment for a form of cancer, as staged by an older, less accurate clinical method and using modern sophisticated imaging techniques. The cure rate for each stage of the disease is higher in those staged with the more modern technique, yet the overall cure rate for the

Table 4.7 Comparison of results of treatment for cancer using an old and a new staging system.

Stage	Old staging systems			New staging systems		
	No. of patients	% Cured	No. cured	No. of patients	% Cured	No. cured
I	30	80	24	25	84	21
II	30	50	15	25	60	15
III	30	20	6	25	28	7
IV	10	10	1	25	12	3
All	100	46	46	100	46	46

entire cohort of patients, at 46 per cent, is identical whichever staging system is used. This illustrates the phenomenon of stage migration, where apparently superior results are produced by the upstaging of patients. This is called 'stage migration' or creep, and is sometimes referred to as the 'Will Rogers' phenomenon'.[54] Will Rogers was an American wit from Oklahoma who stated that every time an Oklahoma man moves to California, the average IQ of both states improves.

FOLLOW-UP POLICIES

Follow up of patients treated for cancer is performed for several reasons which are of different importance. Some of these are for the direct benefit of individual patients, whereas others are for the benefit of future cohorts of patients. Possible reasons for follow up are given below:

- To monitor the primary tumour site and nodal areas after completion of initial radical therapy. This has the aim of detecting residual disease or relapse at an early stage when it is still possible to institute potentially curative salvage treatment.
- To ensure that the patient is being successfully rehabilitated with regard, for example, to speech and swallowing after radical treatments which may have interfered with normal head and neck physiology.
- To reassure the patient that the team which treated them still cares about their progress and wants to know if any problems develop. Patients can be educated about which symptoms should lead to clinical review earlier than planned. Advice given about secondary prevention strategies, such as smoking cessation, can be reinforced and monitored.
- To prevent treatable morbidity, such as dental decay and hypothyroidism, before it becomes clinically significant by the monitoring and early detection of problems.
- To obtain accurate data about important outcome measures for the purposes of medical audit and clinical governance; these include local and regional control, treatment-related morbidity, second malignant neoplasms, functional impairment and survival.
- To provide training opportunities for trainees in surgery and oncology and the professions allied to medicine.

In patients with head and neck squamous carcinoma, the appropriate frequency of routine follow up varies, depending on several of the factors mentioned above, but principally on

Table 4.8 Follow-up frequency after treatment for squamous cancer of the head and neck.

Time after treatment	Good possibility of successful salvage, if local or nodal relapse	Little chance of successful salvage
First year	Monthly	Six-weekly
Second year	Two-monthly	Three-monthly
Third year	Three-monthly	Six-monthly
Fourth year	Six-monthly	Six-monthly
Fifth year	Six-monthly	Six-monthly
After five years	Annually or discharge	Annually or discharge

the likelihood of relapse and the possibility of salvage treatment. For example, a patient with T_2N_0 cancer of the anterior tongue treated with brachytherapy alone, without prophylactic neck irradiation or surgery, has a significant likelihood of nodal relapse which may be subsequently cured by neck dissection if detected early, but which might become inoperable if there is a three-month delay. Similarly, a patient with early laryngeal cancer treated by radiotherapy alone requires frequent follow up, so that salvage surgery can be performed without delay in the event of local failure.

In such patients, follow up should be monthly in the first year after completion of treatment, two-monthly in the second year, three-monthly in the third year, then six-monthly to five years (**Table 4.8**). Subsequently, annual follow up may be deemed appropriate, but in many cases discharge to the care of the general practitioner is a reasonable alternative.

In contrast, a patient who has undergone composite resection of a T_2N_0 oropharyngeal cancer with postoperative radiotherapy to the primary site and both sides of the neck requires less frequent follow up to detect relapse, as there is very little chance of effective salvage. Nonetheless, follow up is still necessary to monitor deglutition, nutrition and dentition. In this case, an appropriate follow-up schedule might be six-weekly for the first year, three-monthly for the second year and then six-monthly to five years, with optional annual follow up after that.

Different follow-up plans may be more appropriate for patients with rare tumours, such as lymphoma or sarcoma. In patients who have a thyroid cancer, follow up is usually lifelong as recurrences can occur many years following initial treatment.

KEY LEARNING POINTS

- The sex and age of the patient, the duration and severity of symptoms and signs, and the presence and severity of intercurrent disease should all be documented.
- Assessment by endoscopy and biopsy should be performed by a senior surgeon and in all cases by the head and neck surgeon responsible for any future procedure.
- Radiological investigations to evaluate the primary site should be performed prior to biopsy to avoid the effect of upstaging from the oedema caused by biopsy trauma.
- Staging of head and neck cancer is a system designed to express the relative severity, or extent, of the disease. It is meant to facilitate an estimation of prognosis and provide useful information for treatment decisions. Classification by anatomical extent of head and neck cancer as determined clinically and histopathologically is the TNM system.
- The UICC and AJCC booklets provide a summary and cornerstone for accurate staging.
- The clinical (pretreatment) classification (cTNM) based on examination, imaging, endoscopy and biopsy should be clearly documented in the case file only when all the information is collated.
- Individual TNM classifications should be assembled into four groups (stages I–IV), each with similar survival outcomes.
- The AJCC or UICC book should be available in every theatre, MDT meeting and clinic to assist in applying the correct stage.

REFERENCES

1. Zubrod CG, Schneiderman M, Frei E. Appraisal of methods for the study of chemotherapy of cancer in man. Comparative therapeutic trial of nitrogen mustards and triethylene thiophosphoramide. *Journal of Chronic Diseases* 1960; **11**: 7–33.
2. Karnofsky DA, Abenmann WH, Craver LF, Burchenall JH. The use of nitrogen mustards in the palliative treatment of carcinoma. *Cancer* 1948; **1**: 634–56.
3. Sobin LH, Gospodarowicz M, Wittekind C. *TNM classification of malignant tumours, UICC,* 7th edn. New York: Wiley-Liss, 2009.
4. Edge SB, Byrd DR, Compton CC *et al.* (eds). *The AJCC cancer staging manual,* 7th edn. New York: Springer, 2009.
5. Alderson D, Jones T, Roland NJ. Intra and inter observer error in assessment of cervical lymph nodes. *Head and Neck* 2001; **23**: 739–43.
6. Roland NJ, Caslin AW, Turnbull LS *et al.* Rapid report of fine needle aspiration cytology of salivary gland lesions in a head and neck clinic. *Journal of Laryngology and Otology* 1993; **107**: 1025–8.
7. Caslin AW, Roland NJ, Turnbull LS *et al.* Immediate report of fine needle aspiration cytology of head and neck lesions in a head and neck clinic. *Clinical Otolaryngology* 1993; **28**: 552–8.
8. Tandon S, Shahab R, Benton J *et al.* FNAC in a regional Head and Neck Center. Comparison with a systematic review and meta-analysis. *Head and Neck* 2008; **30**: 1246–52.
9. Saklad M. Grading of patients for surgical procedures. *Anaesthesiology* 1941; **2**: 281.
10. Houghton DJ, Hughes ML, Garvey C. Role of chest CT scanning in the management of patients presenting with head and neck cancer. *Head and Neck* 1998; **20**: 614–18.
11. Ghosh S, Roland NJ, Kumar A *et al.* Detection of pulmonary tumours in head and neck cancer patients. *European Archives of Otorhinolaryngology* 2007; **264** (Suppl.): S5–S151.
12. Haughey BH, Gates GA, Arfken CL, Harvey J. Meta analysis of second malignant tumours in head and neck cancer: the case for an endoscopic screening protocol. *Annals of Otology, Rhinology, and Laryngology* 1992; **101**: 105–12.
13. Davidson J, Witterick I, Gilbert R *et al.* The role of panendoscopy in the management of mucosal head and neck malignancy. *Head and Neck* 1999; **22**: 1–6.
14. McGavran MH, Bauer WC, Ogura JH. The incidence of cervical lymph node metastases from epidermoid carcinoma of the larynx and their relationship to certain characteristics of the primary tumour. *Cancer* 1961; **14**: 55–66.
15. Michales L. *Ear, nose and throat histopathology.* New York: Springer Verlag, 1987.
16. Graem N, Helwig-Larsen K, Keiding N. Precision of histological grading of malignancy. *Acta Pathologica Microbiologica Scandinavica A* 1980; **88**: 307–17.
17. Roland NJ, Caslin AW, Nash J, Stell PM. The value of grading squamous cell carcinoma of the head and neck. *Head and Neck* 1992; **14**: 224–9.
18. Fortin A, Couture C, Doucet R *et al.* Does histologic grade have a role in the management of head and neck cancers. *Journal of Clinical Oncology* 2001; **19**: 4107–16.
19. Department of Health. *Improving outcomes guidance for cancer of the head and neck,* NHS Cancer Plan. London: Department of Health, 2007. Available from www.nice.org.uk.
20. Jones AS, Roland NJ, Field JK, Phillips D. The level of cervical lymph node metastases: their prognostic relevance and relationship with head and neck squamous carcinoma primary sites. *Clinical Otolaryngology* 1994; **19**: 63–9.

21. Jones AS, Phillips D, Helliwell T, Roland NJ. Occult node metastases in head and neck squamous cell carcinoma. *European Archives of Otorhinolaryngology* 1993; **250**: 446-9.

22. Hibbert J, Marks NJ, Winter PJ, Shaheen OH. Prognostic factors in oral squamous cell carcinoma and their relation to clinical staging. *Clinical Otolaryngology* 1983; **8**: 197-203.

23. Stell PM. Prognosis in laryngeal carcinoma: tumour factors. *Clinical Otolaryngology* 1989; **15**: 68-81.

24. Remacle M, Eckel HE, Antonelli A *et al*. Classification Committee, European Laryngological Society: Endoscopic Cordectomy. Proposal for a European classification. *European Archives of Otorhinolaryngology* 2000; **257**: 221-6.

25. Watkinson JC, Johnston D, James D *et al*. The reliability of palpation in the assessment of tumours. *Clinical Otolaryngology* 1990; **5**: 405-10.

26. Hiranandani LH. Panel on epidemiology and etiology of laryngeal carcinoma. *Laryngoscope* 1975; **851**: 1187.

27. Berlinger NT, Tsakraklides V, Pollak K *et al*. Prognostic significance of lymph node histology in patients with squamous cell carcinoma of the larynx, pharynx and oral cavity. *Laryngoscope* 1976; **86**: 792-803.

28. Gilmore BB, Repola DA, Batsakis JG. Carcinoma of the larynx: lymph node reaction patterns. *Laryngoscope* 1978; **88**: 1333-8.

29. Johnson JT, Myers EN, Bedetti CD *et al*. Cervical lymph node metastases. Incidence and implications of extracapsular carcinoma. *Archives of Otolaryngology* 1985; **111**: 534-7.

30. Puri SK, Fan CY, Hanna E. Significance of extracapsular lymph node metastases in patients with head and neck squamous carcinoma. *Current Opinion in Otolaryngology and Head and Neck Surgery* 2003; **11**: 119-23.

31. Violaris N, Roland NJ, O'Neil D *et al*. Soft tissue cervical metastases of cervical squamous cell carcinoma. *Clinical Otolaryngology* 1994; **9**: 394-9.

32. Kashima HK. The characteristics of laryngeal cancer correlating with cervical lymph node metastases. In: Alberti PW, Bryce DP (eds). *Workshops from the centennial conference in laryngeal cancer*. New York: Appleton Century Crofts, 1976: 855-64.

33. McGavran MH, Bauer WC, Ogura JH. The incidence of cervical lymph node metasases from epidermoid carcinoma of the larynx and their relationship to certain characteristics of the primary tumour. *Cancer* 1961; **14**: 55-66.

34. Staley C, Herzon FS. Elective neck dissection in carcinoma of the larynx. *Otolaryngologic Clinics of North America* 1970; **3**: 543.

35. Jakobsson PA. Histologic grading of malignancy and prognosis in glottic carcinoma of the larynx. In: Alberti PW, Bryce DP (eds). *Workshops from the centennial conference in laryngeal cancer*. New York: Appleton Century Crofts, 1976.

36. Anneroth G, Hansen IS, Silverman JS. Malignancy grading in oral squamous cell carcinomas. *Journal of Oral Pathology* 1986; **15**: 162-8.

37. Crissman JD, Liu WY, Gluckman JL, Cummings G. Prognostic value of histopathological paramaters in squamous cell carcinoma of the oropharynx. *Cancer* 1984; **54**: 2995-3001.

38. Graem N, Helweg-Larsen K, Keiding N. Precision of histologic grading of malignancy. *Acta Pathologica Microbiologica Scandinavica* 1980; **88**: 307-17.

39. Roland NJ, Caslin AW, Bowie GL, Jones AS. Has the cellular proliferation marker Ki67 any clinical relevance in squamous cell carcinoma of the head and neck? *Clinical Otolaryngology* 1994; **19**: 13-18.

40. Jones AS, Roland NJ, Caslin AW *et al*. A comparison of kinetic parameters in squamous cell carcinoma of the head and neck. *Journal of Laryngology and Otology* 1994; **108**: 859-64.

41. Roland NJ, Rowley H, Scraggs M *et al*. MiB1 and involucrin expression in laryngeal squamous carcinoma. *Clinical Otolaryngology* 1996; **21**: 429-38.

42. Rowley H, Helliwell TR, Jones AS *et al*. An immunohistochemical analysis of p53 protein expression in premalignant and malignant tissues of the oral cavity. *Clinical Otolaryngology* 1997; **22**: 23-29.

43. Rowley H, Roland NJ, Helliwell T *et al*. p53 protein expression in tumours from the head and neck subsites, larynx and hypopharynx, and differences in relationship to survival. *Clinical Otolaryngology* 1998; **23**: 57-62.

44. Ambrosch P, Kron M, Freudenberg LS. Clinical staging of oropharyngeal carcinoma. A critical appraisal of a new stage-grouping proposal. *Cancer* 1998; **82**: 1613-20.

45. Hall SF, Groome PA, Rothwell D, Dixon PF. Using TNM staging to predict survival in squamous cell carcinoma of head and neck. *Head and Neck* 1999; **21**: 30-8.

46. Picirillo JF. Purposes, problems, and proposals for prognosis in cancer staging. *Archives of Otolaryngology, Head and Neck Surgery* 1995; **121**: 145-9.

47. Jones GW, Brownman G, Goodyear M *et al*. Comparisons of the additions of T and N integer scores with TNM stage groups in head and neck cancer. *Head and Neck* 1993; **15**: 497-503.

48. Synderman CH, Wagner RL. Superiority of the T and N integer score (TANIS) staging system for squamous cell carcinoma of the oral cavity. *Otolaryngology, Head and Neck Surgery* 1995; **112**: 691-4.

49. Hart AAM, Mak-Kregar S. Hilgers FJM. The importance of correct stage grouping in oncology: results of a nationwide study of oropharyngeal carcinoma. I. The Netherlands. *Cancer* 1996; **77**: 587-90.

50. Kiricuta IC. The importance of correct stage grouping in oncology: results of a nationwide study of oropharyngeal carcinoma I. The Netherlands (letter). *Cancer* 1996; **77**: 587-90.

51. Lydiatt WM, Shah JP, Hoffman HT. AJCC stage groupings for head and neck cancer: should we look at alternatives?

A report of the Head and Neck Sites Task force. *Head and Neck* 2001; **23**: 607–12.

52. Pugliano FA, Picirillo JF, Zequeria MR *et al.* Symptoms as an index of biologic behaviour in head and neck cancer. *Otolaryngology, Head and Neck Surgery* 1999; **120**: 380–6.

53. Picirillo JF. Importance of comorbidity in head and neck cancer. *Laryngoscope* 2000; **110**: 593–602.

54. Feinstein AR, Sosin DM, Wells CK. The Will Rogers phenomenon. Stage migration and new diagnostic techniques as a source of misleading statistics for survival in cancer. *New England Journal of Medicine* 1985; **312**: 1604.

5

Imaging

ALISON PAGE AND JULIE OLLIFF

A picture is worth a thousand words.

attributed to Frederick R Barnard (1921)

INTRODUCTION

Radiology is a continually evolving medical speciality which has witnessed many exciting advances since the discovery of x-rays more than 100 years ago, resulting in the numerous imaging modalities now available. In the last ten years alone, we have witnessed major advances in imaging technology with the introduction of high resolution and 3D ultrasound (US), multidetector computed tomography (MDCT), new contrast agents in magnetic resonance imaging (MRI) and the advent of positron emission tomography (PET) in clinical practice. In addition, the role of the radiologist is evolving, particularly as there is increased awareness now that the management of the patient with cancer is best done within a multidisciplinary team comprising surgeons, oncologists, pathologists, radiologists and all the specialist support services.

Imaging is routinely required at the time of presentation for diagnostic and staging purposes in most oncology patients. It has a major role in ascertaining whether tumours

are operable, and in patients with tumours more appropriately treated with radiotherapy and/or chemotherapy, it has a role in evaluating the clinical response. It may also be required to answer a specific clinical question in an individual patient.

The imaging modality of choice usually depends on the clinical scenario. One should bear in mind that all imaging techniques utilizing ionizing radiation, including plain films, fluoroscopy, computed tomography (CT) and nuclear medicine investigations carry with them a potential increased lifetime risk of developing cancer.[1] Data from the years 1991–6 suggest that about 0.6 per cent of the cumulative risk of cancer to age 75 years in the UK could be attributable to diagnostic x-rays.[2] However, the average annual radiation dose to the general public from all sources is 2.5 mSv, of which medical exposure only contributes 15 per cent.[3]

In young patients, and those patients who may potentially undergo multiple examinations or extended follow up, it may be more appropriate to choose magnetic resonance imaging or ultrasound as the imaging modality.

Knowledge of the normal anatomy as displayed by cross-sectional imaging techniques is the key to understanding the imaging of head and neck cancer. Although some aspects of the disease, such as the mucosal extent of primary head and neck cancers, are far better assessed by the clinician, the deep spread can often only be assessed with CT or MRI.

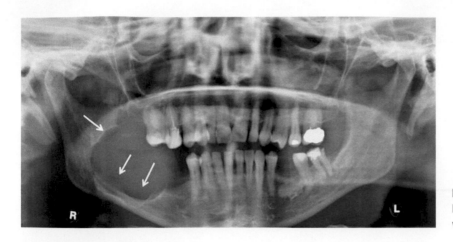

Figure 5.1 Orthopantomogram showing large ameloblastoma in the right mandible with smooth bone erosion (arrows).

PLAIN FILMS

A chest radiograph (chest x-ray) is used as part of the pre-anaesthetic assessment in head and neck cancer patients, but should also be performed to exclude coexistent pathology, such as a bronchogenic carcinoma, and to assess for the presence of pulmonary metastatic disease. However, the sensitivity of a chest x-ray in detecting synchronous primary or metastatic lung tumours is much less than the sensitivity of computed tomography.[4] Thus, if the primary tumour and nodal status place the patient at high risk for pulmonary metastases, then some authors recommend preoperative chest CT in addition.[5]

A retrosternal thyroid goitre may be apparent on the chest radiograph as a superior mediastinal mass which displaces or narrows the trachea. The trachea may also become stenotic following percutaneous tracheostomy insertion. Although additional thoracic inlet views can be acquired to further assess the degree of narrowing, evaluation with multiplanar computed tomography and respiratory flow-volume loops have been shown to be more sensitive than plain films.[6]

An orthopantomogram (OPG) is often performed to assess the dentition. It also evaluates periodontal pathology and focal mandibular lesions (**Figure 5.1**). In patients with oral cancers, particularly those located in the retromolar trigone, it can be useful to assess the extent of mandibular bone involvement (**Figure 5.2**). However, thin section CT is superior for confirming subtle bone destruction.[7]

CONTRAST STUDIES (FLUOROSCOPY)

The barium swallow examines the oesophagus. Double-contrast films are used to demonstrate morphology and mucosal lesions, and the addition of bread to the barium allows assessment of motility. Isotonic iodinated water soluble contrast agent should be used in preference to barium when aspiration is present or suspected, or when anastomoses are being assessed postoperatively, since barium aspiration can be fatal.

The pharynx and upper oesophagus are examined using videofluoroscopy or cinefluoroscopy. Contrast examinations are able to evaluate the act of swallowing by analysing the following features:

- tongue movement;
- soft palate elevation;
- epiglottic tilt;
- laryngeal closure;
- pharyngo-oesophageal segment (cricopharyngeal opening) and pharyngeal peristalsis.

Malignant pharyngeal and oesophageal tumours can be diagnosed by their irregular narrowing of the lumen associated with mucosal destruction, ulceration and shouldering. The length of the tumour can be measured, which is important for staging hypopharyngeal tumours and planning operative intervention for possible free jejunal transfer, as well as radiotherapy field planning. Previous radiotherapy, caustic ingestion and connective tissue disorders can cause smooth oesophageal narrowing.

ULTRASOUND

Ultrasound is an imaging modality utilizing high frequency sound. The probes (transducers) contain piezoelectric crystals which generate pulsed beams of sound in response to either mechanical or electrical stimuli. The crystals also receive the reflected beam which has been attenuated and refracted by tissue interfaces. Recent development in technology, particularly the evolution of high resolution US, has resulted in a greater role for ultrasound in evaluating the neck.

Ultrasound is ideal for examining superficial structures in the neck, but due to attenuation of the sound beam as it passes through the tissues, examination of large necks and deep structures, such as the deep lobe of the parotid, is more difficult. In addition, the ultrasound beam will not readily penetrate bone, cartilage and gas, making it an inappropriate technique for local staging of many primary head and neck cancers.

Ultrasound is extremely useful in differentiating solid from cystic mass lesions, and can detect calcification. An assessment can be made of the size, margin and consistency of a neck mass. Evaluation of the internal structure and the margins of neck nodes will facilitate differentiation between benign and malignant nodes.

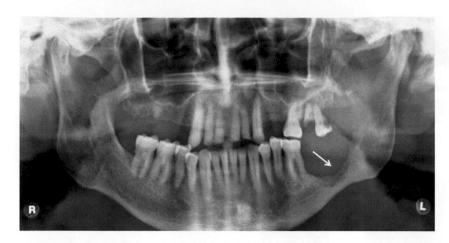

Figure 5.2 Orthopantomogram demonstrating local erosion of the alveolar surface of the left angle of the mandible due to squamous cell carcinoma (arrow).

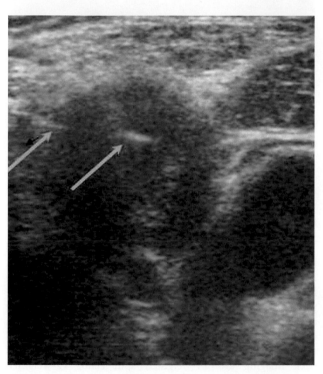

Figure 5.3 Ultrasound image showing a metallic needle (arrows) positioned within a necrotic level I node.

Colour flow and Doppler ultrasound can be used to evaluate the vessels within the neck, the relationship of masses to the major vascular structures, and also vascularity within masses and neck nodes.

The accuracy of core biopsy and fine-needle aspiration cytology of small neck masses and nodes is improved with ultrasound guidance, as the metallic needles are clearly seen passing through the subcutaneous tissues into the lesion or node (**Figure 5.3**).

COMPUTED TOMOGRAPHY

Computed tomography uses ionizing radiation. It has evolved significantly since its inception in 1972. Spiral CT scanners which use a single rotating x-ray tube and a complementary series of rotating x-ray detectors are now being replaced by multislice helical scanners also known as multirow detector computed tomography scanners. MDCT scanners use revolving x-ray tubes and a multiple row detector array that simultaneously acquire a series of 4, 16, 32 and, currently, 64 slices. Images are acquired while the patient passes through the gantry providing a three-dimensional volume block of data. Although images are usually acquired axially, multislice scanning enables the radiologist to manipulate the data to produce both thin section images and multiplanar reformats. As images are more rapidly acquired, there is decreased movement and respiratory artefact.

In addition to potentially inducing a new cancer, exposure to a cumulative high dose of ionizing radiation can induce cataracts within the lens of the eye. Therefore, unless relevant to the examination, the orbits should be excluded from the CT. Axial images are acquired with the patient lying supine. Direct coronal images can be obtained if the patient lies prone with the neck extended. This position can be uncomfortable, and has been replaced in most centres by the use of MDCT with coronal reformats. The larynx is optimally assessed with images reformatted to the plane of the vocal cords. Reformats can also aid assessment when there is artefact from dental amalgam (**Figure 5.4**).

The administration of an iodinated contrast medium results in vascular opacification, enhancement and increased conspicuity of the primary tumour and rim enhancement in pathological nodes. There is a small risk of reaction to the contrast media, including nausea, urticaria and broncho-spasm, but patients rarely develop serious long-term seque-lae. Anaphylactoid reactions, and death as a consequence, are also rarely seen.[8, 9] Iodinated contrast media has been implicated as being nephrotoxic and reported as inducing acute renal failure in 1–6 per cent of unselected patient populations and up to 50 per cent in high-risk patient populations.[10] An iso-osmolar or a low osmolar non-ionic contrast medium is preferred in patients with renal impairment and diabetes, and hydration before and after the examination may be required.[11]

CT scans can be displayed on different settings known as windows. Soft tissue and bone settings are routinely used in the head and neck. The scans of bony and cartilaginous structures, for example the laryngeal cartilages in a patient with suspected laryngeal carcinoma, should also be reconstructed using a bony algorithm which is helpful for

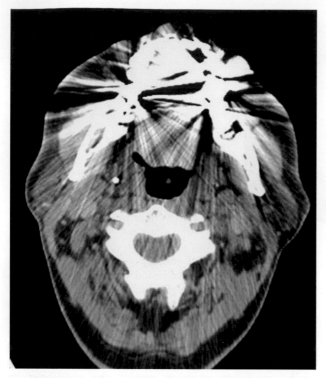

Figure 5.4 Beam hardening artefact from dental amalgam on computed tomography.

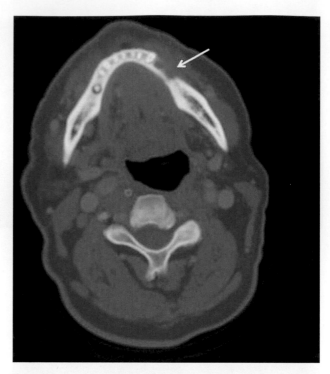

Figure 5.5 Focal erosion of the buccal surface of the left body of mandible on computed tomography (bone windows).

demonstrating bone and cartilage involvement (**Figure 5.5**). Coronal and sagittal reformats allow better evaluation of the skull base. The pulmonary parenchyma should be reviewed at lung window settings if the chest is also being examined. Beam hardening artefact from dental amalgam can significantly degrade images of the oral cavity (see **Figure 5.4**). Similar artefacts can also occur at bone–soft tissue interfaces.

MAGNETIC RESONANCE IMAGING

Magnetic resonance imaging utilizes a homogeneous magnetic field, which in most clinical scanners ranges from 0.5 to 3.0 tesla in strength. Radiofrequency pulses are used to excite the protons within the nuclei of the cells and coils detect the changes in the magnetic field.

The strong magnetic field requires stringent safety measures and all patients complete a questionnaire prior to scanning. MRI is contraindicated in patients with cardiac pacemakers, cochlear implants and metallic intraorbital foreign bodies. All patients in whom a metallic intraorbital foreign body is suspected require imaging of the orbits with conventional radiography to exclude a potential foreign body. Those patients who have iatrogenic foreign bodies *in situ*, such as surgical clips, embolization coils, vascular stents, prosthetic heart valves and joint prostheses may not be suitable for MRI. It is important to establish the timing of surgery and whether the foreign body is ferromagnetic. Dental prostheses can also be problematic (**Figure 5.6a,b**).

The long bore of the conventional magnet has been reported to induce moderate to severe anxiety in up to 25 per cent of patients undergoing examination, occasionally resulting in examination failure.[12] MRI scanning in an interventionally configured (open) magnet may be appropriate in claustrophobic patients who fail examination in a conventional magnet without sedation.[13]

Although CT is superior to MRI in assessment of cortical bone, MRI has superior soft tissue contrast compared to CT, and allows true multiplanar imaging. Scan times are long however and require good patient cooperation as images are prone to movement artefact from coughing, swallowing and dyspnoea. An appropriate coil is placed over the region of interest and scans are performed in at least two orthogonal planes. The most common sequences used in head and neck imaging are T1-weighted spin echo, T2-weighted spin echo and short tau inversion recovery (STIR). The T1-weighted sequence displays anatomy well and is used to assess lymph nodes and medullary bone involvement. T2-weighted sequences demonstrate fluid well and the STIR sequence suppresses the signal from fat allowing easy demonstration of pathology, particularly tumours, inflammation and oedema.

Intravenous gadolinium chelates may be administered to assess for pathological enhancement in patients with suspected recurrent tumour following surgery and radiotherapy, and for abnormal enhancement in involved nodes. It is also useful for assessing perineural spread of the primary tumour. After contrast administration fat-suppressed T1-weighted images are used. Gadolinium is generally well tolerated and is safer than the iodinated CT contrast agents. However, it can also induce acute renal failure in patients with renal impairment.[14] Nephrogenic systemic fibrosis is also now recognized as a serious late complication following administration of gadolinium-based contrast to patients with dialysis-dependent renal failure.[15]

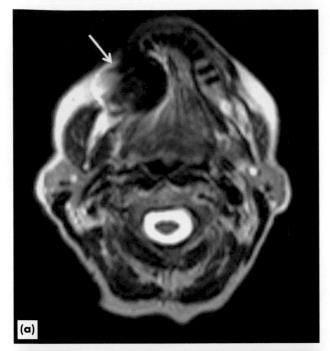

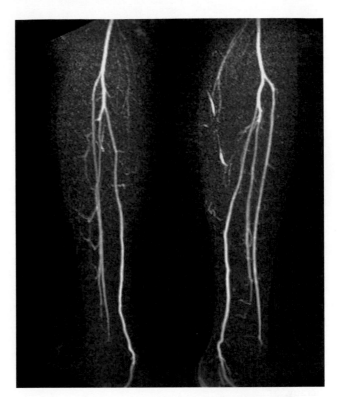

Figure 5.7 Magnetic resonance angiography of distal leg vessels.

provides an anatomical road map of the arterial tree and allows confirmation that the remaining vessels will adequately supply the foot once the flap has been harvested (**Figure 5.7**).

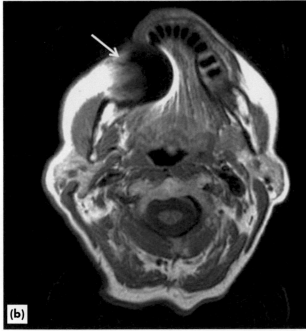

Figure 5.6 T2-weighted (a) and T1-weighted (b) axial magnetic resonance images demonstrating signal loss around a metallic dental bridge.

MAGNETIC RESONANCE ANGIOGRAPHY

Magnetic resonance angiography can demonstrate flow within vessels and evaluate arterial stenoses. All patients in whom a fibula free flap graft would be the most appropriate method of facial reconstruction, even if they have no evidence of peripheral vascular disease and no history of intermittent claudication, ideally should have preoperative assessment of the leg vessels with MR angiography.[16] This

NUCLEAR MEDICINE

Nuclear medicine studies utilize radioactive isotopes that are often bound to physiological molecules (radiopharmaceuticals). These investigations predominantly evaluate function and physiology. Anatomical detail and spatial resolution are poor compared to other imaging modalities.

Radioisotope whole-body bone scanning with the conventional isotope technetium-99m methylene diphosphonate (^{99m}Tc) has a high sensitivity, but a poor specificity in demonstrating bony metastatic disease in patients and can be used to assess for local bone invasion. However, ^{99m}Tc single photon emission computed tomography (SPECT) has a higher specificity than conventional bone scanning and can be used to improve the accuracy of predicting local bone invasion in patients with oral cavity tumours.[17]

Suspected postoperative pulmonary emboli can be confirmed using a ventilation-perfusion scan (VQ scan). These utilize ^{99m}Tc-labelled macroaggregated albumin to demonstrate blood flow within the pulmonary capillary network and either Xenon-127 gas or nebulized ^{99m}Tc to evaluate the ventilation of the lungs.

Iodine-based isotopes are used in the assessment and treatment of thyroid disease. Functioning thyroid nodules take up iodine-123 (^{123}I). Iodine-131 (^{131}I) can be used to treat and image iodine avid differentiated thyroid tumours.

POSITRON EMISSION TOMOGRAPHY

Positron emission tomography is an imaging technique utilizing radioisotopes that emit positrons. Fluorine-labelled deoxyglucose (^{18}F-FDG), a glucose analogue, is the isotope used for 98 per cent of PET imaging. Like other forms of nuclear medicine, PET imaging provides functional information. As the anatomical detail and special resolution of a PET scan alone is relatively poor, anatomical correlation with CT or MRI is necessary.

Combined in-line PET-CT scanners allow accurate co-registration of the functional information from the PET scan and the anatomical information from a non-contrasted relatively low-dose CT scan. PET-CT has a higher accuracy of depicting cancer and evaluating its anatomical localization, than PET alone.[18]

False-positive results in PET-CT can occur due to normal physiological uptake in tissues, such as the tonsils and salivary glands. Tracer also accumulates in metabolically active tissues and in muscles, secondary to contraction, such as phonation, during the uptake phase (**Figure 5.8**). False-negative results are seen in tumours with low metabolic activity, such as salivary gland tumours, in necrotic tumour, and in patients who have undergone recent treatment, particularly PET-CT performed within four months of radiation therapy.[19, 20]

In patients with suspected head and neck cancer ^{18}F-FDG PET-CT is a valuable tool in the preoperative staging of head and neck tumours, as it can evaluate regional lymph node metastases, detect distant metastases and identify unsuspected synchronous primary lesions. It is also useful in evaluating patients with proven pathological cervical adenopathy but an unknown primary lesion (**Figure 5.9**).[21] However, ^{18}F-FDG PET-CT rarely provides additional information regarding the T stage of tumour over initial clinical evaluation and cross-sectional imaging with CT and MR.

^{18}F-FDG PET-CT is useful in the postoperative patient to monitor tumour recurrence (**Figure 5.10a,b**) and, after chemoradiotherapy, it can be used to evaluate the response of lesions to treatment, and aid selection of patients for subsequent neck dissection or salvage surgery.[22]

NASOPHARYNGNEAL CANCER

Squamous cell carcinoma accounts for 70 per cent of superficial malignant tumours in the nasopharynx. Lymphomas account for a further 20 per cent with tumours, such as adenocarcinoma, rhabdomyosarcoma, adenoid cystic carcinoma, melanoma, plasmacytoma, fibrosarcoma and carcinosarcoma making the remainder. Imaging should aim to provide an assessment of the pattern of spread of the tumour especially into areas not easily examined clinically, i.e. deep extension and extension superiorly to the skull base and beyond.

The fossa of Rosenmüller is a common site of origin of nasopharyngeal cancer (**Figure 5.11a,b**). Submucosal lesions will not be detected endoscopically and MRI with its superior soft tissue contrast is the best suited imaging modality to detect these lesions. Both CT and MRI will detect skull base invasion (**Figure 5.12a,b**). CT can detect early cortical

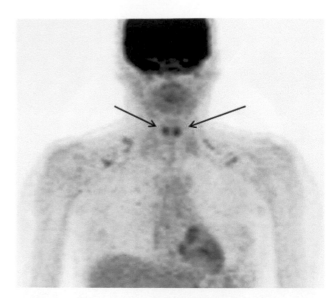

Figure 5.8   ^{18}F-FDG PET-CT demonstrating physiological tracer uptake in the glottis.

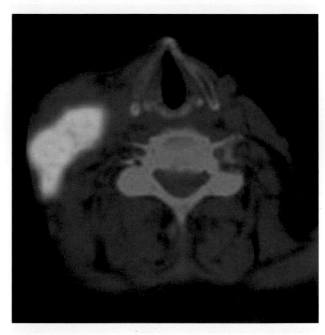

Figure 5.9   Avid tracer uptake within pathological right neck nodes on ^{18}F-FDG PET-CT. Unknown primary.

involvement better than MRI, but MRI is better than CT for the delineation of marrow involvement. It may be necessary to perform both in some patients to accurately determine the disease extent. The pharyngobasilar fascia provides a barrier to disease, but once this is breached, tumour can invade the skull base directly (**Figure 5.13**). High resolution T1-weighted MR images are used to examine the pharyngobasilar fascia which appears as a continuous low signal intensity linear structure.

Lateral extension into the deep structures of the nasopharynx can occur via the sinus of Morgagni, a natural fascial defect sited in the superolateral wall of the nasopharynx which allows passage of the Eustachian tube and levator veli

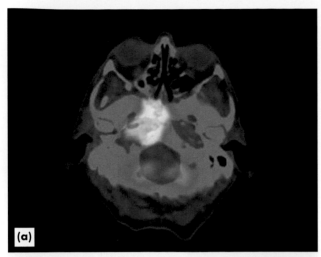

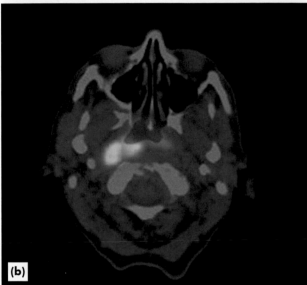

Figure 5.10   (a,b) ^{18}F-FDG PET CT showing recurrent oropharyngeal tumour invading the skull base post-radiotherapy and photodynamic therapy (PDT).

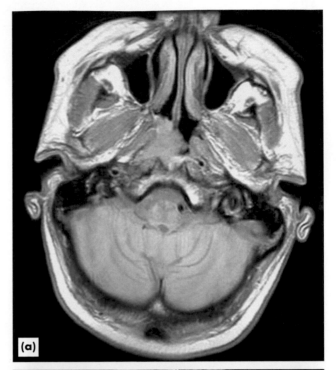

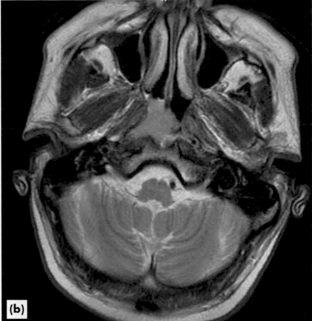

Figure 5.11   Axial T1-weighted (a) and T2-weighted (b) magnetic resonance images demonstrating a right-sided nasopharyngeal tumour filling the fossa of Rosenmüller.

palatini muscle. Tumour can then gain access to the masticator and pre- and post-styloid parapharyngeal spaces. This can result in involvement of the third division of the fifth cranial nerve. Retrograde perineural spread to the skull base can then occur. The most common sites of skull base invasion are the petroclinoid fissure and foramen lacerum. This can result in internal carotid artery encasement and extension into the cavernous sinus. Perineural spread is best imaged with T1-weighted fat suppressed MR scans following intravenous gadolinium. This is seen as expansion and added enhancement of the nerve. Tumour may also directly invade the skull base and involve the foramen ovale. Occult submucosal spread may occur in a caudad direction. The inferior limit of disease is often visualized well on coronal images.

Nodal disease is extremely common (85–90 per cent) at presentation and is likely to be bilateral in half. Retropharyngeal nodes are usually the first affected nodes, but level 2 nodes may be involved without retropharyngeal nodal disease.

MR imaging has been shown to have a higher accuracy (92.1 per cent) than PET-CT for the diagnosis of residual and/or recurrent disease following treatment at the primary site. The combined use of both modalities was more accurate for restaging.[23]

PARAPHARYNGEAL SPACE PATHOLOGY

The parapharyngeal space extends from the skull base to the styloglossus muscle at the level of the angle of the mandible.

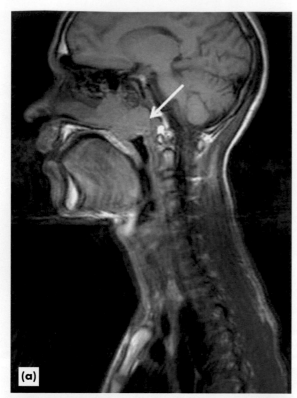

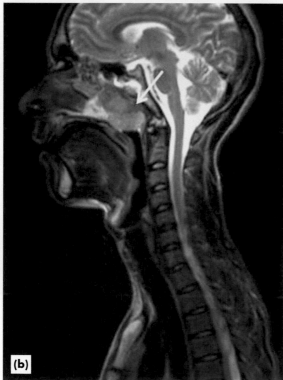

Figure 5.12   Sagittal T1-weighted (a) and T2-weighted (b) magnetic resonance images demonstrating a bulky nasopharyngeal tumour with direct extension into the clivus (arrows).

The prestyloid and post/retrostyloid spaces are divided by the tensor styloid vascular fascia. The carotid sheath lies within the retrostyloid compartment. The deep portion of parotid gland bulges into the lateral aspect of the prestyloid

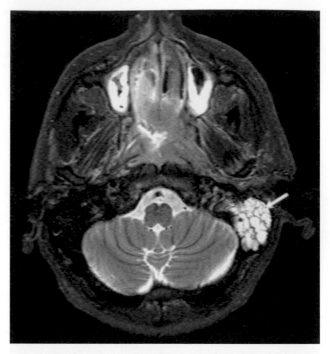

Figure 5.13   Large nasopharyngeal tumour invading the nasal cavity with loss of the pharyngobasilar fascia and obstruction of the left Eustachian tube resulting in opacification of the left mastoid air cells (small arrow).

compartment extending through the stylomandibular tunnel anterior to the styloid process, the styloid muscles and the retrostyloid compartment. The majority of tumours in the parapharyngeal space arise either from the deep lobe of the parotid in the prestyloid compartment (see below) or from neural tumours in the poststyloid compartment. True lesions within the parapharyngeal fat are likely to be salivary tumours from salivary gland rests or much less commonly neural tumours from the sympathetic chain. There may, however, only be a thin isthmus connecting a tumour of the deep lobe of the parotid with the gland itself which may not be apparent on imaging and thus an erroneous diagnosis of a parapharyngeal fat mass may be made which may alter the surgical approach.

MR imaging is thought to be better than CT as the initial imaging investigation. Scans should be obtained with contrast enhancement if a neural tumour is suspected. The origin of a mass related to the parapharyngeal space can be inferred by the pattern of displacement of normal anatomical structures.[24] Parotid and extraparotid salivary gland tumours displace the internal carotid artery (ICA) posteriorly. Paragangliomas and most schwannomas displace the ICA anteriorly.

The most common neurogenic tumour is a schwannoma of the vagus nerve. This will usually displace the ICA anteriorly and medially. Vagal schwannomas also tend to separate the carotid artery from the internal jugular vein, whereas schwannomas arising from the cervical sympathetic chain do not cause this.[25, 26] They are usually well-defined soft tissue masses, but areas of haemorrhage and necrosis can occur. If the tumour arises within the jugular fossa, it may expand the fossa and extend both intracranially as well as into the neck. The bone will however remain well corticated. Although

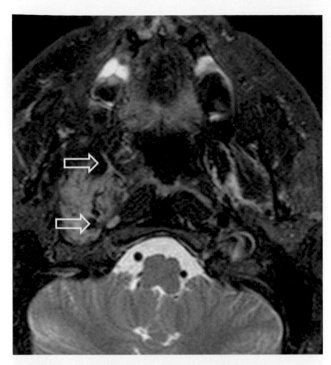

Figure 5.14 STIR (short tau inversion recovery) magnetic resonance image demonstrating flow voids (open arrows) in a large right high T2 signal parapharyngeal paraganglioma.

schwannomas are hypovascular they may demonstrate delayed enhancement following intravenous contrast.

Both glomus vagale and glomus jugulare tumours arise around the vagus nerve and tend to displace the ICA anteriorly. Carotid body tumours will displace the ICA anteriorly, but will generally also splay the carotid bifurcation. Paragangliomas within the parapharyngeal space are usually well-defined oval-shaped lesions with vascular flow voids seen on MRI, particularly in tumours larger than 2 cm in diameter (**Figure 5.14**) and possibly a salt and pepper appearance on T2-weighted images. These tumours enhance avidly following intravenous contrast and if they involve the skull base will cause the bony margins to appear irregular and eroded, similar to a malignant tumour.

Lymph nodes within the parapharyngeal space are those within level 2. Retropharyngeal nodes are outside this anatomical region, although they push into it if enlarged. Necrotic nodes may mimic an abscess on imaging, but clinical correlation will usually differentiate between the two.

ORAL CAVITY

The oral cavity is made up of the lip, upper and lower gingiva, buccal mucosa, hard palate, floor of the mouth, and oral (anterior two-thirds) of the tongue.

Lip

Imaging has little role to play in early lesions which may not be distinguishable from the normal orbicularis oris muscle.

The margins of more advanced infiltrative lesions may be defined more readily with imaging.

Bone erosion which usually occurs along the buccal surface of the mandibular or maxillary alveolar ridge is best detected with CT. Once tumour gains access to the mandible, there is the potential for perineural spread along the inferior alveolar nerve. The presence of bone erosion upstages these lesions to T4 and necessitates bony resection.

The lymphatic drainage is to level 1 nodes (submental and submandibular) and level 2 nodes.

Floor of mouth

Imaging is used to assess the presence of bone erosion and tumour size which may clinically be underestimated if there is submucosal extension. It is important to determine the relationship of the tumour to the midline septum and to the contralateral neurovascular bundle, since this will alter treatment.[27] Midline spread may occur directly across the genioglossus muscle and midline septum or occur via the potential space between the genioglossus and geniohyoid muscles. Ill-defined tumour margins, invasion of the sublingual space and proximity of tumour to neurovascular structures are highly suggestive of neurovascular involvement. Tumours with a mean diameter of 2 cm or greater are also more likely to invade the neurovascular bundle. These patients are at greater risk of cervical nodal involvement.

Thin-section CT is again the imaging modality of choice if bone involvement is suspected, e.g. fixed lateral floor of mouth tumours but otherwise, MRI may give more information about the tumour especially if there is artefact from dental amalgam. The primary tumour is often seen well on unenhanced T1-weighted MR scans (**Figure 5.15a,b**) and tumour involvement of the normal marrow is also well demonstrated by this imaging sequence. The periosteum does provide a barrier to tumour infiltration and tumour may gain access to the marrow via tooth sockets in edentulous patients. The specificity of MR imaging has been shown to be significantly lower than that of CT in the assessment of marrow invasion.[28] A prospective study using the MR detection of tumour signal replacing hypointense cortical rim as the main radiological finding for mandibular invasion had high accuracy (93 per cent), sensitivity (93 per cent) and specificity (93 per cent).[29] Another group,[30] however, found that although MR was sensitive it had a poor positive predictive value for mandibular invasion. In a further study, ^{99m}Tc single photon emission computed tomography (SPECT) (a radioisotope technique) correctly predicted mandibular invasion in 11/12 cases with no false-positives, and CT only 3/12.[31]

Posterior spread can occur along the mylohyoid muscle and tumour can thus gain access to the deep fascial spaces of the neck. Tumour can also extend posteriorly to involve the tongue base. Obstruction of the submandibular ducts will result in dilatation of the ducts (**Figure 5.16**) and probable enlargement of the affected gland which can be mistaken clinically for a nodal mass.

The depth of tumour invasion is related to the probability of nodal spread. The lymphatic drainage is to nodes in levels 1 and 2.

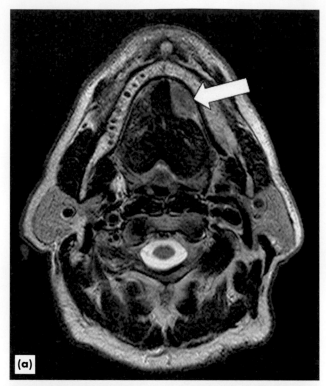

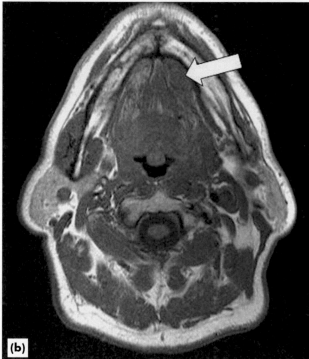

Figure 5.15 Axial T2-weighted (a) and T1-weighted (b) magnetic resonance images of a localized tumour in the anterior left floor of the mouth (solid arrow).

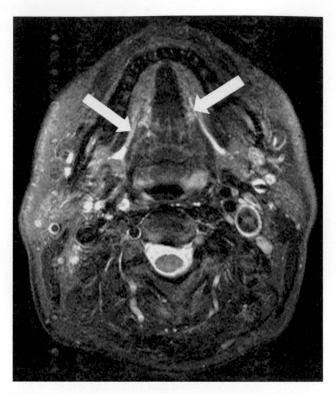

Figure 5.16 Axial STIR magnetic resonance image showing bilateral submandibular salivary gland duct obstruction (white arrows).

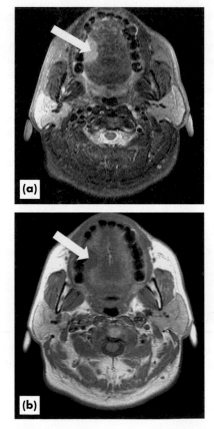

Figure 5.17 STIR (a) and T1-weighted (b) axial magnetic resonance images of a small right lateral tongue tumour (white arrow).

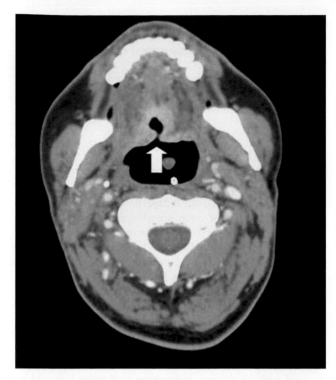

Figure 5.18 Contrast-enhanced computed tomography demonstrates a small superficial tumour of the tongue base crossing the midline (white arrow).

Tongue

The majority of tumours arise from the lateral aspect (**Figure 5.17a,b**) or undersurface of the tongue. Large tumours of the anterior and middle third of the tongue tend to spread to the floor of the mouth and coronal imaging can be useful in the evaluation. Spread to the tongue base may occur from tumours of the posterior third. Imaging should assess the size of the lesion and whether the lesion has crossed the midline (**Figure 5.18**). Identification of the relationship of the mass to the neurovascular bundle is important and will alter management.

Gingiva and buccal mucosa

Buccal mucosa squamous cell carcinoma (SCC) most commonly arises along the lateral walls and spread may occur along the buccinator muscle and into the pterygomandibular raphe with erosion of underlying bone. Lesions involving the lower gingiva may invade the mandible.

Hard palate

Primary SCC of the hard palate is rare and is usually due to tumour spread from adjacent gingiva. Cross-sectional imaging may understage these lesions which are better assessed by endoscopy. Low volume superficial tumours may not be visible on imaging, but more advanced lesions with suspected bone involvement should be examined using CT. Multi-detector CT should be assessed in the coronal plane examining soft tissue and bone windows to stage tumours involving the hard palate.

Adenoid cystic carcinoma commonly shows perineural spread into the pterygopalatine fossa via the greater and lesser palatine nerves. This extension may be better imaged using MRI with gadolinium enhancement.

Retromolar trigone carcinoma

The retromolar trigone is a small triangular area posterior to the last mandibular molar tooth. The pterygomandibular raphe lies deep to the mucosa in this region and attaches superiorly to the hamulus of the medial pterygoid plate. Inferiorly, it attaches to the mylohyoid line of the mandible. Tumour spread inferiorly can therefore involve the floor of the mouth. Tumours arising in this region may grow anteriorly into the buccal region or posteriorly into the tonsil via the superior constrictor muscle. Superior extension may occur deep to the maxillary tuberosity invading the buccal space fat lateral to the maxillary antrum. Tumours can gain access via the mandibular and maxillary nerves, to the cavernous sinus and the skull base. Bone involvement is often not detected clinically and may occur early. This should be assessed with imaging and will alter management.

OROPHARYNGEAL CANCER

The majority of lesions are due to squamous cell carcinoma, but minor salivary gland tumours can present as a mass within the oropharynx particularly involving the palate. Treatment of tonsillar and soft-palate lesions depends upon the size of the tumour and involvement of surrounding structures. There should be a detailed evaluation of submucosal extension into the soft tissues of the neck; pre- and poststyloid parapharyngeal space, the nasopharynx and the tongue base should be assessed. Bone erosion and invasion of the prevertebral muscles can occur in advanced lesions. Submucosal extension may not be visible clinically and bulky disease close to or invading the skull base and evidence of encasement of the internal carotid artery may preclude surgery.[32]

Lesions involving the anterior tonsillar pillar may spread superiorly to involve both the hard and soft palate (**Figure 5.19a,b**). Spread from here can occur to the skull base via the tensor and levator veli palatini muscles. Spread can occur along the superior constrictor muscle to the pterygopalatine raphe and buccinator muscle. Large tumours may extend to involve the tongue base along the palatoglossus muscle. Tumours solely involving the posterior tonsillar pillar are rare. These tumours can extend superiorly to involve the soft palate and inferiorly to involve the posterior aspect of the thyroid cartilage, the middle pharyngeal constrictor and the pharyngoepiglottic fold.

Lesions involving the tonsillar fossa arise either from the mucosal lining or from remnants of the palatine tonsil itself. These lesions may present as a nodal mass within the neck, usually located within level 2 (**Figure 5.20**). The primary lesion may spread anteriorly to the anterior pillar and from here to the sites described previously. Similarly posterior

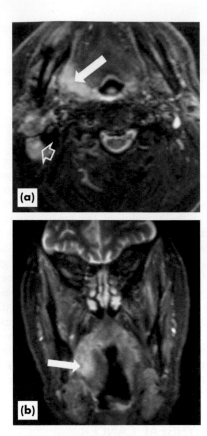

Figure 5.19 STIR axial (a) and STIR coronal (b) magnetic resonance images demonstrating a right tonsillar tumour (white arrows) with pathologically enlarged right level II nodes (arrowhead).

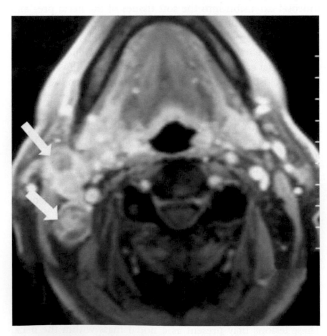

Figure 5.20 T1-weighted fat-saturated contrast enhanced axial magnetic resonance image demonstrating a right tonsillar tumour with pathologically enhancing nodes (white arrows).

spread can occur to the posterior pillar and beyond. Deep extension can occur to the superior constrictor muscle allowing access to the parapharyngeal space and thus to the skull base.

Spread to level 2 nodes is the most common pattern of nodal involvement, but tumours involving the posterior wall can give rise to retropharyngeal and level 5 nodal disease.

LARYNGEAL CANCER

Cross-sectional imaging may not demonstrate small lesions confined to the mucosa, but is superior to clinical assessment for the delineation of submucosal spread of disease. The larynx and pharynx are complex anatomical regions, but it is the knowledge of this anatomy as displayed on CT and MRI that is the key to oncological staging. Treatment options for patients with laryngeal cancer include surgery, radiotherapy and chemotherapy and combinations of these. The choice of treatment will depend upon the location, spread and volume of disease. Removal of part or whole of the larynx will have significant impact upon a patient's ability to communicate and self-image.

Mucosal extension of disease and cord mobility is better assessed with endoscopy, but submucosal spread should be determined with cross-sectional imaging. Tumour volume is one of the critical factors determining tumour-free survival and local control following radiotherapy. Multirow detector computed tomography-calculated tumour volume has been shown to have a high level of agreement with histology, with

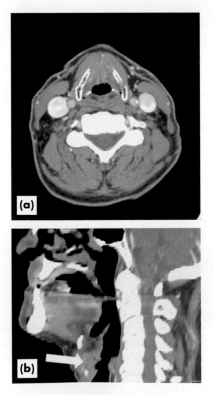

Figure 5.21 Contrast-enhanced axial computed tomography scan (a) with sagittal reformat (b) showing pre-epiglottic spread (arrow).

a slight tendency of MDCT to overestimation proportional to the size of the tumour.[33] Transglottic spread, pre-epiglottic involvement greater than 25 per cent (**Figure 5.21a,b**), extensive paralaryngeal spread and cord mobility are other predictors. Clinical T stage and invasion of the thyroid cartilage by tumour on MR are also predictors of failure of local control by radiotherapy. A study of 80 patients pre-radiotherapy demonstrated that MR findings of abnormal signal intensity within the thyroid cartilage and a tumour volume greater than 5 cc conferred an adverse prognosis.[34] Work performed by Murakami and colleagues[35] using dynamic helical CT suggests that lesions separate from the thyroid cartilage have a 95 per cent probability of local control, whereas those adjacent had 42 per cent local control. Other important factors were clinical T stage, tumour detectability, maximum dimension, tumour volume, anterior commissure involvement (**Figure 5.22**), ventricle involvement and thyroid cartilage involvement. Other authors have, however, questioned the reliability of CT, finding considerable inter-observer variation in the assessment of tumour volume, cartilage invasion and cartilage sclerosis on the basis of CT imaging, apparently limiting its clinical significance.[36] More recently, the findings of intermediate T2 MR signal intensity (SI) in cartilage and hypopharyngeal extension of tumour have been shown to be predictors of a greater likelihood of local failure when glottic tumours are treated by radiotherapy alone.[37]

The paraglottic spaces are paired fatty regions lying deep to the true and false cords. They merge superiorly with the C-shaped pre-epiglottic fat space. These spaces are of high signal intensity on T1-weighted MR images and of low SI on fat-suppressed MR images. They are of low attenuation on CT. Tumour spread into these regions may be underestimated

clinically, but will present as abnormal intermediate SI soft tissue on unenhanced T1-weighted MR images and intermediate to high SI tissue on STIR and T2-weighted MR images. Enhancing tumour is visible on T1-weighted MR images with fat suppression following intravenous gadolinium (**Figure 5.23**). Pre-epiglottic space invasion (**Figure 5.21a,b**) is important in the assessment of extension to the tongue base and the hyoid cartilage. MR imaging has been shown to have a sensitivity of 100 per cent, specificity of 84 per cent and accuracy of 90 per cent in this regard.[38]

The correct prediction of laryngeal cartilage invasion is hampered by the irregular ossification of the thyroid cartilage and the reaction of cartilage to both invasion by and proximity of tumour to the cartilage.

The ossified cartilage contains marrow fat and will therefore be of high signal on T1-weighted MR images and low SI on fat-suppressed MR images. Cortical bone will have very low SI on T1- and T2-weighted images. Non-ossified hyaline cartilage has an intermediate to low SI on T1- and on T2-weighted images. It has a density similar to squamous carcinoma. There is no enhancement of cortical bone, fatty marrow or hyaline cartilage after intravenous gadolinium. On unenhanced T1-weighted images invaded hyaline cartilage and fatty marrow demonstrate a low to intermediate SI. On T2-weighted images hyaline cartilage invaded by tumour has a higher SI than normal cartilage. Although MRI has a high negative predictive value with cartilage invasion being excluded if none of these signs are present, reactive inflammation, oedema and fibrosis in the vicinity of the tumour may display similar appearances to cartilage invaded by tumour causing MRI to have a positive predictive value of 68–71 per cent.[39, 40] Peritumoral inflammatory changes are most commonly seen in the thyroid cartilage causing the specificity of MRI to detect tumour invasion to be lower at this site (56 per cent) than in the cricoid cartilage (87 per cent) or arytenoid cartilage (95 per cent).[39]

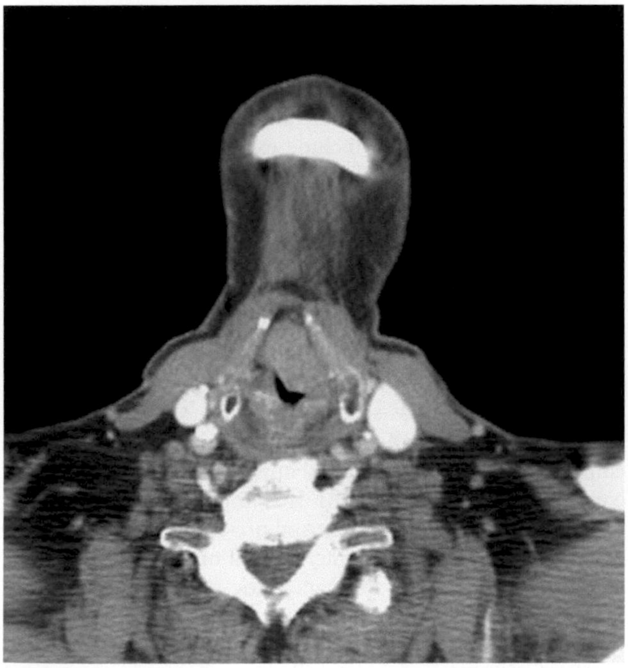

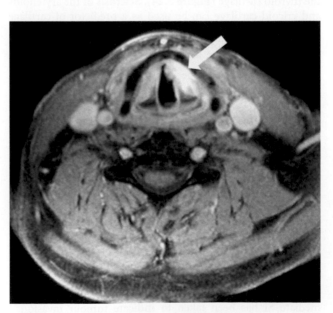

Figure 5.22 T3 left cord tumour with thickening of the anterior commissure on contrast-enhanced computed tomography.

Figure 5.23 Fat-saturated T1-weighted spin echo axial magnetic resonance post-contrast demonstrating a left cord tumour with paraglottic spread (white arrow).

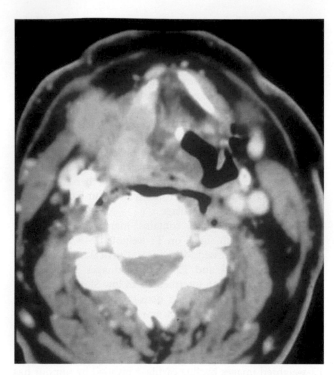

Figure 5.24 Contrast-enhanced axial computed tomography demonstrating extralaryngeal tumour and lysis of the right thyroid lamina.

A study examining 111 laryngeal cartilages comparing CT with histopathology,[41] found that sclerosis of a laryngeal cartilage was the most sensitive criterion for invasion for all laryngeal cartilages, but was not very specific being also due to reactive inflammation. The presence of extralaryngeal tumour and erosion or lysis of the cartilage was the most specific indicator of invasion (sensitivity 71 per cent, specificity 83 per cent and negative predictive value 89 per cent) in the thyroid cartilage (**Figure 5.24**). Sclerosis of the arytenoids and cricoid cartilage can be used as a predictor of cartilage invasion.[41] The presence of arytenoid cartilage sclerosis can be due to invasion or to the presence of tumour adjacent to the perichondrium.[42, 43] Some authors[44] have found that diagnostic accuracy can be improved if sclerosis of the arytenoid cartilage is not taken as an indicator of cartilage involvement.

The high negative predictive value achieved by MRI and its higher sensitivity than CT for cartilage invasion suggests that it should be better than CT for the evaluation of the laryngeal cartilage. The accuracy of MR imaging is better than CT if a meta-analysis is performed,[45] but the use of MR will result in a significant number of false-positive examinations and the positive diagnosis of neoplastic invasion of the cartilage should be made with extreme caution on MRI.[46] The term 'abnormal signal intensity in the cartilage' rather than 'invasion of cartilage' has been suggested.[47] More attention is now being paid to the degree of abnormal SI on T2-weighted MR scans within the thyroid cartilage. Very bright SI is taken as inflammatory change, whereas intermediate SI has been taken to indicate tumour invasion.[37] New criteria have been suggested:[48] SI in cartilage greater than that of adjacent tumour on T2-weighted or post-contrast T1-weighted MR scans is taken to indicate inflammatory change, whereas SI similar to tumour is taken to represent malignant invasion. This has resulted in an improved specificity (82 versus 74 per cent) and was greatest for the thyroid cartilage (75 versus 54 per cent) with no alteration of sensitivity.

CT is used to stage laryngeal cancer in many centres. This is probably due to a number of factors: time, availability and the ease of volumetric studies with MDCT. CT has a higher specificity than MR in all reported studies[45] and the use of MR imaging will, however, lead to a number of false-positive cases where the larynx will be removed and there will be no evidence of cartilage involvement. It may be that a combination of the two imaging modalities would be ideal.

The latest American Joint Committee on Cancer (AJCC) criteria for laryngeal cartilage invasion have now differentiated between the presence of cortical invasion of the inner margin of the thyroid cartilage (T3) versus complete infiltration of laryngeal cartilage (T4a). Full thickness involvement remains an indicator for surgical management, whereas T3 tumours may be treatable with radiotherapy with or without chemotherapy.[49]

Recognition of involvement of the anterior commissure (**Figure 5.22**) is also important. Broyle's ligament lies between the anterior commissure and the thyroid cartilage and invasion of this structure leads to a higher rate of cartilage infiltration. The anterior commissure should not exceed 1 mm in thickness and there should not be any soft tissue in the interthyroidal notch.

Subglottic extension and/or cricoid cartilage involvement is another indicator of a need for a total laryngectomy as the appropriate form of treatment. The presence of an enlarged Delphian node (the node lying anterior to the trachea) is another indicator of subglottic extension or of a subglottic primary (an unusual occurrence).

PHARYNGEAL CANCER

The majority of pharyngeal tumours are squamous cell cancers. The risk factors include excessive alcohol, smoking and previous radiation. The patients present with symptoms of dysphagia and odontophagia. They may present with otalgia due to referred pain along the course of the internal laryngeal nerve from the pyriform sinus and thus to the auricular nerve.

Nodal disease is common in these patients at presentation (75 per cent). A significant number of patients have a synchronous (25 per cent) or metachronous (40 per cent) second primary cancer. Cross-sectional imaging may not identify lesions confined to the mucosa which are best examined clinically. Submucosal spread is, however, better delineated by contrast-enhanced CT or MRI. It is important to understand the anatomy of the paraglottic and pre-epiglottic fat spaces as described previously. The anterior wall of the pyriform sinus is the posterior wall of the paraglottic space. Extension into this space allows tumour to gain access to the larynx and tongue base which may not be clinically apparent. Involvement of the tongue base will generally make a patient inoperable.

The apex of the pyriform sinus is at the level of the true vocal cords and spread from tumour into the larynx at this

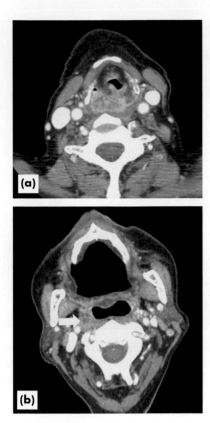

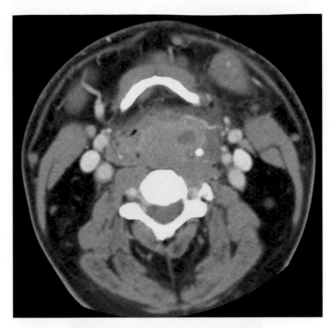

Figure 5.26   Axial-enhanced computed tomography scan showing bulky pharyngeal tumour with retropharyngeal fascia invasion.

Figure 5.25   Contrast-enhanced computed tomography demonstrating a primary posterior pharyngeal wall tumour (a) with a rim enhancing right retropharyngeal node (b).

level should be looked for on cross-sectional imaging. Tumours sited in the lateral wall of the hypopharynx can easily involve the thyroid cartilage. Lesions involving the aryepiglottic fold may spread into the supraglottis and the arytenoid cartilages. The diagnosis of laryngeal cartilage invasion can be made if tumour is seen on the extralaryngeal aspect of the cartilage (**Figure 5.24**) and the cartilage is seen to be destroyed or lytic. Sclerotic change seen in the cartilage on CT may be due to tumour surrounding the cartilage rather than truly invading it. High signal intensity on T2-weighted MR images may be due to peritumoral inflammatory change, rather than true invasion. Involvement of the laryngeal cartilage framework can lead to radiation necrosis if these patients are treated by radiotherapy rather than surgery.

Posterior wall tumours can spread submucosally cranially to involve the posterior tonsillar pillars. The lymphatic drainage of the posterior pharyngeal wall is to retropharyngeal nodes (**Figure 5.25a,b**). These are not assessable clinically. Tumours of the posterior wall of the hypopharynx may be rendered inoperable by the presence of nodal disease encasing vessels at the skull base. Spread into the prevertebral muscles or vertebrae themselves may also make the patient inoperable (**Figure 5.26**). The preservation of a high SI fat stripe on axial or sagittal T1-weighted MR scans has been shown to be a good predictor for excluding prevertebral muscle invasion.[50] The width of this stripe is, however, variable from patient to patient and from superior, where it is wider, to inferior.[49] The diagnosis of prevertebral muscle involvement can be difficult to make with certainty on cross-sectional imaging. Although this will obliterate the normal fat

plane seen posteriorly, it may not always be readily visible in thin patients. Abnormal enhancing tumour extending into and expanding the muscle is a more reliable sign. Overstaging can occur in the presence of a bulky tumour when the fat plane may be effaced but not invaded, but clinical examination may still demonstrate a mobile tumour in these cases. Abnormal muscle contour, T2 MR hyperintensity and enhancement may be present in patients in whom the tumour is mobile and resectable.[51]

True post-cricoid tumours are rare and have a poor prognosis. These patients may present with hoarseness from involvement of the posterior larynx (arytenoid cartilages and posterior aspect of the cricoid cartilage) causing vocal cord paralysis. It is important to estimate the inferior extent of tumour which may be difficult to assess endoscopically and could thus result in positive surgical margins. Submucosal spread will be identified by abnormal enhancement and wall thickening. PET-CT can be helpful in determining the lower extent of metabolically active disease, although small volume tumour may not be recognized. Barium swallow can also be useful in this regard.

NASAL CAVITY AND PARANASAL SINUSES

Plain films, CT and MRI can be used in assessing the paranasal sinuses. CT is superior to plain films and direct coronal CT imaging, with a low radiation dose technique utilizing a low mAs, has been employed for assessing benign inflammatory pathology. However, as it is difficult to distinguish inflammatory conditions from tumour with unenhanced CT then a higher radiation dose enhanced MDCT is necessary when tumour is suspected, and both axial images and multiplanar reformats should be evaluated. MR is superior in this aspect, particularly T2-weighted imaging which can

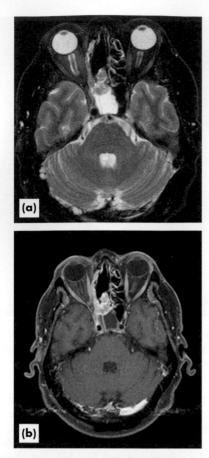

Figure 5.27 Fat-saturated T2-weighted (a) and fat-saturated T1-weighted magnetic resonance following intravenous contrast (b). Recurrent enhancing enthesioneuroblastoma in the right nasal cavity with obstruction of the right sphenoid sinus.

differentiate tumour which appears low signal due to its high cellular content from inflammatory tissue and secretions which have a high water content and thus high T2 signal (**Figure 5.27a,b**). Although inspissated secretions may sometimes demonstrate low T2 signal, they are generally of increased signal on T1-weighted imaging.[52]

Primary malignancy arising in the sinonasal cavity is relatively rare, accounting for only 3 per cent of all head and neck tumours.[53] The tumours are diverse and most lesions are epithelial tumours, including squamous cell carcinomas and melanoma (**Figure 5.28**), and other non-squamous cell epithelial tumours such as salivary gland lesions, neuroectodermal and neural tumours. Metastases, osseous lesions, soft tissue sarcomas and lymphoproliferative disease also involve the sinonasal cavity (**Figure 5.29**).[54]

Early symptoms of sinonasal malignancy are non-specific and can be mistaken for benign pathology, such as sinusitis. Thus tumours often present at a relatively advanced stage locally and up to 20 per cent may have adenopathy, including involvement of retropharyngeal nodes.

Squamous cell carcinomas comprise 80 per cent of all malignant sinonasal tumours, with the majority of these (85 per cent) arising in the maxillary antrum. Both CT and MRI have a role in evaluating the disease extent and assessing operability, and often complement one another. Local bone destruction is superiorly demonstrated on multiplanar

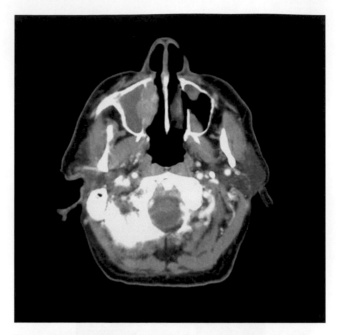

Figure 5.28 Contrast-enhanced axial computed tomography scan demonstrating a destructive enhancing soft tissue mass (melanoma) involving the medial wall and with obstruction of the right maxillary antrum.

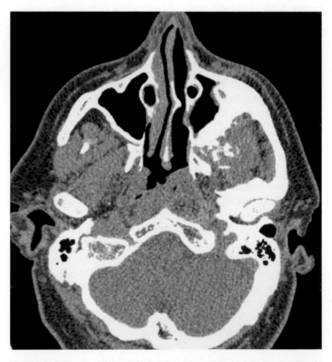

Figure 5.29 Contrast-enhanced axial computed tomography scan showing chondrosarcoma of the posterior wall of the left maxillary antrum extending into the infratemporal fossa.

reformat thin section CT, including erosion of the medial and inferolateral walls of the sinus and destruction of the alveolar ridge of the maxilla. Axial images are best for demonstration of lateral tumour extension into the infratemporal fossa (**Figure 5.29**) and posterior extension into pterygopalatine

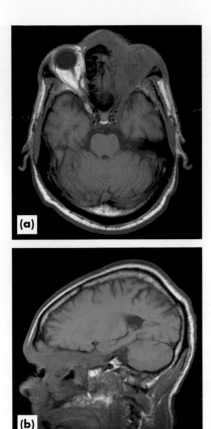

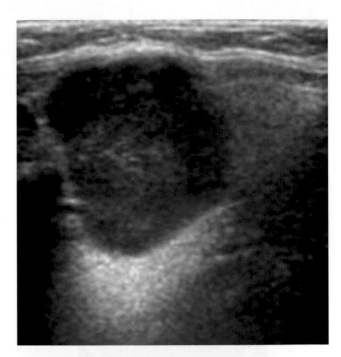

Figure 5.31   Ultrasound of a pleomorphic adenoma demonstrating a well-defined hypoechoic mass with typical through transmission.

Figure 5.30   Axial T1-weighted (a) and sagittal T1-weighted (b) magnetic resonance image demonstrating tumour extension into the orbit and anterior cranial fossa.

fossa, while coronal images are best for spread of tumour superiorly into the orbit and intracranial extension.

Coronal and sagittal MR imaging elegantly demonstrate direct tumour extension into the floor of the anterior and middle cranial fossae, the pterygopalatine fossa and the orbits (**Figure 5.30a,b**). Gadolinium-enhanced MR is used to evaluate perineural spread of tumour which is most commonly seen with adenoid cystic carcinoma, the majority occurring in the maxillary antrum and nasal cavity. The maxillary division of the trigeminal nerve is most often affected, and the nerve may show abnormal enhancement and enlargement.

Non-squamous cell sinonasal tumours are less common than squamous cell tumours. Melanomas account for only 3.5 per cent of sinonasal tumours and more commonly arise from the nasal cavity (**Figure 5.28**). On MRI, melanotic tumours are high signal on T1 and low signal on T2, whereas amelanotic tumours are low signal on T1 and high signal on T2. Enthesioneuroblastomas (olfactory neuroblastomas) (**Figure 5.27**) arise in the nasal vault and can spread into the anterior cranial fossa via the cribiform plate. This is best evaluated with imaging in the coronal and sagittal plane.

SALIVARY GLAND TUMOURS

The salivary glands are divided into two groups: the major salivary glands and the minor salivary glands. The three pairs of major salivary glands are the parotids, submandibular and sublingual glands. The numerous small glands distributed throughout the oral cavity mucosa, the sinonasal cavity, the hard and soft palates, the pharynx and the larynx comprise the minor salivary glands.

Salivary gland tumours account for less than 3 per cent of all head and neck tumours, but despite the low incidence there are a wide variety of benign and malignant lesions. Tumours are most commonly seen in the parotid salivary gland.[55] About 50 per cent of all minor salivary gland tumours are malignant. Most occur in the palate and upper lip region.

Plain films and sialography remain useful for sialadenitis and suspected stone disease, but are no longer used for assessing tumours.

High frequency ultrasound (7–14 mHz) is an ideal tool for examining the superficial lobe of the parotid and the submandibular salivary glands. It can be utilized to guide fine needle aspiration and core biopsies, particularly of small masses that are difficult to palpate. Benign salivary gland lesions are usually well defined and homogeneous on US (**Figure 5.31**). Irregular margins, inhomogeneity and disorganized colour flow are features of malignant tumours.[56]

CT or MRI is required to assess the deep lobe of the parotid gland. Calcification is better demonstrated on CT and tumour extension beyond the ramus of the mandible, the course of the retromandibular vein, extension of deep lobe tumours into the parapharyngeal space and displacement of the vessels are also well demonstrated on CT. The facial nerve is not seen on CT and perineural invasion typically seen in adenoid cystic tumours can only be demonstrated well on MR. Ideally, imaging needs to be in the plane of the nerve, and fat-suppressed T1-weighted images following gadolinium contrast demonstrate this optimally.

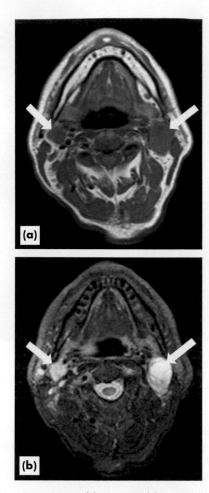

Figure 5.32 T1-weighted (a) and STIR (b) axial images demonstrating a small pleomorphic adenoma within the tail of both parotid glands (arrows).

Pleomorphic adenoma is the most common salivary gland tumour. They are hypoechoic on ultrasound and often display through transmission of sound (**Figure 5.31**). On CT, they are usually of higher attenuation (i.e. denser) than the surrounding fatty parenchyma, with variable enhancement. Small tumours have fairly homogeneous low T1-weighted and high T2-weighted signal intensity on MR (**Figure 5.32a,b**). Larger lesions are heterogeneous on all imaging modalities due to dystrophic calcification, necrosis, cystic change and areas of haemorrhage.

Warthin's tumours (papillary cystadenoma lymphomatosum) are the second most common benign tumour of the parotid (**Figure 5.33**) and classically have a multiseptated cystic architecture on US, although cyst formation is common resulting in an anechoic lesion on US. CT, however, usually demonstrates the tumour nodule within the thin-walled cyst. The cystic component can generally be differentiated from the solid component on MR, although the cystic component is more readily appreciated on CT.

Mucoepidermoid carcinoma accounts for a quarter of malignant salivary gland tumours with almost half involving major salivary glands, predominantly the parotid, and the remainder occur throughout the oral cavity in the palate, retromolar region, buccal mucosal and lips. Imaging appearances depend on the grade of the tumour. Low-grade

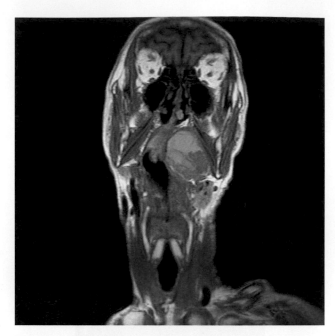

Figure 5.33 T1-weighted coronal magnetic resonance image demonstrating a large haemorrhagic Warthin's tumour in the left parapharyngeal space.

lesions appear similar to pleomorphic adenomas. High-grade lesions can metastasize and are locally infiltrating, destroying salivary gland ducts.

Although acinar cell carcinoma is relatively common, accounting for up to a third of parotid gland malignancies, they have no specific imaging features, often appearing as benign lesions on CT and MR.

Adenoid cystic carcinoma is typically a slow growing, widely infiltrative tumour with a tendency to perineural spread. It accounts for 2–8 per cent of all salivary gland tumours and occurs most commonly in the parotid, submandibular gland and palate. Retrograde tumour extension to the skull base from the parotid gland occurs via the facial and mandibular nerve. If there is extensive infiltration, widening of the bony nerve canal can be seen on CT. Contrast-enhanced MR, however, is more sensitive and reliable at demonstrating nerve enlargement and involvement (**Figure 5.34a,b**).

The parotids contain lymph nodes within the gland capsule and pathology may arise within these, rather than the glandular or stromal tissue.

Reactive lymphoid hyperplasia within intraparotid nodes occurs secondary to infection in the scalp and ear. Intraparotid nodes can also be involved as part of a generalized systemic lymphadenitis due to infections, such as HIV or tuberculosis, and inflammatory conditions, such as sarcoidosis.

Lymphoma and metastases, usually from malignant melanoma or cutaneous or mucosal squamous cell carcinoma can also involve intraparotid nodes.

LYMPH NODES

Radiological identification of lymphatic tumour spread and characterization of cervical lymph nodes is important in

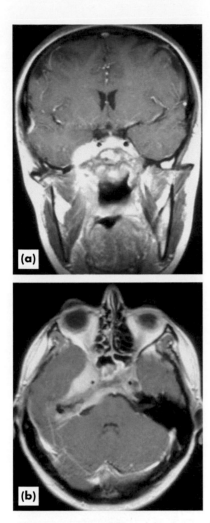

Figure 5.34   Contrast-enhanced T1-weighted coronal (a) and axial (b) magnetic resonance image demonstrating perineural spread from adenoid cystic carcinoma.

patients with newly diagnosed cancer, as neck palpation is known to be an inaccurate technique for assessment of nodes. The presence of nodal metastases indicates a worse prognosis in patients, and modifies the available treatment options. Cervical nodes are also a common site of involvement in patients with lymphoma. However, none of the currently available imaging methods reliably depict small tumour deposits in non-enlarged nodes or differentiate reactively enlarged nodes from metastatic adenopathy.

Ultrasound

Normal cervical lymph nodes are elliptical in shape. Sono-graphically, most normal nodes have an outer hypoechoic cortex and a central echogenic (bright) hilus which is continuous with the surrounding fatty tissue. Normal and reactive cervical lymph nodes may show hilar vascularity or appear avascular.[57] Malignant infiltration results in enlarged, more rounded nodes with disruption of the normal sonographic structure. Loss of the usual sharp outline of an involved node suggests extracapsular spread and correlates with advanced malignancy. Nodal calcification can be seen in metastatic

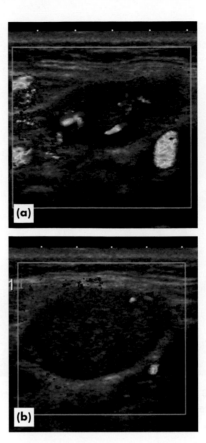

Figure 5.35   Involved nodes with disordered flow (a) and peripheral flow (b) on colour Doppler ultrasound.

nodes from both papillary and medullary carcinoma of the thyroid. Metastatic and lymphomatous infiltration alters the normal vascularity within a node and both peripheral, and mixed peripheral and hilar flow may be demonstrated on colour flow Doppler sonography (**Figure 5.35a,b**).[58] Power Doppler evaluation of lymph node vascularity in addition to sonographic measurement of node size gives a high diagnostic accuracy of metastatic lymph nodes with a sensitivity of 92 per cent and specificity of 100 per cent.[59]

Ultrasound–guided fine needle aspiration cytology

The accuracy of lymph node evaluation is also increased when US is combined with cytology following a fine needle aspiration. A recent large meta-analysis comparing US alone, with US-guided fine needle aspiration cytology (FNAC), CT and MRI demonstrated that US-guided FNAC was the most accurate imaging modality to detect cervical lymph node metastases.[60]

Computed tomography and magnetic resonance imaging

Assessment of lymph nodes with CT and MRI should ideally be done when staging the primary tumour. Normal lymph nodes usually measure <1 cm in short axis diameter and have an oval shape with a smooth well-defined border.

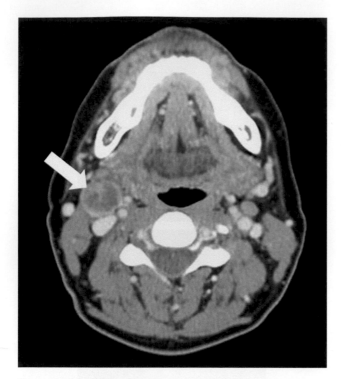

Figure 5.36 Pathological node on contrast-enhanced computed tomography (arrow).

Benign nodes are a uniform density or signal intensity and contain a distinctive fatty hilus.

The CT and MR criteria used to assess nodes for metastatic involvement are node size and shape, the presence of central necrosis and localized grouping of nodes within an expected lymph drainage region for a known tumour.[61] Studies on cancer staging using lymph node size alone on CT or MRI to assess for metastatic involvement report low accuracy with sensitivities of 65 and 88 per cent and specificities of 47 and 41 per cent, respectively, for CT and MRI.[62] The most accurate CT criterion is the presence of central necrosis which is demonstrated as peripheral/rim enhancement in the node following administration of iodinated contrast media (**Figure 5.36**). A similar appearance is seen on fat-suppressed T1-weighted MR images post-gadolinium (**Figure 5.37a,b**). The sensitivity of both MR and CT in detecting necrosis within nodes is similar (93 and 91 per cent, respectively), and better than that of US (77 per cent). However, there is no significant difference in the specificity of the three modalities (89, 93 and 93 per cent, respectively).[63]

Extracapsular spread of tumour beyond the capsule of the lymph node can be very accurately diagnosed on CT and MR when there are poorly defined margins around the node and enhancement of the node capsule.[61]

It was hoped that MR lymph contrast agents could improve the detection of metastatic nodes. In animals, the administration of an ultrasmall superparamagnetic iron oxide (USPIO) preparation intravenously 24–48 hours prior to MR examination of the lymph nodes is beneficial, as there is a decrease in the signal intensity of normal, but not metastatic nodes, on T2-weighted MR sequences.[64] However, the clinical usefulness of USPIO agents is unfortunately limited by technical problems (motion and susceptibility

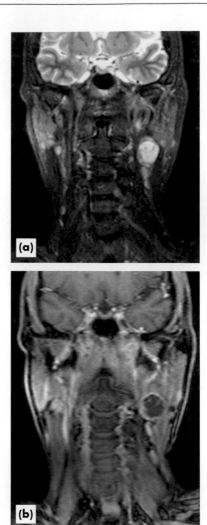

Figure 5.37 STIR coronal image precontrast (a) demonstrating a left level II node and fat-saturated T1-weighted coronal image following gadolinium chelate (b) demonstrating a rim enhancement and central necrosis.

artefacts and spatial resolution) and, although the detection of metastatic lymph nodes on MR following administration of USPIO has a high sensitivity (88 per cent) and specificity (77 per cent), there are false-positive results due to inflammatory nodes and false-negative results from the presence of undetected micrometastases.[65]

Diffusion-weighted MR imaging, which allows visualization of molecular diffusion and perfusion via microcirculation of blood in the capillary network may improve detection of metastatic nodes in the neck. Cancer metastases to regional lymph nodes may be associated with alteration in both water diffusion and microcirculation within the node and calculation of the apparent diffusion coefficient (ADC) can be used as an adjunct tool to help discriminate metastatic neck nodes.[66] In addition, studies have shown a significant difference in diffusion-weighted MR imaging and ADC values for nodes involved by metastatic squamous cell carcinoma, nodes involved by metastatic nasopharyngeal carcinoma and those infiltrated with lymphoma, the ADC value for lymphoma and nasopharyngeal carcinoma being less than that for squamous cell carcinoma. This technique may therefore have the potential of differentiating between the causes of malignant lymphadenopathy.[67]

¹⁸F–FDG PET–CT

Combined ¹⁸F-FDG PET-CT imaging is reported to be more accurate in lymph node evaluation than either PET or contrast-enhanced CT alone in patients with squamous cell carcinoma of the head and neck, with a sensitivity, specificity and accuracy of 92, 99 and 97 per cent, respectively, for predicting metastatic lymph node compared to histopathological findings.[68]

¹⁸F-FDG PET has been shown to be superior to combined CT and MRI in the detection of cervical nodes in patients with squamous cell tumours of the oral cavity. The sensitivity of ¹⁸F-FDG PET for the detection of cervical nodal metastasis on a level-by-level basis was significantly higher than that of CT/MRI, whereas their specificities appeared to be similar.[69]

POST-TREATMENT CHANGES AND RECURRENCE

Knowledge of previous treatment is essential to enable correct interpretation of images. If staging is performed following emergency tracheostomy, there will be soft tissue swelling, distortion and commonly surgical emphysema from the surgery. This can potentially lead to tumour overstaging.

Following total laryngectomy, there will be loss of the thyroid and cricoid cartilages and the hyoid bone. The neopharynx is formed by suturing the two open ends of the hypopharynx together and recurrence at this site should be looked for. The stoma should have walls of uniform thickness and focal areas of nodularity, intraluminal soft tissue masses or necrosis should be regarded with suspicion.[70] There will be variable loss of the thyroid, and asymmetry of tissue here may lead to an erroneous diagnosis of disease recurrence (**Figure 5.38**). A knowledge of the normal imaging appearances of surgical flaps is essential.[71] Denervation of the flap can give rise to enhancement following intravenous

contrast which can be mistaken for disease recurrence (**Figure 5.39a,b**).

Asymmetry of the neck on clinical examination and imaging may be due to previous neck dissection. This can be due to previous resection of one submandibular gland (**Figure 5.40**). There will be loss of the normal fat plane

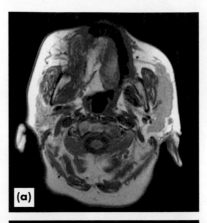

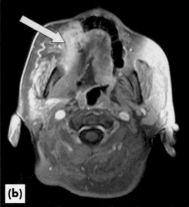

Figure 5.39 Axial T1-weighted magnetic resonance image of a radial free forearm flap reconstruction of the right floor of mouth (a) with enhancement of the denervated muscle (arrow) on fat-saturated axial T1-weighted post intravenous gadolinium (b).

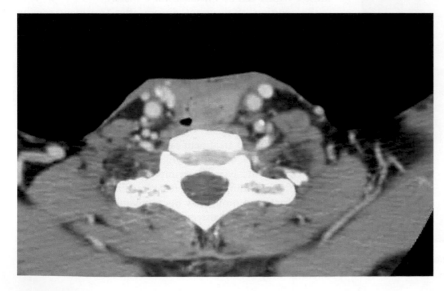

Figure 5.38 Asymmetric thyroid post laryngectomy.

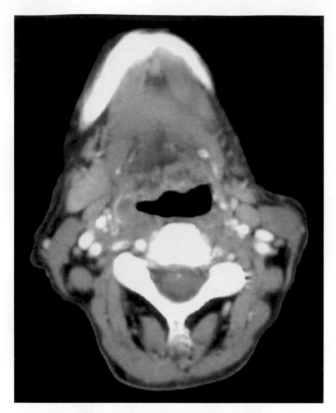

Figure 5.40   Contrast-enhanced computed tomography scan post left neck dissection with resection of the left submandibular gland.

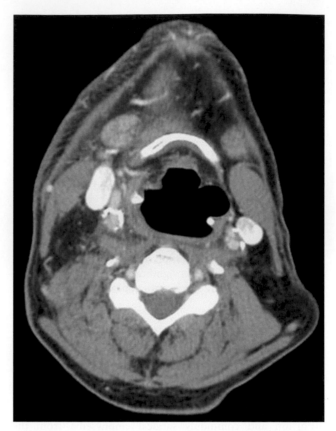

Figure 5.42   Computed tomography scan demonstrating thickening of the right subcutaneous fat and platysma muscle post radiotherapy.

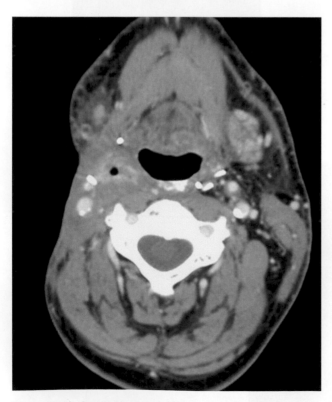

Figure 5.41   Contrast-enhanced computed tomography scan post right neck dissection with loss of fat planes.

around the vascular compartment (**Figure 5.41**). The internal jugular vein may be absent and there may be surgical resection of the sternomastoid muscle. Damage to the accessory and hypoglossal nerves can occur as a result of neck dissection giving rise to abnormality within the tongue with fat infiltration of the affected side (hypoglossal palsy) and abnormal high signal within the affected trapezius muscle on T2-weighted sequences (accessory nerve palsy) and evidence of compensatory muscle hypertrophy of the levator scapulae muscle which can be mistaken for a mass.

Recognition of recurrent disease after treatment can be extremely difficult. The laryngopharynx will become oedematous following radiotherapy. Expected changes occur with generalized oedema of skin, soft tissues and fat (**Figure 5.42**). This leads to high SI changes on T2-weighted MR images. The epiglottis, aryepiglottic folds and arytenoids appear swollen and there is thickening of the anterior commissure.[72] Lack of response on follow-up imaging or a failure of reduction of tumour volume by greater than 50 per cent at four months are likely to be due to treatment failure.

Radionecrosis of the laryngeal cartilages may lead to degeneration and lysis. Superimposed infection may lead to air trapping within the necrotic cartilage. Differentiation from recurrent tumour may be impossible on CT and MRI.

Mandibular radio-osteonecrosis is seen in a small percentage of patients and differentiation between this and recurrent tumour is also difficult. On CT, there are areas of sclerosis, rarefaction and sequestration, and pathological fractures may occur.

Positron emission tomography is increasingly used to identify disease recurrence, although inflammatory change (including radio-osteonecrosis) will give rise to false-positive studies. Endoscopy and biopsy can diagnose mucosal recurrence, but follow-up imaging may be useful for deep disease.

KEY LEARNING POINTS

Advantages of ultrasound

- High definition images of superficial structures
- Assessment of flow in vascular structures
- Guidance for needle aspiration and biopsy

Disadvantages of ultrasound

- Poor penetration

Advantages of computed tomography

- High spatial and contrast resolution
- Assessment of deep tumour spread, local nodes and distant metastases
- Detects subtle cortical bone destruction

Disadvantages of computed tomography

- Uses potentially hazardous ionizing radiation
- Often requires potentially nephrotoxic iodinated contrast media
- Prone to artefact from dental amalgam and metallic implants

Advantages of magnetic resonance imaging

- High spatial and contrast resolution
- Assessment of deep tumour spread and local nodes
- Detects cartilage and bone marrow involvement

Disadvantages of magnetic resonance imaging

- Long scan times
- Requires stringent safety measures
- Prone to artefact from respiration and movement

Role of ^{18}F-FDG PET-CT

- Evaluating patients with pathological cervical nodes and an unknown primary
- Evaluating regional lymph node metastases
- Excluding distant metastases and synchronous primary tumours
- Monitor tumour recurrence in the post-operative neck
- Excluding residual disease after chemoradiotherapy

Imaging issues

- Nasopharynx
  - Normal asymmetry of the lateral pharyngeal recess
  - Variability in normal lymphoid tissue
- Parapharyngeal space
  - Displacement of internal carotid artery and parapharyngeal fat
  - Tumour vascularity and bony margins
- Lip carcinoma
  - Bone erosion
  - Soft tissue invasion
- Floor of mouth carcinoma
  - Extent of bone erosion
  - Deep invasion along the mylohyoid and hyoglossus muscles
  - Relationship to ipsilateral lingual neurovascular bundle
  - Extension across the midline and relationship to contralateral neurovascular bundle
  - Tongue base invasion
  - Extension into the soft tissues of the neck
- Tongue
  - Objective size of tumour
  - Involvement of neurovascular bundle
  - Has tumour crossed midline
- Oropharyngeal tumours
  - Objective size of primary tumour
  - Perineural and deep spread of tumour
  - Soft palate to pterygopalatine fossa (V_2) and foramen rotundum
  - Faucial tonsil to masticator space involving branches of V_3 at skull base (foramen ovale)
  - Lingual tonsil to neurovascular bundle of tongue
  - Posterior oropharyngeal wall to retropharyngeal space
- Laryngeal tumours
  - Tumour volume
  - Laryngeal cartilage involvement
  - Spread beyond the larynx
  - Paraglottic disease volume
- Sinonasal cavity
  - Differentiation of tumour from secretions
  - Bone destruction
  - Local tumour spread
  - Perineural tumour spread
- Salivary gland tumours
  - Ultrasound-guided fine needle aspiration and biopsy
  - Deep lobe of parotid involvement
  - Intraparotid nodal disease
  - Perineural tumour spread

REFERENCES

1. Hall EJ, Brenner DJ. Cancer risks from diagnostic radiology. *British Journal of Radiology* 2008; **81**: 362–78.
2. Berrington de Gonzalez A, Darby S. Risk of cancer from diagnostic x-rays: estimates for the UK and 14 other countries. *Lancet* 2004; **363**: 345–51.

3. Quinn AD, Taylor CG, Sabharwal T, Sikdar T. Radiation protection awareness in non-radiologists. *British Journal of Radiology* 1997; **70**: 102–6.

4. Houghton DJ, Hughes ML, Garvey C *et al.* Role of chest CT scanning in the management of patients presenting with head and neck cancer. *Head and Neck* 1998; **20**: 614–18.

5. Ferlito A, Shaha AR, Silver CE *et al.* Incidence and sites of distant metastases from head and neck cancer. *ORL, Journal for Otorhinolaryngology and its Related Specialties* 2001; **63**: 202–7.

6. Gittoes N, Miller MR, Daykin J *et al.* Upper airways obstruction in 153 consecutive patients presenting with thyroid enlargement. *British Medical Journal* 1996; **312**: 484.

7. Mukherji SK, Isaacs DL, Creager A *et al.* CT detection of mandibular invasion by squamous cell carcinoma of the oral cavity. *American Journal of Roentgenology* 2001; **177**: 237–43.

8. Lasser EC, Lyon SG, Berry CC. Reports on contrast media reactions: Analysis of data from reports to the US Food and Drug Administration. *Radiology* 1997; **203**: 605–10.

9. Wang CL, Cohan RH, Ellis JH *et al.* Frequency, outcome, and appropriateness of treatment of non-ionic iodinated contrast media reactions. *American Journal of Roentgenology* 2008; **191**: 409–15.

10. Waybill MM, Waybill PN. Contrast media-induced nephrotoxicity: identification of patients at risk and algorithms for prevention. *Journal of Vascular and Interventional Radiology* 2001; **12**: 3–9.

11. Kuhn MJ, Chen N, Sahani DV *et al.* The PREDICT study: a randomised double-blind comparison of contrast-induced nephropathy after low- or isoosmolar contrast agent exposure. *American Journal of Roentgenology* 2008; **191**: 151–7.

12. McIsaac HK, Thordarson DS, Shafran R *et al.* Claustrophobia and the magnetic resonance imaging procedure. *Journal of Behavioral Medicine* 1998; **21**: 255–68.

13. Spouse E, Gedrocy WM. MRI of the claustrophobic patient: Interventionally configured magnets. *British Journal of Radiology* 2000; **73**: 146–51.

14. Ergün I, Keven K, Uruç I *et al.* The safety of gadolinium in patients with stage 3 and 4 renal failure. *Nephrology, Dialysis, Transplantation* 2006; **21**: 697–700.

15. Broome DR, Girguis MS, Baron PW *et al.* Gadodiamide-associated nephrogenic systemic fibrosis: why radiologists should be concerned. *American Journal of Roentgenology* 2007; **188**: 586–92.

16. Lorenz RR, Esclamado R. Preoperative magnetic resonance angiography in fibula-free flap reconstruction of head and neck defects. *Head and Neck* 2001; **23**: 844–50.

17. Imola MJ, Gapany M, Grund F *et al.* Technetium 99m single photon emission computed tomography scanning for assessing mandible invasion in oral cavity cancer. *Laryngoscope* 2001; **111**: 373–81.

18. Schöder H, Yeung HWD, Gonen M *et al.* Head and neck cancer: clinical usefulness and accuracy of PET/CT image fusion. *Radiology* 2004; **231**: 65–72.

♦ 19. Blodgett TM, Fukui MB, Snyderman CH *et al.* Combined PET-CT in head and neck: Part 1. Physiological, altered physiological and artifactual FDG uptake. *Radiographics* 2005; **25**: 897–912.

♦ 20. Fukui MB, Blodgett TM, Snyderman CH *et al.* Combined PET-CT in the head and neck: Part 2. Diagnostic uses and pitfalls of oncologic imaging. *Radiographics* 2005; **25**: 913–30.

21. Quon A, Fischbein NJ, McDougall IR *et al.* Clinical role of 18F-FDG PET/CT in the management of squamous cell carcinoma of the head and neck and thyroid carcinoma. *Journal of Nuclear Medicine* 2007; **48**: 58S–67S.

22. Ong SC, Schöder H, Lee NY *et al.* Clinical utility of 18F-FDG PET/CT in assessing the neck after concurrent chemoradiotherapy for locoregioal advanced head and neck cancer. *Journal of Nuclear Medicine* 2008; **49**: 532–40.

23. Comoretto M, Balestreri L, Borsatti E *et al.* Detection and restaging of residual and/or recurrent nasopharyngeal carcinoma after chemotherapy and radiation therapy: comparison of MR imaging and FDG PET/CT. *Radiology* 2008; **249**: 203–11.

♦ 24. Stambuk HE, Patel SG. Imaging of the parapharyngeal space. *Otolaryngologic Clinics of North America* 2008; **41**: 77–101, vi.

25. Furukawa M, Furukawa MK, Katoh K, Tsukuda M. Differentiation between schwannoma of the vagus nerve and schwannoma of the cervical sympathetic chain by imaging diagnosis. *Laryngoscope* 1996; **106**: 1548–52.

26. Saito DM, Glastonbury CM, El-Sayed IH, Eisele DW. Parapharyngeal space schwannomas: preoperative imaging determination of the nerve of origin. *Archives of Otolaryngology, Head and Neck Surgery* 2007; **133**: 662–7.

♦ 27. Stambuk HE, Karimi S, Lee N, Patel SG. Oral cavity and oropharynx tumors. *Radiologic Clinics of North America* 2007; **45**: 1–20.

28. Imaizumi A, Yoshino N, Yamada I *et al.* A potential pitfall of MR imaging for assessing mandibular invasion of squamous cell carcinoma in the oral cavity. *AJNR. American Journal of Neuroradiology* 2006; **27**: 114–22.

29. Bolzoni A, Cappiello J, Piazza C *et al.* Diagnostic accuracy of magnetic resonance imaging in the assessment of mandibular involvement in oral-oropharyngeal squamous cell carcinoma: a prospective study. *Archives of Otolaryngology, Head and Neck Surgery* 2004; **130**: 837–43.

30. Chung TS, Yousem DM, Seigerman HM *et al.* MR of mandibular invasion in patients with oral and oropharyngeal malignant neoplasms. *American Journal of Neuroradiology* 1994; **15**: 1949–55.

31. Jungehülsing M, Scheidhauer K, Litzka N *et al.* [99mTc-MDP-SPECT for detection of subclinical mandibular

infiltration of squamous epithelial carcinoma]. *HNO* 1997; **45**: 702–9 (in German).

32. Yousem DM, Gad K, Tufano RP. Resectability issues with head and neck cancer. *American Journal of Neuroradiology* 2006; **27**: 2024–36.

33. Preda L, Lovati E, Chiesa F *et al.* Measurement by multidetector CT scan of the volume of hypopharyngeal and laryngeal tumours: accuracy and reproducibility. *European Radiology* 2007; **17**: 2096–102.

34. Castelijns JA, van den Brekel MW, Tobi H *et al.* Laryngeal carcinoma after radiation therapy: correlation of abnormal MR imaging signal patterns in laryngeal cartilage with the risk of recurrence. *Radiology* 1996; **198**: 151–5.

35. Murakami R, Furusawa M, Baba Y *et al.* Dynamic helical CT of T1 and T2 glottic carcinomas: predictive value for local control with radiation therapy. *American Journal of Neuroradiology* 2000; **21**: 1320–6.

36. Hoorweg JJ, Kruijt RH, Heijboer RJ *et al.* Reliability of interpretation of CT examination of the larynx in patients with glottic laryngeal carcinoma. *Otolaryngology and Head and Neck Surgery* 2006; **135**: 129–34.

37. Ljumanovic R, Langendijk JA, van Wattingen M *et al.* MR imaging predictors of local control of glottic squamous cell carcinoma treated with radiation alone. *Radiology* 2007; **244**: 205–12.

38. Loevner LA, Yousem DM, Montone KT *et al.* Can radiologists accurately predict preepiglottic space invasion with MR imaging? *American Journal of Roentgenology* 1997; **169**: 1681–7.

39. Becker M, Zbären P, Laeng H *et al.* Neoplastic invasion of the laryngeal cartilage: comparison of MR imaging and CT with histopathologic correlation. *Radiology* 1995; **194**: 661–9.

40. Zbären P, Becker M, Läng H. Pretherapeutic staging of laryngeal carcinoma. Clinical findings, computed tomography, and magnetic resonance imaging compared with histopathology. *Cancer* 1996; **77**: 1263–73.

41. Becker M, Zbären P, Delavelle J *et al.* Neoplastic invasion of the laryngeal cartilage: reassessment of criteria for diagnosis at CT. *Radiology* 1997; **203**: 521–32.

42. Muñoz A, Ramos A, Ferrando J *et al.* Laryngeal carcinoma: sclerotic appearance of the cricoid and arytenoid cartilage – CT-pathologic correlation. *Radiology* 1993; **189**: 433–7.

43. Nix PA, Salvage D. Neoplastic invasion of laryngeal cartilage: the significance of cartilage sclerosis on computed tomography images. *Clinical Otolaryngology and Allied Sciences* 2004; **29**: 372–5.

44. Agada FO, Nix PA, Salvage D, Stafford ND. Computerised tomography vs. pathological staging of laryngeal cancer: a 6-year completed audit cycle. *International Journal of Clinical Practice* 2004; **58**: 714–16.

♦ 45. Yousem DM, Tufano RP. Laryngeal imaging. *Magnetic Resonance Imaging Clinics of North America* 2002; **10**: 451–65.

46. Atula T, Markolla A, Leivo I, Makitie A. Cartilage invasion of laryngeal cancer detected by magnetic resonance. imaging. *European Archives of Otorhinolaryngology* 2001; **258**: 272–5.

47. Castelijns JA, Becker M, Hermans R. The impact of cartilage invasion on treatment and prognosis of laryngeal cancer. *European Radiology* 1996; **6**: 156–69.

48. Becker M, Zbären P, Casselman JW *et al.* Neoplastic invasion of laryngeal cartilage: reassessment of criteria for diagnosis at MR imaging. *Radiology* 2008; **249**: 551–9.

49. Yousem DM, Gad K, Tufano RP. Resectability issues with head and neck cancer. *American Journal of Neuroradiology* 2006; **27**: 2024–36.

50. Hsu WC, Loevner LA, Karpati R *et al.* Accuracy of magnetic resonance imaging in predicting absence of fixation of head and neck cancer to the prevertebral space. *Head and Neck* 2005; **27**: 95–100.

51. Loevner LA, Ott IL, Yousem DM *et al.* Neoplastic fixation to the prevertebral compartment by squamous cell carcinoma of the head and neck. *American Journal of Roentgenology* 1998; **170**: 1389–94.

♦ 52. Connor SEJ, Hussain S, Woo EK-F. Sinonasal imaging. *Imaging* 2007; **19**: 39–54.

53. Yuen HY, Kew J, van Hasselt CA. *Maxilla and sinuses in imaging in head and neck cancer: a practical approach.* London: Greenwich Medical Media, 2003.

54. Resto VA, Deschler DG. Sinonasal malignancies. *Otolaryngologic Clinics of North America* 2004; **37**: 473–87.

♦ 55. Yousem DM, Kraut MA, Chalian AA. Major salivary gland imaging. *Radiology* 2000; **216**: 19–29.

56. Bialek EJ, Jakubowski W, Zajkowski P *et al.* US of the major salivary glands: anatomy and spatial relationships, pathologic conditions, and pitfalls. *Radiographics* 2006; **26**: 745–63.

♦ 57. Ying M, Ahuja A. Sonography of neck lymph nodes. Part I: Normal lymph nodes. *Clinical Radiology* 2003; **58**: 351–8.

♦ 58. Ahuja A, Ying M. Sonography of neck lymph nodes. Part II: Abnormal lymph nodes. *Clinical Radiology* 2003; **58**: 358–66.

59. Ariji Y, Kimura Y, Hayashi N *et al.* Power Doppler sonography of cervical lymph nodes in patients with head and neck cancer. *American Journal of Neuroradiology* 1998; **19**: 303–7.

60. de Bondt RB, Nelemans PJ, Hofman PA *et al.* Detection of lymph node metastases in head and neck cancer: a meta-analysis comparing US, USgFNAC, CT and MR imaging. *European Journal of Radiology* 2007; **64**: 266–72.

61. Som PM. Detection of metastases in cervical lymph nodes: CT and MR criteria and differential diagnosis. *American Journal of Radiology* 1992; **158**: 961–69.

62. Kau RJ, Alexiou C, Laubenbacher C *et al.* Lymph node detection of head and neck squamous cell carcinomas by positron emission tomography with fluorodeoxyglucose F 18 in a routine clinical setting. *Archives of*

Otolaryngology, Head and Neck Surgery 1999; **125**: 1322–8.

63. King AD, Tse GMK, Ahuja AT *et al.* Necrosis in metastatic neck nodes: diagnostic accuracy of CT. MR imaging, and US. *Radiology* 2004; **230**: 720–6.

64. Weissleder R, Elizondo G, Witternberg J *et al.* Ultrasmall superparamagnetic iron oxide: an intravenous contrast agent for assessing lymph nodes with MR imaging. *Radiology* 1990; **175**: 494–8.

65. Sigal R, Vogl T, Casselman J *et al.* Lymph node metastases from head and neck squamous cell carcinoma: MR imaging with ultrasmall superparamagnetic iron oxide particles (Sinerem MR) – results of a phase-III multicenter clinical trial. *European Radiology* 2002; **12**: 1104–13.

66. Sumi M, Sakihama N, Sumi T *et al.* Discrimination of metastatic cervical lymph nodes with diffusion-weighted MR imaging in patients with head and neck cancer. *American Journal of Neuroradiology* 2003; **24**: 1627–34.

67. King AD, Ahuja AJ, Yeung DKW *et al.* Malignant cervical lymphadenopathy: diagnostic accuracy of diffusion-weighted MR imaging. *Radiology* 2007; **245**: 806–13.

68. Jeong H, Baek C, Son Y *et al.* Use of integrated 18F-FDG PET/CT to improve the accuracy of initial cervical nodal evaluation in patients with head and neck squamous cell carcinoma. *Head and Neck* 2007; **29**: 203–10.

69. Ng S-H, Yen T-C, Liao C-T *et al.* 18F-FDG PET and CT/MRI in oral cavity squamous cell carcinoma: a prospective study of 124 patients with histologic correlation. *Journal of Nuclear Medicine* 2005; **46**: 1136–43.

70. Kelsch TA, Patel U. Partial laryngectomy imaging. *Seminars in Ultrasound, CT, and MR* 2003; **24**: 147–56.

71. Wester DJ, Whiteman ML, Singer S *et al.* Imaging of the postoperative neck with emphasis on surgical flaps and their complications. *American Journal of Roentgenology* 1995; **164**: 989–93.

◆ 72. Mukherji SK, Weadock WJ. Imaging of the post-treatment larynx. *European Journal of Radiology* 2002; **44**: 108–19.

FURTHER READING

Adams S, Baum RP, Stuckensen T *et al.* Prospective comparison of ^{18}F-FDG PET with conventional imaging modalities (CT, MRI, US) in lymph node staging of head and neck cancer. *European Journal of Nuclear Medicine and Molecular Imaging* 1998; **25**: 1255–60.

Fischbein NJ, Noworolski SM, Henry RG *et al.* Assessment of metastatic cervical adenopathy using dynamic contrast-enhanced MR imaging. *American Journal of Neuroradiology* 2003; **24**: 301–11.

Hermans R. Staging of laryngeal and hypopharyngeal cancer: value of imaging studies. *European Radiology* 2006; **16**: 2386–400.

6

Head and neck pathology

RAM MOORTHY AND ADRIAN T WARFIELD

> We recognize only what we see; we see only what we know.
>
> JW Goethe (1749–1832)

INTRODUCTION

The head and neck region encompasses skin, soft tissue, upper aerodigestive tract elements including laryngopharynx, nose and paranasal sinuses, plus a number of other organ systems, including the ears, thyroid gland, parathyroid glands and pituitary gland, nodal, thymic and mucosa-associated lymphoid tissue, together with more specialized oral, dental, ocular, bone and joint, peripheral and central nervous system components. Within these fields, diseases of the skin adnexa, major and minor salivary glands, accessory mucus glands, ceruminous glands and lacrimal glands are sometimes encountered. In the presence of such anatomical diversity, it is not surprising that the pathology affecting the region is so varied.

History and examination can, on occasion, provide a diagnosis, but pathological evaluation remains the gold standard, especially in malignant disease as a tissue diagnosis, establishing tumour type, tumour grade and tumour stage, is of paramount prognostic importance and substantially influences further management.

PATHOLOGICAL EVALUATION

There are a number of techniques available to evaluate a lesion in the head and neck, ranging from techniques suitable for outpatients, with or without local anaesthetic, to those undertaken under general anaesthesia.

Common techniques are described below.

Fine needle aspiration cytology

Fine needle aspiration cytology (FNAC) was first described in the mid-nineteenth century, but it only gained popularity in the 1950s and now in many specialist units it constitutes the first-line investigation for patients presenting with cervical lymphadenopathy and other head and neck masses, especially major salivary gland and thyroid gland lesions.[1]

FNAC can be undertaken using palpation alone or with ultrasound or computed tomography (CT) guidance and may be performed with or without suction. FNAC primarily relies upon assessment of cytonuclear morphology, generally yielding little background architectural information, although microbiopsies may occasionally be present.

Fixed smears should be immersed in fixative, usually alcohol or less commonly formalin, without delay and are typically stained with the Papanicolau (Pap) method or sometimes haematoxylin and eosin (H&E). Air-dried smears are best subjected to assisted air flow and/or gentle heat and are usually stained with a Romanowsky type stain, commonly May–Grünwald-Giemsa (MGG) or Diff-Quik variants. Needles and syringe hubs may be rinsed in transport medium in an attempt to maximize the cell yield. The resultant liquor may be handled by a variety of cell concentration techniques, such as filtration or centrifugation, back at the laboratory, dependent upon local preferences and the reliance upon either traditional smear techniques or the availability of newer liquid-based cytology technology. The latter may be semi-automated or fully automated. Any clot material is best processed using conventional histology, because free floating cells tend to be preferentially sequestered in such clots and valuable material may otherwise be discarded (**Figure 6.1**).[2]

Core biopsy

A core biopsy is similar to FNAC, but instead of collecting a few clusters of cells a core biopsy, due to the greater calibre of the biopsy needle, will yield a cylinder of tissue that can undergo histological analysis. The relatively poor visualization of overall tissue architecture inherent in this procedure renders it of limited use in the investigation of primary

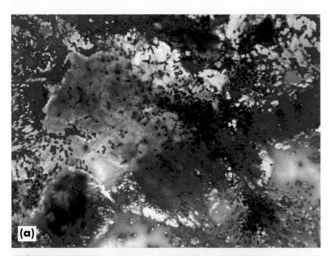

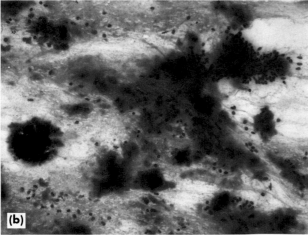

Figure 6.1   Fine needle aspiration cytology (FNAC) preparations from a salivary pleomorphic adenoma. (a) This alcohol-fixed slide depicts weakly stained, feathery stroma intimately admixed with loosely cohesive, isomorphic epithelioid and spindle cells (Pap stain, medium magnification). (b) This air-dried slide from the same tumour at identical magnification highlights the intensely stained myxoid ground substance, which obscures cytological detail in areas (May–Grünwald-Giemsa (MGG) stain, medium magnification).

haematolymphoid disorders, where cautious interpretation is recommended. However, when employed selectively the technique may be more helpful in the investigation of metastatic disease.

This technique can also be undertaken with ultrasound or CT guidance.

Incision biopsy

Incisional biopsy involves taking a representative sample or wedge of a lesion for histological scrutiny. This is a suitable technique for obtaining a diagnosis in accessible tumours affecting the oral cavity, or pharynx, larynx or hypopharynx. In lesions affecting the major salivary glands or in cervical lymphadenopathy, however, incisional biopsy can compromise further treatment.

There are a number of techniques available to obtain an incisional biopsy specimen under local or general anaesthetic depending on both the site of the lesion and patient factors (**Table 6.1**).

A sufficient sample of tissue must be obtained to allow histopathological analysis. Diathermy artefact and mechanical disruption, either crushing (compaction) or stretching (rarefaction), during handling or processing of the specimen can make analysis difficult and occasionally impossible. Certain tissues (e.g. lymphoid tissue) and tumours (e.g. neuroendocrine carcinoma) are more susceptible to this than others. It must be noted that a thick biopsy does not necessarily equate to a deep biopsy – it is often the interface between lesion and native stroma that is critical when seeking evidence of invasion and a thick sample from an exophytic epithelial proliferation may still be too superficial to adequately assess this (**Figure 6.2**).

Excision biopsy

Excision biopsy involves complete removal of the lesion and provides a definitive histological diagnosis. This can range from a small vocal cord nodule or polyp to major en bloc or multipart resection specimens.

Where appropriate, the specimen should preferably be orientated by the surgeon. Placing sutures or marker clips in appropriate positions can do this. Annotated diagrams or digital photographs often aid communication. Specimens can be pinned or clipped on to a cork, foam, polystyrene or even thick cardboard block. Dehydrated cucumber slices are a suitable medium for laryngeal biopsies, which are held in place with tissue adhesive.[9] Resection planes or other structures of particular clinical concern ought to be brought to the pathologist's attention, especially if these may not be immediately obvious following inevitable distortion induced by fixation. It should always be borne in mind that there will be a reproducible reduction in measured mucosal clearance margins of up to circa 50 per cent or so when a fixed, processed, stained and mounted tissue section is compared to the *in vivo* preoperative state due to shrinkage inherent in those histochemical processes (**Figures 6.3** and **6.4**).

Table 6.1 The advantages and disadvantages of commonly used tissue sampling techniques.

Type of sample	Advantages	Disadvantages
Fine needle aspiration	(1) Relatively risk free	(1) Primary cytological diagnosis by FNAC must be confirmed by histology prior to radical treatment for head and neck cancer
	(2) Quick	(2) Diagnostic yield is both lesion sensitive and operator dependent and there can be a high non-diagnostic rate,[3, 5] but this may be improved with the use of ultrasound[3]
	(3) Can be undertaken in outpatients	(3) Analysis is limited by cytopathological expertise and has been a rate-limiting step
	(4) Does not usually compromise future management	(4) Clinicians must be aware of inherent limitations including a risk of false-positives and false-negatives
	(5) In assessment of cervical lymphadenopathy FNAC has been shown to have a sensitivity of 76–98%[3] and a sensitivity typically of >90%.[3] The rates can vary with regards salivary gland and thyroid masses[3, 4, 5]	(5) FNAC is of limited help in the diagnosis of lymphoma. Flow cytometry may be helpful in excluding a diagnosis of lymphoma[5]
Core biopsy	(1) Core biopsy is a simple technique that can be performed in the outpatient setting. It is inexpensive with minimal equipment requirements. The diagnostic yield is higher than for FNAC and the sample undergoes histopathological analysis and therefore specific cytopathological expertise is not required[6]	(1) Appropriate precautions are required in patients on anticoagulation therapy undergoing core biopsy to prevent bleeding and haematoma formation
	(2) The complications of the procedure are relatively minor; the most common being haematoma formation and it does not compromise further treatment, especially surgery, which can occur with open biopsy	(2) There is a theoretical risk of tumour seeding associated with the larger needles used in obtaining a core biopsy, but published case series have rarely encountered this complication[6, 7, 8]
	(3) In contrast to FNAC, a core biopsy sample does in some cases permit a greater chance of sub-classification of a lymphoma and may sometimes obviate the need for an open biopsy[7]	
Incision biopsy	(1) Can provide definitive histological diagnosis	(1) Can affect definitive management of the tumour
		(2) Can require admission as a day-case
		(3) May require a general anaesthetic
		(4) Higher complication rate than FNAC or core biopsy
		(5) Costlier than FNAC or core-biopsy
Excision biopsy	(1) Can provide definitive diagnosis	(1) Higher risk of complication compared to other biopsy techniques
	(2) Can be definitive treatment of the tumour	(2) Can require admission and the need for general anaesthetic
		(3) Costliest method of obtaining a biopsy

FNAC, fine needle aspiration cytology.

Request form

When requesting pathological analysis of a specimen, it is vital that the pathologist is provided with all relevant information to enable a full assessment of the specimen. Required information includes:

- Patient identification and demographics.
- Type of biopsy: FNAC, core biopsy, incision biopsy or excision biopsy.
- Site of biopsy: if biopsies are taken from multiple sites, each site should be clearly labelled and sent separately.
- Relevant history of lesion: duration, symptoms, etc.
- Previous treatment to area: surgery, radiotherapy, trauma, etc.
- History of tobacco, alcohol or other drug use.
- Relevant past medical history, drug history and family history.
- Differential diagnoses based on clinical history and examination.

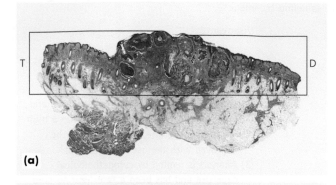

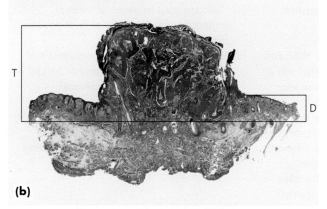

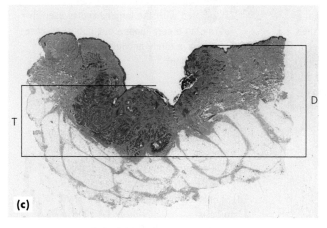

Figure 6.2   The potential discrepancy between tumour thickness and tumour depth. (a) Employing the uppermost granular layer, or actual surface discounting non-vitalized slough if ulcerated, as a fiducial point this relatively flat contoured tumour's thickness is roughly comparable to its depth (H&E stain, ultralow magnification). (b) This fungating exophytic tumour's thickness, however, comfortably exceeds its depth (H&E stain, ultralow magnification). (c) This ulceroinfiltrative, endophytic tumour's depth on the other hand exceeds its maximal thickness in the perpendicular plane (H&E stain, ultralow magnification). (T, tumour thickness; D, tumour depth.)

- If the specimen has been orientated, then an annotated diagram or digital image should be included with the request.
- Any clinical photographs of the lesion can also be helpful.

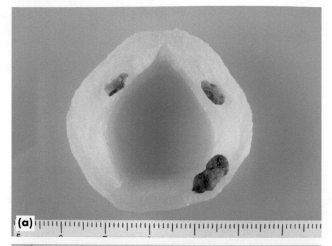

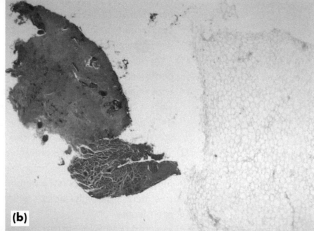

Figure 6.3   Biopsy orientation using a biomount. (a) Three laryngoscopic biopsies glued to a dehydrated cucumber (*Cucumis sativus*) biomount in order to maintain correct orientation in the laboratory. An accompanying endoscopic digital photograph further assists handling of such small biopsies. These may be further inked and/or sliced prior to processing. (b) A correctly embedded, though heavily thermalized, laryngeal biopsy on the left with anucleate cellulosic cucumber biomount to the right (H&E stain, ultralow magnification).

TISSUE PREPARATION

Surgical specimens are ideally fixed immediately in theatre by immersion in formalin, which is the routine fixative of choice. This effectively stops metabolism and arrests autolysis and putrefaction, thereby preserving the tissue structure. The apocryphal maxim is that the minimum ratio by volume of 10 per cent formalin to specimen should be ten to one, although this is somewhat arbitrary and if this was ever evidence based, it is likely to be influenced by intangible factors, such as type of tissue, temperature, agitation and so on – more liberal volumes of fixative are preferable to parsimony in this situation. On rare occasions, alternative fixatives, such as glutaraldehyde or alcohol, may be employed if specialized studies, for example electron microscopy, are contemplated. Fresh unfixed material intended for frozen

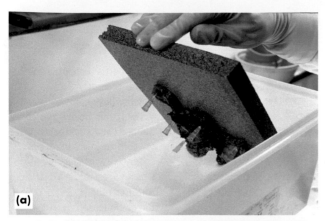

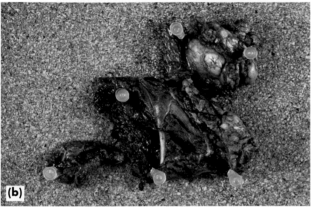

Figure 6.4 Resection specimen orientation utilizing corkboard.
(a) Radical neck dissection specimen pinned to cork block,
inverted and immersed to float in formalin. Hypodermic needles
or other pins should not be pushed completely through the
corkboard to obviate the risk of injury to laboratory personnel.
(b) The fixed specimen as received in the laboratory, ready for
trimming and block selection. This was accompanied by separate
annotation by the surgeon. Alternatively, the surgeon may prefer
to separate the levels in theatre and place them individually in
labelled pots.

section examination, molecular studies or microbiology must
be despatched without delay to the laboratory, cognizant that
it constitutes an infectious biohazard.

Upon receipt in the laboratory, the specimen identity
is corroborated and a unique accession number is allocated.
Following an appropriate period of fixation, either the
pathologist or senior biomedical scientist staff will describe
the specimen macroscopically, dissect and submit representative tissue slices for additional microscopical study,
observing relevant protocols and minimum data set guidelines according to their professional experience and discretion. In most laboratories, these slices are inserted into
proprietary sealable cassettes appropriately labelled.

After a further period of fixation, the tissue slices undergo
cycles of dehydration, clearing, infiltration and embedding
in preparation for microtomy. During dehydration, alcohol
replaces the aqueous fixative within the tissue. Clearing
replaces the alcohol with an antemedium, such as xylene.
Molten paraffin wax then replaces the clearing agent and

infiltrates the tissue. The tissue is subsequently embedded by
encapsulation in paraffin wax in a mould to provide a rigid
support for microtomy. The additional step of decalcification
may be instituted in mineralized tissue, which might otherwise hinder sectioning. Automatic tissue processors enhanced
by pressure, vacuum, heat and microwave facilities in a self-
contained, microprocessor-controlled, programmable unit
are used in many modern laboratories, tailored to local
conditions.

The prechilled, hardened paraffin wax-embedded tissue
block is then sliced, typically at 3–5-µm thick on a microtome. The thin sections are then floated on a warm water
bath prior to transfer on to a glass slide. The sections are then
dried on a hotplate.

The sections may now be stained, typically with haematoxylin and eosin (H&E) and mounted under a glass or
self-adhesive plastic film coverslip to form a permanent
preparation. A wide repertoire of additional histochemical and/or immunohistochemical stains may be similarly
employed, on replicate sections, either manually or by
machine, dependent upon the issues in hand. Finally, the
slides are made available to the pathologist for generation of a
surgical report.

Immunohistochemistry

The principle underpinning all immunohistochemistry (IHC)
is the demonstration of an epitope or antigen via its binding
to a specific antibody, which in turn, is conjugated to a label
that can be visualized histologically. A variety of reporter and
linkage systems to produce a visual signal have been developed
based on fluorescent molecules, alkaline phosphatase and
avidin-biotin, among others.

In general, monoclonal antibodies are more specific than
their polyclonal counterparts. Importantly, no antibody is
absolutely sensitive or 100 per cent specific – immunophenotyping is most intelligently performed using a panel of
expected positive and negative antibodies together with
appropriate positive and negative control sections, mindful of
aberrant cross-reactivity, spurious coexpression, false positive
and false negatives and vagaries of technical quality. Correlation with conventional morphology is imperative.

Among the broad categories of commercially available
diagnostic markers are antibodies directed against intermediate filaments (e.g. cytokeratins, desmin, neurofilament
protein, vimentin), other epithelial markers (e.g. epithelial
membrane antigen, Ber EP4), structural proteins (e.g. calpo-
nin), storage granules/products (e.g. chromogranin, calcitonin,
thyroglobulin), hormone receptors (e.g. oestrogen, progester-
one), nuclear epitopes (e.g. thyroid transcription factor-1,
p16), haematolymphoid epitopes (e.g. the CD system, cyclin
D1), proliferation indices (e.g. Ki67, PCNA), oncoproteins/
tumour suppressor proteins (e.g. bcl-2, p53, p63) and infectious agents (e.g. EBV LMP-1, CMV protein, HHV 8).

A variety of ancillary molecular techniques (e.g. polymerase chain reaction (PCR), *in situ* hybridization (ISH),
genotyping studies) and electron microscopy may be helpful
under selected circumstances.

Multidisciplinary correlation

The cytological and histopathological diagnostic procedure is
a complex process. It cannot be overemphasized that reaching

a final conclusion depends on many factors, including detailed site-specific knowledge coupled with experience of normality, familiarity with the manifold appearances of many disease processes at various stages in their natural history, awareness of mimics and artefacts plus cognizance of the limitations of the technique, in conjunction with patient-specific details and the clinical context. Without consideration of these and appropriate correlation with clinical, radiological and other relevant background information, a pathological slide is in danger of becoming a two-dimensional, brightly stained artefact, which may be as misleading as it can be potentially helpful.

Subsites of the head and neck

The head and neck is divided into a number of subsites as explained in **Table 6.2**.

TUMOURS OF THE HEAD AND NECK

Tumour typing

It follows that there are a multitude of benign and malignant tumours that affect the head and neck region. This section will aim to summarize important pathological features of the more common benign and malignant tumours required by the non-pathologist. For a more in-depth description, especially of less common tumours, a dedicated head and neck pathology or other specialist textbook is recommended.

Benign and malignant tumours can be classified according to the proposed tumour cell origin (histogenesis) and/or its differentiation pathway (**Table 6.3**).

This section is not intended to be an exhaustive account of the pathology of benign and malignant tumours affecting the head and neck, which can be found in any head and neck pathology atlas.[10, 11] We will aim to cover those tumours, both benign and malignant, that are more commonly encountered in clinical practice. Diagnostic cytopathology and histopathology are substantially visual subjects, therefore, illustrations depicting selected examples, but also introducing broader principles, have been chosen to supplement the text.

BENIGN TUMOURS

There is a multitude of benign tumours that affect the head and neck. In this section, a selection of benign tumours will be described.

Benign salivary gland neoplasms

Benign salivary gland classification and tumour-like lesions are largely classified according to WHO criteria and are listed in **Table 6.4**.

Table 6.2 Head and neck site and subsites.

Head and neck site	Subsite
Larynx. From epiglottis to lower border of cricoid cartilage	Supraglottis: epiglottis to false cords
	Glottis: false cords to 5–10 mm below true cords
	Subglottis: 10 mm below true cord to lower border of cricoid cartilage
Oral cavity. From lips to anterior tonsil fauces	Lips
	Anterior tongue
	Buccal mucosa
	Retromolar trigone
	Floor of mouth
Oropharynx. From level of hard palate to hyoid bone	Tongue base
	Tonsils
	Lateral and posterior pharyngeal wall
Hypopharynx	Pyriform fossa/sinus
	Postcricoid region
	Posterior pharyngeal wall
Nasopharynx	
Nasal cavity and paranasal sinuses	Nasal cavity
	Maxillary sinus
	Ethmoid sinus
	Sphenoid sinus
	Frontal sinus
Salivary glands	Parotid
	Submandibular
	Sublingual
	Minor
Thyroid	
Neck	Level I, submandibular IB and submental IA nodes
	Level II, upper jugular nodes including spinal accessory dividing into IIA and IIB
	Level III, middle jugular nodes
	Level IV, lower jugular nodes
	Level V, posterior triangle nodes divided by spinal accessory nerve in to VA and VB
Skin	
Temporal bone	

Salivary pleomorphic adenoma

Salivary pleomorphic adenoma (SPA) (benign mixed salivary tumour) is the most common tumour affecting the salivary glands. It comprises approximately 50 per cent of all salivary gland tumours, 65 per cent of parotid tumours and 40 per cent of intraoral minor salivary gland tumours.[13] The annual incidence is reported as 2.4–3.05/100 000 and shows a slight female preponderance,[11] as do most salivary gland tumours (**Figure 6.5**).

Table 6.3 Classification of tumours by histogenesis with examples.

Cell type		Examples	
		Malignant	**Benign**
Epithelial		Squamous cell carcinoma	Papilloma
		Basal cell carcinoma	
Neuroectodermal	Central	Olfactory neuroblastoma	
	Peripheral	Malignant Melanoma	Paraganglioma
		Neuroendocrine carcinoma	
		Merkel cell tumour	
Mesenchymal	Lymphoproliferative	Lymphoma	
	Vascular	Angiosarcoma	Nasopharyngeal angiofibroma
	Bone	Osteosarcoma	Osteoma
	Odontogenic		Ameloblastoma
	Cartilage	Chondrosarcoma	Chondroma
	Nerve	Nerve sheath tumour	Schwannoma
	Smooth muscle	Leiomyosarcoma	Leiomyoma
	Skeletal muscle	Rhabdomyosarcoma	Rhabdomyoma
	Adipose tissue	Liposarcoma	Lipoma
	Fibrous	Fibrosarcoma	Fibroma
Salivary gland	Epithelial and myoepithelial	Mucoepidermoid carcinoma	Pleomorphic adenoma
		Adenocarcinoma	Warthin's tumour
	Non-epithelial	Lymphoma	Haemangioma
		Sarcoma	Lipoma

Table 6.4 WHO classification of benign salivary gland tumour and tumours-like lesions.[11, 12]

Benign epithelial tumours	Tumour-like lesion
Pleomorphic adenoma	Sialadenosis
Myoepithelioma	Oncocytosis
Basal cell adenoma	Necrotizing sialometaplasia
Warthin's tumour	Benign lymphoepithelial lesion
Oncocytoma	Salivary gland cyst
Canalicular adenoma	Chronic submandibular sialadenitis (Küttner tumour)
Sebaceous adenoma	Cystic lymphoid hyperplasia in AIDS
Lymphadenoma – sebaceous/ non-sebaceous	
Ductal papillomas: inverted ductal papilloma intraductal papilloma sialadenoma papilliferum	
Cystadenoma	

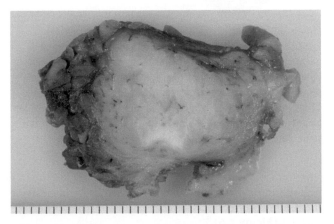

Figure 6.5 Salivary pleomorphic adenoma. The cut surface of a typical salivary pleomorphic adenoma displaying a solid blue/grey hue characteristic of chondromyxoid matrix. More cellular examples tend to be tan or cream/white. Note the localized sessile capsular herniation.

MACROSCOPIC APPEARANCE

SPAs tend to be well demarcated, round or ovoid with broad-based surface bosellations, are firm and freely movable. There may be areas of metaplasia (e.g. lipometaplasia) or retrogression (e.g. cystic change, calcification). They are variably encapsulated and, where present, the capsule may be interrupted, part-circumferential, thick or thin. The cut surface may either be homogeneous or variegated, dependent upon the precise histological pattern. Protuberant pericapsular nodules may be seen, sometimes attached to the main body of the tumour by a slender pedicle, although it may not be apparent in the plane of section examined and with time any such initial connection may regress leading to free lying satellite tumourlets. Simple enucleation of the body of a pleomorphic adenoma risks detaching these nodules, which remain behind forming a nidus for recurrence. Predominantly myxoid examples may be semi-fluid and fluctuant – perioperative capsular rupture and spillage may seed

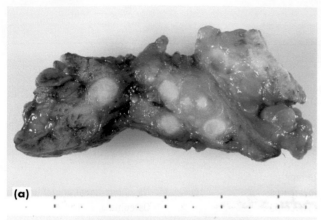

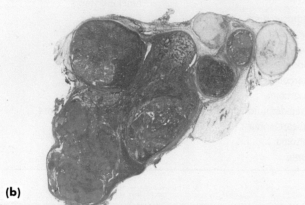

(a)

(b)

Figure 6.6 Recurrent salivary pleomorphic adenoma. (a) Excision of multinodular recurrence of salivary pleomorphic adenoma encompassing the original surgical field, consequent upon incomplete removal at first operation. (b) Whole mount section of another local recurrence showing secondary seeding of fat, residual salivary gland and fibrous tissue. The nodules are clearly of differing composition despite having arisen from the same parent lesion (H&E stain, ultralow magnification).

tumour throughout the operative field, again intensifying the risk of recurrence. Such recurrences are classically multinodular (**Figure 6.6**).[9]

MICROSCOPIC APPEARANCE

SPA arguably presents the greatest morphological diversity of any mammalian neoplasm. Its basic components are epithelium and modified myoepithelium, intermingled with stroma of chondromyxoid appearance and/or mucomyxoid ground substance.[11] The appearances vary widely both between adenomas and within the same tumour. A panoply of other changes may be superimposed or even predominate, e.g. metaplastic differentiation (squamous, lipomatous, osseous, neuroid, angiomatoid), degeneration (cystic change, infarction, mineralization, hyalinization, elastosis), specific growth patterns (e.g. pseudoadenoid cystic, clear cell, epithelial/myoepithelial carcinoma-like, basaloid, giant cell, spindle cell, acinar, plasmacytoid, oncocytoid), crystalloid deposition, dysplasia and malignant transformation.

Table 6.5 Seifert's classification of salivary pleomorphic adenoma.[15]

Subtype	Stromal content
1 (classical SPA)	30–50%
2	80%
3	20–30% and similar epithelial differentiation as subtype 1
4	6% with a relatively monomorphic epithelial structure

Table 6.6 Alternative subclassification system for salivary pleomorphic adenoma.[17, 18]

Subtype	Histological features
Myxoid (stroma-rich)	80% stroma
Cellular	80% cellular
Mixed (classical SPA)	

This heterogeneity can occasionally make diagnosis difficult, especially from limited volume needle core biopsies, incisional biopsies or FNAC.[14]

Subclassification of pleomorphic salivary adenoma into four subtypes has been proposed based on stromal content (**Table 6.5**). A modified version differentiates three subtypes (**Table 6.6**).[15, 16]

This histological classification has limited clinical relevance:

- Myxoid tumours may be more prone to recurrence,[16, 19] but this finding is not consistent.[19, 20]
- Myxoid tumours have more delicate, easily damaged capsules.
- Minor salivary gland pleomorphic adenomas tend to be cellular and unencapsulated.[10]

RISK OF MALIGNANT TRANSFORMATION

Clinical features that are associated with an increased risk of malignant transformation include:[13, 21]

- occurrence in the submandibular gland;
- older patient age;
- tumour size greater than 4.5 cm;
- duration of tumour.

Warthin's tumour

Warthin's tumour (adenolymphoma, papillary cystadenoma lymphomatosum) is the second most common tumour of the salivary glands. It is virtually exclusive to the parotid gland and periparotid lymph nodes[11, 22] and can be multicentric and/or bilateral in 4–10 per cent of cases.[10, 22] It comprises between 3.5 and 30 per cent of primary epithelial salivary gland tumours with geographical variation.[11] It occurs in Caucasians and Asians with a lower incidence in African-Americans and Black Africans.[11]

It can occur over a wide age range, but is common in the sixth decade for women and seventh decade for men.[22] It is more common in males but the male:female ratio has reduced over the last few decades.[11]

There is a link between Warthin's tumour, cigarette smoking[23] and radiation.

MACROSCOPIC APPEARANCE

The tumour is a circumscribed, often thinly encapsulated soft mass that contains multiple cystic and solid/papillary areas, which is white to brown in colour. There may be coagulated tan exudate in the cystic spaces.

MICROSCOPIC APPEARANCE

Warthin's tumour is composed of ciliated, bilayered oncocytic (oxyphilic) epithelium supported by reactive lymphoid stroma. The cystic areas contain amorphous debris.

Warthin's tumour can undergo infarction or degeneration and metaplastic change either spontaneously or secondary to manipulation (e.g. FNAC, incisional biopsy). Benign oncocytic epithelial inclusions are commonly seen in intraparotid and periparotid lymph nodes. When papillary and/or cystic, these have been termed 'embryonal Warthin's tumours' and the phenomenon probably accounts for Warthin's tumour's propensity for multicentricity and bilaterality. Paucilymphocytic Warthin's tumours may closely mimic oncocytic adenoma (oncocytoma) of salivary origin. Malignant transformation, either carcinomatous or lymphomatous is exceptionally rare (**Figure 6.7**).

BENIGN EPITHELIAL NEOPLASMS

Squamous cell papilloma

Papillomas are benign epithelial lesions that can affect the oral cavity, larynx, sinonasal tract, and nasopharynx.

They are typically polypoidal or verrucoid lesions arising from the epithelial surface and can be solitary or multiple lesions depending on site and subtype.

ORAL CAVITY AND OROPHARYNX

The pathological features of oral cavity and oropharynx papillomata are listed in **Table 6.7**.

LARYNX

Squamous cell papilloma (and recurrent respiratory papillomatosis) is the most common benign epithelial neoplasm affecting the larynx. It has a bimodal distribution with a peak before the age of five and a second between 20 and 40 years of age.[11] There is convincing evidence that recurrent respiratory papillomatosis is due to human papillomavirus (HPV) infection, with HPV6 and 11 as the dominant subtypes.[28]

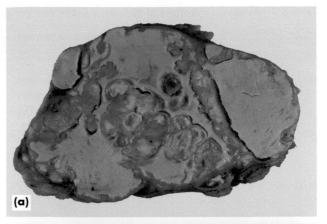

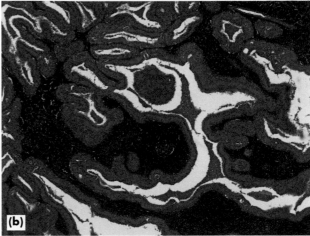

Figure 6.7 Warthin's tumour. (a) The characteristic papillocystic cut surface appearance of Warthin's tumour. Oncocytic epithelium is typically mid-brown. The light tan micronodules correspond to reactive lymphoid follicles. The coagulated cyst contents have retracted slightly during fixation. (b) Well-polarized fronds of oncocytic epithelium supported by hyperplastic lymphoid stroma surrounding cystic lumina are obvious microscopically (H&E stain, ultralow magnification).

Macroscopically, the lesions are exophytic or sessile with a fine lobular surface that can be prone to bleeding when subjected to even minor trauma.

Microscopically, the lesions have a typical papilloma appearance of hyperplastic squamous epithelium overlying a fibrovascular core. Branching papillae covered by thin squamous epithelium may be seen, associated with a basal and parabasal cell proliferation. Koilocytes are often focally present in the upper and superficial zones and contain perinuclear halos.[16]

Immunohistochemical and other studies can confirm evidence of HPV infection, but are not required for diagnosis, treatment or to predict clinical behaviour.

SINONASAL TRACT

Unlike the oral cavity and the larynx, papilloma of the sinonasal tract is relatively uncommon. Sinonasal papillomas arise from the ectodermally derived ciliated epithelium of the nasal cavity, termed the 'Schneiderian membrane'. There are three morphologically distinct types of papillomas.[29]

Table 6.7 Pathological features of oral cavity and oropharynx papillomas.

Subtype	Squamous papilloma or verruca vulgaris	Condyloma acuminatum	Focal epithelial hyperplasia, Heck's disease
HPV status	Approximately half are associated with HPV infection, typically for squamous papilloma HPV6 and 11 and HPV2 and 57 for verruca vulgaris.[24] Other HPV subtypes implicated include 4, 13 and 32[25]	Associated with HPV6, 11.[11, 26, 27] Transmission is venereal or autoinoculation and there is an association with genital condyloma	HPV13 and 32. Disease of children, adolescents and young adults
Macroscopic appearance	Wart-like exophytic lesion	Dome-shaped exophytic nodules which are usually larger than squamous papilloma	Multiple clusters or patches of soft, plaque-like lesions

HPV, human papilloma virus.

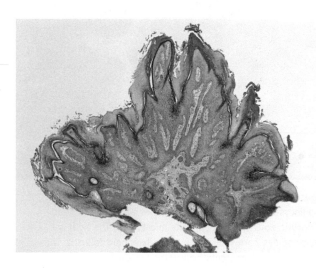

Figure 6.8 Exophytic/fungiform nasal papilloma. Classical exophytic/fungiform nasal papilloma characterized by its radially symmetrical, acrohyperkeratotic outline (H&E stain, ultralow magnification).

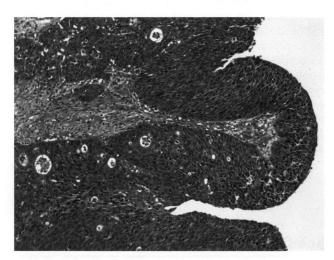

Figure 6.9 Inverted sinonasal papilloma. Inverted sinonasal papilloma illustrating a papilliform surface. This is composed of non-keratinizing squamous and transitional cell-like epithelium with scattered intraepithelial microabscesses. There is no significant cytonuclear atypia in this field (H&E stain, medium magnification).

Exophytic (fungiform) papilloma typically arises on the septum around the nasal vestibule. It closely resembles verruca vulgaris (filiform viral wart) and is associated with HPV6, HPV11, HPV16 and HPV57b. It has no known malignant potential (**Figure 6.8**).

Inverted sinonasal papilloma (Ringertz tumour) may present anywhere within the nose and paranasal sinuses, occasionally elsewhere within the upper aerodigestive tract (e.g. larynx, lacrimal apparatus). It shows a complex, arborescent exoendophytic growth pattern with primary, secondary and tertiary ramifications into underlying stroma. Numerous intraepithelial microabscesses are characteristic and stain for macrophage markers. The epithelium may be squamous (usually non-keratinizing), respiratory glandular, transitional cell-like or a mixture in any combination or permutation. There is historically a contentious association with HPV infection, yet to be conclusively resolved. The tumours may be synchronously or metachronously multicentric, taken as evidence supporting the field

cancerization effect and because it is difficult to achieve adequate surgical clearance, there is a risk of persistence/recurrence. With each recrudescence, the likelihood of dysplasia and ultimately malignant transformation heightens – invasive squamous cell carcinoma, adenosquamous carcinoma and adenocarcinoma in decreasing frequency supervenes (**Figure 6.9**).

Cylindrical cell papilloma (microcystic papillary adenoma, oncocytic Schneiderian papilloma) is unassociated with HPV infection. It comprises exophytic fronds of bilayered, well polarized, oncocytic (oxyphilic) epithelium supported by fibrovascular subintima. Microabscesses confined to the epithelium are invariable, distinguishing it from Rhinosporidiosis with secondary oncocytic metaplasia where subepithelial microcysts are more usually seen. There is a predilection for persistence/recurrence if incompletely excised, but malignant transformation is exceptional.

Benign mesenchymal tumours

SCHWANNOMA

Schwannomas (neurilemmomas) are benign encapsulated tumours that originate from the Schwann cells of the peripheral nerve sheath. Schwannoma in the head and neck may arise from the cranial nerves including Vth and VIIth–XIIth, sympathetic chain, cervical or brachial plexus. It is the most common neoplasm affecting the temporal bone,[11] vestibular schwannoma and a common site of occurrence is the neck,[10] but it is rare in the oral cavity.[30]

NF2 gene is a tumour suppressor gene which is inactivated in 67 per cent of schwannoma, which are in the main sporadic in origin.[31, 32, 33]

Approximately 2 per cent are due to neurofibromatosis 2, which is an uncommon autosomal dominant (mutation on chromosome 22) condition characterized by the presence of bilateral vestibular schwannomas and an increased incidence of extra- and intracranial meningiomas.

Macroscopic appearance

Schwannomas of the upper aerodigestive tract and temporal bone are unencapsulated and those in the soft tissue are encapsulated. The tumour is attached to an identifiable nerve and is firm to rubbery with a tan-white to yellow colour. At operation, it may be mistaken for a lymph node and excised without seeking to preserve or repair the nerve, thereby sustaining unexpected neurological damage.

Microscopic appearance

The tumour consists of alternating fields of:

1. Antoni A areas formed by fasciculated (herringbone-like), closely packed monomorphous spindle cells with fibrillar cytoplasm. The cells sometimes form a palisaded arrangement around acellular, collagenized foci known as Verocay (neuroid) bodies.
2. Antoni B areas where haphazardly orientated, the spindle cells are randomly arranged within a loose myxoid stroma.

Secondary areas of vascular wall hyalinization, microcystic degeneration, haemorrhage, foam cell infiltration and calcification may be seen. Focal bizarre, hyperchromatic and multinucleate giant cell transformation is sometimes encountered. In the absence of increased numbers of mitoses, abnormal mitotic spindles, necrosis or other atypical features, this is designated ancient change, probably a degenerative phenomenon, which is of no known clinical relevance.

Most schwannomas are immunoreactive for S100 protein distinguishing them from neurofibromas, which are less commonly positive, but also show neurofilament protein-positive fibres. Confident distinction may occasionally be impossible invoking the rubric benign peripheral nerve sheath tumour, not further specified (**Figure 6.10**).

Paraganglioma

Paragangliomas are tumours of neuroendocrine origin arising from the extra-adrenal paraganglia of the autonomic

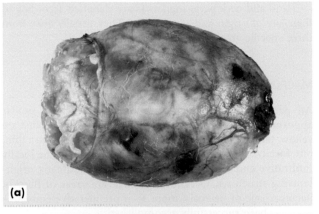

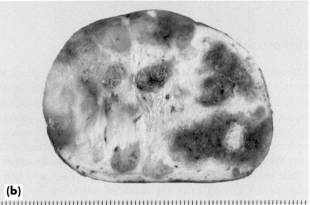

Figure 6.10   Schwannoma. (a) Encapsulated schwannoma from parapharyngeal space giving a smooth surfaced nodal appearance, although the capsule is deficient at one pole. This arises eccentrically from nerve trunk in contrast to neurofibroma, which expands the nerve fibres in a fusiform fashion. (b) The cut surface displays a variegated texture corresponding to areas of Antoni A and Antoni B growth pattern.

nervous system. The extra-adrenal paraganglia can be divided into sympathetic, which occur along the axial region of the trunk, and parasympathetic, which are localized almost entirely in the head and neck region in close association to branches of cranial nerves IX and X. They can also be described as functioning or non-functioning.

Much of the clinical terminology to describe paragangliomas is descriptive and historical (glomus tumours, e.g. glomus jugulare, glomus vagale, glomus tympanicum) and chemodectoma (carotid body tumour) – paraganglioma is now widely accepted as the unifying diagnostic term for these neoplasms.[11]

Head and neck paragangliomas have a familial tendency, which has traditionally been stated as 10 per cent, but with greater understanding of the mode of inheritance, it is felt that 50 per cent or more of head and neck paragangliomas are familial.[34] Head and neck paragangliomas are inherited as an autosomal dominant trait with genetic imprinting, which explains why it is only paternal transmission of the gene that leads to development of a paraganglioma even if the father is unaffected.[34] The affected genes code for subunits of succinate dehydrogenase protein, a mitochondrial enzyme. The genes are found on chromosome 1 and 11.[35]

Head and neck paragangliomas are classified according to their site of origin and innervation. They usually arise from three specific areas (**Table 6.8**).

MACROSCOPIC APPEARANCE

All paragangliomas, irrespective of site have very similar appearance. They are firm well-circumscribed lesions that are yellow, tan, brown or reddish in colour. They can have a thin, but focally thickened, fibrous capsule. They may be locally infiltrative and not easily excised without sacrificing neighbouring structures. Occasionally, there are areas of fibrosis, haemorrhage or necrosis, more so if preoperative embolization has been successfully accomplished.

MICROSCOPIC APPEARANCE

The neoplastic chief cells are arranged in distinctive spherical nests (zellballen) and trabecula within a richly vascularized fibrous stroma. A slender sustentacular cell population typically mantles the cell islands. The chief cells possess cytoplasmic storage granules containing a variety of neuropeptides, whereas the sustentacular cells do not. Chief cells may show random nuclear enlargement and hyperchromasia. While mitoses, necrosis, locally infiltrative growth and lymphovascular emboli raise the index of suspicion for overt malignant behaviour and metastatic risk, conventional histomorphological criteria do not reliably predict aggressive potential in any individual case. They are, therefore, generally all considered to be of borderline malignancy potential.

The chief cells stain positively for neuropeptide products (e.g. chromogranin A, synaptophysin) and CD56. The sustentacular cells are S100 protein immunoreactive. A low Ki67 proliferation fraction is reassuring. With the exception of a proportion of paragangliomas of the cauda equina, all other paragangliomas are epithelial marker negative, which is a useful aid in the differential diagnosis between paraganglioma, carcinoid tumours and pituitary neoplasms.

Preoperative embolization procedures induce a variety of degenerative changes (e.g. hydropic injury, haemorrhage, infarction, necrosis) causing diagnostic difficulty, exacerbated by consequent spurious immunohistochemical profiling (**Figure 6.11**).

The malignant potential of paraganglioma is listed by site in **Table 6.9**.

MALIGNANT DISEASE

Malignant disease of the head and neck is the sixth most common form of cancer with 65 000 new cases and 350 000 cancer deaths worldwide per annum.[38] The group as a whole accounts for over 8000 cases and 2700 deaths per year in England and Wales.[39] The majority of tumours arise from the epithelial-lined upper aerodigestive tract, but can also occur in connective tissue (sarcoma, etc.), lymphoid tissue (lymphoma), skin (melanoma, squamous and basal cell carcinoma) and major and minor salivary glands. The incidence of laryngeal cancer in England during 2007 was 5.7 per 100 000 (1436 cases) in males and 1.1 per 100 000 (278 cases) in females. The incidence rate of cancer of the lip, oral cavity

Table 6.8 Site and features of head and neck paragangliomata.

Name of paraganglion	Location	Features
Carotid body	Carotid bifurcation	Most common site (60%) for paraganglioma in head and neck.[36] They occur primarily in adults typically 40–50 years of age. Hypoxia is a risk factor and explains the gender difference (males:females = 8.3:1) seen in altitudes greater than 2000 m[11] 31% of familial tumours are bilateral compared to 4% of sporadic[36]
Jugulotympanic	Jugular bulb (glomus jugulare) and promontory on medial of middle ear cleft (glomus tympanicum)	Second most common site for head and neck paraganglioma. The sporadic form is more common in females, while the familial form is more common in males[36]
Vagal	Found within or adjacent to the vagus nerve usually near the ganglion nodusum (largest and most inferior of the three ganglia)	Account for less than 5% of head and neck paragangliomas.[36] Most are sporadic, more common in women and occur over a wide age range[11]
Laryngeal	Superior and inferior paraganglia of the larynx	Rare, more common in women and over a wide age-range[11]
Miscellaneous	Orbit[37] Thyroid gland[36] Sinonasal[36]	

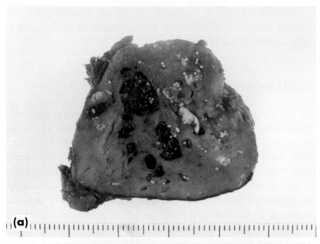

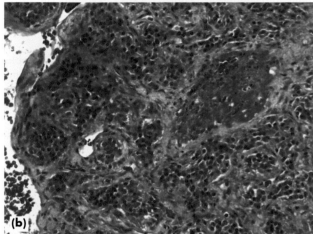

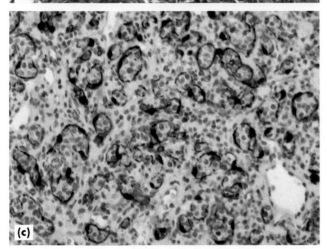

Figure 6.11   Paraganglioma. (a) Cross-section through a recently embolized, subsequently excised paraganglioma. There is early haemorrhagic infarction. Scores of beaded embolization microspheres and fresh intravascular thrombosis are readily apparent. (b) Morphologically bland chief cells in zellballen configuration and trabecular array amidst a richly endowed vascular interstitium. Sustentacular cells are not especially conspicuous (H&E stain, high magnification). (c) The same tumour immunostained for S100 protein highlights a considerable sustentacular cell population outlining groups of chief cells (S100 protein immunohistochemistry (IHC), high magnification).

Table 6.9   Malignant potential of paraganglioma by site.

Paraganglioma	Malignant potential
Carotid body	Varies from 6–12%[11, 36, 37] and sporadic tumours more likely than familial to be malignant[11]
Jugulotympanic	4%[36]
Vagal	16%[36]

and pharynx was 12.8 per 100 000 (3215 cases) in males and 6.6 per 100 000 (1717 cases) in females (www.statistics.gov.uk/statbase/Product.asp?vlnk = 8843). Skin cancer, including cutaneous malignant melanoma (and also primary intracranial tumours) are conventionally excluded from the epidemiological statistics relating to head and neck cancers.

Anatomically, the head and neck is divided into over 30 specific subsites (ICD10 codes) and malignancy at each one individually is relatively uncommon, though many have similar behaviour and progression. Knowledge of the subsite helps determine the likely pattern of spread to cervical lymph nodes and aids in treatment planning for surgery, radiotherapy and/or chemotherapy.

TUMOUR STAGING

Cancer of the head and neck, due to the diversity of pathology and the variation in progression due to anatomical subsites, cannot be meaningfully staged by a single, generic schema.

An ideal staging system has many attributes: precise, site-specific, reproducible, valid, minimal interobserver variability and stable, but must also be simple, easy to use, flexible to account for new advances and widely used.

The TNM system, which evolved from the work of Pierre Denoix in the 1940s, is the only widely accepted staging system available endorsed by both the International Union Against Cancer (UICC) and the American Joint Committee for Cancer Staging (AJCC). There are international expert committees that keep the system under formal continual review and the seventh edition has recently been published by both the AJCC and UICC with implementation from January 2010. There have been some minor changes in TNM staging of the head and neck compared to the sixth edition (2002) and these have been highlighted below (see also Chapter 4, Assessment and staging).

Four categories within the TNM schema are described:

1. **Clinical.** cTNM or TNM is based on findings and assigned prior to starting first definitive treatment.
2. **Pathological.** pTNM is based on the cTNM modified by further information obtained from surgery, especially pathological examination.
3. **Retreatment.** rTNM is used when further treatment is required or recurrence noted after a disease-free interval.
4. **Autopsy.** aTNM is used when the cancer is only classified from the results of post-mortem examination and no evidence of cancer was evident prior to death.

Other descriptors of TNM may occasionally be used and include:

- **'m' suffix**, which is used when there is more than one primary at a single site pT(m)NM;
- **'y' prefix** is used when classification is performed during or after initial multimodality therapy ycTNM or ypTNM.

Tumour differentiation refers to how well developed or mature the malignant cells are. Well-differentiated cells resemble normal cells and tend to grow and spread at a slower rate. There is, however, often morphological heterogeneity both between different tumours of the same type and also within the same tumour. Conventionally, tumours are histologically subtyped according to their best differentiated component. They are graded with reference to their worst differentiated elements on the premise that it is these which will behave most aggressively, and thereby be the major determinant of prognosis.

- Gx, grade cannot be assessed
- G1, well-differentiated
- G2, moderately differentiated
- G3, poorly differentiated.

The presence or absence of residual tumour is classified as:

- Rx, the presence of residual tumour cannot be assessed
- R0, no residual tumour is present
- R1, microscopic residual tumour
- R2, macroscopic residual tumour.

T classification by anatomical subsite

For T classification by anatomical subsite, see **Table 6.10**.[40]

Stage grouping

See Chapter 4, Assessment and staging.

CARCINOMAS

The majority of tumours of the head and neck develop from the epithelial-lined upper aerodigestive tract.

Squamous cell carcinoma

Squamous cell carcinoma (SCC) and its variants represent by far the most common malignant tumour affecting the head and neck region, accounting for approximately 95 per cent of all primary tumours of the oral cavity, oropharynx, larynx, hypopharynx and the most common epithelial tumour of the sinonasal tract, but it is uncommon in the major salivary glands and thyroid, although these may be affected by direct contiguous invasion from neighbouring structures or metastatic spread. Head and neck squamous cell carcinoma (HNSCC) arises from skin or other mucosa-lined tissue.

Typically, HNSCC spreads by direct invasion or via regional lymphatics, although haematogenous spread, especially to the lungs, is possible.

SQUAMOUS EPITHELIAL DYSPLASIA

HNSCC, especially of the oral cavity and larynx, typically originates from a non-invasive (*in situ*) neoplastic epithelial precursor lesion, which may be localized or represent wider field change phenomenon. The stages of preinvasive proliferation, ranging from squamous hyperplasia through to carcinoma *in situ* are cumulatively termed squamous intraepithelial lesion (SIL). Further subclassification denotes proposed 'epithelial dysplasia' or generically 'intraepithelial neoplasia' qualified either by the epithelial type (e.g. squamous intraepithelial neoplasia (SIN), keratinocyte intraepithelial neoplasia (KIN)) or the anatomical subsite (e.g. laryngeal intraepithelial neoplasia (LIN), oral intraepithelial neoplasia (OIN), etc.).

Progression to invasive malignancy is not inevitable, which implies that such lesions may remain stable over time or possess the capacity to regress – indeed most lesions do not proceed to invasive carcinoma in the observed timescale of the studies published to date. The more severe the dysplasia, *pari passu* the greater the risk of transformation into malignant disease. For example, the risk of malignant transformation of oral dysplastic lesions is 10.3 per cent for mild to moderate dysplasia and 24.1 per cent for severe dysplasia and carcinoma *in situ* (CIS, pTis).[41] In the larynx, the risk of progression to invasive carcinoma is 0–11.5 per cent for mild dysplasia, 0–45 per cent for moderate dysplasia, 19–54.5 per cent for severe dysplasia and 15.7–63 per cent for CIS.[42]

It follows that the aetiology of squamous epithelial dysplasia is identical to that of HNSCC and is explained in greater detail below.

Macroscopically, these lesions are irregular, circumscribed lesions with a white (leukoplakia), red (erthyroplakia) or variegated appearance (leukoerythroplakia) (**Figure 6.12**). It can be difficult to differentiate macroscopically between dysplasia and invasive carcinoma, *ergo* microscopical analysis is vital.

Histologically, the diagnosis of squamous epithelial dysplasia is based on both cytonuclear and architectural abnormalities, which are broadly comparable across various sites both within the head and neck and outside (e.g. oral intraepithelial neoplasia (OIN), squamous intraepithelial lesion (SIL), cervical intraepithelial neoplasia (CIN), vulval intraepithelial neoplasia (VIN), anal intraepithelial neoplasia (AIN), penile intraepithelial neoplasia (PIN), etc.), even though the pathogenesis and exact biological implications at each site may differ. This may be further graded according to the degree of epithelial thickness involved (e.g. low/high grade, SIN 1/2/3, mild/moderate/severe/CIS). Full thickness abnormality corresponds to intraepithelial carcinoma (carcinoma *in situ*, pTis) – note that proponents of the SIN nosology merge the categories of SIN 3 and carcinoma *in situ* (intraepithelial carcinoma, pTis).

The grading of dysplasia remains challenging with over 20 systems developed for this purpose, though as yet neither generally ratified criteria nor internationally unified terminology. All the current systems are subjective and, due to the

Table 6.10 T classification by anatomical subsite.[40]

Anatomical site		
Lip and oral cavity	T1	Tumour ≤ 2 cm in greatest dimension
	T2	Tumour > 2 cm, but < 4 cm in greatest dimension
	T3	Tumour > 4 cm in greatest dimension
	T4a	Moderately advanced disease
		Lip – tumour invades through cortical bone, inferior alveolar nerve, floor of mouth or skin (chin and nose)
		Oral cavity – tumour invades cortical bone, deep/extrinsic muscles of tongue, maxillary sinus or skin of face
	T4b	Very advanced disease
		Tumour invades masticator space, pterygoid plates and skull base, or encases internal carotid artery
Oropharynx	T1	Tumour ≤ 2 cm in greatest dimension
	T2	Tumour > 2 cm, but < 4 cm in greatest dimension
	T3	Tumour > 4 cm in greatest dimension
	T4a	Moderately advanced disease
		Tumour invades any of larynx, deep/extrinsic muscles of tongue, medial pterygoid, hard palate and mandible
	T4b	Very advanced disease
		Tumour invades any of lateral pterygoid muscle, pterygoid plates, lateral nasopharynx and skull base or encases internal carotid artery
Hypopharynx	T1	Tumour limited to one subsite of hypopharynx and ≤ 2 cm in greatest dimension
	T2	Tumour invades more than one subsite of hypopharynx or an adjacent site, or measures > 2 cm, but < 4 cm in greatest dimension, without fixation of the hemilarynx
	T3	Tumour > 4 cm in greatest dimension, or with fixation of the hemilarynx
	T4a	Moderately advanced disease
		Tumour invades any of the following: thyroid/cricoid cartilage, hyoid bone, thyroid gland, oesophagus, central compartment soft tissue
	T4b	Very advanced disease
		Tumour invades prevertebral fascia, mediastinal structures or encases internal carotid artery
Larynx – supraglottis	T1	Tumour limited to one subsite of the supraglottis with normal vocal cord mobility
	T2	Tumour invades mucosa of more than one adjacent subsite of supraglottis, glottis or region outside supraglottis without fixation of the larynx
	T3	Tumour limited to larynx with vocal cord fixation and/or invades any of the following: postcricoid area, pre-epiglottic tissues, paraglottic space and/or with minor thyroid cartilage erosion
	T4a	Moderately advanced disease
		Tumour extends through thyroid cartilage, and/or invades tissue beyond the larynx; soft tissues of the neck, deep/extrinsic muscles of the tongue, strap muscles, thyroid gland or oesophagus
	T4b	Very advanced disease
		Tumour invades prevertebral fascia, mediastinal structures or encases internal carotid artery
Larynx – glottis	T1	Tumour limited to the vocal cord(s), including involvement of anterior or posterior commisure with normal mobility
		T1a – Tumour limited to one vocal cord
		T1b – Tumour involves both vocal cords
	T2	Tumour extends to supraglottis and/or subglottis and/or with impaired vocal cord mobility
	T3	Tumour limited to larynx with vocal cord fixation and/or invades paraglottic space and/or with minor thyroid cartilage erosion
	T4a	Moderately advanced disease
		Tumour extends through thyroid cartilage, and/or invades tissue beyond the larynx; soft tissues of the neck, deep/extrinsic muscles of the tongue, strap muscles, thyroid gland or oesophagus
	T4b	Very advanced disease
		Tumour invades prevertebral fascia, mediastinal structures or encases internal carotid artery
Larynx – subglottis	T1	Tumour limited to subglottis.
	T2	Tumour extends to vocal cord(s) with normal or impaired vocal cord mobility
	T3	Tumour limited to larynx with vocal cord fixation
	T4a	Moderately advanced disease

(Continued over)

Table 6.10 T classification by anatomical subsite. (continued)

Anatomical site		
		Tumour extends through cricoid or thyroid cartilage, and/or invades tissue beyond the larynx; soft tissues of the neck, deep/extrinsic muscles of the tongue, strap muscles, thyroid gland or oesophagus
	T4b	Very advanced disease
		Tumour invades prevertebral fascia, mediastinal structures or encases internal carotid artery
Major salivary glands	T1	Tumour ≤2 cm in greatest dimension without extraparenchymal extension
	T2	Tumour >2 cm, but <4 cm in greatest dimension without extraparenchymal extension
	T3	Tumour >4 cm in greatest dimension and/or tumour with extraparenchymal extension
	T4a	Moderately advanced disease
		Tumour invades skin, ear canal, facial nerve or mandible
	T4b	Very advanced disease
		Tumour invades pterygoid plates, skull base or encases internal carotid artery
Nasal cavity and ethmoid sinus	T1	Tumour restricted to one subsite of nasal cavity or ethmoid sinus with or without bony invasion
	T2	Tumour involves two subsites in a single site or extends to involve an adjacent site within the nasoethmoidal complex, with or without bony invasion
	T3	Tumour extends to invade the medial wall or floor of the orbit, maxillary sinus, and palate or cribriform plate
	T4a	Moderately advanced disease
		Tumour invades any of the following: anterior orbital contents, skin of nose or cheek, minimal extension to anterior cranial fossa, pterygoid plates, sphenoid or frontal sinus
	T4b	Very advanced disease
		Tumour invades any of the following orbital apex, dura, brain, middle cranial fossa, cranial nerves other than V2 (maxillary division of trigeminal), nasopharynx and clivus
Maxillary sinus	T1	Tumour limited to mucosa with no erosion or destruction of bone
	T2	Tumour causing bone erosion or destruction, including extension into hard palate and/or middle meatus only
	T3	Tumour invades any of the following: bone of posterior wall of maxillary sinus, subcutaneous tissues, floor or medial wall of orbit, pterygoid fossa and ethmoid sinuses
	T4a	Moderately advanced disease
		Tumour invades any of the following: orbital contents beyond floor and medial wall including anterior orbital contents, skin of cheek, infratemporal fossa, pterygoid plates, cribriform plates, sphenoid or frontal sinus
	T4b	Very advanced disease
		Tumour invades any of the following: orbital apex, dura, brain, middle cranial fossa, cranial nerves other than V2 (maxillary division of trigeminal), nasopharynx and clivus
Nasopharynx	T1	Confined to nasopharynx, oropharynx and/or nasal cavity without parapharyngeal extension
	T2	Tumour with parapharyngeal extension
	T3	Tumour invades bony structures and/or paranasal sinuses
	T4	Tumour with intracranial extension and/or involvement of cranial nerves, infratemporal fossa, hypopharynx, orbit or masticator space
Regional lymphadenopathy		
All sites except nasopharynx	Nx	Regional lymph nodes cannot be assessed
	N0	No regional lymphadenopathy
	N1	Metastasis in a single ipsilateral lymph node ≤3 cm in greatest dimension
	N2a	Metastasis in a single ipsilateral lymph node >3 cm, but <6 cm in greatest dimension
	N2b	Metastasis in multiple ipsilateral lymph nodes, none >6 cm in greatest dimension
	N2c	Metastasis in bilateral or contralateral lymph nodes, none >6 cm in greatest dimension
	N3	Metastasis in a lymph node >6 cm in greatest dimension
Nasopharynx	N1	Unilateral cervical or bilateral retropharyngeal lymph node metastasis above the supraclavicular fossa, ≤6 cm in greatest dimension
	N2	Bilateral cervical lymph node metastasis above the supraclavicular fossa, ≤6 cm in greatest dimension
	N3a	Lymph node metastasis >6 cm in greatest dimension
	N3b	Lymph node metastasis in the supraclavicular fossa

Extracapsular spread (ECS+ or ECS−) is an added descriptor that does not change the nodal staging described above.

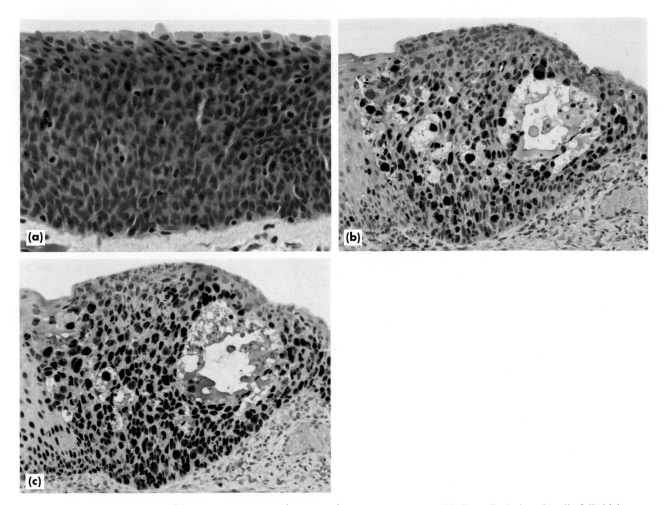

Figure 6.12 Laryngeal dysplasia. (a) Diffusely thickened (acanthotic) surface squamous epithelium displaying virtually full thickness dysmaturation amounting to high-grade dysplasia (i.e. LIN/SIN 3, pTis, carcinoma *in situ*, intraepithelial carcinoma). The basement membrane is thin and intact with no evidence of invasive carcinoma (H&E stain, high magnification). (b) Immunopreparation for Ki67, a proliferation marker, confirms nuclear positivity corresponding to the dysplastic epithelium. Staining is normally confined to the basal/parabasal layers (reserve/germinative cell or progenitor compartment), as seen to the lower left of the photomicrograph (Ki67 immunohistochemistry (IHC), high magnification). (c) Immunopreparation for p63, a tumour suppressor gene product, similarly shows aberrant full thickness staining. Positive nuclei are normally present in the lower third of epithelial thickness (p63 IHC, high magnification).

difficulty in distinguishing between normal and often subtly abnormal epithelium, they are susceptible to discrepant interobserver and intraobserver reproducibility. In reality, dysplasia is a dynamic process manifest as a continuous morphological spectrum, therefore, the rigorous application of discrete categories, whatever their arbitrary histological basis is destined to be problematical. Immunohistochemistry, molecular and other biomarkers are presently of limited assistance in resolving this.

The three most commonly used systems (**Table 6.11**) are:

1. The WHO dysplasia grading system in its present incarnation since 2005, which is similar to that used for precursor lesions in other parts of the body (e.g. uterine cervix, etc.).
2. The similarly based generic squamous intraepithelial neoplasia (SIN) style terminology, loosely modelled on the Bethesda system as originally devised for the uterine cervix.
3. The Ljubljana classification originally proposed in 1971 and refined by a working group of the European Society of Pathology in 1999, which is structured around points of clinical decision, that is minimal follow up, close follow up or surgery.

Aetiology

The main risk factors for HNSCC are tobacco and alcohol use, which either alone or combined, are implicated in 75 per cent of all HNSCC.[44] Tobacco alone increases the risk of cancer occurrence by two- to three-fold, but acts synergistically with alcohol leading to a multiplicative rather than additive increase.[44, 45, 46] Increased duration of exposure to

Table 6.11 Comparison of common grading systems for squamous epithelial precursor lesions (squamous intraepithelial lesion, SIL).[12, 43]

Definition	WHO 2005	Squamous intraepithelial neoplasia (SIN)	Ljubljana classification system
An increase in the number of cells, but with no cellular atypia	Squamous cell hyperplasia		Squamous cell (simple) hyperplasia
Changes are confined to the lower third of the epithelium	Mild dysplasia	SIN1	Basal/parabasal cell hyperplasia[a]
Changes extend to the middle third of the epithelium. Cytological changes can be more marked	Moderate dysplasia	SIN2	Atypical hyperplasia[b]
Changes involve at least two-thirds of the epithelium and atypia is more marked	Severe dysplasia	SIN3[c]	Atypical hyperplasia[b]
Changes involve the full thickness of epithelium, but with no invasion of the basement membrane	Carcinoma *in situ*	SIN 3[c]	Carcinoma *in situ*

[a]Non-neoplastic basal/parabasal ('reserve') cell hyperplasia may histologically mimic mild dysplasia, although the latter is ontogenetically a neoplastic precursor lesion.
[b]Designated 'risky epithelium' – the comparison with moderate and severe dysplasia is approximate.
[c]Most observers employing the SIN schema merge the categories of severe dysplasia and carcinoma *in situ*.

tobacco and/or alcohol increases the risk of developing HNSCC.

Tobacco contains a number of known carcinogens, e.g. polynuclear aromatic hydrocarbons, which cause DNA damage leading to gene mutations.

Alcohol causes DNA damage and gene mutation by a number of mechanisms. These include the effect of acting as a solvent for other carcinogens, nutritional deficiencies, acetaldehyde (a byproduct of alcohol metabolism) and the direct effect of ethanol.

Increasingly, since first described in 1983,[47] it is recognized that the human papilloma virus, especially HPV serotypes 16 and 18, is implicated in oropharyngeal HNSCC independent of tobacco and alcohol. HPV-positive tumours typically affect non-smokers, non-drinkers and younger patients.[48, 49]HPV-related HNSCC behaves in a less aggressive manner than non-HPV HNSCC and has a better long-term prognosis.[50] This HPV effect is less significant in larynx and other subsites.[51]

SCC of the lip is associated with sun exposure and pipe smoking. Sinonasal SCC is linked to nickel and chromate exposure and woodworking. Dietary deficiencies have also been linked to the development of HNSCC, especially vitamins (A, C and E), foods (fruit, vegetables and dairy) and elements (iron especially when associated with iron-deficiency anaemia of Plummer–Vinson–Kelly syndrome, which is associated with postcricoid SCC).[52]

Oral cavity SCC is particularly common in India where a third of all cancers originate in the head and neck. The widespread chewing of betel nut, which causes both oral submucous fibrosis, a recognized premalignant condition, and oral cavity SCC has been implicated, as well as the practice of inverse smoking.

HNSCCs are typically sporadic, but a familial inheritance has been noted in some cases. The risk of HNSCC is also increased in patients with any syndrome associated with an increased risk of cancer. Patients with Fanconi's anaemia have a 700-fold increased risk and the cancer is usually diagnosed in the third decade.

PATHOPHYSIOLOGY

HNSCC is a heterogeneous disease, but a hypothetical progression model has been proposed.[44] Histological progression from normal epithelium to hyperplasia, dysplasia, carcinoma *in situ* and finally invasive carcinoma is related to a number of factors, including genetic changes causing genetic instability leading to cellular change.[44] Genetic changes include the sequential inactivation of tumour suppressor genes and activation of proto-oncogenes by deletions, promoter methylation, gene amplification and point mutations, etc. Carcinogens produced by tobacco, which include nitrosamines and benz-(a)-pyrene, produce mutations in p53 associated with HNSCC.[48]

The molecular changes are due to a number of genetic alterations, which include loss of heterozygosity (LOH) of 9p21, seen in 70–80 per cent of HNSCC. Other abnormalities include LOH 3p, 17p, 11q and 13q.

The E6 and E7 viral oncoproteins on HPV16 and 18 cause inactivation of tumour suppressors p53 and PRb, respectively. The loss of p53-mediated response to DNA damage leads to genomic stability. Loss of PRb causes cell cycle disruption, proliferation and malignant transformation.[53]

MACROSCOPIC APPEARANCE

HNSCC appearance varies depending on subsite, but can be an exophytic or ulcerative lesion with an irregular friable, pale surface. On skin, it typically looks like a non-healing scab or ulcer, which can intermittently bleed. On mucosal surfaces, lesions typically start as whitish or reddish plaque-like lesions

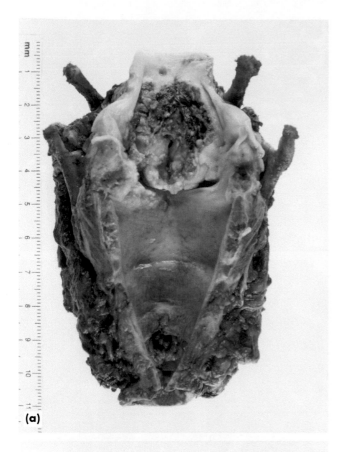

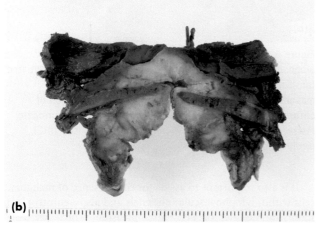

Figure 6.13 Laryngeal squamous cell carcinoma. (a) Total laryngectomy specimen opened in the posterior sagittal plane to disclose advanced, fungating carcinoma effacing much of the epilarynx and supraglottis with local extension on to the left true vocal cord. (b) Transverse section through this confirms bilateral midline tumour herniating through the anterior commissural ligament (Broyles' ligament) into anterior strap musculature without naked eye evidence of laryngeal framework destruction. Other tissue planes (weak spots) allowing tumour to gain access outside the larynx include the paraglottic space and the cricothyroid interspace.

(leukoplakia or erthyroplakia), which then progress to ulcerated, or fungating masses with irregular indurated borders (**Figure 6.13**). Invasive SCC will typically arise within a premalignant lesion and can be difficult to distinguish with

the naked eye and hence the opportunity to biopsy areas of concern even within a previously diagnosed lesion must not be missed.

MICROSCOPIC APPEARANCE

Histologically, mature squamous epithelial cells possess dense haematoxyphilic (purple/blue on H&E) nuclei with a low nucleus–cytoplasmic ratio. The more superficial cells contain smaller, pyknotic nuclei. The cytoplasm is densely eosinophilic (pink on H&E), sometimes orange and finely reticulated owing to keratin intermediate filaments. Mitoses are normally only a feature of the basal/parabasal (reserve/germinative cell or progenitor compartment) layers.

The histological appearance of HNSCC is very similar across all sites in the head and neck (larynx, skin, etc.) and further afield. Well-differentiated SCC characteristically shows cytoplasmic and/or extracellular keratinization plus intercellular prickles (spinous processes corresponding to desmosomes highlighted by cell shrinkage allowing separation between adjacent cell membranes). The term 'epidermoid' is employed for tumours displaying a subjectively squamoid morphology, albeit without this objective evidence of squamous differentiation proper.

Malignant squamous cells display some or all of the following features:

- irregular shape and orientation;
- increased and abnormal mitoses;
- nuclear hyperchromatism;
- coarse and clumped chromatin;
- nuclear pleomorphism;
- elevated nucleus–cytoplasmic ratio;
- prominent nucleoli and macronucleoli;
- premature keratinization (dyskeratosis) or loss of keratin production;
- disordered cell polarity;
- disorganized growth.

The defining feature of invasive HNSCC is breach of the subepithelial basement membrane allowing malignant cells to infiltrate into normal tissue, thereby gaining access to lymphatics, blood vessels and nerves (**Figure 6.14**). Typically, carcinoma *in situ* or areas of dysplasia will surround invasive HNSCC, although this is by no means invariable. This phenomenon of field cancerization reflects the long-term exposure of head and neck mucosa to carcinogens causing genetic alterations, which enable multifocal tumours to arise due to independent genetic events.[54, 55]

Microscopical description includes:

- histological subtype or variant, if applicable;
- histological grade;
- presence or absence of keratinization;
- histological growth pattern;
- quality of advancing margin (cohesive or non-cohesive margin: the latter is associated with a worse prognosis);
- presence of necrosis;
- intensity of host lymphocytic or other inflammatory cell response;
- stromal desmoplasia.

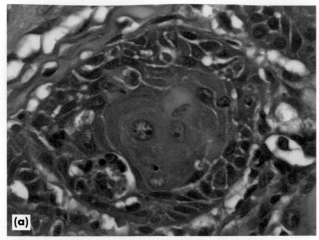

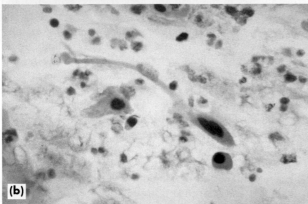

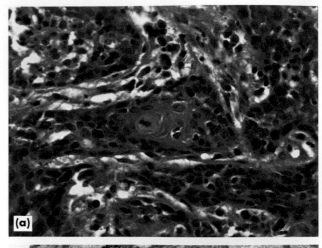

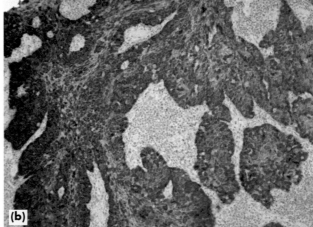

Figure 6.14 Invasive squamous cell carcinoma. (a) Well-differentiated squamous cell carcinoma illustrating definite cytoplasmic keratinization and characteristic intercellular prickles. Note the disordered cell polarity, nuclear pleomorphism (variation in size, shape and intensity of nuclear staining), coarse chromatin and prominent nucleoli (H&E stain, high magnification). (b) This cytology preparation shows several atypical squamous cells amidst a necrolytic milieu (diathesis). Note the large, binucleate caudate ('tadpole') cell, intermediate-sized obovate ('comet') cell and the smaller hyperkeratinizing orangeophilic ('carrot') cell. Other forms commonly seen include fibre ('snake') cells, acanthocytes ('spider') cells and bizarre giant ('monster') cells. Anucleate squamae, dissociated keratotic debris, parakeratotic scale ('sprigs') and keratin whorls ('pearls') may accompany these (Pap stain, high magnification).

The terms 'early stromal invasion', 'minimally invasive carcinoma' and 'microinvasive carcinoma' are sometimes casually used to denote early invasive squamous cell carcinoma of limited infiltration. However, these presently have no agreed, validated definition in the head and neck and are, therefore, potentially confusing. 'Superficial extending carcinoma' implying lack of involvement of deep structures and 'deeply invasive carcinoma' denoting infiltration into muscle and beyond, while biologically valid concepts, are also of limited clinical utility. It is more helpful to measure tumour depth and/or thickness and overall dimensions, and place this within the recognized TNM schema with any relevant subjective descriptive comments, until such time as there is a clinically relevant evidential basis for these other definitions.

Figure 6.15 Human papilloma virus (HPV)-associated oropharyngeal squamous cell carcinoma. (a) Poorly differentiated tonsillar squamous cell carcinoma (H&E stain, medium magnification). (b) Immunohistochemical demonstration of diffuse nuclear and cytoplasmic reactivity for p16, a surrogate marker for HPV infection (p16 immunohistochemistry (IHC), medium magnification).

It is also important to assess for the presence of malignant cells within lymphovascular channels and also neurotropism, signifying vascular or perineural invasion, which are associated with an unfavourable prognosis.

Cytologically, SCC may be so well differentiated that it is impossible to reliably discriminate it from non-neoplastic (hyperplastic, regenerative/reparative, metaplastic, post-irradiation) squamous epithelium, for example in FNAC from inflamed branchiogenic or other benign cysts. Furthermore, the presence of invasion per se cannot be directly evaluated on FNAC – dissociated dysplastic squamous cells may be cytomorphologically indistinguishable from detached invasive carcinomatous squamous cells proper. Paradoxically, extreme reactive atypia may exceed by some degree the limited pleomorphism of a well-differentiated invasive SCC. The presence of inflammation and necrosis (tumour diathesis), marked atypia and abnormal mitoses favour infiltration, but are by no means infallible. Obviously, the context is all important and, in experienced hands, FNAC from a cervical lymph node containing abnormal squamae against a background of proven SCC may be reasonably taken as presumptive evidence of a secondary deposit until otherwise proven.

For these reasons, only under exceptional circumstances should radical cancer treatment be undertaken on the basis of a primary diagnosis reached by FNAC without more definitive tissue diagnosis and even then rigorous clinico-radiological correlation must be exercised.

IMMUNOHISTOCHEMISTRY

The association of HPV and HNSCC (**Figure 6.15**) has become more recognized in the last few years, but testing for evidence of HPV remains difficult and controversial. PCR and/or ISH studies remain the gold standard to identify the presence of high-risk HPV DNA (HPV16 and 18). Semi-quantitative immunohistochemistry for p16 protein is used as a surrogate marker for HPV oncoprotein activity with the caveat that immunostaining is a less sensitive technique, which ought to be validated against PCR/ISH with known positive and negative controls and subject to rigorous quality control.

HNSCC VARIANTS

A number of morphological variants of SCC are recognized, which include among others:

Verrucous carcinoma (VC, Ackerman's tumour) is a controversial manifestation of well-differentiated SCC, typically occurring in the oral cavity but rarely said to occur in the larynx (1–3 per cent of all laryngeal malignancies), hypopharynx, sinonasal tract and nasopharynx plus other sites outside the head and neck.

Verrucous carcinoma, to the naked eye is a warty, exophytic lesion that arises from a broad (sessile) base. It has a superficial spreading growth, but can be deeply destructive extending into muscle, cartilage or bone. Histologically, VC lacks significant atypia and is characterized by blunt incursions and an expansile advancing margin sometimes eliciting brisk lymphocytic response. If adequately sampled, approximately 20 per cent of VCs contain areas of conventional pattern SCC, although often very localized and it is these elements, which determine overall prognosis *ab initio* independent of irradiation – some regard these as hybrid or composite tumours.

Incisional biopsy diagnosis of VC is problematical as its predominant bland morphology may be indistinguishable from benign squamoproliferative lesions on superficial or limited volume material. Typically, three or four biopsies are required, or even excision biopsy, before the overall architecture is appreciated and the diagnosis is seriously entertained. A high index of pathological suspicion and clinical persistence are thus prerequisites.

Spindle cell carcinoma (carcinosarcoma, sarcomatoid carcinoma, carcinoma with sarcomatoid stroma, Lane tumour) (**Figure 6.16**) occurs in the upper respiratory tract or less commonly the oral cavity. Patients are typically elderly males and a significant number will have had previous irradiation.

Spindle cell carcinoma usually has a polypoidal, exophytic configuration with either a broad base or narrow pedicle,

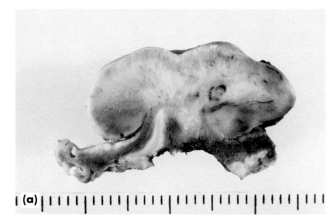

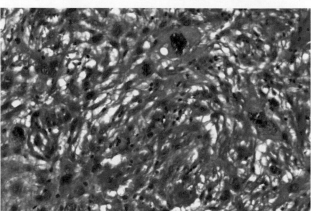

Figure 6.16 Sarcomatoid carcinoma of epilarynx. (a) Cross-section of epiglottic resection specimen, for biopsy-proven sarcomatoid carcinoma. This is ulcerated and polypoidal, but also infiltrates deeper, penetrating into and through epiglottic cartilage. (b) Representative field beneath the tumour surface exhibiting highly pleomorphic spindle and bizarre giant cells with abnormal mitoses reminiscent of undifferentiated pleomorphic sarcoma (H&E stain, high magnification).

which can occasionally autoamputate and be expectorated by the patient. The surface tends to be ulcerated.

It is usually a bimorphic lesion with areas of SCC, either *in situ* or invasive, associated with bizarre spindle cell and/or giant cell proliferation of sarcomatoid appearance. The squamous component can be difficult to identify due to the ulceration and the sarcoma-like component predominates. Immunohistochemistry may be helpful, although the spindle cells are often negative for epithelial markers, sometimes even immunoinert.

Papillary squamous cell carcinoma (confusingly also known as 'verrucous squamous cell carcinoma', apt to be confused with Ackerman's tumour) is an uncommon variant.[56] It may affect most anatomical subsites of the head and neck, including the larynx and hypopharynx.

Macroscopically, the tumour is similar to verrucous carcinoma, but lacks the typical surface keratinization. Microscopically, the lesion is composed of obviously atypical squamous cells overlying fibrovascular papilliform stromal cores. The tumour behaves in a similar manner to conventional HNSCC and management is therefore similar.

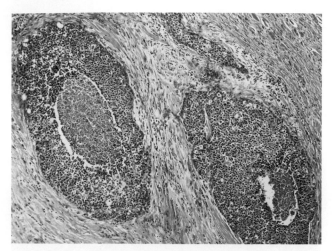

Figure 6.17 Basaloid/basaloid-cystic squamous cell carcinoma of oropharynx. Typical island of poorly differentiated basaloid-cystic squamous cell carcinoma showing central colliquative degeneration and comedo necrosis (H&E stain, medium magnification).

Adenosquamous carcinoma is an uncommon variant of HNSCC, which is considered aggressive and associated with a poor prognosis.[57, 58] It predominantly affects males in the sixth or seventh decade. The larynx, and occasionally the hypopharynx, is the most commonly affected site. Macroscopically, the tumour resembles a typical HNSCC. Microscopically, the tumour is characterized by the presence of conventional squamous cell carcinoma admixed with a variable proportion of true glanduloductal elements indicative of divergent differentiation. Mucin histochemistry and keratin immunoprofiling may aid distinction from acantholytic squamous cell carcinoma with pseudoglandular growth and also from mucoepidermoid carcinoma.

Basaloid/basaloid-cystic squamous cell carcinoma is a high-grade aggressive variant of squamous cell carcinoma typically found in middle-aged male patients affecting the oropharynx, larynx and hypopharynx (**Figure 6.17**).[59, 60] Macroscopically, these are firm to hard tumours with central necrosis and superficial ulceration. Microscopically, the tumour is infiltrating and deeply invasive and presents a typical basaloid appearance consisting of pleomorphic cells arranged in a lobular configuration with palisading.[16, 59] Cystic degeneration with central comedonecrosis is often a feature. There may be minimal objective evidence of squamous cell differentiation.

Other unconventional variants include acantholytic (pseudoadenoidal/pseudoangiosarcomatoid,) small cell, clear cell, giant cell and lymphoepithelial carcinoma. In practice, many SCCs are heterogeneous in pattern at least focally (**Figure 6.18**).

Nasopharyngeal carcinoma

Nasopharyngeal carcinoma (NPC) is a distinct subtype of squamous cell carcinoma that classically originates from nasopharyngeal mucosa, occasionally from other head and neck sites, rarely further afield. Worldwide, it is an uncommon disease with an incidence of less that 1 per 100 000,[61]

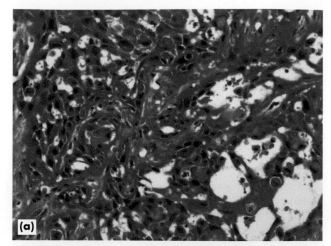

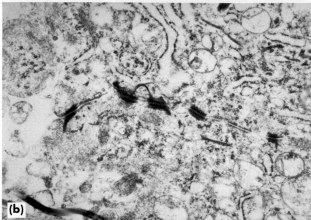

Figure 6.18 Acantholytic/pseudoangiosarcomatoid squamous cell carcinoma. (a) Acantholytic squamous cell carcinoma displaying multifocal loss of intercellular cohesion (acantholysis) forming angulated pseudoglandular interstices, most containing degenerate/apoptotic debris rather than secretions. The lack of glandular differentiation and disorderly polarity surrounding these spaces also militates against adenosquamous carcinoma (H&E stain, high magnification). (b) Transmission electron micrograph (TEM) from a destructive parotid tumour ulcerating through overlying skin. The morphology and immunohistochemistry were equivocal. Electron microscopy, however, clearly identifies five desmosomes along an intercellular junction, diagnostic of epithelial differentiation, thus supportive of squamous cell carcinoma, rather than angiosarcoma proper (TEM, ultra-high magnification).

but has a very distinct geographical distribution. In China, 18 per cent of all adult cancers are NPC and it is especially common in northern provinces, Kwantung and Taiwan, but is uncommon in children (2 per cent).[62] In contrast, 10–20 per cent of all paediatric cancers in northern and central Africa are NPC. Ethnic groups with intermediate risk include Greenland Eskimos and Maghrebin Arabs, but Caucasian populations have the lowest risk. Other factors implicated in the development of NPC include Epstein–Barr virus (EBV) and dietary factors, especially a high intake of salted fish and preserved vegetable products.

Macroscopically, the tumour can be a bulging, exophytic and lobulated, or ulcerative mass. Occasionally, there may be no visible tumour, necessitating blind biopsy of the naso-pharynx.

Microscopically, NPC is classified according to the WHO system, which is dependent on the presence or absence of keratinization. Twenty-six per cent of tumours contain more than one type and are then classified according to the dominant type:

- **I, Keratinizing squamous cell carcinoma** represents approximately 25 per cent of NPC in North America,[61, 62] but only 2 per cent of Chinese patients.[61] This type is rarely found in patients less than 40 years of age. Like HNSCC in other sites, this type of NPC can be classified as well, moderately or poorly differentiated. The cells grow in well-defined nests with easily demonstrable intercellular bridges and keratin pearl formation. The stroma undergoes a desmoplastic response to invasive growth.
- **II, Non-keratinizing NPC**, which is associated with EBV, can be divided into differentiated or undifferentiated, but is of no clinical or prognostic significance:

  - **Differentiated non-keratinizing NPC** which is the least common subtype accounting for 12 per cent worldwide (2 per cent in China).[61, 62] As the name suggests, there is little or no evidence of keratinization, vague intercellular bridges and it may undergo cyst formation. The growth pattern is analogous to transitional cell carcinoma. There is no desmoplastic response to invasive growth.
  - **Undifferentiated non-keratinizing NPC** (undifferentiated carcinoma of nasopharyngeal type, UCNT, lymphoepithelial carcinoma) is the most common subtype accounting for approximately 63 per cent of cases, rising to 95 per cent in China,[61] and is the most common type to affect children. The cells possess round nuclei, prominent eosinophilic nucleoli, and/or dispersed or microvacuolated chromatin with scant cytoplasm.[62] There is generally a prominent non-neoplastic intratumoral and peritumoral lymphoid cell infiltrate, though this may on occasion be sparse. When there is a diffuse, non-cohesive growth pattern, such malignant cells are easily overlooked on cursory inspection. Other recognized growth patterns include cohesive or nested cells. There is no desmoplastic response to invasive growth.

Immunohistochemistry can be helpful in UCNT. Epithelial cell markers highlight the malignant cells and lymphoid cell markers confirm the reactive lymphocytosis and its characteristic distribution. Antibodies against EBV LMP-1 (latent membrane protein 1) are less sensitive than *in-situ* EBER (EBV encoded early RNA) studies. These are more usually positive in Asian than European and North American patients, reflecting the strong association between NPC and EBV (**Figure 6.19**).

Basal cell carcinoma

Basal cell carcinoma (BCC) is the most common skin malignancy, especially in geographical areas with a

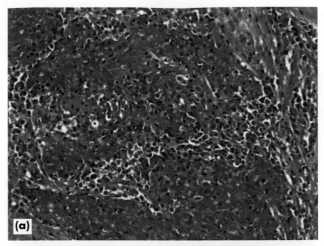

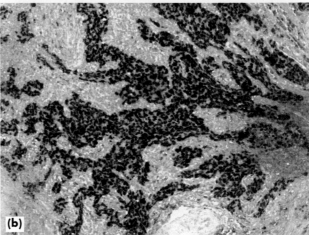

Figure 6.19 Epstein–Barr virus (EBV)-associated undifferentiated carcinoma of nasopharyngeal type. (a) Sheets of poorly differentiated, non-keratinizing malignant cells with ill-defined cytoplasmic borders imparting a syncitial appearance. The nuclei are variously vacuolated or nucleolated. Small lymphocytes are present within and surrounding the tumour cells (H&E stain, medium magnification). (b) *In-situ* hybridization (ISH) for EBER confirms a diffusely positive nuclear signal indicating EBV infection (EBER ISH, medium magnification).

predominantly Caucasian population. Australia accounts for 80 per cent of non-melanoma skin malignancies. The tumour can involve skin in any region, but most commonly affects the head and neck region (85–93 per cent) and very rarely metastasizes (0.1 per cent). There is a high risk (35–50 per cent) of developing further lesions at other sites in the head and neck or distant region.

According to the UICC/AJCC TNM classification, carcinoma of the vermillion border of the lip and commissures qualifies as a head and neck cancer, though in practice there may be some degree of collaboration with the dermato-oncology multidisciplinary team (MDT) in the management of such patients, dependent upon local circumstances.

There are myriads of histological patterns of BCC, although these can be more broadly categorized as low-risk variants (e.g. nodular, nodulocystic, adenoidal, keratotic, pigmented) and high-risk variants (e.g. superficial/multifocal, infiltrative, morphoeic/fibrosing, micronodular, basi-squamous) according to their propensity to locally aggressive behaviour and/or risk of local recurrence. In practice, many BCCs display more than one growth pattern.

EPIDEMIOLOGY

The incidence of BCC has been increasing over the last few decades. There are a number of risk factors associated with the development of BCC, which are listed below.

Risk factors

- Cumulative ultraviolet (UV) exposure including the potentiating effect of some chemicals and severe sunburn during childhood and adolescence.
- Patients with fair skin (Fitzpatrick types I and II), which can be associated with red hair, are at a higher risk than patients with dark skin (Fitzpatrick type VI).
- Exposure to ionizing radiation.
- Patients who are immunosuppressed, e.g. AIDS or transplantation.
- Arsenic and other chemical exposure due to their toxic effect.
- A number of syndromes are associated with the development of BCC, including Gorlin's syndrome, xeroderma pigmentosum, and epidermolysis verruciformis.

MACROSCOPIC APPEARANCE

Growth patterns of basal cell carcinomas are outlined in **Table 6.12**.

MICROSCOPIC APPEARANCE

BCC are composed of hyperchromatic basaloid cells within a fibromucinous stroma. The cells are typically small and uniform. Rarely, they can contain giant tumour cells, clear cells, granular cells and signet ring cells. Mitoses are conspicuous.

Most BCCs are clearly invasive and can infiltrate deeply when located in regions of embryonic fusion planes (e.g. around the nose and ears). Whether superficial BCC represents *in-situ* or early invasive disease remains enigmatic (**Figure 6.20**).

In most cases, BCC is distinctive on routine examination, but occasionally immunohistochemistry is employed to aid

Table 6.12 Basal cell carcinoma growth patterns.

Subtype	Appearance
Nodular	Pearly papule with translucent rolled edges with occasional ulceration
Pigmented	Can be confused with seborrhoeic keratosis or even nodular melanoma
Superficial	Well-demarcated, scaly, erythematous plaque. Typically occurs on the trunk and extremities
Morpheaform	Difficult to diagnose. Ill-defined indurated plaque, [61, 62] which can resemble a scar

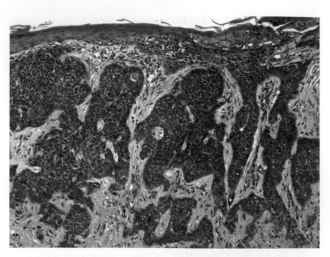

Figure 6.20 Cutaneous basal cell carcinoma. Part of a basal cell carcinoma, nodular subtype showing focal contiguity with overlying stratum basalis and incipient surface ulceration (H&E stain, low magnification).

discrimination from SCC or other neoplasms – both SCC and BCC characteristically express intense and diffuse high molecular weight cytokeratins, cytokeratin 5 (or cytokeratin 5/6) and nuclear p63 staining, thus absence of staining with these markers merits consideration of some other diagnosis. Most SCCs show substantial epithelial membrane antigen (EMA) positivity, whereas BCC is usually negative. BCC is typically immunoreactive for Ber-EP4, unlike cutaneous SCC, which is usually negative though non-cutaneous SCCs may sometimes express this marker. Smooth muscle actin (SMA) positivity is seen in a significant proportion of BCCs, but rarely in cutaneous SCC. BCCs are generally diffusely bcl-2 positive with skin SCCs being negative or only focally staining. bcl-6 is positive in a minority of SCCs, but rarely positive in BCC. p16 immunoreactivity is expressed at a higher frequency in SCC compared to BCC and broadly correlates with the histological grade of SCC.

The status of squamous differentiation in BCC is historically controversial. There is no consensus definition for usage of the term 'basi-squamous carcinoma'. The descriptor 'metatypical' is sometimes used to designate rare tumours with intermediary features between BCC and SCC. Nonetheless, BCCs showing moderate/severe squamous cell atypia portend a higher risk of recurrence and/or metastasis. A minor degree of squamous cell atypia is not unusual in BCCs showing trichogenic differentiation and this is of no known biological significance.

Adenocarcinoma

This is a glandular malignancy that typically affects the sinonasal tract and specifically has no features diagnostic of the various salivary gland adenocarcinomas.

There are two main subtypes of adenocarcinoma:

1. Intestinal type adenocarcinoma
2. Non-intestinal type adenocarcinoma.

EPIDEMIOLOGY

Adenocarcinoma, along with the salivary gland type malignancies, account for 10–20 per cent of sinonasal tumours.[11]

Intestinal-type adenocarcinoma is associated with cumulative exposure to hard wood dust and leather dust and the tumour typically occurs in the ethmoid sinus.[63] The tumour can arise from any sites in the sinonasal tract, usually the upper part of the nasal cavity or maxillary sinus, but in these cases there is usually no association with wood dust exposure.[64]

There does appear to be a male preponderance and this is likely due to occupational exposure.[11]

Sinonasal intestinal-type adenocarcinoma may be morphologically and immunohistochemically indistinguishable from metastatic colorectal adenocarcinoma.

MALIGNANT SALIVARY GLAND DISEASE

Malignant salivary gland tumours are very uncommon and represent approximately 0.5 per cent of all malignancies, 5 per cent of all head and neck cancers and an incidence in the Western world of 2.5–3/100 000/year.[13]

Despite the low incidence, over 40 named malignant salivary gland neoplasms are recognized (**Table 6.13**). This section will describe the pathological characteristics of the more common malignant neoplasms and the authors recommend reference to a specific head and neck pathology atlas for information regarding less common tumours.[11, 18, 31]

Mucoepidermoid carcinoma

Mucoepidermoid carcinoma is the most common malignant salivary gland neoplasm (12–29 per cent of all salivary gland malignancies).[18] It typically affects the parotid gland, but may also occur in the minor salivary glands. The tumour is triphasic comprising goblet cell mucocytes, epidermoid cells (usually with little keratinization) and nondescript cells of intermediate size and shape.

EPIDEMIOLOGY

There is a low frequency of mucoepidermoid tumour in the UK (2 per cent), compared with the rest of Europe (15–20 per cent). It is found more frequently in female patients and can present at any time between the first and ninth decade, but peaks in the fifth decade.[31, 65] The major risk factor for development is previous therapeutic radiation exposure with a latent period of 7–32 years.[31] The growth and outcome is influenced by the histological grade of the tumour.

MACROSCOPIC APPEARANCE

The tumour has a variety of appearances. It can be unencapsulated or incompletely encapsulated, circumscribed or infiltrative. Tumours are predominantly solid, tan-white to pink masses, often cystic filled with a viscous brown fluid. Areas of scarring can also be present and may occasionally prevail.

Table 6.13 WHO classification of salivary gland malignancy.[11, 12]

Malignant epithelial tumours	Haematolymphoid tumours
Acinic cell carcinoma	Hodgkin's lymphoma
Mucoepidermoid carcinoma	Diffuse large B-cell lymphoma
Adenoid cystic carcinoma	Extranodal marginal zone B-cell lymphoma (MALToma)
Polymorphous low-grade adenocarcinoma	
Clear cell carcinoma NOS	
Epithelial/myoepithelial carcinoma	
Basal cell adenocarcinoma	
Sebaceous carcinoma	
Sebaceous lymphadenocarcinoma	
Cystadenocarcinoma	
Low-grade cribriform cystadenocarcinoma	
Mucinous adenocarcinoma	
Oncocytic carcinoma	
Salivary duct carcinoma	
Adenocarcinoma NOS	
Myoepithelial carcinoma	
Carcinoma ex-pleomorphic adenocarcinoma	
Carcinosarcoma	
Metastasizing pleomorphic adenoma	
Squamous cell carcinoma	
Small cell carcinoma	
Large cell carcinoma	
Lymphoepithelial carcinoma	
Sialoblastoma	
Secondary tumours	

MICROSCOPIC APPEARANCE

The tumour consists of varying proportions of admixed mucinous, epidermoid and intermediate type cells. Low-grade tumours are macrocystic and microcystic with plentiful mucocytes, fewer epidermoid cells and infrequent intermediate type cells. Extravasated, dissecting mucin pools may be seen. There may be a sclerosing/fibrosing component. Reactive tumour-associated lymphoproliferation is characteristic.[18] High-grade tumours are more solid and contain fewer mucinous elements with a preponderance of atypical epidermoid cells and epidermoid cells. High-grade tumours are easily mistaken for SCC and recourse to exhaustive sampling augmented by a panel of mucin histochemistry may be diagnostic.

This diversity makes FNAC interpretation challenging.[14] The behaviour of mucoepidermoid carcinoma is very varied and various systems have been proposed to attempt to grade tumours and hence predict outcome. A commonly used system is described in **Table 6.14**.[16, 65]

High-grade tumours tend to be aggressive compared to low-grade tumours, although immaterial of grade

Table 6.14 Grading system for mucoepidermoid carcinoma.[65]

Parameter		Point value
Intracystic component <20%		+2
Neural invasion		+2
Necrosis		+2
Mitotic figures <4/10 HPF		+3
Anaplasia		+4
Grade	Total score	% Death from disease
Low	0–4	3.3%
Intermediate	5–6	9.7%
High	7–14	46.3%

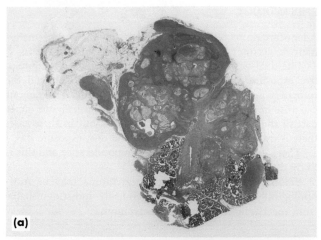

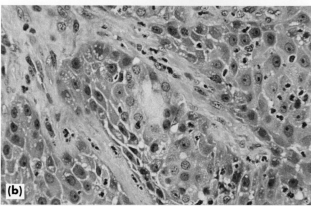

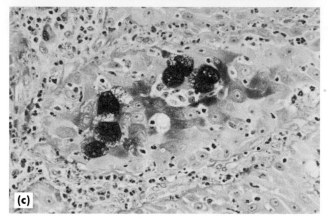

Figure 6.21 Mucoepidermoid carcinoma. (a) Whole mount slide of a low-grade mucoepidermoid carcinoma illustrating an expansile multilobulated architecture, substantial macrocystic and microcystic growth plus peripheral lymphoid tissue response (H&E stain, ultralow magnification). (b) Intermediate-grade tumour depicting epidermoid cells surrounding a rudimentary tubuloductal lumen lined by goblet cell mucocytes, characterized by abundant microvacuolated cytoplasm. It may require a determined search to find these cells in higher grade tumours (H&E stain, high magnification). (c) The same tumour stained for neutral mucosubstances corroborates intracytoplasmic mucin and aids identification of such cells (dPAS stain, high magnification).

mucoepidermoid tumours have a tendency to metastasize, which is not reliably predictable from conventional histomorphological criteria in any individual case.

Central mucoepidermoid carcinoma (**Figure 6.21**) is defined as tumour developing in an area, which normally lacks any salivary gland tissue, typically the mandible near the third molar region and associated with an unerupted tooth or cyst. The tumours are usually low-grade and definitive diagnosis can be difficult until tumour excision.[66]

Acinic cell carcinoma

EPIDEMIOLOGY

Acinic cell carcinoma accounts for 7–17.5 per cent of all malignant salivary gland neoplasms. Approximately 80 per cent arise from the parotid gland and the remaining 20 per cent arising mainly from the minor salivary glands or submandibular glands, and only 1 per cent from the sublingual gland.[18] There is a male preponderance and they usually present in the third decade of life.[67]

MACROSCOPIC APPEARANCE

Macroscopically, the tumours are of a firm to rubbery consistency and range in colour from a tan-grey to yellow or pink mass. They are usually rounded, well circumscribed and can be encapsulated. They can contain areas of haemorrhage or cystic change. Recurrent tumours tend to be less well-demarcated and can appear multinodular.[18, 32]

MICROSCOPIC APPEARANCE

Acinic cell carcinomas recapitulate the serous acinar cell of normal salivary gland tissue, containing zymogen granules in the cytoplasm. Reactive lymphoid stroma is characteristic and may mimic lymph node involvement.[67]

There are a number of recognized growth patterns, which can coexist in a single tumour (**Table 6.15**).

Histochemical stains for zymogen granules may be positive. Immunohistochemically, the most useful stain is alpha-amylase. Reactivity, however, is variable and unpredictable – of note, the papillary-cystic variant is postulated to show

intercalated ductal rather than acinar differentiation and attempts to demonstrate cytoplasmic granules are generally non-contributory (**Figure 6.22**).

Table 6.15 Growth patterns of acinic cell carcinoma.

Growth pattern	Features
Microcystic	The tumour has a lattice-like appearance due to the presence of microcysts
Solid	Cells aggregate into sheets forming lobules or nodules
Papillary–cystic	The tumour contains prominent cysts with intraluminal papillary projections
Follicular	Contain multiple variable-sized cysts loosely resembling thyroid parenchyma

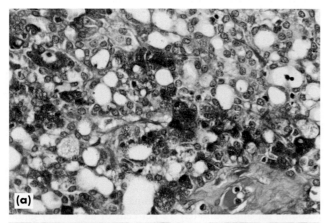

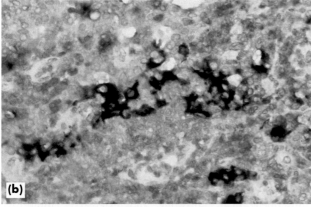

Figure 6.22 Acinic cell carcinoma. (a) Well-differentiated example of solid and follicular growth pattern acinic cell carcinoma composed of serous acinar-like secretory cells containing purple zymogen granules (dPAS stain, high magnification). (b) Immunostaining on the same case confirms alpha-amylase reactivity for these same intracytoplasmic granules (alpha-amylase immunohistochemistry (IHC), high magnification).

Adenocarcinoma not otherwise specified

Adenocarcinoma not otherwise specified (NOS) refers to malignant tumours with glandular or ductal differentiation that do not have specific histologically defining features to enable further subclassification as a recognized subtype.

EPIDEMIOLOGY

Adenocarcinoma NOS is the second[11] or third[32] most common malignant salivary gland neoplasm. It is more common in women and frequently seen in the fifth to eighth decade with a mean age of diagnosis of 58 years[13] and rarely seen in adolescents or children.[11] Sixty per cent occur in the major salivary glands, usually the parotid and 40 per cent occur in the minor salivary glands.

MACROSCOPIC APPEARANCE

Macroscopically, tumours appear as a firm tan-white mass, which can be circumscribed to poorly demarcated with an irregular periphery and potentially infiltrative appearance. There may be areas of haemorrhage, cystic change or necrosis.

MICROSCOPIC APPEARANCE

Adenocarcinoma NOS is a diagnosis of exclusion and therefore tumours that fall within this category can display a variety of features. Common to all tumours in this group is the presence of glandular or ductal features, an invasive growth pattern and the lack of histological characteristics of other salivary adenocarcinomas.

The malignant epithelium can display various architectural features including glandular, ductal, papillary, solid, nest-like, etc. There may be clear cell change and/or mucinous differentiation. The tumours can also be graded into low, intermediate and high based on the degree of gland formation, cellular pleomorphism and mitotic count.

- Low-grade tumours have easily identifiable gland and duct-like structures. There is usually a single cell type with small nucleoli, abundant cytoplasm, distinct cell borders and little nuclear pleomorphism with few mitoses. This can occasionally lead to a benign diagnosis if the invasive growth is not identified.
- Intermediate-grade tumours also have easily identified gland and duct-like structures. Unlike low-grade tumours, there is greater nuclear pleomorphism with more mitoses.
- High-grade tumours tend to be solid, with areas of haemorrhage and necrosis. Unlike low- and intermediate-grade tumours, the gland and duct-like structures are much harder to identify. The cells are much more abnormal and varied. Cellular features include frequent atypical mitoses and enlarged, hyperchromatic, pleomorphic nuclei.

Adenoid cystic carcinoma

EPIDEMIOLOGY

Adenoid cystic carcinoma (ACC) accounts for approximately 10–12 per cent of all malignant salivary gland tumours and is the most common malignant tumour of the submandibular gland. It represents approximately 5 per cent of parotid neoplasms and 30–50 per cent of minor salivary gland neoplasms.[31] There is no sex predilection and it is usually seen in patients in their forties to sixties, rarely in patients less than 20 years old.

Lower-grade ACC pursues a pernicious course typified by relentless, troublesome local recurrence, ultimately presaging wider dissemination after a prolonged interval of years or even decades. Many malignant salivary gland tumours show a proclivity for perineural growth, though this is paradigmatic for ACC with perineural sheath and intraneural growth, the latter commonly visualized microscopically some considerable distance beyond what would be regarded as adequate clearance adjudged by the unaided eye. This neurotropism may radiate in a tentacular fashion well beyond the main body of the tumour. Positive surgical resection planes are, therefore, sometimes an unexpected and unwelcome feature of pathology reports, as this signifies a heightened risk of local recurrence. Obversely, the histological suggestion of clearance from the planes of section usually available examined by routine sampling is not particularly reassuring. High-grade (solid) ACC is an aggressive, destructive malignancy.

MACROSCOPIC APPEARANCE

The tumour is usually a poorly circumscribed solid white tumour. ACC is usually unencapsulated and infiltrates into surrounding soft tissue, muscle and bone sometimes directly through lymph node capsules.

MICROSCOPIC EXAMINATION

Bilroth originally described adenoid cystic carcinoma in 1856 and called it a cylindroma, reflecting the jigsaw arrangement of the cells on microscopical examination.[68]

There are often two recognizable malignant cell subpopulations representing epithelial and myoepithelial components. Three pure growth patterns have been described but many tumours are mixed.[69]

- **Tubular pattern** represents the most differentiated form of adenoid cystic carcinoma.[70] Small nests of cells form few true glandular or tubuloductal spaces and occasional cords.
- **Cribriform pattern** is the most common pattern and most tumours will contain areas displaying this pattern even if not the predominant type.[69] In addition to true gland lumina containing secretions, cells group to form multiple pseudocysts (pseudolumina) containing mucoid basement membrane material. The overall pattern resembles 'Swiss cheese'. This architecture represents an intermediate level of cellular proliferation and biological aggressiveness.[70]
- **Solid pattern** is the least common type and unlike the other two types there are few if any glandular spaces. Cells in the solid type tend to be larger and more pleomorphic with mitoses,[31] interspersed with areas of necrosis.[69] A biphasic cell population may not be apparent and without at least some better-differentiated fields, it may be impossible to arrive at the diagnosis.

ACC may be graded according to the predominant growth pattern:[31]

- I, mostly tubular with some cribriform elements;
- II, either entirely cribriform or cribriform/tubular with less than 30 per cent solid component;
- III, any tumour with more than 30 per cent solid growth.

Histochemistry for mucosubstances may demonstrate both true secretions and basement membrane deposits. Immunohistochemical staining for laminin and type IV collagen duplicates the latter. Staining for epithelial markers typically highlights the luminal secretory cells and myoepithelial cell markers decorate the basally located abluminal cells, which mantle the basement membrane material (**Figure 6.23**).

Carcinoma ex-pleomorphic adenoma

Carcinoma ex-pleomorphic adenoma arises from within a pre-existing salivary pleomorphic adenoma or at the site of a previous pleomorphic adenoma.

EPIDEMIOLOGY

Carcinoma ex-pleomorphic adenoma is not uncommon and accounts for approximately 12 per cent of all salivary gland malignancies and 6.2 per cent of all pleomorphic adenomas.[71] Risk factors for malignant transformation of a pleomorphic adenoma include a submandibular gland site, prolonged duration of tumour, older age of patient (mean, 61 years) and tumour greater than 4 cm.[72] It commonly affects the parotid gland and rarely the sublingual gland.[31]

There is no gender predilection and patients typically present in the sixth to seventh decade.[11]

MACROSCOPIC APPEARANCE

Carcinoma ex-pleomorphic adenoma tends to be larger than its benign counterpart.[11] Tumours tend to be poorly circumscribed, firm, tan-white and extensively infiltrative masses. They can occasionally be well circumscribed and appear encapsulated. The residuum of a pre-existing adenoma is often identified, sometimes alluded to by an effete fibroelastotic, occasionally mineralized vestigial scar. The malignant component tends to radiate centrifugally from this nidus, if present (**Figure 6.24**).

MICROSCOPIC APPEARANCE

The malignant element of a carcinoma ex-pleomorphic adenoma typically comprises high-grade adenocarcinoma or salivary duct carcinoma often with squamoid differentiation, but other specific subtypes of salivary carcinoma are seen and these may on occasion be monotypic rather than mixed.[18] The benign pleomorphic adenoma component can be difficult to identify, may require extensive sampling and in some cases it may never be identified.

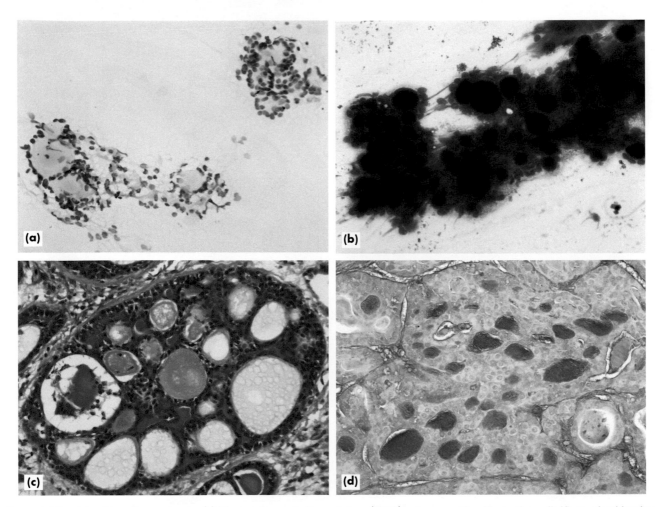

Figure 6.23   Adenoid cystic carcinoma. (a) Fine needle aspiration cytology (FNAC) cytopreparation illustrating cribriform microbiopsies. The characteristic hyaline basement membrane globules are pale in this preparation (Pap stain, medium magnification). (b) FNAC slide showing similar features albeit with striking intense staining of the hyaline globules (May–Grünwald-Giemsa (MGG) stain, medium magnification). (c) Classical cribriform adenoid cystic carcinoma demonstrating pseudolumina filled with variably dense basement membrane type droplets, together with true gland lumina, either empty or containing sparse secretions (H&E stain, high magnification). (d) Histochemical preparation highlighting the basement membrane material. The true gland lumina are negative (Alcian blue, high magnification). (e) Complementary histochemistry confirming true glandular luminal secretions. The pseudolumina have not stained (dPAS stain, high magnification). (f) Immunohistochemical demonstration of abluminal myoepithelial cells delimiting the basement membrane droplets. The luminal cells are negative (S100 protein immunohistochemistry (IHC), high magnification). (g) Immunopreparation showing reciprocal staining of the true glandular epithelial luminal cells. The myoepithelial cells are negative (epithelial membrane antigen IHC, high magnification).

The association of pleomorphic adenoma, carcinoma and sarcoma (carcinosarcoma, true malignant mixed tumour) is very rare, as is the phenomenon of benign metastasizing pleomorphic adenoma, which may be completely indistinguishable histologically from the usual non-metastasizing examples.

Invasion of tumour through the original lesion's capsule carries prognostic significance and has been classified as:[11]

1. **Non-invasive**. Also called dysplasia, intracapsular carcinoma or *in-situ* carcinoma ex-pleomorphic adenoma.
2. **Minimally/microinvasive carcinoma**. <1.5, 5 or 8 mm invasion.
3. **Frankly invasive carcinoma**. >1.5, 5 or 8 mm invasion.

In principle, (1) and (2) have a favourable prognosis compared to (3), although the precise cut-off point to define a category of invasion with minimal metastatic potential is presently unascertained.[73]

Ordinary benign pleomorphic adenomas may show peripheral permeative growth, lymphatic tumour embolus, necrosis and focal internal cytonuclear atypia without signifying malignant transformation. Caution should be exercised in the interpretation of such features if prior FNAC has been attempted. Such tumours are sometimes termed 'atypical pleomorphic adenoma' and generally behave no differently from their more typical counterparts. The wide morphological heterogeneity of pleomorphic adenoma potentially includes localized areas of pseudoadenoid cystic and epithelial/myoepithelial carcinoma-like growth, which may result in overdiagnosis of malignancy on FNAC by the unwary.

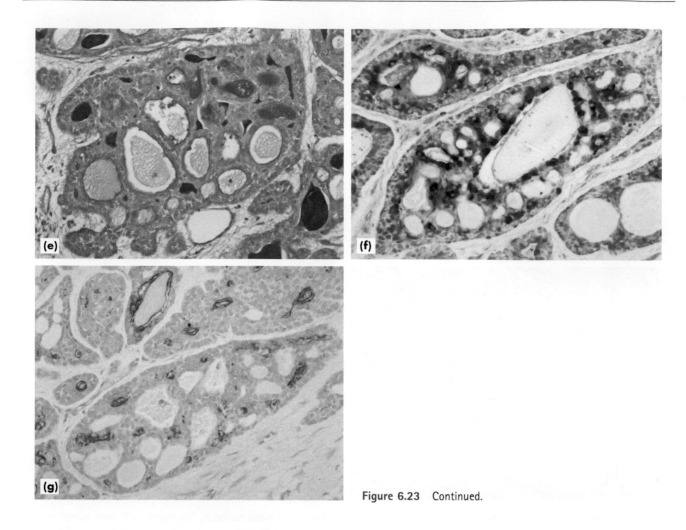

Figure 6.23   Continued.

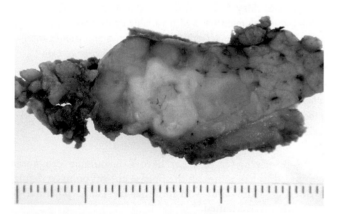

Figure 6.24   Carcinoma ex-salivary pleomorphic adenoma. Cut surface of a longstanding adenoma seen centrally forming a discrete, cream, elastotic scar with focal calcification. This is part-circumferentially surrounded by peripheral lobules of tan carcinoma ex-adenoma, in this example pure acinic cell carcinoma.

NEUROECTODERMAL TUMOURS

Neuroectodermal tumours can be divided into two groups. The first group shows evidence of epithelial differentiation, e.g.

carcinoid tumour of the larynx. The second group is a diverse group of tumours that shows non-epithelial differentiation.

Olfactory neuroblastoma

These are uncommon malignant tumours of the upper nasal cavity affecting specialized olfactory mucosa and arising from the superior turbinate, cribriform plate and superior one third of the nasal septum (**Figure 6.25**).[74] The reported incidence is four cases per million with a bimodal distribution in the second and sixth decade, and no sex or racial predeliction.[11]

MACROSCOPIC APPEARANCE

Macroscopically, olfactory neuroblastoma appears as a soft, polypoidal, highly vascular mucosa-covered mass.

MICROSCOPIC APPEARANCE

The malignant cells are uniform, with small round nuclei, scant cytoplasm and possess finely stippled (salt and pepper) chromatin.[11]

Hyam's classification system divides olfactory neuroblastoma into four types (**Table 6.16**).[9]

The better-differentiated (grade I and II) examples are sometimes termed 'aesthesioneuroblastoma'. Homer–Wright pseudorosettes are formed by cells mantling solid, fibrillary neuropil stroma. Flexner–Wintersteiner rosettes consist of cells surrounding an empty pseudolumen. Other tumours may form perivascular rosettes encircling blood vessel lumina.

Immunohistochemistry may aid discrimination between this and other primitive neoplasms (so-called round blue cell tumours), such as lymphoma, Ewing's tumour, melanoma, Merkel cell tumour, rhabdomyosarcoma, nephroblastoma, retinoblastoma and PNET.[74] There is, however, no single specific positive marker.

Mucosal malignant melanoma

Mucosal malignant melanoma (MMM) is a rare tumour that originates from melanocytes. These are of neuroectodermal derivation and migrate to ectodermally derived mucosa during embryogenesis.[75]

Between 15 and 20 per cent of malignant melanomas arise in the head and neck but the vast majority, over 80 per cent, are of cutaneous or upper aerodigestive tract origin. Mucosal malignant melanoma represents merely 0.5–3 per cent of malignant melanomas from all sites.[10]

Common sites for mucosal malignant melanoma include the sinonasal tract and the oral cavity.[11] Uncommon sites include the nasopharynx, larynx and other sites with non-ectodermally derived mucosa.[75]

It is more common in men, but this finding is not consistent,[11] and the tumour affects a wide age range (20–80 years).

MACROSCOPIC APPEARANCE

Mucosal melanomas are usually pigmented and colour ranges from a light tan to black depending on the amount of melanin production, though amelanotic examples do occur. There is a confounding propensity for primary lesions to spontaneously regress.

MICROSCOPIC APPEARANCE

They typically comprise epithelioid and/or spindle cells. Plasmacytoid, rhabdoid, small cell, giant cell, balloon cell, neurotropic and desmoplastic variants are recognized. The cells are markedly pleomorphic and may contain pigment. Nucleoli are conspicuous and intranuclear inclusions are typical. An adjacent inflammatory infiltrate and necrosis can also be present.[11] Surrounding melanocytic atypia or melanoma *in situ* may mantle vertical growth phase disease.

Histochemical confirmation of brown pigment as melanin may be helpful. With few exceptions, the cells show nuclear and cytoplasmic immunoreactivity for S100 protein. Vimentin, HMB-45, melan A and CD56 are usually positive. Epithelial markers are reciprocally negative, although up to 10 per cent of melanomas may show focal cytokeratin reactivity. Coexpression of CD10 is associated with tumour progression. The desmoplastic variant may be substantially immunoinert.

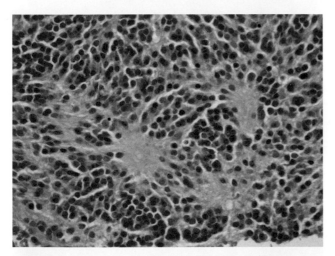

Figure 6.25 Grade I/II olfactory neuroblastoma. Loosely cohesive, uniform, small cells including two Homer–Wright pseudorosettes centred around fibrillary neuropil material. Mitoses are inconspicuous. There is no necrosis (H&E stain, high magnification).

Other neuroectodermal tumours

Other neuroectodermal tumours include Ewing sarcoma, primitive neuroectodermal tumour and melanotic neuroectodermal tumour of infancy.

Table 6.16 Hyam's grading classification of olfactory neuroblastoma.[9]

Histological feature	Grade 1	Grade II	Grade III	Grade IV
Architecture	Lobular	Lobular	May be lobular	May be lobular
Pleomorphism	Absent or slight	Present	Prominent	Marked
Neurofibrillary matrix	Prominent	Present	May be present	Absent
Rosettes	Homer–Wright rosettes (pseudo-rosette) present	Homer–Wright rosettes (pseudo-rosette) present	Flexner–Wintersteiner (true rosettes) may be present	Flexner–Wintersteiner (true rosettes) may be present
Mitoses	Absent	Present	Prominent	Marked
Necrosis	Absent	Absent	Present	Prominent
Glands	May be present	May be present	May be present	May be present
Calcification	Variable	Variable	Absent	Absent

HAEMATOLYMPHOID TUMOURS

Lymphoma is the second most common primary malignancy occurring in the head and neck region. In white populations, lymphoma is a more common cause of cervical lymphadenopathy than metastatic disease. Approximately 25 per cent of all extranodal lymphomas occur in the head and neck. Thus, although in the UK the overwhelming majority of haematolymphoid tumours, predominantly lymphomas and leukaemias, are managed by specialist haemato-oncology multidisciplinary teams, head and neck surgeons are frequently involved in the initial diagnosis of lymphoma. It, therefore, behoves the head and neck pathologist to possess a sound working knowledge of lymphoproliferative conditions

and their differential diagnosis. Access to expert second opinion is inevitable at some point.

It is beyond the ambit of this chapter to delve into the complexities of lymphoma diagnosis and the interested reader is referred to the comprehensive World Health Organization (WHO) classification of tumours of haematopoietic and lymphoid tissues (fourth edition, 2008), which is internationally recognized, periodically reviewed and updated.[76] This takes a multiparameter approach to classification incorporating clinical, morphological and immunophenotypical features plus genetic studies into account with the expectation that the schema will continually evolve and be refined over time.

Lymphomas are broadly divided into Hodgkin's lymphoma (HL) and non-Hodgkin's lymphoma (NHL). HL is characterized by Reed–Sternberg cells and is subdivided into classical HL (incorporating nodular sclerosing, mixed cellularity, lymphocyte-rich and lymphocyte-depleted subtypes) and

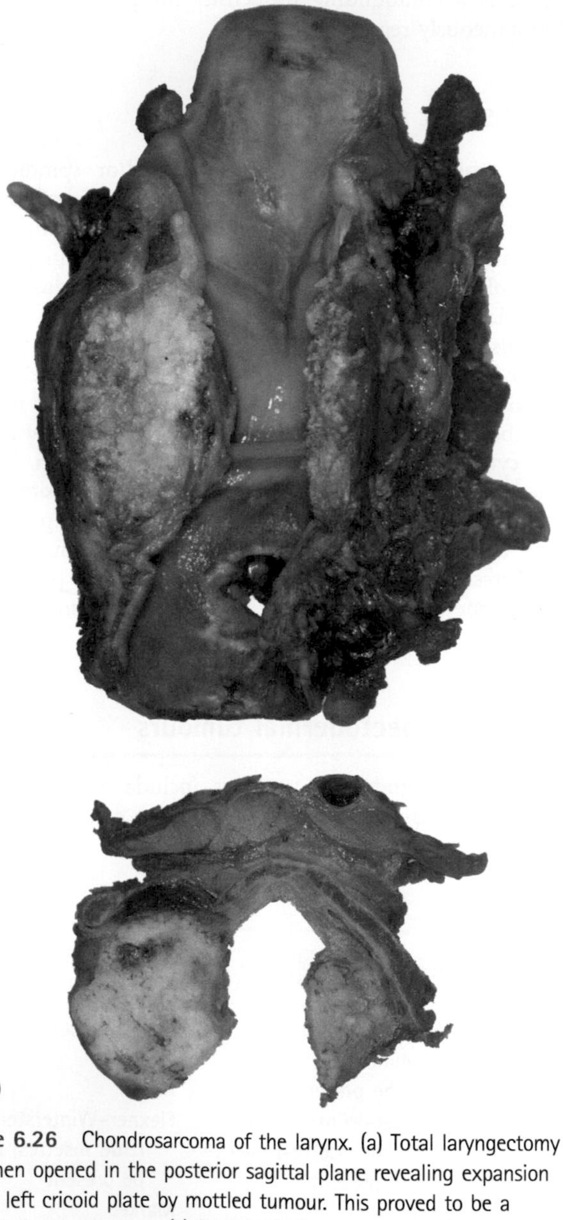

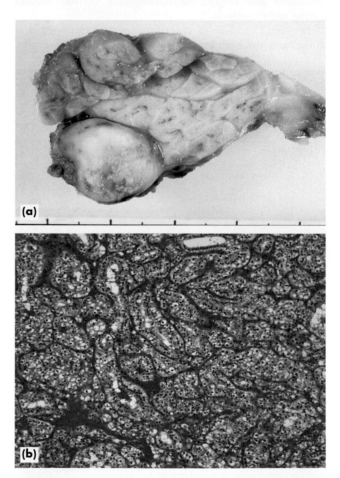

Figure 6.26 Chondrosarcoma of the larynx. (a) Total laryngectomy specimen opened in the posterior sagittal plane revealing expansion of the left cricoid plate by mottled tumour. This proved to be a grade I chondrosarcoma. (b) Representative transverse slice through the subglottis demonstrating a multilobulated contour crossing the midline posteriorly, mottled bluish colouration and speckled calcification imparting a gritty texture.

Figure 6.27 Metastatic disease in the head and neck. (a) Cut surface appearances of metastatic amelanotic malignant melanoma effacing a periparotid lymph node without overt extracapsular spread or direct infiltration into parotid salivary parenchyma. (b) Metastatic clear cell carcinoma from an unsuspected occult renal cell primary site presenting as disseminated malignancy in the head and neck. Renal cell carcinoma has a propensity for spread to a wide variety of sites and metastatic relapse may occur after a lengthy latency–interval period of a decade or more (H&E stain, medium magnification).

nodular lymphocyte predominant HL, according to site of involvement, clinical features, growth pattern, presence of fibrosis, composition of cellular background, number and/or degree of atypia of the tumour cells and frequency of Epstein–Barr virus (EBV) infection. The immunophenotype of the neoplastic cells in these classical HL subtypes is identical.

Roughly 85 per cent of NHLs are B-cell lymphomas, which include follicular lymphoma, marginal zone lymphoma and MALT lymphomas, the latter often extranodal involving the mucosa-associated lymphoid tissue of Waldeyer's ring including the ocular adnexa and thyroid gland (NHL of the thyroid gland is more common than undifferentiated (anaplastic) carcinoma of the thyroid gland). Diffuse large B-cell lymphoma is the most common aggressive NHL. Mantle cell lymphoma and Burkitt's lymphoma are aggressive NHLs sometimes seen in the head and neck. Cutaneous T-cell NHLs (e.g. mycosis fungoides) may be indolent. Peripheral T-cell NHLs, however, may behave more aggressively. Extranodal NK/T-cell lymphoma is strongly associated with EBV and shows a predilection for the upper aerodigestive tract, prototypically the nasal cavity. Its angiocentric and angiodestructive nature may simulate Wegener's granulomatosis and other midline facial necrotizing conditions (so-called 'idiopathic midline destructive disease' in the older literature).

Plasma cell neoplasms, most commonly plasma cell myeloma and extramedullary plasmacytoma, are occasionally encountered in the head and neck region.

Mesenchymal tumours

Apart from the lymphomas, mesenchymal tumours are uncommon malignancies of the head and neck. Malignant mesenchymal tumours (sarcomas) include:

- Fibrosarcoma
- Malignant fibrous histiocytoma
- Leiomyosarcoma
- Rhabdomyosarcoma
- Liposarcoma
- Angiosarcoma
- Kaposi sarcoma
- Malignant peripheral nerve sheath tumour
- Synovial sarcoma
- Chondrosarcoma (**Figure 6.26**)
- Mesenchymal chondrosarcoma
- Osteosarcoma
- Chordoma.

Secondary tumours

Uncommonly, a number of primary tumours can metastasize to the head and neck region (**Figure 6.27**) and include those listed in **Table 6.17**.

Table 6.17 Secondary tumours of head and neck.[11]

Site	Primary tumour
Paranasal sinuses	Kidney
	Lung
	Breast
	Thyroid
	Prostate
Nasopharynx. Very rare. Case reports or small case series	Malignant melanoma
	Kidney
	Lung
	Thyroid
	Colon
	Breast
	Cervix
Hypopharynx and larynx	Melanoma
	Kidney
	Breast
	Lung
	Prostate
	Colon
	Stomach
Oral cavity and oropharynx	Breast
	Kidney
	Lung
	Prostate
	Thyroid
	Colon
Salivary glands. More common accounting for 5% of salivary gland malignancies. Predominantly occur in the parotid glands	80% of parotid gland secondary tumours are from other primary head and neck neoplasms. 85% of submandibular gland secondary tumours are from distant sites including lung, kidney and breast
Ear and temporal bone. Very uncommon, but post-mortem study suggests may be more common especially in patients with disseminated malignant disease	Breast
	Lung
	Head and neck
	Prostate
	Melanoma
	Thyroid
	Kidney

> ### KEY EVIDENCE
>
> - Meticulous and judicious pathological evaluation of head and neck neoplasms is foundational to subsequent effective clinical management and resource utilization.
> - Morphological assessment by light microscopy constitutes the cornerstone of cytological and histological diagnosis, supplemented by ancillary ultrastructural, immunohistochemical, molecular and genetic studies, where relevant.
> - Fine needle aspiration cytology is a comparatively low-risk, cost-effective preliminary investigation in the management of head and neck tumours, subserving both triage and diagnostic roles in experienced hands.

- The histocytopathological diagnostic process is historically heuristic in nature, correlating clinical, pathological, radiological and treatment outcome observations using population and individual case study evidence.

KEY LEARNING POINTS

- The head and neck pathologist must be an accomplished practitioner familiar with perhaps the widest range of organ/tissue-specific malignancies out of all the anatomically defined site-specific specialities.
- In relative terms, head and neck cancer is uncommon, accounting for approximately 8000 new cancer cases (approximately 3 per cent of all cancers) and responsible for approximately 2700 deaths (roughly 5 per cent of all cancer-related deaths) per annum in the UK.
- Tumour site, type, grade and stage are major determinants of survival in head and neck cancer, which is influenced to a lesser degree by a variety of other patient-specific and tumour-specific factors. These are accommodated in the current UICC/AJCC TNM classification.
- Squamous cell carcinoma in its numerous manifestations accounts for upwards of 90 per cent of all malignant head and neck tumours with lymphoma as the second most common malignancy.
- Fine needle aspiration cytology is an established first-line investigation for suspected head and neck cancer. It is rapid, comparatively atraumatic, requires minimal specialized equipment and in experienced hands offers good clinical efficiency, as long as awareness of its inherent limitations and pitfalls is maintained by all concerned.
- The application of immunohistochemistry and molecular markers with deeper understanding of their genetic basis continues to yield insight into the pathogenesis of many head and neck tumours. Their routine use in diagnosis, treatment and prognostication is likely to become more widespread.

REFERENCES

◆ 1. Layfield LJ. Fine-needle aspiration of the head and neck. *Pathology* 1996; **4**: 409–38.

2. Burnett DC, Crocker J (eds). *The science of laboratory diagnosis*, 2nd edn. Chichester: John Wiley & Sons, 2005.

3. Addams-Williams J, Watkins D, Owen S *et al.* Non-thyroid neck lumps: appraisal of the role of fine needle aspiration cytology. *European Archives of Otorhinolaryngology* 2009; **266**: 411–415.

4. Carr S, Visvanathan V, Hossain T *et al.* How good are we at fine needle aspiration cytology? *Journal of Laryngology and Otology* 2010; **124** (7): 765–6.

5. Howlett DC, Harper B, Quante M *et al.* Diagnostic adequacy and accuracy of fine needle aspiration cytology in neck lump assessment: results from a regional cancer network over a one year period. *Journal of Laryngology and Otology* 2007; **121**: 571–9.

6. Howlett DC, Menezes LJ, Lewis K *et al.* Sonographically guided core biopsy of a parotid mass. *American Journal of Roentgenology* 2007; **188**: 223–7.

7. Screaton NJ, Berman LH, Grant JW. Head and neck lymphadenopathy: evaluation with US-guided cutting-needle biopsy. *Radiology* 2002; **224**: 75–81.

8. Taki S, Yamamoto T, Kawai A *et al.* Sonographically guided core biopsy of the salivary gland masses: safety and efficacy. *Clinical Imaging* 2005; **29**: 189–94.

9. Murray CE, Cooper L, Handa KK *et al.* A technique for the orientation of endoscopically resected laryngeal lesions. *Clinical Otolaryngology* 2007; **32**: 197–208.

◆ 10. Wenig B. *Atlas of head and neck pathology.* Oxford: Saunders Elsevier, 2008.

◆ 11. Barnes L, Eveson JW, Reichart P, Sidransky D. *Pathology and genetics of head and neck tumours.* Lyon: IARC, 2005.

◆ 12. Gray WM, McKee G (eds). *Diagnostic cyopathology*, 2nd edn. Oxford: Elsevier Science, 2003.

◆ 13. Speight P, Barrett A. Salivary gland tumours. *Oral Diseases* 2002; **8**: 229–40.

14. Hughes JH, Volk EE, Wilbur DC. Pitfalls in salivary gland fine-needle aspiration cytology: lessons from the College of American Pathologists' Interlaboratory Comparison Program in Nongynecologic Cytology. *Archives of Pathology and Laboratory Medicine* 2005; **129**: 26–31.

15. Seifert G, Langrock I, Donath K. [A pathological classification of pleomorphic adenoma of the salivary glands (author's translation)]. *HNO* 1976; **24**: 415–26.

◆ 16. Zbären P, Stauffer E. Pleomorphic adenoma of the parotid gland: histopathologic analysis of the capsular characteristics of 218 tumors. *Head and Neck* 2007; **29**: 751–7.

17. Thompson L. *Head and neck pathology*, 1st edn. Oxford: Elsevier, 2006.

◆ 18. Eveson J. Malignant neoplasms of the salivary glands. In: Thompson L (ed.). *Head and neck pathology.* Oxford: Elsevier, 2006: 321–71.

19. Stennert E, Wittekindt C, Klussmann JP *et al.* Recurrent pleomorphic adenoma of the parotid gland: a prospective histopathological and immunohistochemical study. *The Laryngoscope* 2004; **114**: 158–63.

◆ 20. Wittekindt C, Streubel K, Arnold G *et al.* Recurrent pleomorphic adenoma of the parotid gland: analysis of 108 consecutive patients. *Head and Neck* 2007; **29**: 822–8.

21. Auclair PL, Ellis GL. Atypical features in salivary gland mixed tumors: their relationship to malignant transformation. *Modern Pathology* 1996; **9**: 652–7.

22. Eveson JW, Cawson RA. Warthin's tumor (cystadenolymphoma) of salivary glands: a clinicopathologic investigation of 278 cases. *Oral Surgery, Oral Medicine, Oral Pathology* 1986; **61**: 256–62.

23. Yu GY, Liu XB, Li ZL, Peng X. Smoking and the development of Warthin's tumour of the parotid gland. *British Journal of Oral and Maxillofacial Surgery* 1998; **36**: 183–5.

24. Syrjänen S. Human papillomavirus infections and oral tumors. *Medical Microbiology and Immunology* 2003; **192**: 123–8.

25. Garlick JA, Taichman LB. Human papillomavirus infection of the oral mucosa. *American Journal of Dermatopathology* 1991; **13**: 386–95.

26. Eversole LR, Laipis PJ, Merrell P, Choi E. Demonstration of human papillomavirus DNA in oral condyloma acuminatum. *Journal of Oral Pathology* 1987; **16**: 266–72.

27. Henley JD, Summerlin DJ, Tomich CE. Condyloma acuminatum and condyloma-like lesions of the oral cavity: a study of 11 cases with an intraductal component. *Histopathology* 2004; **44**: 216–21.

28. Goon P, Sonnex C, Jani P *et al.* Recurrent respiratory papillomatosis: an overview of current thinking and treatment. *European Archives of Otorhinolaryngology* 2008; **265**: 147–51.

29. Hyams VJ. Papillomas of the nasal cavity and paranasal sinuses. A clinicopathological study of 315 cases. *Annals of Otology, Rhinology and Laryngology* 1971; **80**: 192–206.

30. Kanatas A, Mücke T, Houghton D, Mitchell D. Schwannomas of the head and neck. *Oncology Reviews* 2009; **3**: 107–11.

◆ 31. Wenig B (ed.). Neoplasms of the salivary glands. In: *Atlas of head and neck pathology*, 2nd edn. Oxford: Elsevier, 2008: 582–703.

32. Irving RM, Moffat DA, Hardy DG *et al.* Somatic NF2 gene mutations in familial and non-familial vestibular schwannoma. *Human Molecular Genetics* 1994; **3**: 347–50.

33. Begnami MD, Palau M, Rushing EJ *et al.* Evaluation of NF2 gene deletion in sporadic schwannomas, meningiomas, and ependymomas by chromogenic *in situ* hybridization. *Human Pathology* 2007; **38**: 1345–50.

34. Van Der Mey AG, Maaswinkel-Mooy PD, Cornelisse CJ *et al.* Genomic imprinting in hereditary glomus tumours: evidence for new genetic theory. *Lancet* 1989; **2**: 1291–4.

35. Kupferman M, Hanna E. Paragangliomas of the head and neck. *Current Oncology Reports* 2008; **10**: 156–61.

◆ 36. Pellitteri PK, Rinaldo A, Myssiorek D *et al.* Paragangliomas of the head and neck. *Oral Oncology* 2004; **40**: 563–75.

37. Lack EE, Cubilla AL, Woodruff JM, Farr HW. Paragangliomas of the head and neck region. A clinical study of 69 patients. *Cancer* 1977; **39**: 397–409.

38. Parkin DM, Bray F, Ferlay J, Pisani P. Global cancer statistics, 2002. *CA: A Cancer Journal for Clinicians* 2005; **55**: 74–108.

◆ 39. National Institute for Clinical Excellence. *Improving outcomes in head and neck cancers. The manual.* London: NICE, 2004.

40. Sobin LH, Gospodarowicz MK, Wittekind C (eds). *TNM classification of malignant tumours*, 7th edn. Oxford: Wiley-Blackwell, 2009.

◆ 41. Mehanna HM, Rattay T, Smith J, McConkey CC. Treatment and follow-up of oral dysplasia – a systematic review and meta-analysis. *Head and Neck* 2009; **31**: 1600–9.

◆ 42. Sadri M, McMahon J, Parker A. Management of laryngeal dysplasia: a review. *European Archives of Otorhinolaryngology* 2006; **263**: 843–52.

◆ 43. Eversole L. Dysplasia of the upper aerodigestive tract squamous epithelium. *Head and Neck Pathology* 2009; **3**: 63–8.

◆ 44. Argiris A, Karamouzis MV, Raben D, Ferris RL. Head and neck cancer. *Lancet* 2008; **371**: 1695–709.

45. Blot WJ, McLaughlin JK, Winn DM *et al.* Smoking and drinking in relation to oral and pharyngeal cancer. *Cancer Research* 1988; **48**: 3282–7.

46. Vineis P, Alavanja M, Buffler P *et al.* Tobacco and cancer: recent epidemiological evidence. *Journal of the National Cancer Institute* 2004; **96**: 99–106.

47. Syrjanen K. Morphological and immunohistochemical evidence suggesting human papillomavirus (HPV) involvement in oral squamous cell carcinogenesis. *International Journal of Oral Surgery* 1983; **12**: 418–24.

48. Goon P, Stanley M, Ebmeyer J *et al.* HPV and head and neck cancer: a descriptive update. *Head and Neck Oncology* 2009; **1**: 36.

49. Syrjänen S. Human papillomavirus (HPV) in head and neck cancer. *Journal of Clinical Virology* 2005; **32**: S59–S66.

◆ 50. Curado MP, Hashibe M. Recent changes in the epidemiology of head and neck cancer. *Current Opinion in Oncology* 2009; **21**: 194–200.

◆ 51. Hobbs CG, Sterne JA, Bailey M *et al.* Human papillomavirus and head and neck cancer: a systematic review and meta-analysis. *Clinical Otolaryngology* 2006; **31**: 259–66.

52. Teresa R, Andrea A, Liliane C *et al.* Risk factors for oral and pharyngeal cancer in young adults. *Oral Oncology* 2004; **40**: 207–13.

53. Marur S, D'Souza G, Westra WH, Forastiere AA. HPV-associated head and neck cancer: a virus-related cancer epidemic. *Lancet Oncology* 2010; **11**: 781–9.

54. Slaughter DP, Southwick HW, Smejkal W. Field cancerization in oral stratified squamous epithelium; clinical implications of multicentric origin. *Cancer* 1953; **6**: 963–8.

55. Perez-Ordonez B, Beauchemin M, Jordan RC. Molecular biology of squamous cell carcinoma of the head and neck. *Journal of Clinical Pathology* 2006; **59**: 445–53.

56. Ferrer ME, Villanueva E, Lopez A. Papillary squamous cell carcinoma of the oropharynx. *European Archives of Otorhinolaryngology* 2003; **260**: 444–5.

57. Sheahan P, Toner M, Timon CV. Clinicopathological features of head and neck adenosquamous carcinoma. *ORL Journal of Otorhinolaryngology and Related Specialties* 2005; **67**: 10–15.

58. Alos L, Castillo M, Nadal A *et al*. Adenosquamous carcinoma of the head and neck: criteria for diagnosis in a study of 12 cases. *Histopathology* 2004; **44**: 570–9.

59. Banks ER, Frierson HFJ, Mills SE *et al*. Basaloid squamous cell carcinoma of the head and neck: a clinicopathologic and immunohistochemical study of 40 cases. *American Journal of Surgical Pathology* 1992; **16**: 939–40.

60. Ferlito A, Altavilla G, Rinaldo A, Doglioni C. Basaloid squamous cell carcinoma of the larynx and hypopharynx. *Annals of Otology, Rhinology and Laryngology* 1997; **106**: 1024–35.

61. Wei WI, Sham JST. Nasopharyngeal carcinoma. *Lancet* 2005; **365**: 2041–54.

62. Wenig BM. Nasopharyngeal carcinoma. *Annals of Diagnostic Pathology* 1999; **3**: 374–85.

63. Acheson ED, Cowdell RH, Hadfield E, Macbeth RG. Nasal cancer in woodworkers in the furniture industry. *British Medical Journal* 1968; **2**: 587–96.

64. Llorente J, Pérez-Escuredo J, Alvarez-Marcos C *et al*. Genetic and clinical aspects of wood dust related intestinal-type sinonasal adenocarcinoma: a review. *European Archives of Otorhinolaryngology* 2009; **266**: 1–7.

65. Goode RK, Auclair PL, Ellis GL. Mucoepidermoid carcinoma of the major salivary glands. *Cancer* 1998; **82**: 1217–24.

66. Simon D, Somanathan T, Ramdas K, Pandey M. Central mucoepidermoid carcinoma of mandible – a case report and review of the literature. *World Journal of Surgical Oncology* 2003; **1**: 1.

♦ 67. Gomez DR, Katabi N, Zhung J *et al*. Clinical and pathologic prognostic features in acinic cell carcinoma of the parotid gland. *Cancer* 2009; **115**: 2128–37.

♦ 68. Kokemueller H, Eckardt A, Brachvogel P, Hausamen JE. Adenoid cystic carcinoma of the head and neck – 20 years experience. *International Journal of Oral and Maxillofacial Surgery* 2004; **33**: 25–31.

69. Nascimento AG, Amaral ALP, Prado LAF *et al*. Adenoid cystic carcinoma of salivary glands. A study of 61 cases with clinicopathologic correlation. *Cancer* 1986; **57**: 312–19.

70. Matsuba HM, Spector GJ, Thawley SE *et al*. Adenoid cystic salivary gland carcinoma: A histopathologic review of treatment failure patterns. *Cancer* 1986; **57**: 519–24.

♦ 71. Gnepp DR. Malignant mixed tumors of the salivary glands: a review. *Pathology Annual* 1993; **28**: 279–328.

72. McHugh JB, Visscher DW, Barnes EL. Update on selected salivary gland neoplasms. *Archives of Pathology and Laboratory Medicine* 2009; **133**: 1763–74.

♦ 73. Fletcher CDM (ed.). *Diagnostic histopathology of tumours*, 3rd edn. London: Churchill Livingstone Elsevier, 2007.

74. Mills SE. Neuroectodermal neoplasms of the head and neck with emphasis on neuroendocrine carcinomas. *Modern Pathology* 2002; **15**: 264–78.

75. Manolidis S, Donald PJ. Malignant mucosal melanoma of the head and neck. *Cancer* 1997; **80**: 1373–86.

♦ 76. Swerdlow S, Campo E, Harris NL *et al. WHO classification of tumours of haematopoietic and lymphoid tissues*, 4th edn. Lyon: IARC, 2008.

7

Treatment options in head and neck cancer

GRAHAM COX, ROGAN CORBRIDGE AND CHRISTIAN POTTER

It is not worth an intelligent man's time to be in the majority. By definition, there are already enough people to do that.

GH Hardy

INTRODUCTION

Early attempts to control malignant disease of the upper aerodigestive tract by surgical means were hampered by the limitations of anaesthesia, lack of antibiotics and ignorance of the biology of the disease process. Both surgeons and patients showed remarkable heroism in an often futile cause, and the discovery of ionizing radiation at the turn of the twentieth century led to a rapid loss of enthusiasm for surgical excesses. Ever since, the pendulum has swung from one modality to the other as long-term patient survival has increased and concerns, such as functional outcomes and quality of life, have become more prominent.

However, nearly two-thirds of head and neck squamous cell carcinomas (HNSCC) present at an advanced stage and despite many recent advances in medical[1] and surgical[2] oncology, there has been little evidence of an improvement in long-term survival. Novel reconstruction techniques have made radical surgical approaches more feasible, but there has been a significant trend towards organ preservation therapy. However, we must not compromise elimination of the disease in our quest to retain 'function', as an organ containing residual tumour will soon become more of a burden to the patient than the primary radical resection.

This chapter addresses the current treatment options available to the patient with HNSCC and some of the factors involved in the decision-making process. Non-squamous disease and malignancies of the thyroid and salivary glands will not be dealt with in any depth. The reader is directed to the chapters on site-specific disease for a more thorough account of these topics.

THE MULTIDISCIPLINARY TEAM

The sheer complexity and diversity of the anatomy, physiology and pathology of the multiple potential tumour subsites of the head and neck necessitates a team approach to HNSCC. No single clinician can be expected to have the requisite expertise; multiple healthcare specialities have a subspeciality dedicated to HNSCC, and multidisciplinary cooperation across these fields is essential to concentrate expertise at the bedside and clinic. There is no substitute for expert radiological, cytological and histologic opinion and the consequent inclusion of diagnostic and nursing specialists has significantly widened the scope of the multidisciplinary team (MDT).

The benefits of working in a team environment are manifold, with improved consistency and continuity of care. There may be increased opportunities for education, audit and clinical trials and support for patients and colleagues. Inevitably, cancer treatment has become more concentrated in specialist centres in the UK, with a consequent increase in workload which may act to develop and maintain expertise. Guidelines for management have been developed through professional bodies leading to a more consistent approach to HNSCC. It remains to be seen whether this will translate to improved patient outcomes, but the creation of a central database (Data for Head and Neck Oncology, DAHNO) should aid in this endeavour. This central database may also identify outliers in performance and provide a platform for research and clinical outcomes studies on a national level.

TREATMENT CHOICE

Unfortunately, the heterogeneic nature of HNSCC, as well as the diversity of patient characteristics and consequent paucity of level 1 evidence precludes the use of simple algorithms, and each case must be discussed on its own merits. Evidence-based decisions depend more on retrospective outcome studies than randomized controlled trials in most areas, and there are very few trials with a surgical arm.

A large number of factors influence decision-making (**Table 7.1**), and these will be briefly dealt with in turn.

Tumour-related factors

The observation that tumours spread in a predictable manner from the primary to regional nodes to distant systemic metastases was first proposed by Halsted, and forms the cornerstone of our ability to predict outcomes and choose appropriate therapies for cancers. The TNM system was developed as an extension of this concept by Denoix in the 1940s for the Union Internationale Contre le Cancer (UICC). The American Joint Committee on Cancer (AJCC) first met in 1959 with the intention of classifying tumours to aid determination of prognosis and selection of appropriate treatment and evaluation of tumour subgroups in clinical trials. The two

Table 7.1 Factors involved in decision-making in head and neck squamous cell carcinoma.

Factor	
Patient	Age, general medical condition/performance status, especially pulmonary reserve. Occupation, tolerance and compliance with therapy. Socioeconomic background and mobility
Tumour	Site and stage of primary, invasion of adjacent structures. Histology-grade and depth of infiltration. Extent of previous treatment. Presence of nodal or distant metastases
Healthcare	Local expertise in resectional and reconstructive surgery, radiotherapy and medical oncology. Support services for rehabilitation, dentistry and prosthetics. Appropriate nursing support. Cost, convenience, compliance, complications and competence

factions finally agreed on a standard unified TNM system in 1987, and the seventh edition was published in 2009.

The TNM staging system divides patients according to the size and anatomical extent of the primary tumour and its metastatic spread. Thus, patients with similar characteristics can be grouped together to facilitate counselling with regard to prognosis and treatment and the entering of appropriate trials. Unfortunately, HNSCC represents a rather heterogeneous patient and tumour population, and the predictive power of any one tumour stage (**Table 7.2**) leaves a great deal to be desired. There is a constant tension between 'splitters' who would like to subdivide each stage into multiple substages with more accurate prognostic and therapeutic stratification and the 'lumpers' who (perhaps rightly) regard clinicians as rather simple folk, easily bewildered by the various stage partitions and desire the system to be as clinically user-friendly as possible.

The deficiencies of the TNM system are frequently alluded to, and as our understanding of molecular oncology and the behaviour of tumours at a cellular level increases, TNM will require major adjustments or even complete revision. It has been known for decades that the depth of tumour invasion has an adverse effect on prognosis, particularly with regard to tumours of the oral tongue.[4] Endophytic, ulcerative tumours also have a worse prognosis than exophytic tumours with the same T stage.[5] Tumour volume may be of more significance than diameter in certain areas, particularly with respect to response to organ-sparing therapy. The histological nature of the host–tumour interface is also important; 'pushing' interfaces having a better prognosis than infiltrating cords of cells at the edge of the tumour. Perineural spread and lymphovascular invasion of tumour are also highly prognostically significant. Tumour grade, or degree of differentiation, does not appear to be of great significance in HNSCC.

N stage (**Figure 7.1**) is possibly the most significant single clinical indicator of prognosis, but potentially major prognostic factors, such as extracapsular spread and location within the neck, are ignored. The ability of positron emission tomography (PET) scans[6] to delineate occult disease both in the neck and at distant metastatic sites has yet to be taken into account by staging systems. It is likely that a significant proportion of tumours are understaged at diagnosis, but pathological staging data are only available from patients undergoing surgery, further muddying the waters.

The presence of metastases at diagnosis will generally have a major impact on the treatment selected, although some patients with rarer tumours, such as adenoid cystic carcinoma, may survive for many years in these circumstances. In one series of HNSCC patients, PET scanning was found to alter the initial TNM stage in 34 per cent of patients[7] with profound consequences for management plans. Wider availability of this modality may thus be invaluable in treatment planning.

Molecular biomarkers

A biomarker is any characteristic that is objectively measured as an indicator of normal biological processes, pathogenic processes or pharmacologic responses to a therapeutic intervention.[8] The ideal biomarker would be:

- **diagnostic**, used to diagnose cancer and recurrence accurately, as well as screen asymptomatic patients
- **prognostic**, accurately risk-stratifying patients and predicting response to therapies
- **therapeutic**, the marker itself being a target for treatment
- **cost effective**, being easily detectable by a standard, reliable and simple assay on a small sample.

Table 7.2 Historical survival data following standard therapy for head and neck cancer.

	Survival (%) by stage			
	I	II	III	IV
Lip	95	95	50	50
Floor of mouth	69	49	25	7
Bucosal mucosa	75	65	30	20
Alveolar ridge	78	64	35	15
Oral tongue	72	52	39	19
Tonsil	100	90	75	25
Base of tongue	90	90	45	10–40
Piriform sinus	58	50	32	38
Supraglottic larynx	86	100	57	12
Glottic larynx	96	88	65	57
Paranasal sinus	80	54	46	24
Nasopharynx	T1, 52	T2, 45	T3, 39	T4, 10

Reproduced with permission from Jacobs CD, Goffinet DR, Fee WE Jr. Head and neck squamous cancers. *Currrent Problems in Cancer* 1990; **14**: 1–72.[3]

Unsurprisingly, no such marker exists, and no marker is currently contributing significantly to the decision-making process. The increasing use of gene microarray technology is currently producing large amounts of data of questionable clinical relevance. However, there are a couple of interesting markers with significant clinical potential, as follows.

HUMAN PAPILLOMAVIRUS

Epidemiological data have shown a dramatic increase in cancers of the oropharynx, particularly tongue base and tonsil in the younger population.[9] Over the same time, there has been a marked concomitant improval in survival rates for this subgroup of tumours,[10] around 60 per cent of which test positive for HPV-16 infection.[11] These cancers tend to be poorly differentiated with basaloid features, but have an excellent response to therapy.[12] It has been hypothesized that this may be partly explained by the presence of functional wild-type p53 activity in this subset of tumours.[9] Diagnostic testing may involve polymerase chain reaction (PCR) of tumour samples or detection of human papillomavirus (HPV) DNA in plasma, but is likely to be highly sensitive. The recent introduction of widespread vaccination for high-risk HPV subtypes in schoolgirls in the UK will hopefully lead to a rapid decrease in incidence in the near future. It is a sobering thought that much of the improvement in survival data for oropharyngeal carcinomas may be accounted for by this subset of the disease, and not improvements in our treatment regimes.

EPIDERMAL GROWTH FACTOR RECEPTOR

Activation of epidermal growth factor receptor (EGFR) leads to a phosphorylation cascade via a tyrosine kinase pathway

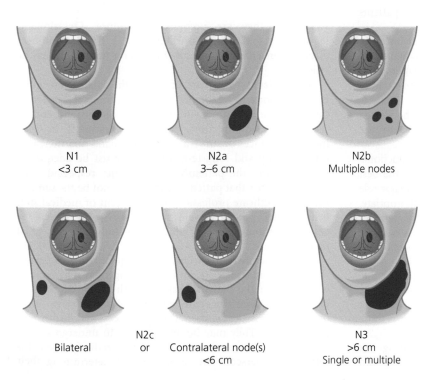

N1	N2a	N2b
<3 cm	3–6 cm	Multiple nodes

Bilateral   **N2c** or   Contralateral node(s) <6 cm   **N3** >6 cm Single or multiple

Figure 7.1 Nodal staging of HNSCC.

with wide effects on cell proliferation, apoptosis, invasion, angiogenesis and metastasis.[13] These EGFR-related molecular pathways are found to be altered in 90 per cent of HNSCC, and elevated EGFR expression is known to be related to poor prognosis.[14] One study has demonstrated overexpression as a biomarker for good response to accelerated fraction radiotherapy.[15] Cetuximab, a monoclonal antibody to EGFR has shown efficacy in treatment of locally advanced HNSCC[16] and other agents are currently in development.

Patient-related factors

The only non-tumour-related factor explicitly mentioned by TNM is age in differentiated thyroid cancer. HNSCC patients typically are of advanced age and have multiple comorbidities as they share risk factor exposure with a number of systemic diseases, such as hypertension, myocardial infarction, cerebrovascular events and chronic pulmonary obstructive disease.[17] Aged patients are more likely to receive substandard treatment of their primary tumour, 38 per cent of those >60 years and 64 per cent >80 years receiving suboptimal treatment in one series,[18] with predictable adverse outcomes.

Immunosuppression by factors such as HIV can have severe adverse effects on prognosis. Fanconi anaemia gives a 500–700-fold increase in the risk of HNSCC, the majority of which are HPV-associated.[19] Patients with head and neck cancer are frequently malnourished, which may have adverse prognostic implications. Although survival benefits of preoperative nutritional supplementation have been demonstrated only in severely malnourished patients,[20] supplementation may correct nutrient deficiencies, minimize malnutrition-related morbidity and mortality, reduce the length and cost of hospitalization, and may prevent alcohol withdrawal syndrome. Nutritional support given preoperatively for 7–10 days decreases postoperative complications by approximately 10 per cent in malnourished patients with weight loss of 10 per cent or more.[21]

Inadequate pulmonary function will preclude many types of partial laryngeal surgery where aspiration is a significant risk. Patients of low socioeconomic status, black patients and those without private medical insurance were shown to have a poorer prognosis in a recent National Cancer Database (NCDB) survey of advanced laryngeal cancer in the United States, which may simply reflect inequalities in access to care in that society.

There are a number of measurement tools of functional status, of which the Karnofsky index (**Table 7.3**) is the best known. The patient's physical condition may play a major role in determining which treatment pathway is most appropriate. One study has shown the considerable impact of the patient's performance status on prognosis in a wide variety of tumours.[22] As comorbidities increase, the proportion of patients receiving no treatment increases in parallel.[23]

The prognostic impact of comorbidities could thus be due to the physiological burden of chronic disease itself or the selection by patient and doctor of suboptimal treatment regimes. For HNSCC at least, it seems that the former is more likely.[24]

The patient's occupation may have a bearing on how much facial disfigurement or alteration in speech and

Table 7.3 Karnofsky index.

General category	%	Specific criteria
Able to carry on normal activity. No special care needed	100	Normal general status, no complaint, no evidence of disease
	90	Able to carry on normal activity. Minor sign of symptoms of disease
	80	Normal activity with effort, some signs or symptoms of disease
Unable to work. Able to live at home and care for most personal needs. Various amount of assistance needed	70	Able to care for self, unable to carry on normal activity or do work
	60	Requires occasional assistance from others, frequent medical care
	50	Requires considerable assistance from others, frequent medical care
Unable to care for self. Requires institutional or hospital care or equivalent. Disease may be rapidly progressing	40	Disabled, requires special care and assistance
	30	Severely disabled, hospitalization indicated, death not imminent
	20	Very sick, hospitalization necessary, active supportive treatment necessary
Terminal states	10	Moribund
	0	Dead

swallowing they are prepared to endure. Occasionally, logistical factors, such as willingness to travel significant distances on a daily basis for 6–7 weeks for treatment, may be crucial.

The patient's wishes are of course the final determining factor in choice of treatment, as they will bear the burden of the disease and treatment-related complications and endure the long-term dysfunctions thereof. The trade-offs between increased chances of survival on the one hand and increased acute toxicity and long-term disability must be adequately explained, and the patient's own priorities respected. One must remember that patient priorities may not be the same as those of healthcare professionals; 46 per cent of medical staff believed their patients would sacrifice survival prospects for better voice and quality of life, whereas only 20 per cent of patients agreed.[25]

Family members and friends also frequently play a part in the decision-making process, and their agendas may conflict with those of the patients. Patients with advanced HNSCC consistently prioritize cure and long-term survival over quality of life issues far more than their peers and health-care professionals. They may be more willing to undergo radical aggressive treatment than we give them credit for, and this serves to underscore the importance of determining their priorities in the initial discussion of treatment options. What may seem an irrational decision to an objective clinician may be anything but when one is confronted by one's own mortality.

Social support networks are critical in the endurance of difficult treatments, and married patients seem to be willing to undergo more aggressive treatment than single patients. It may be that married patients have a perceived sense of responsibility to their loved ones or simply perceive they will have greater support during the recovery phase. There is certainly a positive prognostic effect of marriage, which may be associated with better health habits and social support.

Health-care factors

In the ideal situation, the full range of therapies in terms of surgical modalities, reconstruction, radiotherapy and chemotherapy, should be made available to the patient. In practise, local expertise tends to be stronger in some areas than others, and support services may be inadequate for some of the more demanding options. The recent tend towards centralization of services in the UK and central importance of the MDT approach may mitigate against this. However, the 5 Cs of Cost, Convenience, Compliance, Complications and Competence may in practice play more of a role than we would like to think in the treatment decision.

TREATMENT GOALS

The primary goal of oncologic treatment is either curative or palliative. There are a number of secondary goals, such as preservation of form and function, and, where this is not possible, to restore form and function to a degree that a reasonable quality of life is restored also. Every effort should be made to minimize sequelae of treatment and in the prevention of development of second primary tumours. Cessation of smoking and excessive alcohol intake are cornerstones of the latter.

Resectability

One key issue which may determine the treatment pathway is the feasibility of surgical resection. As anaesthetic, reconstructive and rehabilitive techniques have progressed, the boundaries of what was once thought to be irresectable have been gradually pushed back. In 2002, the TNM staging classification was modified to reflect this by dividing the T4 stage into T4a and T4b (**Table 7.4**) with the latter being generally categorized as unresectable, or at the borders thereof, and thus more suitable for non-surgical therapy. There is obviously a middle ground where resection is still technically feasible, but the likely morbidity or mortality would preclude such an option in all but the most extreme cases. A tumour is only deemed truly unresectable when the surgeon doubts the ability to remove all gross tumour on anatomical grounds or believes local control will not be achieved by surgery followed by adjuvant radiotherapy.

It must be emphasized that the T4b stage does not imply incurability, and in some instances (for example, nasopharyngeal cancer (NPC) extending into the intracranial compartment) concomitant chemoradiotherapy (CCRT) may give excellent results.

There are three criteria repeated across must tumour sites, and these will be examined in turn:

1. **Vascular encasement/invasion.** The presence of disease in intimate relationship with the great arterial

Table 7.4   T4 versus T4b tumour classification for various sites of head and neck cancers.

Site	T4a	T4b
Oral cavity	Tumour invades adjacent structures, bone, muscle of tongue, maxillary sinus, facial skin	Tumour invades masticator space, pterygoid plates, or skull base and/or encases internal carotid artery
Oropharynx	Tumour invades the larynx, deep muscle of tongue, medial pterygoid, hard palate or mandible	Tumour invades lateral pterygoid muscle, pterygoid plates, lateral nasopharynx or skull base or encases carotid artery
Hypopharynx	Tumour invades thyroid/cricoid cartilage, hyoid bone, thyroid gland, oesophagus or central compartment	Tumour invades prevertebral fascia, encases carotid artery or involves mediastinal structures
Supraglottis, glottis, subglottis	Tumour invades through the thyroid cartilage and/or invades tissues beyond the larynx (e.g. trachea or oesophagus)	Tumour invades prevertebral fascia, encases carotid artery or invades mediastinal structures
Maxillary sinus, nasal cavity, ethmoid sinus	Tumour invades anterior orbital contents, skin of cheeks, pterygoid plates, infratemporal fossa, cribriform plate, sphenoid or frontal sinus	Tumour invades orbital apex, dura, brain, middle cranial fossa, cranial nerves other than V2, nasopharynx or clivus
Salivary glands	Tumour invades skin, mandible, ear canal, and/or facial nerve	Tumour invades skull base and/or pterygoid plates and/or encases carotid artery
Thyroid	Tumour grows outside the thyroid capsule into subcutaneous tissue, larynx, trachea, oesophagus, recurrent laryngeal nerve	Tumour invades prevertebral fascia or encases carotid arteries or mediastinal vessels

After Yousem DM, Gad K, Tufano RP. Resectability issues with head and neck cancer. *American Journal of Neuroradiology* 2006; **27**: 2024–36.[26]

vessels of the neck is a not uncommon problem in the N3 neck, and the critical question is whether the carotid can be preserved surgically. Preoperative imaging is usually the key to accurate assessment; the computed tomography (CT) criterion of 180° circumferential attachment has been shown to have lower predictive value than 270° encirclement of the vessel on magnetic resonance imaging (MRI). Actual demonstration of tumour within the vessel lumen is highly specific for vascular involvement, but rarely seen and poorly sensitive. In the case of a non-salvageable artery, temporary transfemoral balloon occlusion of the affected vessel may be attempted, and transcranial Doppler sonography may be used to objectively assess the flow in the ipsilateral middle cerebral artery if resection is still contemplated.

2. **Prevertebral fascia involvement**. Fixation of tumour to the prevertebral musculature may be suspected clinically in extensive pharyngeal or laryngeal tumours which have reduced mobility on the vertebral column. Attempts to strip tumour off the longus colli/capitis muscle complex is rarely a fruitful endeavour, with a high incidence of residual disease and lymphatic spread to inaccessible nodes in the retropharynx and posterior neck. The retropharyngeal space usually contains fat, lymph nodes and connective tissue, and generally provides a stripe of high signal on T1 MRI which is an excellent indicator of resectibility. Effacement of this signal by tumour is a very poor prognostic sign.

3. **Mediastinal invasion**. This rare eventuality is sometimes seen in extensive hypopharyngeal, transglottic and thyroid cancers which may infiltrate mediastinal fat and invade the great vessels at the root of the neck. On occasion, these may be amenable to surgical approach with the aid of a thoracic surgeon, particularly in the case of differentiated thyroid carcinoma. However, obliteration of the periaortic fat and >45° contact with the aorta on CT suggests a dismal prognosis. Transoesophageal ultrasound is gaining popularity in staging of oesophageal cancer and may occasionally be useful in these rarer situations.

INDICATORS OF EXTENSIVE SURGICAL REQUIREMENTS

Selection of the appropriate surgical approach and degree of resection requires adequate preoperative planning including examination under anaesthesia and imaging techniques. Before undertaking potentially mutilational surgery, the patient must be fully informed of the likely consequences; changing the surgical plan mid-operation without adequate consent is to be avoided at all costs.

1. **Laryngeal cartilage invasion**. Recently, the TNM staging for advanced laryngeal cancer has altered, with minor degrees of cortical invasion of the thyroid cartilage restaged as T3 and T4a being reserved for gross invasion through the full width of cartilage. The latter stage is associated with reduced efficacy of medical modalities, and is generally seen as an indication for laryngectomy. In some patients, distortion of the cartilages may be clinically obvious, but radiological findings are often critical. The thyroid cartilage often contains areas of ossification and chondrification in continuity and the latter may be isoattenuated to an adjacent neoplasm. MRI has a high sensitivity, but low specificity and may lead to false positives and inadvertent laryngectomy, whereas the low sensitivity of CT may lead to inappropriate organ-sparing protocols.

2. **Pre-epiglottic fat invasion**. Invasion of pre-epiglottic fat by supraglottic tumours increases the risk of spread of disease to the neck and requires a cuff of tongue base to be resected with consequences for function and attendant reconstructive options. Conservation laryngeal surgery is not possible if the hyoid bone is involved. MRI is an excellent modality for determining the extent of pre-epiglottic involvement.

3. **Mandibular invasion**. Unexpected bony invasion discovered intraoperatively can have major adverse consequences if adequate reconstructive options have not been planned. The periosteum generally forms an effective barrier, but once breached invasion is inevitable. Imaging studies by CT and MRI are complicated by the often dismal state of the patient's dentition, with false positives common from cortical erosion by recent dental extractions, inflammatory odontogenic disease or the sequelae of radiotherapy. CT specificity seems higher than MRI for detection of cortical invasion, marrow involvement and inferior alveolar canal invasion. Specialist dental CT software (DentaScan®) technology may be used to reformat thin axial slices into panoramic and cross-sectional views, and PET/CT fusion studies show great promise in this area. Occasionally, invasion will not become obvious until intraoperative periosteal stripping, and flexibility in surgical planning is essential.

4. **Skull base invasion**. Similar parameters are used as for mandibular invasion – bone thinning, erosion and displacement on CT, and replacement of marrow on T_1-weighted MRI. Involvement of cranial nerves may cause foraminal enlargement on CT or direct enhancement of the nerves on MRI. Muscle denervation may result in secondary fatty replacement and atrophy. Nodular dural enhancement or thickening >5 mm with pial enhancement is highly suggestive of dural invasion, often a preliminary step before parenchymal invasion. Extension of disease into the cavernous sinus makes surgical resection unfeasible.

5. **Orbital invasion**. Infiltration of the orbit is somewhat limited by the tough periorbita, but this is not readily identifiable on imaging. Peritumoral oedema can result in false positives on MRI with abnormal signal within the extraocular muscles. This is less of an issue with CT, and both modalities are best used in combination with clinical assessment.

INFORMED CONSENT

Obtaining informed consent to a procedure is fundamental to good medical practice, ensuring that the provision of treatment is not only legal but ethical. There are three essential requirements in the consent process (**Box 7.1**). The doctor must give sufficient information to the competent patient to enable them to understand the risks and benefits of treatment and a realistic idea of other options that may exist. The competent patient may then use this information to make a voluntary reasoned decision without coercion. If this process is not followed and the surgeon carries out a procedure without adequate consent, the surgeon has committed assault even if the patient comes to no significant harm as a result of the surgery. The competent patient also has the right to refuse treatment in their best interest, no matter how irrational this may appear to others.

The amount of information offered to the patient is critical to the consent process. A reasonable standard of disclosure is the amount of information that a 'reasonable person' would want before agreeing to treatment. It is reasonable to explicitly ask the patient what they would like to know and what questions need to be answered during the consent process. Express consent may be written or verbal, although for obvious medicolegal reasons, the former is preferred. Consent is implied if the patient accepts an investigation or treatment without question or behaviour to suggest non-consent.

The issue of mental capacity is covered by the Mental Capacity Act 2005. A competent patient is capable of understanding, retaining and weighing information relevant to a specific decision. They must also be able to communicate their choice by any means. A patient cannot be deemed to lack capacity simply because the treating clinicians disagree with their decision.

PRINCIPLES OF ONCOLOGIC SURGERY

The importance of preoperative planning cannot be overemphasized, enabling the surgeon to make an explicit surgical plan based on the tumour's biological behaviour, location and extent. Result of biopsies and staging investigations and the outcome of the MDT discussion should be documented in the case notes, and any preoperative imaging studies available in theatre. A thorough medical and anaesthetic assessment of the patient should take place before any

---

> ## Box 7.1   Essential requirements of the consent process
>
> - You must have the capacity (or ability) to make the decision.
> - The medical provider must disclose information on the treatment, test or procedure in question, including the expected benefits and risks, and the likelihood (or probability) that the benefits and risks will occur.
> - You must comprehend the relevant information.
> - You must voluntarily grant consent, without coercion or duress.

---

major procedures are undertaken and any intercurrent illnesses or nutritional problems addressed adequately to optimize the patient's condition. Informed consent should be documented and the entire theatre and anaesthetic teams should be made aware of the nature of the procedure and any likely changes to the operative plan that may become necessary. The anaesthetist should ideally be familiar with the management of potentially difficult airways and have experience of fibreoptic intubation techniques. The type (for example, laser or microlaryngoscopy) and location (transnasal, transoral) of endotracheal tube should be discussed with anaesthetic staff, and if major surgery to the upper airway is planned, an elective covering tracheostomy may be fashioned. The patient should be positioned and attention paid to likely pressure areas. A thorough endoscopic examination of the tumour should also be carried out to confirm the stage of the tumour and the appropriate nature of the surgical plan. If reconstruction is being planned, a template of the likely defect may be fashioned to enable the reconstructive team to plan their procedure. Following this, the neck may be gently extended by means of a sandbag under the shoulders and the head turned away from the side of the operation. Local deep vein thrombosis (DVT) prophylaxis measures should be followed, such as compression stockings and Flowtron® boots.

Wound infection can have potentially dire consequences, and if the aerodigestive tract is to be entered and mucosae breached, the procedure is regarded as clean-contaminated, and appropriate prophylactic antibiotics given on induction of anaesthesia. Due to the frail nature of many patients with cancers of the upper aerodigestive tract and major possible consequences of infection, most surgeons would also give prophylactic antibiotics for clean procedures which may last for more than 90 minutes, such as a neck dissection. The antibiotic regime should be broad-spectrum, and local microbiological protocols should be followed. Typical agents would include co-amoxyclav, ceftriaxone, or clindamycin in combination with metronidazole. There is some evidence to suggest that courses lasting more than 24 hours are potentially counterproductive in altering the general flora of the patient and encouraging the emergence of resistant strains.[27] However, it is common clinical practice to continue the antibiotic course until either the drains are removed or there is good evidence of no anastomotic leak following a contrast swallow. Patients should be screened for MRSA (methicillin-resistant *Staphylococcus aureus*) before major surgery and, if positive, appropriate decontamination and isolation precautions followed after liaison with the infection control team. The prophylactic agent should be selected for its efficacy on MRSA, with teicoplanin or vancomycin generally favoured.

The planned incision should be carefully marked, bearing in mind likely extensions that may be required and relaxed skin tension lines. A long-acting local anaesthetic solution, such as bupivacaine 0.5 per cent with 1:200 000 adrenaline may be infiltrated along the incision line for analgesic and haemostatic purposes, and allowed to have its effect on the tissues while patient preparation continues. In the case of parotid surgery, a nerve monitor may be inserted into the facial muscles at this juncture. The operative site is washed with sterile povidone-iodine solution and draped appropriately, giving good exposure of the surgical site and any likely extensions. Once the entire team is in position and

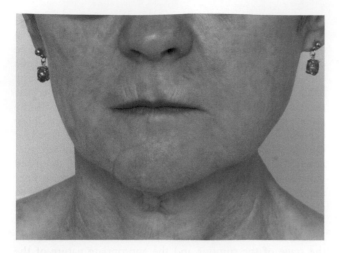

Figure 7.2 Cosmetic outcome of stepped incision for mandibulotomy.

permission sought from the anaesthetist to commence, the surgeon should murmur to themselves the aphorism of Sir Harold Gillies 'seven times seven turn your knife in your hand err you cut the skin of a fellow man' before taking the plunge.

The ideal of a bloodless field is highly dependent on a combination of hypotensive anaesthesia and meticulous surgical technique. Tissues should be handled with precision and care, the assistant providing countertraction as dissection proceeds to better visualize and deal with vessels before they are violated. To gain adequate access to the oropharynx, a mandibulotomy is generally required. The lip incision may be stepped at the vermilion border and should sweep downwards lateral to the symphysis menti to improve cosmesis (**Figure 7.2**). Paramedian mandibulotomy should be carried out just anterior to the mental nerve to preserve sensation to the lower lip. Titanium reconstruction plates should be aligned and their screw holes drilled while temporarily placed. The incision is marked in pencil on the mandible before a reciprocating saw is used to complete the mandibulotomy. At the end of the procedure the mandible is repositioned and aligned by fixing the plates using the predrilled screw holes.

Once adequate access is achieved, the tumour excision should be planned. In the oral cavity and oropharynx, a margin of 10 mm from gross visible or palpable tumour is acceptable, and smaller margins are reasonable in the glottic area.[28] Seventy-five per cent of patients with a positive margin will go on to develop a local recurrence, whereas only 25 per cent with negative pathological margins will do so.[29] In the United States, the reported incidence of positive pathological margins is 16 per cent.[30] The margin should be marked with ink or diathermy spots on the mucosa before excision, as inevitable distortion will occur as resection proceeds. Handling of the tumour should be avoided whenever possible; care and gentle minimal manipulation is advised. Any questions about the complete nature of the resection should result in samples from the resection edges being sent for frozen section pathological assessment. Once the specimen has been examined for completeness, it is oriented for the pathologist. This may be achieved by sewing it to an acetate sheet with the anatomical landmarks and orientation drawn in to aid the pathologist.

The wounds should be thoroughly washed with saline, water or 10 per cent hydrogen peroxide solution, and the contaminated instruments discarded for a fresh set. The surgical team should remove their gowns and gloves and rescrub for the reconstruction or closure of the wound. A nasogatric feeding tube may be placed or percutaneous gastrostomy fashioned according to the likelihood of returning to oral intake. Adequate closed suction drainage should be applied to the wound and maintained on suction during closure to prevent any haematoma formation. Blake drains are ideally suited to the wide skin flaps of neck surgery. There are many ways to close the skin, but good apposition of the superficial cervical fascia over platysma is essential for success, and the use of buried absorbable sutures is ideal for this. The skin itself may be closed by interrupted sutures everting the skin edges or stainless steel clips. Topical chloramphenicol ointment may be applied in place of a dressing for the immediate postoperative period.

The drains are generally removed when producing serous fluid at a rate of <30 mL/day, and sutures removed at day 7 unless the incision area has been irradiated when 10 days should suffice. Antireflux medication, hyoscine patches and regular mouthwashes may be prescribed. If the pharynx has been repaired, the patient should be kept nil by mouth for 7–10 days, when a contrast swallow may be performed to assess any possible anastomotic leaks. Should the area be watertight, oral feeding may be recommenced at this stage.

Early mobilization is the key to rapid successful rehabilitation of the postoperative head and neck patient, and intensive physiotherapy and proactive nursing care may aid this.

THE ROLE OF SURGERY

Curative surgery should be directed primarily towards the extirpation of disease, maximizing the chances of oncologic control and cure before concerning oneself with functional preservation. The latter is of little moment to the patient with an inadequate resection and persistent mutilating disease. Resectability should not be confused with operability, and frequently the patient's overall health or expectations of recovery will preclude surgical intervention. Similarly, demonstrating the extent of one's surgical repertoire by means of a heroic resection as a technical exercise with little prospect of cure or functional recovery does the patient few favours.

Anatomical subsites

Early stage tumours (T1 or 2) with no nodal involvement may be treated by a single modality depending on the level of local expertise and the anatomical location of the disease. There is not a single level I study comparing radiotherapy with surgical resection for the evaluation of local control or survival.[31]

ORAL CAVITY AND OROPHARYNX

Management is highly dependent on the degree of involvement of the oral tongue, tongue base, hard and soft palates.

The majority of T1–3 tumours of oral tongue, floor of mouth and hard palate should be comfortably resectable without significant functional impairment, especially with microvascular tissue transfer reconstruction. Excellent oncological results can be achieved in this way,[32, 33] with disease-specific survival of 65–95 per cent. Bony involvement of the hard palate or mandible is again amenable to composite flap reconstruction, with obturation reserved for major hard palate defects in those with a poor performance status. The functional morbidity of total glossectomy has historically been regarded as too great to warrant primary surgery, and CCRT undoubtedly has a role to play in high-volume T4 tumours of the oral tongue and tongue base. However, if preservation of a lingual artery and hypoglossal nerve are feasible, free flap reconstruction may give acceptable functional results (Galm, unpublished observations).

Tumours requiring resection of more than one-third of the soft palate or more than half of the tongue base are usually considered candidates for chemoradiation, but aggressive surgical approaches via mandibulotomy with free flap reconstruction are oncologically sound and can have surprisingly good functional outcomes.

LARYNX

The earliest attempts to resect the larynx were met with unsurmountable complications and poor surgical outcomes.[34] Of the first 103 total laryngectomies performed, 39 per cent died from the operative procedure and only nine survived for a year, the longest survivor lasting five years.

In 1961, Pressman *et al.* noted the highly compartmentalized nature of the larynx, underpinning the rationale of the subtotal and partial laryngectomy, with the hope of maintaining speech and swallowing without the need for a permanent stoma.[35] In 1972, the CO_2 laser was introduced for transoral resection of early laryngeal tumours with good effect, and more recently this technique has been extended to more advanced tumours.

For early stage glottic cancer (T1–T2 N0), options include transoral laser excision, radiotherapy and open partial laryngectomy. Rates of local control, laryngeal voice preservation and survival seem equivalent between these options, unless there is anterior commissure involvement, when laser treatment appears to provide inferior local control and voice quality. Open partial laryngectomy appears to be best suited to a subset of bulky T2b lesions and to salvage local recurrences from other modalities, as it has greater complication rates and involves greater overall cost. Laser surgery seems best suited to smaller T1a lesions, with radiotherapy effective for all early cancers.

By definition, a T4 laryngeal cancer has already produced an organ that is not functioning adequately with cord fixation, cartilage invasion and loss of structural integrity. Functionally, speech and swallowing will be impaired and frequently the airway will be compromised. Under these circumstances, preservation of the 'organ' is of dubious benefit as return to useful function is highly unlikely and careful surveillance for persistent disease is necessary, with the added morbidities of salvage laryngectomy casting a long shadow over the patient. Survival data suggest a clear benefit to laryngectomy under these circumstances, and quality of life data seem to suggest this is the correct approach.[36]

Most of the debate therefore focuses on the T3 tumour, where the total laryngectomy long represented the gold standard. Conservative laryngeal surgery, designed to retain some degree of laryngeal function, may take the form of transoral laser surgery, supracricoid and near-total laryngectomy. These modalities achieve local control rates similar to primary chemoradiotherapy, with survival rates of 50–65 per cent.[37] The French surgeon Laccoureye pioneered the supracricoid laryngectomy, realizing that impaction of the hyoid bone on the cricoid cartilage could permit restoration of physiologic speech and swallowing via the cricohyodopexy or cricohyoidoepiglottopexy (**Figure 7.3**). At the Laennec Hospital in Paris, the five-year actuarial local control rates for T3 laryngeal tumours was 91.4 per cent, with

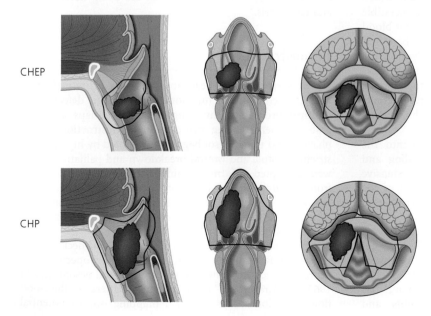

CHEP

CHP

Figure 7.3 The partial laryngeal resections comprising the cricohyoepiglottopexy (CHEP) and cricohyopexy (CHP).

89.8 per cent laryngeal preservation and 98.3 per cent local control.[38] It remains to be seen whether this technique retains such a success rate outside this major centre.

HYPOPHARYNX

T3–4 tumours will typically require a laryngopharyngectomy with either primary closure or flap reconstruction. Involvement of the cricopharyngeus or cervical oesophagus will necessitate the addition of an oesophagectomy. Patients with good performance status and limited T3 disease may be candidates for supracricoid laryngopharyngectomy in centres specializing in this technique. Transoral laser surgery has proven surprisingly effective, with five-year local control rates of 57 per cent for T4 disease.[39] The majority of patients will have nodal disease, and this must be addressed at the time of surgery.

Transoral laser surgery

The CO$_2$ laser was first introduced in the 1970s for laryngeal microsurgery,[40] and was increasingly used for benign conditions, such as papillomatosis. In the 1980s, Steiner[41] popularized its use for malignant disease, and expanded its indications throughout the upper aerodigestive tract. Initially popular for debulking obstructive disease and removing limited early glottic cancers, laser surgery is now used in organ preservation in a wide variety of HNSCCs. A number of specialized gags and instruments have been designed to aid exposure in difficult areas and the precision and haemostatic properties of the laser enable tumour resection with accuracy and speed. The small focal diameter of the CO$_2$ laser enables minimal carbonization with low rates of infection, swelling and scarring.

There are technical differences compared to traditional open oncological surgery. For instance in larger tumours, incisions may be made through the tumour to better delineate its depth. Judicious use of the operating microscope aids the distinguishing of normal tissues from tumour, which may be resected piecemeal from particularly inaccessible areas, such as the pyriform fossae or areas where major blood vessels may be encountered, such as the tongue base and tonsil. Steiner claims that the laser acts to seal lymphatics, preventing dissemination of micrometastases during this process. It is obviously important to maintain topographic accuracy for pathological assessment of surgical margins using this technique, and an experienced pathologist is invaluable.

Blindly following deeply infiltrating tumours into the tissues of the neck is highly technically demanding and should only be carried out by surgeons with extensive exposure to this technique. Open surgical treatment of the neck, if indicated, is generally carried out by Steiner after an interval of 1 week.

Defects following resection are typically allowed to granulate or covered in collagen mesh and fibrin glue. Larger oral cavity defects may be covered by a split skin graft to prevent excessive scarring and reduction in tongue mobility.

Whereas transoral surgery to early laryngeal tumours has rapidly become widely accepted and its results and

indications well understood, the more extensive laser resections are still subject to debate. Excellent results have been reported by the specialist centre, but we await widespread replication by other units.[42] Certainly, the prospect for organ-sparing without the morbidities of CCRT or long post-operative recovery from open resections remains of great interest.

Neck dissection

Crile first described en bloc dissection of the cervical lymphatics in 1906[42, 43] and improvements in anaesthesia, blood transfusion and the development of antibiotics led to its further popularization by Hayes Martin, who reported a series of 1450 radical neck dissections (RND) in a landmark 1951 paper.[43] He included the sternocleidomastoid and internal jugular vein in the resection and condemned Crile's preservation of the accessory nerve as oncologically unsound. Such an extensive resection was regarded as excessive for the N0 neck, but by the early 1960s regional failure rates of >50 per cent were reported in early tongue cancers treated surgically. The technique of modified radical neck dissection with preservation of the non-lymphatic structures was popularized by Bocca and colleagues as a less morbid procedure more suitable for the N0 neck,[44] and became the treatment of choice for patients whose occult metastasis rate would be expected to exceed 20 per cent.

The discovery of predictable patterns of cervical metastatic spread by Lindberg in Texas then Shah at Memorial-Sloan Kettering[45] has led to the concept of selective dissection of the high risk areas of the N0 neck as an alternative to MRND, and these procedures are now being increasingly used in selected situations in the N+ neck.[46] Elective dissection of the N0 neck is also valuable in staging the neck for occult metastases, aiding the decision-making process for adjuvant therapy provision.

In the future, sentinel lymph node biopsy, long a standard of care in melanoma and breast cancer, may lead to even more conservative and selective surgical approach, and endoscopic approaches to the neck are being developed in animal models.[47]

Reconstruction

Heroic surgery to the head and neck was in its early days characterized by major functional and cosmetic defects, with multiple procedures involving local tissue flaps and skin grafts frequently being inadequate. Reconstruction of the pharynx and upper oesophagus was blighted by high rates of stricture, fistula and wound breakdown and palliative efforts were attempted to form skin-lined local flaps to divert saliva from the great vessels. It is not surprising that surgery was not for the faint-hearted, and frequently led to abysmal quality of life for the brief period before locoregional residual disease asserted its presence.

The modern era of reconstructive head and neck surgery began with Bakamjian's introduction of the deltopectoral flap for reconstruction of the pharynx and cervical oesophagus in 1965.[48] McCraw et al.[49] recognized axial patterns of the blood flow in regional flaps in 1977, mapping out 13 potential myocutaneous flaps, and soon after Ariyan[50] introduced the pectoralis major 'workhorse' flap. In the 1980s, microvascular free flaps were popularized, in particular the radial forearm fasciocutaneous flap of Yang,[51] which revolutionized reconstruction of the oral cavity and oropharynx. Composite flaps, such as the free fibular flap, permitted reliable mandibular reconstruction for the first time,[52] ending the era of the 'Andy Gump' deformity.

Head and neck surgery often has dramatic functional effects on speech, respiration and alimentation and the surgical site is often highly visible, leading to unique challenges for the reconstructive surgeon. Some surgeons are willing to partake both in resection and reconstruction, which requires a heroic stamina and degree of technical versatility. Others prefer to work as part of two surgical teams, with the oncological resection not being compromised by thoughts of potential reconstructive challenges. Advanced tumours leaving sizeable defects will usually undergo further adjuvant treatment, and this must be borne in mind when the mode of reconstruction is selected. The ability of the patient to withstand the prolonged operative and postoperative course of a free flap reconstruction may also be a limiting factor.

The first choice for repair of a sizeable defect will usually be a free microvascular tissue transfer due to the wide range of options available, as long as there are reasonable donor and recipient vessels available. In contrast, pedicled flaps have a limited mobility and often excessive bulk. Cutaneous defects of the face are ideally suited to primary closure by local tissue flaps, with undermining of adjacent wound edges to allow for tension-free closure. Larger local flaps, such as the nasolabial or glabellar, can allow for closure of larger defects.

Defects created in the neck are more amenable to reconstruction by pedicled flaps, such as the pectoralis major or latissimus dorsi. These flaps are limited by their vascular pedicle, and the temptation to overstretch or manipulate them to cover higher defects must be resisted. They are also extremely bulky and will only offer limited contouring over the facial skeleton. They are, however, ideal in covering the great vessels of the neck following fistula formation or post-radiotherapy necrosis.

Small oral and pharyngeal defects may be closed directly by primary closure, for instance following wedge resection of the tongue. Excessive tension and scarring may lead to tethering of the tongue, with impaired speech and swallow. Following partial glossectomy, skin or mucosal grafts may be applied to the exposed muscle, but the best functional result probably comes from use of the free radial forearm flap which restores bulk and mobility.

For larger defects, pedicled flaps have the advantage of relatively short operative time and there is no requirement for microsurgical operative skills or equipment. However, there is a higher rate of flap necrosis, dehiscence and fistula formation compared to the use of free flaps in the pharynx. Indeed, studies have suggested the overall costs of pedicled flaps to be greater than free flap transfer in this situation. The radial forearm and anterolateral thigh flaps are now the workhorses of this area. The latter is somewhat bulkier than the former, and its donor site may be closed primarily, but its elevation is somewhat more technically demanding. Both provide thin pliable tissue that can be easily contoured or even tubed or folded to reconstruct the hypopharynx or soft palate.

Circumferential defects in the cervical oesophagus may be reconstructed via the jejunal free flap (which requires a laparotomy), pedicled pectoralis flaps or a gastric pull up. Total glossectomy results in significant and much feared functional deficits. The dynamic features of the tongue have been lost and this must be made up for by increased bulk to allow the reconstructed tongue to contact the palate during the propulsive phase of deglutition. Therefore for tongue defects greater than two-thirds, the rectus abdominis or anterolateral thigh are preferred to the radial forearm free flap.

Appropriate reconstruction of the mandible depends on the location of the defect. The anterior region, comprising the symphysis and parasymphysis is subjected to the greatest forces during mastication, and thus gives the greatest functional deficit when resected and has the highest propensity for mechanical failure when reconstructed. The fibular free flap is the cornerstone of anterior mandibular repair, providing a long segment of robust bone capable of tolerating multiple osteotomies. Donor-site morbidity is relatively low, and the graft is potentially long enough to reach from condyle to condyle. However, the skin paddle is relatively small and unreliable, and the blood supply may be tenuous in those patients with peripheral vascular disease. In this eventuality, the scapular flap, with its potential for two independent skin paddles may be more appropriate. The iliac crest free flap provides a large amount of bone stock shaped in the contour of a hemimandible, but its use has been limited by its bulk, the unreliable immobile skin paddle and the risk of donor site pain and hernia formation. The radial forearm osteocutaneous flap is limited by its poor bone stock which will not withstand multiple osteotomies, but may have some use in small segmental defects with larger overlying mucosal deficits.

Massive soft tissue defects in association with extensive mandibular resections may necessitate multiple free flaps, for example a fibular osteocutaneous in combination with an anterolateral thigh fasciocutaneous flap. Smaller defects of the anterior mandible alone without major soft tissue loss may be repaired by neovascularized bone grafts if less than 5 cm in length.

Lateral mandibular defects are functionally less disabling and segmental defects may be repaired by a reconstruction plate if adequate soft tissue cover is possible. Reconstruction of the posterior mandible can be technically demanding, and the overall function provided by soft-tissue repair alone with a rectus abdominis flap is often surprisingly well tolerated despite some inevitable malocclusion.

Radiotherapy

Ionizing radiation may cause DNA damage at a cellular level by direct interactions from secondary electrons generated within the tissues, or by an indirect effect of free radical formation. This damage may be affected by factors in the tumour microenvironment, such as temperature and degree of hypoxia. The biological consequences of this DNA damage are a loss of reproductive ability and cellular function; it is thought to be the former which is more important in HNSCC.

If a cell is unable to repair its DNA damage before mitosis, cell death will occur. In general, malignant cells have a lower capacity for repair and a shorter cell cycle than normal tissues. This is the basis of the therapeutic ratio in terms of radiosensitivity of tumours compared to neighbouring healthy tissues.

Tissues may be broadly divided into early-responding (including mucosae and tumour) and late-responding (such as muscle, nerve, bone and fat), where the complications of treatment only become apparent weeks to months after cessation of therapy. The size of dose fraction is thought to be critical in determining this late response.

The basic principle of radiotherapy is to achieve as high a dose to the tumour and any occult extensions as possible, while minimizing the dose to surrounding normal tissues. Unfortunately, HNSCC is biologically rather radioresistant and usually in close juxtaposition to critically radiosensitive organs such as the eye, brain, salivary glands and spinal cord.

Ionizing radiation is either particulate (usually electrons) or high-energy electromagnetic radiation (short wavelength x-rays or gamma-rays). X-rays may be classified by their energy level, measured in volts.

The early enthusiasm which greeted radium implants and orthovoltage generators (producing about 100 kV) in the first half of the twentieth century as a 'magic bullet' was soon tempered by the long-term side effects experienced by survivors. External beam therapy was characterized by poor tissue penetration, with severe skin damage and poor cure rates for deep tumours. In the 1950s with the advent of linear accelerator and telecobalt units generating supervoltage (2–6 MV) radiation and deeper tissue penetration with skin sparing, the popularity of radiotherapy began to recover.

Linear accelerator beams also produce a better edge definition, with less of a penumbra, or shadow edge, allowing for narrower treatment margins of normal tissue. Cobalt sources emit megavoltages of gamma rays and were extremely popular for many years due to their relative simplicity of use, but the physical properties and safety issues are inferior to those of a linear accelerator.

Radiation dose is prescribed using the SI units of absorbed dose, the gray (Gy), named after the pioneering radiobiologist LH Gray. The previous unit was the rad, equivalent to 1 centigray (0.01 Gy).

Planning of treatment involves careful delineation of the primary tumour and any neck fields to be included along with the exclusion of local critical tissues, such as the orbit and central nervous system (CNS) from the fields. Close liaison with a radiation physicist is often useful at the time of planning in determination of the treatment pattern. To ensure patient immobility during treatment, a thermoplastic mesh shell (Orfit) is moulded to the contours of the patient's head and neck as they lie on the treatment simulator. Holes may be cut for the eyes and nose, and the mesh fixed to a base-board to ensure replication of positioning for each treatment session.

Radiotherapy is less effective in hypoxic tumours, particularly those with bony or cartilaginous involvement. It is also unsuitable for patients with fistula, exposed bone or inadequate wound healing. Various patient factors may also play a part in the treatment decision. Claustrophobia, an inability to lie flat or neck problems may prevent adequate positioning. Good patient compliance and motivation must be assured as missing just a single fraction can have severe adverse consequences in terms of the overall outcome. The patient's nutritional and immune status also need to be optimized prior to treatment and support staff need to monitor nutritional input and local skin/mucosal care during and immediately following the treatment. A full dental assessment is also mandatory if the mandible is within the radiotherapy field, as post-radiotherapy there is a high incidence of osteoradionecrosis following infections or extraction of diseased teeth.

During the course of treatment, the patient should be monitored by a multidisciplinary team on a weekly basis.

PRIMARY RADIOTHERAPY

For early stage HNSCC, no level I evidence exists comparing primary radiotherapy with other modalities, in particular conservative surgery. For early stage mucosal disease, cure rates of 70–90 per cent would be expected from this modality alone from prospective and retrospective cohort studies.[31] Involvement of bone or muscle will drop the cure rate to 50–70 per cent[53] and hence combined modality therapy is recommended in these circumstances.

Primary radiotherapy has been commonly used to treat early tumours of the base of tongue, hypopharynx and larynx due to the surgical morbidity of accessing these areas adequately for resection. Advances in surgical techniques and reconstructive options have resulted in a great variation in local practices in these areas. Oral cavity lesions are more surgically accessible and only brachytherapy is useful in this region in avoiding the morbidity of mucositis, trismus and xerostomia associated with external beam irradiation.

Similarly in treatment of the neck, radiotherapy may be curative for N1 disease, but total response rates in the N2 neck are only around 50–70 per cent with poor long-term outcomes.[53] Thus, if external beam irradiation is being used to treat the primary tumour, it is generally also used to treat the high risk N0 and N1 neck. On occasion, radiotherapy may be used to treat the primary site (if early stage) following a neck dissection, for example in early hypopharyngeal cancer with extensive neck disease.

Conventional external beam radiotherapy would typically involve a dose of 60–67 Gy to the primary tumour and gross adenopathy delivered in single fractions of 1.8–2 Gy per day, 5 days per week for 6–7 weeks.

PREOPERATIVE RADIOTHERAPY

The uninterrupted preoperative blood supply to a tumour was thought to make the cells potentially more radiosensitive, and it was hoped that larger tumours may be shrunk to an easily resectable size and the possibility of intraoperative embolization of tumour would be reduced.

In the 1960s, a number of clinical trials examined the combined effects of radiotherapy and surgery in an effort to improve locoregional control of advanced HNSCC, and promising results were found with a view to reduction of regional recurrence, but the surgical morbidity was increased. Vandenbrouk's 1977 study compared preoperative and postoperative radiotherapy (PORT) in hypopharyngeal cancer, with reported five-year survivals of 20 and 56 per cent, respectively. Such unfavourable results led to the discontinuation of preoperative irradiation in favour of PORT.

POSTOPERATIVE (ADJUVANT) RADIOTHERAPY

The purpose of PORT is to address clinical and pathological findings that are known to lead to increased failure rates at the primary and regional sites. Following surgery, only microscopic well-vascularized normoxic islands of tumour should remain, which should theoretically be relatively radiosensitive.

Numerous studies have demonstrated improvements in locoregional control of HNSCC when PORT is used appropriately.[54] Indications include positive (or close) margins, perineural spread, lymphovascular invasion, bone invasion, extension into soft tissues, multiple involved nodes, extracapsular spread and involved nodes >3 cm in diameter. The interval between surgery and irradiation is critical, and most retrospective studies indicate that a delay of no greater than 4–6 weeks is preferable.[55] The increasing use of microvascular tissue transfer has improved the attainment of this goal.

There is no significant dose–response relationship for total doses from 57.6 to 68.4 Gy unless there is evidence of extracapsular spread (ECS) within the neck, when 63 Gy was found to be more beneficial than 57.6 Gy.[56] There is thus a consensus that a dose of 60–66 Gy should be delivered to the surgical bed and all anatomical sites at risk of recurrence.

A recent review of 8795 patients in the Surveillance, Epidemiology and End-Results (SEER) US database has shown a 10 per cent absolute increase in five-year cancer-specific survival and overall survival in patients with N+ disease treated with PORT.[57] There is no level I evidence for the use of PORT, but there is a broad consensus to its efficacy and a prospective trial would now be considered unethical.

SALVAGE RADIOTHERAPY

Traditionally, surgery has been the major modality in the context of recurrent disease, but radiotherapy has a role in those who have not previously been irradiated. Many patients in this situation are simply not surgical candidates due to tumour extent or comorbidities.

Reirradiation is gaining in popularity with modalities such as intensity-modulated radiotherapy (IMRT) allowing for improved sparing of local tissues. The likelihood of success is heavily dependent on the location and extent of disease. Inadequate previous treatment, whether surgical or by radiotherapy, also may have a favourable prognosis.[58] Patients with multifocal locoregional recurrences have a very poor prognosis and are unlikely to benefit from retreatment. Survival rates remain very poor, and distant metastatic disease is not infrequent.

Radiotherapy may be beneficial in the palliative setting for control of local symptoms, such as pain, bleeding and fungation.

INTERSTITIAL RADIOTHERAPY (BRACHYTHERAPY)

Interstitial radiotherapy refers to the implantation of a radioactive source directly into the treatment field providing specific intense local irradiation with a very rapid fall off in dose from the surface of the source. It is highly operator-dependent and relies on local expertise to produce optimum results. Most published series originate in highly specialist centres and their applicability to less expert units is questionable.

This technique thus allows an increased concentration of radiation at the implant site while minimizing the dose to surrounding tissues. In some units, it is the treatment of choice for small tumours of the oral cavity (<30 mm) without bony involvement. Significantly less serious side effects, in terms of mucositis, trismus and xerostomia, are achievable with this technique. Brachytherapy is also occasionally used postoperatively in the oral cavity or oropharynx for positive or close resection margins in unfavourable tumours. It may provide particular benefit in the context of previously irradiated unresectable recurrent disease of the oral cavity, nasopharynx and oropharynx. Recent studies have suggested a potential role in the postoperative neck in high risk or recurrent disease.[31]

LOW-DOSE RATE IMPLANTS

Low-dose rate (LDR) implants have a relatively long half-life and thus longer overall treatment times. Radiation exposure to medical staff may be minimized by the use of remote afterloader techniques. Under a general anaesthetic, fine needles are placed through the tumour site and hollow plastic tubes threaded over these to remain in place. These hollow applicators are then afterloaded remotely by machine without direct clinician exposure to the radioactive source. The patient must be nursed in isolation in a shielded room until the course is completed, generally after a week. The treatment time is thus much shorter than conventional external beam radiotherapy, countering the risk of tumour repopulation.

HIGH-DOSE RATE IMPLANTS

With high-dose rate (HDR) implants, temporary implantation of iridium-192 sources can give an adequate local dose in minutes, so there is little opportunity for migration of the source and the treatment is relatively cheap. The actual radiation dose tends to be higher than with LDR, giving some concern as to the risk of late effects. The novel technique of pulsed-dose brachytherapy (PDR) combines the two techniques to give a pulse of high dose for 10–30 minutes each hour amounting to approximately the same dose as in LDR.

ALTERED FRACTIONATION

Radiotherapy schedules have conventionally been given as daily fractions 5 days per week for 5–7 weeks for historical reasons of convenience. The rationale for departing from this scheme is to increase the biological dose without increasing the risk of late normal tissue damage.

HYPERFRACTIONATION

Hyperfractionation is defined as dividing the treatment into smaller than conventional doses per fraction without altering the overall treatment duration to increase the therapeutic differentiation between late-responding normal tissue and tumour; for example, a regime of 1.2 Gy given twice daily over 7 weeks for a total of 81.6 Gy, increasing the dose while keeping the treatment time constant. Locoregional control rates have been improved by about 15 per cent over historical controls in HNSCC by this method,[59] without any overall increase in late complications.

ACCELERATED FRACTIONATION

This involves shortening the overall treatment duration using conventional doses to minimize tumour growth during treatment fractions, for example 1.6 Gy twice daily for 6 weeks. A range of different regimens have been devised and once again locoregional control rates have been improved[60] at the expense of increased acute toxicity, but it has proven difficult to demonstrate an improvement in overall survival.

The Meta-analysis of Radiotherapy in Carcinomas of the Head and Neck collaborative group (MARCH)[61] have demonstrated an 8 per cent survival benefit at five years for hyperfractionated therapy, and an overall five-year survival benefit of 3.4 per cent for all altered fractionation schedules in the 15 randomized trials assessed. There was a more significant benefit in locoregional control, again most pronounced in the hyperfractionated group and in younger patients with good performance status. It is possible that the latter are better able to tolerate the increased early side effects.

HIGHLY CONFORMAL RADIOTHERAPY

In an effort to further minimize damage to normal tissue, efforts have been made to increase the conformity of the radiation dose to the tumour morphology. With standard radiotherapy techniques, a large safety margin of normal tissue is irradiated along with tumour. In IMRT, CT images are used to provide a 3D reconstruction of the tumour and specific target doses to the tumour and maximum tolerable doses to surrounding tissues planned on a slice-by-slice basis. A computer-derived algorithm then determines the beam parameters to provide the desired dose distribution to what is often a highly irregular target. A large number of radiation portals with dynamic multileaf collimators (MLC) are required to achieve this highly tailored dose distribution. The MLC are Tungsten plates only a few millimetres thick whose position is controlled by small electric motors controlled by the planning computer.

Tomotherapy is a new variant of IMRT which combines a highly sophisticated computer-controlled radiation beam collimation with an on-board CT scanner to create an image of the treatment site. It therefore combines planning, patient positioning and treatment delivery into one system. Helical tomography integrates a linear accelerator into a spiral CT scanner which continuously rotates around the patient on a gantry.

The use of PET/CT fusion images for IMRT planning may better delineate tumour from normal contiguous tissues. This may be particularly useful in reirradiation of recurrent disease.[62]

Excellent local control rates have been reported in naso- and oropharyngeal primary sites with this technique, with

potential for preservation of salivary tissue and reduced xerostomia.[63] However, long-term outcome data are understandably sparse.

STEREOTACTIC RADIOSURGERY

This highly conformal technique allows for the delivery of relatively large doses in a single or a few fractions, and is being increasingly used in the treatment of recurrent HNSCC, particularly in inaccessible areas such as the skull base. Multiple low-dose radiation beams are delivered in a pattern that allows them to overlap at the target lesion. The dose provided results in significant cell damage regardless of cell cycle phase, and to a degree does away with the classical concept of radiosensitivity. Fractionation of the dose may be useful in treating larger targets in close proximity to vital structures.

PARTICLE RADIOTHERAPY

High energy protons may be focused with magnetic fields to produce a very narrow beam with little scatter, and thus highly conformal therapy is possible. Most energy deposition comes towards the end of the particle's track, thus sparing superficial tissues, and the range of the protons may be adjusted by varying the energy of the beam. Current clinical uses are mastly restricted to NPC.

Carbon ions are relatively heavy charged particles used in tumours otherwise thought to be poorly radiosensitive, such as chordomas and chondrosarcomas of the skull base.

Neutron beams are less dependent on tumour oxygenation for efficacy and have been extensively investigated in salivary gland malignancies with mixed results.[64]

Chemotherapy

HNSCC has proven much more resistant to cure by chemotherapy than many other solid tumours, such as the lymphomas and sarcomas. However, although indications for single modality treatments are very limited, much attention has recently been paid to combination regimes with both radiotherapy and surgery. Medical oncology is a highly technical specialty requiring a significant amount of supportive care for the patients in terms of clinical nurse specialists experienced in recognizing and treating the complications of these often highly toxic regimens.

Since the advent of platinum-based agents in the 1970s, the role of chemotherapy has gradually evolved from producing short-lived local responses in the palliative setting to the widely used curative multimodality regimes for advanced HNSCCs. Its use has been spurred on by the observation that even when locoregional control has been achieved in advanced HNSCC, the long-term prognosis is still disappointing, with second primaries and metastatic disease accounting for a large proportion of treatment failures.

Chemotherapeutic agents (**Table 7.5**) typically act by interfering with basic cellular processes, usually associated with mitosis, thus selectively affecting those tissues with high turnover. There is thus a degree of synergy with radiotherapy,

Table 7.5 Classes of agents.

Class	
Alkylating agents	Cyclophosphamide, chlorambucil, melphelan: bind covalently to DNA, forming crosslinks and inhibiting replication
Antimetabolites	Methotrexate: antifolate agent which inhibits dihydrofolate reductase
	5-fluorouracil-pyrimidine antagonist: inhibits DNA synthesis
Plant derivatives	Vincristine: derived from rosy periwinkle, prevents tubulin spindle formation during mitosis
	Paclitaxel/docetaxel: yew tree derivatives, prevent microtubule disassembly
Antibiotics	Actinomycin D, doxorubicin, bleomycin: intercalate between DNA base-pairs, preventing mitosis
Miscellaneous	Carboplatin: cisplatin-platinum derivatives, crosslink DNA

and scope for combinations of agents with differing mechanisms to work synergistically.

INDUCTION (NEOADJUVANT) CHEMOTHERAPY

Neoadjuvant therapy is used prior to definitive therapy with the intention of improving the success rate of the primary therapy. It was hoped that initial debulking of tumour by this means might improve the efficacy of local therapy, and drug delivery to tumour would be optimal before the blood supply was reduced by local therapies. The potential to eradicate micrometastatic disease before clinical presentation was also a hope. Response to induction therapy may also be used to assess prognosis and select the definitive course of treatment. Many pilot studies in the 1980s appeared to suggest high response rates of HNSCC to cisplatin with acceptable toxicity, but it has proved difficult to translate this into an overall survival benefit.

However, several studies demonstrated that tumour response to induction chemotherapy predicted a beneficial response to further treatment, and a better overall prognosis. This finding led the Veterans Affairs (VA) Laryngeal Cancer Study Group to investigate non-surgical laryngeal preservation. In their landmark study, patients with advanced laryngeal cancer were randomized to receive either standard treatment (laryngectomy+PORT) or two cycles of induction cisplatin. Those who showed a good clinical response to the induction agent then underwent radiotherapy, whereas non-responders underwent laryngectomy.[65] The European Organisation for Research and Treatment of Cancer (EORTC) designed a similar study for patients with hypopharyngeal cancer, with similar outcomes.[66]

Both studies showed comparable survival rates for radical surgery compared to organ preservation by induction chemotherapy followed by radiotherapy, with preservation of the larynx in approximately two-thirds of survivors of the VA trial and 42 per cent of survivors of the EORTC trial.

A follow-up randomized trial (RTOG91-11) further evaluated the optimum organ-sparing protocol in advanced resectable laryngeal cancer. Patients were randomized to receive radical radiotherapy alone, sequential induction chemotherapy followed by radiotherapy or concurrent chemoradiotherapy. Treatment failures underwent salvage laryngectomy, and again there was no significant overall survival difference between the three arms. However, the concomitant chemoradiotherapy had significantly higher rates of locoregional control and preservation of the larynx. High volume T4 tumours invading cartilage or tongue base were excluded from this trial, somewhat limiting its impact.

HNSCC appears to be exquisitely sensitive to platinum-based induction chemotherapy, with response rates of up to 80–90 per cent reported, but translating this into a gain in overall survival has proven frustratingly difficult. One must remember that a complete response is defined as complete disappearance of the primary tumour. Partial response occurs when the product of two perpendicular diameters decreases by more than 50 per cent of the original. The clinical significance of this is clearly rather limited.

The Meta-analysis of Chemotherapy on Head and Neck Cancer collaborative group have demonstrated a non-significant survival improvement of just 2 per cent at five years for induction regimes, leading to the search for other more biologically active regimens. Addition of a taxane, such as docetaxel, is currently under investigation in multiple trials.[67]

ADJUVANT CHEMOTHERAPY

A randomized controlled trial of PORT followed by chemotherapy versus PORT alone in high-risk HNSCC patients failed to demonstrate a survival advantage in the face of high toxicity and poor patient compliance of this prolonged treatment plan.[68] In view of the perceived success of concurrent chemoradiotherapy, this approach has been sidelined.

SALVAGE/PALLIATIVE CHEMOTHERAPY

Chemotherapy has long been the standard of care for patients presenting with recurrent or advanced disease not suitable for radical treatment. Cisplatin and 5FU are the standard agents in combination, but although they have a high initial response rate with tolerable toxicity, this has not translated into a significant prolongation of survival. Patients with a poor performance status may be more suited to a single agent therapy or the use of targeted therapy, such as cetuximab. In any case, the marginal benefits of treatment must be carefully weighed against the potential impact on quality of life.

Patients with bulky locoregional disease or high tumour volume and prior treatment of recurrence are likely to respond poorly to chemotherapy and may be more suited to supportive care.

CONCURRENT CHEMORADIOTHERAPY

The rationale behind combining the two non-surgical modalities lies in their potential synergies. Chemotherapy has both a potential radiosensitizing effect for locoregional disease and also has a systemic antimetastatic effect. Concurrent regimens are rapidly increasing in scope and popularity and in many units represent the primary treatment of locally advanced disease and the adjuvant of choice for high-risk surgical pathology.

DEFINITIVE CONCURRENT CHEMORADIATION

The first randomized controlled trial demonstrating improved survival of CCRT over radiotherapy alone in advanced resectable HNSCC was published in 1997. The CCRT arm also showed a reduction in distant metastases in the face of increased local and systemic toxicity.

The MACH-NC meta-analysis of 63 trials,[69] including almost 11 000 patients showed the addition of chemotherapy to locoregional treatment conferred an overall survival benefit of 4 per cent at five years, but the benefit of CCRT was 8 per cent at five years. Adjuvant and neoadjuvant regimens showed no survival benfit. A similar meta-analysis of nasopharyngeal carcinoma showed a significant survival advantage for CCRT

The RTOG91-11 study strongly indicated the superiority of CCRT to other methods of combined therapy administration,[70] leading to a marked increase in popularity of this organ-preserving strategy. It is now routinely used as the standard of care in many centres for all locally advanced subsites within the head and neck.

The Groupe d'Oncologie Radiotherapie Tête et Cou (GORTEC) randomly assigned 226 patients with advanced oropharyngeal disease to either CCRT or radiotherapy alone, with observed improvement in overall survival at three years for the CCRT arm at the cost of increased toxicity.[71]

The management of locally advanced nasopharyngeal carcinoma (NPC) has altered radically in recent years following publication of the US Intergroup Nasopharynx study.[72] Patients with stage III or IV disease showed a significant five-year survival benefit from CCRT compared to radiotherapy alone, a finding confirmed by the Meta-analysis of Chemotherapy in NPC study.[73]

However, the MACH-NC demonstrated a non-significant increase in death for laryngeal preservation protocols combined with classical laryngectomy followed by PORT (6 per cent at five years).[69] Also, the US National Cancer Database analysis of cancer deaths has shown survival from laryngeal cancer decreasing over the 1990s compared to the 1980s, the only common cancer to show such a finding.[74] Further analysis of the data from 1995–8 has shown a definite survival advantage for those patients treated surgically rather than via an organ-sparing approach for advanced laryngeal cancer, most notably those with stage IV disease. This was not clinical trial data and as such are subject to extremes of selection bias, but one might expect those selected for organ preservation therapy to have performance scores comparable to, if not in excess of, those undergoing laryngectomy. Some have suggested that this calls into question the applicability of findings from major referral centre-structured trials to general clinical practice, a sobering thought indeed.

ADJUVANT CCRT

Locoregional recurrence and distant metastases are not infrequent after surgical resection of advanced HNSCC, especially in tumours with adverse pathological features.

Two major phase 3 trials have examined the efficacy of CCRT in the postoperative setting in the context of high-risk pathological findings, such as multiple lymph node involvement, ECS and positive resection margins.[75, 76] Both studies showed improved local control by CCRT and disease-free survival compared to conventional PORT with no effect on distant metastases and an observed increase in toxicity. Comparative analysis of the trials revealed that ECS and positive resection margins were the most powerful predictors of additional benefit from adjuvant CCRT. However, a five-year updated analysis of the RTOG trial no longer showed statistical significance for any end point. The performance status of the patient and availability of appropriate supportive care are critical to adequate compliance to this approach.[77] Compounds that reduce treatment toxicity, such as amifostine to protect salivary output or palifermine to alleviate mucositis, need further evaluation in this setting.

Targeted therapies

The epidermal growth factor receptor is a member of the ErbB growth factor receptor tyrosine kinase family and is overexpressed in around 95 per cent of all HNSCC. Overexpression of EGFR has been associated with disease recurrence and worse patient survival, and several strategies have been developed to target this molecule. Cetuximab is a chimerical monoclonal antibody directed to the EGFR. In combination with radiotherapy, it has shown increased survival in advanced HNSCC patients compared to radiotherapy alone.[16] It does not cause significant myelosuppression or mucositis, and may represent an alternative to CCRT for those who cannot withstand the toxicity of platinum-based chemotherapy regimes. Cetuximab has yet to be directly compared with CCRT in a randomized clinical trial.

Other targeted agents include panitumumab, a fully human monoclonal antibody to the EGFR, and erlotinib, which inhibits the tyrosine kinase downstream from the EGFR. Bevacizumab is a monoclonal antibody to the vascular endothelial growth factor (VEGF), thought to be essential for angiogenesis in rapidly growing tumour tissues. Tirapazamine is a hypoxic sensitizer currently being evaluated in phase II studies.[78]

Salvage surgery

As CCRT has played an increasing role in the primary management of advanced HNSCC, surgeons are increasingly being called upon in the context of locoregionally recurrent or persistent disease. NCDB data in the United States show a doubling in rates of primary CCRT use for advanced oropharyngeal and laryngeal primaries between 1985 and 2001. This effect was most pronounced in teaching hospitals, strongly suggesting that the trend will continue when current trainees become independent practitioners.

The surgeon is thus increasingly confronted with diagnostic dilemmas, the clinical picture being confused by the inevitable tissue oedema, necrosis and chondritis secondary to CCRT. The post-treatment patient also commonly complains of hoarseness, dysphagia, respiratory distress and pain; these are often the symptoms which brought them to medical attention in the first instance. Patients with suspected recurrent disease are generally subjected to examination under anaesthesia and biopsies. There is a relatively high rate of false negatives due both to difficulties in interpreting histological changes and the growth pattern of recurrent tumours. Recurrence is often multifocal, dispersed throughout the treated region and often beneath an intact mucosa.

Imaging studies are notoriously difficult to interpret without an adequate post-treatment baseline study. However, the baseline study itself may be confused by the presence of residual disease, which may be difficult to tell apart from progression of CCRT-related tissue changes. CT[79] and MRI findings have been compared with salvage laryngectomy specimens with disappointing results. PET scans appear to show significant benefits in this regard as non-tumour FDG uptake appears unaffected by treatment,[80] whereas recurrent disease shows significantly higher uptake rates. Differentiation between inflammatory changes and recurrent tumour remains a significant problem. Diffusion-weighted MRI gives an indication of the cellularity of tissues by measuring the apparent diffusion coefficient (ADC) of water molecules. Recurrent tumour tends to have a low ADC in comparison to necrosis, which exhibits a high ADC secondary to the loss of membrane integrity. Thus, a combination of imaging modalities may be useful in guiding further biopsies.

In the case of the N+ neck treated with CCRT, there is ongoing debate as to the wisdom of a planned neck dissection. Those patients with an N1 neck and good clinical response to CCRT[81] generally may be closely observed. Those with N2/3 necks and residual palpable disease or suspicious radiological findings on completion of treatment will generally undergo a neck dissection of some description. However, the specimen obtained is not uncommonly free of obvious tumour and there is a high chance of overtreating these patients.[82] In this situation, PET once again would appear to be of value, with a surveillance scan three to four months following treatment completion to direct biopsies.[83] Earlier scans have a high false-negative rate as FDG uptake is suppressed by the treatment and the number of viable tumour cells drops. Later scans may compromise the success of salvage surgery.

If salvage resections are deemed possible by the MDT and desirable by the patient, a number of issues need to be examined before proceeding. Complication rates are significantly increased in this patient population;[84] a meta-analysis of historical series (1980–98) found a weighted mortality rate of 5.2 per cent, and a major complication rate of 27 per cent. The vast majority of these patients had undergone irradiation alone with no CCRT and had not undergone free flap reconstruction. The RTOG91-11 trial found a pharyngocutaneous fistula rate of 30 per cent post-CCRT versus 15 per cent for radiation alone, and a later smaller study had similar figures of 31.6 and 15.6 per cent, respectively.[85] Thus, the poor quality of tissue in the local surgical site may preclude optimal wound healing, and it is probably advisable to utilize free tissue transfer to optimize recovery in these conditions. However, prolonged operative time and increased rate of systemic postoperative complications may limit this option.

Tumours that survive the challenge of CCRT may be expected to be more aggressive and resilient in the face of other treatment modalities. The overall five-year survival in the historical meta-analysis was 39 per cent, with the stage at recurrence having a major impact on prognosis. T3 and T4 recurrences in a further series had a two-year survival of 31 per cent and a five-year survival of 15 per cent, a fairly gloomy prospect.[86] The authors found that a disproportionate number of survivors had undergone inadequate primary treatment, and there were very few successful salvages in patients who had undergone radical initial therapy. It would appear that the best chance of a cure is at the first attempt.

In contrast, the two-year survival post-salvage laryngectomy in the RTOG91-11 trial was 76 per cent, but one must remember that high volume and T4 tumours were excluded from this study, as were patients with a Karnofsky score <60. A more recent (and realistic) series of 38 patients with biopsy-proven recurrence post-CCRT showed a two-year survival of 27 per cent.[87]

A further challenge to the surgeon is the extent of resection. CCRT does not appear to kill tumour cells concentrically, leaving a neater, smaller tumour, but cells appear to die in diffuse patterns throughout the tumour, and thus the resection should probably be based on the initial pretreatment tumour volume rather than the palpable residual volume.[88]

PALLIATIVE CARE

Palliative care is interdisciplinary care that provides support for the physical, emotional and psychological suffering of patients with any advanced illness regardless of age, diagnosis or life expectancy. The goal is to prevent or alleviate suffering and to improve the quality of life for people facing severe, complex illness. The complex nature and often uncertain prognosis of HNSCC may lead to situations where radical treatments are given with palliative intent, and there is a spectrum of palliation from the primary treatment through salvage treatment to end-of-life terminal care. Patients with HNSCC often have a relapsing course with periods of freedom from disease and symptoms interspersed with bouts of serious illness, debility and physical or psychological symptoms. Whereas treatment modalities have increased the disease-free interval for patients with advanced HNSCC, cure rates have not significantly changed and patients are often living longer with quiescent subclinical disease.

During the period when treatment aims are altering from eradication of disease to symptom control, it is important to involve the specialist palliative care staff at an early stage. However, the patient must not feel they are being abandoned by their clinical team and it must be emphasized that active medical care will continue albeit with different aims.

Ideally, the patient should be cared for in a home situation by the family and community health service. Macmillan, Ian Rennie or Marie Curie cancer nurses can be invaluable in providing support under these circumstances and direct contact with palliative care physicians through attendance at a day hospice may be useful.

Admission to hospice care is not necessarily permanent and discharge is common after admission for respite, convalescence or short periods to optimize symptom control. Of course, if home social support networks are lacking then institutional care may be the only sensible option. On occasion, a strong relationship has been built up between the patient and the surgical or oncology staff where they have been treated, and it may be suitable for continued care to be provided in the hospital environment with input from the palliative care team.

Symptom control

PAIN

Intractable pain is unacceptable in the palliative care setting and utmost effort should be made to determine the underlying cause. A full pain history and examination should be sought rather than simply reaching for the drug chart to increase the opiates. In HNSCC, pain may have aetiologies and pathophysiological mechanisms different from other malignancies. Nociceptive pain from destruction of local tissues is common, but also neuropathic pain from the tumour damaging or travelling along nerves should be recognized. Nociceptive pain may be treated according to the WHO pain relief ladder (**Figure 7.4**). For mild pain, non-opioid agents, such as paracetamol, aspirin or ibuprofen, may be appropriate. Failure to control pain should result in prescription of a mild opiate in conjunction with a simple analgesic, such as paracetamol and codeine. If this proves inadequate then, by definition, the pain is severe and strong opiates, such as morphine or diamorphine, are indicated. Many patients, relatives and even some health-care professionals are unduly concerned about making this final step to a strong opiate due to fears of addiction or severe side effects, but the patient should not be denied the undoubted benefits these drugs offer.

Long-acting agents should be used on a regular basis to avoid breakthrough pain, and there is no place for PRN (pro re nata, or as needed) prescribing. The initial dose can be titrated with a shorter acting agent, such as oramorph 4-hourly, before switching to a slow-release preparation, such as MST. Gentle laxatives and antiemetics should be prescribed to prevent constipation and excessive nausea, respectively. If the oral route is unavailable then transdermal patches containing fentanyl are available. Alternatively subcutaneous opiates may be administered, and towards the end of life these may be given by syringe driver.

Neuropathic pain from raised intracranial pressure or direct nerve damage may be more responsive to anticonvulsants, steroids, local anaesthetics and tricyclic antidepressants.

SKIN

Following radiotherapy, dermatitis and soft tissue damage is not uncommon in the face and neck. A progression from erythema to blistering to ulcerations and slough is commonly seen. The acute changes will generally settle around 2 weeks after treatment. The scalp should be washed very gently with mild shampoo if involved. Topical low-potency steroid creams and aloe vera have been used prophylactically and as treatment for skin damage, but a systematic review has shown no benefits.[89] A plain lanolin-free nonscented hydrophilic cream may be helpful as long as the skin remains intact. Itching may be treated with low-potency steroid cream with close clinical observation for further skin damage.

XEROSTOMIA

On occasion, surgery to the oral cavity and mandible can cause difficulty with oral continence of secretions and sialorrhoea. Speech therapy input and the judicious use of hyoscine patches may alleviate this. A much more common problem in those who have undergone radiotherapy is xerostomia, particularly if CCRT has been used. This can lead to difficulties with eating and swallowing, dental caries and decreased quality of life.[90] Frequent sips of water, ice cubes, sugar-free chewing gum and artificial saliva may all prove useful. Pilocarpine is a parasympathomimetic sialogogue, but its side effects (including sweating, rhinorrhoea and urinary frequency) may prevent its wider use in this patient population.

DYSPHAGIA AND ODYNOPHAGIA

Artificial hydration and nutrition via the nasogastric or gastrostomy route is commonly used as a temporary measure during the recovery phase from treatment. However, the requirement may become lifelong if swallowing difficulties do not settle with time. Alterations in smell and taste also often have an adverse effect on the appetite, and nutritional supplements may be necessary.

PSYCHOLOGICAL SYMPTOMS

Patients are often understandably frustrated by the many setbacks experienced during their clinical pathway, and

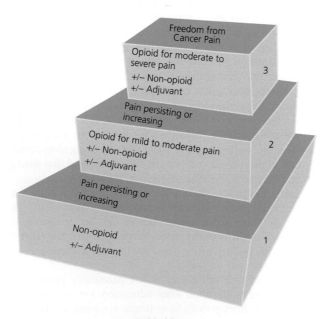

Figure 7.4 WHO pain relief ladder.

changes in outward appearance and essential functions may be difficult to bear. Even small cosmetic alterations can have a huge adverse impact on patient body-image and self-esteem.[91] Between 20 and 50 per cent of patients with HNSCC experience moderate to severe depression at some point after diagnosis,[92] and the use of antidepressants is often helpful under these circumstances.[93]

The high rate of locoregional recurrence in HNSCC is also a source of considerable anxiety which may be particularly pervasive. Benzodiazepines and selective serotonin reuptake inhibitors (SSRI) may be helpful in the short term, and many centres have a psychologist with an interest in the psychosocial impact of HNSCC. Patients may experience guilt and self-blame about the toll the illness is taking on their loved ones, and alterations in their ability to leave the house and interact socially with others can lead to difficult changes in the dynamics of long-term relationships. The Macmillan clinical nurse specialist is invaluable in this situation, and can provide the patient with access to patient-support groups and facilities, such as Maggie's Centres, which may provide supportive information and counselling.

END-OF-LIFE ISSUES

Predicting the terminal phase of a patient's illness may be difficult. Late signs include the patient becoming bed-bound and comatose, only able to take sips of fluid and unable to take oral medications or tolerate artificial hydration or nutrition. Clear communication with patient and family is essential to ensure they understand that the terminal phase has arrived. Issues such as the emergency management of the airway or the potential for major vessel erosion must be considered by the medical staff and discussed with patient and family if they are likely to arise imminently. A supply of opiates or benzodiazepines should be rapidly available at the bedside and all carers informed if asphyxiation or a carotid blowout seem likely.

Artificial hydration and nutrition may become burdensome and inappropriate towards the end of life and may prolong the dying process unnecessarily.

THE FUTURE

Caution must be exercised in the extrapolation of clinical findings in highly expert tertiary centre-structured trials to general clinical practice in units where local expertise and clinical support networks may fall short of our highest aspirations.

Advances in robotic surgery and fibreoptic carbon dioxide lasers may soon allow for surgical laryngeal functional preservation in more extensive tumours without the local and systemic morbidity of CCRT.[94]

Whereas preservation of function is crucial to the success of many interventions in HNSCC, we must not lose sight of the fact that in a curative context successful extirpation of disease must not be sacrificed for short-lasting secondary benefits. Also preservation of a functionless organ which may be harbouring residual disease is of no benefit to the patient. The top priorities of the patient with HNSCC are almost

universally cure and prolongation of life, with functional and cosmetic considerations much lower down the list of priorities than clinicians might be tempted to suppose.

> ### KEY EVIDENCE
>
> - Head and neck cancer is the most complex 'organ site' for treatment decision-making and thus a specialist multidisciplinary team is required for optimal patient management.[93]
> - Adequate initial assessment of the primary, nodal sites and potential distant metastases is essential for the decision-making process.[94]
> - New standards of patient care for locally advanced disease employ cisplatin-based chemotherapy with radiation with the intent of preserving speech and swallowing.[68]

> ### KEY LEARNING POINTS
>
> - Head and neck cancer is the most complex 'organ site' for treatment decision-making and thus a specialist multidisciplinary team is required for optimal patient management.[95]
> - Adequate initial assessment of the primary, nodal sites and potential distant metastases is essential for the decision-making process.[96]
> - New standards of patient care for locally advanced disease employ cisplatin-based chemotherapy with radiation with the intent of preserving speech and swallowing.[69]

REFERENCES

◆ 1. Bernier J. Current state-of-the-art for concurrent chemoradiation. *Seminars in Radiation Oncology* 2009; 19: 3–10.
2. Scher RL, Esclamado RM. Organ and function preservation: the role of surgery as the optimal primary modality or as salvage after chemoradiation failure. *Seminars in Radiation Oncology* 2009; 19: 17–23.
3. Jacobs CD, Goffinet DR, Fee WE Jr. Head and neck squamous cancers. *Currrent Problems in Cancer* 1990; 14: 1–72.
4. Fukano H, Matsuura H, Hasegawa Y, Nakamura S. Depth of invasion as a predictive factor for cervical lymph node metastasis in tongue carcinoma. *Head and Neck* 1997; 19: 205–10.

5. Weber RS, Gidley P, Morrison WH *et al.* Treatment selection for carcinoma of the base of the tongue. *American Journal of Surgery* 1990; **160**: 415–19.

6. Agarwal V, Branstetter BF, Johnson JT. Indications for PET/CT in the head and neck. *Otolaryngologic Clinics of North America* 2008; **41**: 23–49, v.

7. Connell CA, June Corry J, Milner AD *et al.* Clinical impact of, and prognostic stratification by, F-18 FDG PET/CT in head and neck mucosal squamous cell carcinoma. *Head and Neck* 2007; **29**: 986–95.

8. Chang SS, Califano J. Current status of biomarkers in head and neck cancer. *Journal of Surgical Oncology* 2008; **97**: 640–3.

9. Gillison ML. Human papillomavirus-associated head and neck cancer is a distinct epidemiologic, clinical, and molecular entity. *Seminars in Oncology* 2004; **31**: 744–54.

10. Li G, Sturgis EM. The role of human papillomavirus in squamous carcinoma of the head and neck. *Current Oncology Reports* 2006; **8**: 130–9.

11. Kreimer AR, Clifford GM, Boyle P *et al.* Human papillomavirus types in head and neck squamous cell carcinomas worldwide: a systematic review. *Cancer Epidemiology, Biomarkers and Prevention* 2005; **14**: 467–75.

12. Fakhry C, Westra WH, Sigui L *et al.* Improved survival of patients with human papillomavirus-positive head and neck squamous cell carcinoma in a prospective clinical trial. *Journal of the National Cancer Institute* 2008; **100**: 261–9.

13. Loeffler-Ragg J, Schwentner I, Sprinzl GM, Zwierzina H. EGFR inhibition as a therapy for head and neck squamous cell carcinoma. *Expert Opinion on Investigational Drugs* 2008; **17**: 1517–31.

14. Kim S, Grandis JR, Rinaldo A *et al.* Emerging perspectives in epidermal growth factor receptor targeting in head and neck cancer. *Head and Neck* 2008; **30**: 667–74.

15. Bentzen SM, Atasoy BM, Daley FM *et al.* Epidermal growth factor receptor expression in pretreatment biopsies from head and neck squamous cell carcinoma as a predictive factor for a benefit from accelerated radiation therapy in a randomized controlled trial. *Journal of Clinical Oncology* 2005; **23**: 5560–7.

• 16. Bonner JA, Harari PM, Giralt J *et al.* Radiotherapy plus cetuximab for squamous-cell carcinoma of the head and neck. *New England Journal of Medicine* 2006; **354**: 567–78.

17. Syrigos KN, Karachalios D, Karapanagiotou EM *et al.* Head and neck cancer in the elderly: an overview on the treatment modalities. *Cancer Treatment Reviews* 2009; **35**: 237–45.

18. Derks W, de Leeuw JR, Hordijk GJ *et al.* Reasons for non-standard treatment in elderly patients with advanced head and neck cancer. *European Archives of Otorhinolaryngology* 2005; **262**: 21–6.

19. Lowy DR, Gillison ML. A new link between Fanconi anemia and human papillomavirus-associated malignancies. *Journal of the National Cancer Institute* 2003; **95**: 1648–50.

20. Snyderman CH. Nutrition and head and neck cancer. *Current Oncology Reports* 2003; **5**: 158–63.

21. Bertrand PC, Piquet MA, Bordier I *et al.* Preoperative nutritional support at home in head and neck cancer patients: from nutritional benefits to the prevention of the alcohol withdrawal syndrome. *Current Opinion in Clinical Nutrition and Metabolic Care* 2002; **5**: 435–40.

22. Piccirillo JF, Tierney RM, Costas I *et al.* Prognostic importance of comorbidity in a hospital-based cancer registry. *Journal of the American Medical Association* 2004; **291**: 2441–7.

23. Desch CE, Penberthy L, Newschaffer CJ *et al.* Factors that determine the treatment for local and regional prostate cancer. *Medical Care* 1996; **34**: 152–62.

24. Piccirillo JF. Importance of comorbidity in head and neck cancer. *Laryngoscope* 2000; **110**: 593–602.

25. List MA, Stracks J, Colangelo L *et al.* How do head and neck cancer patients prioritize treatment outcomes before initiating treatment? *Journal of Clinical Oncology* 2000; **18**: 877–84.

26. Yousem DM, Gad K, Tufano RP. Resectability issues with head and neck cancer. *American Journal of Neuroradiology* 2006; **27**: 2024–36.

27. Skitarelić N, Morović M, Manestar D. Antibiotic prophylaxis in clean-contaminated head and neck oncological surgery. *Journal of Craniomaxillofacial Surgery* 2007; **35**: 15–20.

28. Bradley PJ, MacLennan K, Brakenhoff RH, Leemans CR. Status of primary tumour surgical margins in squamous head and neck cancer: prognostic implications. *Current Opinion in Otolaryngology and Head and Neck Surgery* 2007; **15**: 74–81.

29. Jones AS, Bin Hanafil Z, Nadapalan V *et al.* Do positive resection margins after ablative surgery for head and neck cancer adversely affect prognosis? A study of 352 patients with recurrent carcinoma following radiotherapy treated by salvage surgery. *British Journal of Cancer* 1996; **74**: 128–32.

30. Jacobs JR, Ahmad K, Casiano R *et al.* Implications of positive surgical margins. *Laryngoscope* 1993; **103**: 64–8.

♦ 31. Corvo R. Evidence-based radiation oncology in head and neck squamous cell carcinoma. *Radiotherapy and Oncology* 2007; **85**: 156–70.

32. Sessions DG, Spector GJ, Lenox J *et al.* Analysis of treatment results for floor-of-mouth cancer. *Laryngoscope* 2000; **110**: 1764–72.

33. Sessions DG, Spector GJ, Lenox J *et al.* Analysis of treatment results for oral tongue cancer. *Laryngoscope* 2002; **112**: 616–25.

34. Weir NF. Theodore Billroth: the first laryngectomy for cancer. *Journal of Laryngology and Otology* 1973; **87**: 1161–9.

35. Pressman JJ, Simon MB, Monell C. Anatomical studies related to the dissemination of cancer of the larynx. *Transactions – American Academy of Ophthalmology and Otolaryngology* 1960; **64**: 628–38.

36. Major MS, Bumpous JM, Flynn MB *et al.* Quality of life after treatment for advanced laryngeal and hypopharyngeal cancer. *Laryngoscope* 2001; **111**: 1379–82.

37. Sessions DG, Lenox J, Spector GJ. Supraglottic laryngeal cancer: analysis of treatment results. *Laryngoscope* 2005; **115**: 1402–10.

38. Dufour X, Hans S, De Mones E *et al.* Local control after supracricoid partial laryngectomy for 'advanced' endolaryngeal squamous cell carcinoma classified as T3. *Archives of Otolaryngology – Head and Neck Surgery* 2004; **130**: 1092–9.

39. Martin A, Jäckel MC, Christiansen H *et al.* Organ preserving transoral laser microsurgery for cancer of the hypopharynx. *Laryngoscope* 2008; **118**: 398–402.

40. Strong MS, Jako GJ. Laser surgery in the larynx. Early clinical experience with continuous CO_2 laser. *Annals of Otology, Rhinology and Laryngology* 1972; **81**: 791–8.

41. Steiner W. Results of curative laser microsurgery of laryngeal carcinomas. *American Journal of Otolaryngology* 1993; **14**: 116–21.

42. Silver CE, Rinaldo A, Ferlito A. Crile's neck dissection. *Laryngoscope* 2007; **117**: 1974–7.

43. Rinaldo A, Ferlito A, Silver CE. Early history of neck dissection. *European Journal of Otorhinolaryngology* 2008; **265**: 1535–8.

44. Bocca E, Pignataro O, Sasaki CT. Functional neck dissection. A description of operative technique. *Archives of Otolaryngology* 1980; **106**: 524–7.

45. Shah JP, Andersen PE. The impact of patterns of nodal metastasis on modifications of neck dissection. *Annals of Surgical Oncology* 1994; **1**: 521–32.

46. Ferlito A, Silver CE, Rinaldo A. Neck dissection: present and future? *European Archives of Otorhinolaryngology* 2008; **265**: 621–6.

47. Cote V, Kost K, Payne RJ *et al.* Sentinel lymph node biopsy in squamous cell carcinoma of the head and neck: where we stand now, and where we are going. *Journal of Otolaryngology* 2007; **36**: 344–9.

48. Bakamjian VY, Long M, Rigg B. Experience with the medially based deltopectoral flap in reconstructive surgery of the head and neck. *British Journal of Plastic Surgery* 1971; **24**: 174–83.

49. McCraw JB, Dibbell DG, Carraway JH. Clinical definition of independent myocutaneous vascular territories. *Plastic and Reconstructive Surgery* 1977; **60**: 341–52.

50. Ariyan S. The pectoralis major for single-stage reconstruction of the difficult wounds of the orbit and pharyngoesophagus. *Plastic and Reconstructive Surgery* 1983; **72**: 468–77.

51. Yang GF. [Free grafting of a lateral brachial skin flap]. *Zhonghua Wai Ke Za Zhi* 1983; **21**: 272–4.

52. Gilbert A. Free vascularized bone grafts. *International Surgery* 1981; **66**: 27–31.

53. Laskar SG, Agarwal JP, Srinivas C *et al.* Radiotherapeutic management of locally advanced head and neck cancer. *Expert Review of Anticancer Therapy* 2006; **6**: 405–17.

54. Fletcher GH. The evolution of the basic concepts underlying the practice of radiotherapy from 1949 to 1977. *Radiology* 1978; **127**: 3–19.

55. Ang KK, Trotti A, Brown BW *et al.* Randomized trial addressing risk features and time factors of surgery plus radiotherapy in advanced head-and-neck cancer. *International Journal of Radiation Oncology, Biology, Physics* 2001; **51**: 571–8.

56. Peters LJ, Goepfert H, Ang KK *et al.* Evaluation of the dose for postoperative radiation therapy of head and neck cancer: first report of a prospective randomized trial. *International Journal of Radiation Oncology, Biology, Physics* 1993; **26**: 3–11.

57. Kao J, Lavaf A, Teng MS *et al.* Adjuvant radiotherapy and survival for patients with node-positive head and neck cancer: an analysis by primary site and nodal stage. *International Journal of Radiation Oncology, Biology, Physics* 2008; **71**: 362–70.

58. Mendenhall WM, Mendenhall CM, Malyapa RS *et al.* Re-irradiation of head and neck carcinoma. *American Journal of Clinical Oncology* 2008; **31**: 393–8.

59. Parsons JT, Mendenhall WM, Cassisi NJ *et al.* Hyperfractionation for head and neck cancer. *International Journal of Radiation Oncology, Biology, Physics* 1988; **14**: 649–58.

60. Fu KK, Pajak T, Trotti A *et al.* A Radiation Therapy Oncology Group (RTOG) phase III randomized study to compare hyperfractionation and two variants of accelerated fractionation to standard fractionation radiotherapy for head and neck squamous cell carcinomas: first report of RTOG 9003. *International Journal of Radiation Oncology, Biology, Physics* 2000; **48**: 7–16.

61. Bourhis J, Overgaard J, Audry H *et al.* Hyperfractionated or accelerated radiotherapy in head and neck cancer: a meta-analysis. *Lancet* 2006; **368**: 843–54.

62. De Neve W, De Gersem W, Derycke S *et al.* Clinical delivery of intensity modulated conformal radiotherapy for relapsed or second-primary head and neck cancer using a multileaf collimator with dynamic control. *Radiotherapy and Oncology* 1999; **50**: 301–14.

63. Lee N, Xia P, Quivey JM *et al.* Intensity-modulated radiotherapy in the treatment of nasopharyngeal carcinoma: an update of the UCSF experience. *International Journal of Radiation Oncology, Biology, Physics* 2002; **53**: 12–22.

64. Douglas JG, Einck J, Austin-Seymour M *et al.* Neutron radiotherapy for recurrent pleomorphic adenomas of major salivary glands. *Head and Neck* 2001; **23**: 1037–42.

65. The Department of Veterans Affairs Laryngeal Cancer Study Group. Induction chemotherapy plus radiation

compared with surgery plus radiation in patients with advanced laryngeal cancer. *New England Journal of Medicine* 1991; **324**: 1685–90.

66. Lefebvre JL, Chevalier D, Luboinski B *et al.* Larynx preservation in pyriform sinus cancer: preliminary results of a European Organization for Research and Treatment of Cancer phase III trial. EORTC Head and Neck Cancer Cooperative Group. *Journal of the National Cancer Institute* 1996; **88**: 890–9.

67. Vermorken JB, Remenar E, van Herpen C *et al.* Cisplatin, fluorouracil, and docetaxel in unresectable head and neck cancer. *New England Journal of Medicine* 2007; **357**: 1695–704.

68. Laramore GE, Scott CB, Al-Sarraf M *et al.* Adjuvant chemotherapy for resectable squamous cell carcinomas of the head and neck: report on Intergroup Study 0034. *International Journal of Radiation Oncology, Biology, Physics* 1992; **23**: 705–13.

69. Pignon JP, Bourhis J, Domenge C, Designé L. Chemotherapy added to locoregional treatment for head and neck squamous-cell carcinoma: three meta-analyses of updated individual data. MACH-NC Collaborative Group. Meta-Analysis of Chemotherapy on Head and Neck Cancer. *Lancet* 2000; **355**: 949–55.

70. Weber RS, Berkey BA, Forastiere A *et al.* Outcome of salvage total laryngectomy following organ preservation therapy: the Radiation Therapy Oncology Group trial 91-11. *Archives of Otolaryngology, Head and Neck Surgery* 2003; **129**: 44–9.

71. Calais G, Alfonsi M, Bardet E *et al.* [Stage III and IV cancers of the oropharynx: results of a randomized study of Gortec comparing radiotherapy alone with concomitant chemotherapy]. *Bulletin of Cancer* 2000; **87**: 48–53.

72. Al-Sarraf M, Pajak TF, Cooper JS *et al.* Chemoradiotherapy versus radiotherapy in patients with advanced nasopharyngeal cancer: phase III randomized Intergroup Study 0099. *Journal of Clinical Oncology* 1998; **16**: 1310–17.

73. Pignon JP, le Maitre A, Maillard E, Bourhis J. Meta-analysis of chemotherapy in head and neck cancer (MACH-NC): an update on 93 randomised trials and 17,346 patients. *Radiotherapy and Oncology* 2009; **92**: 4–14.

74. Hoffman HT, Porter K, Karnell LH *et al.* Laryngeal cancer in the United States: changes in demographics, patterns of care, and survival. *Laryngoscope* 2006; **116** (Suppl. 111): 1–13.

75. Cooper JS, Pajak TF, Forastiere AA *et al.* Postoperative concurrent radiotherapy and chemotherapy for high-risk squamous-cell carcinoma of the head and neck. *New England Journal of Medicine* 2004; **350**: 1937–44.

76. Bernier J, Domenge C, Ozsahin M *et al.* Postoperative irradiation with or without concomitant chemotherapy for locally advanced head and neck cancer. *New England Journal of Medicine* 2004; **350**: 1945–52.

77. Benasso M, Bonelli L, Numico G *et al.* Treatment with cisplatin and fluorouracil alternating with radiation favourably affects prognosis of inoperable squamous cell carcinoma of the head and neck: results of a multivariate analysis on 273 patients. *Annals of Oncology* 1997; **8**: 773–9.

78. Rischin D, Peters L, Fisher R *et al.* Tirapazamine, cisplatin, and radiation versus fluorouracil, cisplatin, and radiation in patients with locally advanced head and neck cancer: a randomized phase II trial of the Trans-Tasman Radiation Oncology Group (TROG 98.02). *Journal of Clinical Oncology* 2005; **23**: 79–87.

79. Zbáren P, Christe A, Caversaccio MD *et al.* Pretherapeutic staging of recurrent laryngeal carcinoma: clinical findings and imaging studies compared with histopathology. *Otolaryngology, Head and Neck Surgery* 2007; **137**: 487–91.

80. Rigo P, Paulus P, Kaschten BJ *et al.* Oncological applications of positron emission tomography with fluorine-18 fluorodeoxyglucose. *European Journal of Nuclear Medicine* 1996; **23**: 1641–74.

81. Gourin CG, Williams HT, Seabolt WN *et al.* Utility of positron emission tomography-computed tomography in identification of residual nodal disease after chemoradiation for advanced head and neck cancer. *Laryngoscope* 2006; **116**: 705–10.

82. Yao M, Smith RB, Graham MM *et al.* Pathology and FDG PET correlation of residual lymph nodes in head and neck cancer after radiation treatment. *American Journal of Clinical Oncology* 2007; **30**: 264–70.

83. Fleming AJ Jr, Johansen ME. The clinician's expectations from the use of positron emission tomography/computed tomography scanning in untreated and treated head and neck cancer patients. *Current Opinion in Otolaryngology, Head and Neck Surgery* 2008; **16**: 127–34.

84. Goodwin WJ Jr. Salvage surgery for patients with recurrent squamous cell carcinoma of the upper aerodigestive tract: when do the ends justify the means? *Laryngoscope* 2000; **110**: 1–18.

85. Ganly I, Patel S, Matsuo J *et al.* Postoperative complications of salvage total laryngectomy. *Cancer* 2005; **103**: 2073–81.

86. Gleich LL, Ryzenman J, Gluckman JL *et al.* Recurrent advanced (T3 or T4) head and neck squamous cell carcinoma: is salvage possible? *Archives of Otolaryngology Head and Neck Surgery* 2004; **130**: 35–8.

87. Richey LM, Shores CG, George J *et al.* The effectiveness of salvage surgery after the failure of primary concomitant chemoradiation in head and neck cancer. *Otolaryngology, Head and Neck Surgery* 2007; **136**: 98–103.

88. Zbaren P, Nuyens M, Curschmann J, Stauffer E. Histologic characteristics and tumor spread of recurrent glottic carcinoma: analysis on whole-organ sections and comparison with tumor spread of primary glottic carcinomas. *Head and Neck* 2007; **29**: 26–32.

89. Bolderston A, Lloyd NS, Wong RK *et al*. The prevention and management of acute skin reactions related to radiation therapy: a systematic review and practice guideline. *Supportive Care Cancer* 2006; **14**: 802–17.

90. Brosky ME. The role of saliva in oral health: strategies for prevention and management of xerostomia. *Journal of Supportive Oncology* 2007; **5**: 215–25.

91. Callahan C. Facial disfigurement and sense of self in head and neck cancer. *Social Work and Health Care* 2004; **40**: 73–87.

92. Duffy SA, Ronis DL, Valenstein M *et al*. Depressive symptoms, smoking, drinking, and quality of life among head and neck cancer patients. *Psychosomatics* 2007; **48**: 142–8.

93. Block SD. Assessing and managing depression in the terminally ill patient. ACP-ASIM End-of-Life Care Consensus Panel, American College of Physicians, – American Society of Internal Medicine. *Annals of Internal Medicine* 2000; **132**: 209–18.

94. Jackel MC, Martin A, Steiner W. Twenty-five years experience with laser surgery for head and neck tumors: report of an international symposium, Gottingen, Germany, 2005. *European Archives of Otorhinolaryngology* 2007; **264**: 577–85.

95. British Association of Otorhinolaryngology Head and Neck Surgery. Effective head and neck cancer management. Third Consensus Document, ENT-UK. London: BAOHNS, 2002.

96. Scottish Intercollegiate Guidelines Network. Guideline 90, Diagnosis and management of head and neck cancer. Edinburgh: SIGN, 2006.

8

Principles of conservation surgery

IAN GANLY AND JATIN P SHAH

To live is to function. That is all there is in living.

Oliver Wendell Holmes, Jr (1849–1935)

INTRODUCTION

Surgery for head and neck cancer can have significant effects on function such as speech and swallowing, as well as major effects on aesthetic appearance. There is therefore much interest in developing alternative strategies in the treatment of head and neck cancer. Organ-preserving radiation and chemoradiation is an example of this. Improvements in radiation delivery techniques, such as hypo- and hyperfractionation regimes and conformal 3D radiation, intensity-modulated radiation therapy (IMRT), dose painting and image-guided radiotherapy have led to radiation doses being concentrated to the tumour with limitation in damage to surrounding normal tissue. New chemotherapeutic agents and regimes have also led to chemoradiation being introduced as an alternative to radical surgery, especially for cancers of the larynx, hypopharynx and oropharynx. In addition, our greater understanding of tumour biology related to local progression and its behaviour and spread has led to the development of modified surgical approaches to head and neck cancers, which previously would have been removed with radical surgery. The introduction of the CO_2 laser has led to the development of transoral resection of cancers of the larynx, hypopharynx and oropharynx, whereas the introduction of endoscopes, image

guidance systems and powered instrumentation now allows nasal cavity and paranasal sinus tumours to be removed by an endoscopic approach in selected cases, where previously open surgery, such as craniofacial resection, was used. This chapter will focus only on the conservation surgical approaches in head and neck cancer. Chemoradiation will be discussed in Chapter 45, Chemoradiation in head and neck cancer. Conservation surgery of the skin is discussed in Chapter 38, Non-melanoma and melanoma skin cancer, and conservation surgery of the thyroid in Chapter 23, Surgical management of differentiated thyroid cancer.

DEFINITION

The aim of conservation or functional head and neck surgery is to preserve form or function without compromising oncological resection. Therefore, conservation surgery is any operation which gives the same oncological result as radical surgery – long thought to be the most effective treatment – but allows preservation of function or aesthetic appearance.

Sites of conservation

Conservation surgery applies most commonly to the neck and larynx. However, conservation surgical procedures for the oral cavity, oropharynx, hypopharynx, paranasal sinuses and parotid gland have now been reported.

CONSERVATION SURGERY FOR THE NECK

Introduction

The single most important factor affecting prognosis for squamous cell carcinoma of the head and neck is the status of the cervical lymph nodes. Metastasis to the regional lymph nodes reduces the five-year survival rate by 50 per cent compared to that of patients with early stage disease. The American Cancer Society has reported that 40 per cent of patients with squamous carcinoma of the oral cavity and pharynx present with regional metastases. Therefore, management of the cervical lymph nodes is an important component in the overall treatment plan for patients with squamous cell carcinoma of the head and neck.

Regional cervical lymph nodes are grouped into several levels. Lymph node levels of the neck were first described by Memorial Sloan-Kettering Cancer Center and were classified into levels I–VII (**Figure 8.1**, **Table 8.1**). The gold standard operation for removal of cervical lymph nodes in both patients with clinically negative and clinically positive necks was the classical radical neck dissection. This involves removal of all five levels (I–V) of the neck, including the sternocleidomastoid muscle, internal jugular vein and accessory nerve, and submandibular salivary gland. However, with our greater understanding of the patterns of lymph node spread, it is now possible to carry out more modified neck dissections to preserve form and function. This is through our understanding that the location of metastases is mainly determined by the location of the primary site. Cancers of the oral cavity typically spread first to the nodes in levels I, II and III, whereas cancers of the oropharynx, hypopharynx and larynx spread first to the nodes in levels II, III and IV (**Figure 8.2**). This observation is based on the philosophy that nodal spread of cancer proceeds in an orderly and predictable fashion as determined by the lymphatic drainage pattern in the neck.[1, 2] To determine lymph node levels at risk from a particular primary site, Shah[3] analysed pathology specimens from 1119 classical radical neck dissections (RND) for squamous cell carcinoma of the upper aerodigestive tract.

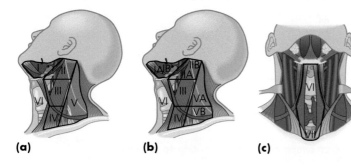

(a)   **(b)**   **(c)**

Figure 8.1 (a) Memorial Sloan-Kettering Cancer Center levelling system of cervical lymph nodes; (b) current modification of levelling system; (c) levels VI and VII. Redrawn with permission from Shah JP, Patel SG. *Head and neck surgery and oncology*, 3rd edn. New York: Mosby CV, 2003.

Table 8.1 Clinical and surgical landmarks for neck node levels.

Node level	Clinical landmarks	Surgical landmarks
Level I	Submental and submandibular triangles	Superior-lower border of the body of the mandible Posterior-posterior belly of digastric Inferior-hyoid bone
Level II	Upper jugular lymph nodes	Superior-base of skull Posterior-posterior border of sternocleidomastoid muscle Anterior-lateral limit of sternohyoid Inferior-hyoid bone
Level III	Middle jugular lymph nodes	Superior-hyoid bone Posterior-posterior border of sternocleidomastoid muscle Anterior-lateral limit of sternohyoid Inferior-cricothyroid membrane
Level IV	Lower jugular lymph nodes	Superior-cricothyroid membrane Posterior-posterior border of sternocleidomastoid muscle Anterior-lateral limit of sternohyoid Inferior-clavicle
Level V	Posterior triangle lymph nodes	Posterior-anterior border of trapezius muscle Anterior-posterior border of sternocleidomastoid muscle Inferior-clavicle
Level VI	Anterior compartment of the neck	Superior-hyoid bone Inferior-suprasternal notch Lateral-medial border of carotid sheath on either side
Level VII	Superior mediastinal lymph nodes	Superior-suprasternal notch

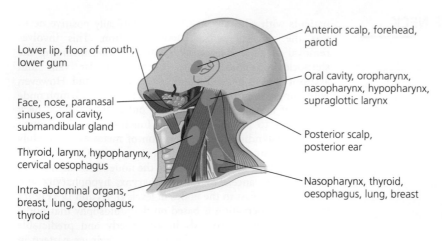

Lower lip, floor of mouth, lower gum

Face, nose, paranasal sinuses, oral cavity, submandibular gland

Thyroid, larynx, hypopharynx, cervical oesophagus

Intra-abdominal organs, breast, lung, oesophagus, thyroid

Anterior scalp, forehead, parotid

Oral cavity, oropharynx, nasopharynx, hypopharynx, supraglottic larynx

Posterior scalp, posterior ear

Nasopharynx, thyroid, oesophagus, lung, breast

Figure 8.2 Regional lymph nodes draining a specific primary site. Redrawn with permission from Shah JP, Patel SG. *Head and neck surgery and oncology*, 3rd edn. New York: Mosby CV, 2003.

Table 8.2 Percentage of positive lymph nodes in the cN+ neck.

Primary site	Percentage positive nodes at each lymph node level according to primary site				
	I	II	III	IV	V
Oral cavity	61	57	44	20	4
Oropharynx	17	85	50	33	11
Hypopharynx	10	78	75	47	11
Larynx	8	68	70	35	5

Table 8.3 Percentage of positive lymph nodes in the cN0 neck.

Primary site	Percentage positive nodes at each lymph node level according to primary site				
	I	II	III	IV	V
Oral cavity	58	51	26	9	2
Oropharynx	7	80	60	27	7
Hypopharynx	0	75	75	0	0
Larynx	14	52	55	24	7

This consisted of 343 RNDs for the clinically negative neck (N0) and 776 RNDs for the clinically positive neck. From this study, the incidence of pathological positive neck specimens was 82 per cent for the clinically positive neck and 33 per cent for the clinically negative neck. **Tables 8.2** and **8.3** show the percentage of patients with pathological positive nodes at each level for cN+ and cN0 disease. In the cN+ setting (**Table 8.2**), patients with primary oral cavity tumours had the majority of positive nodes in levels I–III, levels IV and V were involved in 20 and 4 per cent of specimens, respectively. In patients with primary oropharyngeal tumours, the majority of positive nodes were in levels II–IV, levels I and V were involved in 17 and 11 per cent of specimens, respectively. In patients with hypopharyngeal tumours, most positive nodes were in levels II–IV, levels I and V were involved in 10 and 11 per cent of specimens, respectively. In patients with primary tumours of the larynx, most positive nodes were in levels II–IV, levels I and V were involved in 8 and 5 per cent, respectively.

In the cN0 setting (**Table 8.3**), patients with primary oral cavity tumours had the majority of positive nodes in levels

I–III, levels IV and V were involved in 9 and 2 per cent of specimens, respectively. In patients with primary oropharyngeal tumours, the majority of positive nodes were in levels II–IV; levels I and V were involved in 7 per cent. In patients with hypopharyngeal tumours, most positive nodes were in levels II–IV, levels I and V were not involved. In patients with primary tumours of the larynx, most positive nodes were in levels II–IV, levels I and V were involved in 14 and 7 per cent, respectively.

The question of level V metastases was addressed in a separate study on 1277 RNDs by Davidson *et al.*[4] Metastases were found in 40 (3 per cent) patients. Level V metastases were highest in patients with hypopharyngeal and oropharyngeal primary sites (7 and 6 per cent, respectively). Only three of 40 patients with a cN0 neck had a positive level V lymph node. The incidence of level V metastases is small and extremely unlikely in the cN0 setting.

Therefore, in the N0 setting, selective neck dissection removing lymph nodes selectively draining the lymph node basin most at risk can now be done. In the N+ setting, however, comprehensive neck dissection of all five levels is necessary.

The highest functional morbidity of a comprehensive radical neck dissection removing all five levels of lymph nodes results from compromise of shoulder function due to loss of the spinal accessory nerve. Andersen et al.[5] studied the oncological safety of a comprehensive modified neck dissection preserving the spinal accessory nerve in the N+ setting. The regional failure rates and disease-specific survival rates in patients with N+ disease were comparable for classical radical neck dissection and modified comprehensive neck dissection type I, preserving the accessory nerve as long as the nerve was not directly infiltrated by tumour.

Conservation neck dissection for N0 disease (selective neck dissection)

Selective neck dissection spares all non-lymphatic tissue, including the sternocleidomastoid muscle, internal jugular vein and spinal accessory nerve. However, it removes only selected levels of lymph nodes on the involved side of the neck, unlike a comprehensive neck dissection. The extent of selective node dissection is determined by the predictive pattern of metastases based on the location of the primary tumour. It is based on the clinical observation that squamous cell carcinomas of the upper aerodigestive tract metastasize in a predictable and sequential pattern. Selective neck dissections are therefore generally carried out for the clinically negative neck (N0) where there is at least a 15–20 per cent risk of occult metastatic disease. Common selective neck dissections, and their indications are shown in **Figures 8.3** and **8.4** and **Table 8.4**. These include the supraomohyoid neck dissection (SOHND) in which lymph nodes in levels I–III and the submandibular salivary gland are removed (**Figure 8.3a**); the extended supraomohyoid neck dissection in which lymph nodes in levels I–IV and the submandibular gland are removed (**Figure 8.3b**); the anterolateral neck dissection (LND) in which lymph nodes in levels II–IV are removed (**Figure 8.3c**); posterolateral neck dissection (PLND) in which lymph nodes in levels II–V and also the suboccipital and retroauricular lymph nodes are removed (**Figure 8.3d**); central or anterior compartment neck dissection in which lymph nodes at level VI in the prelaryngeal, pretracheal and paratracheal regions are removed (**Figure 8.3e**).

- **Supraomohyoid neck dissection.** Supraomohyoid neck dissection is recommended for squamous cell carcinoma of the oral cavity with a high risk of micrometastases in a clinically negative neck. Byers[6] reported a recurrence rate of 5.8 per cent in 154 N0 patients treated with supraomohyoid neck dissection. Similar recurrence rates were reported by Spiro et al.[7] and O'Brien.[8]
- **Extended supraomohyoid neck dissection.** Extended supraomohyoid neck dissection is recommended for squamous cell carcinoma of the lateral tongue. This is based on the observation that patients with primary carcinoma of the lateral border of the oral tongue have a small, but increased risk of skip metastases to level IV compared to other sites in the oral cavity. Therefore, selective treatment of the N0 neck in lateral tongue cancer should include level IV.

- **Anterolateral neck dissection.** Anterolateral neck dissection (LND) is recommended for squamous cell carcinoma of the larynx or pharynx with a high risk of micrometastases in a clinically negative neck. If the primary tumour crosses the midline, this procedure is carried out bilaterally. LND is indicated for cancer of the oropharynx when the primary tumour is treated with surgery for a clinically negative neck. If postoperative radiation therapy is indicated, it is not necessary to perform bilateral LND because radiation alone is effective in treating the node negative contralateral neck. Cancers of the hypopharynx frequently metastasize to both sides of the neck. Therefore, bilateral LND is recommended in the cN0 setting. In supraglottic and advanced glottic cancer bilateral neck dissection is generally recommended. LND is not indicated for early glottic lesions.
- **Posterolateral neck dissection.** Posterolateral neck dissection is recommended for primary cutaneous malignancies of the posterior scalp, e.g. melanoma and squamous cell carcinoma.
- **Central compartment neck dissection.** Central compartment neck dissection is recommended for differentiated thyroid carcinoma in which the disease is limited to the pretracheal and paratracheal nodes (level VI).

Conservation neck dissection for N+ disease

MODIFIED RADICAL NECK DISSECTION FOR N+ DISEASE

Comprehensive neck dissections involve the removal of all lymphatic tissue in the lateral neck (levels I–V) and are generally carried out for the clinically positive neck (N+). They can be classified into radical and modified radical neck dissection (**Figure 8.5**), depending on what other structures are excised. The gold standard operation is the radical neck dissection which involves the removal of lymph nodes in levels I–V, as well as the sternocleidomastoid muscle, internal jugular vein, spinal accessory nerve and submandibular salivary gland. Modified radical neck dissection is divided into types I, II or III, depending on the structures which are conserved. Type I MRND involves preservation of one structure: the spinal accessory nerve. Type II involves preservation of two structures: the spinal accessory nerve and the sternocleidomastoid muscle. Type III involves preservation of the spinal accessory nerve, internal jugular vein and the sternocleidomastoid muscle. Type I MRND is the most commonly employed neck dissection for squamous cell carcinoma of the upper aerodigestive tract with clinically positive neck disease. Type III MRND is most commonly employed for metastatic differentiated carcinoma of the thyroid. Bocca coined the term 'functional neck dissection' and employed this type of operation for squamous cell carcinoma, mostly in patients with larynx cancer. The operation was safe and successful in patients with cN0 neck, but in patients with cN+ neck, regional failure with recurrence occurred in 29 per cent.[9] Based on what we know today regarding the patterns of neck metastases, dissection of all five levels of lymph nodes in the cN0 neck is unnecessary. Furthermore, in the cN+ setting, the operation is unsafe due

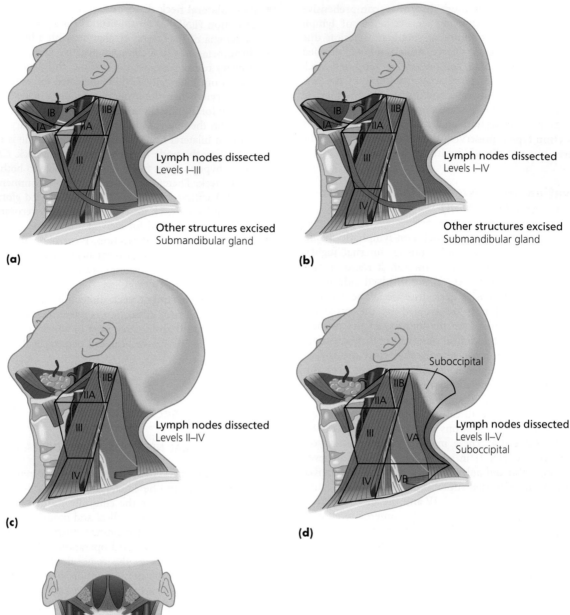

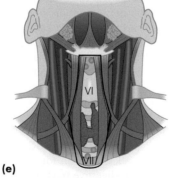

Figure 8.3 Classification of selective neck dissection. (a) Supraomohyoid neck dissection; (b) extended supraomohyoid neck dissection; (c) jugular (anterolateral) neck dissection; (d) posterolateral neck dissection; (e) central compartment node dissection. Redrawn with permission from Shah JP, Patel SG. *Head and neck surgery and oncology*, 3rd edn. New York: Mosby CV, 2003.

to high failure rates. Thus, the 'functional neck dissection' has fallen out of the repertoire of contemporary head and neck surgery. A modification of the type III mRND is that described by Ballantyne, where level V is removed using an anterior approach. With this technique, the medial aspect of level V is removed, preserving the accessory nerve and cervical plexus. This offers better functional results and quality of life. However, the operation is not recommended if there is evidence of level V disease clinically or radiologically, for the

N3 neck, fixed nodal disease or when multiple levels are involved. It is also not recommended after radiotherapy.

SELECTIVE NECK DISSECTION FOR N+ DISEASE

The use of selective neck dissection in patients with clinically positive neck disease is controversial. Some studies have recommended that it may be used for nodal metastases

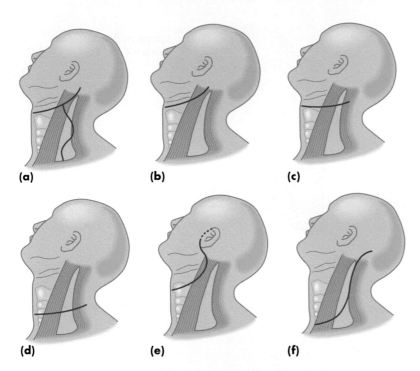

(a)   **(b)**   **(c)**

(d)   **(e)**   **(f)**

Figure 8.4   Skin incisions for various types of neck dissection. (a) Comprehensive; (b) supraomohyoid; (c) jugular; (d) comprehensive (thyroid); (e) modified (parotid); (f) posterolateral. Redrawn with permission from Shah JP, Patel SG. *Head and neck Surgery and Oncology*, 3rd edn. New York: Mosby CV, 2003.

Table 8.4   Classification of different types of neck dissection with clinical indications.

Comprehensive	Nodal levels removed	Structures preserved	Indications
Radical neck dissection	Levels I–V	None	N+ neck for SCC where SAN involved
Modified radical neck dissection type I	Levels I–V	SAN	N+ neck for SCC where SAN free of disease
Modified radical neck dissection type II	Levels I–V	SAN, SCM	N+ neck for SCC where IJV involved but SAN free of disease
Modified radical neck dissection type III	Levels I–V	SAN, SCM, IJV	Metastatic differentiated thyroid carcinoma
Selective			
Supraomohyoid neck dissection	Levels I–III	SAN, SCM, IJV	N0 neck for SCC of oral cavity and oropharynx (include level 4);
			N0 neck malignant melanoma where primary site is anterior to ear (include parotidectomy for face and scalp)
Lateral neck dissection	Levels II–IV	SAN, SCM, IJV	N0 neck for SCC of larynx and hypopharynx
Posterolateral neck dissection	Levels II–V, suboccipital, retroauricular nodes	SAN, SCM, IJV	N0 neck malignant melanoma where primary site is posterior to ear

confined to the first echelon nodes (usually N1) when the primary is being treated by surgery. However, it is important to point out that postoperative radiation therapy to the neck is required in this setting.[6, 7, 10, 11, 12, 13, 14] For node-positive disease, the results of selective supraomohyoid neck dissection are more variable. In 1985, Byers[6] reported a regional recurrence rate of 15 per cent. In 1997, Pellitteri et al.[11] reported a regional recurrence rate of 11 per cent. In 1999, Byers[14] reported that the regional recurrence rate was 36 per cent in patients with pN1 neck disease who had not received

radiation therapy, but was 5.6 per cent among those who had received postoperative radiation. For pN2b disease, the failure rate was 8.8 per cent with radiation and 14 per cent without. In 1996, Spiro et al.[7] reported a recurrence rate of 6 per cent in patients who had received postoperative radiation following supraomohyoid neck dissection. Andersen et al.[15] reported a ten-year retrospective of 106 previously untreated clinically and pathologically node-positive patients undergoing 129 selective neck dissections; regional metastasis was clinically staged as N1 in 58 patients

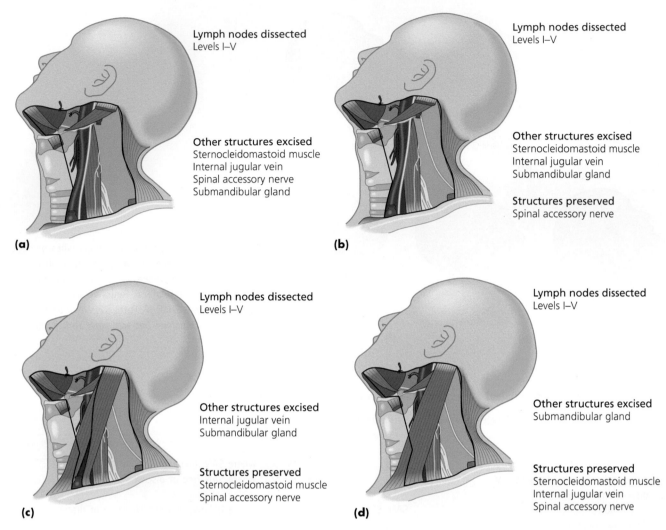

Figure 8.5   Classification of comprehensive neck dissection: (a) classic radical neck dissection; (b) modified radical neck dissection, type I; (c) modified radical neck dissection, type II; (d) modified radical neck dissection, type III. Redrawn with permission from Shah JP, Patel SG. *Head and neck surgery and oncology*, 3rd edn. New York: Mosby CV, 2003.

(54.7 per cent), N2a in five (4.7 per cent), N2b in 28 (26.4 per cent), N2c in 14 (13.2 per cent) and N3 in one (0.9 per cent). Extracapsular extension of tumour was present in 36 patients (34.0 per cent) and postoperative radiation therapy was administered to 76 patients (71.7 per cent). Overall, nine patients experienced disease recurrence in the neck for a regional control rate of 94.3 per cent illustrating that in highly selective patients selective neck dissection for node-positive disease is possible.

NECK DISSECTION FOR N+ DISEASE POST-CHEMORADIATION

Organ-preserving chemoradiotherapy is an emerging alternative in the treatment of laryngopharyngeal carcinoma. Management of the clinically positive neck in such patients remains controversial. It is generally accepted that patients with N0 and N1 disease can be treated by chemoradiation (CTRT) alone. However, for N2/3 disease, there is insufficient data to determine when to perform a neck dissection. Many investigators recommend neck dissection for all patients

with N2a or N3 disease, regardless of response or if persistent disease is present as determined clinically or by computed tomography (CT) or magnetic resonance imaging (MRI). Brizel *et al.*[16] reported a four-year disease-free survival of 75 per cent for N2/N3 for those with a CR in the neck who had neck dissection, compared to 53 per cent in those with CTRT who did not have a neck dissection ($p = 0.08$). They therefore recommended a mRND for N2/3 disease irrespective of neck response. This suggests that clinical/radiographic response in the neck is a crude predictor of the pathologic response and supports the idea that mRND eradicates residual disease that would otherwise recur regionally and/or seed distant sites. Evidence for residual disease was reported by Grabenbauer *et al.*,[17] who found, in patients who had a neck dissection following a complete response in the neck, an incidence of 23 per cent residual disease – the rate of positive histology being 20 per cent for N1, 20 per cent for N2a/b and 54 per cent for N2c/N3 disease. However, other investigators have reported no detectable disease following a complete response to CTRT.[18] The reason for this variation in pathological positive nodes in neck dissection specimens is related to the pathologic processing; meticulous step sectioning is more likely to identify residual disease than a sampling of one or two sections from the node. Another argument put forward for neck dissection post-CTRT is that if patients develop recurrence, very few can be salvaged. For example, in the University of Florida[19] experience in 139 patients with positive neck disease treated by radiotherapy (RT) alone, 35 developed neck recurrence, salvage was attempted in nine patients and only successful in two. However, one must also balance the benefits of neck dissection against possible sequelae since wound complications are increased post-CTRT. Acute events such as chyle leak, wound breakdown, and flap necrosis occur in 17 per cent of patients and late complications, such as soft tissue fibrosis, can be severe, causing reduced neck movement, tightness and pain.[18, 20] Therefore, to improve the utility of neck dissection in patients with a complete response post-CTRT, we need to identify those patients who have residual disease. One possible approach is to use quantitative positron emission tomography (PET), an area of current research.[21]

Alternatively, one could adopt a policy of performing a neck dissection in all patients, but reducing morbidity by carrying out a selective neck dissection rather than a comprehensive neck dissection. Several authors have now reported such an approach with no significant negative impact on regional recurrence rates.[22, 23, 24, 25]

CONSERVATION SURGERY FOR CANCER OF THE LARYNX

The choice of therapy for early stage squamous cell cancer of the larynx is determined by patient- and tumour-related factors, as well as physician preference. Opinions on therapy vary across disciplines and between countries because both surgery and radiotherapy are equally effective.[26, 27, 28, 29, 30, 31] Conservation laryngeal operations are historically the original organ preservation techniques; the first hemilaryngectomy was carried out by Billroth in 1874. With the availability of the laser, operating microscope and sophisticated endoscopes, transoral laser resections of laryngeal and pharyngeal lesions have gained popularity. The main aim of all conservation procedures is to maintain speech and swallowing and avoid a tracheostomy. Conservation laryngeal surgery options thus may be classified into open partial laryngeal surgical procedures and transoral endoscopic laser surgical procedures. In both types of surgery, the principles of resection are the same, and securing negative margins is crucial to the success of the procedure.

Principles of organ preservation laryngeal surgery

LOCAL CONTROL

Local control is the most important principle, since survival will be compromised if local failure occurs. This is because early detection of the recurrence is difficult due to alteration in the anatomy following index treatment. Therefore, organ preservation surgery should only be used when resection of the tumour can be confidently achieved.

ACCURATE ASSESSMENT OF TUMOUR EXTENT

The surgeon must be able to confidently predict the degree of tumour extension. This requires a comprehensive knowledge of laryngeal anatomy. Clinical examination using flexible laryngoscopy allows for assessment of vocal cord and arytenoid mobility, which helps to determine what deeper structures are invaded. Cancers involving the glottis and supraglottis have different effects on vocal cord mobility and arytenoid mobility. In glottic cancer, impaired cord mobility may be due to the bulk of the tumour on the cord surface or superficial thyroarytenoid muscle invasion.[32] If the cord is fixed, studies have shown that this is due to invasion of the thyroarytenoid muscle.[33, 34, 35] In supraglottic cancer, cancer invasion into the thyroarytenoid muscle is less likely and the most common cause of cord fixation is deep arytenoid cartilage invasion superiorly.[33] For arytenoid mobility, there are two types of arytenoid impairment: pseudofixation due to the weight of the tumour and actual fixation due to cancer invasion of the intrinsic laryngeal muscles, the cricoarytenoid joint or both. All patients should also have an examination under anaesthesia so that the tumour can be assessed by direct laryngoscopy using angled telescopes to visualize the ventricle, anterior commissure and subglottis. Palpation of the vallecula is also important in the case of supraglottic cancers to assess the extent of submucosal invasion.

Clinical examination may be aided by imaging, such as CT and MRI. Coronal T_1-weighted MRI is useful to assess subglottic extension. The cricoarytenoid area is best assessed by axial CT scans which will show sclerosis if perichondrial or direct arytenoid cartilage invasion has occurred. Sagittal MRI is good for the assessment of pre-epiglottic space invasion. MRI is also highly sensitive for assessment of thyroid cartilage invasion; enhancement into cartilage on postgadolinium fat-suppressed scans are highly sensitive to invasion. PET has also gained popularity. The most promising role for this is in the assessment of post-treatment effects and the detection of early recurrence.

CRICOARYTENOID UNIT

The cricoarytenoid unit is the basic functional unit of the larynx. The cricoarytenoid unit consists of an arytenoid cartilage, the cricoid cartilage, the associated musculature and the nerve supply from the superior and recurrent laryngeal nerves for that unit. It is the cricoarytenoid unit, not the vocal folds, that allows for physiologic speech and swallowing without the need for a tracheostome. Therefore, preservation of at least one functional unit allows organ preservation laryngeal surgery.

Open partial laryngeal surgery

CLINICAL ASSESSMENT

When considering a patient for conservation laryngeal surgery, the following general principles should be considered:

- The patient must be able to tolerate a general anaesthetic.

- The patient should not have any medical problems that may impair wound healing, e.g. transplantation patients or those with diabetes mellitus.
- The patient should have good pulmonary function to tolerate the postoperative course, which often involves a period of aspiration. This is the main problem of conservation laryngeal surgery. The amount of postoperative aspiration varies with the type of surgery. Vertical hemilaryngectomy typically causes little impact on swallowing function, whereas supraglottic laryngectomy results in dysphagia and aspiration.[36] A percutaneous gastrostomy tube may be required for patients with a significant prolonged period of aspiration.
- The patient should play an active role in speech and swallowing rehabilitation. All patients should have a speech and swallowing assessment preoperatively and both the patient and family should participate in the work required for rehabilitation.
- Any patient undergoing partial laryngectomy should be informed of the complexities of salvage conservation procedures, and must give consent for total laryngectomy. Any patient who cannot do this is not a good candidate for conservation laryngeal surgery. Careful preoperative planning will reduce the incidence of conversion to total laryngectomy.

CONSERVATION SURGERY FOR GLOTTIC LARYNGEAL CANCER

The possible surgical options include vertical partial laryngectomy and supracricoid partial laryngectomy with cricohyoidoepiglottopexy.

Vertical partial laryngectomy

Technique

This procedure may be a lateral or an anterolateral vertical partial laryngectomy. The technique involves vertical cuts through the laryngeal cartilage (**Figure 8.6**). The majority of the ipsilateral thyroid cartilage, true vocal cord, portions of the subglottic mucosa and false cord are removed. The extent of resection depends on the preoperative and intraoperative assessment of tumour extent. The strap muscles are closed over the residual perichondrium to form a pseudocord. A tracheostomy is generally required for 3–7 days.

If the anterior commissure is involved, a frontolateral partial laryngectomy can be performed.

Criteria for the selection of a lesion suitable for vertical partial laryngectomy

There are certain criteria which must be met before a patient is considered suitable for a vertical partial laryngectomy. These are shown in **Box 8.1**, and are general guidelines. However, these criteria are not absolute and may be extended.

Oncological results

For T1 glottic cancers, local recurrence rates are reported to be less than 10 per cent.[37, 38, 39] If the anterior commissure is not involved, local control of 93 per cent has been reported, whereas if the anterior commissure is involved, the local control rate is reduced to 75 per cent[38] due to subglottic recurrence. Therefore, when the anterior commissure is involved, a wide surgical margin in the subglottis is indicated.

For T2 glottic cancers, higher local failure rates of 4–26 per cent are reported.[38, 39, 40, 41] This is due to subglottic and supraglottic invasion. Subglottic extension is associated with cricoid cartilage invasion, which is not resected in the standard vertical partial laryngectomy. Extension into the supraglottis through the ventricle may result in thyroid cartilage invasion.

For T3 glottic cancers, local recurrence rates are higher, ranging from 11 to 46 per cent.[42, 43, 44]

Box 8.1   Criteria for selection of a lesion suitable for vertical partial laryngectomy

- Lesion of mobile cord extending to anterior commissure
- Lesion of mobile cord involving vocal process and anterosuperior portion of arytenoid
- Subglottic extension should not be more than 5 mm
- Select patients with fixed vocal cord lesion not extending across the midline
- A unilateral transglottic lesion not violating the above criteria
- True cord/anterior commissure lesion not involving more than anterior third of the opposite cord

---

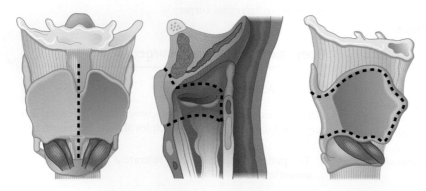

Figure 8.6 Vertical partial laryngectomy.

Excellent oncologic results can therefore be expected for T1 glottic carcinomas, although once the anterior commissure is involved or if there is extension beyond the glottis, vertical partial laryngectomy should be used with caution. It is not recommended for advanced T2 or T3 lesions.

Functional results and complications

Following partial laryngectomy, there is some degree of hoarseness. More impairment to the voice occurs if there is no reconstruction, whereas the best voice is associated with replacement of the glottis with an adjacent false cord flap.[45] Complications are uncommon and include delay in decannulation, stenosis and dysphagia. Laryngocutaneous fistula is uncommon.

Supracricoid partial laryngectomy with cricohyoidoepiglottopexy

Technique

Supracricoid partial laryngectomy with cricohyoido-epiglottopexy (CHEP) operation involves resection of both true cords, both false cords, the entire thyroid cartilage, paraglottic spaces bilaterally and a maximum of one arytenoid (**Figure 8.7**). Reconstruction is performed using the epiglottis, hyoid bone, cricoid cartilage and tongue. A temporary tracheostomy and feeding tube is required. This procedure is mainly used for T1b glottic carcinomas with anterior commissure involvement, selected T2 and T3 glottic carcinomas.

Oncologic results

The local recurrence rate for T2 glottic cancers is 4.5 per cent (three of 67),[46] whereas the local recurrence rate for T3 glottic cancers is 10 per cent (two of 20).[47] The consistently low recurrence rates are mainly due to the complete resection of the entire thyroid cartilage and bilateral paraglottic spaces.

Transglottic lesions (i.e. lesions which extend across the laryngeal ventricle involving both the true cord and false cord) have a failure rate of 23 per cent for conservative procedures which involve either extended vertical partial laryngectomy or extended supraglottic partial laryngectomy.

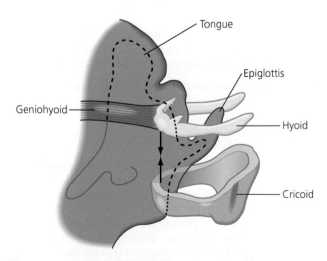

Figure 8.7 Supracricoid partial laryngectomy with cricohyoidoepiglottopexy (CHEP).

Supracricoid partial laryngectomy with cricohyoidoepiglotto-pexy does not result in complete removal of the supraglottis. Therefore for transglottic carcinomas, a supracricoid partial laryngectomy with cricohyoidopexy is recommended.

Functional results and complications

Temporary dysphagia and aspiration is expected. Nasogastric feeding is therefore required postoperatively and the time to removal ranges from 9 to 50 days. The need for removal of the larynx for intractable aspiration is low and ranges from 0 to 4 per cent. The voice quality is poor initially, but improves over several months.[48] Complications include hyoid necrosis and neolaryngeal stenosis.

CONSERVATION SURGERY FOR SUPRAGLOTTIC LARYNGEAL CANCER

Surgical treatment of tumours of the supraglottic larynx creates a significant physiologic disturbance in the act of deglutition. Almost every patient aspirates to a varying degree following surgery. Most patients handle this with little difficulty and can handle most types of foods without significant pulmonary complications. However, patients with a poor pulmonary reserve, advanced stage of emphysema, and those of advanced age are poor candidates for conservation surgery. The conservative open surgical options available for supraglottic cancers include the supraglottic horizontal partial laryngectomy and the supracricoid laryngectomy with cricohyoidopexy.

Horizontal supraglottic partial laryngectomy

Technique

In this procedure, the epiglottis, hyoid bone, pre-epiglottic space, thyrohyoid membrane, upper half of the thyroid cartilage and the supraglottic mucosa are removed (**Figure 8.8**). The vallecula is transected superiorly, the ventricles inferiorly and the aryepiglottic folds laterally. Closure is by approximating the base of tongue to the lower half of the thyroid cartilage and closing the posterior false cord mucosa to the medial pyriform sinus mucosa. A temporary tracheostomy is required. Bilateral selective neck dissection is carried out at the same time. In this procedure, it is important to identify and preserve the internal and external branches of the superior laryngeal nerve. The tongue base sutures are placed in the midline and 1 cm off to avoid damage to the hypoglossal nerves and lingual arteries.

Criteria for the selection of a lesion suitable for supraglottic partial laryngectomy

Several criteria related to tumour factors must be met in patients considered suitable for supraglottic partial laryngectomy. These are shown in **Box 8.2**. These criteria give good general guidelines, but the indications for the operation expand as the experience of the surgeon increases. A supraglottic partial laryngectomy may also be necessary for the surgical treatment of highly selected patients with primary tumours of the base of the tongue and secondary extension to the supraglottic larynx, tumours of the pyriform sinus involving its medial wall, and bulky tumours of the

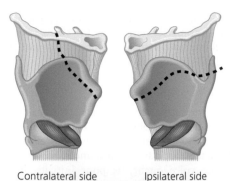

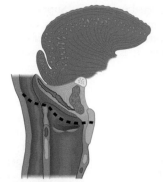

Contralateral side   Ipsilateral side

Figure 8.8 Horizontal supraglottic partial laryngectomy.

Box 8.2   Criteria for selection of a lesion suitable for supraglottic partial laryngectomy

- At least 5 mm margin at anterior commissure
- True vocal cords must be mobile
- Only one arytenoid may be removed
- No cartilage invasion by tumour
- Tongue mobility should be normal
- No extension to interarytenoid or post-cricoid area
- Apex of pyriform sinus should be free
- Generally lesions should be <3 cm

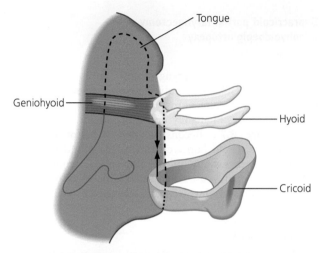

Figure 8.9 Supracricoid partial laryngectomy with cricohyoidopexy (CEP).

pharyngeal wall and secondary extension to the supraglottic larynx.

Oncologic results

When local recurrence is analysed by T stage, high local control is obtained for selected T1 and T2 tumours, but extremely variable results are obtained for T3 and T4 lesions with local recurrence of 75 per cent for T3 and 67 per cent for T4. Therefore, supraglottic laryngectomy should be considered with extreme caution in T3 and T4 lesions.[49, 50, 51, 52, 53, 54] Lee *et al.*[52] reported that improved local control is obtained if postoperative radiotherapy is given, although poorer functional results may occur as a consequence. Extension of supraglottic lesions below the false cord and impaired cord mobility are contraindications for supraglottic laryngectomy.

Functional results and complications

Normal to mild breathiness in voice occurred in 87 per cent of patients, and 67 per cent had mild to no evidence of hoarseness.[55] Aspiration is common and complete swallowing rehabilitation may take up to three months.[56] Hirano *et al.*[57] noted that 84 per cent of patients had removal of the nasogastric tube within 30 days, whereas the rest required feeding for up to three months. Factors which were significant for duration of nasogastric tube removal were the extent of removal of the arytenoid cartilage[57, 58] and the preservation of the superior laryngeal nerves.[56] Resection of the hyoid and tongue base was not related to swallowing outcome. Laryngocutaneous fistula rates are more common than vertical hemilaryngectomy and range from 0 to 12 per cent. Other complications include aspiration pneumonia

(0–10.8 per cent) and inability to decannulate the tracheostomy (0–5.5 per cent).[59]

Supracricoid partial laryngectomy with cricohyoidopexy

Technique

Supracricoid partial laryngectomy with cricohyoidopexy (CHP) is suitable for supraglottic carcinomas not amenable to supraglottic laryngectomy due to one of the following:

- glottic level involvement through the anterior commissure or ventricle;
- pre-epiglottic space invasion;
- decreased cord mobility;
- limited thyroid invasion.

These lesions are not rare; the incidence of spread to the glottis may be between 20 and 54 per cent. This is due to spread within the paraglottic space.[60] This operation involves resection of both true cords, both false cords, the entire thyroid cartilage, both paraglottic spaces bilaterally, and a maximum of one arytenoid, thyrohyoid membrane and epiglottis (**Figure 8.9**). Reconstruction is performed using the hyoid bone, cricoid cartilage and tongue. A temporary tracheostomy and feeding tube is required.

Criteria for the selection of a lesion suitable for supracricoid partial laryngectomy

Indications and contraindications for supracricoid partial laryngectomy with CHP and CHEP are shown in **Box 8.3**.

Oncologic results

Laccourreye *et al.*[61] have reported no local recurrences of supraglottic carcinomas treated this way in 68 patients (T1-1, T2-40, T3-26, T4-1) over a follow-up period of 18 months. Chevalier and Piquet[62] reported a local recurrence rate of 3.3 per cent. In tumours with pre-epiglottic space invasion, Laccourreye *et al.*[63] reported a local control of 94 per cent in 19 patients with a five-year follow-up period. The reason for such good results is due to the en bloc resection of bilateral paraglottic spaces, pre-epiglottic space and thyroid cartilage.

Contraindications to this procedure are the following:[61]

- subglottic extension > 10 mm anteriorly and 5 mm posteriorly because of cricoid cartilage involvement;
- arytenoid fixation;
- massive pre-epiglottic space involvement with invasion of the vallecula;
- extension to the pharyngeal wall, vallecula, base of tongue, postcricoid region, interarytenoid region;
- cricoid cartilage invasion.

Functional results and complications

Swallowing and speech problems are to be expected in this procedure. Success in this operation is dependent on careful patient selection, intraoperative technique and postoperative rehabilitation. Nasogastric feeding is required from 30 to 365 days[63, 64] and total laryngectomy may be required in up to 10 per cent of patients. Dysphagia is more common if one arytenoid is resected. Voice studies have shown these patients have poorer voice due to instability of the neoglottis resulting from a wide surgical resection.[65]

Box 8.3   Criteria for selection of a lesion suitable for supracricoid partial laryngectomy

Indications for supracricoid laryngectomy

- T1 and supraglottic lesions with ventricle extension
- T2 infrahyoid epiglottis or posterior one-third of the false cord
- Supraglottic lesions extending to glottis or anterior commissure, with or without vocal cord mobility
- T3 transglottic carcinoma with limitation of the vocal cord
- Selective T4 lesions invading the thyroid cartilage

Contraindications for supracricoid laryngectomy

- Bulky pre-epiglottic space involvement
- Gross thyroid cartilage destruction
- Interarytenoid or bilateral arytenoids involvement
- Fixed arytenoids
- Subglottic extension > 10 mm anteriorly or > 5 mm posteriorly
- Inadequate pulmonary reserve

CONSERVATION LARYNGEAL SURGERY FOR RADIATION FAILURE

Patients who fail radiotherapy for glottic cancer who were originally suitable for vertical partial laryngectomy may still be eligible for this surgery provided the tumour has not progressed. Local control in such patients may be from 80 to 90 per cent.[66] Of those with supraglottic carcinoma treated with radiotherapy who fail, only 30 per cent may still be suitable for conservation surgery. Sorenson *et al.*[67] reported poor oncologic and functional results in such patients and advocated total laryngectomy in these patients.

Contraindications to hemilaryngectomy after RT failure include:

- tumour involving the arytenoid;
- subglottic extension > 10 mm anteriorly and 5 mm posteriorly because of cricoid cartilage involvement;
- cartilage invasion of the thyroid or cricoid.

One alternative for larger lesions is to use either supracricoid laryngectomy with cricohyoidopexy or cricohyoidoepiglottopexy as the salvage procedure. This can give local control rates of 83.3 per cent.[68]

Transoral endoscopic laser resection

INTRODUCTION

In recent years, transoral endoscopic laser resection has become accepted as an alternative to open partial laryngeal surgery and radiotherapy.[69, 70, 71, 72, 73, 74, 75, 76, 77, 78] Oncologic results are comparable between all techniques, but transoral laser microsurgery has potential advantages over both open surgery and radiotherapy which are summarized in **Box 8.4**. In this technique, the cancer is removed via a transoral route using specialized rigid laryngoscopes to expose the tumour and then using the CO_2 laser and microlaryngeal instruments to remove the tumour under microscopic visualization (**Figure 8.10**). The technique relies on removal of cancer in a blockwise method, resulting in several resection specimens. This requires cutting through cancerous tissue, which of course is against the principles of conventional oncologic surgery. However, with microscopic laser surgery, it is possible to see the structure of the cut surface of the tumour, allowing exposure of the superficial and deep extension of the tumour more precisely and allowing one to differentiate between malignant and non-malignant structure (**Figure 8.11**). This way the surgeon can individually adjust the safety margin. The microscope can also facilitate the detection of any further dysplastic or neoplastic changes of the mucosa surrounding the tumour (field cancerization). The technique also has several other advantages over traditional surgery. Dissection through healthy tissue to reach the tumour is not required and contributes to limited surgical trauma and limited blood loss. This means that the need for reconstruction is usually not necessary as the resulting defect is smaller and heals spontaneously. This also has a major impact on function of speech and swallowing. By preserving functionally important structures, such as cartilage, muscle and nerves, a more rapid and effective rehabilitation of the patient is achieved.

Box 8.4　Transoral laser microsurgery compared to open surgery and radiotherapy

Transoral laser microsurgery compared to open surgery for early vocal cord carcinoma

- Outpatient procedure possible
- Shorter operating time
- Less overtreatment
- Better voice quality
- Lower morbidity
- No feeding tube
- No trachestomy
- Fewer complications
- Similar oncologic results

Transoral laser microsurgery compared to radiotherapy for early vocal cord carcinoma

- Similar oncologic results
- Similar functional results
- Shorter treatment time
- Lower costs
- May give repeated laser treatments
- Radiotherapy still treatment option if laser unsuccessful

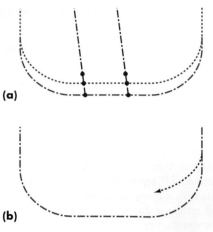

(a)

(b)

Figure 8.11　Blockwise resection of tumours by laser microsurgery (a) as opposed to en bloc resection (b).! Reproduced with permission from Wolfgang S, Ambrosch P. *Endoscopic laser surgery of the upper aerodigestive tract.* Stuttgart: Thieme.

larynx and pharynx, however, is quite steep. Significant experience with a large number of patients is required to gain the expertise, technical dexterity and judgement for a successful outcome. Large experience, therefore, is reported only from a few centres.

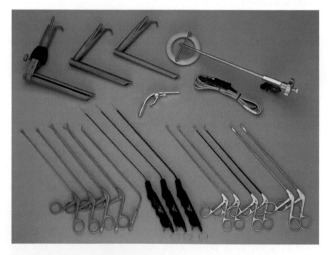

Figure 8.10　Instruments for transoral endoscopic laser resection. Reproduced with permission from Wolfgang S, Ambrosch P. *Endoscopic laser surgery of the upper aerodigestive tract.* Stuttgart: Thieme.

Tracheostomy is rarely indicated, patients are able to swallow sooner and often experience very little or even no pain postoperatively. As a result, the length of operation, hospital stay and duration of illness are markedly shortened and therefore costs are reduced accordingly. Lastly, during and after laser surgery, all surgical options still remain open. For example, during the operation, the procedure can be changed to an open approach at any time. Postoperatively, further laser resections can be done or an open conventional surgery performed. Laser surgery can be repeated many times for local recurrences, as well as second primary tumours. The learning curve for transoral laser surgery of tumours of the

TRANSORAL ENDOSCOPIC LASER RESECTION FOR GLOTTIC CARCINOMA

T1, T2 tumours

Transoral laser resection of early T1 and T2 glottic cancers has been reported with excellent oncologic results. Steiner et al.[79] reported on 158 patients with T1a and 30 patients with T1b cancers, with five-year local control rates of 96 and 85 per cent, respectively, and a larynx preservation rate of 97.6 and 99 per cent, respectively. For T2a glottic cancers ($n = 129$) and T2b cancers ($n = 115$), five-year local control rates were 84 and 70 per cent, respectively, with larynx preservation rates of 96 and 86 per cent. Excellent results have been reported by Ledda et al.[80] (five-year local control of 98 per cent for 103 patients with T1 or T2 cancers).

T3, T4 tumours

For large volume T2, T3 and T4 tumours, organ-preserving chemoradiation is now the standard treatment. The surgical treatment is total laryngectomy. However, conservation surgery by endoscopic laser resection is possible for T3 tumours. Steiner et al.[79] have reported on 95 patients with T3 glottic cancers with a five-year local control rate of 69 per cent, larynx preservation rate of 84 per cent, overall survival of 58 per cent and recurrence-free survival of 60 per cent.

TRANSORAL ENDOSCOPIC LASER RESECTION FOR SUPRAGLOTTIC CARCINOMA

T1, T2 tumours

Endoscopic laser resection of supraglottic laryngeal cancer can be carried out for all T-stage tumours. For tumours

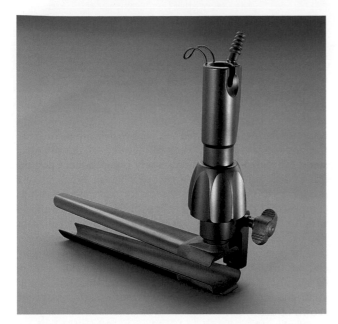

Figure 8.12   Distending laryngoscope for endoscopic resection of supraglottic tumours and tumours of the pyriform sinus. Reproduced with permission from Wolfgang S, Ambrosch P. *Endoscopic laser surgery of the upper aerodigestive tract.* Stuttgart: Thieme.

located in the supraglottis, exposure for laser microsurgery is dependent upon the use of a distending laryngoscope (**Figure 8.12**). Steiner (personal communication) has reported five-year local control rates for T1 ($n = 23$) and T2 ($n = 72$) cancers of 95 and 85 per cent with larynx preservation rates of 96 and 99 per cent, respectively. Overall survival rates were 87 and 73 per cent, respectively. These results are comparable to open supraglottic laryngectomy, but functional results are superior since clinically relevant aspiration did not occur in the laser-treated patients.

T3, T4 tumours

For large volume T2, T3 and T4 tumours, organ-preserving chemoradiation is now the standard treatment. This is because open surgery is radical and involves either a total laryngectomy, total laryngopharyngectomy and flap, or total laryngectomy and glossectomy. However, many institutions have now advocated conservation surgery in this setting by transoral endoscopic laser resection, allowing larynx and pharynx preservation. No tracheostomy is required, but patients require percutaneous endoscopic gastroscopy (PEG) feeding in the postoperative period. Adjuvant PORT (postoperative radiotherapy) is required. In supraglottic cancer, it is important to treat both sides of the neck. For the clinically negative neck, either separate or synchronous selective neck dissection can be performed or both necks can be treated with PORT bilaterally. For the clinically positive neck, either separate or synchronous comprehensive neck dissections should be performed with transoral laser resection. Steiner (personal communication) has reported the five-year local control rates for T3 ($n = 76$) and T4 ($n = 45$) cancers of 79 and 69 per cent with larynx preservation rates of 95 and 84 per cent, respectively. Overall survival rates were 67 and 54

per cent, respectively. Again, patient selection is important, as good pulmonary function and patient motivation is required for the entire time it takes to rehabilitate the patient. This surgery may not be possible if there is extensive field change.

CONSERVATION SURGERY FOR RECURRENT EARLY STAGE LARYNGEAL CANCER

Between 10 and 40 per cent of patients with early stage laryngeal cancer treated with radiotherapy recur after treatment. Many of these patients recur with higher T-stage disease and require salvage total laryngectomy. However, some patients still have T1 or T2 tumours which are amenable to salvage partial laryngectomy (PL). In many institutions, salvage surgery is often by total laryngectomy due to lack of experience in conservation surgery of the larynx, as well as the belief that increased complications are associated with partial laryngectomy of irradiated cartilage and that negative tumour margins are difficult to achieve in a fibrotic oedematous larynx. However, salvage partial laryngectomy is possible in select patients who do not progress on therapy or who recur with early stage disease. Such patients require careful endoscopic and radiologic assessment. Salvage partial laryngectomy may be by frontolateral vertical PL, supracricoid PL or by transoral laser resection. For frontolateral vertical PL, Shah et al.,[81] emphasized the importance of excluding patients in whom the recurrent tumour has extended beyond its original site, thereby making it unsuitable for a conservation operation, and of checking resection margins by intraoperative frozen sections. McLaughlin et al.[82] also highlighted the importance of CT scanning to determine if salvage was possible, recommending total laryngectomy if cartilage invasion, vocal cord fixation, extensive subglottic disease or recurrence beyond the original is seen on CT scan. Local control rates of 66–96 per cent have been reported for PL in early stage glottic laryngeal tumours.[81, 82, 83, 84, 85, 86, 87, 88, 89]

Salvage supracricoid partial laryngectomy with cricohyoidepiglottopexy for radio-recurrent glottic cancer involves removal of the thyroid cartilage and both paraglottic spaces with preservation of the cricoid cartilage, hyoid bone, epiglottis and one or both arytenoids cartilage and recurrent laryngeal nerves. It has been advocated as a better operation than the frontolateral vertical partial laryngectomy, where patients often end up with a small glottis and poor voice. In the supracricoid partial laryngectomy (SCPL) with CHEP, rehabilitation takes time and patients require a temporary tracheostomy and PEG due to aspiration. Therefore, patient motivation and support are essential, as well as good pulmonary function in patients treated this way. Salvage by endoscopic laser resection has also been advocated. Local control rates are reported to be 60–70 per cent.[75] Patients have to be selected and monitored carefully afterwards.

For supraglottic cancers, salvage partial laryngectomy by horizontal supraglottic partial laryngectomy[90] or supracricoid partial laryngectomy and cricohyoidopexy (CHP)[70, 91] is possible if the tumour has not extended beyond the original site as assessed endoscopically and by CT imaging. However, in general, salvage surgery for supraglottic cancer often requires a total laryngectomy.

CONSERVATION SURGERY FOR CANCER OF THE HYPOPHARYNX

Carcinoma of the hypopharynx includes cancer of the pyriform sinus (70 per cent), postcricoid region (15 per cent) and posterior pharyngeal wall (15 per cent). Of all head and neck sites, hypopharyngeal cancer has the poorest prognosis with an overall five-year survival of less than 20 per cent. This is because patients usually present with advanced stage disease (stage III/IV) either due to advanced T stage or neck metastases. Approximately 66 per cent of patients have nodal disease at first presentation, and of the remaining, 34 per cent present with N0 disease and 41 per cent present with occult neck metastases. Therefore, management of hypopharyngeal cancer involves not only treatment of the primary, but also the neck.

T1 and small volume T2 tumours without neck metastases

Patients are usually treated with radiation to the primary and the neck bilaterally. However, partial pharyngectomy and bilateral selective neck dissection can also be performed.

T1 and small volume T2 tumours with neck metastases

Patients may be treated with comprehensive neck dissection for the neck and radiation to the primary. Alternatively, partial pharyngectomy and comprehensive neck dissection with PORT can be carried out.

Large volume T2, T3 and T4 tumours with/without neck metastases

RADICAL SURGERY

Patients may require radical surgery. If the larynx is not involved, surgery involves resection of the primary tumour (preserving larynx) with reconstruction, neck dissection and postoperative radiation therapy. If the larynx is involved, surgery entails excision of the primary tumour with laryngectomy and reconstruction, and neck dissection followed by postoperative radiation therapy. Reconstruction of the pharynx may be by free jejunum or tubed free radial forearm flaps for circumferential defects and by free radial forearm flaps, anterolateral thigh flaps or pedicled pectoralis myocutaneous flaps for partial pharyngeal defects. This type of surgery is radical and associated with significant effects both on speech and swallowing. For this reason, organ-preserving chemoradiation has now been advocated and has largely superseded radical surgery for this disease. For cancer of the pyriform sinus, five-year survival figures of 25 per cent are comparable to surgery with larynx preservation rates of 35 per cent.[92] However, many of these patients suffer the long-term sequelae of chemoradiation which include swallowing difficulty from stenosis of the hypopharynx and aspiration from a nonfunctioning larynx. For this reason, alternative surgical conservation approaches have been advocated by some investigators using transoral endoscopic laser resection.

CONSERVATIVE TREATMENT BY TRANSORAL ENDOSCOPIC LASER RESECTION OF PYRIFORM SINUS TUMOURS

Endoscopic laser resection of patients with pyriform sinus tumours can now be carried out with synchronous or separate neck dissection. For tumours located in the pyriform sinus, exposure for laser microsurgery is dependent upon the use of the distending laryngoscope (**Figure 8.12**). Steiner et al.[93] have reported their results for 129 patients which comprised 24 patients with T1, 74 with T2, 17 with T3 and 14 with T4 tumours. Seventy-five per cent of patients had stage III/IV disease and 25 per cent stage I/II disease. Forty-two per cent of patients had surgery alone and 58 per cent surgery and postoperative radiotherapy. With a median follow up of 44 months, 87 per cent of patients were controlled locally. Local and locoregional recurrence rates for each T stage are shown in **Table 8.5**.

Of the 17 patients with either local or locoregional recurrence, ten were able to be salvaged; eight had further laser microsurgery ± radiotherapy, one had partial pharyngectomy with laryngeal preservation and one had partial pharyngectomy with total laryngectomy. Six patients had palliative treatment and one patient was unknown. The five-year overall survival was 71 per cent for stage I/II and 47 per cent for stage III/IV disease. The five-year recurrence-free survival was 95 and 69 per cent, respectively. These are extremely high cure rates reported for hypopharynx cancer, and are not duplicated by other authors in the literature.

The EORTC organ preservation chemoradiation study[92] reported on 100 patients with stage III/IV disease; a 25 per cent disease-free survival and 35 per cent organ preservation rate was reported. In contrast, Steiner et al.[93] have reported a five-year overall survival of 47 per cent, recurrence-free survival of 69 per cent and an organ preservation rate of 99 per cent for patients with pyriform sinus tumours treated by laser resection. In addition, functional results were excellent compared with radical surgery and chemoradiation with 27 per cent of patients requiring no feeding tube and 73 per cent requiring a feeding tube for a median duration of 7 days (range 1–25 days). Excellent oncologic results have also been published by Vilaseca et al.[94] who reported on 28 patients with hypopharyngeal carcinomas with a four-year overall and disease-specific survival of 43 and 59 per cent, respectively, and a larynx preservation rate of 78 per cent. These data suggest that function-preserving laser surgery for pyriform sinus cancer has a definite role to play in the management of these patients.

Table 8.5 Local and locoregional recurrence rates.

No. patients (n = 129)	Local recurrence	Locoregional recurrence
T1 (24)	2 (8.3%)	0 (0%)
T2 (74)	5 (6.7%)	3 (4.1%)
T3 (17)	2 (11.8%)	0 (0%)
T4 (14)	3 (21.4%)	2 (14.3%)

CONSERVATION SURGERY FOR CANCER OF THE ORAL CAVITY

Limited resection of oral cavity cancers is to be condemned. However, it is possible to carry out conservation surgery to the mandible during resection of oral cavity and oropharynx cancers. To determine if the mandible is invaded by cancer, careful assessment of the mandible is best carried out by bimanual palpation under anaesthetic. Radiographic imaging should be used to supplement the clinical evaluation; CT is effective at assessing cortical erosion, whereas MRI is particularly useful for determining marrow involvement and involvement of the inferior alveolar nerve.

Tumour invasion of the mandible

In order to assess the extent and need for mandible resection it is necessary to understand the process of invasion of the mandible.[95, 96, 97, 98] Tumours do not invade directly through intact periosteum and cortical bone towards the cancellous part of the mandible because the periosteum acts as a protective barrier.[96, 97, 99] Instead, the tumour advances along the attached gingiva towards the alveolus. In patients with teeth, the tumour extends up to the alveolar process and then invades the mandible via the dental sockets to extend into the cancellous part of the mandible. In edentulous patients, the tumour extends up to the alveolar process and then infiltrates the dental pores to extend into the cancellous part of the mandible. In the irradiated mandible, the periosteal barrier is weak and therefore direct invasion through the lingual plate may occur.[96, 97]

Mandibulotomy approach for access for oral cavity and oropharynx cancers

Previously, resection of oral cavity lesions in regions with limited access, such as the retromolar trigone and posterior tongue, were resected with a segment of mandible. However, there are no lymphatic channels passing through the mandible and therefore there is no need for an in continuity composite resection. Segmental mandibulectomy should be carried out if there is:

* gross invasion by oral cancer;
* tumour close to mandible in a previously irradiated patient;
* invasion of the inferior alveolar nerve or canal by tumour;
* massive soft tissue disease adjacent to the mandible.

If none of these criteria is present, then access to the primary tumour can be with a mandibulotomy approach. Mandibulotomy can be performed in one of three locations: lateral (through the body or angle of the mandible), midline or paramedian. Access is best by a paramedian approach due to the disadvantages of the lateral and midline approach (**Box 8.5**).[100, 101, 102]

The paramedian mandibulotomy avoids all of the disadvantages outlined in **Box 8.5**.[103] The preferred site is between the lateral incisor and canine teeth since the roots of these two teeth diverge. Therefore, bone cuts can be performed without damaging the teeth. Only the myohyoid muscle is

---

Box 8.5 Disadvantages of lateral and midline mandibulotomy

Lateral mandibulotomy

* Mandibulotomy site under stress due to unequal muscular pull on the two segments resulting in delayed healing
* Denervation of the teeth distal to the mandibulotomy site
* Disruption of the endosteal blood supply resulting in devascularization of the distal teeth and distal mandible
* If postoperative radiation is required, the mandibulotomy site is direcly within the field leading to delayed healing

Midline mandibulotomy

All the disadvantages of the lateral mandibulotomy are avoided. However, specific disadvantages are:

* Requires extraction of one central incisor tooth which alters the aesthetic appearance of the lower dentition
* Division of the muscles arising from the geneal tubercle, i.e. geniohyoid and genioglossus muscles. This results in delayed recovery of mastication and swallowing

---

divided, the genioglossus and geniohyoid muscles are preserved. This results in minimal problems with swallowing.

Marginal mandibulectomy

If the periosteum or superficial aspect of the cortical mandible bone is involved, it is possible to carry out a marginal mandibulectomy rather than segmental mandibulectomy. In the dentate patient, marginal mandibulectomy is possible since the cortical part of the mandible inferior to the roots of the teeth remains uninvolved by tumour. However, in edentulous patients, the feasibility of mandibulectomy depends on the vertical height of the body of the mandible. With ageing, the alveolar process recedes and the mandibular canal comes closer and closer to the surface of the alveolar process. This eventually leads to a pipestem mandible and in these circumstances it may be impossible to carry out a marginal mandubulectomy with iatrogenic fracture.

Marginal mandibulectomy is contraindicated when there is gross invasion into the cancellous part of the mandible or when there is massive soft tissue disease. It is also contraindicated in the irradiated mandible or in the edentulous patient with a pipestem mandible.

CONSERVATION SURGERY FOR CANCER OF THE OROPHARYNX

Cancer of the oropharynx includes the soft palate, tonsil, base of tongue and posterior pharyngeal wall.

T1 and T2 tumours with/without neck metastases

The primary is usually treated with radiotherapy. If the neck is clinically negative, radiation therapy is usually used as well. If clinically positive, the neck is treated with comprehensive neck dissection and PORT. Surgery can also be used to treat the primary tumour either by open resection or transoral laser resection.

T3 and T4 tumours with/without neck metastases

RADICAL SURGERY

Radical surgery of cancer of the tonsil or base of tongue involves a paramedian mandibulotomy for access, resection of the primary, comprehensive neck dissection and reconstruction with free tissue (usually free radial forearm flap, anterolateral thigh, free rectus muscle or occasionally pedicled myocutaneous pectoralis major flap). Such surgery has significant effects on speech and swallowing and because of this organ-preserving chemoradiation is now often advocated. However, even chemoradiation has both acute and chronic toxicity associated with it, also affecting speech and swallowing. Recently, conservation surgery using transoral laser resection has been used by some investigators.[104]

CONSERVATIVE SURGERY BY TRANSORAL LASER RESECTION

An alternative to chemoradiation or radical surgery is transoral laser resection followed by PORT. This technique requires appropriate usage of retractors and distending pharyngoscopes to give adequate access and the CO_2 laser to resect the tumour. A temporary tracheostomy may be required, as well as a temporary PEG tube for feeding. Such a technique has a learning curve. As in laryngeal cancer, this technique relies on resection in blocks of tissue and this poses problems with margin assessment by the pathologist. Because of this, postoperative radiotherapy is generally recommended in all such patients. As in all conservation surgery, selection of patients is paramount in the success of the technique. In particular, the patient must play an active role both in speech and swallowing rehabilitation. The technique does have limitations and these are listed below:

- extension to the retromolar trigone;
- lateral spread to the internal carotid artery and masticator space;
- field change;
- inferolateral spread to the soft tissue of the neck;
- contralateral lingual artery involvement.

The largest series to date is by Steiner et al.[104] who reported on 48 patients with base of tongue cancer (T1, 2 per cent; T2, 25 per cent; T3, 15 per cent; T4, 58 per cent; 94 per cent had stage III/IV disease). Selective neck dissection was carried out in 43 patients and 23 patients had postoperative radiotherapy. The five-year local control rate was 85 per cent,

recurrence-free survival 73 per cent and overall survival 52 per cent. Swallowing was normal in 92 per cent of patients and 88 per cent had understandability of speech. These results suggest that organ-preserving laser microsurgery has a role to play in the management of selected patients with base of tongue cancer both in terms of oncologic control and functional results.

Recently, transoral robotic surgery (TORS) has been employed by some with the claims of improved visualization, better assessment and manoeuvrability, and more accurate resection with satisfactory margins.[105] However, the role of robotic surgery in conservation procedures in the head and neck is evolving and requires further experience.

CONSERVATION SURGERY FOR CANCER OF THE NASAL CAVITY AND PARANASAL SINUSES

Malignant and benign tumours of the paranasal sinuses and skull base are resected by open procedures which allow for complete en bloc resection. Several facial incisions have been described to approach these types of tumours (**Figure 8.13**). Lateral rhinotomy alone can be used for anteriorly located nasal lesions. A Weber–Ferguson incision is used for tumours involving the medial wall of the maxillary sinus requiring medial maxillectomy. The Weber–Ferguson incision with a Lynch extension is used for tumours of the ethmoid sinus. For more advanced tumours of the maxillary sinus requiring subtotal or total maxillectomy, a Weber–Ferguson incision with subciliary extension is used. For tumours with anterior skull base involvement, an anterior craniofacial approach is required (**Figure 8.14**). This involves both a transfacial and transcranial incision for complete en bloc removal of tumour. All of these approaches result in a facial incision which may be cosmetically unacceptable to some patients, but also may result in disfigurement of the facial skeleton when large bony resections are required. Craniofacial surgery is also associated with significant morbidity and mortality, with an overall complication rate of 33 per cent and mortality of 4–6 per cent.[106] The advent of rigid endoscopes has revolutionized the management of paranasal sinus inflammatory disease by functional endoscopic sinus surgery (FESS). More complex intranasal pathology can now be managed; for example, dacrocystrhinotomy can be carried out for nasolacrimal duct obstruction, orbital decompression for exophthalmos of hyperthyroidism and endoscopic repair of cerebrospinal fluid leaks. Recently, endoscopic techniques have been successfully used to manage benign tumours, such as inverted papilloma,[107, 108, 109, 110, 111] angiofibromas[112, 113, 114, 115] and hypophyseal tumours.[116, 117] Certainly, the endoscopic approach for benign disease has advantages over open surgical resection. As there is no facial incision, resection of normal tissue is avoided, resulting in better function as well as cosmesis, and improved visualization of the tumour can be obtained using angled endoscopes, as well as increasing microscopic visualization of the tumour by magnification of images obtained. The availability of real-time image guidance, neuro-navigation and intraoperative MRI has further improved the safety and accuracy of endoscopic resections.

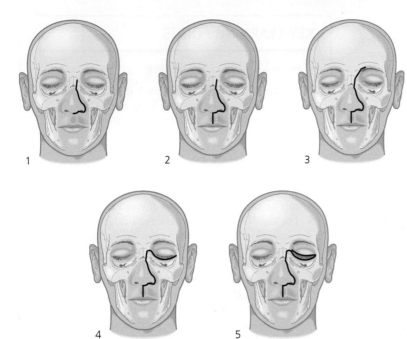

Figure 8.13   Different incisions used for resection of paranasal sinus tumours. (1) Lateral rhinotomy; (2) Weber–Ferguson; (3) Weber–Ferguson with Lynch extension; (4) Weber–Ferguson with subciliary extension; (5) Weber–Ferguson with subciliary and supraciliary extension.

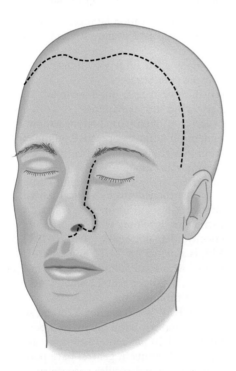

Figure 8.14   Skin incision used for anterior craniofacial resection.

Box 8.6   Criteria for selection of a lesion suitable for endoscopic resection of paranasal sinus tumours

Possible indications

- Midline lesions with limited lateral extension
- Benign tumours, such as inverted papilloma and angiofibroma
- Low-grade malignant tumours
- Resection for palliative intent
- Medical comorbidity limiting open surgical approach

Possible contraindications

- Lateral extension of tumour
- Intracranial invasion involving brain ± dura
- Intraorbital invasion
- High-grade malignant tumours

However, whether or not endoscopic resection can be safely and successfully carried out for malignant sinonasal disease still remains questionable. A recent report by the international collaborative group encompassing 17 international sites reported on the prognostic factors important in sinonasal tumours with skull base invasion.[118] This study reported that intracranial involvement, comorbidity, surgical resection margins and pathology were the main factors predicting survival. Endoscopic approaches do not allow for complete en bloc removal of tumour, and therefore resection margins remain a controversial area. Random biopsies of the resection bed following excision may be used to check for completeness of endoscopic removal. Another area of controversy is whether or not the endoscopic technique can be used for tumours with intracranial extension; for tumours invading periosteum or bone, endoscopic removal of tumour may be possible with resection of bone provided the tumour is mainly in the midline with no lateral extension. However, reconstruction of the resultant bony defect is then required. For open surgery, the galealpericranial flap[119, 120] is used, but this is not possible with the endoscopic approach. Reconstruction with non-vascularized tissue, such as fascia lata and tissue glue, has been reported, but this remains an area of uncertainty. For tumours requiring dura excision this is also possible, but again reconstruction is the main area of concern.[121] When intracranial extension into brain occurs, endoscopic resection is contraindicated. Histology of the malignant tumour is also a significant predictor of survival; therefore more aggressive types of tumours, such as sinonasal undifferentiated carcinoma, melanoma, high-grade sarcomas, high-grade squamous and adenocarcinomas are best treated with open surgery. However, for benign tumours or low-grade malignant tumours, such as low-grade sarcomas, small central esthesioneuroblastomas or salivary gland tumours, endoscopic approaches may be possible. Lastly, endoscopic resection may be the treatment of choice when the objective of surgery is palliation or when the patient has significant comorbidity which precludes an open surgical approach. A summary of possible indications and contraindications for endoscopic surgery for paranasal sinus tumours is shown in **Box 8.6**.

CONSERVATION SURGERY FOR TUMOURS OF THE PAROTID GLAND

Warthin's tumour excision without parotidectomy

Surgery is the mainstay for treatment for both benign and malignant parotid tumours. The most common benign tumours are pleomorphic adenoma and Warthin's tumours (adenolymphoma). Conservation surgery, i.e. enucleation for pleomorphic adenoma, is not recommended due to the high incidence of local recurrence. This is due to the presence of pseudopodia.[122,123] Treatment of recurrent pleomorphic adenoma results in a higher incidence of facial nerve paresis and Frey's syndrome.[124] However, enucleation is possible in Warthin's tumours where there are no pseudopodia. Heller and Attie[125] reported on 162 patients with Warthin's tumours, of whom 112 were amenable to a simple enucleation. In only two patients did an additional tumour develop. No permanent facial nerve injuries occurred.

Preservation of facial nerve for malignant tumours

For early stage parotid cancers, superficial parotidectomy with facial nerve preservation is advocated. However, for late stage cancer or cancers, the resection may need to involve removal of the mandible, zygoma and temporal bone, as well as part or all of the facial nerve. In the last decade, there has been a trend to a more conservative approach to the facial nerve. Most surgeons now advocate preservation of the facial nerve branches unless they are adherent to or directly invaded by tumour. This approach, however, relies on the use of postoperative radiation to control for microscopic residual disease.[126] If major branches or the main trunk are involved, then immediate cable grafts should be done using branches of the cervical plexus or sural nerve.

KEY LEARNING POINTS

Conservation surgery for the neck

- For the N0 neck, selective neck dissection can be done. The type of neck dissection is determined by the location of the primary tumour.
- For the N+ neck, radical neck dissection is the old standard. Modified radical neck dissection type I can be done preserving function to the shoulder. Type II–III modified neck dissection can be done for metastatic thyroid cancer.
- For the N+ neck, selective neck dissection is controversial. Recurrence rates up to 36 per cent have been reported. This can be reduced to 5–8 per cent if postoperative radiotherapy is given.
- Neck dissection for residual neck disease following chemoradiation is associated with significant morbidity. Selective neck dissection can be done provided the residual disease is localized to one level of the neck.

Conservation surgery for cancer of the larynx

- The aim of conservation laryngeal surgery is to maintain speech and swallowing and avoid tracheostomy.
- It may be by open surgery or transoral endoscopic laser surgery.
- Preservation of at least one functional cricoarytenoid unit is required.
- The success of open partial laryngectomy is dependent on good preoperative pulmonary function and good postoperative speech and swallowing rehabilitation.
- Open partial laryngectomy for glottic cancer:
  - It can be carried out by vertical partial laryngectomy (VPL) or by supracricoid partial laryngectomy with cricohyoidepiglottopexy (SCPL-CHEP).
  - VPL is suitable for T1,T2 and select T3 lesions with local failure occurring in 7 per cent T1, 4–26 per cent T2 and 11–46 per cent T3 tumours.
  - SCPL-CHEP is suitable for T1b and select T2,T3 tumours. Local failure of 5 per cent for T2 and 10 per cent T3 tumours is reported. Patients in general have poor quality voice and require nasogastric tube feeding for several weeks due to aspiration.
- Open partial laryngectomy for supraglottic cancer:
  - It can be carried out by horizontal supraglottic partial laryngectomy (HSGPL) or by supracricoid partial laryngectomy with cricohyoidpexy (SCPL-CHP).
  - HSGPL is suitable for T1,T2 supraglottic cancers. It is contraindicated if there is extension below the false cord or there is impaired vocal cord mobility. Aspiration is

common. Preservation of the superior laryngeal nerve is important. Nasogastric feeding and delayed tracheostomy decannulation is not uncommon.
- SCPL-CHP is suitable for T1,T2 and select T3 tumours. It is suitable if the vocal cord is invaded or there is pre-epiglottic space invasion.
- Transoral endoscopic laser surgery:
  - Transoral endoscopic laser surgery involve blockwise removal of cancer allowing an individualized approach to surgery.
  - It has comparable oncological results to open surgery and radiotherapy.
  - Compared to open surgery, it is a short operation, can be done as an outpatient procedure, with better voice, and avoids tracheostomy and nasogastric feeding.
  - Compared to radiotherapy, it is of lower cost, can be repeated and radiotherapy still remains an option should laser treatment fail.

Conservation surgery for recurrent early stage laryngeal cancer

- Provided there is no progression of disease, conservation surgery for early glottic cancer can be done by VPL, SCPL-CHEP or transoral laser surgery.
- Local control rates of 66–96 per cent for VPL and 60–70 per cent for transoral laser surgery have been reported.
- In general, salvage surgery for recurrent supraglottic laryngeal surgery is not amenable to partial laryngectomy and requires total laryngectomy.

Conservation surgery for cancer of the hypopharynx

- Conservation surgery with open partial pharyngectomy is possible for T1,T2 pyriform sinus cancer.
- Transoral endoscopic laser resection for T1–T3 pyriform sinus cancer is possible, but over 50 per cent require postoperative radiotherapy. Oncological results are comparable to chemoradiation. Functional results are superior to chemoradiation.

Conservation surgery for cancer of the oral cavity

- Limited resection of oral cancers is to be condemned.
- However, conservation surgery of the mandible is possible.
- Marginal mandibulectomy can be done rather than segmental mandibulectomy if invasion is limited to the periosteum or superficial bone cortex.
- Marginal mandibulectomy is contraindicated in the edentulous patient, irradiated mandible or if there is extensive soft tissue cancer.

Conservation surgery for cancer of the oropharynx

- Conservation surgery for T1–T3 tumours of the tonsil and base of tongue can be carried out by transoral endoscopic laser resection or transoral robotic surgery. Postoperative radiation is required.
- Surgery is dependent on careful patient selection, adequate exposure and visualization via specialized retractors and the use of endoscopic laser or robotic instrumentation.

Conservation surgery for cancer of the nasal cavity and paranasal sinuses

- Conservation surgery by endoscopic surgery is possible for benign tumour and centrally located low-grade malignancies.
- Surgery is assisted by real-time image guidance, intraoperative magnetic resonance imaging (MRI) and neuronavigation.
- Surgery is not en bloc and therefore is dependent on intraoperative frozen section margins to ensure completeness of resection.

Conservation surgery for tumours of the parotid gland

- Conservation surgery by enucleation for pleomorphic adenoma is to be condemned. Enucleation is acceptable for Warthin's tumour.

REFERENCES

1. Rouviere H. *Anatomy of the human lymphatic system.* Ann Arbor, MI: Edward Brothers 1938.
2. Fisch UP, Sigel ME. Cervical lymphatic system as visualized by lymphography. *Annals of Otology, Rhinology, and Laryngology* 1964; **73**: 870–82.
3. Shah JP. Patterns of lymph node metastases from squamous cell carcinomas of the upper aerodigestive tract. *American Journal of Surgery* 1990; **160**: 405–9.
4. Davidson BJ, Kulkarny V, Delacure MD, Shah JP. Posterior triangle metastases of squamous cell carcinoma of the upper aerodigestive tract. *American Journal of Surgery* 1993; **166**: 395–8.
5. Andersen PE, Shah JP, Cambronero E, Spiro RH. The role of comprehensive neck dissection with preservation of the spinal accessory nerve in the clinically positive neck. *American Journal of Surgery* 1994; **168**: 499–502.
6. Byers RM. Modified neck dissection: A study of 967 cases from 1970 to 1980. *American Journal of Surgery* 1985; **150**: 414–21.
7. Spiro RH, Morgan GJ, Strong EW *et al.* Supraomohyoid neck dissection. *American Journal of Surgery* 1996; **172**: 650–3.
8. O'Brien CJ. A selective approach to neck dissection for mucosal squamous cell carcinoma. *Australia and New Zealand Journal of Surgery* 1994; **64**: 236–41.

9. Bocca E, Pignatato O, Oldini C, Cappa C. Functional neck dissection: an evaluation and review of 843 cases. *Laryngoscope* 1984; **94**: 942–5.

10. Traynor SJ, Cohen JI, Gray J *et al.* Selective neck dissection and the management of the node positive neck. *American Journal of Surgery* 1996; **172**: 654–7.

11. Pellitteri PK, Robbins KT, Neuman T. Expanded application of selective neck dissection with regard to nodal status. *Head and Neck* 1997; **19**: 260–5.

12. Simental AA Jr, Duvvuri U, Johnson JT, Myers EN. Selective neck dissection in patients with upper aerodigestive tract cancer with clinically positive nodal disease. *Annals of Otology, Rhinology, and Laryngology* 2006; **115**: 846–9.

13. Bradford CR. Selective neck dissection is an option for early node-positive disease. *Archives of Otolaryngology – Head and Neck Surgery* 2004; **130**: 1436.

14. Byers RM, Clayman GL, McGill D *et al.* Selective neck dissections for squamous carcinoma of the upper aerodigestive tract: patterns of regional failure. *Head and Neck* 1999; **21**: 499–505.

15. Andersen PE, Warren F, Spiro J *et al.* Results of selective neck dissection in management of the node-positive neck. *Archives of Otolaryngology – Head and Neck Surgery* 2002; **128**: 1180–4.

16. Brizel DM, Prosnitz RG, Hunter S *et al.* Necessity for adjuvant neck dissection in setting of concurrent chemoradiation for advanced head and neck cancer. *International Journal of Radiation Oncology, Biology, Physics* 2004; **58**: 1418–23.

17. Grabenbauer GG, Rodel C, Ernst-Stecken A *et al.* Neck dissection following chemoradiotherapy of advanced head and neck cancer – for selected cases only? *Radiotherapy and Oncology* 2003; **66**: 57–63.

18. Robbins KT, Wong FS, Kumar P *et al.* Efficacy of targeted chemoradiation and planned selective neck dissection to control bulky nodal disease in advanced head and neck cancer. *Archives of Otolaryngology – Head and Neck Surgery* 1999; **125**: 670–5.

19. Mendenhall WM, Million RR, Cassisi NJ. Squamous cell carcinoma of the supraglottic larynx treated with radical irradiation: analysis of treatment parameters and results. *International Journal of Radiation Oncology, Biology, Physics* 1984; **10**: 2223–30.

20. Narayan K, Crane CH, Kleid S *et al.* Planned neck dissection as an adjunct to the management of patients with advanced neck disease treated with definitive radiotherapy: For some or for all? *Head and Neck* 1999; **21**: 606–13.

21. Wong RJ, Lin DT, Schoder H *et al.* Diagnostic and prognostic value of [(18)F]fluorodeoxyglucose positron emission tomography for recurrent head and neck squamous cell carcinoma. *Journal of Clinical Oncology* 2002; **20**: 4199–208.

22. Boyd T, Harari P, Tannahil S *et al.* Planned postradiotherapy neck dissection in patients with advanced head and neck cancer. *Head and Neck* 1998; **20**: 132–7.

23. Stenson KM, Haraf DJ, Pelzer H. The role of cervical lymphadenopathy after aggressive concomitant chemoradiotherapy: the feasibility of selective neck dissection. *Archives of Otolaryngology – Head and Neck Surgery* 2000; **126**: 950–6.

24. Robbins KT, Ferlito A, Suarez C *et al.* Is there a role for selective neck dissection after chemoradiation for head and neck cancer? *Journal of the American College of Surgeons* 2004; **199**: 913–16.

25. Robbins KT, Doweck I, Samant S, Vieira F. Effectiveness of superselective and selective neck dissection for advanced nodal metastases after chemoradiation. *Archives of Otolaryngology – Head and Neck Surgery* 2005; **131**: 965–9.

26. Ton-Van J, Lefebvre JL, Stern JC *et al.* Comparison of surgery and radiotherapy in T1 and T2 glottic carcinomas. *American Journal of Surgery* 1991; **162**: 337–40.

27. Pellitteri PK, Kennedy TL, Vrabec DP *et al.* Radiotherapy: the mainstay in the treatment of early glottic carcinoma. *Archives of Otolaryngology – Head and Neck Surgery* 1991; **117**: 297–301.

28. Mendenhall WM, Parson JT, Stringer SP *et al.* T1–T2 vocal cord carcinoma: a basis for comparing the results of radiotherapy and surgery. *Head and Neck* 1988; **10**: 373–7.

29. Dey P, Arnold D, Wight R *et al.* Radiotherapy versus open surgery versus endolaryngeal surgery (with or without laser) for early laryngeal squamous cell cancer. *Cochrane Database of Systematic Reviews*: 2002; **(2)**: CD002027.

30. Mendenhall WM, Werning JW, Hinerman RW *et al.* Management of T1–T2 glottic carcinomas. *Cancer* 2004; **100**: 1786–92.

31. Jones AS, Fish B, Fenton JE, Husband DJ. The treatment of early laryngeal cancers (T1–T2N0): surgery or irradiation? *Head and Neck* 2004; **26**: 127–35.

32. Kirchner JA. Two hundred laryngeal cancers: patterns of growth and spread as seen in serial section. *Laryngoscope* 1977; **87**: 474–82.

33. Hirano M, Kurita S, Matsuoka H, Tateishi M. Vocal fold fixation in laryngeal carcinomas. *Acta Otolaryngologica* 1991; **111**: 449–54.

34. Kirchner JA, Som ML. Clinical significance of fixed vocal cord. *Laryngoscope* 1971; **81**: 1029–44.

35. Olofsson J, Lord IJ. van Nostrand AWP. Vocal cord fixation in laryngeal carcinoma. *Acta Otolaryngologica* 1973; **75**: 496–510.

36. Rademaker AW, Logemann JA, Pauloski BR *et al.* Recovery of postoperative swallowing in patients undergoing partial laryngectomy. *Head and Neck* 1993; **15**: 325.

37. Rothfield RE, Johnson JT, Myers EN *et al.* The role of hemilaryngectomy in the management of T1 vocal cord cancer. *Archives of Otolaryngology – Head and Neck Surgery* 1989; **115**: 677–80.

38. Laccourreye O, Weinstein G, Brasnu D *et al*. Vertical partial laryngectomy: a critical analysis of local recurrence. *Annals of Otology, Rhinology, and Laryngology* 1991; **100**: 68–71.

39. Mohr RM, Quennelle J, Shumrick DA. Vertico-frontolateral laryngectomy. *Archives of Otolaryngology* 1983; **109**: 384–95.

● 40. Johnson JT, Myers EN, Hao S *et al*. Outcome of open surgical therapy for glottic carcinoma. *Annals of Otology, Rhinology, and Laryngology* 1993; **102**: 752–5.

41. Biller HF, Lawson W. Hemilaryngectomy for T2 glottic cancers. *Archives of Otolaryngology* 1971; **93**: 238–43.

42. Biller HF, Lawson W. Partial laryngectomy for vocal cord cancer with marked limitation or fixation of the vocal cord. *Laryngoscope* 1986; **96**: 61–4.

43. Kessler DJ, Trapp TK, Calcaterra TC. The treatment of T3 glottic carcinoma with vertical partial laryngectomy. *Archives of Otolaryngology – Head and Neck Surgery* 1987; **113**: 1196–9.

44. Mendenhall WM, Million RR, Sharkey DE, Cassisi NJ. Stage T3 squamous cell carcinoma of the glottic larynx treated with surgery and/or radiation therapy. *International Journal of Radiation Oncology, Biology, Physics* 1984; **10**: 357–63.

45. Liu C, Ward PH, Pleet L. Imbrication reconstruction following partial laryngectomy. *Annals of Otology, Rhinology, and Laryngology* 1986; **95**: 567–71.

46. Laccourreye O, Weinstein G, Brasnu D *et al*. A clinical trial of continuous cisplatin-fluorouracil induction chemotherapy and supracricoid partial laryngectomy for glottic carcinomaclassified as T2. *Cancer* 1994; **74**: 2781–90.

47. Laccourreye O, Salzer SJ, Brasnu D *et al*. Glottic carcinoma with a fixed true vocal cord: outcome after neoadjuvant chemotherapy and supracricoid partial laryngectomy with cricohyoidoepiglottopexy. *Otolaryngology – Head and Neck Surgery* 1996; **114**: 400–6.

48. Crevier-Buchman L, Laccourreye O, Weinstein G *et al*. Evolution of speech and voice following supracricoid partial laryngectomy. *Journal of Laryngology and Otology* 1995; **109**: 410.

49. Burstein FD, Calcaterra TC. Supraglottic laryngectomy: series report and analysis of results. *Laryngoscope* 1985; **95**: 833–6.

◆ 50. Coate HL, DeSanto LW, Devine KD, Elveback LR. Carcinoma of the supraglottic larynx. A review of 221 cases. *Archives of Otolaryngology* 1976; **102**: 686–9.

◆ 51. DeSanto LW. Cancer of the supraglottic larynx: a review of 260 patients. *Otolaryngology – Head and Neck Surgery* 1985; **93**: 705–11.

52. Lee NK, Goepfert H, Wendt CD. Supraglottic laryngectomy for immediate stage cancer: UT MD Anderson Cancer Center experience with combined therapy. *Laryngoscope* 1990; **100**: 831–6.

◆ 53. Som ML. Conservation surgery for carcinoma of the supraglottis. Dissertation, University of London, 1969.

54. Spaulding CA, Constable WC, Levine PA, Cantrell RW. Partial laryngectomy and radiotherapy for supraglottic cancer: a conservative approach. *Annals of Otology, Rhinology, and Laryngology* 1989; **98**: 125–9.

55. Klein AD, Wasserstrom JP, Sessions DG *et al*. Rehabilitation of partial laryngectomy patients. *Transactions of the American Academy of Ophthalmology and Otolaryngology* 1977; **84**: 324–34.

56. Padovan IF, Oreskovic M. Functional evaluation after partial resection in patients with carcinoma of the larynx. *Laryngoscope* 1975; **85**: 626–39.

57. Hirano M, Kurita S, Tateishi M, Matsuoka H. Deglutition following supraglottic horizontal laryngectomy. *Annals of Otology, Rhinology, and Laryngology* 1987; **96**: 7–11.

58. Flores TC, Wood BG, Levine HL *et al*. Factors in successful deglutition following supraglottic laryngeal surgery. *Annals of Otology, Rhinology, and Laryngology* 1982; **91**: 579–83.

59. Biustein FD, Calcaterra TC. Supraglottic laryngectomy: series report and analysis of results. *Laryngoscope* 1985; **95**: 833.

60. Weinstein GS, Laccourreye O, Brasnu D. Reconsidering a paradigm: the spread of supraglottic carcinoma to the glottis. *Laryngosope* 1995; **105**: 1129–33.

● 61. Laccourreye H, Laccourreye O, Weinstein GS *et al*. Supracricoid laryngectomy with cricohyoidopexy: a partial laryngeal procedure for selected supraglottic and transglottic carcinomas. *Laryngoscope* 1990; **100**: 735–41.

62. Chevalier D, Piquet JJ. Subtotal laryngectomy with cricohyoidopexy for supraglottic carcinoma: review of 61 cases. *American Journal of Surgery* 1994; **168**: 472–3.

63. Laccourreye O, Brasnu D, Merite-Drancy A *et al*. Cricohyoidopexy in selected infrahyoid epiglottic carcinomas presenting with pathological preepiglottic space invasion. *Archives of Otolaryngology – Head and Neck Surgery* 1993; **119**: 881–6.

64. Laccourreye O, Cauchois R, Menard M *et al*. Deglutition and partial supracricoid laryngectomie. *Annales d'Otolaryngologie et de Chirurgie Cervicofaciale* 1992; **109**: 73–5.

65. Laccourreye O, Crevier-Buchmann L, Weinstein G *et al*. Duration and frequency characteristics of speech and voice following supracricoid partial laryngectomy. *Annals of Otology, Rhinology, and Laryngology* 1995; **104**: 516–21.

● 66. Biller HF, Barnhill FR, Ogura JH *et al*. Hemilaryngectomy following radiation failure for carcinoma of the vocal cords. *Laryngoscope* 1970; **80**: 249–53.

67. Sorenson H, Hansen HS, Thomsen KA. Partial laryngectomy following irradiation. *Laryngoscope* 1980; **90**: 1344–9.

68. Laccourreye O, Weinstein G, Brasnu D et al. Supracricoid partial laryngectomy after failed laryngeal radiation therapy. Laryngoscope 1996; 106: 495–9.

69. Wolfensberger M, Dort JC. Endoscopic laser surgery for early glottic carcinoma: a clinical and experimental study. Laryngoscope 1990; 100: 1100–5.

70. Steiner W. Results of curative laser microsurgery of laryngeal carcinomas. American Journal of Otolaryngology 1993; 14: 209–17.

71. Csanády M, Czigner J, Sávay L. Endolaryngeal CO$_2$ laser microsurgery of early vocal cord cancer. A retrospective study. Advances in Otorhinolaryngology 1995; 49: 219–21.

72. Eckel HE. Local recurrences following transoral laser surgery for early glottic carcinoma: frequency, management and outcome. Annals of Otology, Rhinology and Laryngology 2001; 110: 7–15.

73. Pradhan SA, Pai PS, Neeli SI, D'Cruz AK. Transoral laser surgery for early glottic cancers. Archives of Otolaryngology – Head and Neck Surgery 2003; 129: 623–5.

74. Peretti G, Piazza C, Bolzoni A et al. Analysis of recurrences in 322 Tis, T1 or T2 glottic carcinomas treated by carbon dioxide laser. Annals of Otology, Rhinology, and Laryngology 2004; 113: 853–8.

75. Steiner W, Vogt P, Ambrosch P, Kron M. Transoral carbon dioxide laser microsurgery for recurrent glottic carcinoma after radiotherapy. Head and Neck 2004; 26: 477–84.

76. Motta G, Esposito E, Testa D et al. CO$_2$ laser treatment of supraglottic cancer. Head and Neck 2004; 26: 442–6.

77. Motta G, Esposito E, Motta S et al. CO$_2$ laser surgery in the treatment of glottic cancer. Head and Neck 2005; 27: 566–73.

78. Ansarin M, Zabrodsky M, Bianchi L et al. Endoscopic CO$_2$ laser surgery for early glottic cancer in patients who are candidates for radiotherapy: Results of a prospective nonrandomized study. Head and Neck 2006; 28: 121–5.

79. Steiner W, Ambrosch P, Rodel RM, Kron M. Impact of anterior commissure involvement on local control of early glottic carcinoma treated by laser microresection. Laryngoscope 2004; 114: 1485–91.

80. Ledda GP, Puxeddu R. Carbon dioxide laser microsurgery for early glottic carcinoma. Otolaryngology – Head and Neck Surgery 2006; 134: 911–15.

81. Shah JP, Loree TR, Kowalski L. Conservation surgery for radiation failure carcinoma of the glottic larynx. Head and Neck 1990; 12: 326–31.

82. McLaughlin MP, Parsons JT, Fein DA et al. Salvage surgery after radiotherapy failure in T1–T2 squamous cell carcinoma of the glottic larynx. Head and Neck 1996; 18: 229–35.

83. Lydiatt WM, Shah JP, Lydiatt KM. Conservation surgery for recurrent carcinoma of the glottic larynx. American Journal of Surgery 1996; 172: 662–4.

84. Lavey RS, Calcaterra TC. Partial laryngectomy for glottic cancer after high-dose radiotherapy. American Journal of Surgery 1991; 162: 341–4.

85. DelGaudio JM, Fleming DJ, Esclamado RM. Hemilaryngectomy for glottic carcinoma after radiation therapy failure. Head and Neck 1994; 120: 959–63.

86. Watters GWR, Patel SG, Rhys-Evans PH. Partial laryngectomy for recurrent laryngeal carcinoma. Clinical Otolaryngology 2000; 25: 146–52.

87. Makeieff M, Venegoni D, Mercante G et al. Supracricoid partial laryngectomies after failure of radiation therapy. Laryngoscope 2005; 115: 353–7.

88. Sewnaik A, Meeuwis CA, Van der Kwast TH, Kerrebijn JD. Partial laryngectomy for recurrent glottic carcinoma after radiotherapy. Head and Neck 2005; 27: 101–7.

89. Ganly I, Patel SG, Matsuo J et al. Results of surgical salvage after failure of definitive radiation therapy for early-stage squamous cell carcinoma of the glottic larynx. Archives of Otolaryngology – Head and Neck Surgery 2006; 132: 59–66.

90. Nichols RD, Mickelson SA. Partial laryngectomy after irradiation failure. Annals of Otology, Rhinology, and Laryngology 1991; 100: 176–80.

91. Spriano G, Pellini R, Romano G et al. Supracricoid partial laryngectomy as salvage surgery after radiation failure. Head and Neck 2002; 24: 759–65.

92. Lefebvre JL, Chevalier D, Luboinski B et al. Larynx preservation in pyriform sinus cancer: preliminary results of a European Organization for Research and Treatment of Cancer phase III trial. Journal of the National Cancer Institute 1996; 34: 890–9.

93. Steiner W, Ambrosch P, Hess CF, Kron M. Organ preservation by transoral laser microsurgery in piriform sinus carcinoma. Otolaryngology – Head and Neck Surgery 2001; 124: 58–67.

94. Vilaseca I, Blanch JL, Bernal-Sprekelsen M, Moragas M. CO$_2$ laser surgery: a larynx preservation alternative for selected hypopharyngeal carcinomas. Head and Neck 2004; 26: 953–9.

95. Brown JS, Browne RM. Factors influencing the patterns of invasion of the mandible by oral squamous cell carcinoma. International Journal of Oral and Maxillofacial Surgery 1995; 24: 417–26.

96. McGregor AD, MacDonald DG. Patterns of spread of squamous cell carcinoma to the ramus of the mandible. Head and Neck 1993; 15: 440–4.

97. McGregor AD, MacDonald DG. Routes of entry of squamous cell carcinoma to the mandible. Head and Neck Surgery 1988; 10: 294–301.

98. Barttelbort SW, Ariyan S. Mandible preservation with oral cavity carcinoma: rim mandibulectomy versus sagittal mandibulectomy. American Journal of Surgery 1993; 166: 411–15.

99. Marchetta FC, Sako K, Murphy JB. The periosteum of the mandible and intraoral carcinoma. American Journal of Surgery 1971; 122: 711–13.

● 100. Spiro RH, Gerold FP, Shah JP *et al.* Mandibulotomy approach to oropharyngeal tumors. *American Journal of Surgery* 1985; **150**: 466–9.

101. Shaha AR. Mandibulotomy and mandibulectomy in difficult tumours of the base of tongue and oropharynx. *Seminars in Surgical Oncology* 1991; **7**: 25–30.

102. Dubner S, Spiro RH. Median mandibulotomy: a critical assessment. *Head and Neck* 1991; **13**: 389–93.

103. Sullivan PK, Fabian R, Driscoll D. Mandibular osteotomies for tumor extirpation: the advantages of rigid fixation. *Laryngoscope* 1992; **102**: 73–80.

● 104. Steiner W, Fierek O, Ambrosch P *et al.* Transoral laser microsurgery for squamous cell carcinoma of the base of the tongue. *Archives of Otolaryngology – Head and Neck Surgery* 2003; **129**: 36–43.

● 105. O'Malley BW Jr, Weinstein GS, Snyder W, Hockstein NG. Transoral robotic surgery (TORS) for base of tongue neoplasms. *Laryngoscope* 2006; **116**: 1465–72.

● 106. Ganly I, Patel S, Singh B *et al.* Complications of craniofacial resection for malignant skull base tumors. Report of an International Collaborative Study. *Head and Neck* 2005; **27**: 445–51.

◆ 107. Karkos PD, Fyrmpas G, Carrie SC, Swift AC. Endoscopic versus open surgical interventions for inverted nasal papilloma: a systematic review. *Clinical Otolaryngology* 2006; **31**: 499–503.

108. Minovi A, Kollert M, Draf W, Bockmuhl U. Inverted papilloma: feasibility of endonasal surgery and long-term results of 87 cases. *Rhinology* 2006; **44**: 205–10.

109. Busquets JM, Hwang PH. Endoscopic resection of sinonasal inverted papilloma: a meta-analysis. *Otolaryngology – Head and Neck Surgery* 2006; **134**: 476–82.

● 110. Wolfe SG, Schlosser RJ, Bolger WE *et al.* Endoscopic and endoscope-assisted resections of inverted sinonasal papillomas. *Otolaryngology – Head and Neck Surgery* 2004; **131**: 174–9.

111. Wormald PJ, Ooi E, van Hasselt CA, Nair S. Endoscopic removal of sinonasal inverted papilloma including endoscopic medial maxillectomy. *Laryngoscope* 2003; **113**: 867–73.

112. Carrau RL, Snyderman CH, Kassam AB, Jungreis CA. Endoscopic and endoscopic-assisted surgery for juvenile angiofibroma. *Laryngoscope* 2001; **111**: 483–7.

113. Fagan JJ, Snyderman CH, Carrau RL, Janecka IP. Nasopharyngeal angiofibromas: selecting a surgical approach. *Head and Neck* 1997; **19**: 391–9.

● 114. Hofmann T, Bernal-Sprekelsen M, Koele W *et al.* Endoscopic resection of juvenile angiofibromas – long term results. *Rhinology* 2005; **43**: 282–9.

◆ 115. Mann WJ, Jecker P, Amedee RG. Juvenile angiofibromas: changing surgical concept over the last 20 years. *Laryngoscope* 2004; **114**: 291–3.

116. Kelley RT, Smith JL 2nd, Rodzewicz GM. Transnasal endoscopic surgery of the pituitary: modifications and results over 10 years. *Laryngoscope* 2006; **116**: 1573–6.

◆ 117. Sethi DS, Leong JL. Endoscopic pituitary surgery. *Otolaryngologic Clinics of North America* 2006; **39**: 563–83.

● 118. Patel SG, Singh B, Polluri A *et al.* Craniofacial surgery for malignant skull base tumors. *Cancer* 2003; **98**: 1179–87.

● 119. Jackson IT, Adham MN, March WR. Use of galeal frontalis myofacial flap in craniofacial surgery. *Plastic and Reconstructive Surgery* 1986; **77**: 905–10.

120. Snyderman CH, Janecka IP, Sekhar LN *et al.* Anterior cranial base reconstruction: role of galeal and pericranial flaps. *Laryngoscope* 1990; **100**: 60–64.

121. Kassam A, Snyderman CH, Mintz A *et al.* Expanded endonasal approach: the rostrocaudal axis. Part I. Crista galli to the sella turcica. *Neurosurgery Focus* 2005; **19**: E3.

● 122. Lam KH, Wei WI, Ho HC, Ho CM. Whole organ sectioning of mixed parotid tumors. *American Journal of Surgery* 1990; **160**: 377–81.

123. Clairmont AA, Richardson GS, Hanna DC. The pseudocapsule of pleomorphic adenomas (benign mixed tumors): the argument against enucleation. *American Journal of Surgery* 1977; **134**: 242–3.

124. Laskawi R, Schott T, Schroder M. Recurrent pleomorphic adenomas of the parotid gland: clinical evaluation and long term follow-up. *British Journal of Oral and Maxillofacial Surgery* 1998; **36**: 48–51.

● 125. Heller KS, Attie JN. Treatment of Warthin's tumor by enucleation. *American Journal of Surgery* 1988; **156**: 294–6.

● 126. Armstrong JG, Harrison LB, Spiro RH *et al.* Malignant tumors of major salivary gland origin: a matched pair analysis of the role of combined surgery and postoperative radiotherapy. *Archives of Otolaryngology – Head and Neck Surgery* 1990; **116**: 290–3.

9

Measures of treatment outcomes

JANET A WILSON AND HELEN COCKS

There are two ways to live your life, one is as though nothing is a miracle, the other is as though everything is a miracle.

Albert Einstein

INTRODUCTION

Health-care resources are rationed throughout the world. All clinicians therefore share a responsibility to ensure that their treatment is effective and efficient. Efficacy implies that a treatment actually achieves what it sets out to do, for example, cure a given proportion of patients of their disease. Efficiency incorporates concepts of cost efficiency, that is to say could the resources be obtained more cheaply? The costs include not only the health-care resources required to provide the treatment, but also the costs to the patient in terms of treatment-related morbidity – and the resultant cost of not treating another condition because of the expenditure.[1] Modern health-care systems demand robust outcome measures. These should be disease specific and reflect the concerns of the patient. Their measurement is compounded by the fact that patients and carers, as well as patients and healthy 'observers', have different opinions as to what constitutes the most favourable outcome.[2]

The traditional end point for assessing outcomes of treatment of patients with head and neck cancer (HNC) – survival, local and regional disease control have been expanded in recent years to include measurements of functional status and quality of life (QOL). This chapter will address functional outcome as opposed to QOL per se, to which Chapter 10, Quality of life, is devoted.

MORTALITY

For most cancers, the reporting of mortality remains the cornerstone of outcomes assessment (**Box 9.1**). Nonetheless, despite the many advances in the method of cancer treatments, it must be accepted that there are many cancers, including most head and neck cancers, where these treatment developments have not been mirrored by changes in mortality rates which have remained static over the last three or four decades. It is important, however, not to let a lack of improvement in mortality obscure the value of a genuine therapeutic advance. For example, modern techniques of head and neck resection with skillful reconstruction often result in a far superior cosmetic and functional outcome and quality of life, even if the cure rate is no greater than with older, more morbid procedures. It is also important to monitor mortality rates of those patients receiving the relatively recently introduced organ preservation treatments.

SURVIVAL ANALYSIS

Survival analysis is a technique for analysing 'time to event' and can be used for many outcomes not simply death (**Box 9.2**). Problems with survival analysis are the

---

Box 9.1   Advantages and disadvantages of death as an outcome

Advantages

- It is undeniably the most important outcome to both doctor and patient
- There are only two categories: alive or dead
- The distinction cannot be fudged

Disadvantages

- Insensitive in diseases with low mortality
- Usually delay before manifest
- Inaccuracies in recording the cause of death
- Disregards functional outcome/quality of life

Box 9.3   Instruments to assess comorbidity

Self-reporting

- Charlson-based
- Cardiopulmonary Comorbidity Index
- Seattle index of comorbidity
- American Society of Anesthesiologists (ASA) Risk Classification

Notes review

- Kaplan–Feinstein Index (KFI)
- Adult Comorbidity Evaluation (ACE-27)
- Charlson Comorbidity Index (CCI)
- Index of Coexistent Disease (ICED)

Box 9.2   Survival analysis

- Disease-specific survival
- Actuarial survival
- Median survival time
- Kaplan–Meier survival curve
- Log rank test

---

non-parametric distribution of the data and the fact that the time to event is not always observed, it is not appropriate to wait for all patients in the study to die. Also, a number of patients may be lost to follow up, termed 'censored events'. The Kaplan–Meier survival curve is the most common means of expressing survival in a study group.[3] It is used to estimate survival rates and hazards from such incomplete data assuming that those censored subjects have the same prospect of survival as uncensored subjects. The median survival time is the survival time at which the cumulative survival is equal to 0.5.

The log rank test provides methods for comparing two or more survival curves, but is only appropriate where relative mortality does not change over time (proportional hazards assumption).

COMORBIDITY

Comorbidity refers to disease that coexists with and is unrelated to the index disease and has been shown to play a major role in the treatment, outcome and prognosis of a number of malignancies. There is significant comorbidity in head and neck cancer patients due to the long-term effects of smoking and alcohol lying second only to lung or colorectal cancer. Several studies have shown the importance of comorbidity on outcome and the prognosis of head and neck cancer.[4, 5, 6, 7, 8] It is an independent prognostic indicator even when age and TNM stage have been controlled for, hence its inclusion here.[5]

In 1948, the first attempt to quantify the performance status of patients with advanced cancer was made by

Karnofsky.[9] Since then, there has followed the evolution of a variety of instruments to measure comorbidity (**Box 9.3**). Information can be obtained from patient questionnaires, patient-based interviews and from reviewing the medical notes. The most widely used are discussed below.

Kaplan–Feinstein index

The Kaplan–Feinstein index (KFI) was developed for assessment of comorbidity on outcome in diabetes mellitus and has been used to study the impact of comorbidity in several cancers.[10] Specific diseases are classified and a score given of mild, moderate or severe according to severity of organ decompensation. Where multiple comorbities are present, an overall score is assigned according to the highest ranked illness, and where there are two or more moderate outcomes the overall score is defined as severe.

Adult comorbidity evaluation

Adult comorbidity evaluation (ACE-27)[5] is a modification of the KFI, validated and especially designed for comorbidity evaluation in patients with cancer. It includes conditions such as diabetes, dementia and AIDS, which were not included in the original KFI. An overall score of 1, 2 or 3 is assigned according to the highest ranked single condition, except where two or more grade 2 illnesses occur in different organ systems where a score of 3 is given.

Charlson comorbidity index

The Charlson comorbidity index (CCI)[11] is a weighted sum of the presence or absence of each of 19 conditions. Each condition is assigned a weight from 1 to 6, where a higher value indicates more severe disease. The index is the sum of all the weights.

Most data on comorbidity in head and neck cancer relate to use of one of these three indices. The KFI has been found to be most successful in stratification of survival analysis in patients with squamous cell cancer of the head and neck

Table 9.1 Advantages and disadvantages of patient-based and case-review approaches.

	Advantages	Disadvantages
Patient-based approach	Functional impact of disease more accurate	Patients may have limited insight into illnesses Can only be obtained prospectively
Case-review approach	Allows for both prospective and retrospective evaluation More accurate	Severity of comorbidity may be difficult to determine Only positive comorbidities may be documented Time required to review notes

when compared with the Charlson index, and two other scales not discussed here, the cumulative rating scale and the index of co-existent disease.[12] The CCI is simple to use and has been used to evaluate comorbidity in laryngeal cancer[13] and thyroid cancer,[14] and has been validated against the ACE-27 for use in head and neck cancer.[15] However, because answers evaluate the presence or absence of disease rather than severity, it has been found to be less sensitive than the ACE-27 in assessing comorbidity.[16, 17]

The ACE-27 has been widely used in the head and neck cancer population and is applicable in the UK setting.[17] It can be used to grade comorbidity retrospectively from case notes showing reliability and good interrater agreement. Some comorbidity items on the ACE-27, such as adrenal disease and pancreatitis, are not routinely asked about and may be missed from case note review. In addition, severity of symptoms may also be lacking from the patient record (**Table 9.1**).[16] The use of operative pre-assessment enhances data capture, but only for surgical patients.

The use of the ACE-27 has shown the correlation of comorbidity grade with morbidity and mortality following surgery for all head and neck cancer patients.[18] One study looking at patients undergoing major surgery in the oral cavity or oropharynx with microvascular soft tissue reconstruction showed moderate to severe comorbidity associated with a much higher major complication rate (55 per cent compared with 4 per cent in patients with no or mild comorbidity scores).[19] The ACE-27 has also been used to show comparative comorbidity – patients with supraglottic cancer have a higher comorbidity burden compared with those with glottic tumours, which might in part account for their poorer prognosis.[20]

Overall, comorbidity data add valuable prognostic information that may influence treatment modality. Use of single sources alone may result in some misclassification of comorbidity. Enhancing data extracted from notes with a patient self-report questionnaire can improve the accuracy of comorbidity grading.[21]

Collection of comorbidity data using the ACE-27 is part of the data set for the Database for Head and Neck Oncology (DAHNO). Some units are enhancing this information with a patient questionnaire.

PATIENT PRIORITIES FOR TREATMENT OUTCOMES

An early classic paper on the cost utility analysis of the treatment of advanced laryngeal cancer by radiotherapy and laryngectomy presented a trade off of quality of life (retention of laryngeal speech) versus quantity of life (improved survival after primary laryngectomy) to a group of healthy (non-medical) volunteers. In order to maintain natural speech, approximately 20 per cent of those questioned would have chosen radiation instead of surgery.[22] This paper was innovative and influential in suggesting that for some people quality, not quantity, of life was more important. In a later paper by De Santo et al.,[23] 20 per cent of patients expressed themselves willing to accept a reduced lifespan in order to preserve their larynx and quality of life. In contrast, 46 per cent of the health-care professionals questioned had felt that the patients would accept this trade off. A recent study published by List et al.[24] showed that both patients and non-patients ranked 'being cured of cancer', 'living as long as possible' and 'having no pain' most frequently in the top three of 12 statements.[24]

There are also differences in the perception of the relative importance of different categories of symptom between patients and carers. In 1992, Mohide et al.[2] demonstrated that carers ranked impaired communication and self-image/self-esteem as the two most important QOL outcome domains following laryngectomy. The patients themselves ranked the physical symptoms of tracheal mucus production and interference with social activities as the two most important items. It is important to bear this lack of correlation between patient and carer priorities in mind when counselling patients about treatment options.

IMPACT OF HEAD AND NECK CANCER ON OUTCOME

Treatment for head and neck cancer is likely to affect some of the most basic human functions – verbal communication, social interaction, eating and breathing. Traditional treatment for many advanced head and neck cancers has been surgical excision with or without adjuvant radiotherapy. It is easy to see how speech and swallowing can be affected in patients undergoing resection for large oral cavity or oropharyngeal lesions and in the most extreme case of the laryngectomee. Recently, much emphasis has been placed on organ preservation by the use of combined modality chemoradiotherapy showing approximately the same long-term survival as surgery and adjuvant radiotherapy.[25] Therefore, the clinical trade off is no longer the length of life, but functional outcome and quality of life. Anatomic preservation does not guarantee that function will remain intact; patients experience a number of significant debilitating side effects. Vocal quality is reduced and swallowing problems are common due to the stiffening of tissues in the pharynx and upper oesophagus. A disease-specific quality of life survey covering five domains (speech, eating, aesthetics, pain/discomfort and social/role functioning) demonstrated that speech and eating had the most impact on well-being.[26] It is essential that these outcomes are measured in addition to survival to validate the use of these regimes and so that clinicians can provide patients with evidence and information regarding the potential effects of their treatments.

Impairment, disability and handicap

The World Health Organization has proposed an International Classification of Impairment Disabilities and Handicaps (ICIDH).[27] This was most recently modified in 1997. Most self-assessment questionnaires have been developed with the purpose of measuring psychosocial handicapping effects of voice disorders as referred to by the WHO in their definition of disability and handicap: 'the social, economic or environmental disadvantage resulting from an impairment or disability'.

VOICE AND SPEECH

Outcome measures: the tools available

Choosing the most appropriate outcome measure is essential for the efficacy of any study. Many tools exist for the measurement of outcomes of voice and speech. Most have been developed from a diverse population of dysphonic and dysarthric patients, but are applicable to the study of the head and neck cancer patient (see **Table 9.2**). Some of the most commonly used will be discussed here in more detail.

ASSESSING OUTCOME OF VOICE

In 1989, Hirano[29] identified over 50 techniques being used for the evaluation of voice throughout the world. Still today,

there exists no established voice outcome package. Measurements of voice available that are useful for measuring vocal change over time can broadly be divided into subjective or perceptual measurements and 'objective' or instrumental measurements (although not truly objective because interpretation is required). In addition, recent years have seen the development of tools to measure the functional effects of voice disorders from a patient's perception (self-assessment).

Self-assessment

VOICE HANDICAP INDEX

Voice Handicap Index (VHI)[30] is a standardized, self-assessment scale that measures patient perception of the impact of dysphonia on various aspects of routine living. It was derived retrospectively from symptoms identified from review of written case histories from a seven-year period. Initially, 85 items were identified. These were refined by responses from a group of 65 subjects who presented varied voice pathology, but of whom 84 per cent had either a mass lesion or neurogenic disorder, including 26 per cent laryngectomee patients.

The authors report good internal consistency with good test–retest reliability. They also found that VHI scales correlated well with patients' perceptions of voice disorder severity; however, there is little information on validity of the VHI

The VHI is the most widely used of the self-assessment questionnaires. It consists of 30 statements on voice-related aspects in daily life each with a score of 0 to 4, where 0 stands for never, 1 for almost never, 2 for sometimes, 3 for almost always and 4 for always. The maximum score is therefore 120, values above 60 indicate a severe disability, those between 40 and 60 moderate disability and less than 40 mild or no disability. The questions are divided into three subscales or domains: physical, functional and emotional, with ten questions in each.

The VHI has been used as an outcome assessment tool in laryngeal cancer in both patients with a laryngeal and

Table 9.2   Tools available for the assessment of outcome of voice and speech.

Parameter	Perceptual measures	Instrumental measures
Voice		
Patient rating of function/acceptability	Vocal Handicap Index (VHI)	
	Voice Symptom Score (VoiSS)	
	Vocal Performance Questionnaire (VPQ)	
	Voice Activity and Participation Profile (VAPP)	
Voice quality	GRBAS	Acoustic analysis
		Laryngograph
Laryngeal function	Fibreoptic and stroboscopic profiles	Flow volume loops
Speech		
Speech intelligibility	Speech Intelligibility Test	Spectography
	Assessment of Intelligibility of Dysarthric Speech (ASSIDS)	
Range, strength, accuracy of articulation	Frenchay Dysarthria Assessment	Spectography
		Electropalatography

Adapted from Ref. 28

alaryngeal voice, but overall there is a paucity of outcome data of this nature. Several studies have explored post-treatment outcomes for early glottic cancer. A meta-analysis identified six studies between 1966 and 2005 with 208 patients (202 T1a) treated with laser excision and 91 (85 T1a) with external beam radiotherapy, showing VHI scores of the two groups to be similar.[31] In the assessment of laser excision of the T1a larynx, Brondbo et al.[32] reported favourable results showing no impact of voice on daily life.

In the assessment of voice following partial laryngectomy, the VHI has also been used to compare endoscopic laser excision with open resection[33] and in outcome assessment of supracricoid partial laryngectomy.[34, 35]

One study used a modification of the VHI in the assessment of voice in the laryngectomee; they showed that voice handicap severity is moderate in this group of patients and in the range of 'common' dysphonia.[36] Another showed the VHI to be significantly higher in the laryngectomy than in patients with functional voice disorders, but differing only slightly from patients with organic laryngeal dysphonia.[37]

A study from the Veterans Affairs Group compared the surgically voice-restored laryngectomee and patients undergoing radiotherapy for laryngeal cancer. Physical voice handicap scores did not differ significantly, but emotional and functional handicap scores were higher in the laryngectomee. However, there was considerable diversity of scores for the laryngectomy group, with some scoring less than the radiotherapy group. It is difficult to draw too many conclusions here since laryngectomy patients had more advanced stage disease.[38]

There does not appear to be any data looking at voice outcome in patients treated with chemoradiotherapy as a primary modality, but a recent paper from London's Royal Marsden Hospital showed that in the laryngectomee there was a wide variation in the handicap reported on the VHI with functional aspects of the voice significantly affected by age, radiotherapy and chemotherapy. Physical aspects were significantly affected by age and chemotherapy and only age significantly affected the emotional aspects of the voice.[39]

One study has looked at partner perception of voice handicap using a modification of the VHI. This showed good agreement among all three of the VHI subscales. However, whether these proxy ratings can be extrapolated to the head and neck cancer population is not known.[40]

VOICE SYMPTOM SCALE

The Voice Symptom Scale (VoiSS)[41] is the most rigorously evaluated and psychometrically robust measure currently available for self-assessment of voice quality. Unlike the other voice rating tools available, it is patient derived. It originated in an open-ended questionnaire, resulting in 467 problems reported by 133 consecutive patients with voice disorders from a British non-cancer population.[42] A prototype summary list of all these problems was administered to 168 voice patients and these underwent principal component analysis. Third, a modified 44-item scale was administered to 180 new subjects and with further analysis the final VoiSS 30-item questionnaire was born which was further tested on 319 subjects including a few with malignancy.[43] It has good

reliability. The VoiSS consists of 15 items, eight relating to impairment to emotional response and seven to physical symptoms and is unique in that it addresses other symptoms, which may arise from the laryngopharynx, such as sore throat and phlegm.

The VoiSS has not yet been widely used in the head and neck cancer population, but a study looking at a population of patients treated by endoscopic resection or radiotherapy for early glottic cancer produced similar results for three self-report vocal performance questionnaires – VHI, VoiSS or Voice Performance Questionnaire (VPQ). The exception was the emotional subscale of the VoiSS, which gave better results for those treated with radiotherapy and in addition reflected the concurrent pharyngeal symptoms.[44]

VOICE ACTIVITY AND PARTICIPATION PROFILE

Voice Activity and Participation Profile (VAPP)[45] was developed in Hong Kong and was developed as a means to investigate perception of voice problem, activity limitation and participation restriction. Initial items were selected by consultation with 45 dysphonic patients and ten speech and language pathologists, resulting in a 28-item questionnaire consisting of five sections: self-perception of voice (one item), effect on job (four items), effect on daily communication (12 items), effect on social communication (four items) and effect on emotion (seven items). Each item uses a visual analogue scale 10 cm long ranging from not affected at the left end to always affected at the right. This was then tested on 40 further dysphonic patients with benign disease and 40 controls. This study showed good internal consistency and test–retest reliability and good correlation with the VHI. The authors also compute an activity limitation score and a participation restriction score, which seems to have been fairly arbitrarily assigned.

Short-form self-assessment questionnaires

Both the VHI and the VoiSS are 30-point questionnaires and can be time consuming to complete and score and may provide a degree of redundant information. Although these are extremely useful as research tools, in the clinical setting concise, clinically useful self-report questionnaires are of more use. Two short-form, voice-related scales have been reported, the Vocal Handicap Index-10 item questionnaire (VHI-10) and the Vocal Performance Questionnaire (VPQ).

VOCAL HANDICAP INDEX-10 ITEM QUESTIONNAIRE

Item analysis carried out on the VHI by patients with voice disorders and controls identified the ten most robust VHI items resulting in the creation of the Vocal Handicap Index-10 item questionnaire (VHI-10).[46] Statistical analysis comparing validity with the VHI on a large number of patients with a wide spectrum of voice disorders showed good correlation. As for the VHI, a five-point item scale is used, resulting in a total score of between 0 and 40.

VOCAL PERFORMANCE QUESTIONNAIRE

The VPQ[47] was designed for evaluation of voice therapy in non-organic dysphonia. It is a 12-item questionnaire which examines the physical symptoms and socioeconomic impact of the voice disorder. The patient selects a statement that best answers each question. The statements are graded in terms of severity of vocal performance. A numerical score of 1–5 is assigned to each answer and these are summed to provide an overall score of vocal severity – maximum score 60 and minimum score 12.

These two short-form voice-related scales (VPQ and VHI-10) use a single total score. This has been found to be valid and there is high internal consistency. In addition, the two questionnaires correlate highly with one another.[48]

PERCEPTUAL ASSESSMENT: CLINICIAN RATED

GRBAS

The GRBAS rating scheme[49] is considered as a practical minimum standard for the perceptual rating of voice.[50, 51] It has established inter- and intrarater reliability with trained expert raters.[52] It consists of five domains: grade (representing overall voice quality), roughness (which looks at fluctuations in fundamental frequency, indicative of vocal edge abnormalities), breathiness (which assesses air escape), asthenia (a general decrease in power of or weakness of the voice) and strain (which assesses hyperfunctionality). All are assessments of laryngeal function.

Assessment is made on a recording of a voice reading an established phonetically balanced passage, such as the 'rainbow passage' or on current conversational speech. Each aspect of the GRBAS scale is given a score of 0–3, where 0 is normal, 1 shows slight deviance, 2 moderate deviance and 3 severe deviance. This scale has been shown to be reliable across all parameters except strain.[53]

Patients' self-assessment using the GRBAS scale has been evaluated and patients appear to have good validity and consistency using the scale as a self-assessment tool, however, correlation with clinician assessment is poor.[54]

Correlation between self-assessment using the VHI and clinician-rated perceptual data using the GRBAS has also shown little correlation, with patients indicating only mild functional and emotional consequences, but GRBAS scores showed severely dysphonic voice with supracricoid laryngectomy VHI mean values of 29.9.[34]

The GRBAS scale has been used in the assessment of voice in the head and neck cancer population, in partial laryngeal surgery and in the comparison of radiotherapy and laser excision in the treatment of early glottic lesions. Interestingly, it has also been used as a tool to assess alaryngeal speech.[55, 56] It has not been developed for or validated in this group of highly specialized patients and whether it really is of clinical use is questionable.

PERCEPTUAL ASSESSMENT OF ALARYNGEAL SPEECH

Although attempts have been made to develop a scale for perceptual evaluation of alaryngeal speech, a reliable, reproducible perceptual rating system developed for assessment of voice in the laryngectomee does not seem to exist.

Van As *et al.*[57] report the use of a semantic bipolar seven-point scale (e.g. ugly–beautiful, deviant–normal, low–high), for both untrained and trained raters, initially consisting of 19 or 20 items. They describe wide ranging inter- and intra-rater reliability, (e.g. better for deviant–normal than creaky–not creaky) and overall better for trained listeners. Finally, they attempt to reduce the number of items into subsets representing underlying perceptual dimensions – quality and pitch for untrained listeners and quality, tonicity, pitch and tempo for trained listeners. However, this scale has not been used subsequently.

Eadie and Doyle[58, 59, 60] report the use of direct magnitude estimation (continuous) and equally appearing interval (interval) scales for the auditory perceptual rating of naturalness, severity, acceptability and pleasantness of tracheo-oesophageal voice. When rated by naive listeners, they have found that female voice is considered less acceptable and natural when gender is known and not correctly identified when gender is not known.

Instrumental measures

A large number of instrumental voice measurements can be used to diagnose and determine the extent of disease and evaluate nature and severity of dysphonia. Only a few are useful in measuring changes in voice quality with time, and most have little use in the assessment of outcome in the head and neck cancer patient, although measurements may help with targeting rehabilitation. Discussed here are a few of the more common and potentially more useful measures.

MAXIMAL PHONATION TIME

Maximal phonation time (MPT) is the time for the production of a prolonged /a/, for as long as possible after maximal inspiration at a spontaneous comfortable pitch and loudness measured in seconds. Generally, three measurements are made and the longest taken.

FLOW VOLUME LOOPS

These are sensitive tests of upper airway flow and are useful where problems are associated with laryngeal or tracheal obstruction. They are obtained with forced inspiration and expiration.

ACOUSTIC MEASURES OF SPEECH SIGNAL

Acoustic analysis is widely used in testing vocal function because it is objective and reproducible, as long as the same equipment is used on each occasion. A prerequisite is a voice sample recorded on to digital audiotape (DAT). Standard protocols exist from the National Centre for Voice and Speech for the recording of speech samples.

From these recordings, acoustic measurements of the speech signal can be made, including frequency, amplitude, jitter (pertubation/stability of pitch), shimmer (pertubation/stability of amplitude), and noise to harmonic ratio.

The main use of acoustic measurements in the literature of head and neck cancer patients has been to compare outcomes for treatments for early glottic tumours,[61, 62] in the assessment of voice after supracricoid laryngectomy[34] and in the assessment of speech therapy following treatment for such lesions.[63] These measurements have also been assessed in the laryngectomy group of patients. Measurements of jitter and shimmer require a speech signal near to periodicity to allow the software to produce any measure of cycle-to-cycle variation. In the laryngectomy voice is often aperiodic, making assessment of these acoustic measures problematic; Van As-Brooks et al.[64] describe the use of visual inspection of narrow-band spectrogram to enhance acoustic measures in the laryngectomee.

SPEECH

Speech sounds are produced by regulating air flow from the lungs. The role of the oral cavity is in articulation, oronasal separation and resonance. The utterance of most consonants requires the closing off of the nose and articulation relies on movements of the tongue, pharynx, palate, lip and jaw. Consequently, many speech disorders result from treatment for oral cavity, oropharynx and maxillofacial tumours.[65] These can be divided into those due to inadequate oronasal separation and articulation disorders. Speech and language therapists are highly trained in listening and identifying abnormalities in speech and are best placed to assess hyper- and hyponasality.

Articulation is usually evaluated by intelligibility tests, the most significant measure of speech being how well it is understood. Analysis of articulation can determine the source of speech disorder, regardless of the language in which the test is carried out. Because of this, most scales for assessment of speech are clinician-rated, rather than self-assessment tools.

Self-assessment tools

THE FUNCTIONAL INTRAORAL GLASGOW SCALE

This is a self-assessment tool described by one group used to study 196 patients undergoing surgery for oral cavity cancer. It consists of an ordinal five-grade scale: always understandable (5), needing repetition sometimes (4), needing repetition many times (3), understandable only by relatives (2), incomprehensible (1). This very simple scale showed good correlation with a conversational understandability test performed by speech and language therapists and with an objective computer-based method of speech analysis.[66]

Clinician-rated tools

A vast array of clinician-rated intelligibility tests exist and are naturally language specific; in practice, they are the domain of the expert speech and language therapist.

SPEECH INTELLIGIBILITY TEST

The simplest measure seems to be the Speech Intelligibility Test.[67] Patients are required to read a phonetically selected passage, the rainbow passage, which is recorded. These recordings are graded by experienced listeners according to the number of words written correctly by the listeners.

ASSESSMENT OF INTELLIGIBILITY OF DYSARTHRIC SPEECH

The Assessment of Intelligibility of Dysarthric Speech (ASSIDS)[68] is used by the speech and language therapist and contains assessment of single word and sentence intelligibility. It requires a recording of either 50 single words or sentences of 5–15 words selected at random. Each sample is judged by a pool of scorers (one scorer can be used if improvement is being sought in an individual patient). The recording is listened to and transcribed by the scorer and an intelligibility score given as a percentage of responses that were correct. In addition to percentage intelligibility, scores can be calculated for speaking rate, rate of (un)intelligible speech and a communication efficiency ratio. These calculations are based on a healthy person speaking a 220-word paragraph at a rate of 190 words per minute.

Scales designed specifically for the head and neck patient population

There are a couple of tools that have been specifically designed for the assessment of the head and neck cancer patient.

PERFORMANCE STATUS SCALE FOR HEAD AND NECK CANCER PATIENTS

The Performance Status Scale for Head and Neck (PSSHN)[69] is designed to assess unique areas of dysfunction experienced by this group of patients. It has three domains: (1) understanding of speech, (2) normalcy of diet and (3) eating in public. There is a score from 0 to 100 for each domain. The higher the score, the better the ability of the patient to function.

VOICE PROSTHESIS QUESTIONNAIRE

The Voice Prosthesis Questionnaire[70] looks specifically at the surgically voice-restored laryngectomy. It has recently been published and shows good reliability and validity and is the first designed specifically for the valved laryngectomy patient. It is a self-administered 45-point questionnaire and has sections relating to speech, leakage, valve changing, maintenance, QOL, humidification and hand free issues.

DYSPHAGIA

Introduction

Dysphagia has always been an important functional outcome of the treatment of larger head and neck cancer tumours.[71]

Over the past few years, it has become increasingly apparent that non-surgical therapy while organ sparing, may not be so sparing of function, particularly swallow competency. There seems reasonably convincing evidence of a direct relationship between total radiation dose and severity of dysphagia. In one early study, a substantial majority of patients receiving more than 74 Gy were still gastrostomy dependent at 12 months compared with fewer than the one in five who had received only 60 Gy.[72] Conversely, larger doses of ionizing radiation and/or chemotherapy are equally likely to improve overall survival rates. Thus, there is increasing hope that more precisely distributed radiation might prove 'dysphagia sparing'. Intensity modulated radiotherapy (IMRT) remains under assessment in this respect. IMRT has been shown to preserve salivary function and hence reduce the distressing xerostomia which remains a substantial factor contributing to dysphagia in many patients treated non-surgically.[73] The ability of IMRT schedules to reduce aspiration remains more controversial. One study suggests that sparing of the pharyngeal constrictors significantly improves swallow competency.[74]

The impact of swallow dysfunction in head and neck cancer patients may be considered under three principal headings:

1. Aspiration and recurring pulmonary infection
2. Poor nutritional status with secondary impact on healing and probably prognosis
3. Quality of life issues around resumption of what is one of the most fundamental of human and human social activities – the ability to eat a meal.

Nonetheless, we lack sufficient high quality research.[75]

Dysphagia assessments fall broadly into two categories: those that assess the severity of the swallowing disorder and those which try to establish its cause. In head and neck cancer patients, issues of causation generally relate to the biomechanics of the altered swallow mechanism, whether sensory or motor.

A management challenge experienced by most head and neck cancer centres is that dysphagia tends to be a long-lasting problem, persisting for many months after treatment and therefore for considerable periods of time following patient discharge from hospital. Given the relative rarity and heterogeneous nature of head and neck cancers, it is likely that many patients do not find community services adequate for their assessment and therapy needs. Radiological evidence suggests that the biomechanics of persistent post-chemoradiotherapy dysphagia are centred on reduced laryngeal elevation and cricopharyngeal opening.[76] At a median follow up of 26 months following treatment, one disease-free cohort were found to have established normal swallowing in fewer than 10 per cent of patients. Twenty per cent suffered from increasing dysphagia, although others responded to dilatation of pharyngeal stenosis.[77]

In the longer term, surrogate measures of swallow performance, such as nutritional status and method of intake, whether oral, partial oral or total reliance on tube feeding are valuable, albeit relatively insensitive, indicators. Recently, more interest has been focused on the longer-term dysphagia impact on patient and carer psychological well-being.[78]

Swallowing remains one of the most complex, partially reflex phenomena in the human body and its vulnerability in

Box 9.4   Requirements for efficient swallowing

- Facial tone
- Rotatory and lateral movement of mandible
- Fine motor control tongue
- Adequate saliva
- Sensate oral mucosa
- Pharyngo-oesophageal wave
- Competent, mobile larynx

the face of anatomical and physiological changes is perhaps therefore not surprising. The many requirements for a competent swallow are shown in **Box 9.4**.

Equally, there are numerous specific causes for head and neck cancer dysphagia, but these can be grouped as follows.

Major causes of dysphagia in head and neck cancer patients

Xerostomia is recognized as one of the most unpleasant side effects of radiotherapy and has been the subject of considerable research over the years.[79] More recently, attempts have been made to assess the functional impact of tongue dysfunction. Impairment of tongue base movement disables the tongue base thrust, which forms the key to bolus propulsion during the normal swallow. Food accumulates in the hypopharynx, resulting in overspill and aspiration. Tongue strengthening exercises have therefore been developed to reduce this side effect.[80] Silicone strain gauge tongue pressure measuring devices have been developed to pursue tongue power over time. The research requires further development, but at present it has been shown that a fixed position array of sensors is a more reliable assessment method of tongue function.[81]

Because of the life-threatening potential of aspiration, it remains the focus of much assessment, intervention and research.[82] One chemoradiotherapy study demonstrated a 59 per cent incidence of aspiration, with a 9 per cent fatality rate.[83] Swallowing therapy does improve certain grades of aspiration, but the most severe categories of aspiration show a disappointing response. More conspicuous is the development of a pharyngo-oesophageal stricture following non-surgical therapy due to a combination of severe mucositis and scarring of the fibromuscular wall of the pharynx.[84] Dilatation does improve swallow performance in the presence of such a stricture, but a majority of stricture patients require permanent gastrostomy feeding.[85]

The most simple assessments are direct bedside clinical assessments. The dysphagia parameters were originally established by John and Enderby.[86] The therapy outcome measure categories are fairly broad, and acceptably reliable after a short period of training.

Attempts have been made to define swallow performance (**Table 9.3**) in terms of the volume and speed of the swallow mechanism, although conventionally such quantitative swallow performance measures at the bedside have tended to

Table 9.3 Swallowing assessments.

Assessment	References
Direct	
Specialist clinical assessment	Nathadwarawala et al.[87]
Evan's blue dye test	Winklmaier et al.[88]
Videofluoroscopy, including OPSE	Logemann et al.[89]
Functional Endoscopic Evaluation of Swallowing	Bastian[90] and Aviv et al.[91]
Electromyography	Crary et al.[92] and Carnaby-Mann and Crary[93]
Observer-rated questionnaire	
Performance Status Scale for Head and Neck	List et al.[69]
Therapy Outcome Measures	John and Enderby[86]
Self-report questionnaires	
MD Anderson Dysphagia Inventory (MDADI)	Kulbersh et al.[94]
University of Washington QoL (UW-QOL)	Lovell et al.[95]
Swal-QOL	McHorney et al.[96]
Indirect	
Nutritional status/route of feeding	Lees[97] and Oates et al.[98]
Patient/partner distress/general quality of life	Verdonck de-Leeuw et al.[78] and Rogers et al.[99]

be applied more in neurological rather than head and neck cancer patients.[87] One advantage of bedside assessment is that it provides personal contact with the patient. As with other direct assessments, it has the added benefit of being able to address severity, causation and to some extent possible therapeutic manoeuvres.

Traditionally, patients aspirating more than around 10 per cent of any bolus should be restricted from taking the relevant consistency orally. More recent advice, however, suggests a more pragmatic approach may be appropriate, allowing clinicians to incorporate other parameters, such as age, oral health, reflux and cough reflex. Up to 30 per cent of chemotherapy patients being tube fed rather than being fed by gastrostomy may aspirate.[100]

Evans blue dye test can be added to the bedside assessment in patients with suspected fistula or with a tracheostomy. The test has undergone recent studies to evaluate its sensitivity and specificity in predicting aspiration. Comparison of the modified Evans blue dye test with check endoscopy via a tracheostomy site in an acute rehabilitation hospital demonstrated an overall false-negative rate of 50 per cent. However, a superior sensitivity – 82 per cent – was demonstrated in a subsequent survey of long-term tracheotomized patients.[101] A further extension of clinical assessment is to perform a direct instrumental observation, i.e. functional endoscopic evaluation of swallowing. This can be used in isolation or in conjunction with the blue dye test to detect more subtle levels of aspiration that may not otherwise be detectable.

VIDEOFLUOROSCOPY

Videofluoroscopy remains the most frequently applied assessment of complex swallow problems as it allows assessment of anatomy (although to a lesser extent than direct endoscopic observation, see below under Functional endoscopic evaluation of swallowing), coordination in movements

of the oropharyngeal and oesophageal stages of swallowing and it is therefore a very helpful tool in assessing dysphagia of unknown origin.[102, 103] However, videofluoroscopy is a relatively expensive and time-consuming investigation involving transportation of the patient to the radiology department, usually the involvement of a multiprofessional team and with limited opportunities for repeat assessments. Many units provide such a service no more than weekly, some with lesser frequency. In the head and neck cancer patient, a definite distinction cannot be made between cancer, oedema and irradiation fibrosis. Post-surgical reconstruction is more easily assessed by, for example, flexible endoscopy.

As with any swallow assessment, the procedure is not entirely natural. With videofluoroscopy, the substances ingested are not entirely normal foodstuffs. The timing of the swallow has to be directed by the examining clinicians, i.e. the patient is usually required to await the command to swallow. Typically, the volumes involved are considerably smaller than the normal bolus volume. Assessments of the reliability of videofluoroscopy show superior accuracy for aspiration than for determination of pathophysiology. The situation is improved with group discussion. The application of protocols and use of frame-by-frame analysis seems inconsistent.[104, 105, 106]

In the most expert of hands, videofluoroscopy can be applied using timing parameters and also other semi-quantitative estimates of swallow performance. The most usual of these is the oropharyngeal swallow efficiency (OPSE). This is calculated as:

$$\frac{\% \text{ Bolus transfer to upper oesophagus}}{\text{Oropharyngeal transit time}}$$

This composite time–volume estimate of swallow performance has been used in head and neck cancer patients.[107] Interestingly, the lack of recovery of this ratio did not correlate with ongoing dysphagia and nutritional deficit. In other words, it is likely to be too sensitive a test to be of

Table 9.4   Penetration–Aspiration Scale.[108]

Score	Criteria
1	Material does not enter the airway
2	Material enters the airway, remains above the vocal folds, and is ejected from the airway
3	Material enters the airway, remains above the vocal folds and is not ejected from the airway
4	Material enters the airway, contacts the vocal folds and is ejected from the airway
5	Material enters the airway, contacts the vocal folds and is not ejected from the airway
6	Material enters the airway, passes below the vocal folds and is ejected into the larynx or out of the airway
7	Material enters the airway, passes below the vocal folds and is not ejected from the trachea despite effort
8	Material enters the airway, passes below the vocal folds and no effort is made to eject

clinical value in assessing rehabilitation of head and neck cancer patients.

In contrast, the penetration–aspiration scale (**Table 9.4**) assesses the presence and depth of invasion of material entering the airway, and the patient response to the aspiration and the ability to eject any misdirected material.[108, 109] However, the reliability of this assessment is disappointing.[110] In the United States, the costs of videofluoroscopy for a head and neck cancer patient are over $450. It may well have a larger part to play, therefore, in the clinical research setting to evaluate the impact of still novel treatment approaches, such as chemoradiation: in one study, 54 per cent of chemoradiation patients aspirated compared with only 33 per cent undergoing radiation alone. The significance of this relatively small study is not clear since it was the larger tumours that had undergone chemoradiotherapy.[111] Nonetheless, the findings underline the ongoing importance of videofluoroscopy in assessing silent aspiration, particularly in a group of patients undergoing immunosuppressive systemic therapy. Indeed, a longer-term follow up of non-laryngectomy survivors of head and neck cancer at five years, showed an ongoing 44 per cent aspiration. Aspirators had lost a mean of 10 kg from their pretreatment status, while non-aspirators had a small weight gain. Aspiration was also found to be associated with lower scores on a number of quality-of-life scales.[82]

Functional endoscopic evaluation of swallowing

Fibreoptic endoscopic evaluation of swallowing has emerged over the past two decades as not only a complement to videofluoroscopy, but as a useful investigation in its own right. Endoscopic evaluation can assess in some detail atypical anatomical arrangements following surgery, plus ancillary features such as vocal cord movement. It is readily repeated at the patient's bedside as often as should be required and is therefore a more flexible option than videofluoroscopy. There is no doubt, however, that there are certain parameters which videofluoroscopy alone can address, such as oral transit time or indeed oropharyngeal swallowing efficiency. However, whether these translate to important clinical sequelae in the head and neck cancer population remains in doubt. Aviv[112] found no statistical difference in pneumonia in a group of diverse dysphagia patients assessed either by videofluoroscopy or endoscopic evaluation of swallowing. Patients with absent pharyngeal motor function combined with poor pulmonary reserve and diminished or absent laryngeal sensation are expected to aspirate.[113]

Flexible endoscopic evaluation of swallowing with sensory testing (FEESST) allows more specific assessment of sensory and motor components than in a standard endoscopic evaluation. A review of over 1300 patients undergoing FEESST including 207 with head and neck cancer found it to be a safe examination with epistaxis incidence of less than 0.1 per cent.[91] Any patient with completely insensate laryngopharynx is at extremely high risk of aspiration. Moderate sensory deficits will also result in aspiration if there is a coexisting motor dysfunction.[113]

Aspiration occurring during a swallow cannot be detected on FEESST as there is a 'white out' during contact between the tongue base and the posterior pharyngeal wall as the bolus is propelled out of the oropharynx. Fortunately, aspiration during the swallow reflex itself is not a common occurrence, as most aspiration occurs before or after the swallow has taken place. Endoscopic evaluation of swallowing has variable reliability in different series. However, one study found that combining the technique with the penetration aspiration scale developed for videofluoroscopy could achieve concurrence by different raters on events of penetration and aspiration in 97 per cent of instances.[114] Sharing the video image with the patient being examined offers additional therapeutic opportunities through visual biofeedback as the patient observes the impact of swallowing manoeuvres or head positions on their swallow performance. Endoscopic swallow evaluation is relatively cheap yet only a small minority of speech and language therapists in North America have access to the procedure.[103]

In the head and neck cancer population, endoscopic evaluation of the response of the upper aerodigestive tract to therapy is carried out routinely and regularly following therapy.

In a multidisciplinary team setting, therefore, it is a straightforward matter to combine such a structural assessment with a functional swallowing assessment, for example by the speech and language therapist team members. This is not only a pragmatic approach to swallow evaluation, but clinically sensible, as it allows the twin objectives of eradication of disease and maximal preservation of function to be monitored in parallel.

In addition, the introduction of endoscopic swallow evaluation on a much more regular basis has opened up new areas of relevant research to trace their response to non-surgical therapy, such as the quantification of laryngopharyngeal oedema.[115]

Electromyography

Surface electromyography (sEMG) signals have been used to identify swallow events.[92] The full application of sEMG has yet to be established as the interrater reliability of a method has only recently been established. There is, not surprisingly, higher agreement among more experienced assessors, but even novices achieve a 0.51 kappa coefficient.

At least in the short term, the principal value of the technique in head and neck patients probably is as an adjunct to biofeedback and rehabilitation manoeuvres.

Observer-rated questionnaires

Two brief observer ratings are in fairly regular use to assess both speech and swallowing. The Performance Status Scale for Head and Neck has been referred to above in the context of speech outcome.[69] Understandability of speech is scaled 1 to 5. Swallow performance is assessed by (1) eating in public (scale 1–5) and (2) normalcy of diet (scale 1–10). These two scales have been shown to show a strong correlation with the head and neck subscale of the FACT (Functional Assessment of Cancer Therapy, head and neck scale) health status questionnaire, while also providing additional information not reflected by FACT. The Therapy Outcome Measure (TOM) is a practical tool to measure care outcomes simply and quickly in a wide variety of clinical settings.[86] There is only one TOM scale specific to head and neck patients (laryngectomy); three other scales cover voice, dysarthria and phrenology and one addresses dysphagia.

Self-report questionnaires

MD ANDERSON DYSPHAGIA INVENTORY

The MD Anderson Dysphagia Inventory (MDADI)[94] presents 20 items self-scored on a scale of 1 to 5. A global assessment examines overall daily routine, the emotional subscale has six items on the distress caused by dysphagia; the functional subscale has five items addressing ease of food preparation and eating in public. An eight-item physical subscale assesses dietary consistency, aspiration, weight maintenance and fatigue. The higher the MDADI score, the better the day-to-day functioning for quality of life. Pretreatment swallowing exercises may improve swallowing in patients treated non-surgically.[94]

UNIVERSITY OF WASHINGTON QOL

The University of Washington Quality of Life (UW-QoL) questionnaire version 4 has 12 domains including pain, appearance, activity, recreation, swallowing, chewing, speech, shoulder, taste, saliva, mood and anxiety. The patient scores each from 0 (poorest function) to 100 (highest or near normal function). Additionally, the questionnaire asks patients to nominate up to three domains as being particularly important to them in the previous 7 days. Patients also rate global health-related quality of life. The UW-QoL was the most popular questionnaire in a UK survey.[116]

The ability for patients to be able to prioritize their most personally important quality of life domains is important, not only because it promotes a patient-focused analysis of treatment outcome, but also because it enables clinicians to attempt to weigh up the differential impact of different

therapies. For example, in nasopharyngeal carcinoma patients, the UW-QoL demonstrated the three most important issues in a Singapore population were swallowing (59 per cent), hearing (45 per cent) and xerostomia (41 per cent).[95]

Patients frequently rate problems, such as interference with social activities, as more troublesome than speech disturbance. Survival and being cured of cancer are most important for more than three-quarters of patients at all time points (except in the oldest cohort). Next important was being pain free followed by having energy and being able to return to normal activities.

The SWAL-QoL outcomes tool for oropharyngeal dysphagia in adults was developed in 2000 by McHorney et al.[96] McHorney's team eventually reduced a 93-item instrument into two separate tools, the SWAL-QoL, which has 44 items encompassing ten quality-of-life domains, and the SWAL-CARE, a 15-item tool relating to quality of care and patient satisfaction. The SWAL-QoL aims to provide quality-of-life and quality-of-care outcomes for dysphagia researchers and clinicians. It remains the most comprehensive assessment of swallow performance to date.

There is no single 'best fit' self-report outcome tool. From the patient's point of view, there is merit in having a single questionnaire, which addresses both functional outcome and general quality of life. Separate tools, one to assess the number of key functional outcomes and one for generic quality of life are likely to be more sensitive to change. Very specialist, extensive, single function instruments (even those that do encompass general quality of life items) might best be reserved for a research setting.

Indirect functional outcomes of swallowing

The most conspicuous impact of swallow dysfunction, after aspiration pneumonia, is that of nutritional status. Over half of head and neck cancer patients are likely to be malnourished at diagnosis of their head and neck cancers and nutritional assessment is important not only at base line, but also prior to replacement or removal of feeding tubes and at the time of recommendation for recommencing oral feeding. Nutritional status is affected by general quality of life issues, such as fatigue, loss of appetite and problems with social eating in addition to more specific swallowing problems, dental disease, trismus, xerostomia and cough.[98] Physician-scored rating correlates poorly with quality-of-life scores further emphasizing the importance of including quality of life as part of the overall functional assessment.

A number of techniques can be used to assess nutritional status. All methods have limitations and consequently measuring a combination of variables is usually carried out in most cases.[117] Nutritional screening must be reliable, practical and easy to perform, simple to interpret and low in cost. Screening tools must correlate well with more sophisticated techniques for assessing body composition.[118] Effective nutritional screening will also anticipate nutritional depletion and allow action to be taken to prevent its onset or correct it before it becomes clinically significant.

This is particularly true in head and neck cancer patients where weight loss, low body weight, loss of appetite and a reduction in oral intake (due to, for example, nausea or dysphagia) are common markers of nutritional deficiency.[119]

Different nutritional parameters yield differences in the number of head and neck surgical subjects classed as malnourished: the most powerful predictor of major postoperative complications is a weight loss of >10 per cent in the six months before surgery. Patients with severe nutritional deficit appear to have a reduced two-year survival, perhaps linked to abnormal cell-mediated immunity. There is some evidence that so-called 'immune enhancing' nutritional formulas (e.g. arginine, nucleic acids and fish-oil derivatives) can reduce the incidence of postoperative infectious complications compared with standard supplements.[120]

The relevance and inseparable nature of general quality of life to head and neck cancer functional outcomes has already been alluded to. Consideration should also be given to the distress caused to spouses, carers and significant friends and family members. The impact of head and neck cancer and its treatment on those around the patient is a very new area of research, but one recent paper found that the frequency of distress (20 per cent) in partners was so high as to suggest the need for a routine psychological screening for those caring for patients.[78]

KEY EVIDENCE

- Comorbidity is an independent prognostic indicator for outcome and prognosis for head and neck cancer, even when TNM stage is controlled for.[4, 5, 6, 7, 8]
- Disease-specific quality of life surveys show speech and eating have the most impact on well-being.[26] Measurement of these outcomes is essential to validate use of new treatment regimes.
- Voice outcome for early glottic cancer as measured by the VHI is similar for laser excision and external beam radiotherapy.[31]
- The total radiation dose received is directly related to severity of dysphagia. Significantly more patients receiving more than 74 Gy are gastrostomy dependent than those receiving only 60 Gy.[72]

KEY LEARNING POINTS

Impact of head and neck cancer

- Voice, speech intelligibility, social communication
- Swallowing, diet, social eating
- Disrupted body image, depression, anxiety
- Work impairment, social isolation
- Airway: aspiration, swimming, bathing

Acoustic measurements of voice

- Frequency

- Amplitude
- Jitter
- Shimmer
- Noise-to-harmonic ratio

Causes of head and neck cancer dysphagia

- Oral incompetence/loss of articulators, trismus
- Loss of tongue control/propulsion
- Pharyngo-oesophageal hold up – functional/mechanical
- Gastro-oesophageal reflux

Bedside classification of dysphagia

- Within normal limits
- **Mild** – slight delay in reflex, good oropharyngeal motor function
- **Moderate** – delayed reflex, suspected pooling before swallow, heavy coating in the pharynx post-swallow
- **Severe dysphagia** – trace of aspiration, delayed swallow reflex and probable pooling
- **Profound dysphagia** – absent swallow/cough reflex and poor oral pharyngeal motor function

---

REFERENCES

1. Bosanquet N, Sikora K. The economics of cancer care in the UK. *Lancet Oncology* 2004; **5**: 568–74.
2. Mohide EA, Archibald SD, Tew M *et al.* Postlaryngectomy quality of life dimensions identified by patients and health care professionals. *American Journal of Surgery* 1992; **164**: 619–22.
3. Kaplan EL, Meier P. Nonparametric estimation from incomplete observations. *Journal of the American Statistical Association* 1958; **53**: 457–81.
4. Piccirillo JF. Importance of comorbidity in head and neck cancer. *Laryngoscope* 2000; **110**: 593–602.
5. Lacy PD, Piccirillo JF, Merritt MG, Zequeira MR. Head and neck squamous cell carcinoma: better to be young. *Otolaryngology and Head and Neck Surgery* 2000; **122**: 253–8.
6. Singh B, Bhaya M, Zimbler M *et al.* Impact of comorbidity on outcome of young patients with head and neck squamous cell carcinoma. *Head and Neck* 1998; **20**: 1–7.
7. Hall SF, Groome PA, Rothwell D. The impact of comorbidity on the survival of patients with squamous cell carcinoma of the head and neck. *Head and Neck* 2000; **22**: 317–22.
8. Stein M, Herberhold C, Walther EK, Langenberg A. Influence of comorbidity on the prognosis of squamous cell carcinoma in the head and neck. *Laryngorhinootologie* 2000; **79**: 345–9.
9. Karnofsky DA, Abelman WH, Cravel LF, Burchenal JH. The use of nitrogen mustards in the palliative treatment of carcinoma. *Cancer* 1948; **1**: 634–56.

10. Kaplan MH, Feinstein AR. The importance of classifying initial comorbidity in evaluating the outcome of diabetes mellitus. *Journal of Chronic Diseases* 1974; **27**: 387–404.

11. Charlson ME, Pompei P, Ales KL, MacKenzie CR. A new method of classifying prognostic comorbidity in longitudinal studies: development and validation. *Journal of Chronic Diseases* 1987; **40**: 373–83.

12. Hall SF, Rochon PA, Streiner DL *et al.* Measuring comorbidity in patients with head and neck cancer. *Laryngoscope* 2002; **112**: 1988–96.

13. Sabin SL, Rosenfeld RM, Sundaram K *et al.* The impact of comorbidity and age on survival with laryngeal cancer. *Ear, Nose and Throat Journal* 1999; **78**: 581–4.

14. Kuijpens JLP, Janssen-Heijnen MLG, Lemmens VE *et al.* Comorbidity in newly diagnosed thyroid cancer patients: a population-based study on prevalence and the impact on treatment and survival. *Clinical Endocrinology* 2006; **64**: 450–5.

15. Singh B, Bhaya M, Stern J *et al.* Validation of the Charlson comorbidity index in patients with head and neck cancer: a multi-institutional study. *Laryngoscope* 1997; **107**: 1469–75.

16. Rogers SN, Aziz A, Lowe D, Husband DJ. Feasibility study of the retrospective use of the Adult Comorbidity Evaluation index (ACE-27) in patients with cancer of the head and neck who had radiotherapy. *British Journal of Oral and Maxillofacial Surgery* 2006; **44**: 283–8.

17. Paleri V, Wight RG. Applicability of the adult comorbidity evaluation 27 and the Charlson indexes to assess comorbidity by notes extraction in a cohort of United Kingdom patients with head and neck cancer: a retrospective study. *Journal of Laryngology and Otology* 2002; **116**: 200–5.

18. Ferrier M, Spuesens EB, Le Cessie S, Baatenburg de Jong RJ. Comorbidity as a major risk factor for mortality and complication in head and neck surgery. *Archives of Otolaryngology and Head and Neck Surgery* 2005; **131**: 27–32.

19. Borggreven PA, Kuik DJ, Quak JJ *et al.* Comorbid condition as a prognostic factor for the complications in major surgery of the oral cavity and oropharynx with microvascular soft tissue reconstruction. *Head and Neck* 2003; **25**: 808–15.

20. Paleri V, Wight RG, Davies GR. Impact of comorbidity on the outcome of laryngeal squamous cancer. *Head and Neck* 2003; **25**: 1019–26.

21. Paleri V, Wight RG. A cross-comparison of retrospective notes extraction and combined notes extraction and patient interview in the completion of a comorbidity index (ACE-27) in a cohort of United Kingdom patients with head and neck cancer. *Journal of Laryngology and Otology* 2002; **116**: 937–41.

22. McNeil BJ, Weichselbaum R, Pauker SG. Speech and survival: tradeoffs between quality and quantity of life in laryngeal cancer. *New England Journal of Medicine* 1981; **305**: 982–7.

23. De Santo LW, Olsen KD, Perry WC *et al.* Quality of life after surgical treatment of cancer of the larynx. *Annals of Otology, Rhinology, and Laryngology* 1995; **104**: 763–9.

24. List MA, Rutherford JL, Stracks J *et al.* Prioritizing treatment outcomes: head and neck cancer patients versus non-patients. *Head and Neck* 2004; **26**: 163–70.

25. The Department of Veterans Affairs. Induction chemotherapy plus radiation compared with surgery plus radiation in patients with advanced laryngeal cancer. *New England Journal of Medicine* 1991; **324**: 1685–90.

26. Hynds-Karnell L, Funk GF, Hoffman HT. Assessing head and neck cancer patient's outcome domains. *Head and Neck* 2002; **22**: 6–11.

27. World Health Organization. *International classification of impairment, disability and handicap. Beta-1: A manual of dimensions of disablement and participation.* Geneva: WHO, 1997.

28. British Association of Otorhinolaryngologists Head and Neck Surgeons. Effective head and neck cancer management. Third Consensus Document. London: BAO-HNS, 2002.

29. Hirano M. Objective evaluation of the human voice; clinical aspects. *Folia Phoniatrica* 1989; **41**: 89–144.

30. Jacobson BH, Johnson A, Grywalski C *et al.* The Voice Handicap Index (VHI): development and validation. *American Journal of Speech and Language* 1997; **6**: 66–70.

31. Cohen SM, Garrett CG, Dupont WD *et al.* Voice-related quality of life in T1 glottic cancer: irradiation versus endoscopic excision. *Annals of Otology, Rhinology, and Laryngology* 2006; **115**: 581–6.

32. Brondbo K, Benninger MS. Laser resection of T1a glottic carcinomas: results and postoperative voice quality. *Acta Otolaryngologica* 2004; **124**: 976–9.

33. Peretti G, Piazza C, Cattaneo A *et al.* Comparison of functional outcomes after endoscopic versus open-neck supraglottic laryngectomies. *Annals of Otology, Rhinology, and Laryngology* 2006; **115**: 827–32.

34. Schindler A, Favero E, Nudo S *et al.* Voice after supracricoid laryngectomy: subjective, objective and self-assessment data. *Logopedics, Phoniatrics, Vocology* 2005; **30**: 114–19.

35. Makeieff M, Venail F, Garrel R *et al.* Voice handicap evaluation after supracricoid partial laryngectomy. *Revue de Laryngologie, Otologie, Rhinologie* 2004; **125**: 313–17.

36. Moerman M, Martens JP, Dejonckere P. Application of the Voice Handicap Index in 45 patients with substitution voicing after total laryngectomy. *European Archives of Otorhinolaryngology* 2004; **261**: 423–8.

37. Schuster M, Lohscheller J, Hoppe U *et al.* Voice handicap of laryngectomees with tracheoesophageal speech. *Folia Phoniatrica et Logopaedica* 2004; **56**: 62–7.

38. Stewart MG, Chen AY, Stach CB. Outcomes analysis of voice and quality of life in patients with laryngeal cancer. *Archives of Otolaryngology – Head and Neck Surgery* 1998; **124**: 143–8.

39. Kazi R, De Cordova J, Singh A et al. Voice-related quality of life in laryngectomees: assessment using the VHI and VRQOL Symptom scales. *Journal of Voice* 2007; **21**: 728–34.

40. Zraick RI, Risner BY, Smith-Olin de L et al. Patient versus partner perception of voice handicap. *Journal of Voice* 2007; **21**: 485–94.

● 41. Deary IJ, Wilson JA, Carding PN, MacKenzie K. A patient-derived Voice Symptom Scale. *Journal of Psychosomatic Research* 2002; **54**: 483–9.

42. Scott S, Robinson K, Wilson JA et al. Patient reported problems associated with dysphonia. *Clinical Otolaryngology* 1997; **22**: 37–40.

43. Wilson JA, Webb A, Carding PN et al. The Voice Symptom Scale (VoiSS) and Vocal Handicap Index (VHI): a comparison of structure and content. *Clinical Otolaryngology* 2004; **29**: 169–74.

44. Loughran S, Calder N, MacGregor FB et al. Quality of life and voice following endoscopic resection or radiotherapy for early glottic cancer. *Clinical Otolaryngology* 2005; **30**: 42–7.

45. Ma EP, Yiu EM. Voice Activity and Participation Profile: assessing the impact of voice disorders on daily activity. *Journal of Speech, Language, and Hearing Research* 2001; **44**: 511–24.

● 46. Rosen CA, Lee AS, Osborne J et al. Development and validation of the voice handicap index-10. *Laryngoscope* 2004; **114**: 1549–56.

47. Carding PN, Horsley IA. An evaluation of study of voice therapy in non-organic dysphonia. *European Journal of Disorders of Communication* 1992; **27**: 137–58.

48. Deary IJ, Webb A, MacKenzie K et al. Short, self-report voice symptom scales: psychometric characteristics of the voice handicap index-10 and the Vocal Performance Questionnaire. *Otolaryngology and Head and Neck Surgery* 2004; **131**: 232–5.

● 49. Hirano M. Clinical examination of voice. In: Arnold GE, Wikle F, Wyke BD (eds). *Disorders of human communication*. New York: Springer Verlag, 1981: 83–4.

∗ 50. De Jonckere PH, Crevier-Buchman L, Marie JP et al. Implementation of the European Laryngological Society (ELS) basic protocol for assessing voice treatment effect. *Revue de Laryngologie, Otologie, Rhinologie* 2003; **124**: 279–83.

51. Carding P, Carlson E, Epstein R et al. Formal perceptual evaluation of voice quality in the United Kingdom. *Logopedics, Phoniatrics, Vocology* 2000; **25**: 133–8.

52. De Bodt MS, Wuts FL, van de Heyning PH et al. Test-retest study of the GRBAS scale: influence of experience and professional background on perceptual ratings of voice quality. *Journal of Voice* 1997; **11**: 74–80.

53. Webb AL, Carding PN, Deary IJ et al. The reliability of three perceptual evaluation scales for dysphonia. *European Archives of Otorhinolaryngology* 2004; **261**: 429–34.

54. Lee M, Drinnan M, Carding P. The reliability and validity of patient self-rating of their own voice. *Clinical Otolaryngology* 2005; **30**: 357–61.

55. Kazi R, Singh A, Mullan GP et al. Can objective parameters derived from videofluoroscopic assessment of post-laryngectomy valved speech replace current subjective measures? An e-tool-based analysis. *Clinical Otolaryngology* 2006; **31**: 518–24.

56. Kazi R, Kiverniti E, Prasad V et al. Multidimensional assessment of female tracheoesophageal prosthetic speech. *Clinical Otolaryngology* 2006; **31**: 511–17.

57. Van As CJ, van Beinum K, Pols LC, Hilgers FJ. Perceptual evaluation of tracheoesophageal speech by naïve and experienced judges through the use of semantic differential scales. *Journal of Speech, Language and Hearing Research* 2003; **46**: 947–59.

58. Eadie TL, Doyle PC. Direct magnitude estimation and interval scaling of naturalness and severity in tracheoesophageal speakers. *Journal of Speech, Language and Hearing Research* 2002; **45**: 1088–96.

59. Eadie TL, Doyle PC. Scaling of voice pleasantness and acceptability in tracheoesophageal speakers. *Journal of Voice* 2005; **19**: 373–83.

60. Eadie TL, Doyle PC, Hamen K, Beaudin PG. Influence of speaker gender on listener judgements of tracheoesophageal speech. *Journal of Voice* 2008; **22**: 43–57.

61. Caminero Cueva MJ, Senaris Gonzalez B, Lopez Llames A et al. Voice quality assessment after laryngeal cancer radiotherapeutic treatment at initial stages. *Clinical and Translational Oncology* 2006; **8**: 284–9.

62. Schindler A, Palonta F, Preti G et al. Voice quality after carbon dioxide laser and conventional surgery for T1A glottic cancer. *Journal of Voice* 2004; **18**: 545–50.

63. Van Gogh CD, Verdonck-de Leeuw IM, Boon-Kamma BA et al. The efficacy of voice therapy in patients after treatment for early glottic carcinoma. *Cancer* 2006; **106**: 95–105.

64. Van As-Brooks CJ, van Beinum K, Pols LC, Hilgers FJ. Acoustic signal typing for evaluation of voice quality in tracheoesophageal speech. *Journal of Voice* 2005; **20**: 355–68.

◆ 65. Michi K. Functional evaluation of cancer surgery in oral and maxillofacial region: speech function. *International Journal of Clinical Oncology* 2003; **8**: 1–17.

66. Nicolatti G, Soutar DS, Jackson MS et al. Objective assessment of speech after surgical treatment for oral cancer: experience from 196 selected cases. *Plastic and Reconstructive Surgery* 2004; **113**: 114–25.

67. Plank DM, Weinberg B, Chalian VA. Evaluation of speech following prosthetic obturation of surgically acquired maxillary defects. *Journal of Prosthetic Dentistry* 1981; **45**: 626–38.

68. Yorkston KM, Beukelman DR. *Assessment of intelligibility of dysarthric speech*. Austin, TX: Pro-Ed, 1981.

69. List MA, Ritter-Sterr C, Lansky SB. A performance status scale for head and neck cancer patients. *Cancer* 1990; **66**: 564–9.

70. Kazi R, Singh A, De Cordova J *et al.* Validation of a voice prosthesis questionnaire to assess valved speech and its related issues in patients following total laryngectomy. *Clinical Otolaryngology* 2006; **31**: 404–10.

71. List MA, Bilir SP. Functional outcomes in head and neck cancer. *Seminars in Radiation Oncology* 2004; **14**: 178–89.

72. Smith RV, Kotz T, Beitler JJ, Wadler S. Long-term swallowing problems after organ preservation therapy with concomitant radiation therapy and intravenous hydroxyurea: initial results. *Archives of Otolaryngology – Head and Neck Surgery* 2000; **126**: 384–9.

73. Eisbruch A, Schwartz M, Rasch C *et al.* Dysphagia and aspiration after chemoradiotherapy for head and neck cancer: which anatomic structures are affected and can they be spared by IMRT? *International Journal of Radiation Oncology, Biology, Physics* 2004; **60**: 1425–39.

74. Feng FY, Kim HM, Lyden TH *et al.* Intensity-modulated radiotherapy of head and neck cancer aiming to reduce dysphagia: early dose–effect relationships for the swallowing structures. *International Journal of Radiation Oncology, Biology, Physics* 2007; **68**: 1289–98.

75. Frowen JJ, Perry AR. Swallowing outcomes after radiotherapy for head and neck cancer: a systematic review. *Head and Neck* 2006; **28**: 932–44.

76. Pauloski BR, Rademaker AW, Logemann JA *et al.* Relationship between swallow motility disorders on videofluorography and oral intake in patients treated for head and neck cancer with radiotherapy with or without chemotherapy. *Head and Neck* 2006; **28**: 1069–76.

77. Nguyen NP, Moltz CC, Frank C *et al.* Evolution of chronic dysphagia following treatment for head and neck cancer. *Oral Oncology* 2006; **42**: 374–80.

78. Verdonck-de Leeuw IM, Eerenstein SE, Van der Linden MH *et al.* Distress in spouses and patients after treatment for head and neck cancer. *Laryngoscope* 2007; **117**: 238–41.

79. Jellema AP, Slotman BJ, Doornaert P *et al.* Impact of radiation-induced xerostomia on quality of life after primary radiotherapy among patients with head and neck cancer. *International Journal of Radiation Oncology, Biology, Physics* 2007; **69**: 751–60.

80. Lazarus C. Tongue strength and exercise in healthy individuals and in head and neck cancer patients. *Seminars in Speech and Language* 2006; **27**: 260–7.

81. Ball S, Idel O, Cotton SM, Perry A. Comparison of two methods for measuring tongue pressure during swallowing in people with head and neck cancer. *Dysphagia* 2006; **21**: 28–37.

82. Nguyen NP, Frank C, Moltz CC *et al.* Aspiration rate following chemoradiation for head and neck cancer: an underreported occurrence. *Radiation Oncology* 2006; **80**: 302–6.

83. Franzmann EJ, Lundy DS, Abitbol AA *et al.* Complete hypopharyngeal obstruction by mucosal adhesions: a complication of intensive chemoradiation for advanced head and neck cancer. *Head and Neck* 2006; **28**: 663–70.

84. Campbell BH, Spinelli K, Marbella AM *et al.* Aspiration, weight loss, and quality of life in head and neck cancer survivors. *Archives of Otology – Head and Neck Surgery* 2004; **130**: 1100–3.

85. Nguyen NP, Smith HJ, Sallah S. Evaluation and management of swallowing dysfunction following chemoradiation for head and neck cancer. *Current Opinion in Otology, Head and Neck Surgery* 2007; **15**: 130–3.

86. John A, Enderby P. Reliability of speech and language therapists using therapy outcome measures. *International Journal of Language and Communication Disorders* 2000; **35**: 287–302.

87. Nathadwarawala KM, Nicklin J, Wiles CM. A timed test of swallowing capacity for neurological patients. *Journal of Neurology, Neurosurgery, and Psychiatry* 1992; **55**: 822–5.

88. Winklmaier U, Wust K, Schiller S, Wallner F. Leakage of fluid in different types of tracheal tubes. *Dysphagia* 2006; **21**: 237–42.

89. Logemann JA, Roa Pauloski B, Rademaker A *et al.* Impact of the diagnostic procedure on outcome measure of swallowing rehabilitation in head and neck cancer patients. *Dysphagia* 1992; **7**: 179–86.

90. Bastian RW. The videoendoscopic swallowing study: an alternative and partner to the videofluoroscopic swallow study. *Dysphagia* 1993; **8**: 359–61.

91. Aviv JE, Murry T, Zschommler A *et al.* Flexible endoscopic evaluation of swallowing with sensory testing: patient characteristics and analysis of safety in 1,340 consecutive examinations. *Annals of Otorhinolaryngology* 2005; **114**: 173–6.

92. Crary MA, Carnaby-Mann GD, Groher ME, Helseth E. Functional benefits of dysphagia therapy using adjunctive sEMG biofeedback. *Dysphagia* 2004; **19**: 160–4.

93. Carnaby-Mann GD, Crary MA. Examining the evidence on neuromuscular electrical stimulation for swallowing: a meta-analysis. *Archives of Otolaryngology – Head and Neck Surgery* 2007; **133**: 564–71.

94. Kulbersh BD, Rosenthal EL, McGrew BM *et al.* Pretreatment, preoperative swallowing exercises may improve dysphagia quality of life. *Laryngoscope* 2006; **116**: 883–6.

95. Lovell SJ, Wong HB, Loh KS *et al.* Impact of dysphagia on quality-of-life in nasopharyngeal carcinoma. *Head and Neck* 2005; **27**: 864–72.

96. McHorney CA, Martin-Harris B, Robbins J, Rosenbek J. Clinical validity of the SWAL-QOL and SWAL-CARE outcome tools with respect to bolus flow measures. *Dysphagia* 2006; **21**: 141–8.

97. Lees J. Incidence of weight loss in head and neck cancer patients on commencing radiotherapy treatment at a

regional oncology centre. *European Journal of Cancer Care* 1999; **8**: 133-6.

98. Oates JE, Clark JR, Read J *et al.* Prospective evaluation of quality of life and nutrition before and after treatment for nasopharyngeal carcinoma. *Archives of Otolaryngology – Head and Neck Surgery* 2007; **133**: 533-40.

99. Rogers SN, Laher SH, Overend L. Importance-rating using the University of Washington quality of life questionnaire in patients treated by primary surgery for oral and oropharyngeal cancer. *Journal of Craniomaxillofacial Surgery* 2002; **30**: 125-32.

100. Magne N, Marcy PY, Foa C *et al.* Comparison between nasogastric tube feeding and percutaneous fluoroscopic gastrostomy in advanced head and neck cancer patients. *European Archives of Otorhinolaryngology* 2001; **258**: 89-92.

101. Belafsky PC, Blumenfeld L, LePage A, Nahrstedt K. The accuracy of the modified Evan's blue dye test in predicting aspiration. *Laryngoscope* 2003; **113**: 1969-72.

102. Murray J. *Manual of dysphagia assessment in adults*. San Diego: Singular Publishing Group, 1999.

103. Mathers-Schmidt BA, Kurlinski M. Dysphagia evaluation practices: inconsistencies in clinical assessment and instrumental examination decision making. *Dysphagia* 2003; **18**: 114-25.

104. Kuhlemeier KV, Yates P, Palmer JB. Intra- and interrater variation in the evaluation of videofluorographic swallowing studies. *Dysphagia* 1998; **13**: 142-7.

105. Scott A, Perry A, Bench J. A study of interrater reliability when using videofluoroscopy as an assessment of swallowing. *Dysphagia* 1998; **13**: 223-7.

106. Martino R, Pron G, Diamant NE. Oropharyngeal dysphagia: surveying practice patterns of the speech-language pathologist. *Dysphagia* 2004; **19**: 165-76.

107. Tei K, Maekawa K, Kitada H *et al.* Recovery from post surgical swallowing dysfunction in patients with oral cancer. *Journal of Oral and Maxillofacial Surgery* 2007; **65**: 1077-83.

● 108. Rosenbek JC, Robbins JA, Roecker EB *et al.* A penetration–aspiration scale. *Dysphagia* 1996; **11**: 93-8.

109. Robbins J, Coyle J, Rosenbek J *et al.* Differentiation of normal and abnormal airway protection during swallowing using the penetration-aspiration scale. *Dysphagia* 1999; **14**: 228-32.

110. McCullough GH, Wertz RT, Rosenbek JC *et al.* Inter- and intrajudge reliability for videofluoroscopic swallowing evaluation measures. *Dysphagia* 2001; **16**: 110-18.

111. Nguyen NP, Moltz CC, Frank C *et al.* Aspiration rate following nonsurgical therapy for laryngeal cancer. *Journal for Otorhinolaryngology and its Related Specialties* 2007; **69**: 116-20.

112. Aviv JE. Prospective, randomised outcome study of endoscopy versus modified barium swallow in patients with dysphagia. *Laryngoscope* 2000; **110**: 563-74.

113. Setzen M, Cohen MA, Perlman PW *et al.* The association between laryngopharyngeal sensory deficits, pharyngeal motor function, and the prevalence of aspiration with thin liquids. *Otolaryngology and Head and Neck Surgery* 2003; **128**: 99-102.

114. Colodny N. Interjudge and intrajudge reliabilities in fibreoptic endoscopic evaluation of swallowing (FEES) using the penetration–aspiration scale; a replication study. *Dysphagia* 2002; **17**: 308-15.

115. Patterson JM, Hildreth A, Wilson JA. Measuring edema in irradiated head and neck cancer patients. *Annals of Otology, Rhinology, and Laryngology* 2007; **116**: 559-64.

116. Kanatas AN, Rogers SN. A national survey of health-related quality of life questionnaires in head and neck oncology. *Annals of the Royal College of Surgeons of England* 2004; **86**: 6-10.

117. Baker JP, Detsky AS, Wesson DE, Jeejeebhoy KN. Nutritional assessment: a comparison of clinical judgement and objective measurements. *New England Journal of Medicine* 1982; **306**: 969-72.

118. Elia M (ed.). *Guidelines for detection and management of malnutrition*. Malnutrition Advisory Group. Maidenhead: BAPEN, 2000.

119. Grobbelaar EJ, Owen S, Torrance AD, Wilson JA. Nutritional challenges in head and neck cancer. *Clinical Otolaryngology* 2004; **29**: 307-13.

120. Snyderman CH, Kachman K, Molseed L *et al.* Reduced postoperative infections with an immune-enhancing nutritional supplement. *Laryngoscope* 1999; **109**: 915-21.

10

Quality of life

SIMON ROGERS

> Health is a large word. It embraces not the body only, but the mind and spirit as well ... and not today's pain or pleasure alone, but the whole being and outlook of a man.
>
> James H West

INTRODUCTION

For patient and their carers, quality of life (QOL) following head and neck cancer (HNC) is a crucially important issue. The treatment of HNC is more than cure and survival. The cancer and its treatment affect functions that are integral to human existence – for example, communication, eating, socialization and interpersonal contacts. Over the last decade, there has been a tremendous increase in the number of publications on this subject, which reflects the importance of the patient perspective as an outcome parameter in addition to survival, recurrence and complication rates.

This chapter is written in two sections. The first section explores the general topic of QOL assessment and covers definitions, why, when and how to measure, and perceived barriers. The second section looks at the QOL in patients with HNC and covers outcomes, predictors and carers.

QUALITY OF LIFE ASSESSMENT

Definition of quality of life and health–related quality of life

Quality of life is a concept that has become increasingly important in relation to patient outcomes following treatment for cancer. Nevertheless, it is a concept that is difficult to define and measure because it is broad and individual to each person (**Box 10.1**).

There are many definitions, but the following are particularly useful:

- 'An individual's perceptions of their position in life taken in the context of the culture and value systems in which they live and in relation to their goals, standards and concerns.' Quality of life as defined by the World Health Organization.[1]
- A person's sense of well-being that stems from satisfaction or dissatisfaction with the areas of life that are important.[2]
- The measure between age expectations or present experience, and the perceived and actual goals (Calman-gap theory).[3, 4]

Box 10.1 Quality of life

Quality of life is not:

- a single entity which can be simply measured
- the same as toxicity
- absolute or static, but relative and variable

Quality of life questionnaires are:

- subjective
- always an approximation
- a pale reflection of what we all think of as quality of life

---

It is the third definition that has become more widely used in clinical practice as it addresses how a patient perceives problems as a consequence of the illness and its treatment and how much this differs from what they expected.[5] This difference can be measured.

Because QOL is such a broad, multidimensional concept, efforts have been made to focus on certain issues and the term 'health-related quality of life (HRQOL)' has evolved. This is a more restricted concept and does not, for example, include satisfaction or well-being. It is restricted to those factors that are part of an individual's health. Aaronson et al.[6] have defined HRQOL as 'the assessment of the impact of the disease and its treatment on the physical, psychological and social aspects of quality of life'. It is essential that the assessment includes the perceived effects of cancer and treatment (disease specific) and where possible is patient-derived and assessed in a cultural setting.

The enormous breadth of QOL makes it impossible to summarize all the issues in one chapter and, unfortunately, it is likely that certain aspects have regrettably been omitted. Only some of the key aspects have been covered and further reading around the subject is recommended.

Why measure HRQOL

In the management of HNC, outcome is more than just cure and survival. Clinicians are very familiar with the traditional outcomes, such as laboratory test (e.g. infection rates), imaging (e.g. videofluoroscopy), clinical measurement (e.g fistula rates), process indicators (e.g. length of stay), recurrence and mortality. However, clinicians are less aware of outcomes based on patient experience, symptoms, function/ dysfunction, satisfaction, importance and quality of life. A combination of both the objective and subjective can give additional insight into the issue, as shown in the assessment of speech and swallowing following soft palate reconstruction using a radial forearm free flap in conjunction with a superiorly based pharyngeal flap and radial forearm free tissue transfer. In this study, both questionnaire data and speech intelligibility and videofluoroscopy were used to demonstrate the benefit of using a superiorly based flap in patients having more than half their soft palate resected.[7] In addition to being used in combination if the relationship between the objective and subjective scoring is strong, it is possible to use only one as a surrogate for the other. An example of this is when reporting HRQOL using a permanent gastrostomy feeding tube as an indicator of HRQOL, as the presence of a long-term gastrostomy strongly indicates a poor HRQOL outcome.[8]

The value of patient-derived outcome following treatment was recognized in the policy framework for the commissioning of cancer services.[3] It recognized the need for information on the quality and outcome of care and it emphasized that, in the critical appraisal of outcome, it is imperative to include the patient's perspective of function/dysfunction and well-being/distress. The measurement of QOL has been suggested as a national outcome parameter by the British Association of Head and Neck Oncologists in the national dataset and also is often a mandatory secondary outcome to any randomized control trials.

Another reason to include HRQOL as an outcome is when two methods of treatment produce equivalent cure rates. In this situation, one of the major factors determining which treatment should be chosen is the post-treatment quality of life.[9]

It can be assumed that clinicians appreciate the patient's perspective and with experience it is possible to recognize patients' concerns and to address these. However, differences in perspectives between doctors and patients can easily occur with doctors overestimating the objective symptoms and underestimating more subjective problems.[10] This was highlighted in a survey of 278 patients regarding appearance issues after surgery. Worst appearance scores were reported in those with advanced disease, free flaps, segmental jaw resection and neck dissection. One hundred and fourteen patients (41 per cent) were identified as having a potential appearance problem based on their University of Washington Head and Neck Cancer Questionnaire domain score. However, only seven (6 per cent) had the issue mentioned in the case notes or letters. Of these, five had intervention. Given the important problem of appearance following HNC, it raises the potential for unrecognized patient and care needs that are not identified in a busy clinical setting.[11]

Other advantages in measuring HRQOL include providing a baseline against which effectiveness of an intervention can be measured. Measurement may enable priority to be given to those particular patients who appear to be making poor progress, and providing valuable information for subsequent patients and give a good idea of the likely impairment they can expect following surgery. This can then help the patient and clinician in the decision-making process before and after treatment.[12] Higginson et al. suggest the following additional value of HRQOL measurement, which may facilitate communication, screen for hidden problems (e.g. psychological distress), identify preference, train new staff, be useful in clinical audit and clinical governance.[13] There is evidence that routine HRQOL assessment has a positive impact on patient–doctor communication and could actually improve HRQOL and emotional functioning.[14] Its measurement and analysis encourage multidisciplinary team working, can help to identify poor outcome groups, give better insight as to the expectations of patients and carers, and can give information about cancer journey.[15]

Given sufficient information, patients can make a choice between treatments and can engage in discussion of trade offs between the burden and the HRQOL outcome. This was demonstrated in a retrospective chart analysis of 140 patients with stage I and II glottic cancer in the study period 1990–8. The premise was that both options were offered based on equivalent control rates. Their choice was between (1) transoral microendoscopic laser surgery as a single stage, short duration of definitive treatment with histological assessment of margins and radiotherapy for recurrence or second primaries or (2) percutaneous radiotherapy which they were advised had a superior expected voice quality. In this cohort, 75 patients chose radiotherapy and 65 surgery.[16]

When to measure HRQOL

There is relatively little benefit in measuring HRQOL on every patient without a very clear purpose. Usually, the

HRQOL hypothesis being tested is part of a clinical trial or an explicit objective in a clinical study. HRQOL can have a major role in treatment decisions in certain situations, such as (1) when two treatments both have a very good chance of cure; (2) when two treatments have equivalent survival outcome, but different HRQOL outcomes; (3) when either treatment is very unlikely to give cure; (4) if the HRQOL outcome is very poor; or (5) the intention is non-curative and the sole consideration is the quality of time the patient and carer have remaining. HRQOL is an important additional factor in treatment decisions in some cases, for example, when there is a 'meaningful' difference in HRQOL between two treatments but the HRQOL benefit is counter to the expected survival advantage. In this situation, the patient has to trade off survival benefit against additional HRQOL burden. HRQOL is of little value when there is no meaningful difference between HRQOL between different treatments or when survival is 'significantly' better with one treatment than another.

When measuring HRQOL, there are two study designs, cross-sectional or longitudinal. Cross-sectional assessment allows the recruitment of many patients as they are at different time points in their cancer journey. This design has been frequently used in the past,[17] particularly for questionnaire validation and predictors of HRQOL outcome and patient-derived function. Cross-sectional surveys are limited by dropout and response shift. Over time, there is a survivorship effect. Also, patients cope and adapt and this makes differences between patient groups less noticeable.[18, 19] The term used for data collected over a period of time on a group of patients is 'longitudinal'. This might be pretreatment and at intervals following this, such as six months and one year, or it might be related to an intervention where the timing of the assessment is of critical importance if a change is to be adequately detected. Longitudinal data have distinct advantages as they capture the change in the patient's HRQOL during the cancer journey and also reflect greater changes in domain scores.

How to measure HRQOL

Health-related quality of life is usually measured by questionnaire.[20] Depending on the scope of enquiry, and the number and complexity of the items contained, questionnaires can be delivered in a variety of ways. If the questionnaire is relatively simple, patients can be sent postal questionnaires or asked to fill out questionnaires in the clinic. If a battery of questionnaires is needed to test a hypothesis, they can form the basis of a semistructured interview. In this situation, patients can be given time and encouragement to complete all the items. Also, semistructured interviews are a useful approach for patient-generated index or utility assessment as these approaches need to be carefully explained to patients and tend to be more time consuming. On some occasions, open interview is better, for example, in item generation, where little is known about an issue or where the quality of life construct is much wider and rapidly changing, such as in palliative care.

THE PROPERTIES OF AN IDEAL QUESTIONNAIRE

There are many different questionnaires available (**Box 10.2**). As an introduction to this area, the ideal features of

---

> **Box 10.2 Questionnaires[21]**
>
> - Purpose: Target phase of illness
> - Number of items: Summary Score
> - Self-administered: Patient item generation
> - Patient item reduction: Internal reliability
> - Test–retest reliability: Face validity
> - Content validity: Concurrent validity
> - Responsiveness: Cross-cultural input

questionnaires will first be discussed, and then focus will move to commonly used HRQOL questionnaires.

There are certain ideal properties of a questionnaire and these include reliability, validity, responsiveness, precision, interpretability, acceptability and feasibility.[13] The following criteria are helpful in identifying an appropriate questionnaire:[22]

- disease specific;
- functional status included;
- represents global construct of quality of life;
- patient self-administered;
- short, easily understood questions;
- sensitive to change over short time periods;
- sensitive to changes in dysfunction due to illness and treatment;
- clinical relevance;
- adequate validity and reliability.

Sadura et al.[23] suggested that the high compliance rate found in a study they carried out to demonstrate the implementation of HRQOL data collection on cancer clinics was due to the fact that patients filled in the questionnaires in clinic, rather than taking them home with them. A second factor in achieving high patient compliance was that patients could complete the questionnaire within 10 minutes. Additionally, they suggested that patients appreciated the interest being shown in aspects of their disease; this appreciation seems to create a positive feedback loop within the patient–health-care worker team.

TYPES OF QUESTIONNAIRE AVAILABLE

Questionnaires can be broadly classified into six different groups:

1. The performance measures such as Karnofsky or ECOG. These have been used for a long time and essentially report level of physical function. They were used to help validate the newer questionnaires when no other measures were available, but essentially their enquiry is very limited and does not address the facets of HRQOL.
2. The global or generic questionnaire, such as SF36, HAD, CESD, EQ-5D. These questionnaires can be used in other disease states and in the normative population. Comparison to the non-cancer group is of value when assessing the impact of HNC.
3. The general cancer questionnaires, such as EORTC C30 and FACT G. These can be used in any cancer

as the items contained are germane to cancer and its treatment. These items include broad concepts that are affected by cancer, such as cognitive level or pain.

4. The HNC cancer-specific questionnaires, such as EORTC H&N and UW-QOL. These focus on the problems encountered specifically in patients with cancer of the head and neck and its treatment. This enquiry is highly relevant as key issues are addressed, such as speech, swallowing and shoulder function.

5. The H&N function-specific questionnaires, such as PSSHN. These are limited in their enquiry and focus on certain elements of function only. However, because the questionnaire is focused on only one domain, the enquiry can have more depth. Newer questionnaires have emerged aimed at being more sensitive and responsive; examples include dysphagia,[24] pace of oral rehabilitation,[25] PEG feeding tube,[26] shoulder[27] and xerostomia.[28]

6. Finally, there is a whole raft of other 'quality of life' issues that can be tested using questionnaires. Examples include emotion, coping/distress, pain, family/social support, appearance/body image, fatigue, self-esteem, satisfaction, sexual function, personality and spirituality. If enquiry extends into these fields, it is better to take advice from colleagues with wider experience in the use of these measures, such as a clinical psychologist.[29, 30]

CHOICE OF QUESTIONNAIRE

It must be recognized that although there is a wide choice of questionnaires (**Box 10.3**), they all have their unique features, strengths and limitations. There is no perfect questionnaire. Careful consideration must be given before embarking on developing a new questionnaire. It might be better to use several questionnaires so that the area of interest has been captured. The process of validation is time consuming and lengthy, and there is agreement that no new general cancer or head and neck-specific questionnaires are needed for general use. However, there is scope for additional specific questionnaires to better assess in detail certain issues, such as dysphagia in laryngectomy patients. However, it must be recognized that validation takes a long time.

In choosing a questionnaire, it is important to identify the domains of interest relevant to the purpose of the HRQOL data collection. It is essential to identify why the data are being collected as this shapes the study design and the use of one or several questionnaires. It is possible to use a modular questionnaire, where one group has developed several questionnaires for both general cancer and HNC (e.g. FACT, EORTC, or alternatively to use a single questionnaire that covers the HRQOL construct, e.g. UW-QOL).

Patients tend to answer similar domains in the different questionnaires in the same way (e.g. swallowing questions), thus it is possible to draw inferences from domain scores in different questionnaires. There can be strong correlation between questionnaires, e.g. the UW-QOL cluster paper, also items in UW-QOL shoulder, CES D, etc.[43]

HRQOL should be included as an outcome when there is a need to test a specific hypothesis. The collection of HRQOL is time consuming and hence routine collection for the sake of it has limited value.

Barriers to measuring HRQOL in clinical practice

Although there are many perceived benefits to measuring HRQOL, there are several difficulties (**Table 10.1**).

Patients are happy to complete questionnaires in clinic, as it would help them describe their health problems to their doctor. Although questionnaire length is not a major issue, most prefer a short questionnaire of less than 20 items.[44] It seems that patients assume that this information from the

Box 10.3 Examples of head and neck questionnaire commonly used in the literature

- Functional Assessment of Cancer Therapy-Head and Neck Subscale[31]
- EORTC Quality of Life Head and Neck 35[32]
- University of Washington Head and Neck Cancer Questionnaire v 4[33]
- Performance Status Scale for H&N Cancer[34]
- Less often reported
- Quality of life Questionnaire[35]
- McMaster Univ H&N Radiotherapy Q[36]
- Functional Status in H&N Cancer[37]
- H&N Cancer-Specific Quality of Life[8]
- H&N Oncology health status assessment[38]
- Head and Neck Survey[39]
- Self-Evaluation of Communication Experiences after Laryngeal cancer[40]
- Liverpool University Questionnaire[41]
- Structured QOL 34 item[42]

Table 10.1 Difficulties and benefits to measuring HRQOL.

	%
Perceived difficulties	
Lack of resources	57
Not convinced of value	16
Not part of departmental practice	11
Lack of information about questionnaires	7
Unable to process the data collected	6
Forgot to distribute	3
Benefits	
More information about the patient	28
Identification of problems	22
Research	10
Quality of life as an outcome	10
Terminate aggressive surgery	4
None	20

Data from Kanatas AN, Rogers SN. A national survey of health-related quality of life questionnaires in head and neck oncology. *Annals of the Royal College of Surgeons of England* 2004; **86**: 6–10.

Box 10.4   Factors to take into account when reporting quality of life in clinical trials

- Recruitment bias
- Dropout – survivorship effect
- Non responders
- Sufficient power – rare diverse cancer
- Allow for other variables e.g martial status, comorbidity, personality
- Lack of blindness – informal intervention
- Cross-cultural validity
- Agreed standard of analysis and reporting
- Establishing clinical meaning and a clinically relevant difference

questionnaire will be used to improve care for other patients, hence value the enquiry. Computer network support and the use of touch screen technology perhaps offers the key to allowing HRQOL data to be available in routine clinics to help inform the decision process and also identify problem issues that could then be amenable to intervention.

Health-related quality of life outcomes have become a standard component of secondary outcomes in randomized control trials. By including the patient perspective, there is supplementary information on clinical benefit that gives the study added relevance. When using HRQOL data in clinical trials, various points need to be considered (**Box 10.4**).

QUALITY OF LIFE IN HEAD AND NECK CANCER

The issue of survival

Survival and cure are of primary importance. This supports aggressive treatment; however, there is high individual variability and the primacy of survival is influenced by treatment.[45, 46]

Comparison with normative data and other disease states

There are several articles in the literature that give a review of QOL in HNC. Of those published more recently, several address general issues,[47, 48, 49, 50, 51] three have focused on psychosocial aspects,[52, 53, 54] one on neck dissection,[55] and three on the issue of questionnaires.[21, 56, 57]

The HRQOL of patients with HNC can be compared to normative reference data and other disease states. There are reference data for many general questionnaires, such as the Medical Outcomes Short Form 36 (SF 36). Patients with HNC scored lower than norms, particularly for physical role limitation, mental role limitation and social functioning. There was a strong association found between tumour stage and severity of pain. At three months following surgery, there was a considerable deterioration in physical functioning, limitation of physical role, energy and general health perception. There was little change in domains between three

and six months. By 12 months postoperatively, patients approached pretreatment scores. Patients with posterior sites tended to have a bigger deterioration in scores to one year than patients with anterior sites, most notably in social function.[58] Using the EQ-5D compared to national reference data, patients under 60 years of age fared significantly worse than expected for their age, but this was not so for older patients. Older patients had a QOL similar to what would have been expected for their non-cancer peers and the fall in QOL over time in the cancer group seems to mirror the expected age-related changes.[59] Also, comparison has been made using head and neck cancer-specific questionnaires in a general population. Compared to a group of patients attending for a check up at their dentist, the key differences at baseline were anxiety, pain, swallowing, chewing and mood. At one year, there were big differences in all domains with deterioration in the oral cancer group. The difference was least notable in pain, shoulder, mood and anxiety. Eighty-three per cent of the people attending their dentist, compared to 78 per cent of the cancer group at one year, either reported good, very good or outstanding QOL.[60]

It is possible to compare HNC with other disease states by using general questionnaires. For example, comparison using the EQ-5D mean VAS score suggests that HNC patients fit in the middle of a range from no illness, psoriasis, liver transplant, cystic fibrosis, HNC, irritable bowel syndrome, HIV, chronic liver disease, dementia and chronic fatigue syndrome.

HRQOL outcome in general in different HNC sites

There is a great deal of published data from which an indication can be gleaned as to the difference in HRQOL between different sites.[61, 62, 63, 64]

Papers have either reported HRQOL in a mixture of head and neck patients or specific to a subsite, such as oral cavity, oropharynx and larynx. There were a few sites excluded, as they are not usually considered in the main group. Specific examples include parotid,[65] oesophageal,[66] thyroid,[67] skull base[68] and non-melanoma cervicofacial skin cancer.[69]

It is often easier to use a graph to depict the data contained in tables (**Figure 10.1**). This shows that the HRQOL is similar across the different subsites at presentation, that there is a dip in the first three to six months following treatment, and a plateau over the longer term. It has been suggested that outcome at one year reflects the long-term situation.[70] The graph also demonstrates that the HRQOL outcome is potentially better for laryngeal and oral cavity subsites compared to oropharynx and hypopharynx. In clinical practice, the poor HRQOL in oropharynx and pharynolarynx has influenced the treatment protocols aimed at organ preservation. However, it must be considered that HRQOL outcome and individual domains are significantly affected by the stage of the cancer and the use of combined treatment modalities. Also, domains can move in different directions (get better or worse). For example, from pretreatment to follow up, anxiety, mood and pain can improve following primary surgery for oral and oropharyngeal cancer, while the other function domains deteriorate.[71] What the patients

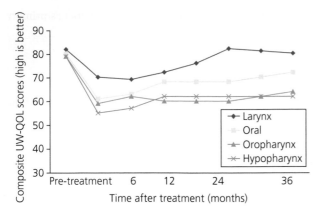

Figure 10.1   Health-related quality of life (HRQOL) over time from diagnosis comparing larygeal, oral, oropharyngeal and hypopharyngeal sites.

consider as important domains can differ and hence the impact on their HRQOL as a result of changes in different domains can influence outcome if those domains considered most important are most severely affected.[33]

Patients most at risk of a poor HRQOL outcome

There are a number of different patient and treatment factors that are associated with HRQOL. These include age, gender, site, stage, emotional status, smoking and alcohol, marital status and income, performance status, method of reconstruction, access, mandibular resection, neck dissection, percutaneous endoscopic gastrostomy and postoperative radiotherapy.[8, 51] It is possible to postulate some of the patient characteristics which are associated with poor outcome (**Box 10.5**). In recognizing this, it might be appropriate to discuss different treatment strategies that should be the standard protocol or it might be possible to arrange additional support for the patient and their carer. The rationale for identifying this group as having potential problems with HRQOL is explained further in the next section.

Key HRQOL issues

In this section, the most common HRQOL issues in patients with HNC will be explored (**Box 10.6**). Focus will be on the more recent literature.

COPING

The patient might find it difficult to cope and, if cured, may become less satisfied with the residual level of dysfunction. The appreciation and promotion of coping strategies is an important facet of optimizing HRQOL, as at times there is very little to be done to improve a handicap following such surgery. Family and carer support is vital. As much as possible should be done to assist the patient's carers in the cancer journey. It has been said that 'learning to live with cancer is no easy task … learning to live with someone else's cancer

> **Box 10.5   Possible problem pool**
>
> - Alcohol abuse
> - Deprivation
> - Personality
> - Pre-existing distress
> - Single with poor family support structure
> - Site: Oropharynx and hypopharynx
> - Stage IV disease
> - Younger patient
> - Unknown factors

> **Box 10.6   Key issues**
>
> - Coping
> - Dental status
> - Disfigurement
> - Emotion
> - Fear of recurrence
> - Function
> - Oral rehabilitation
> - Pain
> - Personality
> - Sociodemographic
> - Speech
> - Swallowing
> - Shoulder
> - Xerostomia

may be even more difficult'. Denial, alcohol and fatalism are examples of poor coping styles.[72] An avoidance-focused coping style was generally associated with lowered HRQOL. There seems to be a stronger association between HRQOL and coping style, which in part relates to cognitive and emotional function.[73] Interventions aimed at improving coping can be effective in improving quality of life and reduce depressive symptoms in HNC patients. A short-term psychoeducational coping strategies intervention showed that compared with their baseline scores, the intervention group had improved physical and social functioning, global quality of life, fatigue, sleep disturbance than the matched control subjects.[74]

Dental status

Although there is a limited research base, some studies in the non-HNC population show significant associations between oral health status and HRQOL[75] Teeth are important for the appearance of a smile, as well as chewing, and optimal dental care is essential for both dentate and edentulous patients. It is recognized that there is a deterioration in masticatory efficiencies following treatment of oral cancer.[76] In oral cancer in particular, dental status is important, as patients tend to be limited to semisolid diets postoperatively and have difficulty wearing dentures.[77] Dental status is important in HRQOL. Partially dentate individuals without dentures fair worse and tend to report a poorer HRQOL and also more 'problems with their teeth', 'trouble eating', and 'trouble enjoying meals'.[78] It is helpful before treatment starts to have an understanding of the patient's dental expectations and motivation so that appropriate dental care can be planned on an individual basis.

DISFIGUREMENT

In HNC, disfigurement has been identified as a key HRQOL domain for many years.[79, 80] The domain is common to the head and neck-specific HRQOL questionnaires. Following HNC, there can be overt alteration in body structure, loss of function and its implications for social interaction have been associated with depression.[81] Any additional burden of communication difficulties and social rejection greatly confounds the problems experienced.[82] Appearance concerns can be missed in a busy clinical setting[11] and efforts should be made to identify problems as simple advice, counselling therapy, camouflage and possible revision surgery might help alleviate distress.

EMOTION

Several studies over the years have reported a high incidence of psychological distress in this patient population.[83, 84] Anxiety is at its highest before treatment, and both anxiety and depression tend to improve from this baseline. Some patients have pre-existing psychological distress and this group find the cancer diagnosis much harder to deal with. Depression is also common along with worry, anxiety, mood disorders and fatigue.[85] Psychological interventions have a role in reducing this distress. Early detection and appropriate specialist referral are integral components of patient care. It is possible to screen for psychological morbidity relatively easily using the HAD. In addition, single item domain measures would appear to be effective.[86]

FEAR OF RECURRENCE

Recurrence following HNC tends to occur within the first two years following treatment. This is a particularly stressful time for patient and carers. One study reported that at three months post-treatment, over 80 per cent of patients expressed concern over the possibility of recurrence and that this level reduced to 72 per cent at seven months.[87, 88] Fears of recurrent disease remain for some time following initial treatment and are not necessarily related to the stage of disease or radicality of treatment. There is an association with psychological morbidity, especially anxiety. Therefore, an attempt should be made to identify patients who have a notable fear of recurrence and they should be offered appropriate support.

FUNCTION

The importance of function in HNC is reflected in the number of domains that tap into these issues in the HNC questionnaires. In most situations, the better the functional outcome following treatment the better the HRQOL as function and HRQOL are inextricably linked.[89] With better function, the patient perceives fewer consequences as a result of cancer and this leads to better acceptance of the situation and QOL. There are many ways of limiting the functional deficits following surgery[90] and ways of preserving function in laryngeal malignancy.[91] Good function has many components and its precise HRQOL 'value' in clinical practice remains elusive, as function is strongly influenced by the extent of disease at presentation where the patient's primary concern is for cure.

ORAL REHABILITATION

Oral rehabilitation is a key aspect of HRQOL by virtue of the importance to human existence of social interaction, eating and drinking. A patient's HRQOL is improved if they are successfully rehabilitated.[92] There are many aspects to oral rehabilitation which by necessity are beyond the scope of this chapter; however, there are notable positive effects on eating,[93] effective restoration of the mandible,[94, 95] appropriate use of obturation,[96, 97] benefit of osseointegrated implants in allowing rehabilitation to be achieved[98, 99] and minimizing trismus.[100]

PAIN

Pain has been considered a critical aspect of HRQOL and indeed uncontrolled pain is of major significance in the patient's well-being.[101] Head and neck pain is heterogeneous in nature and influenced by other factors such as distress or dysfunction.[102] It would appear that patients having both surgery and radiotherapy were significantly more likely to have troublesome pain.[103] However, better analgesia regimes tend to mean that pain is well controlled following successful treatment and hence functional disorders play the more dominant role.[104]

PERSONALITY

Personality is a predictor of HRQOL in HNC patients. It has been suggested that before treatment, optimists report better role, cognitive and emotional function, less pain and fatigue and a better global rating of HRQOL than did pessimists. Following treatment, optimists report better role and cognitive functioning, less pain and better global HRQOL than did pessimists. Pessimists reported a greater deterioration in the role domain following treatment than did optimists.[105] High neuroticism, but not extraversion, has been associated with a lowered QOL.[106] A sense of humour is beneficial to HRQOL.[107] Interestingly, neuroticism has been associated with a risk of HNC as a result of increased alcohol consumption implicating a link between personality trait and the prognosis.[108] Personality has also been associated with one-year survival independent of other sociodemographic and clinical variables.[109]

SOCIODEMOGRAPHIC

Deprivation influences the incidence and outcome of patients with cancer. At presentation, HRQOL was not linked to deprivation, however, following surgery patients from more deprived areas reported poorer HRQOL especially in the pain domain. Living alone, and heavy alcohol and smoking consumption were associated with lower HRQOL scores and, as these are linked with deprivation, they could be used to heighten awareness among the head and neck team of a patient at risk.[110] In patients with oral cancer treated with microvascular free-flap reconstruction, sociodemographic factors have been shown to predict quality of life. In addition, heavy drinking and unemployment have been associated with an increase in risk of death[111] and can influence cognitive functioning.[112] Marital status may influence prognosis through mechanisms of health behaviour and/or social support mechanisms.[112]

SPEECH

Speech is a key HRQOL domain in HNC. As a functional issue, it is repeatedly cited as one of the most important aspects by patients.[33, 86] In the oral cavity and oropharynx, primary closure when feasible is a better option than free flap reconstruction, in relation to postoperative swallowing and speech function.[113] There are several recent papers that address the issue of HRQOL and speech and specialist assessment and intervention is essential in order to help address the needs of HNC patients.[71, 114, 115, 116, 117, 118, 119, 120]

SWALLOWING

In the oropharynx, surgical resection seems to affect swallowing more than speech.[113] Chemoradiation rather than surgery, followed by radiation, for oropharyngeal primaries has been associated with significantly better emotional and functional scores. The difference is much less noticeable for laryngeal and hypopharyngeal primaries.[40] Nutritional support is paramount and, when comparing patients with dysphagia from a variety of medical conditions, long-term nutrition via the feeding tube maintained the patients' quality of life.[121] However, for HNC patients, the presence of a feeding tube was found to be the strongest negative predictor of QOL.[8] In patients with long-term feeding tubes following surgery for oral and oropharyngeal cancer, those with PEGs reported significant deficits in all UW-QOL domains compared to non-PEG or PEG-removed patients, and also reported a much poorer quality of life. The major PEG-related problems were not those of discomfort, leakage or blockage, but interference with family life, intimate relationships, social activities, and hobbies. More can be done to counsel and support patients with long-term PEG placement.[26]

SHOULDER

There is an appreciation of the significant detrimental impact on shoulder function following a modified radical and radical neck dissection.[122, 123] This has led to a change in practice toward more selective approaches.[55] The problems are much less following function preserving neck dissections, but radiotherapy might cause additional problems.[124, 125] However, even after a unilateral selective level 1 to 3 clearance, there was significant loss of shoulder flexion and abduction in the operated side compared to the non-operated side, but not in regard to the other cervical spine and shoulder measurements.[126] The benefit of performing sentinel node biopsy on HRQOL is yet to be fully evaluated. Physiotherapists have a role in screening patients with shoulder dysfunction postoperatively, thus allowing early intervention.

XEROSTOMIA

Xerostomia can have a significant impact on the quality of life of patients treated by radiation therapy. Treatment can result in a profoundly dry mouth which causes additional problems with eating, swallowing, dental health and speech. In a study by Wijers et al.,[127] 64 per cent of the long-term survivors still experienced a moderate to severe degree of permanent xerostomia after treatment by conventional two-dimensional radiation therapy. Adjuvant radiotherapy after primary surgery is identified as one of the biggest detrimental factors to HRQOL,[70] but is used on the premise that cure rates are improved.[92] Recently, there has been a great deal of interest in ways of reducing xerostomia and its potential beneficial impact on HRQOL.[28, 128, 129, 130, 131, 132, 133] Early results are proving very encouraging.

CONCLUDING REMARKS

In conclusion, the evaluation of HRQOL in patients with head and neck cancer is integral to optimal patient care. Survival is usually the initial primary concern of patients, however after treatment there is a shift towards HRQOL and living with the consequences of head and neck cancer treatment (survivorship). It is feasible for HRQOL evaluation to be part of routine clinical practice and this supports holistic care for individual patients and their carers.

KEY EVIDENCE

- HRQOL information can change clinical practice both in terms of treatment protocols and strategies and also in terms of individualized patient care.[134]
- The patient's perspective of outcome is a critical component of healthcare evaluation.[34]
- There is a tremendous amount of HRQOL literature available to allow the clinical team to inform both patient and carers.[135]

KEY LEARNING POINTS

- HRQOL outcomes can help to provide a holistic assessment integrated into clinical practice.
- The problems patients report following treatment for head and neck cancer (survivorship issues) can be addressed through interventions. Interventions need to include couple therapy and family therapy and practitioners need to be trained in these approaches, as well as individual counselling.
- Patient Report Outcomes measures combined with objective evaluation provide a much better evaluation than either alone.

> • There are still inadequate outcomes data on the late effects of treatment and the comparison between surgical approach and 'organ preservation'.

REFERENCES

1. World Health Organization. What quality of life? The WHOQOL Group. In: World Health Forum vol. 17. Geneva: WHO, 1996: 354–6.

2. Ferrans CE. Quality of life: conceptual issues. *Seminars in Oncology Nursing* 1990; **6**: 248–54.

3. Calman KC. Definitions and dimensions of quality of life In: Aaronson NK, Beckmann J (eds). *The quality of life of cancer patients*. New York: Raven Press, 1987: 1–9.

4. Morton RP. QOL measures in head and neck cancer. Capabilities and caveats. *Current Oncology* 1995; **2**: 77–83.

5. Morton RP, Izzard ME. Quality of life in head and neck cancer patients. *World Journal of Surgery* 2003; **27**: 884–9.

6. Aaronson NK, Ahmedzai S, Bergman B *et al*. The European Organisation for Research and Treatment of Cancer QLQ-C30: a quality-of-life instrument for use in international clinical trials in oncology. *Journal of the National Cancer Institute* 1993; **85**: 365–76.

7. Brown JS, Zuydam A, Jones C *et al*. Soft palate reconstruction using a radial forearm free flap in conjunction with a superiorly based pharyngeal flap and radial forearm free tissue transfer. *Head and Neck* 1997; **19**: 524–34.

8. Terrell JE, Ronis DL, Fowler KE *et al*. Clinical predictors of quality of life in patients with head and neck cancer. *Archives of Otolaryngology – Head and Neck Surgery* 2004; **130**: 401–8.

9. Rider WD, Harwood AR. The Toronto philosophy of management in head and neck cancer. *Journal of Otolaryngology* 1982; **11**: 14–16.

10. Maher EJ, Jefferis AF. Decision making in advanced cancer of the head and neck: variations in the views of medical specialists. *Journal of the Royal Society of Medicine* 1990; **83**: 356–9.

11. Millsopp L, Brandom L, Humphris G *et al*. Facial appearance after operations for oral and oropharyngeal cancer: A comparison of casenotes and patient-completed questionnaire. *British Journal of Oral and Maxillofacial Surgery* 2006; **44**: 358–63.

12. Hopkins A. *Measures of the quality of life and the uses to which such measures may be put*. London: Royal College of Physicians of London, 1992.

13. Higginson IJ, Carr AJ. Measuring quality of life: using quality of life measures in the clinical setting. *British Medical Journal* 2001; **322**: 1297–300.

14. Velikova G, Booth L, Smith AB *et al*. Measuring quality of life in routine oncology practice improves communication and patient well-being: a randomized controlled trial. *Journal of Clinical Oncology* 2004; **22**: 714–24.

15. Hammerlid E, Persson LO, Sullivan M, Westin T. Quality-of-life effects of psychosocial intervention in patients with head and neck cancer. *Otolaryngology and Head and Neck Surgery* 1999; **120**: 507–16.

16. Stoeckli SJ, Schnieper I, Huguenin P, Schmid S. Early glottic carcinoma: treatment according patient's preference. *Head and Neck* 2003; **25**: 1051–6.

17. Rogers SN, Fisher SE, Woolgar JA. A review of quality of life assessment in oral cancer. *International Journal of Oral and Maxillofacial Surgery* 1999; **28**: 99–117.

18. Allison PJ, Locker D, Feine JS. Quality of life: a dynamic construct. *Social Science and Medicine* 1997; **45**: 221–30.

19. Breetvelt IS, Van Dam FS. Underreporting by cancer patients: the case of response-shift. *Social Science and Medicine* 1991; **32**: 981–7.

20. Maguire P, Selby P. Assessing quality of life in cancer patients. *British Journal of Cancer* 1989; **60**: 437–40.

21. Ringash J, Bezjak A. A structured review of quality of life instruments for head and neck cancer patients. *Head and Neck* 2001; **23**: 201–13.

22. Varricchio CG. Relevance of quality of life to clinical nursing practice. *Seminars in Oncology Nursing* 1990; **6**: 255–9.

23. Sadura A, Pater J, Osoba D *et al*. Quality-of-life assessment: patient compliance with questionnaire completion. *Journal of the National Cancer Institute* 1992; **84**: 1023–6.

24. Chen AY, Frankowski R, Bishop-Leone J *et al*. The development and validation of a dysphagia-specific quality-of-life questionnaire for patients with head and neck cancer: the M.D. Anderson dysphagia inventory. *Archives of Otolaryngology, Head and Neck Surgery* 2001; **127**: 870–6.

25. Pace-Balzan A, Cawood JI, Howell R *et al*. The Liverpool Oral Rehabilitation Questionnaire: a pilot study. *Journal of Oral Rehabilitation* 2004; **31**: 609–17.

26. Rogers SN, Thomson R, O'Toole P, Lowe D. Patients experience with long-term percutaneous endoscopic gastrostomy feeding following primary surgery for oral and oropharyngeal cancer. *Oral Oncology* 2007; **43**: 499–507.

27. Taylor RJ, Chepeha JC, Teknos TN *et al*. Development and validation of the neck dissection impairment index. *Archives of Otolaryngology – Head and Neck Surgery* 2002; **128**: 44–9.

28. Henson BS, Inglehart MR, Eisbruch A, Ship JA. Preserved salivary output and xerostomia-related quality of life in head and neck cancer patients receiving parotid-sparing radiotherapy. *Oral Oncology* 2001; **37**: 84–93.

29. Rabin R, de Charro F. EQ-5D: a measure of health status from the EuroQol Group. *Annals of Medicine* 2001; **33**: 337–43.

30. Ware JE, Sherbourne CD. A 36-item short-form health survey (SF36): conceptual framework and item selection. *Medical Care* 1992; **30**: 473–83.

31. List MA, Ritter-Sterr C, Lansky SB. A performance status scale for head and neck cancer patients. *Cancer* 1990; **66**: 564–9.

32. Bjordal K, Kaasa S. Psychometric validation of the EORTC Core Quality of Life Questionnaire, 30-item version and a diagnosis-specific module for head and neck cancer patients. *Acta Oncologica* 1992; **31**: 311–21.

33. Rogers SN, Laher SH, Overend L, Lowe D. Importance-rating using the University of Washington Quality of Life questionnaire in patients treated by primary surgery for oral and oro-pharyngeal cancer. *Journal of Craniomaxillofacial Surgery* 2002; **30**: 125–32.

◆ 34. Rogers SN. Quality of life perspectives in patients with oral cancer. *Oral Oncology* 2010; **46**: 445–7.

35. Rathmell AJ, Ash DV, Howes M, Nicholls J. Assessing quality of life in patients treated for advanced head and neck cancer. *Clinical Oncology* 1991; **3**: 10–16.

36. Browman GP, Levine MN, Hodson DI et al. The Head and Neck Radiotherapy Questionnaire: a morbidity/quality-of-life instrument for clinical trials of radiation therapy in locally advanced head and neck cancer. *Journal of Clinical Oncology* 1993; **11**: 863–72.

37. Baker C, Schuller DE. A functional status scale for measuring quality of life outcomes in head and neck cancer patients. *Cancer Nursing* 1995; **18**: 452–7.

38. Funk GF, Karnell LH, Dawson CJ et al. Baseline and post-treatment assessment of the general health status of head and neck cancer patients compared with United States population norms. *Head and Neck* 1997; **19**: 675–83.

39. Gliklich RE, Goldsmith TA, Funk GF. Are head and neck specific quality of life measures necessary? *Head and Neck* 1997; **19**: 474–80.

40. Gillespie MB, Brodsky MB, Day TA et al. Swallowing-related quality of life after head and neck cancer treatment. *Laryngoscope* 2004; **114**: 1362–7.

41. Young PE, Beasley NJ, Houghton DJ et al. A new short practical quality of life questionnaire for use in head and neck oncology outpatient clinics. *Clinical Otolaryngology* 1998; **23**: 528–32.

42. Ackerstaff AH, Lindeboom JA, Balm AJ et al. Structured assessment of the consequences of composite resection. *Clinical Otolaryngology and Allied Sciences* 1998; **23**: 339–44.

43. Rogers SN, Rajlawat B, Goru J et al. Comparison of the domains of anxiety and mood of the University of Washington Head and Neck Cancer Questionnaire (UW-QOL V4) with the CES-D and HADS. *Head and Neck* 2006; **28**: 697–704.

44. Mehanna HM, Morton RP. Patients' views on the utility of quality of life questionnaires in head and neck cancer. *Clinical Otolaryngology* 2006; **31**: 310–6.

● 45. Sharp HM, List M, MacCracken E et al. Patients' priorities among treatment effects in head and neck cancer: evaluation of a new assessment tool. *Head and Neck* 1999; **21**: 538–46.

46. List MA, Stracks J, Colangelo L et al. How do head and neck cancer patients prioritize treatment outcomes before initiating treatment? *Journal of Clinical Oncology* 2000; **18**: 877–84.

47. Ferlito A, Rogers SN, Shaha AR et al. Quality of life in head and neck cancer. *Acta Otolaryngologica* 2003; **123**: 5–7.

48. Baliga MD. Re: Anderson G, Lewthwaite A, Yeats N. Quality of life following surgery for oral and pharyngeal malignancy. *British Journal of Oral and Maxillofacial Surgery* 2001; **39**: 163.

49. Langenhoff BS, Krabbe PF, Wobbes T, Ruers TJ. Quality of life as an outcome measure in surgical oncology. *British Journal of Surgery* 2001; **88**: 643–52.

50. Stoikova MS, Maslinkova JG. A review of scales for assessment of the quality of life (QOL) in patients with oral cavity cancer. *Folia Medica (Plovdiv)* 2001; **43**: 160–3.

51. Chandu A, Smith AC, Rogers SN. Health-related quality of life in oral cancer: a review. *Journal of Oral and Maxillofacial Surgery* 2006; **64**: 495–502.

52. Ledeboer QC, Velden LA, Boer MF et al. Physical and psychosocial correlates of head and neck cancer: an update of the literature and challenges for the future. *Clinical Otolaryngology* 2005; **30**: 303–19.

53. Llewellyn CD, McGurk M, Weinman J. Are psycho-social and behavioural factors related to health related-quality of life in patients with head and neck cancer? A systematic review. *Oral Oncology* 2005; **41**: 440–54.

54. Owen C, Watkinson JC, Pracy P, Glaholm J. The psychosocial impact of head and neck cancer. *Clinical Otolaryngology and Allied Sciences* 2001; **26**: 351–6.

55. Rogers SN, Ferlito A, Pellitteri PK et al. Quality of life following neck dissections. *Acta Otolaryngologica* 2004; **124**: 231–6.

56. Fung K, Terrell JE. Outcomes research in head and neck cancer. *Journal of Otorhinolaryngology and Related Specialties* 2004; **66**: 207–13.

57. Hecker DM, Wiens JP, Cowper TR et al. American Academy of Maxillofacial Prosthetics. Can we assess quality of life in patients with head and neck cancer? A preliminary report from the American Academy of Maxillofacial Prosthetics. *Journal of Prosthetic Dentistry* 2002; **88**: 344–51.

58. Rogers SN, Humphris G, Lowe D et al. The impact of surgery for oral cancer on quality of life as measured by the Medical Outcomes Short Form 36. *European Journal of Cancer and Oral Oncology* 1998; **34**: 171–9.

59. Rogers SN, Miller RD, Ali K et al. Patients perceived health status following primary surgery for oral and oropharyngeal cancer. *International Journal of Oral and Maxillofacial Surgery* 2006; **35**: 913–19.

60. Rogers SN, O'Donnell JP, Williams-Hewitt S et al. Health-related quality of life measured by the UWQOL – reference values from a general dental practice. *Oral Oncology* 2006; **42**: 281–7.

61. Bjordal K, de Graeff A, Fayers PM *et al.* A 12 country field study of the EORTC QLQ-C30 and head and neck specific module (EORTC QLQ-H&N35). *European Journal of Cancer* 2000; **36**: 1796–807.

62. de Graeff A, de Leeuw JR, Ros WJ *et al.* A prospective study on quality of life of patients with cancer of the oral cavity or oropharynx treated with surgery with or without radiotherapy. *Oral Oncology* 1999; **35**: 27–32.

63. Rogers SN, Lowe D, Brown JS, Vaughan ED. The University of Washington Head and Neck cancer measure as a predictor of outcome following primary surgery for oral cancer. *Head and Neck* 1999; **21**: 394–401.

● 64. Weymuller EA, Yueh B, Deleyiannis FW *et al.* Quality of life in patients with head and neck cancer: lessons learned from 549 prospectively evaluated patients. *Archives of Otolaryngology – Head and Neck Surgery* 2000; **126**: 329–35.

65. Nitzan D, Kronenberg J, Horowitz Z *et al.* Quality of life following parotidectomy for malignant and benign disease. *Plastic and Reconstructive Surgery* 2004; **114**: 1060–7.

66. Viklund P, Lindblad M, Lagergren J. Influence of surgery-related factors on quality of life after esophageal or cardia cancer resection. *World Journal of Surgery* 2005; **29**: 841–8.

67. Dagan T, Bedrin L, Horowitz Z *et al.* Quality of life of well-differentiated thyroid carcinoma patients. *Journal of Laryngology and Otology* 2004; **118**: 537–42.

68. Gil Z, Abergel A, Spektor S *et al.* Development of a cancer-specific anterior skull base quality-of-life questionnaire. *Journal of Neurosurgery* 2004; **100**: 813–19.

69. Rhee JS, Loberiza FR, Matthews BA *et al.* Quality of life assessment in nonmelanoma cervicofacial skin cancer. *Laryngoscope* 2003; **113**: 215–20.

70. Rogers SN, Hannah L, Lowe D, Magennis P. Quality of life 5–10 years after primary surgery for oral and oro-pharyngeal cancer. *Journal of Craniomaxillofacial Surgery* 1999; **27**: 187–91.

71. Radford K, Woods H, Lowe D, Rogers SN. A UK multi-centre pilot study of speech and swallowing outcomes following head and neck cancer. *Clinical Otolaryngology and Allied Sciences* 2004; **29**: 376–81.

72. Dropkin MJ. Anxiety, coping strategies, and coping behaviors in patients undergoing head and neck cancer surgery. *Cancer Nursing* 2001; **24**: 143–8.

73. Aarstad AK, Aarstad HJ, Bru E, Olofsson J. Psychological coping style versus disease extent, tumour treatment and quality of life in successfully treated head and neck squamous cell carcinoma patients. *Clinical Otolaryngology* 2005; **30**: 530–8.

74. Vilela LD, Nicolau B, Mahmud S *et al.* Comparison of psychosocial outcomes in head and neck cancer patients receiving a coping strategies intervention and control subjects receiving no intervention. *Journal of Otolaryngology* 2006; **35**: 88–96.

75. Naito M, Yuasa H, Nomura Y *et al.* Oral health status and health-related quality of life: a systematic review. *Journal of Oral Science* 2006; **48**: 1–7.

76. Namaki S, Matsumoto M, Ohba H *et al.* Masticatory efficiency before and after surgery in oral cancer patients: comparative study of glossectomy, marginal mandibulectomy and segmental mandibulectomy. *Journal of Oral Science* 2004; **46**: 113–17.

77. Finlay PM, Dawson F, Robertson AG, Soutar DS. An evaluation of functional outcome after surgery and radiotherapy for intra-oral cancer. *British Journal of Maxillofacial Surgery* 1992; **30**: 14–17.

78. Allison PJ, Locker D, Feine JS. The relationship between dental status and health-related quality of life in upper aerodigestive tract cancer. *European Journal of Cancer and Oral Oncology* 1999; **35**: 138–43.

79. Dropkin MJ. Disfigurement and dysfunction with head and neck cancer surgery. *Head and Neck Nursing* 1998; **16**: 28–9.

80. Katz MR, Irish JC, Devins GM *et al.* Psychosocial adjustment in head and neck cancer: the impact of disfigurement, gender and social support. *Head and Neck* 2003; **25**: 103–12.

81. D'Antonio LL, Long SA, Zimmerman GJ *et al.* Relationship between quality of life and depression in patients with head and neck cancer. *Laryngoscope* 1998; **108**: 806–11.

82. Dropkin MJ. Body image and quality of life after head and neck cancer surgery. *Cancer Practice* 1999; **7**: 309–13.

83. de Leeuw JR, de Graeff A, Ros WJ *et al.* Prediction of depression 6 months to 3 years after treatment of head and neck cancer. *Head and Neck* 2001; **23**: 892–8.

84. Katz MR, Kopek N, Waldron J *et al.* Screening for depression in head and neck cancer. *Psycho-oncology* 2004; **13**: 269–80.

85. de Boer MF, McCormick LK, Pruyn JF *et al.* Physical and psychosocial correlates of head and neck cancer: a review of the literature. *Otolaryngology and Head and Neck Surgery* 1999; **120**: 427–36.

86. Rogers SN, Gwanne S, Lowe D *et al.* The addition of mood and anxiety domains to the University of Washington quality of life scale. *Head and Neck* 2002; **24**: 521–9.

87. Humphris GM, Rogers SN, McNally D *et al.* Fear of recurrence and possible cases of anxiety and depression in orofacial cancer patients. *International Journal of Oral and Maxillofacial Surgery* 2003; **32**: 486–91.

88. Humphris GM, Rogers SN. The association of cigarette smoking and anxiety, depression and fears of recurrence in patients following treatment of oral and oropharyngeal cancer. *European Journal of Cancer Care* 2004; **13**: 328–35.

89. Rogers SN, Lowe D, Fisher SE *et al.* Health related quality of life and clinical function in patients treated by primary surgery for oral cancer. *British Journal of Oral and Maxillofacial Surgery* 2002; **40**: 11–18.

90. Rogers SN. Surgical principles and techniques for functional rehabilitation after oral cavity/oropharyngeal

oncological surgery. *Current Opinion in Otolaryngology and Head and Neck Surgery* 2001; **9**: 114–19.

91. Lefebvre JL. Laryngeal preservation in head and neck cancer: multidisciplinary approach. *Lancet Oncology* 2006; **7**: 747–55.

92. Rogers SN, McNally D, Mahmood M *et al.* The psychological response of the edentulous patient following primary surgery for oral cancer: a cross-sectional study. *Journal of Prosthetic Dentistry* 1999; **82**: 317–21.

93. Beeken L, Calman F. A return to 'normal eating' after curative treatment for oral cancer. What are the long-term prospects? *European Journal of Cancer, B Oral Oncology* 1994; **30B**: 387–92.

94. Wilson KM, Rizk NM, Armstrong SL, Gluckman JL. Effects of hemimandibulectomy on quality of life. *Laryngoscope* 1998; **108**: 1574–7.

95. Rogers SN, Devine J, Lowe D *et al.* Longitudinal health-related quality of life following mandibular resection for oral cancer: A comparison between rim and segment. *Head and Neck* 2004; **26**: 54–62.

96. Moroi HH, Okimoto K, Terada Y. The effect of an oral prosthesis on the quality of life for head and neck cancer patients. *Journal of Oral Rehabilitation* 1999; **26**: 265–73.

97. Rogers SN, Lowe D, McNally D *et al.* Health-related quality of life after maxillectomy: a comparison between prosthetic obturation and free flap. *Journal of Oral and Maxillofacial Surgery* 2003; **61**: 174–81.

98. Shaw RJ, Sutton AF, Cawood JI *et al.* Oral rehabilitation following treatment for head and neck malignancy. *Head and Neck* 2005; **27**: 459–70.

99. Rogers SN, Panasar J, Pritchard K *et al.* A survey of oral rehabilitation in a consecutive series of 130 patients treated by primary surgery for oral and oro-pharyngeal squamous cell carcinoma. *British Journal of Oral and Maxillofacial Surgery* 2005; **43**: 23–30.

100. Cohen EG, Deschler DG, Walsh K, Hayden RE. Early use of a mechanical stretching device to improve mandibular mobility after composite resection: a pilot study. *Archives of Physical Medicine and Rehabilitation* 2005; **86**: 1416–19.

101. Keefe FJ, Brantley A, Manuel G, Crisson JE. Behavioural assessment of head and neck cancer pain. *Pain* 1985; **23**: 327–36.

102. Connelly ST, Schmidt BL. Evaluation of pain in patients with oral squamous cell carcinoma. *Journal of Pain* 2004; **5**: 505–10.

103. Whale Z, Lyne PA, Papanikolaou P. Pain experience following radical treatment for head and neck cancer. *European Journal of Oncology Nursing* 2001; **5**: 112–20.

104. Gellrich NC, Schimming R, Schramm A *et al.* Pain, function, and psychologic outcome before, during, and after intraoral tumor resection. *Journal of Oral and Maxillofacial Surgery* 2002; **60**: 772–7.

105. Allison PJ, Guichard C, Gilain L. A prospective investigation of dispositional optimism as a predictor of health-related quality of life in head and neck cancer patients. *Quality of Life Research* 2000; **9**: 951–60.

106. Aarstad HJ, Aarstad AK, Birkhaug EJ *et al.* The personality and quality of life in HNSCC patients following treatment. *European Journal of Cancer* 2003; **39**: 1852–60.

107. Aarstad HJ, Aarstad AK, Heimdal JH, Olofsson J. Mood, anxiety and sense of humor in head and neck cancer patients in relation to disease stage, prognosis and quality of life. *Acta Otolaryngologica* 2005; **125**: 557–65.

108. Aarstad HJ, Heimdal JH, Aarstad AK, Olofsson J. Personality traits in head and neck squamous cell carcinoma patients in relation to the disease state, disease extent and prognosis. *Acta Otolaryngologica* 2002; **122**: 892–9.

109. Allison PJ, Guichard C, Fung K, Gilain L. Dispositional optimism predicts survival status 1 year after diagnosis in head and neck cancer patients. *Journal of Clinical Oncology* 2003; **21**: 543–8.

110. Woolley E, Magennis P, Shokar P *et al.* The correlation between indices of deprivation and health-related quality of life in patients with oral and oropharyngeal squamous cell carcinoma. *British Journal of Oral and Maxillofacial Surgery* 2006; **44**: 177–86.

111. Markkanen-Leppanen M, Makitie AA, Haapanen ML *et al.* Quality of life after free-flap reconstruction in patients with oral and pharyngeal cancer. *Head and Neck* 2006; **28**: 210–16.

112. de Graeff A, de Leeuw JR, Ros WJ *et al.* Sociodemographic factors and quality of life as prognostic indicators in head and neck cancer. *European Journal of Cancer* 2001; **37**: 332–9.

113. Zuydam AC, Lowe D, Brown JS *et al.* The speech and swallowing aspect of health-related quality of life following primary surgery for oral and oropharyngeal cancer. *Clinical Otolaryngology* 2005; **30**: 428–37.

114. Loughran S, Calder N, MacGregor FB *et al.* Quality of life and voice following endoscopic resection or radiotherapy for early glottic cancer. *Clinical Otolaryngology* 2005; **30**: 42–7.

115. Sewnaik A, van den Brink JL, Wieringa MH *et al.* Surgery for recurrent laryngeal carcinoma after radiotherapy: partial laryngectomy or total laryngectomy for a better quality of life? *Otolaryngology and Head and Neck Surgery* 2005; **132**: 95–8.

116. Meyer TK, Kuhn JC, Campbell BH *et al.* Speech intelligibility and quality of life in head and neck cancer survivors. *Laryngoscope* 2004; **114**: 1977–81.

117. Plouin-Gaudon I, Lengele B, Desuter G *et al.* Conservation laryngeal surgery for selected pyriform sinus cancer. *European Journal of Surgical Oncology* 2004; **30**: 1123–30.

118. Smith JC, Johnson JT, Cognetti DM *et al.* Quality of life, functional outcome, and costs of early glottic cancer. *Laryngoscope* 2003; **113**: 68–76.

119. Alves CB, Loughran S, MacGregor FB *et al.* Bioplastique medialization therapy improves the quality of life in

terminally ill patients with vocal cord palsy. *Clinical Otolaryngology and Allied Sciences* 2002; **27**: 387–91.

120. Finizia C, Bergman B. Health-related quality of life in patients with laryngeal cancer: a post-treatment comparison of different modes of communication. *Laryngoscope* 2001; **111**: 918–23.

121. Klose J, Heldwein W, Rafferzeder M *et al.* Nutritional status and quality of life in patients with percutaneous endoscopic gastrostomy (PEG) in practice: prospective one-year follow-up. *Digestive Diseases and Sciences* 2003; **48**: 2057–63.

122. Kuntz AL, Weymuller EA Jr. Impact of neck dissection on quality of life. *Laryngoscope* 1999; **109**: 1334–8.

123. van Wilgen CP, Dijkstra PU, van der Laan BF *et al.* Shoulder and neck morbidity in quality of life after surgery for head and neck cancer. *Head and Neck* 2004; **26**: 839–44.

124. Laverick S, Lowe D, Brown JS *et al.* The impact of neck dissection on health-related quality of life. *Archives of Otolaryngology – Head and Neck Surgery* 2004; **130**: 149–54.

125. Rogers SN, Scott B, Lowe D. An evaluation of the shoulder domain of the University of Washington quality of life scale. *British Journal of Oral and Maxillofacial Surgery* 2007; **45**: 5–10.

126. Scott B, Lowe D, Rogers SN. An evaluation of shoulder and cervical spine movements after head and neck cancer: clinician rated and questionnaire assessment. *Physiotherapy* 2007; **93**: 102–9.

127. Wijers OB, Levendag PC, Braaksma MM *et al.* Patients with head and neck cancer cured by radiation therapy: a survey of the dry mouth syndrome in long-term survivors. *Head and Neck* 2002; **24**: 737–47.

128. Jabbari S, Kim HM, Feng M *et al.* Matched case-control study of quality of life and xerostomia after intensity-modulated radiotherapy or standard radiotherapy for head-and-neck cancer: Initial report. *International Journal of Radiation Oncology, Biology, Physics* 2005; **63**: 725–31.

129. Ng MK, Porceddu SV, Milner AD *et al.* Parotid-sparing radiotherapy: does it really reduce xerostomia? *Clinical Oncology* 2005; **17**: 610–17.

130. Roesink JM, Schipper M, Busschers W *et al.* A comparison of mean parotid gland dose with measures of parotid gland function after radiotherapy for head-and-neck cancer: Implications for future trials. *International Journal of Radiation Oncology, Biology, Physics* 2005; **63**: 1006–9.

131. Parliament MB, Scrimger RA, Anderson SG *et al.* Preservation of oral health-related quality of life and salivary flow rates after inverse-planned intensity-modulated radiotherapy (IMRT) for head-and-neck cancer. *International Journal of Radiation Oncology, Biology, Physics* 2004; **58**: 663–73.

132. Braaksma MM, Wijers OB, van Sornsen de Koste JR *et al.* Optimisation of conformal radiation therapy by intensity modulation: cancer of the larynx and salivary gland function. *Radiotherapy and Oncology* 2003; **66**: 291–302.

133. Eisbruch A, Ship JA, Dawson LA *et al.* Salivary gland sparing and improved target irradiation by conformal and intensity modulated irradiation of head and neck cancer. *World Journal of Surgery* 2003; **27**: 832–7.

134. Rogers SN. Quality of life of head and neck cancer patients. Has treatment planning altered? *Oral Oncology* 2009; **45**: 435–9.

♦ 135. Rogers SN, Ahad SA, Murphy AP. A structured review and theme analysis of papers published on 'quality of life' in head and neck cancer: 2000 to 2005. *Oral Oncology* 2007; **43**: 843–68.

FURTHER READING

Fitzpatrick R, Davey C, Buxton MJ, Jones DR. Evaluating patient-based outcome measures for use in clinical trials. *Health Technology Assessment* 1998; **2**: i–iv, 1–74.

Staquet MJ, Hays RD, Fayers PM. *Quality of life assessment in clinical trials. Methods and practice.* Oxford: Oxford University Press, 1998.

Streiner D, Norman G. *Health measurement scales: a practical guide to their development and use.* Oxford: Oxford Medical Publications, 2008.

11

Complications and their management

KIM AH-SEE AND MRINAL SUPRIYA

You are a true surgeon from the moment you are able to deal with your complications.

Owen H Wangensteen

INTRODUCTION AND DEFINITION

A complication following head and neck surgery can be defined as an adverse event that impacts on the patient's recovery, alternatively described as a possible 'side effect' of surgery.

An awareness of the possible complications enables the surgeon to provide informed consent when discussing surgery with the patient. While not all conceivable complications can be covered, particular emphasis may be placed on certain outcomes depending on the individual and their comorbidities. As a general rule, minor but frequently occurring problems, such as auricular paraesthesia after parotidectomy, should be discussed in addition to rarer but more significant complications, such as facial nerve damage. Remember that clear documentation of such preoperative discussions will mitigate possible future medicolegal issues.

The incidence of complications will vary from surgeon to surgeon. Some of this variation may be due to differing definitions. For example, what do we mean by a wound infection? However, underpinning the ability to quote our own complication rates is personal audit of our work. All surgeons, including trainees, must be active in this regard.

This chapter cannot be all inclusive, but basic principles will be highlighted. A careful preoperative assessment, meticulous surgical technique, high quality postoperative care and appropriate rehabilitation are the cornerstones of preventing and managing complications.

General and specific complications will be discussed in some detail with emphasis, where appropriate, on elements of prevention, identification and management.

CLASSIFICATION

These can be initially classified as general or specific. General relates to the risks of undergoing any surgical procedure while specific relates to the particular operation in question. These will be discussed below.

In addition, complications may be classified as: early, occurring during or within 24 hours of surgery; intermediate complications arise during the early days or weeks postoperatively; and finally, late complications generally occur months or years after surgery (**Table 11.1**).

PREVENTION AND EVALUATION

Patients undergoing head and neck surgery usually have a history of tobacco and alcohol consumption. As such they are

Table 11.1 Classification of complications.

Classification of complications
General and specific
Early, intermediate and late
Local and systemic
Major and minor

likely to suffer from both cardiovascular and respiratory disease.[1] These have a significant impact on recovery from surgery and are therefore an important part of the pre-operative evaluation.[2] Advice should be sought from the anaesthetist involved who may recommend further medical assessment. Smoking cessation has a positive effect on post-operative wound healing.[3] Several tools exist for the global assessment of a patient's fitness. The ASA and CEPOD scores are outlined in **Tables 11.2** and **11.3**, respectively. Two commonly used measures of performance status are described in **Tables 11.4** and **11.5**.

Control of coexisting medical conditions is required for optimal outcome (**Table 11.6**).

A successful operation will only remain so with optimal postoperative care, whether this is on the ward, in high dependency or in intensive care. General guidelines exist for postoperative care and all surgeons should be familiar with these as part of good medical care.[4]

Optimal postoperative care requires:

- clinical assessment and monitoring;
- respiratory management;
- cardiovascular management;
- fluid, electrolyte and renal management;

- control of sepsis;
- nutrition.

MANAGEMENT: GENERAL

Mortality rates in head and neck surgery are fortunately low. However, the development of medical complications is associated with a longer hospital stay and increased mortality rates.[5] Likewise the presence of pre-existing comorbidities requires prompt management to reduce the incidence of subsequent major surgical complications.[6]

Cardiovascular

The risk factors for deep vein thrombosis (DVT) in hospitalized patients are described in **Box 11.1**.[7] Identification of these risk factors will require consideration of DVT prophylaxis, such as TED stockings, pneumatic compression and low molecular weight heparin preoperatively. Recent NICE guidelines recommend the screening of all patients admitted to hospital according to the list

Table 11.2   ASA score.

Class	Physical status	Example
I	A completely healthy patient	A fit patient for tonsillectomy
II	A patient with mild systemic disease	Essential hypertension, mild diabetes without end organ damage
III	A patient with severe systemic disease that is not incapacitating	Angina, moderate to severe COPD
IV	A patient with incapacitating disease that is a constant threat to life	Advanced COPD, cardiac failure
V	A moribund patient who is not expected to live 24 hours with or without surgery	Ruptured aortic aneurysm, massive pulmonary embolism
E	Emergency case	

COPD, chronic obstructive pulmonary disorder.

Table 11.3   CEPOD scores.

Grade	
1	Elective – Operation at time to suit both surgeon and patient
2	Scheduled – Operation within 24 hours. Delayed operation after resuscitation
3	Urgent – Operation between 1 and 3 weeks. Early surgery preferred, but not life saving
4	Emergency – Operation within 1 hour. Immediate operation or resuscitation simultaneous with surgical treatment

Table 11.4   WHO performance scale.

Scale	
0	Able to carry out all normal activity without restriction
1	Restricted in physically strenuous activity, but ambulatory and able to carry out light work
2	Ambulatory and capable of all self-care, but unable to carry out work; up and about more than 50% of waking hours
3	Capable only of limited self-care; confined to bed more than 50% of waking hours
4	Completely disabled; cannot carry out any self-care; totally confined to bed or chair

Table 11.5   Karnofsky performance scale.

Karnofsky performance scale	
100	Normal, no complaints, no evidence of disease
90	Able to carry on normal activity: minor symptoms of disease
80	Normal activity with effort: some symptoms of disease
70	Cares for self: unable to carry on normal activity or active work
60	Requires occasional assistance but is able to care for needs
50	Requires considerable assistance and frequent medical care
40	Disabled: requires special care and assistance
30	Severely disabled: hospitalization is indicated, death not imminent
20	Very sick, hospitalization necessary: active treatment necessary
10	Moribund, fatal processes progressing rapidly

Table 11.6   Medical comorbidities.

Comorbidity	Possible investigations
Cardiovascular disease	BP, pulse, ECG, echocardiogram
Respiratory disease	CXR, PFTs, blood gases
Endocrine disease	Thyroid function, glucose,
Renal disease	Urea and electrolytes, GFR
Haematological disease	FBC and blood film, coagulation studies

BP, blood pressure; CXR, chest x-ray; ECG, electrocardiogram; GFR, glomerular filtration rate; PFT, pulmonary function test.

of recognized risk factors for venous thromboembolic events.[8]

Patients can be further categorized into low, medium or high risk depending on the number of risk factors present.[9] Fortunately, the rate of DVT and subsequent pulmonary embolism (PE) in head and neck surgery is low (<1 per cent).[9] Symptoms of DVT and PE are as mentioned in **Box 11.2**. Definitive diagnosis may require V/Q scanning or D-dimer test.

Ischaemic heart disease is common in patients with head and neck cancer. Preoperative optimization is required as described above to minimize risk, however postoperative cardiac failure or myocardial infarction (MI) may occur and require treatment. Commonly, in surgical patients, MI occurs due to an imbalance between myocardial oxygen supply and demand in the presence of pre-existing coronary artery disease. Myocardial oxygen supply may be diminished by anaemia or hypotension, whereas oxygen demand may be increased by tachycardia and hypertension resulting from postoperative pain, withdrawal of anaesthesia or shifts in intravascular volume. Perioperative myocardial infarction usually occurs 1–4 days after surgery when the effects of anaesthesia have dissipated and perioperative pain and fluid shifts are occurring.[10]

Respiratory

PNEUMONIA

Preoperative respiratory status in head and neck cancer patients may be poor with a history of chronic obstructive

---

Box 11.1   DVT risk factors

Assessment of individual risk factors should include:

- Age over 60
- Obesity (BMI >30)
- Varicose veins
- Dehydration
- Previous VTE
- Thrombophilia
- Cancer
- Heart failure
- Recent MI or stroke
- Oestrogen therapy (including HRT)
- High dose progestogen
- Pregnancy
- Puerperium
- Immobility
- Inflammatory bowel disease
- Nephrotic syndrome

---

pulmonary disease (COPD) being common.[11] Additional risk factors for respiratory complications are previous myocardial infarction and American Society of Anesthesiologists (ASA) grade.[12] Optimizing pulmonary function preoperatively is important and may require input from physiotherapy and respiratory physician colleagues.

The creation of a tracheostomy or tracheotomy significantly increases the patient's vulnerability to postoperative pneumonia[11] and demands meticulous postoperative stoma care with humidification and regular suctioning of secretions.

Impaired postoperative swallowing with aspiration will eventually lead to bronchopneumonia. Strict adherence to a 'nil by mouth' policy with an alternative nutritional route is necessary. Careful monitoring during rehabilitation of swallowing will require input from speech and language therapy with videofluoroscopic and endoscopic evaluation.[13] The presence of thoracic and abdominal wounds, as may be required for total laryngopharyngo-oesophagectomy, further restricts patient mobilization and respiratory function.

The diagnosis of bronchopneumonia is made clinically and supported by further investigations, including full blood

---

Box 11.2   Features of DVT and PE

- Symptoms and signs of DVT:
  - Swelling of the leg or swelling along the vein in the leg.
  - Pain or tenderness in the leg. The pain is usually only in one leg. Pain might only occur when standing or walking.
  - Feeling of increased warmth in the area of the leg that is swollen or tender.
  - Red or discolored skin on the affected leg.

Common symptoms and signs of pulmonary embolism:

- Sudden onset of:
  - Unexplained shortness of breath
  - Pleuritic chest pain
  - Haemoptysis
- General, less specific signs and symptoms:
  - Anxiety or feelings of dread
  - Lightheadedness
  - Fainting
  - Rapid breathing
  - Increased heart rate
  - Sweating

Box 11.3   Symptoms and signs of pneumonia

- Pleuritic chest pain
- Shortness of breath
- Cough
- Production of sputum
- Rigors or night sweats
- Confusion
- Raised respiratory rate
- Fever of >38 °C
- Focal chest signs:
  - Decreased chest expansion; dullness on percussion; decreased entry of air; bronchial breathing; and crackles

---

Table 11.7   Features of pneumothorax.

Features	
Symptoms	Breathlessness
	Sudden onset chest pain
	Cough
Signs	Tachycardia
	Hypotension
	Hypoxia
	Cyanosis
	Decreased breath sound
	Hyper-resonant chest on percussion
	Decreased vocal resonance and tactile fremitus
	Deviation of trachea (if under tension)

Small iatrogenic pneumothoraces in clinically stable patients may be carefully observed. Clinical instability, significant symptoms, or a larger pneumothorax should prompt placement of a small bore chest drain.[14] Haemothorax or pleural effusion can be difficult to diagnose even with radiology in a supine patient. Chest x-ray should, if possible, be in an upright position to demonstrate the fluid. Aspiration and/or drainage may be required, especially if the patient is symptomatic.

Nutrition

The nutritional state of a head and neck cancer patient should be addressed preoperatively to facilitate wound healing in the postoperative period and to reduce complication rates.[15] Simple measures of nutritional status are weight, body-mass index (BMI), skin fold measurements (e.g. triceps) and serum albumin and lymphocyte count. Patients undergoing major head and neck surgery are at risk of malnutrition and close collaboration with the dietician is important.[16]

REFEEDING SYNDROME

Rapid refeeding in a patient with malnutrition can result in the potentially fatal 'refeeding syndrome'. This condition is seen in an undernourished patient, who is fed (enterally or parenterally) over a short period of time and results from metabolic and hormonal changes. Typically this condition is manifest by hypophosphataemia as well as low potassium, magnesium and thiamine deficiency. Slow and measured feeding over the first week, accompanied by close electrolyte monitoring and vitamin supplementation, prevent development of this condition.[17]

Technical problems related to the provision of nutrition can occur. These include problems with nasogastric (NG) tube placement, percutaneous endoscopic gastromy (PEG) tube procedures and long-line and total parenteral nutrition (TPN) related problems. The position of a NG tube should be confirmed both clinically and radiologically prior to initiating feeding. Aspiration of feed from a misplaced or displaced NG tube is a serious complication requiring immediate cessation of tube feeding and urgent physiotherapy. If long-term tube feeding is anticipated, then PEG tube

count, chest x-ray and culture of purulent secretions. Symptoms and signs of pneumonia are shown in **Box 11.3**.

Management of bronchopneumonia requires rigorous physiotherapy and appropriate antibiotic therapy; microbiology advice for the latter is advisable.

PNEUMOTHORAX/HAEMOTHORAX

Damage to the pleura during surgery, for example when dissecting low in the neck or when mobilizing the oesophagus, will result in pneumothorax.

Clinical features are shown in **Table 11.7**.

Treatment choice is dictated by the degree of collapse. An iatrogenic pneumothorax ≥3 cm (from chest apex to lung) or >15 per cent in size by chest x-ray should be considered for drainage using a smaller bore chest tube.[14]

feeding should be considered. This is aesthetically more convenient for the patient and, although complications such as cellulites, ileus, tube extrusion, tube blockage and peristomal leakage can occur, is more acceptable to patients than long-term NG tube placement.[18, 19]

MANAGEMENT: SPECIFIC METABOLIC COMPLICATIONS

Shock

Shock in a postoperative patient can have a significantly adverse outcome, therefore every effort should be made to prevent it, while the surgeon should actively aim for early diagnosis if it does happen. Shock is defined as a state where the circulation is unable to meet the metabolic requirements of the body. For clinical purpose this can be either due to lack of circulatory fluid (hypovolaemic shock), or due to failing heart (cardiogenic shock), or because of increased metabolic needs of the body (septic shock). Initial management involves the administration of oxygen and volume infusion with isotonic crystalloids. Intubation and mechanical ventilation, with appropriate sedation and paralysis, decreases the basal metabolic rate by about 30 per cent and should be considered early. A urinary catheter is vital to measure urinary output, an excellent measure of tissue perfusion (normal in adult is about 0.5 mL/kg per hour or about 30–50 mL/h for most adults). Patients refractory to a crystalloid fluid bolus of 1–2 L should be considered for central venous (CV) catheter.

HYPOVOLAEMIC SHOCK

Hypovolaemic shock can occur after extensive head and neck surgery, especially if involving free tissue transfer. Early compensatory circulatory response includes increased heart rate and progressive vasoconstriction. Tachycardia is the earliest measurable circulatory sign of shock.[20] Vasoconstriction leads to increased diastolic pressure, reduced pulse pressure and cool peripheries. Assessing severity of shock as proposed by ATLS can help institute appropriate therapy. It is important to note that a consistent drop in systolic pressure occurs late, after loss of more than 30 per cent of circulating blood volume. As mentioned before, establishing a patent airway, obtaining adequate intravenous access, controlling obvious haemorrhage and assessing tissue perfusion should be initiated. Ringer's lactate or normal saline is the initial fluid of choice, 1–2 L given as an initial fast bolus. The total amount of fluid needed is roughly 3 mL for each millilitre of estimated blood loss.[20] Indicators of end-organ perfusion, i.e. urinary output, mental state and peripheral perfusion, should be monitored. Patients showing transient response should be considered for blood transfusion. Patients not responding should be considered for early surgical intervention as ongoing blood loss is likely to be the underlying problem. The possibility of non-haemorrhagic shock should also be considered in these cases. Central venous pressure (CVP) monitoring or cardiac ultrasonography can help differentiate shock in these selected patients (see **Table 11.8**).

SEPTIC SHOCK

Postoperative infection can result in a spectrum of disease ranging from strictly localized lesion to massive systemic inflammatory response syndrome (SIRS). High risk patients should be closely monitored for evidence of SIRS. Elderly persons, those with comorbid conditions and those who are immunocompromised are especially at high risk, including those with cancer on chemotherapeutic agents, those with end-stage renal or liver disease, those with advanced HIV or those on steroids for chronic conditions. Indwelling catheters (vascular, urinary) also place patients at high risk. Sepsis is the presence of SIRS in the setting of infection. Severe sepsis is defined as sepsis with evidence of end-organ dysfunction as a result of hypoperfusion. Septic shock is defined as sepsis along with persistent hypotension despite fluid resuscitation and resulting in tissue hypoperfusion.[21] Bacteraemia is defined as the presence of viable bacteria within the liquid component of blood and is seen in fewer than 50 per cent of cases of sepsis.[22]

SIRS is defined by the presence of at least two of the following four criteria:[21]

1. Temperature higher than 38 °C or lower than 36 °C.
2. Heart rate greater than 90 beats per minute.
3. Respiratory rate greater than 20 breaths per minute.
4. WBC count higher than 12 000/mm^3 or lower than 4000/mm^3 or with more than 10 per cent immature forms (bands).

Table 11.8   Management of haemorrhagic shock: the ATLS protocol.

	Class I	Class II	Class III	Class IV
Blood loss (mL)	Up to 750	750–1500	1500–2000	>2000
Blood loss (% blood volume)	Up to 15%	15–30%	30–40%	>40%
Pulse rate	<100	>100	>120	>140
Blood pressure	Normal	Normal	Decreased	Decreased
Pulse pressure	Normal or increased	Decreased	Decreased	Decreased
Respiratory rate	14–20	20–30	30–40	>35
Urine output (mL/h)	>30	20–30	5–15	Negligible
CNS/Mental state	Slightly anxious	Mildly anxious	Anxious, confused	Confused, lethargic
Fluid replacement	Crystalloid	Crystalloid	Crystalloid and blood	Crystalloid and blood

Complications from sepsis include central nervous system dysfunction, adult respiratory distress syndrome (ARDS), liver failure, acute renal failure (ARF) and disseminated intravascular coagulation (DIC). In septic shock, ARDS has been observed in about 18 per cent of cases, DIC in about 38 per cent and renal failure in about 50 per cent.[22]

The reported mortality rate in sepsis and septic shock varies according to the underlying host condition, infecting organism, aggressiveness of treatment and the subsequent development of complications. The mortality rate for severe sepsis is quoted as anywhere between 30 and 50 per cent.[22] Therefore, every effort should be made to diagnose these early.

Altered mental status is perhaps the most consistent clinical feature in sepsis. Narrow pulse pressure and tachycardia are the earliest signs of shock. Early sepsis is characterized by warm shock, i.e. tachycardia, warm extremities and adequate capillary refill. Laboratory investigations should include white blood cell (WBC) count, haemoglobin, comprehensive chemistry panel, coagulation studies, blood culture and other cultures and sensitivities dictated by clinical examination.

Patients with severe sepsis and septic shock require admission to an intensive care unit for careful monitoring and goal-directed therapy. Antibiotics are given parenterally in adequate doses to achieve bactericidal serum levels and must have a broad spectrum covering Gram-positive, Gram-negative and anaerobic bacteria because all classes of these organisms produce identical clinical pictures.

CARDIOGENIC SHOCK

Cardiogenic shock in the postoperative set up is usually due to myocardial ischaemia or infarction. This results in decreased pumping ability of the heart that causes global hypoperfusion. This is defined as sustained hypotension (systolic blood pressure less than 90 mmHg lasting more than 30 minutes) with evidence of tissue hypoperfusion (oliguria/cold peripheries) in the presence of adequate left ventricular filling pressure.[23] The usual symptoms of acute cardiac ischaemia (e.g. chest pain, shortness of breath, diaphoresis, nausea, vomiting) may be absent in these patients due to ongoing medications. However, as in any shock, circulation is markedly impaired leading to tachycardia, delayed capillary refill, hypotension, diaphoresis and poor peripheral pulses. Breathing may be laboured and presence of audible coarse crackles with or without wheezing points towards left ventricular failure while right ventricular failure is marked by jugular venous distention. An ECG is helpful if it reveals an acute injury pattern consistent with an MI. A normal ECG, however, does not rule out the possibility. The usual work up also includes tests for cardiac enzymes (e.g. creatine kinase, troponin, myoglobin), complete blood count (CBC), electrolytes, coagulation profile and arterial blood gas (ABG). All patients require intravenous access, high-flow oxygen and cardiac monitoring. The key is involving a cardiologist at the earliest opportunity because their expertise is invaluable for facilitating transfer to more definitive care (e.g. cardiac catheterization suite, intensive care unit, operating room).

Acid–base imbalance

The extracellular pH is tightly controlled within 7.35–7.45 as cellular enzymes need a strictly controlled biochemical environment to function normally. Any change in the pH triggers a compensatory mechanism through buffers which include bicarbonate, protein, haemoglobin and phosphate. Of these the bicarbonate system is the most important and is represented by the Henderson–Hasselbach equation:

$$pH = 6.1 + \log[HCO3^-]/PaCO_2 \times 0.03.$$

The respiratory system is able to regulate pH by modulating alveolar ventilation in the presence of constant metabolic production of CO_2. An increase in alveolar ventilation (e.g. tachypnoea) will decrease the $PaCO_2$ and vice versa. Brainstem respiratory centres which are sensitive to H+ concentration respond rapidly. In contrast, the renal control is slow and maximum effect takes place only after several days. This principally involves controlling the secretion of H+ relative to the amount of filtered HCO_3. A modern portable gas analyser can easily measure pH, $PaCO_2$ and PaO_2, which are usually carried out on arterial blood taken from the radial, brachial or femoral artery. Acidosis means an increase in arterial hydrogen ion concentration and can be due to respiratory failure leading to CO_2 retention (respiratory acidosis) or relative lack of bicarbonate due to GI loss (metabolic acidosis). Conditions leading to hyperventilation wash off alveolar CO_2 and lead to a rise in pH (respiratory alkalosis) while loss of body acids is the usual cause for raised plasma bicarbonate and hence the pH (metabolic alkalosis).

Lactic acidosis is usually implicated in postoperative acid-base imbalance. Inadequate tissue perfusion due to any form of shock results in anaerobic metabolism leading to lactic acid production and subsequent metabolic acidosis. Patients with an arterial lactate level of more than 5 mmol/L and a pH of less than 7.35 are critically ill and have a very poor prognosis. Multicentre trials have shown a mortality rate of 75 per cent in these patients.[24] Therefore, it is important to consider intensive unit care early on. Lactate acidosis should always be suspected in the presence of elevated anion gap metabolic acidosis (anion gap = sodium − (chloride + bicarbonate); the gap is usually between 6 and 12 mEq/L). The normal value for anion gap must be adjusted in patients with hypoalbuminaemia. Reduction in serum albumin by 10 g/L reduces the normal value for anion gap by 2.5 mmol/L. Mechanical ventilation should be initiated early on as initial tachypnoea results in ventilatory muscle fatigue. Normal saline should be used for fluid replacement, avoiding solutions containing lactate. Antibiotics, surgical drainage and debridement of a septic focus are of obvious importance in appropriate cases. Controversy continues to surround the use of alkali in treating lactic acidosis.[25] Sodium bicarbonate ($NaHCO_3$) breaks down into carbon dioxide and water in the tissues. Therefore, if its use is being considered, it is important to ensure that patients have effective ventilation to eliminate carbon dioxide and are able to handle additional sodium and volume load. In addition, dialysis may be needed in patients with coexisting renal failure or congestive heart failure.[26]

Calcium balance

Hypoparathyroidism is predictable after total thyroidectomy, less so after laryngectomy or hemi/subtotal thyroidectomy. Intraoperative mobilization and postoperative fibrosis can impact the blood supply to a preserved parathyroid leading to their insufficiency. The incidence rises if radiotherapy to the neck is given, before or after surgery. It can also happen due to tumour invasion or combined therapy. Having said that, most patients in whom all parathyroid tissue has been removed do not develop permanent hypoparathyroidism, presumably due to ectopic parathyroid.

Patients undergoing total thyroidectomy performed for benign pathology should commence thyroxine prior to discharge from hospital.[27] Likewise, monitoring diabetic control will be required to avoid complications related to abnormal glucose homeostasis, although there is little evidence that the presence of diabetes contributes to higher wound infection rates.[28]

Postoperative monitoring of serum calcium and thyroid function tests is required and will need correction if abnormal. Circumoral tingling, peripheral tingling and numbness, carpopedal spasm, hyperreflexia, positive Chvostek's sign (tapping the facial nerve just anterior to the ear results in contraction of the facial muscles, seen in 10 per cent of normals) and Trousseau's sign (elicited by inflating a blood pressure cuff for 3–5 minutes 10–20 mmHg above the level of systolic blood pressure leading to mild ischaemia that unmasks latent neuromuscular hyperexcitability, and carpal spasm is observed) are all classic pointers to this diagnosis. The early symptom of paraesthesia can be subtle and, if untreated, can result in severe hypocalcaemia leading to tetany (may include laryngospasm), focal or generalized seizures and cardiac arrhythmia. Therefore, all patients undergoing the above-mentioned procedures must have baseline calcium level estimated (corrected to albumin level) followed by a repeat test for calcium and albumin in the first postoperative day. Some authorities recommend more frequent assessment, starting in the recovery room, followed by a test every 8 hours following total thyroidectomy. The critical period for determining the need for supplemental calcium has been demonstrated to be in the first 24–72 postoperative hours.[29]

Patients having hypocalcaemic tetany should be managed with an initial slow intravenous injection of 10–20 mL of 10 per cent calcium gluconate (providing approximately 2.25–4.5 mmol of calcium), with plasma-calcium and ECG monitoring (risk of arrhythmias if given too rapidly). This can be repeated as required or, if only temporary improvement, followed by a continuous intravenous infusion to prevent recurrence.[30] If magnesium deficiency is present, add 20 mL (~40 mmoL) of 50 per cent magnesium sulphate solution to 230 mL N saline (10 g/250 mL). Infuse 50 mL of this (equivalent to 2 g MgSO$_4$, 8 mmoL) over 10 minutes, and at 25 mL/h thereafter. Chronic hypocalcaemia is best managed with oral calcium together with either vitamin D, or activated (hydroxylated) vitamin D. Lack of parathyroid hormone (PTH) dampens vitamin D activation (1,25 hydroxylation). Activated vitamin D is responsible for calcium absorption from the small intestine and therefore enteral calcium supplements alone are less effective in elevating serum calcium. Ergocalciferol (vitamin D$_2$) is the most frequently administered preparation because of its safety margin

and low cost. The usual dose is 50 000–150 000 U per day. However, to be active it must be 25-hydroxylated in the liver and 1-hydroxylated in the kidney. Therefore, significant liver or renal disease limits its use.[31] Vitamin D preparations that act more rapidly are also available. Alfacalcidol (1α-hydroxycholecalciferol) at a dose of 1 μg daily is useful in patients with existing renal impairment. Calcitriol (1,25-dihydroxycholecalciferol) given at a dose of 0.25–1.00 μg per day is also available. These preparations have shorter half-lives than vitamin D but are more potent and more expensive. If the patient is unable to receive oral medication, these vitamin D preparations can be administered parenterally.[30] All patients on supplemental vitamin D must have their serum calcium level checked at intervals (initially weekly). Loss of PTH impairs calcium absorption in the nephrons and therefore high serum calcium level can lead to nephrolithiasis.

Bleeding

Vascular injury giving rise to bleeding is one of the commonly encountered problems in head and neck surgery. The presence of major neurovascular bundles in the neck makes thorough anatomical knowledge indispensable, along with experience in using vascular instruments. Traditionally, postoperative haemorrhage has been classified as immediate, reactionary (within 24 hours of the operation) or secondary. Using this classification, immediate haemorrhage is said to occur when there has been inadequate control of bleeding by the end of the surgical procedure, whereas in reactionary bleeding the haemorrhage is typically attributed to the opening up of a vessel in spasm or an inadequately applied tie or clip to a vessel as the blood pressure rises after anaesthesia or patient coughing. In practice, the difference between the immediate and reactionary classifications is of little relevance. It is much more important to appreciate the possibility of haemorrhage after head and neck surgery, diagnose the complication at an early stage, commence appropriate resuscitation and stop the bleeding together with addressing any underlying causes. Such causes may include anticoagulant therapy, unrecognized bleeding disorder, a recent large transfusion or sepsis and disseminated intravascular coagulation. General considerations include monitoring full blood count, coagulation screen and electrolytes. One should also assess the need for blood transfusion, vitamin K (if elevated PT), protamine sulphate (if heparin or low molecular weight heparin (LMWH) overdose) and clotting factors/fresh frozen plasma (**Figure 11.1**).

MANAGEMENT OF BLEEDING

- Diagnose the problem.
- Resuscitate the patient.
- Stop the bleeding.
- Treat the cause.

The haemorrhage may present with bleeding via the sutured incisional wounds, either in the skin or from a mucosal surface in the mouth, pharynx or larynx. It is important to appreciate that bleeding into the oral cavity and pharynx may compromise the airway, either by obstruction or as a result of

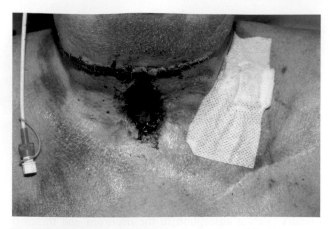

Figure 11.1 Primary postoperative haematoma following laryngectomy.

aspiration of blood into the lower respiratory tract. In patients who have had a temporary tracheotomy performed at the time of their major resection of a head and neck carcinoma, this complication is avoided provided the tracheotomy tube cuff is inflated. For those without such airway protection there is even more urgency to return to the operating room swiftly, with the added problems of securing the compromised airway for the surgical team and anaesthetist. Haemorrhage into the neck wound space may also compromise the airway. This complication is noted particularly with thyroid surgery but can arise with neck dissections.

The source of the bleeding may be the wound edges themselves, from tissue transferred into the wound either on a pedicle or by free transfer, or from vessels in the wound. The most notable major vessels with potential for bleeding during and after neck dissection are the carotid artery and the branches of the external carotid, the thyrocervical trunk, the transverse cervical artery and the internal jugular vein. A bleed following a major neck operation, for example neck dissection or parotid surgery, usually manifests by swelling of the wound site. This may be preceded by ongoing filling of a surgical drain that becomes unable to remove the collecting blood. Drainage may also fail if the drain is of insufficient calibre, it becomes blocked by a clot or the vacuum seal fails and suction is lost. Thus, an empty or non-filling drain cannot be interpreted as ruling out the presence of bleeding.

Postoperative haematoma can be avoided by meticulous haemostasis and closed suction drains. An expanding haematoma needs a return to theatre with re-exploration and control of the site of bleeding. Stable haematomas can be aspirated with application of a pressure dressing, while organized non-fluctuant haematoma can be managed conservatively.

Patients with evidence of bleeding following major head and neck surgery are acutely ill. Immediate management is required. Intravenous access of appropriate calibre is needed. A significant active haemorrhage requires two large bore (e.g. 14G) cannulas situated in non-peripheral sites (e.g. the antecubital fossa). At the time of placing the cannulas, blood must be taken for cross-matching to allow for possible transfusion unless this has been arranged preoperatively. Management is as discussed above under Shock. A neck pressure dressing is very unlikely to stop a haemorrhage and simply delays definitive management of the situation while further compromising the haemodynamic status of the patient. Ongoing bleeding requires prompt return to theatre. The wound is reopened and irrigated with saline. Points of haemorrhage are identified and controlled.

Secondary haemorrhage is less predictable in terms of onset and severity. It commonly occurs 5–10 days after surgery and the cause is attributed to infection, producing breakdown of clot leading to bleeding. It may be unheralded and unexpected resulting in late presentation. In these situations the wound is explored and proximal vascular control is required to control the haemorrhage.

Internal jugular vein injury

To avoid troublesome bleeding from the internal jugular vein (IJV), it should be mobilized circumferentially using a spreading motion perpendicular to the vessel wall. In the event of a large accidental IJV rent, this can be repaired using a running 6-0 vascular suture. It is good practice to tie off tributaries away from the IJV wall to avoid eddy currents and subsequent thrombosis formation. Injury to vagus, hypoglossal and accessory nerves should be avoided while ligating the vessel.

Troublesome bleeding can ensue if either end of the IJV retracts. Packing with haemostatic sponge may control bleeding if the superior pole retracts into the temporal bone, failing which one may need to skeletonize the jugular vein or sigmoid sinus to control the bleed. Similarly, a sternal split may rarely be needed if the lower stump retracts into the mediastinum.

In cases of a slipped ligature or venous tear, one must consider the possibility of air embolism. This serious problem can be identified by a 'sucking' noise and can cause acute cardiovascular collapse. Placing the patient in the Trendelenburg position can reduce this risk. Direct pressure, aspiration from the tip of a CVP catheter if *in situ*, stopping nitrous oxide from the anaesthetic circuit, increasing venous pressure and turning the patient into the left lateral Trendelenburg position are all accepted management steps for this potentially lethal complication. Blind clamping may extend the rent and should not be attempted.

Carotid artery rupture

Cases with prior radiation, significant atheromatous disease, tumour adherence and extensive deep scarring, are all prone to carotid artery rupture intraoperatively. The incidence ranges from 3 to 4 per cent in patients undergoing neck dissection.[32] This risk is raised seven-fold in irradiated patients. The mortality and neurological sequelae more than double in cases with non-elective carotid resection compared to elective ligation.[33] Intraoperative repair of tears in stable patients can be performed using vascular nylon sutures with or without shunting. Similarly, if tumour invasion necessitates carotid resection, the saphenous vein or synthetic patches can be used as a graft. The assistance of a vascular colleague will be required.

Irradiation, flap necrosis, mucocutaneous cervical salivary fistula and deep neck space infection all place patients at higher risk of postoperative carotid blow out due to arterial wall necrosis. In all cases stabilizing the patient with control of airway (consider cuffed tube), fluid resuscitation (crystalloids and blood) and direct pressure application always comes first. Any other intervention can be considered only after the patient is stabilized from a respiratory and cardiac standpoint. Debridement and wound toilet along with vascular tissue cover of a threatened carotid blowout can prevent this condition from developing into an impending or acute carotid blowout. In the presence of impending or acute carotid blowout, after stabilization, all such patients should be referred for angiography which is both diagnostic as well as therapeutic.[32] Adequacy of contralateral carotid to the circle of Willis can be assessed by temporary balloon occlusion, while monitoring neurological status and measuring back flow pressure. If judged adequate, ligation or embolization is associated with a lower risk of cerebrovascular accident. If collateral supply is insufficient, the options include stenting or arterial bypass surgery. In circumstances where no acute intervention radiology support is available, the accepted management has been exploration, debridement and ligation with a transfixion suture through a healthy vessel wall with a reported mortality rate of 9–100 per cent (median 40 per cent) and major neurological complication of 9–84 per cent (median 60 per cent).[32]

Chyle leak

Neck dissection, mostly of the left side, carries a risk of chylous fistulae, occurring in 1–3 per cent of cases[33] with some papers reporting incidence as high as 5.8 per cent.[34]

The thoracic duct is located to the right of and behind the left common carotid artery and the vagus nerve. From here, it arches upward, forward and laterally, passing behind the IJV and in front of the anterior scalene muscle and the phrenic nerve. It then opens into the IJV, the subclavian vein or the angle formed by their junction. The duct is anterior and medial to the thyrocervical trunk and the transverse cervical artery. Precise knowledge of these anatomic relationships is important to avoid injuring the duct during a neck dissection. One must also remember that the thoracic duct may be multiple in its upper end and that at the base of the neck it usually receives a jugular, a subclavian and usually other minor lymphatic trunks, which must be ligated or clipped individually.[35]

Chyle leak is apparent as clear fluid intraoperatively and is confirmed by increased flow on Valsalva manoeuvre by the anaesthetist. This involves changing the ventilation circuit to manual (in an intubated patient), closing the expiratory valve and increasing the circuit pressure to about 30 mmHg. Persistent chyle leak can cause serious nutritional, immunological and electrolyte imbalance. It is generally not advisable to try and identify this vessel specifically during surgery as this may increase the probability of damaging it.[36] The vessel is quite fragile and surrounded by fatty tissue, which makes it prone to tearing. Therefore, direct clamping and ligating may be counterproductive. If a leak is identified during surgery the duct is ligated, without going through the vessel wall, along with surrounding tissue with a non-absorbable suture or vascular clips. If this fails, fibrin sealant and collagen felt or vicryl mesh may be used; muscle flaps can be used in severe cases.[29, 36] Diathermy does not seal the fragile lymphatic vessels.

Postoperative presence of milky appearance in the neck drain after starting feed points towards chylous fistula. This can be confirmed either by identifying triglycerides greater than 100 mg/dL or chylomicrons more than 4 per cent in the drained fluid.[37] Alternatively, a reduction in the volume of drain fluid on stopping enteral feed supports a diagnosis of chyle leak.[36] The management is controversial, however most authors favour medical management as the initial step. A low output leak will usually close spontaneously and can be managed with aspiration, pressure dressing and low fat elemental diet supplemented with medium chain triglyceride (MCT) delivered enterally. MCTs are thought to be absorbed directly into blood rather than the thoracic duct. Unresponsive cases may benefit from TPN and decrease the need for surgical intervention.[3] Close monitoring of volume, electrolytes and nutritional status is of vital importance in managing these cases.

Surgical re-exploration and ligation of the duct is advised in the presence of complications (e.g. flap necrosis), deteriorating general condition or a 'high output leak' (>300 mL/day suggested by Scott-Brown, >500 mL/day by Kassel et al.,[37] and >1000 mL by Nussenbaum et al.[38]). Identifying the duct in these circumstances is usually very difficult due to oedematous and friable tissue. The Trendelenburg position, continuous positive pressure ventilation and a high fat preoperative feed all can help locate the duct.[39, 40] Sclerosants such as tetracycline have also been advocated though they make subsequent exploration extremely difficult. Thoracoscopic ligation of the thoracic duct is needed if neck exploration fails in its identification or the patient develops chylothorax.

Infection

Infection following head and neck surgery can be either local or systemic.

Systemic infection is fortunately rare but may arise if local infection is inadequately treated.

Localized infections can occur around intravenous access sites, while prolonged urethral catheterization will predispose to urinary tract infection. Early mobilization will prevent skin breakdown and development of cutaneous infection.

Local wound infection is uncommon after clean procedures when no mucosal surface is open (e.g. neck dissection). In these circumstances prophylactic antibiotics are not required and careful wound care will suffice. However, in clean-contaminated operations, such as laryngectomy, prophylactic antibiotic use is indicated. Standard practice usually involves a single intraoperative dose of a broad-spectrum antibiotic followed by 24–48 hours of antibiotic. There is little evidence in the literature to support the use of longer courses of antibiotics.[28, 40]

Preoperative risk factors are related to patient factors, such as diabetes mellitus, nutritional deficiency, excessive tobacco and alcohol intake and poor oral hygiene. Tumour factors include stage and site, while previous treatments (prior radiotherapy, chemotherapy) can have a detrimental effect on wound healing.[41] In addition, the presence of a tracheostomy increases the risk of wound infection rates.[41]

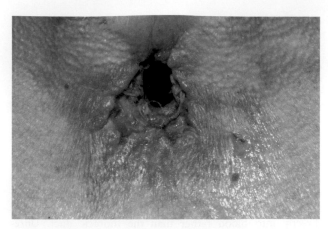

Figure 11.2 Local wound infection around stoma following laryngectomy.

Intraoperative risk factors are related to the type of surgical procedure (composite resection, partial or total pharyngolaryngectomy, reconstruction with regional or distant flaps) and surgical technique (inadequate haemostasis and drainage, poor pharyngeal closure, duration of the procedure or inadequate sterile surgical technique).

Postoperative risk factors are related to wound care, the nutritional and metabolic state of the patient, and the healing of the mucosal repair (**Figure 11.2**).

Increasing prevalence of methicillin-resistant *Staphylococcus aureus* (MRSA) is an important source of wound infection complicating the postoperative recovery.[42] This is a particularly difficult infection to eradicate and can lead to devastating, potentially fatal, infection.[43] Early advice from microbiology is paramount in helping control this infection. Monitoring the patient's MRSA status requires regular swabs from wound sites, along with strict barrier nursing to avoid transmission to other patients.

Clostridium difficile infection is also an increasing problem that surgeons must be aware of. Widespread use of broad-spectrum antibiotics in an increasingly elderly group of patients is a risk factor. Most of the steep rise in *C. difficile* infection is in patients aged over 65 years. Age is an independent risk factor as natural immunity to the organism reduces with advancing years. Likewise, patients with malignancy, sepsis, multi-organ failure, or those who stay in intensive care or high dependency units for prolonged periods (where there can be surrounding environmental contamination), are particularly vulnerable.[44] Diagnosis is made on the presence of gastrointestinal symptoms and stool culture. Again, advice from microbiology is recommended for appropriate treatment, while strict patient isolation and meticulous hygiene standards are paramount to prevent further spread.[45]

Neurological

NERVE INJURY

The nerves at risk of injury during head and neck surgery are listed in **Box 11.4**.

Box 11.4   Nerves at risk

- Cranial nerves VII–XII
- Brachial plexus
- Phrenic nerve
- Recurrent laryngeal nerve
- Superior laryngeal nerve
- Sympathetic chain

Three degrees of nerve injury are recognized.

1. Neuropraxia consists of damage to the myelin sheath without damage to the axon fibres. Microsurgical intervention is not indicated, as function spontaneously returns.
2. Axonotmesis is characterized by combined damage to the axon and the nerve sheath. Subsequent proliferation of the Schwann cells and nerve fibre regeneration takes place and surgical intervention is not necessary.
3. Neurotmesis is complete interruption of all structures of the nerve. Because of the elasticity of the nerve, a gap between the nerve ends develops; spontaneous regeneration therefore is rarely observed. The regenerative capacity of the axons leads to the development of neuromas at the proximal nerve stump. Microsurgical intervention is indicated.

Prevention of nerve injury demands excellent anatomical knowledge and awareness of variations thereof. Meticulous surgical technique when handling and working in the vicinity of nerves is required.

Intraoperative nerve monitoring is increasingly popular with surgeons in an attempt to avoid nerve injury.[46] Intraoperative nerve injury will require direct end-to-end repair, if possible, or the use of cable grafts if a significant gap exists between cut ends.

Development of postoperative palsy may indicate external pressure on nerves from oedema or bleeding. Late recognition of nerve deficit may require future exploration with a view to reconstruction with or without cable grafting.[47]

INCREASED INTRACRANIAL PRESSURE

The intracranial pressure (ICP) rises three-fold when one internal jugular vein is divided and five-fold when both are tied. Symptoms are likely to arise if both veins are tied simultaneously, but may also occur even if staged procedures result in both veins being sacrificed or if a dominant jugular is divided.

Measures to help reduce the risk of raised ICP include:

- no constricting dressings around the neck;
- avoid hyperextension of neck (especially after bilateral dissection);
- nurse upright.

Signs and symptoms of increased ICP include:

- restlessness and headache;

- bradycardia;
- increasing blood pressure;
- facial cyanosis and swelling.

Treatment includes inducing an osmotic diuresis using intravenous mannitol, 200 mL of 25 per cent initially. A prompt diuresis will occur within 10–15 minutes and the ICP will start to reduce and the symptoms will improve. It is rare for mannitol to be needed again.

Airway

Upper airway obstruction should always be anticipated in head and neck surgery. The old aphorism 'when you think about a tracheostomy, that's the time to perform it' still stands. Therefore, an elective tracheostomy should be considered prior to surgery in which there is a risk of significant tissue oedema or bleeding. This controlled procedure is a more attractive scenario than an emergency tracheostomy under difficult circumstances, with progressive airway obstruction.

A system of staging upper airway obstruction can be used and may help determine best treatment. The staging system is clinically based and ranges from stage I: in which there are no subjective signs of shortness of breath, respiratory rate is normal and no stridor is present, to stage IV: in which the patient is cyanotic, has severe stridor and may eventually have cardiac arrest.[48, 49] In the presence of acute upper airway obstruction following head and neck surgery, initial medical treatment include humidified oxygen, systemic corticosteroids and nebulized adrenaline. Failure to improve or progression requires urgent airway intervention including either intubation, if considered safe and feasible, emergency cricothyroidotomy or tracheostomy. Signs of upper airway obstruction are shown in **Box 11.5**.

A critical part of tracheostomy is meticulous aftercare either on the ward, high-dependency unit or intensive care unit. Clearly document the type and fixation of the tube and the placement of tracheal stay-sutures (in case of tube displacement), as well as postoperative instructions including, suctioning and oxygen therapy (**Figure 11.3**).

WOUND HEALING

Many patients with a head and neck lesion have high risk factors, i.e. malnutrition, preoperative radiation, poor oral hygiene, chronic infection, advanced age, necrotic tumour mass, anaemia and exposure to non-sterile cavities

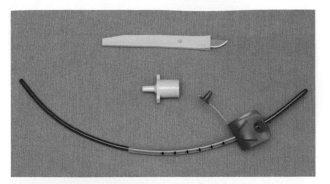

Figure 11.3   Minitracheostomy kit.

intraoperatively. This makes careful preoperative planning necessary to optimize these risk factors and minimize the problems associated with wound healing. Adherence to good basic surgical principle help decrease this risk, for example maintaining a sterile operative field, gentle tissue handling, precise use of cautery, keeping the flaps moist and careful drain placement. Gentle curved skin crease incisions and including platysma in the skin flap helps achieve good cosmesis and flap viability. Antibiotic prophylaxis confined to the perioperative period is recommended for contaminated/clean-contaminated head and neck surgery[40] and usually consists of cephalosporin with or without metronidazole.

Postoperative erythema and induration are common, especially in cases with previous irradiation, and in most cases resolve over a few days. Cases with wound dehiscence need good nursing care in the form of wound culture, appropriate antibiotic therapy, regular saline dressing and optimizing nutritional status. We now have a wide variety of dressings which can be tailored for individual wounds to encourage healing.[50] The principle in dealing with these wounds is to have a stepwise approach of initially clearing the infection, then encouraging granulation and finally inducing epithelialization. Chronic wound environment is characterized by disequilibrium between matrix-degrading enzymes and their inhibitors.[50] Studies of basic fibroblast growth factor (bFGF) on irradiated endothelial cell cultures suggest that bFGF can be a potent inducer of repair. This has sparked interest in utilizing various growth factors for chronic wounds though clinical trials have shown mixed results.[50]

Pharyngocutaneous fistula

The risk of pharyngocutaneous fistula remains high in cases undergoing laryngeal/hypopharyngeal/floor of mouth tumour resection, especially if they have had irradiation to these areas. Its incidence in the past ranged from 5 to 65 per cent while recent series have rates from 9 to 23 per cent. It remains the most common complication after major hypopharyngeal or laryngeal ablation (**Figure 11.4**).[51] Early (<48 hours) postoperative fever has been shown to be a good predictor of future fistula and wound infection.[52] This is clinically apparent 7–11 days after surgery as a tender erythematous lower skin incision/flap with or without pyrexia and leukocytosis. Nasogastric/PEG feed, antiseptic absorbing dressings, antibiotic and minimal debridement (if needed) leads to spontaneous healing of the majority (50–80 per cent)

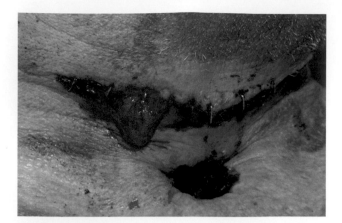

Figure 11.4 Pharyngocutaneous leak following laryngectomy.

of small fistulas by secondary intention.[51] A cuffed tracheostomy tube may be needed if the fistula tract is close to the tracheostome. Contrast swallow or methylene blue dye swallow is performed to assess the leak (**Figure 11.5**). Conservative management may fail due to residual/recurrent tumour, massive fistula with extensive mucosal dehiscence, poor general status or concomitant metabolic problems of the patient. After addressing the general health of the patient, one can consider delayed closure in the presence of healthy granulation tissue. Pectoralis major or latissimus dorsi myocutaneous flaps remain the preferred option for this though free flaps can also be used (**Figure 11.6**). Patients with exposed major vessels are an exception as they need urgent cover with vascularized local, pedicled or free flap to prevent vascular blow out.

FLAPS: GENERAL CONSIDERATIONS

Economic and functional analysis of patients undergoing head and neck surgery suggests that the best outcome results from primary closure wherever possible.[53]

However, in situations where this is impractical, the modern surgeon has an option of wide ranging flaps. Reconstruction of head and neck defect with pedicled flap or microvascular free tissue transfer has become commonplace in the last two decades, but unfortunately has also led to an increase in complications particular to them. Not surprisingly, patients with poor cardiopulmonary or vascular health undergoing tissue transfer can translate into longer intensive care, total hospital stay, increased medical complications and higher rates of mortality.[53] Given these issues the optimum management of flap complications remains their prevention.[53]

Local skin flaps

Most local (except nasolabial) and free skin flaps are based on a random-pattern blood supply referring to anastomoses found within the dermis and subdermal plexus. These have AV shunts (precapillary communications between the arterial and venous circulations) that allow blood to bypass the capillary bed. However, complete opening of these AV shunts

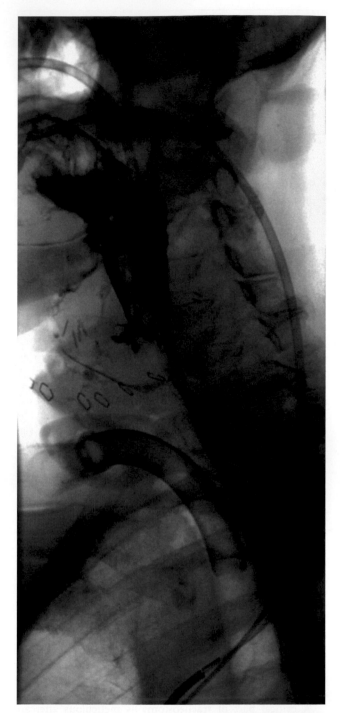

Figure 11.5 Contrast study demonstrating pharyngeal leak in soft tissue of neck anteriorly.

can direct blood away from the nutrient capillary bed and compromise the viability of the distal flap despite normal or even increased total blood flow. The previously taught length–width ratio is only a rough guideline, and it cannot be relied on as an absolute determinant of flap success.[54] A variety of factors may cause a skin flap to fail, with necrosis of all or part. The most common cause of flap failure is vascular insufficiency due to excessive length (with a random blood supply) or excessive tension. Vasoconstrictors such as nicotine (hence consider delaying surgery in smokers),

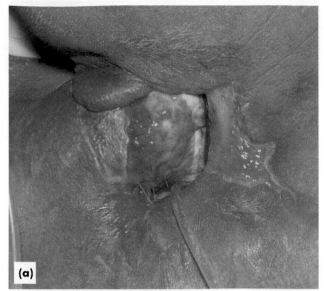

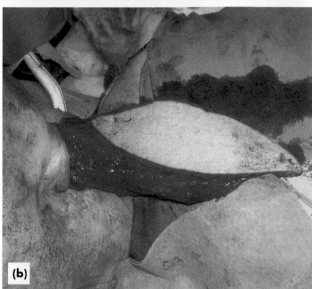

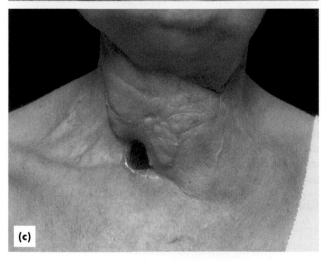

Figure 11.6 (a) Pharyngocutaneous fistula; (b) mobilized pectoralis major flap; (c) healed pectoralis major flap in place post-operatively.

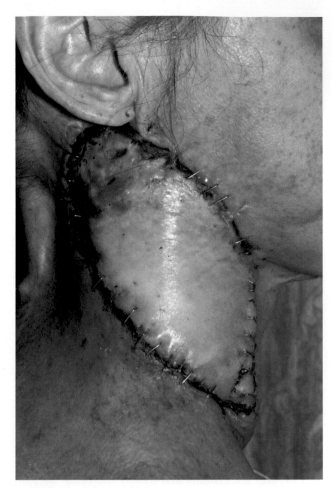

Figure 11.7 Failing distal end of pectoralis major myocutaneous flap. Notice the bluish mottled appearance.

epinephrine and dopamine may also affect viability.[54] Underlying haematoma or seroma can cause flap necrosis due to increased wound tension, pressure on feeding vessels and vasoconstriction resulting from breakdown products. Therefore, ensuring adequate haemostasis and securing a dressing (e.g. acroflavin soaked cotton wool) with overlying ties can help prevent this complication. It is also important to control factors such as diabetes, hypertension and infection, and avoid compression of the flap pedicle as these are known to affect viability.

Locoregional myocutaneous flap

Historically, locoregional flaps (LRF) such as pectoralis, trapezius and latissimus dorsi were commonly used and often described as the 'workhorse' of reconstruction. Pectoralis major myocutaneous flap remains the most commonly used LRF and a large series reported a complication rate of 35 per cent including dehiscence, haematoma and infection in relation to a number of comorbidities, smoking and oral cavity reconstruction.[55] Partial muscle or cutaneous necrosis can result as the distal portion of an LRF is one angiosome distal to its vascular territory and is seen in 14–29 per cent of cases[53] (**Figure 11.7**). However, complete flap loss is rare, occurring in less than 10 per cent of cases.[33] Partial or total loss can result in dehiscence, frequently leading to fistula.[53] Irrespective of the choice of any flap, pedicled or free, a comprehensive understanding of vascular anatomy is essential to ensure flap survival and achieving the best possible functional and aesthetic results. Minimizing skin and subcutaneous tissue avulsion, avoiding inwardly bevelled skin incisions, and identifying and preserving vascular pedicle are all essential towards this end. It is critical to avoid undue compression, tension or kinking of vascular pedicle when insetting the flap.[33]

Free tissue transfer

The development of microvascular techniques has led to the frequent use of free tissue transfer (FTT) in reconstructing head and neck defects. Compared to LRF, any advantage in terms of functional and aesthetic outcome still remains a topic of debate. Overall complication rates between LRF and FTT have recently been shown to be equivalent. LRFs tend to have late wound breakdown while FTTs are associated with early complications.[56] Recent series have shown failure rates for FTT ranging from 1 to 8 per cent.[57] Prior radiation, atherosclerosis, smoking, sepsis, advanced age and poor surgical technique are associated with failure of FTT.[33] Use of the operating microscope or surgical loupes helps achieve good microvascular anastomosis and some authors have reported comparable results while utilizing anastomotic coupling devices.[58] Ensuring adequate donor and recipient vessels is important. LRFs are typically associated with minimal donor site morbidity while this varies considerably for FTT, skin graft failures and sensory loss being the most commonly encountered problems.[53] Preoperative clinical (e.g. objective Allen's test) and/or noninvasive vascular assessment (colour flow Doppler evaluation) can dramatically improve donor site morbidity during FTT. Monitoring free flaps is critical as timely intervention is directly related to successful salvage.[58] The gold standard for non-buried flap monitoring is clinical observation. Cold, white and non-blanching flaps are indicators of arterial insufficiency while the more common venous insufficiency is marked by a swollen, bluish flap with dark blood on pin-prick testing. Objective tests for monitoring flaps include hand-held Doppler, surface temperature probe, impedance plethysmography, photoplethysmography, micro-lightguide spectrophotometer and more recently implantable Cook–Swartz Doppler probes. Early recognition of a failing flap with return to theatre within 24 hours postoperatively has superior salvage rates than cases delayed beyond 24 hours.[59] Timely re-exploration and revascularizing of a failing flap is critical for its salvage. One series reported the median time of return to theatre is 60 minutes in successful salvage, while this was 105 minutes for failed ones.[59] Venous congestion has also been managed with leeches.[60]

LASERS

Meticulous safety precautions during use of the CO_2 laser in head and neck surgery will minimize the risk of laser complications. The use of laser-safe anaesthetic tubes, clear

---

communication with your anaesthetist and protection of the patient with moist towels and swabs is imperative.[61] The complications from CO_2 laser arise either directly from the laser beam itself or from the reflected beam. In addition, late effects of laser surgery can occur.

A laser fire occurs if the three components of fire exist together: a source of ignition (laser); flammable material (tubes, swabs); and oxygen (air and anaesthetic gases).

Strict precautions as above should be taken prior to laser use. In the event of an airway fire consider the steps in **Box 11.6**.[62] Direct laser damage to other tissues, such as skin or eyes, requires appropriate topical treatment such as antibiotic cream or ointment.

Early postoperative complications of laser use include the development of oedema with possible airway compromise. Close monitoring of the airway is required and administration of intravenous steroids (e.g. dexamethasone 8 mg twice a day) for the first 24 hours postoperatively. Progressive airway obstruction may require reintubation or indeed tracheostomy.

Late complications from the laser include web formation and airway stenosis.[63] Management of webs and stenoses can be very challenging and may require resection and reconstructive procedures. Some success has been reported with the use of topical mitomycin C following division of webs and stenotic segments in the upper airway.[64]

COMPLICATIONS OF RADIOTHERAPY AND CHEMOTHERAPY

The use of radical radiotherapy with or without additional chemotherapeutic agents is commonly associated with significant morbidity and occasionally mortality. The basic principle of treatment with radiotherapy is to maximize the chance of cure by delivering a high dose of ionizing radiation to the tumour and any occult extension. Allowance is made for microscopic extension not seen on planning imaging by incorporating a margin of presumed extension together with a further margin of expected normal tissue. It is inevitable that normal cells will be unavoidably affected by the treatment, producing unwanted toxicities. Generally, these complications can be considered as acute (early complications arising during or shortly after treatment has ended) or late (generally permanent) (see **Box 11.7**).

The normal tissues affected most by chemotherapy and radiotherapy are those with the highest rate of cellular

---

Box 11.7   Complications of radiotherapy and chemotherapy

- Acute effects
  - Occur during or immediately after treatment
  - Usually settle spontaneously
- Late effects
  - Occur months or years after treatment
  - May be progressive or irreversible

Box 11.8   Acute mucositis grading

- Injection
- Patchy mucositis
- Confluent fibrinous mucositis
- Ulceration, haemorrhage or necrosis
- Death resulting from mucositis

---

turnover. Radiation of the head and neck can cause irreversible damage to skin, mucosal surfaces, salivary gland tissue, vasculature, muscle and bone.

Skin effects

With conventional fractionated radiation therapy, cutaneous erythema develops in the irradiated area about 2–3 weeks into the treatment regime. This may progress to skin peeling or dry desquamation. Pruritis is common and the induced scratching may result in skin breakdown with infection. With higher doses to the skin, blistering can occur with moist desquamation. This usually settles within one month of completion of the treatment. Secondary infection may occur in areas of moist desquamation. It is important to keep these areas clean and avoid abrasion. Hair loss occurs in the treated area after about 3 weeks. This is usually transient unless the radiation dose to the skin is above 50 Gy with regrowth expected to start in the region of three months after the end of the treatment. Increased suntan-like pigmentation may occur in the treated area. It is important to warn patients what to expect and thus to avoid rubbing, scrubbing or scratching. Soaps and cosmetics should not be applied to the treated areas and washing should be with lukewarm water only. Wet shaving is not recommended but use of an electric razor is permitted. Skin should be protected from sun exposure both during the treatment and lifelong afterwards.

The late effects of radiotherapy on the skin include atrophy, telangiectasia, hypopigmentation and fibrosis. The risk of a skin cancer developing in a radiotherapy field is increased permanently.

Mucosal effects

The upper aerodigestive tract mucosa is highly susceptible to toxicity from radiotherapy and chemotherapy because of the high cellular turnover, the diverse and complex microflora and trauma associated with normal mastication and swallowing.[65] The early reaction of mucosa to treatment is similar to skin. Mucositis is the term devised for the inflammatory response which has been graded by the Radiation Therapy Oncology Group (see **Box 11.8**).

Virtually all patients undergoing radiotherapy (with or without additional chemotherapy) will develop a grade 1 or 2 mucositis. High grade toxic effects are greater with concurrent chemotherapy regimes and, in particular, mucosal toxicity of concurrent radiotherapy and cisplatin is almost twice as much compared with radiotherapy given as a single modality or with induction chemotherapy.[66] The first signs of mucosal damage with chemotherapy arise within the first few days of therapy but with radiation alone the changes are seen after 1–2 weeks. The mucosa becomes reddened and oedematous. Pain is initially mild, becoming more severe and requiring analgesia with the inflammatory serosanguinous discharge associated with grade 2 mucositis. Grade 3 mucositis may require opioid analgesia. The onset of significant pain results in compromised chewing and swallowing and adequate analgesia is very important. Otherwise, the pain effects on oral intake may lead to significant dehydration and weight loss. Taste disturbance and altered, unpleasant oral sensation is common and may enhance the anorexic effects of the pain. Swallowing is also compromised by the xerostomia due to salivary gland dysfunction arising from the direct effects of radiotherapy on these tissues. Input from the dietetic service is essential. Initially, the patient may have to change from a solid to soft diet and oral nutritional supplements may be required. It is common practice in those receiving chemoradiotherapy to have a PEG inserted prior to treatment in anticipation of significant compromise in oral feeding with the need for an alternative route for enteral nutrition. Severe mucosal toxicity can compromise treatment protocols. At times the reactions are so severe as to require a temporary unplanned break in the therapy or even complete cessation. Any reduction in treatment or alteration in the schedule because of severe mucosal morbidity adversely affects patient survival rates.

Acute mucosal reaction with oedema in the larynx may lead to hoarseness of the voice where it is not already compromised by disease. The mucositis may also result in a compromised airway in a patient where there is already narrowing produced by a tumour. This should be anticipated by the surgeon with possible intervention by laser debulking in advance of definitive treatment and awareness that a tracheostomy may become necessary.

Management of these early complications requires appropriate patient education, the optimization of the oral region by pretreatment intervention and prompt treatment of acute lesions resulting from the treatment. Pretreatment interventions include dental assessment and intervention to ensure optimal dental status and oral hygiene (that may include extraction of carious teeth if repair is not possible), input from dieticians and possible placement of a PEG tube.

Dental effects

The risk of dental caries increases following radiotherapy and chemotherapy. This is due to altered saliva production, a change in the oral flora and loss of mineralizing components.

When radiotherapy doses exceed 54 Gy the resulting xerostomia is often irreversible. The saliva that is produced is more viscous and some of the lubricating effects of saliva are lost. The buffering capacity of saliva is reduced and the oral flora becomes more pathogenic. Patients must maintain excellent oral hygiene to avoid plaque accumulation and avoid periodontal disease. Plaque removal by brushing and flossing is essential. The use of high concentration fluorides is advocated and topical antimicrobial rinses are available. Saliva substitutes are available to help the symptom of xerostomia. The patient should attend a dental practitioner to ensure elimination of oral disease before cancer therapy.

Vascular effects and tissue necrosis

Initial effects of vascular inflammation and fibrosis associated with therapy may lead to long-term problems with tissue hypovascularity and hypoxia. Trauma and injury, including surgical and dental procedures, may result in non-healing areas with necrosis and there is a risk of secondary infection. The mandible is susceptible to osteoradionecrosis because of the unilateral nature of its blood supply compared with the maxilla.[67] The need for pre-therapy and subsequent dental care has been highlighted above. When bone exposure occurs, coverage with mucosal or vascularized tissue is required. Presenting features of osteoradionecrosis include pain, reduced sensation, fistula, infection and pathologic fracture. Hyperbaric oxygen therapy has been used to treat bone necrosis and is thought to help by increasing tissue oxygenation and increase angiogenesis.[68] Availability of this treatment is often limited and patients may have to travel considerable distances to have their therapy. In non-responsive or severe cases a partial mandibular resection of sequestered bone may be required with free tissue reconstruction to maintain function and help cosmesis. Radionecrosis may also affect the skull base. Fortunately this is a rare, but potentially very serious, complication. Presentations include cacosmia, epistaxis, ear discharge and headache. This can progress to meningitis, blindness, lower cranial nerve dysfunction and carotid artery haemorrhage.

Where soft tissue fibrosis occurs in the region of the mandible the functional result may be significant trismus. These changes should be anticipated or identified as early as possible to limit progression of the trismus. Patient interventions include mandibular stretching exercises and the use of prosthetic aids.

The cartilages of the larynx may also develop chondroradionecrosis as a delayed complication (**Figure 11.8**). The incidence of this complication has reduced over time to approximately 1 per cent.[69] Radiotherapy to the larynx may result in oedema, perichondritis and frank cartilage necrosis. Symptoms mimic those of cancer recurrence and this may present a diagnostic dilemma. Conservative treatments include use of antibiotics and steroids with humidification. There appears to be a role for hyperbaric oxygen therapy which may avoid the need for total laryngectomy.[70]

Hypothyroidism

Hypothyroidism can develop years after radiotherapy to the neck in up to 25 per cent of patients treated. This possibility

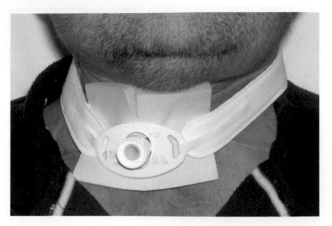

Figure 11.8 Non-cuffed Shiley tracheostomy tube *in situ*.

is increased if there has also been some surgical intervention that included partial removal of the thyroid gland. It is wise to check thyroid function routinely in those at risk. Thyroid replacement therapy should be started if the TSH level is elevated, even if the free thyroxine level is normal, as compensated hypothyroidism may lead to overt myxoedema.

Visual effects

The lens of the eye is one of the most radiosensitive structures in the body and doses of radiation as low as 6 Gy may result in cataract formation. Radiation planning takes account of this fact, however it may not be possible to avoid this dosage and if this is the case then the patient should be warned beforehand and made aware that this can be corrected surgically. The retina is relatively radioresistant but the optic nerve and chiasm are sensitive to radiation. Ultimately there is a trade off between maximizing cure and avoiding blindness. Fortunately irreversible visual loss is unusual in head and neck malignancies but can arise, for example, when treating sinonasal tumours invading the orbit.

KEY EVIDENCE

- Smoking cessation has a positive effect on postoperative wound healing.[3]
- The creation of a tracheostomy or tracheotomy significantly increases the patients' vulnerability to postoperative pneumonia.[11]
- Patients undergoing total thyroidectomy should commence thyroxine prior to discharge from hospital.[27]
- Increasing prevalence of methicillin-resistant *Staphylococcus aureus* (MRSA) and *Clostridium difficile* infection are important sources of infection complicating the postoperative recovery.[40, 41, 42, 43]
- The intracranial pressure (ICP) can rise threefold when one internal jugular vein is divided and five-fold when both are tied.

- Antibiotic prophylaxis confined to the perioperative period is recommended for contaminated/clean-contaminated head and neck surgery.[38]
- The severity of mucosal toxicity from concurrent radiotherapy and cisplatin is almost double that of radiotherapy given as a single modality or with induction chemotherapy.[64]

KEY LEARNING POINTS

- Clinicians managing patients with head and neck pathology must be aware of the potential complications arising from treatment and their appropriate management.
- Complications arise due to interplay of patient factors, disease complexity and the treatment instituted.
- The ability to recognize the complications at an early stage in order to initiate prompt and effective management is critical for favourable outcome. This, in turn, depends on awareness and careful postoperative assessment.
- Rigorous audit of complications is imperative for identifying areas in patient care that could improve outcome.

REFERENCES

1. McCulloch TM, Jensen NF, Girod DA et al. Risk factors for pulmonary complications in the postoperative head and neck surgery patient. Head and Neck 1997; 19: 372–7.
2. Farwell DG, Reilly DF, Weymuller EA Jr et al. Predictors of perioperative complications in head and neck patients. Archives of Otolaryngology – Head and Neck Surgery 2002; 128: 505–11.
3. Kuri M, Nakagawa M, Tanaka H et al. Determination of the duration of preoperative smoking cessation to improve wound healing after head and neck surgery. Anesthesiology 2005; 102: 892–6.
4. Scottish Intercollegiate Guideline Network. Postoperative management in adults. August 2004. Available from: www.sign.ac.uk/pdf/sign77.pdf.
5. Bhattacharyya N, Fried MP. Benchmarks for mortality, morbidity and length of stay for head and neck surgical procedures. Archives of Otolaryngology – Head and Neck Surgery 2001; 127: 127–32.
6. Ferrier MB, Spuesens EB, Le Cessie S, Baatenburg de Jong RJ. Comorbidity as a Major Risk Factor for Mortality and Complications in Head and Neck Surgery. Archives of Otolaryngology – Head and Neck Surgery 2005; 131: 27–32.
7. Scottish Intercollegiate Guideline Network. Prophylaxis of venous thromboembolism. October 2002. Available from: www.clinicalguidelines.scot.nhs.uk/NationalGuidelines/sign62.pdf.
8. NICE Guideline 92. Venous thromboembolism: reducing the risk. January 2010. Available from: www.org.uk/CG92.
9. Moreano EH, Hutchison JL, McCulloch TM et al. Incidence of deep venous thrombosis and pulmonary embolism in otolaryngology–head and neck surgery. Otolaryngology – Head and Neck Surgery 1998; 118: 777–84.
10. Grayburn PA, Hillis LD. Cardiac events in patients undergoing non cardiac surgery: shifting the paradigm from noninvasive risk stratification to therapy. Annals of Internal Medicine 2003; 138: 506–11.
11. Rao MK, Reilley TE, Schuller DE, Young DC. Analysis of risk factors for postoperative pulmonary complications in head and neck surgery. Laryngoscope 1992; 102: 45–7.
12. Buitelaar DR. Cardiovascular and respiratory complications after major head and neck surgery. Head and Neck 2006; 28: 595–602.
13. Denk DM, Kaider A. Videoendoscopic biofeedback: a simple method to improve the efficacy of swallowing rehabilitation of patients after head and neck surgery. ORL; Journal of Oto-Rhino-Laryngology and its Related Specialties 1997; 59: 100–5.
14. Baumann MH, Strange C, Heffner JE et al. Management of spontaneous pneumothorax: an American College of Chest Physicians Delphi consensus statement. Chest 2001; 119: 590–602.
15. van Bokhorst-de van der Schueren MA, van Leeuwen PA, Sauerwein HP et al. Assessment of malnutrition parameters in head and neck cancer and their relation to postoperative complications. Head and Neck 1997; 19: 419–25.
16. Wiel E, Costecalde ME, Séguy D et al. [Perioperative evolution of the nutritional status in head and neck surgical patients. Prospective and descriptive case series]. Annales Francaises d'Anesthesie et de Reanimation 2005; 24: 600–6.
17. Mehanna HM, Moledina J, Travis J. Refeeding syndrome: what it is, and how to prevent and treat it. British Medical Journal 2008; 336: 1495–8.
18. Lin HS, Ibrahim HZ, Kheng JW et al. Percutaneous endoscopic gastrostomy: strategies for prevention and management of complications. Laryngoscope 2001; 111: 1847–52.
19. Magne N, Marcy PY, Foa C et al. Comparison between nasogastric tube feeding and percutaneous fluoroscopic gastrostomy in advanced head and neck cancer patients. European Archives of Oto-Rhino-Laryngology 2001; 258: 89–92.
20. American College of Surgeons Committee on Trauma. ATLS Advanced trauma life support program for doctors, 7th edn. Chicago: American College of Surgeons, 2004.
21. ACCP. American College of Chest Physicians/Society of Critical Care Medicine Consensus Conference: definitions for sepsis and organ failure and guidelines for the use of

innovative therapies in sepsis. *Critical Care Medicine* 1992; **20**: 864–74.

22. Filbin MR, Stapczynski JS. Shock, septic. In: Dire DJ, Talavera F, Weiss EL *et al.* (eds). *Infectious diseases.* February 2006. Available from: www.emedicine.com/ EMERG/topic533.htm.

23. Brandler E, Sinert R. Cardiogenic shock In: Plantz S, Adler J (eds). *E medicine – online textbook of emergency medicine.* Boston: Medical Publishing, 2007.

24. Gunnerson KJ, Saul M, He S, Kellum JA. Lactate versus non-lactate metabolic acidosis: a retrospective outcome evaluation of critically ill patients. *Critical Care* 2006; **10**: R22.

25. Cooper DJ, Walley KR, Wiggs BR, Russell JA. Bicarbonate does not improve hemodynamics in critically ill patients who have lactic acidosis. A prospective, controlled clinical study. *Annals of Internal Medicine* 1990; **112**: 492–8.

26. Sharma S. Lactic acidosis. eMedicine. March 2007. Available from: www.Emedicine.medscape.com/article/ 167027.

27. British Association of Endocrine Surgeons. Guidelines for the surgical management of endocrine disease and training requirements for endocrine surgery, p 5. Available from: www.baets.org.uk/pages/baets%20guidelines.pdf.

28. Coskun H, Erisen L, Basut O. Factors affecting wound infection rates in head and neck surgery. *Otolaryngology – Head and Neck Surgery* 2000; **123**: 328–33.

29. Bailey BJ (ed.). *Head and neck surgery,* 3rd edn, vol. 2. Chapter 115. Philadelphia, PA: Lippincott Williams & Wilkins, 2001: 1410.

30. Joint Formulary Committee (ed.). British National Formulary 62. London: British Medical Association/Royal Pharmaceutical Society of Great Britain, March 2008. Available from: http://bnf.org/bnf/bnf/current/ 5030.htm#_5030.

31. Baran DT, Arnonin N. Disorders of mineral metabolism. In: Irwin Rs, Rippe JM (eds). *Irwin and Rippe's intensive care medicine,* 6th edn. Philadelphia, PA: Lippincott, Williams & Wilkins, 2008: 1287.

32. Cohen J, Rad I. Contemporary management of carotid blowout. *Current Opinion Otolaryngology – Head and Neck Surgery* 2004; **12**: 110–15.

33. Curran AJ, Irish JC, Gullane PJ. Complications in head and neck surgery. In: Rhys Evans PH, Montgomery PQ, Gullane P (eds). *Principles and practice of head and neck oncology.* London: Martin Dunitz, 2003: 843.

34. Gregor RT. Management of Chyle fistulization in association with neck dissection. *Otolaryngology Head and Neck Surgery* 2000; **122**: 434–9.

35. Robbins K, Samant S, Ronen O. Neck dissection. In: Cummings CW, Haughey BH, Thomas JR (eds). *Cummings otolaryngology: head and neck surgery,* 5th edn. Philadelphia, PA: Mosby Elsevier, 2010.

36. Hehar SS, Bradley PJ. Management of Chyle leaks. *Current Opinion Otolaryngology – Head and Neck Surgery* 2001; **9**: 120–5.

37. Kassel RN, Havas TE, Gullane PJ. The use of topical tetracycline in the management of persistent chylous fistulae. *Journal of Otolaryngology* 1987; **16**: 174–8.

38. Nussenbaum B, Liu JH, Sinard RJ. Systematic management of chyle fistula: the Southwestern experience and review of the literature. *Otolaryngology – Head and Neck Surgery* 2000; **122**: 31–8.

39. Gregor RT. Management of Chyle Fistulization in association with neck dissection. *Otolaryngology Head and Neck Surgery* 2000; **122**: 434–9.

40. Scottish Intercollegiate Guidelines Network. Antibiotic prophylaxis in surgery, Guideline number 104, July 2008. Available from: www.sign.ac.uk/pdf/sign104.pdf.

41. Penel N, Fournier C, Lefebvre D, Lefebvre JL. Multivariate analysis of risk factors for wound infection in head and neck squamous cell carcinoma surgery with opening of mucosa. Study of 260 surgical procedures. *Oral Oncology* 2005; **41**: 294–303.

42. Shiomori T, Miyamoto H, Makishima K. Significance of airborne transmission of methicillin-resistant Staphylococcus aureus in an otolaryngology-head and neck surgery unit. *Archives of Otolaryngology – Head and Neck Surgery* 2001; **127**: 644–8.

43. Parton M, Beasley NJ, Harvey G *et al.* Four cases of aggressive MRSA wound infection following head and neck surgery. *Journal of Laryngology and Otology* 1997; **111**: 874–6.

44. Bradbury AW, Barrett S. Surgical aspects of Clostridium difficile colitis. *British Journal of Surgery* 1997; **84**: 150–9.

45. Van Dalen T, van Dijk Y, Kaan JA *et al.* Clostridium difficile outbreak in surgical wards. *Nederlands Tijdschrift voor Geneeskunde* 1998; **142**: 253–5.

46. Edwards BM, Kileny PR. Intraoperative neurophysiologic monitoring: indications and techniques for common procedures in otolaryngology-head and neck surgery. *Otolaryngologic Clinics of North America* 2005; **38**: 631–42.

47. Hausamen JE, Schmelzeisen R. Current principles in microsurgical nerve repair. *British Journal of Oral and Maxillofacial Surgery* 1996; **34**: 143–57.

48. Bradley PJ. Treatment of the patient with upper airway obstruction caused by cancer of the larynx. *Otolaryngology – Head and Neck Surgery* 1999; **120**: 737–41.

49. Friedman M. Upper airway obstruction: an avoidable cause of death. *Operative Techniques in Otolaryngology-Head and Neck Surgery* 1992; **3**: 149.

50. Hom DB, Adams G, Koreis M, Maisel R. Choosing the optimal dressing for irradiated soft tissue wounds. *Otolaryngology – Head and Neck Surgery* 1999; **121**: 591–8.

51. Mäkitie AA, Irish J, Gullane PJ. Pharyngocutaneous fistula. *Current Opinion in Otolaryngology – Head and Neck Surgery* 2003; **11**: 78–84.

52. Friedman M, Venkatesan TK, Yakoviev A *et al.* Early detection and treatment of postoperative pharyngocutaneous fistula. *Otolaryngology – Head and Neck Surgery* 1999; 121: 378–80.

53. Rosenthal EL, Dixon SF. Free flap complication: When is enough enough. *Current Opinion in Otolaryngology – Head and Neck Surgery* 2003; 11: 236–9.

54. Eugene A, Patrick B, Rick M, George S. Skin flap physiology and wound healing. In: Cummings CW, Haughey BH, Thomas JR (eds). *Cummings otolaryngology: head and neck*, 5th edn. Philadelphia, PA: Mosby Elsevier, 2010.

55. Liu R, Gullane P, Brown D, Irish J. Pectoralis major myocutaneous flap in head and neck reconstruction: retrospective review of indications and results in 244 consecutive cases at the Toronto General hospital. *Journal of Otolaryngology* 2001; 30: 34–40.

56. Richard GL, Jonathan ZB. Improving outcomes of locoregional flaps: An emphasis on anatomy and basic science. *Current Opinion Otolaryngology – Head and Neck Surgery* 2006; 14: 260–4.

57. Blackwell KE. Unsurpassed reliability of free flaps for head and neck reconstruction. *Archives of Otolaryngology – Head and Neck Surgery* 1999; 125: 295–9.

58. Smith RB, Sniezek JC, Weed DT *et al.* Utlization of free tissue transfer in head and neck surgery. *Otolaryngology – Head and Neck Surgery* 2007; 137: 182–91.

59. Brown JS, Devine JC, Magennis P *et al.* Factors that influence the outcome of salvage in free tissue transfer. *British Journal of Oral and Maxillofacial Surgery* 2003; 41: 16–20.

60. Weinfeld AB, Yuksel E, Boutros S *et al.* Clinical and scientific considerations in leech therapy for the management of acute venous congestion: an updated review. *Annals of Plastic Surgery* 2000; 45: 207–12.

61. De Vane GG. Laser initiated endotracheal tube explosion. *AANA Journal* 1990; 58: 188–92.

62. Oswal VH. *Carbon dioxide laser in otolaryngology and head and neck surgery.* Oxford: Butterworth-Heinemann, 1988.

63. Perkins JA, Inglis AF Jr, Richardson MA. Iatrogenic airway stenosis with recurrent respiratory papillomatosis. *Archives of Otolaryngology – Head and Neck Surgery* 1998; 124: 281–7.

64. Ubell ML, Ettema SL, Toohill RJ *et al.* Mitomycin-c application in airway stenosis surgery: analysis of safety and costs. *Otolaryngology – Head and Neck Surgery* 2006; 134: 403–6.

65. Eisbruch A, Rhodus N, Rosenthal D *et al.* The prevention and treatment of radiotherapy-induced xerostomia. *Seminars in Radiation Oncology* 2003; 13: 302–8.

66. Forastiere AA, Goepfert H, Maor M *et al.* Concurrent chemotherapy and radiotherapy for organ preservation in advanced laryngeal cancer. *New England Journal of Medicine* 2003; 349: 2091–8.

67. Jereczek-Fossa BA, Orecchia R. Radiotherapy-induced mandibular bone complications. *Cancer Treatment Reviews* 2002; 28: 65–74.

68. Marx RE, Ehler WJ. Relationship of oxygen dose to angiogenesis induction in irradiated tissue. *American Journal of Surgery* 1990; 160: 519–24.

69. Hermans R, Pameijer FA, Mancuso AA *et al.* CT findings in chondroradionecrosis of the larynx. *American Journal of Neuroradiology* 1998; 19: 711–18.

70. Narozny W, Sicko Z, Kot J *et al.* Hyperbaric oxygen therapy in the treatment of complications of irradiation in head and neck area. *Undersea and Hyperbaric Medicine* 2005; 32: 103–10.

PART **TWO**

BENIGN DISEASE

Section editor: Patrick Bradley

12

Benign neck disease

RICARD SIMO AND JEAN-PIERRE JEANNON

To study the phenomenon of disease without books is to sail an unchartered sea, while to study books without patients is not to go to sea at all.

Sir William Osler

INTRODUCTION

Neck masses present commonly to clinicians. In the adult population, approximately 80 per cent of non-thyroid neck masses are neoplastic, and of these 80 per cent are metastatic, and in 75 per cent of these metastatic masses, the primary index tumours is located above the clavicle. In children under 15 years, 90 per cent of neck masses are benign and of these up to 55 per cent may be congenital.

Benign neck masses can be classified as congenital and acquired. The latter group are often enlarged lymphadenopathies, but there may be a wide range of different pathologies involved causing their swelling. The introduction of the fine needle aspiration biopsy/cytology (FNAB/FNAC) with or with out the use of ultrasound scanning (USS) guidance has revolutionized the management of neck lumps and has now become the gold standard investigation.

The evaluation and management of patients who present with a neck lump, should have a systematic and uncompromising clinical approach. This must include a thorough history, examination of the external and internal head and neck, followed by relevant investigations, which may include bloods tests and radiological imaging.

History

The history should include the age, sex, past medical history, travel abroad, the mode of onset and duration of the mass, associated symptoms including dysphonia, dysphagia, odynophagia, sore throat, referred otalgia, nasal obstruction, cranial nerve neuropathies, weight loss, anorexia, malaise and night sweats.

Examination

The examination should include an inspection of the skin over the skull, face and neck, and of the ears, nose, oral cavity and oropharynx. The fibreoptic endoscope should be used to inspect the nasal cavity, nasopharynx, oropharynx, larynx and hypopharynx. The neck should be examined in a systematic fashion and the number, size, site, shape, texture and involvement of the skin and the deep cervical structures noted. Additionally, while concentrating on the head and neck as a source to explain the presence of a neck mass, it is frequently worth extending the general physical examination to include the chest and breasts in women, including the axillae.

Investigations

The investigations of patient with neck lumps should be tailored to each individual case and it would not be appropriate for all patients to have all possible available investigations. All patients with neck lumps should have as a minimum a full blood count (FBC), chest x-ray and FNAB/FNAC.

If an inflammatory mass is suspected, especially in a young patient, the above investigations together with an erythrocyte sedimentation rate (ESR), C-reactive protein (CRP), Epstein–Barr virus and cytomegalovirus titres, liver function tests, lactic dehydrogenase (LDH) test, brucella and toxoplasma serology may be advisable.

Once a clinical or tissue diagnosis has been made, it is possible to determine what if any further tests or imaging is required. If the diagnosis is infective or inflammatory a plain chest x-ray or no further imaging may be required. If a neoplastic lesion is diagnosed, computed tomography (CT) scanning, magnetic resonance imaging (MRI) and positron emission tomography (PET) scanning alone or a combination may be performed to determine the exact anatomical location, extent and radiological staging of the lesion.[1]

A basic understanding of the different pathologies in patients presenting with a neck lump is essential to direct adequate investigations and conclude an accurate working diagnosis without compromising the patient's clinical outcome. Occasionally, one needs to be very conscious that a working diagnosis may be incorrect, so it is paramount that patients are reviewed frequently during the early stages, to ensure resolution of the mass, if that is what is anticipated, or refer onwards to a specialist or second opinion if the anticipated diagnosis has not be confirmed, or doubt of diagnostic accuracy persists.[1, 2, 3, 4, 5, 6, 7, 8, 9, 10, 11, 12]

CONGENITAL NECK DISEASES AND MASSES

Lymphangiomas

Lymphangiomas are degenerative lesions arising from lymphatics, and can be classified as simple lymphangiomas, cavernous lymphangiomas and cystic hygromas.

- **Lymphangioma simplex** are also called 'capillary lymphangiomas'. They are composed of thin-walled, capillary-sized lymphatic channels, usually asymptomatic and present as pale, small vesicle-like lesions visible on the skin or oral cavity.
- **Cavernous lymphangioma** represent 40 per cent of all lymphangiomas, composed of dilated lymphatic spaces, often with a fibrous adventitia, typically occuring in the tongue, cheeks and lips, and present as a painless diffuse swelling.
- **Cystic hygroma** are composed of cysts and sinuses, varying in size from a few millimetres to several centimetres in diameter, usually presenting as a cystic mass of varying diameter, containing eosinophilic acellular lymph fluid.

Aetiology

The lymphatic system arises from five primitive sacs (two jugular sacs, two posterior sciatic sacs and a single retroperitoneal sac) developed from the venous system. From these, endothelial buds extend centrifugally to form the peripheral lymphatic system. Two principal theories have been postulated to explain the origin of the lymphangiomas:

1. **Sequestration of lymphatic tissue** derived from segments of the primitive sacs which retain the proliferative growth potential and bear no connection with the normal lymphatic system.
2. **Endothelial fibrillar membrane proliferation** from the walls of the cyst, penetrate the surrounding tissue along the lines of least resistance between muscles and vessels, canalize and produce more cysts.

Clinical features

Although congenital and in the majority of cases present at birth, sometimes they can manifest for the first time in young adults. They can appear anywhere in the head and neck. To palpation, they feel cystic and transilluminate. They may remain static or involute, but in some cases they may gradually increase in size and occasionally, especially after internal haemorrhage or infection, can grow rapidly potentially risking pressure on the respiratory system possibly leading to a life-threatening airway compromise or obstruction.

Diagnosis and investigations

The diagnosis is usually made on clinical grounds, but CT and MRI scanning will more accurately determine the size, the exact anatomical location, its relationship with important structures and aid the surgical planning.

Treatment

The treatment of these lesions is difficult and challenging and many methods of treatment have been described over the years. The treatment strategy varies depending on the anatomical location, size and involvement of the surrounding structures. Observation has been proposed by Broomhead (1964) as up to 15 per cent of patients may have spontaneous regression.[13] Repeated aspirations may be helpful in the event of rapid increase in size causing pressure symptoms, while awaiting definitive treatment. Injection of sclerosants, such as bleomycin, tetracyclines and alcohol, has been suggested, but internal scarring is reported to be unpredictable resulting in difficulty with any subsequent surgery and it is not currently recommended. The intralesion injection of OK-432 (Picibanil®) has shown promising results. It causes an inflammatory reaction thrombosis with subsequent necrosis. Surgical excision remains the treatment of choice, but it is challenging and it should be therefore, best undertaken by experienced surgeons in specialist centres. Surgery can be helped by the injection of tissue blue into the lymphatic spaces (**Figure 12.1**).[14, 15, 16, 17, 18, 19, 20, 21, 22]

Dermoid cysts

Dermoid cysts are classified as epidermoid, true dermoid and teratoid cysts depending on the types of tissues identified pathologically within them. Twenty per cent of all dermoid cysts are found in the neck and 30 per cent of these in the face. They make up 28 per cent of all midline cysts, with no sex predominance.

- **Epidermoid cysts** contain only skin, but no other adnexal structures. They are lined with squamous epithelium with or without keratinous material. These are the most commonly encountered variety.

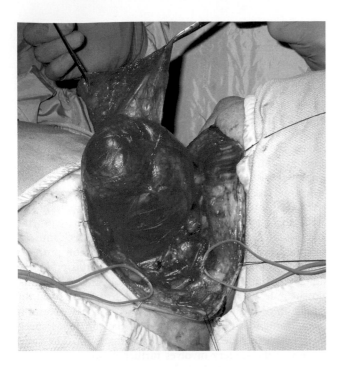

Figure 12.1 Operative picture of a lymphangioma of the supraclavicular region.

- **True dermoids cysts** are lined with squamous epithelium and contain skin with appendages such as hair, hair follicles, sebaceous glands and sweat glands.
- **Teratoid cysts** are lined either with squamous or respiratory epithelium. They contain all three embryological elements: ectodermal, endodermal and mesodermal elements, such as nails, teeth, brain and glandular tissue.

Aetiology

These lesions develop as a consequence of ectodermal differentiation of multipotential cells trapped at the time of closure of the anterior neuropore, especially along the lines of fusion, hence their being located along the midline of the neck. In the head and neck, other areas of tissue fusion may present with dermoid cysts, outer angular dermoids and the nasal dorsum.

Clinical features

The peak age of incidence is usually the second and third decade. They can present as cystic or solid painless mass, usually in the submental region, above or below the mylo-hyoid muscle. More infrequently, they can manifest as an inflammatory swelling (**Figure 12.2**).

Diagnosis and investigations

The diagnosis is usually based on the patient's age, the clinical location and presentation. Ultrasound-guided fine needle aspiration cytology (FNAC) may be useful in the diagnosis of these lesions. Cross-sectional imaging, such as CT and MRI may be useful when there is a large lesion, to aid surgical planning.

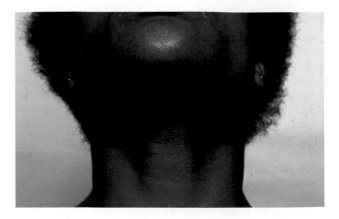

Figure 12.2 Dermoid cyst.

Treatment

Complete surgical excision is the treatment of choice.[23, 24]

Thyroglossal duct cysts

Thyroglossal cysts are the most common upper neck midline lesions. They can present as a mass or a lump, at any level between the foramen caecum and the upper mediastinum, with the majority presenting about the level of the hyoid bone. They are usually sporadic, but a rare familial variant has been documented, identified as an autosomal dominant in prepubertal girls. Thyroglossal duct carcinoma, although rare, may present and be identified by the pathologist in a thyroglossal duct cyst (see Chapter 23, Surgical treatment of differentiated thyroid cancer).

Aetiology

Embryologically, the thyroid gland originates from the floor of the primitive pharynx between the first and second pharyngeal pouches. In addition to the major median enlage, there are smaller paired lateral enlages, which contribute to the parafollicualr or calcitonin-secreting C cells. The median enlage loses its lumen at about the 5th week of gestation and breaks into fragments, the lower end dividing into two portions that become the lobes of the thyroid gland. Thyroglossal duct cysts arise from epithelial cells when they cease to remain inactive. The stalk should atrophy during the 6th week, but should it persist as a patent tract, then it becomes a thyroglossal duct along which cysts can develop. It may run from the thyroid gland inferiorly, upwards and in the region of the hyoid bone, the tract may be located behind, through or in front of the bone, ending deeply in the junction of the anterior two-thirds and posterior third of the tongue, at the foramen caecum area of the tongue. The methods involved for the development of cystic changes is not fully understood.[25] A fistula is usually caused by spontaneous drainage of an abscess or more commonly resulting following an attempted drainage of a misdiagnosed midline neck abscess or resulting from an inadequate attempt at excision usually associated with leaving an intact hyoid bone.

Clinical features

Ninety-five per cent of thyroglossal cysts present as an asymptomatic cystic mass at or about the level of the hyoid bone. The mass moves on swallowing or on protrusion of the tongue. Up to 5 per cent of these cysts present as an acute inflammatory episode with or without an infection, and 15 per cent may have an associated discharging fistula. There is no sex preponderance. The mean age of presentation is five years with a range between four months to old age. Ninety per cent are in the midline, but 10 per cent may be to one or other side, with 95 per cent of these being in the left side. Seventy-five per cent are prehyoid, with the remaining 25 per cent being located above or below the hyoid, and can sometimes be found within the mediastinum (**Figure 12.3**).

Diagnosis and investigations

Patients with suspected thyroglossal duct cysts should be investigated with thyroid-stimulating hormone (TSH) estimation and ultrasound-guided FNAC. TSH and T4 will determine the thyroid status of the patient. Ultrasound scanning may help with the location and diagnosis of the cyst, and will also confirm the presence of a normal thyroid gland in its anatomical position. FNAC will demonstrate cystic contents containing colloid. Isotope scan either ^{99}Tc or ^{123}I may be useful if the cyst is located above the hyoid or in the posterior tongue or to identify and exclude the possibility of a lingual thyroid. CT scanning or MRI should be considered in the presence of large cysts, when malignancy is suspected and when the possibility of a lingual thyroid has been considered.

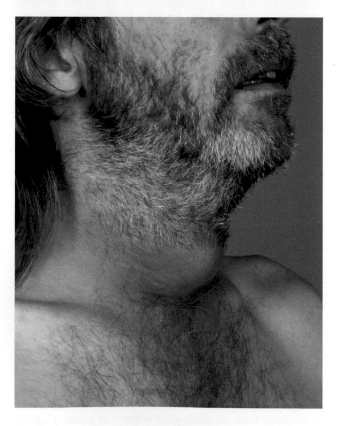

Figure 12.3 Infected thyroglossal duct cyst.

Treatment

Surgical excision is the treatment of choice, as there is always a risk that these cysts could become infected, resulting in scarring of the neck skin and development of recurrent episodes of the cyst enlarging, causing patient discomfort. The Sistrunk procedure was described in 1920, which resulted in cure in the majority of cases. Previously, the hyoid bone was not excised which resulted in a large percentage of recurrences associated with infections. A modification of Sistrunk's technique is currently being employed as the standard surgical procedure without the need to excise the tongue base epithelium. The excision is performed through a transverse midline neck incision just below the cyst. In the common thyroglossal duct cyst, the lesion is dissected from the infrahyoid strap neck muscles and the laryngeal cartilages. Then, the dissection proceeds upwards to the region of the hyoid bone. At this point, the suprahyoid muscles, mylohyoid, geniohyoid and genio-glossus muscles, are detached from the hyoid bone and the middle third of the hyoid bone between the lesser cornu is cut and mobilized in continuity with the soft tissue specimen, which includes the thyroglossal duct cyst. The completion of the surgery involves further dissection upwards, into the tongue base to include an excision of a core of tissue which should include a tissue tract or raphe between the mylohyoid muscles, a portion of each genioglossus muscle and up to the area of the foramen caecum. This technique has resulted in a significant reduction of the recurrence rates when compared with a simple excision or removal of the cyst alone (Shalang procedure).[25, 26, 27, 28, 29, 30, 31, 32, 33, 34]

Treament of recurrent cysts and fistulae

Up to 8 per cent of thyroglossal cysts may recur following adequate surgical excision. If a substandard excision, with no excision of the hyoid bone, has been carried out, a full Sistrunk's procedure should be undertaken. However, if a full Sistrunk's procedure has been carried out, further surgery may be difficult. In these cases, the previous incision scar should be excised, with a full central compartment neck dissection and excision of the scar tissue up to the foramen caecum.[25, 26, 27, 28, 29, 30, 31, 32, 33, 34]

Branchial cysts

The word 'branchial' is derived from the Greek *bragchia* meaning gills. Branchial cysts appear as a developmental failure of the branchial apparatus. Branchial anomalies account for up to 17 per cent of all paediatric cervical masses. They often manifest in young adults with an incidence peak in the third decade. Cysts are usually lined by stratified squamous epithelium, except in 10 per cent of cases where they may have respiratory epithelium. Eighty per cent have lymphoid tissue in their outer wall and they contain straw-coloured fluid in which cholesterol crystals are found.

Aetiology

Four theories have been suggested to explain the origin of branchial cysts.

1. **Branchial apparatus theory**. This theory suggests that branchial cysts represent the remains of pharyngeal pouches or branchial clefts, or a fusion of these two elements. The development of the branchial apparatus extends from the 3rd to the 8th week of gestation. This theory should suggest that cysts should be present at birth, whereas the peak of incidence is usually the second to third decade.
2. **Cervical sinus theory**. This theory advocates that branchial cysts represent the remains of the cervical sinus of His, which is formed by the second arch growing down to meet the fifth arch. The second arch mesoderm almost covers the neck entirely and forms the platysma muscle.
3. **Thymopharyngeal duct theory**. This theory suggests that the cysts are remnants of the original connection between the thymus and the third branchial pouch from which it originates. However, a persistent thymic duct has never been described and there has never been a branchial cyst found deep to the thyroid gland.
4. **Inclusion theory**. This theory postulates that branchial cysts are epithelial inclusions within a lymph node. This theory is supported by the fact that most branchial cysts have lymphoid tissue in their wall and have been reported in the parotid and the pharynx. This theory also explains why most branchial cysts have no internal opening, that the peak of age incidence is later than for a congenital lesion and that it is almost unknown in neonates.

Clinical features

Sixty per cent of branchial cysts are located in the upper third of the neck, at the anterior margin of the sternocleidomastoid muscle, although they have been reported in any site of the neck or parotid gland. Eighty per cent are said to present as persistent and 20 per cent are intermittent swelling. Seventy per cent are clinically cystic, although up to 30 per cent may feel solid. In up to 40 per cent of cases, patients may have had an upper respiratory tract infection prior to noticing the mass. Inflamed cysts may complicate with abscess formation with the possibility of rupture (**Figure 12.4**).

Diagnosis and investigations

All patients with a suspected branchial cyst should be investigated with at least an FBC and ultrasound-guided FNAC. Ultrasound-guided FNAC yields acellular fluid with cholesterol crystals on microscopy examination. However, cytological findings should be taken with caution as squamous debris may suggest the possibility of malignancy. If lymph nodes are necrotic, as is seen in squamous cell carcinoma and tuberculosis, they may be difficult to distinguish sonographically from a second branchial cleft cyst, but FNAB is usually helpful. CT scanning and MRI are useful investigations in large cysts (**Figure 12.5**) to allow surgical planning.

Treatment

Surgical excision is the treatment of choice. This is indicated as cysts have a tendency to become infected, can enlarge to a large size causing local discomfort, pressure symptoms and obvious cosmetic deformity. The procedure is initiated by a transverse cervical incision made on the neck skin crest overlying the cyst. The platysma is incised and subplatysmal flaps are elevated. The cervical fascia is incised over the anterior border of the sternocleidomastoid muscle, which is retracted laterally. The cyst is then identified and dissected from its fascial attachments and capsule, ensuring that the cyst wall is not ruptured. During the dissection, the carotid sheath and its contents should be identified and mobilized out of the surgical area. Also, the marginal branch of the facial nerve, vagus, accessory and hypoglossal nerves should be identified and preserved. The cyst is excised completely and there is usually no need to look for a tract, although the tail of the cyst may need to be dissected from the tail of the parotid gland or parapharyngeal space.[35, 36, 37, 38, 39, 40, 41, 42]

Branchial fistulae and sinuses

Branchial fistulae are congenital defects consisting of a skin-lined tract, opening internally as a slit on the anterior aspect of the tonsillar fossa if it is of second arch origin. The external

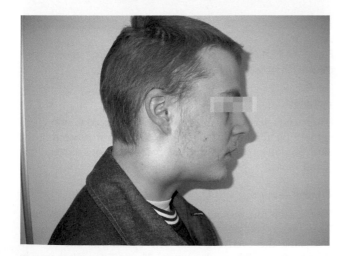

Figure 12.4 Right branchial cyst.

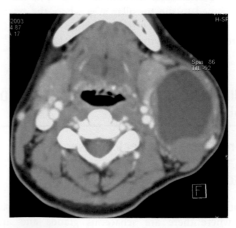

Figure 12.5 Computed tomography scan, demonstrating a large left branchial cyst.

opening is at the anterior border of the sternocleidomastoid muscle, at the junction of its middle and lower thirds.

Branchial sinuses or branchial pits open along a line between the tragus and the sternoclavicular joint at the anterior border of the sternocleidomastoid muscle, but with no internal opening.

Aetiology

They arise as a failure of completion of development of the branchial apparatus including the first, second, third and fourth arches. During the 4th week of intrauterine life, six branchial arches develop as neural crest cells migrate cranially. During the 5th week, the second branchial arch grows over the third and fourth branchial clefts, which form a cervical sinus. Failure of the cervical sinus to close may therefore potentially communicate with the second branchial pouch in the area of the tonsil fossa, the third pouch in the area of the larynx and the fourth pouch opening in the piriform fossa.

Clinical features

They present almost always in young infants as a discharging sinus which may or may not have an internal fistulous opening. Clinically, second branchial cleft fistulae are the most common. They have a cutaneous opening along the anterior border of the sternocleidomastoid, usually at the junction of the middle and lower thirds, tracking up between the internal and external carotid arteries ending in the tonsillar fossa. Third and fourth branchial fistulae are more rare, opening low in the neck and ending in the piriform sinus.

Diagnosis and investigations

The diagnosis is made on clinical grounds. A CT fistulogram may be helpful to determine the pathway of the tract, differentiate a sinus from a fistula and aid surgical planning (**Figure 12.6**).

Treatment

Surgical excision is the treatment of choice. The excision is performed in a stepladder fashion, removing the mouth of the sinus with an ellipse of neck skin. The tract is followed upwards as high as possible and then another transverse cervical or cervicofacial incision is made. The dissection is then continued to the tonsillar area where the tract usually disappears and should be ligated before it avulses to minimize a recurrence of symptoms (**Figure 12.7**).[43, 44, 45]

ACQUIRED BENIGN NECK DISEASES AND MASSES

Non-inflammatory neck masses

SEBACEOUS CYSTS

Sebaceous cysts are skin appendages or lesions occurring mainly where there are sebaceous glands and are most common in hairy skins, particularly in the beard region and scalp.

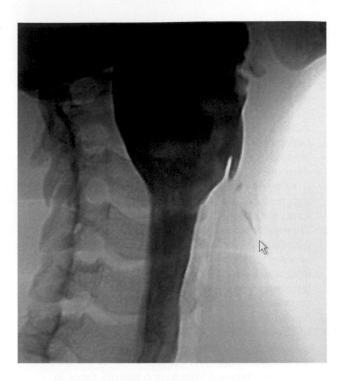

Figure 12.6 Fistulogram of a left branchial fistula.

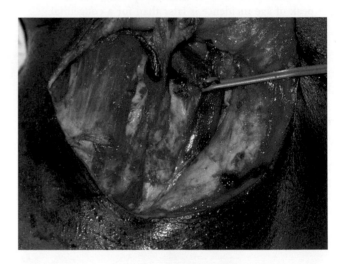

Figure 12.7 Left branchial fistula tract emerging between the constrictor muscles.

Aetiology

These cysts develop when the duct of a sebaceous skin gland responsible for the production of oily sebum protecting the skin becomes blocked. The retained secretions distend the gland causing a progressive enlargement of the cyst.

Clinical features

The lesions can be single or multiple and of different size. They tend to be spherical, smooth and well-defined, stretching the overlying skin. The opening of the blocked duct is often visible as a 'punctum'. The cyst may discharge, in which case the creamed secreted dry material may accumulate in the centre to form a sebaceous horn and they also have a tendency to become infected.

Diagnosis and investigations

Sebaceous cysts often display very distinct clinical features and rarely require investigations. They have a non-specific sonographic appearance and FNAB/FNAC is best avoided.

Treatment

Surgical excision is the treatment of choice as they are unsightly, have a tendency to grow, burst, become infected and reoccur. The excision should be performed very carefully ensuring that the punctum – and the scar if they have been previously incised and drained due to infection – is excised with a small elipse of healthy skin to avoid leaving part of the capsule of the cyst which will lead to the recurrence of the lesion.[46]

ACQUIRED DERMOID CYSTS (IMPLANTATION DERMOIDS)

Dermoid cysts are usually solitary, with solid and cystic areas containing skin appendages.

Aetiology

Acquired dermoids occur due to a penetrating injury or following surgery resulting in the implantation of dermal or skin structures deep into the subcutaneous tissue.

Clinical features

These cysts present at the site of a penetrating injury and often display solid and cystic areas containing sebaceous material.

Diagnosis and investigations

The diagnosis is often made on clinical grounds; however, ultrasound-guided FNAC may be helpful in some cases where the history of injury is not clear.

Treatment

Surgical excision is the treatment of choice. The incision should include the injury tract which should be completely excised in continuity with the cyst to avoid recurrence.[47]

PILOMATRIXOMA OR CALCIFIYING EPITHELIOMA OF MALHERBE

Pilomatrixoma is a benign tumour of the prickle cell layer of the skin, first described by Malherbe and Chenantais in 1880 as a calcified epithelioma. It is most frequently seen in the first two decades of life with two-thirds of these occurring in patients under ten years of age and it is more common in females with a female to male ratio of 3:2. The majority of these tumours (68 per cent) occur in the head and neck region. Malignant transformation has been described, but is very rare.

Aetiology

The aetiology is unknown, although an episode of local inflammation or trauma may precede their development.

Clinical features

Pilomatrixomas are usually solitary and present as a firm, nodular superficial lesion measuring up to 3 cm in size. There is usually no discoloration, but if situated very superficially a blue-red colour may be seen (**Figure 12.8**).

Diagnosis and investigations

Pilomatrixomas have very distinct clinical features. If the diagnosis is suspected, FNAC can be performed. Cytopathological features include the identification of basaloid and squamous cells, calcium deposits and foreign body giant cells.

Treatment

Surgical excision is the treatment of choice if the lesion is bothersome or there is doubt about diagnosis. The excision must be carefully performed in the same manner as for an epidermoid cyst, as leaving part of the capsule will result in the recurrence of the lesion.[48, 49]

LIPOMAS

Lipomas are benign lesions of the adipose layer. The adipose cells are organized into large lobules divided by loose fibrous septa. Lipomas can be multiple and occasionally can be painful (Dercum disease). Although the majority of lipomas are sporadic, a minority can be familial. The most common familial lipomatosis affecting the head and neck is Madelug's lipomatosis. In the neck region, lipomas may be subfascial or arising from the muscles. They grow very slowly and have a very low risk of malignant transformation.

Aetiology

The aetiology is unknown; however, history of preceding trauma which leads to the breakdown of the adipose layer and abnormal growth has been suggested.

Clinical features

Lipomas usually occur in adults and have a variable size. The tumour has a smooth, lobulated surface with a well-defined edge. They tend to be soft and as they lie in the dermis the skin over the lesion can be moved over it.

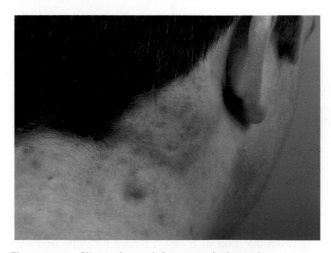

Figure 12.8 Pilomatrixoma left post-auricular region.

Diagnosis and investigations

Lipoma has a very characteristic appearance on USS and does not require FNAC. In large lipomas, CT scanning and MRI may be useful in assessing the anatomy of the lesions and aid surgical planning.

Treatment

Surgical excision is the treatment of choice when the lesion is of large size causing an obvious cosmetic deformity, when there is suspicion of malignancy or by patient's choice.[50, 51, 52]

Inflammatory neck masses

ACUTE CERVICAL LYMPHADENITIS

Acute cervical lymphadenitis is common especially in the paediatric population. It results as a consequence of a viral or bacterial infective process in the upper aerodigestive tract, the ears or the skin of the head and neck.

Clinical features

The mass is usually painful and can result in an abscess, which will become fluctuant. The patient is usually toxic and the primary infective process is usually evident, although in small children it may not be clear.

Diagnosis and investigations

The diagnosis is made on clinical grounds. If the episode is severe and the child requires admission, then basic haematological investigation may aid diagnosis. Usually, no other investigations are required unless there is clinical suspicion that the patient is developing an abscess or it may be a neoplastic underlying process. In these cases, ultrasound-guided FNAC may aid the diagnosis.

Treatment

If a bacterial infection is suspected or diagnosed, treatment is initially empiric with supportive therapy and broad-spectrum antibiotic therapy.[53, 54]

INFECTIOUS MONONUCLEOSIS

Infectious mononucleosis or glandular fever is a viral infection caused by Epstein–Barr virus (EBV) that usually affects adolescents and younger adults. EBV infection is also associated with the development of EBV-associated lymphoid or epithelial cell malignancies, such as Hodgkin's lymphoma, Burkitt's lymphoma, nasopharyngeal carcinoma and multiple sclerosis.

Aetiology

Epstein–Barr virus is a gamma-herpes virus that infects over 90 per cent of the human population worldwide. It is usually transmitted between individuals in saliva, and establishes replicative infection within the oropharynx, as well as life-long latent infection of B cells. Primary EBV infection generally occurs during early childhood.

Clinical features

Primary EBV infection generally occurs during early childhood and is asymptomatic or results in a mild self-limiting illness characterized by fever, tonsillitis and lymphadenopathy. If delayed until adolescence or later, it can be associated with the clinical syndrome of infectious mononucleosis, which is characterized by fever, pharyngitis, lymphadenopathy especially cervical and malaise. Five per cent of patients develop a maculopapular rash and up to 50 per cent of patients may develop palatal petechiae, acute bacterial tonsillitis usually with a grey fibrinous medial exudate, splenomegaly and hepatomegaly. In severe cases or in immunocompromised patients, autoimmune haemolytic anaemia, thrombocytopenia, splenic rupture, encephalitis, cranial nerve paralysis and acute upper airway obstruction as a result of significant tonsillar hypertrophy can develop.

Diagnosis and investigations

The diagnosis is made on clinical grounds. The full blood count will show more than 50 per cent of monocuclear cells and more than 10 per cent atypical lymphocytes. The ESR and CRP will be elevated. Monospot and Paul Bunnell tests will be positive, although may be negative especially in the first 2 weeks of the disease. Hepatic enzymes may also be elevated.[55, 56, 57, 58, 59, 60]

Treatment

The treatment is largely supportive with conservative measures, including rest and hydration. Avoidance of contact sports and heavy lifting is advised for at least 6 weeks and alcohol should also be avoided while the liver function tests remain abnormal.

Broad-spectrum antibiotic therapy may be useful in cases of secondary bacterial infective tonsillitis but ampicillin and its derivates should be avoided, as patients may develop a maculopapular rash. Corticosteroid therapy is advisable in cases of impending airway obstruction, thrombocytopenia and haemolytic anaemia, as well as other complications such as cranial nerve paralysis. Antiviral chemotherapy with acyclovir or famcyclovir has been reported to help in some cases.[55, 56, 57, 58, 59, 60]

CAT SCRATCH DISEASE

Cat scratch disease mainly affects children and young adults with a peak of incidence between two and 14 years. The disease appears to be very common in the United States where over 24 000 people may be affected every year, but also affects Europe, Africa, Australia and Japan.

Aetiology

Cat scratch disease is caused by the Rickettsia Bartonella sp. *Bartonella henselae* is the most common species to cause the widest spectrum of diseases in humans, and cats, especially kittens, are the main reservoir.

Clinical features

Cervical lymphadenopathy is preceded by an erythematous papula at the site of inoculation. Systemic symptoms, such as fever, malaise, anorexia, headache and splenomegaly, can occur but tend to be more common in immunocompromised patients.

Diagnosis and investigations

Serological testing for *Bartonella henselae* is both sensitive and specific of cat scratch disease. More recently polymerase chain reaction RNA of this bacteria has been used in its diagnosis.

Treatment

Several antibiotics, such as gentamicin, rifampicin, ciprofloxacin and especially azithromycin, which is associated with rapid resolution, have been advocated. However, the use of antibiotics in cat scratch disease with no systemic symptoms remains controversial as many infections may resolve without treatment.[61, 62]

CERVICAL NECROTIZING FASCIITIS

This is a rare, but life-threatening, infection that causes progressive necrosis of the skin and subcutaneous tissue, such as the fat and fasciae.

Aetiology

It results from an odontogenic or tonsillar bacterial infection or complicates a deep space neck infection or surgery. *Streptoccocus milleri* or *S. viridans* and mixed anaerobes are the most common aetiological agents.

Clinical features

The diagnosis is made on clinical grounds and the picture is very characteristic with initial cellulitis of the skin with disproportionate pain which progresses to necrosis of the subcutaneous tissues and skin.

Diagnosis and investigations

The white cell count and inflammatory parameters are raised. The ultrasound scan and CT scan may show oedema and air pockets of the skin, which are diagnostic features.

Treatment

If untreated, cervical necrotizing fascitis can be fatal, so early diagnosis and treatment are essential. Intravenous high-dose antibiotic therapy, against aerobic and anaerobic bacteria, with debridement of all necrotic areas, are mandatory.[63, 64, 65]

CHRONIC CERVICAL LYMPHADENITIS

There are a wide range of chronic inflammatory conditions that may present with enlarged lymph nodes or lymphadenopathy. They are often associated with systemic symptoms, such as malaise, weight loss, anorexia and night sweats, and therefore history taking is very important. These include HIV and AIDS, sarcoidosis, toxoplasmosis, actinomycosis and tuberculosis. In all of them, except tuberculosis, the enlargement of the lymph nodes may be very non-specific and therefore a clinical diagnosis may be difficult.

HIV–AIDS

Acquired immunodeficiency syndrome (AIDS) is a viral disease caused by human immunodeficiency virus (HIV). The infection is classified as:

- acute infection or seroconversion illness
- asymptomatic infection
- persistent generalized lymphadenopathy (PGL)
- full blown AIDS.

Aetiology

HIV-AIDS results from the HIV virus being transmitted via contaminated blood or human secretions. It is prevalent in homosexuals, promiscuous heterosexuals and intravenous drug abusers.

Clinical features

Up to 30 per cent of seroconverted patients develop PGL and it may be the first manifestation of the disease. As with the acute seroconversion illness, it tends to be non-specific. It is characterized by multiple diffuse lymphadenopathy involving two or more extrainguinal sites for greater that three months. It may be an early sign of HIV infection with 70 per cent of patients developing diffuse lymphadenopathy within the first few months after seroconversion. PGL can also present associated with other manifestations of the disease (**Box 12.1**).

Investigations

When suspected, HIV serology is indicated and diagnostic. FNAC will help the diagnosis of PGL and will also assist to identify other causes of infection, such as tuberculosis (TB), Kaposi's sarcoma (KS) or non-Hodgkin's lymphoma (NHL).

Treatment

The CD4$^+$ lymphocyte count is the most important reference factor for initiating antiretroviral therapy (ART) in asymptomatic patients. The large number of available drugs, the increased sensitivity of tests to monitor viral load, and the possibility of determining viral resistance is leading to a more individualized approach to therapy.[66, 67, 68, 69, 70, 71]

Box 12.1   Otorhinolaryngological manifestations of HIV infection

- Candidiasis
- Hairy leukoplakia
- HIV-gingivitis
- Necrotizing ulcerative gingivitis
- Kaposi's sarcoma
- Non-Hodgkin's lymphoma
- Benign lymphoepithelial cyst parotid gland
- Benign hyperplasia of the lymphoid tissue
- Pneumocystic carinii pneumonia
- Tuberculosis
- Opportunistic infections

TUBERCULOUS ADENITIS

Tuberculosis is the oldest documented infectious disease. It is the leading cause of death from a single infective agent and is on the increase. Among the factors associated with reversal of a previous decline are increased world travel and a rising incidence of immunodeficiency through HIV infections or intravenous drug abuse. Pulmonary tuberculosis is the most common manifestation, but extrapulmonary disease is likewise on the increase with tuberculous adenitis or historically named 'scrofula' being the most common. The word 'scrofula' comes from the Latin *scrofulae* meaning brood sow. In the Middle Ages, it was believed that the 'royal touch' of the sovereign of England or France could cure the disease. It was therefore known as the King's Evil. The kings were thought to have received this power by descent from Edward the Confessor who some legends said had received the power from St Remigius. Tuberculous adenitis can affect any lymph node group of the head and neck, including the salivary glands and thyroid. It is therefore imperative to have a high index of suspicion especially in certain ethnic groups.

Aetiology

Mycobacterium tuberculosis is an obligate aerobe, non-spore forming slender rod. Humans are the only reservoir and it is usually acquired from contact from a TB-infected patient via air-borne transmission. After a short period of replication in the lungs, silent dissemination occurs through the lympho-hematogenous system to extrapulmonary sites, including the cervical lymph nodes. This pathophysiological process differs from non-tuberculous atypical mycobacterial adenitis (NTM) which is addressed later in this chapter.

Clinical features

Ninety per cent of patients have unilateral involvement mainly of the jugular chain, followed by the submandibular triangle and the posterior triangle. The lymph nodes are usually firm, painless and they present with a characteristic erythematous skin discoloration. If the disease has progressed without being diagnosed, they tend to fistulae, present an obvious discharging sinus or form a 'cold' abscess, which

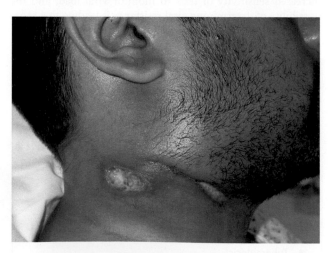

Figure 12.9 Right cervical tuberculous adenitis with central necrosis (scrofula).

suggests the clinical diagnosis. TB can also affect the ear, nose, pharynx, larynx, salivary and the thyroid gland and this may be particularly difficult to diagnose as patients often present with a discrete mass resembling a neoplastic lesion (**Figure 12.9**).

Diagnosis and investigations

Head and neck tuberculosis can be very difficult to diagnose as the clinical features may resemble neoplastic disease especially when presenting as a single-organ involvement. Full blood count is non-specific and may be normal. ESR is often elevated. Chest x-ray is mandatory, but only up to 20 per cent of patients will have positive changes. Soft tissue x-rays of the neck may be helpful as they will show dystrophic calcification characteristic of TB infection. Mantoux and Heaf test may not be diagnostic if the patient has been vaccinated against TB, but a grade IV skin reaction on this test may suggest active infection. Ultrasound scanning of the nodes will often show multiple matted nodes, but may be unspecific. FNAC can reveal mycobacteria, but may be positive in only 40 per cent of patients; however, the use of FNAC and polymerase chain reaction allows a quick and accurate diagnosis with high specificity (84 per cent) and sensitivity (100 per cent). If possible, excision biopsy (although this may be very difficult as matted and neurologic damage and bleeding may be excessive) or incision biopsy (if there is already skin involvement of the affected nodes) should be undertaken. Samples should be sent for microbiology as well as histological analysis and this should provide the definitive diagnosis. The microbiology cultures may take up to 6 weeks to grow mycobacteria and may delay treatment. HIV testing is advised in all patients.

Treatment

The treatment of active tuberculous adenitis, once suspected or proven, is by the use of antituberculous therapy. Increasing resistance is currently a significant problem and therefore chemotherapy should be adjusted according to sensitivity. Surgery has a limited role and should only be used as a diagnostic tool or in cases of residual disease.[72, 73, 74, 75]

NON–TUBERCULOUS ATYPICAL MYCOBACTERIAL ADENITIS

Non-tuberculous atypical mycobacteria is increasing in the Western world and, contrary to tuberculous infection, affects otherwise healthy immunocompetent children of middle-class families.

Aetiology

Mycobacterium avium and *Mycobacterium avium intracellulare* are the main two pathogens. The route of entry is usually through the oropharynx or the eye from injection of contaminated soil leading to superficial lymphadenopathy in the neck.

Clinical features

Patients affected by NTM are usually young healthy children without symptoms or signs of systemic illness and with multiple cervical lymphadenopathy. The lymphadenopathy often adheres to the skin causing a characteristic red-purple

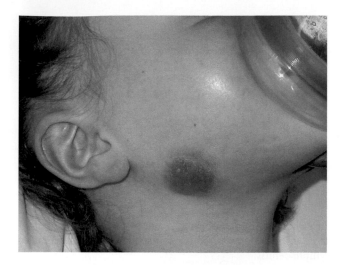

Figure 12.10   Child with right parotid non-tuberculous lesion.

discoloration and occasionally causing abscess with sinus formation and scarring (**Figure 12.10**).

Diagnosis and investigations

The diagnosis is made on clinical suspicion and the definitive diagnosis relies on isolating the organisms in culture either from microbiological swabs, FNAC or incisional biopsy.

Treatment

Most children may eventually develop their own immunity, so a period of observation may be advisable, especially if the lesion is in the parotid gland. Antibiotic therapy with macrolides, such as clarythromycin or azithromycin, with or without antituberculous therapy has been suggested. In some studies, up to 67 per cent of resolution has been experienced without surgical excision. Surgical curettage with or without antibiotic therapy may be an option and has been advised with some success in selected cases especially if a full surgical excision may lead to significant morbidity. Surgical excision is the ultimate treatment of choice and it appears to be more effective than antibiotic therapy alone.[76, 77, 78, 79, 80, 81]

BRUCELLOSIS

Brucellosis is primarily a disease of the domestic animals and causes contagious abortion or other reproductive problems in cattle (*Brucella abortus*), pigs (*B. suis*), goats (*B. melitensis*), dogs (*B. canis*) and sheep (*B. ovis*). Current pasteurization, other hygienic preventive measures and adequate animal vaccinations have greatly reduced the incidence of the disease in Western countries.

Aetiology

Human spread by *Brucella* sp. occurs by direct contact of infected tissue with conjunctiva or broken skin, by ingestion of contaminated meat or dairy products and by inhalation of contagious aerosols.

Clinical features

The clinical features are often non-specific and some infections are subclinical. When the infection is clinically evident,

most patients complain of night sweats, chills, undulating pyrexia and malaise. Up to 20 per cent of patients will develop cervical lymphadenopathies and a similar percentage will have splenomegaly.

Diagnosis and investigations

When the diagnosis is suspected, blood cultures will often isolate the bacteria and provide definitive diagnosis. Serology will also provide the diagnosis in those cases in which the clinical picture is less obvious.

Treatment

The treatment is done by multiple antibiotic therapy, as treatment with single agents is associated with a 30 per cent chance of relapse. The current recommendation by the World Health Organization (WHO) is the use of doxycycline 200 mg with rifampicin 900 mg daily for 6 weeks.[82]

TOXOPLASMOSIS

Aetiology

Toxoplasmosis is a worldwide infection cause by *Toxoplasma gondii*, a protozoon transmitted by the ingestion of cysts excreted in the faeces of infected cats, or from eating undercooked beef or lamb.

Clinical features

Congenital infection usually causes hydrocephalus or microphaly. Aquired infections present with generalized malaise, myalgia, fever, cough and maculopapular rash. If not treated, a chronic phase will develop, which may be asymptomatic or present with isolated cervical lymphadenopathy. In immunocompromised patients especially with HIV-AIDS, it may cause encephalitis.

Diagnosis

The diagnosis is made on clinical history and complemented by serology which will confirm diagnosis. The white cell count will show lymphocytosis with atypical mononuclear cells. FNAC may suggest the diagnosis, although may be non-specific.

Lymph node biopsy will reveal features supporting the diagnosis of toxoplasmosis. Cerebrospinal fluid (CSF) analysis may demonstrate the parasite and confirm the diagnosis if there is central nervous system involvement.

Treatment

Where treatment is indicated, a combination of sulphadimidine, pyrimethamine and folic acid is used and the blood count should be monitored regularly until it becomes normal.[83, 84, 85]

ACTINOMYCOSIS

Aetiology

Actinomycosis is a bacterial infection caused by *Actinomyces israelii*, an anaerobic organism which is a commensal in the healthy oral cavity. The organism may become pathogenic when the mucous membrane is injured. Infection is usually associated with severe dental caries and periodontitis.

Clinical features

Patients present with a firm indurated mass with ill-defined edges usually lateral to the mandible. If left untreated, the infection may spread to the adjacent tissues and may become bony hard. Once the infection is established, multiple sinus may develop which discharge pus and watery fluid characteristically containing sulphur granules.

Diagnosis and investigations

The diagnosis may be suspected on clinical grounds which is usually very characteristic. The FNAC may show sulphur granules which are diagnostic. The biopsy will again show the characteristic colonies of sulphur granules, but the organism may be difficult to culture.

Treatment

The treatment is with intravenous benzylpenicillin or cephalosporins in high doses that may require to be continued for at least 6 weeks. However, longer courses of antibiotic therapy up to a year may be necessary in resistant cases or immunocompromised patients. Removal of carious teeth is imperative to excise the site of origin of the infection.[86]

Neck abscesses

SUPERFICIAL SOFT TISSUE NECK ABSCESSES

Cervical abscesses are relatively uncommon in comparison with the number of acute and chronic lymphadenitis cases in the paediatric and adult population. However, small children under the age of four years and immunocompromised patients appear to be more susceptible.

Aetiology

Failure of patients to localize the organism at the site of attachment to nasal or pharyngeal epithelium will result in the spread of infection via lymphatics causing suppuration. The most common pathogens are *Staphyloccoccus aureus*, *Streptococcus pyogenes* and, in the paediatric population, atypical mycobacteria.

Clinical features

The development of the abscess is often preceded by an upper respiratory tract infection, although sometimes this may not be obvious from the history especially in the young paediatric population.

Diagnosis and investigations

The diagnosis is based on the clinical suspicion. FBC, ESR and CRP are useful to ascertain the inflammatory origin and to monitor progress. Ultrasound and CT scanning will be useful to determine whether the mass has a central area of necrosis that may require incision and drainage.

Treatment

The treatment involves a combination of supportive therapy, broad-spectrum antibiotic therapy until culture and sensitivity results are available, and surgical incision and drainage. Repeated needle aspiration is not usually helpful unless the abscess arises from a thyroglossal duct cyst, in which case incision and drainage is reserved as last resort and only antibiotic therapy and repeated aspiration has failed.[87]

RETROPHARYNGEAL SPACE ABSCESS

Retropharyngeal space abscess is less common than in the past, but still represents a life-threatening infection that can result in airway obstruction and death if not recognized.

Aetiology

In infants, aetiology is usually due to an upper respiratory tract infection and in adults is usually due to tuberculous lymphadenitis.

Clinical features

Children with retropharyngeal abscesses have or recently had an upper respiratory tract infection or dental sepsis. They appear ill, unwell, toxic and with pyrexia of 38–39 °C. The abscess swelling may obstruct the posterior nares and push on the soft palate, potentially with a risk of respiratory obstruction. In adults, the clinical features are those of an insidious onset with low-grade fever, mild oropharyngeal discomfort and low risk of obstruction.

Diagnosis and investigations

The diagnosis is made on clinical grounds and investigations should not be advised if airway obstruction is present or an imminent risk. The white cell count and inflammatory markers, such as ESR and CRP, are usually raised. A plain lateral soft tissue neck x-ray will often show the abscess, but must be interpreted with caution. CT scanning will delineate the abscess (**Figure 12.11**).

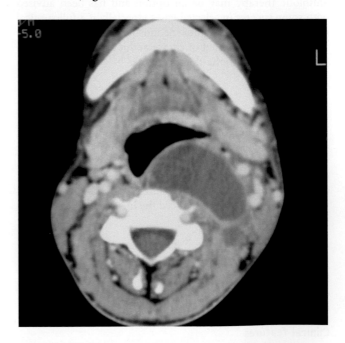

Figure 12.11 Computed tomography scan demonstrating a retropharyngeal abscess.

Treatment

In children, retropharyngeal abscesses represent a real emergency. In this situation, the children should be taken to the operating theatre and, once the airway is secured, the pus should be incised and drained. It may be necessary to keep the child intubated and ventilated until the drainage has subsided and the infection resolved. The insertion of a tracheostomy is currently rarely needed. In adults, once the pus is drained and the diagnosis confirmed, antituberculous chemotherapy should be commenced.[88, 89, 90, 91, 92, 93, 94, 95, 96, 97]

PARAPHARYNGEAL SPACE ABSCESS

Parapharyngeal space abscesses tend to be more common in adults than in children. They often result from an infective process of the upper aerodigestive tract, especially tonsillitis or tonsillectomy in 60 per cent of cases or a dental infection in 30 per cent of patients. This, however, may be trivial or it might have occurred and resolved a few days prior to the onset. In the remaining 10 per cent, the cause is otogenic.

Aetiology

Streptococcus viridans was the most common pathogen (39 per cent of positive cultures), followed by *Staphylococcus epidermidis* (22 per cent) and *Staphylococcus aureus* (22 per cent).

Clinical features

Patients are usually unwell, pyrexial and toxic. They present with trismus due to the affection of the pterygoid muscles and the tonsil may be displaced medially. It usually displaces the upper third of the sternocleidomastoid muscle, especially posteriorly.

Diagnosis and investigations

The diagnosis is based on the history and examination and made on clinical grounds. The white cell count and the inflammatory markers, such as ESR and CRP, are usually raised. The ultrasound or CT scan will delineate the abscess and confirm diagnosis. Needle aspiration under ultrasound or CT guidance should be considered.

Treatment

Small loculated abscesses or cellulites can be managed conservatively with intravenous broad-spectrum antibiotics covering aerobic, as well as anaerobic bacteria for 12–24 hours. Needle aspiration under ultrasound or CT guidance should be considered and may be helpful in small collections. However, large collections will require formal incision and drainage via an external approach. The collection is accessed medial to the carotid sheath and the insertion of a drain is mandatory to prevent recollection.[88, 89, 90, 91, 92, 93, 94, 95, 96, 97]

SUBMANDIBULAR SPACE ABSCESS OR LUDWIG'S ANGINA

The word 'angina' comes from the Greek *ankhon* meaning 'strangling'. Ludwig's angina is the cellulitis of the submandibular space that can lead to a compromise of the airway due to easy spread of the infection through the sublingual soft tissue. It is named after the German physician Willhem Frederick von Ludwig, who first described the condition in 1836. Over 80 per cent of patients have a dental infection and the rest usually have an upper respiratory tract infection.

Aetiology

Streptococcus viridans was the most common pathogen (39 per cent of positive cultures), followed by *Staphylococcus epidermidis* (22 per cent), *Staphylococcus aureus* (22 per cent) and *Escherichia coli*.

Clinical features

Patients are often elderly or young children, and they are unwell and toxic. There is trismus and excessive salivation. The swelling is diffuse, and there is erythema and cellulitis of the skin. The floor of the mouth appears oedematous, brown in colour with the tongue pushed upwards and back which can cause a potential airway obstruction (**Figure 12.12**).

Diagnosis and investigations

The diagnosis is based on the history and examination, and made on clinical grounds. The white cell count and the inflammatory markers, such as ESR and CRP, are usually

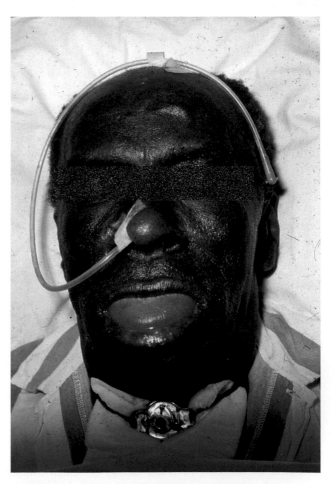

Figure 12.12 Patient with submandibular space abscess or Ludwig's angina who required a tracheostomy.

raised. The ultrasound or CT scan will delineate the abscess and confirm diagnosis, although abscess formation is rare.

Treatment

Ludwig's angina is a cellulitis rather than abscess. Airway management is paramount and high-dose intravenous antibiotic therapy targeted to the causing bacteria should be commenced. Needle aspiration under ultrasound or CT guidance should be considered and may be helpful in some circumstances. However, established collections will require formal incision and drainage via an external approach. The collection is best accessed through a lateral transverse cervical incision at the level of the hyoid bone, and a drain should be inserted. Tracheostomy may be required for airway management in a significant proportion of patients with well-established Ludwig's angina.[88, 89, 90, 91, 92, 93, 94, 95, 96, 97]

MISCELLANEOUS RARE CAUSES OF NECK MASSES

Organized haematomas

Aetiology

Aetiology involves blunt or penetrating trauma of the neck.

Clinical features

Patients present with a neck mass that usually causes local discomfort and occasionally constant pain.

Diagnosis and investigations

A history of trauma is usually present, although not always obvious. Ultrasound-guided FNAC will suggest diagnosis, but the sonographic appearances depend on the age of the haematoma. If in the liquid state, the blood can be aspirated. CT scan and MRI will display distinct radiological features and determine the anatomy. The sonographic appearance depends on the age of the haematoma. If in the liquid state, the blood can be aspirated. Follow-up ultrasound may be helpful to ensure that there is no underlying lesion.

Treatment

Surgical excision is the treatment of choice, although it may be difficult due to the surrounding fibrosis of the lesions.[98, 99]

Castleman disease

Castleman disease is a rare entity, which is characterized by hyperplasia of lymph nodes and capillary proliferation that usually affects adolescents and young adults. Three histological patterns has been described: hyaline vascular type, plasma cell type and mixed type. Two clinical types have been identified: a localized type (ECL) usually of benign clinical course and a multicentric type (ECM), which has a worse prognosis and may lead to the development of non-Hodgkin's lymphoma.

Aetiology

It is unknown, although up to 50 per cent of multicentric variants are caused by Kaposi sarcoma-associated virus (KSHV), a gammaherpes virus that causes Kaposi sarcoma and primary effusion lymphoma.

Clinical features

Patients usually present with a progressive enlarging lateral cervical lymphadenopathy often associated with autoimmune iron-deficiency anaemia. ECM may present with B symptoms, such as fever, anorexia and weight loss.

Diagnosis and investigations

Full blood count shows iron-deficiency anaemia and the ESR is elevated. FNAC often shows a lymphocytic aspirate and it is not normally diagnostic, therefore surgical excision is advised for histological diagnosis. Imaging studies are often not useful.

Treatment

The anaemia is difficult to treat as it often does not respond to iron supplement. Surgical excision is usually therapeutic in ECL, although it may be difficult in ECM. Treatment with ganciclovir or the anti-CD20 B cell monoclonal antibody, may improve the outcome in some patients with ECM. In ECM, long-term follow up is advised in association with haemato-oncology teams.[100, 101, 102]

Kikuchi disease

Kikuchi disease (KD) is a self-limiting disease of the lymph nodes that usually affects young women. It is also known as Kikuchi–Fujimoto disease and was first described by Kikuchi in Japan in 1972. Histologically, it is characterized by a histiocytic necrotizing lymphadenitis.

Aetiology

It is unknown, however an autoimmune aetiology has been proposed as some human leukocyte antigen (HLA) class II genes are more frequent in patients with KD. An association with systemic lupus erythematosus (SLE) has also been reported.

Clinical features

The disease often presents with persistently intermittent fever and tender enlarged cervical lymph nodes. It is self-limiting, but it may take up to three months to resolve.

Diagnosis and investigations

The diagnosis can be confirmed by histopathological findings of the lymph node in open biopsy.

Treatment

The disease is usually self-limiting and does not respond to antibiotic therapy. Supportive therapy with non-steroidal anti-inflammatory drugs may help to alleviate the lymphadenopathy tenderness and pyrexia.[103, 104]

Kawasaki disease

Kawasaki disease (KWD) is an acute, self-limiting vasculitis of childhood, although it may also occur in adults. It was first described by Tomisaku Kawasaki in Japan in 1967. In some countries, Kawasaki disease has now surpassed acute rheumatic fever as the leading cause of acquired heart disease in children.

Aetiology

The aetiology is unknown; however, the acute presentation and the clustering of cases may indicate an infectious aetiology.

Clinical findings

The illness is characterized by fever, bilateral non-exudative conjunctivitis, erythema of the lips and oral mucosa, changes in the extremities, rash and cervical lymphadenopathy. Coronary artery aneurysms or ectasia develop in approximately 15–25 per cent of untreated children and may lead to myocardial infarction and sudden death.

Diagnosis and investigations

The diagnosis is based on the recognition of this characteristic sequence of clinical events, none of which are pathognomonic. Establishing the diagnosis may be further complicated by the occurrence of other, seemingly unrelated, clinical features, such as irritability, neck stiffness, sterile pyuria, pneumonitis and hepatitis. There is no laboratory test that can help in confirming a diagnosis.

Treatment

Treatment is with intravenous gammaglobulin therapy and high doses of aspirin.[105, 106]

Other rare causes of cervical neck masses

Other rare causes of cervical neck masses include sarcoidosis, fibromatosis colli, Rosai–Dorfman disease, Kimura disease, dermatofibroma and prominent transverse process of atlas.[107, 108]

VISCERAL BENIGN NECK DISEASES

Pharyngeal pouch

Pharyngeal pouch, also known as Zenker's diverticulum, is a unilateral pulsion diverticulum of the pharyngeal mucosa. It occurs at the interface of the inferior constrictor of the pharynx and the upper oesophageal sphincter. This potential space is known as Killian's dehiscence and lies between the fibres of cricopharyngeous and thyropharyngeous. Although this potential anatomical weakness in the pharyngeal wall is present in everyone, this condition only occurs in a small proportion of the population and presents late in life. Therefore it is thought to be an acquired condition.[1]

Aetiology

The aetiology of pharyngeal pouch has not been fully established. The two factors which appear to be the most important in the aetiology of pharyngeal pouch are:

1. **Cricopharyngeal hypertonicity**: failure of relaxation of the cricopharyngeous muscle is thought to raise intraluminal pressure within the pharynx promoting pouch formation.[2]
2. **Pharyngeal/oesophageal incoordination**: dysmotility of the reflex bolus has been identified as an important factor in production of the pouch.[3, 4] This may or may not be associated with gastro-oesophageal reflux.

Pharyngeal pouches usually enlarge in a posterolateral direction displacing the oesophagus, although it appears that right-handed individuals have left-sided pouches and left-handed ones have right-sided pouches.

Clinical features

Pharyngeal pouches may be found as an incidental finding in the asymptomatic patient being investigated for other symptoms. If there are no adverse effects relating to this incidental finding and the patient is asymptomatic, then the pouch can be ignored.

Symptoms usually present in the elderly. Dysphagia is the most common presenting symptom of a pharyngeal pouch. The dysphagia may be progressive as the pouch enlarges. Weight loss may result from prolonged dysphagia. Regurgitation of food after meals may occur as the pouch empties itself. Chronic cough may be a symptom of aspiration which can be a feature of this condition. Silent aspiration may result from the pharyngeal pouch, and respiratory assessment is important if surgical intervention is to be contemplated. Very rarely, a pharyngeal pouch may present as a lateral neck mass.

Diagnosis and investigations

The diagnosis is often suspected from the history. Initial physical examination is indicated including fibreoptic nasolaryngoscopy. This is essential to exclude any other laryngeal or hypopharyngeal pathology. Occasionally, the pouch can be seen when asking the patient to perform a valsalva manoeuvre during the laryngoscopic examination. If a pharyngeal pouch is suspected, then a water-soluble contrast swallow study is indicated and is usually diagnostic (**Figure 12.13**). Direct laryngoscopy and pharyngoscopy under general anaesthetic may be appropriate if the contrast swallow studies are negative.

Treatment

If the pharyngeal pouch is asymptomatic and there are no respiratory complications, then it can be managed conservatively. In patients with obvious gastro-oesophageal reflux, treatment with proton-pump inhibitors may help their symptoms. Management of pharyngeal pouches has changed considerably over the last decade.[5] Endoscopic approaches are now favoured, as they are quick, safe and well established. However, the traditional open approaches are still practised as they have specific indications, and there will be a proportion of patients in whom the endoscopic approach is not possible due to unfavourable anatomy or in cases of recurrence. The two approaches have been compared

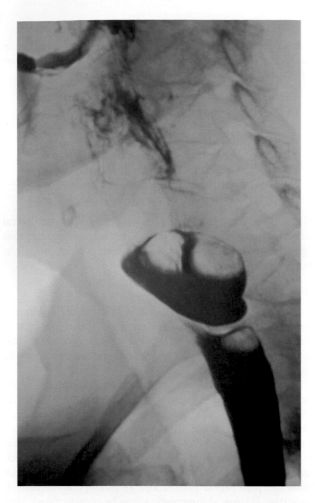

Figure 12.13 Contrast swallow demonstrating a pharyngeal pouch.

in terms of results and morbidity. The endoscopic diverticulotomy has been shown to be superior due to shorter inpatient stay and faster return to oral diet. However, there is little evidence using objective measurements comparing the two procedures and little evidence to show which has a higher recurrence rate. The open procedure is almost always followed up by a contrast study prior to commencement of oral diet, to ensure that pharyngeal healing has occurred. The endoscopic procedure usually does not have a follow-up contrast study. In those cases where one is performed postoperatively, there is usually a small residual pouch visible. The open approach is the only one to perform a cricopharyngeal myotomy which, is thought to be the most important factor in pouch formation. The advantages of the endoscopic procedure over the open approach, in terms of shorter operative time, ease of procedure, short inpatient stay and fast return to oral diet make it more cost effective, even though its superiority in terms of efficacy has not been demonstrated. The endoscopic procedure can easily be repeated for recurrences.

Endoscopic approaches

In the past, the endoscopic diathermy diverticulectomy or Dohlman's procedure was popular and indicated in patients who had a poor anaesthetic risk. Currently, however, endoscopic stapling and transoral CO_2 laser diverticulotomy have substituted this approach. Endoscopic stapling is possibly the most popular procedure and it is now established as the recommended treatment of choice in the majority of patients with symptomatic pharyngeal pouches.

Endoscopic stapling diverticulotomy

The procedure is performed as follows: a distraction distending diverticuloscope is introduced into the pharynx. This instrument has two limbs, one is introduced into the lumen of the oesophagus and the other in the pouch. The diverticuloscope is opened up in order to visualize the pouch. The pouch contents are aspirated in order to empty the pouch. A rigid endoscope is introduced to inspect the mucosal lining of the pouch. Any necessary biopsies should be taken. A stapling gun is introduced under direct vision with the aid of a rigid endoscope. The staple gun is then activated and divides and seals the bar which separates the pouch and the oesophagus.[7] The advantages of the endoscopic approach are that it results in a short anaesthetic time, short inpatient stay and quick return to oral diet. It is, therefore, suitable for the elderly patient with comorbidity.

Open approaches

Open techniques are currently less rarely performed and reserved for recurrent cases and those unsuitable for endoscopic approach. They include surgical inversion, diverticulopexy with or without cricopharyngeal myotomy and in cases in which the pouch is small, cricopharyngeal myotomy alone.

Open surgical excision or one-stage diverticulectomy

Initially, it is necessary to perform an endoscopic assessment of the pouch so it can be identified and inspected. This will also allow the pouch to be packed with gauze, such as BIPP, so it facilitates the identification of the pouch in the neck. At the time, a rigid dilator is also inserted in the oesophagus to facilitate the cricopharyngeal myotomy performed at the time of the procedure. Pharyngeal pouches are accessed via a lateral pharyngotomy approach. This involves a horizontal skin crease incision at the level of the cricoid cartilage. The sternocleidomastoid muscle is mobilized and retracted laterally. The neurovascular bundle of the carotid sheath is also mobilized and retracted posterolaterally. The middle thyroid vein often needs to be divided in order to access the pouch. The pouch is excised and pharyngeal defect repaired by suturing in layers. A cricopharyngeal myotomy is also performed to facilitate swallowing and to prevent the recurrence of the pouch.[109, 110, 111, 112, 113, 114, 115, 116, 117, 118, 119, 120, 121]

PHARYNGEAL POUCH CARCINOMA

It is a recognized sequelae of this condition. It is thought to result due to chronic inflammation of the pouch due to the effect of its contents. Dysplasia and metaplasia is thought to result as a consequence. This condition is usually associated with a poor prognosis due to late presentation and coexistence of comorbidity.[109, 110, 111, 112, 113, 114, 115, 116, 117, 118, 119, 121, 122]

Laryngoceles

A laryngocele is an abnormal cystic dilatation of the saccule of the larynx. The saccule is a small mucosal pouch which lies between the vestibular fold of the larynx and the inner surface of the thyroid cartilage. It is thought to be an anatomical vestigial remnant within the ventricle of the larynx and contains numerous mucinous glands. Laryngoceles can be internal (within the larynx), external (outside the larynx) or mixed (both). They are usually unilateral and can rarely be bilateral. Laryngoceles can contain either air or mucous and, if they become infected, they are called 'laryngopyoceles'.

Aetiology

The aetiology of laryngoceles is unknown. They may be congenital or acquired. Intraluminal laryngeal pressure has been postulated as the causative factor in producing laryngoceles. The association with activities, such as glass blowing and playing wind instruments, has only been made in case reports. There is, therefore, little evidence to suggest causation. A small proportion of laryngoceles has been identified to coexist with laryngeal carcinomas. External laryngoceles have been found in up to 16 per cent of laryngectomy specimens for laryngeal carcinomas, as opposed to 2 per cent in laryngectomy specimens for pyriform sinus carcinoma. It has been suggested that the neoplastic growth results in increased luminal pressure in the larynx precipitating laryngocele formation. Other laryngeal pathologies, such as amyloidosis, scleroderma and SLE, have also been associated with the formation of laryngoceles. The above associations, however, are subject to significant reporting bias and therefore should be considered with caution.

Clinical features

Laryngoceles may often be asymptomatic and have been identified to be a prevalent incidental autopsy finding. Dysphonia is the most common presenting symptom. A lateral neck mass may result due to pathological enlargement through the thyrohyoid ligament. Acute airway obstruction may result in stridor if the laryngocele enlarges and obstructs the larynx. Securing the airway and resection of the laryngocele is indicated. Laryngoceles can also become infected and produce laryngopyoceles. These behave as abscesses and require incision and drainage if external, or endoscopic decompression and drainage if internal.

Diagnosis and investigations

Full physical examination including fibreoptic nasolaryngoscopy is essential to rule out any coexisting laryngeal pathology, especially in those high-risk patients with carcinoma of the larynx. Cross-section imaging with a contrasted CT scan is the investigation of choice for laryngoceles (**Figure 12.14**). If patients are found with any mucosal lesions, endoscopic assessment under general anaesthesia with biopsies should be undertaken.

Treatment

As the majority of laryngoceles are asymptomatic and are not associated with any pathology, treatment may not be necessary. However, as there is a potential risk of infection and pyocele formation, advice should be given to patients to

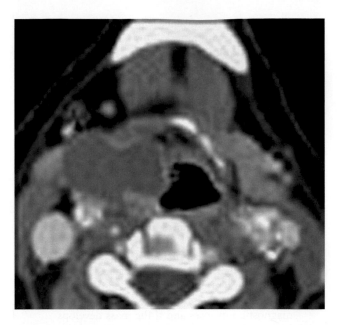

Figure 12.14 Computed tomography scan demonstrating a large laryngocele arising from the right laryngeal ventricle.

make an informed decision with regards to surgical intervention. Internal laryngoceles can be treated with transoral laser resection. The CO_2 laser can be used to marsupialize or excise the pouch. External laryngoceles can be approached via a lateral pharyngotomy/thyrotomy approach. The lateral surface of the larynx is exposed, the external component of the laryngocele is mobilized and resected and the mucosal defect repaired. A covering tracheostomy may be necessary for large lesions.[123, 124, 125, 126, 127]

KEY EVIDENCE

- This is a diverse chapter addressing multiple benign disorders.
- There is a lack of substantive high level of evidence due to the intrinsic nature of the disorders addressed in most areas with most evidence being level 2 or below.
- Congenital abnormalities of the head and neck are best treated with surgical excision whenever possible.[45]
- Head and neck tuberculosis should be treated with systemic antituberculous therapy and surgery has a limited role in its management.[72, 73, 74, 75]

KEY LEARNING POINTS

- Benign neck masses and visceral benign neck diseases are common and represent a diverse group of disorders.

- The evaluation and management of patients who present with a neck lump should have a systematic and uncompromising clinical approach.
- The examination of these patients should be comprehensive and always include a fibre-optic endoscopic examination of the upper aero-digestive tract.
- All patients with neck lumps should be investigated with ultrasound-guided fine needle aspiration as an initial investigation whenever possible.
- The great majority of congenital neck masses can be treated with surgical excision if indicated, however surgery requires meticulous technique to avoid recurrence.
- Acquired non-inflammatory neck masses are mainly treated with surgical excision.
- Acquired inflammatory neck masses should be treated medically and surgery is reserved for diagnostic purposes and if the mass develops into an abscess.
- Head and neck acquired neck abscess requires incision and drainage in most instances.
- Pharyngeal pouch surgery has evolved and the majority of these can be dealt with endoscopic rather than open surgery.
- Laryngoceles are rare but when developed, primary laryngeal cancer should always be excluded.

REFERENCES

1. Simo R, Leslie A. Differential diagnosis and management of neck lumps. *Surgery* 2006; **24**: 312–22.
2. Watkinson JC, Gaze MN, Wilson JA. *Stell and Maran's head and neck surgery*, 4th edn. Oxford: Butterworth and Heineman, 2000.
3. Homer JJ, Silva P. Management of neck lumps. *Practitioner* 2003; **247**: 726–34.
4. Prakash PK, Hanna FW. Differential diagnosis of neck lumps. *Practitioner* 2002; **246**: 252–4, 256–7, 259.
5. Smith OD, Ellis PD, Bearcroft PW *et al.* Management of neck lumps – a triage model. *Annals of the Royal College of Surgeons of England* 2000; **82**: 223–6.
6. Karcher AM, Zaman A, Brewis C, Fahmy T. Neck lumps: expect the unexpected. *Lancet* 2000; **355**: 1070.
7. Fife DG. The management of lumps in the neck. *British Journal of Hospital Medicine* 1997; **57**: 522–6.
8. Premachandra DJ, McRae D, Prinsley P. Biopsy of neck lumps in adults should be preceded by examination of the upper aerodigestive tract. *Postgraduate Medical Journal* 1990; **66**: 113–15.
9. Siodlak MZ, Grainger JM, Gleeson MJ, Wengraf CL. Fine needle aspiration biopsy of neck lumps in a district hospital. *Clinical Otolaryngology and Allied Sciences* 1986; **11**: 131–5.
10. Gleeson MJ, Herbert A, Richards A. Management of lateral neck masses in adults. *British Medical Journal* 2000; **320**: 1521–4.
11. Layfield LJ. Fine-needle aspiration in the diagnosis of head and neck lesions: A review and discussion of problems in differential diagnosis. *Diagnostic Cytopathology* 2007; **35**: 798–805.
12. Sack MJ, Weber RS, Weinstein GS *et al.* Image-guided fine-needle aspiration of the head and neck: five years' experience. *Archives of Otolaryngology – Head and Neck Surgery* 1998; **124**: 1155–61.
13. Broomhead IW. Cystic hygroma of the neck. *British Journal of Plastic Surgery* 1964; **17**: 225–44.
14. Al-Khateeb TH, Al Zoubi F. Congenital neck masses: a descriptive retrospective study of 252 cases. *Journal of Oral and Maxillofacial Surgery* 2007; **65**: 2242–7.
15. Orvidas LJ, Kasperbauer DK. Pediatric lymphangiomas of the head and neck. *Annals of Otology, Rhinology and Laryngology* 2000; **109**: 411–12.
16. Hamoir M, Plouin-Gaudon I, Rombaux P *et al.* Lymphatic malformations of the head and neck: a retrospective review and support for staging. *Head and Neck* 2001; **23**: 326–37.
17. Renton JP, Smith RJ. Current treatment paradigms in the management of lymphatic malformations. *Laryngoscope* 2011; **121**: 56–9.
18. de Serres LM, Sie KC, Richardson MA. Lymphatic malformations of the head and neck: A proposal for staging. *Archives of Otorhinolaryngology Head and Neck Surgery* 1995; **121**: 577–82.
19. Godin DA, Guarisco JL. Cystic hygromas of the head and neck. *Journal of the Louisiana State Medical Society* 1997; **149**: 224–8.
20. Brewis C, Pracy JP, Albert DM. Treatment of lymphangiomas of the head and neck by intralesional injection of OK-432 (Picibanil). *Clinical Otolaryngology and Allied Sciences* 2000; **25**: 130–4.
21. Laranne J, Keski-Nisula L, Rautio R *et al.* OK-432 (Picibanil) therapy for lymphangiomas in children. *European Archives of Otorhinolaryngology* 2002; **259**: 274–8.
22. Ozen IO, Moralioglu S, Karabulut R *et al.* Surgical treatment of cervicofacial cystic hygromas in children. *Journal for Otorhinolaryngology and its Related Specialties* 2005; **67**: 331–4.
23. Pryor SG, Lewis JE, Weaver AL, Orvidas LJ. Pediatric dermoid cysts of the head and neck. *Otorhinolaryngology – Head and Neck Surgery* 2005; **132**: 938–42.
24. Filston HC. Hemangiomas, cystic hygromas, and teratomas of the head and neck. *Seminars in Pediatric Surgery* 1994; **3**: 147–59.
25. Todd NW. Common congenital anomalies of the neck. Embriology and surgical anatomy. *Surgical Clinics of North America* 1993; **73**: 599–610.

26. Folley DS, Fallat ME. Thyroglossal duct cysts and other congenital midline cervical anomalies. *Seminars in Pediatric Surgery* 2006; **15**: 70–5.

27. Dedivitis RA, Camargo DL, Peixoto GL *et al.* Thyroglossal duct: a review of 55 cases. *Journal of the American College of Surgeons* 2002; **194**: 274–7.

28. Lev S, Lev MH. Imaging of cystic lesions. *Radiologic Clinics of North America* 2000; **38**: 1013–27.

29. Shah R, Gow K, Sobol SE. Outcome of thyroglossal duct cyst excision is independent of presenting age or symptomatology. *International Journal of Pediatric Otorhinolaryngology* 2007; **71**: 1731–5.

30. Ghaneim A, Atkins P. The management of thyroglossal duct cysts. *International Journal of Clinical Practice* 1997; **51**: 512–3.

31. Ostlie DJ, Burjonrappa SC, Snyder CL *et al.* Thyroglossal duct infections and surgical outcomes. *Journal of Pediatric Surgery* 2004; **39**: 396–9.

32. Perkins JA, Inglis AF, Sie KC, Manning SC. Recurrent thyroglossal duct cysts: a 23 year experience and new method of management. *Annals of Otology, Rhinology and Laryngology* 2006; **115**: 850–6.

33. Kim MK, Pawel BR, Isaacson G. Central neck dissection for the treatment of recurrent thyroglossal duct cysts in childhood. *Otolaryngology – Head and Neck Surgery* 1999; **121**: 543–7.

34. Patel NN, Hartley BE, Howard DJ. Management of thyroglossal tract disease after failed Sistrunks procedure. *Journal of Laryngology and Otology* 2003; **117**: 710–12.

35. Roback SA, Telander RL. Thyroglossal duct cysts and branchial cleft anomalies. *Seminars in Pediatric Surgery* 1994; **3**: 142–6.

36. Folley DS, Fallat ME. Thyroglossal duct cysts and other congenital midline cervical anomalies. *Seminars in Pediatric Surgery* 2006; **15**: 70–5.

37. Kadhim AL, Sheahan P, Colreavy MP, Timon CV. Pearls and pitfalls in the management of branchial cyst. *Journal of Laryngology and Otology* 2004; **118**: 946–50.

38. Nicollas R, Guelfucci B, Roman S, Triglia JM. Congenital cysts and fistulas of the neck. *International Journal of Pediatric Otorhinolaryngology* 2000; **55**: 117–24.

39. Nicollas R, Ducroz V, Garabedian EN, Triglia JM. Fourth branchial pouch anomalies: a study of six cases and review of the literature. *International Journal of Pediatric Otorhinolaryngology* 1998; **44**: 5–10.

40. Golledge J, Ellis H. The aetiology of lateral cervical (branchial) cysts: past and present theories. *Journal of Laryngology and Otology* 1994; **108**: 653–9.

41. Regauer S, Gogg-Kamerer M, Braun H, Beham A. Lateral neck cysts – the branchial theory revisited. A critical review and clinicopathological study of 97 cases with special emphasis on cytokeratin extresion. *Acta Pathologica, Microbiologica, et Immunologica Scandinavica* 1997; **105**: 623–30.

42. Wasson J, Blaney S, Simo R. A third branchial pouch cyst presenting as stridor in a child. *Annals of the Royal College of Surgeons of England* 2007; **89**: W12–14.

43. Acierno SP, Waldenhausen JH. Congenital cervical cysts, sinuses and fistulae. *Otolaryngologic Clinics of North America* 2007; **40**: 161–76.

44. Choi SS, Zalzal GH. Branchial anomalies: a review of 52 cases. *Laryngoscope* 1995; **105**: 909–13.

45. Nicoucar K, Giger R, Jaecklin T *et al.* Management of congenital third branchial arch anomalies: a systematic review. *Otolaryngology – Head and Neck Surgery* 2010; **142**: 21–8.

46. Golden BA, Zide MF. Cutaneous cysts of the head and neck. *Journal of Oral and Maxillofacial Surgery* 2005; **63**: 1613–19.

47. Ro EY, Thomas RM, Isaacson GC. Giant dermoid cyst of the neck can mimic a cystic hygroma: using MRI to differenciate neck lesions. *International Journal of Pediatric Otorhinolaryngology* 2007; **71**: 653–8.

48. Trivedi PM, Black M, Mitchell DB, Simo R. Pathology quiz – What is your diagnosis? Pilomatrixoma (Malherbes's Tumour). CME Bulletin. *Otorhinolaryngology, Head and Neck Surgery* 2004; **8**: 61–2.

49. Pirouzmawesh A, Reinish JF, Gonzalez-Gomez I *et al.* Pilomatrixoma: a review of 346 cases. *Plastic and Reconstructive Surgery* 2003; **112**: 1784–9.

50. Keskin D, Eziemik N, Celik H. Familial multiple lipomatosis. *Israel Medical Association Journal* 2002; **4**: 1121–3.

51. Copcu E, Sivrioglu NS. Post-traumatic lipoma: analysis of 10 cases and explanation of possible mechanisms. *Dermatologic Surgery* 2003; **29**: 215–20.

52. El-Monem MH, Gaarfar AH, Magdy EA. Lipomas of the head and neck: presentation variability and diagnostic work-up. *Journal of Laryngology and Otology* 2006; **120**(1): 47–55.

53. Luu TM, Chevalier I, Gaurthier M *et al.* Acute adenitis in children: clinical course and factors predictive of surgical drainage. *Journal of Paediatrics and Child Health* 2005; **41**: 273–7.

54. Gosche JR, Vick L. Acute subacute, and chronic cervical lymphadenitis in children. *Seminars in Pediatric Surgery* 2006; **15**: 99–106.

55. Auwaerter PG. Recent advances in the understanding of infectious mononucleosis: are prospects improved for treatment or control? *Expert Review of Anti-infective Therapy* 2006; **4**: 1039–49.

56. Vetsika EK, Callan M. Infectious mononucleosis and Epstein–Barr virus. *Expert Reviews in Molecular Medicine* 2004; **6**: 1–16.

57. Cantani A, Mastrantoni F. Recent advances on Epstein–Barr virus infectious mononucleosis. *Rivista Europea per le Scienze Mediche e Farmacologiche* 1989; **11**: 41–4.

58. Ganzel TM, Goldman JL, Padhya TA. Otolaryngologic clinical patterns in pediatric infectious mononucleosis.

American Journal of Otolaryngology 1996; **17**: 397–400.

59. Chan SC, Dawes PJ. The management of severe infectious mononucleosis tonsillitis and upper airway obstruction. *Journal of Laryngology and Otology* 2001; **115**: 973–7.

60. White PD, Thomas JM, Kangro HO *et al.* Predictors and associations of fatigue syndromes and mood disorders that occur after infectious mononucleosis. *Lancet* 2001; **358**: 1946–54.

61. Capponeti G, Pantanowitz L. Cat-cratch disease lymphadenitis. *Ear Nose and Throat Journal* 2007; **86**: 449–50.

62. Conrad DA. Treatment of cat scratch disease. *Current Opinion in Pediatrics* 2001; **13**: 56–9.

63. Richter GT, Bower CM. Cervical complications following routine tonsillectomy and adenoidectomy. *Current Opinion in Otolaryngology and Head and Neck Surgery* 2006; **14**: 375–80.

64. Hohlweg-Majert B, Weyer N, Metzger MC, Schön R. Cervicofacial necrotizing fasciitis. *Diabetes Research and Clinical Practice* 2006; **72**: 206–8.

65. McMahon J, Lowe T, Koppel DA. Necrotizing soft tissue infections of the head and neck: case reports and literature review. *Oral Surgery, Oral Medicine, Oral Pathology, Oral Radiology, and Endodontics* 2003; **95**: 30–7.

66. Burton F, Patete ML, Goodwin WJ Jr. Indications for open cervical node biopsy in HIV-positive patients. *Otolaryngology – Head and Neck Surgery* 1992; **107**: 367–9.

67. Hadfield PJ, Birchall MA, Novelli V, Bailey CM. The ENT manifestations of HIV infection in children. *Clinical Otolaryngology and Allied Sciences* 1996; **21**: 30–6.

68. Deb T, Singh NB, Devi HP, Sanasam JC. Head and neck manifestations of HIV infection: a preliminary study. *Journal of the Indian Medical Association* 2003; **101**: 93–5.

69. Barzan L, Tavio M, Tirelli U, Comoretto R. Head and neck manifestations during HIV infection. *Journal of Laryngology and Otology* 1993; **107**: 133–6.

70. Burton F, Patete ML, Goodwin WJ. Jr Indications for open cervical node biopsy in HIV patients. *Otolaryngology and Head and Neck Surgery* 1992; **107**: 367–9.

71. Singh A, Georgalas C, Patel N, Papesch M. ENT presentations in children with HIV. *Clinical Otolaryngology and Allied Sciences* 2003; **28**: 240–3.

72. Penfold CN, Revington PJ. A review of 23 patients with tuberculosis of the head and neck. *British Journal of Oral and Maxillofacial Surgery* 1996; **34**: 508–10.

73. Choudhury N, Bruch G, Kothari P *et al.* 4 years' experience of head and neck tuberculosis in a south London hospital. *Journal of the Royal Society of Medicine* 2005; **98**: 267–9.

74. Al Serhani AM. Mycobacterial infection of the head and neck: Presentation and diagnosis. *Laryngoscope* 2001; **111**: 2012–16.

75. Morad NA. Tuberculous cervical lymphadenopathy; should antituberculous therapy be proceeded by histological proof? *Tropical Doctor* 2000; **30**: 18–20.

76. Denielides V, Patriakakos G, Moerman M *et al.* Diagnosis, management and surgical treatment of non-tuberculous mycobacterial head and neck infection in children. *Journal for Otorhinolaryngology and its Related Specialties* 2002; **64**: 284–9.

77. Tunkel DE, Romaneschi KB. Surgical treatment of cervicofacial nontuberculous mycobacterial adenitis in children. *Laryngoscope* 1995; **105**: 1024–8.

78. Saggese D, Compradretti GC, Burnelli R. Nontuberculous mycobacterial adenitis in children: diagnostic and therapeutic management. *American Journal of Otolaryngology* 2003; **24**: 79–84.

79. Hazra R, Robson CD, Perez-Atayde AR, Husson RN. Lymphadenitis due to nontuberculous mycobactera in children: presentation and response to therapy. *Clinical Infectious Diseases* 1999; **28**: 123–9.

80. Luong A, McClay JE, Jafri HS, Brown O. Antibiotic therapy for nontuberculous mycobacterial cervicofacial lymphadenitis. *Laryngoscope* 2005; **115**: 1746–51.

81. Tunkel DE. Surgery for cervicofacial nontuberculous mycobacterial adenitis in children: an update. *Archives of Otolaryngology – Head and Neck Surgery* 1999; **125**: 1109–13.

82. Andriopoulos P, Tsironi M, Deftereos S *et al.* Acute brucellosis: presentation, diagnosis and treatment of 144 cases. *International Journal of Infectious Diseases* 2007; **11**: 52–7.

83. Montoya JG, Liesenfield O. Toxoplasmosis. *Lancet* 2004; **363**: 1965–76.

84. Durlach RA, Kaufer F, Carral L, Hirt J. Toxoplasmic lymphadenitis – clinical and serologic profile. *Clinical Microbiology and Infection* 2003; **9**: 625–31.

85. Tuzuner N, Dugusay G, Demirkesen C *et al.* Value of lymph node biopsy in the diagnosis of acquired toxoplasmosis. *Journal of Laryngology and Otology* 1996; **110**: 348–52.

86. Burns BV, al-Ayoubi A, Ray J *et al.* Actynomicosis of the posterior triangle: A case report and review of the literature. *Journal of Laryngology and Otology* 1997; **111**(11): 1082–5.

87. Simo R, Hartley C, Rapado F *et al.* Microbiology and antibiotic treatment of head and neck abscesses in children. *Clinical Otolaryngology and Allied Sciences* 1998; **23**: 164–8.

88. Brook I. Microbiology and management of peritonsillar, retropharyngeal and parapharyngeal abscesses. *Journal of Oral and Maxillofacial Surgery* 2004; **62**: 1545–50.

89. Perhiscar A, Har-El G. Deep neck abscess: A retrospective review of 210 cases. *Annals of Otology, Rhinology and Laryngology* 2001; **110**: 1051–4.

90. Gidley PW, Ghorayeb BY, Steirnberg CM. Contemporary management of deep neck space infections. *Otolaryngology – Head and Neck Surgery* 1997; **116**: 16–22.

91. Poe LB, Petro GR, Matta I. Percutaneous CT-guided aspiration of deep neck abscess. *American Journal of Neuroradiology* 1996; **17**: 1359–63.

92. Plaza Mayor G, Martinez San Millan J, Martinez Vidal A. Is conservative treatment of deep neck space infections appropriate? *Head and Neck* 2001; **23**: 126–33.

93. Daya H, Lo S, Papsin B *et al.* Retropharyngeal and parapharyngeal infections in children: the Toronto experience. *International Journal of Pediatric Otorhinolaryngology* 2005; **69**: 81–6.

94. Larawin V, Naipao J, Dubey SP. Head and neck space infections. *Otolaryngology – Head and Neck Surgery* 2006; **135**: 889–93.

95. Huang TT, Liu TC, Chen PR *et al.* Deep neck infections: analysis of 185 cases. *Head and Neck* 2004; **26**: 854–60.

96. Boscolo-Rizzo P, Marchiori C, Montolli F *et al.* Deep neck infections: a constant challenge. *Journal for Otorhinolaryngology and its Related Specialties* 2006; **68**: 259–65.

97. Sethi DS, Stanley RE. Deep neck abscesses – changing trends. *Journal of Laryngology and Otology* 1994; **108**: 138–43.

98. Helidonis E, Myers EN. Organized hematoma of the neck simulating carotid body tumor. *International Surgery* 1975; **60**: 519–20.

99. DiFrancesco RC, Escamilla JS, Sennes LU *et al.* Spontaneous cervical hematoma: a report of two cases. *Ear, Nose and Throat Journal* 1999; **78**: 168, 171, 175.

100. Beraldo S, Altavilla G, Bernante P, Pelizzo MR. Castleman's disease as an uncommon cause of a neck mass. *Acta Otolaryngologica* 2006; **126**: 108–11.

101. Song JJ, Jung MH, Woo JS *et al.* Castleman's disease of the head and neck. *European Archives of Otorhinolaryngology* 2006; **263**: 160–3.

102. Coca Prieto I, Ortega Jimenez MV, Fernandez Ruiz E *et al.* Localized Castleman's disease: description of a case and review of the literature. *Anales de Medicina Interna* 2003; **20**: 534–6.

103. Phelan E, Lang E, Gormley P, Lang J. Kikuchi-Fujimoto disease: a report of 3 cases. *Ear, Nose and Throat Journal* 2007; **86**: 412–13.

104. Payne JH, Evans M, Gerrard MP. Kikuchi-Fujimoto disease: a rare but important cause of lymphadenopathy. *Acta Paediatrica* 2003; **92**: 261–4.

105. Yoskovitch A, Tewfik TL, Duffy CM, Moroz B. Head and neck manifestations of Kawasaki disease. *International Journal of Pediatric Otorhinolaryngology* 2000; **52**: 123–9.

106. Kao HT, Huang YC, Lin TY. Kawasaki disease presenting as cervical lymphadenitis or deep neck infection. *Otolaryngology – Head and Neck Surgery* 2001; **124**: 468–70.

107. Sharp JF, Rodgers MJ, MacGregor FB *et al.* Angiolymphoid hyperplasia with eosinophilia. *Journal of Laryngology and Otology* 1990; **104**: 977–9.

108. Gumbs MA, Pai NB, Saraiya RJ *et al.* Kimura's disease: a case report and literature review. *Journal of Surgical Oncology* 1999; **70**: 190–3.

109. Siddiq MA, Sood S, Strachan D. Pharyngeal pouch (Zenker's diverticulum). *Postgraduate Medical Journal* 2001; **77**: 506–1.

110. Zanninoto G, Costantini M, Boccu C *et al.* Functional and morphological study of the cricopharyngeal muscle in patients with Zenker's diverticulum. *British Journal of Surgery* 1996; **83**: 1263–7.

111. Van Oveerbeeck JJ. Meditation on the pathogenesis of hypopharyngeal (Zenker's) diverticulum and a report of endoscopic treatment in 545 patients. *Annals of Otology, Rhinology and Laryngology* 1994; **103**: 178–85.

112. Siddiq MA, Sood S. Current management in pharyngeal pouch management by UK otolaryngologists. *Annals Royal College of Surgeons of England* 2004; **86**: 247–52.

113. National Institute for Health and Clinical Excellence. Interventional Procedure Guidance 22: Endoscopic stapling of the pharyngeal pouch. London: NICE, 2003.

114. Chang CY, Payyapilli RJ, Scher RL. Endoscopic staple diverticulotomy for Zenker's diverticulum: review of literature and experience in 159 consecutive case. *Laryngoscope* 2003; **113**: 957–65.

115. Koay CB, Commins D, Bates GJ. The role of endoscopic stapling diverticulotomy in recurrent pharyngeal pouch. *Journal of Laryngology and Otology* 1998; **112**: 954–5.

116. Chang CY, Payyapilli RJ, Scher RL. Endoscopic staple diverticulostomy for Zenker's diverticulum: review of literature and experience in 159 consecutive cases. *Laryngoscope* 2003; **113**: 957–65.

117. Krespi Y, Kacker A, Remacle M. Endoscopic treatment of Zenker's diverticulum using CO_2 laser. *Otolaryngology – Head and Neck Surgery* 2002; **127**: 309–14.

118. Dauer E, Salassa J, Iuga L, Kasperbauer J. Endoscopic laser vs open approach for cricopharyngeal myotomy. *Otolaryngology – Head and Neck Surgery* 2006; **134**: 830–5.

119. Lawson G, Remacle M. Endoscopic cricopharyngeal myotomy: indications and technique. *Current Opinion in Otolaryngology and Head and Neck Surgery* 2006; **14**: 437–41.

120. Stafford ND, Moore-Gillon V, McKelvie P. Handedness and the side on which pharyngeal pouches occur. *British Medical Journal* 1984; **288**: 815–16.

121. Thaler ER, Weber RS, Goldberg AN, Weinstein GS. Feasibility and outcome of endoscopic staple-assisted esophagodiverticulostomy for Zenker's diverticulum. *Laryngoscope* 2001; **111**: 1506–8.

122. Bradley PJ, Kochaar A, Quraishi MS. Pharyngeal pouch carcinoma: real or imaginary risks? *Annals of Otology, Rhinology and Laryngology* 1999; **108**: 1027–32.

123. Gray H. *Anatomy of the human body.* Philadelphia: Lea & Febiger, 1918 (Bartleby.com, 2000).

124. Stell PM, Maran AG. Laryngocele. *Journal of Laryngology and Otology* 1975; **89**: 915–24.

125. Dursum G, Ozgursoy OB, Beton S, Batikhan H. Current diagnosis and treatment of laryngocele in adults. *Otolaryngology – Head and Neck Surgery* 2007; **136**: 211–15.

126. Martinez Devesa P, Ghufoor K, Lloyd S, Howard D. Endoscopic CO_2 laser management of laryngocele. *Laryngoscope* 2002; **112**: 1426–30.

127. Weissler MC, Fried MP, Kelly JH. Laryngocele as a cause of airway obstruction. *Laryngoscope* 1985; **95**: 1348–51.

13

Benign tumours of the mouth and jaw

JULIA A WOOLGAR AND GILLIAN L HALL

Benign: (*adj.*) harmless, non-malignant, non-cancerous, innocent.

INTRODUCTION

This chapter deals with benign tumours of the oral cavity and jaws. The first section covers the common soft tissue hyperplasias and benign neoplasms. The second section deals with bony lesions – odontogenic neoplasms, a group of lesions unique to the jaws; reactive and neoplastic fibro-osseous lesions and true benign neoplasms of bone and cartilage. Clinical presentation, radiological findings and salient histological features are outlined. The chapter is an introduction to these diverse lesions and a source of reference for more detailed study. In most cases, simple conservative excision is sufficient management, but for some lesions, such as the ameloblastoma, treatment is controversial. Some benign lesions may be the presenting feature of a more serious systemic condition and although rare, they merit discussion.

COMMON SOFT TISSUE SWELLINGS: HYPERPLASIAS AND BENIGN NEOPLASMS

The vast majority of soft tissue masses occurring in the oral cavity are hyperplastic inflammatory responses to local, often chronic, trauma or infection. They may be predominantly of epithelial or connective tissue origin or a combination. These hyperplastic lesions are found in 3 per cent of adults and account for more than 80 per cent of diagnostic oral pathology specimens.[1] In other lesions, such as some squamous papillomas, the aetiopathology is less certain and the

distinction between reactive hyperplasia and benign neoplasia is somewhat arbitrary. True benign neoplasms of diverse histogenesis may occur within the mouth, but most are rare. The following account considers lesions mainly according to their cell of origin rather than the pathological process.

Squamoproliferative (epithelial) lesions

The squamous cell papilloma is the main benign neoplasm derived from oral epithelium, but a variety of virally induced epithelial hyperplasias (such as verruca vulgaris, the common wart) present similar clinical features. At least 16 types of human papilloma virus (HPV) have been isolated from oral lesions.[2] There is no evidence that oral viral hyperplasias and papillomas are premalignant.

SQUAMOUS CELL PAPILLOMA, VERRUCA VULGARIS AND OTHER VIRAL WARTS

These are common oral lesions with a prevalence of 0.1–0.5 per cent.[3] They occur at all ages with the highest incidence in children and young adults with a slight male predominance. Typical presentation is a localized sessile or pedunculated cauliflower-like growth which rapidly grows to around 6 mm, then remains a constant size. The colour may appear pink or white depending on the degree of keratinization. Anterior oral sites are mainly affected and lesions may be multiple, since transmission is often from lesions on the fingers. Histologically, folds of hyperplastic epithelium are supported by vascular cores. Coarsely granular keratohyaline and koilocytes within the upper prickle cell layer are typical of HPV infection and the virus can be identified by immunohistochemistry or *in situ* hybridization.[2] Papillomas respond to simple excision or ablation by laser or cryosurgery. Verruca vulgaris may regress spontaneously.

CONDYLOMA ACUMINATUM

The oral counterpart of anogenital condyloma acuminatum (HPV types 6, 11, 16 and 18) tends to be larger than the papilloma, with a broad base and pink nodular surface.[4] Histologically, the fronds are short and blunt with prominent clusters of koilocytes. Lesions tend to recur, but unlike the anogenital lesions, there is no documented malignant transformation.

FOCAL EPITHELIAL HYPERPLASIA (HECK'S DISEASE)

Multiple soft, rounded, pink swellings on the lips, cheek and tongue, induced by HPV 13 and 32, are found mainly in children and young adults. The condition is rare in the United Kingdom, but up to 40 per cent of children are reportedly affected in some regions of the world.[5] Histologically, sharply defined areas of acanthosis with 'mitosoid bodies' are seen. Lesions resolve spontaneously.

PAPILLOMAS IN IMMUNODEFICIENCY

Florid HPV-induced lesions are common, especially in HIV infection and may coalesce as widespread papillomatosis. Multiple, and unusual, HPV subtypes are typical. White hairy leukoplakia seen on the lateral tongue in 20–25 per cent of HIV-infected patients[6] contains the Epstein–Barr virus.

KERATOACANTHOMA

This benign tumour of hair follicle epithelium is seen on the lips.[7] Aetiology is unknown. It is characterized by rapid growth followed by slow, spontaneous involution. The mature lesion, a nodule with a central crater, mimics squamous carcinoma clinically and histologically. Simple excision, often necessary for diagnosis, is curative.

VERRUCIFORM XANTHOMA

This wart-like lesion is seen mainly on the gingiva of female adults[8] and may be a response to local trauma. The histological characteristic is epithelial papillomatosis with foamy histiocytes filling the connective tissue papillae. Recurrence is rare after simple excision.

Fibroepithelial hyperplasias

These common lesions result from an overgrowth of both surface epithelium and one or more element of the supporting connective tissues. There are several clinical subtypes, affecting both the lining mucosa, gingivae and mucoperiosteum (**Box 13.1**).

Box 13.1   Fibroepithelial hyperplasia

Localized gingival hyperplasia

- Fibrous epulis
- Ossifying fibrous epulis
- Vascular epulis
- Giant cell epulis (peripheral giant cell granuloma)

Generalized gingival hyperplasia

- Idiopathic plaque-induced
- Hereditary autosomal-dominant (gingival fibromatosis)
- Fibrous enlargement of the maxillary tuberosity
- Drug-induced
  - epanutin
  - cyclosporin
  - nifedipine and verapamil

Mucosal fibroepithelial hyperplasias

- Fibroepithelial polyp
- Denture-irritation fibroepithelial hyperplasia (denture granuloma)
- Leaf fibroma
- Papillary hyperplasia of the palate
- Giant cell fibroma
- Cowden syndrome

LOCALIZED GINGIVAL HYPERPLASIA

Minor localized swellings of the gingivae (epulides) are commonplace and many resolve following a 'scale and polish' and improvement of oral hygiene measures. Persistent or symptomatic lesions may appear as painless, triangular swellings of the interdental papilla which gradually increase in size. Histologically, four main types are recognized on the basis of the predominant component of the core. The composition influences the clinical appearance and may also reflect differences in aetiology and pathogenesis.

Fibrous epulis

This is the most common type, accounting for more than 50 per cent. Typically, it presents as a firm, smooth-surfaced, broadly pedunculated or sessile mass. The colour is often similar to the adjacent gingiva, but depends on the vascularity of the core and the thickness and integrity of the surface epithelium. Typically, lesions occur on the labial or buccal aspect of the tooth, most commonly an incisor or canine. Males and females are equally affected, with no strong age predilection.

Histologically, the proportion of fibroblasts to collagen fibres varies and may reflect the maturity of the lesion, age of the patient and nature of the irritation. Highly cellular lesions are more common in adolescents.

Simple surgical removal is curative and the lesion is unlikely to recur if initiating factors are removed and a good standard of oral hygiene is maintained.

Ossifying fibrous epulis

Mineral deposits or bone are seen in 30 per cent of fibrous epulides. Some show droplets of dystrophic mineral, while others develop well-formed trabeculae of metaplastic woven, or even lamellar, bone. Cementum-like material is also seen occasionally.[9] Ossifying fibrous epulides tend to occur in adolescents and young adults and show a greater tendency to recur than their non-ossifying counterparts.

Vascular epulis

Highly vascularized epulides are more common in females and are linked to pregnancy.[10] Lesions may grow rapidly during pregnancy and may regress postpartum or become more fibrous. Vascular epulides present as red, soft lesions with a glazed or ulcerated surface and may bleed spontaneously or on minimal trauma. Histologically, the core consists of solid sheets of non-canalized endothelial cells and/ or masses of thin-walled blood vessels in an oedematous stroma. Ulceration and associated inflammation are common. A minority display a lobular architecture similar to the pyogenic granuloma.

Giant cell epulis (peripheral giant cell granuloma)

This accounts for around 10 per cent of epulides, and predominantly affects females.[11] Occurrence is usually anterior to molars, and mainly mandibular, but lesions may occur in edentulous areas. Typically, it presents as a purplish, hourglass swelling extending from the buccal to lingual aspect and may cause pressure erosion of the underlying interdental bone. The histological appearances are distinct with abundant multinucleated osteoclast-like giant cells lying in highly vascular stroma of oval to spindle-shaped mononuclear cells. Dilated blood vessels and haemosiderin-laden macrophages are seen at the periphery, particularly in the zone of dense fibrous tissue that separates the lesion from the surface epithelium. The aetiology is uncertain and the lesion appears distinct from the central giant cell granuloma and brown tumour of hyperparathyroidism which arise within the jaw bone. If the origin – peripheral or central – is in doubt, then x-rays and serum biochemistry are necessary.

GENERALIZED GINGIVAL HYPERPLASIA

Four categories of generalized gingival fibrous hyperplasia are recognized (**Box 13.1**). It arises as an exaggerated response to dental plaque, resulting in fibroblastic proliferation and increased collagen production. Idiopathic cases are generally seen at puberty suggesting a hormonal influence. Between 10 and 60 per cent of patients on epanutin are affected.[12] Fibrous enlargement of the maxillary tuberosity usually presents in adults, but appears to have a genetic basis. In all categories, surgical removal tends to be followed by recurrence, unless excellent plaque control is maintained.

MUCOSAL FIBROEPITHELIAL HYPERPLASIAS

These may be seen as a distinct polyp, either broad-based or on a peduncle, or as a more diffuse overgrowth (**Box 13.1**). The lip and buccal mucosa are the usual sites. The surface is usually the same colour as the surrounding mucosa, unless trauma has resulted in ulceration or frictional keratosis. The hyperplasias associated with ill-fitting dentures typically affect the mandibular labial and buccal sulci and have an elongated shape indented by the denture flange. 'Leaf fibroma' is the term given to pedunculated palatal lesions. More generalized papillary hyperplasia of the palate presents as an eythematous, pebbled area often beneath an ill-fitting denture associated with chronic candidal infection. All forms share similar histological features of hyperplastic surface epithelium covering a core of collagenous connective tissue with variable inflammation and vascularity. Conservative excision is curative provided the irritating factors are removed. The giant cell fibroma[13] is a histological variant of the fibroepithelial polyp characterized by the presence of stellate, multinucleated fibroblasts of no clinical significance.

Cowden syndrome, a rare autosomal disorder, is characterized by multiple hamartomas and benign and malignant neoplasms at almost any body site.[14] Oral manifestations include multiple papules consisting of a fibrovascular core covered by acanthotic epithelium. Facial lesions include cysts and adnexal tumours.

Tumours of fibrous tissue

Nodular fasciitis, often referred to as a pseudotumour, presents as a subcutaneous/submucosal soft tissue mass that often grows rapidly over a period of 1–2 weeks causing suspicion of a malignancy.[15] Preceding minor trauma is probably an important aetiological factor. Mainly labial and buccal, although any mucosal site may be affected, lesions are typically 2–5 cm. Affected individuals are usually young adults (<30 years) with no gender predilection.

The histological features can be worrisome, with richly cellular areas of plump myofibroblasts, readily detected mitotic activity and sometimes apparent infiltration of adjacent tissues. The loose myxoid stroma, extravasated erythrocytes and scattering of chronic inflammatory cells aid the diagnosis. Recurrence following even incomplete surgical removal is rare and should prompt re-evaluation of the diagnosis.

There are no true benign purely fibrous soft tissue tumours of the oral cavity. Benign fibrous histiocytoma and myofibroma are rarely reported.[16] Benign fibrous histiocytoma is analogous to its counterpart in the skin and presents as a subepithelial, firm, circumscribed nodule. Myofibroma occurs both as a soft tissue lesion and less commonly as an intraosseous lesion. Occurrence over a wide age range including infants as young as nine months is reported. Diagnosis in infants should prompt examination for multiple lesions (myofibromatosis) which has a poor prognosis when multiple vital organs are involved. In solitary cases, conservative excision is curative.

FIBROMATOSIS

Fibromatosis shows locally aggressive behaviour and frequent recurrence,[17] but does not metastasize. Presentation is usually in the first decade with a painless slowly growing mass. The cheeks, tongue and submandibular region are favoured oral sites. Lesions may cause erosion of bone. Intraosseous lesions of both maxilla and mandible are also described. Histologically, differentiation from a low-grade fibrosarcoma may be difficult. Lower mitotic count and nuclear staining with beta-catenin immunohistochemical stain may help. Recurrence rate in one oral series[17] was 24 per cent, significantly lower than that for other body sites (50–70 per cent). Treatment is surgical with the aim of establishing disease-free margins. Given the poorly defined periphery of the lesion and large size, this is often difficult. Chemotherapy and radiotherapy have been used, but the latter is not desirable in a young patient.

Vascular lesions

PYOGENIC GRANULOMA

Pyogenic granuloma, an exuberant mass of granulation tissue, arises following acute or chronic trauma or infection. All ages and both genders are susceptible.[18] Lesions present as exophytic, red soft lesions that may ulcerate or bleed spontaneously. Histologically, they consist of lobular proliferations of endothelial cells and young capillaries in an oedematous, inflamed stroma. Conservative surgical excision is usually curative, but around 15 per cent of cases recur.

CALIBRE–PERSISTENT ARTERY

This is a developmental anomaly affecting the lower lip in 80 per cent of cases with the remaining lesions affecting the upper lip and hard palate. In the lower lip, it arises when the inferior alveolar artery retains its large size and muscular wall, even in its terminal portion within the orbicularis oris muscle.[19] Symptoms of persistent ulceration, non-healing lip fissure or a pulsatile nodule usually occur after the age of 40 years. Removal of the abnormal vessel during diagnostic biopsy is curative, although excessive haemorrhage may be a surgical problem.

HAEMANGIOMAS

These common tumours are generally accepted as hamartomas rather than true neoplasms. They occur more commonly in the head and neck than any other body site. Oral lesions account for 14 per cent and reportedly are found in 0.5 per cent of adults.[20] Most are present at birth or arise in early childhood, but some present in old age. The lips, tongue, cheek or palate are the most common intraoral sites and lesions vary in size, shape and surface appearance. Most are dark reddish-purple, soft and either smooth and flat or raised and globular. Typically, they blanch on pressure. Larger lesions often contain phleboliths which may be detected radiologically. Trauma may cause haemorrhage or lead to a sudden increase in size due to thrombosis and inflammation. The facial muscles, jaw bones and major salivary glands may also be affected and the juvenile haemangioma is the most common tumour affecting salivary glands in children.

Haemangiomas are classified according to the ratio of endothelial cells to vessels and the calibre and thickness of the vessel walls into capillary, cavernous, arteriovenous and mixed. Capillary haemangiomas include sheets of non-canalized endothelial cells sometimes arranged in lobules similar to the pyogenic granuloma. Other histological variants, such as epithelioid and sclerosing, are unusual in the mouth. Haemangiomas may be treated by conservative surgical excision or debulking, intralesional injection of sclerosing chemicals, cryosurgery, laser ablation and ligation of the feeder vessel.[20] Congenital capillary haemangiomas usually spontaneously regress by six years of age.

VARICOSITIES AND VENOUS LAKES

Sublingual varicosities affecting the ranine veins and venous anomalies of the lips increase in frequency with age and rarely require treatment.

STURGE–WEBER SYNDROME

This congenital disorder is characterized by haemangiomas of the face with a distribution over one or more branches of the trigeminal nerve, oral mucosa and ipsilateral leptomeninges over the cerebral cortex.

HEREDITARY HAEMORRHAGIC TELANGIECTASIA

Transmitted as an autosomal dominant trait, this is characterized by multiple knots of dilated malformed capillaries (telangiectases) in skin, oral and nasal mucous membranes and internal organs.

LYMPHANGIOMA

Lymphangiomas, hamartomatous malformations of lymph vessels, are less common than haemangiomas and generally present in infancy and early childhood.[21] The tongue is the most common intraoral site and a frequent cause of macroglossia. Typically, lesions have a pebbled or verrucous surface due to the superficially located lymphatic vessels abutting on to the surface epithelium and often, hyperkeratosis. Histologically, lesions are poorly circumscribed and composed of capillary and cavernous lymph sinuses lined by cytologically bland endothelium.

CYSTIC HYGROMA

This lymphangiomatous malformation typically affects the submandibular region and neck, and presents at birth with a large, fluctuant swelling often ramifying into the base of tongue and floor of mouth.[21] The extensive cystic dilatation of the vessels accounts for the progressive growth. The cystic fluid is straw-coloured with low protein content. Lack of a discrete margin and growth along tissue planes and neurovascular bundles hamper removal, and early intervention when the lesion is smaller offers the best chance of cure.

Tumours of adipose tissue

'FIBROLIPOMA'

Some fibroepithelial polyps – reactive fibroepithelial hyperplasias – include mature adipose cells within their fibrous core and are sometimes referred to as 'fibrolipomas'.[22] It is uncertain whether the adipose tissue represents entrapped fat cells or degenerative metaplasia.

HERNIATED BUCCAL FAT PAD

Acute trauma from cheek biting may rupture the buccal fat pad allowing a portion to herniate as a yellowish-coloured sessile or peduculated submucosal mass, 3–4 cm in diameter. Once formed, the mass does not increase further in size, but surgical removal is necessary to prevent fresh trauma.[23] Histologically, the herniated mass is composed of normal mature adipose tissue supported by fibrovascular septae.

LIPOMA

The lipoma, a benign neoplasm of adipocytes, presents mainly in adults as a soft, smooth submucosal mass, often with a yellowish surface discoloration. The cheek, tongue and floor of mouth are the usual sites, but cases have been reported within maxillary bones and paranasal sinuses.[22] Magnetic resonance imaging is more useful than computed tomography and ultrasonography in preoperative diagnosis. Histologically, mature adipocytes are supported by fibrovascular septae with variable circumscription and encapsulation. As in lipomas at other body sites, several histological variants are recognized including intramuscular (infiltrating), fibrolipoma, angiolipoma, myxolipoma, spindle cell, pleomorphic, myolipoma and angiomyolipoma. In addition, hibernomas and lipoblastomas have been reported. Recurrence after conservative surgical removal is rare. Intramuscular lipomas are typically more diffuse and are generally managed by debulking. 'Lipomatosis' is applied to extensive involvement of a wide area of stromal connective tissue.

MULTIPLE HEAD AND NECK LIPOMAS

Multiple lipomas are seen in several syndromes including neurofibromatosis, Gardner syndrome, Proteus syndrome and hemifacial hypertrophy.

Tumours of peripheral nerves

Reactive and benign neoplasms of peripheral nerves are listed in **Box 13.2**.

TRAUMATIC (AMPUTATION) NEUROMA

The traumatic neuroma is a disorganized overgrowth of nerve fibres, Schwann cells and scar tissue associated with the proximal end of a severed nerve.[24] Small lesions may affect the oral mucosa following minor trauma, but rarely develop in tooth extraction sockets. Lesions arising following parotid gland surgery and within skin flaps may be misdiagnosed clinically as recurrent neoplasm.

Box 13.2   Lesions of peripheral nerves

- Traumatic (amputation) neuroma
- Lingual subgemmal neurogenic plaque
- Mucosal neuroma
- Palisaded encapsulated neuroma
- Schwannoma
- Neurofibroma
- Granular cell tumour

LINGUAL SUBGEMMAL NEUROGENIC PLAQUE

This is a hyperplastic neural lesion arising adjacent to taste buds of foliate papillae which has distinctive histological features that may be misinterpreted as neurofibroma or neuroma of multiple endocrine neoplasia syndrome.[25]

MUCOSAL NEUROMA

These usually present as sessile, painless nodules and may be mistaken clinically for simple fibroepithelial polyps. Lesions tend to be multiple (between two and eight) and may also involve perioral and perinasal skin. Their correct diagnosis is important since they are pathognomonic of the multiple endocrine neoplasia syndromes (MEN)[26, 27] and are most frequently associated with MEN IIb (**Box 13.3**). Initial presentation with oral lesions is usual. Prompt referral to an endocrinologist is indicated if the diagnosis is suspected in an otherwise asymptomatic youngster. Prophylactic total thyroidectomy is performed early since medullary carcinoma is inevitable and particularly aggressive in MEN IIb.

The histological differentiation between mucosal neuroma and benign neural lesions, such as palisaded encapsulated neuroma and neurofibroma is subtle.[28] In the mucosal neuroma, connective tissues are expanded by a proliferation of hyperplastic nerves, intertwined with each other and embedded in a loose fibrous stroma. Inflammatory cells are lacking and the perineural sheath is characteristically thickened.

PALISADED ENCAPSULATED NEUROMA

This presents as a solitary mucosal polyp rarely affecting facial skin.[29] Trauma is a likely aetiological factor. The diagnosis is usually made in elderly adults and hence, clinical features are helpful in differentiation from mucosal neuroma. Histologically, the lesion is circumscribed but without a well-defined capsule. Interlacing bundles of Schwann cells form the bulk and axonal processes can be identified on careful examination. Simple conservative excision is curative.

SCHWANNOMA

This relatively common benign nerve sheath tumour has a distinct predilection for head and neck.[30] Lesions are usually solitary unless associated with neurofibromatosis 2. The slow-growing discrete lump is usually asymptomatic. Because of their origin from nerve sheath cells, schwannomas

Central giant cell lesion

Central giant cell lesion (CGCL), a reactive, reparative lesion, mainly affects the posterior mandible of young adult females.[79] Most cases are sporadic, but some are related to systemic conditions, including Noonan syndrome. Lesions may be incidental findings or present with pain, paraesthesia, swelling and loose teeth. Radiography shows an expansile, multilocular radiolucency with well-defined, scalloped borders and intralesional wavy septae. Tooth displacement, loss of lamina dura and root resorption are typical. Histology shows osteoclast-like, multinucleated giant cells supported by a highly vascular stroma containing spindle-shaped fibroblasts and trabeculae of metaplastic bone. Enucleation may be followed by recurrence, and calcitonin, glucocorticoids and interferon alpha have been advocated for persistent lesions.[80]

The brown tumour of hyperparathyroidism is morphologically similar to CGCL and parathormone levels should be determined especially in elderly patients and when lesions are multifocal.

CGCL must be distinguished from the giant cell tumour (GCT) of bone. GCT mainly affects long bones with occasional cases in the sphenoid, ethmoid and temporal bones. Subtle histological differences are described.[81] GCT is locally aggressive and malignant forms, capable of lung metastases, may occur sporadically or in Paget's disease.

Cherubism

This autosomal dominant inherited condition (mapped to chromosome 4p16.3) presents in early childhood with symmetrical swelling of the maxilla, mandibular angle and ramus, delayed eruption and tooth displacement, visual impairment and cervical lymphadenopathy.[82] Affected bones are expanded by well-demarcated 'soap bubble' radiolucencies followed by progressive sclerosis. Microscopy resembles central giant cell lesion with the addition of characteristic perivascular collagenous cuffs. Lesions regress after puberty, and surgery should only be carried out to improve function in severe cases.

BENIGN TUMOURS OF BONE

Osteoma and other bony overgrowths

Exostoses (localized overgrowths) are more common than neoplasms. Most exostoses consist of lamellae of compact bone, although larger ones may have a cancellous core. Torus palatinus develops in the midline of the palate. Torus mandibularis forms bilaterally on the lingual aspect of the mandible in the premolar region. Tori and other exostoses present as hard, rounded swellings covered by mucosa of normal appearance unless traumatized.

Osteomas are more common in the paranasal sinuses than the jaw bones. Lesions may arise on the surface of the bone presenting clinically as slow-growing, hard swellings, or be confined within the substance of the cancellous bone. Radiologically, a sharply defined, densely radiopaque mass is typical. Osteomas resemble mature bone. Compact (ivory) osteomas consist of dense lamellae arranged in layers. Cancellous osteomas consist of slender trabeculae supported by fatty marrow surrounded by a cortical shell. Generally, exostoses and osteomas are only removed if they interfere with dentures or for cosmesis.

Multiple jaw osteomas raise the possibility of Gardner's syndrome (familial adenomatous polyposis).[83] The osteomas may be present for a decade or more before intestinal malignancy develops and their correct diagnosis can lead to early recognition of the syndrome and the opportunity for prophylactic colectomy.

Osteochondroma (cartilage-capped osteoma) grow by ossification beneath a cartilaginous cap. Most maxillofacial lesions affect the condyle and coronoid process and may interfere with joint function. Their status – developmental versus neoplastic – is uncertain and some may be difficult to distinguish from condylar hyperplasia.

OSTEOID OSTEOMA AND OSTEOBLASTOMA

These two benign tumours show identical histological features, but subtle clinicoradiological differences. In the jaws, osteoblastoma is more common than osteoid osteoma.[84] Both tumours typically affect patients <30 years and present with localized pain that is particularly severe at night and relieved by aspirin. The osteoid osteoma is always <2 cm in maximum dimension. Osteoblastoma has a greater tendency for growth and thus may present with swelling.

Radiologically, both present as well-defined lucent lesions with a sclerotic rim and sometimes speckled intralesional calcification. At operation, a nidus of soft tissue with gritty areas that easily shells out from the surrounding bone is typical.

The histological features (a cellular and vascular stroma with active formation of osteoid and woven bone) can be worrying and reminiscent of malignant osteosarcoma. Peripheral maturation into lamellar bone, as well as precise clinical and radiological information, is important in determining the correct diagnosis. Recurrence following conservative treatments, such as curettage, is reported in the range of 10–20 per cent.

Cartilaginous tumours

Benign cartilage tumours of the jaws are rare, and many ultimately prove to be malignant. Typically, chondromas present as firm nodules, <3 cm in diameter, in the anterior maxilla and posterior mandible. They consist of hyaline cartilage often with focal calcification/ossification accounting for the variable radiographic appearances. The histological distinction from a low-grade chondrosarcoma is notoriously difficult. Chondroblastomas and chondromyxoid fibromas are also encountered.[85, 86] Cartilaginous tumours can grow in the soft tissues as a result of seeding of tumour cells at operation and the treatment of choice is wide excision and prolonged follow up.

Synovial chondromatosis is rare in the temporomandibular joint[87] and is usually diagnosed by the characteristic radiological images produced by the multiple metaplastic nodules of cartilage within the synovial connective tissue.

KEY LEARNING POINTS

- Most oral swellings are a hyperplastic response to chronic irritation.
- Biopsy diagnosis is necessary since hyperplastic and benign neoplasms may have similar clinical manifestations.
- The range of epithelial and connective tissue benign lesions is wide.
- Lesions may herald or represent part of a systemic, sometimes serious, condition.
- Odontogenic tumours are unique to the jaws and include the ameloblastoma.
- Treatment of ameloblastoma is controversial in view of its variable invasive potential.

REFERENCES

1. Jones AV, Franklin CD. An analysis of oral and maxillofacial pathology in adults over a 30-year period. *Journal of Oral Pathology and Medicine* 2006; **35**: 392–401.
2. Praetorius F. HPV-associated diseases of oral mucosa. *Clinics in Dermatology* 1997; **15**; 399–413.
3. Tay AB. A 5-year survey of oral biopsies in an oral surgical unit in Singapore. *Annals of the Academy of Medicine, Singapore* 1999; **28**: 665–71.
4. Kui LL, Xiu HZ, Ning LY. Condyloma acuminatum and human papilloma virus infection in the oral mucosa of children. *Pediatric Dentistry* 2003; **25**: 149–53.
5. Carlos R, Sedano HO. Multifocal papilloma virus epithelial hyperplasia. *Oral Surgery, Oral Medicine, and Oral Pathology* 1994; **77**: 631–5.
♦ 6. Greenspan D, Greenspan JS. HIV-related oral disease. *Lancet* 1996; **348**: 729–33.
7. Ghadially FN. Keratoacanthoma In: Freedberg IM, Eisen AZ, Wolff K *et al.* (eds). *Fitzpatrick's dermatology in general medicine.* New York: McGraw-Hill, 2003: 766–72.
8. Philipsen HP, Reichart PA, Takata T, Ogawa I. Verruciform xanthoma: biological profile of 282 oral lesions based on a literature survey with nine new cases from Japan. *Oral Oncology* 2003; **39**: 325–36.
9. Bouquot JE, Crout RJ. Odd gums: The prevalence of common gingival and alveolar lesions in 23,616 white Americans over 35 years of age. *Quintessence International* 1988; **19**: 747–53.
10. Sills ES, Zegerelli DJ, Hoschander MM, Strider WE. Clinical diagnosis and management of hormonally responsive oral pregnancy tumor (pyogenic granuloma). *Journal of Reproductive Medicine* 1996; **41**: 467–70.
11. Mighell AJ, Robinson PA, Hume WJ. Peripheral giant cell granuloma: a clinical study of 77 cases from 62 patients, and literature review. *Oral Diseases* 1995; **1**: 12–19.
12. Dongari A, McDonnell HT, Langlais RP. Drug-induced gingival overgrowth. *Oral Surgery, Oral Medicine, and Oral Pathology* 1993; **76**: 543–8.
13. Magnusson BC, Rasmusson LG. The giant cell fibroma. A review of 103 cases with immunohistochemical findings. *Acta Odontologica Scandinavica* 1995; **53**: 293–6.
14. Requena L, Gutierrez J, Sanchez-Yus E. Multiple sclerotic fibromas of the skin: A cutaneous marker of Cowden's disease. *Journal of Cutaneous Pathology* 1991; **19**: 346–51.
15. DiNardo LJ, Wetmore RF, Potsic WP. Nodular fasciitis of the head and neck in children. A deceptive lesion. *Archives of Otolaryngology – Head and Neck Surgery* 1991; **117**: 1001–2.
16. Bielamowicz S, Dauer MS, Chang B, Zimmerman MC. Noncutaneous benign fibrous histiocytoma of the head and neck. *Otolaryngology – Head and Neck Surgery* 1995; **113**: 140–6.
♦ 17. Fowler CB, Hartman KS, Brannon RB. Fibromatoses of the oral cavity and paraoral region. *Oral Surgery, Oral Medicine, and Oral Pathology* 1994; **77**: 373–86.
18. Mooney MA, Janniger CK. Pyogenic granuloma. *Cutis* 1995; **55**: 133–6.
19. Lovas JGL, Rodu B, Hammond HL, Allen CM. Caliber-persistent labial artery: A common vascular anomaly. *Oral Surgery, Oral Medicine, Oral Pathology, Oral Radiology, and Endodontics* 1998; **86**: 308–12.
20. Rossiter JL, Hendrix RA, Tom LW, Potsic WP. Intramuscular haemangioma of the head and neck. *Otolaryngology – Head and Neck Surgery* 1993; **108**: 18–26.
21. Kennedy TL. Cystic hygroma-lymphangioma: A rare and still unclear entity. *Laryngoscope* 1989; **99**: 1–10.
22. De Visscher JGAM. Lipomas and fibrolipomas of the oral cavity. *Journal of Maxillofacial Surgery* 1982; **10**: 177–81.
23. Clawson JR, Kline KK, Armbrecht EC. Trauma-induced avulsion of the buccal fat pad into the mouth: Report of a case. *Journal of Oral Surgery* 1968; **26**: 546–7.
24. Sist TC, Greene GW. Traumatic neuromas of the oral cavity: Report of thirty-one new cases and review of the literature. *Oral Surgery, Oral Medicine, and Oral Pathology* 1981; **51**: 394–402.
25. Triantafyllou A, Coulter P. Structural organization of subgemmal neurogenous plaques in foliate papillae of tongue. *Human Pathology* 2004; **35**: 991–9.
26. Morrison PJ, Nevin NC. Multiple endocrine neoplasia type 2B (mucosal neuroma syndrome, Wagenmann-Froboese syndrome). *Journal of Medical Genetics* 1996; **33**: 779–82.
27. Carney JA. Familial multiple endocrine neoplasia: the first 100 years. *American Journal of Surgical Pathology* 2005; **29**: 254–74.

♦ 28. Fletcher CD. Distinctive soft tissue tumors of the head and neck. *Modern Pathology* 2002; **15**: 324–30.

29. Magnusson B. Pallisaded encapsulated neuroma (solitary circumscribed neuroma) of the oral mucosa. *Oral Surgery, Oral Medicine, Oral Pathology, Oral Radiology, and Endodontics* 1996; **82**: 302–4.

30. Williams HK, Cannell H, Silvester K, Williams DM. Neurilemmoma of the head and neck. *British Journal of Oral and Maxillofacial Surgery* 1993; **31**: 32–5.

♦ 31. Shapiro SD, Abramovitch K, Van Dis ML. Neurofibromatosis: Oral and radiographic manifestations. *Oral Surgery, Oral Medicine, and Oral Pathology* 1984; **58**: 493–8.

32. Junquero LM, de Vicente JC, Vega JA. Granular-cell tumours: An immunohistochemical study. *British Journal of Oral and Maxillofacial Surgery* 1997; **35**: 180–4.

33. Fanburg-Smith JC, Meis-Kindblom JM, Fante R, Kindblom LG. Malignant granular cell tumor of soft tissue: diagnostic criteria and clinicopathological correlation. *American Journal of Surgical Pathology* 1998; **22**: 779–94.

34. Reinshagen K, Wessel LM, Roth H, Waag KL. Congenital epulis: a rare diagnosis in paediatric surgery. *European Journal of Pediatric Surgery* 2002; **12**: 124–6.

35. Kapadia SB, Meis JM, Frisman DM. Adult rhabdomyoma of the head and neck: A clinicopathologic and immunophenotypic study. *Human Pathology* 1993; **24**: 608–17.

36. Kaugars GE, Heise AP, Riley WT *et al.* Oral melanotic macules. A review of 353 cases. *Oral Surgery, Oral Medicine, and Oral Pathology* 1993; **76**: 59–61.

37. Ide F, Shimoyama T, Horie N. Glial choristoma in the oral cavity: Histopathologic and immunohistochemical features. *Journal of Oral Pathology and Medicine* 1997; **26**: 147–50.

38. Nelson ZL, Newman L, Loukota RA. Melanotic neuroectodermal tumour of infancy: An immunohistochemical and ultrastructural study. *British Journal of Oral and Maxillofacial Surgery* 1995; **33**: 375–80.

♦ 39. Slootweg P. Odontogenic tumours – an update. *Current Diagnostic Pathology* 2006; **12**: 54–65.

40. Barnes L, Eveson JW, Reichart P, Sidransky D (eds). *World Health Organization classification of tumours. Pathology and genetics of head and neck tumours.* Lyon: IARC Press, 2005.

41. Shear M, Singh S. Age-standardized incidence rates of ameloblastoma and dentigerous cyst on the Witwatersrand, South Africa. *Community Dentistry and Oral Epidemiology* 1978; **6**: 195–9.

42. Chidzonga MM. Ameloblastoma in children. The Zimbabwean experience. *Oral Surgery, Oral Medicine, Oral Pathology, Oral Radiology, and Endodontics* 1996; **81**: 168–70.

♦ 43. Reichart PA, Philipsen HP, Sonner S. Ameloblastoma: biological profile of 3677 cases. *European Journal of Cancer Part B, Oral Oncology* 1995; **31B**: 86–99.

44. Sachs S. Surgical excision with peripheral ostectomy; a definitive, yet conservative, approach to the surgical management of ameloblastoma. *Journal of Oral and Maxillofacial Surgery* 2006; **64**: 476–83.

45. Carlson E, Marx R. The ameloblastoma: primary curative surgical management. *Journal of Oral and Maxillofacial Surgery* 2006; **64**: 484–94.

♦ 46. Ghandi D, Ayoub A, Pogrel MA *et al.* A surgeon's dilemma. *Journal of Oral and Maxillofacial Surgery* 2006; **64**: 1010–14.

47. Ord RA, Blanchaert RH, Nikitakis NG, Sauk JJ. Ameloblastoma in children. *Journal of Oral and Maxillofacial Surgery* 2002; **60**: 762–70.

48. Newman L, Howells GL, Coghlan KM *et al.* Malignant ameloblastoma revisited. *British Journal of Oral and Maxillofacial Surgery* 1995; **33**: 47–50.

49. Laughlin EH. Metastasizing ameloblastoma. *Cancer* 1989; **64**: 776–80.

50. Reichart HP, Philipsen P. Unicystic ameloblastoma. A review of 193 cases from the literature. *Oral Oncology* 1998; **34**: 317–25.

51. Gardner DG. Some current concepts on the pathology of ameloblastomas. *Oral Surgery, Oral Medicine, Oral Pathology, Oral Radiology, and Endodontics* 1996; **82**: 660–9.

52. Philipsen HP, Reichart PA, Nikai H *et al.* Peripheral ameloblastoma: biological profile based on 160 cases from the literature. *Oral Oncology* 2001; **37**: 17–27.

53. Manor Y, Mardinger O, Katz J *et al.* Peripheral odontogenic tumours – differential diagnosis in gingival lesions. *International Journal of Oral and Maxillofacial Surgery* 2004; **33**: 268–73.

♦ 54. Philipsen HP, Reichart PA, Praetorius F. Mixed odontogenic tumours and odontomas. Considerations on interrelationship. Review of the literature and presentation of 134 new cases of odontomas. *Oral Oncology* 1997; **33**: 86–99.

55. Takeda Y. Ameloblastic fibroma and related lesions: current pathologic concept. *Oral Oncology* 1999; **35**: 535–40.

56. Batra P, Prasad S, Parkash H. Adenomatoid odontogenic tumour: a review and case report. *Journal of the Canadian Dental Association* 2005; **71**: 250–3.

57. Woolgar JA, Rippin JW, Browne RM. A comparative study of odontogenic keratocysts in basal cell naevus syndrome and control patients. *Journal of Oral Pathology* 1987; **16**: 75–80.

♦ 58. Shear M. The aggressive nature of the odontogenic keratocyst: is it a benign cystic neoplasm? *Oral Oncology* 2002; **38**: 219–26.

59. Philipsen HP, Reichart PA. Calcifying epithelial odontogenic tumour: biological profile based 181 cases from the literature. *Oral Oncology* 2000; **36**: 17–26.

60. Philipsen HP, Reichart PA. Squamous odontogenic tumour (SOT): A benign neoplasm of the periodontium. *Journal of Clinical Periodontology* 1996; **23**: 922–6.

61. Toida M. So-called calcifying odontogenic cyst: Review and discussion on the terminology and classification. *Journal of Oral Pathology and Medicine* 1998; **27**: 49–52.

62. Li TJ, Yu SF. Clinicopathologic spectrum of the so-called calcifying odontogenic cysts: a study of 21 intra-osseous cases with reconsideration of the terminology and classification. *American Journal of Surgical Pathology* 2003; **27**: 372–84.

63. Lo Muzio LL, Nocini PF, Favia G. Odontogenic myxoma of the jaws. A clinical, radiologic, immunohistochemical, and ultrastructural study. *Oral Surgery, Oral Medicine, Oral Pathology, Oral Radiology, and Endodontics* 1996; **82**: 426–33.

64. Dunlap CL. Odontogenic fibroma. *Seminars in Diagnostic Pathology* 1999; **16**: 293–6.

65. Gardner DG. Central odontogenic fibroma: current concepts. *Journal of Oral Pathology and Medicine* 1996; **25**: 556–61.

66. Siar CH, Ng KH. Clinicopathological study of peripheral odontogenic fibromas (WHO-type) in Malaysians (1967–95). *British Journal of Oral and Maxillofacial Surgery* 2000; **38**: 19–22.

67. El-Mofty S. Cemento-ossifying fibroma and benign cementoblastoma. *Seminars in Diagnostic Pathology* 1999; **16**: 302–7.

68. Eversole LR. Malignant epithelial odontogenic tumours. *Seminars in Diagnostic Pathology* 1999; **16**: 317–24.

69. Slater LJ. Odontogenic sarcoma and carcinoma. *Seminars in Diagnostic Pathology* 1999; **16**: 325–32.

70. Slootweg PJ. Maxillofacial fibro-osseous lesions: Classification and differential diagnosis. *Seminars in Diagnostic Pathology* 1996; **13**: 104–12.

71. Slootweg PJ, Panders AK, Koopmans R, Nikkels PG. Juvenile ossifying fibroma. An analysis of 33 cases with emphasis on histopathological aspects. *Journal of Oral Pathology and Medicine* 1994; **23**: 385–8.

72. Williams HK, Maugham C, Speight PM. Juvenile ossifying fibroma. An analysis of eight cases and a comparison with other fibro-osseous lesions. *Journal of Oral Pathology and Medicine* 2000; **29**: 13–18.

73. El-Mofty S. Psammatoid and trabecular juvenile ossifying fibroma of the craniofacial skeleton: Two distinct clinicopathological entities. *Oral Surgery, Oral Medicine, Oral Pathology, Oral Radiology, and Endodontics* 2002; **93**: 296–304.

74. Cohen MM, Howell RE. Etiology of fibrous dysplasia and McCune–Albright syndrome. *International Journal of Oral and Maxillofacial Surgery* 1999; **28**: 366–71.

◆ 75. Waldron CA. Fibro-osseous lesions of the jaws. *Journal of Oral and Maxillofacial Surgery* 1993; **51**: 828–35.

76. Su L, Weathers DW, Waldron CA. Distinguishing features of focal cemento-osseous dysplasias and cemento-ossifying fibromas I. A pathologic spectrum of 316 cases. *Oral Surgery, Oral Medicine, Oral Pathology, Oral Radiology, and Endodontics* 1997; **84**: 301–9.

77. Su L, Weathers DW, Waldron CA. Distinguishing features of focal cemento-osseous dysplasias and cemento-ossifying fibromas. II. A clinical and radiological spectrum of 316 cases. *Oral Surgery, Oral Medicine, Oral Pathology, Oral Radiology, and Endodontics* 1997; **84**: 540–9.

78. Ackerman GL, Altini M. The cementomas – a clinicopathological reappraisal. *Journal of the Dental Association of South Africa* 1992; **47**: 187–94.

79. Betts NJ, Stewart JC, Fonseca RJ, Scott RF. Multiple central giant cell lesions with a Noonan-like phenotype. *Oral Surgery, Oral Medicine, Oral Pathology, Oral Radiology, and Endodontics* 1993; **76**: 601–7.

80. de Lange J, Rosenberg AJ, van den Akker HP et al. Treatment of central giant cell granuloma of the jaw with calcitonin. *International Journal of Oral and Maxillofacial Surgery* 1999; **28**: 372–6.

81. Auclair PL, Cuenin P, Kratochvil FJ et al. A clinical and histomorphic comparison of the central giant cell granuloma and the giant cell tumor. *Oral Surgery, Oral Medicine, Oral Pathology, Oral Radiology, and Endodontics* 1988; **66**: 197–208.

82. Mangion J, Rahman N, Edkins S. The gene for cherubism maps to chromosome 4p-16.3. *American Journal of Human Genetics* 1999; **65**: 151–7.

83. Antoniades K, Eleftheriades I, Karakasis D. The Gardner syndrome. *International Journal of Oral and Maxillofacial Surgery* 1987; **16**: 480–3.

84. Lucas DR, Unni KK, McLeod RA et al. Osteoblastoma: clinicopathologic study of 306 cases. *Human Pathology* 1994; **25**: 117–34.

85. Kurt AM, Unni K, Sim FH, McLeod RA. Chondroblastoma of bone. *Human Pathology* 1989; **20**: 965–78.

86. Zilman DA, Dorfman HD. Chondromyxoid fibroma of bone: thirty-six cases with clinicopathologic correlation. *Human Pathology* 1989; **20**: 952–64.

87. Milgram JW. Synovial osteochondromatosis: a histopathological study of thirty cases. *Journal of Bone and Joint Surgery* 1977; **59**: 792–801.

14

Paragangliomas

RICHARD M IRVING AND THOMAS PC MARTIN

But hark! My pulse, like a soft drum
Beats my approach, tells thee I come.

Henry King, *An Exequy* (1657)

INTRODUCTION

While paragangliomas of the head and neck will usually present to otolaryngologists, they demand a multidisciplinary approach, and are best managed by teams with an up-to-date knowledge of these complex lesions. The genetics of paragangliomas is an intriguing and emerging field, and in some cases, genetic investigation and appropriate referral to a clinical geneticist may be indicated. In virtually all cases, accurate diagnosis can be achieved preoperatively by appropriate imaging and skilled radiological interpretation. Treatments are becoming more conservative with an increasing acceptance of 'watch and wait' and radiotherapy as viable therapeutic options. Where surgery is being advocated, the emphasis is on function preservation, modifying traditional approaches in order to achieve this. Postoperatively, cranial nerve rehabilitation with the assistance of a dedicated team of therapists will often be a vital part of management.

NOMENCLATURE

Historically, paragangliomas have been described according to their histological appearance (glomus tumours), their staining characteristics (non-chromaffin paraganglioma) or their physiological function (receptoma or chemodectoma).[1] Currently, the accepted nomenclature supported by the World Health Organization[2] describes paragangliomas according to their anatomical location (carotid paraganglioma, vagal paraganglioma, etc.).

THE PARAGANGLION SYSTEM

Anatomy

In 1903, because of their morphological approximation to neural ganglia, Kohn[3] coined the term 'paraganglion' to describe the 'organs of Zuckerandl': disc-like aggregations of tissue in the adventitia of the aorta. These (usually microscopic) paraganglia are found throughout the body, usually closely associated with neural and vascular structures, and have been classified anatomically by Glenner and Grimley[4] into four main groups: (1) branchiomeric (associated with the vasculature of the head and neck extending to the arch of the aorta), (2) intravagal, (3) aorticosympathetic (associated with the sympathetic chain in the thorax and abdomen) and (4) visceral-autonomic. Abdominal (aorticosympathetic and visceral autonomic) paraganglia are anatomically associated with the sympathetic autonomic system, while paraganglia of the head and neck (branchiomeric and intravagal) are more closely associated with the parasympathetic system.[5]

The most well-known head and neck paraganglion is the carotid paraganglion, but paraganglia are also recognized throughout the neurovasculature of the region, with the most common illustrated in **Figure 14.1**. Carotid paraganglia are

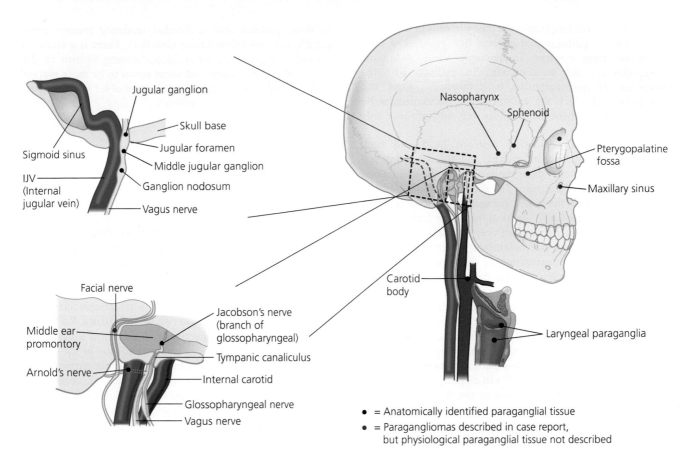

Figure 14.1 Drawing depicting different positions of paraganglia and paragangliomas in the head and neck.

located at the adventitia of the bifurcation of the common carotid artery, and associated with the nerve of Hering, a branch of the glossopharyngeal nerve. Paraganglia in the jugulotympanic region are much smaller than carotid paraganglia (0.5 mm versus 2.5 mm) but well described: in 1953, Guild's examination of 88 temporal bones revealed a total of 248 paraganglia, of which 135 were associated with Jacobson's nerve (the tympanic branch of the glossopharyngeal nerve), and 113 were associated with Arnold's nerve (the auricular branch of the vagus nerve) and the adventitia of the dome of the jugular bulb.[6] Vagal paraganglia are described at all three ganglia along the suprahyoid course of the Xth nerve, namely the superior jugular ganglion, the middle ganglion, and the inferior nodose ganglion.[7] There are two recognized pairs of laryngeal paraganglia: a superior paraganglion situated in the false cord and associated with the superior laryngeal vessels, and an inferior paraganglion closely associated with the cricoid cartilage in the subglottis.[8] The fact that paragangliomas have been identified in the orbit, pterygopalatine fossa, thyroid, nasopharynx and sphenoid and maxillary sinuses, suggests that these locations also harbour paranganglia, although normal paraganglial tissue has not been found at these sites.[9, 10, 11, 12, 13, 14]

Microstructure of paraganglia

All paraganglia are characteristically composed of two distinct cell types: type I and type II cells. Type I cells have the capacity for the synthesis and storage of catecholamines and

are characterized by a rich concentration of cytoplasmic organelles, and by hormone-containing granules. Type II cells are sustentacular cells and are similar to Schwann cells morphologically. A feature of paraganglial cells that is relevant to their investigation and management is their rich density of somatostatin receptors (SSR2 in particular): this can be exploited by the use of somatostatin analogues in the radiological investigation and treatment of paragangliomas (see below under Radionuclide techniques and ^{18}F-DOPA-PET). In common with other endocrine tissue, paraganglionic tissue is richly vascularized.[15]

Physiology

In terms of function, the paraganglion system forms part of the physiologically important, but generally poorly understood, diffuse neuroendocrine system (DNES). This term describes a wide variety of cells throughout the body that are anatomically associated with neural structures and are functionally active, secreting hormones, neurotransmitters and other regulatory proteins to exert either endocrine, paracrine (i.e locally active) or autocrine (i.e autoregulatory) effects. Examples of cells within the DNES include thyroid 'C' cells, gastroenteropancreatic hormone-producing cells, and pituitary endocrine cells. Cells within this family share a common embryological origin (the neural crest), a common biochemistry (the amine precursor and uptake decarboxylase (APUD) system), common histological features, and are primarily homeostatic in function.

The most active biochemical pathway in cells of the DNES is the synthetic pathway that governs the synthesis of catecholamines from tyrosine. Interestingly, while abdominal paraganglia are able to complete this pathway with the conversion of norepinephrine to epinephrine, head and neck paraganglia lack the enzyme (phenylehanolamine-N-methyltransferase) necessary for this step, and produce only norepinephrine.[16]

The anatomical distinction between head and neck (i.e. branchiomeric and intravagal) and thoracoabdominal (i.e. aorticosympathetic) paraganglia seems to be maintained in their physiological function. The adrenal medulla could be loosely described as 'the largest paraganglion in the body' in that it is microscopically identical to other 'extra-adrenal paraganglia'. The function of aorticosympathetic paraganglia seems to be to secrete catecholamines in infancy and early childhood during the maturation of the adrenal medulla, a theory supported by the fact that these paraganglia degenerate in early childhood.[17]

The fundamental role of the carotid paraganglion is well understood and was the subject of the Nobel Prize for Physiology and Medicine awarded to Heymans et al. in 1938.[18] The carotid paraganglion acts as a chemoreceptor stimulated by hypoxic blood chemistry (low PaO_2, an increase in pCO_2 and a low pH). Stimulation results in discharging of Hering's nerve, with reflex communication to the respiratory centre in the medulla oblongata and a consequent increase in respiratory rate and depth. The exact mechanisms of chemoreception are only poorly understood, but it has been postulated that the mitochondrial respiratory chain in type I cells is sensitive to hypoxia, and triggers a release of catecholamine to Hering's nerve.[19]

The physiological role of other head and neck paragangliomas is less clear, but it may be reasonable to suggest that they also play a part in respiratory regulation. This contention, proposed by Lack,[20] is supported by the fact that the anatomy of head and neck paraganglia suggests an atavistic relation to gill arches of aquatic species. Further evidence is provided by the close proximity of paraganglia to structures that might allow detection of hypoxia (the jugular bulb), or its correction (the vagus nerve and the larynx).

PATHOLOGY OF PARAGANGLIOMAS

Epidemiology

Paragangliomas are rare tumours and most general otolaryngologists will not expect to see more than one tumour each year. The true incidence is difficult to calculate with estimates ranging from 1:30 000[21] to 1:500 000[22] but it is important to recognize that calculations are hampered by confusion over nomenclature as discussed above.[23] In terms of frequency, carotid paragangliomas are the most common, followed by jugulotympanic, vagal and laryngeal in descending order of frequency, the latter two being exceedingly rare, with only 190 and 81 cases identified in the English language literature, respectively.[24, 25]

A large series of 236 patients with paragangliomas reported a mean age of presentation of 47 years with a range of ± 16 years (1 s.d.).[26] A younger age of presentation occurs in those patients with a familial tendency towards paragangliomas (see below under Genetics). There is a tendency towards a higher rate of incidence among women in this series (60 per cent), and this trend seems to be more marked in the less common tumours, with ratios of 6:1 F:M described in jugulotympanic paragangliomas.[27]

ASSOCIATION WITH HYPOXIA

No carcinogens are particularly associated with paragangliomas, but there is a well-recognized association between hypoxia and carotid paraganglion hypertrophy. This is manifested by increased rates of carotid paraganglion hypertrophy at altitude, and in patients affected by conditions that induce hypoxia (chronic obstructive pulmonary disease, cystic fibrosis and cyanotic heart disease).[28, 29] In these cases, however, caution should be exercised in management, with great care taken to recognize a distinction between neoplasia and hypertrophy – the latter is likely to be self-limiting and harbours no risk of malignancy. Rodriguez-Cuevas et al.[30] describe a series of 40 natives of Mexico City, in which surgical treatment was carried out in 27 patients with enlarged carotid paraganglia with some surgical morbidity (seven permanent cranial nerve palsies): none of the patients had presented with any functional impairment, none of the 'tumours' showed any malignant behaviour, and histological findings were consistent with type I cell hyperplasia, rather than neoplasia. In such populations and locations, it would seem sensible to pursue a conservative, rather than aggressive management strategy.

BIOLOGICAL ACTIVITY, MALIGNANCY AND FUNCTIONALITY

The majority of paragangliomas are slow-growing, benign, but locally invasive and destructive lesions. Spread is centrifugal, following paths of least resistance, and can lead to extensive bony destruction at the skull base. Growth is slow, with a median increase in dimension of 0.83 mm/year and a median tumour doubling time of ten years.[31] Malignancy is defined by regional spread (WHO classification)[2] and is rare in head and neck paragangliomas. A recent National Cancer Database report from the United States identified only 59 cases of malignant tumours, representing the largest published series in the literature.[32] In the majority of cases (69 per cent), metastatic spread was limited to regional lymph nodes, although distant metastasis to liver, lung, bone and skin are also reported.[33, 34] Five-year survival was 77 per cent for regional disease and 11 per cent for distant metastasis. In this series, only one case of malignancy with distant spread arose from a carotid paraganglioma, suggesting that lesions from other sites may be more aggressive.[32] The National Cancer Database report concludes that the rate of malignancy in paragangliomas is approximately 10 per cent, other large series suggest slightly lower figures of 4–6 per cent.[35, 36] There is no formal staging system.

Production of catecholamines is unusual in head and neck paragangliomas, in contrast to phaeochromocytomas and, to a lesser extent, extra-adrenal abdominal paragangliomas. Paraganglion cells have the capacity to produce norepinephrine (see above under Physiology), and in some this physiological activity can lead to classical symptoms of catecholamine excess (palpitations, diaphoresis and headaches) associated with hypertension in patients with paragangliomas. One study reporting on a series of 297 patients with paragangliomas (204/297 were located in the head and neck), found rates of catecholamine excess as measured by urinary catecholamines in 9.7 per cent of patients with levels measured ($n = 93$).[26] This level falls to 4.5 per cent if the whole group is included, and a true figure is likely to be closer to this level, given that the study is from a tertiary referral centre (the Mayo Clinic), and that those patients who did not have levels measured were likely to have been asymptomatic.

HISTOPATHOLOGY

Paragangliomas of the head and neck demonstrate the same cell types as normal paraganglia: type I and II cells, and a profuse capillary network; they are also indistinguishable from paragangliomas in the thorax and abdomen. Tumours are encapsulated by a dense fibrous pseudocapsule. The characteristic histopathological feature they demonstrate are 'zellballen' (literally, cell balls), a nesting arrangement of type I cells that is demonstrated to a lesser degree in normal paraganglion tissue. These zellballen are surrounded by fibrovascular stromal tissue, and as they grow, may develop central degeneration or necrosis.

Malignancy is not reliably detected on histopathological grounds. The type I cells may be heterogenous in shape and size, and demonstrate nuclear atypia and pleomorphism, but these features are not clear indicators of malignancy. Similarly, the fibrous pseudocapsule may often be breached at points within the specimen, but equally, this feature should not be seen as evidence of capsular invasion and aggressive tumour behaviour.[37]

Immunohistochemistry may offer potential for more reliable differentiation between benign and malignant variants of paragangliomas than histopathology. Edström Elder et al.[38] analysed 32 phaeochromocytomas and abdominal paragangliomas, using a number of immunohistochemical markers and gene expression techniques. The combined use of the monoclonal antibody MIB-1 (a marker for the nuclear protein Ki-67), with the measurement of telomerase activity (hTERT), were highly sensitive markers for malignancy. While these techniques have not been employed with head and neck parangangliomas, the biological similarities between disease at the two sites would certainly suggest that these techniques warrant further investigation.

GENETICS

Approximately 10 per cent of paragangliomas of the head and neck are thought to be familial in aetiology, and the study of the genetics of these lesions has been a very fertile area of research during the past decade. Patients with familial paragangliomas tend to present earlier than those with sporadic tumours (mean age of presentation, 30 years), and they are prone to the development of multiple paragangliomas at different sites. For an example of aggressive bilateral familial paragangliomas, see **Figure 14.2**. Significantly, patients with some variants of familial paragangliomas are also more likely

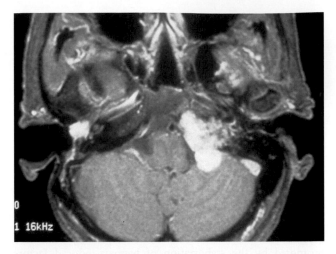

Figure 14.2 Axial T_1 Gd magnetic resonance image demonstrating bilateral paragangliomas. A recurrent tympanicum is seen on the right and a larger jugulare with intracranial extension seen on the left.

to develop malignant tumours, and to develop phaeochromocytomas.[39, 40, 41]

Historical background

An awareness of the familial nature of some paragangliomas dates back as far as 1933, when carotid body tumours were described in two sisters.[42] By the 1960s, it was well understood that head and neck paragangliomas were found in clusters in some families, and that within these families, tumours were often multiple.[43] In the early 1990s, Dutch researchers investigated a five-generation pedigree with evidence of familial paragangliomas (16/95 individuals affected), and mapped a locus of homozygosity (PGL1) in affected family members to chromosome 11q23.[44] Subsequent studies identified the loci PGL2, 3 and 4.[45, 46, 47] Interestingly, while the latter families demonstrate an autosomal dominant pattern of inheritance, the PGL1 families are characterized by maternal imprinting, whereby the phenotype is only expressed if inherited from the paternal side.

Identification of SDHD, B and C

Subsequent research identified the gene defined by PGL1 as SDHD, a gene encoding a subunit of succinate-ubiquinone oxidoreductase (mitochondrial complex II), a component of the mitochondrial electron transport chain involved in the Krebs cycle.[48] Further studies have revealed that the genes implicated by the loci PGL3 and 4 (SDHC and SDHB) also encode for subunits of the same protein complex. The relative frequency of different gene mutations varies with geographical location: in the Netherlands, where two founder mutations are implicated, there is a strong tendency towards SDHD-associated disease, representing 97 per cent of 32 Dutch families investigated. In central Europe (Germany and Poland),[40] and the United States, SDHD and SDHB are found in almost equal proportions, with SDHC a rare occurrence. As yet, no gene has been identified associated with the PGL2 locus.

Possible pathogenetic mechanisms suggested by molecular genetics

The close association between familial paragangliomas and the SDHX family of genes has led to speculation about the pathogenesis of the lesions. As noted above, it has long been recognized that chronic hypoxia due to disease (i.e. chronic obstructive pulmonary disease (COPD)), or the physiological strain of living at high altitude lead to an increased rate of carotid paraganglion hypertrophy.[28, 29] The link between SDHX and hypoxia lies in the role played by mitochondria in oxidative respiration and their role as oxygen sensors. Normal cells generate vascular endothelial growth factor (VEGF), and other growth factors (i.e. erythropoietin) in response to hypoxia – a process mediated by production of reactive oxygen species by the mitochondrial respiratory chain and promoted by the stabilization of hypoxia-induced factors (HIF-1 and -2). It has been demonstrated *in vitro* that SDH inactivation leads to a stabilization of HIF-1 and -2, with subsequent downstream activation of VEGF and erythropoietin.[49] This theory is supported by functional studies using immunohistochemistry and measurements of enzyme activity to analyse MCII function and vascular growth factor expression in paragangliomas.[50, 51, 52]

Although these studies offer interesting insights into the tumorigenesis of familial paragangliomas, it is not clear how significant the mechanism of inappropriate hypoxic drive is in the more common sporadic form of paraganglioma. Studies that have sought genetic defects in SDHX genes in sporadic paragangliomas have not found mutations in these genes,[53] but it may be that in these tumours there is epigenetic modification of gene function, leading to MCII dysfunction.[54]

Differing clinical characteristics of SDHX varieties of familial paraganglioma syndromes

In counselling patients and determining management, it is important to recognize differences between the various SDHX types of familial paragangliomas. These are summarized in **Table 14.1**, with information drawn from a study based upon a central European (Germany and Poland) registry of head and neck paragangliomas (HNPG) ($n = 121$) and phaechromocytomas ($n = 371$).[33] This study identified and investigated a total of 66 carriers of SDHD ($n = 34$) and SDHB ($n = 32$) mutations and assessed clinical characteristics related to the two genes. A later study from the same group used the same registries and expanded their search to other centres in Europe to identify 22 patients with the SDHC mutation to provide similar clinical information.[34]

Table 14.1 demonstrates that SDHX genetic defects are far from homogenous. While both SDHD and SDHB tend to present at the age of 30 and have a similar penetrance, in other respects they differ quite markedly. The SDHB mutation is associated with a high rate of malignancy, and is more likely to be associated with other malignancies presenting at a young age. SDHD presents a more benign phenotype, although these patients are more likely to develop multiple tumours. SDHC is particularly characterized by a phenotype that is restricted to the head and neck. The association of SDHD and SDHB with phaeochromocytoma and extra-adrenal paraganglioma deserves special attention. It should be noted that in the case of SDHB, patients with the genetic defect are more likely to present with a phaeochromocytoma than with a paraganglioma.

SCREENING FOR FAMILIAL PARAGANGLIOMAS

The identification of patients and their relatives carrying SDHX genes is of importance for genetic counselling and further management. In the case of patients with subclinical phaeochromocytoma, this could be a life-saving intervention. In considering whether to submit a patient presenting with a paraganglioma for genetic testing, it is important to recall that even a thorough family history may not reveal hidden disease. This is particularly true in families with an SDHD mutation, where maternal imprinting can cause a mutation to apparently skip generations (while the phenotype is only expressed if inherited from the paternal side, genotype

Table 14.1 Clinical characteristics of SDHX varieties.

	SDHD ($n = 34$)	SDHB ($n = 32$)	SDHC ($n = 22$)
Mean/median age at diagnosis (years)	31 (mean)	29 (mean)	46 (median)
Penetrance	50% by 31 years, 86% by 50 years	50% by 35 years, 77% by 50 years	N/A
No. with multiple tumours	25 (74%)	10 (31%)	2 (9%)
No. with HNPG	27 (79%)	10 (31%)	22 (100%)
No. with phaeochromocytoma	18 (53%)	9 (32%)	0 (0%)
No. with extra-adrenal abdominal paragangliomas	7 (21%)	16 (50%)	0 (0%)
No. with malignant tumours	0 (0%)	11 (34%)	0 (0%)
Carriers with other cancers	1 (3%)[a]	3 (9%)[b]	0 (0%)

Reproduced with permission from Ref. 39.

Information presented here is derived from information drawn from studies based upon a central European (Germany and Poland) registry of HNPG ($n = 121$) and phaechromocytomas ($n = 371$), extending to other centres in Europe.[6, 16]

[a]One patient (age 26) also showed a papillary carcinoma of the thyroid.

[b]One patient (age 14) also showed a papillary carcinoma of the thyroid, two patients from one family demonstrated clear cell renal carcinoma (age 21 and 26).

transmission is unaffected by imprinting). **Figure 14.3** illustrates this phenomenon with a sample pedigree.

All patients with a family history of paragangliomas or phaeochromocytoma should be offered genetic testing, and referred to a clinical geneticist. Apparently isolated patients with multiple paragangliomas or paragangliomas and phaeochromocytoma should also be referred for genetic testing. The case for investigating patients with unifocal disease and no positive family history is less clear cut. Those studies that have reported screening for SDHX mutations in such patients[40, 55, 56] have found various positive rates (8, 9 and 19 per cent, respectively). Given that the mean age of presentation in mutation-positive cases is 30 years compared to 47 years in paraganglioma patients as a whole,[26, 40] it would seem reasonable to prioritize younger patients for screening. In Neumann's study,[40] the only one to specify age at presentation, nine of ten mutation-positive patients from a total of 77 individuals screened were under 50 years old. Screening all those patients with unifocal disease and no clear family history who were under 50 years old would lead to genetic testing of a little over half the presenting population, with an estimated detection rate of approximately 20 per cent.

Patients who are identified as carriers of SDHX genes should be thoroughly investigated, including screening of potentially susceptible relatives. The radiological investigation of paragangliomas will be discussed below under Radiological investigations, but clearly, these patients should be followed up in the long term, preferably with the involvement of a clinician with a special interest in this rare condition and the involvement of a clinical geneticist. The management of familial paragangliomas is an evolving subject, but a distinction must be made between SDHD and SDHC variants,

where a relatively conservative approach might be adopted to prevent excessive iatrogenic morbidity, and SDHB variant, where a more aggressive approach would be warranted by the inherent increased risk of malignancy.

ANATOMICAL CLASSIFICATION SYSTEMS EMPLOYED

Carotid paragangliomas

Carotid paragangliomas are most commonly classified according to size (see **Figure 14.4**), in a system initially proposed by Shamblin *et al.*[57] This system categorizes tumours by the degree to which they encase the carotid arteries, and also reflects the degree to which the tumour adheres to the vascular adventitia. Group I tumours are relatively easy to excise surgically, but larger lesions can prove particularly difficult to remove without vascular grafting.

Jugular and tympanic paragangliomas

Uncertainty about the anatomical origins of paraganglial tissue in the middle ear and the proximity of 'tympanic' and 'jugular' paraganglia have led to these two lesions being conflated into 'jugulotympanic' paragangliomas by the WHO classification, and in classification systems such as the one advocated by Oldring and Fisch.[58] The Glasscock–Jackson system[59] expands the tympanic subclassification. The salient distinction between jugulare and tympanicum lies in the bony integrity of the jugular bulb: if the lesion is in the middle ear and the jugular bulb is intact, then it is a tympanic paraganglioma – if the bulb is eroded, then the origin of the tumour is most likely to be jugular, and will need neurotological expertise if surgery is undertaken. For examples of tympanic and jugulotympanic tumours, see **Figures 14.5 and 14.6**.

Vagal paragangliomas

Arising from paraganglia associated with the vagal ganglion, these lesions arise below the skull base. As they enlarge, they may extend into the jugular foramen and are then subject to the same classification system as jugulare tumours.

CLINICAL FEATURES OF PARAGANGLIOMAS

The clinical features associated with paragangliomas differ according to their location.

Carotid paragangliomas

Carotid paragangliomas typically present with a slowly enlarging, pulsatile, painless, soft mass at the angle of the mandible. Classically, the mass is expansile, mobile only laterally, and can be emptied of blood by gentle pressure;

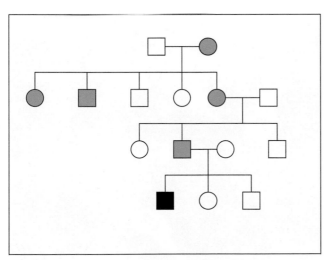

Legend:

■ ● Male/Female disease carrier

■ Affected individual

Figure 14.3 Sample family tree in SDHD illustrating how disease can be hidden within families due to maternal imprinting. The susceptibility gene is carried and transmitted by females, but only manifests as disease when inherited from a father. Reproduced with permission from Ref. 39.

Sagittal view   Axial view

Group I

Group II

Group III

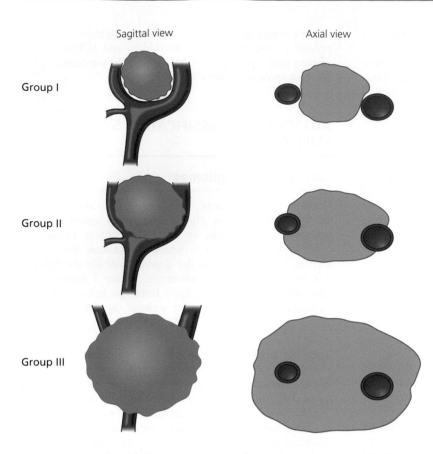

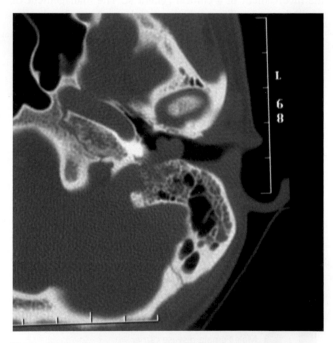

Figure 14.4 Shamblin classification of carotid paragangliomas.

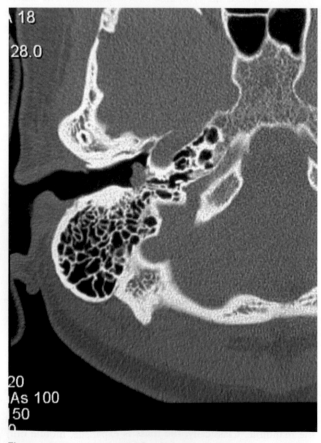

Figure 14.5 An example of a tympanic tumour.

Figure 14.6 An example of a jugulotympanic tumour.

releasing the tumour will allow it to refill slowly. A bruit may be heard over the mass and this can be silenced with pressure. Occasionally, the mass will project into the lateral oropharynx, displacing the tonsil, soft palate and uvula. Some 10 per cent of patients present with neurological symptoms associated with the mass, most frequently affecting the Xth nerve, but symptoms related to the VIIth, IXth and XIIth nerves have also been reported. There may also be an associated Horner's syndrome due to the involvement of the cervical sympathetic chain, or carotid sinus syndrome, characterized by bradycardia and syncopal episodes.[60, 61, 62, 63] In functional paragangliomas, patients may present with symptoms of headache, palpitations or diaphoresis.

Tympanic paragangliomas

Tympanic paragangliomas present typically with pulsatile tinnitus, which is present in approximately 80 per cent of patients, and is the primary symptom in over half of patients. Hearing loss is the primary presenting symptom in some 30 per cent, and a symptom in a total of 60 per cent.[64, 65] Hearing loss is predominantly conductive in character, but can be sensorineural if the labyrinth is involved by tumour. The tympanic membrane can be eroded, leading to a patient presenting with bleeding from the ear, but this is a late sign. Typically, the clinician will find a bluish-red mass on otoscopy (**Figure 14.7**): if the inferior border of the lesion can be seen, this is a Glasscock–Jackson type I tumour; if not, then involvement of the jugular bulb cannot be ruled out. Important differential diagnoses are a high jugular bulb (this will usually be darker in colour), and an aberrant internal carotid artery (this will normally be placed in the anterior mesotympanum). For these reasons, and because of the vascularity of paraganglioma tissue, myringotomy and biopsy should not be undertaken due to the risk of haemorrhage.

Jugular paragangliomas

These lesions, while they may extend to the middle ear and cause similar symptoms to tympanic paragangliomas, are likely to produce neurological signs and symptoms in addition to those described above. In Sanna's series of 55 patients with jugular paragangliomas,[66] 45 per cent presented with pulsatile tinnitus as a primary presenting complaint, while tinnitus and hearing loss were symptoms in 72 and 77 per cent of cases, respectively. Significantly, 43 per cent of the patients had at least one cranial nerve deficit at presentation. The most commonly affected nerves were the IXth and Xth,

with 38 per cent of cases affected in each case; 13 per cent of patients had paralysis of all four lower cranial nerves. As might be expected, the degree of cranial nerve impairment increased as the size of the tumour increased, with intracranial extension being strongly associated with cranial nerve deficits. A similar incidence of preoperative cranial nerve deficit (46 per cent) is found in Jackson's series of 152 patients.[65] Intracranial extension (to the posterior cranial fossa via the medial wall of the jugular bulb) is common in jugular paragangliomas, affecting 62 per cent of 55 patients in Sanna's series, and 36 per cent in Jackson's series. It is important to recognize that these two authors define 'intracranial' slightly differently. Sanna et al.[66] include both intra- and extradural extension, whereas Jackson[65] considers only intradural extension as significant.

Vagal paragangliomas

Vagal paragangliomas present most commonly as a mass in the neck, usually a little more cranial than a carotid paraganglioma. In common with carotid paragangliomas, vagal tumours can project into the lateral oropharynx. As noted above, the three suprahyoid ganglia can all contain paraganglion tissue, and paragangliomas can arise from any of these sites. The most common site is the inferior, nodose ganglion, located some 2 cm caudal to the jugular foramen. Tumours at the jugular foramen can develop into dumb-bell lesions with both intracranial and cervical components.[67] If cranial nerve impairment is present, the pattern of impairment is likely to reflect the anatomy described: lesions at the jugular foramen risk involvement of all four lowest cranial nerves, while lesions originating at the nodose ganglion may only impair vagal function. Netterville et al.[68] described the largest series of vagal paragangliomas in the literature (46 cases), and found a neck mass to be the most common presenting symptom, with tinnitus, hoarseness and a pharyngeal mass also common; 36 per cent of patients presented with at least one cranial nerve impaired.

Laryngeal paragangliomas

Laryngeal paragangliomas are exceedingly rare. Lesions in the supraglottis (the more common type) present with hoarseness, shortness of breath and dysphagia. Hoarseness usually recovers after treatment, and for this reason is generally considered to be due to a mass effect rather than a neurological impairment. Infraglottic paragangliomas represent only 15 per cent of laryngeal paragangliomas and present with hoarseness, haemoptysis and dyspnoea due to tracheal obstruction.[8]

INVESTIGATIONS

The issue of genetic investigation of patients with paragangliomas has been discussed. Further specialized investigations are endocrine and radiological, with the aim of establishing any functionality and determining the extent of disease.

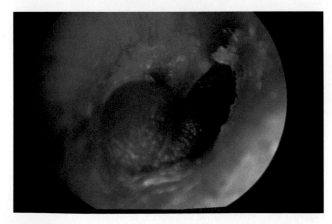

Figure 14.7 Otoscopic view of a tympanic paraganglioma.

Endocrine investigations

The purpose of endocrine investigations is two-fold: to identify those patients with a functioning paraganglioma, and to screen for subclinical phaeochromocytoma. While the majority of patients with functioning tumours will be hypertensive and have at least one symptom of catecholamine excess, it is reasonable to screen all patients with a paraganglioma. It is important to recognize that prior to investigation, β-blockade should be ceased for at least 7 days. Combined 24-hour urinary collection of metanephrine, norepinephrine, epinephrine and dopamine is highly sensitive and specific for tumoral catecholamine excess, with measurement of norepinephrine alone sensitive in 89 per cent of cases.[26] In a study of nine functioning head and neck paragangliomas from a pool of 205, the range of abnormal results for norepinephrine was from 2019 to 2331 nmol, with a normal range of <1005 nmol (<170 µg), emphasizing the specificity of this test. Patients in whom abnormally elevated levels of catecholamines are detected should be investigated radiologically for evidence of synchronous paragangliomas (in particular extra-adrenal abdominal paragangliomas) and phaeochromocytomas. Synchronous tumours should provoke genetic investigation.

Radiological investigations

A wide array of radiological tools play an important role in both the investigation and management of paragangliomas, and close collaboration with radiological colleagues is advised to ensure the maximal use of available local facilities.

COMPUTED TOMOGRAPHY AND MAGNETIC RESONANCE IMAGING

Paragangliomas are detectable with both contrast-enhanced computed tomography (CT) and magnetic resonance imaging (MRI), but these two modalities have different strengths in different anatomical sites. The particular strength of CT scanning is in the evaluation of paragangliomas of the temporal bone, allowing accurate estimation of tumour size, bony destruction and detailed assessment of surgical landmarks. MRI is particularly valuable in assessing intracranial extension and in the assessment of soft tissues (for example in detecting encroachment and encasement of the internal carotid artery and internal jugular veins). A further benefit of MRI lies in the ability to distinguish tumour from surrounding inflammatory tissue or fluid (for example, in the mastoid cavity).[69] Classical radiological appearances are well established: Olsen originally described the 'salt-and-pepper' pattern seen on T_2-weighted magnetic resonance images in paragangliomas that are more than 2 cm in diameter (the pattern arises because of tumour vascularity);[70] the 'lyre' sign, is produced by the splaying of the branches of common carotid artery by a carotid paraganglioma. In addition to standard imaging techniques, both CT and MRI venography and arteriography can be employed to determine the involvement of the vascular structures related to the lesion under investigation.

Screening protocols for pulsatile tinnitus

Tympanic and jugular paragangliomas typically present with pulsatile tinnitus, and this presentation should encourage radiological screening. The presence of objective tinnitus (in which the pulsation is audible to a second party in addition to the patient) is of importance, and should be sought: these patients are more likely to yield positive results.[71] Differential diagnoses include vascular malformations, other rare neoplastic lesions (facial nerve haemangioma and cavernous haemangioma) and acoustic neuromas (although these only rarely present with pulsatile tinnitus).[72] For the purposes of screening, both CT and MRI will detect the presence of paragangliomas in the temporal bone, as described above, but as a first-line screening tool, MRI would be a preferable choice in terms of radiation exposure, the ability to image the internal acoustic meatus, and a reduced likelihood of contrast reaction.[69]

Angiography

Once an important tool in the diagnosis of paragangliomas, angiography has been largely superseded by non-invasive imaging modalities. Nevertheless, angiography plays an important role in evaluating the important feeder vessels preoperatively prior to tumour embolization. **Figure 14.8** represents a vagal paraganglioma imaged in this manner. Temporary balloon occlusion testing, to assess cerebral perfusion, may be indicated in certain large carotid paragangliomas or in order to determine whether the patient will tolerate common carotid clamping to enable tumour removal. This test can also evaluate whether or not a patient will tolerate internal carotid artery sacrifice, which is rarely indicated when removing extensive jugulare tumours.

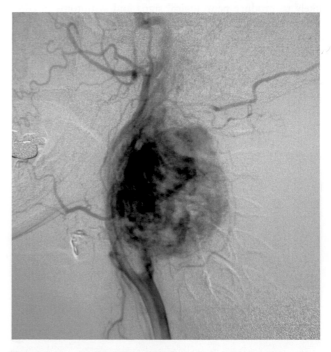

Figure 14.8 Preoperative angiogram demonstrating the 'tumour blush' of a glomus vagale tumour.

Ultrasonography

Ultrasound has a role in the diagnosis and assessment of neck masses and in the cost-effective follow up of carotid and low vagal paragangliomas that are being managed conservatively. Grey-scale ultrasound can be employed to demonstrate the size of carotid lesions, and can also assess encasement of carotid vessels; colour Doppler flow imaging will demonstrate the hypervascularity of paragangliomas.[73] Ultrasound is ineffective at imaging bony structures and neck lesions that extend to the skull base will require further imaging with CT or MRI.

Radionuclide techniques and ^{18}F–DOPA–PET

While imaging modalities, such as MRI and CT, allow very accurate assessment of the anatomical relations of tumours, radionuclide techniques have a place in confirming diagnoses when other radiological findings are equivocal, in whole-body screening for occult disease and in postoperative assessment to ensure tumour control when postsurgical tissue changes can make other imaging difficult.[69] Paranglial tissue is richly supplied with somatostatin, and this is the basis for ^{111}In-pentetreotide scanning, which employs the radiolabelled somatostatin analogue octreotide to target paraganglioma tissue. ^{123}I-metaiodobenzylguanidine (MIBG) scanning is another technique that depends upon the uptake of radiolabelled material by the APUD system.[74] ^{18}F-DOPA-PET ([18]fluorine-dihydroxyyphenylalanine positron emission tomography) is a relatively new whole-body technique that identifies neuroendocrine cells due to their uptake of dopamine, a technique that also exploits an understanding of the APUD system. Of these three techniques, MIBG is recognized to be the least sensitive, with rates of detection low (in a study of eight paragangliomas, only four were detected by this method, while all eight were detected with ^{111}In-pentetreotide scanning).[75] ^{18}F-DOPA-PET appears to be the most sensitive technique, and in one study of patients with familial paragangliomas, a number of lesions were identified that were not detectable on magnetic resonance scanning, even (in a small number of cases) after retrospective review, rendering this technique ideal for the screening of subclinical disease.[76] Radionuclide techniques also have a role to play in the management of metastatic disease.

MANAGEMENT

The management of paragangliomas is a controversial and complex issue. The mainstay of treatment is surgery, but in a number of cases, other modalities have their place. Radiotherapy has long been employed in the management of skull base tumours, and perhaps will have an increasing role in the management of paragangliomas in the future. The slow rate of growth of these tumours also makes them amenable to a conservative 'watch and wait' approach, and this is appropriate for those who may not tolerate extensive surgery and its complications due to age or medical comorbidities. A further group in which a conservative approach is demanded is those patients with familial tumours that are likely to be multifocal.

Radiotherapy

Prior to the development of microsurgical techniques in the 1970s, radiotherapy was the mainstay of treatment of temporal bone neoplasms.[77] As techniques pioneered by Fisch[78] increasingly permitted access to the infratemporal fossa, surgeons enthusiastically adopted surgical management of these challenging tumours. Radiotherapy does not usually lead to a reduction in tumour volume, but can halt tumour progression resulting in tumour control. Radiotherapy can be either fractionated external beam, with a typical dose of 45 Gy in 25 fractions given once daily; stereotactic radiosurgery, in which one high dose of radiation is administered in a highly focused region concentrated on the tumour mass; or stereotactic radiotherapy, a fractionated adaption of stereotactic radiosurgery.[79]

Studies that have addressed questions of local control in radiotherapy predominantly describe treatment with external beam (stereotactic radiosurgery is a relatively recent phenomenon with limited follow up at present). Krych et al.[80] described 33 patients with a median follow up of 13 years and a ten-year control rate of 92 per cent. Complications included xerostomia, loss of smell and taste, hearing loss (two patients), and dysphagia. A rate of local control with radiotherapy in 90–95 per cent of patients is found in other large series, with similar complications quoted.[81, 82] Major complications of radiotherapy are rare, but include osteonecrosis (1.7 per cent) and brain necrosis (0.84 per cent).[83] In many historical cases of radiation-induced complications, doses administered were much higher than those currently given. The risk of radiation-induced malignancy is a more serious complication: Krych et al.[80] identified three reported cases of radiation-induced malignancy reported in the world literature between 1966 and 2005. Two of these tumours were fibrosarcomas, while one was an anaplastic astrocytoma: the time of onset of disease post-radiotherapy ranged from eight to 25 years. Taking these three reported malignancies into account, the rate of radiation-induced malignancy is likely to stand at between 0.5 and 1 per cent.

Surgery

Lesions at different locations require different surgical approaches, and each site will be considered individually. In all cases, with the exception of tympanic paragangliomas, surgical management is often multidisciplinary, involving vascular and interventional radiological colleagues. A further observation is that due to the complications involved in surgery at the skull base, the low rate of malignancy and the slow growth of these lesions, a policy of tumour removal at all costs is often inappropriate. Subtotal resection with cranial nerve preservation is being increasingly adopted as an acceptable treatment plan. Functioning tumours should have been identified preoperatively and appropriately controlled prior to and during surgery.

PREOPERATIVE EMBOLIZATION AND ASSESSING CROSSFLOW

Preoperative embolization on the day prior to surgery has become a standard procedure in larger paraganglioma surgery. Studies that have compared embolized with non-embolized procedures have observed highly significant reductions in intraoperative haemorrhage and operation time. Embolization must be superselective, in that only the artery feeding the tumour is embolized, and in the temporal bone, multiple cannulations may be required to ensure that all compartments of the tumour are devascularized.[84, 85] While uncommon (approximately 1 per cent), complications of embolization include intracranial stroke and cranial nerve neuropathy (often temporary, due to tissue oedema or due to partial occlusion of the vasa nervorum),[69] and for this reason, it is reserved for larger tumours. Even when preoperative embolization is employed, patients often lose in excess of 2 units of blood during the resection of a large jugular paraganglioma.

In rare instances, it may be necessary to determine the feasibility of carotid sacrifice, which can be assessed by preoperative balloon occlusion testing.

CAROTID PARAGANGLIOMAS

Traditionally, in the United Kingdom, resection of carotid paragangliomas is performed by vascular surgeons, and given the importance of vascular control – and the potential for vascular trauma – it would be recommended to undertake this surgery in partnership with a vascular surgeon. In large tumours, temporary occlusion of the common carotid artery with heparinization may be necessary to facilitate removal. The structures most at risk in the procedure are the hypoglossal nerve and the superior laryngeal nerve. Preoperative cranial nerve lesions suggest tumour involvement and do not bode well for postoperative preservation. The vagus nerve, and the external carotid artery, which may need to be ligated to facilitate resection, may be at risk in larger tumours.

The patient is positioned with neck extended and rotated to allow maximum exposure to the upper neck. Subcutaneous injection with 40 mL of 1:100 000 adrenaline will aid haemostasis. The incision should follow a skin crease 2 cm below the mandible to prevent injury to the marginal mandibular branch of the facial nerve and should be continued through platysma. Superior and inferior flaps should be raised in order to maximize exposure, and this can be achieved in the upper neck without damage to the marginal mandibular nerve by incising the fascia overlying the submandibular gland and reflecting this over the nerve in a cuff. With the flaps raised, the anterior border of the sternocleidomastoid is incised and retracted to allow exposure of the carotid sheath.

Vascular control is vital to the success of this operation, and early control with sloops of the common carotid artery is achieved after exposure and dissection of the contents of the carotid sheath. The hypoglossal nerve will be seen running lateral to the paraganglioma, and this should be mobilized from the tumour and reflected superiorly. The tumour should also be freed from the vagus nerve laterally, and, as much as possible, the superior laryngeal nerve posteriorly. If possible, ligation of the ascending pharyngeal artery, the principal feeding vessel for the tumour, can aid controlled dissection, which should follow the tumour's mobilization.

The tumour is dissected in an adventitial plane from the caudal pole cranially, using careful bipolar dissection to limit bleeding as much as possible. The extreme vascularity of paragangliomas can make this dissection difficult, particularly in larger (type 2 and 3) tumours. Van der Mey et al.[86] recommend temporary occlusion of the common carotid artery with heparinization if preoperative balloon occlusion testing suggests the patient will tolerate this. If not, the use of a Javed shunt can be helpful. On rare occasions, the tumour can extend to the skull base, and the surgeon must be prepared to undertake an infratemporal approach to the jugular foramen. With the excision of the tumour complete, meticulous attention should be paid to haemostasis, and a drain sited under two-layer closure.

Results for carotid paraganglioma surgery are generally good. In a series of 45 tumours, Plukker et al.[87] reported only three permanent cranial nerve palsies and three vascular complications – all occurring in type 3 tumours.

TYMPANIC PARAGANGLIOMAS

The excision of tympanic paragangliomas is determined by their size. Small tumours (i.e. Glasscock–Jackson type 1), in which all borders of the tumour can be visualized through the tympanic membrane, can be removed via a tympanotomy approach. The vascularity of the tumour can make dissection difficult, but gentle mobilization and the identification of the feeding vessel (the tympanic branch of the ascending pharyngeal artery) should facilitate excision. Larger tumours that fill the middle ear cleft or extend to the mastoid cavity will need more extensive exposure and, to this end, an extended facial recess approach is recommended.[88] Some authors have recommended the use of laser instruments (Nd-YAG and KTP) in excising tympanic paragangliomas, arguing that relatively large lesions can be safely removed via a simple tympanotomy approach using this technique,[89, 90] although our preference is for an extended facial recess approach for larger tumours even when the laser is being used. Surgical complications are unusual, but include tympanic membrane perforation and conductive hearing loss following disruption of the ossicular chain.

JUGULAR PARAGANGLIOMAS

The resection of jugular paragangliomas is a considerable surgical challenge: the lesions are difficult to access, highly vascular, and are closely related to, if not adherent to, vital neurological and vascular structures. A tailored, multidisciplinary approach is vital, involving vascular and neurosurgical colleagues as appropriate. In all cases, preoperative embolization is recommended. Multiple cranial nerve monitoring is also recommended with facial and vagal recording as a minimum standard with additional monitoring of IX, XI and XII as indicated. A lumbar drain to enable intraoperative reduction in intracranial pressure can be used in tumours with a large intracranial extension.[65]

The challenge of surgery is to remove the lesion, while preserving preoperative neurological function (**Figure 14.9a,b**). The extent of the surgery is tailored to the individual case, the basis of which is an infratemporal fossa approach to the jugular foramen. Where possible, middle ear function is preserved by performing an extended facial recess

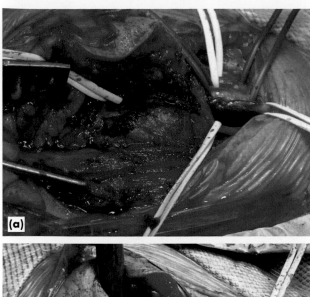

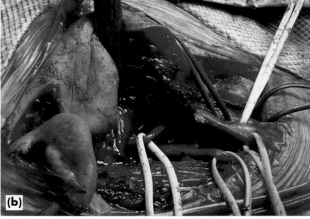

Figure 14.9 (a) Pre- and (b) postsurgical removal pictures of a rare case of a glomus tumour arising from the cervical sympathetic chain. The jugular was pushed anteriorly and laterally in this case and the tumour could be removed maintaining the vagus nerve in continuity.

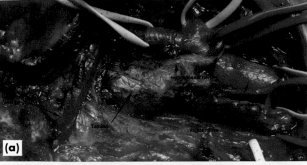

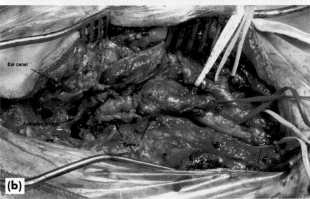

Figure 14.10 Demonstration of infratemporal fossa type A approach to a large glomus vagale showing the upper neck exposure of the tumour (a) and jugular foramen exposure with intact canal wall and VII within fallopian bridge (b).

approach. In situations where there is a significant pre-operative sensorineural loss or access to the petrous apex is required, then sacrifice of the inner ear should be considered. Functioning bulbar nerves are preferably left undisturbed even if this requires some tumour to be left behind. Carotid sacrifice is rarely indicated, but if this is being considered then preoperative occlusion testing should have been carried out.

The surgery commences with a postauricular incision that extends in a skin crease into the neck. A wide mastoidectomy is performed, with decompression of the sigmoid sinus and removal of the mastoid tip. The inferior tympanic bone should be removed to skeletonize the external auditory canal and improve access to the distal internal carotid artery. Access to the jugular foramen is hampered laterally by the facial nerve and, traditionally, the nerve has been anteriorly rerouted from the fallopian canal and implanted into the anterior epitympanum,[91] but in most cases, this can be avoided by skeletonizing the fallopian canal (the 'fallopian bridge' technique) (for an illustration, see **Figure 14.10a,b**):[92] an intermediate solution is to perform a 'short mobilization'.[65] The vertical portion of the facial nerve below the posterior semicircular canal is in the authors' experience

the site most commonly involved by tumour. If the nerve is functioning normally prior to surgery, the nerve is probably best left *in situ* with the tumour attached, whereas if the nerve is paralysed prior to surgery resection and interposition nerve grafting is indicated. Exposure in the neck is facilitated by retraction or division of the sternomastoid muscle. Vascular control is achieved with slooping of the proximal internal carotid artery, and exposure distally; the internal jugular vein is ligated distally, and the sigmoid sinus packed extraluminally. The tumour within the jugular bulb is then carefully dissected from the internal carotid artery and lower cranial nerves, remembering that the inferior petrosal sinus drains into the anteromedial jugular bulb, and has not yet been controlled: this is packed intraluminally once the tumour has been removed.

Extensive anterior exposure of the tumour may require transection of the external auditory canal, and the ear to be reflected forwards. The mandible is dislocated from the tympanic bone, and may be retracted or partially excised; further exposure anteriorly can be achieved with resection of the zygoma. Access to and mobilization of the entire intrapetrous carotid can be achieved by this approach.

Intracranial extension can be either intra- or extradural. The tumour may be resected in one stage with the extracranial component, or removed at a later date. Sanna *et al.*[66] advocate a staged resection for tumours with >2 cm intracranial extension, employing the upper portion of the original incision. They argue that the tumour excision is less problematic because the remnant has devascularized, and that closure of the dural defect is less prone to failure when the surgical wound is less extensive. Jackson[65] advocates a one stage procedure with extensive local and, if necessary, free tissue flap closure and the protection of a lumbar drain. Both authors achieve similar results in terms of cerebrospinal fluid leak rates (3.7 and 4.5 per cent, respectively).

The results of surgery for jugular paragangliomas vary considerably according to the size and location of the tumour, but it should be recognized that complications, particularly in terms of cranial nerve injuries, are common. Death is a rare but recognized complication: in Jackson's series of 182 patients, five patients died following surgery due to internal carotid artery resection (three) or pulmonary embolus (two, this occurred in functioning tumours). Tumour control rates, defined as complete removal of tumour without recurrence, are 85 per cent (Jackson) and 83 per cent (Sanna). Cranial nerve defects are often present preoperatively, but further deficits postoperatively are also common: in Sanna's series, new cranial nerve deficits occurred in 33, 30, 25 and 12 per cent of cranial nerves IX, X, XI and XII, respectively. Jackson's rates of new cranial nerve deficit are slightly higher, with the same nerves affected in 57, 40, 62 and 56 per cent of cases, respectively.

VAGAL PARAGANGLIOMAS

Many of the issues and surgical approaches previously described with reference to carotid and jugular paragangliomas apply to vagal paragangliomas. As previously described, vagal paragangliomas can arise at different points along the vagus nerve as it leaves the jugular foramen. Those lower lesions may be approached through the neck, in an approach similar to that described for carotid surgery, while higher lesions that extend to the skull base will require an infratemporal approach as described for jugular disease. Particular challenges relate to the involvement of the internal carotid artery, to which the tumour can be tightly adherent, or even encasing, and to vagal rehabilitation of the patient following surgery. In Netterville et al.'s series of 40 operated patients,[68] 37 patients underwent sacrifice of the vagal nerve, requiring extensive rehabilitation: clearly, in patients without a pre-existing palsy of the vagus nerve or one of its branches, alternative treatment strategies such as 'watch and wait' or radiotherapy should be very carefully considered.

LARYNGEAL PARAGANGLIOMAS

The surgical treatment of laryngeal paragangliomas is conservative, but due to the high degree of local recurrence, open, rather than endoscopic techniques are generally advocated.[93] In most cases, the tumour, which is generally located in the false cord, can be excised by a lateral pharyngotomy approach, in cases of larger tumours, supraglottic laryngectomy may be necessary. Subglottic paragangliomas should be excised by a laryngofissure approach.

CRANIAL NERVE REHABILITATION

Postsurgical cranial nerve injury is common in paraganglioma management, and the rehabilitation of cranial nerves is a vital component of treatment. The success of rehabilitation is dependent upon the nerves affected and the age, comorbidities and motivation of the patient. Enthusiastic and aggressive swallowing rehabilitation is key, and a number of surgical adjuncts can also be useful. Netterville et al.[68] advocate primary medialization surgery (with silastic implants) in the event of complete vagal sacrifice. In addition, they describe unilateral palatal adhesion (in which the paralysed soft palate is sutured to the posterior pharyngeal wall) to reduce nasal regurgitation of liquids in patients who suffer from this persistently following vagal paralysis. Rehabilitation is undertaken in a multidisciplinary setting, and if possible, patients who are likely to need postoperative rehabilitation should be introduced to speech and language therapists before they undergo surgery. Rehabilitation for facial paralysis is occasionally required and can be complicated by the inability to use the hypoglossal nerve, which may have been damaged either by the tumour or the treatment. Accessory nerve lesions can also be troublesome and are best treated by physiotherapy. Surgery to the shoulder musculature is rarely indicated.

Management of malignant disease

Malignancy is rare in paragangliomas, with spread to local lymphatics most commonly found. If lymph node involvement is suspected clinically and confirmed with imaging, surgical excision should be accompanied with neck dissection. Radiotherapy has been demonstrated to lead to residual viable tissue in lesions that are effectively 'controlled' in terms of local spread,[65] and for this reason is not recommended as a sole modality for treatment of malignant lesions. Lee et al.[32] note a trend in recent years towards the use of adjuvant radiotherapy in these patients and draw a tentative conclusion that this combination therapy is likely to offer an increased survival next to single modality treatment with surgery, an assertion tempered by the small numbers of patients involved. Traditional chemotherapy has little role in the treatment of malignant paragangliomas as might be suggested by the slow rate of growth in these tumours.

KEY EVIDENCE

- Studies of a five-generation pedigree in the Netherlands identified a locus of homozygosity to chromosome 11.[44] Subsequent in vitro studies have demonstrated an association between hypoxia-induced growth factors and the proteins (SDHD, B and C) associated with this and other affected loci.[49]
- ^{18}F-DOPA-PET appears to be the most sensitive imaging modality available for paragangliomas, and may provide useful for the identification of subclinical lesions, particularly in familial cases.[76]

KEY LEARNING POINTS

- Paragangliomas are rare, usually benign vascular lesions that can be found at many locations in the head and neck, but primarily affect the carotid body, tympanum and jugular bulb.
- The lesions predominantly affect patients in their fifth and sixth decades with a female sex bias.
- A small but significant proportion of tumours are familial. In this group, there is an important association with phaeochromocytoma. Patients with germline abnormalities of the SDH family of genes will often suffer multiple tumours during their lifetime, and are at greater risk of malignancy (SDHB). Any patients with multiple tumours, a positive family history or an early presentation should be referred for genetic investigations.
- Management of paragangliomas is focused upon disease removal or control, with an emphasis upon preservation of neurological function. Treatment can be conservative ('watch and wait'), surgical or radiotherapeutic, depending upon patient and tumour factors.

REFERENCES

1. Martin TPC. What we call them: the nomenclature of head and neck paragangliomas. *Clinical Otolaryngology* 2006; **31**: 185–6.
2. Barnes L, Everson J, Reichart P, Sidransky D (eds). *WHO classification of tumours: pathology and genetics of tumours of the head and neck.* Lyon: IARC Press, 2005.
3. Kohn A. Die paraganglien. *Archiv fur Mikroskopische Anatomie* 1903; **62**: 263–365.
4. Glenner GG, Grimley PM. Tumours of the extra-adrenal paraganglion system (including chemoreceptors). In: Firminger HI (ed.). *Atlas of tumour pathology.* Washington DC: Armed Forces Institute of Pathology, 1974: 1–90.
5. Lack EE. Paraganglia of the head and neck region. In: Firminger HI (ed.). *Atlas of tumour pathology.* Washington DC: Armed Forces Institute of Pathology, 1997: 303.
6. Guild SR. The glomus jugulare, a nonchromaffin paraganglion, in man. *Annals of Otology, Rhinology, and Laryngology* 1953; **62**: 1045–71.
7. Lack EE. Vagal paraganglioma. In: Firminger HI (ed.). *Atlas of tumour pathology.* Washington DC: Armed Forces Institute of Pathology, 1997: 355.
8. Myssiorek D, Halaas Y, Silver C. Laryngeal and sinonasal paragangliomas. *Otolaryngologic Clinics of North America* 2001; **34**: 971–82.
9. Sharma MC, Epari S, Gaikwad S *et al.* Orbital paraganglioma: report of a rare case. *Canadian Journal of Ophthalmology* 2005; **40**: 640–4.
10. Walker PJ, Fagan PA. Catecholamine-secreting paraganglioma of the pterygopalatine fossa: case report. *American Journal of Otology* 1993; **14**: 306–8.
11. Corrado S, Montanini V, De Gaetini C *et al.* Primary paraganglioma of the thyroid gland. *Journal of Endocrinological Investigation* 2004; **27**: 788–92.
12. Chambers EF, Norman D, Dedo HH, Ferrell LD. Primary nasopharyngeal chemodectoma. *Neuroradiology* 1982; **23**: 285–8.
13. Talbot AR. Paraganglioma of the maxillary sinus. *Journal of Laryngology and Otology* 1990; **104**: 248–51.
14. Koegel L Jr, Levine HL, Waldman SR. Paraganglioma of the sphenoid sinus appearing as labile hypertension. *Otolaryngology – Head and Neck Surgery* 1982; **90**: 704–7.
15. Wasserman PG, Savargaonkar P. Paragangliomas: classification, pathology, and differential diagnosis. *Otolaryngologic Clinics of North America* 2001; **34**: 837–44.
16. McCaffrey TV, Myssiorek D, Marrinan M. Head and neck paragangliomas: physiology and biochemistry. *Otolaryngologic Clinics of North America* 2001; **34**: 837–44.
17. Coupland RE. Postnatal fate of the abdominal para-aortic bodies in man. *Journal of Anatomy* 1954; **88**: 455–64.
18. De Castro F. The discovery of sensory nature of the carotid bodies. *Advances in Experimental Medicine and Biology* 2009; **648**: 1–18.
19. Biscoe TJ, Duchen MR. Responses of type I cells dissociated from the rabbit carotid body to hypoxia. *Journal of Physiology* 1990; **428**: 39–59.
20. Lack EE. Paraganglia of the head and neck region. In: Firminger HI (ed.). *Atlas of tumour pathology.* Washington DC: Armed Forces Institute of Pathology, 1997: 303.
21. Bikhazi PH, Roeder E, Attaie A, Lalwani AK. Familial paragangliomas: the emerging impact of molecular genetics on evaluation and management. *American Journal of Otology* 1999; **20**: 639–43.
◆ 22. Roman S. Phaeochromocytoma and functional paraganglioma. *Current Opinion in Oncology* 2003; **16**: 8–12.
23. Myssiorek D. Head and neck paragangliomas: an overview. *Otolaryngologic Clinics of North America* 2001; **34**: 829–36.
24. Urquhart AC, Johnson JT, Mers EN *et al.* Glomus vagale: paraganglioma of the vagus nerve. *Laryngoscope* 1994; **104**: 440–5.
25. Barnes L. Paraganglioma of the larynx. A critical review of the literature. *Journal of Otorhinolaryngology and Related Specialties* 1991; **53**: 220–34.
● 26. Erickson D, Yogish CK, Ebersold MJ *et al.* Benign paragangliomas: clinical presentation and treatment outcomes in 236 patients. *Journal of Clinical Endocrinology and Metabolism* 2001; **86**: 5210–16.

27. Brown JS. Glomus jugulare tumours revisited: a ten year statistical follow-up of 231 cases. *Laryngoscope* 1985; **95**: 284–8.

28. Arias-Stella J, Valcarcel J. Chief cell hyperplasia in the human carotid body at high altitudes. *Archives of Pathology and Laboratory Medicine* 1976; **100**: 636–9.

29. Heath D. Post-mortem size and structure of the human carotid body. *Thorax* 1970; **25**: 129–40.

30. Rodriguez-Cuevas H, Lau I, Rodriguez HP. High altitude paragangliomas, diagnostic and therapeutic considerations. *Cancer* 1986; **57**: 672–6.

31. Jansen JC, van den Berg R, Kuiper A *et al.* Estimation of growth rate in patients with head and neck paragangliomas influences the treatment proposal. *Cancer* 2000; **88**: 2811–16.

● 32. Lee JH, Barich F, Karnell LH *et al.* National cancer data base report on malignant paragangliomas of the head and neck. *Cancer* 2002; **94**: 730–7.

33. Martin CE, Rosenfeld L, McSwain B. Carotid body tumours: a 16-yr follow-up of seven malignant cases. *Southern Medical Journal* 1973; **66**: 1236–43.

34. Argiris A, Mellott A, Spies S. PET scan assessment of chemotherapy response in metastatic paraganglioma. *American Journal of Clinical Oncology* 2003; **26**: 563–6.

35. Borsanyi SJ. Glomus jugulare tumours. *Laryngoscope* 1962; **72**: 1336–45.

36. Manolidis S, Shohet JA, Jackson CG, Glasscock ME 3rd. Malignant glomus tumours. *Larygoscope* 1999; **109**: 30–4.

37. Lack EE. Carotid body paraganglioma. In: Firminger HI (ed.). *Atlas of tumour pathology.* Washington DC: Armed Forces Institute of Pathology, 1997: 328–39.

● 38. Edström Elder E, Xu D, Höög A *et al.* KI-67 and hTERT expression can aid in the distinction between malignant and benign pheochromocytoma and paraganglioma. *Modern Pathology* 2003; **16**: 246–55.

◆ *39. Martin TPC, Irving RM, Maher ER. The genetics of paragangliomas: a review. *Clinical Otolaryngology* 2007; **32**: 7–11.

● 40. Neumann HP, Pawlu C, Peczkowska M *et al.* Distinct clinical features of paraganglioma syndromes associated with SDHB and SDHD gene mutations. *Journal of the American Medical Association* 2004; **292**: 943–51.

41. Schiavi F, Boedeker CC, Bausch B *et al.* Predictors and prevalence of paraganglioma syndrome associated with mutations of the SDHC gene. *Journal of the American Medical Association* 2005; **294**: 2057–63.

● 42. Chase W. Familial and bilateral tumours of the carotid body. *Journal of Pathology and Bacteriology* 1933; **36**: 1–12.

43. Resler DR, Snow JB Jr, Williams GR. Multiplicity and familial incidence of carotid body and glomus jugulare tumors. *Annals of Otology, Rhinology, and Laryngology* 1966; **75**: 114–22.

● 44. Heutink P, van der Mey AG, Sandkuijl LA *et al.* A gene subject to genomic imprinting and responsible for hereditary paragangliomas maps to chromosome 11q23-qter. *Human Molecular Genetics* 1992; **1**: 7–10.

45. Mariman EC, van Beersum SE, Cremers CW *et al.* Analysis of a second family with hereditary non-chromaffin paragangliomas locates the underlying gene at the proximal region of chromosome 11q. *Human Genetics* 1993; **91**: 357–61.

46. Niemann S, Steinberger D, Muller U. PGL3 a third, not maternally imprinted locus in autosomal dominant paraganglioma. *Neurogenetics* 1999; **2**: 167–70.

● 47. Astuti D, Latif F, Dallol A *et al.* Gene mutations in the succinate dehydrogenase subunit SDHB cause susceptibility to familial pheochromocytoma and to familial paraganglioma. *American Journal of Human Genetics* 2001; **69**: 49–54.

● 48. Baysal BE, Ferrell RE, Willett-Brozick JE *et al.* Mutations in SDHD, a mitochondrial complex II gene, in hereditary paraganglioma. *Science* 2000; **287**: 848–51.

49. Selak MA, Armour SM, MacKenzie Ed *et al.* Succinate links TCA cycle dysfunction to oncogenesis by inhibiting HIF-alpha prolyl hydroxylase. *Cancer Cell* 2005; **7**: 77–85.

50. Douwes Dekker PB, Hogendoorn PC, Kuipers-Dijkshoorn N *et al.* SDHD mutations in head and neck paragangliomas result in destabilization of complex II in the mitochondrial respiratory chain with loss of enzymatic activity and abnormal mitochondrial morphology. *Journal of Pathology* 2003; **201**: 480–6.

51. Gimenez-Roqueplo AP, Favier J, Rustin P *et al.* The R22X mutation of the SDHD gene in hereditary paraganglioma abolishes the enzymatic activity of complex II in the mitochondrial respiratory chain and activates the hypoxia pathway. *American Journal of Human Genetics* 2001; **69**: 1186–97.

52. Jyung RW, LeClair EE, Bernat RA *et al.* Expression of angiogenic growth factors in paragangliomas. *Laryngoscope* 2000; **110**: 161–7.

53. Astuti D, Hart-Holden N, Latif F *et al.* Genetic analysis of mitochondrial complex II subunits SDHD, SDHB and SDHC in paraganglioma and phaeochromocytoma susceptibility. *Clinical Endocrinology* 2003; **59**: 728–33.

54. Gimm O, Armanios M, Dziema H *et al.* Somatic and occult germ-line mutations in SDHD, a mitochondrial complex II gene, in nonfamilial pheochromocytoma. *Cancer Research* 2000; **60**: 6822–5.

● 55. Baysal BE, Willett-Brozick JE, Lawrence EC *et al.* Prevalence of SDHB, SDHC, and SDHD germline mutations in clinic patients with head and neck paragangliomas. *Journal of Medical Genetics* 2002; **39**: 178–83.

56. Bayley JP, van Minderhout I, Weiss MM *et al.* Mutation analysis of SDHB and SDHC: novel germline mutations in sporadic head and neck paraganglioma and familial paraganglioma and/or phaeochromocytoma. *BMC Medical Genetics* 2006; **7**: 1.

57. Shamblin WR, ReMine WH, Sheps SG, Harrison EG Jr. Carotid body tumour (chemodectoma). Clinicopathologic analysis of ninety cases. *American Journal of Surgery* 1971; **122**: 732–9.

58. Oldring D, Fisch U. Glomus tumours of the temporal region. *Archives of Otolaryngology* 1981; **107**: 209.

59. Glasscock ME, Jackson CG, Harria PF. Glomus tumours: diagnosis, classification, and management of large lesions. *Archives of Otolaryngology* 1982; **108**: 401.

60. Bernard RP. Carotid body tumours. *American Journal of Surgery* 1992; **163**: 494–6.

61. Wax MK, Briant DR. Carotid body tumours: a review. *Journal of Otolaryngology* 1992; **21**: 277–84.

62. Van der Mey AG, Frijns JH, Cornelisse CJ *et al.* Does intervention improve the natural course of glomus tumours? A series of 108 patients seen in a 32 year period. *Annals of Otology, Rhinology, and Laryngology* 1992; **101**: 635–42.

63. Rosenkrantz L, Schell AR. Carotid body tumour as a reversible cause of recurrent syncope. *New York State Journal of Medicine* 1984; **84**: 38–9.

64. O'Leary MJ, Shelton C, Giddings NA *et al.* Glomus tympanicum tumors: a clinical perspective. *Laryngoscope* 1991; **101**: 1038–43.

◆ 65. Jackson CG. Glomus tympanicum and glomus jugulare tumors. *Otolaryngologic Clinics of North America* 2001; **34**: 941–70.

66. Sanna M, Jain Y, De Donato G *et al.* Management of jugular paragangliomas: the Gruppo Otologico experience. *Otology and Neurotology* 2004; **25**: 797–804.

◆ 67. Sniezek JC, Netterville JL, Sabri AN. Vagal paragangliomas. *Otolaryngologic Clinics of North America* 2001; **34**: 925–39.

68. Netterville JL, Jackson CG, Miller FR *et al.* Vagal paraganglioma: a review of 46 patients treated during a twenty-year period. *Archives of Otolaryngologyogy – Head and Neck Surgery* 1998; **124**: 1133–40.

◆ 69. Lustrin ES, Palestro C, Vaheesan K. Radiographic evaluation and assessment of paragangliomas. *Otolaryngologic Clinics of North America* 2001; **34**: 881–906.

70. Olsen WL, Dikon WP, Kelly WM *et al.* MR imaging of paragangliomas. *American Journal of Roentgenology* 1987; **148**: 201–4.

71. Brunberg JA. What MR sequences should be used in the evaluation of pulsatile tinnitus? *American Journal of Roentgenology* 1995; **165**: 226.

72. Weissman JL, Hirsch BE. Imaging of tinnitus: a review. *Radiology* 2000; **216**: 342–9.

73. Derchi LE, Seraffini G, Rabbia C *et al.* Carotid body tumours: US evaluation. *Radiology* 1992; **182**: 457–9.

74. Brink I, Hoegerle S, Klisch J, Bley TA. Imaging of pheochromocytoma and paraganglioma. *Familial Cancer* 2005; **4**: 61–8.

75. Muros MA, Llamas-Elvira JM, Rodriguez A *et al.* [111]Inpentetreotide scintigraphy is superior to ^{123}I-MIBG scintigaphy in the diagnosis and location of chemodectoma. *Nuclear Medicine Communications* 1998; **19**: 735–42.

● 76. Hoegerle S, Ghanem N, Altehoefer C *et al.* ^{18}F-DOPA positron emission tomography for the detection of glomus tumours. *European Journal of Nuclear Medicine and Molecular Imaging* 2003; **30**: 689–94.

77. Sharma PD, Johnson AP, Whitton AC. Radiotherapy for jugulo-tympanic paragangliomas (glomus jugulare tumours). *Journal of Laryngology and Otology* 1984; **98**: 621–9.

✳ 78. Fisch U. Infratemporal fossa approach for extensive tumors of the temporal bone and base of the skull. In: Silverstein H, Norrel H (eds). *Neurological surgery of the ear*, vol. 2. Birmingham, AL: Aesculapius, 1977: 34–53.

79. Mendenhall WM, Hinerman RW, Amdur RJ *et al.* Treatments of paragangliomas with radiation therapy. *Otolaryngologic Clinics of North America* 2001; **34**: 1007–21.

● 80. Krych AJ, Foote RL, Brown PD *et al.* Long-term results of irradiation for paraganglioma. *International Journal of Radiation Biology and Related Studies in Physics, Chemistry, and Medicine* 2006; **65**: 1063–6.

81. Cole JM, Beiler D. Long-term results of treatment for glomus jugulare and glomus vagale tumors with radiotherapy. *Laryngoscope* 1994; **104**: 1461–5.

82. Hinerman RW, Mendenhall WM, Amdur RJ *et al.* Definitive radiotherapy in the management of chemodectomas arising in the temporal bone, carotid body, and glomus vagale. *Head and Neck* 2001; **23**: 363–71.

◆ 83. Boedeker CC, Ridder GJ, Schipper J. Paragangliomas of the head and neck: diagnosis and treatment. *Familial Cancer* 2005; **4**: 55–9.

84. Young NM, Wiet RJ, Russell EJ, Monsell EM. Superselective embolisation of glomus jugulare tumors. *Annals of Otology, Rhinology, and Laryngology* 1988; **97**: 613–20.

85. Tikkakoski T, Luotonen J, Leinonen S *et al.* Preoperative embolisation in the management of neck paragangliomas. *Laryngoscope* 1997; **107**: 821–6.

86. Van der Mey AGL, Jansen JC, van Baalen JM. Management of carotid body tumours. *Otolaryngologic Clinics of North America* 2001; **34**: 907–24.

87. Plukker JT, Brongers EP, Vermey A *et al.* Outcome of surgical treatment for carotid body paraganglioma. *British Journal of Surgery* 2001; **88**: 1382–6.

88. Forest JA, Jackson GC, McGrew BM. Long-term control of surgically treated glomus tympanicum tumours. *Otology and Neurotology* 2001; **22**: 232–6.

89. Robinson PJ, Grant HR, Brown SG. Nd-YAG laser treatment of a glomus tympanicum tumour. *Journal of Laryngology and Otology* 1993; **107**: 236–7.

90. Molony NC, Salto-Tellez M, Grant WE. KTP laser assisted excision of glomus tympanicum. *Journal of Laryngology and Otology* 1998; **112**: 956–8.

91. Jenkins HA, Fisch U. Glomus tumours of the temporal region. *Archives of Otolaryngology* 1981; **107**: 209–14.

* 92. Pensak ML, Jackler RK. Removal of jugular foramen tumours: the fallopian bridge technique. *Otolaryngology – Head and Neck Surgery* 1997; **117**: 586.

93. Myssiorek D, Halaas Y, Silver C. Laryngeal and sinonasal paragangliomas. *Otolaryngologic Clinics of North America* 2001; **34**: 971–82.

Tracheostomy

J PAUL M PRACY AND MARIA ROGERS

If it were done, when 'tis done, then 'twere well it were done quickly.

William Shakespeare, *Macbeth*, Act 1 Scene 7

INTRODUCTION

Tracheostomy is one of the oldest surgical procedures.[1] There are references to the creation of a surgical airway in many ancient texts.[2] Until the end of the nineteenth century and the introduction of asepsis, together with the development of safe anaesthetic techniques, the procedure was extremely hazardous. Tracheostomy was seen as a last resort in hopeless cases and was the cause of great anxiety for the patient and surgeon alike. Chevalier Jackson established the principles of the operation at the beginning of the twentieth century and these remain in place today.[3] The development of percutaneous tracheostomy over the past 15 years has taken surgical airway management out of the exclusive province of the otolaryngologist. There are now a wide variety of clinicians confronted by the challenges of tracheostomy care and decannulation strategies.

A tracheotomy is a surgical opening in the trachea, while a tracheostomy is the creation of a stoma at the skin surface which leads into the tracheal lumen.

TEMPORARY TRACHEOSTOMY

A temporary tracheostomy may be either an elective or an emergency procedure. The most common use of an elective temporary tracheostomy is for prolonged ventilatory support in a ventilated patient. A temporary tracheostomy may also be planned as part of a major surgical procedure in which there are concerns about postoperative swelling or bleeding, which may precipitate upper airway obstruction. A temporary tracheostomy may be short term, long term or permanent.

An emergency tracheostomy is a rare procedure, perhaps only indicated in cases of severe trauma. In all other cases, it could be argued that the performance of an emergency tracheostomy is indicative of an underestimation of the severity of the breathing problem. The majority of cases can be dealt with by carrying out an urgent procedure under local anaesthesia with the patient awake. In extremis, it should be possible to perform a cricothyroidotomy and maintain ventilation via a wide bore cannula until conversion to a formal tracheostomy can be undertaken.

A permanent or 'end' tracheostomy is an elective procedure carried out as part of a surgical procedure involving the removal of the larynx, such as a laryngectomy or pharyngolaryngectomy. A permanent tracheostomy is also created in laryngeal diversion procedures used to prevent aspiration. The continuity between the laryngopharynx and the trachea is permanently disrupted and the cut end of the trachea is sutured to the skin.

The effects of a tracheostomy include:

- laryngeal bypass – loss of cough and phonation;
- reduction in respiratory dead space;
- loss of nasal mucosa filtration and humidification;
- increased risk of infection;
- tube acts as foreign body leading to local inflammation;
- sump above tracheostome and below larynx, when mucus collects.

INDICATIONS

Indications for tracheostomy are the following:

- upper airway obstruction;
- removal of secretions;
- prolonged ventilation;
- part of another procedure.

Upper airway obstruction

When confronted by a patient with an upper airway obstruction, it is essential to carry out a rapid but complete assessment of the patient's overall condition. There may be coexisting medical problems which are contributory to their breathing problems and the management of such problems may need to be incorporated into the solution of the airway problem.[4] It is important to ascertain the precise level of obstruction so that any intervention provides relief at the lowest level of obstruction. With the advent of improved intubating laryngoscopes and advanced techniques, such as fibreoptic intubation or the use of oesophageal airways, upper airway obstruction is no longer the most common indication for tracheostomy.

Prolonged ventilation

Tracheostomy is the safest means of assisting ventilation where prolonged positive pressure is needed. It is easier to secure a tracheostomy tube than either an orotracheal or nasotracheal tube and the reduced dead space assists weaning of respiratory support. It has been demonstrated that the introduction of percutaneous tracheostomy has led to a doubling in the number of tracheostomies being carried out. It may be that the ease of access to tracheostomy has resulted in reduced duration of intubation.[5] With the introduction of low pressure cuffs for endotracheal tubes, a longer period of intubation has become acceptable. There are studies showing an increased rate of subglottic stenosis if intubation continues for more than 10 days,[6] although there are those who would argue that intubation can be prolonged for up to 3 weeks.[7] There is evidence that early tracheostomy in trauma patients reduces the length of ventilation and hospital stay[8] and it may be that the same applies for general intensive treatment unit (ITU) patients.

Removal of secretions

The accumulation of secretions in the lower respiratory tract is responsible for a reduction in gas diffusion within the alveoli. This results in respiratory failure. A tracheostomy reduces the dead space, so reducing the work of breathing and also makes it easier to aspirate secretions with less upset to the patient.

Part of another procedure

A permanent tracheostomy is an unavoidable consequence of a major head and neck procedure in which it is necessary to remove the whole of the larynx. A temporary tracheostomy should be regarded as mandatory for all major resections involving the oral cavity or pharynx. In these cases, the tracheostomy allows protection of the lower airway from aspiration of blood, in the event of a haemorrhage, as well as guarding against upper airway obstruction from postoperative swelling. Percutaneous tracheostomy is probably not appropriate in these cases, as the pretracheal tissues fit tightly around the tube.[9] In the event of tube displacement, the tissues can collapse inwards, closing the airway with a potentially fatal outcome.[10]

ANATOMY

As with any surgical procedure, when performing a tracheostomy, it is essential to have a sound knowledge of the relevant applied anatomy of the upper trachea. Problems are likely to happen if the surgeon strays from the midline. The recurrent laryngeal nerve runs in the tracheo-oesophageal groove and the great vessels are lateral to this within the carotid sheath. It is rare in a straightforward tracheostomy to lose sense of where the midline is, but in obese patients and small children, it is possible to lose the anatomical landmarks and stray laterally. The thyroid isthmus crosses in front of the trachea covering a variable number of the tracheal cartilaginous rings. It is a highly vascular structure and inadvertent damage during dissection or friction from the tube may result in postoperative haemorrhage. The innominate artery crosses the front of the trachea, from left to right, at a variable height. In cases of a high innominate artery, it may be encountered during dissection or may suffer erosion from the tracheostomy tube with potentially fatal postoperative haemorrhage.[11]

CONTRAINDICATIONS

There are no absolute contraindications to tracheostomy. However, in the case of terminal patients, very careful consideration must be given to the psychological effects on the patient and the quality of life aspects. There is no right or wrong answer and each patient must be approached on an individual basis.

PREOPERATIVE CONSIDERATIONS

In the elective setting, it is imperative that adequate consent is received from the patient or their relatives. As part of this process, it is necessary to cover the risks and benefits of the procedure in some detail. This must be a frank and open discussion and the potential complications and sequelae of tracheostomy must be pointed out. This is particularly true of paediatric tracheostomy.

OPERATIVE PROCEDURE

Cricothyroidotomy/minitracheostomy

In an emergency, rapid control of the upper airway can be achieved by use of an airway inserted through the cricothyroid membrane. Once an incision has been made through the membrane, a minitracheostomy tube or a wide bore cannula can be used to keep the tract open and provide an alternative airway.

The patient is positioned with the neck extended over a pillow. The cricothyroid membrane can be palpated and the area is infiltrated with local anaesthetic and epinephrine. The cricothyroid membrane can be incised either with a scalpel or a wide bore cannula attached to a syringe half filled with saline. In the former case, once the airway has been opened, the blunt handle of the scalpel can be inserted and rotated to create space for a tube to be passed into the trachea. In the latter case, the needle of the cannula is used to breach the membrane and as the needle and cannula are inserted, the plunger of the syringe is withdrawn. Once air bubbles into the syringe, the trachea has been entered, the cannula can then be introduced over the needle. The cannula can be connected via a universal connector to an ambubag and the patient can be ventilated for a short period of time. Using this system, CO_2 is not cleared and so conversion to a formal tracheostomy should be undertaken as soon as possible.

A minitracheostomy tube should not be left in situ for more than a short time as there will inevitably be some friction between it and the cricoid cartilage which will predispose the patient to subglottic stenosis.

Percutaneous tracheostomy

First described over 50 years ago,[12, 13] this technique has grown in popularity and is now the most common procedure for the provision of an alternative airway for ITU patients. The growth of the procedure followed the introduction over the last 10–15 years of commercial kits based on well-defined techniques.[14, 15] In the United Kingdom, the most commonly employed kit depends on the dilatation technique originally described by Ciaglia et al.[14]

The patient should be positioned as for a formal surgical tracheostomy (see below under Open surgical tracheostomy). The trachea is punctured, using a needle and cannula, just below the first tracheal cartilage ring. A syringe half filled with saline is attached to the cannula. Gentle aspiration allows correct positioning of the cannula, because air is aspirated through the saline as the needle passes into the trachea. The needle is withdrawn and a guide wire is inserted through the cannula, which is itself withdrawn to allow for either a single or graded serial dilators to be passed over the guide wire. The dilators create a passage which is wide enough for the insertion of a standard tracheostomy tube,

which is passed over the largest of the dilators and secured in position within the trachea. It is advisable to view the internal lumen of the trachea during this procedure by using a flexible bronchoscope, as this is likely to reduce complications.[16]

Open surgical tracheostomy

Although there are many variations in the technique of open surgical tracheostomy, they are all based on the same fundamentals. The technique described is that preferred by the author. The procedure should, when possible, be carried out in an operating theatre, under sterile conditions. It is usual for the patient to have a general anaesthetic but, where this is deemed hazardous, the procedure can be carried out under local anaesthetic.

The patient should be positioned supine, with the neck extended by placing a sandbag under the shoulders. It is important that the patient is positioned square on the table with the shoulders at the same level. This will ensure that the midline structures of the neck are truly in the midline throughout the operation. When operating under local anaesthesia, it may be necessary to compromise on the degree of neck extension as overextension may further restrict the airway.

A horizontal incision is sited halfway between the sternal notch and the lower border of the cricoid cartilage. Once the skin has been incised, dissection continues through the subcutaneous tissues to the strap muscles, which are retracted laterally, following blunt dissection in the midline to separate them. Following this manoeuvre, the thyroid isthmus should be visible. The isthmus should be clamped, divided and transfixed. At this point, the anterior tracheal wall is encountered. It is useful to identify the cricoid cartilage so as to plan the point of entry into the trachea. Ideally, the tracheotomy should be made between the second and fourth tracheal rings. Before entering the trachea, it is important to select an appropriately sized tracheostomy tube and check that the cuff and all the connecting equipment works properly, so that ventilation can continue uninterrupted following the tracheostomy. There needs to be good communication between the surgeon and the anaesthetist.

Having informed the anaesthetist that the trachea is about to be opened, the tracheotomy can be performed. The guiding principle should be to cause as little disruption to the trachea as possible, maintain cartilage and prevent damage to the cricoid cartilage. These aims are best achieved by the use of a vertical slit between silk stay sutures. Once the trachea has been opened, the anaesthetist should withdraw the endotracheal tube under the direction of the surgeon who can visualize the tube being withdrawn. When the tip of the endotracheal tube is immediately above the tracheotomy, withdrawal can stop and the tracheostomy tube should be inserted. The cuff should be inflated and the tube connected to the ventilator.

The incision should be closed loosely and the tracheostomy tube secured in position with tapes, sutures or both.

CHOICE OF TUBE

There is a wide variety of tracheostomy tubes available, made from different materials and with different features.

The choice of tube depends on the indication for the tracheostomy, the postoperative needs of the patient, as well as the anatomy of the patient, while also taking into account patient comfort and management of the tracheostomy.

Where possible the tracheostomy tube chosen should feature an inner tube, as described below, as this promotes a safe airway, reducing the risk of obstruction. Consequently, the tracheostomy tube can stay in place for up to 29 days without disrupting the airway. The first tube inserted at the time of the procedure should be a cuffed tube. The most commonly used tubes are polyvinylchloride (PVC) tubes available with or without cuffs and fenestrations.

Cuff

Cuffed tracheostomy tubes are used to provide a seal to allow positive pressure ventilation or to prevent aspiration. The pressure of air within the cuff must be high enough to provide an adequate seal, but not so high as to damage the tracheal mucosa resulting in subglottic stenosis. It is therefore imperative that cuffs are not overinflated where the pilot balloon feels solid. The use of modern low-pressure cuffs has for the most part reduced this problem where the recommended cuff pressure of 15–25 cmH$_2$O can be easily monitored.

Inner tube

Several tubes are now supplied with an inner tube, which fits snugly inside the main tube. The tip of the inner tube projects a few millimetres beyond the distal end of the main tube. This means that secretions will collect in the inner tube, which can be removed, cleaned and replaced without disruption to the patient or their airway. The process for cleaning the inner tubes is determined through local guidelines.

With a strong focus on hospital decontamination processes, manufacturers are now developing inner tube systems, which are disposable.

Fenestration

The fenestration is sited at the point of maximum curvature in the tube and may be in the form of a single hole or a number of small holes. The fenestration allows air to pass from the tube through the larynx, so increasing the air available for phonation and increasing the volume of the voice. Fenestrated tubes feature an inner tube which is fenestrated, as well as one that is non-fenestrated, so that the clinical needs of the patient can be met without disrupting the airway. The differences between the inner tubes are usually identified by the colour of the 15 mm connector or the inner tube itself.

Flexibility

In some cases, a rigid tracheostomy tube will not conform to the anatomy of the patient and will lie at an awkward angle or in a position which results in tracheal trauma from the tip of the tube rubbing against the tracheal wall. In these circumstances, it may be better to use a softer more flexible tube usually made from silicone. If the use of a softer tube results in obstruction of the tube due to kinking, it may be necessary to use an armoured flexible tube. Armoured tubes are reinforced with metal wire along the shaft of the tube, which needs to be considered in terms of imaging and radiotherapy.

Adjustable flange

An adjustable flange allows the intratracheal length of the tube to be altered to take account of the depth of the stoma, which may be increased by alterations in anatomy, such as a huge thyroid mass, or to bypass intratracheal obstruction. These tubes can be flexible or predetermined in that they are suitable for depth of stoma only.

In most cases, hyperflexible tracheostomy tubes and adjustable flange tubes do not feature an inner tube and so meticulous postoperative care in terms of airway assessment, suction and humidification is required. These tubes can block easily and may require changing after 7–10 days if there are any difficulties with secretions. The Uniperc^{TM} adjustable flange tracheostomy tube (Portex) has been developed for the larger neck and may be inserted surgically or percutaneously. It features an inner tube which may be removed, cleaned and replaced, hence it may stay in place for 29 days.

Extra length tubes with disposable inner tubes are also available which are predetermined with a choice of either distal or proximal extensions, however, these are not adjustable. Although inner tubes are featured with some adjustable and extra length tubes, secretions may still build up at the distal end of the tube, so continuous nursing care and monitoring is required to prevent obstruction.

It is not recommended that patients are discharged home with single lumen tubes. The Moores tube (Kapitex$^®$) is flexible, features an inner tube system and is very useful when a long, soft, flexible tube is needed and the cuff is no longer necessary.

Flexible and adjustable flange tubes can be customized where patients have specific needs.

POSTOPERATIVE CONSIDERATIONS

On their return to the ward, it is important that the patient is looked after by a nurse who is experienced in the care of tracheostomy patients and knowledgeable about the potential complications, as well as the different types of tubes. Local guidelines, procedures or protocols should be in place for the management of patients with a tracheostomy. Communication materials must be available for the patient.

The original tracheostomy tube must be secured in position for at least 3 days to allow a good tract to form. The tube may be changed after 7 days, if this is clinically indicated, and any sutures can then be removed. Tubes should be secured with tapes fastened by a secure knot on both sides of the neck, with the neck in a neutral position. If the neck is extended when the tapes are fastened, then the tapes will be too long and will not hold the tube in the appropriate position so that it may be coughed out. Alternatively, Velcro tracheostomy tubes holders can be used and can be adjusted quite easily around the neck.

The cuff should be deflated once the risk of aspiration has passed, in most cases there is no need for cuff inflation after the first 12 hours.

Following tracheostomy, the inspired air passes directly into the trachea without being warmed and humidified by the upper airway. As a result, the air is irritant to the trachea and there is an increase in the quantity and viscosity of the tracheal secretions. The patient may require frequent suctioning in the early postoperative period and the use of humidified oxygen, nebulizers or heat and moisture exchangers is essential to reduce the risk of tube obstruction due to crust formation. As the trachea becomes accustomed to the presence of the tube and the patient learns to clear the secretions by coughing through the tube, so the need for suctioning decreases.

Swallowing problems are common following tracheostomy. These are usually due to the sensation of pressure in the upper oesophagus because of an inflated cuff and because the movement of the larynx during swallowing is reduced because of a tethering effect of the tube.

If at any stage there are doubts regarding the position of the tube, or whether the lumen of the tube is obstructed, a flexible nasendoscope can usually be passed through the tube to inspect the lumen of the tube and the trachea.

COMPLICATIONS

Complications of tracheostomy are listed in **Table 15.1**.

Immediate

Haemorrhage is the most common fatal complication of tracheostomy,[17] as well as the most common complication. Bleeding is usually due to damage to the thyroid veins or the thyroid isthmus. If there is significant bleeding at the end of the procedure, the wound should be explored and any bleeding vessel ligated. Packing the tracheostomy wound to tamponade the bleeding is widely practised, but should be seen as little more than a temporary procedure prior to re-exploration of the wound.

While life threatening, air embolism is fortunately rare following tracheostomy. If the large veins of the neck are

opened during the procedure, air may be sucked into the venous system and pass into the right atrium.

Damage to structures in the vicinity of the operative field is often the result of altered anatomy or inattention to good surgical technique. Inexperienced surgeons may inadvertently stray from the midline and so cause damage to the contents of the carotid sheath, oesophagus or recurrent laryngeal nerve. In emphysematous patients, the apex of the lung may extend into the lower neck and can be damaged as a result of lateral dissection. An inadequate incision, poor retraction or poor haemostasis can result in less than ideal exposure and consequent damage to the tracheal walls or cricoid cartilage. Damage to the cricoid is particularly serious and if recognized at the time of surgery, the tracheostomy should be resited lower in the trachea and the damage repaired.

Immediate complications are best prevented by good haemostasis during surgery and meticulous attention to surgical technique.

Intermediate

Accidental extubation is easily avoided provided that the tube is adequately secured at the time of the procedure, by suturing the flanges of the tube to the skin. If the tube is displaced and comes to lie in the pretracheal space, the complication may not become immediately apparent. The patient can continue to breathe and the soft tissues gradually prolapse around the tracheal opening which slowly begins to seal. Dyspnoea slowly increases and, by the time the displacement is apparent, the tube may be impossible to replace as the tracheotomy has virtually closed. An experienced nurse will pick up on the early warning signs. Any difficulty breathing through the tube must be fully investigated. The use of a flexible scope passed through the lumen of the tube may identify displacement or obstruction of the tube due to crusting, granulation tissue or poor placement of the tube tip with respect to the tracheal wall.

If the tracheostomy tube or the trachea is obstructed and the skin incision has been closed tightly, then air may be forced out into the soft tissues of the neck during expiration resulting in subcutaneous emphysema. Surgical emphysema, under these circumstances, can track up to the lower eyelids and down into the upper chest. In severe cases, the swelling may cause displacement of the tube.

Tracheo-oesophageal fistulae may be the result of intra-operative damage to the posterior wall of the trachea or persistent rubbing of the tip of the tube on the posterior wall in the early postoperative period. The fistula usually presents when the patient starts to show signs of aspiration, in spite of the cuff being inflated. Tracheoarterial fistulae present most commonly in previously irradiated patients, particularly if a low tracheostomy has been carried out. There is rarely any premonitory sign and the usual presentation is with sudden massive haemorrhage. The tracheostomy tube must be changed immediately for a cuffed tube, the cuff should be inflated to prevent further aspiration of blood and compression applied to any bleeding vessel via the tracheostome. The wound should be explored immediately as there is a very high mortality associated with this complication. The most common artery affected is the innominate, although there are reports of tracheocarotid fistulae.[11, 18]

Table 15.1   Complications of tracheostomy.

Immediate	Intermediate	Late
Haemorrhage	Extubation	Tracheocutaneous fistula
Air embolism	Obstruction	Tracheal stenosis
Local damage	Subcutaneous emphysema	
	Infection	
	Fistulae	

Late

Epithelialization of the tract is a normal event in the evolution of a tracheostomy. The longer the tracheostomy has been present, the more established the process is and the more likely the tract is to persist following decannulation. The incidence can be reduced if great attention is paid to ensuring an airtight seal is maintained once the stoma has been occluded. If there is evidence of granulation tissue in the fistula, simple cautery with silver nitrate may effect a closure. A small number of cases will require formal surgical closure. This involves excision of the tract all the way down to the anterior tracheal wall and closure in several layers.

Tracheal stenosis is almost always the result of damage to the cricoid or first tracheal ring at the time of surgery or damage to the trachea from the rubbing of a poorly positioned tube, resulting in mucosal inflammation.

Decannulation

If the patient is able to breathe around the tube when it is occluded, then there is no need to downsize the tube. This is usually the case, if the initial cuffed tube has been replaced with an uncuffed fenestrated tube. Decannulation should take place in an ordered sequence and local protocol should be followed. The tube should be blocked during the day and unblocked at night for the first 24 hours. If the patient tolerates this, then the tube can be occluded for a full 24-hour period and if this is tolerated then the tube can then be removed. If the patient is unable to tolerate this occlusion of the tube, then it may be necessary to downsize the tube to give more room around the tube. Patients who have been dependent on the tracheostomy for a long time may require a more prolonged decannulation process as it may take some time for them to overcome their anxiety about being unable to breathe without the tube in place.

Once the tube has been removed, an airtight dressing must be applied to occlude the stoma. In most cases, several gauze squares covered with an occlusive dressing will be sufficient. The dressing should be changed whenever an air leak appears to improve the chance of full closure of the fistula. Where possible, the patients should be encouraged to support the tracheostomy site while talking and coughing to promote healing.

LONG-TERM TRACHEOSTOMY

Certain clinical situations are such that the patients will require a tracheostomy long term or permanently. Discharge plans and continuing care issues need to be addressed at the earliest opportunity and action plans put in place. For patients with an end tracheostomy (following total laryngectomy), physical, psychological and social assessments and preparation should be made in the preoperative phase to ensure the best outcomes for the patients and their families. This is best achieved through a combination of multidisciplinary pretreatment assessment clinics, home visits and patient visitors.

Careful consideration of the discharge destination, immediate support and communication needs is required to ensure patient safety. Where possible, patients are encouraged to maintain independence and need focused education to acquire skills in self-care in terms of their tracheostomy. Patients, their partners and families need to be included in the education programme at the earliest opportunity in order to gain proficiency and confidence in what is required.

Community care teams need to be included and good communication across the care boundaries is required to provide support to patients where care issues can be complex and challenging. Community-based teams require specific education in terms of tracheostomy care and the ongoing supply of specialist equipment.

After discharge, it is essential that strategies are put in place for trouble shooting and the management of complications arising. This can be achieved through clinical nurse specialists, Macmillan nurses or key workers who have expertise in altered airways, who can assess patients and advise on treatments as soon as problems arise reducing the need for emergency admission to hospital.

Patients with end tracheostomy will undergo continuing voice rehabilitation programmes and so become very familiar with maintenance of their voice prosthesis and problem-solving strategies.

RESUSCITATION

The aim of trachesotomy care is to prevent complications arising from the tracheostomy itself. This can be achieved through constant vigilance and attention to detail, taking into account the needs for suction, humidification, stoma care and specific tube care.

Airflow through the tube should be checked regularly to identify problems early and prevent emergency situations.

Patients with a tracheostomy can experience breathing difficulties at any time which may be very distressing. Nurses and the medical team should be alert to this and investigate any changes immediately.

It is essential that specific equipment is kept at the patient's bedside (**Box 15.1**), so that emergency events can be dealt with much more effectively and efficiently, ensuring the patient's safety.

Box 15.1   Bedside equipment

- Oxygen apparatus
- Suction apparatus (in working order)
- Tracheal dilators
- Two spare tracheostomy tubes
  - one the same size and type as worn by the patient
  - one a size smaller
- Stitch cutter
- Endotracheal tube tapes/tracheostomy tube holders
- Lubricating gel
- 10 mL syringe

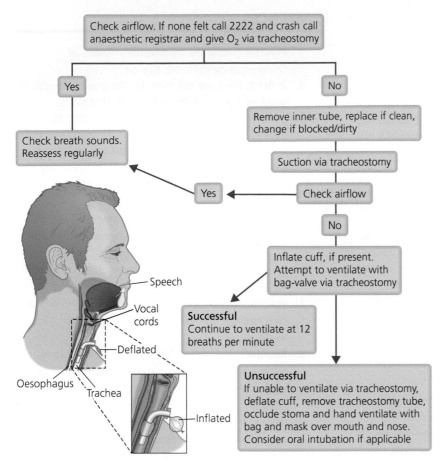

Check airflow. If none felt call 2222 and crash call anaesthetic registrar and give O₂ via tracheostomy

Yes

No

Check breath sounds. Reassess regularly

Remove inner tube, replace if clean, change if blocked/dirty

Suction via tracheostomy

Check airflow

Yes

No

Inflate cuff, if present. Attempt to ventilate with bag-valve via tracheostomy

Successful
Continue to ventilate at 12 breaths per minute

Unsuccessful
If unable to ventilate via tracheostomy, deflate cuff, remove tracheostomy tube, occlude stoma and hand ventilate with bag and mask over mouth and nose. Consider oral intubation if applicable

Speech

Vocal cords

Deflated

Oesophagus

Trachea

Inflated

Figure 15.1 Guidelines for emergency care of tracheostomy patients.

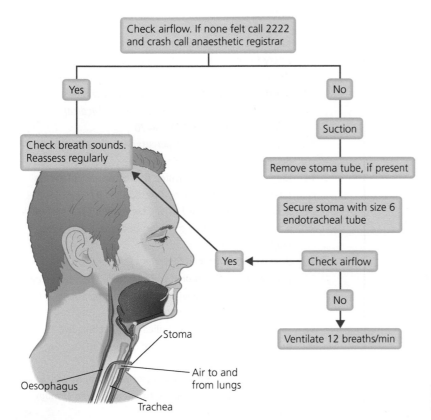

Check airflow. If none felt call 2222 and crash call anaesthetic registrar

Yes

No

Check breath sounds. Reassess regularly

Suction

Remove stoma tube, if present

Secure stoma with size 6 endotracheal tube

Yes

Check airflow

No

Ventilate 12 breaths/min

Stoma

Air to and from lungs

Oesophagus

Trachea

Figure 15.2 Guidelines for emergency care of laryngectomy patients.

In the event of respiratory or cardiopulmonary arrest, the procedure as stated in the local resuscitation policy should be followed. The presence of a tracheostomy tube or an end tracheostomy may sometimes cause anxiety for members of the resuscitation team not familiar with the anatomy of the altered airway. In the first instance, it is essential to ensure that there is no obstruction of the airway or within the trachea. This can be assessed by feeling for airflow through the tracheostomy by placing a hand in front of it, inspecting the inner tube and performing tracheal suction to ensure the easy passage of the catheter.

For patients with a tracheostomy, it is essential that resuscitation is given using the tracheostomy and not the mouth, and the guidelines outlined in **Figure 15.1** may be followed.

Patients with laryngectomy will require mouth-to-stoma resuscitation, rather than mouth-to-mouth resuscitation, as the stoma is the only point of entry to the lower airway. The stoma should be examined for any obstruction and tracheal suction performed to determine airway patency. Resuscitation can be given more effectively following the insertion of a tracheostomy tube or an endotracheal tube (**Figure 15.2**).

KEY EVIDENCE

- The evidence in support of this chapter is from retrospective observational and cohort studies. There have been few publications in the past 30 years related to open surgical procedures and the majority of publications in the past 15 years have been concerned with the impact of the introduction of percutaneous techniques, primarily in the intensive care setting.

KEY LEARNING POINTS

- Effects of tracheostomy: laryngeal bypass, reduced respiratory dead space, loss of nasal functions, increased risk of infection.
- Indications for tracheostomy: upper airway obstruction, removal of secretions, prolonged ventilation, part of another procedure.
- Complications of tracheostomy: *immediate* (haemorrhage, air embolism), *intermediate* (accidental extubation, tube obstruction, tracheo-oesophageal fistula), *late* (persistent tract, stenosis).
- Resuscitation: for patients with a tracheostomy, the stoma is likely to be the easiest means of access to the airway and may be the only route of access to the airway. Local guidelines should be followed.

REFERENCES

1. Frost EA. Tracing the tracheostomy. *Annals of Otolaryngology* 1976; **85**: 618–24.
2. Porter R. Medicine and faith. In: *The greatest benefit to mankind.* London: Fontana Press, 1997: 83–105.
3. Jackson C. Tracheostomy. *Laryngoscope* 1909; **19**: 285–90.
4. Weymuller E. Acute airway management. In: Cummings CW, Fredrickson JM, Harker LA (eds). *Otolaryngology – head and neck surgery.* St Louis: Mosby, 1998: 2368–81.
5. Simpson TP, Day CJE, Jewkes CF, Manara AR. The impact of percutaneous tracheostomy on intensive care unit practice and training. *Anaesthesia* 1999; **54**: 172–97.
6. Whited RE. Posterior commissure stenosis post long-term intubation. *Laryngoscope* 1983; **93**: 1314–18.
7. Watson CB. A survey of intubation practices in critical care medicine. *Ear, Nose and Throat* 1983; **62**: 494–501.
8. Rodriguez JL, Steinberg SM, Luchetti FA *et al.* Early tracheostomy for primary airway management in the surgical critical care setting. *Surgery* 1990; **108**: 655–9.
9. Gysin C, Dulguerov P, Guyot J-P *et al.* Percutaneous versus surgical tracheostomy. *Annals of Surgery* 1999; **230**: 708–14.
10. Van Heerden PV, Webb SAR, Power BM, Thompson WR. Percutaneous dilatational tracheostomy – a clinical study evaluating two systems. *Anaesthesia and Intensive Care* 1996; **24**: 56–9.
11. Kapural L, Sprung J, Glunic I *et al.* Tracheo-innominate artery fistula after tracheostomy. *Anesthesia and Analgesia* 1999; **88**: 777–80.
12. Sheldon CH, Pudenz RH, Tichy FY. Percutaneous tracheostomy. *Journal of the American Medical Association* 1957; **165**: 2068–70.
13. Toye FJ, Weinstein JD. A percutaneous tracheostomy device. *Surgery* 1969; **65**: 384–9.
14. Ciaglia P, Firsching R, Syniec C. Elective percutaneous dilatational tracheostomy. *Chest* 1985; **87**: 715–19.
15. Schaner A, Ovil Y, Sidi J *et al.* Percutaneous tracheostomy – a new method. *Critical Care Medicine* 1989; **17**: 1052–6.
16. Winkler WB, Karnik R, Seelmann O *et al.* Bedside percutaneous dilatational tracheostomy with endoscopic guidance: experience with 71 ICU patients. *Intensive Care Medicine* 1994; **20**: 476–9.
17. Hardy KL. Tracheostomy: Indications, techniques, and tubes. *American Journal of Surgery* 1973; **126**: 300–7.
18. Bradley PJ. Bleeding around a tracheostomy wound: what does it all mean? *Journal of Laryngology and Otology* 2009; **123**: 952–6.

16

Trauma of the larynx and cervical trachea

PATRICK J GULLANE, CARSTEN E PALME AND RALPH W GILBERT

> However beautiful the strategy, you should occasionally look at the results.
>
> Winston Churchill

INTRODUCTION

The structures within the laryngotracheal region provide vital function in terms of ventilation, swallowing and voice. Because of the complex anatomy within this region, traumatic injuries can produce significant acute dysfunction, create a life-threatening condition and/or result in long-term upper aerodigestive tract morbidity. Comprehensive assessment and prompt management are essential to minimize the likelihood of perioperative complications and long-term morbidity and thus optimize patient outcome.

ANATOMY AND AETIOLOGY

The laryngotracheal complex consists of soft tissue structures (laryngeal ligaments, intrinsic and extrinsic musculature) housed within an intricate cartilaginous framework. This structure is vulnerable to significant dysfunction with any minor alteration that may be caused by a variety of traumatic mechanisms. The larynx is located in the midline of the neck and is a soft and mobile structure, which can sustain a significant traumatic force before injury occurs.[1] It is protected anteriorly by the mandible and posteriorly by the vertebral column and can be divided into three subsites: the supraglottis, glottis and subglottis. The cricoid cartilage is a rigid circumferential structure located in the upper airway, which provides support to the airway and articulates with the arytenoid cartilages.

The aetiology of injuries in this region varies and may be divided into traumatic, inhalational, post-intubation and iatrogenic causes. The reported overall incidence of traumatic laryngeal injuries is relatively low and ranges between 1 in 5000 to 1 in 137 000 emergency room admissions.[1, 2, 3] These injuries occur most commonly in young males (80 per cent) ranging in age from 24 to 37 years[1, 2, 4] and usually result from blunt trauma or a penetrating wound. The majority of blunt traumatic injuries are related to motor vehicle accidents, contact sports, strangulation, punching, hanging or 'clothesline-type injuries' which are commonly seen in motorcycle and snowmobile accidents.[1, 5, 6, 7] Penetrating trauma is most often due to gunshot or stab wounds. In previous reports, the majority of accidental injuries which resulted in significant laryngeal damage was blunt trauma.[1] However, a change in urban violence has seen an increasing number of patients with penetrating injuries.[3, 6, 8, 9, 10, 11] In a recent series of 1562 patients presenting with neck trauma, gunshot and knife wounds accounted for 14.8 per cent of all cases of significant upper aerodigestive tract injury, while blunt trauma was responsible for only 1.2 per cent.[10] Mandatory seat belt laws have contributed to a dramatic reduction of blunt cervical trauma.[3, 12, 13] Mortality rates from injury involving the laryngotracheal complex range from 2 to 18 per cent.[2, 10] Although blunt laryngeal trauma is associated with significant sequelae, Chagnon and Mulder[12] reported that penetrating wound injuries were more likely to result in death. This mortality rate may be related to the higher likelihood of concomitant injury involving critical organs or tissues including the chest, skull base and/or critical neurovascular structures from gun or knife injuries.[8, 9, 10, 14] This is in contrast to the review by Bhojani et al.[11] who reported a higher mortality rate in patients with blunt trauma. These patients were also older and more likely to require emergency airway management compared to those with penetrating wounds.[11] The variability in reported injury outcome may relate to the referral pattern and geographical diversity.

Inhalation-type injuries involving the laryngotracheal complex occur following exposure to fires and/or noxious gases or ingestion. Airway oedema commonly occurs following these exposures and in the majority of cases, it resolves without sequelae. However, inhalational injuries or ingestion of corrosive agents, such as bleaches or acids, may cause full thickness burns that result in scar formation with potentially devastating morbidity to the upper aerodigestive tract.

Laryngotracheal complex injuries may occur following a cricothyroidotomy, a translaryngeal tracheostomy, a high tracheostomy or other therapeutic procedures including upper aerodigestive tract endoscopy, endolaryngeal surgery (cold steel, laser), routine tracheostomy (percutaneous or open) or as a result of prolonged placement of a nasogastric tube.[15, 16, 17, 18] Most commonly, these lesions occur after orotracheal intubation resulting in chronic inflammation, granulation tissue, fibrosis and resultant stenosis. In the past three decades, modifications in the tracheostomy cuff and avoidance of a high tracheostomy have reduced the incidence of tracheal stenosis, but have not significantly reduced the rate of subglottic stenosis. Stenosis in this region may be related to the intubation (multiple insertions, prolonged duration or traumatic intubation), the tube utilized and patient factors.[19, 20] Comorbidities, such as diabetes and vascular disease, may increase the risk of developing laryngotracheal stenosis. To minimize the injury to the local tissue associated with intubation, it is recommended that a low cuff pressure and the smallest diameter polyvinyl chloride tube be used.

In recent years, a greater awareness and recognition of this problem, in addition to improved technique, better instrumentation, development of modern materials and timely intervention, have significantly decreased the development of adverse laryngotracheal complex sequelae after routine airway management.

PATHOPHYSIOLOGY

The degree of pathology following injury to the laryngotracheal complex will vary and is largely dependent upon the mechanism of injury (**Figure 16.1**).

External trauma to the laryngotracheal complex in both the adult and paediatric population can lead to rapid asphyxiation due to aspiration of blood, intrapulmonary haemorrhage, cricotracheal separation and/or recurrent laryngeal nerve palsy. In cases of external trauma, concomitant cervical spine injury (8–14 per cent), closed head injury (13–28 per cent), chest trauma (13 per cent), fractured ribs

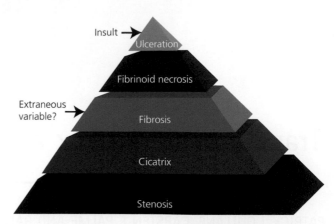

Figure 16.1 The pathophysiology in the development of a stenotic lesion is depicted in this pyramid. (Reproduced with permission from Patrick J Gullane.)

or sternum, pneumothorax, haemothorax, or disruption of the oesophagus (3–14 per cent) may occur and should be included in the evaluation.[2, 9]

The compression force of blunt trauma may result in a fracture of the thyroid and/or cricoid cartilage and/or laceration of associated endolaryngeal soft tissue structures (**Figure 16.2a–e**). The majority of fractures in this region involve the thyroid lamina (median or paramedian location) and are usually longitudinal in nature.[21] These injuries occur in patients of all ages, despite the common belief that ossified cartilages are at an increased risk of fracture from external trauma.[22, 23] With penetrating injuries, compound wounds may develop and lead to significant disruption of the laryngotracheal complex. These injuries may result in varying degrees of oedema, haematoma, inflammation, displacement of laryngeal structures and scar tissue formation. Perichondritis may occur with the long-term possibility of chondronecrosis and major laryngeal dysfunction. Cricotracheal separation caused by a 'clothesline-type injury' is a rare injury that emergency personnel should consider when treating these patients (**Figure 16.3**). These injuries are associated with significant disruption of the laryngotracheal complex and unilateral or bilateral recurrent laryngeal nerve avulsion. Cricoarytenoid joint dislocation or subluxation may occur with all mechanisms of accidental trauma.

In the paediatric population, laryngotracheal injuries have a somewhat different pathophysiology due to the decreased prevalence of violent trauma compared to the adult population. However, seemingly minimal trauma can lead to a devastating injury with the associated consequences of airway obstruction and loss of normal phonatory function. Minor anterior neck trauma can result in airway oedema, haematoma formation and even rupture of the membranous trachea.[24] Due to the loose attachment of submucosal tissue to the underlying perichondrium and a relative paucity of fibrous tissue, the elasticity of the trachea prevents fracture, but minor traumatic forces are often translated to the laryngotracheal complex leading to vocal cord avulsion, arytenoid dislocation or subluxation and/or significant soft tissue injury.[24, 25]

Simple airway manipulation, as seen in endotracheal intubation, may cause laceration of endolaryngeal soft tissue, haematoma formation, dislocation/subluxation of the

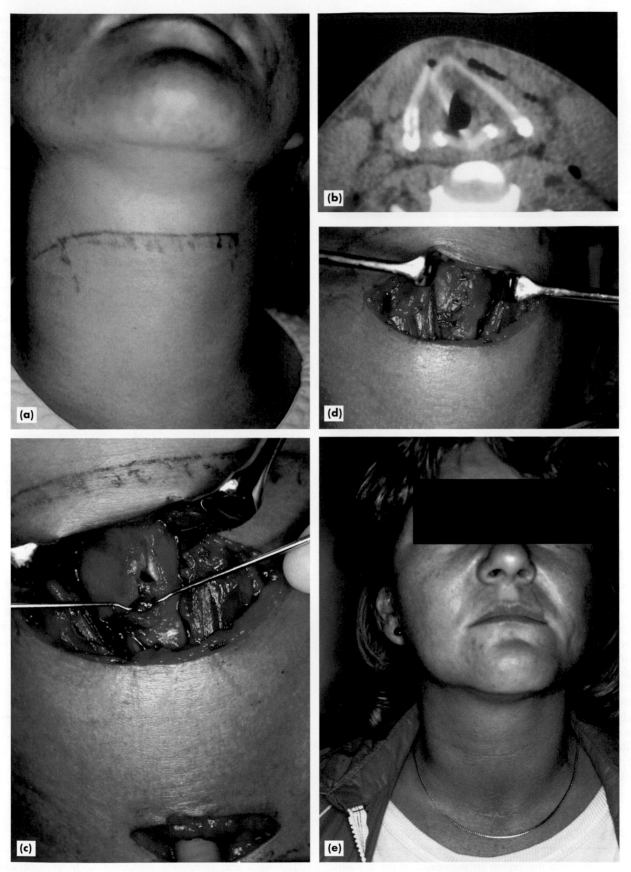

Figure 16.2 This case involved external trauma from a motor vehicle accident. (a) Soft tissue hallmark of blunt trauma. (b) CT scan demonstrates a paramedian thyroid cartilage fracture. (c) Intraoperative exposure demonstrates the laryngeal fracture. (d) Fracture reduction and repair using 28-gauge wire. (e) Patient at one-year follow up with a normal voice and well-healed incision. (Reproduced with permission from Patrick J Gullane).

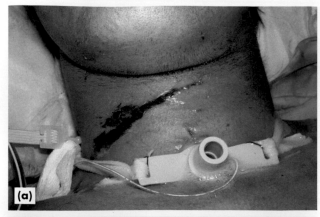

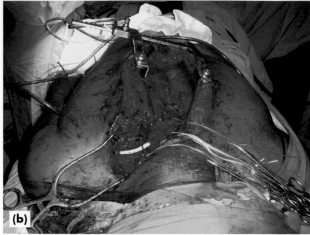

Figure 16.3   'Clothesline' injury with tracheal separation. (Reproduced with permission from Patrick J Gullane.)

cricoarytenoid joint or laryngeal nerve palsy.[26, 27] Similarly, endolaryngeal surgery using either cold steel instruments or carbon dioxide (CO_2) laser, is associated with a variety of injuries which may cause significant laryngotracheal dysfunction (synechia, cricoarytenoid joint ankylosis, subglottic stenosis). Prolonged intubation is associated with significant inflammation, formation of granulation tissue, the development of secondary infection and scar formation and the development of 'laryngeal bed sores' as described by Benjamin[28] particularly in the posterior glottic and subglottic region. The long-term sequelae include glottic and/or subglottic stenosis with airway compromise and/or vocal cord dysfunction. In addition to the duration of intubation, factors such as patient age, concomitant medical illness (diabetes, vascular disease, immunosuppression, gastro-oesophageal reflux disease), endotracheal tube material and the level of care are associated with the development of complications after endotracheal intubation.

CLASSIFICATION OF STENOTIC LESIONS

Stenotic lesions in this region are delineated by the anatomic location (i.e. supraglottic, subglottic and posterior glottic) and associated structures. To assist in the management of posterior glottic stenosis, Bogdasarian and Olsen[29] developed

a four-tier classification system based on the structures involved (**Figure 16.4a–d**): type I includes an isolated interarytenoid band; type II stenosis is more extensive and includes a posterior glottic mucosal tunnel, but no arytenoid cartilage ankylosis; type III has ankylosis of one arytenoid joint; and in type IV both arytenoid joints are fixated.

CLASSIFICATION OF TRAUMATIC LARYNGOTRACHEAL INJURY

A number of classification systems have been developed to assist in the evaluation and management of patients with traumatic laryngotracheal complex injuries.[4, 30, 31] Trone et al.[31] developed one of the first classification systems to describe injury involving the upper airway in order to facilitate the development of an appropriate treatment plan. This classification system (**Table 16.1**) utilizes physical examination, fibreoptic laryngoscopy and computed tomography (CT) scanning. Patients are divided into four groups according to the extent of the injury: group 1, minor endolaryngeal haematoma and no detectable cartilage fracture; group 2, oedema, haematoma, minor mucosal disruption, non-exposed cartilage and/or non-displaced fractures on CT scan; group 3, massive oedema, mucosal tears, exposed cartilage and/or vocal cord immobility; group 4, as with group 3 with the addition of more than two fracture lines or massive mucosal trauma. Fuhrman et al.[4] modified this classification to include complete cricotracheal separation as a fifth group. Trone et al.'s classification system[31] does not stress the independent prognostic importance of injury involving the anterior commissure, cricoarytenoid joint dislocation/subluxation, cricoid fracture and unilateral or bilateral recurrent laryngeal nerve palsy.[1] However, this classification has provided criteria for tracheostomy and/or surgical exploration, demonstrated prognostic merit and its simplicity has permitted wide application to the management of laryngotracheal injuries.[1, 4, 32, 33] Other classification systems that describe disruption of the laryngotracheal complex have been presented by Ogura et al.[30] and Richardson,[34] but do not help to differentiate between a non-operative or operative approach. The classification system therefore should be based on the underlying cause, the type and degree of injury and its sequelae.

ASSESSMENT

Successful management of the patient following cervical trauma requires a multidisciplinary team approach that includes an emergency physician, a trauma surgeon, an anaesthesiologist, radiology and appropriate ancillary staff (**Figure 16.5**).

Signs and symptoms

The signs and symptoms associated with laryngotracheal injury will vary depending on the mechanism and severity of the injury. Symptoms may present acutely or develop slowly over time and rapidly escalate to a medical emergency. This is

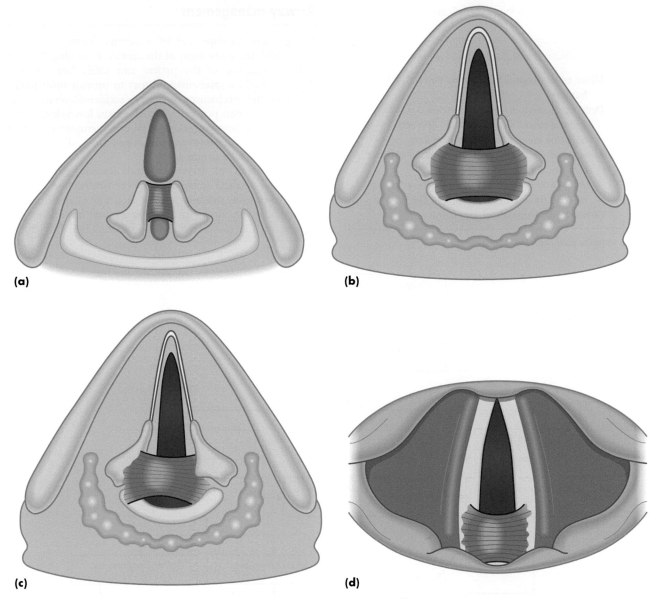

Figure 16.4 This classification system was introduced by Bogdasarian and Olsen.[29] (a) Type I stenosis involves an interarytenoid band alone. (b) Type II stenosis, a posterior glottic mucosal tunnel is formed with no artytenoid cartilage ankylosis. (c) Type III stenosis involves fixation of one arytenoid joint. (d) Type IV stenosis both arytenoid joints are ankylosed and non-mobile. (Reproduced with permission from Patrick J Gullane.)

in sharp contrast to the presentation following intubation, which produces inflammatory changes that occur over a prolonged period of time with a slow onset of airway symptoms.

The clinical manifestations of injury following intubation commonly present weeks after extubation with symptoms and signs of chronic airway dysfunction and/or loss of normal phonation. Patients may present with stridor and dyspnoea. Depending on the degree of stenosis, the dyspnoea may be minimal at rest and significantly worsen with exertion. Patients may also complain of a dry cough and have difficulty handling their secretions.

Following acute trauma to the cervical region and laryngotracheal complex, patients may be asymptomatic for the first 24–48 hours after the injury and therefore these cases

must be managed with a high degree of suspicion and expert level of care.[35, 36] Dysphonia and shortness of breath are the two most common symptoms encountered followed by dysphagia, odynophonia and an inability to lie supine.[4] The clinical signs include those associated with acute airway obstruction (stridor, tachypnoea, sweating, tachycardia and the use of the accessory muscles of respiration), neck ecchymosis, loss of the normal laryngeal prominence, tenderness, subcutaneous emphysema, grossly displaced cartilage fractures, tracheal deviation and/or haemoptysis.[1] Cricotracheal separation should be suspected when the mechanism of injury is a 'clothesline-type' of trauma and with the presence of aphonia, cervical ecchymosis, extensive subcutaneous emphysema and elevation of the hyoid (**Figure 16.6**).[12]

Table 16.1 Laryngotracheal injury classification according to Trone *et al.*[31]

Group	
1	Minor endolaryngeal haematoma without detectable fracture
2	Oedema, haematoma, minor mucosal disruption without exposed cartilage, non-displaced fractures noted on computed tomography scan
3	Massive oedema, mucosal tears, exposed cartilage, cord immobility
4	As group 3, with more than two fracture lines or massive trauma to laryngeal mucosa
5[a]	Complete laryngotracheal separation

[a]Group 5 added by Fuhrman *et al.*[4]

Airway management

The primary management of accidental laryngeal trauma begins with the assessment of the airway. Providing that it is stable, evaluation of the patient can safely begin with a thorough and comprehensive history to provide information regarding the mechanism of injury (accidental versus iatrogenic, blunt versus penetrating, high versus low velocity) and the extent of laryngotracheal complex disruption. Past or present medical illnesses (cardiac, respiratory, diabetes) and medications are also noted.

Management of laryngotracheal trauma requires the ability to recognize impending airway obstruction and the ability to expedite safe and prompt care. The establishment of a safe and stable airway is the primary goal in patients presenting with any degree of airway obstruction. This should

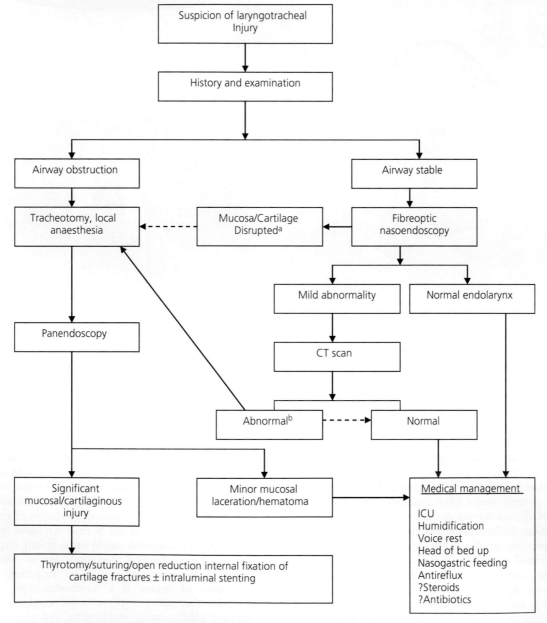

Figure 16.5 Management algorithm for patients following laryngotracheal injury. [a]Minor mucosal disruption and [b]minimally/non-displaced cartilage fracture can be managed conservatively.

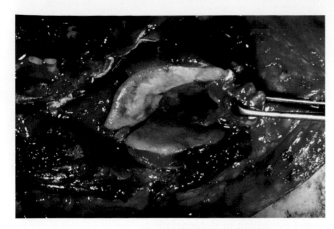

Figure 16.6 Intraoperative view of posterior cricoid plate fracture with associated tracheal disruption. (Reproduced with permission from Patrick J Gullane.)

precede a comprehensive history, fibreoptic examination, imaging or other investigations.

Once the patient is stabilized, the cervical spine and any concomitant neurovascular injury can be assessed and a complete systems review performed. X-rays may be limited to a routine trauma series within the Accident and Emergency Department. Precise and comprehensive assessment of any potential laryngotracheal injury requires knowledge of the anatomy and the ability to complete the examination without causing any additional discomfort or disruption to the airway. Careful palpation for any evidence of subcutaneous emphysema, haematoma or possible cartilage fractures should be performed. Evaluation of the endolarynx using fibreoptic nasoendoscopy is a key component of the examination in order to assess airway patency, mucosal lacerations, haematoma, arytenoid position, cartilage exposure or vocal cord mobility.[37]

Treatment for primary airway control includes simple endotracheal intubation, fibreoptic awake intubation and/or tracheostomy under local anaesthesia. Occasionally, an emergency cricothyroidotomy may be required and/or an open tracheostomy to secure the airway and to exclude any significant injury, such as cricotracheal separation.[1] Gussack *et al.* recommend that endotracheal intubation is performed by the most experienced anaesthesiologist using a small-sized tube under direct visualization for minor laryngotracheal disruption and/or a supraglottic haematoma.[38] This study reported successful intubation in eight of 11 patients with acute laryngeal trauma. Because endotracheal intubation is extremely challenging and difficult in these patients, Schaefer[39] recommends a tracheostomy under local anaesthesia in patients with signs or symptoms of potential airway obstruction. A failure rate as high as 76 per cent of cases of laryngotracheal injury has been reported with intubation.[40] There is also a significant risk of iatrogenic injury to the already compromised airway and/or other neurovascular structures (cervical spine), which may lead to potentially devastating sequelae.[39] In cases of cricotracheal separation, 'blind' placement of an endotracheal tube across the area of separation can convert a stable situation to one that is life threatening. Those that advocate endotracheal intubation for primary airway management, generally do so with significant

expertise within the setting of a tertiary referral centre.[38] We recommend tracheostomy under local anaesthesia as the gold standard for primary airway management in adults with acute laryngeal trauma.[1, 3, 4, 39, 40, 41, 42]

In paediatric patients, primary airway management requires a different approach and includes a gaseous induction with spontaneous ventilation and securing the airway with rigid bronchoscopy followed by tracheostomy. Cricothyroidotomy is rarely used in paediatric patients as it may compound any injury present and may not provide an adequate airway.[12]

The indications for tracheostomy under local anaesthesia include any evidence of airway obstruction, inability to lie supine, significant upper aerodigestive tract oedema or when open surgical exploration is indicated. The tracheostomy is optimally performed in the operating theatre with the availability of airway instrumentation, suction and lighting, an experienced surgical assistant and with the support of anaesthesia and nursing. Placement of the tracheostomy incision should be slightly lower than usual to avoid the area of laryngotracheal injury. A horizontal incision, midway between the cricoid cartilage and the sternal notch is most frequently used and if necessary, lateral extension of the incision will allow adequate exposure of all structures within the neck region to assess and repair any other injury that is present.

Once the airway has been established, further evaluation of the laryngotracheal injury can be performed. A variety of laryngoscopes, microlaryngeal instruments and rigid telescopes facilitate the precise examination of the endolarynx, which should include the mucosal surfaces, the cartilaginous framework, including the integrity and mobility of the cricoarytenoid joint. Video equipment can provide precise and careful documentation for future comparison. A thorough evaluation of the oesophagus and tracheobronchial tree is also necessary for complete assessment.

IMAGING

With the advancement in imaging technology and instrumentation, CT scans and magnetic resonance imaging (MRI) are now the gold standard for examination of the laryngotracheal region.

In patients with stenotic upper airway obstruction, CT scans and MRI provide details regarding the location and dimensions of the stenotic segment. Endoscopy with a flexible bronchoscope will assist in visualizing the lesion, to identify the precise size, extent and location of the stenotic area relative to the true vocal cords. Rigid bronchoscopy may be used to assess the stiffness of the lesion and will help to determine the usefulness of non-operative interventions, such as laser vaporization or dilatation.

In the assessment of laryngotracheal complex trauma, CT scanning and MRI has replaced traditional imaging methods including laryngeal tomography and laryngograms.[1] CT scans and MRI provide comprehensive assessment of the cartilaginous laryngeal framework and associated soft tissue structures and can assist in identifying cartilage fractures (single, multiple, angulated, displaced, undisplaced), haematoma, cricoarytenoid joint dislocation/subluxation and stenosis. It can provide excellent assessment of the nature and extent of laryngotracheal disruption to assist in treatment planning and operative intervention if necessary.

Some surgeons have recommended CT scanning for all patients with trauma involving the laryngotracheal complex to adequately assess and to assist in the surgical planning for reconstruction.[5] However, Schaefer contends that a more selective approach is warranted and that CT scanning does not provide additional information when clear indications for surgical exploration exist and may potentially delay treatment.[4, 43] A CT scan should never be performed in a patient with an unsecured airway and since a CT scan requires the patient to lie supine for an extended period of time, the patient's airway status should be monitored. It is therefore essential that experienced staff and resources are available to respond to any deterioration of the airway during imaging. In patients with cervical neck trauma, we prefer to obtain a CT scan with contrast, but this should not be performed at the expense of safe airway management.

Because of the high prevalence of associated occult vascular or oesophageal injury, angiography and swallowing studies (with or without contrast) may also be indicated in patients presenting with penetrating cervical trauma.[6, 8, 44]

MANAGEMENT

Non-operative and operative interventions are available for the treatment of patients with pathology involving the laryngotracheal complex and a comprehensive patient evaluation will provide the necessary information regarding the best management. The challenge is to select the most efficacious treatment, which will maximize functional outcome and minimize additional morbidity from unnecessary surgery or delayed treatment.

Non-operative approach

The mechanism of injury, the severity of symptoms and other patient factors, such as comorbidities, will determine the available options for non-operative treatment ranging from medical management to dilatation and/or stents.

In patients with subglottic stenosis, non-operative treatment including corticosteroid injections, airway dilatation, laser vaporization and stents usually precedes consideration of surgical intervention. Dilatation may provide temporary relief of symptoms, but it is rarely a definitive therapy. In some cases, aggressive dilatation may cause trauma to the region thus worsening the stenosis and increasing airway dysfunction. Mitomycin-C has been used following dilatation to prevent recurrence of the stenosis;[45] however, others[46] have reported no improvement. When non-operative treatment has failed to improve airway function or with continued decline in patient symptoms, surgical intervention is usually recommended.

In patients with acute traumatic injuries, the goal of treatment is to stabilize the fracture and to promote normal soft tissue healing. Schaefer and Close[3] reported good functional outcome following a non-operative approach in patients with minor mucosal lacerations (excluding the anterior commissure region or free edge of the vocal fold) and undisplaced, single fractures of the laryngeal cartilaginous framework.

Bent et al.[1] reported normal airway and phonatory function in patients with non-displaced thyroid cartilage fractures and minimal intralaryngeal injury who were treated without surgery. This approach included at least 24 hours of close observation in an intensive care or high dependency unit, constant humidification, voice rest and elevation of the head of the bed. A subset of patients may require establishment of a safe airway (intubation or tracheostomy) and a panendoscopy to rule out concomitant injury to structures within the upper aerodigestive tract. If this examination is negative and no other indication for surgical exploration is found, these patients can be effectively managed non-operatively. Close observation and frequent reassessment by those experienced in managing these patients are required to ensure satisfactory healing and successful extubation or decannulation.

Specific treatment with medication for these injuries is limited, but there is some evidence for antireflux therapy to prevent irritation of mucosal injuries and subsequent development of laryngeal stenosis, especially in patients with gastro-oesophageal reflux disease.[47] Occasionally, nasogastric tube feeding is required, however this may potentiate gastro-oesophageal reflux and may cause added insult to the injured larynx. The use of corticosteroids remains controversial and there are no definitive studies regarding its efficacy in the treatment of patients with trauma to the upper airway. Potentially, corticosteroids may reduce soft tissue oedema, but must be administered within hours of the injury. Similarly, the role of antibiotics in preventing sequelae of uncontrolled infection leading to perichondritis, impaired wound healing, cartilage destruction and loss of airway function, is controversial. The use of broad-spectrum antibiotics (penicillin, cephalosporin) is recommended for comminuted injuries and those requiring surgical exploration and repair.[4, 23]

Operative approach

The goal of surgical intervention involving the laryngotracheal complex is to restore primary function, including ventilation, airway protection and phonation. Significant debate and controversy exists in the literature regarding the indications for surgery, its timing, method of repair and the use of intraluminal stenting.

CRICOTRACHEAL STENOSIS

Because of the unique function and complex anatomy in this region, many surgical techniques have been described for treatment of subglottic stenosis.[48] We have found that circumferential tracheal or combined cricotracheal resection with primary anastomosis provides optimal outcome in the appropriately selected patients, based upon preoperative evaluation of the stenotic region and patient comorbidities.[49, 50, 51] Several principles should be followed to ensure a successful result and to minimize the risk of postoperative complications with simple resection and primary anastomosis. The segment of excised trachea should not exceed 5 cm to ensure that there is no tension on the anastomosis. The proximal margin of the resected segment must be at least 5 mm distal to the true vocal cords because more proximal lesions will require a complex reconstruction to restore function. Similarly, patients who present with cricoarytenoid ankylosis and fixed vocal cords should be selected carefully and may require an associated laryngofissure with laryngeal repair. This surgery should be approached with caution in patients with diabetes, severe vascular dysfunction, poor pulmonary function, prior radiation treatment to the trachea or larynx and in patients who are being treated with immunosuppressive drugs, including corticosteroids. The risks associated with poor wound healing may be minimized with preoperative treatment of comorbidities, complete excision of the stenotic tissue, an adequate thyrotracheal repair and support of the airway postoperatively.

To optimize patient outcome following cricotracheal resection with thyrotracheal anastomosis, a few key surgical details are outlined. A low collar incision is used and the airway is exposed from the hyoid bone to the manubrium. The region of stenosis is identified, the margins delineated and an en bloc resection of the stenotic region is performed. To avoid injury to the recurrent laryngeal nerves, the dissection is limited to the inner aspect of the cricoid cartilage and to minimize the risk of tracheal ischaemia, minimum lateral dissection is used. If the stenosis extends close to the vocal cords, a laryngofissure may be necessary to improve the exposure for the resection and anastomosis (**Figure 16.7a,b**). If a laryngofissure is performed, the posterior aspect of the cricoid plate is thinned and at least 50 per cent of the plate is maintained to retain the vertical height. The trachea is mobilized to the level of the carina and lateral stay sutures are used to elevate the proximal margin of the trachea. The anastomosis between the trachea and the subglottis is completed using a running No. 4-0 PDS suture posteriorly and No. 4-0 vicryl laterally and anteriorly. To prevent irritation of the oesophagus, the posterior knots are placed inside the airway and to minimize granulation tissue within the airway, the vicryl sutures are tied exterior to the airway. A T-tube is used to support the airway and is positioned approximately 6–7 mm cephalad to the vocal cords. At the proximal end of the T-tube, a bronchial blocker (**Figure 16.8a,b**) is placed transorally to permit ventilation through the horizontal arm of the T-tube and is required to complete the anastomosis. A T-tube is used to protect the anastomosis and to stent the airway. A distal tracheostomy is rarely necessary.

TRAUMA

In cases of major disruption of the cartilaginous and/or soft tissue framework of the larynx, suture repair, rigid internal fixation and/or intraluminal stenting may be required. Stanley et al.[52] reported that spontaneous healing with normal phonatory function will not occur with non-operative treatment alone and the result will be a permanent dysfunction of the larynx. However, the optimal approach to minimally or non-displaced fractures is controversial and there are no definitive studies detailing the absolute indications for internal fixation versus non-operative management.[5] Other factors that must be considered in the selection of the most beneficial approach include the presence of concomitant major injuries (i.e. neurovascular, chest, abdomen), associated medical morbidity, time from injury and individual patient factors.[5]

The ideal timing for surgical intervention is associated with significant controversy and debate in the literature.

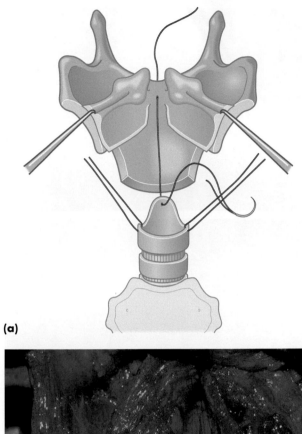

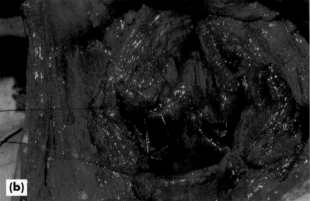

Figure 16.7 (a,b) High cricotracheal resection with laryngofissure and repair using a membranous tracheal mucosal flap. (Reproduced with permission from Patrick J Gullane.)

Some recommend that a period of observation is required prior to surgery to allow any significant oedema in the upper aerodigestive tract to subside. However, others recommend exploration within 24 to 48 hours, to avoid the establishment of active infection and early scar formation.[3, 53] The potential long-term result of significant delay are airway and voice dysfunction.[38, 54] A recent multi-institutional review of 392 patients with external laryngeal trauma reported that 80 per cent of surgical interventions were performed within 48 hours of the injury, supporting early surgical exploration as the preferred standard of care.[2]

Surgical loupes and a headlight will allow precise delineation of the injury and surrounding anatomic detail. The patient is positioned supine with a shoulder roll to slightly extend the cervical spine, and a horizontal cervical collar incision in line with any tracheostomy is employed. Superior and inferior subplatysmal flaps extending from the sternal notch to the level of the hyoid are then made. The strap muscles are divided in the midline and then division of the thyroid isthmus is performed. This approach facilitates

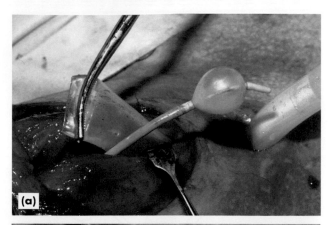

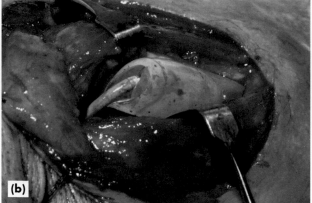

Figure 16.8 (a,b) Intraoperative view of bronchial blocker placed within the proximal end of the T-tube to permit ventilation during the repair. (Reproduced with permission from Patrick J Gullane.)

excellent exposure of the laryngotracheal complex and if more distal exposure is required, a partial sternotomy or a right thoracotomy can be employed. In general, an anterior approach to the laryngotracheal complex should be used to avoid excessive lateral dissection or circumferential mobilization due to the risk of devascularization. In addition, exploration and dissection of the recurrent laryngeal nerves should be minimized to avoid the possibility of additional injury to these structures.[55] The endolarynx can be exposed via a laryngofissure incision or using any fracture line that is located within 2–3 mm of the midline.[23] If a midline thyrotomy is required, an oscillating saw using the thinnest available blade should be utilized. Care is taken to stay in the midline and we prefer to divide the anterior commissure region using Potts scissors under direct vision. Similarly, access to posterior tracheal lacerations can be gained via an anterior midline tracheal incision.[55] Once the endolarynx is exposed, repair of a significant mucosal tear, a subluxed or dislocated arytenoid or fractured cartilaginous structures can be performed. Because of the delicate surrounding tissue, any excessive and unnecessary handling should be avoided to prevent additional injury. Mucosal tears can be primarily repaired with fine monofilament sutures (5/0 monocryl). For large defects, local rotation flaps or free tissue transfer using either buccal mucosa or skin may be employed.[56] These reconstructions must be secured with sutures and supported by intraluminal stenting.

Successful functional outcome after trauma requires that the cartilaginous fractures are anatomically reduced and stabilized. Adequate exposure to the fracture line is essential to achieve a good outcome and, in general, we prefer to elevate the outer perichondrial layer 1–2 cm lateral to any median or paramedian thyroid cartilage fracture. However, if the fracture is located more laterally along the lamina, the outer perichondrial layer is incised in the midline and then elevated in continuity with the overlying strap muscles.[33] A similar approach can be used for the management of fractures involving the cricoid cartilage. Historically, a number of techniques including simple suturing of perichondrium or wiring of cartilage segments (24- or 26-gauge wire) have been described with varying success.[5] Mini-reconstruction adaptation plates are now frequently utilized for the management of laryngotracheal complex injuries and permit immediate fixation and stabilization of these cartilage fractures.[57] The main disadvantages with using this technique are the increased cost, ease of stripping the screw, additional skill required by the surgeon and potential for infection.[57] However, the advantages in allowing primary tissue healing and being able to recreate normal laryngeal framework dimensions, make this technique an excellent alternative to traditionally described methods in the management of laryngotracheal complex fractures.[32]

Reconstruction of the anterior commissure region either after fracture or laryngofissure requires precise suturing of the anterior aspect of each vocal fold to the corresponding outer perichondrial layer.[39] Cartilage loss can be easily managed using local tissue including strap muscle flaps sutured into the defect. More extensive loss can be repaired using free cartilage grafts from a variety of sites, including the septum or more commonly the rib. All repairs should have a temporary tracheostomy sufficient for ventilation, placed two to three rings distal to the area of repair to avoid contamination and potential delay in wound healing.

Indications for the use of airway stenting include disruption of the anterior commissure, massive mucosal trauma and/or significant destruction or loss of the cartilaginous laryngotracheal complex. The ideal stent should consist of a material which is inert, of sufficient strength and length to stabilize the cartilaginous structures from the supraglottic to the subglottic region, has a shape that mirrors the internal structure of the larynx and does not cause any added injury due to excess movement and pressure. Contemporary advances in the development of alloplastic materials have seen the emergence of a variety of softer and more inert intraluminal stents. In patients with significant traumatic laryngeal disruption, we prefer to use a Montgomery laryngeal stent secured with prolene sutures. In general, the adolescent size is sufficient for the adult larynx and can be removed endoscopically approximately 2–4 weeks following surgery (**Figure 16.9**). Other alternative stents include the Aboulker stent, a T-tube or silastic sheeting individually fashioned to promote mucosalization and prevent the formation of endolaryngeal synechia. The anterior commissure, the interarytenoid area and the subglottis are at significant risk of excessive scarring. Regardless of the material that is used, stenting the upper airway represents a risk–benefit analysis with the need for stabilizing the airway being balanced with the possible negative effects of added endolaryngeal injury and/or infection.[23]

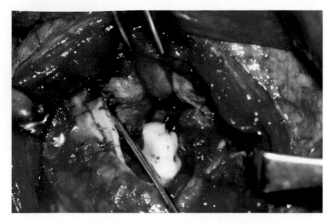

Figure 16.9 Intraoperative view of thyroid and cricoid cartilage fracture with repair and Montgomery laryngeal stent. (Reproduced with permission from Patrick J Gullane.)

CRICOARYTENOID JOINT DYSFUNCTION

Injury to the cricoarytenoid joint is a rare phenomenon and it is most commonly caused by routine endotracheal intubation, but can be due to blunt or penetrating cervical trauma. The true incidence of this condition is unknown, however, it is estimated to occur in less than 1 in 1000 cases of routine intubation.[17] The gender distribution is approximately equal and it can occur at any age.[58] There is some controversy about the mechanism of injury that leads to either anterior or posterior displacement. Historically, anterior dislocation was thought to be due to inappropriate placement of the laryngoscope blade or the arytenoid cartilage being caught up within the lumen of the endotracheal tube.[59] Quick and Mervin[60] postulated that posterior dislocation was caused most commonly on the left-hand side by a right-handed physician potentially directing the endotracheal tube against the arytenoids. However, Dudley et al.[61] reported that posterior dislocation was more likely to occur due to premature extubation with an incompletely deflated cuff. Paulsen et al.[27] demonstrated in a human laryngeal model that it was not possible to dislocate or sublux the arytenoid cartilage in this method and more likely it was the development of hemarthroses (secondary to a variety of external and internal traumatic mechanisms) involving the joint space which leads to ankylosis and subsequent dysfunction of the cricoarytenoid joint. Underlying systemic conditions, including chronic renal disease, acromegaly and chronic steroid use, may lead to degeneration of the ligaments or joint spaces and can place these patients at an increased risk to traumatic cricoarytenoid joint dysfunction.[60] The majority of these patients present with a clear history of endolaryngeal manipulation (intubation, microlaryngeal surgery) or external trauma. The most common symptoms include dysphonia (hoarseness, breathiness) or airway obstruction and on physical examination and/or strobovideolaryngoscopy, there is poor mobility of the vocal cords and/or a displaced arytenoid (anterior, posterior, lateral or combination). Evaluation with CT imaging is helpful to assess the relationship of the arytenoids and the underlying cricoid cartilage. However, the diagnosis is confirmed with electromyography (EMG) of the laryngeal muscles which demonstrates normal neural function of the recurrent laryngeal nerve despite poor vocal cord mobility.[58, 59, 62] The differential diagnosis should include ankylosis of the cricoarytenoid joint and posterior synechia caused by prolonged intubation, inflammatory disease, local infection or longstanding unrecognized recurrent laryngeal nerve palsy.

Standard treatment combines reduction of the cricoarytenoid joint and ideally it should be performed within one month after symptom onset.[63, 64] The role of speech pathology remains to be established with some advocating its routine use, while others feel it has no place in the acute management of patients with traumatic cricoarytenoid joint dysfunction.[58] Failed reduction is approached in a manner similar to vocal cord paralysis to return the vocal fold to a more functional position. Techniques include vocal fold injection (silicone, fat), medialization thyroplasty and/or arytenoid adduction procedures.[65, 66] Arytenoidectomy has been advocated if symptoms of significant airway obstruction predominate, however, this should be preceded by a sufficient trial of non-operative interventions.[67] The outcome after therapy for traumatic cricoarytenoid joint dysfunction is generally excellent in terms of airway patency, however, return to normal phonation is relatively uncommon.[68, 69]

CONCLUSION

Advancements in the assessment and management of patients with trauma to the laryngotracheal region have lead to enhanced patient outcome and health-related quality of life. Improvements in imaging and fibreoptic endoscopy have facilitated the evaluation of patients with acute trauma and more chronic stenotic lesions. Successful outcome following traumatic laryngotracheal injuries depends upon patient, injury and treatment-specific factors. However, in our experience, early repair of mucosal and cartilaginous injury has led to improved functional outcome with a normal airway, no dysphagia and acceptable voice in the majority of patients, and the extent and severity of injury remain strong predictors of patient outcome. Good function following surgical management of stenotic lesions requires appropriate patient selection, complete resection of the pathologic tissue, an acceptable thyrotracheal anastomosis and support of the airway postoperatively. Patient comobidities may increase the risk of complications in the perioperative period and should be assessed and if possible treated preoperatively to minimize this risk. Patient and family counselling is essential to provide patients with realistic expectations after complex surgery, which may require prolonged periods of rehabilitation and recovery.

KEY EVIDENCE

- Traumatic laryngeal and tracheal injuries are complex, potentially devasting and uncommon.
- Following these types of traumatic injuries, chronic upper aerodigestive tract dysfunction is common and requires prolonged rehabilitation.

> - The best outcome is achieved with a multidisciplinary team approach in centres with significant expertise in managing complex head and neck disease.

KEY LEARNING POINTS

- Understand the functional anatomy of the larynx and trachea.
- Be aware of the pathophysiology of laryngeal and subglottic stenosis.
- Be familiar with the classification systems of laryngotracheal complex injuries.
- Comprehensive assessment and prompt management are essential to minimize the likelihood of perioperative complications and long-term morbidity.
- Understand the presentation and management both closed and open of acute and chronic laryngeal and tracheal trauma and stenosis.

ACKNOWLEDGEMENTS

Thank you to Christine B Novak, PhD (Research Associate Wharton Head and Neck Centre, and Scientist, Toronto Rehabilitation Institute, University Health Network, Toronto, Canada) for her assistance and contributions to this manuscript.

REFERENCES

1. Bent JP 3rd, Silver JR, Porubsky ES. Acute laryngeal trauma: a review of 77 patients. *Otolaryngology – Head and Neck Surgery* 1993; **109**: 441–9.
2. Jewett BS, Shockley WW, Rutledge R. External laryngeal trauma analysis of 392 patients. *Archives of Otolaryngology – Head and Neck Surgery* 1999; **125**: 877–80.
* 3. Schaefer SD, Close LC. Acute management of laryngeal trauma. *Annals of Otology, Rhinology, and Laryngology* 1989; **98**: 98–104.
4. Fuhrman GM, Stieg FH, Buerk CA. Blunt trauma: classification and management protocol. *Journal of Trauma* 1990; **30**: 87–92.
5. Bent JP 3rd, Porubsky ES. The management of blunt fractures of the thyroid cartilage. *Otolaryngology – Head and Neck Surgery* 1994; **110**: 195–202.
6. Irish JC, Hekkenberg R, Gullane PJ et al. Penetrating and blunt neck trauma. *Canadian Journal of Surgery* 1997; **40**: 33–8.
7. Kleinsasser NH, Priemer FG, Schulze W, Kleinsasser O. External trauma to the larynx: classification, diagnosis,

therapy. *European Archives of Otorhinolaryngology* 2000; **257**: 439–44.
8. Grewal H, Rao PM, Mukerji S, Ivatury RR. Management of penetrating laryngotracheal injuries. *Head and Neck* 1995; **17**: 494–502.
9. Minard G, Kudsk KA, Croce MA et al. Laryngotracheal injuries. *American Journal of Surgery* 1992; **58**: 181–7.
10. Vassiliu P, Baker J, Henderson S et al. Aerodigestive tract injuries of the neck. *American Journal of Surgery* 2001; **67**: 75–9.
11. Bhojani RA, Rosenbaum DH, Dikman E et al. Contemporary assessment of laryngotracheal trauma. *Journal of Thoracic and Cardiovascular Surgery* 2005; **130**: 426–32.
12. Chagnon FP, Mulder DS. Laryngotracheal trauma. *Chest Surgery Clinics of North America* 1996; **6**: 733–48.
13. Yen PT, Lee HY, Tsai MH et al. Clinical analysis of external laryngeal trauma. *Journal of Laryngology and Otology* 1994; **108**: 221–5.
14. Mathisen DJ, Grillo HC. Laryngotracheal trauma. *Annals of Thoracic Surgery* 1987; **43**: 254–62.
15. Blanc VG, Tramblay NAG. The complications of endotracheal intubation with a review of the literature. *Anesthesia and Analgesia* 1974; **53**: 202–13.
16. Hotchkiss KS, McCaffrey JC. Laryngotracheal injury after percutaneous dilational tracheostomy in cadaver specimens. *Laryngoscope* 2003; **113**: 16–20.
17. Kambic V, Radsel Z. Intubation lesions of the larynx. *British Journal of Anaesthesia* 1978; **50**: 587–90.
18. Maktabi MA, Hoffman H, Funk G. Laryngeal trauma during awake fiberoptic intubation. *Anesthesia and Analgesia* 2002; **95**: 1112–14.
19. Santos PM, Afrassiabi A, Weymuller EA Jr. Risk factors associated with prolonged intubation and laryngeal injury. *Otolaryngology – Head and Neck Surgery* 1994; **111**: 453–9.
20. Weymuller EA Jr. Prevention and management of intubation injury of the larynx and trachea. *American Journal of Otolaryngology* 1992; **13**: 139–44.
21. Lee SY. Experimental blunt injury to the larynx. *Annals of Otology, Rhinology, and Laryngology* 1992; **101**: 270–4.
22. Austin JR, Stanley RB, Cooper DS. Stable internal fixation of fractures of the partially mineralized thyroid cartilage. *Annals of Otology, Rhinology, and Laryngology* 1992; **101**: 76–80.
23. Schaefer SD. The treatment of acute external laryngeal injuries. *Archives of Otolaryngology, Head and Neck Surgery* 1991; **117**: 35–9.
24. Corsten G, Berkowitz RG. Membranous tracheal rupture in children following minor blunt cervical trauma. *Annals of Otology, Rhinology, and Laryngology* 2002; **111**: 197–9.
25. Gold SM, Gerber ME, Shott SR, Myer CM. Blunt laryngeal trauma in children. *Archives of Otolaryngology, Head and Neck Surgery* 1997; **123**: 83–7.
26. Cavo JW. True vocal cord paralysis following intubation. *Laryngoscope* 1985; **95**: 1352–9.

* 27. Paulsen FP, Rudert HH, Tillman BN. New insights into the pathomechanism of postintubation arytenoids subluxation. *Anesthesiology* 1999; **91**: 659–65.

* 28. Benjamin B. Prolonged intubation injuries of the larynx: endoscopic diagnosis, classification and treatment. *Annals of Otology, Rhinology, and Laryngology* 1993; **160** (Suppl.): 1–15.

29. Bogdasarian RS, Olsen NR. Posterior glottic laryngeal stenosis. *Otolaryngology – Head and Neck Surgery* 1980; **88**: 765–72.

30. Ogura JH, Hennemann H, Spector GJ. Laryngotracheal trauma: diagnosis and treatment. *Canadian Journal of Otolaryngology* 1973; **2**: 112–18.

* 31. Trone TH, Schaefer SD, Corder HM. Blunt and penetrating laryngeal trauma: a 13 year review. *Otolaryngology – Head and Neck Surgery* 1980; **88**: 257–61.

32. de Mello-Filho FV, Carrau RL. The management of laryngeal fractures using internal fixation. *Laryngoscope* 2000; **110**: 2143–6.

33. Pou AM, Shoemaker DL, Carrau RL *et al.* Repair of laryngeal fractures using adaptation plates. *Head and Neck* 1998; **20**: 707–13.

34. Richardson MA. Laryngeal anatomy and mechanism of trauma. *Ear, Nose and Throat Journal* 1981; **60**: 346–51.

35. Back MR, Baumgartner FJ, Klein SR. Detection and evaluation of aerodigestive tract injuries caused by cervical and transmediastinal gunshot wounds. *Journal of Trauma* 1997; **42**: 680–6.

36. Myers EM, Iko BO. The management of acute laryngeal trauma. *Journal of Trauma* 1987; **27**: 448–52.

37. Gullane PJ, Witterick I, Novak CB, O'Dell MJ. Endoscopic evaluation of the larynx. In: Patterson GA, Cooper JD, Rice TW (eds). *Pearson's thoracic and esophageal surgery.* Philadelphia, PA: Elsevier, 2008: 81–8.

38. Gussack GS, Jurkovich GJ, Luterman A. Laryngotracheal trauma: a protocol approach to a rare injury. *Laryngoscope* 1986; **96**: 660–5.

39. Schaefer SD. The acute management of external laryngeal trauma: a 27 year experience. *Archives of Otolaryngology, Head and Neck Surgery* 1992; **118**: 598–604.

40. Reece CP, Shatney CH. Blunt injuries of the cervical trachea: a review of 51 patients. *Southern Medical Journal* 1988; **81**: 1542–7.

41. Camnitz PS, Sheperd SM, Henderson RA. Acute blunt laryngeal and tracheal trauma. *American Journal of Emergency Medicine* 1987; **5**: 157–62.

42. Snow JB. Diagnosis and therapy of acute laryngeal and tracheal trauma. *Otolaryngologic Clinics of North America* 1984; **17**: 101–6.

43. Schaefer SD, Brown OE. Selective application of CT in the management of laryngeal trauma. *Laryngoscope* 1983; **93**: 1473–5.

44. Roon AJ, Christensen N. Evaluation and treatment of penetrating cervical injuries. *Journal of Trauma* 1979; **19**: 391–7.

45. Rahbar R, Valdez TA, Shapshay SM. Preliminary results of intraoperative mitomycin-C in the treatment and prevention of glottic and subglottic stenosis. *Journal of Voice* 2000; **14**: 282–6.

46. Koshkareva Y, Gaughan JP, Soliman AMS. Risk factors for adult laryngotracheal stenosis: a review of 74 cases. *Annals of Otology, Rhinology, and Laryngology* 2007; **116**: 206–10.

47. Koufman JA. The otolaryngologic manifestations of gastroesophageal reflux disease (GERD). *Laryngoscope* 1991; **101** (Suppl.): 1–78.

48. Thurnher D, Moukarbel RV, Novak CB, Gullane PJ. The glottis and subglottis: an otolaryngologist's perspective. *Thoracic Surgery Clinics* 2007; **17**: 549–60.

* 49. Pearson FG, Cooper JD, Nelems JM, Van Nostrand AW. Primary tracheal anastomosis after resection of the cricoid cartilage with preservation of recurrent laryngeal nerves. *Journal of Thoracic and Cardiovascular Surgery* 1975; **70**: 806–16.

* 50. Pearson FG, Gullane PJ. Subglottic resection with primary tracheal anastomosis: including synchronous laryngotracheal reconstructions. *Seminars in Thoracic and Cardiovascular Surgery* 1996; **8**: 381–91.

51. Maddaus MA, Toth JL, Gullane PJ, Pearson FG. Subglottic tracheal resection and synchronous laryngeal reconstruction. *Journal of Thoracic and Cardiovascular Surgery* 1992; **104**: 1443–50.

52. Stanley RB Jr, Cooper DS, Florman SH. Phonatory effects of thyroid cartilage fractures. *Annals of Otology, Rhinology, and Laryngology* 1987; **96**: 493–6.

53. Leopold DA. Laryngeal trauma. A historical comparison of treatment methods. *Archives of Otolaryngology. Head and Neck Surgery* 1983; **109**: 106–12.

54. Downey WL, Owen RC, Ward PH. Traumatic laryngeal injury – its management and sequelae. *Southern Medical Journal* 1977; **60**: 756–60.

55. Mussi A, Ambrogi MC, Menconi G. *et al.* Surgical approaches to membranous tracheal wall lacerations. *Journal of Thoracic and Cardiovascular Surgery* 2000; **120**: 115–18.

56. Schaefer SD. Laryngeal and esophageal trauma. In: Cummings CW, Fredrickson JM, Harker LA (eds). *Otolaryngology – head and neck surgery.* St Louis: Mosby, 2005: 2001–2.

57. Woo P. Laryngeal framework reconstruction with minimplates. *Annals of Otology, Rhinology, and Laryngology* 1990; **99**: 772–7.

58. Sataloff RT, Bough D, Spiegel JR. Arytenoid dislocation: diagnosis and treatment. *Laryngoscope* 1994; **104**: 1353–61.

59. Close LC, Merkel M, Watson B, Schaefer SD. Cricoarytenoid subluxation, computed tomography and electromyography findings. *Head and Neck Surgery* 1987; **9**: 341–8.

60. Quick CA. Mervin GE. Arytenoid dislocation. *Archives of Otolaryngology* 1978; **104**: 267–70.

61. Dudley JP, Manusco AA, Fonkalsrud EW. Arytenoid dislocation and computed tomography. *Archives of Otolaryngology* 1984; **110**: 483–4.

62. Miller RH, Rosenfeld DB. The role of electromyography in clinical laryngology. *Otolaryngology – Head and Neck Surgery* 1984; **92**: 287–91.

63. Hoffman HT, Brunberg JA, Winter P *et al.* Arytenoid subluxation: diagnosis and treatment. *Annals of Otology, Rhinology, and Laryngology* 1991; **100**: 1–9.

64. Rudert H. Uncommon injuries of the larynx following intubation. Recurrent paralysis, torsion and luxation of the cricoarytenoid joints. *HNO* 1984; **32**: 393–8.

65. Ishiki N, Okamura H, Ishikawa T. Thyroplasty type I (lateral compression) for dysphonia due to vocal cord paralysis and atrophy. *Acta Otolaryngologica* 1975; **80**: 465–73.

66. Prasertwanitch Y, Schwartz JJ, Vandam LD. Arytenoid cartilage dislocation following prolonged endotracheal intubation. *Anesthesiology* 1974; **41**: 516–17.

67. Tolley NS. Chessman TD, Morgan D, Brookes DB. Dislocated arytenoid: an intubation induced injury. *Annals of the Royal College of Surgeons of England* 1990; **72**: 353–6.

68. Maragos NE. Arytenoid fixation surgery for the treatment of arytenoid fractures and dislocations. *Laryngoscope* 1999; **109**: 834–7.

69. Rubin AD, Hawkshaw MJ, Moyer CA *et al.* Arytenoid cartilage dislocation: a 20-year experience. *Journal of Voice* 2005; **19**: 687–701.

17

Penetrating neck injuries

ANDREW J NICOL AND JOHANNES J FAGAN

There are 4 degrees of intra-operative hemorrhage:

1. Why did I get involved in this operation?
2. Why did I become a surgeon?
3. Why did I study to become a doctor?
4. Why was I born?

Alexander Artemiev, *Aphorisms and Quotations for the Surgeon*

INTRODUCTION

The patient presenting to the Accident and Emergency Department with massive bleeding from a penetrating neck injury requires haemostatic surgery. The question, however, is how to manage the stable patient with penetrating neck trauma. The past two decades have seen a major shift in management of such patients from mandatory surgical exploration towards a more selective, conservative approach, based on clinical findings and special investigations. The advent of diagnostic tools, such as oesophagography, flexible endoscopy, angiography, colour flow Doppler imaging and multislice helical computed tomography (CT) has resulted in an increasing confidence in our ability to better evaluate injuries to the neck. The fact that certain of these injuries

can safely be managed conservatively or more effectively by endovascular intervention has further swung the pendulum towards a selective, conservative approach. Groote Schuur Hospital Trauma Centre currently treats 220 patients with penetrating neck trauma per annum.[1] In such a busy centre, it is essential that patients be assessed expeditiously, but safely.

RESUSCITATION

Resuscitation is performed according to the guidelines of the Advanced Trauma Life Support (ATLS) course.[2] The main priority on admission of a patient to the Accident and Emergency Department is to exclude conditions that can cause death within the ensuing few minutes.

AIRWAY CONTROL AND CERVICAL SPINE PROTECTION

A definitive airway is required in patients presenting with massively bleeding wounds, rapidly expanding haematomas, stridor, acute respiratory distress, airway obstruction from blood and secretions, and unconscious patients who are unable to protect the airway. This might require placement of a cuffed endotracheal tube in the adult patient. With a large, open wound communicating directly with the trachea, the endotracheal tube may be inserted directly through the wound. Airway control in the majority of patients with penetrating neck injuries can be safely achieved with rapid sequence induction and direct laryngoscopy.[3] A tracheostomy performed in the Accident and Emergency Department is not advisable due to the bleeding that can be encountered, making visualization difficult. Fibreoptic laryngoscopy is not usually appropriate in the emergency setting, but can be considered in more stable patients where there is not an immediate threat to the airway. Blind, awake intubations are also inappropriate in penetrating neck wounds, as patients are often intoxicated and combative, and deaths have been attributed to this method of intubation.[3, 4]

The position of the cricothyroid membrane should be established prior to attempted intubation, as an emergency cricothyroidotomy might be required should intubation be unsuccessful. Cricothyroidotomy may be technically difficult due to a haematoma displacing the airway. The skin should be incised over the cricothyroid membrane and the anatomical structures again palpated to identify the membrane. A blade is inserted through the membrane and then twisted through 90° to open the incision. An arterial forceps is placed into the airway prior to removal of the blade and the tract enlarged. A size 6 endotracheal tube can then be inserted and the cuff inflated. The endotracheal tube is secured with tape and is cut shorter to ensure that the tube does not kink when attached to the ventilator. Correct placement is confirmed by auscultating the chest.

An unstable cervical spine without an obvious neurological injury is extremely rare in the penetrating neck setting. Gunshot wounds to the neck have a high rate of concomitant cervical spine fracture, but unstable cervical spines tend to be associated with a spinal cord injury. A hard cervical collar should not be maintained at the expense of delaying life-saving airway manoeuvres or attempts at obtaining haemostasis in the neck. Once such procedures have been completed, then the cervical collar should be fitted and spinal precautions resumed.[5]

ASSESSMENT OF BREATHING

A tension pneumothorax or haemothorax should be excluded by palpating whether the trachea is central and by auscultating the chest. Acute respiratory distress accompanied by decreased breath sounds and low oxygen saturation recordings is an indication for insertion of a chest drain on the ipsilateral side. This is performed by blunt dissection through the fifth intercostal space in the anterior axillary line. A tension pneumothorax is a clinical diagnosis and should not have to be diagnosed by chest x-ray (CXR).

ADEQUACY OF CIRCULATION

Two high-flow lines with 14-gauge cannulae should be inserted into the antecubital fossae. Two litres of warmed crystalloid should be infused rapidly in the event of hypovolaemic shock. This is followed with emergency blood in the event of the blood pressure not stabilizing. Digital pressure can be applied to a bleeding neck wound, or a 20-FG Foley urinary catheter can be inserted into the neck wound and the balloon inflated with 5 mL of water, to stem bleeding. The lumen of the Foley catheter is cross-clamped with arterial forceps to prevent blood haemorrhaging through the urinary port. In the authors' experience, Foley catheter balloon tamponade has been extremely effective in the haemostasis of bleeding, penetrating neck wounds.[1] The patient should remain recumbent, or the neck wound must be covered with an occlusive dressing to prevent air embolism. Blood should be sent for crossmatch and a haemoglobin level. The patient is monitored with precordial electrocardiogram (ECG) leads and a non-invasive blood pressure cuff. Should the blood pressure not stabilize, neurogenic shock should be excluded as a result of a penetrating spinal cord injury. The telltale signs of neurogenic shock are an unexplained bradycardia, absence of limb movement, paradoxical respiration and priapism. A central venous line should be inserted if there is doubt about the type of shock.

ASSESSMENT OF DISABILITY

A rapid assessment of the patient's Glasgow Coma Score (GCS) and pupil size is made. Power in the limbs should be assessed to exclude an ischaemic stoke from carotid artery injury.

EXPOSURE OF PATIENT

All the clothes are removed, and the patient is fully examined to avoid overlooking injuries. The patient should be log-rolled to examine the back for penetrating injuries. The patient is kept warm.

PLACEMENT OF TUBES AND ESSENTIAL X-RAYS

A nasogastric tube and a urinary catheter are inserted. Anteroposterior and lateral cervical spine x-rays are requested to determine the presence of spinal column injury and prevertebral air that could signify a pharyngeal or oesophageal injury. Chest x-ray is done to exclude mediastinal air, pneumo- or haemothorax, and a widened mediastinum. A widened mediastinum may indicate intrathoracic great vessel or oesophageal injury.

REASSESSMENT OF PATIENT

Haemodynamically unstable patients are taken to the operating theatre. If the patient's condition is stabilizing, then a more thorough examination is undertaken in the secondary survey.

Secondary survey

A detailed head-to-foot examination is performed. In gunshot injuries, the entrance and exit wounds are noted, as the tract of the projectile would indicate which anatomical structures might have been injured. In the absence of an exit wound, anteroposterior and lateral cervical x-rays are requested to locate the bullet and determine the course of the tract. The wound should not be probed as this could result in massive bleeding from a vascular injury. Drainage from the wound, such as saliva, lymphatic or cerebrospinal fluid, is noted. The neck is palpated for the presence of subcutaneous emphysema. The presence of 'hard signs' of vascular injury, such as a peripheral pulse deficit, bruit or a large haematoma are noted. A full neurological examination is performed, and Horner's syndrome, cranial nerve, spinal cord and brachial plexus injury are excluded.

Full history

A full history should be recorded with specific reference to the nature of the trauma. Symptoms related to oesophageal injury, such as haematemesis, dysphagia and odynophagia are noted. Dysphonia is suggestive of a vagal or recurrent laryngeal nerve injury. The past medical and surgical history is recorded.

Further investigations

Female patients of child-bearing age must have a pregnancy test done prior to further radiological examination. Special investigations such as angiography, CT scan, ultrasound and contrast studies may now be ordered in the haemodynamically stable patient.

MANDATORY OPERATION VERSUS MANDATORY IMAGING VERSUS SELECTIVE PHYSICAL EXAMINATIONS AND INTERVENTION

A patient who presents with massive bleeding from a cervical wound, an expanding haematoma or a large blowing wound from a large tracheal wound clearly needs immediate exploration. But what of the patient who is haemodynamically stable and does not fulfil these criteria for immediate exploration? The optimum management of such haemodynamically stable patients has been controversial for a number of years. However, evidence-based medicine is providing a means to resolve these arguments and the clinical management of these neck injuries is becoming clearer.

Non-operative management of penetrating neck injuries was the norm prior to the Second World War, and had an associated mortality rate of 15–18 per cent.[6] In 1944, Bailey[7] proposed early operative intervention for penetrating neck trauma, and with the introduction of antibiotics and tracheostomy, the mortality rate was reduced to 7 per cent. In 1957, Fogelman and Stewart[8] reported that the mortality for patients not promptly explored was 35 per cent versus 6 per cent for those undergoing immediate exploration.

This led to mandatory exploration of the neck becoming the standard of care for penetrating cervical trauma that had breached the platysma muscle. Proponents of mandatory surgery believed that the risk of missing a vascular or aerodigestive injury outweighed the morbidity and cost of a negative exploration. They argued that clinical evaluation was unreliable and diagnostic studies used to detect oesophageal and vascular injuries were not 100 per cent sensitive. In 1963, Stone and Callahan[9] questioned the need for mandatory exploration for civilian injuries. Yet mandatory surgical exploration remained the standard of care for the next few decades. This policy was associated with a high incidence (30–89 per cent) of unnecessary neck exploration.[10, 11, 12, 13]

Proponents of selective exploration allude to the high rate of negative findings with mandatory neck exploration and the excellent specificity of special investigations such as angiography, oesophagography, oesophagoscopy and flexible laryngotracheobronchoscopy to exclude clinically significant injuries. Also many of the injuries, such as thyroid, pharyngeal and selected venous trauma, may be treated conservatively. Four prospective studies on a selective conservative approach to penetrating cervical injuries have confirmed the safety of such an approach. Demetriades et al.[14] reported successful conservative management in 80 per cent of 335 patients in the largest published series. There were no deaths attributed to this policy. The combination of clinical and selective investigations yielded a sensitivity of 100 per cent and a specificity of 85 per cent for significant vascular and aerodigestive tract injury. Patients were clinically assessed and the direction of the tract taken into account, as well as potential structures that may have been injured. Further investigations were considered on the basis of clinical symptoms and signs. They did not consider 'soft signs', such as shock responding to resuscitation, non-expanding haematoma, dyspnoea, subcutaneous emphysema, hoarseness, dysphagia or minor haematemesis to be absolute indications for exploration. They concluded that the decisions about selective exploration can be made on the basis of careful initial and repeated clinical examination.

The success of this selective approach has ranged from 29 to 97 per cent in other studies.[14, 15, 16, 17] The mortality reported in the studies by Campbell and Robbs[15] and Ngakane et al.[17] was not attributable to the cervical trauma, but was due to associated injuries (**Table 17.1**).

Clinical examination and adjunctive investigations (based on clinical examination) have been shown to be able to exclude clinically significant injury at several other large trauma centres.[18, 19, 20]

Therefore, the issue at hand concerning penetrating neck injuries is no longer about the safety of non-operative management, but now centres on the indications for investigations and which investigations should be performed.

CLINICAL EVALUATION

Vascular injury

The reported accuracy of clinical evaluation to detect vascular injury varies widely. 'Hard' signs of vascular injury include

Table 17.1 Prospective studies of selective conservative management.

	Patients	Observed	Explored	Negative findings	Mortality
Demetriades et al.[14]	335	80%	20%	15%	0%
Campbell and Robbs[15]	108	82%	24%	0%	1.2%
Narrod and Moore[16]	77	29%	62%	15%	0%
Ngakane et al.[17]	109	97%	3%	0%	1.8%

external haemorrhage, expanding haematoma, pulse deficit, bruit and a pulsatile haematoma. Sclafani et al.[21] reported a sensitivity of 61 per cent and specificity of 80 per cent and Meyer et al.[12] reported an accuracy of 68 per cent suggesting that physical examination alone was a poor predictor of vascular injury.

Others have reported that clinical examination is a reliable means of detecting vascular neck trauma. Demetriades et al.[22] reported a sensitivity of 100 per cent for clinical detection of significant vascular injury, and Beitsch et al.[23] found that negative findings on physical examination are highly predictive of an absence of an arterial injury.

In a recent prospective study of 59 patients undergoing routine angiography for cervical gunshot wounds, Mohammed et al.[24] reported that ten patients without clinical signs of vascular injury had an injury on angiography. This finding questioned the validity of physical examination alone in the management of the stable patient presenting with a gunshot wound to the neck. Routine angiography was recommended for all gunshot wounds to the neck, even where the entrance wound is in zone 2.

Eddy[25] reported on 138 patients with penetrating injuries to zone 1 of the neck in whom routine angiography was performed. The negative predictive value of a normal chest x-ray and a normal physical examination was 100 per cent in this series.

The authors' current practice is to perform angiography in stable patients only in the presence of a large haematoma, bruit, pulse deficit, widened mediastinum on chest x-ray, or when bleeding has been tamponaded with a Foley's catheter (see **Figure 17.1**). All high velocity gunshot wounds to the neck undergo surgical exploration.

Pharyngeal and oesophageal injury

Clinical evaluation of penetrating oesophageal injury has a reported sensitivity of 80 per cent, specificity of 64 per cent and accuracy of 72 per cent.[26] In our own series of 52 patients with a penetrating oesophageal injury over an eight-year period at Groote Schuur Hospital, the most sensitive sign, present in 48 per cent of patients, was prevertebral air on lateral cervical spine x-ray.[27] The symptoms, signs and radiological findings encountered in these patients are listed in **Table 17.2**. The most common symptoms were dysphagia (29 per cent) and odynophagia (21 per cent).

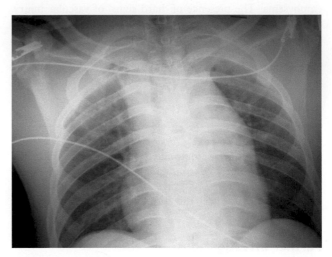

Figure 17.1 Gunshot wound to zone 1 left neck with widened mediastinum on chest x-ray.

Table 17.2 Clinical features of penetrating oesophageal injury.[27]

Symptom/sign	Patients	(%)
Prevertebral air	25	48
Subcutaneous emphysema	24	46
Haemothorax	17	33
Dysphagia	15	29
Odynophagia	11	21
Blood in nasogastric tube	5	10
Hoarse voice	5	10
Widened mediastinum	5	10
Mediastinal air	5	10
Haematemesis	3	6
Haemoptysis	3	6

DIAGNOSTIC INVESTIGATIONS

Angiography

A four vessel arch angiogram with selective catheterization is the gold standard for the investigation of vascular trauma. Angiography has the benefits of identifying the site of injury

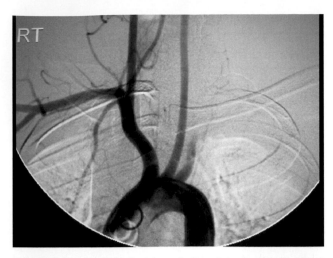

Figure 17.2 Angiogram with occlusion of the first part of the subclavian artery following gunshot wound to zone 1 left neck.

and hence assisting with decision-making regarding proximal and distal control, delineation of crossover circulation through the circle of Willis, and identification of injuries that are amenable to endovascular management, with particular reference to the vertebral artery.

Routine angiography has been recommended for patients with zones 1 and 3 injuries, as it has been stated that these areas are difficult to assess clinically.[21, 28] Yet two studies with a combined total of 535 patients demonstrated that all patients with vascular injuries requiring treatment presented with symptoms[18, 29] (see **Figure 17.2**).

Most authors are in agreement that clinical examination and ancillary investigations should replace mandatory surgical exploration for zones 1 and 3 injuries.[30] It also appears logical that if there is a suspicion of an injury in zone 2 in the haemodynamically stable patient, an angiogram should be performed to identify vertebral artery injury that can be managed by endovascular technique. Naidoo et al.[31] reported on 41 patients with injuries to non-critical vessels treated by endovascular procedures with excellent results.

Colour flow duplex Doppler

Colour flow Doppler (CFD) imaging is being used for the evaluation of cervical vascular injury. It is non-invasive, relatively inexpensive and does not require ionizing radiation. It is, however, operator dependent and expertise may not always be available out of hours.

In a prospective study of CFD, Ginzburg et al.[32] reported 100 per cent sensitivity, but there were some false-positive reports. Demetriades et al.[33] compared CFD with angiography in 82 patients. CFD identified 10 out of 11 angiographically detected injuries. CFD does miss some vascular injuries and ultrasound has limitations in the evaluation of zones 1 and 3 of the neck. Arterial visualization may also be poor in the presence of subcutaneous emphysema, and acoustic shadows of the transverse processes limit evaluation of the vertebral arteries. Similarly, the clavicle can obscure injury to the subclavian and axillary arteries.

Endoscopy and contrast studies

Contrast oesophagography is an excellent means to detect oesophageal and pharyngeal injury, but is ideally suited to the awake, haemodynamically stable and cooperative patient. The sensitivity of contrast oesophagography for traumatic perforation varies from 48 to 100 per cent.[34, 35] In the unconscious, stable, intubated patient, the contrast can be passed via a nasogastric tube which is then pulled back into the pharynx in order to image the oesophagus. A water-soluble contrast medium should be used initially. If no obvious leak is detected, then barium should be administered. Gastrograffin can cause serious pulmonary problems if aspirated and is no longer used.

Rigid oesophagoscopy requires a general anaesthetic and provides limited visibility. Sensitivity of flexible oesophagoscopy is reported as 40–90 per cent.[34, 35] Weigelt et al.[26] showed in a prospective study that barium swallow had 89 per cent sensitivity and 100 per cent specificity, but that flexible oesophagoscopy was unreliable in the proximal oesophagus. Wood et al.[36] reported 100 per cent sensitivity of oesophagography, and 96 per cent specificity. They also cautioned that oesophageal and vascular injuries can be missed on neck exploration. Flowers et al.[37] and Srinivasan et al.[38] more recently reported 100 per cent sensitivity for flexible oesophagoscopy to detect a penetrating injury of the oesophagus.

Computed tomographic scan

A small prospective study of 14 patients with penetrating zone 2 neck injuries who all underwent CT scan followed by mandatory neck exploration, concluded that neck injuries could be accurately evaluated by high resolution CT scan of the neck.[39] There were no oesophageal injuries in that study. The authors' experience has been that CT scan is not reliable for the detection of oesophageal injuries. CT scan can provide information about the tract of a gunshot wound and the need for further investigations.

Helical CT angiography (HCTA) is rapid, does not require arterial puncture and is less expensive than conventional angiography. Several prospective series comparing HCTA with conventional angiography for diagnosing arterial injuries in the neck have reported a sensitivity and specificity as high as 90–100 per cent.[40, 41, 42] The pitfalls of HCTA are the presence of artefacts, caused by bullet fragments or the shoulders of large patients, which may resemble intimal tears. Evaluation of the subclavian artery is also limited. In cases of doubtful or non-diagnostic HCTA, patients must undergo conventional angiography (see **Figure 17.3**).

GUNSHOT WOUNDS VERSUS KNIFE WOUNDS

A higher incidence of a therapeutic operation is required in a gunshot wound to the neck as opposed to stab wounds. Even so, the majority of patients presenting with a gunshot wound to the neck can be safely managed non-operatively. Although 73 per cent of transcervical gunshot wounds to the neck are

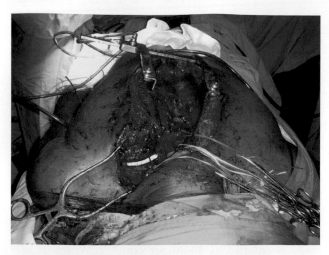

Figure 17.3 Sternotomy and supraclavicular exposure of subclavian artery and insertion of polytetrafluoroethylene (PTFE) graft.

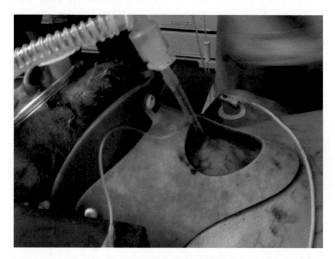

Figure 17.4 Cricothyroidotomy in gunshot wound to the neck.

associated with injuries to vital structures, only 21 per cent of these will require operative intervention[43] (see **Figure 17.4**).

RETAINED SHARP OBJECTS

Patients may present with a sharp foreign body, such as a knife or screwdriver that is still *in situ*. These must not be removed in the Accident and Emergency Department. An anteroposterior and a lateral x-ray must be obtained to identify what vital structures may have been injured. A CT scan is very useful to provide information about the proximity of the foreign body to the oesophagus, trachea and arteries, even though there will be scatter. CT can guide the need for further investigations, but proximity of a retained sharp object to a large artery is an indication for an angiogram. Retained foreign bodies must be removed in theatre under a general anaesthetic.

SPECIFIC INJURIES

Pharyngeal injury

Hypopharyngeal injury should be suspected in all zones 1 and 2 penetrating neck injuries, particularly in the presence of dysphagia, odynophagia, dysphonia, haemoptysis, haematemesis and surgical emphysema. Oedema, blood in the pharynx, or a visible perforation may be noted on flexible nasopharyngoscopy. Oesophagography is unreliable, but direct pharyngoscopy should reveal all injuries.[44] Hypopharyngeal perforations with minimal leakage on contrast study can be managed conservatively. Yugueros *et al.*[45] prospectively managed 14 patients with perforations of the hypopharynx non-operatively. All patients were managed with nasogastric tube feeding, antibiotics for 7 days and kept nil by mouth. All isolated pharyngeal injuries are managed non-operatively at the authors' institution, as this is safe and effective management. The neck wound should not be sutured, but be left open to drain into a drainage bag. A contrast study is repeated on day 7, and if there is no persistent leak, the patient is fed.

Penetrating oesophageal injury

Penetrating oesophageal injury is relatively rare, and only between one and nine new patients present to major level 1 trauma centres per annum.[28, 46, 47, 48, 49, 50, 51] This may be due to the proximity of the oesophagus to vital vascular structures resulting in lethal vascular injury, as well as its relatively protected anatomical position.

Haemodynamically unstable patients must be taken directly to theatre to obtain haemostasis. The oesophagus can be directly examined at the time of neck exploration. Endoscopy may also be performed in theatre once bleeding has been controlled.

Haemodynamically stable patients with symptoms of odynophagia, dysphagia, haematemesis, or signs of subcutaneous emphysema, blood in the nasogastric tube, leakage of saliva from the wound, prevertebral air on lateral neck x-ray, or pneumomediastinum must be investigated with a contrast oesophagogram. It should initially be a water-soluble study. In the absence of an obvious leak or a tracheo-oesophageal fistula, it can be followed by a barium oesophagogram. The sensitivity of the oesophagogram is reported to be in the region of 93 per cent.[27] If the oesophagogram is negative, but there is still a strong suspicion of an injury, then this should be followed by flexible oesophagoscopy, as these two modalities combined give a sensitivity of almost 100 per cent[26] (see **Figure 17.5**).

CT scan may be employed as a screening tool to decide on the need for contrast oesophagography. CT can indicate the course of a bullet through the neck and demonstrate the proximity of the tract to the oesophagus. However, CT scan should not be used alone to diagnose an oesophageal injury, as sensitivity is poor.

The authors' institution has reported on the management of 52 patients with penetrating oesophageal injuries over eight years (23 cervical, 23 thoracic and 4 abdominal).[27] Primary single layer repair with wide drainage remains the

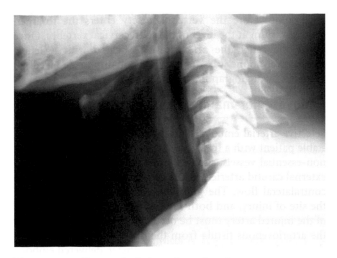

Figure 17.5 Prevertebral air on lateral neck x-ray.

procedure of choice even after delayed diagnosis in stable patients. Primary repair maintains oesophageal continuity and avoids the need for multiple operations. With concomitant tracheal injury, a sternocleidomastoid muscle buttressing flap is interposed to prevent the development of a tracheo-oesophageal fistula. In the septic patient, a 'damage control' approach is adopted. Sepsis is initially controlled by proximal oesophagostomy, stapling of the distal oesophagus and external drainage. A feeding jejunostomy and gastrostomy can then be performed 24 hours later, once the patient has been stabilized in the intensive care unit. At a later stage, an oesophagectomy may be required, followed by reconstruction with a gastric pull up, colonic interposition or jejunal interposition.

The risk of complications related to oesophageal injury is directly related to the time interval between the trauma and definitive management of the oesophageal injury. It is therefore important to keep this time period as short as possible (see **Figure 17.6**).

Tracheal injury

Cervical tracheal injury is relatively uncommon and is frequently associated with oesophageal, vascular or spinal injury. Symptoms of tracheal injury include a blowing wound, surgical emphysema, haemoptysis and hoarseness. If the tracheal injury communicates with the mediastinum, then the patient may present with pneumomediastinum. If there is communication with the pleural space, then the patient may present with a tension pneumothorax. CXR may reveal surgical emphysema, a pneumomediastinum or a pneumothorax.

The initial priority is to secure an airway. Minor tracheal injuries in patients not requiring cervical exploration can be managed expectantly. The trachea can sometimes be intubated through a blowing wound in the neck. Earlier teaching that nasotracheal or orotracheal intubation should be avoided as it may aggravate an existing tracheal injury or cause a false passage appears to have been an overcautious approach.[52] Distal tracheobronchial disruptions can be

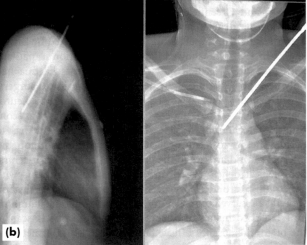

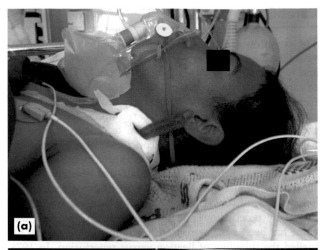

Figure 17.6 (a) Screwdriver in neck. (b) Anteroposterior and lateral x-ray to determine position of screwdriver.

bypassed under vision with an introducer passed through a rigid bronchoscope, or by intubating over a flexible bronchoscope.

Tracheotomy is appropriate for laryngeal trauma to protect the injured larynx when it is not possible to safely pass an endotracheal tube, or in the presence of quadriplegia requiring ventilatory support. In cases of massive surgical emphysema, a tracheotomy might expedite recovery. In cases where there is communication with the pleural space and a large air leak after placement of an intercostal drain, patients will require operative intervention. Tracheal repair is achieved with interrupted sutures. When there is an associated oesophageal injury, the repair must be bolstered with a muscle flap. A sternocleidomastoid muscle flap should be used. The muscle may be pedicled either superiorly or inferiorly. The superior vascular pedicle is a branch of the occipital artery that crosses the hypoglossal nerve and enters on the deep aspect of the upper third of the muscle, while the inferior pedicle is a branch of the suprascapular artery.[53] A tracheotomy or an endotracheal tube may be used to protect the tracheal repair in selected cases.

28. Klyachkin ML, Rohmiller M, Charash WE *et al*. Penetrating injuries of the neck: selective management evolving. *American Surgeon* 1997; **63**: 189–94.

29. Biffl WL, Moore EE, Rhese DH *et al*. Selective management of penetrating neck trauma based on cervical level of injury. *American Journal of Surgery* 1997; **174**: 678–82.

30. Rao PM, Ivatury RR, Sharma P *et al*. Cervical vascular injuries: a trauma center experience. *Surgery* 1993; **114**: 527–31.

31. Naidoo NM, Corr PD, Robbs JV *et al*. Angiographic embolisation in arterial trauma. *European Journal of Vascular and Endovascular Surgery* 2000; **19**: 77–81.

32. Ginzburg E, Montalvo B, LeBlang S *et al*. The use of duplex ultrasonography in penetrating neck trauma. *Archives of Surgery* 1996; **131**: 691–3.

33. Demetriades D, Theodorou D, Cornwell E *et al*. Penetrating injuries of the neck in patients in stable condition; physical examination, angiography or color flow Doppler. *Archives of Surgery* 1995; **130**: 971–5.

34. Bishara RA, Pasch AR, Douglas DD *et al*. The necessity of mandatory exploration of penetrating zone II neck injuries. *Surgery* 1986; **100**: 655–60.

35. Dunbar L, Adkins RB, Waterhouse G. Penetrating injuries to the neck. Selective management. *American Surgeon* 1984; **50**: 198–204.

36. Wood J, Fabian TC, Mangiante EC. Penetrating neck injuries: recommendations for selective management. *Journal of Trauma* 1989; **29**: 602–5.

37. Flowers JL, Graham SM, Ugarte MA *et al*. Flexible endoscopy for the diagnosis of esophageal trauma. *Journal of Trauma* 1996; **40**: 261–6.

38. Srinivasan R, Haywood T, Horwitz B *et al*. Role of flexible endoscopy in the evaluation of possible esophageal trauma after penetrating injuries. *American Journal of Gastroenterology* 2000; **95**: 1725–9.

* 39. Mazolewski PJ, Curry JD, Browder T, Fildes J. Computed tomographic scan can be used for surgical decision making in zone II penetrating neck injuries. *Journal of Trauma* 2001; **51**: 315–19.

40. Leblang SD, Nunez DB, Rivas LA *et al*. Helical computed tomographic angiography in penetrating neck trauma. *Emergency Radiology* 1997; **4**: 200–6.

41. Munera F, Soto JA, Palacio D *et al*. Diagnosis of arterial injuries caused by penetrating trauma to the neck: comparison of helical CT angiography and conventional angiography. *Radiology* 2000; **216**: 356–62.

42. Gracias VH, Reilly PM, Philpott J *et al*. Computed tomography in the evaluation of penetrating neck trauma: a preliminary study. *Archives of Surgery* 2001; **136**: 1231–5.

43. Demetriades D, Theodorou D, Cornwell E *et al*. Transcervical gunshot wounds: mandatory operation is not necessary. *Journal of Trauma* 1996; **40**: 758–60.

44. Fetterman BL, Shindo ML, Stanley RB *et al*. Management of traumatic hypopharyngeal injuries. *Laryngoscope* 1995; **105**: 8–13.

* 45. Yugueros P, Sarmiento J, Garcia A, Ferrada R. Conservative management of penetrating hypopharyngeal wounds. *Journal of Trauma* 1996; **40**: 267–9.

46. Glatterer MS, Toon RS, Ellestad C *et al*. Management of blunt and penetrating external esophageal trauma. *Journal of Trauma* 1985; **25**: 784–92.

47. Symbas PN, Tyras DH, Hatcher CR, Perry B. Penetrating wounds of the esophagus. *Annals of Thoracic Surgery* 1972; **13**: 552–8.

48. Shama DM, Odell J. Penetrating neck trauma with tracheal and oesophageal injuries. *British Journal of Surgery* 1984; **71**: 534–6.

49. Weiman DS, Walker WA, Brosnan KM *et al*. Noniatrogenic esophageal trauma. *Annals of Thoracic Surgery* 1995; **59**: 849–50.

50. Jones WG, Ginsberg RJ. Esophageal perforation: a continuing challenge. *Annals of Thoracic Surgery* 1992; **53**: 534–43.

51. Asensio JA, Berne J, Demetriades D *et al*. Penetrating esophageal injuries: time interval of safety for preoperative evaluation – how long is safe? *Journal of Trauma* 1997; **43**: 319–24.

52. Levy RD, Degiannis E, Hatzitheophilou C *et al*. Management of penetrating injuries of the cervical trachea. *Annals of the Royal College of Surgeons of England* 1997; **79**: 195–7.

53. Losken A, Rozycki GS, Feliciano DV. The use of the sternocleidomastoid muscle flap in combined injuries to the oesophagus and carotid artery or trachea. *Journal of Trauma* 2000; **49**: 815–17.

54. Bradley EL. Management of penetrating carotid injuries: an alternative approach. *Journal of Trauma* 1973; **13**: 248–55.

55. Liekweg WG, Greenfield LJ. Management of penetrating carotid arterial injury. *Annals of Surgery* 1978; **188**: 587–92.

56. Brown MF, Graham JM, Feliciano DV *et al*. Carotid artery injuries. *American Journal of Surgery* 1982; **144**: 748–53.

* 57. Navsaria P, Omoshoro-Jones J, Nicol A. An analysis of 32 surgically managed penetrating carotid artery injuries. *European Journal of Vascular and Endovascular Surgery* 2002; **24**: 349–55.

58. Stain SC, Yellin AE, Weaver FA, Pentecost MJ. Selective management of nonocclusive arterial injuries. *Archives of Surgery* 1989; **124**: 1136–40.

59. Frykberg ER, Crump JM, Vines FS *et al*. A reassessment of the role of arteriography in penetrating proximity extremity trauma: a prospective study. *Journal of Trauma* 1989; **29**: 1041–52.

60. Meier DE, Brink BE, Fry WJ. Vertebral artery trauma: acute recognition and treatment. *Archives of Surgery* 1981; **116**: 236–9.

61. Golueke P, Sclafani S, Phillips T *et al.* Vertebral artery injury – diagnosis and management. *Journal of Trauma* 1987; **27**: 856–65.

62. McLaughlin DJ, Modic M, Masaryk T *et al.* A new approach to the treatment of penetrating injuries to the vertebral artery. *Vascular Surgery* 1998; **32**: 639–46.

63. Beningfield S. Radiology. In: Nicol A, Steyn E (eds). *Oxford handbook of trauma for Southern Africa*. Oxford: University Press, 2004: 104.

64. Du Toit DF, Leith JG, Strauss DC *et al.* Endovascular management of traumatic cervicothoracic arteriovenous fistula. *British Journal of Surgery* 2003; **90**: 1516–21.

PART THREE

ENDOCRINE DISEASE

Section editor: John C Watkinson

PART THREE

ENDOCRINE DISEASE

Section editor: John C. Watkinson

ENDOCRINE DISEASE

Section editor: John C Watkinson

ENDOCRINE DISEASE

Section editor: John C Watkinson

18

Molecular biology and genetic testing of endocrine head and neck tumours

DAE KIM AND NEIL GITTOES

We can't plan life. All we can do is be available for it.

Lauryn Hill

INTRODUCTION

Over the last decade, advances in molecular biology and bio-technology have provided unprecedented insights into human disorders, most notably in human cancer biology. Neoplasms arise as a result of an accumulation of inherited and/or somatic mutations of genes involved in the control of cellular growth and differentiation. Further understanding of the critical genes involved have helped to clarify pathogenetic mechanisms important in thyroid and parathyroid tumours, and thus provided novel therapeutic targets, prognostic and diagnostic markers, and are helping to identify asymptomatic individuals at risk of future cancer development through genetic screening.

This chapter aims to provide an overview of the current knowledge of molecular biology in thyroid and parathyroid tumorigenesis, and genetic testing that is available for screening and diagnosis.

THYROID TUMOURS

Aetiology of thyroid cancer

The aetiology of thyroid cancer is known to be multifactorial. Several risk factors are known to be of importance in the causation of thyroid cancer. Prolonged hyperstimulation with thyroid stimulating hormone (TSH) is believed to be important in malignant change within multinodular goitres.[1] The presence of a solitary thyroid nodule is also a risk factor for malignancy.[2] The prevalence of malignancy within a solitary thyroid nodule is approximately 10 per cent.[1] Another well-recognized aetiological factor in thyroid cancer is ionizing radiation. Studies have consistently demonstrated significantly increased risk of thyroid cancer in children following radiation exposure (both therapeutic and as a consequence of nuclear fallout).[3] Genetic factors are also important. There is a definite tendency for thyroid carcinoma to occur in members of the same family.[4]

In common with most solid tumours, thyroid tumorigenesis is believed to be a complex multistep phenomenon involving the acquisition of multiple genetic lesions that confer a growth advantage to cells.[5] Unlike many other highly specialized cells, thyroid epithelial cells are not terminally differentiated and are thus able to proliferate in response to certain growth factors. Mutations causing altered regulation of growth factors and abnormal receptor function may play a critical role in thyroid tumour progression. Genes acting at multiple steps along growth signalling pathways can function as oncogenes when their structure is disrupted. Several oncogenes have been shown to be significantly associated with the development of differentiated thyroid cancer.[6] Loss-of-function mutations of genes coding for growth inhibitory proteins, involved in cell cycle checkpoints or cell survival, may also contribute significantly to thyroid tumorigenesis.[7]

During the transformation from a normal to a cancerous cell it is widely agreed that several fundamental properties have to be acquired as a result of new genetic lesions.[8] Genetic instability and tumour angiogenesis are critical factors in tumour progression, and have been demonstrated to play an important role in thyroid tumorigenesis.[9]

Growth factors in pathogenesis of thyroid tumours

Unregulated growth signals result in cell transformation. These may arise as a result of constitutive synthesis of growth factors, constitutive activation of their receptors or the intracellular signal transduction pathways. Thyrotropin or TSH induces human thyroid cell growth and proliferation. Chronic TSH stimulation in goitres is believed to be an important factor in the development of thyroid tumours within long-standing nodular goitres.[1] Epidermal growth factor (EGF) has also been shown to induce thyroid cell proliferation.[10] Increased EGF and EGF receptor expression has been demonstrated in cancers compared with normal thyroid tissues.[11] Indeed, the highest level of EGF receptor expression was observed in aggressive anaplastic tumours,[12] and elevated EGF expression has been demonstrated to be prognostic for tumour recurrence.[13]

Thyrocytes secrete many other growth factors (including vascular endothelial growth factor (VEGF) and fibroblast growth factor (FGF)-2), and growth promoting cytokines such as interleukin 1 (IL-1), IL-8 and transforming growth factor b (TGF-b). One study demonstrated TGF-b expression in 58 per cent of malignant thyroid tumours but not in benign tumours or normal thyroid epithelium.[14] Further, receptors to many of these growth factors and novel receptors such as platelet-derived growth factor (PDGF) are expressed by thyroid cancer cells.[15] Expression of both growth factor and its receptor (for example FGF-2 and its receptor FGFR1) suggests existence of mitogenic autocrine pathways that might promote autonomous cell divisions.

Receptor defects

TYROSINE KINASE RECEPTORS

Chromosomal rearrangements leading to inappropriate expression of a fusion onco-protein containing a tyrosine kinase domain (ret and trk tyrosine receptors) appear to be an important and common oncogenic mechanism in differentiated thyroid cancers. What is more interesting is the yet still unexplained specificity of this fusion mechanism for a papillary rather than a follicular subtype (for further detailed discussion see below under Ret and trk gene rearrangements).

G–PROTEIN AND G-PROTEIN COUPLED RECEPTORS

The G-proteins are a subfamily of GTP-binding proteins, which include ras. They are heterodimers, composed of α-, β- and γ-subunits, each encoded by distinct genes. G-proteins couple a diversity of receptors (including the TSH receptor, TSH-R) with their effectors by acting as molecular switches. Gsα is utilized widely as a positive transducer for the activation of adenylate cyclase and calcium channels.

The TSH receptor (TSH-R), a member of the seven transmembrane G-protein associated receptors, can be activated by point mutations leading to amino-acid substitutions that either abrogate the requirement for ligand or enhance responses to ligand-mediated activation.[16] Mutations of the *TSH-R* are observed in many autonomously functioning thyroid nodules (AFTNs), which are characterized by progressive growth and the ability to synthesize hormones in the absence of TSH stimulation.

Activating mutations in the critical domains of both Gsα and *TSH-R* result in the mimicking of TSH stimulation and upregulation of adenylate cyclase activity. Transgenic studies with mice have shown persistently elevated cAMP levels (as a result of TSH driven adenylate cyclase activity) to induce thyroid hyperplasia and goitre formation.[17]

Defects in either the *TSH-R* or Gsα genes are present in 50–80 per cent of solitary AFTNs.[18, 19] Recent studies have also demonstrated *gsp* mutations in non-functioning thyroid tumours. Goretzki *et al.* found *gsp* mutations in 75 per cent of thyroid tumours from Germany and 20 per cent from the United States.[20] A few thyroid carcinomas with activating point mutations of the *TSH-R* gene[21] have been reported, but these are relatively rare.

Constitutive upregulation of adenylate cyclase activity resulting from gsp and THS-R mutations may play a potentially important role in thyroid tumour formation, but their exact contribution remains unclear (see **Figure 18.1**). From these findings, it is likely that these alterations are early events in thyroid tumorigenesis.

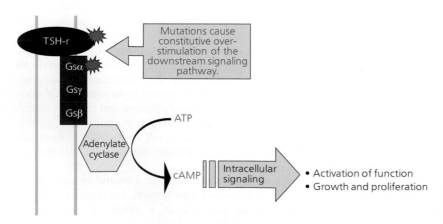

Figure 18.1 TSH-R and Gsα mutations causing follicular cell proliferation and hyperfunction.

NUCLEAR RECEPTORS

Peroxisome proliferator-activated receptors (PPARs) are nuclear receptors that bind to DNA as heterodimers with the retinoid X receptors. PPARγ has been shown to play an important role in regulating genes involved in adipocyte differentiation and lipid metabolism.[22] An involvement of this nuclear receptor in thyroid cancer was discovered by the characterization of a translocation in a subset of thyroid follicular carcinomas which results in fusion of the DNA binding domains of thyroid transcription factor PAX8 to PPARγ1.[23] PAX8-PPARγ1 rearrangements are detectable in 10 per cent of follicular adenomas and 41 per cent of follicular carcinomas, suggesting a role for this fusion protein in malignant transformation.[24]

6More recently, mutations in the thyroid hormone receptor (TR) α1 and β1 transcripts have been reported in papillary thyroid cancers.[25] Furthermore, gene-targeted mice with a mutant TRβ (TRβPV mice) develop invasive thyroid cancers later in life, suggesting a role for TRβ in thyroid cancer progression.[26]

Oncogenes and tumour suppressor genes in the pathogenesis of thyroid cancer

Cancer is a complex, multistep process. However, recent years have seen major advances in understanding the role of two classes of genes that are of particular importance in carcinogenesis that provide a more substantive picture. These are oncogenes and tumour suppressor genes. By definition, an oncogene refers to an abnormal gene with a 'gain-in-function' when a normally present proto-oncogene becomes inappropriately activated through mutation. This contrasts with 'tumour suppressor genes' that represent 'loss-in-function' because of the loss or inactivation of a proto-oncogene. Proto-oncogenes are normal genes involved in cell cycle control, growth factor regulation and cell receptor function and are normally silent but can become activated or inactivated by chromosomal translocations, gene deletions or mutations, and promote uncontrolled cell growth.

Several of the known oncogenes have been consistently detected in differentiated thyroid neoplasms. Some are more strongly associated than others and, interestingly, few are limited to specific forms of thyroid tumours. The role of oncogenes in specific human cancers are developing rapidly and their biology are providing key insights into thyroid cancer biology.

RAS

The *ras* proto-oncogene codes for a G-protein, p-21, which is found within cell membranes and hydrolyses GTP to GDP. P21 plays a critical intermediate role in connecting the stimulatory signal from tyrosine kinases such as EGF receptor and via Raf-1 to a mitogenic cascade involving the MAP kinases.[27] Final products act upon nuclear transcriptional factors such as *c-fos* and *c-jun*. The *ras* proto-oncogene appears to be part of a growth-promoting pathway in normal human thyroid as well as nodular goitre formation. Three

families of ras oncogenes have been identified (*K-ras*, *H-ras* and *N-ras*), each located in separate chromosomal locations.

Ras mutations are found in 30 per cent of human cancers, making this the most widely mutated human proto-oncogene. Activated *ras* has been detected previously in 20 per cent of papillary carcinomas and 53 per cent of follicular carcinomas.[28] The consistently higher prevalence in the more aggressive and dedifferentiated follicular-type cancers may be relevant and adds further weight to the potentially important role of the *ras* oncogene in thyroid tumorigenesis. However, no consistent correlation between the level of *ras* overexpression and the degree of dedifferentiation or metastatic tendency has been observed.

Supportive evidence of the role of *ras* in thyroid cancer is available from *in vitro* cell line studies. Fusco *et al.* demonstrated *K-ras-* and *H-ras-*transfected cells undergo morphological transformation and loss of differentiation.[29] Furthermore, injection of these cells into syngenic rats induced tumour formation.[29]

The prevailing view is that *ras* activation probably represents an early event in thyroid tumorigenesis and is itself not sufficient for malignant transformation. Studies have shown *ras* to be present in a high proportion of the earliest forms of thyroid tumours. One study noted 50 per cent of microfollicular adenomas to contain activated *ras* oncogene.[30] Others have noted normal cells immediately adjacent to RAS-containing tumour cells also harbour RAS.[31] Furthermore, it seems that up-regulated RAS is an important feature in goitre formation.[32]

B–RAF MUTATION

B-Raf (encoded by *BRAF*) is a serine/threonine kinase and is a member of the mitogen-activated protein kinase pathway, involved in the transduction of mitogenic signals from the cell membrane to the nucleus within. *BRAF* gene mutations have been shown to be common in human cancers.[33] Several studies have recently identified the most common *BRAF* mutation, T1796A transverse mutation, in 29–69 per cent of papillary thyroid cancers.[34, 35, 36, 37, 38] In contrast to classical genetic mutations in thyroid cancers such as *RET-PTC* and *ras* mutations, which are also apparent in some benign thyroid lesions, remarkably to date this mutation has consistently been reported to be 100 per cent specific for papillary thyroid carcinomas (PTC), with no benign thyroid neoplasms having been found to harbour *BRAF* mutations. Consequently, *BRAF* mutation has been proposed as a specific molecular marker with relatively good sensitivity for the diagnosis of PTC. Moreover, a *BRAF* mutation has been demonstrated to be a novel prognostic biomarker that predicts poor clinicopathological outcomes.[37, 38] Namba *et al.* reported a significant association of *BRAF* mutation with distant metastases and advanced pathological stages of PTC.[37] Nikiforova *et al.* reported a significant association of *BRAF* mutations with extrathyroidal invasion and advanced pathological stages of PTC.[38] Xing *et al.* demonstrated, using a novel colorimetric mutation detection method, that *BRAF* mutations were readily detectable in thyroid fine needle aspiration cytology (FNAC) aspirates. In a series of 48 patients undergoing thyroidectomies for cancer or suspected malignancy, they showed that 50 per cent of the nodules that proved to be

PTC on final histology were correctly diagnosed by *BRAF* mutation analysis on FNAC samples performed preoperatively; there were no false positives.[39] They also reported a statistically significant association of *BRAF* mutation with neck lymph node metastases and higher incidence of recurrence. With multivariate analysis, presence of *BRAF* mutation was shown to be an independent prognostic factor for poor survival in PTCs. Detection of *BRAF* mutation in thyroid FNAC samples could be a useful diagnostic adjunctive technique in the evaluation of thyroid nodules with indeterminate cytological findings, although this requires further definition by larger studies. Further, detection of *BRAF* mutation-positive patients may help identify those patients who are likely to have a poorer prognosis, allowing appropriate referral and planning for more extensive treatment.

C–MYC AND C–FOS

Mutations of several other proto-oncogenes, such as *c-myc* (nuclear transcriptional factor family), *c-fos* and *c-jun* (immediate early genes), have also been demonstrated in differentiated thyroid cancers.[6, 9]

The *c-myc* proto-oncogene encodes a nuclear protein that binds to DNA and acts as a transcriptional factor for genes involved in growth and differentiation. Normally, *c-myc* expression steadily declines as the cell cycle progresses and eventually shuts off with full differentiation and is important in inhibition of uncontrolled proliferation.[40] Oncogenic activation leads to the inappropriate upregulation of this important growth/differentiation gene and has been detected in various human cancers including some thyroid tumours. *c-fos* is an immediate/early gene that regulates the expression of specific target genes by binding to their regulatory sequence of DNA. Aberrant activation of this transcriptional regulator has been demonstrated in thyroid tumours.[41]

Del Senno *et al.* studied six thyroid carcinomas and demonstrated increased expression of *c-myc* in three out of six thyroid cancers and an abnormal *c-myc* product in four out of six.[42] No increase in *c-fos* was detected in this study. Terrier *et al.* studied 23 cases of thyroid carcinoma for alterations in the expression or structure of *c-myc* and *c-fos* proto-oncogenes. They provided a similar figure of 57 per cent of thyroid cancers with increased expression levels of *c-myc*, as well as 61 per cent of upregulation of *c-fos*. They also demonstrated a prognostic correlation with the expression level of *c-myc*. Those cancers with an unfavourable clinical and histological prognosis were twice as likely to demonstrate increased c-Myc levels than those with better prognosis, a finding which has been repeated in other studies.[43] These initial findings need further and more thorough evaluation.

MET

MET protein is a transmembrane receptor with tyrosine kinase activity. Its natural ligand is known to be HGF/SF (multifunctional cytokine hepatocyte growth factor/scatter factor). The oncogene is constitutively activated by amplification of the gene or through mutational change.[44] Oncogene activation is associated with mitogenesis, as well as motogenesis, and has been suggested to contribute to tumour aggressive and metastatic behaviour.[45] MET oncogene is seen in various cancer human types, including up to 70 per cent of papillary and 25 per cent of follicular carcinomas, although it is not detected either in medullary thyroid cancer (MTC) or in normal thyroid tissues.[46]

C–ERBB

c-erbB codes for the EGF receptor. EGF is a known mitogenic and de-differentiative agent which is present in normal thyroid tissue. A recent study revealed increased *c-erbB2/neu* and *c-erbB* RNA in three of five papillary carcinomas.[47] These and other similar data suggest that the excessive expression of *c-erbB* may be an important factor in the initiation and/or maintenance of the neoplastic phenotype in some papillary carcinomas.

RET AND TRK GENE REARRANGEMENTS

The *ret* proto-oncogene is located on chromosome 10q11-2 and codes for a transmembrane protein with tyrosine kinase activity, the activity of which is normally restricted to a subset of cells derived from embryonic neural crest cells.[48] It is believed to be important in neuronal cell differentiation and found to be commonly amplified in neuroendocrine tumours. This makes *ret* a natural oncogene candidate for tumours of the thyroid C-cells. Indeed, point mutation of *ret* is now recognized as the basis for most forms of hereditary and sporadic MTCs[49] (discussed in further detail below under Medullary thyroid cancer).

The thyroid carcinoma gene, *PTC*, is an oncogene found in 25 per cent of papillary thyroid cancers, which was initially described by Fusco *et al.*[50] Subsequently, it was discovered to be a fusion between a gene of unknown function (D10S170) and the TK domain of the *ret* proto-oncogene as a result of a chromosomal rearrangement that involves a paracentric inversion of the long arm of chromosome 10.[51] It is now evident that *ret* may undergo fusion arrangements with gene sequences other than D10S17, resulting in the constitutive activation of the RET protein kinase.

Although the *ret* proto-oncogene is not expressed in normal thyroid follicular cells, the rearranged *ret/PTC* oncogene is highly expressed in papillary thyroid cancer cells,[52] undetectable in over 250 non-thyroidal tumours.[48] *PTC/ret* rearrangements are specific for papillary carcinomas and have been found in 5–40 per cent of PTCs in adults and are more common in paediatric PTC, as well as in cancers from children exposed to ionizing radiation.[7, 53, 54, 55, 56]

One prospective study examined thyroid FNAC aspirates for the presence of *RET-PTC* rearrangements in comparison with final histology following surgery. They reported only 50 per cent of papillary cancers to be positive for *RET-PTC*.[57] No false positive results were obtained for the 39 benign thyroid conditions, including adenomas, hyperplasia and thyroiditis. Interestingly, identification of such mutations was shown to assist in the correct diagnosis in nine of 15 cases that would otherwise have been considered indeterminate or insufficient for cytological diagnosis.[57] Other studies have reported supportive data suggesting *RET-PTC* detection as a marker for papillary thyroid cancers.[58, 59]

Somatic rearrangements of another member of the tyrosine kinase receptor gene family, the proto-oncogene *NTRK1* which is normally restricted to neural-crest-derived cells, are also seen in papillary thyroid cancers, albeit with far lower prevalence.[60] The proto-oncogene *trk* is similar in many ways to ret and also codes for the transmembrane tyrosine kinase receptor for neural growth factor (NGF receptor). The *trk* oncogene is also a fusion protein because of chromosomal rearrangement: inversion on the long arm of chromosome 1.[61] As is the case with other TK-type oncogenes, *trk* is found in a small percentage of papillary tumours, but not detected in follicular carcinomas.

It is now evident that both *ret* and *trk* may undergo fusion arrangements with various gene sequences.[62] All rearrangements result in constitutive activation of the normally functioning tyrosine kinase domain as a result of the active tyrosine kinase domain becoming spliced with a non-oncogenic gene that is normally highly expressed in the cytoplasm of thyroid follicular cells. This delivers a signal via incompletely defined pathways, which have been shown to contribute to the de-differentiation and transformation of rodent thyroid cell lines.[63] As with *ras*, there is compelling evidence for the ability of *ret* (and by implication *trk*) to initiate human thyroid tumorigenesis, which in this case is along the pathway of papillary carcinoma (as opposed to follicular tumour development).

Chromosomal rearrangements leading to inappropriate expression of a fusion oncoprotein containing a tyrosine kinase domain appear to be an important and common oncogenic mechanism in differentiated thyroid cancers. What is more interesting is the yet still unexplained specificity for this fusion mechanism for a papillary rather than a follicular subtype. Complimenting this observational evidence, gene transfer experiments transfecting activated *ret* gene into normal follicular cells have demonstrated proliferating colonies of thyrocytes with major phenotypic differences from those induced by *ras*, and which consist of a pattern of growth characteristic of papillary tumour.[64] It seems that the 'choice' of initiating oncogene (e.g. *ret* versus *ras*) may determine the eventual resulting tumour phenotype and is an interesting observation warranting further investigation.

Loss of heterozygosity and tumour suppressor genes

Oncogenesis also frequently involves the loss of so-called tumour suppressor genes (TSGs). These genes are critical to normal cell growth and division. Loss of gene expression through mutation events allows the cell to undergo uncontrolled cell division. *P53* and *Rb* genes are classical examples of TSGs, and the loss of either gene function has been shown to be associated with most human cancer development, including thyroid cancers. Inactivating point mutations of the *p53* tumour suppressor gene are highly prevalent in anaplastic and poorly differentiated thyroid tumours but not in well-differentiated thyroid cancers.[65, 66] Overall, a meta-analysis reported 14 per cent of thyroid cancers to exhibit *p53* mutations.[65] Mutations of the retinoblastoma (*Rb*) gene were demonstrated in 55 per cent of thyroid carcinomas but none in benign tumours.[67] Twelve per cent of thyroid malignancies have been shown to harbour both *p53* and *Rb* mutations.[67]

Loss of chromosomal material in tumour cells are detected using PCR techniques, so called LOH, and these provide clues to potential TSG locations. These events also occur in thyroid cancers, in particular in follicular tumours. Several groups have examined thyroid tumours for loss-of-heterozygosity (LOH) to identify other potential tumour suppressor genes. There is little evidence for LOH in papillary thyroid tumours.[9, 68] However, a variety of chromosomal regions have been incriminated in the aetiology of follicular tumours. LOH involving chromosome 3p was shown to be specific to follicular tumours,[69] and up to 14 per cent of follicular adenomas exhibited LOH at 11q13.[70]

Genetic instability and thyroid cancer

Chromosomal aberrations, both in number and integrity, were shown to be associated with tumours by pathologists over 100 years ago and have been used since to identify and stratify the aggressiveness of cancers.[71] With the exception of a few haematological tumours, the majority of these chromosomal defects are not specific to tumour type but may indicate the underlying genetic instability in the cancer cells.

Several groups of researchers[72, 73] proposed that the low mutation rate in normal cells cannot account for the hundreds of gene defects detected in cancer cells. In 1974, Loeb *et al.* postulated the 'mutator phenotype' theory to explain this biological discrepancy. They proposed that cancer cells acquire a degree of 'genetic instability' as a result of mutations in certain genes involved in the maintenance of DNA integrity and fidelity during replication. The manifested increase in mutation rate in cancer cells also helps to explain the variations in gene defects seen even within specific tumour types and in part the observed heterogeneity in the subpopulation of cells seen within most solid tumours. Advances in genetic and molecular technology have provided compelling evidence for 'mutator phenotype' theory in human cancers. It is now widely accepted that cancer results from the accumulation of many mutations and that an underlying genetic instability is necessary for the generation of the multiple mutations that underlie cancer.

Thyroid cancers have been demonstrated to exhibit both chromosomal and intra-chromosomal instability using several molecular techniques. Allelic deletions are an indication of chromosomal instability and, in several studies of tumour LOH patterns, specific chromosomal regions such as 3p, 2p, 2q and 11q appear more susceptible to allelic loss in thyroid tumours[68, 74] compared with normal thyroid tissue. Aneuploidy is a common feature of thyroid follicular adenomas (29 per cent) and carcinomas (56 per cent), as well as of many human thyroid carcinoma cell lines[75, 76] and, in thyroid papillary cancer, aneuploidy has been shown to be associated with higher death rates.[77] A comprehensive analysis of LOH studies revealed a higher tendency to lose genetic material in follicular neoplasms, particularly follicular carcinomas, in comparison with papillary cancers, and it was suggested that a fundamental difference may exist for mechanisms controlling chromosomal instability in these two forms of thyroid tumours.[68] Further, development of chromosomal instability has been suggested to underlie the progression to more aggressive phenotypes of thyroid cancer.

Microsatellite instability (MSI) has been demonstrated in thyroid cancers. One group reported 21 per cent of thyroid tumours to exhibit MSI.[78] MSI was seen significantly more frequently in follicular tumours than in papillary variants. However, no difference was detected between benign versus malignant tumours. Using inter-simple sequence PCR, thyroid cancers have been shown to exhibit a high degree of genetic instability compared with colorectal tumours.[79] Genetic instability was shown to be higher in younger patients (<43 years) compared with patients older than 43 years. Further, the level of genetic instability measured using this technique has been suggested to differentiate between benign and malignant thyroid tumours.[80] Additionally, as an indirect measure of genetic instability, marked hypermutability of p53 has been demonstrated in thyroid cancer.[65]

Therefore, genetic instability is a major feature in the initiation and progression of thyroid neoplasms. Further understanding of this process would provide critical insights into thyroid tumorigenesis.

Angiogenesis in thyroid cancer

Angiogenesis is the sprouting of new blood vessels from pre-existing capillaries and is a key rate-limiting step in tumour progression and critical for metastatic spread.[8, 81] Solid tumours gain access to the host blood supply and induce their own microcirculation by stimulating in-growth of endothelial cells from the surrounding stroma.[82] In response to appropriate stimuli, the normally quiescent vasculature becomes activated to grow new capillaries.

Thyroid cancers are more vascular than normal thyroid glands. Assessment of angiogenesis in 128 papillary thyroid cancers demonstrated a three-fold increase in vascularity in tumours compared with normal thyroid tissues,[83] and greater mean vessel density (MVD) in malignant tumours compared with benign thyroid lesions.[84] Further, increased risk of recurrence and shorter survival was demonstrated in those with the more vascular thyroid tumours.[85, 86] The finding of greater vascularization in follicular tumours compared with papillary tumours, particularly adjacent to or in areas penetrating the capsule, is consistent with the hypothesis that angiogenesis may play a more prominent role in tumour spread in follicular tumours.[84] This is important because follicular tumours tend to spread via the blood stream, whereas papillary thyroid tumour spread occurs via the lymphatic system.

Increased VEGF expression, a potent pro-angiogenic growth factor, has been demonstrated in thyroid cancer when compared with normal gland and benign tumours.[87, 88, 89] VEGF has also been shown to be related to thyroid tumour behaviour. Higher VEGF expression been shown to be present in metastatic thyroid cancer compared with non-metastatic disease.[88] Also, nodal metastases showed increased VEGF expression with respect to the primary tumour.[90] Further, high VEGF expression has been shown to be associated with disease recurrence and poorer survival.[91] Increasing VEGF expression parallels increases in cell proliferation, as assessed using Ki-67 labelling index, suggesting that areas of increased cell division may be due to increased VEGF secretion, perhaps allowing increased local angiogenesis.[88]

Taken together, angiogenesis represents an important process in thyroid tumour progression. However, further studies focusing on angiogenesis involved specifically in thyroid tumorigenesis are necessary in the hope that these will allow novel thyroid-specific therapies to be developed.

Medullary thyroid cancer

MTC arises from the parafollicular or C-cells that produce calcitonin (CT), and accounts for 5–10 per cent of all thyroid cancers. MTC may be sporadic or hereditary. MTC is hereditary in about 25 per cent of cases. Hereditary MTC is transmitted as an autosomal dominant trait and may be either transmitted alone (FMTC) or as part of a multiple endocrine neoplasia (MEN) type 2A or 2B syndrome.[92]

In all MTCs, there is positive immunohistochemical staining for calcitonin and carcinoembryonic antigen (CEA). Calcitonin is a small 32-amino acid peptide present in the blood. Modern immunoradiometric (IMRA) assay offers high specificity and sensitivity and are now used routinely to detect levels in the blood. Elevated basal CT levels are found in subjects with MTC, C cell hyperplasia, and rarely in patients without any C-cell abnormality. In patients with C-cell disease, CT basal levels are raised early in the disease process and the highest concentrations are observed in patients with greatest tumour burden. However, there are exceptions and there is no strict relationship between CT levels and tumour burden. Indeed, basal CT levels may be normal in some patients with MTC. In these patients, pentagastrin provocation testing is sometimes used to detect abnormal CT levels. The main clinical interest in pentagastrin stimulation testing is in subjects belonging to an MTC family in whom it may allow to schedule appropriate surgery, and to ascertain cure in MTC patients in whom basal serum CT levels is undetectable postoperatively. Measurement of serum CEA concentration may also be useful during follow up because high concentrations or rapidly rising levels indicate disease progression or recurrence.[93]

The genetic abnormalities that may be responsible for MTC development have been mainly derived from studies in hereditary MTC syndromes. Hereditary cancers are due to germline mutations of a given gene and every cell in the body will harbour the mutation. In contrast, sporadic cancers are due to somatic mutation occurring in the same gene in a single cell that becomes neoplastic. Only the tumour cells would therefore harbour the mutation and is tumour tissue specific. Germline mutations of the ret proto-oncogene has been identified in MEN 2A, FMTC and MEN 2B (see below under Inherited cancer syndromes and genetic testing).

The ret gene has 21 exons and encodes a membrane bound tyrosine kinase receptor. Upon ligand binding and activation of the receptor, autophosphorylation of the tyrosine kinase motifs results in the stimulation of numerous downstream intracellular signalling pathways. Approximately 98 per cent of all mutations causing MEN 2A are known. Further, there is a close relationship between the genotype and phenotype.[94] The screening for these mutations, therefore, provides effective diagnostic and prognostic information (see below under Inherited cancer syndromes and genetic testing for further discussion). Mutations at known codons have been described for MEN 2B and FMTC. In MEN 2B, a mutation at codon 918 account for 95 per cent of the patients.[95] *De novo* mutations (i.e. germline mutations that do not exist in parents) have been found in 4–10 per cent of index cases with MEN 2A and FMTC, and in most cases of MEN 2B.[96]

Somatic activation of oncogenes is also seen in MTC, although because of its relative rarity, they are less well-characterized in comparison to papillary and follicular carcinomas. Somatic mutation (found exclusively in the tumour) in codon 918 of the ret proto-oncogene have been identified in 25–33 per cent of sporadic MTC.[97] Other codon mutations have been described. It therefore appears that loss of normal *ret* allele or duplication and amplification of the mutant allele contributes to transformation in a high percentage of MTCs.

Studies have demonstrated consistent associations with at least two other oncogenes, *ras* and *myc*. Elevated levels of *H-ras*, *c-myc* and *N-myc* have been found in primary tumour and in lymph node metastases by Northern analysis and *in situ* hybridization.[98] Terrier *et al*. have also shown significant levels of another oncogene, *c-fos*, in their two cases of MTC studied, as well as in mouse MTC lines.[43] In a recent study of 21 MTC specimens by Boultwood *et al*., elevated levels of *N-myc* were seen in six of 21 and *c-myc* in one of 21 samples.[99] These oncogenes were not detected in normal thyroid C-cells. It is evident that more extensive studies are needed for a more complete understanding of oncogenic events in MTC development.

Anaplastic thyroid cancer

Anaplastic carcinomas represent one of the most aggressive human cancers. Patients have a mean survival rate that ranges from four to 12 months and a five-year survival rate that ranges from 1.0 to 7.1 per cent.[100] Its rarity and rapidly fatal clinical course have made it a difficult cancer to study and treat. Early studies have suggested that both hyper-TSH stimulation and irradiation may be important cofactors in this process. However, Abe *et al*. have demonstrated that growth and metabolic activity of undifferentiated thyroid tumours is independent of TSH function.[101] Also, only a small minority of individuals with anaplastic cancer have a history of radiation exposure.

Whether anaplastic tumours arise *de novo* or require a pre-existing differentiated thyroid carcinoma (DTC) for their evolution ('anaplastic transformation') is an ongoing issue of controversy. Despite a limited understanding, anaplastic transformation or the intra-tumoural evolution of anaplastic carcinoma from pre-existing differentiated cancer has become well accepted.[100] Many clinicians now believe that the development of anaplastic thyroid cancer is part of the natural history of untreated differentiated thyroid cancer.

Clinical evidence for the occurrence of 'anaplastic transformation' comes from the fact that anaplastic tumour evolution occurs in older individuals and often with a long history of a thyroid tumour, or a history of a previously incompletely resected tumour.

Pathological studies provide the most convincing evidence of anaplastic transformation. Multiple large cohort studies have reported significant associations of anaplastic tumours with a DTC component. Up to 90 per cent of anaplastic cancers have been found in association with DTC.[100, 102]

Papillary carcinoma is the most commonly DTC found, although follicular and Hurthle cell tumours have also been documented.

Allelotyping studies suggest that papillary and follicular carcinomas have different genetic pathways of anaplastic transformation. Papillary tumours have a much lower prevalence of LOH than either follicular and anaplastic tumours.[68] This suggests a fundamental difference in the underlying mechanism maintaining chromosomal stability in these tumours. LOH hotspots have been located to chromosome 16p and a tumour suppressor gene located at this locus may play an important role in anaplastic transformation.[103]

Molecular research in anaplastic cancer has been limited and relies mainly on *in vitro* cell line studies. Anaplastic tumour cell lines in culture, or as xenografts in athymic mice, have provided investigators with an experimental model to study the disease biology. Mutations of the *p53* gene in human neoplasia are generally regarded as late events, and appear to be relevant to the development and progression of malignant thyroid cancer. Studies have reported very low prevalence of *p53* mutations in differentiated thyroid tumours whereas *p53* mutations were seen predominantly or exclusively in anaplastic cancers.[104] Codon positions 273 and 248 appear to be mutational hotspots in anaplastic thyroid cancer. This provides strong evidence that mutational inactivation of *p53* may be a critical transitional step leading to progression to these aggressive undifferentiated cancers.

The important role of *p53* in anaplastic tumour development has also been demonstrated in experimental studies in which reintroduction of wild-type *p53* into anaplastic thyroid cancer cells led to inhibition of cellular proliferation and the induction of differentiation and cellular responsiveness to TSH stimuli.[105]

Mutant *Rb* alleles have been reported in 55 per cent of thyroid cancers, but none in benign tumours.[106] The rates of *Rb* mutations were similar in anaplastic and differentiated thyroid carcinomas. However, 12 per cent of cancers harboured both *Rb* and *p53* mutations. Such double mutations appeared more frequently in advanced disease stage.[106] It appears that Rb is an important factor in thyroid cell transformation and possibly, with *p53*, in tumour progression. Other genes that have been investigated and are believed to play a role in anaplastic transformation include *blc-2*, *β-catenin*, *c-myc* and *Nm23*.[9]

Much of the information on the molecular determinants of thyroid tumour progression remains unclear. Understanding of the underlying biology of anaplastic tumour evolution is critical for insights fundamental to the emergence of new and more effective treatments for individuals diagnosed with this lethal malignancy.

Summary

Based upon current understanding of molecular events in thyroid carcinogenesis (see **Box 18.1**), we may postulate a schematic picture of the sequential molecular changes which determine thyroid tumour development and progression (see **Figure 18.2**). The role for *gsp* and *TSH-R* mutations in thyroid cell hyperplasia and follicular adenoma formation has been well established. *ras* mutations appear to be an early event, as they are common to benign and malignant tumours. The pathways leading to follicular or papillary carcinoma are divergent. Mutational activation of *ret* and *trk* oncogenes are specific to papillary carcinomas. Conversely, loss of function of a gene on chromosome 11q13, possibly MEN1 gene, may direct the tumour clone towards a follicular phenotype. Loss of heterozygosity at chromosome 3p is specific for follicular carcinoma and implies the involvement of an important tumour suppressor gene mapping to that chromosomal region. Mutations of *p53* are highly prevalent in anaplastic thyroid carcinomas and, together with mutations in the *Rb*

gene, may represent the critical transitional step in the progression of well-differentiated tumours into these aggressive thyroid cancers. However, much of the information on the molecular determinants of thyroid tumour initiation and progression remains rather sketchy.

PARATHYROID TUMOURS

Primary hyperparathyroidism is a commonly detected endocrine disorder and is the most common cause of hypercalcaemia. By far the most common lesion found in patients with primary hyperparathyroidism is the solitary parathyroid adenoma, occurring in 80 per cent of patients.[107] Multiple adenomas have been reported in 2–4 per cent of cases.[108, 109] Parathyroid adenomas may be sporadic or inherited as part of MEN syndromes, familial hyperparathyroidism or hereditary hyperparathyroidism with jaw tumours (HPT-JT).

Genetic abnormalities in parathyroid tumours

Several candidate genes have been described to be causal in this disorder. Investigations of the *PTH* gene, which is located on chromosome 11q15 detected restriction fragment length polymorphism (RFLP) abnormalities in sporadic parathyroid adenomas.[110] Further analysis demonstrated the rearrangement of part of the *PTH* gene onto chromosome location 11q13. The protein that was overexpressed as a result of this rearrangement was designated PRAD 1 (parathyroid adenoma 1), and is a novel member of the cyclin-D family of cell-cycle regulatory proteins. The rearrangement leads to the transcriptional activation and overexpression of cyclin D1 by bringing this gene into close proximity with the regulatory region of PTH. Therefore, upon *PTH* gene activation, cyclin D1 gene is also stimulated, leading to growth of the clone that harbours the genetic abnormality. As many as 15 per cent of sporadic parathyroid adenomas has been shown to overexpress cyclin D1.[111]

Box 18.1　Summary of molecular events in thyroid tumorigenesis (see Figure 18.2)

- A role for *gsp* and *TSH-R* mutations in thyroid cell hyperplasia and follicular adenoma formation.
- *ras* mutations appear to be an early event as they are common to benign and malignant tumours.
- Unclear of the earliest molecular changes that are responsible for the initiation of thyroid cancer development.
- The pathways leading to follicular or papillary carcinoma are divergent.
- Mutational activation of *B-raf*, *ret* and *trk* oncogenes are specific to papillary carcinomas.
- Loss of function of a gene on chromosome 11q13, possibly *MEN1* gene, and chromosome 3p may direct the tumour clone towards a follicular phenotype.
- Mutations of *p53* are highly prevalent in anaplastic thyroid carcinomas and, together with mutations in the *Rb* gene, may represent the critical transitional step in the progression of well-differentiated tumours into these aggressive thyroid cancers.
- Angiogenesis and genetic instability are important processes in tumour progression.

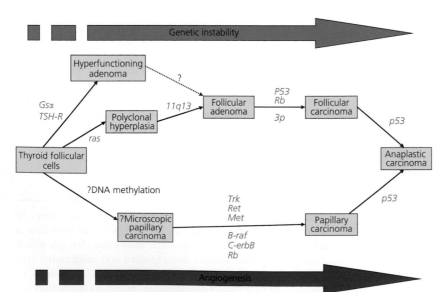

Figure 18.2　Summary of molecular events in thyroid tumorigenesis.

The *Rb* tumour suppressor gene responsible for the pathogenesis of retinoblastomas is involved in the pathogenesis of various other human tumours. Allelic deletion of *Rb* gene has also been demonstrated in parathyroid carcinomas and in 10 per cent of parathyroid adenomas.[112] Abnormal histological staining patterns for Rb protein in 50 per cent of carcinomas but none in the adenomas.[112] Together, these observations demonstrate an important role for the *Rb* gene in the development of parathyroid carcinomas, and may help in the histological distinction of parathyroid adenoma from carcinoma.

LOH studies have revealed allelic loss of chromosome 1q32 in 40 per cent of sporadic parathyroid adenomas.[113] Within this region of DNA, which represents about 110 million base pairs of DNA, there appears to be an important tumour suppressor gene playing a role in many sporadic adenomas.

Another genetic abnormality that appears to be important in the aetiology of parathyroid adenoma is the tumour suppressor gene associated with MEN type 1. Twelve to 20 per cent of patients with sporadic parathyroid adenomas have been shown to harbour bi-allelic defects in the *MEN1* gene, which encodes a 610 amino acid protein referred to as MENIN.[114] The 164 reported somatic mutations of *MEN1* are as diverse in nature and location as observed for germline mutations responsible for the inherited MEN1 syndrome.

Parathyroid adenomas are also associated with MEN syndrome type 2a. Although *c-ret* mutations are responsible for MEN2a, a search for the most common mutation at codon 634 has proved to be negative, suggesting a different mechanism responsible for the development of sporadic and inherited parathyroid adenomas.

The gene causing hyperparathyroidism-jaw tumour syndrome, *HRPT2*, encodes for a ubiquitously expressed protein called parafibromin.[115] As parathyroid tumours are malignant at a higher frequency in HPT-JT than in MEN1 or MEN2, mutations in *HRPT2* are probably an important factor in increased risk of parathyroid carcinoma. Shattuck *et al.* directly sequenced the *HRPT2* gene in 21 parathyroid carcinomas from 15 patients who had no known family history of primary hyperparathyroidism or the HPT-JT syndrome at presentation.[116] Parathyroid carcinomas from 10 of the 15 patients had *HRPT2* mutations, all of which were predicted to inactivate the encoded parafibromin protein. Howell *et al.* detected somatic *HRPT2* mutations in four of four sporadic parathyroid carcinoma samples, and germline mutations were found in five of five HPT-JT parathyroid tumours (in two families) and two parathyroid tumours from one family with familial isolated primary hyperparathyroidism. 'Two hits' – either double mutations or one mutation and loss of heterozygosity at 1q24-q32 – affecting *HRPT2* were found in two sporadic carcinomas.[117] These findings suggest that *HRPT2* mutation is an early event that may lead to parathyroid malignancy and that intragenic mutation of *HRPT2* may be a marker of malignant potential in both familial and sporadic parathyroid tumours.

However, recent studies have demonstrated that in the majority of benign parathyroid tumours, mutations of *HRPT2* are not evident and the expression of parafibromin remains unaltered. The role of *HRPT2* gene and its protein parafibromin in tumorigenesis remains to be further investigated (see **Box 18.2** for a summary of genes postulated to be involved in parathyroid tumorigenesis).

> ## Box 18.2   Genes postulated to be involved in parathyroid tumorigenesis
>
> - *PTH* rearrangements and over-expression of PRAD1.
> - Retinoblastoma tumour suppressor gene deletions seen in parathyroid carcinomas and 10 per cent of adenomas.
> - LOH in the chromosomal region of 1q32 suggest putative TSG is important in the development of 40 per cent of parathyroid adenomas.
> - Allelic defects in *MEN1* gene found in up to 20 per cent of parathyroid adenomas.
> - Parathyroid adenomas are associated with MEN2a. However, the *ret* mutation at codon 634 responsible for MEN2a is negative in sporadic adenomas, suggesting a different mechanism is responsible for hereditary and non-hereditary forms of parathyroid adenomas.
> - Mutations of the gene *HRPT2*, responsible for HPT-JT syndrome, has been detected in parathyroid carcinomas and may represent a marker of malignant potential in parathyroid adenomas.

INHERITED CANCER SYNDROMES AND GENETIC TESTING

Members of some families are prone to developing specific types of malignancies in the absence of identifiable carcinogen exposure. Affected members of these families may represent clustering of sporadic occurrences, multifactorial inheritance or the presence of low penetrance genes. These groupings are classified as familial cancers. Close relatives are at moderately increased risk of developing certain malignancies. However, the average age of onset is usually similar to that observed in the general population.

In contrast, in about 5–10 per cent of individuals, predisposition to a specific group of cancers is the result of a heritable mutation in a cancer predisposing gene, so called germline mutation. The at-risk individuals tend to develop tumours at an earlier age than usual and are at risk of developing more than one primary tumour. In addition, the siblings and offspring of an affected individual each have a 50 per cent chance of inheriting the cancer predisposing mutation, consistent with autosomal dominant inheritance.

Multiple endocrine neoplasia type 1

MEN1 syndrome represents the combination of over 20 different endocrine and non-endocrine tumours. Thus, there is no simple definition of MEN1. A practical definition is a case with two or three main MEN1-related endocrine tumours: parathyroid adenoma, enteropancreatic endocrine tumour and pituitary tumour. MEN1 syndrome is usually inherited, although in 10 per cent of cases arise *de novo*.

Parathyroid tumours occur in 95 per cent of MEN1 patients. Pancreatic islet cell tumours occur in about 40 per cent of patients and gastrinomas (leading to the Zollinger Ellison syndrome (ZES)) are the most common type and also the most important cause of morbidity and mortality in MEN1 patients. However, with improved metabolic management deaths from ZES or HPT in MEN1 have been virtually eliminated. Approximately one-third of deaths in MEN1 cases are caused by MEN1-associated malignancies. Anterior pituitary tumours occur in about 30 per cent of MEN1 patients, with prolactinomas representing the most common type. Unlike thyroid cancer in MEN2, the MEN1-related cancers have no effective prevention or cure. The principal cancer host organs (pancreas and lung) are difficult to screen for early tumours and are not appropriate for ablative surgery.

Primary HPT is the most common endocrinopathy and is usually the first clinical expression of MEN1 in up to 90 per cent of patients, with a typical age of onset of 20–25 years (reaching nearly 100 per cent penetrance by the age of 50 years): this is 30 years earlier than that from sporadic parathyroid adenoma.[118] In contrast, MEN1 is rare and represents only 2–4 per cent of all cases of primary HPT.[119] Biochemical testing for HPT in MEN1 is central in the recognition of parathyroid tumours, and it has occasional application in ascertainment of MEN1 carriers. Patients with MEN1 generally have parathyroid tumours in three or all four parathyroid glands.[118] These tumours are asymmetric in size and are regarded as independent clonal adenomas. The issue of which operation is optimal remains controversial.

The gene causing MEN1 was localized to chromosome 11q13 by genetic mapping studies. Further studies defined the MEN1 gene in 1997, consisting of ten exons that codes a novel 610 amino acid protein named MENIN.[114] The precise function of MENIN still remains to be elucidated. Preliminary studies have shown MENIN to play a role in a large number of cellular functions through its interactions with other proteins, most notably in transcriptional regulation and genome stability.[120]

Over 600 germline mutations of MEN1 gene has been described and the majority (>80 per cent) of these are inactivating, and are consistent with its role as a tumour suppressor gene. More than 10 per cent of the MEN1 gene germline mutations arise de novo and may be transmitted to subsequent generations.[120] Importantly, 5–10 per cent of MEN1 patients do not harbour mutations in the coding region of MEN1 gene, and these individuals may have mutations in the promoter and untranslated regions, which remains to be clarified. The mutations are diverse in their type and are scattered throughout the 1830 bp coding region with no evidence for mutation clustering as observed in MEN2. Correlations between MEN1 mutations and the clinical manifestations are absent, and this contrasts with the situation in MEN2 and ret gene (**Table 18.1**). Further, the MEN1-related tumours behave similarly to sporadic tumour counterparts.

MEN 1 genetic testing for familial MEN1 syndrome

The first step in the analysis is to identify the specific MEN1 mutation in the germline DNA derived from a peripheral blood sample (leukocytes DNA best represents the germline DNA) from the affected index case using direct DNA

Table 18.1   Contrasts between MEN1 and MEN2 (ret) germline mutation tests.[121]

Test feature	*MEN1* gene	*Ret* gene
Informative to patient and clinician	Yes	Yes
Guides intervention to prevent of cancer	No	Yes
Guides intervention to cure cancer	No	Yes
Recommended for child	Maybe	Yes
Chromosomal locus of gene	11q13	10cen
Mutation type	Inactivate	Activate
Genotype/phenotype correlation	No	Yes
False negative rate	10–20%	2–5%

sequencing strategies. Because MEN1 gene somatic mutation is found in common endocrine cancers, tumour DNA is rarely used as an index of the uncommon MEN1 germline mutation (responsible for MEN1 syndrome). In most index cases of familial MEN1, a germline mutation of MEN1 will be identified. Subsequent analysis of other family members at risk is simplified by testing selectively for the MEN1 germline mutation that has already been found to be specific for that family. However, many large studies have failed to find a MEN1 germline mutation in 10–20 per cent of index cases for familial MEN1.[122] Such failures are believed to be due to mutations in untested parts of the MEN1 gene or large deletions that are transparent to PCR methods. In such families with no identifiable germline mutation, haplotype analysis or genetic linkage analysis around the MEN1 locus can allow for screening for MEN1 carrier status.

When DNA-based testing for MEN1 carrier state is not helpful, individuals at a 50 per cent risk of being an MEN1 carrier (first degree relatives of an MEN1 case) should have biochemical testing (calcium, PTH and PRL) for MEN1 carrier ascertainment.

Indications for germline MEN1 testing are still under development. Testing can be offered to index cases with MEN1 or with atypical MEN1 and to their relatives. A careful assessment must be made of sporadic cases with multiple endocrine tumours to exclude those that prove unexpectedly to have familial MEN1. Candidates for testing should include any sporadic cases with two or more MEN1-related tumours. There are limited data on the frequency of an MEN1 germline mutation among the common cases with apparently sporadic tumour in one organ: parathyroid adenoma (1 per cent), gastrinoma (5 per cent) and prolactinoma (1 per cent).[119] The likelihood of MEN1 mutation is higher with younger onset age for the tumour type or with tumour multiplicity in that organ. These preliminary data suggest importance should be given to testing the presumably sporadic gastrinoma (see **Box 18.3** for summary guidelines for the genetic testing of MEN1 patients).

Multiple endocrine neoplasia type 2

The MEN2 syndrome describes the association of MTC, pheochromocytoma, and parathyroid tumours. MEN2 is an

Box 18.3   Summary guidelines for genetic testing of MEN1 patients

- Surgery has not been shown to prevent or cure MEN1-related cancers.
- HPT develops in over 90 per cent of *MEN1* carriers.
- *MEN1* germline mutation testing is recommended for *MEN1* carrier identification. All kindred with MEN1 are likely to have a mutation in the *MEN1* gene.
- However, MEN1 germline mutation testing has a false negative rate of 10–20 per cent.
- If a family lacks an identifiable *MEN1* mutation, 11q13 haplotype testing about the *MEN1* locus or genetic linkage analysis can identify carriers.
- The main candidates for *MEN1* mutation analysis include index cases with MEN1, their clinically apparent unaffected relatives and some cases with features atypical for MEN1.
- *MEN1* carrier analysis should be used mainly for information. It should rarely determine major intervention.
- MEN1 tumour patterns in families do not have clear variants or specific correlations with an *MEN1* germline mutation pattern. Thus, the *MEN1* carriers in a family with either typical or atypical expression of MEN1 should be monitored similarly.
- Biochemical and imaging test should be used for periodic screening of tumours in *MEN1* carriers.

autosomal dominant syndrome, and all variants show a high penetrance for medullary thyroid cancer; 90 per cent of MEN2 carriers will eventually show evidence for MTC. Three clinical variants of MEN2 are recognized: MEN2a, MEN2b and MTC-only (FMTC). MEN2a is the most common variant, and the development of MTC (almost 100 per cent) is associated with pheochromocytoma (50 per cent) and parathyroid adenomas (20 per cent). MEN2b, which represents 5 per cent of all MEN2 cases, is characterized by the occurrence of MTC, pheochromocytoma in association with Marfanoid habitus, mucosal neuromas and intestinal autonomic ganglion dysfunction leading to multiple diverticulae and megacolon. Parathyroid tumours do not usually occur in MEN2b. MEN type 2b is the most aggressive of the MEN2 variants. MTC-only is a variant in which only MTC is the sole manifestation. MTC is the first neoplastic manifestation in most MEN2 patients because of its earlier and overall higher penetrance. Earlier studies reported mortality of 15–20 per cent when treatment was initiated after identification of a thyroid nodule.[123] However, carrier diagnosis before adulthood allowing early thyroidectomy has lowered the mortality from hereditary MTC to less than 5 per cent.[124]

A single gene is responsible for all three syndromes, and is located on chromosome 10q11.2.[94] The *c-ret* proto-oncogene encodes a tyrosine kinase receptor. Specific activating mutations of *c-ret* have been described for each of the three MEN2 variants. Thus, in 95 per cent of patients, MEN2a is associated with mutation of the cystein-rich extracellular domain of the protein receptor, with missense mutation in codon 634 (Cys → Arg) accounting for 85 per cent of MEN2a mutations.

MTC-only is also associated with missense mutations in the extracellular domain, and most mutations are in codon 618. In contrast, 95 per cent of MEN2b is associated with mutations in codon 918 (Met → Thr) of the intracellular tyrosine kinase domain.

The aggressiveness of MTC correlates with the MEN2 variant syndrome and with the mutated *ret* codon.[94] Prevention or cure of inevitable MTC is by surgery, and should be performed before the age of possible malignant progress.

MEN2 genetic testing

MEN2 carrier determination is one of the few examples of a genetic test that mandates a highly effective clinical intervention. Sequencing DNA for *ret* mutation is effective and widely available. In 1997, a consensus was reached that the decision to perform prophylactic thyroidectomy in MEN2 should be based predominantly on the result of *ret* mutation testing, rather than CT testing.[125] There were several unique features of MEN2 that formed this recommendation.[121] First, early detection and subsequent surgical intervention alters the clinical course of MTC. Second, treatment of early MTC by thyroidectomy is well tolerated, even by most infants. This contrasts with complex issues involved in surgical removal of organs MEN1-associated malignancies. Third, the use of abnormal CT tests to dictate thyroidectomy led to a low (5–10 per cent), but still problematic, incidence of false positive tests. Fourth, the *ret* test has a higher rate of true positives and lower rates of false negatives and false positives than the CT test. Also, it facilitates even earlier thyroidectomy. Fifth, the specific *ret* codon mutation correlates well with clinical behaviour and guides stratified treatment.

The general issues for carrier screening is the same for MEN1 mutation testing. There are also unique features in MEN2 relevant to genetic testing (see **Box 18.4**). Up to 98 per cent of MEN2 index cases have an identified *ret* mutation. Extensive research has demonstrated a limited number of MEN2-associated mutations involving the *ret* exons 10, 11, 13, 14, 15 and 16. Therefore, only these exons must be tested routinely. Only if this is negative should the remaining 15 exons be sequenced (currently only available in research laboratories and large endocrine centres). If this extended *ret* testing is negative in the index case, haplotype analysis or genetic linkage analysis about the *ret* locus can be considered if the family history is suggestive of inherited MEN2. Periodic tumour monitoring should be performed in such suspected but unconfirmed MEN2 carrier patients. CT testing remains applicable for diagnosis of the carrier state in these unusual situations.

The likelihood of a *ret* germline mutation in a patient with apparently sporadic MTC is 1–7 per cent.[126] Despite the modest mutation yield, all cases of sporadic MTC should be tested for germline *ret* mutation because of the critical clinical implications of finding a *ret* mutation. A germline *ret* mutation is more likely if the sporadic MTC is of early age onset or there is multiplicity in the thyroid gland. If there is clinical suspicion, these cases should be offered extended mutation analysis if the test for the standard exon sequencing is negative. Analysis for *ret* mutation in tumour tissue from an apparently sporadic case of MTC has limited value. Mutations at codon 883 and 918 (25 per cent) occur

---

Box 18.4 MEN2 genetic testing consensus guideline summary

- Three clinical variants of MEN2 are recognized: MEN2a, MEN2b and MTC-only (FMTC). MEN2a is the most common variant.
- The main morbidity from MEN2 is now MTC (with improved recognition and management of pheochromocytoma). MEN2 variants differ in aggressiveness of MTC: MEN2b > MEN2a > FMTC.
- To avoid missing a diagnosis of MEN2a with its risk of pheochromocytoma, clinicians should only diagnose FMTC from rigorous criteria.
- MEN2 carrier detection should be the basis for recommending thyroidectomy to prevent or cure MTC. This carrier testing is mandatory for all children at 50 per cent risk.
- When performed rigorously, *ret* germline mutation testing reveals a ret mutation in over 95 per cent of MEN2 index cases. It has replaced CT testing as the basis for carrier diagnosis in MEN2 families.
- The *ret* codon mutations can be stratified into three categories of risk from MTC. These three categories predict the MEN2 syndromic variant, the age of onset of MTC and the aggressiveness of MTC.
- Blood leukocyte testing for germline *ret* mutation should be performed in all cases of apparent sporadic MTC (or pheochromocytoma in young patients < 40) due to the critical implications of a positive test.
- Periodic screening for other tumours in MEN2 carriers is based upon the MEN2 variant, as characterized by the *ret* codon mutation and by manifestations in the rest of the family.

- Level 1 (least risk for MTC): children with *ret* codon 609, 768, 790, 791, 804 and 891 mutations have the least risk for MTC. The biological behaviour of MTC in these patients is variable, but, in general, grows more slowly and develops at a later age. There is little consensus upon the management of these patients. Some recommend treatment as for the high risk group (level 2), others suggest thyroidectomy by ten years of age, and still others recommend periodic pentagastrin-stimulated CT testing with thyroidectomy at the first abnormal test result.

Hyperparathyroidism–jaw tumour syndrome

The HPT-JT syndrome is an autosomal dominant disorder characterized by the development of parathyroid adenomas and carcinomas and fibro-osseous jaw tumours. In addition, some patients can develop many other tumour types (renal, pancreatic and testicular).

The jaw tumours are different to the brown tumours observed in some patients with primary hyperparathyroidism, and do not resolve after parathyroidectomy. Ossifying fibromas of the jaw are an important distinguishing feature of HPT-JT and the occurrence of these can precede the development of hypercalcaemia by several decades. However, it is important to note that the parathyroid tumours may occur in isolation and without any evidence of jaw tumours. This can cause diagnostic confusion with other hereditary disorders such as MEN1. In HPT-JT, patients usually have single adenoma or a carcinoma, while MEN1 patients will often have multigland disease.

The gene causing HPT-JT, *HRPT2*, is located on chromosome 1q25 and encodes for an ubiquitously expressed 531 amino acid protein PARAFIBROMIN.[115] To date, 13 different heterozygous mutations translating truncated forms of parafibromin have been reported in HPT-JT families. Although no consensus clinical guideline exists for *HRPT2* genetic testing, testing for germline HRPT2 mutations are available commercially (see GeneTests, www.genetests.org).

Cowden's disease

Cowden's disease (CD), also known as multiple hamartoma syndrome, is a rare autosomal dominantly inherited disease characterized by the formation of hamartomas in various organs, including skin, thyroid, breast and gastrointestinal (GI) tract. Multiple trichilemmomas of the skin and mucocutaneous papillomatosis are common diagnostic features found in > 90 per cent of affected individuals. Other frequent lesions are goitre and adenomas of the thyroid gland. In addition, patients with CD have an increased risk for the development of malignant tumours, including most commonly carcinomas of the breast and thyroid. People with Cowden syndrome have up to a 10 per cent lifetime risk of follicular or papillary thyroid cancer; follicular thyroid cancer is most common. Approximately 70 per cent of people with Cowden syndrome will have benign thyroid changes, including multinodular goitre, adenomatous nodules and follicular adenomas.

---

somatically in sporadic MTC and therefore provide a false positive testing.[127]

ret mutation testing is not indicated for sporadic HPT in the absence of other clinical suspicion for hereditary MEN2. Even in those subjects with family history of HPT, several other hereditary disorders are more likely.

The mutated codon of *ret* correlates with the MEN2 variant, including the aggressiveness of MTC. Genetic information allows stratification of MTC risk and provides a basis for a three-level stratified thyroid management:[121]

- Level 3 (highest risk for aggressive MTC): children with MEN2b and/or *ret* codon 883, 918 or 922 mutation. The finding of microscopic MTC within the first year in this setting is common, and metastases in the first of life have been described. These children should have a thyroidectomy within the first six months of life (first month preferably). Thyroid surgery for MEN2b should include a central node dissection.
- Level 2 (high risk for MTC): children with *ret* codon 611, 618, 620, 634 mutations are at high risk of MTC and should have thyroidectomy performed before the age of five years.

In the vast majority of patients with CD, the disease is caused by germline mutation in the tumour suppressor gene *PTEN*. *PTEN* is mapped to chromosome 10q23 and encodes a lipid phosphatase involved in the PI3/Akt intracellular signalling pathway. PTEN protein regulates important cellular functions including cell proliferation, cell cycle control, apoptosis and cell migration.

Approximately 133 germline *PTEN* and 332 cancer-associated somatic mutations have been reported in the literature to date. *PTEN* germline mutations are also found in patients with Bannayan–Riley–Ruvalcaba syndrome, Lhermitte–Duclos syndrome, VATER syndrome, proteus and proteus-like syndromes. It is evident that *PTEN* mutations are responsible for a variety of hereditary syndromes, all with overlapping clinical features.

Marsh *et al.* identified *PTEN* mutations in 30 of 37 (81 per cent) CD families, including missense and nonsense point mutations, deletions, insertions, a deletion/insertion and splice site mutation.[128] Genetic heterogeneity of CD was suggested by the fact that Tsou *et al.* found no coding sequence mutations in 23 CD families for whom linkage to the *PTEN* locus had never been established.[129]

Cowden syndrome and Bannayan–Ruvalcaba–Riley syndrome share clinical characteristics such as hamartomatous polyps of the gastrointestinal tract, mucocutaneous lesions and increased risk of developing neoplasms. Furthermore, both conditions and several other distinctive phenotypes are caused by mutations in the *PTEN* gene. For this reason, some have suggested that the spectrum of disorders be referred to as PTEN hamartoma tumour syndrome (PHTS).

Although no consensus clinical guideline exists for PTEN genetic testing, testing for germline PTEN mutations are available commercially (see GeneTests, www.genetests.org).

Other inherited syndromes

People with familial adenomatous polyposis (FAP) have a 2 per cent lifetime risk of developing papillary thyroid cancer. The average age at thyroid cancer diagnosis is 28 and women with FAP appear to be at greater risk than men. FAP is most commonly associated with an increased risk of colorectal cancer and accounts for about 1 per cent of colorectal cancer cases. People with FAP typically develop hundreds to thousands of colon polyps (small growths). The polyps are initially benign, but there is nearly a 100 per cent chance that the polyps will develop into cancer if left untreated. In FAP, colorectal cancer usually occurs by the age of 40. Individuals with FAP are also at risk for other types of cancer including stomach, small bowel, pancreas and hepatoblastoma (liver cancer seen mainly in early childhood).

Although FAP is inherited in an autosomal dominant pattern, approximately 30 per cent of people with FAP have no family history of the condition. Mutations in the *APC* gene cause FAP and attenuated familial adenomatous polyposis (AFAP).

Gardner syndrome, colonic polyposis with extra bowel tumours, especially osteomas, and a rather characteristic retinal lesion, is now known to be a phenotypic variant of FAP, caused by mutation in the *APC* gene. Herve *et al.* reported a case of papillary carcinoma in a 16-year-old girl with Gardner syndrome. They reviewed the literature and estimated that the incidence of thyroid carcinoma in patients with Gardner syndrome approached 100 times that of the general population.[130] Genetic testing for mutations in the APC gene is available.

Genetic counselling

Although variable, depending upon the syndrome and mutation, inherited cancer risk can approach 85–100 per cent over a lifetime. There are complex medical, psychosocial and ethical ramifications of identifying individuals at risk through genetic testing. Cancer genetic risk assessment and genetic counselling is the process of identifying and counselling individuals at risk for familial and hereditary cancer. The purpose of cancer genetic counselling is to educate patients about their chance of developing cancer, help them derive personal meaning from cancer genetic information, and empower them to make educated, informed decisions about genetic testing, cancer screening and cancer prevention. Informed decision making and informed consent requires understanding and integrated genetic, medical and psychosocial information. Because of the number of issues involved, comprehensive cancer genetic risk assessment and counselling benefits from a multidisciplinary approach including genetic counsellors, medical geneticists, surgeons, oncologists, and other relevant professionals that can help the patient address the different informational, medical and psychosocial needs.

Cancer genetic counselling process includes:

- **Personal, medical and family history**: The first step begins with the collection of a patient's personal and family history. This is often done using a questionnaire.
- **Psychosocial assessment**: An individual's decision to seek and utilize information regarding cancer genetics is based upon a variety of factors. Assessment of the psychosocial issues is the optimal method for the clinician to appreciate all of the factors that affect risk perception and ultimately, utilization of the cancer genetic information.[131] Further, this process also enlightens the provider on the potential impact of cancer genetic information on the client's quality of life, educational and career goal, and other aspects of their lives.
- **Molecular testing for hereditary cancer syndromes**: Consider offering molecular testing for hereditary cancer susceptibility only when a patient has a significant personal or family history of cancer, the test can be adequately interpreted, the results will affect medical management, the clinician can provide or make available adequate genetic education and counselling, and the patient can provide informed consent.[132] However, testing is not recommended in situations where there is a low probability of carrying a mutation given the potential psychosocial ramifications.
- **Pre-test genetic counselling and informed consent**: Informed consent is necessary for molecular testing, and involves a thorough discussion of the possible outcomes of testing, a review of the potential benefits, risks, and limitations, and a discussion of alternative testing to genetic testing. Elements of informed consent in cancer genetic risk assessment are detailed by Geller *et al.*[133] In

general, genetic cancer susceptibility testing is not performed on people under the age of 18 for consent reasons. The exception includes cases where medical intervention is warranted in childhood, such as MEN2 ret testing.

The pre-test counselling required for informed consent must include a discussion about the cancer risks associated with gene mutations, including the concepts of penetrance and variable expressivity. Further, accuracy of the genetic testing for the given gene should be discussed together with possible test outcome. An important issue that must be considered is genetic discrimination. The patients considering genetic testing need to be aware of the potential consequences on insurability, and whether the results will be disclosed to any third party (such as relatives). Further information about genetic discrimination and current legislation can be found at the following websites: www.thomas.loc.gov, www.tgac.org and www.nationalpartnership.org. Some life/disability insurers now include questions regarding genetic testing on the application form. There is also the possibility of employment discrimination.

- **Disclosure of test result and post-test counselling**: Together with the delivery of the result a review of the significance of the test must be provided. Given the specificity and sensitivity of the genetic test, a discussion of how the result affects the patient's cancer risk. Further, there must be a review of the screening recommendations and options of cancer reduction, prophylactic surgery and long-term monitoring, including the benefits, risks and limitations of these options. Appropriate referrals to other medical professionals for further discussions should be made as required.
- **Informing other relatives**: A discussion of cancer risks to other relatives and the importance of informing the appropriate family members about the genetic test result must be made. Only after written consent can the test result be shared with relatives. However, if a high-risk patient refuses to consent at-risk relatives, an ethics committee should be consulted ('duty to warn').

CANCER GENETICS AND GENETIC TESTING RESOURCES

GeneTests and GeneReviews: www.genetests.org
American Society of Clinical Oncology: www.asco.org
National Society of Genetic Counsellors: www.nsgc.org

KEY LEARNING POINTS

- There have been major advances in our understanding of the molecular basis for thyroid cancer. Key genes and their mutations have been demonstrated to be important in thyroid cancer biology. However, there remains much to be further elucidated.
- Our understanding of parathyroid tumour biology is less developed. Several genes have

been studied (*MEN1, PTH* and *HRPT2*) and have been postulated to play an important role in the development of parathyroid tumours. However, much of this information has been gathered from the study of hereditary diseases.
- Genetic testing in endocrine disease relates to the MEN syndromes. Genetic testing plays a key role in the management of MEN type 2 and less prominent role in MEN type 1.
- *ret* mutational analysis is now a key investigation in the management of patients with MEN type 2. *ret* analysis offers a risk stratification based on the codons mutated and guides clinical management.
- Genetic counselling is important prior to any genetic testing. Informed consent is integral to genetic counselling, which aims to provide the maximum benefit both for the clinician and the patient.

REFERENCES

◆ 1. Schlumberger MJ. Papillary and follicular thyroid carcinoma. *New England Journal of Medicine* 1998; **338**: 297–306.

2. Belfiore A, La Rosa GL, La Porta GA *et al*. Cancer risk in patients with cold thyroid nodules: relevance of iodine intake, sex, age, and multinodularity. *American Journal of Medicine* 1992; **93**: 363–9.

3. Heidenreich R, Machein M, Nicolaus A *et al*. Inhibition of solid tumor growth by gene transfer of VEGF receptor-1 mutants. *International Journal of Cancer* 2004; **111**: 348–57.

4. Schneider AB, Ron E. Carcinoma of the follicular epithelium: epidemiology and pathogenesis. In: Braverman LE, Utiger RD (eds). *The thyroid: a fundamental and clinical text*, 9th edn. Philadelphia, PA: Lippincott, Williams and Wilkins, 2005: 889–906.

5. Aeschimann S, Kopp PA, Kimura ET *et al*. Morphological and functional polymorphism within clonal thyroid nodules. *Journal of Clinical Endocrinology and Metabolism* 1993; **77**: 846–51.

6. Kim DS, McCabe CJ, Buchanan MA, Watkinson JC. Oncogenes in thyroid cancer. *Clinical Otolaryngology* 2003; **28**: 386–95.

◆ 7. Fagin JA. Minireview: branded from the start-distinct oncogenic initiating events may determine tumor fate in the thyroid. *Molecular Endocrinology* 2002; **16**: 903–11.

◆ 8. Hanahan D, Weinberg RA. The hallmarks of cancer. *Cell* 2000; **100**: 57–70.

◆ 9. Farid NR, Shi Y, Zou M. Molecular basis of thyroid cancer. *Endocrine Reviews* 1994; **15**: 202–32.

10. Dumont JE, Maenhaut C, Pirson I. Growth factors controlling the thyroid gland. *Baillière's Best Practice and Research Clinical Endocrinology and Metabolism* 1991; **5**: 727–54.

11. Hashimoto T, Matsubara F, Mizukami Y. Tumour markers and oncogene expression in thyroid cancer using biochemical and immunohistochemical studies. *Endocrine Journal* 1990; **37**: 247–54.

12. Di Carlo A, Mariano A, Pisano G. Epidermal growth factor receptor and thyrotropin response in human tissues. *Journal of Endocrinological Investigation* 1990; **13**: 293–9.

13. Mizukami Y, Nonomura A, Hashimoto T. Immunohistochemical demonstration of epidermal growth factor and c-myc oncogene product in normal, benign and malignant thyroid tissues. *Histopathology* 1991; **18**: 11–18.

14. Jasani B, Wyllie FS, Wright PA. Immunocytochemically detectable TGF-beta associated with malignancy in thyroid epithelial neolasia. *Growth Factors* 1990; **2**: 149–55.

15. Heldin NE, Gustavasson B, Claesson-Welsh L. Aberrant expression of receptors for platelet-derived growth factor in an anaplastic thyroid carcinoma cell line. *Proceedings of the National Academy of the United States of America* 1988; **85**: 9302–6.

16. Parma J, Duprez L, van Sande J *et al.* Somatic mutations in the thyrotropin receptor gene cause hyperfunctioning thyroid adenomas. *Nature* 1993; **365**: 649–51.

17. Ledent C, Dumont FE, Parmentier M *et al.* Thyroid expression of an A2 adenosine receptor transgene induces thyroid hyperplasia and hyperthyroidism. *EMBO Journal* 1992; **11**: 537–42.

◆ 18. Mazzaferri EL. Management of a solitary thyroid nodule. *New England Journal of Medicine* 1993; **328**: 553–9.

19. Vanvooren V, Uchino S, Duprez L *et al.* Oncogenic mutations in the thyrotropin receptor of autonomously functioning thyroid nodules in the Japanese population. *European Journal of Endocrinology* 2002; **147**: 287–91.

20. Goretzki PE, Lyons J, Stacey-Phipps S *et al.* Mutational activation of Ras and Gsp oncogenes in differentiated thyroid cancer and their biological implications. *World Journal of Surgery* 1992; **16**: 576–82.

21. Camacho P, Gordon D, Chiefari E *et al.* A Phe 486 thyrotropin receptor mutation in an autonomously functioning follicular carcinoma that was causing hyperthyroidism. *Thyroid* 2000; **10**: 1009–12.

22. Evans RM, Barish GD, Wang YX. PPARs and the complex journey to obesity. *Nature Medicine* 2004; **10**: 355–61.

23. Kroll TG, Sarraf P, Pecciarini L *et al.* PAX8-PPARgamma1 fusion oncogene in human thyroid carcinoma [corrected]. *Science* 2000; **289**: 1357–60.

24. Cheung L, Messina M, Gill A *et al.* Detection of the PAX8-PPAR gamma fusion oncogene in both follicular thyroid carcinomas and adenomas. *Journal of Clinical Endocrinology and Metabolism* 2003; **88**: 354–7.

25. Puzianowska-Kuznicka M, Krystyniak A, Madej A *et al.* Functionally impaired TR mutants are present in thyroid papillary cancer. *Journal of Clinical Endocrinology and Metabolism* 2002; **87**: 1120–8.

26. Suzuki H, Willingham MC, Cheng SY. Mice with a mutation in the thyroid hormone receptor beta gene spontaneously develop thyroid carcinoma: a mouse model of thyroid carcinogenesis. *Thyroid* 2002; **12**: 963–9.

27. Marshall CJ. Ras effectors. *Current Opinion in Cell Biology* 1996; **8**: 197–204.

28. Wright PA, Lemoine NR, Mayall ES *et al.* Papillary and follicular thyroid carcinomas show a different pattern of ras oncogene mutation. *British Journal of Cancer* 1989; **60**: 576–7.

29. Fusco A, Pinto A, Tramontano D *et al.* Block in the expression of differentiation markers of rat thyroid epithelial cells by transformation with Kirsten murine sarcoma virus. *Cancer Research* 1982; **42**: 618–26.

◆ 30. Fagin J. Molecular defects in thyroid gland neoplasia. *Journal of Clinical Endocrinology and Metabolism* 1992; **75**: 1398–400.

31. Schark C, Fulton N, Kaplan EL *et al.* N-ras 61 oncogene mutations in Hurthle cell tumours. *Surgery* 1990; **108**: 994–9.

32. Studer H, Gerber H, Peter HJ *et al.* Histomorphological and immunohistochemical evidence that human nodular goitres grow by episodic replication of multiple clusters of thyroid follicular cells. *Journal of Clinical Endocrinology and Metabolism* 1992; **75**: 1151–8.

● 33. Davies H, Bignell GR, Cox C *et al.* Mutations of the *BRAF* gene in human cancer. *Nature* 2002; **417**: 949–54.

34. Kimura ET, Nikiforova MN, Zhu Z *et al.* High prevalence of *BRAF* mutations in thyroid cancer: genetic evidence for constitutive activation of the RET/PTC-RAS-*BRAF* signaling pathway in papillary thyroid carcinoma. *Cancer Research* 2003; **63**: 1454–7.

35. Cohen Y, Xing M, Mambo E *et al.* *BRAF* mutation in papillary thyroid carcinoma. *Journal of the National Cancer Institute* 2003; **95**: 625–7.

36. Soares P, Trovisco V, Rocha AS *et al.* *BRAF* mutations and RET/PTC rearrangements are alternative events in the etiopathogenesis of PTC. *Oncogene* 2003; **22**: 4578–80.

37. Namba H, Nakashima M, Hayashi T *et al.* Clinical implication of hot spot *BRAF* mutation, V599E, in papillary thyroid cancers. *Journal of Clinical Endocrinology and Metabolism* 2003; **88**: 4393–7.

38. Nikiforova MN, Kimura ET, Gandhi M *et al.* BRAF mutations in thyroid tumors are restricted to papillary carcinomas and anaplastic or poorly differentiated carcinomas arising from papillary carcinomas. *Journal of Clinical Endocrinology and Metabolism* 2003; **88**: 5399–404.

39. Xing M, Tufano RP, Tufaro AP *et al.* Detection of *BRAF* mutation on fine needle aspiration biopsy specimens: a new diagnostic tool for papillary thyroid cancer. *Journal of Clinical Endocrinology and Metabolism* 2004; **89**: 2867–72.

40. Eilers M, Schirm S, Bishop JM. The Myc protein activates transcription of the alpha-prothymosin gene. *EMBO Journal* 1991; **10**: 133–41.

41. Curran T. *The fos oncogene*. New York: Elsevier, 1988.
42. Del Senno L, Gambari R, Degli Uberti E *et al*. c-myc oncogene alterations in uman thyroid carcinomas. *Cancer Detection and Prevention* 1987; **10**: 159–66.
43. Terrier P, Sheng ZM, Schlumberger M *et al*. Structure and expression of c-myc and c-fos proto-oncogenes in thyroid carcinomas. *British Journal of Cancer* 1988; **57**: 43–7.
44. Comoglio PM. Structure, biosynthesis and biochemical properties of the HGF receptor in normal and malignant cells. *EXS* 1993; **65**: 131–65.
45. Matsumato K, Nakamura J. Hepatocyte growth factor: molecular structure, roles in liver regeneration and other biological functions. *Critical Reviews in Oncogenesis* 1992; **3**: 27–54.
46. Di Renzo MF, Narsimhan RP, Olivero M *et al*. Expression of the Met/HGF receptor in normal and neoplastic human tissues. *Oncogene* 2003; **6**: 1997–2003.
47. Aasland R, Lillenhaug JR, Male R *et al*. Expression of oncogenes in thyroid tumours: co-expression of c-erbB2/neu and c-erb. *British Journal of Cancer* 1988; **57**: 358–63.
48. Santoro M, Carlomagno F, Hay ID *et al*. Ret oncogene activation in human thyroid neoplasms is restricted to the papillary cancer subtype. *Journal of Clinical Investigation* 1992; **89**: 1517–22.
49. Mulligan LM, Kwok JB, Ponder BA *et al*. Germ-line mutations of the Ret proto-oncogene in multiple endocrine neoplasia type 2A. *British Journal of Cancer* 1993; **363**: 458–60.
• 50. Fusco A, Grieco M, Jenkins RB *et al*. A new oncogene in human papillary thyroid carcinomas and their lymph-nodal metastases. *Nature* 1987; **328**: 170–2.
51. Pierotti MA, Santoro M, Jenkins RB. Characterization of an inversion on the long arm of chromosome 10 juxtaposing D10S170 and Ret and creating the oncogene sequence ret/PTC. *Proceedings of the National Academy of the United States of America* 1992; **89**: 1616–20.
• 52. Grieco M, Santoro M, Vecchio G *et al*. PTC is a novel rearranged form of the ret proto-oncogene and is frequently detected *in vivo* in human thyroid papillary carcinomas. *Cell* 1990; **60**: 557–63.
53. Santoro M, Melillo RM, Carlomagno F *et al*. Molecular mechanisms of RET activation in human cancer. *Annals of the New York Academy of Sciences* 2002; **963**: 116–21.
54. Nikiforov YE, Rowland JM, Bove KE *et al*. Distinct pattern of ret oncogene rearrangements in morphological variants of radiation-induced and sporadic thyroid papillary carcinomas in children. *Cancer Research* 1997; **57**: 1690–4.
55. Fugazzola L, Pilotti S, Pinchera A *et al*. Oncogenic rearrangements of the RET proto-oncogene in papillary thyroid carcinomas from children exposed to the Chernobyl nuclear accident. *Cancer Research* 1995; **55**: 5617–20.
56. Bongarzone I, Fugazzola L, Vigneri P *et al*. Age-related activation of the tyrosine kinase receptor protooncogenes RET and NTRK1 in papillary thyroid carcinoma. *Journal of Clinical Endocrinology and Metabolism* 1996; **81**: 2006–9.
57. Cheung CC, Carydis B, Ezzat S *et al*. Analysis of ret/PTC gene rearrangements refines the fine needle aspiration diagnosis of thyroid cancer. *Journal of Clinical Endocrinology and Metabolism* 2001; **86**: 2187–90.
58. Elisei R, Romei C, Vorontsova T *et al*. RET/PTC rearrangements in thyroid nodules: studies in irradiated and not irradiated, malignant and benign thyroid lesions in children and adults. *Journal of Clinical Endocrinology and Metabolism* 2001; **86**: 3211–16.
59. Chiappetta G, Toti P, Cetta F *et al*. The RET/PTC oncogene is frequently activated in oncocytic thyroid tumors (Hurthle cell adenomas and carcinomas), but not in oncocytic hyperplastic lesions. *Journal of Clinical Endocrinology and Metabolism* 2002; **87**: 364–9.
60. Bongarzone I, Pierotti MA, Monzini N *et al*. High frequency of activation of tyrosine kinase oncogenes in human papillary thyroid carcinoma. *Oncogene* 1989; **4**: 1457–62.
61. Grieco A, Pierotti MA, Della Porta G *et al*. Trk-T1 is a novel oncogene formed by the fusion of TPR and Trk genes in human papillary thyroid carcinomas. *Oncogene* 1992; **7**: 237–42.
62. Lanzi C, Borrello MG, Bongarzone T *et al*. Identification of the product of two oncogenic re-arranged forms of the ret proto-oncogene in papillary thyroid carcinomas. *Oncogene* 1992; **7**: 2189–94.
63. Santoro M, Meilillo RM, Fusco A *et al*. The Trk and Ret tyrosine kinase oncogenes cooperate with ras in the neoplastic transformation of a rat thyroid epithelial cell line. *Cell Growth and Differentiation* 1993; **4**: 77–84.
64. Bond JA, Wyllie AH, Wynford-Thomas D *et al*. In vitro reconstruction of tumour initiation in a human epithelium. *Oncogene* 1994; **9**: 281–90.
65. Shahedian B, Shi Y, Zou M, Farid NR. Thyroid carcinoma is characterized by genomic instability: evidence from p53 mutations. *Molecular Genetics and Metabolism* 2001; **72**: 155–63.
• 66. Fagin JA, Matsuo K, Karmakar A *et al*. High prevalence of mutations of the p53 gene in poorly differentiated human thyroid carcinomas. *Journal of Clinical Investigation* 1993; **91**: 179–84.
67. Zou MJ, Shi YF, Farid NR. Retinoblastoma gene defects are central to thyroid carcinogenesis. *Endocrine Journal* 1994; **2**: 193–8.
68. Ward LS, Brenta G, Medvedovic M, Fagin JA. Studies of allelic loss in thyroid tumors reveal major differences in chromosomal instability between papillary and follicular carcinomas. *Journal of Clinical Endocrinology and Metabolism* 1998; **83**: 525–30.

69. Herrmann MA, Hay ID, Bartelt DH. Cytogenetic and molecular genetic studies of follicular and papillary thyroid cancers. *Journal of Clinical Investigation* 1991; **88**: 1596–604.

70. Matsuo K, Tang SH, Fagin JA. Allelotype of human thyroid tumors: loss of chromosome 11q13 sequences in follicular neoplasms. *Molecular Endocrinology* 1991; **5**: 1873–9.

71. Cheng K, Loeb L. Genetic instability and tumour progression: mechanistic considerations. *Advances in Cancer Research* 1993; **60**: 121–56.

72. Renan M. How many mutations are required for tumourigenesis? Implications from human cancer data. *Molecular Carcinogenesis* 1993; **7**: 139–46.

73. Loeb L. Mutator phenotype may be required for multistage carcinogenesis. *Cancer Research* 1991; **51**: 3075–9.

74. Zedenius J, Wallin G, Svensson A *et al.* Allelotyping of follicular thyroid tumors. *Human Genetics* 1995; **96**: 27–32.

75. Joensuu H, Klemi P, Eerola E. DNA aneuploidy in follicular adenomas of the thyroid gland. *American Journal of Pathology* 1986; **124**: 373–6.

76. Joensuu H, Klemi PJ. Comparison of nuclear DNA content in primary and metastatic differentiated thyroid carcinoma. *American Journal of Clinical Pathology* 1988; **89**: 35–40.

77. Sturgis CD, Caraway NP, Johnston DA *et al.* Image analysis of papillary thyroid carcinoma fine-needle aspirates: significant association between aneuploidy and death from disease. *Cancer Research* 1999; **87**: 155–60.

78. Lazzereschi D, Palmirotta R, Ranieri A *et al.* Microsatellite instability in thyroid tumours and tumour-like lesions. *British Journal of Cancer* 1999; **79**: 340–5.

79. Wiseman SM, Loree TR, Rigual NR *et al.* Papillary thyroid cancer: high inter-(simple sequence repeat) genomic instability in a typically indolent cancer. *Head and Neck* 2003; **25**: 825–32.

80. Stoler DL, Datta RV, Charles MA *et al.* Genomic instability measurement in the diagnosis of thyroid neoplasms. *Head and Neck* 2002; **24**: 290–5.

81. Folkman J. What is the evidence that tumors are angiogenesis dependent? *Journal of the National Cancer Institute* 1990; **82**: 4–6.

82. Bergers G, Benjamin LE. Tumorigenesis and the angiogenic switch. *National Reviews Cancer* 2003; **3**: 401–10.

83. Akslen LA, Livolsi VA. Increased angiogenesis in papillary thyroid carcinoma but lack of prognostic importance. *Human Pathology* 2000; **31**: 439–42.

84. Segal K, Shpitzer T, Feinmesser M *et al.* Angiogenesis in follicular tumors of the thyroid. *Journal of Surgical Oncology* 1996; **63**: 95–8.

85. Dhar DK, Kubota H, Kotoh T *et al.* Tumor vascularity predicts recurrence in differentiated thyroid carcinoma. *American Journal of Surgery* 1998; **176**: 442–7.

86. Ishiwata T, Iino Y, Takei H *et al.* Tumor angiogenesis as an independent prognostic indicator in human papillary thyroid carcinoma. *Oncology Reports* 1998; **5**: 1343–8.

87. Katoh R, Miyagi E, Kawaoi A *et al.* Expression of vascular endothelial growth factor (VEGF) in human thyroid neoplasms. *Human Pathology* 1999; **30**: 891–7.

88. Klein M, Picard E, Vignaud JM *et al.* Vascular endothelial growth factor gene and protein: strong expression in thyroiditis and thyroid carcinoma. *Journal of Endocrinology* 1999; **161**: 41–9.

89. Soh EY, Duh QY, Sobhi SA *et al.* Vascular endothelial growth factor expression is higher in differentiated thyroid cancer than in normal or benign thyroid. *Journal of Clinical Endocrinology and Metabolism* 1997; **82**: 3741–7.

90. Bunone G, Vigneri P, Mariani L *et al.* Expression of angiogenesis stimulators and inhibitors in human thyroid tumors and correlation with clinical pathological features. *American Journal of Pathology* 1999; **155**: 1967–76.

91. Fellmer PT, Sato K, Tanaka R *et al.* Vascular endothelial growth factor-C gene expression in papillary and follicular thyroid carcinomas. *Surgery* 1999; **126**: 1056–61; discussion 61–2.

92. Gagel RF, Marx SJ. Multiple endocrine neoplasia. In: *Williams textbook of endocrinology*, 11th edn. Philadelphia: Saunders, 2007.

93. Mendelsohn G, Wells SA, Baylin SB. Relationship of carcinoembryonic antigen and calcitonin to tumor virulence in medullary thyroid carcinoma. *Cancer* 1984; **54**: 657–62.

94. Eng C, Clayton D, Schuffenecker L *et al.* The relationship between specific RET proto-oncogene mutations and disease phenotype in multiple endocrine neoplasia type 2. International RET mutation consortium analysis. *Journal of the American Medical Association* 1996; **276**: 1575–9.

95. Hofstra RM, Landsvater RM, Ceccherini I *et al.* A mutation in the RET proto-oncogene associated with multiple endocrine neoplasia type 2B and sporadic medullary thyroid carcinoma. *Nature* 1994; **367**: 375–6.

96. Schuffenecker I, Ginet N, Goldgar D *et al.* Prevalence and parental origin of de novo RET mutations in MEN 2a and FMTC. *American Journal of Human Genetics* 1997; **60**: 233–7.

97. Romei C, Elisei R, Pinchera A *et al.* Somatic mutations of the ret proto-oncogene in sporadic medullary thyroid carcinoma are not restricted to exon 16 and are associated with tumor recurrence. *Journal of Clinical Endocrinology and Metabolism* 1996; **81**: 1619–22.

98. Klimpfinger M, Ruhri C, Putz B *et al.* Oncogene expression in medullary thyroid cancer. *Virchows Archiv. B: Cell Pathology* 1988; **54**: 256–9.

99. Boultwood J, Wyllie FS, Williams ED *et al.* N-myc expression in neoplasia of human thyroid cells. *Cancer Research* 1988; **48**: 4073–7.

100. Wiseman SM, Loree TR, Rigual NR *et al.* Anaplastic transformation of thyroid cancer: review of clinical, pathologic, and molecular evidence provides new insights into disease biology and future therapy. *Head and Neck* 2003; **25**: 662–70.

101. Abe Y, Ichikawa Y, Muraki T *et al.* Thyrotropin (TSH) receptor and adenylate cyclase activity in human thyroid tumors: absence of high affinity receptor and loss of TSH responsiveness in undifferentiated thyroid carcinoma. *Journal of Clinical Endocrinology and Metabolism* 1981; **52**: 23–8.

102. Wada N, Duh QY, Miura D *et al.* Chromosomal aberrations by comparative genomic hybridization in hurthle cell thyroid carcinomas are associated with tumor recurrence. *Journal of Clinical Endocrinology and Metabolism* 2002; **87**: 4595–601.

103. Kadota M, Tamaki Y, Sakita I *et al.* Identification of a 7-cM region of frequent allelic loss on chromosome band 16p13.3 that is specifically associated with anaplastic thyroid carcinoma. *Oncology Reports* 2000; **7**: 529–33.

104. Donghi R, Longoni A, Pilotti S *et al.* Gene p53 mutations are restricted to poorly differentiated and undifferentiated carcinomas of the thyroid gland. *Journal of Clinical Investigation* 1993; **91**: 1753–60.

105. Fagin JA, Tang SH, Zeki K *et al.* Reexpression of thyroid peroxidase in a derivative of an undifferentiated thyroid carcinoma cell line by introduction of wild-type p53. *Cancer Research* 1996; **56**: 765–71.

106. Zou MJ, Shi YF, Farid NR. Frequent inactivation of the retinoblastoma gene in human thyroid carcinoma. *Endocrine Journal* 1993; **39**: 269–74.

107. Silverberg SJ, Bilezikian JP. *Primary hyperparathyroidism.* Philadelphia: Lippincott-Willliams and Wilkins, 2001.

108. Attie JN, Bock G, Auguste L. Multiple parathyroid adenoomas: report of thirty-three cases. *Surgery* 1990; **108**: 1014–102.

109. Verdonk CA, Edis AJ. Parathyroid 'double adenomas': fact or fiction? *Surgery* 1981; **90**: 523–6.

110. Arnold A, Kim HG, Gaz RD *et al.* Molecular cloning and chromosomal mapping of DNA rearranged with the parathyroid hormone gene in a parathyroid adenoma. *Journal of Clinical Investigation* 1989; **83**: 2034–40.

111. Hsi ED, Zukerberg LR, Yang WI, Arnold A. Cyclin D1/PRAD1 expression in parathyroid adenomas: an immunohistochemical study. *Journal of Clinical Endocrinology and Metabolism* 1996; **81**: 1736–9.

112. Cryns VL, Thor A, Xu HJ *et al.* Loss of the retinoblastoma tumor suppressor gene in parathyroid carcinoma. *New England Journal of Medicine* 1994; **330**: 757–61.

113. Cryns VL, Yi SM, Tahara H *et al.* Frequent loss of chromosome arm 1p DNA in para-thyroid adenomas. *Genes, Chromosomes and Cancer* 1995; **13**: 9–17.

114. Chandrasekharappa SC, Guru SC, Manickam P *et al.* Positional cloning of the gene for multiple endocrine neoplasia-type 1. *Science* 1997; **276**: 404–7.

115. Carpten JD, Robbins CM, Villablanca A *et al.* HRPT2, encoding parafibromin, is mutated in hyperparathyroidism-jaw tumor syndrome. *Nature Genetics* 2002; **32**: 676–80.

116. Shattuck TM, Valimaki S, Obara T *et al.* Somatic and germ-line mutations of the HRPT2 gene in sporadic parathyroid carcinoma. *New England Journal of Medicine* 2003; **349**: 1722–9.

117. Howell VM, Haven CJ, Kahnoski K *et al.* HRPT2 mutations are associated with malignancy in sporadic parathyroid tumours. *Journal of Medical Genetics* 2003; **40**: 657–63.

118. Marx SJ. *Multiple endocrine neoplasia type 1*, 8th edn. New York: McGraw-Hill, 2001.

119. Uchino S, Noguchi S, Sato M *et al.* Screening of the MEN1 gene and discovery of germ-line and somatic mutations in apparently sporadic parathyroid tumors. *Cancer Research* 2000; **60**: 5553–7.

◆ 120. Thakker RV. Genetics of endocrine and metabolic disorders: parathyroid. *Reviews in Endocrine and Metabolic Disorders* 2004; **5**: 37–51.

121. Brandi ML, Gagel RF, Angeli A *et al.* Guidelines for diagnosis and theyapy of MEN type 1 and type 2. *Journal of Clinical Endocrinology and Metabolism* 2001; **86**: 5658–71.

122. Bassett JH, Forbes SA, Pannett AA *et al.* Characterization of mutations in patients with multiple endocrine neoplasia type I. *American Journal of Human Genetics* 1998; **62**: 232–44.

123. Kakudo K, Carney JA, Sizemore GW. Medullary carcinoma of thyroid. Biologic behavior of the sporadic and familial neoplasm. *Cancer* 1985; **55**: 2818–821.

124. Gagel RF, Tashjian AH Jr, Cummings T *et al.* The clinical outcome of prospective screening for multiple endocrine neoplasia type 2a: an 18-year experience. *New England Journal of Medicine* 1988; **318**: 478–84.

◆ 125. Lips CJM. Clinical management of the multiple endocrine neoplasia syndromes: results of a computerized opinion poll at the Sixth International Workshop on Multiple Endocrine Neoplasia and von-Hippel-Lindau disease. *Journal of Internal Medicine* 1998; **243**: 589–94.

126. Eng C, Mulligan LM, Smith DP *et al.* Low frequency of germline mutations in the RET proto-oncogene in patients with apparently sporadic medullary thyroid carcinoma. *Clinical Endocrinology* 1995; **43**: 123–7

127. Zedenius J, Larsson C, Bergholm U *et al*. Mutations of codon 918 in the RET proto-oncogene correlate to poor prognosis in sporadic medullary thyroid carcinomas. *Journal of Clinical Endocrinology and Metabolism* 1995; **80**: 3088–90.

128. Marsh DJ, Coulon V, Lunetta KL *et al*. Mutation spectrum and genotype-phenotype analyses in Cowden disease and Bannayan-Zonana syndrome, two hamartoma syndromes with germline PTEN mutation. *Human Molecular Genetics* 1998; **7**: 507–15.

129. Tsou HC, Teng DH-F, Ping XL *et al*. The role of MMAC1 mutations in early-onset breast cancer: causative in association with Cowden syndrome and excluded in BRCA1-negative cases. *American Journal of Human Genetics* 1997; **61**: 1036–43.

130. Herve R, Farret O, Mayaudon H *et al*. Association syndrome de Gardner et carcinome thyroidien. *La Presse Médicale* 1995; **24**: 415.

131. Biesecker BB. Psychological issues in cancer genetics. *Seminars in Oncology Nursing* 1997; **13**: 129–34.

◆ 132. American Society of Clinical Oncology. Statement of the American Society of Clinical Oncology: Genetic testing for cancer susceptibility. *Journal of Clinical Oncology* 1996; **14**: 1730–40.

133. Geller G, Botkin JR, Green MJ *et al*. Genetic testing for susceptibility to adult-onset cancer. The process and content of informed consent. *Journal of the American Medical Association* 1997; **277**: 1467–74.

19

Thyroid and parathyroid gland pathology

RAM MOORTHY AND ADRIAN T WARFIELD

Send a slide to five different pathologists and receive six different answers.

Anon

INTRODUCTION

The endocrine pathology discussed in this chapter is that affecting the extracranial endocrine system, that is the thyroid and parathyroid glands found in the anterior triangle of the neck bilaterally. This section is not intended to be an encyclopaedic treatise, more a summary overview with selective consideration of clinically important differential diagnoses. Surgical pathology is a visual subject, therefore no apology is offered for the liberal use of illustrations to supplement the text.

THYROID GLAND

The normal thyroid gland

The term 'thyroid gland' was first coined by Thomas Wharton in the seventeenth century to describe the gland in close proximity to the 'shield-shaped' thyroid cartilage.[1]

Embryologically, the thyroid gland develops from the median anlage and the two lateral anlagen. The median anlage starts as a thickening of the endodermal epithelium in the foregut between the first and second branchial arches at the base of the tongue close to the developing myocardium,[1,2] which in later life constitutes the foramen caecum. The cells proliferate to form the thyroid bud and then a diverticulum, which expands and migrates from the base of tongue to lie anterior to the trachea. The track between the thyroid gland and base of tongue typically disappears by birth. The two lateral anlagen (known as the 'ultimobranchial bodies') develop from the caudal aspect of the fourth pharyngeal pouch supplemented by migratory neural crest elements and fuse with the median anlage as the thyroid gland descends in the neck. The median anlage forms the thyroid follicular cells and the lateral anlagen form the clear parafollicular cells (C-cells).[3]

The thyroid gland is the largest of the discrete endocrine organs typically weighing between 15 and 25 g (roughly 0.4 per cent of body mass), being slightly larger in women,[1] dependent upon age, nutritional and hormonal status. Macroscopically, the normal thyroid gland presents a bilobate structure with a reddish-brown colour. The two lobes are connected by a central isthmus. A vestigial, accessory pyramidal lobe is present superiorly in 40 per cent of the population. There is a thin investing fibrous capsule, which is continuous with the pretracheal fascia. This capsule, however, is discontiguous or focally interrupted in approximately 60 per cent of individuals and extracapsular thyroid tissue is present in almost 90 per cent of glands. A variety of pericapsular inclusions, such as parathyroid tissue, heterotopic thymus, lymph nodes and autonomic paraganglia, are considered normal. Mesenchymal derived inclusions within the thyroid gland include stromal adipocytic, skeletal muscular and cartilaginous elements.[4]

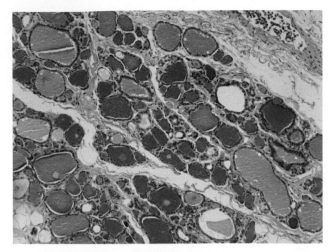

Figure 19.1   Normal thyroid gland demonstrating a lobular architecture with uniform, round/ovoid follicles. The latter contain plentiful stored colloid with fine marginal vacuolation. The parallel linear marks in the colloid ('ripple' or 'wave' effect) are an artefact of microtomy. The C-cell population is typically inconspicuous (H&E stain, low magnification).

Microscopically, the functional unit of the thyroid gland is the follicle, which in the euthyroid state consists of a monolayer of cuboidal or flattened epithelial cells (thyrocytes) surrounding a central lumen containing stored colloid. The follicles are loosely aggregated into lobules (thyromeres), each containing circa 20 to 50 follicles separated by slender connective tissue septula (**Figure 19.1**). Intracolloidal birefringent oxalate crystals, brown cytoplasmic lipofuscin ('wear and tear') pigment and haemosiderin pigment are usually of incidental portent, though may be increased with age and in certain disease states. The C-cells form a minor cell subpopulation, accounting for less than 10 per cent by number, and are typically concentrated at the junction between the middle and upper thirds of the lateral lobes in a hypothetical central longitudinal axis through each lobe, corresponding to the planes of medial and lateral anlagen fusion – solid cell nests, C-cell hyperplasia and medullary thyroid carcinoma, therefore, do not ordinarily occur in the isthmus. C-cells are usually larger, more rounded, polyhedral or fusiform in shape, with paler cytoplasm than follicular epithelium.

SOLID CELL NESTS

So-called solid cell nests (SCN) are collections of non-follicular cells, found in approximately 25 per cent of resected thyroid glands, which probably represent remnants of the ultimobranchial apparatus. They are present in greater numbers in infants and children and gradually decline with advancing age. The role of SCN in the normal structure and function of the thyroid gland is incompletely understood and their biological significance remains a source of controversy and debate. Solid cell nests may harbour minimal properties of a stem cell phenotype with capacity for self-renewal and end differentiation.

Solid cell nests comprise irregularly shaped clusters of interfollicular cells delineated by basal lamina. The dominant

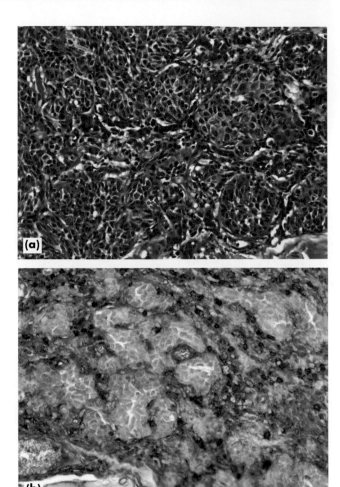

Figure 19.2   (a) Ultimobranchial apparatus rests (solid cell nests) disposed as discrete congeries of squamoid (epidermoid) cells without keratinization, discovered incidentally in a thyroidectomy specimen indicated for partially treated Graves' disease (H&E stain, medium magnification). (b) Such cell rests typically express pan-neuroendocrine immunomarkers, but not thyroglobulin and are thus shown here in negative relief (thyroglobulin IHC, medium magnification).

cell component (main cell) comprises polygonal to fusiform cells disposed in solid array sometimes with an epidermoid appearance, though generally non-keratinizing and devoid of intercellular bridges ('prickles'). They less commonly show a glandular morphology and may paradoxically be microcystic, micropapillary and/or mucinous. SCN coexpress cytokeratins, carcinoembryonic antigen (CEA, CD66e), galectin-3 and many pan-neuropeptides, such as chromogranin A, synaptophysin and somatostatin, but are negative for markers of terminal differentiation, such as thyroglobulin (TG), thyroid transcription factor-1 (TTF-1) and calcitonin (**Figure 19.2**). They may also contain a minor subpopulation of C-cells, which show a partially differentiated immunophenotype. SCN consistently stain for p63, a homologue of p53, a nuclear transcription factor that induces expression of cytokeratin 5 (CK5) and cytokeratin 14 (CK14). The gene for p63 is universally expressed in basal cells of stratified epithelia and plays a major role in triggering the maturation of these into squamous epithelium. Solid cell nests are postulated to be precursors of certain thyroid gland neoplasms, notably papillary thyroid carcinoma. They may also play a role in the histogenesis of Hashimoto's thyroiditis, which is also associated with papillary thyroid carcinoma. Papillary thyroid carcinoma and Hashimoto's thyroiditis, therefore, may be linked in pathogenesis via a common population of pluripotent p63 positive embryonal stem cell remnant progenitors.[5]

FINE NEEDLE ASPIRATION CYTOLOGY

Fine needle aspiration cytology (FNAC) is generally recognized as an effective first-line investigation in the evaluation of a thyroid swelling.[6, 7, 8, 9] In experienced hands, FNAC of the thyroid gland is accurate with a sensitivity of 65–98 per cent, a specificity of 72–100 per cent, a false-positive rate of 1–8 per cent and false-negative rate of 1–11 per cent.[7, 10] The non-diagnostic or inadequate rate can be as high as 28 per cent,[10] but targeting by ultrasound (US) guidance can reduce the incidence of a non-diagnostic FNAC.[11] US guidance is recommended in nodules with a higher chance of non-diagnostic FNAC by simple palpation. These include cystic nodules and smaller or non-palpable lesions.[9] Thus, FNAC as a screening test is highly sensitive, though lacks specificity – circa 15–30 per cent of aspirates designated suspect of a follicular neoplasm are ultimately malignant, ergo the remaining majority 70–85 per cent or so of nodules are benign in the final analysis.

FNAC is substantially a screening/triage procedure for follicular carcinoma, identifying those patients who require further investigation and a primary diagnostic test for other thyroid malignancies, principally papillary carcinoma, medullary carcinoma, undifferentiated (anaplastic) carcinoma and lymphoma. The traditional wet-fixed and air-dried direct smear methodology supplemented by cell concentration techniques, such as centrifugation, filtration and cell blocks, generally remains the gold standard in thyroid FNAC in preference to the newer liquid-based technology, though with ongoing development and experience this may shift. The cytopathologist, however, can only ever be as good as the aspiration sample that he or she receives.

In spite of acknowledged cytodiagnostic pitfalls, some outlined below, the use of FNAC in the preliminary evaluation of solitary or dominant nodules reduces the use of surgery by approximately one-third, doubles the proportion of malignancies among surgical resections and increases cost-effectiveness. Serious diagnostic delay due to false-negative FNAC is uncommon where there is appropriate clinical follow up.[12]

Historically, the diagnostic criteria and reporting nomenclature employed have varied widely, although these have evolved to broad consensus, as epitomized by the North American National Cancer Institute (Bethesda) terminology (2007)[13] stratified into six subdivisions and the parallel UK Royal College of Physicians/British Thyroid Association guidelines (2002 and 2007), the latter updated in 2009 by the Royal College of Pathologists in consultation with the British Society for Clinical Cytology and other interested parties.[14] These schemata are outlined in **Table 19.1**.

The Italian Society of Pathology and Cytopathology/Italian Section of the International Academy of Pathology classification (2007)[15] substantially mirrors the UK five-tier system with a single category encompassing all borderline lesions (designated 'follicular proliferation' and 'follicular lesion', respectively). The shorthand numerical diagnostic coding intrinsic to these systems is not intended to replace a full narrative cytology report. Furthermore, the vernacular habit of grouping non-diagnostic/unsatisfactory and non-neoplastic/benign aspirates under the rubric 'negative reports' should be dispelled. As a fundamental principle, it is emphasized that while the presence of malignant cells is diagnostic, the absence of malignant cells can never be wholly exclusionary. The WHO classification schema (2004) for carcinoma of the thyroid gland[8] is widely endorsed.

The technique for specimen preparation is summarized in Chapter 6, Head and neck pathology.

Limitations of FNAC of the thyroid gland

The follicular patterned lesion is the most commonly encountered type of thyroid FNAC specimen in clinical practice. Distinction between a hyperplastic (adenomatoid) nodule in a multinodular goitre and a follicular neoplasm may not always be achievable. The presence of dispersed colloid, monolayered sheets of bland thyrocytes and normofollicular or macrofollicular structures are more typical of hyperplasia. Dense colloid globules, paucity or absence of colloid and microfollicular configuration (**Figure 19.3**) tend to support neoplasia. It is necessary to focus on the predominant cytoarchitectural pattern, rather than a minor subpopulation of microfollicles, with the proviso that this approach is predicated upon adequate cell sampling. The agreed criterion for this is that samples from solid lesions should contain at least six groups of thyroid follicular epithelial cells across all the submitted slides, each composed of at least ten well-visualized epithelial cells. Note that this constitutes a minimum standard, though the degree of diagnostic confidence should increase with higher yield samples and that this threshold does not necessarily preclude a positive diagnosis of malignancy if a lesser quantum of characteristic cells is present.

Reliable discrimination between a benign adenoma and differentiated follicular carcinoma on subjective morphological grounds is now realized to be always difficult, often impossible. While the presence of high cellularity, cell crowding, tridimensional (acervate) groups, nucleomegaly, cytonuclear atypia, three or more nucleoli per cell, irregular karyoplasm and necrosis are individually not absolute, in aggregate they tend to favour a diagnosis of malignancy. Follicular variant of papillary thyroid carcinoma (FVPTC) enters the differential diagnosis, where a scrupulous search for its characteristic nuclear morphology is indicated. The separation of minimally invasive from widely invasive follicular carcinoma on FNAC, contingent upon extent of extracapsular invasion, is obviously untenable *ab initio*.

Oncocytic (oxyphil) cell lesions are problematical on FNAC. Hashimoto's thyroiditis and oncocytic (oxyphil) metaplasia in multinodular hyperplasia are generally separated by conspicuous lymphocytosis in the former

Table 19.1   Comparison of the BTA/RC/RCPathP[6, 14] and Bethesda[15, 16] classification systems for reporting thyroid gland fine needle aspiration cytology (FNAC) specimens together with their clinical implications.

BTA/RCP/RCPath	Bethesda	Risk of malignancy (based on Bethesda classification)
Thy1, non-diagnostic for cytological diagnosis	I, non-diagnostic or unsatisfactory Virtually acellular specimen Other (obscuring blood, clot, etc.)	1–4%
Thy1c, non-diagnostic for cytological diagnosis in a cystic lesion	Cyst fluid only	Up to 10% of cystic lesions harbour malignancy
Thy2, non-neoplastic	II, benign Consistent with a benign follicular nodule (includes adenomatoid or colloid nodule) Consistent with lymphocytic (Hashimoto's) thyroiditis in the proper clinical context Consistent with granulomatous thyroiditis Other	0–3%
Thy2c, non-neoplastic cystic lesion		
Thy3a, neoplasm possible – atypia/non-diagnostic	III, atypia of undetermined significance or follicular lesion of undetermined significance	5–15%
Thy3f, neoplasm possible, suggesting follicular neoplasm	IV, follicular neoplasm or suspicious for a follicular neoplasm	15–30%
	Specify if oncocytic (Hürthle) cell type	15–45%
Thy4, suspicious of malignancy	V, suspicious for malignancy (papillary, medullary, metastatic, lymphoma, other)	60–75%
Thy5, malignant	VI, malignant (papillary, poorly differentiated, undifferentiated/anaplastic, medullary, squamous cell carcinoma, carcinoma with mixed features (specify), non-Hodgkin's lymphoma, metastatic, other)	97–99%

(**Figure 19.4**), although the degree of inflammatory cell infiltrate varies with the natural history of the disease and paucilymphocytic variants are described. The cytological distinction between Hürthle cell adenoma and carcinoma is unreliable – benign oncocytic (oxyphil) cells may display extreme pleomorphism and, paradoxically, there is often less cytonuclear variation in Hürthle cell neoplasms. Confident recognition of the rare oncocytic (oxyphil) variant of papillary thyroid carcinoma on FNAC is extremely difficult. The conclusion oncocytic (oxyphil) cell lesion or neoplasm, not otherwise specified is occasionally the best that can be achieved with a recommendation for excision, as clinically indicated. A solitary thyroid nodule composed predominantly of oncocytes on FNAC merits excision because oncocytic (oxyphil) thyroid neoplasms show on average a 30 per cent malignancy rate based on histology. Moreover, the larger an oncocytic tumour, the greater the likelihood of invasive malignancy – there is a 65–80 per cent chance of malignancy in oncocytic neoplasms exceeding 4 cm maximum dimension.

Aspirates from cystic lesions may not be fully diagnostic, particularly if there is limited or degenerate epithelial sampling. Cysts of any type tend to contain variform inflammatory cells, foam cells, pigmented macrophages and cytolytic debris (**Figure 19.5**). Copious dispersed colloid favours benignity, though in the absence of adequate epithelial cell content the possibility of a cystic neoplasm or cystic degeneration in a neoplasm, of which papillary thyroid carcinoma is paradigmatic, cannot be completely ruled out on FNAC microscopical appearances in isolation – up to 10 per cent of thyroid carcinomas missed on FNAC harbour a cystic component.

The diagnosis of high-grade non-Hodgkin's lymphoma is generally straightforward with adequate FNAC material. Recognition of low-grade non-Hodgkin's lymphoma, typically extranodal marginal zone lymphoma ('MALToma'), however, is sometimes fraught especially if arising in the context of autoimmune thyroiditis where monomorphism of the neoplastic lymphocytes, which triggers the suspicion of neoplasia, is diluted or obscured by reactive lymphoproliferative elements. Histological examination is typically advised, particularly if more definitive subclassification is desired.

FNAC-induced iatrogenic change

Although FNAC is popularly considered to be a comparatively atraumatic procedure, the technique is known to induce histological changes, which may modulate or even obscure the underlying pathology and potentially mislead the unwary.

Several studies propose an incidence for FNAC-induced iatrogenic changes of close to 100 per cent.[18] Relevant factors

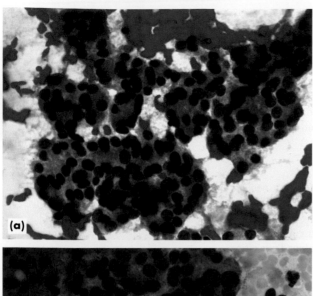

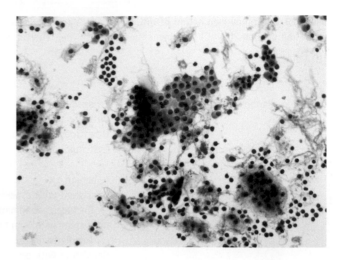

Figure 19.4 FNAC (Thy2) from Hashimoto's thyroiditis depicting loosely cohesive, monolayered clusters of mildly pleomorphic oncocytic (oxyphil) thyrocytes admixed with polymorphous small lymphocytes. Oncocytes often show a prominent 'cherry pink' macronucleolus and their cytoplasm may appear orange, green, blue or even clear with the Papanicolau stain (Pap stain, medium magnification).

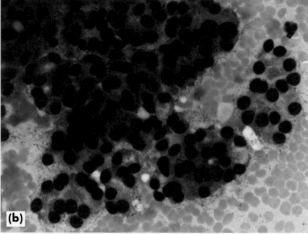

Figure 19.3 (a) Cellular fine needle aspiration cytology (FNAC) (Thy3f) specimen suggestive of a follicular neoplasm. Note several microfollicular structures (defined as 12 or less circumferential thyroid epithelial cells, in contrast to macrofollicles composed of 20 or more peripheral cells (Pap stain, high magnification).[17] (b) Similar microfollicles seen on its companion air-dried smear. There is sparse colloid in some of the follicles (MGG stain, high magnification).

include the nature and size of the target lesion, the calibre of the needle used, the number of passes attempted, the precise FNAC technique employed, how conscientiously such effects are sought and the interval between FNAC and excision surgery. The retrospective nature of such audit is prone to underestimate the true frequency.

The resultant secondary damage may broadly be classified into tissue damage and repair effects, tumour and tissue infarction and epithelial dislodgement/displacement phenomena. The acronym WHAFFT ('worrisome histologic alterations following fine needle aspiration of the thyroid gland') was originally proposed and has further been divided into acute WHAFFT and chronic WHAFFT.[19]

Tissue damage and repair artefact includes haemorrhage, fibrovascular granulation tissue organization and regenerative/degenerative atypia. Haemorrhagic needle tracks and associated proliferation of fibroblasts/myofibroblasts are typically pericapsular and radiate to the centre of the lesion,

perpendicular to the capsule. The influx of inflammatory cells, siderophages, linear fibrosis/hyalinization, cholesterol granulomata, dystrophic mineralization, epithelial metaplasia and epithelial and endothelial atypia may on occasion be so exuberant and kaposiform as to closely mimic a sarcoma (so-called 'post-FNAC spindle cell nodule') (**Figure 19.6**).

The thyroid gland is a richly vascularized organ (receiving approximately 2 per cent of total cardiac output) and post-FNAC vascular effects include venous thrombosis, recanalization and papillary endothelial hyperplasia, sometimes to an extent to resemble angiosarcoma ('pseudo-angiosarcomatoid'). Mitochondrion-rich oncocytic (oxyphil) cell lesions are exquisitely sensitive to ischaemia, therefore, characteristically susceptible to partial or global infarction, either spontaneously or post-FNAC. Where extensive, such infarction may render definitive histological evaluation difficult or impossible and a diagnosis of oncocytic neoplasm, not further specified may be the best that can be proffered under these circumstances. However, a minor population of better preserved tissue, the ghost-like outlines of papillae, necrotic cells or psammoma bodies, together with review of the original FNAC material may yield some insight into the underlying pathology. Immunocytochemical positivity for certain epitopes persists for a surprising time after infarction – leukocyte common antigen (CD45) and CD20 staining, for example, may reproducibly define lymphoproliferation long after tumour cells are devitalized, although antibodies such as carcinoembryonic antigen (CD66e) are more capricious and stain fields of necrotic tissue and abscess cavitation indiscriminately.

Angulated follicles and reparative stromal response, accompanied by nuclear hyperchromasia, fusiform epithelial morphology and squamous metaplasia may appear infiltrative ('pseudoinfiltration'), and thereby merit serious consideration of follicular carcinoma, squamous cell carcinoma or mucoepidermoid carcinoma.

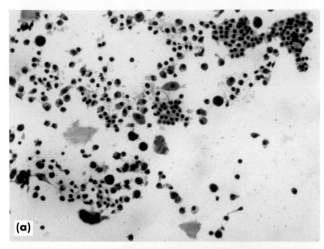

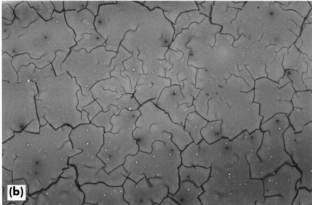

Figure 19.5 (a) Fine needle aspiration cytology (FNAC) (Thy2c) from a benign thyroid cyst showing monolayered sheets ('honeycomb') of cohesive, isomorphic epithelial cells amidst foam cells and pigmented macrophages with minimal necrolytic debris ('dirty background') (Pap stain, medium magnification). (b) FNAC (Thy1c) of the contents of a benign colloid cyst/nodule illustrating abundant, evenly dispersed, tessellated ('cracked') colloid ('parched earth' sign). There is no cell sampling in this field (MGG stain, low magnification).

Epithelial displacement and/or tumour implantation along the FNAC needle tracks into soft tissues or skin does occur, although apart from the uncommon sarcomas such deposits usually disintegrate and viable tumour seeding is rarely of serious clinical importance. Fields of reactive papillary endothelial hyperplasia (Masson's pseudotumour) in pericapsular vasculature may closely mimic lymphovascular involvement by papillary thyroid carcinoma. Mechanical tumour cell dislodgement into blood vessels may resemble vascular invasion. Rigorous criteria are recommended, notably the presence of a protruberant connection with the vessel wall, partial or complete endothelialization of the tumour tissue and/or admixture of tumour cells with blood/thrombus, all indicative of a vital response. Opinion is divided as to whether immunostaining (e.g. CD31, CD34 for vascular and D2-40 for lymphatic endothelium) ought to be routinely or selectively used. Pericapsular defects in various stages of healing must not be misinterpreted as capsular infiltration ('pseudoinvasion').

DEVELOPMENTAL CONDITIONS

Developmental conditions involve the presence of normal thyroid tissue in sites outside the normal thyroid gland (heterotopia or ectopia, hamartoma and choristoma). This includes lingual thyroid, mediastinal thyroid, benign lymph node inclusions, so-called 'lateral aberrant thyroid gland' and sequestrated ('parasitic') thyroid nodules. Mature adult cystic teratoma (dermoid cyst) of the ovary may show a preponderance of thyroid tissue (struma ovarii) sometimes with carcinoid elements (strumal carcinoid). The same repertoire of pathological conditions that affect eutopic thyroid gland may also be rarely encountered at these other sites (Figure 19.7).

Thyroglossal tract anomalies

Thyroglossal duct remnants persist due to failure of involution of the thyroglossal duct following embryological descent of the thyroid gland. They are the most common cause of a congenital neck mass and the second most common cause of a cervical mass in childhood.[20]

Thyroglossal duct remnants can occur at almost any site from the base of tongue to the suprasternal region, predominantly at four locations, namely intralingual, suprahyoid, thyrohyoid and suprasternal (Figure 19.8).[21] Cysts predominate with fewer sinuses and fistulae. Counterintuitively, follicular thyroid tissue is not a prerequisite for diagnosis. Thyroglossal duct carcinoma is rare, estimated as occurring in no more than 1 per cent of thyroglossal duct cysts and, when it supervenes, it is usually a subtype of papillary thyroid carcinoma.

ACQUIRED CONDITIONS

Squamous differentiation

The presence of squamous epithelium is not uncommon. It is usually either an acquired, adaptive response (metaplasia) due to inflammation, or related to developmental rests of cells (heteroplasia),[22, 23] although may also occur in some neoplasms (differentiation) (Table 19.2 and Figure 19.9).

Non-neoplastic squamous epithelium is usually microscopically bland though may sometimes show an alarming degree of reactive/reparative cytonuclear atypia. Benign squamous epithelium generally presents the same immunophenotype as elsewhere, that is cytokeratins (notably CK5 and CK14), epithelial membrane antigen (EMA) and p63 positivity, usually with thyroglobulin, TTF-1 and carcinoembryonic antigen (CEA, CD66e) negativity. Malignant squamous differentiation, however, may not conform to this profile and anomalous epitope expression may be confounding.

Oncocytic change

Oncocytic (oxyphilic) cells are characterized by swollen, granular, mitochondrion-rich cytoplasm and may occur in both endocrine tissues and non-endocrine organs, including pituitary, parathyroid, thyroid, adrenal, lacrimal and salivary

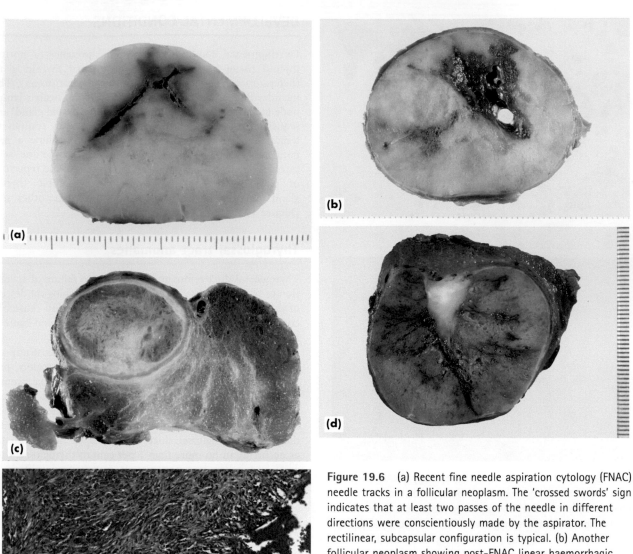

Figure 19.6 (a) Recent fine needle aspiration cytology (FNAC) needle tracks in a follicular neoplasm. The 'crossed swords' sign indicates that at least two passes of the needle in different directions were conscientiously made by the aspirator. The rectilinear, subcapsular configuration is typical. (b) Another follicular neoplasm showing post-FNAC linear haemorrhagic infarction with early macrocystic change. (c) Globally infarcted oncocytic (oxyphil) cell neoplasm, not further subclassifiable, following FNAC displaying complete yellow ischaemic type necrosis. (d) Obvious healing rectilinear FNAC artefact perpendicular to the capsule with a retracted, cuneiform, fibrous pericapsular scar in an otherwise minimally invasive follicular carcinoma. (e) Post-FNAC, spindle cell nodule composed of richly vascularized myofibroblastic ('kaposiform') stroma bordering encysted haematoma (H&E stain, medium magnification).

glands, kidney, intestine, pancreas, lung and sinonasal tract. The incidence of oncocytic change increases with advancing age and may be extensive at any one site (oncocytosis). When such cells occur in the thyroid gland, they are termed 'Hürthle cells' (Askanazy cells). It is a purely descriptive term and does not in itself indicate biological potential – oncocytic cells occur in both non-neoplastic and neoplastic (benign and malignant) conditions ('mitochondriomas') (**Table 19.3**). Oncocytic change is a cellular adaptive process, which is believed to occur in response to pathological or physiological stress and the oxygen-sensitive nature of the mitochondria renders the cells unusually susceptible to traumatic/ischaemic injury. There is ongoing debate as to whether such oncocytic

transformation is a form of metaplasia or more correctly represents a process of transdifferentiation.[24] The pathogenetic basis underpinning oncocytic change is complex. The genetic events driving oncocytic change involve mutations in mitochondrial DNA and somatic mutations that affect mitochondrial function. Importantly, these changes are largely unrelated to the genetic events that result in proliferation and neoplastic transformation of thyroid follicular epithelial cells.

There is hallmark concomitant nuclear enlargement often with striking nuclear pleomorphism, coarse karyoplasm and conspicuous macronucleolation, even in benign oncocytes. The distinction between oncocytic hyperplasia and neoplasia

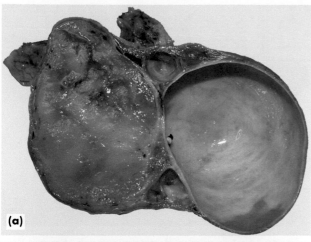

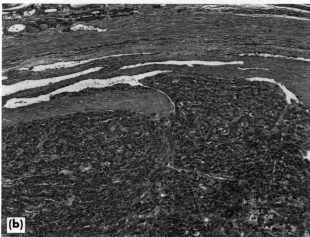

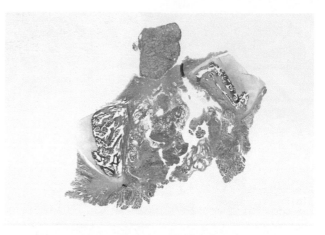

Figure 19.8 Whole mount preparation of a Sistrunk's procedure specimen showing hyoid bone, closely associated connective tissue plus a nubbin of normofollicular thyroid tissue representing thyroglossal duct remnants (H&E stain, ultralow magnification).

Table 19.2 Conditions associated with squamous epithelium in the thyroid gland.

Non-neoplastic	Neoplasms
Nodular hyperplasia (goitre)	Papillary carcinoma
Chronic lymphocytic thyroiditis and variants	Squamous cell carcinoma, primary or secondary
Hashimoto's thyroiditis	Mucoepidermoid carcinoma, primary or secondary
Following FNAC, core biopsy or contralateral lobectomy	Carcinoma with thymus-like elements (CASTLE)
Developmental solid cell nests and thymic rests	Teratoma

FNAC, fine needle aspiration cytology.

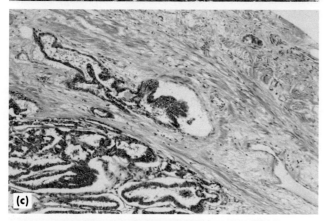

Figure 19.7 (a) Adult cystic ovarian teratoma (dermoid cyst). The solid component is substantially follicular thyroid tissue with clinically unsuspected fields of minimally invasive (angioinvasive) follicular carcinoma microscopically. (b) Minimally invasive follicular carcinoma ex-ovarian teratoma. The endothelialized tongue-like angioinvasion is identical to that seen in such tumours occurring in eutopic thyroid gland (H&E stain, medium magnification). (c) Lymphovascular invasion in well-differentiated papillary thyroid carcinoma, classical pattern ex-struma ovarii. Again, this is identical to that occurring in eutopic thyroid gland proper (H&E stain, medium magnification).

can be difficult, particularly in the context of thyroiditis. Note that in autoimmune thyroid disease, oncocytic change is not restricted to Hashimoto's thyroiditis, but it may also be encountered in long-standing Graves' disease. Oncocytic change occurring in follicular nodules and/or multinodular goitre, is conventionally regarded as hyperplastic, whereas clonality studies have demonstrated that many of the larger nodules are in fact monoclonal, thus the biologically correct approach would be to regard these as follicular adenomas.

The mitochondria themselves stain with the phosphotungstic acid haematoxylin (PTAH) method. Positive cytoplasmic immunostaining for cytokeratins (notably CK14), vimentin, antimitochondrial antibody and weakly for thyroglobulin (TG) is typical. Carcinoembryonic antigen (CEA, CD66e) reactivity is variable. Electron microscopy demonstrates abnormally configured mitochondria (**Figure 19.10**).

Thyroiditis

The various manifestations of thyroiditis are summarized in **Table 19.4**. These may be either non-autoimmune or

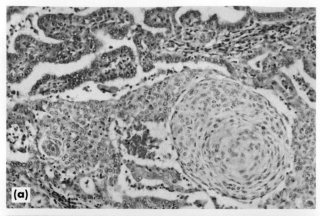

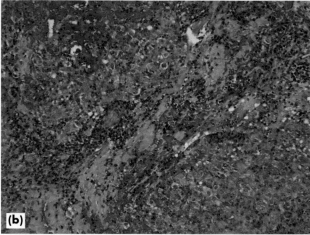

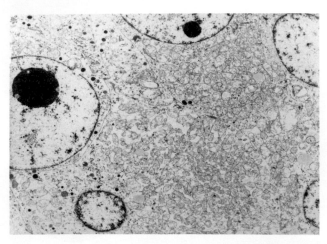

Figure 19.10 Transmission electron micrograph of several tumour cells from a poorly differentiated oncocytic (oxyphil) carcinoma of the thyroid gland. Note the cytoplasmic expansion by scores of swollen mitochondria and paucity of other cell organelles. Two prominent osmiophilic macronucleoli are also plainly seen (transmission electron microscope (TEM), ultra-high magnification).

Figure 19.9 (a) Papillary thyroid carcinoma exhibiting isolated areas of squamous differentiation (squamous morulae), which are seen focally in up to 50 per cent of cases (H&E stain, medium magnification). (b) Carcinoma with thymus-like elements (CASTLE) showing smooth contoured lobules of non-keratinizing squamoid epithelial cells demarcated by a central broad fibrous septum, percolated by lymphocytes and plasma cells (H&E stain, medium magnification).

Table 19.3 Conditions associated with oncocytic (oxyphilic) epithelium in the thyroid gland.[23, 24]

Non-neoplastic	Neoplastic
Hashimoto's thyroiditis	Follicular adenoma
Nodular hyperplasia	Follicular carcinoma
Long-standing Graves' disease	Papillary thyroid carcinoma
Post-irradiation	Medullary carcinoma
Post-chemotherapy	Poorly differentiated thyroid carcinoma
Ageing	Undifferentiated (anaplastic) carcinoma

autoimmune, the latter typified by Hashimoto's thyroiditis and Graves' disease and their variants. Drug-induced thyroiditis is associated with the use of a number of drugs including amiodarone, lithium, interferon-alpha and interleukin-2.

Lateral aberrant thyroid tissue

Lateral aberrant thyroid (LAT) tissue or gland describes anomalous deposits of follicular thyroid tissue in the lateral neck. Originally believed to indicate persistent lateral thyroid anlage, the modern view is that the overwhelming majority, but not all, actually represent metastatic follicular thyroid carcinoma or FVPTC, the cytonuclear morphology of which may be so deceptively bland as to be virtually indistinguishable from normal or hyperplastic thyroid parenchyma proper.[26]

Pragmatically, any such deposits lateral to the carotid sheath ought to be regarded as metastatic disease until otherwise proven. Those extracapsular deposits medial to the carotid sheath may either represent benign sequestrated ('parasitic') thyroid nodules, which generally recapitulate the appearances in the body of the main gland proper, or metastatic tumour. Benign thyroid tissue inclusions in cervical lymph nodes are rarely encountered and are difficult to confirm with certainty.

Hyperplastic nodules

Historically, multiple nodules as part of multinodular goitre, either incompletely capsulated or unencapsulated, are designated hyperplastic (adenomatoid or cellular colloid) nodules. One or more may predominate, thereby simulating a solitary nodule clinically and/or radiologically (**Figure 19.11**). They do not normally compress the adjacent gland, which often displays a similar growth pattern. Secondary retrogressive changes frequently present, sometimes extensive, include coarse fibrosclerosis (sometimes resembling a 'radial scar'), cystic degeneration, calcification, infarction, fresh haemorrhage, haemosiderosis, siderophages, foam cells, cholesterol granulomata, endarteritis obliterans and localized inflammation. Squamous, lipocytic, chondroid, osseous and oncocytic (oxyphil) metaplasia are occasionally

Table 19.4 Classification and features of thyroiditis.[23, 25]

	Age	Sex ratio	Cause	Thyroid function	TPO status	ESR	Gross pathological features
Hashimoto's thyroiditis (chronic lymphocytic or chronic autoimmune thyroiditis)	All ages, peak 30–50	8–9:1	Autoimmune	Hypothyroidism	High	Normal	Symmetrical diffuse enlargement of the thyroid gland. Firm consistency, pale colour and multilobulated
(Painless). Postpartum thyroiditis (subacute lymphocytic thyroiditis)	Childbearing age		Autoimmune	Can be thyrotoxic, hypothyroid or both	High	Normal	Firm to hard, tan white appearance and nodules of varying size
(Painless). Sporadic thyroiditis (subacute lymphocytic thyroiditis)	All ages peak, 30–40	2:1	Autoimmune	Can be thyrotoxic, hypothyroid or both	High	Normal	Firm to hard, tan white appearance and nodules of varying size
Painful. Subacute thyroiditis (de Quervain's, giant-cell, pseudo-granulomatous thyroiditis)	20–60	5:1	Unknown	Can be thyrotoxic, hypothyroid or both	Low	High	Firm to hard, tan white appearance and nodules of varying size
Suppurative. Thyroiditis (infectious, bacterial, pyogenic thyroiditis)	20–40	1:1	Infectious	Euthyroid	Absent	High	Variable appearance including focal or diffuse enlargement and abscess formation. Can appear normal
Riedel's thyroiditis	30–60	3–4:1	Unknown, sometimes part of the spectrum of IgG4 sclerosing diseases	Euthyroid	Present	Normal	Thyroid replaced by dense, tan-white, firm to hard tissue, often extending into neighbouring structures

seen. Simple papillae (papillary hyperplastic nodule) do rarely occur and the papillae tend to radiate towards the centre of the lesion (centripetal growth) (**Figure 19.12**).[27] Exhaustive efforts to exclude papillary thyroid carcinoma must be pursued under these circumstances.

The concept of thyroid follicular epithelial dysplasia remains theoretical. Up to 70 per cent of hyperplastic nodules are in fact clonal proliferations and can express various markers of malignant follicular-patterned thyroid tumours. However, no morphological, immunohistochemical or molecular study to date has been able to discriminate between adenomatoid nodules, follicular adenoma and follicular carcinoma with absolute sensitivity and specificity.[28]

TUMOURS OF FOLLICULAR EPITHELIUM

Follicular adenoma

Follicular adenoma classically occurs as a solitary benign, encapsulated tumour, which shows follicular epithelial differentiation[8] with no evidence of either capsular or vascular invasion and neither architectural nor cytonuclear features of papillary thyroid carcinoma (**Figure 19.13**). It possesses a circumferential, smooth contoured or gently undulating, slender, fibrous delimiting capsule usually displaying little variation in thickness – fields of capsular augmentation warrant a conscientious search to exclude a carcinoma. Surrounding native gland may be compressed and/or atrophic.[8, 23] Internally, there may be a variety of growth patterns, such as normofollicular, microfollicular (fetal), macrofollicular (colloid), solid, trabecular and organoid, though the architecture tends to be fairly uniform within any individual example. Mitoses are few. Degenerative stromal changes, particularly post-FNAC, are identical to multinodular hyperplasia, but squamous metaplasia is uncommon and, where present, merits consideration of papillary thyroid carcinoma, follicular variant (FVPTC).

Histological subtypes of adenoma include solid, fetal, oxyphilic (oncocytic), clear cell, signet ring cell and lipoadenoma, defined according to the predominant growth pattern (accounting for over 75 per cent of the overall tumour). These, however, do not differ clinically or in biological behaviour from conventional follicular adenoma.

Atypical adenoma (follicular tumour of uncertain malignant potential, FTUMP) is used by some to describe follicular neoplasms, which display some worrisome microscopic features although falling short of unequivocal capsular or vascular infiltration.[29] These include irregularly thickened capsule, partial thickness incursions into, but not completely

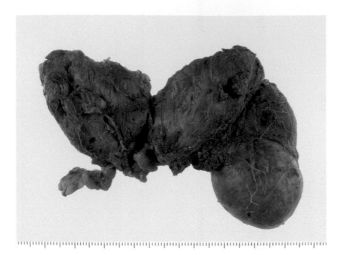

Figure 19.11 Total thyroidectomy specimen showing a protruberant, well-circumscribed, ovoid mass arising from the left lower pole, clinically excised as a solitary thyroid nodule. This proved to be a dominant hyperplastic (adenomatoid) nodule arising in chronic lymphocytic (Hashimoto's) thyroiditis with several smaller intraparenchymal nodules throughout the main body of the gland bilaterally.

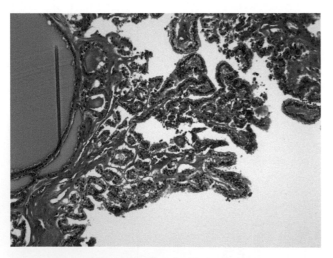

Figure 19.12 Part of a papillary hyperplastic nodule illustrating arborescent, centrifugally projecting papillae. The epithelial cells are monolayered, well polarized and bland. There were no cytoarchitectural features to indicate papillary thyroid carcinoma despite a rigorous search (H&E stain, medium magnification).

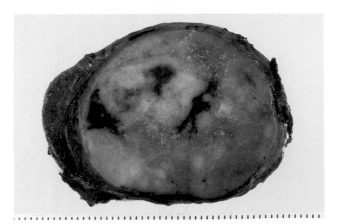

Figure 19.13 The cut surface of a benign follicular adenoma showing a largely solid, fleshy texture with localized cystic change. The perimeter is evenly contoured and the investing capsule is uniformly slender.

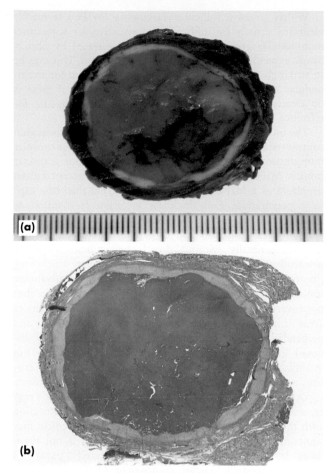

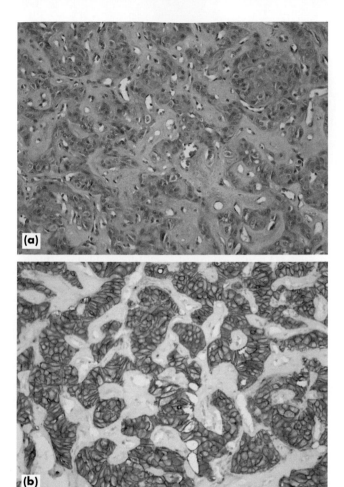

Figure 19.14 (a) A cross-sectional slice through an atypical adenoma (follicular tumour of uncertain malignant potential, FTUMP). Despite the widespread capsular fibrosis and multiple, irregular, virtually full thickness internal incursions, at no point can convincing complete transcapsular infiltration be demonstrated. (b) Whole mount preparation of the same lesion. Circumferentially, tumour does not invade beyond the original capsular contour (H&E stain, ultralow magnification).

through the capsule, hypercellularity, increased mitoses and/or abnormal forms and nuclear atypia (**Figure 19.14**).

Hyalinizing trabecular tumours

Hyalinizing trabecular tumours (HTT) are a group of neoplasms originally regarded as adenomas (hyalinizing trabecular adenoma (HTA), paraganglioma-like adenoma of the thyroid (PLAT)). It has subsequently transpired that the supposed characteristic organoid growth pattern with interstitial perivascular hyalinization may also be seen focally in nodular hyperplasia plus a number of other benign and malignant thyroid neoplasms many, although not all, showing histological features of papillary thyroid carcinoma, including *RET/PTC* gene rearrangements. In those cases of pure HTT architecture without papillary carcinomatous morphology there appears to be a spectrum of biological potential ranging from adenoma to carcinoma, both minimally invasive and widely invasive by conventional criteria.[30] A proportion of such

Figure 19.15 (a) Minimally invasive hyalinizing trabecular carcinoma demonstrating the typical organoid nested and trabecular architecture separated by hyalinized interstitium, richly endowed with blood vessels. Elsewhere, this example showed mushrooming transcapsular growth. There are no features to suggest papillary thyroid carcinoma in this neoplasm, but there was synchronous classical papillary thyroid carcinoma separately in the specimen (H&E stain, medium magnification). (b) The same tumour illustrating universal Ki67 (MIB-1) immunoreactivity – note that this is peculiarly membraneous and cytoplasmic in distribution. Ki67 is conventionally used as a proliferation marker where in other circumstances it stains the nuclei only of those cells in certain phases of the cell cycle (Ki67 IHC, medium magnification).

neoplasms exhibit characteristic, peculiar, avid cytoplasmic Ki67 (MIB-1) immunostaining (**Figure 19.15**). Immunopositivity for cytokeratins, thyroglobulin and vimentin generally with negative pan-neuroendocrine marker and calcitonin staining discriminates HTT from paraganglioma proper and medullary thyroid carcinoma.

Follicular carcinoma of the thyroid

Follicular thyroid carcinoma (FTC) is a malignant epithelial tumour arising in both eutopic thyroid gland and/or heterotopic thyroid tissue, showing follicular cell differentiation and is bereft of the characteristic features of papillary thyroid carcinoma (PTC). It accounts for 5–15 per cent of all thyroid cancers in iodine-sufficient regions. It spreads via haematogenous routes, preferentially to bone and lung with metastatic disease as a presenting feature in 11 per cent of patients. It is divided into two basic categories defined by the extent of capsular infiltration and/or presence of vascular invasion – meticulous examination of the tumour capsule and interface with native gland is consequently of paramount importance.

Minimally invasive follicular carcinoma (MIFC) is the more common variant and is characterized by microscopical transcapsular invasion and/or pericapsular vascular infiltration.[31] With experience, subtle capsular transgression and/or accompanying fibrous capsular thickening may be appreciated in the gross specimen by the unaided eye (**Figure 19.16**), but not microinvasive capsular violation or vascular permeation.

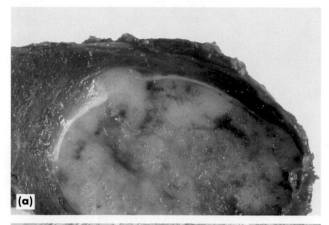

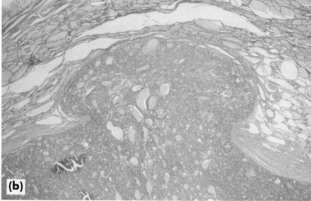

Figure 19.16   (a) Obvious mushrooming, full thickness, transcapsular herniation qualifying as minimally invasive follicular carcinoma, easily discernible to the unaided eye during dissection. There is slight lateral capsular buttressing, but negligible neocapsule formation along the advancing margin in this example. Note that there is no universally endorsed maximum size limit for this phenomenon. (b) The same area viewed histologically corroborates prolapsing impingement into perilesional native gland with no tentacular/permeative infiltration and neither significant host inflammatory nor stromal response (H&E stain, low magnification).

Widely invasive follicular carcinoma (WIFC) is readily identified grossly by infiltrative, destructive, or sometimes multinodular growth, the latter often separated by fibrous bands, expanding into surrounding native gland. This may be so strikingly obviously nodular as to be mistaken for multinodular hyperplasia by the unwary, particularly if there is no clearly identifiable vestige of pre-existing capsule for reference.

The interpretation of capsular invasion remains somewhat controversial. Most authorities require full thickness capsular transgression beyond the original lesional contour (capsular invasive MIFC), whereas a minority of authors accept a given neoplasm as a MIFC if it shows only partial thickness capsular penetration. Full thickness violation is manifest as multiple foci, less commonly a single nidus, of mushrooming herniation bulging into and displacing surrounding native follicles, generally without direct, tentacular, infiltrative/permeative growth. Lateral fibrous capsular thickening ('buttressing') and neocapsule formation along the advancing tumour to native gland interface are paradigmatic, but not invariable. Incomplete capsular encroachment includes areas of irregular or serratiform inner capsular contour and perpendicular dentate capsular incursions. Horizontally disposed ('entrapped') intracapsular follicles usually do not qualify, although they should prompt further detailed scrutiny, as should any unexplained area of capsular expansion. Circumscribed extracapsular nodules ('satellite tumour') may represent MIFC visualized outside the plane of connection with the body of the tumour (although such a pedicle may sometimes be impossible to demonstrate and is not mandated by some observers) or a sequestrated ('parasitic') congerie of benign follicles; comparison of the cytonuclear features with the main tumour bulk may aid discrimination. Artefactual capsular puncture, healing and distortion following FNAC should be interpreted with caution and the entry/exit site of perforating capsular blood vessels, where there is normally curvilinear capsular interruption, not misconstrued. Well-sampled tumours that fall short of these criteria are termed 'follicular tumour of uncertain malignant potential' (FT-UMP) in alternative terminology.

There is relatively good consensus as to what defines angioinvasion or lymphovascular invasion, to wit tumour penetration into medium calibre or large calibre intracapsular or extracapsular blood vessels. There should be polypoidal intraluminal growth either endothelialized with/or without thrombus, although not necessarily adherent (**Figure 19.17**). The point of attachment of tumour to vessel wall is a prerequisite for some observers. Free-lying endoluminal nests of tumour cells may represent artefactual dislodgement of cells by surgeon or pathologist and are disallowed. Tumour cells occupying capillary-sized intracapsular vessels are of no proven clinical importance and should be discounted. Tumour within intralesional or subcapsular vessels does not qualify. Reactive vascular endothelial hyperplasia may simulate angioinvasion and, when recognized, ought to prompt a rigorous search for vascular invasion proper. Immunostaining for vascular endothelial markers (e.g. CD31, CD34) and lymphatic endothelium (e.g. D2-40) may be helpful in selected instances. Cognizant that absolute discrimination between blood vessel invasion and lymphatic space infiltration may ultimately be impossible, the current College of American Pathologists (CAP)

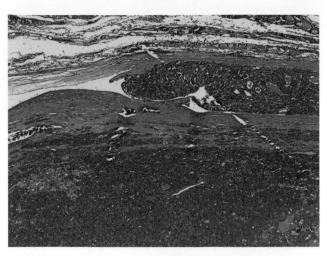

Figure 19.17 Pericapsular angioinvasion qualifying as encapsulated (angioinvasive) minimally invasive follicular carcinoma. There is a broad tongue of endothelialized tumour unequivocally protruding into a large-calibre intracapsular vessel (H&E stain, low magnification).

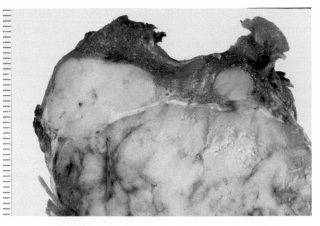

Figure 19.18 The cut surface of a widely invasive follicular carcinoma demonstrating successive generations of capsular transgression to the point where the original lesional capsule becomes almost obscured.

protocol (2009) recommends merging the two and reporting under the unifying designation of 'lymphovascular invasion'.[32]

Capsular invasive MIFC without lymphovascular infiltration portends an extremely low risk of metastasis (less than 1 per cent). Some surgeons pursue a conservative management approach and treat these cancers by lobectomy alone with surveillance, acknowledging that there is a small risk of undertreatment in a minority of cases. The term 'grossly encapsulated angioinvasive follicular carcinoma' has been proposed for encapsulated tumours with any foci of lymphovascular invasion, based on the premise that access to even one or a few endothelial lined vessels confers the capacity for more aggressive behaviour with perceived higher risk of recurrence, thereby negating a designation of 'minimal invasion'. Some authors base their definition of MIFC on the number of foci of invasion. Those tumours with a total of two foci of capsular or vascular invasion are said to show a low risk of metastasis, whereas those with four or more blood vessels involved have a higher likelihood of recurrence (47 per cent for follicular oncocytic tumours) and of metastasis (roughly 18 per cent),[3] invoking the designation of 'grossly encapsulated follicular carcinoma with extensive angioinvasion' for the latter.[32]

Widely invasive follicular carcinoma (WIFC) is an aggressive neoplasm with a high risk of distant secondaries (29–66 per cent). It displays infiltrative growth within and beyond the anatomical thyroid capsule proper, sometimes in the form of successive generations of herniating capsular transgression (**Figure 19.18**). Vascular penetration is common and typically widespread. A tumour size greater than 3.5 cm portends a less favourable prognosis.

Extrathyroidal extension (ETE) describes involvement of perithyroidal soft tissues by a primary thyroid carcinoma. This may be further subdivided into minimal ETE and extensive ETE. As previously noted, the thyroid capsule, though continuous with the pretracheal fascia is not a discrete anatomical structure, is incomplete or focally absent in

the majority of individuals, is additionally fenestrated by lymphovascular channels and contains small nerve radicles. The histological evaluation of minimal ETE is consequently sometimes vexatious and subjective. Importantly, both adipocytes and skeletal muscle bundles may be normally encountered within the thyroid gland and may also be a component of a variety of pathological thyroid conditions. The identification of desmoplastic response, adipocytic and/or muscular impingement in close proximity to large calibre, thick-walled vessels and/or large nerve trunks, on the other hand, may be more helpful as such would not be expected within the confines of thyroid gland proper. Extensive ETE is characterized by direct infiltration well beyond the limits of the thyroid gland into subcutis, neighbouring viscera, including larynx, trachea, oesophagus, recurrent laryngeal nerve, carotid artery or mediastinal vasculature. Extensive ETE is invariably obvious, typically identified by the surgeon perioperatively.

The prognosis for those carcinomas with minimal ETE worsens referenced against those without ETE. Similarly, the survival prospects for those suffering carcinomas with extensive ETE are significantly diminished in comparison with minimal ETE.

There is a dearth of evidence-based information addressing the influence of resection margin status and clinical outcome in the international literature. While knowledge of a positive margin is intuitively meritorious, scrupulous studies in large series of patients with long-term follow up analysing this have yet to be published. Similarly, there is presently no data validating the exercise of measuring the distance of tumour to closest resection margin and/or documenting close margins as an independent or co-variable prognostic index.[33]

Oncocytic (oxyphil) cell tumours

Follicular neoplasms comprising 75 per cent or more oncocytic (oxyphil) cells are designated as such and are subclassified according to the same criteria as their non-oncocytic counterparts based upon morphology, immunohistochemical profiling and molecular markers into oncocytic (oxyphil) adenoma, oncocytic (oxyphil) tumour of uncertain malignant potential, minimally or widely invasive oncocytic (oxyphil) carcinoma (Hürthle cell carcinoma). Oncocytic variants of papillary thyroid carcinoma, poorly differentiated thyroid carcinoma (PDTC), undifferentiated (anaplastic) carcinoma and medullary thyroid carcinoma are recognized. Focal clear cell change is common in oncocytic tumours and, where this constitutes over 75 per cent of the lesion, it is traditionally designated clear cell carcinoma. Under such circumstances, it is imperative to exclude metastatic carcinoma (renal or adrenal),[34] malignant melanoma, intrathyroidal parathyroid gland neoplasms and clear cell variant of medullary thyroid carcinoma.

Grossly, they are usually single nodules (solitary oxyphil follicular tumour, SOFT) (**Figure 19.19**), although they may be multiple (multiple oxyphil follicular tumours, MOFT) and are sometimes associated with Hashimoto's thyroiditis and/or conventional papillary thyroid carcinoma. A higher proportion of oncocytic (oxyphil) tumours are malignant than other follicular lesions, although when staged comparably there are reportedly no significant differences in outcome between the two. The incidence of malignancy in oncocytic (oxyphil) cell neoplasms increases with size, that is, 17, 23 and 65 per cent or more associated with maximum dimensions of less than 1 cm, between 1 and 4 cm and larger than 4 cm, respectively.[35] Most examples are sporadic. Familial examples are rare and exceptionally indicate a germline mutation.[36]

Macroscopically, they are classically mahogany brown tumours with a propensity for ischaemic infarction, either spontaneously or post-FNAC. They may show numerous histological patterns, including papillary areas, which may morphologically overlap with oncocytic (oxyphil) papillary thyroid carcinoma. They are typified by cytonuclear atypia and mitoses, though in isolation these do not reproducibly predict biological behaviour.

Oncocytic (oxyphil) parathyroid gland neoplasms should always be considered when evaluating a potential oncocytic (oxyphil) thyroid neoplasm, as they may be indistinguishable by routine orthodox microscopy without recourse to immunostaining.

Papillary thyroid carcinoma

Papillary thyroid carcinoma is a malignant epithelial tumour showing follicular cell differentiation with characteristic nuclear features. It accounts for approximately 80 per cent of all thyroid cancer and is also the most common paediatric thyroid malignancy. In adults it typically occurs between the ages of 20 and 50 years, with a female preponderance, with less pronounced gender bias in patients over 50 years old. It normally carries an excellent prognosis, especially in younger patients. In areas of adequate dietary iodine, papillary thyroid carcinoma usually presents as a solitary thyroid nodule. In regions of iodine insufficiency, multinodular goitre is common and papillary thyroid carcinoma can present as a more prominent or distinctive nodule. It has a propensity for lymphatogenous spread, initially to locoregional lymph nodes.

The potential macroscopical and microscopical manifestations of PTC are protean. Prototypically, it is invasive with irregular outline and either a scirrhous or granular, gritty texture often with multiloculated cystic change and colloid contents (**Figure 19.20**). The encapsulated follicular variant of PTC (Lindsay tumour) is usually well-circumscribed possessing a solid, fleshy cut surface, closely resembling an adenoma.

The principal defining feature of PTC is its nuclear morphology by light microscopy (**Figure 19.21**), thus the diagnosis of PTC is sustainable even in the absence of invasive growth. Crucially, however, the distinctive nuclear appearances may be very localized and, in an appropriate context, the diagnosis may still be entertained in their absence. Ordinarily, there is at least focal nuclear enlargement (nucleomegaly), nuclear crowding and nuclear overlap ('basket of eggs'). Homogenization of karyoplasm ('ground

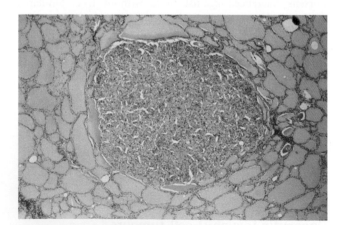

Figure 19.19 A small, benign solitary oncocytic (oxyphil) cell follicular tumour (SOFT), occurring sporadically in a background of chronic lymphocytic (Hashimoto's) thyroiditis. Despite its lack of capsule and occasional rudimentary papillae, there were no diagnostic features to suggest papillary thyroid carcinoma (H&E stain, low magnification).

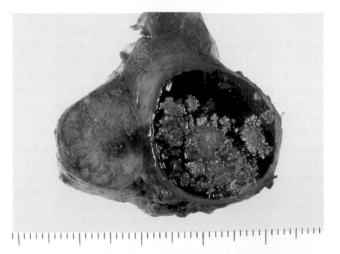

Figure 19.20 The cut surface of a classical papillary thyroid carcinoma illustrating a solid, granular appearance with adjoining encysted elements distended by inspissated colloid. The yellow punctate structures represent psammoma calcification and imparted a gritty texture.

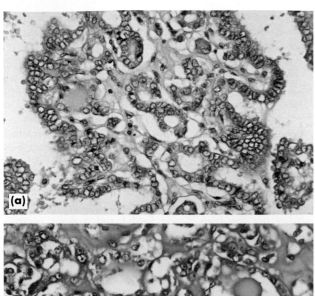

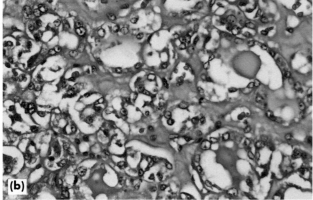

Figure 19.21 (a) The characteristic nuclear enlargement, nuclear crowding, nuclear overlap ('basket of eggs') and optically clear karyoplasm ('Orphan Annie eye') of papillary thyroid carcinoma. A few nuclear grooves ('coffee beans') and isolated intranuclear pseudo-inclusions ('vacuoles') are also present. (b) For comparison, this depicts pseudo-clear ('bubbly') nuclear artefact consequent upon suboptimal tissue fixation and processing. Superficially, these resemble the nuclei of papillary carcinoma and, although there is some anisonucleosis, there is no real nuclear crowding or overlap. The nucleoplasm is polyvacuolated with conspicuous nucleolation. There is patchy retraction cleft formation due to exaggerated tissue shrinkage. These changes were seen towards the centre of a multinodular goitre and gradually merged with reassuringly better preserved follicles more peripherally (H&E stain, high magnification).

glass') with margination of chromatin (likened to the empty looking, pupil-less eyes of Harold Gray's cartoon strip characters, most famously the waif 'little orphan Annie' and her canine companion 'Sandy') is characteristic, but not pathognomonic – it is not invariable, it is rarely present in FNAC and frozen sections, it may be encountered in other non-neoplastic conditions, it may be simulated by suboptimal tissue fixation ('bubbly' or pseudoclear artefact) and is subject to vagaries of interobserver and intraobserver reproducibility. Longitudinal nuclear grooves ('coffee bean') formed by redundant, folded nuclear membrane and intranuclear cytoplasmic inclusions (pseudoinclusions, vacuoles) formed by cytoplasmic herniation are typical and may be visualized on both FNAC and frozen section **Figure 19.22**), but again are not exclusive and may also be mimicked by intranuclear bubble artefact ('pseudopseudoinclusions').[27]

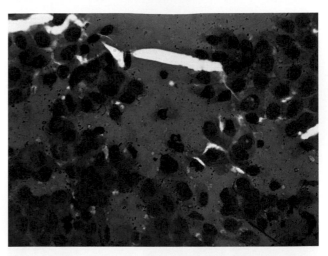

Figure 19.22 Fine needle aspiration cytology (FNAC) preparation illustrating numerous rounded intranuclear cytoplasmic inclusions and several longitudinal nuclear grooves in papillary thyroid carcinoma (May–Grunwald-Giemsa (MGG) stain, high magnification).

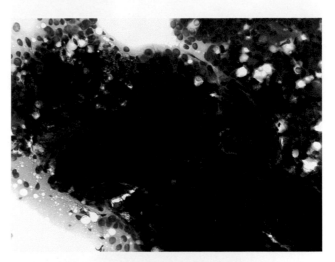

Figure 19.23 Fine needle aspiration cytology (FNAC) tissue microbiopsy from a papillary thyroid carcinoma. Despite its thickness, obscuring much cytonuclear detail (a few nuclear pseudo-inclusions and nuclear grooves are nonetheless visible), the branching vascularized fronds are a useful diagnostic feature. Colloid, where present, tends to be globular or in strands ('chewing gum' or 'stringy') (Pap stain, medium magnification).

A papillary architecture is typical, although by no means universal. The papillae are often well vascularized and complexly arborescent, sometimes oedematous (hydropic), hyalinized, fibrocellular, calcified or micropapillary in configuration (**Figure 19.23**). Follicles are usually present, albeit with an elongated, tortuous or crenated outline, sometimes with rudimentary or abortive papillae and colloid is often densely hypereosinophilic. Intrafollicular multinucleated giant cells of macrophage/histiocyte lineage phagocytosing colloid (colloidophagy) are more often seen in PTC than in other lesions.

Psammoma bodies (laminated calcospherites) are present in roughly 50 per cent of PTCs histologically, less frequently on FNAC and are virtually pathognomonic – they must, however, be stromal in location in contradistinction to calcified, inspissated intrafollicular colloid (psammomatoid bodies or pseudopsammoma calcification) seen in normality and other disease states (**Figure 19.24**). Importantly, psammoma bodies may also be seen in other neoplastic and non-neoplastic conditions, both within and outside the thyroid gland. Rarely, psammoma bodies or linear scoring artefact following microtomy provide the only presumptive evidence

of regressed or infarcted PTC. Multicentric PTC is common and represents either intrathyroidal lymphatic spread or synchronous primary tumorigenesis with different *RET/PTC* translocations.

Numerous variants of PTC have been described, none mutually exclusive within an individual tumour (**Table 19.5**). A single tumour is classified according to its predominant histological pattern. Most subtypes are of no prognostic significance, although tall cell, diffuse sclerosing, diffuse follicular, solid, trabecular and dedifferentiated variants (**Figure 19.25**) are biologically more aggressive in contrast to the encapsulated variant (where conventional infiltrative growth may not be apparent), which portends a highly favourable outcome. Increased mitoses (over two mitoses per ten high power fields) and tumour necrosis signify worse survival in PTC. PTCs measuring less than 1 cm are associated with an excellent prognosis and the outlook worsens for those tumours exceeding 4 cm. Positive lymph nodal metastasis in PTC is usually an indication for radioactive iodine therapy and the presence of extranodal

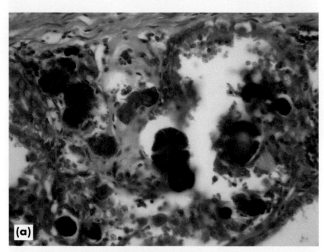

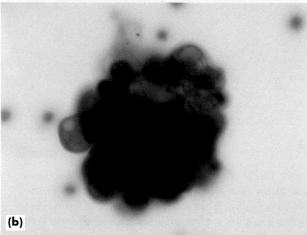

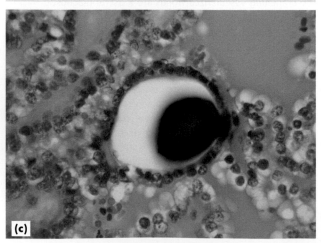

Table 19.5 Histological variants of papillary thyroid carcinoma.[23]

Variant	
Classical	Tall cell
Follicular	Columnar cell
Solid	Oncocytic (oxyphil)
Encapsulated	Warthin tumour-like
Diffuse sclerosing	Clear cell
Diffuse follicular	Macrofollicular
Trabecular	Cribriform-morular (including FAP-associated)
Lipomatous stroma	Exuberant nodular fasciitis-like stroma
Spindle cell	Dedifferentiated

FAP, familial adenomatous polyposis.

Figure 19.24 (a) Psammoma bodies in papillary thyroid carcinoma. These concentrically laminated concretions are stromal in location. They are often said to represent mineralized 'tombstones' to a mummified cell, the latter forming the initial nidus for mineral encrustation and may occasionally be large and complex in configuration. Some of these have splintered during microtomy. Any calcified deposits or other hard objects are prone to dislodgement by the microtome blade and being swept across the tissue section to give parallel linear score artefact (H&E stain, medium magnification). (b) Fine needle aspiration cytology (FNAC) from a papillary thyroid carcinoma showing two concentrically lamellated psammoma bodies mantled by vacuolated epithelial cells. Psammoma bodies are seen in 40–60 per cent of papillary thyroid carcinomas in histological sections, but in only 20 per cent of cases in FNAC specimens (H&E stain, high magnification).[37] (c) A psammomatoid or pseudo-psammoma body composed of inspissated, partially mineralized intrafollicular colloid (H&E stain, high magnification).

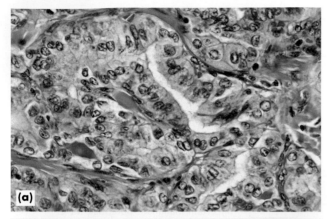

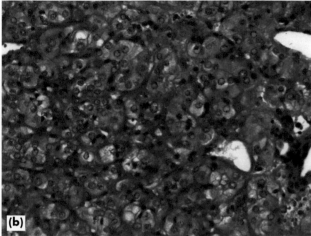

Figure 19.25   (a) Tall cell variant of papillary thyroid carcinoma. The cells are columnar, their height being at least three times greater than their width and they are not hyperstratified, in contradistinction to columnar cell carcinoma (H&E stain, high magnification). (b) Solid variant of papillary thyroid carcinoma. The small cell nests demonstrate the distinctive nuclear features. This example behaved extremely aggressively (H&E stain, high magnification).

extension heightens the risk of distant metastasis and death. Areas of squamous differentiation (morulae) occur in approximately 50 per cent of cases and the distinctive PTC nuclear morphology is absent from such areas. The WHO definition of tall cells in PTC is merely a preponderance of tumour cells whose height is at least three-fold (previously two-fold) greater than their width and this pattern should not be confused with columnar cell carcinoma.

PTC stains immunohistochemically for cytokeratins (CK), thyroglobulin and thyroid transcription factor-1, but not pan-neuroendocrine markers. Areas of squamous differentiation lose their thyroglobulin and thyroid transcription factor-1 reactivity. A plethora of markers has been proposed to aid discrimination between follicular variant of PTC and other follicular lesions, notably high molecular weight cytokeratins (HMWCK), cytokeratin 19, mesothelium-associated antibody (HBME-1), galectin-3, Leu7 (CD57), LeuM1 (CD15), fibronectin-1, platelet-derived growth factor (CD44) and *RET* among others. None, individually or in combination, are entirely sensitive or specific for PTC – they may

be capricious even in classical PTC. Moreover, a number of inflammatory and other neoplastic conditions may yield overlapping results.

Three independent molecular pathways are recognized in the tumorigenesis of PTC with distinct gene expression profiles, namely activation of the proto-oncogene receptor tyrosine (*RET*) kinase, mutation of the gene for B-raf (*BRAF*) and *ras* mutation. *RET* kinase activation consequent upon chromosomal translocation is collectively referred to as *RET/PTC* translocation and occurs in up to 60 per cent of PTCs. *RET/PTC* 1 fusion correlates to classical PTC and papillary microcarcinoma. *RET/PTC* 3 fusion is seen in tall cell and solid PTC variants plus irradiation-induced tumours. *RET/PTC* expression is not a feature of follicular carcinoma, poorly differentiated carcinoma or undifferentiated (anaplastic) carcinoma. Mutation of the gene for B-raf (*BRAF*) accompanies 29–69 per cent of PTCs, more prevalent in classical PTC, tall cell, Warthin tumour-like and oncocytic (oxyphil) variants. Follicular variant PTC harbours *ras* gene mutations and may show *PAX8/PPARγ* translocation, but rarely *RET/PTC* translocation or *BRAF* mutations, a profile akin to that of follicular adenoma and follicular carcinoma.[3]

Difficulty in classifying follicular patterned lesions of the thyroid gland

The histomorphological differential diagnosis of follicular patterned lesions of the thyroid gland remains a controversial area of current diagnostic surgical pathology, hampered by relative lack of objective criteria and limited follow-up data, compounded by subjective interpretation with well-recognized interobserver and intraobserver variation, occasionally necessitating an *ipse dixit* diagnosis based on pragmatic constraints and experience.[26]

A belief among some experts that there is overdiagnosis of FVPTC[38] draws some support from molecular and genetic observations. Furthermore, *RET/PTC* expression in some cases of follicular variant PTC show multicentric rather than diffuse alterations, suggestive of carcinomatous transformation ex-adenoma, although by convention it is recommended that the entire encapsulated lesion is arbitrarily regarded as PTC for staging purposes.[28]

Alternative nomenclature has been proposed to accommodate this diagnostic uncertainty and is summarized here (**Figure 19.26**). This provides a more descriptive schema, which may be invoked in the minority of cases where diagnostic equivocation is irresolvable by conventional morphology and the stigma of malignancy is undesired.[29] Where diagnostic distinction between follicular carcinoma and papillary thyroid carcinoma is difficult, the generic rubric 'well-differentiated thyroid carcinoma' may be employed, although every effort to subclassify more precisely should still be made.[39]

Papillary thyroid microcarcinoma

Papillary thyroid microcarcinomas (papillary microtumours) are by definition less than 10 mm in diameter. They may be an incidental finding in thyroid glands removed for other

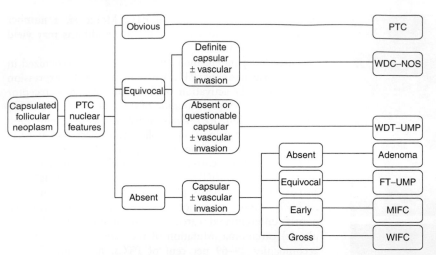

Figure 19.26 Diagnostic algorithm for resolution of the differential diagnosis of encapsulated follicular lesions of the thyroid gland. PTC, papillary thyroid carcinoma; WDC-NOS, well-differentiated carcinoma, not otherwise specified; WDT-UMP, well differentiated tumour of uncertain malignant potential; FT-UMP, follicular tumour of uncertain malignant potential; MIFC, minimally invasive follicular carcinoma; WIFC, widely invasive follicular carcinoma.

pathology or serendipitously detected on imaging of the thyroid gland (latent carcinoma).[40] Alternatively, they may be found retrospectively in patients presenting with metastatic disease from an initially unsuspected small primary lesion (occult or covert carcinoma). Further subdivision into tumours less than 5 mm ('minute') and 5–10 mm ('tiny') maximum dimension is of no clinical relevance. Occult and latent papillary carcinomas may or may not be microcarcinomas.

Most studies report a prevalence for latent papillary microcarcinomas of circa 5–10 per cent, but figures as high as 30 per cent or so are acknowledged. Despite their propensity for multifocality in one lobe (23 per cent), bilaterality (17 per cent) and locoregional lymph node metastasis (16 per cent), they almost always pursue an indolent clinical course with excellent prognosis, usually not requiring additional intervention.[3] Exceptionally, however, papillary thyroid microcarcinomas behave more aggressively and the presence of two or more foci, lymphovascular invasion, extrathyroidal extension and higher risk morphology (e.g. tall cell features) may prompt more comprehensive treatment, despite tenuous long-term vindication for this. A significant number of subcentimetre papillary carcinomas occurring in children and adolescents harbour extrathyroidal extension and/or distant metastasis, prompting the CAP recommendation to restrict use of the term 'papillary thyroid microcarcinoma' to those over 19 years of age.[33]

Morphologically, papillary microcarcinomas are usually either infiltrative and sclerotic or circumscribed but unencapsulated, located between native follicles without discernible host response (**Figure 19.27**). Such microscopical foci, therefore, are easily missed on cursory histological screening and are apt to mimic solid cell nests or even heterotopic thymic rests on scanning magnification.

Poorly differentiated thyroid carcinoma

Poorly differentiated thyroid carcinoma encompasses a spectrum of heterogeneous tumours showing limited evidence of follicular cell differentiation associated with biological behaviour intermediate between differentiated (follicular and papillary) thyroid carcinoma and undifferentiated (anaplastic) carcinoma.[41] PDTC typically arise *de novo*, but may occur through transformation of differentiated carcinoma

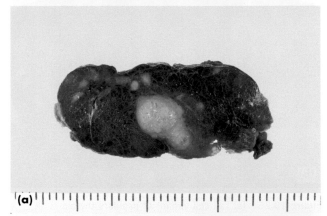

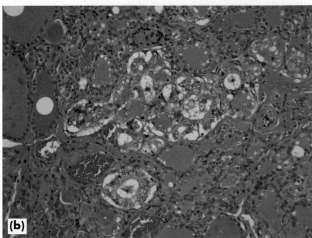

Figure 19.27 (a) Multicentric papillary thyroid microcarcinoma (UICC/TNM pT1(m)), each deposit measuring less than 10 mm diameter. These show a sclerotic morphology. (b) Microscopical deposit of papillary microcarcinoma. This is poorly demarcated and is eliciting no stromal or inflammatory response whatsoever. Such foci are readily overlooked on cursory or low power examination (H&E stain, medium magnification).

(**Figure 19.28**). They may progress to undifferentiated (anaplastic) carcinoma either *ab initio* or after recurrence.

PDTC may be defined mainly on the basis of growth pattern. Insular (primordial) carcinoma represents the archetype

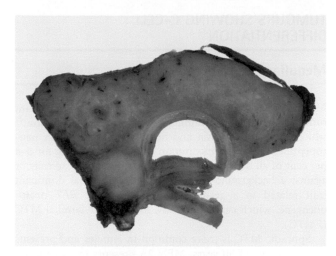

Figure 19.28 Transverse slice through a total laryngopharyngectomy and bilateral radical neck dissection specimen for advanced stage, poorly differentiated thyroid carcinoma. The bulk of the specimen comprises heterogeneous tumour largely enclaving upper trachea and cervical tubular oesophagus. Microscopically, this showed intermingled areas of papillary thyroid carcinoma, follicular carcinoma and insular carcinoma with localized squamous differentiation.

Figure 19.29 Classical poorly differentiated (insular) thyroid carcinoma displaying the characteristic solid tumour cell islands (insulae) separated by narrow fibrovascular septa. There is no hint of follicular or other differentiation here (H&E stain, medium magnification).

and is composed of large solid nests (insulae) punctuated by occasional primitive follicles (**Figure 19.29**). Minor elements of classical papillary thyroid carcinoma and/or follicular carcinoma may be recognized. Obversely, an insular growth pattern is by no means exclusive to poorly differentiated carcinoma and important differential diagnoses include medullary thyroid carcinoma, solid variant papillary thyroid carcinoma and undifferentiated (anaplastic) carcinoma.

Alternatively, PDTC may be specified according to mitotic state (exceeding five mitoses per ten high power fields, × 400) and/or comedo-like tumour necrosis. These portend

a survival rate of 60 per cent at five years, irrespective of tumour architecture. Furthermore, the combination of solid growth and the presence of at least one of the following: convoluted nuclei, tumour necrosis and/or over three mitoses per ten high power fields, × 400, is a powerful predictor of poor outcome. This group constitutes the major cause of radioiodine (RAI) refractory, positron emission tomography (PET)-positive incurable thyroid carcinomas.[33]

Confusingly, the term 'poorly differentiated carcinoma' is also applied by some observers to differentiated carcinomas showing a solid, trabecular or scirrhous pattern, to tall cell papillary carcinomas and to columnar cell carcinomas. This lack of consensus may explain conflicting data as to whether a minority component of insular carcinoma in an otherwise differentiated carcinoma is an independent prognostic factor or not and, if so, at what threshold this begins to be a clinically valid observandum.

Unsurprisingly, the tumour cells demonstrate cytokeratins, thyroglobulin and thyroid transcription factor-1 immunopositivity, but negative pan-neuroendocrine markers and calcitonin.

Columnar cell carcinoma

Columnar cell carcinoma is a rare thyroid neoplasm, which once invasive pursues a more aggressive course than other differentiated thyroid carcinomas. Where it remains encapsulated, however, there appears to be little risk of metastasis.[41] There is disagreement as to whether it is best classified as a distinct entity rather than a variant of papillary thyroid carcinoma. There is indeed morphological overlap between columnar cell carcinoma, the cribriform-morular variant of papillary thyroid carcinoma and also so-called familial adenomatous polyposis (FAP)-associated thyroid carcinoma (remembering that thyroid carcinomas of conventional pattern also occur in FAP patients).

This notwithstanding, the typical architecture resembles that of intestinal and endometrioid carcinomas with complex glandular, cribriform and solid growth. The individual cells are tall and columnar, but striking nuclear hyperstratification and hyperchromasia enable separation from tall cell variant of papillary thyroid carcinoma (**Figure 19.30**). Immunohistochemically, it is usually cytokeratin, thyroglobulin and thyroid transcription factor-1 positive.

Undifferentiated carcinoma

Undifferentiated (anaplastic) carcinoma is a highly malignant tumour typically seen in elderly patients with a female preponderance. It accounts for approximately 2–10 per cent of all malignant thyroid neoplasms,[42] with a predilection for iodine-deficient regions although its overall incidence is declining.[43] Undifferentiated (anaplastic) thyroid carcinoma is usually widely invasive at presentation and inoperable in roughly half of cases. It carries a high mortality and accounts for nearly a half of all deaths associated with thyroid malignancy.[8] The overall median survival is four months and the five-year survival rate is less than 10 per cent. All undifferentiated thyroid carcinomas are arbitrarily UICC/TNM staged as pT4 due to their anticipated aggressive behaviour, classically showing widespread infiltration of

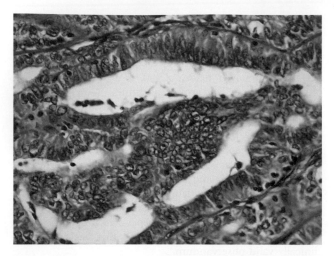

Figure 19.30 Columnar cell carcinoma illustrating the classical, complex glandular growth pattern resembling gastric, colorectal or endometrial adenocarcinoma. The tumour cells are columnar with prominent nuclear hyperstratification (H&E stain, high magnification).

surrounding structures, regional lymph node metastases and distant metastasis to any site.[8] Presentation with early, intracapsular anaplastic carcinoma, which is more amenable to surgical extirpation, portends a slightly more favourable outlook but is uncommon.

Undifferentiated (anaplastic) carcinoma can arise *de novo*, but the presence of synchronous better differentiated carcinomatous elements in over 50 per cent of cases is taken as evidence of dedifferentiation of a pre-existing neoplasm.[44] Thus, there may be a history of longstanding thyroid disease complicated by a recent phase of accelerated growth. The histological features are tremendously variable with two main patterns being pleomorphic epithelioid (giant cell) and spindle cell (sarcomatoid) (**Figure 19.31**). A variety of other microscopical patterns are recognized and are renowned for troublesome differential diagnosis (**Table 19.6**). Angiolymphatic penetration is characteristic and a brisk inflammatory response is often encountered.

While the term 'carcinoma' is applied, compelling proof of epithelial differentiation is not always forthcoming and the diagnosis ultimately rests upon an acceptable morphological pattern in an appropriate clinicoradiological context. Immunohistochemical staining for cytokeratin and vimentin are at least focally positive in approximately 90 per cent of cases with epithelial membrane antigen reactivity in 50 per cent of examples. Thyroglobulin, thyroid transcription factor-1, calcitonin and pan-neuroendocrine epitopes are typically negative. Diffusion of thyroglobulin from destroyed non-neoplastic follicles, however, may give rise to spurious immunopositivity. Endothelial markers (CD31, CD34 and factor VIII) may be focally demonstrated in some tumours presenting an angiosarcomatoid morphology, which may rarely prevail. Occasional cases are completely immunoinert and ultrastructural studies are seldom rewarding. Where appropriate, a haematolymphoid immunopanel should always be considered, particularly on FNAC and needle core biopsies, so as not to overlook high-grade or anaplastic non-Hodgkin's lymphoma.

TUMOURS SHOWING C-CELL DIFFERENTIATION

Medullary thyroid carcinoma

Medullary thyroid carcinoma (MTC) is a malignant tumour displaying parafollicular C-cell differentiation,[45] which secretes calcitonin and often a variety of other neuropeptides.[46] It is an uncommon tumour accounting for 5–8 per cent of all thyroid cancers.[47] It may occur sporadically or against a background of an inherited autosomal dominant trait related to a germline mutation of the *RET* proto-oncogene, which cause MEN 2A, MEN 2B or familial MTC (FMTC).

Sporadic MTC is more common in females and presents at a mean age of 50 years. MEN 2A presents in adolescence or young adults, while MEN 2B presents in infancy or childhood.[8] Sporadic tumours are usually single, whereas hereditary tumours are often multicentric and/or bilateral. FMTC arises from C-cell hyperplasia, which is considered a precursor lesion and can be identified histologically with due diligence.

Regional lymph node metastasis and distant lymphatogenous spread are found in 20 and 8 per cent of cases at presentation, respectively. Secondary sites of predilection include lung, liver, adrenal and bone. MEN 2B MTC generally pursues a more aggressive course than MEN 2A MTC, which in turn portends a less favourable prognosis than sporadic MTC, although for those with neoplasms confined to within the thyroid gland, overall long-term survival approaches 95 per cent, indeed many patients survive for years despite secondary systemic involvement.[3] Micro-MTCs detected through screening are associated with a better outcome than those examples over 1 cm.

MTCs may be well demarcated or infiltrative, sometimes encapsulated (**Figure 19.32**). They are commonly located in the middle third of the lateral lobes, where C-cell concentration is greatest. Microscopically, they comprise solid sheets, nests and trabecula of cells separated by slender fibrovascular septa (**Figure 19.33**). A panoply of histological variants are seen, most of no clinical importance other than they may masquerade as other tumours (**Table 19.7**). There is usually only modest nuclear pleomorphism, but necrosis may be a feature. Amyloid protein deposition is present in up to 80 per cent or so of cases (**Figure 19.34**) and may mineralize or elicit a foreign body granulomatous response.

The usual immunophenotype is positive for cytokeratins, calcitonin, thyroid transcription factor-1, carcinoembryonic antigen (CEA, CD66e) and pan-neuroendocrine markers. Calcitonin-depleted tumours may behave more aggressively, but almost invariably stain for CEA (**Figure 19.35**). Other neuropeptides may be demonstrated, including calcitonin gene-related peptide, somatostatin, ACTH, serotonin, gastrin, bombesin and histaminase, among others. A S100 protein positive subpopulation of sustentacular cells is more commonly seen in hereditary cases (**Figure 19.36**), potentially overlapping morphologically with paraganglioma, although paragangliomas (with the rare, anomalous exception of those involving the cauda equina) are cytokeratin negative. It is wise to be aware that neuroendocrine

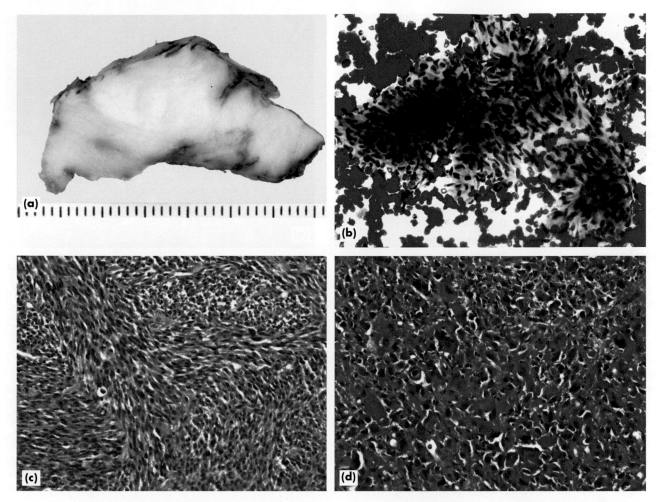

Figure 19.31 (a) A cross-sectional slice through a thyroid lobectomy specimen substantially replaced by undifferentiated (anaplastic) thyroid carcinoma. The solid, dense, featureless and infiltrative nature is paradigmatic. (b) Fine needle aspiration cytology (FNAC) specimen from undifferentiated (anaplastic) thyroid carcinoma showing a tridimensional, acervate clump of pleomorphic, high-grade malignant spindle cells (Pap stain, medium magnification). (c) A field of fibrosarcoma-like undifferentiated (anaplastic) thyroid carcinoma composed of fasciculated, malignant fusiform cells (H&E stain, medium magnification). (d) Undifferentiated (anaplastic) thyroid carcinoma showing highly pleomorphic epithelioid tumour cells with numerous bizarre giant cells and monster cells ('monstrocytes'), some polykaryocytic (H&E stain, medium magnification).

neoplasms other than MTC may sometimes express aberrant calcitonin immunoreactivity, for example laryngeal and bronchopulmonary atypical carcinoid tumours, although the latter are typically immunonegative for carcinoembryonic antigen (CEA, CD66e) and there is more often than not normocalcaemia.

Electron microscopy identifies membrane-bound electron-dense storage granules ranging from 100 to 300 nm in diameter with augmented rough endoplasmic reticulum and Golgi apparatus (**Figure 19.37**).

C-cell hyperplasia and neoplasia

FMTC develops in a milieu of C-cell hyperplasia and there is no recognized benign C-cell adenoma counterpart. Reactive (physiological) C-cell hyperplasia occurs with advancing age, in thyroiditis, in hyperparathyroidism, in close proximity to other thyroid neoplasms or solid cell nests and in

hypergastrinaemia. There is no unanimously accepted definition of nodular (neoplastic, 'MTC *in situ*') C-cell proliferation, but over 50 C-cells per × 100 field has been proposed,[48] where there is obliteration of follicular spaces by solid, intrafollicular C-cell growth delimited by basement membrane, as demonstrated by immunostaining for collagen IV (**Figure 19.38**). Once there is violation of basement membrane and/or tumour-derived basal lamina reduplication, that intuitively constitutes MTC proper – the distinction between micro-MTC and intrathyroidal spread of MTC, however, may be impossible.

C-cells cannot be reliably identified by morphology on routine histological slides without recourse to calcitonin, carcinoembryonic antigen (CEA, CD66e) or pan-neuroendocrine immunophenotyping. This has, however, assumed less importance with the advent of more sensitive and specific molecular analysis looking for *RET* proto-oncogene germline mutations in the diagnosis of hereditary MTC syndromes.

Table 19.6   Recognized histological variants of undifferentiated (anaplastic) thyroid carcinoma and their mimics.

Pattern	Major differential diagnosis
Epithelioid	Poorly differentiated carcinoma
	Papillary carcinoma, solid variant
	Metastatic carcinoma
Sarcomatoid	Sarcoma proper
Angiomatoid	Angiosarcoma
Osteoclastic	Pleomorphic sarcoma
Rhabdoid	Rhabdomyosarcoma
Lympho-epithelioma-like	CASTLE
Paucicellular	Riedel's thyroiditis
Carcino-sarcomatoid	Osteosarcoma
	Rhabdomyosarcoma
Adenosquamous	Metastatic carcinoma
	Sclerosing mucoepidermoid with eosinophilocytosis
Squamous cell carcinoma	Metastatic disease
	Direct extension
	Papillary thyroid carcinoma
	CASTLE

Note that any individual tumour may present a mixture of appearances in any combination or permutation.

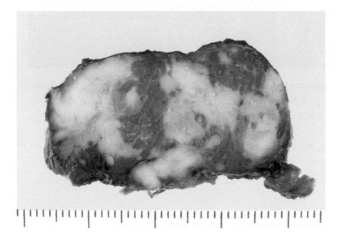

Figure 19.32   The cut surface of multicentric medullary thyroid carcinoma occurring in MEN 2B demonstrating widespread effacement of thyroid tissue by infiltrative, solid, white tumour, which abuts and focally violates anatomical thyroid capsule.

Tumours displaying joint follicular and C-cell differentiation

The concept of mixed follicular-parafollicular carcinoma is enigmatic. Collision (combined) tumours include follicular carcinoma plus MTC and papillary carcinoma plus MTC. True follicular-parafollicular carcinoma (differentiated carcinoma of intermediate type) occurring as a genuine hybrid (composite) neoplasm is exceptionally rare. The two cell populations may either share origin from a common stem cell or be of dual clonality. The follicular component is

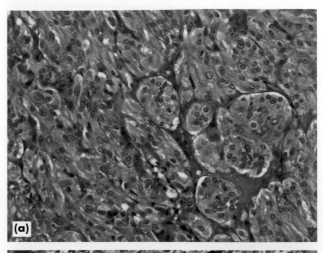

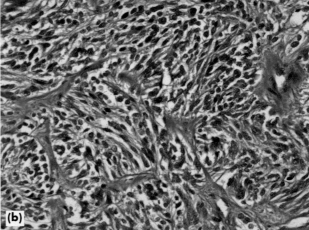

Figure 19.33   (a) The typical nested or pseudoalveolar ('zell ballen') architecture of medullary thyroid carcinoma, type ordinaire. These tumour cells are largely epithelioid and monotonous (H&E stain, high magnification). (b) This field shows mild pleomorphism and a more fusiform cell morphology (H&E stain, high magnification).

Table 19.7   Histological variants of MTC.

Variant	
Follicular/glandular	Small cell
Oncocytic (oxyphilic)	Clear cell
Giant cell (anaplastic)	Spindle cell
Pigmented	Squamous
Papillary	Pseudoangiosarcomatoid
Neuroblastoma-like	Carcinoid-like
Paraganglioma-like	Medullary microcarcinoma (latent carcinoma)

There is often a mixed pattern in any individual example.

sometimes non-neoplastic, thereby raising the possibility of implicated follicles within a slowly growing MTC. False-positive thyroglobulin staining may result from passive diffusion out of nearby native follicles or following active

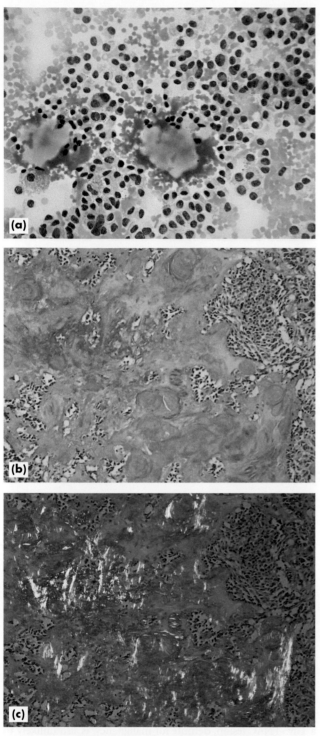

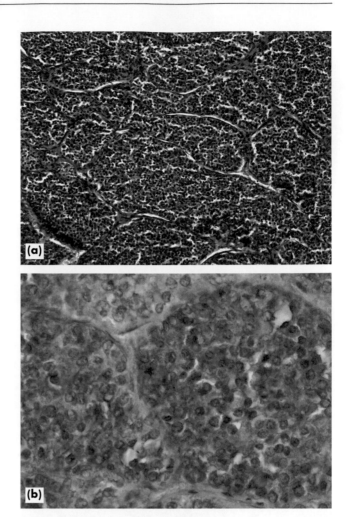

Figure 19.35 (a) Calcitonin poor, small cell variant of medullary thyroid carcinoma. Note the insular growth pattern (H&E stain, intermediate magnification). (b) The same tumour exhibiting carcinoembryonic antigen (CEA, CD66e) positivity. This example was negative for calcitonin and only weakly positive for chromogranin A, reflecting a paucity of intracytoplasmic storage granules, despite raised circulating serum calcitonin levels (CEA IHC, high magnification).

Figure 19.34 (a) Fine needle aspiration cytology (FNAC) preparation from medullary thyroid carcinoma, depicting loosely cohesive, moderately pleomorphic, plasmacytoid tumour cells together with several globules of amorphous amyloid protein (May–Grunwald-Giemsa (MGG) stain, high magnification). (b) Medullary thyroid carcinoma with conspicuous amorphous, dense, pink/red amyloid protein stroma separating groups of tumour cells (Congo red stain, low magnification). (c) The identical field viewed under high intensity, cross-polarized light corroborates anomalous red/green colouration (sometimes incorrectly termed 'apple green birefringence') characteristic of amyloid protein. Similar anomalous colours are also often seen on routine H&E staining, though more weakly so. (Congo red stain, high magnification).

pinophagocytosis by tumour cells, rather than endogenous synthesis proper. The conventional ontogenetic explanation proposing different origins for follicular cells and C-cells, however, fails to reconcile the observation of apparent genuine coexpression of both thyroglobulin and calcitonin in the same tumour cell.[3]

OTHER NEOPLASMS AND TUMOUR–LIKE LESIONS

There are very many other less common or incredibly rare neoplasms affecting the thyroid gland of epithelial, mesenchymal, haematolymphoid, thymic, parathyroid gland and developmental origin, together with a few tumour-like lesions (**Box 19.1**).

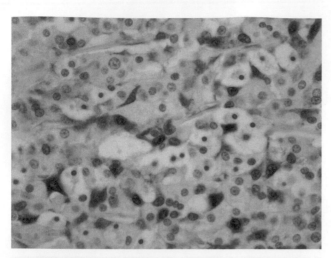

Figure 19.36 Medullary thyroid carcinoma in MEN 2 showing typical S100 protein reactive, spindly sustentacular cells mantling small nests of secretory tumour cells (S100 IHC, high magnification).

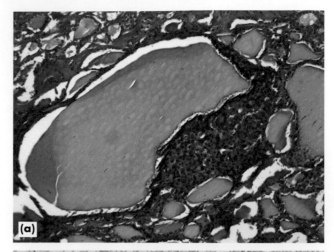

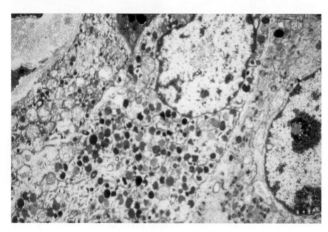

Figure 19.37 Transmission electron micrograph depicting several tumour cells from a medullary thyroid carcinoma, occurring in a child with known MEN 2B. Numerous dense, membrane-bound neurosecretory vesicles are present in the cytoplasm (transmission electron microscope (TEM), ultra-high magnification).

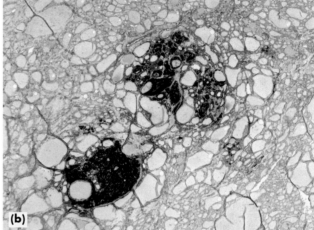

Figure 19.38 (a) Early nodular (neoplastic) C-cell hyperplasia in MEN 2, readily identified on routine staining. There is expansion of C-cells within the follicular basement membrane, but no destructive or infiltrative growth (H&E stain, medium magnification). (b) More marked and multicentric nodular (neoplastic) C-cell proliferation with follicular obliteration and interstitial expansion. This probably amounts to at least medullary carcinoma *in situ*, if not medullary thyroid microcarcinoma ('microtumour') proper (calcitonin IHC, high magnification).

Metastatic tumours

The thyroid gland is commonly affected by metastases either by direct extension from neighbouring structures, haematogenous or lymphatic spread. Local structures include the larynx or lymph nodes and common non-head and neck primary sites include bronchopulmonary, breast, malignant melanoma and renal cell carcinoma (**Figure 19.39**). The latter may occur metachronously following an interval of up to 19 years or be a synchronous presenting feature of the disease.[34]

INTRAOPERATIVE FROZEN SECTION EXAMINATION

The use of perioperative frozen section examination to assist in the diagnosis of thyroid lesions has dwindled in recent years.

The widespread adoption of FNAC has enabled broad preoperative categorization of many lesions, which by their very nature cannot be further refined by frozen section assessment, for example Thy3 follicular lesion, follicular neoplasm and oncocytic (oxyphil) neoplasm. Frozen section examination on a Thy5 FNAC lesion, definite for malignancy, is also unlikely to confer any significant benefit other than perhaps evaluation of resection margins. If the distinction between high-grade lymphoma and undifferentiated (anaplastic) carcinoma has not already been made on FNAC or needle core biopsy, then frozen section is equally unlikely to resolve this. Fleshy, solitary encapsulated lesions are likely to represent follicular adenoma or minimally invasive follicular carcinoma, but attempts to comprehensively sample the capsule in the fresh state should be resisted pending tissue fixation with a view to proper paraffin sections in order to obviate artefactual disruption and distortion of the all important pericapsular tissue planes. The indications for perioperative frozen section examination of

Box 19.1 Uncommon or rare tumours and tumour-like lesions described in the thyroid gland

- Squamous cell carcinoma
- Mucoepidermoid carcinoma
- Mucoepidermoid carcinoma with eosinophilocytosis
- Mucinous carcinoma
- Spindle cell tumour with thymus-like differentiation (SETTLE)
- Carcinoma showing thymus-like differentiation (CASTLE)
- Malignant lymphomas and leukaemias
- Langerhan's cell histiocytosis
- Angiosarcoma
- Solitary fibrous tumour
- Smooth muscle neoplasms
- Peripheral nerve sheath tumours
- Paraganglioma
- Teratoma
- Inflammatory pseudotumour
- Fibromatosis
- Granular cell tumour
- Synovial sarcoma
- Haemangiopericytoma
- Lipoma
- Liposarcoma
- Chondrosarcoma
- Osteosarcoma
- Haemangioma
- Lymphangioma
- Epithelioid haemangioendothelioma
- Small cell neuroendocrine carcinoma

The list is not exhaustive and a few may arguably be reclassified differently in the light of modern thinking.

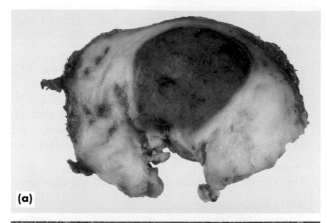

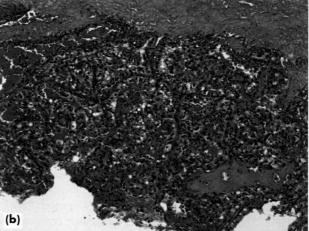

Figure 19.39 (a) Thyroid lobectomy specimen corticated by squamous cell carcinoma, secondary to direct contiguous infiltration from an advanced stage, upper aerodigestive tract primary site. (b) Needle core biopsy of metachronous, metastatic clear cell renal carcinoma presenting as a mass in the thyroid gland some 13 years after nephrectomy for clear cell carcinoma. Its true nature was completely unsuspected clinically – there was no mention of a previous operation in the clinical records. Nonetheless, the pathological findings were unequivocal and the kidney specimen was eventually retrieved from the archives for comparison and review (H&E stain, medium magnification).

thyroid gland lesions are best agreed by the relevant multidisciplinary team at a local level, taking into consideration local circumstances, individual experience and preferences together with clinical expectations.[49]

THYROID CANCER STAGING

The UICC/AJCC TNM classification of malignant tumours is internationally ratified, currently in its seventh edition (**Box 19.2**).[50]

PARATHYROID GLANDS

The normal parathyroid glands

Most individuals possess at least two pairs of parathyroid glands (PTG). The cephalad pair are embryologically derived from the fourth branchial cleft and are usually located over the posterior surface of the thyroid gland close to the point of entry of the inferior thyroid artery. The caudad glands are of

third branchial pouch origin and typically lie over the lower thyroid gland pole, although they are more variably placed and may be found within the mediastinum or even the pericardium, consequent upon comigration with the thymus, which is similarly of third branchial pouch ontogeny. Supernumerary or heterotopic (ectopic) glandular tissue may consist of less well-formed, more diffuse cell aggregates within cervical soft tissues (parathyromatosis) often in close proximity to eutopic glands and this pattern also characterizes surgically implanted gland tissue.[4]

The parathyroid glands secrete parathyroid hormone (parathormone, PTH), which elevates serum calcium via direct effects on kidney and bone and indirectly through the intestine. To the unaided eye, the glands are a yellow-brown colour. At operation, brown fat, yellow fat, sequestrated thyroid tissue, thymus, lymph node and autonomic ganglia may all mimic these appearances and such are not infrequently submitted for frozen section examination in

---

Box 19.2   UICC/AJCC TNM classification of malignant tumours of the thyroid gland (7th edn).[50]

Rules for classification

The classification applies to carcinomas. There should be microscopic confirmation of the disease and division of cases by histological type.

The following are the procedures for assessing T, N and M categories:

T categories	Physical examination, endoscopy and imaging
N categories	Physical examination and imaging
M categories	Physical examination and imaging

Regional lymph nodes

The regional lymph nodes are the cervical and upper/superior mediastinal nodes.

TNM clinical classification

T, Primary tumour

Tx	Primary tumour cannot be assessed
T0	No evidence of primary tumour
T1	Tumour 2 cm or less in greatest dimension, limited to the thyroid
T1a	Tumour 1 cm or less in greatest dimension, limited to the thyroid
T1b	Tumour more than 1 cm, but not more than 2 cm in greatest dimension, limited to the thyroid
T2	Tumour more than 2 cm, but not more than 4 cm in greatest dimension, limited to the thyroid
T3	Tumour more than 4 cm in greatest dimension, limited to the thyroid or any tumour with minimal extrathyroid extension (e.g. extension to sternothyroid muscle or perithyroid soft tissues)
T4a	Tumour extends beyond the thyroid capsule and invades any of the following: subcutaneous soft tissues, larynx, trachea, oesophagus, recurrent laryngeal nerve
T4b	Tumour invades prevertebral fascia, mediastinal vessels or encases carotid artery

All anaplastic carcinomas are considered T4 tumours

T4a*	(anaplastic carcinoma only) Tumour (any size) limited to the thyroid
T4b*	(anaplastic carcinoma only) Tumour (any size) extends beyond the thyroid capsules

Notes: Multifocal tumours of all histological types should be designated (m) (the largest determines the classification), e.g. T2(m).

N, Regional lymph nodes

NX	Regional lymph nodes cannot be assessed
N0	No regional lymph node metastasis
N1	Regional lymph node metastasis
N1a	Metastasis in level VI (pretracheal, paratracheal and prelaryngeal/Delphian lymph nodes)
N1b	Metastasis in other unilateral, bilateral or contralateral cervical (levels I, II, IV or V) or retropharyngeal or superior mediastinal lymph nodes

M, Distant metastasis

M0	No distant metastasis
M1	Distant metastasis

pTNM pathological classification

The pT and pN categories correspond to the T and N categories.

pN0	Histological examination of a selective neck dissection specimen will ordinarily include six or more lymph nodes. If the lymph nodes are negative, but the number ordinarily examined is not met, classify as pN0.

Histological types

The four major histopathological types are:

- Papillary carcinoma (including those with follicular foci)
- Follicular carcinoma (including so-called Hürthle cell carcinoma)
- Medullary carcinoma
- Anaplastic/undifferentiated carcinoma

Stage grouping

Separate stage groupings are recommended for papillary and follicular (differentiated), medullary and anaplastic (undifferentiated) carcinomas:

Papillary or follicular, under 45 years

Stage I	Any T	Any N	M0
Stage II	Any T	Any N	M1

Papillary or follicular, 45 years and older

Stage I	T1a, T1b	N0	M0
Stage II	T2	N0	M0
Stage III	T3	N0	M0
	T1, T2, T3	N1a	M0
Stage IVA	T1, T2, T3	N1B	M0
	T4a	N0, N1	M0
Stage IVB	T4b	Any N	M0
Stage IVC	Any T	Any N	M1

Medullary

Stage I	T1a, T1b	N0	M0
Stage II	T2, T3	N0	M0
Stage III	T1, T2, T3	N1a	M0
Stage IVA	T1, T2, T3	N1b	M0
	T4a	Any N	M0
Stage IVB	T4b	Any N	M0
Stage IVC	Any T	Any N	M1

Anaplastic carcinoma

All anaplastic carcinoma are stage IV

Stage IVA	T4a	Any N	M0
Stage IVB	T4b	Any N	M0
Stage IVC	Any T	Any N	M1

Summary, thyroid gland

Papillary, follicular and medullary carcinoma

T1	≤2 cm, intrathyroidal
T2	>2–4 cm, intrathyroidal
T3	>4 cm or minimal extrathyroidal extension
T4a	Subcutaneous, larynx, trachea, oesophagus, recurrent laryngeal nerve
T4b	Prevertebral fascia, mediastinal vessels, carotid artery

Anaplastic/undifferentiated carcinoma

T4a	Tumour limited to thyroid
T4b	Tumour beyond thyroid capsule

All types

Na1	Level VI
N1b	Other regional

lieu of parathyroid gland proper. Microscopically, in the normal state, the glands are lobulated, richly vascularized and composed of nests and/or trabecula of polygonal parenchymal cells, that is a mixture of chief (principal) cells, water-clear cells and oncocytic (oxyphil) cells, interspersed with adipocytes (**Figures 19.40** and **19.41**). The number, size and composition of the glands, however, are subject to wide normal and abnormal variation (**Table 19.8**) influenced by age, gender, nutritional and hormonal status. With advancing age, congeries of oncocytic (oxyphil) cells are increasingly encountered.

Hyperparathyroidism

Hyperparathyroidism is defined by elevated serum PTH and is the most common pathological condition affecting the parathyroid glands. It is classified into primary, secondary and tertiary forms dependent upon the identification of a driving stimulus (**Table 19.9**), although the end result is an absolute increase in parenchymal cell mass affecting one or more glands (**Figure 19.42**).

In primary parathyroid gland hyperplasia, all of the parathyroid glands are enlarged, albeit unevenly in some cases. In

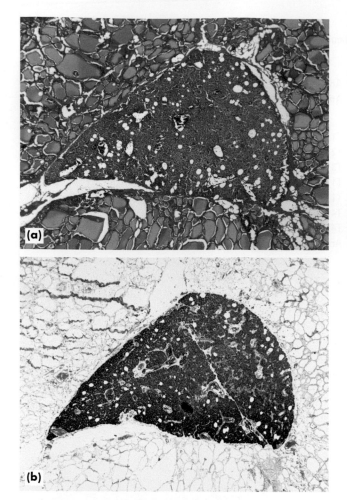

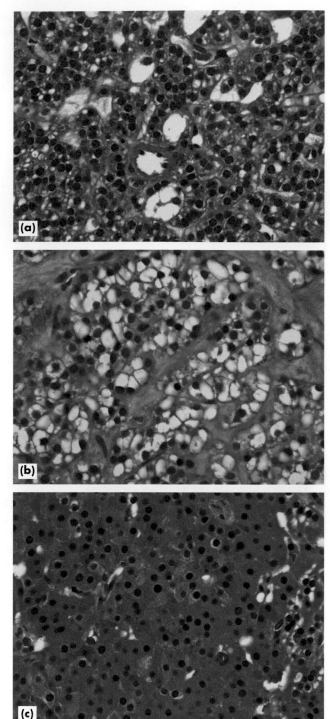

Figure 19.40 (a) An intrathyroidal parathyroid gland presenting a normal vascularized, lobular microarchitecture comprising parenchymal cells interspersed with a normal complement of mature fat cells – these are of haphazard distribution and density. Note its clear circumscription and delicate fibrous capsule (H&E stain, low magnification). (b) A replicate section immunostained with anti-PTH antibody showing intense parenchymal positivity, in sharp contrast to the surrounding negative thyroid gland follicles acting as an internal negative control (PTH IHC, low magnification).

parathyroid gland adenoma, only a single gland is enlarged, the remaining glands being of normal size or small. This is typically accompanied by marked diminution in intraglandular adipocytes and reduced or absent intracytoplasmic lipid droplets (**Figure 19.43**), although rarely the latter may paradoxically be more abundant in chief cells located between hyperplastic nodules. Additionally, foci of irregularly distributed stromal fat cells may persist recapitulating a rim of normal glandular tissue, which when juxtaposed to a fat-depleted hyperplastic nodule, may lead to erroneous interpretation as an adenoma – the most reliable discrimination between hyperplasia and adenoma is achieved through histological examination of multiple glands augmented by multiple sections through larger glands. If only one parathyroid gland is available for examination and proves to be enlarged and/or hypercellular, definitive pathological distinction between hyperplasia and adenoma cannot be reliably achieved.

Figure 19.41 (a) Nests and trabecula of isomorphic chief cells forming occasional glandular lumina or so-called microfollicular/pseudofollicular growth pattern (H&E stain, high magnification). (b) Clusters of water-clear cells displaying their characteristic clear, generally univacuolar cytoplasm with eccentrically displaced nuclei (H&E stain, high magnification). (c) Nodular sheets of oncocytic (oxyphil) cells illustrating their hallmark, copious, granular and densely eosinophilic cytoplasm, attributable to plentiful mitochondria. A minor degree of random nuclear pleomorphism is often encountered (H&E stain, high magnification).

Table 19.8 Attributes of normal and abnormal parathyroid glands in man.[3]

Characteristic	Normal range	Abnormal
Number	Usually 4, but ranges from 1–12	
Size	Length 3–6 mm	>6 mm in any plane
	Width 2–4 mm	
	Depth 0.5–2 mm	
Weight	Each gland approximately 30 mg – the inferior glands are often heavier than the superior ones	Any individual gland >60 mg
	Total parathyroid gland mass 120 ± 3.5 mg in males	
	142 ± 5.2 mg in females	
Percentage fat	17–50%	Complete absence or very marked reduction
	Male average 20.5%	
	Female average 15.6%	
Intracytoplasmic lipid	Abundant	Absent or sparse

Only primary and tertiary hyperparathyroidism are associated with hypercalcaemia and its attendant systemic sequelae, but all three forms may manifest with bone disease. Aberrant parathyroid hormone-related peptide (PTHrP) secretion may occur as a paraneoplastic phenomenon (humoural hypercalcaemia of malignancy) in some malignant neoplasms, notably squamous cell carcinoma of primary

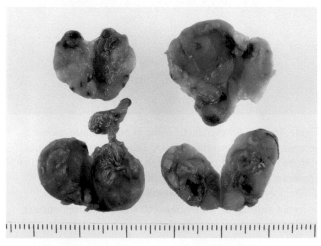

Figure 19.42 Left and right upper and lower parathyroid glands in quadriglandular hyperplasia of secondary hyperparathyroidism following renal transplantation. These each weighed between 0.5 and 1.2 g and were incised bivalvate peroperatively to disclose the variegated, multinodular cut surfaces seen here to be irregular, both within and between glands. The lower glands are often asymmetrically larger than the upper glands.

Table 19.9 Classification of hyperparathyroidism.

Type	Definition	Causes	Pathological changes
Primary	Over-production of PTH due to intrinsic abnormality of one or more glands causing elevated serum calcium with depressed serum phosphate	PTG adenoma 85% PTG carcinoma 1% PTG hyperplasia 14% Sporadic MEN 1 MEN 2 Familial isolated hyperparathyroidism Familial hypocalcuric hypercalcaemia	Adenoma or carcinoma changes Chief cell hyperplasia Reduced or absent intra-parenchymal fat Diffuse or nodular changes
Secondary	Compensatory hyperplasia of parathyroid glands due to decreased serum calcium usually resulting in normocalcaemia	Chronic renal failure Malabsorption Vitamin D deficiency Renal tubular acidosis	Hyperplasia of all glands. May be indistinguishable from primary hyperparathyroidism. Multinodular or diffuse
Tertiary	Autonomous parathyroid gland hyperfunction following secondary hyperparathyroidism	Any cause of secondary hyperparathyroidism	Very similar to secondary hyperparathyroidism, although glands are typically larger and multinodular May rarely be associated with adenoma or carcinoma

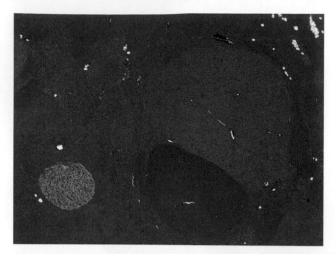

Figure 19.43 A hyperplastic gland in hyperparathyroidism, secondary to chronic renal disease, displaying hypercellularity with hugely reduced stromal fat cell content. The multinodular appearance is due to proliferation of groups of cells with different cytological features, mostly chief cells here with, unevenly distributed, water-clear cell and oxyphil cell nodules (H&E stain, ultralow magnification).

bronchopulmonary, upper aerodigestive tract and female genital tract origin, sometimes with renal cell carcinoma. Approximately 50 per cent of metastatic prostatic adenocarcinoma deposits evince anomalous PTH immunopositivity, crossreacting with PTHrP, which may prove to be a source of differential diagnostic confusion. Hypercalcaemia directly related to the osteolytic effects of bone metastasis, independent of PTHrP, may occur in mammary carcinoma and haematological malignancies. Lithium therapy prescribed for psychiatric disorders may induce a form of primary hyperparathyroidism, which abates on cessation of the drug, although parathyroidectomy may still be indicated.

Parathyroid gland adenoma

Parathyroid gland adenoma is the predominant cause of primary hyperparathyroidism. It may occur spontaneously or within the context of various syndromes. Irradiation of the neck is a potential risk factor. Excision of the abnormal gland is curative and results in normalization of biochemical indices and increased bone mineral density. Up to 10 per cent of patients relapse, sometimes after an interval of many years.

The morphological spectrum of parathyroid adenomas occurring in heterotopic sites, e.g. mediastinum, thyroid gland or oesophagus, is identical to that in eutopic locations. However, not only may they lead to unsuccessful cervical exploration, they may mimic thyroid gland adenomas or medullary thyroid carcinoma histologically.

Double adenomas may rarely occur (responsible for between 1.7 and 12 per cent of cases of primary hyperparathyroidism) and are usually bilateral. All of the patients are symptomatic and show a higher PTH level and tumour weight compared to solitary adenoma and parathyroid gland hyperplasia. Distinction from asymmetrical parathyroid gland hyperplasia, particularly in the context of MEN, is extremely difficult. The diagnosis is, therefore, only considered conclusive when follow

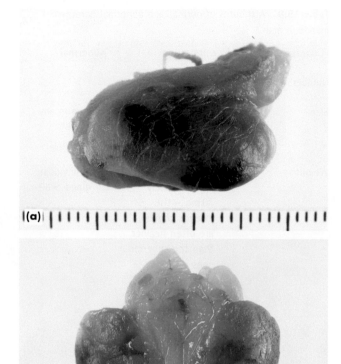

Figure 19.44 (a) The external surface of a parathyroid gland adenoma, weighing 1.2 g in primary hyperparathyroidism, demonstrating a delicate capsule with ramifying surface blood vessels. (b) When transected, its variegated, multinodular texture is very similar to a hyperplastic gland, although in this instance it was the only abnormal gland of those recovered at operation.

up after removal of two abnormal glands shows no recurrence. Gene-profiling studies indicate that multiple gland neoplasia represents a distinct molecular entity.

Parathyroid gland adenomas occur more frequently in the lower parathyroid glands. The mean weight is 0.55 g, but tumours weighing as much as 53 g are recorded and, generally, the more severe the hypercalcaemia, the bulkier the adenoma. Macroscopically, parathyroid gland adenomas are well marginated, soft and vary from yellow-red to orange-brown in colour (**Figure 19.44**). The oncocytic (oxyphil) cell variant presents a so-called mahogany brown cut surface, characteristic of such mitochondria-rich tumours at many sites. Secondary haemorrhage and/or cystic change (**Figure 19.45**) may be encountered, either spontaneously occurring or post-FNAC. The remaining, uninvolved parathyroid glands should be normal or reduced in size.

Microscopically, parathyroid gland adenomas are circumscribed and may be lobulated or nodular. They are hypercellular and substantially or completely bereft of intraglandular adipocytes, with the exception of lipoadenoma. An attenuated, part-circumferential mantle of normal or compressed parathyroid gland tissue is identified in 50 per cent

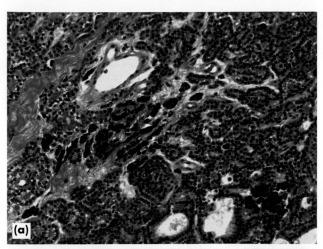

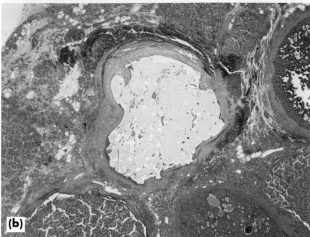

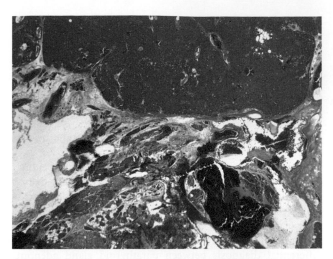

Figure 19.46 View of the edge of a parathyroid gland adenoma. Note its sharp demarcation, hypercellularity and absence of intratumoral lipocytes. There is a peripheral nubbin of attenuated looking parathyroid glandular tissue typically present close to the vascular hilum of the gland with preserved intraglandular fat cells for comparison (H&E stain, ultralow magnification).

Figure 19.45 (a) This adenoma shows scattered collections of interstitial siderophages containing phagocytosed coarsely granular, golden brown haemosiderin pigment, indicative of antecedent haemorrhage (H&E stain, intermediate magnification). (b) Another example displays focal cystic change with accompanying fibrocollagenous scar tissue plus part-circumferential, dystrophic, mural calcification (H&E stain, low magnification).

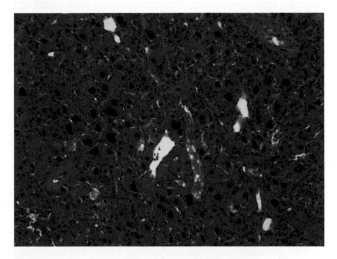

Figure 19.47 The presence of occasionally numerous bizarre giant or monster cells, some plurinucleate, possessing enlarged hyperchromatic nuclei, albeit without mitoses or other worrisome features, against a background of bland-looking cells should not be taken as evidence of malignancy. The cells illustrated here are predominantly oxyphilic (H&E stain, intermediate magnification).

or so of cases, dependent upon the planes of section examined (**Figure 19.46**), often near the hilum of the gland. The tumour cells may be disposed in solid sheets, cords, acini, follicles and/or microcysts. Glandular structures may contain eosinophilic colloid-like secretions and these are dPAS-positive but immunonegative for thyroglobulin. Intrafollicular or interstitial amyloid protein may rarely be deposited.

Most adenomas are composed of chief cells, though oncocytic (oxyphil) cells and/or water-clear cells are often present, either dispersed or in nodular aggregates. The chief cells of an adenoma are usually larger than their non-neoplastic counterparts present in the uninvolved rim of parathyroid tissue, where present, and in the remaining, non-neoplastic glands. They also typically possess less intracellular fat than the uninvolved tissue and the other suppressed glands. Mitoses usually number less than one per ten high power fields without abnormal forms. There may be random nuclear pleomorphism and/or multinucleation sometimes with bizarre, hyperchromatic giant cells (**Figure 19.47**), although in the absence of other indicators of potential malignancy these should not be

misconstrued as evidence portending aggressive behaviour. Flow cytometry is of limited assistance in discriminating between parathyroid gland adenoma and carcinoma because aneuploidy is found in up to 25 per cent of histologically and clinically benign tumours.

VARIANTS OF PARATHYROID GLAND ADENOMA

Lipoadenoma (parathyroid hamartoma) is a very rare occurrence showing admixture of parenchymal cells with copious mature adipocytes, the latter accounting for 20–90 per cent of the tumour. Approximately 50 per cent of such cases are associated with hypercalcaemia. The uninvolved parathyroid glands are normal.

Papillary variant is rare and apt to be mistaken for papillary thyroid carcinoma.

Water-clear adenoma is substantially or wholly composed of water-clear cells. It may be confused with clear cell neoplasms of the thyroid gland, including metastasis.

Follicular variant shows a predominant follicular (acinar) architecture often with intraglandular secretions and may be misinterpreted as a follicular thyroid neoplasm.

Oxyphil adenoma (oncocytic adenoma) is composed entirely of mitochondria-rich oncocytic (oxyphil) cells and may or may not be functional. It must be distinguished from nodular oxyphilic cell change with advancing age and, when intrathyroidal, from oxyphil (Hürthle) cell neoplasms of the thyroid gland.

Immunohistochemistry is occasionally valuable in the differential diagnosis between parathyroid gland adenoma and other neoplasms, notably of the thyroid gland. Parathyrocytes are cytokeratin positive and stain for many pan-neuroendocrine markers, both membrane-bound peptide products, such as PTH, chromogranin A, synaptophysin, etc., and cytosol epitopes including neurone specific enolase. Chief cells show nuclear immunoreactivity for TTF-1. Reciprocally negative staining for thyroglobulin may also be helpful. Immunostaining for antimitochondrial antibody highlights oncocytic (oxyphil) differentiation, but in itself does not discriminate between oncocytic parathyroid gland tissue and oncocytic change in other tissues. Staining for fat on frozen section is seldom of diagnostic help.

Molecular genetic studies by X-linked restriction fragment length polymorphism provide evidence for monoclonality in many parathyroid gland adenomas. Tumour-specific DNA alterations are present in the PTH gene in some cases. A minority of cases demonstrate pericentric inversion of chromosome 11, which causes translocation of the cyclin D1 gene with the PTH gene resulting in overexpression of cyclin D1 and cell proliferation. Cyclin D1 expression is identified by immunohistochemistry more frequently than this cyclin D1 gene rearrangement suggesting that other molecular factors are operant in cyclin D1 deregulation. Cyclin D1 is also common in parathyroid hyperplasia and parathyroid carcinoma.

The germline mutation underlying MEN 1 is associated with some sporadic parathyroid gland adenomas. The *RET* proto-oncogene germline mutation underlying MEN 2 does not appear to be involved in the genesis of sporadic parathyroid gland adenomas. Other chromosomal abnormalities are detected by comparative genomic hybridization and fluorescent *in situ* hybridization (FISH) techniques.

PARATHYROID CARCINOMA

This is defined as a malignant neoplasm of parathyroid parenchymal cells and is responsible for approximately 0.5 to 2 per cent of all cases of primary hyperparathyroidism, although some series report as high as 5 per cent. It occurs most frequently in the fifth and sixth decades (i.e. roughly a decade younger than adenomas) with no gender predilection. Most patients are severely hypercalcaemic with active bone and renal disease at presentation, they tend to suffer worse symptoms attributable to this compared to those with adenoma and there is more often a palpable neck mass, although this presentation is by no means

invariable. Initial designation as adenoma may be revised at a later time following recurrence and/or metastasis.[51]

Parathyroid carcinoma tends to invade local structures, is slow growing and metastasizes late. Complete surgical excision at first operation affords the best opportunity for cure, although this relies upon early recognition of its malignant nature, which cannot always be achieved. Following surgery, approximately 30 per cent of patients suffer local recurrence, usually within three years. Roughly 30 per cent develop metastasis, typically late in its course, generally to regional lymph nodes (30 per cent), lungs (40 per cent), liver (10 per cent) and bone. Survival is 60–85 per cent and 40–70 per cent at five years and ten years, respectively, with an average survival following recurrence of seven to eight years. Non-functioning examples may behave more aggressively than functioning ones. Death is usually attributable to the metabolic complications of hypercalcaemia rather than overwhelming tumour burden. Repeated surgery may palliate and adjuvant radiotherapy has a limited role. The response to chemotherapy is poor. The hypercalcaemia may become refractory to medical management and specialist anti-PTH immunotherapy has proven beneficial in very severe cases (**Figure 19.48**), occasionally eliciting a direct antitumour effect.[52]

The tumour size is generally larger than that of parathyroid gland adenoma with an average weight between 6.7 and 12 g, although smaller tumours are currently being identified earlier. It may be encapsulated or obviously infiltrative. There may be a soft, brown appearance indistinguishable from adenoma, or a firm, grey-white texture. Troublesome intraoperative dissection, owing to adherence to contiguous structures, should alert the perceptive surgeon to a possibility of malignancy.

Parathyroid carcinomas may be deceptively bland or overtly malignant and anything in between – it is the biological behaviour, however, which ultimately defines parathyroid carcinoma. In rare cases, there may be no histomorphological clues to indicate potential aggressiveness. Nonetheless, first-order morphological criteria of malignancy (absolute criteria) include

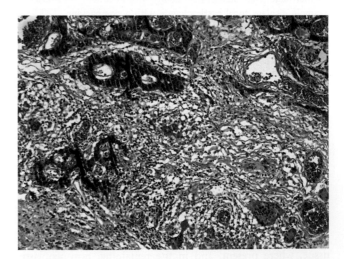

Figure 19.48 Metastatic parathyroid carcinoma in the lung, following anti-parathormone (PTH) immunotherapy for refractory, severe hypercalcaemia. Note the vigorous granulomatous inflammatory response, secondary to Freund's complete adjuvant, which used to intensify the immune response, closely associated with the nests of residual tumour cells (H&E stain, medium magnification).

Table 19.10 Microscopical criteria for the diagnosis of parathyroid carcinoma.[3, 49]

First order criteria	Second order criteria
Presence of either/or:	In the absence of first order criteria at least two or more of the following:

1. Invasion into surrounding tissues
    Thyroid
    Oesophagus
    Nerves
    Connective tissue
2. Histologically documented locoregional or distant metastasis
	1. Capsular invasion
	2. Vascular invasion
	3. Mitoses >5 per 10/hpf
	4. Broad intralesional fibrous septa with division into nodules
	5. Coagulative type necrosis
	6. Diffuse growth with elevated nucleus to cytoplasmic ratio
	7. Diffuse cellular atypia
	8. Abundant macronucleoli

invasion into adjacent tissues and/or histologically documented metastasis. When these are absent or inconclusive, a combination of second-order facultative features (features associated with malignancy), each in themselves not fully diagnostic, are invoked (**Table 19.10**).

Microscopically, the capsule is often thickened and is classically contiguous with broad internal fibrous septula, dividing the tumour into irregular nodular compartments (this must be differentiated from scarring in an adenoma, secondary to spontaneous infarction, FNAC or previous surgery). Invasion beyond the delimiting capsule (**Figure 19.49**) may or may not be obvious (and can be mimicked by pseudoinfiltration, sequestration/benign entrapment and/or implantation of benign tissue following rupture of a parathyroid adenoma capsule). Fibrosis and haemosiderin deposition may be encountered in hyperplasia, degenerate adenomas and carcinomas. Pericapsular vascular invasion (**Figure 19.50**) is virtually diagnostic of malignancy (although artefactual dislodgement of cells simulating tumour embolus must be considered) but is present in only 10 to 15 per cent of cases. Perineural infiltration is also diagnostic of malignancy, but is similarly an uncommon finding. There may be a variety of growth patterns and a trabecular or rosettoid architecture favours malignancy (but is not common and not entirely specific). Diffuse growth of isomorphic cells with elevated nucleus–cytoplasmic ratio is a tocsin (**Figure 19.51**), as is generalized nuclear pleomorphism (in contrast to focal, random cytonuclear atypia). Macronucleolation may be conspicuous. Areas of coagulative necrosis may be seen (and should not be mistaken for ischaemic damage or haemorrhage). The interpretation of mitoses has proven controversial – mitoses are present in both hyperplasia and adenoma, although generally below one mitosis per ten high power fields (obversely, mitotic figures may be completely absent in some metastasizing carcinomas and care must be taken to distinguish mitoses in endothelial and other stromal elements from those in tumour cells). The presence of very many mitoses and/or abnormal forms, however, is usually taken as presumptive evidence of malignant potential. There is currently no UICC/AJCC TNM staging classification for parathyroid carcinomas.[53]

The immunohistochemical proliferation marker Ki67 (MIB-1) is slightly higher in parathyroid carcinoma than adenoma, although there is overlap, with a proliferative index greater than 5 per cent suggestive of malignancy. Ki67 may also help in discriminating genuine mitotic figures from pyknotic nuclei (mitosoid bodies) in equivocal cases.

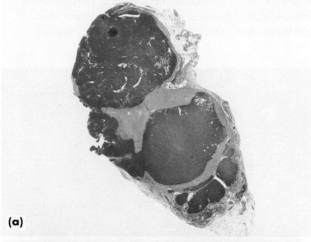

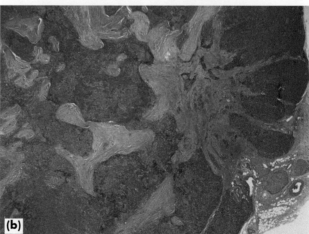

Figure 19.49 (a) Whole mount preparation of an oncocytic parathyroid carcinoma in a patient with MEN 2 demonstrating irregular, thick fibrous capsulation contiguous with conspicuous internal fibrous septa. This gland was adherent to surrounding structures at operation and dissected out with some difficulty (H&E stain, ultralow magnification). (b) The edge of another parathyroid carcinoma depicting an irregular, thick peripheral capsule, together with coarse intratumoral fibrous bands separating the expansile tumour nodules. This presents a broad advancing margin with surrounding soft tissues, rather than direct tentacular, permeative infiltration (H&E stain, low magnification).

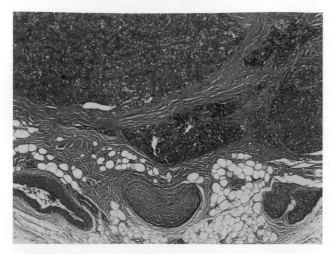

Figure 19.50 A pericapsular neurovascular bundle showing endothelialized intravascular tumour invasion characteristic of parathyroid carcinoma (H&E stain, medium magnification).

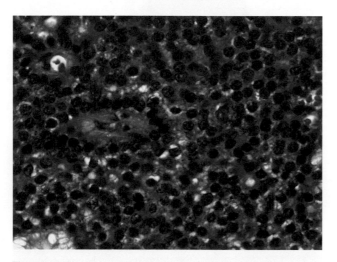

Figure 19.51 Parathyroid carcinoma composed of monotonous tumour cells showing raised nucleus–cytoplasmic ratio, nuclear hyperchromasia, coarse chromatin, macronucleolation and focal multinucleolation. A solitary mitosoid body is present towards the upper left hand corner (H&E stain, high magnification).

Galectin-3, cyclin D1, parafibromin, retinoblastoma protein and p27 immunostaining may be of limited assistance. Cytokeratin 14 (CK14) immunoreactivity has been reported as positive in oncocytic (oxyphil) adenomas, but not in oncocytic carcinomas.

An increased incidence of parathyroid carcinoma is reported in some hereditary hyperparathyroidism syndromes. Familial hyperparathyroidism represents a clinically and genetically heterogeneous group of disorders that includes multiple endocrine neoplasia 1 (MEN 1), multiple endocrine neoplasia 2 (MEN 2), familial hypocalciuric hypercalcaemia (FHH), hyperparathyroidism-jaw tumour (HPT-JT) syndrome and familial isolated hyperparathyroidism (FIHP). Parathyroid carcinoma is seen in 10–15 per cent of the autosomal dominant HPT-JT syndrome, but it is exceptionally rare in MEN 1 and MEN 2. Early studies of FIHP

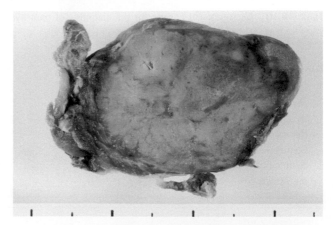

Figure 19.52 This atypical parathyroid gland adenoma is macroscopically indistinguishable from adenoma type ordinaire. The cut surface displays subtle capsular irregularity and localized fibrous thickening. First order criteria of malignancy were absent.

suggested an increased risk of parathyroid carcinoma, although the inclusion of some patients with HPT-JT syndrome casts doubt upon this conclusion. There are no reported cases of parathyroid carcinoma with FHH.

ATYPICAL PARATHYROID GLAND ADENOMA

Atypical parathyroid gland adenoma (parathyroid neoplasm of uncertain malignant potential or 'equivocal') is a diagnostic term attributed to a parathyroid gland tumour, which displays worrisome features, although falls short of fulfilling the first-order criteria for a confident designation of malignancy. This rubric acknowledges the limitations of predicting the behaviour of an individual tumour based upon conventional histomorphological assessment (it is the pathologist, who is uncertain, not the tumour) and it is not proffered as a distinct clinicopathological entity. Only a small minority of such atypical adenomas are expected to recur and/or metastasize and the rank importance of second-order criteria in quantifying this small risk of more aggressive behaviour has yet to be established.

Atypical parathyroid gland adenomas are generally indistinguishable from adenoma type ordinaire by the unaided eye (**Figure 19.52**). The most common microscopical features, ranked according to frequency, however, include intracapsular entrapment (87 per cent), intratumoral fibrosis (75 per cent), haemosiderosis (58 per cent), cyst formation (50 per cent), mitoses (25 per cent) and peritumoral fibrosis (25 per cent). The Ki67 proliferative index typically lies intermediate between adenoma and frank carcinoma. The value of ploidy studies in predicting local recurrence is based upon small studies.

Nonetheless, the use of this terminology serves to highlight those patients who merit closer surveillance, such as regular serum calcium measurements, while avoiding the stigma of a firm label of malignancy, wholly unjustified in most cases.[3]

OTHER PARATHYROID GLAND TUMOURS

Paraganglioma may rarely occur at this site. Tumour-like lesions, which may on occasion enter the differential diagnosis, include parathyroid cysts, branchiogenic cysts and amyloidosis. Secondary neolasms may be the result of direct extension from adjacent structures, such as larynx or thyroid, or from distant metastatic disease, most commonly of primary mammary, haematolymphoid, malignant melanoma or bronchopulmonary derivation.

FROZEN SECTION EXAMINATION

Intraoperative frozen section examination of parathyroid gland tissue in cases of hyperparathyroidism is intended to establish the nature of the excised tissue and ascertain whether it is normal or abnormal. Without knowledge of the status of the remaining glands, a more definitive diagnosis of hyperplasia or adenoma (very rarely carcinoma) cannot be proffered. Incisional biopsies render the task more difficult, as do freezing ('ice crystal') artefact, other technical

constraints and sampling error. The process is inevitably subject to interobserver variation. Some workers advocate routine lipid stains as an adjunct to assessing intracytoplasmic fat, others do not. Oncocytic (oxyphil) cells, however, contain minimal lipid and occasional non-oncocytic hyperplastic and adenomatous parathyrocytes may retain significant lipid content. This notwithstanding, the overall accuracy of frozen section evaluation is extremely high and demonstrates good concordance with subsequent paraffin sections in experienced hands (**Figure 19.53**). The frozen section diagnosis of parathyroid carcinoma is understandably seldom sustainable, although alerting the surgeon to the possibility may alter peroperative management should there be other suspicious features.

The number of intraoperative frozen section examination requests in many centres has fallen, coincident with the development and refinement of preoperative imaging studies. Minimally invasive parathyroidectomy assisted by

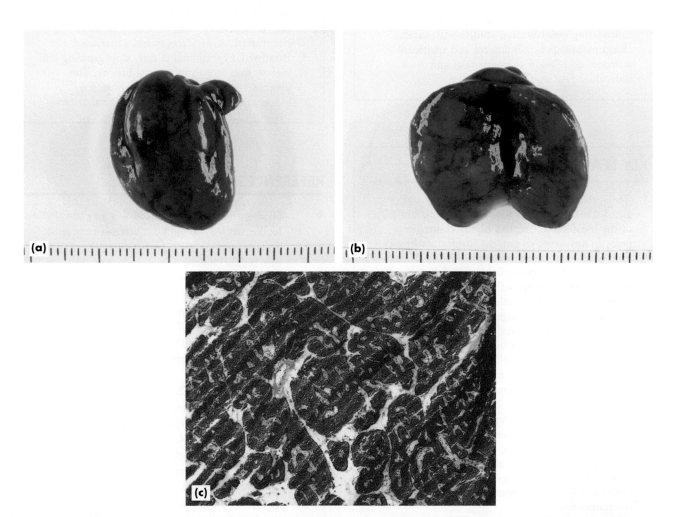

Figure 19.53   (a) The external surface of a fresh parathyroid gland nodule, weighing 1.8 g, sent for intraoperative frozen section examination – see **Figure 19.5**, for comparison with the appearances of a similar fixed specimen. (b) The same nodule bivalved in the unfixed state to demonstrate ill-defined parenchymal multinodularity. (c) Frozen section histology confirms hypercellular parathyroid gland tissue devoid of intraglandular fat. The entire consultation was completed in less than 5 minutes following receipt of the specimen in the laboratory. The linear striations and folds/rents in the section are artefactual. Without knowledge of the status of the remaining parathyroid glands, this could represent either an adenoma or hyperplasia. This notwithstanding, the findings supported the clinical impression of an adenoma. Subsequent paraffin sections on routinely processed tissue serve as a quality audit (H&E stain, medium magnification).

intraoperative PTH assay has shown promising results and also reduces the burden of frozen section evaluation.

KEY EVIDENCE

- Accurate and timely pathological tumour subtyping, tumour grading and tumour staging underpin subsequent effective clinical management of thyroid gland and parathyroid gland neoplasia.
- Morphology remains the gold standard of histocytological diagnosis, increasingly facilitated, but not yet supplanted, by advances in ultrastructural, immunohistochemical, molecular and genetic understanding of normality and disease states.
- Advancement in diagnostic pathology has traditionally evolved along heuristic lines, assimilating observational studies with careful clinicopathologico-radiological and treatment outcome correlation at population and individual case study levels.

KEY LEARNING POINTS

- The apparently limited repertoire of thyroid gland disease belies its subtlety, masking some of the most subjective and highly contentious fields in any arena of current surgical pathology.
- Fine needle aspiration cytology (FNAC) of the thyroid gland is a generally accepted first-line investigation for triage of solitary thyroid nodules, is helpful in evaluating diffuse, non-toxic goitre, aids the diagnosis of clinically suspected malignancy and facilitates discrimination between treatable lymphomas and poor prognosis anaplastic carcinoma.
- Papillary thyroid carcinoma in its numerous guises accounts for approximately 80 per cent of all thyroid malignancies. It generally portends an excellent prognosis, particularly in younger patients, modulated by both patient-specific and tumour-specific variables.
- The capsule of any follicular neoplasm should be extensively sampled specifically searching for both capsular and lymphovascular microinvasion.
- Oncocytic (oxyphil, Hürthle cell) change is a cellular adaptive process occurring in a wide variety of non-neoplastic and neoplastic conditions. It is subject to its own molecular basis, independent to that of any underlying tumour.
- There remain several unresolved issues in the histopathological diagnosis of thyroid

carcinomas. Large clinicopathological studies subject to long-term follow up are still required with the anticipation that many of these controversial areas will ultimately be resolved. Until such time, traditional morphological techniques underpin the diagnosis of thyroid cancer.
- The role of ancillary immunohistochemical, molecular and genetic studies in the determination of malignancy of the thyroid gland is evolving and has yet to be fully realized in routine diagnostic practice.
- All patients newly diagnosed with medullary thyroid carcinoma should be offered genetic testing given its association with multiple endocrine neoplasia syndromes.
- The value of perioperative frozen section examination of thyroid gland lesions is disputed among pathologists and surgeons. The indications for such are best agreed by the multidisciplinary team according to local circumstances, preferences and experience.
- Parathyroid carcinoma is rare, slow growing and metastasizes late in its natural history. The diagnosis is predicated upon clinical, biochemical, imaging and pathological criteria.

REFERENCES

◆ 1. McGlashan J. The thyroid gland: anatomy and physiology. In: Gleeson MB, Burton GG, Clarke MJ et al. (eds). *Scott-Brown's otorhinolaryngology, head and neck surgery*, 7th edn. London: Hodder Arnold, 2008: 314–27.
◆ 2. De Felice M, Di Lauro R. Thyroid development and its disorders: genetics and molecular mechanisms. *Endocrinology Reviews* 2004; **25**: 722–46.
◆ 3. Chan JKC. Tumours of the thyroid and parathyroid glands In: Fletcher CDM (ed.). *Diagnostic hisopathology of tumours*, 3rd edn. London: Churchill Livingstone Elsevier, 2007.
◆ 4. Wenig BH, Heffess CS, Adair CF. *Atlas of endocrine pathology*. Philadelphia: WB Saunders, 1999.
◆ 5. Akhtar MS, Scognamiglio T. Solid cell nests: role in thyroid disease. *Advances in Anatomic Pathology* 2007; **14**: 141–2.
◆ 6. British Thyroid Association/RCoP. Guidelines for the management of thyroid cancer. Report of the thyroid cancer guideline update group, 2nd edn. London: Royal College of Physicians, London, 2007.
   7. Gharib H, Goellner JR. Fine-needle aspiration biopsy of the thyroid: an appraisal. *Annals of Internal Medicine* 1993; **118**: 282–9.
◆ 8. DeLellis RA, Lloyd RV, Heitz PU et al. (eds). *Pathology and genetics of tumours of endocrine organs*. Lyon: IARC Press, 2004.
◆ 9. Cooper DS, Doherty GM, Haugen BR et al. Revised American Thyroid Association management guidelines for

patients with thyroid nodules and differentiated thyroid cancer. *Thyroid* 2009; **19**: 1167–214.

10. Carr S, Visvanathan V, Hossain T *et al*. How good are we at fine needle aspiration cytology? *Journal of Laryngology and Otology* 2010; **124**: 765–6.

11. Carmeci C, Jeffrey RB, McDougall IR *et al*. Ultrasound-guided fine-needle aspiration biopsy of thyroid masses. *Thyroid* 1998; **8**: 283–9.

◆ 12. Buley I. Problems in fine needle aspiration of the thyroid. *Current Diagnostic Pathology* 1995; **2**: 23–31.

◆ 13. Cibas ES, Ali SZ. The Bethesda system for reporting thyroid cytopathology. *American Journal of Clinical Pathology* 2009; **132**: 658–65.

14. Cross P, Chandra A, Giles T *et al*. *Guidance on the reporting of thyroid cytology specimens*. London: Royal College of Pathologists, 2009.

15. Crippa S, Mazzucchelli L. The Bethesda system for reporting thyroid fine-needle aspiration specimens. *American Journal of Clinical Pathology* 2010; **134**: 343–5.

16. Schmitt FC. Thyroid cytology: is FNA still the best diagnostic approach? *International Journal of Surgical Pathology* 2010; **18**(3 Suppl.): 201S–204S.

◆ 17. Layfield LJ. *Cytopathology of the head and neck*. Chicago: American Society of Clinical Pathology, 1997.

◆ 18. Chau YC, Chan JKC. Fine needle aspiration induced changes. *Current Diagnostic Pathology* 2003; **9**: 78–88.

◆ 19. LiVolsi VA, Merino MJ. Worrisome histologic alterations following fine-needle aspiration of the thyroid (WHAFFT). *Pathology Annual* 1994; **29**: 99–120.

20. Sturgis EM, Miller RH. Thyroglossal duct cysts. *Journal of the Louisiana State Medical Society* 1993; **145**: 459–61.

21. Shahin A, Burroughs FH, Kirby JP, Ali SZ. Thyroglossal duct cyst: A cytopathologic study of 26 cases. *Diagnostic Cytopathology* 2005; **33**: 365–9.

22. Harcourt-Webster JN. Squamous epithelium in the human thyroid gland. *Journal of Clinical Pathology* 1966; **19**: 384–8.

◆ 23. Wenig B. *Atlas of head and neck pathology*. Oxford: Saunders Elsevier, 2008.

◆ 24. Mete O, Asa S. Oncocytes, oxyphils, Hürthle, and Askanazy cells: morphological and molecular features of oncocytic thyroid nodules. *Endocrine Pathology* 2010; **21**: 16–24.

25. Pearce EN, Farwell AP, Braverman LE. Thyroiditis. *New England Journal of Medicine* 2003; **348**: 2646–55.

26. Watson MG, Birchall JP, Soames JV. Is 'lateral aberrant thyroid' always metastatic tumour? *Journal of Laryngology and Otology* 1992; **106**: 376–8.

◆ 27. Rosai J, Kuhn E, Carcangiu ML. Pitfalls in thyroid tumour pathology. *Histopathology* 2006; **49**: 107–20.

◆ 28. Baloch ZL, LiVolsi VA. Our approach to follicular-patterned lesions of the thyroid. *Journal of Clinical Pathology* 2007; **60**: 244–50.

29. Williams ED, Abrosimov V, Bogdanova T. Guest editorial: Two proposals regarding the terminology of thyroid tumors. *International Journal of Surgical Pathology* 2000; **8**: 181–3.

30. LiVolsi VA. Hyalinizing trabecular tumor of the thyroid: adenoma, carcinoma, or neoplasm of uncertain malignant potential? *American Journal of Surgical Pathology* 2000; **24**: 1683–4.

◆ 31. LiVolsi VB, Baloch ZW. Follicular neoplasms of the thyroid. Views, biases and experiences. *Advances in Anatomic Pathology* 2004; **11**: 279–87.

◆ 32. Ghossein R, Asa SL, Barnes L *et al*. Protocol for the examination of specimens from patients with carcinomas of the thyroid gland. Version Thyroid 3.0.0.0. Washington DC: College of American Pathologists, 2009.

33. Ghossein R. Update to the College of American Pathologists reporting on thyroid carcinomas. *Head and Neck Pathology* 2009; **3**: 86–93.

34. Wada N, Hirakawa S, Rino Y *et al*. Solitary metachronous metastasis to the thyroid from renal cell carcinoma 19 years after nephrectomy: report of a case. *Surgery Today* 2005; **35**: 483–7.

35. Chen H, Nicol TL, Zeiger MA *et al*. Hürthle cell neoplasms of the thyroid. Are there features predictive of malignancy? *Annals of Surgery* 1998; **227**: 542–6.

◆ 36. Katoh R, Harach HR, Williams ED. Solitary, multiple, and familial oxyphil tumours of the thyroid gland. *Journal of Pathology* 1998; **186**: 292–9.

37. Galera-Davidson H. Diagnostic problems in thyroid FNAs. *Diagnostic Cytopathology* 1997; **17**: 422–8.

38. Renshaw AA, Gould EW. Why there is the tendency to 'overdiagnose' the follicular variant of papillary thyroid carcinoma. *American Journal of Clinical Pathology* 2002; **117**: 19–21.

39. Baloch ZL, Livolsi VA. Follicular-patterned lesions of the thyroid. *American Journal of Clinical Pathology* 2002; **117**: 143–50.

40. Grodski S, Delbridge L. An update on papillary microcarcinoma. *Current Opinion in Oncology* 2009; **21**: 1–4.

◆ 41. Baloch ZL, Livolsi VA. Newly described tumours of the thyroid. *Current Diagnostic Pathology* 2000; **6**: 151–64.

42. Lang B, Lo C-Y. Surgical options in undifferentiated thyroid carcinoma. *World Journal of Surgery* 2007; **31**: 969–77.

43. Hodgson N, Button J, Solorzano C. Thyroid cancer: is the incidence still increasing? *Annals of Surgical Oncology* 2004; **11**: 1093–7.

44. Lo CY, Lam KY, Wan KY. Anaplastic carcinoma of the thyroid. *American Journal of Surgery* 1999; **177**: 337–9.

45. Williams ED. Histogenesis of medullary carcinoma of the thyroid. *Journal of Clinical Pathology* 1966; **19**: 114–18.

46. Bussolati G, Foster GV, Clark MB, Pearse AG. Immunofluorescent localisation of calcitonin in medullary C-cell thyroid carcinoma, using antibody to the pure porcine hormone. *Virchows Archives B Cellular Pathology* 1969; **2**: 234–8.

47. Pacini F, Castagna MG, Cipri C, Schlumberger M. Medullary thyroid carcinoma. *Clinical Oncology* 2010; **22**: 475–85.

♦ 48. McNicol A. The role of the pathologist. In: Mazzaferri ELH, Mallick C, Kendall-Taylor P (eds). *Practical management of thyroid cancer. A multidisciplinary approach.* London: Springer-Verlag, 2006: 95–107.

♦ 49. Anderson CE, McLaren KM. Best practice in thyroid pathology. *Journal of Clinical Pathology* 2003; **56**: 401–5.

♦ 50. Sobin LH, Gospodarowicz MK, Wittekind C (eds). *TNM classification of malignant tumours*, 7th edn. Oxford: Wiley-Blackwell, 2009.

♦ 51. DeLellis R. Parathyroid carcinoma. An overview. *Advances in Anatomic Pathology* 2005; **12**: 53–61.

52. Betea D, Bradwell A, Havey T *et al.* Hormonal and biochemical normalisation and tumour shrinkage induced by parathyroid hormone immunotherapy in a patient with metastatic parathyroid carcinoma. *Journal of Clinical Endocrinology and Metabolism* 2004; **89**: 3413–20.

♦ 53. Johnson S, Stephenson TJ. *Dataset for parathyroid cancer histopathology reports.* London: Royal College of Pathologists, 2010.

Endocrine imaging

JULIE OLLIFF

What a lot of information, all in shades of grey...

THE THYROID

There have been many advances in imaging in the last decade. Most hospitals now have access to ultrasound equipment with high spatial resolution and colour Doppler. Multislice CT has enabled the acquisition of thin section scans in a 3D data block enabling manipulation of the data to give high resolution images in any plane. Functional imaging using nuclear medicine, and in particular positron emission tomography, can assess tumour metabolism with FDG glucose positron emission tomography (PET) combined with computed tomography (CT) demonstrating areas of increased glucose metabolism with anatomical correlation.

Imaging may be used to assess thyroid morphology and function. There is no single imaging modality available presently that can adequately perform both. Ultrasound (US) is the best technique to use if the texture of the gland needs to be examined. Ultrasound penetrates bone and gas poorly. Retrosternal extension of the gland is therefore better demonstrated by CT or magnetic resonance imaging (MRI). The laryngeal cartilage framework is also poorly penetrated by US and therefore formal staging of a thyroid cancer is better performed by CT which can examine both the neck and chest. CT will however use iodinated contrast agents intravenously. MRI can be used to evaluate the neck and mediastinum with an unenhanced CT performed to stage pulmonary metastatic disease, if an iodine load will affect clinical management. The administration of intravenous

iodinated contrast agents will affect radioactive iodine uptake for up to 6 weeks.

US may be used to guide fine needle aspiration of a focal thyroid mass. It can also be used to guide aspiration or biopsy of a suspicious neck node.

Thyroid scintigraphy is most commonly performed using technetium pertechnate or iodine 123 or 131. Nodules that do not take up radio-isotope are termed cold nodules. Those that are equivalent to surrounding thyroid tissue are described as warm and those that take up more radio-isotope than surrounding tissue are described as hot.

NORMAL THYROID

The normal thyroid appears of homogenous even intermediate reflectivity on ultrasound (**Figure 20.1a and b**). The two lobes of the thyroid can be identified with the bridging isthmus. Small hypoechoic areas which can simulate nodules are seen due to blood vessels. The flow within these structures can readily be delineated by examination using colour or power Doppler.

The thyroid is of higher attenuation than soft tissue on CT, causing it to appear brighter than adjacent muscle (**Figure 20.2**). This is because the iodine located within the gland has a higher atomic number than soft tissue. Calcium within bone and cartilage, or within a thyroid nodule, has a higher atomic number than iodine and will appear denser than surrounding normal thyroid tissue. The gland will enhance homogenously and thus appear brighter following intravenous contrast.

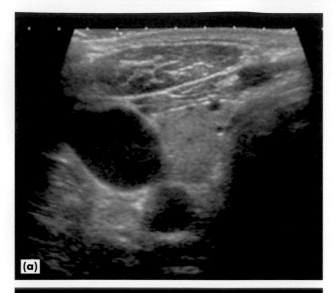

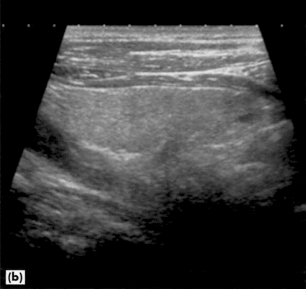

Figure 20.1 Transverse (a) and longitudinal (b) US scans of the normal thyroid.

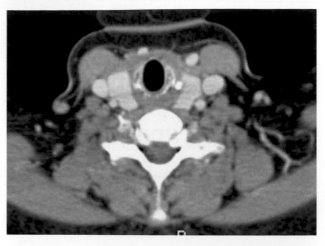

Figure 20.2 CT scan demonstrating normal thyroid of similar attenuation (density) to adjacent contrast enhanced vessels and of higher attenuation than muscle.

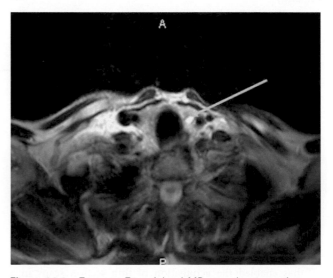

Figure 20.3 Trasverse T2 weighted MR scan demonstrating normal right lobe. The left lobe contains a small cyst (arrow).

The normal thyroid on MRI has a signal intensity slightly higher than that of the adjacent strap muscles on T1-weighted sequences and is hyperintense compared to those on T2-weighted sequences (**Figure 20.3**). Gadolinium-based contrast agents given intravenously will enhance normal thyroid tissue causing it to appear hyperintense to muscle on T1-weighted sequences.

PATHOLOGY

Palpable thyroid nodules are present in 4–10 per cent of the adult population. However, less than 1 per cent of all cancers occur in the thyroid gland. The differentiation of a benign nodule which may require no specific treatment from a malignant nodule presents a diagnostic dilemma. At present, there is no firm consensus as to the correct evaluation of

thyroid nodules. Imaging is playing an increasing role in the diagnostic evaluation of patients who either present with a thyroid swelling or with an incidentally discovered thyroid nodule. The increased incidence of neck ultrasound for other conditions has resulted in the increased diagnosis of non-palpable thyroid nodules in patients who are euthyroid and asymptomatic. The diagnostic work-up of these patients presents a particular challenge.

True cysts within the thyroid are uncommon. Cystic change may be seen within benign and malignant conditions. The presence of fluid can be identified readily on ultrasound appearing anechoic. The phenomenon of posterior enhancement will be present which is seen as a band of increased reflectivity behind the fluid containing structure (**Figure 20.4**). The morphology of a cyst is better demonstrated with US (**Figure 20.5**) than with CT or MRI. Cystic lesions will appear as areas of low attenuation (dark) on CT and will appear of low SI (dark) on T1W sequences and high signal intensity

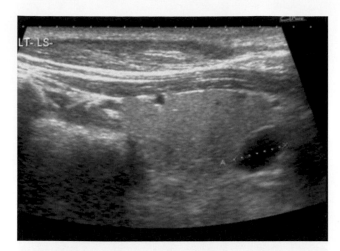

Figure 20.4 Ultrasound scan demonstrating a cyst in the lower pole of the thyroid.

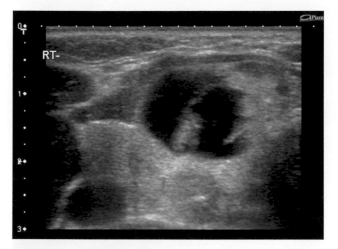

Figure 20.5 Ultrasound demonstrates a complex cystic mass with internal strucure.

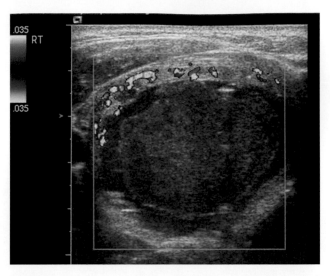

Figure 20.6 Ultrasound of clot within a cystic nodule that had been aspirated. The clot does not demonstrate colour Doppler flow.

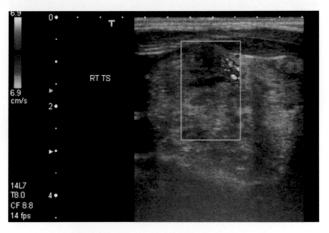

Figure 20.7 Thyroid ultrasound demonstrating many nodules within a multinodular gland.

(bright) on T2W (**Figure 20.3**) and STIR scans. Internal structure and wall thickness can be assessed with US (**Figure 20.5**). Colour flow Doppler may be used to interrogate any soft tissue nodules to try and differentiate between viable tissue and clot or debris (**Figure 20.6**).

A simple goitre will appear enlarged on ultrasound and may be of homogenous reflectivity but may be diffusely heterogenous and of increased or decreased reflectivity. A multinodular goitre may be generally heterogenous with more focal areas of altered reflectivity due to the nodules (**Figure 20.7**). These are often hypoechoic compared to adjacent normal thyroid tissue. Cystic change will result in areas of fluid causing regions of anechoic change if the fluid is simple. The presence of colloid causes multiple small foci of increased reflectivity to occur within the cyst which have bright comet tails (**Figure 20.8**). Haemorrhage can be seen with layering of blood products within the cyst. Colloid and haematoma will not have any abnormal colour blood flow within them. Areas of increased reflectivity can also be identified on US due to the presence of calcification (**Figure 20.9**) or haemorrhage (**Figure 20.6**). Calcification can be recognized by the apparent shadowing behind it, seen on US scan (**Figure 20.9**).

There are no certain ways on imaging of differentiating a benign from a malignant thyroid nodule. Radio-isotope imaging has been used to stratify the likelihood of malignancy with hot nodules being benign in over 90 per cent of cases. These are likely to be due to adenomas or hyperplasia. The risk of cancer in a cold nodule is four times that of a hot nodule but it is still more likely to be a benign lesion.

The role of ultrasound in the assessment of thyroid nodules and cervical lymph nodes to determine the likelihood of malignancy within a thyroid mass is evolving. Several features can be assessed.

Nodule size

The size of a nodule should be measured by placing callipers outside of any visible halo (**Figure 20.10**). Nodule size is not a predictor of malignancy,[1, 2, 3, 4] or of stage of disease. Kang et al.[5] found malignancy in 57 of 198 nodules <1.5 cm and 20 per cent of these cancers were stage III. The lack of

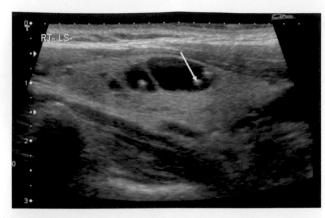

Figure 20.8 Cystic mass within the thyroid containing small bright regions with comet tails due to colloid (arrow).

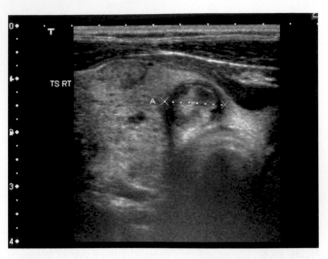

Figure 20.10 Callipers are placed outside any visible halo.

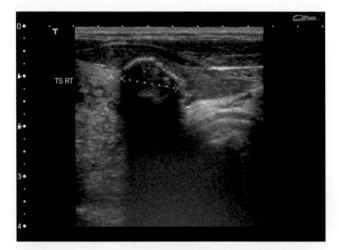

Figure 20.9 Thyroid ultrasound demonstrating a bright curvilinear band with posterior shadowing due to peripheral calcification.

relationship of size to stage was also found in a study that looked at 99 patients undergoing surgery for papillary cancer with primary tumours measuring <1.5 cm. Over one-third of this group of patients had disease outside the thyroid including distant metastatic involvement.

Consistency

Several US features have been shown to be associated with an increased risk of malignancy but none have been shown to be reliable indicators. The feature which has the highest sensitivity is a solid composition. A solid nodule, however, has a fairly low (15.6–27 per cent) chance of being malignant.

Calcification should not be confused with the small reflective foci with posterior comet tail artefact (**Figure 20.8**) which indicate the presence of colloid.[6] The presence of microcalcifications (**Figure 20.11**) has the highest positive predictive value of malignancy, of 41.8–94.2 per cent. The sensitivity of this sign is low because microcalcification is only found in 26.1–59.1 per cent of cancers. A predominantly solid (<25 per cent cystic change) nodule containing

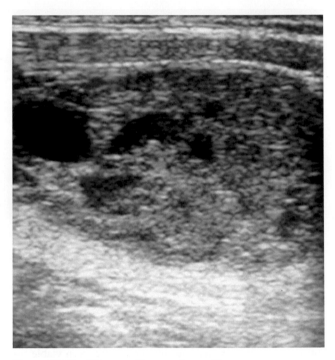

Figure 20.11 UltrasoundS scan of a papillary cancer demonstrating microcalcification and cystic change.

microcalcification has a 31.6 per cent likelihood of being cancer whereas a predominantly cystic nodule (>75 per cent cystic change) with no calcification has a 1 per cent likelihood of being cancer.[7] Predominantly solid nodules containing coarse calcification (**Figure 20.12**) are twice as likely to be malignant as those without any calcification. The significance of rim calcification is uncertain.

Number of nodules

More than one nodule is present in many patients. The presence of multiple nodules within the thyroid does not confer benignity. Each nodule should be evaluated on its own

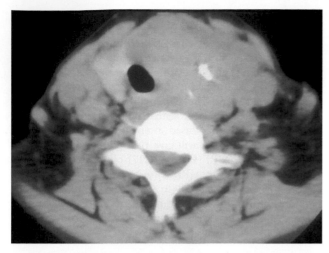

Figure 20.12 Computed tomography scan demonstrating coarse calcification within a papillary thyroid cancer.

individual US characteristics.[7] A recent paper studied almost 3000 patients who underwent US-guided fine needle aspiration cytology (FNAC). Multiple nodules were biopsied in 360 patients. These authors concluded that the cancer risk is similar for patients with one or two nodules measuring greater than 1 cm and decreases with three or more thyroid nodules.[8]

Blood flow

Colour Doppler can be used to assess blood flow in relation to thyroid nodules. Flow which is mainly internal or central is said to increase the chance of a nodule being malignant (**Figure 20.13**). Flow at the periphery (**Figure 20.14**) is suggestive of benign pathology. Some authors have suggested a grading system[9] and combine 2D US findings with colour flow Doppler characteristics to identify those nodules that should undergo US-guided FNAC.

Interval growth

A rapid increase in size may be due to true growth of a nodule or may be due to haemorrhage or cystic change. Ultrasound can differentiate solid from cystic components within a mass. Both benign and malignant nodules will grow over time but rapid growth of a nodule indicates an increased risk of malignancy.[10, 11] There is, however, no good evidence base to quantify the rate of growth that is significant.

Abnormal lymph nodes

Ultrasound can also assess the morphology of cervical lymph nodes. The shape and size of a lymph node can be examined. Lymph nodes with a short axis diameter of more than 7 mm should be regarded with suspicion. The presence of an abnormal texture with loss of the normal reflective hilum, microcalcification, cystic change or abnormal colour Doppler blood flow (**Figure 20.15**) should prompt US-guided FNAC

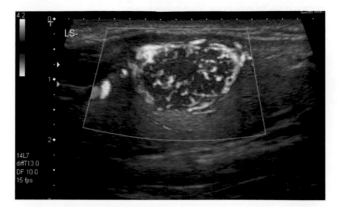

Figure 20.13 Thyroid nodule exhibiting marked internal colour flow on Doppler interrogation.

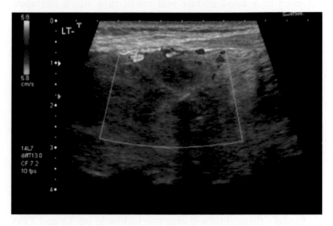

Figure 20.14 Nodule with peripheral flow and little central colour flow.

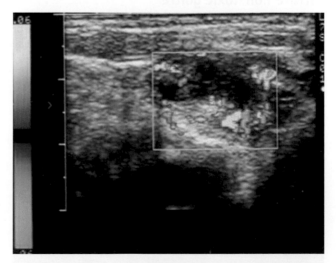

Figure 20.15 Abnormal lymph node involved by papillary cancer.

of that node. Any nodule within the ipsilateral thyroid lobe should also undergo fine needle aspiration. Lymph node metastases may be bigger and more conspicuous than the primary thyroid malignancy.

BENIGN THYROID DISORDERS

Graves' disease

The thyroid appears diffusely hyper-reflective on US without nodules. An increase in vascularity is seen on Doppler interrogation (**Figure 20.16**). The gland appears enlarged with avid enhancement on MRI and CT. It is of decreased attenuation (density) on unenhanced CT. It will demonstrate increased tracer uptake.

Toxic multinodular goitre

Nodules and cystic change will result in areas of increased and decreased density on CT and MRI with areas of increased and decreased tracer uptake on radio-isotope studies. The presence of a toxic nodule will result in a single hot spot. Decreased uptake will be seen in the remainder of the gland elsewhere if the nodule is autonomous.

Hashimoto's thyroiditis

The thyroid may be of normal size or enlarged. Diffuse heterogenous echotexture is present on US. Numerous poorly defined hyporeflective regions separated by fibrous bands may be seen. The presence of large nodules raises the possibility of lymphoma. The gland will appear atrophic and heterogenous due to fibrosis eventually. A heterogenous texture is seen on CT and MRI. There may be areas of increased SI on T2W images.

Riedel's thyroiditis will give rise to low SI on T1 and T2W MRI images.

Diffuse non-toxic goitre

There is diffuse glandular enlargement with diffuse uniform or irregular reflectivity that may be increased or decreased on US.

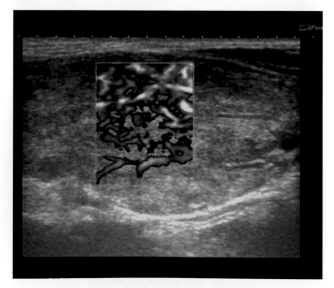

Figure 20.16 Diffusely increased reflectivity and abnormal increased colour flow in Graves' disease.

Nodular goitre

The presence of cystic change, haemorrhage, necrosis or calcification result in diffuse heterogenous echotexture or in multiple focal nodules of decreased reflectivity. Calcifications appear as discrete areas of increased reflectivity with shadowing behind them. The gland will appear enlarged on CT and may be heterogenous, with the larger nodules seen as individual areas of decreased attenuation. The presence of colloid or haemorrhage will give rise to areas of high signal intensity on T1W MRI (**Figure 20.17b**) images. Calcification is not seen as well on MRI as on US and CT. The role of imaging in these patients is to demonstrate any significant extension into the mediastinum and the relationship of the goitre to the great vessels (**Figure 20.17a** and **b**). Although

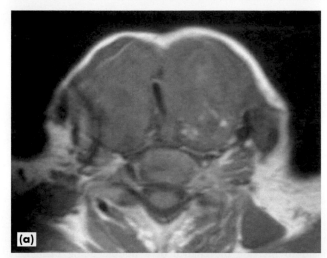

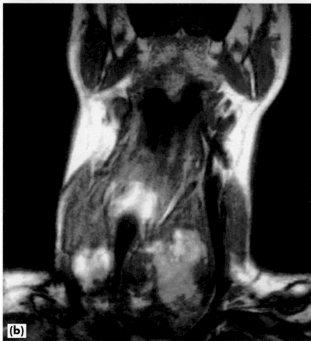

Figure 20.17 (a) Axial T1W magnetic resonance (MR) scan. There is marked compression of the trachea by enlarged thyroid. (b) Coronal T1W MR scan demonstrates the extent and heterogeneity of the goitre.

tracheal displacement and compression are clearly seen, they do not appear to necessarily correlate well with the degree of airways obstruction.

Thyroid neoplasms

Benign adenoma usually slowly increase in size. A sudden increase is likely to be due to haemorrhage within the lesion. Cystic degeneration is not uncommon.

THYROID CANCER

Papillary carcinoma is frequently multifocal and small in size. The primary lesion may therefore result in a multinodular appearance or diffuse alteration in texture or not be seen on imaging. Histologically these tumours may have calcification, haemorrhage or cystic change within them. The presence of psammoma bodies in over one-third of patients results in microcalcification which can be appreciated on US as multiple small hyper-reflective areas similar to colloid but without the comet tail (**Figure 20.18**). Larger solitary tumours will be appreciated as a solitary nodule. The imaging appearances are therefore variable.

The incidence of nodal metastases at presentation is higher than other thyroid tumours, occurring in up to 50 per cent of patients at presentation. These are also often small in size at presentation but, like the primary tumour, can have areas of cystic change, haemorrhage or calcification within them (**Figures 20.15** and **20.18**). This enables the diagnosis of a pathological node even if it is within normal size limits. The most common pattern of spread is to nodes within the anterior and posterior cervical chains but spread to the

retropharyngeal nodes may be rarely seen and papillary cancer can present as a retropharyngeal/parapharyngeal mass. Metastatic spread to the lungs, bone and brain occurs less commonly.

On CT the primary and involved nodes may be of higher density due to calcification, haemorrhage or colloid (**Figure 20.12**). They will also enhance more than surrounding soft tissue (**Figure 20.19**). Cystic change will result in a reduced density. Occasionally, cystic change will result in a thin-walled cystic mass within the neck which may be mistaken for a benign cyst. CT is currently the most sensitive imaging modality for the detection of pulmonary metastases.

On MRI the nodes can have low to intermediate signal intensity on T1- and T2-weighted scans or high signal intensity (**Figure 20.20**) on both T1- and T2-weighted scans.[12] The latter is thought to reflect high thyroglobulin content. Takashima and colleagues[13] assessed 50 patients with papillary carcinoma of the thyroid, metastatic disease was present in 68 per cent of patients. Using the combined criteria of a cystic node or size of 13 mm or more (short axis

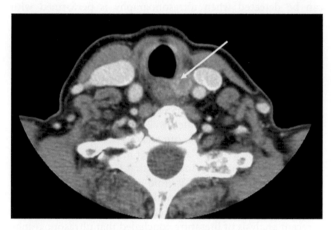

Figure 20.19 Contrast-enhanced computed tomography scan demonstrating an abnormal enhancing node involved by papillary thyroid cancer within the tracheo-oesophageal groove.

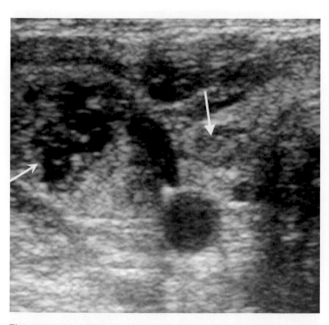

Figure 20.18 Ultrasound scan demonstrating a small primary papillary cancer within the right lobe of the thyroid (arrow) with a larger nodal deposit (arrow). Both lesions contain small bright foci due to microcalcification.

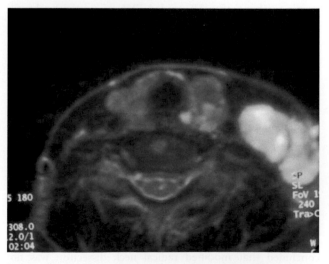

Figure 20.20 Magnetic resonance scan demonstrating a small left lobe papillary cancer with enlarged heterogeneous left level IV/V nodes.

diameter) the specificity was 100 per cent, and accuracy of 82 per cent (PPV 100 per cent) but a sensitivity of only 59 per cent. A comparison study between MRI and US for staging papillary cancer was performed prospectively in 14 patients.[14] These authors recommended the use of US as the first staging investigation because it can identify punctuate calcification and small abnormal nodes although both tests failed to identify metastatic nodes in the central group but correctly identified 14 of the 15 nodal groups outside the central group. MRI findings may contain prognostic importance in patients with locally advanced papillary thyroid cancer.[13] Recurrence was seen in 18 of 66 patients. Multivariate analysis determined that MRI findings of tumour size and nodal metastasis were significant independent variables for disease-free survival. MRI has also been shown to be a sensitive and accurate technique for the detection of well-differentiated thyroid cancer, particularly papillary cancer (PPV 86 per cent, accuracy 85 per cent) metastatic to cervical lymph nodes in a retrospective study of 26 patients.[15]

There is no doubt that pathological nodes may be diagnosed with US.[16] Lymph node metastases as small as 2–3 mm can be detected when ultrasonography is performed with a high frequency probe. The majority (81.2 per cent) of malignant nodes in 20 patients with papillary carcinoma were found to be homogenous and hyperechoic (87.5 per cent) compared to adjacent sternomastoid muscle with peripheral punctuate calcification seen in 68.7 per cent.[17] Cystic change seen on US is said to be highly suggestive of papillary thyroid cancer[18] and cystic lymph nodes are well characterized by US and have a thickened outer wall, internal echoes, internal nodularity and septations, but may appear as a simple cyst and thus mimic a branchial cleft cyst in younger patients.[12, 19] Some authors have demonstrated that US can be used in the follow up of patients with thyroid carcinoma, demonstrating that US can reveal occult nodal disease in patients with normal serum thyroglobulin measurements.[20, 21, 22, 23, 24, 25, 26] A recent analysis of literature concluded that ultrasonography performed by an experienced operator is the most sensitive means of detecting neck recurrences of differentiated thyroid cancer.[27] Some authors recommend the detection of recurrent papillary cell cancer by thyroglobulin assessment in the needle washout after US-guided FNA of suspicious lymph nodes.[28, 29] Preoperative neck US mapping has also been recommended for persistent/recurrent papillary thyroid cancer improving surgical outcomes.[30]

The role of US in the initial staging of patients with differentiated thyroid cancer is not well documented. Some units suggest that neck ultrasonography should be performed routinely in all patients with differentiated thyroid carcinoma at presentation[31] and that the examination should include not only level VI but the 'at risk' levels in the lateral compartment (levels III, IV and V). A study performed some years ago[32] concluded that ultrasound was useful for preoperative investigation of thyroid papillary carcinoma but that several limitations existed, especially in evaluating extracapsular extension and regional lymph node metastasis which were underestimated in 48.1 per cent of cases. A more recent study of 590 patients[33] with papillary microcarcinoma concluded that modified radical neck dissection was not necessary in patients without lateral node metastasis detected on US preoperatively and patients with preoperatively detected lateral node metastasis are more likely to develop recurrence in lymph nodes so careful modified neck dissection (MND) should be performed.

Follicular cancer

These tumours unlike papillary cancer are usually solitary lesions. On US these tumours may be iso- or hypoechoic compared to adjacent normal thyroid. The margins may be ill defined if there is extensive extracapsular invasion. There are no definite distinguishing features on imaging unless invasion into adjacent structures such as the trachea (**Figure 20.21**) or larynx can be identified. Vascular invasion may be seen. Lymphatic spread is uncommon, occurring in less than 8 per cent.[34] Distant metastatic spread to lung and bone is more commonly seen. These tumours also concentrate iodine and I^{131} may be used to treat and follow up these tumours.

Recurrent disease

A rising serum thyroglobulin necessitates investigation of disease recurrence. Initial investigation is performed with a radioiodine scan but tumour dedifferentiation may lead to decreased or lost iodine-accumulating ability. FDG PET-CT has emerged as the investigation of choice in patients with a negative radioiodine scan and raised thyroglobulin. Good anatomical imaging does however retain an important role since small volume recurrence may not be demonstrated by FDG PET.

Medullary cell cancer

Medullary cell tumours are derived from parafollicular or C-cells which are thought to be derived from neural crest

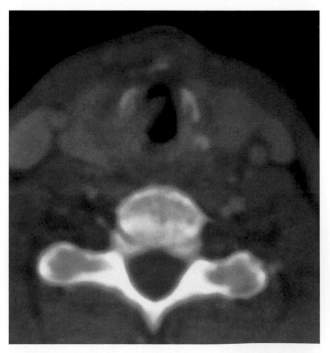

Figure 20.21 Computed tomography scan – there is invasion of the right side of the trachea by follicular thyroid cancer.

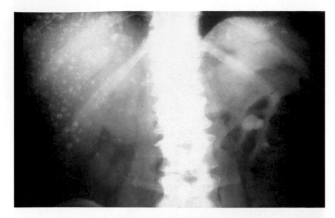

Figure 20.22 Calcified liver metastases from medullary thyroid cancer.

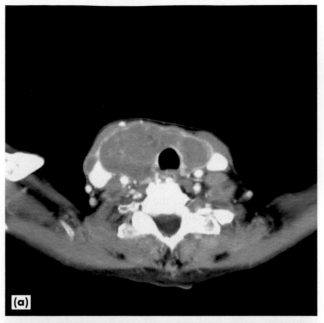

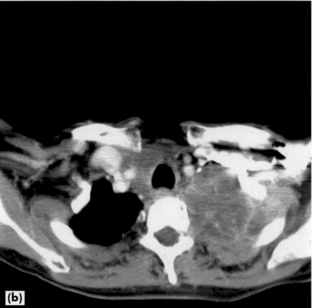

Figure 20.23 Computed tomography scans demonstrate extensive low density tumour due to a necrotic anaplastic thyroid cancer replacing the thyroid (a) and involving the left lung apex and supraclavicular fossa (b).

tissue. Many tumours express calcitonin. The tumours themselves and their metastases may calcify. They may invade locally and may spread to regional lymph nodes. Metastatic spread occurs to lungs, bone and liver (**Figure 20.22**). Some cases are associated with multiple endocrine neoplasia (MEN) types IIA and IIB. Medullary carcinoma does not concentrate radio-iodine and follow up is by serial serum calcitonin and carcinoembryonic antigen (CEA) measurements. Anatomical imaging is performed if recurrent disease is suspected. These neoplasms may be gallium or thallium avid. Metaiodobenzylguanidine (MIBG) may also be useful. More recently FDG PET has been shown to be useful in the demonstration of recurrent or metastatic disease, with a sensitivity of 70–76 per cent.[35, 36] It has been demonstrated to have a superior sensitivity and specificity compared to indium-111 pentetreotide (SMS), pentavalent technetium-99m dimercaptosuccinic acid (DMSA), technetium-99m sestamibi (MIBI), CT and MRI.[37]

Ultrasound has been shown to be superior to other imaging modalities in the detection of primary lesions within the thyroid in gene carriers of MENIIA and familial medullary thyroid cancer (FMTC). Whole body PET-CT is being used to stage metastatic disease.[38]

Hürthle cell tumour

These uncommon tumours arise from follicular epithelium. There are no distinguishing imaging features. Both nodal and haematogenous spread occurs. It generally has lower iodine avidity than other differentiated thyroid neoplasms. 18F-FDG PET has been shown to have excellent diagnostic accuracy in Hürthle cell thyroid cancer patients, improving on CT and radio-iodine scintigraphy. Intense 18F-FDG is said to be associated with a worse prognosis.[39, 40]

Anaplastic carcinoma

This aggressive and rapidly fatal tumour usually presents in elderly women. They often occur in people with long-standing goitre. They grow rapidly and compress and invade the airways and oesophagus. The primary tumour is usually hyporeflective on US but often contains punctuate

calcification and areas of necrosis (**Figure 20.23**). Lymph node involvement is common also with nodal necrosis.

Thyroid lymphoma

This is an uncommon condition. The thyroid may be the primary site of disease or may be involved secondarily. Patients may have a previous history of Hashimoto's thyroiditis. Tumours are not iodine avid but take up gallium. Presentation is usually with a rapidly enlarging thyroid mass causing symptoms of airway compression and/or dysphagia.

A solitary mass is more commonly seen than multifocal involvement.[41]

THE PITUITARY

Imaging techniques and normal anatomy

MRI is the optimal technique to image the pituitary. It has several advantages when compared to CT. Multiplanar images can be obtained with the pituitary best visualized in the coronal and sagittal planes. Multislice CT remains the imaging modality of choice in the patients unable to undergo MRI. Reconstructions can then be performed in axial, sagittal and coronal planes.

Scans need to be of high spatial resolution which necessitates thin slices with both CT (1 mm) and MRI (<3 mm). Coronal MRI allows evaluation of the sella and parasellar structures and the sagittal scans (**Figure 20.24**) demonstrate the midline structures well. T1 WSE MRI scans are the most commonly used. MRI scans are often obtained pre- and post-intravenous paramagnetic contrast agent administration. The intravenous contrast agents enhance areas in which the blood–brain barrier is absent or poorly developed (pituitary gland, infundibulum, median eminence, tuber cinereum and cavernous sinus). Inflammatory processes or tumour may destroy the blood–brain barrier.

The anterior lobe of the pituitary derives from Rathke's pouch. On T1-weighted MRI it is of intermediate signal intensity similar to white matter. The smaller posterior lobe of the pituitary and pituitary stalk form the neurohypothesis which is derived from a neural downgrowth of the fetal brain. It is usually of high signal intensity on T1-weighted MRI. This is best seen on midline sagittal scans (**Figure 20.24**). This high signal is related to the concentration of vasopressin stored in the posterior lobe.[42, 43, 44] The pars intermedia is a caudal pharyngeal outgrowth which is not well developed in humans but may be present as a small cystic space. The infundibulum or pituitary stalk extends from the mid aspect of the top of the gland towards the median eminence of the hypothalamus traversing the suprasellar cistern. The infundibulum is slightly wider at the hypothalamus and gradually narrows as it joins the pituitary gland (**Figure 20.24**). The width of the normal infundibulum may increase during pregnancy but should not exceed 4 mm in diameter.[45, 46] It should not exceed the diameter of the basilar artery.

The size of the pituitary is variable. The average dimensions in adults are 12 mm in width, 8 mm in anteroposterior diameter and 3–8 mm in height. Normal physiological hypertrophy increases its size in adolescents and pregnant women. At puberty the pituitary gland enlarges and may reach a height of 10 mm in girls and 8 mm in boys.[47, 48, 49] In pregnancy the gland increases progressively in size, reaching its maximum dimensions immediately postpartum, reaching up to 12 mm in height.[50] The gland returns to normal in the second week postpartum.

The pituitary enhances homogenously following intravenous administration of contrast agent. The adjacent cavernous sinus will also enhance but fast flowing blood in the carotid arteries causes these structures to remain of very low signal intensity pre- and post-contrast (**Figure 20.25**).

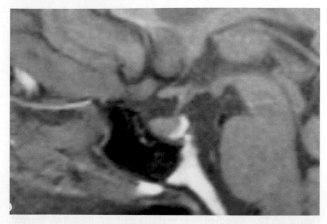

Figure 20.24 T1W magnetic resonance image sagittal scan of a normal pituitary gland.

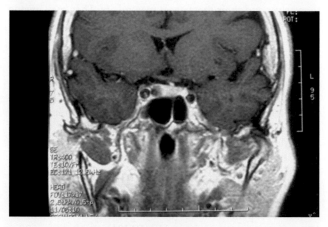

Figure 20.25 Contrast-enhanced coronal T1W magnetic resonance scan with a microadenoma in the right side of the gland displacing the pituitary stalk to the left. The carotid arteries within the cavernous sinuses are seen as low signal intensity structures due to flow void.

If scans are obtained rapidly following i.v. contrast then the posterior pituitary will be seen to enhance approximately 4 seconds before the infundibulum, with the anterior lobe enhancement occurring 10–15 seconds later.[51] This is due to the differing blood supply, the neurohypophysis being supplied by the inferior hypophyseal artery which arises from the cavernous portion of the internal carotid artery. The anterior lobe of the pituitary is supplied from the portal system which is derived from branches of the superior hypophyseal artery. This artery arises more distally from the supraclinoid portion of the internal carotid artery.

PITUITARY TUMOURS

Adenoma

Pituitary adenomas account for 10–15 per cent of all intracranial tumours.[45] They are usually tumours of adults and are almost always benign. Tumours measuring less than 1 cm in size are termed microadenomas (**Figure 20.25**) and are more of a diagnostic challenge on imaging than macroadenomas (tumours measuring >10 mm in diameter). Approximately 25 per cent of tumours have no hormone activity. These tumours are usually diagnosed later than secretory lesions and are often diagnosed because they compress adjacent structures such as the optic chiasm producing field defects or the pituitary itself. Extension into the cavernous sinus may give rise to cranial nerve deficits. The presence of cavernous sinus invasion may be difficult to diagnose because the dural reflection of the medial wall of the cavernous sinus is thin, unlike the lateral dural reflection. Cavernous sinus invasion can be inferred[52] if tumour extends to the lateral reflection (**Figure 20.26**). Asymmetry of the cavernous sinus in association with high prolactin levels has also been shown to be a good indicator of sinus invasion.[53, 54] Narrowing or occlusion of the carotid arteries by tumour is rare.[55] Pituitary adenomas may expand inferiorly to present as a mass within the sphenoid sinus (**Figure 20.26**). Superior extension rarely causes hydrocephalus from

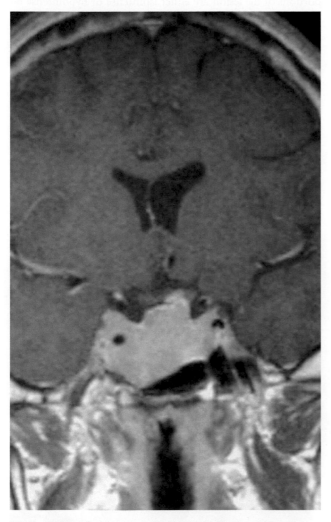

Figure 20.26 Contrast-enhanced coronal T1W magnetic resonance image demonstrates a macroadenoma involving the right cavernous sinus and extending into the sphenoid sinus. Suprasellar extension is displacing the stalk to the left and abutting the left side of the optic chiasm.

distortion of the third ventricle and obstruction of the foramen of Munro.

An MRI grading system for pituitary adenomas has been suggested by Edal and colleagues.[56] They have added to the Knosp–Steiner classification.[57] They have devised five grades of suprasellar extension: grade 0 – no bulging of the adenoma into the suprasellar space; grade 1 – the adenoma bulges upwards into the suprasellar cistern but without reaching the optic chiasm; grade 2 – it reaches the optic chiasm but without displacing it; grade 3 – the adenoma displaces and usually stretches the chiasm to a variable degree; grade 4 – obstructive hydrocephalus of one or both lateral ventricles caused by tumour extension.

Infrasellar extension is described by three grades. Grade 0 – intact floor of sellar. The inferior contour of the adenoma is smooth and rounded. The floor may be expanded but there is no sign of penetration into the sphenoid sinus. Grade 1 – there is focal bulging of the adenoma as an indirect sign of perforation of the dura and floor of the sella. There may be variable filling of the sphenoid sinus. Grade 2 – tumour penetration beneath the sphenoid sinus to the rhinopharynx and/or forward to the ethmoid area and nasal cavity.

Parasellar extension is graded by these authors using the Knosp–Steiner classification[57] in this a medial tangent – the intercarotid line (a line through the cross-sectional centres of the intercavernous carotid artery) is used to distinguish five grades: grade 0 – the normal condition; grade 1 – tumour extends up to the line; grade 2 – tumour extends to the lateral margin of the carotid artery; grade 3 – tumour extends beyond the lateral margins of the carotid artery; grade 4 – there is total encasement of the intracavernous carotid artery.

Moderate hyperprolactinaemia may be seen from stalk deviation (**Figures 20.25** and **20.26**) by a non-functioning tumour. Diabetes insipidus occurs very rarely.[58]

Prolactin secreting tumours are the most common functioning adenomas. They may cause amenorrhoea, galactorrhoea, infertility, loss of libido or impotence. These signs are more apparent in premenopausal women and these tumours are more likely to present at a smaller size than in men and postmenopausal women. The next most common tumours are those that produce ACTH and growth hormone. Tumours secreting growth hormone cause the clinical syndromes of giantism in children and acromegaly in adults. ACTH secreting tumours produce Cushing's disease. There are no imaging features to differentiate between the differing secretory adenomas but ACTH secreting adenomas are on average the smallest of all adenomas[58] with a mean size of 3 mm. The position of the adenoma within the pituitary does to some extent depend upon that of the normal secretory cells with prolactinomas and growth hormone secreting tumours tending to be located laterally, and ACTH, TSH and LH/FSH secreting tumours lying centrally.

The most reliable imaging sign of a pituitary adenoma is a focal area of abnormal signal intensity (**Figure 20.25**). Pituitary adenomas are typically hypointense compared to the normal pituitary on non-contrast-enhanced T1-weighted images. A small number of lesions are iso- or hyperintense. The presence of high signal intensity within the lesion (**Figure 20.27**) is thought to be due to old blood within the tumour and occurs in 20–30 per cent of tumours.[58] This is more likely to occur in macroadenomas and in patients receiving bromocriptine.[59] Pituitary adenomas may present with symptoms and signs of pituitary apoplexy. Tumours which are hyperintense on T2-weighted images may be soft or partially necrotic.[58] The acquisition of T2-weighted scans does not usually aid in the diagnosis of a microadenoma.[60] There are several secondary and less reliable signs of a pituitary adenoma. The stalk may be deviated away from the side of the tumour (**Figure 20.25**). However, there have been reports of stalk deviation towards the tumour.[61, 62, 63] The normal pituitary stalk may not lie in the midline and the presence of stalk deviation alone should not be taken to indicate the presence of a pituitary adenoma with almost one-half of patients having MRI of the pituitary having tilt of the pituitary stalk.[64, 65] There may be focal bone erosion if the tumour lies on the inferior aspect of the gland or adjacent to the dorsum sellae or a focal bulge of the superior surface of the gland.

Pituitary adenomas enhance to a lesser degree than the normal pituitary on early post-contrast scans but they may demonstrate increased signal intensity within the tumour on delayed scans making the lesion either isointense or hyperintense compared to the normal pituitary.[66, 67] Imaging following the administration of gadolinium-containing contrast agents has been shown to increase the sensitivity to a small degree[67, 68, 69] with the majority of microadenomas being visible on pre-contrast studies.[60] Contrast-enhanced studies are particularly useful in patients suspected of having an ACTH secreting tumour.[67, 70, 71, 72, 73] Dynamic scanning may diagnose a small number of small lesions not seen pre-contrast or on scans obtained on a routine post-contrast scan and very delayed scans (30–60 minutes post-injection) have been shown to demonstrate otherwise undetectable lesions, with contrast being concentrated within the tumour.[71]

The accuracy of MRI in the detection of pituitary adenomas is difficult to establish with not all patients having surgical correlation and there being a high incidence of small incidental lesions being found in pituitary glands on imaging in asymptomatic patients and at autopsy.

DIFFERENTIAL DIAGNOSIS

Craniopharyngioma

These tumours are derived from embryonic squamous cell nests of Rathke's cleft. Most craniopharyngiomas present as a calcific cystic suprasellar mass, only rarely is the mass completely intrasellar. The calcific components of the mass may be difficult to identify on MRI but may have a mottled appearance.[74] The cystic components of the tumour often demonstrate a high signal intensity on T1-weighted images (**Figure 20.28**) as well as T2-weighted images due to a higher protein content or haemorrhage within the cyst. The solid portions of the lesion are either isointense or hypointense on T1-weighted images and of high signal intensity on T2-weighted scans. The solid components show enhancement following intravenous contrast agents.[58]

Meningioma

Meningiomas arising from the parasellar region can project into the sellar turcica and may thus mimic a pituitary adenoma. Intrasellar meningiomas are rare but have been reported.[75] Typically, these lesions appear isointense on T1- and T2-weighted images. They enhance avidly and

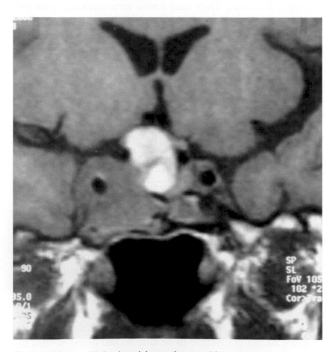

Figure 20.27 High signal intensity on this non-contrast magnetic resonance image is due to haemorrhagic products.

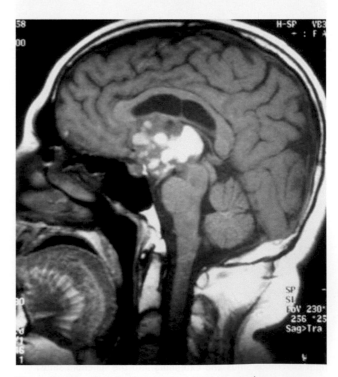

Figure 20.28 Unenhanced sagittal T1W magnetic resonance image of a craniopharyngioma.

homogeneously. A tapered extension of an intracranial dural base or 'tail' is suggestive of a meningoma.[76, 77] On CT, hyperostosis of the underlying bone or dense calcification of associated dural structures is also suggestive of meningomas. The pituitary fossa is usually normal in size. The normal pituitary gland may be visible on MRI lying separate to the mass.

Other tumours

Hypothalamic hamartomas can occur in the sella and parasellar areas. Contrast enhancement should not occur in these lesions.[58] Other rare tumours, such as parasellar granular cell tumours including myoblastomas and choristomas and infundibulomas, can present with visual loss and some degree of endocrine dysfunction. These are rare tumours originating from the neurohypophysis.[75]

An important differential diagnosis is that of an aneurysm from the cavernous, infraclinoid or supraclinoid internal carotid artery. These may present signs of visual loss depending upon the location of the aneurysm. They may also extend into the sella and cause direct pituitary compression with resultant endocrine dysfunction.[78] In these cases MRI is more usual than CT since CT cannot reliably distinguish an adenoma from an aneurysm or other pituitary lesion. On MRI the rapid blood flow through the aneurysm lumen causes the phenomenon of 'flow void'. There may also be heterogeneously increased signal caused by the presence of blood products and calcification within the aneurysm.[79]

THE PARATHYROIDS

The parathyroid glands are derived from the third (lower pair of parathyroid glands) and fourth (upper pair) pharyngeal pouches. The majority of people have four glands but 25 per cent have more than this. The superior glands are more constant in position, lying along the dorsal aspect of the superior pole of the thyroid laterally near the recurrent laryngeal nerve. The lower glands have more varied positions, lying along the dorsal aspects of the lower poles of the lobes of the thyroid but they can lie further away at the cervicothoracic junction and even within the superior mediastinum. The normal parathyroids are difficult to visualize with US.

The main indication for imaging the parathyroid glands is during the investigation of hyperparathyroidism which is either caused by an adenoma usually affecting one gland, parathyroid hyperplasia in which all glands are involved or parathyroid carcinoma. Primary hyperparathyroidism is caused by an adenoma in 80 per cent, hyperplasia in approximately 20 per cent and carcinoma is rare, occurring in 1 per cent. In many institutions the parathyroids are not routinely imaged before the first surgical exploration. In good hands this will have a success rate of over 90 per cent.

Generally, the abnormal parathyroid gland is of lower reflectivity than the normal thyroid and the echogenic capsule will separate one from the other (**Figure 20.29**). Calcification is rare in parathyroid adenomas but may be seen in hyperplastic parathyroid glands and in parathyroid

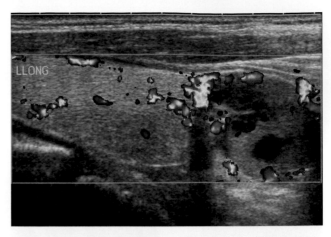

Figure 20.29 Colour flow Doppler examination demonstrating a lesion inferior to the thyroid.

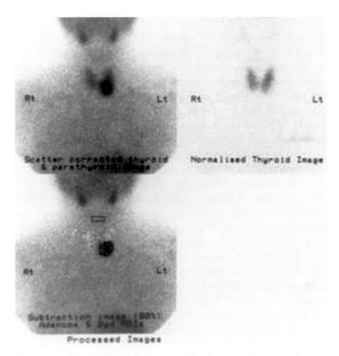

Figure 20.30 Left-sided parathyroid adenoma shown well on subtracted study.

carcinomas. Cystic change may be seen. Most lesions (90 per cent) are hypervascular unless they are small, measuring less than 1 cm in diameter, or show cystic change.[80] US and CT scan demonstrate high sensitivity but low specificity and are not used as the first imaging investigation.

Functional imaging of parathyroid tissue using thallium was introduced in the 1980s but has largely been superceded by the use of ^{99m}Tc-labelled isonitriles. The optimum technique at present uses ^{99m}Tc-sestamibi with subtraction imaging or washout imaging. A recent systematic review[81] reported the percentage sensitivity (95 per cent confidence intervals) for sestamibi in the identification of solitary adenomas as 88.44 (87.48–89.40), multigland hyperplasia 44.46 (41.13–47.8), double adenomas 29.95 (−2.19 to 62.09), and carcinoma 33. This review does not separate the wash-

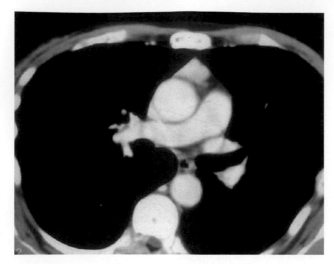

Figure 20.31 Mediastinal parathyroid adenoma.

out and subtraction techniques. The subtraction technique (**Figure 20.30**) using ^{99m}Tc-sestamibi and ^{123}I allows the recognition of the site to be related to the thyroid tissue when the parathyroid gland is in a normal position in the neck. If there is an equivocal scan then high resolution ultrasound should be used in addition. With ectopic glands, the combined use of single-photon emission computed tomography may then provide anatomical information to enable localization of the functional abnormality.[82] Ultrasound will not identify an ectopic gland located within the mediastinum. In these patients CT (**Figure 20.31**) or MRI may provide additional information if nuclear medicine investigations are equivocal. In patients who have had surgical exploration by an experienced parathyroid surgeon in a unit with an experienced nuclear medicine team and negative sestamibi imaging, it is reasonable to image the patient with ^{11}C methionine. It is debatable whether patients with a high likelihood of secondary hyperparathyroidism should be imaged. The only possible justification is when the glands are thought to be ectopic in position.[82] Smaller-volume parathyroid adenomas measuring less than 1 cm, those histologically poor in oxyphils and those in the upper position are less likely to be localized with sestamibi scans.[83]

being tailored to each patient using imaging to direct individual patient care.

KEY LEARNING POINTS

Normal thyroid

- No single imaging modality can assess both morphology and function.
- Thyroid nodules are commonly seen on all imaging.
- The management of thyroid nodules remains a challenge.
- Imaging cannot confidently distinguish benign nodules from malignant nodules.

Thyroid cancer

- US is used to assess thyroid nodules.
- Magnetic resonance and CT is used to stage known thyroid malignancy.
- PET-CT is emerging as an important investigation for recurrence and possibly in initial staging.

Pituitary tumours

- MRI is the investigation of choice for suspected pituitary pathology.
- Deviation of the pituitary stalk does not necessarily imply the presence of a pituitary mass.
- Calcification within a mass may not be visible on MRI.
- Meningioma and craniopharyngioma may mimic a pituitary adenoma.

The parathyroids

- US and CT are not used as the first imaging investigation.
- Ectopic glands may be located within the mediastinum.

CONCLUSION

The next decade will see the further development of functional and molecular imaging. The use of PET-CT scanners to delineate tumour can potentially lead to more selective targeting and intensification of treatment of head and neck cancer, while reducing critical normal tissue doses. At present, tissue hypoxia may be imaged using MRI giving an insight into the likely susceptibility of tumour to radiotherapy treatment. Novel tracers are being developed such as 19F thymidine (FLT) PET which gives tumour proliferation maps and Cu (II)-diacetyl-bis(N4-methylthiosemicarbazone) (Cu-ATSM), F–MISO PET which can provide tumour hypoxia maps. These developments will lead to treatments

REFERENCES

1. Kim EK, Park CS, Chung WY *et al.* New sonographic criteria for recommending fine-needle aspiration biopsy of nonpalpable solid nodules of the thyroid. *AJR. American Journal of Roentgenology* 2002; **178**: 687–6.
2. Papini E, Guglielmi R, Bianchini A *et al.* Risk of malignancy in nonpalpable thyroid nodules: predictive value of ultrasound and color Doppler features. *Journal of Clinical Endocrinology and Metabolism* 2002; **87**: 1941–6.
3. Peccin S, de Castro JA, Furlanetto TW *et al.* Ultrasonography: is it useful in the diagnosis of cancer in

thyroid nodules. *Journal of Endocrinological Investigation* 2002; **25**: 39–43.

4. Frates MC, Benson CB, Doubilet PM *et al*. Likelihood of thyroid cancer based on sonographic assessment of nodule size and composition [abstr]. In: *Radiological Society of North America Scientific Assembly and Annual Meeting Program*. Oak Brook, IL: Radiological Society of North America, 2004: 395.

5. Kang H, No J, Chung J *et al*. Prevalence, clinical and ultrasonographic characteristics of thyroid incidentalomas. *Thyroid* 2004; **14**: 29–33.

6. Ahuja A, Chick W, King W, Metreweli C. Clinical significance of the comet-tail artifact in thyroid ultrasound. *Journal of Clinical Ultrasound* 1996; **24**: 129–33.

◆ 7. Frates MC, Benson CB, Charboneau JW *et al*. Society of Radiologists in Ultrasound Management of thyroid nodules detected at US: Society of Radiologists in Ultrasound consensus conference statement. *Radiology* 2005; **237**: 794–800.

8. Barroeta JE, Wang H, Shiina N *et al*. Is fine-needle aspiration (FNA) of multiple thyroid nodules justified? *Endocrine Pathology* 2006; **17**: 61–5.

9. Chammas MC, Gerhard R, de Oliveira IR *et al*. Thyroid nodules: evaluation with power Doppler and duplex Doppler ultrasound. *Otolaryngology – Head and Neck Surgery* 2005; **132**: 874–82.

10. Grant CS, Hay ID, Gough IR *et al*. Long-term follow-up of patients with benign thyroid fine-needle aspiration cytologic diagnoses. *Surgery* 1989; **106**: 980–6.

11. Alexander EK, Hurwitz S, Heering JP *et al*. Natural history of benign solid and cystic thyroid nodules. *Annals of Internal Medicine* 2003; **138**: 315–18.

12. Som PM, Brandwein M, Lidov M *et al*. The varied presentations of papillary thyroid carcinoma cervical nodal disease: CT and MR findings. AJNR. *American Journal of Neuroradiology* 1994; **15**: 1123–8.

13. Takashima S, Matsushita T, Takayama F *et al*. Prognostic significance of magnetic resonance findings in advanced papillary thyroid cancer. *Thyroid* 2001; **11**: 1153–9.

14. King AD, Ahuja AT, To EW *et al*. Staging papillary carcinoma of the thyroid: magnetic resonance imaging vs ultrasound of the neck. *Clinical Radiology* 2000; **55**: 222–6.

15. Gross ND, Weissman JL, Talbot JM *et al*. MRI detection of cervical metastasis from differentiated thyroid carcinoma. *Laryngoscope* 2001; **111**(11 Pt 1): 1905–9.

16. Ahuja A, Ying M. An overview of neck node sonography. *Investigative Radiology* 2002; **37**: 333–42.

17. Ahuja AT, Chow L, Chick W *et al*. Metastatic cervical nodes in papillary carcinoma of the thyroid: ultrasound and histological correlation. *Clinical Radiology* 1995; **50**: 229–31.

18. Kessler A, Rappaport Y, Blank A *et al*. Cystic appearance of cervical lymph nodes is characteristic of metastatic papillary thyroid carcinoma. *Journal of Clinical Ultrasound* 2003; **31**: 21–5.

19. Wunderbaldinger P, Harisinghani MG, Hahn PF *et al*. Cystic lymph node metastases in papillary thyroid carcinoma. AJR. *American Journal of Roentgenology* 2002; **178**: 693–7.

20. Simeone JF, Daniels GH, Hall DA *et al*. Sonography in the follow-up of 100 patients with thyroid carcinoma. AJR. *American Journal of Roentgenology* 1987; **148**: 45–9.

21. Franceschi M, Kusic Z, Franceschi D *et al*. Thyroglobulin determination, neck ultrasonography and iodine-131 whole-body scintigraphy in differentiated thyroid carcinoma. *Journal of Nuclear Medicine* 1996; **37**: 446–51.

22. Antonelli A, Miccoli P, Ferdeghini M *et al*. Role of neck ultrasonography in the follow-up of patients operated on for thyroid cancer. *Thyroid* 1995; **5**: 25–8.

23. Antonelli A, Miccoli P, Fallahi P *et al*. Role of neck ultrasonography in the follow-up of children operated on for thyroid papillary cancer. *Thyroid* 2003; **13**: 479–84.

24. de Rosário PW, Guimarães VC, Maia FF *et al*. Thyroglobulin before ablation and correlation with posttreatment scanning. *Laryngoscope* 2005; **115**: 264–7.

25. Pagano L, Klain M, Pulcrano M *et al*. Follow-up of differentiated thyroid carcinoma. *Minerva Endocrinologica* 2004; **29**: 161–74.

26. Torlontano M, Attard M, Crocetti U *et al*. Follow-up of low risk patients with papillary thyroid cancer: role of neck ultrasonography in detecting lymph node metastases. *Journal of Clinical Endocrinology and Metabolism* 2004; **89**: 3402–7.

◆ 27. Schlumberger M, Pacini F, Wiersinga WM *et al*. Follow-up and management of differentiated thyroid carcinoma: a European perspective in clinical practice. *European Journal of Endocrinology* 2004; **151**: 539–48.

28. Baskin HJ. Detection of recurrent papillary thyroid carcinoma by thyroglobulin assessment in the needle washout after fine-needle aspiration of suspicious lymph nodes. *Thyroid* 2004; **14**: 959–63.

29. Uruno T, Miyauchi A, Shimizu K *et al*. Usefulness of thyroglobulin measurement in fine-needle aspiration biopsy specimens for diagnosing cervical lymph node metastasis in patients with papillary thyroid cancer. *World Journal of Surgery* 2005; **29**: 483–5.

30. Binyousef HM, Alzahrani AS, Al-Sobhi SS *et al*. Preoperative neck ultrasonographic mapping for persistent/recurrent papillary thyroid cancer. *World Journal of Surgery* 2004; **28**: 1110–4.

31. Schlumberger M, Pacini F. *Thyroid tumours*, 2nd edn. Paris: Nucleon, 2003: 127–46.

32. Shimamoto K, Satake H, Sawaki A *et al*. Preoperative staging of thyroid papillary carcinoma with ultrasonography. *European Journal of Radiology* 1998; **29**: 4–10.

33. Ito Y, Tomoda C, Uruno T *et al*. Preoperative ultrasonographic examination for lymph node metastasis:

usefulness when designing lymph node dissection for papillary microcarcinoma of the thyroid. *World Journal of Surgery* 2004; **28**: 498–501.

34. Franssila KO, Ackerman LV, Brown CL, Hedinger CE. Follicular carcinoma. *Seminars in Diagnostic Pathology* 1985; **2**: 101–2.

35. Brandt-Mainz K, Muller SP, Gorges R *et al.* The value of fluorine-18 fluorodeoxyglucose PET in patients with medullary thyroid cancer. *European Journal of Nuclear Medicine* 2000; **27**: 490–6.

36. Schoder H, Yeung HW. Positron emission imaging of head and neck cancer, including thyroid carcinoma. *Seminars in Nuclear Medicine* 2004; **34**: 180–97.

37. Diehl M, Risse JH, Brandt-Mainz K *et al.* Fluorine-18 fluorodeoxyglucose positron emission tomography in medullary thyroid cancer: results of a multicentre study. *European Journal of Nuclear Medicine* 2001; **28**: 1671–6.

38. Boer A, Szakall SJr, Klein I *et al.* FDG PET imaging in hereditary thyroid cancer. *European Journal of Surgical Oncology* 2003; **29**: 922–8.

39. Lowe VJ, Mullan BP, Hay ID *et al.* 18F-FDG PET of patients with Hurthle cell carcinoma. *Journal of Nuclear Medicine* 2003; **44**: 1402–6.

40. Pryma DA, Schoder H, Gonen M *et al.* Diagnostic accuracy and prognostic value of 18F-FDG PET in Hurthle cell thyroid cancer patients. *Journal of Nuclear Medicine* 2006; **47**: 1260–6.

41. Takashima S, Ikezoe J, Morimoto S *et al.* Primary thyroid lymphoma: evaluation with CT. *Radiology* 1988; **168**: 765–8.

42. Fujisawa I, Asato R, Kawata M *et al.* Hyperintense signal in the posterior pituitary on T1W MR: experimental study. *Journal of Computer Assisted Tomography* 1989; **13**: 371–7.

43. Kucharczyk J, Kucharczyk W, Berry I *et al.* Histochemical characterization and functional significance of the hyperintense signal of MR images of the posterior pituitary. *AJNR. American Journal of Neuroradiology* 1989; **152**: 153–7.

44. Sato N, Endo K, Kawai H *et al.* Haemodialysis relationship between signal intensity of posterior pituitary gland MR imaging and level of plasma antidiuretic hormone. *Radiology* 1995; **194**: 277–80.

45. Elster A. Modern imaging of the pituitary. *Radiology* 1993; **187**: 1–14.

46. Korogi Y, Takahashi M. Current concepts in imaging patients with pituitary and hypothalamic dysfunction. *Seminars in Ultrasound, CT and MR* 1995; **16**: 270–8.

47. Konishi Y, Kuriyama M, Sudo M *et al.* Growth patterns of the normal pituitary gland and in pituitary adenoma. *Developmental Medicine and Child Neurology* 1990; **32**: 69–73.

48. Elster AD, Chen MYM, Williams DW III, Key LL. Pituitary gland: MR imaging of physiologic hypertrophy in adolescence. *Radiology* 1990; **174**: 681–5.

49. Doraiswamy PM, Tts JM, Figiel GS *et al.* MRI imaging of physiologic pituitary gland hypertrophy in adolescence. *Radiology* 1991; **178**: 284–5.

50. Elster AD, Sanders TG, Vines FS. Chen MYM. Size and shape of the pituitary gland during pregnancy and post partum: measurement with MR imaging. *Radiology* 1991; **181**: 531–5.

51. Yuh WT, Fisher DJ, Nguyen HD *et al.* Sequential MR enhancement pattern in normal pituitary gland and in pituitary adenoma. *AJNR. American Journal of Neuroradiology* 1994; **15**: 101–8.

52. Ahmadi J, North CM, Segall HD *et al.* Cavernous sinus invasion by pituitary adenomas. *AJR. American Journal of Roentology* 1986; **146**: 257–62.

53. Scotti G, Yu C, Dillon W *et al.* MRI imaging of cavernous sinus involvement by pituitary adenomas. *AJNR. American Journal of Neuroradiology* 1988; **9**: 657–64.

54. Scotti G, Yu CY, Dillon WP *et al.* MRI of cavernous sinus involvement by pituitary adenomas. *AJR. American Journal of Roentology* 1988; **151**: 799–806.

55. Chong BW, Newton TH. Hypothalamic and pituitary pathology. *Radiologic Clinics of North America* 1993; **31**: 1147–53.

56. Edal AL, Skjodt K, Nepper-Rasmussen HJ. SIPAP. A new MR classification for pituitary adenomas. *Acta Radiologica* 1997; **38**: 30–6.

57. Knosp E, Steiner E, Kitz K *et al.* Pituitary adenomas with invasion of the cavernous sinus space. A magnetic resonance imaging classification compared with surgical findings. *Neurosugery* 1993; **33**: 610–7.

58. Kucharczyk W, Montanera WJ, Becker LE. The sella turcica and tera para-sella region. In: Atlas SW (ed.). *Magnetic resonance imaging of the brain and spine*. Philadelphia: Lippincott-Raven, 1996: 871–930.

59. Yousem DM, Arrington JA, Zinreich SJ *et al.* Pituitary adenomas: possible role of Bromocriptine in intra-tumoural haemorrhage. *Radiology* 1989; **170**: 239–43.

60. Sanders WT, Chundi VV. Extra-axial tumours including pituitary and para-sella. In: Orrison WW Jr (ed.). *Neuroimaging*. Philadelphia: WB Saunders Company, 1998: 612–717.

61. Chambers E, Turski P, LaMasters D, Newton T. Regions of low density in the contrast enhanced pituitary gland: normal and pathologic processes. *Radiology* 1982; **144**: 109–13.

62. Wolpert S. The radiology of pituitary adenomas. *Seminars in Roentgenology* 1984; **19**: 53–69.

63. Hemminghytt S, Kalkhoss R, Daniels D *et al.* Computed tomographic study of hormones secreting microadenomas. *Radiology* 1983; **146**: 65–9.

64. Ahmadi H, Larsson E, Jinkins J. Normal pituitary gland: coronal MR imaging of infundibular tilt. *Radiology* 1990; **177**: 389–92.

65. Bergland R, Ray B, Torack R. Anatomic variations in the pituitary gland and adjacent structures in 225 human autopsy cases. *Journal of Neurosurgery* 1968; **28**: 93–9.

66. Doppman J, Frank J, Dwyer A et al. Gadolinium DTPA enhanced MR imaging of ACTH secreting macroadenomas of the pituitary gland. *Journal of Computer Assisted Tomography* 1988; **12**: 728–35.

67. MacPherson P, Hadley D, Teasdal E, Teasdal G. Pituitary microadenomas. Does Gadolinium enhance their demonstration? *Neuroradiology* 1989; **31**: 293–8.

68. Stadnik T, Stevenaert A, Beckers A et al. Pituitary microadenomas: diagnosis with 2 and 3 dimensional MR imaging at 1.5 T before and after injection of Gadolinium. *Radiology* 1990; **176**: 419–28.

69. Steiner E, Imhof H, Knosp E. Gd-DTPA enhanced high resolution MR imaging of pituitary adenomas. *Radiographics* 1989; **9**: 587–98.

70. Doppman JL, Frank JA, Dwyer AJ et al. Gadolinium DTPA enhanced MR imaging of ACTH-secreting microadenomas of the pituitary gland. *Journal of Computer Assisted Tomography* 1988; **12**: 728–35.

71. Dwyer AJ, Frank JA, Doppman JL et al. Pituitary adenomas in patients with Cushing disease: initial experience with GD DTPA-enhanced MR imaging. *Radiology* 1987; **163**: 421–6.

72. Nakamura T, Schorner W, Bittner RC et al. Value of para-magnetic contrast agent Gadolinium DTPA in the diagnosis of pituitary adenomas. *Neuroradiology* 1988; **30**: 481–6.

73. Steiner E, Imhof H, Knosp E. Gd-DTPA enhanced high resolution MR imaging of pituitary adenomas. *Radiographics* 1989; **9**: 587–98.

74. Tsuchiya K, Makita K, Surui S et al. MRI appearances of calcified regions within intra-cranial tumours. *Neuroradiology* 1993; **35**: 341–4.

75. Freda PU, Post KD. Differential diagnosis of sellar masses. *Endocrinology and Metabolism Clinics of North America* 1999; **28**: 81–117.

76. Goldsher D, Litt AW, Pinto RS et al. Dural tail associated with meningiomas on GD-DTPA-enhanced MR images: characteristics, differential diagnostic value and possible implications for treatment. *Radiology* 1990; **176**: 447–50.

77. Taylor SL, Barakos JA, Harsh GR et al. Magnetic resonance imaging of tuberculum sellae meningiomas: preventing pre-operative mis-diagnosis of pituitary macroadenoma. *Neurosurgery* 1992; **31**: 621–7.

78. Weir B. Pituitary tumours and aneurysms: case report and review of the literature. *Neurosurgery* 1992; **30**: 585–91.

79. Johnsen DE, Woodruff WW, Allen IS et al. MR imaging of the sellar and juxta sellar regions. *Radiographics* 1991; **11**: 727–58.

80. Ahuja AT, Wong KT, Ching AS et al. Imaging for primary hyperparathyroidism – what beginners should know. *Clinical Radiology* 2004; **59**: 967–76.

81. Ruda JM, Hollenbeak CS, Stack BC Jr. A systematic review of the diagnosis and treatment of primary hyperparathyroidism from 1995 to 2003. *Otolaryngology – Head and Neck Surgery* 1322005: 359–72.

82. Kettle AG, O'Doherty MJ. Parathyroid imaging: how good is it and how should it be done? *Seminars in Nuclear Medicine* 2006; **36**: 206–11.

83. Stephen AE, Roth SI, Fardo DW et al. Predictors of an accurate preoperative sestamibi scan for single-gland parathyroid adenomas. *Archives of Surgery* 2007; **142**: 381–6.

21

Benign thyroid disease

KRISTIEN BOELAERT, LORRAINE M ALBON AND JAYNE A FRANKLYN

Diagnosis precedes treatment

Rusell John Howard, 1875–1942

INTRODUCTION

Benign thyroid disease is common with thyroid dysfunction affecting around 2 per cent of women and 0.2 per cent of men in the UK. Hyperthyroidism is a pathological syndrome in which tissue is exposed to excessive amounts of circulating thyroid hormone, leading to a clinical picture of thyrotoxicosis. Hypothyroidism results from insufficient production and secretion of thyroid hormones. Our understanding of the effects of thyroid hormones under physiological circumstances, as well as in pathological conditions, has increased dramatically over the last two centuries and it has become clear that overt thyroid dysfunction is associated with significant morbidity and mortality. Although the evidence suggests that successful treatment of overt thyroid dysfunction significantly improves overall survival, the issue of treating mild or subclinical hypo- and hyperthyroidism remains controversial. In addition to thyroid dysfunction, enlargement of the thyroid gland affects up to 60 per cent of the population, with higher frequencies in women and the elderly. Most patients with thyroid enlargement can be managed conservatively after malignancy is ruled out, the challenge to the clinician being to identify the minority of patients with thyroid cancer who therefore require surgical intervention and additional therapies.

This chapter aims to provide an overview of the current knowledge of the management of patients presenting with thyroid dysfunction or enlargement.

HYPERTHYROIDISM

Epidemiology

In patients with hyperthyroidism, tissues are exposed to excessive amounts of thyroid hormones resulting in thyrotoxicosis.[1] Primary thyrotoxicosis is the most common and results from pathology of the thyroid itself; secondary thyrotoxicosis results from abnormalities in the anterior pituitary gland, the site of thyroid stimulating hormone (TSH) production.

The prevalence of hyperthyroidism, defined as reduced serum TSH concentrations with raised free T4 (fT4) and free T3 (fT3) concentrations is about 2 per cent in the female UK population.[2] The annual incidence is 0.8/1000 per year in women; much lower incidence rates are observed in men.[3] Additionally, subclinical hyperthyroidism, defined as serum TSH concentrations below the normal reference range with normal concentrations of fT4 and fT3, is even more common. A UK survey of 1210 subjects aged over 60 years registered with a single general practice, indicated that 6.3 per cent of women and 5.5 per cent of men in the UK had low TSH levels.[4] In the US, investigators noted hyperthyroidism in 0.5 per cent of randomly selected individuals, with subclinical disease evident in 0.8 per cent of subjects rising to 3 per cent in those aged over 80 years.[5]

Aetiology

Hyperthyroidism has many causes. Graves' disease, an auto-immune condition caused by stimulation by antibodies directed against the TSH receptor, is the cause in most patients. The development of one or more autonomously functioning thyroid nodules that produce excessive amounts of thyroid hormones is also a common problem. Various forms of thyroiditis or thyroidal inflammation are less common but clinically important.[1] A number of other conditions can result in hyperthyroidism and are displayed in **Table 21.1**. Most of these conditions have specific pathophysiological features, clinical presentation and treatment strategies.

Clinical features

The diverse effects of thyroid hormones account for the numerous and varied symptoms of hyperthyroidism. Although there is a rough correlation between the severity of symptoms and circulating amounts of thyroid hormone, patients often have greatly differing symptoms, especially elderly individuals who often have no symptoms whatsoever. In the most extreme case, this absence of symptoms has been termed apathetic or masked thyrotoxicosis.[6]

Typical symptoms of hyperthyroidism indicate the action of excess thyroid hormone in the cell, as well as enhanced β-adrenergic activity. Patients usually have fatigue, nervousness or anxiety, tremor, weight loss, palpitations and heat sensitivity. Women may have irregular menses and decreased fertility, although frank amenorrhoea is rare.[7] Men also can have reduced libido and sometimes painful gynaecomastia.[8]

Clinical findings include tachycardia, warm moist skin, the presence of an enlarged thyroid and a slight tremor. Less frequent neurological findings include poor concentration and personality changes.[1] Elderly individuals have less obvious symptoms and signs than younger patients, including a lower frequency of goitre and a higher prevalence of cardiac manifestations such as atrial fibrillation (AF), and more rarely congestive cardiac failure. About 15 per cent of elderly individuals with new onset AF have thyrotoxicosis.[9, 10] Conversely, a high proportion (as many as 25–35 per cent) of elderly people with thyrotoxicosis will develop AF that is resistant to treatment until the underlying thyroid disorder has been corrected.[11] Classical symptoms and signs may not be present in all patients and the elderly in particular may present atypically. A low threshold for performing thyroid function tests is therefore appropriate.

Other indicators of hyperthyroidism include osteoporosis, hypercalcaemia, congestive cardiac failure, shortness of breath, muscle weakness, anxiety or amenorrhoea. There may be symptoms and signs suggestive of ophthalmopathy and a goitre may be present. Hyperthyroidism may also present as thyroid storm, a life-threatening situation with signs including tachycardia, AF, congestive cardiac failure, hyperpyrexia, agitation, psychosis or coma.[12] This syndrome

Table 21.1 Causes of hyperthyroidism.

Causes of hyperthyroidism	Pathophysiological features	Frequency
Circulating thyroid stimulators		
Graves' disease	Thyroid stimulating immunoglobulins	Common
TSH secreting tumour	Pituitary adenoma	Rare
Hyperemesis gravidarum	Human chorionic gonadotrophin (HCG) secretion	Uncommon
Choriocarcinoma	Human chorionic gonadotrophin (HCG) secretion	Rare
Thyroidal autonomy		
Toxic multinodular goitre	Activating mutations in the TSH receptor or G proteins	Common
Toxic solitary adenoma	Activating mutations in the TSH receptor or G proteins	Common
Destruction of thyroid follicles (thyroiditis)		
Subacute thyroiditis	Probable viral infection	Uncommon
Postpartum thyroiditis	Autoimmune	Common
Drug (amiodarone) induced thyroiditis	Direct toxic drug effects	Uncommon
Acute (infectious) thyroiditis	Thyroid infection (bacterial, fungal, etc.)	Uncommon
Exogenous thyroid hormone		
Iatrogenic	Excess ingestion of thyroid hormone	Common
Factitious	Excess ingestion of thyroid hormone	Rare
Ectopic thyroid tissue		
Struma ovarii	Ovarian teratoma containing thyroid tissue	Rare
Metastatic follicular thyroid cancer	Large tumour mass capable of secreting thyroid hormone autonomously	Rare
Other		
Pituitary resistance to thyroid hormone (RTH)	Mutated thyroid hormone β receptor with greater expression in the pituitary compared with peripheral tissues	Rare

typically occurs after a precipitating event, such as trauma, childbirth, infection or surgery, in a known hyperthyroid subject, but may also arise in patients not previously diagnosed with thyroid disease. Thus, the diagnosis of thyrotoxicosis should always be considered in any patient with fever and altered mental status.[1]

Diagnosis of hyperthyroidism

LABORATORY DIAGNOSIS

The single most important test is the measurement of serum TSH concentration. If this is within the normal range, then hyperthyroidism can be ruled out. The exceptions to this rule are very rare pituitary causes of thyrotoxicosis such as TSH-oma or syndromes of thyroid hormone resistance. In these cases, there may be a modest rise in TSH accompanied by a rise in fT3 and fT4.

A low TSH is not specific for thyrotoxicosis and 'non-thyroidal' illness or treatment with a variety of drugs may lower the TSH below the normal range, although it is still usually detectable in these circumstances. For these reasons, it is preferable to measure the TSH in conjunction with serum fT4 and, in specific cases, fT3 as well.

In most cases of hyperthyroidism, the typical picture is of undetectable serum TSH with elevated serum concentrations of fT4 and fT3. A low TSH and normal fT4 should prompt fT3 measurement as 10 per cent of cases of thyrotoxicosis are so called 'T3 toxicosis', with a rise in fT3 alone. This is most commonly seen in mild cases of toxic nodular hyperthyroidism or early in relapse of Graves' disease.[1] It should be noted that not all laboratories perform T3 assays unless specifically requested.

Patients with hyperthyroidism often have non-specific changes in commonly requested laboratory tests. Indices of liver function are slightly raised in a minority of patients. Hypercalcaemia is present in about 10 per cent of patients, because of increased bone turnover and subsequent suppression of parathyroid hormone in serum.[1] **Table 21.2** details the laboratory abnormalities found in thyrotoxicosis.

Table 21.2 Laboratory investigations in suspected thyrotoxicosis.

Thyroid function tests	Elevated free T4 and/or free T3	
	Suppressed TSH	Unless TSH-oma/RTH
Immunology	Positive thyroid autoantibodies	Typical of Graves' disease
Biochemistry	Elevated alkaline phosphatase	
	Elevated calcium	
Haematology	Normochromic normocytic anaemia	Long standing cases
	Raised ESR	Subacute thyroiditis

THYROID SCINTIGRAPHY

The 24 h radioactive iodine uptake is a measure of the iodine avidity of the thyroid gland. In most hyperthyroid states, including Graves' disease, toxic multinodular goitre and toxic adenoma, the results are at the higher end of normal or raised. However, the test lacks specificity, since values can be high in individuals with normal thyroids and with iodine deficiency or in hypothyroid patients with Hashimoto's thyroiditis. Also, thyroid scintigraphy lacks sensitivity because low values are seen in the various forms of destructive thyroiditis that cause hyperthyroidism (subacute and postpartum thyroiditis), as well as in hyperthyroid patients exposed to pharmacological doses of iodine. In some cases where the aetiology of thyroid hyperfunction is unclear, diagnosis can be aided by the use of scintigraphy. This imaging modality can be used to differentiate between 'hot' and 'cold' areas of increased and decreased function, respectively. There are specific scintigraphic appearances associated with different conditions (**Figure 21.1**).

Graves' disease

In iodine replete parts of the world, Graves' disease is the most common cause of thyrotoxicosis. It is defined as a syndrome consisting of hyperthyroidism, moderate goitre, ophthalmopathy and dermopathy. In many patients, hyperthyroidism and goitre are the only features. It is more common in women than men (ratio 5:1), men are often affected later and the disease may be more severe. Its peak incidence is in the 20s and 30s, but it can occur at any age, although is uncommon before puberty. Graves' disease is more common in smokers (whose risk of the disease is almost doubled) and smoking is an even stronger risk factor for the development of thyroid eye disease.[13]

PATHOGENESIS

Graves' disease is an autoimmune disorder characterized by antibodies in the circulation that are directed against the TSH receptor. These antibodies mimic the effects of pituitary TSH, thereby stimulating thyroid growth and function. Whether the disease is triggered by abnormal clones of auto-reactive T cells, or abnormal antigen presentation by thyroid follicular cells, either independently or in response to cytokines released by infiltrating T cells, is uncertain.[13] The cause of Graves' ophthalmopathy and dermopathy is also unknown, but cross-reactivity between thyroidal antigens and antigens in orbital and extra-orbital tissues (especially preadipocyte fibroblasts) is a strong possibility. The TSH receptor is a strong candidate, since it seems to be expressed in connective tissues in the orbit and elsewhere.[14, 15] A concordance rate of only 20 per cent in monozygotic twins indicates that environmental factors trigger the development of Graves' disease in genetically susceptible individuals. These factors include life stresses,[16] sex steroids, smoking,[17] dietary iodine intake and immune modulators such as interferon α.[18]

CLINICAL MANIFESTATIONS AND NATURAL HISTORY

Although Graves' disease can occur rapidly over a few weeks, in most the onset is gradual and insidious. Patients exhibit

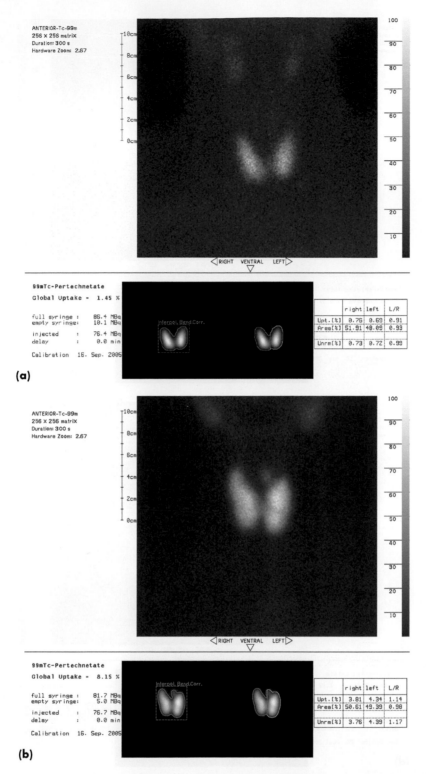

(a)

(b)

Figure 21.1   Scintigraphic appearances: (a) normal thyroid; (b) Graves' disease with pyramidal lobe; (c) dominant hot nodule; (d) multinodular goitre. Image courtesy of Portsmouth Hospitals NHS Trust.

many typical features of thyrotoxicosis and may have 'extra-thyroidal' signs that are not seen in other forms of thyrotoxicosis. A diffuse goitre is present in the majority of cases but the thyroid may be of normal size in around 3 per cent.[1, 13] The goitre is usually symmetrical; there may be an overlying palpable thrill and a bruit may often be heard. The thrill and bruit result from the increased blood flow to the thyroid.[1, 13]

Graves' disease is usually treated with anti-thyroid medication in the first instance. During the administration of adequate therapy, the disease may be quiescent but may return if compliance diminishes or dosage is inappropriately reduced. As with many autoimmune conditions, Graves' disease is sometimes self-limiting and around 30 per cent of patients experience lasting remission after treatment.

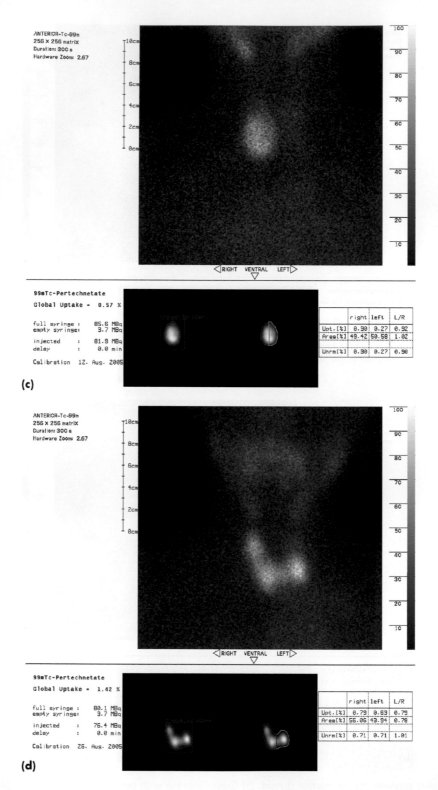

(c)

(d)

Figure 21.1 Continued.

EXTRA–THYROIDAL MANIFESTATIONS OF GRAVES' DISEASE

Ophthalmopathy

Many patients with Graves' disease have involvement of the eyes. Clinically evident ophthalmopathy occurs in about 50 per cent of patients, in 75 per cent of whom the eye signs appear within a year before or after the diagnosis of hyperthyroidism[13] (**Figure 21.2**). However, imaging studies reveal evidence of ophthalmopathy, in the form of enlarged extraocular muscles in most patients without clinical signs.[19] Patients who smoke are more likely to suffer eye disease of greater severity that non-smokers and hypothyroidism may exacerbate it.[20] About 90 per cent of patients with ophthalmopathy have hyperthyroidism;

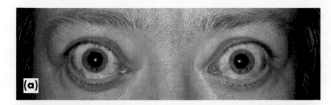

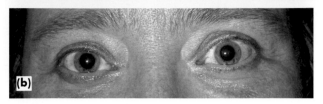

Figure 21.2 Patient with thyroid eye disease and optic neuropathy. (a) Pre-corrective surgery. Note the upper lid retraction, corneal injection, periorbital fat deposition and proptosis. (b) After surgical decompression. With kind permission from Mr J Uddin, Moorfields Hospital, London, UK.

Box 21.1 Signs of thyroid eye disease

- A feeling of grittiness and discomfort in the eye
- Retrobulbar pressure or pain
- Eyelid lag or retraction
- Periorbital oedema, chemosis, scleral injection
- Exophthalmos (proptosis)
- Extra-ocular muscle dysfunction
- Exposure keratitis
- Optic neuropathy

Box 21.2 Activity and severity assessments in Graves' orbitopathy (GO)[22]

- Activity measures based on classical features of inflammation: clinical activity score (CAS) is the sum of all items present:
  - Spontaneous retrobulbar pain
  - Pain on attempted up- or down-gaze
  - Redness of the eyelids
  - Redness of the conjunctiva
  - Swelling of the eyelids
  - Inflammation of the caruncle and/or plica
  - Conjunctival oedema

A CAS $\geq 3/7$ indicates active GO.

- Severity measures:
  - Lid aperture
  - Swelling of the eyelids (absent/equivocal, moderate, severe)
  - Redness of the eyelids (absent/present)
  - Conjunctival oedema (absent, present)
  - Inflammation of the caruncle or plica (absent, present)
  - Exopthalmos (measured in mm using the same Hertel exopthalmometer and same intercanthal distance for an individual patient)
  - Subjective diplopia score (0 = no diplopia; 1 = intermittent, i.e. when tired; 2 = inconstant, i.e. diplopia at extremes of gaze; 3 = constant)
  - Eye muscle involvement (ductions in degrees)
  - Corneal involvement (absent/punctuate keratopathy/ulcer)
  - Optic nerve involvement

---

the remainder have autoimmune hypothyroidism or are euthyroid at presentation.[21]

The ophthalmopathy is characterized initially by swelling of the extraocular muscles, proliferation of periorbital fat and later fibrosis leading to muscle tethering.[13] The lesions develop due to an accumulation of glycosaminoglycans and a lymphocytic infiltration of the orbital and retro-orbital tissues.[13] The most frequent signs of ophthalmopathy (**Box 21.1**) are eyelid retraction or lid lag and periorbital oedema. Although a minor degree of eyelid retraction (1–2 mm) may be due to sympathetic overactivity, and can occur in patients with any type of hyperthyroidism, more marked retraction is likely to be due to Graves' ophthalmopathy. Exophthalmos (proptosis) occurs in up to a third of patients and diplopia occurs in 5–10 per cent. Compression of the optic nerve at the apex of the orbit may cause visual loss but is rare.

Clinicians can estimate the activity and severity of thyroid eye disease using an internationally accepted scoring system. The criteria used in the most widely accepted scoring system from the European Group on Graves' Orbitopathy (EUGOGO) is displayed in **Box 21.2**. Decreasing visual acuity and a loss of colour vision are ominous signs and may be caused by pressure on the optic nerve by the swollen extraocular rectus muscles or – less commonly – sheer stretch of the optic nerve. Urgent treatment is needed if permanent visual loss is to be avoided. **Box 21.3** lists the indications for urgent ophthalmology referral.

Mild to moderate ophthalmopathy often improves spontaneously, and only simple measures are needed. Severe ophthalmopathy, in particular impaired vision, improves in about two-thirds of patients who are treated with high doses of glucocorticoids, orbital irradiation or both.[23] Orbital decompression is effective in patients with optic neuropathy and exophthalmos, either as the initial treatment or after the failure of glucocorticoid treatment.[24] The place of other medical treatments is unclear. **Box 21.4** summarizes the treatment of Graves' ophthalmopathy.[13]

Dermopathy

This occurs in about 1–2 per cent of patients with Graves' disease, almost always accompanied by severe eye disease. Usually occurring as a localized area of indurated non-pitting oedema over the skin of the shins and known as pretibial myxoedema, it may affect other areas of the body and areas of trauma.[25] The skin appears raised, oedematous, nodular and discoloured with a pink or brownish tinge. Dermopathy is characterized by lymphocytic infiltration of the dermis, the accumulation of glycosaminoglycans and oedema[13, 26] (**Figure 21.3**).

Box 21.3   Indications for urgent ophthalmology referral

- Rapid deterioration in visual acuity
- Ocular nerve palsies
- Unacceptable cosmetic appearance
- Visual acuity of less than 6/18
- Decreased colour vision
- Corneal ulceration

Box 21.4   Treatment of Graves' ophthalmopathy

Mild or moderate disease

- Maintenance of euthyroidism
- Cessation of smoking
- Avoidance of bright light and dust
- Sleeping with head raised
- Use of artificial tears
- Use of simple eye ointment at night
- Diuretic therapy

Severe disease

- Glucocorticoids (e.g. 40–80 mg of prednisolone daily, with the dose tapered over a period of at least three months with or without initial intravenous pulses of methylprednisolone)
- Radiotherapy
- Surgical decompression of the orbits
- Experimental treatments: immunosuppressive drugs, i.v. immune globulins, octreotide, plasma exchange

Stable disease

- Surgery on extraocular muscles to correct diplopia
- Cosmetic surgery to repair retraction of eye lids
- Orbital decompression to correct exophtalmos

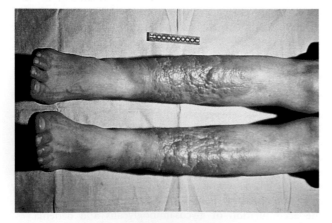

Figure 21.3   Pretibial myxoedema.

Acropachy

This is very rare, occurring in fewer than 1 per 1000 patients and presents as clubbing of the fingers with sub-periosteal new bone formation seen on plain x-ray.[27] Again, thought to arise from glycosaminoglycan accumulation, it occurs in conjunction with ophthalmopathy or dermopathy. There is no treatment.

LABORATORY DIAGNOSIS

In most patients with Graves' disease, serum fT3 and fT4 are raised and serum TSH is undetectable. The 24-hour radio-iodine uptake test usually indicates raised values, but is usually not needed to make the diagnosis. Three thyroid autoantibodies may be measured in clinical practice, those against thyroid peroxidase (TPO), thyroglobulin and the TSH-receptor. In a study of the prevalence and usefulness of thyroid autoantibodies, TPO antibodies were positive in 90 per cent of cases of Graves' disease, thyroglobulin antibodies in 49 per cent, while TSH-R antibodies were found only in 45 per cent.[28] Thyroid peroxidase antibodies are thus the most commonly measured antibodies in UK clinical practice.

Toxic multinodular goitre

A toxic multinodular goitre is a thyroid gland that has at least two autonomously functioning thyroid nodules that secrete excess thyroid hormone, producing typical signs and symptoms of hyperthyroidism.[29] Most patients in the UK are more than 50 years old, although the condition is much more frequent in younger age groups in other parts of the world because of iodine deficiency. The exact cause of multinodular goitre is not known, but is probably related to mutations in individual cells that lead to clonal expansion of individual nodules with autonomous thyroid function.[30] Due to the long natural history, an elderly patient presenting with a toxic multinodular goitre may describe the presence of the goitre many years before the thyrotoxicosis develops.[31] In patients with underlying non-toxic multinodular goitre, pharmaco-logical doses of iodine (e.g. from iodinated contrast agents), can lead to hyperthyroidism (iodine-induced hyperthyroidism or Jod–Basedow effect). This type of hyperthyroidism is common in areas of the world with iodine deficiency.[32]

Patients with toxic multinodular goitre present with typical signs and symptoms of hyperthyroidism, although they may not all be present since the degree of thyroid hyperfunction is typically less marked in these subjects. It is the cardiovascular effects that predominate and these include palpitations, AF and other tachyarrhythmias. Most patients will have a goitre and multiple nodules may be palpable. Subclinical hyperthyroidism is often recorded. Compressive symptoms such as dysphagia, dyspnoea and neck pressure may occur.[1]

Solitary toxic thyroid nodules

Solitary autonomous thyroid nodules that produce enough thyroid hormones to suppress the secretion of TSH from the pituitary, with consequent suppression of the contralateral thyroid lobe are called toxic nodules. They usually grow to least 3 cm in diameter before they result in overt hyperthyroidism and accounts for only around 5 per cent of cases with hyperthyroidism.[33] Autonomous function has been linked to activating mutations in the thyroid receptor,[34] or further downstream in the stimulatory G protein pathway linked to cyclic AMP production.[35]

The frequency increases with age, and they are more common in women. Often, subclinical hyperthyroidism is evident on biochemical testing.[36] Radionuclide scanning typically shows a focus of isotope accumulation with no uptake in other areas of the thyroid (**Figure 21.1c**).

Treatment of hyperthyroidism

The initial approach to the hyperthyroid patient is to minimize symptoms (often with a beta-adrenergic blocking drug) and to reduce the synthesis of thyroid hormones. Three modalities of treatment exist: drug therapy, radioiodine treatment and surgery. The advantages and disadvantages of the various treatment modalities are summarized in **Table 21.3**. The selection of treatment depends on many factors, including the underlying aetiology, the preferences of patients and clinicians, availability of a skilled surgeon, cost and local restrictions on the use of radioisotopes.[1] All three treatment modalities are associated with similar improvements in quality of life and satisfaction for patients,[37] and are equally effective.[38] Overt hyperthyroidism always needs treatment to avoid subsequent cardiovascular, skeletal or psychological secondary effects.

Table 21.3 Advantages and disadvantages of the different treatment modalities for thyrotoxicosis.

Treatment	Advantages	Disadvantages
Thionamides	Rapid symptom relief	Risk of severe side effects
	Inexpensive	Frequent clinic visits
	Chance of remission	Common mild side effects
	No exposure to radioactivity	Long course of treatment
		High chance of relapse
Radioiodine	Definitive treatment	Risk of hypothyroidism
	Outpatient procedure	Radiation protection measures
		Radiation thyroiditis
Surgery	Definitive treatment	Inpatient procedure
	Histological diagnosis	Risk of surgery
		Permanent hypothyroidism
		Risk of hypocalcaemia

ANTI-THYROID DRUGS

The thionamides (carbimazole and propylthiouracil) represent the mainstay of drug treatment of thyrotoxicosis in the UK. They disrupt the thyroid's incorporation of iodine and thus control thyroid hormone synthesis. Carbimazole has a faster effect than propylthiouracil (PTU)[39] and is given once daily, leading to better compliance.[40] In general, PTU should only be used if patients develop adverse reactions to carbimazole or during the first trimester of pregnancy (including in women trying to become pregnant).

Patients should be started on treatment after diagnosis of hyperthyroidism is made and while awaiting specialist advice. All patients diagnosed with hyperthyroidism should be referred to a specialist.[41] The starting dose of carbimazole should be 20 mg daily in a single dose, except in severe disease (i.e. fT3 and fT4 levels more than twice the upper limit of the normal reference range), when treatment should start at 30 mg daily. PTU is given in divided doses and 200 mg of PTU is approximately equivalent to 20 mg carbimazole. In general, after treatment with either drug, values of fT4 and fT3 gradually decrease to normal values over 4–6 weeks.

If a diagnosis of Graves' disease has been established, then the patient may be offered a full course of thionamide therapy in the hope of inducing remission. Optimal duration of treatment is 12–18 months[42, 43] and drug doses are titrated according to the serum concentration of fT4. This should be measured regularly, ideally every 4–6 weeks initially, then 8–12-weekly once control is achieved. Most patients require a maintenance dose of 5–10 mg carbimazole and 50–100 mg PTU. Larger dose requirements are suggestive of poor compliance. Thionamides do not induce remission or cure of thyrotoxicosis that is due to nodular disease. They may be used in the short term to induce euthyroidism prior to proceeding to definitive treatment with radioiodine or surgery.

Although most clinicians use thionamides alone to treat Graves' disease, some prefer the 'block and replace' regimen which uses thionamides to completely block endogenous thyroid hormone production which is then replaced with thyroxine. There is no substantial evidence that the block and replace approach has any advantages in terms of remission of Graves' disease. There is clear evidence for increased side effects (some serious), which are probably related to the higher doses of thionamides required.[44]

Remission rates with thionamide drugs are less than 50 per cent, although they may be slightly higher in the elderly.[38, 45] Relapse usually occurs within 3–6 months of thionamide withdrawal, in which case patients should be offered definitive treatment. Retrospective and prospective data indicate that a number of factors are associated with a poor prognosis although age, gender and goitre size appear to be the most important predictors (**Box 21.5**).[1, 45] Once remission has been achieved, cure is likely if the patient remains euthyroid for six months, although relapse may occur after several years.[46]

Side effects can occur with both carbimazole and PTU; mild side effects occur in 1–5 per cent of patients. The most common side effects are pruritic eruptions, fever, gastro-intestinal upset and arthralgias. Occasionally, the rash necessitates a swap from one drug to the other and cross-reactivity in this context is typically not a problem.[1]

Box 21.5 Poor prognostic factors for relapse of medically treated Graves' disease

- Male gender
- Age <40 years
- Presence of large goitre
- Severe biochemical disease
- Greatly increased ratio of serum T3/T4
- Repeated episodes of relapse
- Very high levels of TSH receptor antibodies

Agranulocytosis, vasculitis and liver damage are the major side effects of anti-thyroid drugs. Agranulocytosis arises in 0.2–0.5 per cent of patients,[47] and it is essential that all patients are warned (preferably in writing) of the risk of agranulocytosis and that clear instructions are given to present urgently for a full blood count if they develop a fever or sore throat. The agranulocytosis is usually transient and resolves after thionamide withdrawal but can be fatal, particularly if there is delay by either patient or doctor. Vasculitis associated with anti-cytoplasmic neutrophil antibodies in the circulation occurs mainly in patients receiving propylthiouracil.[48] Cholestatic and hepatitic forms of liver damage have been described with thionamide drugs.[49, 50] Recently, there have been significant concerns regarding propylthiouracil-induced liver failure and this drug is now no longer recommended as first-line treatment, except in specific circumstances. Agranulocytosis, along with hepatitis and vasculitis, are absolute contraindications to the further use of thionamides.

β-adrenergic blockers (e.g. propranolol 40 mg twice daily) are useful adjuncts to thionamides in the treatment of thyroid hormone excess. They act promptly to reduce symptoms such as tremor, palpitation and tachycardia and reduce the risk of tachyarrhythmias.[51] They should be used cautiously in the elderly where heart failure may be present.

In patients who develop AF, anticoagulation with warfarin should be considered due to the risk of embolic complications. There have been no controlled trials of the use of anticoagulants in thyrotoxic AF, but overwhelming evidence of their efficacy in other settings argues in favour of their use unless clear contraindications exist. Approximately half of those with thyrotoxic AF will revert spontaneously to sinus rhythm; this typically occurs within three months of initiation of anti-thyroid therapy. For those who remain in AF, joint cardiological management involving specific therapy to restore sinus rhythm may be considered when the patient is euthyroid.

RADIOIODINE (^{131}I) TREATMENT

Radioiodine is the treatment of choice for relapsed Graves' disease and toxic nodular hyperthyroidism and is increasingly used as first-line therapy in Graves' disease.[21] Additionally, ^{131}I treatment is used in the treatment of autonomous thyroid nodules and to induce shrinkage of benign goitres.[52]

Radioiodine is administered orally as sodium ^{131}I in a single capsule in the outpatient setting. It is incorporated into thyroid tissue and the β-emissions result in lasting thyroid tissue damage. There is a lag effect with the maximum thyroid ablation occurring over 6 weeks to four months. Depending on the administered dose, 50–85 per cent of patients achieve euthyroidism and shrinkage of goitre around two months after therapy.[1, 21] Fifteen to 20 per cent of patients require a second or (rarely) third dose, given 6–12 months after initial treatment.

Many studies have shown ^{131}I treatment to be safe and cost-effective and in terms of cancer (a concern for many patients), long-term safety has been well demonstrated.[21, 53, 54] National radiation protection policies exist and include measures to avoid contamination of the home or work place with ^{131}I including avoidance of close contact with small children, avoiding sharing utensils and sleeping alone. Although there is no national consensus regarding the most appropriate dose of radioiodine,[55] most centres will administer a fixed dose of 400–600 MBq, which is large enough to induce cure in the majority of patients.[21] Permanent hypothyroidism results in most patients, though this may be many years later; the incidence of ^{131}I-induced hypothyroidism is dose dependent.[1, 56]

Unless the hyperthyroidism is very mild, patients should receive pretreatment with anti-thyroid drugs and ^{131}I treatment is given when biochemical euthyroidism is restored. Thionamides are often restarted temporarily following ^{131}I therapy to avoid exacerbation of hyperthyroidism due to radiation-related thyroiditis. The frequency of this complication is low but pretreatment to lower thyroid hormone concentrations is advisable in the elderly and those with cardiac disease.[57] If pretreatment is necessary then carbimazole may be preferable to propylthiouracil, as there is some evidence to suggest that there is a higher failure rate of a given dose of radioiodine in patients receiving PTU around the time of ^{131}I therapy.[58] Whichever thionamide is used, the drug must be discontinued 1 week before radioiodine administration to allow maximum uptake into the gland. Success rates fall from over 90 per cent to under 50 per cent if the drug is continued at the time of radioiodine administration.[59, 60] Most centres advise discontinuing thionamides for a week before radioiodine is given and many recommend that the drug is restarted afterwards.

Following ^{131}I administration, patients should have 4–6-weekly TSH and fT4 measurements. If biochemical hyperthyroidism persists after a six month period, it is likely that a further dose of radioiodine will be necessary. Those treated with low-dose radioiodine, males, those with severe hyperthyroidism and those with a medium to large goitre are less likely to be cured after a single dose of ^{131}I.[56] All patients who have received radioiodine require long-term biochemical follow up with an annual serum TSH measurement. Effectively achieved with a computerized recall system, this is essential as the incidence of hypothyroidism is significant many years after treatment with radioiodine and eventually up to 90 per cent may become hypothyroid.

Radioiodine may worsen ophthalmopathy, especially in smokers,[61] and adjunctive treatment with corticosteroids may ameliorate or even prevent this.[61] Most physicians delay administration of radioiodine until moderate or severe eye disease has been stable for 12 months. Those with mild eye disease are given radioiodine at the same time as a course of steroid prophylaxis.[61, 62]

SURGERY

Although most experts agree that surgery has little part to play in the initial management of thyrotoxicosis, there are instances where total thyroidectomy is a safe and effective treatment for thyroid over-activity. These include patient preference (often relating to radiation protection issues), poor response to anti-thyroid drugs, especially in pregnancy; presence of a very large goitre and presence of a coexisting potentially malignant lesion. Surgery should be performed by a skilled surgeon;[63] complications include bleeding, infection as well as transient or permanent hypoparathyroidism and recurrent laryngeal nerve damage which occurs in 1–2 per cent of patients.[64]

Thyroiditis

Thyroiditis refers to any inflammatory condition of the thyroid.[1] The classification of thyroiditis is confusing but may be divided into those processes in which pain and tenderness develop, and those which do not have pain as a predominant feature (**Box 21.6**). Generally, the former rarely result in permanent hypothyroidism, but the latter often do.

Subacute thyroiditis is probably caused by a viral infection.[65] Patients present with systemic symptoms, including malaise, fever and thyroidal pain, as well as tremor and heat intolerance. The thyroid gland is usually extremely tender, firm and irregular. Laboratory tests show raised inflammatory markers (ESR, CRP) and initial thyroid function tests show thyrotoxicosis with a suppressed TSH and an elevated serum T4. After 12–16 weeks, there may be a hypothyroid phase during which the damaged tissue is unable to generate thyroid hormone following which euthyroidism is generally restored.[66] The course of serum TSH concentrations during subacute thyroiditis is shown in **Figure 21.4**. Radioactive iodine uptake is low, indicating damage to the thyroid gland. Treatment of subacute thyroiditis is supportive and includes the use of aspirin and other non-steroidal anti-inflammatory drugs. β-adrenergic blockers are useful if symptomatic in 66the thyrotoxic phase, but anti-thyroid drugs per se are not indicated. Permanent thyroid damage and recurrences are rare.

Subclinical hyperthyroidism

This is essentially a biochemical diagnosis consisting of low or undetectable serum TSH concentration with a normal serum fT4 and fT3 concentration. Subclinical hyperthyroidism may be exogenous as a consequence of treatment with thyroxine, or endogenous as a result of nodular thyroid disease or undetected early Graves' disease. Exogenous subclinical hyperthyroidism is by far the most common with over 20 per cent of patients on thyroxine having low TSH values on at least one occasion.[67]

Potential complications of subclinical hyperthyroidism include an increased risk of AF and cardiovascular disease and loss of bone mineral density. Evidence that subclinical hyperthyroidism is a risk factor for AF is clear, indeed it has been suggested that those aged over 60 with an undetectable TSH have a three-fold increase in relative risk.[68] Low

---

Box 21.6   Classification of thyroiditis

1. Associated with pain and tenderness
   a. Subacute granulomatous thyroiditis (De Quervains' or giant cell thyroiditis)
   b. Infectious thyroiditis
   c. Radioiodine-induced thyroiditis

2. Not associated with pain and tenderness
   a. Subacute lymphocytic thyroiditis (silent)
      i. Postpartum thyroiditis
      ii. Drug-induced thyroiditis (e.g. lithium)

   b. Chronic lymphocytic thyroiditis
      i. Hashimoto's thyroiditis
      ii. Postpartum thyroiditis

   c. Fibrous thyroiditis (Riedel's thyroiditis)
   d. Amiodarone-induced thyroiditis

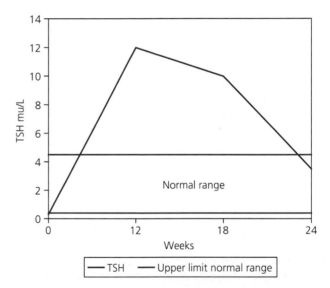

Figure 21.4   Course of subacute thyroiditis.

TSH appears to affect long-term survival, since in the elderly population an increased mortality due to cardiovascular causes can be predicted by a single low TSH measurement.[69] There is evidence that subclinical hyperthyroidism is associated with osteoporosis, especially in post-menopausal women,[70] but clear evidence for an increased risk of fracture is lacking.[71]

The treatment of subclinical hyperthyroidism remains controversial. The increasing evidence for associated morbidity and mortality, especially in terms of cardiovascular risk, has lent support to the view that anti-thyroid treatment should be considered in those with persistent suppression of TSH and evidence for underlying thyroid disease (nodular thyroid disease or Graves' disease), especially if associated with AF or known cardiac disease.[72, 73] Crucial evidence for a beneficial effect of such treatment, i.e. reduction in AF incidence or vascular mortality in those with subclinical hyperthyroidism, awaits the results of randomized controlled clinical trials.[71]

Practically, it is sensible to repeat thyroid function tests on a six-monthly basis in those who have endogenous subclinical hyperthyroidism. Where AF and osteoporosis may have been exacerbated by excess thyroid hormone, treatment is prudent. As these patients are usually elderly, radioiodine is the treatment of choice unless contraindications exist.

HYPOTHYROIDISM

Epidemiology

Hypothyroidism results from insufficient production and secretion of thyroid hormones. This is most commonly due to disturbance within the thyroid gland itself, (primary hypothyroidism) or within the hypothalamic-pituitary-thyroid axis (secondary hypothyroidism).[74] **Box 21.7** lists the causes of primary hypothyroidism.

The prevalence of hypothyroidism in the UK is estimated at around 2 per cent of adult women and 0.2 per cent of men,[2] rising to 5–10 per cent in women over 65.[4]

Clinical features

An insufficiency of thyroid hormone affects every organ system in the body and the effects of hypothyroidism can be broadly divided into[1] the generalized slowing of all metabolic processes leading to, among others, fatigue, cold intolerance and weight gain,[2] and the tissue accumulation of glycosaminoglycans which leads to the characteristic changes such as coarse dry skin, hair loss and doughy peripheral oedema. **Box 21.8** lists the manifestations of hypothyroidism.

The onset of symptoms can be insidious (particularly in the elderly), such that severe myxoedema may result. The typical patient complains of lethargy and fatigue; these complaints plus the accompanying apathy and listlessness means that ability to work is impaired. There may be a slow increase in weight despite a reduction in appetite and constipation is a common feature. Cold intolerance is typical. Patients may have a husky gruff voice attributed to 'laryngitis', but resulting from oedema of the vocal cords. Women may complain of dry coarse hair and brittle nails. Menstrual periods may be heavy and a desired conception elusive.[74] Myopathy can cause difficulty in walking upstairs or rising from a chair and numbness and paraesthesia in the hands may develop as carpal tunnel syndrome results from peripheral oedema. Occasionally, neuropsychiatric complications may develop with bizarre behaviour, so called 'myxoedema madness'. A low threshold for thyroid function testing is necessary, since few patients have a full set of symptoms. Current consensus, however, is that routine screening is not indicated.[73]

Aetiology of hypothyroidism

CHRONIC AUTOIMMUNE HYPOTHYROIDISM/HASHIMOTO'S THYROIDITIS

This condition is the most common cause of hypothyroidism in iodine-replete areas. It is a typical autoimmune condition, more common in females and running in families where a history of Graves' disease may feature along with other autoimmune conditions such as vitiligo, pernicious anaemia, rheumatoid arthritis and type 1 diabetes mellitus.[75] Although it is most common in older women, it can occur in infants as young as two years of age and is the major cause of hypothyroidism in children.[74] The role of autoimmunity in its pathogenesis is supported by the histological finding of diffuse lymphocytic infiltration of the thyroid gland and presence of circulating thyroid autoantibodies.[76]

Box 21.7 Causes of primary hypothyroidism

Associated with goitre

- Hashimoto's thyroiditis (chronic thyroiditis)
- Iodine deficiency
- Inherited defects of biosynthesis
- Drug induced (amiodarone, lithium, phenylbutazone)
- Maternal transmission (e.g. anti-thyroid drugs)

Not associated with goitre

- Atrophic thyroiditis
- Iatrogenic (e.g. radioiodine, surgery, neck irradiation)
- Congenital anomaly (e.g. thyroid agenesis)

Self-limiting

- Transient thyroiditis
- Post partum thyroiditis
- Iatrogenic (overtreatment with anti-thyroid medication)

Box 21.8 Manifestations and laboratory findings in hypothyroidism

Symptoms: Weakness/fatigue, coarse dry skin, pale skin/flush (peaches and cream), periorbital oedema, loss/drying of hair, coarse facial features, constipation, cold intolerance, decreased appetite with weight gain, myopathy, peripheral oedema, intellectual impairment, slow/hoarse speech, carpal tunnel syndrome, neuropsychiatric problems, menorrhagia, ovulatory failure, galactorrhoea.

Signs: Pale cool skin, characteristic facial features, peripheral/facial oedema, bradycardia, slow relaxing tendon reflexes, hoarse voice, goitre.

Laboratory findings: Low serum free T4 concentration, mild hyponatraemia, raised TSH concentration (if TSH concentration suppressed, consider central lesion), positive thyroid microsomal autoantibodies. Normochromic normocytic anaemia, raised serum cholesterol, triglycerides, LDL, lowered HDL (atherogenic lipid profile), raised serum prolactin.

Initially, the thyroid hypofunction may be subclinical, but may become overt with a rate of developing hypothyroidism at a rate of around 5 per cent per year. The typical goitre is moderate in size and smooth. The presence of the goitre may predate the development of overt hypothyroidism, and generally the goitre remains static or may decrease in size. Some patients present without a palpable goitre and are said to have atrophic autoimmune thyroiditis, which is thought to represent the end point of Hashimoto's thyroiditis.[77]

IATROGENIC HYPOTHYROIDISM

Iatrogenic hypothyroidism may result from surgery, treatment with radioactive iodine and external beam radiotherapy in patients who have undergone treatment for head and neck malignancy. Occasionally, hypothyroidism can result from overtreatment of hyperthyroidism with anti-thyroid medication, but with close monitoring this is not common.[74] Patients who have undergone thyroidectomy should commence thyroid hormone replacement before leaving hospital. In addition, the majority of patients treated with 400–600 MBq doses of ^{131}I will develop hypothyroidism.[21] External beam radiotherapy given to the neck may result in both hypothyroidism and an increased risk of thyroid malignancy, especially in children and adolescents. For patients who have had more than 25 Gy, there may be a slow onset dose dependent development of hypothyroidism.[78] Such patients should be carefully monitored both for hypothyroidism which may initially be subclinical, and for nodular thyroid disease which may herald a thyroid malignancy.

IODINE DEFICIENCY AND THE THYROID

Worldwide, the most common cause of hypothyroidism remains iodine deficiency.[79] In iodine-replete regions, neonatal hypothyroidism is routinely screened for in the post-natal period.[74] Causes of neonatal hypothyroidism include thyroid gland agenesis or dysgenesis, inherited defects in thyroid hormone biosynthesis and transplacental transmission of anti-TSH antibodies (causing transient neonatal hypothyroidism).

CENTRAL HYPOTHYROIDISM

Lack of hypothalamic thyrotropin releasing hormone (TRH) or pituitary TSH may lead to hypothyroidism, although central hypothyroidism accounts for less than 1 per cent of all cases of hypothyroidism. The most common causes are pituitary tumours and the surgery/radiotherapy used to treat them.[80] Such central causes may be distinguished from primary hypothyroidism by a normal or low serum TSH concentration that is inappropriate given a low serum fT3 and fT4 concentration. Specialist advice is required in these patients.

Treatment of hypothyroidism

Thyroxine is the drug of choice for the treatment of hypothyroidism.[81] It is absorbed from the upper small bowel with about 80 per cent efficiency, and has a long enough half-life (7 days) to allow for daily or even weekly dosing if compliance is an issue. Thyroxine is a pro-hormone which is de-iodinated in peripheral tissues to the active hormone T3.

The aim of treatment is to return the patient to a euthyroid state both clinically, as judged from symptoms, and biochemically as judged from serum TSH estimations. The majority of patients require 100–125 µg daily to achieve euthyroidism but variation exists. In those less than 50 years of age with no evidence of ischaemic heart disease, a moderate dose (typically 100 µg) may be started immediately. In older patients, or those with known cardiac disease, a starting dose of 25 µg is prudent due to the risk of exacerbating or precipitating cardiac disease because of the rise in cardiac output associated with initiation of therapy. Increments of 25 µg can be added every 4–6 weeks until TSH concentrations are within the normal range. Due to slow response of serum TSH concentrations, 4–6 weeks should elapse before measuring TSH concentration after initiating therapy or after dose adjustment. Once stable, serum TSH needs to be checked on an annual basis to ensure on-going compliance.[74]

In those with central hypothyroidism, it is imperative that hypoadrenalism be excluded before initiating thyroxine therapy. An adrenal crisis may be precipitated if hypoadrenalism is not treated before thyroxine therapy is commenced. In central hypothyroidism, the serum TSH concentration is of no value in monitoring therapy, thus dose adjustments should be made on serum fT4 and fT3 levels alone.

A minority of subjects feel that their symptoms of hypothyroidism are not controlled on thyroxine therapy despite normal concentrations of TSH and T4. Some choose to take T3 in addition to or instead of thyroxine, although due to its rapid absorption and short half-life, it must be taken three times a day and fluctuations in thyroid hormone levels exist. At present there is no evidence to suggest advantage over T4 therapy and combination therapy with T4 and T3 is best avoided.[82, 83]

Subclinical hypothyroidism

This is essentially a biochemical diagnosis consisting of raised serum TSH concentrations with normal fT4 concentrations. Subclinical hypothyroidism is common, with data from population surveys estimating a prevalence of 7–8 per cent in women and 2–4 per cent in men.[71] The prevalence rises with age to about 15 per cent in women aged over 60 years.

The aetiology may be clear from the history, e.g. previous ^{131}I treatment or thyroidectomy. Around 60 per cent of women with subclinical hypothyroidism have positive antibodies to thyroid peroxidise.[84] Prospective studies have confirmed that those with both positive antibodies and elevated TSH concentration are at risk of developing overt hypothyroidism at the rate of around 5 per cent per year, the risks being higher for those aged over 60 years.[3]

Controversy exists as to who should be treated and at what point, as the potential risks of inappropriate overtreatment to bone and cardiovascular system resulting from T4 treatment have been outlined. Recent guidelines state that apart from the data relating raised TSH to cholesterol, data showing clear benefits of treatment is lacking. Many clinicians would treat if there were a persistently raised TSH over 10 mU/L and positive autoantibodies, due to the high risk of progression to overt hypothyroidism. For asymptomatic patients with a modestly raised TSH (below 10 mU/L) or with a low or negative titre of microsomal antibodies, six-monthly or annual retesting is advised.[73]

THYROID DISEASE IN PREGNANCY

Hyperthyroidism and pregnancy

Postpartum, around 5 per cent of women develop thyroid dysfunction. Of those who develop postpartum thyroid dysfunction, around one-third have postpartum thyroiditis, with symptoms of thyrotoxicosis at around 12 weeks post delivery followed by a period of hypothyroidism at around 3–6 months. In some women, only the hypothyroid phase is evident and eventually there will be a return to a euthyroid state.[1] About 25 per cent of such women develop permanent hypothyroidism. Recurrent postpartum thyroiditis develops in up to 80 per cent of subsequent pregnancies. Referral for specialist monitoring is advised, and annual thyroid function tests are subsequently indicated.[1]

Transient thyrotoxicosis may be seen in cases of hyperemesis gravidarum, the likely mechanism being stimulation of the TSH receptor by raised β-HCG levels resulting in increased production of T3 and T4. Management is supportive and anti-thyroid medication should be avoided.

Pregnancy is complicated by Graves' disease in about 1 in 500 women.[85] Recognition of Graves' disease in pregnancy is important since untreated hyperthyroidism is associated with miscarriage, premature labour, low birthweight and pre-eclampsia.[86] Diagnosis of thyrotoxicosis may be delayed as symptoms and signs may be wrongly attributed to physiological changes occurring in pregnancy.[1] Treatment of thyrotoxicosis in pregnancy aims to achieve rapid biochemical euthyroidism whilst alleviating symptoms. Propranolol may be used as an adjunct but the mainstay of treatment is anti-thyroid medication, as radioiodine is contraindicated in this situation. Propylthiouracil is preferred to carbimazole as it crosses the placenta less and is associated with fewer potential teratogenic side-effects. In the rare instance of a serious adverse reaction to thionamides, surgery may be performed, preferably in the second trimester.[1] Joint management with the endocrinologist, obstetrician and paediatrician is important, as there is a risk of fetal and neonatal thyrotoxicosis indicated by low birth weight, irritability and tachycardia.

Hypothyroidism and pregnancy

Overt hypothyroidism can have adverse effects on both mother and fetus with increasing risks of pre-eclampsia, placental abruption, low birth weight and an increased perinatal mortality. Considerable debate surrounds the potential effect of subclinical hypothyroidism on the unborn fetus. Recent studies have shown mild but statistically significant adverse neuropsychological effects in children born to mothers with mildly raised TSH in the first trimester.[87, 88, 89, 90] Current opinion is that only targeted screening should be undertaken in high-risk patients, for example those with a personal or family history of thyroid dysfunction, a personal history of other autoimmune conditions such as diabetes mellitus, or obstetric complications known to be associated with hypothyroidism (i.e. recurrent miscarriage and preterm labour).[73]

During pregnancy, the requirement for thyroid hormone increases and around 75 per cent of women with treated hypothyroidism will need an increased dose during pregnancy, often by around 50 per cent. It is recommended to measure thyroid function tests around 4–6 weeks' gestation, 6 weeks after any increase in dose of T4 and at least once per trimester. Specialist monitoring of thyroid function is indicated. Post-delivery, the dose can be reduced to pre-pregnancy levels and checked to ensure it remains sufficient.

THYROID ENLARGEMENT

Epidemiology and aetiology

Thyroid enlargement is common. The Framingham study in the United States indicated a 5–10 per cent life-time risk of developing a thyroid nodule,[91] and the Whickham survey in the north-east of England reported a 15 per cent prevalence of goitres or thyroid nodules.[2] Additionally, high resolution ultrasound can detect thyroid nodules in 19–67 per cent of individuals, with higher frequencies in women and the elderly, even when the gland is normal to palpation.[52]

In contrast, thyroid cancer is rare, accounting for approximately 1 per cent of all new malignant disease (0.5 per cent of cancers in men and 1.5 per cent in women), although thyroid cancer is one of the most rapidly increasing malignancies.[92] Because of its favourable prognosis, thyroid carcinoma causes an even lower percentage of cancer deaths, reported at 0.21 and 0.3 per cent for men and women, respectively.[93] The majority of thyroid cancers are papillary carcinomas (72–85 per cent), with the remainder comprising follicular (10–20 per cent), medullary (1.7–3 per cent), anaplastic (<1 per cent) and other carcinomas (1–4 per cent). Papillary and follicular carcinomas are termed differentiated thyroid cancers.[93] Most patients with thyroid enlargement can be managed conservatively after malignancy is ruled out, the challenge to the clinician being to identify the minority of patients with thyroid cancer who therefore require surgical intervention and additional therapies.[52]

Assessment of patients with thyroid enlargement

Most patients with thyroid enlargement need no treatment after biochemical euthyroidism is confirmed and malignancy is excluded.[52]

CLINICAL EVALUATION

The history and clinical examination remain the diagnostic cornerstones in evaluating patients with thyroid enlargement, and in some cases may be suggestive of thyroid carcinoma.[94] The physical examination should focus on inspection of the neck (including regional lymph nodes) and the upper thorax and palpation of the nodule/goitre to determine its size and nodularity. Notably, there is considerable inter- and intra-observer variation regarding size and morphology of the thyroid.[52]

In many cases, however, thyroid glands harbouring malignancy are clinically indistinguishable from those that do not, and there is substantial variation among practitioners in evaluating nodules – a finding that may explain why an increasing number of thyroid specialists use imaging as part of the evaluation of thyroid nodules.[52, 94] The presence of discomfort in the neck, jaw or ear and dysphagia, hoarseness or dyspnoea can occur in patients with benign thyroid nodules, and particularly in those with large multinodular goitres, but this may also indicate thyroid carcinoma. A hard and fixed nodule is suggestive of thyroid carcinoma, as is vocal cord paralysis and ipsilateral lymphadenopathy, but these clinical features are absent in the vast majority of patients with this diagnosis.[52, 94]

The risk of harbouring thyroid cancer is highest in men, and in those at the extremes of age.[52, 94] Nodular thyroid disease is 5–10 times more common in females, whereas the rates of thyroid carcinoma are nearly equal in men and women. Therefore, the presence of a thyroid nodule in a man is more likely to reflect an underlying carcinoma.[52, 94] In addition, head and neck irradiation in infancy or childhood is associated with subsequent development of carcinoma and epidemiological studies have observed increased rates of childhood papillary thyroid cancer in Belarus and Ukraine following the Chernobyl nuclear reactor accident.[52, 94] Rate of growth is of importance; thyroid carcinomas are generally slow growing entities and rapid enlargement during thyroid hormone therapy is particularly worrisome.[52]

Overall, when the clinical suspicion of malignancy is high, thyroidectomy should be advocated irrespective of benign cytology, because the likelihood of malignancy is high. **Box 21.9** lists clinical criteria suggestive of the diagnosis of thyroid cancer.

LABORATORY INVESTIGATIONS

Determination of the serum thyrotropin (TSH) concentration is the most used test by thyroidologists in the evaluation

---

Box 21.9   Factors suggesting the diagnosis of thyroid carcinoma in patients presenting with thyroid enlargement

- Rapid tumour growth
- Very firm nodules
- Fixation to adjacent structures
- Vocal cord paralysis
- Regional lymphadenopathy
- Family history of medullary thyroid cancer (MTC) or multiple endocrine neoplasia (MEN)
- Age <20 or >60 years
- Male sex
- Solitary nodule
- Elevated TSH
- History of head or neck irradiation
- Compression symptoms: dysphagia, dysphonia, hoarseness, dyspneoea, cough

---

of patients presenting with thyroid enlargement and recent guidelines form the American Thyroid Association (ATA) and British Thyroid Association (BTA) state that serum TSH should be measured in the initial evaluation of a patient with a thyroid nodule.[95, 96, 97, 98] If the TSH is below the laboratory reference range, assays for fT3 and fT4 are required in order to exclude overt hyperthyroidism (raised free T4 and free T3) or 'T3-toxicosis' (raised serum free T3 alone). Similarly, if TSH is raised then overt hypothyroidism must be excluded (this being indicated by low fT4 with a raised TSH concentration). Results from surveys have indicated that when TSH levels are within the normal range, subsequent assessment of circulating free thyroid hormone levels is more favoured by European physicians when compared with North American thyroidologists.[52, 95, 96] Although virtually all patients with thyroid carcinoma are euthyroid, the presence of a suppressed serum TSH level (generally indicative of subclinical or overt thyrotoxicosis) does not rule out the presence of malignancy.[52]

Interestingly, recent studies have indicated that the presenting serum TSH concentration is an independent predictor of thyroid malignancy. The first study, evaluating 1500 patients presenting with thyroid enlargement and investigated with fine needle aspiration cytology (FNAC), indicated significantly increased odds ratios for malignancy in males, in those of younger age, in those with solitary nodules and in those with serum TSH >0.9 mU/l.[99] A further study confirmed that the likelihood of thyroid cancer increases with higher serum TSH concentration in 843 patients undergoing surgery for suspected thyroid malignancy. Moreover, the mean presenting serum TSH concentration was significantly higher in patients with stage III/IV disease compared with those with less advanced stage differentiated thyroid cancer (stage I/II).[100]

Anti-thyroid peroxidase measurements are measured by more than half of clinicians, but it is notable that thyroid autoantibodies are found in approximately 10 per cent of the population and autoimmunity may coexist with a thyroid nodule or goitre.[52] The role of routine measurement of serum calcitonin remains controversial. This hormone is a marker of medullary thyroid carcinoma, which accounts for less than 10 per cent of all thyroid cancers and is reported to be elevated in less than 0.5 per cent of all patients with thyroid nodules.[52] Early detection of medullary thyroid cancer is important but due to the presence of heterophilic antibodies, the immunometric calcitonin assay has a high false-positive rate. Again, European physicians tend to use this assay more routinely than their American counterparts.[52, 95, 96] and it seems clear that if the plasma calcitonin level is found to be above 10 pg/mL, this must elicit further investigation. The routine use of measurement of serum thyroglobulin is of little value in the initial laboratory assessment of patients with thyroid enlargement because of marked overlap of measurements in those with benign and malignant disease. Guidelines from the ATA and BTA therefore state that routine measurement of serum thyroglobulin for initial evaluation of thyroid nodules is not recommended.[97, 98]

DIAGNOSTIC IMAGING

The number of imaging modalities available to determine size and thyroid gland morphology is growing rapidly. These include ultrasonography, scintigraphy, computed tomography (CT) scanning, magnetic resonance (MR) imaging and, most recently, positron emission tomography (PET).

The most widely used form of imaging is ultrasonography, which has many favourable features including detection of non-palpable nodules, estimation of nodule size/goitre volume (e.g. to monitor the effect of therapy) and guidance of FNAC[52, 101] These advantages have led to changes in the attitude of clinicians and 80 per cent of ETA (European Thyroid Association) members, as well as 60 per cent of ATA members now routinely include ultrasonography in the initial management of patients presenting with a goitre.[95, 96] Some ultrasonographic characteristics, such as hypoechogenicity, solid nodules, microcalcifications, irregular margins, increased intranodular flow visualized by Doppler, increased ratio of anterior/posterior dimensions in transverse and longitudinal views (more tall than wide) and especially the evidence of invasion or regional lymphadenopathy, are associated with increased cancer risk.[94] However, the high sensitivity of this test can also lead to the detection of clinically insignificant nodules resulting in unnecessary work-up and anxiety.[52, 101] Furthermore, the low specificity of findings in most studies disqualifies ultrasound scanning from the differentiation between benign and malignant lesions and is clearly inferior to FNAC in this setting.[52, 101]

Thyroid isotope imaging/scintigraphy has been used for many years and is helpful in the determination of the functionality of thyroid nodules. This technique allows the differentiation between 'hot' (functional) and 'cold' (non-functional) nodules with the risk of malignancy in cold nodules being reported as high as 8–25 per cent. However, compared with FNAC, this diagnostic tool is significantly less sensitive and specific in distinguishing benign from malignant lesions and has therefore been largely abandoned in routine practice.[52, 98]

CT scanning and MRI provide high-resolution three-dimensional imaging of the thyroid gland, but neither of these methods provides advantages over ultrasound scanning in terms of detailed visualization of intrathyroidal structure. Furthermore, these methods have little value in the differentiation between benign and malignant lesions.[52] Newer techniques, such as 2-deoxy-2-fluoro-D glucose (FDG-PET), are more promising in this respect but their use is limited by considerations of cost and accessibility. Tracheal imaging appears to be of limited value in the routine diagnostic work up of patients presenting with thyroid enlargement although respiratory flow loop determination is helpful in the assessment of patients with large goitres.[102] Overall, FNAC is far superior to any of these diagnostic techniques and remains the current gold standard in the evaluation of patients presenting with thyroid enlargement.[52, 95, 96]

FINE NEEDLE ASPIRATION CYTOLOGY

FNAC provides the most direct and specific information about the pathology of thyroid nodules, has an extremely low complication rate, is inexpensive and easy to learn, therefore remaining the preferred diagnostic tool by the majority of thyroidologists.[95, 96] Most centres using this procedure have achieved a 35–75 per cent reduction in the number of patients requiring surgery, while at the same time doubling or tripling the malignancy yield at thyroidectomy.[103]

The efficacy of this investigative tool has been evaluated in several large series which have confirmed it to be an accurate test in the diagnosis of thyroid cancer, its sensitivity and specificity ranging between 65–98 and 72–100 per cent, respectively.[92, 104] The recent ATA guidelines state that FNAC is the procedure of choice in the evaluation of thyroid nodules.[97]

Despite its effectiveness and diagnostic accuracy, the non-diagnostic smear (approximately 15 per cent of all specimens) remains a management dilemma. Although criteria to consider a specimen 'adequate' vary among institutions, a commonly accepted definition for a diagnostic sample is one that includes six or more groups of 10–20 well-preserved follicular epithelial cells per group on at least two slides.[103] Inadequate sampling has been cited as the most common cause of false-negative biopsy results but repeat aspiration can augment the accuracy of the procedure.[103]

Several studies have demonstrated that ultrasound guidance, compared with palpation-guided FNAC, reduces the number of non-diagnostic aspirates, thereby increasing its sensitivity and specificity.[52, 94] Ultrasound-guided FNAC may be necessary for non-palpable or very small thyroid nodules, but there are no studies to demonstrate that the routine use of ultrasonography guidance improves outcome in terms of overall diagnostic rate or long-term outcome from thyroid cancer.

Guidance upon classification of cytological aspirates is provided by the BTA and ATA, as displayed in **Table 21.4**.[97, 98] The action to be undertaken following cytological diagnosis of fine needle aspirates is also displayed. Cystic nodules that repeatedly yield non-diagnostic aspirates need close observation or surgical excision and if the nodule is solid surgery should be more strongly considered.[97] When cytology is benign but patients belong to a high clinical risk group (**Box 21.9**), the decision to proceed to lobectomy may even be made with a benign FNAC diagnosis. This decision might also be made if there are pressure symptoms or rapid growth. In addition, the patient should have the choice to have the lesion removed if they so wish.[98] Indeterminate cytology can be found in 15–30 per cent of FNA specimens. While certain clinical features such as gender or nodule size[105] or cytological features such as presence of atypia[106] can improve the diagnostic accuracy in patients with indeterminate cytology, overall predictive values remain low. Although many molecular markers have been evaluated in the hope of improving diagnostic accuracy for indeterminate specimens, at present none is recommended, because of insufficient data.[97]

ATA guidelines state that diagnostic ultrasound should be performed in those patients presenting with multiple thyroid nodules as sonographic characteristics are superior to nodule size in identifying malignancy.[97] Aspiration is recommended in the presence of two or more thyroid nodules larger than 1–1.5 cm, and those with suspicious sonographic features. If none of the nodules has a suspicious appearance, the likelihood of malignancy is low and it is reasonable to aspirate the largest nodule(s) only.[97] **Figure 21.5** displays a practical guide to the evaluation of patients with thyroid enlargement.

Table 21.4 Classification of cytological classification of fine needle aspirates according to BTA and ATA guidance. The action required following cytological diagnosis is also displayed.[75, 76]

Type of lesion	BTA diagnostic category	ATA diagnostic category	Required action
Any inadequate specimen	Thy1 Non-diagnostic	Non diagnostic aspirate	Repeat FNAC US-guided FNAC if required Close observation Consider surgery if solid lesion
Nodular goitre or thyroiditis	Thy2 Non-neoplastic	Benign cytology	Repeat aspirate after 3-6 months No further diagnostic tests required
Follicular lesions	Thy3 Follicular lesions	Indeterminate cytology	Lobectomy or total thyroidectomy Discussion between surgeon and endocrinologist required
Suspicious but not diagnostic of thyroid carcinoma	Thy4 Suspicious of malignancy	Indeterminate cytology	Surgical intervention for differentiated tumour Further investigation for anaplastic carcinoma, lymphoma, metastatic tumour
Thyroid carcinoma	Thy5 Diagnostic of malignancy	Aspirates diagnostic of malignancy	Surgical intervention for differentiated tumour Further investigation, radiotherapy or chemotherapy for anaplastic carcinoma, lymphoma, metastatic tumour

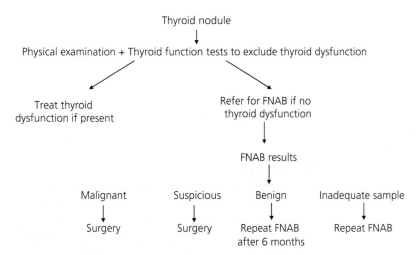

Figure 21.5 A diagnostic strategy to evaluate the solitary or dominant thyroid nodule.

Medical management of patients with thyroid enlargement

NON-TOXIC MULTINODULAR GOITRE

Surgery is the treatment of choice where there is evidence of moderate to severe compressive symptoms, where FNAC of a dominant nodule is suspicious of malignancy, or where the patient prefers surgery for cosmetic reasons. Medical treatment of goitre involves the administration of radioactive iodine; the other medical option of administration of suppressive thyroid hormone is now considered outdated.[52, 131]I treatment is given if surgery is not an option either due to age, frailty or other comorbid conditions, or because the patient refuses surgery.

Radioiodine will cause a reduction in goitre size (up to 60 per cent) in most patients, with shrinkage occurring soon after treatment. The majority of patients experience relief from obstructive symptoms with dyspnoea improving in 75 per cent of those with the largest goitres, accompanied by an increase in cross-sectional area of the trachea of 36 per cent.[107] Factors suggesting a favourable outcome include smaller goitres in younger patients, a shorter history of goitre and higher doses of radioiodine. In those with large goitres, large doses of radioiodine may be necessary, which, due to radiation protection legislation, can entail the hospitalization and isolation of the patient. An alternative is to fractionate therapy over a course of some months in an outpatient setting.

Side effects include hypothyroidism, which is common, the risk increasing if multiple doses are administered. The prevalence varies according to the amount of radiation exposure, with figures quoted ranging between 8 and 40 per cent at 1–2 years.[52] Radiation thyroiditis (neck pain and tenderness) occurs in 3–13 per cent and Graves' type hyperthyroidism associated with development of TSH receptor antibodies may occur in around 5 per cent.

There has been concern over the risk of deterioration in respiratory function in those with tracheal compression after ^{131}I administration due to a transient increase in goitre size immediately after therapy. Studies have shown only a small decrease in tracheal cross-sectional area after therapy with no increase in upper airways obstruction. Some recommend the use of prednisolone peri- and post I[131] to minimize any risks in those with severe tracheal compression but there is no evidence base for this practice.[52]

Recombinant TSH may be used in this setting. The logic is that the higher the serum TSH, the greater the stimulus for radioiodine uptake into the goitre and the greater the chance of efficacy with a lower overall dose of radioiodine. Although preliminary results are encouraging,[108] evidence for efficacy in volume reduction is not yet available, so recombinant TSH is not widely used at present.

Suppressive T4 treatment has historically been used to reduce goitre size. Although some studies have shown benefit, growth of thyroid nodules or goitres often resumes after discontinuation of thyroxine, meaning therapy may need to be life-long. Suppressive therapy necessarily induces a state of subclinical hyperthyroidism (suppression of TSH) with risks of atrial fibrillation and reduced bone density as previously outlined. For these reasons the use of suppressive therapy has been abandoned by most thyroidologists.[52]

SOLITARY NON-TOXIC NODULE

Management is effectively similar to the treatment of multinodular goitre and surgery remains the treatment of choice in those who desire it for cosmetic reasons and in those in whom malignancy is suspected, either on clinical grounds or on the basis of cytological changes suggestive or suspicious of neoplasia. Suppressive therapy with thyroid hormones is not recommended for solitary nodules for reasons previously discussed.

[131]I therapy is a simple, safe and cost effective treatment for those with solitary thyroid nodules which take up iodine (hot nodules) and a thyroid volume reduction of 40 per cent may be seen after a single dose of I[131]. Hypothyroidism is relatively uncommon with a prevalence of around 10 per cent at five years and is higher in those with pre-existing thyroid autoimmunity.

Ten to 15 per cent of solitary thyroid nodules are cystic and simple aspiration is the treatment of choice, however, recurrence rates may be as high as 80 per cent with larger lesions. For this reason, and the fact that many cysts resolve spontaneously over time, an expectant approach may be taken with small cysts less than 3 mL. Larger ones should be aspirated with FNAC performed on any residual nodule and surgery considered, as around 10 per cent of large lesions may harbour thyroid cancer.

The advent of high resolution ultrasonography has led to the discovery of small, asymptomatic and previously unrecognized thyroid nodules. These thyroid incidentalomas are usually smaller that 1.5 cm and are often diagnosed during ultrasonographic evaluation for non-diagnostic neck disorders, posing a management dilemma for the clinician.[97, 103] A recent consensus statement by the Society of Radiologists in Ultrasound on the management of thyroid nodules detected at sonography states that highly suspicious ultrasonographic features, such as microcalcifications, prompt a biopsy in nodules 1 cm or larger. Other suspicious features such as solid consistency prompt biopsy at 1.5 cm or larger, while less suspicious appearances such as mixed solid and cystic consistency should be considered for biopsy only if nodules measure 2 cm or larger.[109] These guidelines remain controversial with endocrinologists as it has been reported that patients undergoing surgery for papillary cancers <1.5 cm have been found to have distant metastasis.[110] Others recommend observation for nodules smaller than 1 cm, in the absence of sonographic features of malignancy and fine needle aspiration biopsy (FNAB) for larger incidentalomas and those with features suspicious of malignancy.[103]

The management of these incidentalomas remains controversial and clinical, as well as sonographic, follow up is generally recommended. FNAC should be performed in rapidly enlarging lesions as well as in those which exhibit suspicious sonographic features, including irregular margins and increased intranodular flow visualized by Doppler.[52, 103] US-guided FNAC may be necessary as the majority of nodules will be impalpable.

CONCLUSION

Benign thyroid disease is common with thyroid dysfunction affecting up to 2 per cent of the population. The underlying aetiology of thyroid disease in iodine-replete areas is usually autoimmune in nature. Determination of serum concentrations of TSH, fT3 and fT4 are the most important diagnostic tests to evaluate thyroid dysfunction. While there is clear evidence that overt thyroid dysfunction required treatment, the management of subclinical thyroid dysfunction remains controversial. The treatment of thyrotoxicosis is with antithyroid drugs or the administration of radioactive iodine. Hypothyroidism is treated with thyroxine replacement, the aim being to restore clinical and biochemical euthyroidism. In addition to thyroid dysfunction, thyroid enlargement is very common. Following clinical examination, all patients should have their serum TSH measured. Thyroid ultrasound is increasingly used in the assessment of thyroid neoplasia but remains inferior to fine needle aspiration biopsy in the specific detection of thyroid cancer. When thyroid malignancy is excluded, patients with thyroid nodules require further follow up and repeat FNAB 3–6 months after the initial FNAB is recommended for benign nodules. Several clinical, biochemical and sonographic criteria can serve as an adjunct to cytological diagnosis in the prediction of thyroid malignancy and can help in the identification of patient groups who require earlier surgical referral or more regular follow up.

DEFICIENCIES IN CURRENT KNOWLEDGE AND DIRECTIONS FOR FUTURE RESEARCH

Further work on the long-term sequelae of thyroid disease, both in the fetus and in adulthood, may add to the debate on screening for thyroid dysfunction, especially in women of childbearing age. Human and mouse databases have provided powerful tools to probe many unanswered questions in thyroidology. The genetic basis for autoimmune thyroid disease is being unravelled by discovery of genetic variations associated with risk for autoimmune disease and important molecules in the disorder's pathogenesis.[111] Already major progress has been achieved in identifying the role of specific components of the HLA system and other immune regulatory genes such as CTLA-4 and CD40 which have functional consequences. Better understanding of the genetic mechanisms leading to autoimmune thyroid disease may lead to targeted therapies for immune modulation. Such understanding may also allow better prediction of treatment outcomes, for example response to anti-thyroid drugs and hence better tailoring of therapies for individual patients. The ability to predict outcome in Graves' disease would be of immense clinical value.

Current research into Graves' ophthalmopathy attempts to elucidate the precise aetiology of the condition. Newly developed animal models may have a positive impact in this field. Research into new approaches for treatment of thyroid eye disease has focused on the use of cytokine antagonists, somatostatin analogues and also on the use of antioxidants.[112] In future, it would be expected that double blind trials involving some of these agents may begin.

Importantly we are beginning to understand the long-term morbidity, and indeed mortality, associated with thyroid dysfunction, largely vascular. This understanding will drive the development of more intensive and effective clinical management strategies and identification of those at particular risk. The relationship between subclinical thyroid dysfunction cardiovascular morbidity and mortality is a further area in need of large randomized controlled trials to guide clinicians in the management of this condition.

Future research in nodular thyroid disease will focus on ways of improving the diagnostic pathway to reduce the number of patients undergoing lobectomy for what proves to be benign disease. Current research into ultrasound and colour Doppler criteria for identification of malignancy may have a positive impact. More likely, however, is a major impact of gene expression studies allowing discrimination, perhaps on biopsy specimens, of benign from malignant disease, as well as identification of genetic and molecular markers in resected tumours which will predict potential recurrence and hence the need for intensive therapy.

KEY EVIDENCE

- The most important initial test to evaluate thyroid dysfunction is measurement of serum TSH concentration.
- Treatment of hyperthyroidism is with antithyroid drugs, radioactive iodine or surgery.
- Overt hypothyroidism requires treatment with thyroxine, the aim being to restore euthyroidism both clinically and biochemically.
- FNAB remains the diagnostic procedure of choice to detect thyroid malignancy.

KEY LEARNING POINTS

- Thionamides represent the mainstay of drug treatment of hyperthyroidism in the UK.
- Radioactive iodine administration is the treatment of choice in patients with toxic nodular goitre and in those with relapsed Graves' disease.
- The treatment of subclinical thyroid disease remains controversial.
- All patients with thyroid nodules or enlargement should undergo serum TSH measurement.
- Patients presenting with thyroid enlargement require regular follow up.
- Some clinical, biochemical and ultrasonographic characteristics may aid in the prediction of thyroid malignancy.

REFERENCES

1. Cooper DS. Hyperthyroidism. *Lancet* 2003; **362**: 459–68.
2. Tunbridge WM, Evered DC, Hall R *et al.* The spectrum of thyroid disease in a community: the Whickham survey. *Clinical Endocrinology* 1977; **7**: 481–93.
3. Vanderpump MP, Tunbridge WM, French JM *et al.* The incidence of thyroid disorders in the community: a twenty-year follow-up of the Whickham Survey. *Clinical Endocrinology* 1995; **43**: 55–68.
4. Parle JV, Franklyn JA, Cross KW *et al.* Prevalence and follow-up of abnormal thyrotrophin (TSH) concentrations in the elderly in the United Kingdom. *Clinical Endocrinology* 1991; **34**: 77–83.
5. Hollowell JG, Staehling NW, Flanders WD *et al.* Serum TSH, T(4), and thyroid antibodies in the United States population (1988 to 1994): National Health and Nutrition Examination Survey (NHANES III). *Journal of Clinical Endocrinology and Metabolism* 2002; **87**: 489–99.
6. Lahey FA. Nonactivated (apathetic) type of hyperthyroidism. *New England Journal of Medicine* 1931; **204**: 747–8.

7. Krassas GE. Thyroid disease and female reproduction. *Fertility and Sterility* 2000; **74**: 1063–70.

8. Carlson HE. Gynecomastia. *New England Journal of Medicine* 1980; **303**: 795–9.

9. Cobler JL, Williams ME, Greenland P. Thyrotoxicosis in institutionalized elderly patients with atrial fibrillation. *Archives of Internal Medicine* 1984; **144**: 1758–60.

10. Trivalle C, Doucet J, Chassagne P *et al.* Differences in the signs and symptoms of hyperthyroidism in older and younger patients. *Journal of the American Geriatrics Society* 1996; **44**: 50–3.

11. Shimizu T, Koide S, Noh JY *et al.* Hyperthyroidism and the management of atrial fibrillation. *Thyroid* 2002; **12**: 489–93.

12. Burch HB, Wartofsky L. Life-threatening thyrotoxicosis. Thyroid storm. *Endocrinology and Metabolism Clinics of North America* 1993; **22**: 263–77.

13. Weetman AP. Graves' disease. *New England Journal of Medicine* 2000; **343**: 1236–48.

14. Bahn RS. Thyrotropin receptor expression in orbital adipose/connective tissues from patients with thyroid-associated ophthalmopathy. *Thyroid* 2002; **12**: 193–5.

15. Wiersinga WM, Prummel MF. Pathogenesis of Graves' ophthalmopathy – current understanding. *Journal of Clinical Endocrinology and Metabolism* 2001; **86**: 501–3.

16. Matos-Santos A, Nobre EL, Costa JG *et al.* Relationship between the number and impact of stressful life events and the onset of Graves' disease and toxic nodular goitre. *Clinical Endocrinology* 2001; **55**: 15–19.

17. Vestergaard P, Rejnmark L, Weeke J *et al.* Smoking as a risk factor for Graves' disease, toxic nodular goiter, and autoimmune hypothyroidism. *Thyroid* 2002; **12**: 69–75.

18. Wong V, Fu AX, George J, Cheung NW. Thyrotoxicosis induced by alpha-interferon therapy in chronic viral hepatitis. *Clinical Endocrinology* 2002; **56**: 793–8.

19. Villadolid MC, Yokoyama N, Izumi M *et al.* Untreated Graves' disease patients without clinical ophthalmopathy demonstrate a high frequency of extraocular muscle (EOM) enlargement by magnetic resonance. *Journal of Clinical Endocrinology and Metabolism* 1995; **80**: 2830–3.

20. Bartalena L, Bogazzi F, Tanda ML *et al.* Cigarette smoking and the thyroid. *European Journal of Endocrinology* 1995; **133**: 507–12.

21. Weetman AP. Radioiodine treatment for benign thyroid diseases. *Clinical Endocrinology* 2007; **66**: 757–64.

22. Bartalena L, Baldeschi L, Dickinson A *et al.* Consensus statement of the European Group on Graves' orbitopathy (EUGOGO) on management of GO. *European Journal of Endocrinology* 2008; **158**: 273–85.

23. Bartalena L, Marcocci C, Pinchera A. Treating severe Graves' ophthalmopathy. *Baillière's Clinical Endocrinology and Metabolism* 1997; **11**: 521–36.

24. Garrity JA, Fatourechi V, Bergstralh EJ *et al.* Results of transantral orbital decompression in 428 patients with severe Graves' ophthalmopathy. *American Journal of Ophthalmology* 1993; **116**: 533–47.

25. Schwartz KM, Fatourechi V, Ahmed DD, Pond GR. Dermopathy of Graves' disease (pretibial myxedema): long-term outcome. *Journal of Clinical Endocrinology and Metabolism* 2002; **87**: 438–46.

26. Peacey SR, Flemming L, Messenger A, Weetman AP. Is Graves' dermopathy a generalized disorder? *Thyroid* 1996; **6**: 41–5.

27. Vanhoenacker FM, Pelckmans MC, De Beuckeleer LH *et al.* Thyroid acropachy: correlation of imaging and pathology. *European Radiology* 2001; **11**: 1058–62.

28. Kumar H, Daykin J, Betteridge J *et al.* Prevalence and clinical usefulness of thyroid antibodies in different disease states of the thyroid. *Clinical Endocrinology* 1999; **50**: 679–80.

29. Siegel RD, Lee SL. Toxic nodular goiter. Toxic adenoma and toxic multinodular goiter. *Endocrinology and Metabolism Clinics of North America* 1998; **27**: 151–68.

30. Tonacchera M, Agretti P, Chiovato L *et al.* Activating thyrotropin receptor mutations are present in nonadenomatous hyperfunctioning nodules of toxic or autonomous multinodular goiter. *Journal of Clinical Endocrinology and Metabolism* 2000; **85**: 2270–4.

31. Vitti P, Rago T, Tonacchera M, Pinchera A. Toxic multinodular goiter in the elderly. *Journal of Endocrinological Investigation* 2002; **25** (10 Suppl.): 16–18.

32. Roti E, Uberti ED. Iodine excess and hyperthyroidism. *Thyroid* 2001; **11**: 493–500.

33. Hamburger JI. Solitary autonomously functioning thyroid lesions. Diagnosis, clinical features and pathogenetic considerations. *American Journal of Medicine* 1975; **58**: 740–8.

34. van Sande J, Parma J, Tonacchera M *et al.* Somatic and germline mutations of the TSH receptor gene in thyroid diseases. *Journal of Clinical Endocrinology and Metabolism* 1995; **80**: 2577–85.

35. Spiegel AM. Mutations in G proteins and G protein-coupled receptors in endocrine disease. *Journal of Clinical Endocrinology and Metabolism* 1996; **81**: 2434–42.

36. Burch HB, Shakir F, Fitzsimmons TR *et al.* Diagnosis and management of the autonomously functioning thyroid nodule: the Walter Reed Army Medical Center experience, 1975–1996. *Thyroid* 1998; **8**: 871–80.

37. Ljunggren JG, Torring O, Wallin G *et al.* Quality of life aspects and costs in treatment of Graves' hyperthyroidism with antithyroid drugs, surgery, or radioiodine: results from a prospective, randomized study. *Thyroid* 1998; **8**: 653–9.

38. Torring O, Tallstedt L, Wallin G *et al.* Graves' hyperthyroidism: treatment with antithyroid drugs, surgery, or radioiodine – a prospective, randomized study. Thyroid Study Group. *Journal of Clinical Endocrinology and Metabolism* 1996; **81**: 2986–93.

39. Homsanit M, Sriussadaporn S, Vannasaeng S *et al.* Efficacy of single daily dosage of methimazole vs. propylthiouracil in the induction of euthyroidism. *Clinical Endocrinology* 2001; **54**: 385–90.

40. Nicholas WC, Fischer RG, Stevenson RA, Bass JD. Single daily dose of methimazole compared to every 8 hours propylthiouracil in the treatment of hyperthyroidism. *Southern Medical Journal* 1995; **88**: 973–6.

41. Vanderpump MP, Ahlquist JA, Franklyn JA, Clayton RN. Consensus statement for good practice and audit measures in the management of hypothyroidism and hyperthyroidism. The Research Unit of the Royal College of Physicians of London, the Endocrinology and Diabetes Committee of the Royal College of Physicians of London, and the Society for Endocrinology. *British Medical Journal* 1996; **313**: 539–44.

42. Allannic H, Fauchet R, Orgiazzi J *et al.* Antithyroid drugs and Graves' disease: a prospective randomized evaluation of the efficacy of treatment duration. *Journal of Clinical Endocrinology and Metabolism* 1990; **70**: 675–9.

43. Maugendre D, Gatel A, Campion L *et al.* Antithyroid drugs and Graves' disease – prospective randomized assessment of long-term treatment. *Clinical Endocrinology* 1999; **50**: 127–32.

44. Wiersinga WM. Immunosuppression of Graves' hyperthyroidism – still an elusive goal. *New England Journal of Medicine* 1996; **334**: 265–6.

45. Allahabadia A, Daykin J, Holder RL *et al.* Age and gender predict the outcome of treatment for Graves' hyperthyroidism. *Journal of Clinical Endocrinology and Metabolism* 2000; **85**: 1038–42.

46. Hedley AJ, Young RE, Jones SJ *et al.* Antithyroid drugs in the treatment of hyperthyroidism of Graves' disease: long-term follow-up of 434 patients. Scottish Automated Follow-Up Register Group. *Clinical Endocrinology* 1989; **31**: 209–18.

47. Tajiri J, Noguchi S, Murakami T, Murakami N. Antithyroid drug-induced agranulocytosis. The usefulness of routine white blood cell count monitoring. *Archives of Internal Medicine* 1990; **150**: 621–4.

48. Gunton JE, Stiel J, Clifton-Bligh P *et al.* Prevalence of positive anti-neutrophil cytoplasmic antibody (ANCA) in patients receiving anti-thyroid medication. *European Journal of Endocrinology* 2000; **142**: 587.

49. Arab DM, Malatjalian DA, Rittmaster RS. Severe cholestatic jaundice in uncomplicated hyperthyroidism treated with methimazole. *Journal of Clinical Endocrinology and Metabolism* 1995; **80**: 1083–5.

50. Williams KV, Nayak S, Becker D *et al.* Fifty years of experience with propylthiouracil-associated hepatotoxicity: what have we learned? *Journal of Clinical Endocrinology and Metabolism* 1997; **82**: 1727–33.

51. Geffner DL, Hershman JM. Beta-adrenergic blockade for the treatment of hyperthyroidism. *American Journal of Medicine* 1992; **93**: 61–8.

52. Hegedus L, Bonnema SJ, Bennedbaek FN. Management of simple nodular goiter: current status and future perspectives. *Endocrine Reviews* 2003; **24**: 102–32.

53. Franklyn JA, Maisonneuve P, Sheppard M *et al.* Cancer incidence and mortality after radioiodine treatment for hyperthyroidism: a population-based cohort study. *Lancet* 1999; **353**: 2111–15.

54. Hall P, Lundell G, Holm LE. Mortality in patients treated for hyperthyroidism with iodine-131. *Acta Endocrinologica (Copenh)* 1993; **128**: 230–4.

55. Vaidya B, Williams GR, Abraham P, Pearce SH. Radioiodine treatment for benign thyroid disorders: results of a nationwide survey of UK endocrinologists. *Clinical Endocrinology* 2008; **68**: 814–20.

56. Allahabadia A, Daykin J, Sheppard MC *et al.* Radioiodine treatment of hyperthyroidism-prognostic factors for outcome. *Journal of Clinical Endocrinology and Metabolism* 2001; **86**: 3611–17.

57. Tamagna EI, Levine GA, Hershman JM. Thyroid-hormone concentrations after radioiodine therapy for hyperthyroidism. *Journal of Nuclear Medicine* 1979; **20**: 387–91.

58. Imseis RE, Vanmiddlesworth L, Massie JD *et al.* Pretreatment with propylthiouracil but not methimazole reduces the therapeutic efficacy of iodine-131 in hyperthyroidism. *Journal of Clinical Endocrinology and Metabolism* 1998; **83**: 685–7.

59. Koroscil TM. Thionamides alter the efficacy of radioiodine treatment in patients with Graves' disease. *Southern Medical Journal* 1995; **88**: 831–6.

60. Sabri O, Zimny M, Schulz G *et al.* Success rate of radioiodine therapy in Graves' disease: the influence of thyrostatic medication. *Journal of Clinical Endocrinology and Metabolism* 1999; **84**: 1229–33.

61. Bartalena L, Marcocci C, Bogazzi F *et al.* Relation between therapy for hyperthyroidism and the course of Graves' ophthalmopathy. *New England Journal of Medicine* 1998; **338**: 73–8.

62. Wiersinga WM, Bartalena L. Epidemiology and prevention of Graves' ophthalmopathy. *Thyroid* 2002; **12**: 855–60.

63. Alsanea O, Clark OH. Treatment of Graves' disease: the advantages of surgery. *Endocrinology and Metabolism Clinics of North America* 2000; **29**: 321–37.

64. Sosa JA, Bowman HM, Tielsch JM *et al.* The importance of surgeon experience for clinical and economic outcomes from thyroidectomy. *Annals of Surgery* 1998; **228**: 320–30.

65. Volpe R. The management of subacute (DeQuervain's) thyroiditis. *Thyroid* 1993; **3**: 253–5.

66. Fatourechi V, Aniszewski JP, Fatourechi GZ *et al.* Clinical features and outcome of subacute thyroiditis in an incidence cohort: Olmsted County, Minnesota, study. *Journal of Clinical Endocrinology and Metabolism* 2003; **88**: 2100–5.

67. Parle JV, Franklyn JA, Cross KW *et al.* Thyroxine prescription in the community: serum thyroid stimulating

hormone level assays as an indicator of undertreatment or overtreatment. *British Journal of General Practice* 1993; **43**: 107–9.

68. Sawin CT, Geller A, Wolf PA *et al.* Low serum thyrotropin concentrations as a risk factor for atrial fibrillation in older persons. *New England Journal of Medicine* 1994; **331**: 1249–52.

69. Parle JV, Maisonneuve P, Sheppard MC *et al.* Prediction of all-cause and cardiovascular mortality in elderly people from one low serum thyrotropin result: a 10-year cohort study. *Lancet* 2001; **358**: 861–5.

70. Faber J, Galloe AM. Changes in bone mass during prolonged subclinical hyperthyroidism due to L-thyroxine treatment: a meta-analysis. *European Journal of Endocrinology* 1994; **130**: 350–6.

71. Boelaert K, Franklyn JA. Thyroid hormone in health and disease. *Journal of Endocrinology* 2005; **187**: 1–15.

72. Fatourechi V. Adverse effects of subclinical hyperthyroidism. *Lancet* 2001; **358**: 856–7.

73. Surks MI, Ortiz E, Daniels GH *et al.* Subclinical thyroid disease: scientific review and guidelines for diagnosis and management. *Journal of the American Medical Association* 2004; **291**: 228–38.

74. Roberts CG, Ladenson PW. Hypothyroidism. *Lancet* 2004; **363**: 793–803.

75. Neufeld M, Maclaren NK, Blizzard RM. Two types of autoimmune Addison's disease associated with different polyglandular autoimmune (PGA) syndromes. *Medicine (Baltimore)* 1981; **60**: 355–62.

76. Amino N, Hagen SR, Yamada N, Refetoff S. Measurement of circulating thyroid microsomal antibodies by the tanned red cell haemagglutination technique: its usefulness in the diagnosis of autoimmune thyroid diseases. *Clinical Endocrinology* 1976; **5**: 115–25.

77. Zimmerman RS, Brennan MD, McConahey WM *et al.* Hashimoto's thyroiditis. An uncommon cause of painful thyroid unresponsive to corticosteroid therapy. *Annals of Internal Medicine* 1986; **104**: 355–7.

78. Hancock SL, Cox RS, McDougall IR. Thyroid diseases after treatment of Hodgkin's disease. *New England Journal of Medicine* 1991; **325**: 599–605.

79. Delange F, de Benoist B, Pretell E, Dunn JT. Iodine deficiency in the world: where do we stand at the turn of the century? *Thyroid* 2001; **11**: 437–47.

80. Rose SR. Cranial irradiation and central hypothyroidism. *Trends in Endocrinology and Metabolism* 2001; **12**: 97–104.

81. Toft AD. Thyroxine therapy. *New England Journal of Medicine* 1994; **331**: 174–80.

82. Bunevicius R, Kazanavicius G, Zalinkevicius R, Prange AJ Jr. Effects of thyroxine as compared with thyroxine plus triiodothyronine in patients with hypothyroidism. *New England Journal of Medicine* 1999; **340**: 424–9.

83. Walsh JP, Ward LC, Burke V *et al.* Small changes in thyroxine dosage do not produce measurable changes in hypothyroid symptoms, well-being, or quality of life:

results of a double-blind, randomized clinical trial. *Journal of Clinical Endocrinology and Metabolism* 2006; **91**: 2624–30.

84. Rosenthal MJ, Hunt WC, Garry PJ, Goodwin JS. Thyroid failure in the elderly. Microsomal antibodies as discriminant for therapy. *Journal of the American Medical Association* 1987; **258**: 209–13.

85. Masiukiewicz US, Burrow GN. Hyperthyroidism in pregnancy: diagnosis and treatment. *Thyroid* 1999; **9**: 647–52.

86. Davis LE, Lucas MJ, Hankins GD *et al.* Thyrotoxicosis complicating pregnancy. *American Journal of Obstetrics and Gynecology* 1989; **160**: 63–70.

87. Haddow JE, Palomaki GE, Allan WC *et al.* Maternal thyroid deficiency during pregnancy and subsequent neuropsychological development of the child. *New England Journal of Medicine* 1999; **341**: 549–55.

88. Pop VJ, de Vries E, van Baar AL *et al.* Maternal thyroid peroxidase antibodies during pregnancy: a marker of impaired child development? *Journal of Clinical Endocrinology and Metabolism* 1995; **80**: 3561–6.

89. Pop VJ, Kuijpens JL, van Baar AL *et al.* Low maternal free thyroxine concentrations during early pregnancy are associated with impaired psychomotor development in infancy. *Clinical Endocrinology* 1999; **50**: 149–55.

90. Pop VJ, Brouwers EP, Vader HL *et al.* Maternal hypothyroxinaemia during early pregnancy and subsequent child development: a 3-year follow-up study. *Clinical Endocrinology* 2003; **59**: 282–8.

91. Vander JB, Gaston EA, Dawber TR. The significance of nontoxic thyroid nodules. Final report of a 15-year study of the incidence of thyroid malignancy. *Annals of Internal Medicine* 1968; **69**: 537–40.

92. Sherman SI. Thyroid carcinoma. *Lancet* 2003; **361**: 501–11.

93. Schneider AB, Ron E. Carcinoma of the follicular epithelium: epidemiology and pathogenesis, In: Braverman LE, Utiger RD (eds). *The thyroid: a fundamental and clinical text.* Philadelphia, PA: Lippincott, Williams & Wilkins, 2005: 889–906.

94. Hegedus L. Clinical practice. The thyroid nodule. *New England Journal of Medicine* 2004; **351**: 1764–71.

95. Bennedbaek FN, Perrild H, Hegedus L. Diagnosis and treatment of the solitary thyroid nodule. Results of a European survey. *Clinical Endocrinology* 1999; **50**: 357–63.

96. Bennedbaek FN, Hegedus L. Management of the solitary thyroid nodule: results of a North American survey. *Journal of Clinical Endocrinology and Metabolism* 2000; **85**: 2493–8.

97. Cooper DS, Doherty GM, Haugen BR *et al.* Management guidelines for patients with thyroid nodules and differentiated thyroid cancer. *Thyroid* 2006; **16**: 1–33.

98. British Thyroid Association and Royal College of Physicians 2002. Guidelines for the management of

thyroid cancer in adults. Available from: www.british-thyroid-association.org.

99. Boelaert K, Horacek J, Holder RL *et al.* Serum thyrotropin concentration as a novel predictor of malignancy in thyroid nodules investigated by fine-needle aspiration. *Journal of Clinical Endocrinology and Metabolism* 2006; **91**: 4295–301.

100. Haymart MR, Repplinger DJ, Leverson GE *et al.* Higher serum thyroid stimulating hormone level in thyroid nodule patients is associated with greater risks of differentiated thyroid cancer and advanced tumor stage. *Journal of Clinical Endocrinology and Metabolism* 2008; **93**: 809–14.

101. Hegedus L. Thyroid ultrasound. *Endocrinology and Metabolism Clinics of North America* 2001; **30**: 339–60.

102. Gittoes NJ, Miller MR, Daykin J *et al.* Upper airways obstruction in 153 consecutive patients presenting with thyroid enlargement. *British Medical Journal* 1996; **312**: 484.

103. Castro MR, Gharib H. Continuing controversies in the management of thyroid nodules. *Annals of Internal Medicine* 2005; **142**: 926–31.

104. Gharib H, Goellner JR. Fine-needle aspiration biopsy of the thyroid: an appraisal. *Annals of Internal Medicine* 1993; **118**: 282–9.

105. Tuttle RM, Lemar H, Burch HB. Clinical features associated with an increased risk of thyroid malignancy in patients with follicular neoplasia by fine-needle aspiration. *Thyroid* 1998; **8**: 377–83.

106. Kelman AS, Rathan A, Leibowitz J *et al.* Thyroid cytology and the risk of malignancy in thyroid nodules: importance of nuclear atypia in indeterminate specimens. *Thyroid* 2001; **11**: 271–7.

107. Huysmans DA, Hermus AR, Corstens FH *et al.* Large, compressive goiters treated with radioiodine. *Annals of Internal Medicine* 1994; **121**: 757–62.

108. Huysmans DA, Nieuwlaat WA, Erdtsieck RJ *et al.* Administration of a single low dose of recombinant human thyrotropin significantly enhances thyroid radioiodide uptake in nontoxic nodular goiter. *Journal of Clinical Endocrinology and Metabolism* 2000; **85**: 3592–6.

109. Frates MC, Benson CB, Charboneau JW *et al.* Management of thyroid nodules detected at US: Society of Radiologists in Ultrasound consensus conference statement. *Radiology* 2005; **237**: 794–800.

110. Baskin HJ, Duick DS. The endocrinologists' view of ultrasound guidelines for fine needle aspiration. *Thyroid* 2006; **16**: 207–8.

111. Ridgway EC, Tomer Y, McLachlan SM. Update in thyroidology. *Journal of Clinical Endocrinology and Metabolism* 2007; **92**: 3755–61.

112. Bartalena L, Wiersinga WM, Pinchera A. Graves' ophthalmopathy: state of the art and perspectives. *Journal of Endocrinological Investigation* 2004; **27**: 295–301.

22

Surgery for benign thyroid disease

TADHG P O'DWYER AND CONRAD V TIMON

Learn the duty as well as taste the pleasure of original work.

Robert J Graves (1796–1853)

INTRODUCTION

The thyroid gland derives its name from the Greek *thyreos* or shield, whereas enlargement or goitre is derived from *guttur* the Latin term for throat.

A goitre is defined as an enlargement of the thyroid. The term is somewhat arbitrary as there is no objective measurement of size or weight that is standardized in the definition. A form of thyroidectomy was first described in China over one thousand years ago.[1] The procedure was recognized as potentially fatal in view of the tendency to result in torrential haemorrhage. In 1866, Samuel Gross wrote that thyroid surgery should be considered as horrible butchery and that no sensible and honest surgeon would be engaged in its practice. It was not until the early twentieth century that Kocher popularized the operation. He reduced bleeding by meticulous haemostatic technique and subsequently received the Nobel Prize for his work in this area. He reported a 0.2 per cent haemorrhage rate in 1898 for the over 5000 thyroidectomies which he performed.[2]

Thyroidectomy is performed in the treatment of, or exclusion of, thyroid cancer and in addition where benign disease gives rise to compression of the oesophagus or trachea, causing dysphagia or stridor, respectively, the treatment of thyrotoxicosis and occasionally for cosmesis.

CLASSIFICATION OF GOITRE

The World Health Organization has classified goitres according to clinical appearance into three grades:

- **Grade 0**: no palpable or visible abnormality of the thyroid.
- **Grade 1**: palpable thyroid mass that is not visualized with the neck in neutral position.
- **Grade 2**: a visual apparent mass with the neck in neutral position.

See also **Box 22.1**.

Multinodular goitre (MNG) is the most common endocrine disorder worldwide and affects 500–600 million people.[3] The natural history of untreated, sporadic, non-toxic goitre is variable and not completely understood, but slow

---

Box 22.1   Classification of goitre

- Epidemiology (sporadic, endemic and familial)
- Aetiology (iodine deficiency, thyroiditis, malignant, drug-induced and genetic)
- Morphology (multinodular or diffuse)
- Functional (non-toxic and toxic)

growth and nodule formation is to be expected. It has been estimated that a 10–20 per cent volume increase occurs per year.[4] As it enlarges, multiple areas of focal nodularity typically form. Some 5–10 per cent of MNG with continued growth may develop hyperthyroidism over a five-year period.[5] Iodine deficiency is probably the most common cause, but even in iodine-deficient areas, patients are generally euthyroid with normal thyroid-stimulating hormone (TSH) and therefore it is likely that a genetic element coexists. Although the prevalence of MNG is decreasing with the use of iodine, there is still a prevalence of sporadic goitres in the United States of about 4–7 per cent and 10 per cent in the UK.[6, 7] Growth may be accelerated by ingestion of goitrogens, iodine deficiency, pregnancy, malignant change and the development of hyperthyroidism. Most recently, a gene located on chromosome 14 has been associated with familial non-toxic MNG and a polymorphism of codon 727 has been associated with toxic MNG.[8, 9]

Although MNG is relatively common in the general population, the majority of patients are asymptomatic. Generally, the growth is slow, but may occur more acutely with excessive iodine, e.g. radiographic contrast, or with medication, e.g. amiodarone. In general, surgery is necessary in extremely large MNG particularly where there is substernal extension with or without evidence of tracheal or oesophageal compression, suspicion of malignancy or the development of a toxic multinodular goitre.

DEVELOPMENT OF SUBSTERNAL GOITRE

There are many proposed classification systems of substernal goitre based on clinical size, relative percentage of thyroid tissue in the mediastinum, radiological appearance or pathological findings.[10] None, however, is completely satisfactory or widely accepted. One accepted definition is that substernal goitre occurs when 50 per cent or more of the gland extends below the thoracic inlet.[11] Although massive cervical goitres may cause tracheal displacement and narrowing, in the majority of cases the main compression of the trachea or oesophagus occurs at or below the thoracic inlet when the goitrous enlargement has resulted in substernal extension.

Substernal goitres were more common at the beginning of the last century (about 18 per cent of cases), but the widespread use of iodized salt has lead to a significant decrease.[12] Currently, the incidence is of the order of 4–6 per cent in patients undergoing thyroid surgery.[13] Its prevalence may yet increase due to the increased use of fine needle aspiration (FNA) for investigation of thyroid swellings and a corresponding decrease in thyroid surgery.

Initially, thyroid enlargement occurs in the neck, but when the pretracheal muscles can no longer stretch, further growth proceeds inferiorly along the path of least resistance. This may be facilitated by negative intrathoracic pressure from swallowing and inspiration, downward traction caused by normal deglutition and the pull of gravity. This mediastinal extension would appear to be more commonly seen in patients with short necks, a tendency for obesity and barrel-shaped emphysematous chest shapes. Once the mediastinal component has enlarged sufficiently to become trapped in the chest, unrestricted growth is possible because of minimal intrathoracic pressure. Thyroid nodules in the substernal component may involute resulting in cysts or haemorrhagic lesions with the potential for rapid increase in size often with pain. Rarely, this may present with acute airway obstruction.

ASSESSMENT OF NON–TOXIC MNG

A thorough history and physical examination is essential. In a large proportion of patients with non-toxic MNG, the patient is unaware of any problem until it is brought to their attention by a friend or relative or doctor on routine clinical examination. Symptoms may initially be non-specific, such as an irritating cough or globus-type sensation, features which will be elicited in a good history. The patient should be asked about a family history of thyroid disease, the area where the patient lives and any history of previous irradiation. Symptomatic patients may complain of symptoms related to pressure and compression of the trachea and oesophagus, and typical ones include dyspnoea, dysphagia or a tightness in the throat. Since the trachea is directly in contact with the thyroid and relatively firm and immobile, symptoms related to the airway are more common. The oesophagus is more mobile and as the goitre increases in size tends to be displaced, but not typically compressed unless the goitre affects both lobes and the oesophagus is trapped between the posterior thyroid lobes laterally, the spinal column posteriorly and the trachea anteriorly. In this situation, the patient may note significant swallowing difficulties.

The patient should be examined supine in good light with the neck fully exposed. Inspection may show an obvious goitre. In general, thyroid nodules greater than 1 cm are palpable. Typically in MNG, multiple nodules involving both thyroid lobes are apparent, but often one lobe is more affected. Clinically, the surgeon should attempt to palpate below the lower extent of the thyroid lobe to determine whether substernal extension has occurred. The development of flushing, neck vein compression and shortness of breath on raising the hands above the head for 1 minute (Pemberton's sign) is suggestive of significant substernal extension with venous compression, although false negatives are common. The use of percussion over the sternum to determine mediastinal involvement, although well documented, has not been of significant clinical value in the authors' practice. As the thyroid lobe increases in size, it tends to displace surrounding structures and the relationship to the trachea (particularly any tracheal deviation) should be noted. In large benign goitres, the carotid artery is displaced posteriorly (Berry's sign). A neck scar indicating previous thyroid surgery may be apparent and is important in deciding further management. The finding of cervical lymphadenopathy, fixation of the mass to the surrounding structures and vocal cord paralysis should alert the physician to the possibility of malignancy.

Finally, a fibreoptic examination of the larynx should be performed. Although recurrent laryngeal nerve damage may occur due to traction by a large thyroid gland, this is a rare event and nerve palsy should suggest thyroid malignancy. Laboratory and diagnostic tests to be performed include thyroid function tests (TFT), antithyroid antibodies and serum calcium.

Ultrasound is the most commonly used investigative procedure. It provides information on the location, consistency and size of nodules. Clinically, even though a solitary nodule may be suspected, ultrasound has demonstrated that in 50 per cent of cases there are multiple nodules present.[14] Fine needle aspiration can be performed more accurately when used in conjunction with ultrasound. Serial follow up of nodule growth can be provided by ultrasound and changes in nodular characteristics may point to possible malignancy where ultrasound-guided FNA should be of benefit. Ultrasound examination is more user dependent than other forms of imaging, such as magnetic resonance imaging (MRI) and computed tomography (CT), but is of limited value in assessing thyroids with significant substernal extension because of its inability to image contents behind the sternum.

Radionuclide thyroid scanning (scintigraphy), although less commonly used, is useful in the evaluation of a dominant nodule in a MNG as a possible focus of malignancy and to assess function of a nodule as a cause of hyperthyroidism. These scans are poorly sensitive in determining substernal extension, but may assist in determining gland functionality.

CT and MRI are useful in the assessment of the large thyroid gland where there is substernal extension and to provide information about the relationship of the gland to surrounding structures in the event of malignancy. It is important not to give iodine contrast with CT imaging, if there is concern regarding the possibility of toxic MNG as this may precipitate an acute toxic state. Similarly, an iodine load in cases of thyroid cancer may delay the ability to image and treat these tumours with radioactive iodine therapy post-surgery, although in practice this is not usually a problem.

Chest x-ray is routinely carried out and may be helpful in looking for tracheal deviation and retrosternal extension. Pulmonary function tests including flow volume loop to confirm airway obstruction are occasionally used, but not usually by experienced physicians as the other investigations used, such as CT, will provide such information.

MANAGEMENT OF MULTINODULAR GOITRE

The majority of patients with MNG are unaware of the condition, and are only diagnosed after a relative or doctor notices and comments on it.

Many will not require therapy if euthyroid, but merely followed by the patient's physician or surgeon. For the larger asymptomatic goitres, without evidence of compression, serial clinical evaluation with imaging (often ultrasound) is performed on a six-month or yearly basis. Any significant growth or radiological signs characteristic of change in the nature of the mass, or development of objective symptoms, should prompt consideration of operative intervention.

A trial of thyroid hormone therapy may be of value in patients with non-toxic MNG who are otherwise well. The response to suppressant thyroxine therapy is variable and there is a tendency for the goitre to return to its previous size when therapy is discontinued. Its use should be avoided in the elderly and in those with cardiac disease, and if the patient is not hypothyroid, use of exogenous thyroxine may on occasion precipitate a thyrotoxic state. If there is no

significant reduction in goitre size after six months of therapy, the treatment should be discontinued.

Radioactive iodine therapy may be used in the management of multinodular goitre to reduce the size of the thyroid gland and/or to treat or prevent obstructive symptoms. It is important to realize, however, that initially acute thyroid swelling in the first week or two after therapy may worsen the airway compromise and require high-dose steroids. This makes its routine use in this condition less attractive, and it is usually restricted to symptomatic patients in whom surgery is contraindicated. In the longer term, hypothyroidism may develop, but is easily managed with thyroxine replacement.

The surgical treatment of MNG is variable from country to country and resource issues also play a role. Patients with MNG who are symptomatic or where there is clinical or radiological evidence of compression or substernal extension should be considered for surgical treatment. Patient concerns about the possibility of malignancy should also be taken into account when considering surgery.

INDICATIONS FOR SURGICAL TREATMENT OF A MULTINODULAR GOITRE

Mechanical obstruction

MNGs generally increase in size in a slow but progressive fashion. Patients may be asymptomatic despite a significant tracheal shift. Rapid enlargement, however, may occur due to haemorrhage into a cyst or with cystic degeneration. Under these circumstances, patients may complain of a feeling of suffocation, odynophagia, dysphagia or airway distress. Symptoms of acute airway obstruction may not occur until up to 70 per cent of the tracheal lumen is obstructed. Tracheal shift with no palpable goitre suggests substernal extension and, under these circumstances, the patient requires a thorough evaluation including a CT scan of the neck and thorax.

Suspicion of malignancy

The presence of a lump in the neck frequently gives rise to concern about the possibility of malignancy. MNGs are continuously changing in size and character and despite physician reassurance, patients may be anxious to have the mass removed. Despite such concerns, the incidence of malignancy is of the order of 5–10 per cent in MNG and is similar to that in a solitary nodule.[15]

Cosmetic issues

Surgery for cosmesis is controversial and is not generally recommended because of the potential complications of the procedure together with the fact that an enlarged thyroid is being replaced with a neck scar.

Hyperthyroidism

Hyperthyroidism is caused by an increase in the circulating level of thyroid hormones, independent of normal thyroid-stimulating hormone (TSH) control. All MNG patients have a potential to become hyperthyroid. Long-term follow up suggests that this toxic potential occurs in at least 20–30 per cent of cases.[16, 17] It usually has a slow onset and the typical signs and symptoms of hyperthyroidism may be absent or modified in this patient cohort.

SURGICAL TREATMENT

Surgical anatomy of multinodular goitre

Surgical removal of a large goitre can be difficult and poses a number of problems for the surgeon. The gland surface is nodular and frequently displaces the surrounding structures. The trachea is normally relatively firm, but despite this, significant enlargement of the thyroid will lead to variable displacement to one side and even a narrowing due to pressure effects. This may be compounded by softening of the tracheal wall with the potential for airway collapse secondary to tracheomalacia. The oesophagus, although more pliable, is less likely to be displaced due to its posterior location in relation to the thyroid. The recurrent laryngeal nerves are commonly elongated and typically displaced laterally and posteriorly as the thyroid expands, however, particularly in revision cases, the nerve may lie more superficially than expected. The parathyroid glands may also be displaced and difficult to locate because of the nodularity of the gland. The enlarging thyroid will tend to displace the carotid sheath contents laterally and safe access to this area may be difficult and require division of the strap muscles. The superior and inferior vascular pedicles may also be significantly displaced, compressed and elongated. The goitre may extend between the trachea and the oesophagus and, on occasion, may extend behind the oesophagus. Goitres as they enlarge may extend into the mediastinum and therefore, knowledge of the anatomy of this region is especially necessary. After the operation, displaced structures, such as the trachea, typically shift back to a more midline position on removal of the compressing mass. Tracheal lumen narrowing due to tracheomalacia may only manifest itself following removal of the splinting effect of the enlarged thyroid leading to potential airway collapse on inspiration following extubation. Tracheomalacia is, however, uncommon.

Surgical technique

PRE-OPERATIVE ASSESSMENT

Hyperthyroidism is controlled medically prior to surgery (see below under Treatment options for hyperthyroidism, p. 414). The thyroid surgeon should review relevant radiology (usually CT scans or MRI) to determine altered anatomy in each case. Radiological analysis should confirm that a mediastinal mass is thyroid in origin and shows the relationship of the goitre to the trachea, oesophagus and great vessels. These investigations will, most importantly, help to determine the ability to resect the thyroid through a transcervical approach. A substernal goitre gets its blood supply from the neck, and transcervical delivery is usually possible even with significant mediastinal involvement once there is a clear line of demarcation between thyroid tissue and surrounding structures. The possibility of a sternal split being required should always be considered with a substernal goitre and discussed with thoracic surgical colleagues before thyroidectomy, understanding that in some cases a final decision can only be made at surgery.

SURGICAL INCISION AND EXPOSURE

An anaesthetist experienced in management of the difficult airway is required. In the majority of cases, although the larynx may be distorted to one side transoral intubation is relatively easy to perform. If the trachea is narrow, an appropriate smaller calibre reinforced endotracheal tube should be used. For patients with significant airway compromise who are unable to lie supine, an awake intubation over a fibreoptic laryngoscope may be appropriate.

The patient is positioned supine with the neck extended using a suitable-sized sandbag transversely placed behind the shoulders. A transverse neck incision above the suprasternal notch in a convenient skin crease is made. The incision size may vary according to the size of the goitre, but usually extends from the anterior border of the sternomastoid muscles and typically is 6–8 cm in length. Greater incision length does not tend to improve exposure to any great extent. The surgeon should avoid placing the incision over the clavicle or on the chest wall as these scars can become unsightly with time.

The skin flaps are raised in a subplatysmal plane superiorly to the thyroid notch and inferiorly to the sternal notch. If significant compression is present, the anterior jugular veins and tributaries are larger and more prominent than usual and care has to be taken not to damage these vessels inadvertently to prevent significant bleeding. The strap muscles are opened in the midline and raised, usually by blunt dissection, off the underlying thyroid gland. Often with a large asymmetrical MNG, the midline is difficult to identify and the dissection should start at the cricoid cartilage level as this facilitates localization of the avascular plane between the strap muscles and underlying thyroid. In larger goitres, the innermost strap muscle, the sternothyroid muscle is stretched and thinned over the thyroid and it is important to delineate the medial border of this muscle to allow dissection in the correct plane between the strap muscles and thyroid capsule. An atraumatic technique is particularly important for these large obstructive goitres, since the venous system may be compressed and significant bleeding from surface thyroid vessels may occur which is difficult to control. Access laterally and to the superior thyroid pedicle may be improved by division of the sternothyroid muscle. Although not a routine step, for access and thyroid mobilization, complete division of the strap muscles on one or both sides may be required. This is best performed by first freeing the anterior border of the sternomastoid muscles, followed by opening, by blunt and sharp dissection, the potential so-called viscerovascular space between the carotid sheath laterally and the thyroid gland and upper aerodigestive structures medially. Only the omohyoid muscle crosses this space and serves as an excellent landmark to help identify the carotid sheath contents, particularly the internal jugular vein.

This muscle may be dissected and reflected superiorly or divided and the carotid sheath contents are retracted laterally to prevent damage during division of the strap muscles. The strap muscles are usually divided more superiorly to preserve the laterally placed motor nerve supply (ansa hypoglossus). The anterior jugular veins should be ligated and divided prior to division of the strap muscles, and care must be take not to damage branches of the middle thyroid vein laterally which may lie just below the muscle. Following division of the strap muscles, the middle thyroid vein and branches are identified and carefully ligated.

MOBILIZATION OF THE THYROID INTO THE WOUND

Many surgeons, after exposure of the thyroid gland, prefer then to identify the recurrent laryngeal nerve when performing a routine thyroidectomy. Identification of the recurrent laryngeal nerve, however, is not possible for large goitres without first mobilizing the enlarged thyroid into the wound. To accomplish delivery of the thyroid, the superior thyroid pedicle is usually exposed, and mobilized by ligation of the superior thyroid vein and artery. Visualization is helped with partial or completed division of the strap muscles. Division of the pedicle vessels is best achieved by putting the pedicle on stretch with ligation and division of the vessels individually as close to the superior thyroid pedicle as possible to prevent damage to the superior laryngeal nerve.

Delivery of the thyroid proceeds mostly by finger dissection, which is used to disimpact the goitre trapped in the inlet and in the superior mediastinum. Gentle finger dissection is used to free the goitre circumferentially, from the surrounding soft tissues, starting anteriorly at the thoracic outlet and proceeding laterally, posteriorly and inferiorly. The dissection is facilitated by simultaneous traction on the previously mobilized superior thyroid pole. This finger dissection is, to a large extent, blind particularly when mobilizing the deeper substernal portion of the gland. It is extremely important for successful haemostatic delivery that the surgeon stays in the same capsular plane as the thyroid mass that is being mobilized. Blunt blind dissection risks inadvertent tearing of branches of the inferior thyroid vein with significant bleed and must be done in a gentle manner. It is also possible to damage the recurrent laryngeal nerve particularly by traction. Usually, the recurrent laryngeal nerve has been stretched by the thyroid enlargement, and displaced laterally and posteriorly. In cases of revision surgery, however, the nerve may be far more superficially placed in relation to the remnant thyroid swelling, having been displaced by enlargement of the so-called tubercle of Zuckerlandl. Gentle but continuous traction is the key to successful delivery of the goitre from the mediastinum. The use of spoon-like instruments may be helpful in facilitating delivery by breaking negative intrathoracic pressure. This instrument is particularly suited for deeper-placed goitres whose lower border is inaccessible with finger dissection. Morselization has been suggested and more recently the use of microdebriders has been described, but there is a concern regarding uncontrollable bleeding.[18] Further mobilization and/or division of the isthmus from the underlying trachea will help in difficult delivery cases. If blunt dissection is not possible because of significant difficulties opening the planes due to adhesions, or

<table>
<tr><td colspan="2">Box 22.2 Sternotomy</td></tr>
<tr><td>
• Rates from 2 to 8%
• Most likely if malignant
• Recurrent disease
• Immobile substernal goitres
• Posterior mediastinal goitres
• Thyroiditis (Hashimoto's or Graves')
</td></tr>
</table>

direct thyroid extension is present suggesting malignancy, then a partial sternotomy needs to be considered (**Box 22.2**).

IDENTIFICATION AND PRESERVATION OF IMPORTANT STRUCTURES

Parathyroid glands

The parathyroid glands require even more meticulous attention than usual when surgery is undertaken for the management of multinodular goitres because of the increased difficulties encountered in their localization, as well as the increased risk of avascular necrosis. The superior parathyroid gland position, even with extremely large goitres, is not usually significantly displaced and it is of paramount importance, particularly if total thyrodectomy is contemplated, that this gland is identified and preserved. The authors prefer to identify this gland early in the operation after the superior pedicle has been completely mobilized. The gland is identified, deep in the wound, on the undersurface of the superior thyroid pole. It is brought into view by grasping the thyroid gland with an artery forceps at the site of the ligated vascular stump, with retraction of the gland inferiorly and laterally. The superior parathyroid gland is usually surrounded by a variable amount of adipose tissue, but has a characteristic caramel colour and is attached to the overlying thyroid tissue by variable-sized blood vessels. Dissection of the plane between the parathyroid and thyroid is usually deferred until the thyroid gland has been delivered into the wound to allow better visualization and to avoid damaging the closely related recurrent laryngeal nerve at the cricothyroid joint.

The inferior parathyroid gland is more subject to variable anatomy and displacement by the goitre. As the goitre enlarges, this gland is often found intimately attached high on the thyroid lobe. In this position, it has a more flattened appearance and may give the appearance of being embedded, due to thyroid growth, within the lobe. Careful dissection will, however, show a plane of dissection between the thyroid and parathyroid. This, together with a longer and more tenuous vascular pedicle, makes it more difficult to preserve with a viable blood supply. Identification is helped by a dry surgical field and the use of magnification loupes (2.5 power). It is important to avoid pinching, clamping or squeezing the parathyroid gland to avoid damage, which is suggested by a change in colour to a darker appearance.

As many parathyroid glands as possible should be identified and preserved before the goitre is removed from the neck. Since the vast majority of parathyroid glands receive their blood supply from the inferior thyroid artery, its main trunk should not be ligated, but its branches are ligated medially as close to the thyroid gland as possible. In those circumstances where the parathyroid glands cannot be preserved *in situ*, because the vascular pedicle to the parathyroid gland is compromised during surgery, they should be removed and preserved for reimplantation at the end of the operation. The parathyroid glands that require reimplantation should be divided into segments of 2 mm blocks and then implanted into a suitable muscle (usually the sternomastoid muscle). Implantation requires a meticulous technique to prevent haematoma formation within the recipient muscle, and also to avoid extrusion of parathyroid fragments from the recipient muscle before the fascia overlying the muscle is closed. The site of implantation into the recipient muscle should be marked with a non-absorbable suture. Preservation of the parathyroids *in situ* with an intact blood supply is preferable to reimplantation because transplanted glands do not always survive.

SUPERIOR AND RECURRENT LARYNGEAL NERVE IDENTIFICATION

The superior laryngeal nerve usually enters the larynx 1 cm superior to the entrance of the superior thyroid artery into the upper pole. Keeping the dissection close to the thyroid capsule will ensure that the nerve is not injured. It is not always necessary to expose or identify the superior laryngeal nerve; however, every attempt should be made to preserve it by dividing and ligating the superior thyroid vessels close to or on the superior thyroid lobe.

Thomusch, in a multicenter study with multivariate analysis of over 7000 patients, found that recurrent laryngeal nerve injury is associated with a number of factors including extent of surgery, repeated operations for recurrent goitres and failure to identify the recurrent laryngeal nerve at operation.[19] Identification of the recurrent laryngeal nerve is therefore mandatory during thyroidectomy. It is usually not possible to search for the recurrent laryngeal nerve until the gland is disimpacted and delivered into the wound. To identify the nerve, a thorough knowledge of the anatomical structures and their relationship to the recurrent laryngeal nerve is required. The trachea, inferior thyroid artery, carotid artery and parathyroid glands are particularly important in nerve identification. The normally located nerve bisects the angle between the inferior thyroid artery and the trachea. It may run superiorly, inferiorly or between branches of the inferior thyroid artery and the nerve may divide into several branches particularly as it approaches the criocothyroid joint before entering the larynx. Identification of the recurrent nerve may be made more difficult due to displacement and stretching from enlargement of the thyroid. In these more difficult cases, it may be best to find the recurrent laryngeal nerve higher than usual beneath Berry's ligament, at the cricothyroid joint, where it is has a constant position even with thyroid enlargement. The recurrent laryngeal nerve is dissected free using fine mosquito forceps. Absolute haemostasis in the region of the nerve will aid in its preservation. Any overlying small branches of the inferior thyroid vein should be ligated with small clips. Use of bipolar cautery should be discouraged, while working close to the nerve as damage of the recurrent laryngeal nerve can occur from heat trauma from cautery or from traction, rather than direct division of the nerve. While tracing the nerve, care should be taken to preserve the inferior thyroid artery laterally to preserve the blood supply to the ipsilateral parathyroids. The use of intraoperative nerve monitoring may be of help to confirm the presence of the nerve, but does not take the place of careful atraumatic surgical dissection. Despite improvement in monitoring, the best results for the resection of substernal thyroid disease are obtained by an experienced thyroid surgeon rather than the occasional operator.

EXTENT OF THYROIDECTOMY

Controversy exists as to the extent of surgery for multinodular goitre. Three different surgical options exist varying according to the extent of thyroid gland removal, namely total, near total and subtotal thyroidectomy. Near total thyroidectomy leaves 2–4 g of thyroid tissue or a 2 × 1 cm piece of thyroid tissue in the tracheo-oesophageal groove. Subtotal thyroidectomy involves the removal of one lobe and the isthmus. More recently, there has been a trend towards total thyroidectomy as the surgical procedure of choice in the management of large MNGs. This prevents recurrence and it is both diagnostic and therapeutic for previously undiagnosed thyroid cancers present in the goitre. Total thyroidectomy by definition, requires life-long thyroxine therapy and has a potential for bilateral vocal cord paralysis and permanent hypocalaemia. However, if performed in a meticulous fashion with the knowledge of the altered surgical anatomy the risks to the recurrent laryngeal nerves (RLNs) and parathyroid glands can be kept to a minimum. This is of particular importance since the surgeon is dealing with a benign condition in an asymptomatic patient.

Most surgeons would concur that total thyroidectomy is warranted where the patient presents with bilateral substernal disease. The decision is more difficult if only unilateral thyroid disease is present with little or no change on the controlateral side. Kraimps et al.[20] have suggested a selectively aggressive surgical plan based on extent of thyroid disease, with the extent of surgery tailored to the extent of thyroid pathology. For bilateral thyroid disease, a total thyroidectomy is performed. If at the time of surgery difficulty is experienced in preservation of the parathyroids on the initial larger side then a near total is performed, leaving a rim of thyroid tissue posteriorly on the smaller side to protect the blood supply of parathyroid glands. For unilateral disease, a total lobectomy and isthmusectomy (partial thyroid) may be preferred, but the surgeon should realize that this operation carriers an overall high rate of contralateral recurrence (in the range of 15–42 per cent) on long-term follow up, and potentially significant more complications if revision surgery is required.[21] In view of this, more aggressive surgery, either total or near-total is particularly indicated in the younger age group and especially female patients with a family history of multinodular goitre.

Sternotomy

Sternotomy is reserved for goitres that cannot be delivered safely through a cervical skin incision, but is rarely required.

Table 22.1 Classification and approach retrosternal goitre.

Grade	Anatomical location	Approach
1	Above aortic arch (above T4)	Cervical
2	Aortic arch to pericardium	Manubriotomy
3	Below right atrium	Full sternotomy

Although the size of the substernal goitre may make it impossible to deal with the thyroid mass through a conventional incision, more frequently the size of the goitre combined with radiological and surgical evidence of poor mobility and adherence of the goitre to mediastinal structures are what lead to the use of a sternotomy. In this procedure, a vertical incision from the midportion of the cervical incision is made vertically on the chest wall. The incision is carried down to the manubrium which is then split with an oscillating saw. Care is taken not to damage underlying manubrial contents particularly if there has been previous surgery in the area. A full sternotomy is not usually required and the sternotomy is usually angled into the second intercostal space avoiding the internal thoracic artery. The retrosternal fascia is divided exposing the mediastianal structures. The goitre can now be dissected out of the mediastinum under direct vision (**Table 22.1**).

PREVENTING COMPLICATIONS

The surgical wound resulting from a large MNG is much more extensive than that seen following the removal of a relatively normal-sized thyroid gland. There is usually extensive dissection of the tissue planes into the superior mediastinum, prevertebral space and into both sides of the neck. Accordingly, special attention is paid to intraoperative haemostasis. The wound is irrigated, and haemostasis is best accomplished by using bipolar diathermy, ligaclips and, on occasion, fine suture ligatures. Small amounts of oozing, particularly near the entrance of the recurrent laryngeal nerve into the larynx at the cricothyroid joint, is best managed conservatively to prevent injury. The authors prefer to use surgical haemostatic agents, such as Surgicell®, rather than risk damage from cautery. Potential venous bleeding areas may become more obvious with valsalva performed by the anaesthetist by increasing intrathoracic pressure.

For larger goitres where a large dead space is left, closed suction drains are commonly used. The wound is closed in layers, with partial opposition of the strap muscles with an absorbable suture leaving a gap inferiorly to allow bleeding from beneath the strap muscle to become obvious on postoperative clinical examination. Neck dressing, which may obscure the wound and haematoma formation, should be avoided.

POSTOPERATIVE CARE

In most instances, the patient is extubated at the end of the operative procedure. Tracheal palpation at operation may suggest tracheomalacia with the endotracheal tube being easily palpated with softening and collapse on palpation of the trachea. If there is significant concern, this should be conveyed to the anaesthetist. Any difficulty with extubation at the end of the procedure may suggest tracheal collapse and in this case the patient may be reintubated and the tube left *in situ* for 24 hours. In this situation, high dependence care management is usually required. Rarely is a tracheostomy required and if possible should be avoided as it may result in further weakening of the trachea.

The surgical drains are usually left in place for a minimum of 36–48 hours, and longer if the drainage is copious. Calcium metabolism is monitored carefully both clinically and biochemically, twice daily, until it has stabilized. Transient hypocalcaemia is commonly due to the initial vascular shock on the preserved parathyroid tissue and may require calcium supplementation. Factors playing a role in hypocalcaemia postoperatively include the extent of surgery, experience of the operator and the number of functioning glands left *in situ*. Most surgeons feel that at least two functioning glands with an intact blood supply should be left to avoid prolonged low calcium.

The majority of patients will have had a significant amount of thyroid tissue removed which results in a hypothyroid state, and thyroxine replacement therapy is usually started upon discharge from hospital. Patients undergoing partial thyroidecomy may be started on thyroxine if subclinically euthryoid, but the routine use is of dubious value in the prevention of recurrence. If carcinoma is present, thyroxine may be withheld in preparation for a whole body iodine scan to search for residual or metastatic disease.

Risk factors for recurrent nodular goitre after thyroidectomy include younger age of patient, the finding of multiple nodules (but not bilateral disease) during surgery and the extent of such surgery. Morbidity was greater after surgery for recurrent disease than for surgery for non-recurrent disease implying that total thyroidectomy in all patients with bilateral MNG, particularly younger patients, avoids many potential complications.[22, 23]

SURGICAL TREATMENT OF HYPERTHYROIDISM

Introduction

Hyperthyroidism is a condition in which the body is exposed to excessive amounts of circulating thyroid hormone. This increase in circulating level of thyroid hormones is independent of normal TSH feedback control. This unregulated release of thyroid hormone is more commonly found in females, and may develop suddenly or more gradually. The overt condition is usually easily diagnosed, but gradual onset hyperthyroidism in the older age group causing mainly cardiac difficulties may not be so clinically obvious. The most common cause of this condition is Graves' disease, followed by toxic multinodular goitre and solitary hyperfunctionaing thyroid nodules.

Autoimmune thyrotoxicosis (Graves' disease) is the most common cause of hyperthyroidism, usually seen in a young age group (30–60 years) making up 70 per cent of all cases. Toxic multinodular goitre is the second most common condition accounting for between 10 and 30 per cent of cases, and is characterized by the development of hyperfunctional thyroid nodules developing in a previous non-toxic multinodular goitre. The least common pathological process is a toxic adenoma which is a solitary hyperfunctional lesion. The incidence of toxic multinodular goitre and toxic adenoma varies considerably, being particularly common in iodine-deficient regions and sometimes referred to as Plummer's disease.

Other forms of overactivity include transient states which may be a feature of a number of thyroid conditions, including subacute thyroiditis (De Quervain's disease), early Hashimoto's disease and postpartum hyperthyroidism. This may also be seen in patients who take large amounts of iodide or thyroxine; struma ovarii, thyrotropin-secreting tumours, choriocarcinoma and amiodarone-induced thyrotoxicosis are particularly rare and may be especially difficult to diagnose and manage.

The majority of patients with hyperthyroidism are treated medically or with radioactive iodine, but surgery now plays an ever increasing part in the management of this condition.

Graves' disease

Graves' disease is commonly attributed to a Dublin-based physician Robert Graves who described the condition in 1835, but Caleb Hillier Parry, a Bath physician, probably described the first case in 1786.[24]

Graves' disease is by far the most common cause of hyperthyroidism. It is an autoimmune disease underlined by the presence of an antibody to the TSH receptor which is present in up to 90 per cent of patients. Elevated free T4 and low TSH levels are present together with a high level of antithyroid autoantibodies. Although stress or medications, such as amiodarone and radiopaque media, may precipitate the condition in susceptible subjects, there are genetic factors involved in its aetiology.[25] Pathologically, the thyroid gland is diffusely enlarged, fleshy and vascular. Microscopically, the follicular epithelium is hyperplastic and a focal lymphocytic infiltration is not an uncommon finding.

As with other autoimmune diseases, Graves' disease is most commonly found in middle-aged females, but may be seen in males and females of all ages including children. Previous history of other autoimmune diseases, and particularly a family history of Graves' disease, predisposes to the condition. Clinical findings may vary, but commonly include features of overactivity, a diffuse goitre and ophthalmopathy.[26] Classically, the patient complaints include irritability, sleeplessness, palpitations, excessive sweating, heat intolerance and weight loss. Typically, patients have tachycardia and palpitations even during sleep. On examination, patients may demonstrate exophthalmos, lid lag and a diffuse bilateral goitre which may have a palpable and audible bruit due to high vascularity. Other manifestations including exophthalmos and pretibial myxoedema (present in 4 per cent of cases) help in differentiating between Graves' and other hyperthyroid conditions.

Ophthalmopathy may be seen alone, or appear before, during or after the patient's thyrotoxic state becomes apparent. It is due to lymphocytic infiltration of the intraorbital muscles, possibly as a cross-reactivity between ocular muscle antibodies and thyroid antigens. Six stages of ophthalmopathy are described from lid lag and retraction (stage 1) to loss of sight from optic nerve damage in the most severe cases.[27]

The natural history of Graves' disease is variable. The disease may undergo spontaneous remission, however, this may not take place for many months or even years, meaning control of the conditions usually with medical therapy is required. Patients who fail to show spontaneous remission often require other forms of treatment, usually radioactive iodine or surgical intervention.

Toxic multinodular goitre

This is the second most common form of thyrotoxicosis after Graves' disease. The patients are older than the typical patient with Graves' disease, but are predominantly female, as with Graves' disease and toxic thyroid adenoma. The history is of a long-standing multinodular goitre, and the condition develops insidiously. It is caused by autonomous hyperactivity of one or more pre-existing thyroid nodules. Symptoms are not those classically associated with thyrotoxicosis, and are commonly cardiac, particularly atrial fibrillation. Although autoimmune antibodies may be present, the titres are usually low and the condition may be differentiated from Graves' clinically by the relatively older age group, long-standing goitre, slower onset and the absence of autoimmune manifestations, such as ophthalmopathy. Differentiation is important since, unlike Graves' disease, spontaneous remission is not a feature, so radioactive therapy and surgery are more attractive than long-term medical therapy.

Toxic thyroid adenoma

Toxic adenoma accounts for approximately 5 per cent of thyrotoxic cases. The peak age incidence is between 40 and 60 years and is more common in females. Clinically, a solitary nodule is found in contrast to the diffuse thyroid gland swelling seen in Graves'. Pathologically, they are autonomously functioning solitary thyroid neoplasms. Rarely spontaneously infarcts may occur, but otherwise the condition will persist and always requires management. After controlling thyrotoxic symptoms, partial thyroidectomy removing the hyperfunctioning adenoma is curative. Radioactive iodine is occasionally used in patients who refuse or are poor candidates for surgery.[28]

INVESTIGATIONS

Suppressed TSH together with an abnormally raised T3 or T4 level is characteristic of thyrotoxicosis. A positive thyroid autoantibody level makes an autoimmune process such as Graves' more likely, but is not an absolute requirement. Scintigraphy using technetium or iodine may be of some help in differentiating between the three common conditions associated with thyrotoxicosis. With Graves' disease, a diffuse homogenous uptake is typical. If a cold area is seen, a fine needle aspirate possibly under ultrasound-guided conditions is warranted to rule out neoplasia. With a toxic MNG, a patchy picture is more characteristic, and with a toxic adenoma a hot nodule against a suppressed background is the usual finding.

Treatment options for hyperthyroidism

Appropriate treatment of hyperthyroidism relies on the identification of the underlying cause. In general, there are three treatment modalities used in the management of hyperthyroidism, namely medical therapy (thionamides, beta-blockers), radioactive iodine and surgery (**Box 22.3**). There is no proven superior management protocol, but all patients, no matter the underlying aetiology, will require control of their toxic condition initially using medical therapy. The antithyroid drugs used most commonly are thiouracil derivatives or imidazole compounds, both of which are relatively slow in onset. Other medications may be required initially, such as beta-blockers, which control the sympathetic overdrive symptoms, such as tachycardia, sweating and tremors. Further treatment depends on the natural history of the underlying condition. With Graves' disease, the condition may vary considerably in different patients from a condition that undergoes spontaneous resolution in a relatively short period of time to life-long hyperthyroidism. Spontaneous recovery may occur in up to half of the cases, so the initial treatment of choice in the United Kingdom is usually long-term medical therapy.[29] The drugs used fall into two main categories, namely uracil derivatives (propylthiouracil) and imidazole compounds (carbimazole). The latter in a dose of 30–60 mg daily is the most commonly used therapy, given until the patient becomes euthyroid. At that stage, the medication is reduced to a maintenance dose and continued for a variable period, usually up to 18 months to allow the thyroid to recover. Adverse reactions to medication include potential for serious bone marrow depression. A beta-blocker may also be used in the short term to control hyperthyroid symptoms.

In those patients who are poorly controlled or relapse despite adequate medical therapy, ablative therapy either radioactive iodine or thyroidectomy is considered.

Radioactive iodine is a common therapy used particularly in patients with Graves' disease who fail or cannot tolerate medical therapy. Indeed, in some countries such as the United States, it may be the first line of treatment, and has potential advantages of cost-effectiveness and avoidance of surgical morbidity, hospitalization and loss of work time.[30, 31] The therapy is given as a capsule which is swallowed, is taken up selectively by active thyroid tissue and destroys the cells of the overactive gland. One or more courses of treatment may be required. The dose given may vary between institutes. A large percentage of patients following radioactive iodine therapy will subsequently become hypothyroid which is an expected side effect and not a complication. It is not recommended for young women who are or wish to become pregnant.

Although most patients with Graves' disease are best treated initially with medical management, surgical intervention is sometimes the preferred treatment for children, and for young women who may have reproductive concerns. Coincident carcinoma, large bulky glands, and patient preference to avoid radioactive iodine or antithyroid medications or where compliance with other treatment modalities are also reasons for surgical removal of the gland.[32, 33, 34] The effect of I^{131} treatment on severe ophthalmopathy remains controversial, but presents another potential indication for gland removal.[27, 35, 36]

In the 1990s, a different therapeutic approach was introduced, using intralesional injection of ethanol. This treatment form is relatively inexpensive, but between four and eight successive treatments are usually required to achieve success. Potential complications include exacerbation of thyrotoxicosis, fever, pain at the injection site and haematoma. Also, the treatment carries a high failure rate in bulky thyroids, all of which has meant that this therapy has not become as popular as more conventional treatments.[37, 38, 39, 40, 41, 42, 43]

Spontaneous resolution is not a feature of toxic multinodular goitre or toxic thyroid goitre, and these conditions require definitive therapy. In toxic multinodular goitre, this is usually radioactive iodine followed by surgery. Occasionally, surgery is indicated as initial treatment (once the patient is euthyroid) when the goitre is large, the patient is fit and presents with obstructive symptoms, such as superior vena caval obstruction. For toxic thyroid adenoma, partial thyroidectomy is curative.

In multinodular goitre and in toxic adenoma, spontaneous or long-term medical therapy-induced remissions are much less likely to occur, making ablative therapy the treatment of choice. Radioactive iodine is a viable option to surgery, but MNG often requires multiple doses of iodine to control toxicity due to larger volume of tissue and poorer uptake. As a result, surgery is often preferred over iodine in patients who have large goitres and compression symptoms. This is especially true in younger patients.

In patients with toxic adenoma, although radioactive iodine may be given, it requires high doses of iodine and this is undesirable in younger patients. A unilateral lobectomy for toxic adenoma is curative and has minimal complications, while for multinodular goitre, total or near total thyroidectomy is required.

> ### Box 22.3   Treatment options for hyperthyroidism
>
> - Antithyroid drugs
> - Radioiodine
> - Surgery is an important aspect of therapy in all types of hyperthyroidism. It may be complementary to other treatments

---

Indications for the surgical treatment of Graves' disease

Thyroidectomy is an important therapeutic option in patients with Graves' disease who have failed medical therapy (**Boxes 22.4 and 22.5**). It is also indicated in children or young woman of reproductive age where there is a general reluctance to give radioactive therapy.[32] It has potential benefit in patients who relapse with thyrotoxicosis after failed radioiodine therapy.[44, 45, 46] It is also considered the

Box 22.4   Indications for surgical treatment of Graves' disease

- Failed medical therapy
- Relapse of thyrotoxic state after radioactive iodine therapy
- In children or other patients where compliance may be difficult
- Large bulky thyroid glands
- Young women of reproductive age
- Proptosis

Box 22.5   Potential advantages of surgery

- Offers permanent cure in most cases
- Achieves results rapidly (good for non-compliant patients)
- Provides tissue for diagnosis
- Renders child-bearing immediately possible
- Allows absolute titration of thyroid hormone

procedure of choice in large bulky thyroid glands, particularly those with compression symptoms and/or substernal extension or where there is a potential for malignancy. It should also be considered in thyrotoxic patients where compliance with other treatments may be an issue and may be preferred to radioactive iodine in patients of male gender, smokers, those with bulky glands and exophthalmos.

Another less common indication for surgery is the treatment of thyroid storm unresponsive to medical therapy. This is a rare, but potentially fatal, event. Amiodaraone is a potent antiarrhythmic drug that is used to treat a variety of cardiac arrhythmias and is structurally related to thyroxine.[47] Its use may lead to amiodarone-induced thyrotoxicosis, which is an unwelcome condition in these already compromised patients.[48, 49, 50] Thyroidectomy for some patients with this condition may be extremely beneficial and allows the continued use of the drug. Surgery has the distinct advantage of a rapid onset of control compared to radioactive therapy which may require many months before control of the condition is seen. It is therefore advantageous in patients who are non-compliant with their medical therapy. Adequate surgery also offers permanent and durable control in the majority of cases of Graves' disease. The cure rate is proportionate to the extent of thyroidectomy; the more thyroid tissue left *in situ*, the more likely is a recurrence of hyperthyroidism. In a meta-analysis by Palit et al.,[51] all patients undergoing total thyroidectomy were controlled, while 7.9 per cent of patients with a subtotal thyroidectomy suffered recurrent disease. Another advantage of surgery is that it provides a pathological specimen to confirm the diagnosis and rule out undiagnosed thyroid cancer. The incidence of thyroid cancer in Graves' disease varies, but does occur in up to 5 per cent of patients.[52, 53, 54, 55]

A concern of any surgical procedure is the safety. The main complications associated with thyroidectomy are vocal cord paralysis and hypocalcaemia. In the literature, the incidence of vocal cord paralysis in experienced surgical hands is minimal.[56, 57, 58, 59, 60, 61] We believe that an acceptable rate of vocal cord paralysis should be less than 2 per cent for all surgeons. With the change in emphasis from partial to total or near total thyroidectomy, the potential for transient and permanent hypocalcaemia has increased. Factors associated with an increase in incidence include extent of disease, previous surgery, extent of surgery and experience of the surgeon. The literature would suggest that the likelihood of permanent hypocalcaemia is minimal in experienced hands (less than 5 per cent).[62, 63, 64, 65, 66]

The cost of therapy is also an issue. Patel *et al.* in a study to determine cost-effectiveness of treating thyrotoxicosis using the three modalities found that the cost per 'cure' was better for radioiodine (£13 753 or US$21 470) compared to thionamides (£3763 or US$5874) and surgery (£6551 or US$10 227). However, only five patients underwent surgery in this study.[67]

Advantages and disadvantages of surgery for Graves' disease

TYPE OF SURGERY FOR HYPERTHYROIDISM

The overall objective in patients undergoing thyroid surgery for hyperthyroidism is to control the toxic condition, without significant morbidity and in particular nerve damage or hypocalcaemia. There is no universally accepted treatment protocol, each patient is treated on an individual basis after assessment and explanation of the risks and benefits of the procedure. For Graves' disease, which is by far the most common and important cause of hyperthyroidism, the present day recommendations are to remove all or near all of the thyroid tissue accepting that the patient will require treatment for hypothyroidism. This policy recognizes that the more extensive the surgery, the more likely that the disease process would be cured. However, this has to be balanced by the potential for complications. Partial surgical resection with the treatment goal to achieve a euthyroid state is not recommended, except for toxic adenoma, because of the high chance of failure to control the toxic state.

In general, there are four choices of operation:

1. Total thyroidectomy removing all gross thyroid tissue.
2. Total lobectomy on one side with a contralateral subtotal lobectomy leaving only the smallest possible remnant of thyroid tissue posteriorly with intact blood supply to the preserved parathyroid glands (near-total thyroidectomy).
3. Unilateral lobectomy and isthmectomy. This procedure is only suitable for hyperthyroidism caused by a toxic adenoma.
4. Bilateral subtotal thyroidectomy leaving bilateral variable amounts of thyroid remnants in an attempt to have a euthyroid patient. This procedure is mostly of historical interest and is rarely performed at this time.

The literature suggests that total thyroidectomy is the most effective surgery for control of Graves' disease. Palit *et al.*

performed a meta-analysis involving 35 studies of over 7000 patients with Graves' disease treated with surgery and follow up for on average 5.6 years.[51] Patients treated with less than total thyroidectomy had a persistent or recurrent hyperthyroidism in 8 per cent of cases.

Hypothyroidism following total thyroidectomy is not a complication, but a natural sequelae. The main complications associated with thyroidectomy include recurrent laryngeal nerve damage and potentially life-long hypocalcaemia. Permanent recurrent laryngeal nerve damage did not statistically differ between different types of surgery for hyperthyroidism.[44] Similarly, the incidence of permanent hypocalcaemia showed no statistical difference with an incidence of 1.6 per cent for total and 1 per cent for subtotal thyroidectomy.[62, 63, 64, 65, 66] These statistics are from international tertiary care centres with significant surgical expertise. The individual surgeon must make the decision as to the extent of surgery taking into account a number of factors, which include surgical experience and personal complication rates with regard to hyperthyroidism. The occasional surgeon should not expect similar excellent outcomes with total thyroidectomy and should consider the lesser subtotal operation or, possibly more correctly, referral to an experienced thyroid surgeon.

Experienced surgeons treating Graves' hyperthyroidism and diffuse toxic multinodular goitre will plan a total thyroidectomy, understanding that as long as a thyroid remnant is present, recurrence of the toxic state is possible. The surgeon will pay particular attention to identifying and preserving both parathyroid glands with an intact blood supply on the initial side dissected. If the thyroid surgeon is not happy that two parathyroid glands have been preserved then a more flexible approach to the type of thyroid surgery is applied. The initial total lobectomy on one side is usually followed by a subtotal lobectomy on the opposite side. This approach leaves a small posterior thyroid remnant, the objective of which is that by preserving this thyroid remnant, the blood supply to the parathyroid glands will be preserved. Regarding recurrent laryngeal nerve preservation, total thyroidectomy, total lobectomy and contralateral subtotal lobectomy should have the same low rate of permanent damage with an experienced surgeon who identifies the nerve prior to removal of the gland.

Surgery for hyperthyroidism

Thyroidectomy for hyperthyroidism requires a similar operation as for other conditions requiring thyroid surgery. The operation may be somewhat more difficult because of increased vascularity and/or inflammation of the thyroid. Preoperative control of the toxic state is essential together with an atraumatic technique. In particular, attention has to be given by the surgeon to identify and preserve the parathyroid glands which may be more intimately attached to the thyroid than usual. In general, although the sequence of steps for the surgery may vary, all have similar broad objectives.

PREPARATION OF THE PATIENT WITH HYPERTHYROIDISM FOR SURGERY

It is of paramount importance, particularly in poorly controlled Graves' disease, that the effects of thyroid overactivity are controlled before surgery to reduce the possibility of thyroid storm. This is caused by a massive increase in the level of free thyroid hormones in the bloodstream. Symptoms are those of extreme hyperthyroidism and may be life threatening. Reduction of thyroid vascularity is also of benefit to help the surgical procedure.

Control is probably best achieved with the input of endocrinology expertise. Initially, a relatively high initial dose of thionamide drugs is used. Once the patient is euthyroid, the dosage may be reduced or thyroxine introduced.[45]

Propranolol may also be started to control symptoms of hyperthyroidism and stopped after surgery.[46] Beta-blockers are of particular importance in patients requiring emergency thyroidectomy where there is no time to render the patient euthyroid with thionamides.

Iodine administration, such as Lugol's iodine 5–10 drops three times daily for 7–10 days, may be used to reduce vascularity. Its effects start within 24 hours and have a maximum effect after 2 weeks. Beyond this, prolonged use of iodine will result in a worsening of hyperthyroidism.[68, 69]

REASONS FOR FAILED CONTROL AFTER SURGERY

Following total or near-total thyroidectomy, recurrent disease suggests that thyroid tissue may have been unintentionally left behind. The locations of this tissue should be known by the thyroid surgeon to prevent recurrent disease. The most likely sites include a missed pyramidal lobe. Other sites of thyroid tissue missed include tissue associated with the superior pole, posterior to Berry's ligament, anterior tracheal wall and adjacent to the parathyroid gland.

MINIMALLY INVASIVE THYROID SURGERY

The majority of patients who undergo thyroidectomy have surgery because of possible or definite cancer. Even with fine needle aspiration cytology used as a screening tool, two-thirds of patients prove to have benign pathology and are undergoing an unnecessary excision biopsy of the thyroid, although with the potential for cure if cancer is present, and the diagnosis may not be certain until definite pathology is available. Since thyroid pathology is relatively more common in the female population, a large proportion of these patients are young women who do not appreciate an unsightly neck scar.

Recent improvements in technology have led to minimal invasive surgery becoming the standard of care as with other surgical procedures, such as cholecystectomy. The potential advantages include less dissection, small incisions, less pain and a shorter hospital stay. Huscher et al.[70] were the first to describe a case report of endoscopic thyroid lobectomy in 1997. Since then, a number of centres particularly in Italy and Japan have described and published on a number of endoscopic parathyroid and thyroid techniques.[71, 72, 73]

In general, two main types have been popularized. The first is the 'closed' videoscopic thyroidectomy, where no neck incisions are performed. The thyroid is approached through multiple ports in the axilla, chest or breast using insufflation and similar techniques perfected in laparoscopic abdominal operations.[74, 75] This procedure is lengthy and involves significant dissection in areas distant from the thyroid bed and, as a consequence is hardly 'minimally invasive'. These difficulties have meant that this type of procedure has not become popular outside a handful of centres primarily in Asia.

The second type of operation is known as 'minimally invasive video-assisted thyroidectomy' (MIVAT) (**Boxes 22.6** and **22.7**). This is performed through a small (1.5–2 cm) suprasternal midline incision or lateral neck incision, and does not use gas insufflation.[76, 77, 78, 79, 80, 81, 82]

Selection criteria for patients undergoing this procedure include thyroid nodules less than 3.5 cm with a volume of less than 25 mL based on ultrasound to allow successful removal. The restriction on size means that only approximately 9 per cent of patients having thyroidectomy are potential candidates for this procedure. Recently, Ruggieri et al.[83] suggested that inclusion criteria can be increased to include thyroid swelling with a volume up to 50 mL, if the neck incision size is increased to 3.5 cm.

There is no generally accepted definition of minimal invasion. The authors have found that once skin incisions for thyroidectomy are less than 3 cm, visualization and access is severely restricted. In particular with these smaller incisions, it is more difficult to identify the recurrent laryngeal nerve and parathyroids. Depending on the level of the incision, safe access and mobilization of the superior thyroid pedicle is particularly difficult. In this situation, the introduction of the endoscope allows visualization of these structures and safe delivery of the thyroid.

Thyroidectomy involves a certain number of set surgical steps. Individual surgeons may prefer to perform these in different sequences, for example delivering the thyroid gland before division of the superior pedicle, or dividing the isthmus of the thyroid before exposure of the gland.

In our opinion, MIVAT should not be considered as a separate thyroid procedure when compared to the classical 'open' procedure. It should be viewed as one end of a spectrum of thyroid procedures all with similar surgical manoeuvres and objectives, but approached through a smaller incision using the endoscope to allow identification and preservation of important structures. This restriction in surgical exposure puts a priority on an atraumatic technique with little or no bleeding.

The use of the endoscope is important in the identification of important structures and mobilization of the gland. It is not used during delivery or final removal of the thyroid.

The thyroid size is the most important criteria for MIVAT inclusion, because the working space provided by the technique is limited. Miccoli et al. have popularized the midline incision less than 2 cm. Using this technique, only thyroid lesions less than 3.5 cm with a volume of less than 20 mL per lobe on preoperative ultrasound (normal size 12 mL) are suitable.[40] Miccoli et al. also exclude patients who are found to have significant adhesions from thyroiditis. Using these criteria, Miccoli et al. found that only 10 per cent of patients undergoing thyroidectomy were eligible.[79, 80, 81, 82] The authors use less stringent criteria for inclusion. Thyroid lesions clinically less than 3.5 cm are considered for the procedure. If after mobilization of the thyroid difficulties with thyroid delivery are experienced, the incision may be extended up to 3 cm to allow safe delivery without spillage of thyroid contents. Using these criteria, up to 18 per cent of patients may be potential candidates for MIVAT. More experience with this procedure has led to the realization that excessive body mass index is also an important criteria in selection. Excessive adiposity means an increase in working distance from the skin edge, with more difficult dissection and identification of important structures, such as the parathyroid glands. The authors would also suggest that in the older patient with lax skin and well-formed skin creases, there is cosmetically little to be offered between a conventional 4 cm skin crease incision and a 2 cm incision not in a skin crease. Although Miccoli has described central neck dissection, the authors do not practise this routinely and in their hands it is a relative contraindication to the technique.

MEN carriers are uncommon, but current recommendations are that they undergo total thyroidectomy at an early stage, usually by the age of five years to avoid the potential for metastatic nodal disease and central neck dissection. Thus, MIVAT has become our procedure of choice for this condition.

Disadvantages include a learning curve, inability to palpate during the operation, a second assistant is required and the procedure is restricted to a minority of patients with thyroid pathology.

Although this procedure makes day-case thyroidectomy a possibility, the potential for life-threatening postoperative haematoma, as with any thyroid procedure, has lead to the patient being observed overnight.

Complications of surgery relating to benign thyroid disease

Complications of surgery relating to benign thyroid disease are listed below:

1. Laryngeal nerve damage:
   a. recurrent laryngeal nerve. Temporal paresis seen in approximately 6 per cent, while permanent paresis is

---

Box 22.6   Potential advantages of MIVAT

- Small incision
- Better cosmesis
- Less pain
- Short hospital stay
- Less soft tissue dissection
- MEN carriers

Box 22.7   Disadvantages of MIVAT

- Learning curve
- Suitability
- Two assistants required and they need to be experienced
- Special instruments
- Lack of feel
- Hypertrophied scar

seen in <1 per 500 in experienced hands and should be <2 per cent for all comers.
  b. superior laryngeal nerve.

2. Hypocalcaemia associated with:
   a. extent of resection
   b. recurrent goitres
   c. age
   d. gender female more likely
   e. volume of thyroid surgery
   f. Graves' disease.

Hypocalcaemia occurs in 1–6 per cent of cases in experienced hands and the community rate is of the order of 13 per cent.

3. Haematoma occurs in 1–2 per cent of cases.
4. Wound infection occurs in 1–2 per cent of cases.
5. Tracheomalacia.

Prevention of wound haematoma

Haematoma is a potential life-threatening complication of thyroidectomy, the frequency of which is 1–2 per cent in large institutions, but may be higher. Preoperatively, correction of any bleeding tendencies is important and the patient should stop potential problematic medications, such as aspirin, for more than 10 days before operation. An atraumatic technique with fastidious control of bleeding is mandatory. Washing the wound copiously to get rid of clot, and the use of the Valsalva manoeuvre routinely is commonly performed to identify potential bleeding sites before completion of the operation.

Routine neck drains do not decrease the incidence of wound haematoma. Wound haematomas following thyroidectomy usually occur within 12 hours of the surgical procedure. Common sites of bleeding are from vessels associated with Berry's ligament, but a definite bleeding point may not be found at exploration. Probably the most important aspect in the treatment of wound haematoma is early detection. In this regard, the education of nurses and junior doctors, who are most likely to first see the compromised patient, regarding the clinical features and management is of special importance. We routinely use small amounts of Surgicell to help with haemostasis. Early identification is mandatory and the patient should be returned to theatre expediently to allow evacuation of the haematoma. An expanding haematoma has the potential to cause anoxia in a short period of time. In this situation, bedside decompression is required. To allow this, a clip remover and scissors should be at the bedside to allow opening of the skin, subcutaneous tissue and critically opening the strap muscles in the midline. This prevents further expansion and compromise of the airway. The patient should then be returned to theatre and undergo gas induction by an experienced anaesthetist before formal exploration and control of bleeding.

TRACHEOMALACIA

Postoperative airway compromise may arise after extubation due to tracheomalacia and collapse of the trachea. This may require PEEP (positive end expiratory pressure) and/or reintubation for 24–48 hours. Tracheomalacia is rare and occurs in <1.5 per cent of cases. It is important to differentiate this condition from bilateral vocal cord palsy. In most cases, despite significant compression of the trachea on removal of the offending goitre, the trachea settles back into a midline position with normal dimensions. Occasionally, an anchor suture is used to hold the trachea in position. Should the trachea remain narrowed, with the lumen less than 70 per cent its original size, consideration should be given to stenting. In rare circumstances, a tracheostomy may have to be performed (**Box 22.8**).

Box 22.8 Key points in reducing complications

- Preoperative evaluation
- Understanding anatomy
- Routine identification of the recurrent laryngeal nerve and parathyroid glands
- Meticulous haemostasis
- Most important – patience and perseverance

KEY EVIDENCE

- Patients with Graves' disease treated with less than total thyroidectomy have a significant persistent relapse rate. This, together with the fact that revision thyroid surgery is associated with potentially more postoperative complications,[21] suggests that total thyroidectomy is the preferred surgery of choice for Graves' disease, while for nontoxic MNG, total thyroidectomy should be particularly considered with bilateral disease and in younger patients.

KEY LEARNING POINTS

- Multinodular goitre (MNG) is common and often asymptomatic.
- Surgery for MNG is indicated if there is evidence of compression, significant substernal extention or concern of malignancy.
- Sternal split is rarely required.
- Cosmesis is not a good indication for surgery.
- Graves' disease is by far the most common cause of hyperthyroidism.
- Spontaneous resolution is not a significant feature of natural history in toxic MNG or toxic adenoma.
- Initial medical therapy is always indicated to control the hyperthyroid state.

- Surgery is indicated for Graves' disease in children, women of child-bearing age, large bulky glands and for cancer concern.

REFERENCES

◆ 1. Welbourn RB. *The history of endocrine surgery.* New York: Praeger, 1990: 19–82.

2. Talbott JH. *A biographical history of medicine: excerpts and essays on the men and their work.* New York: Grune & Stratton, 1970: 1012–14, 1044–6.

3. Matovinevic J. Endemic goitre and cretinism at the dawn of the 3rd millennium. *Annual Review of Nutrition* 1983; 3: 341–412.

4. Berghout A, Wiersinga WM, Drexhage HA *et al.* Comparison of placebo with L-thyroxine or with carbimazole for treatment of sporadic non-toxic goitre. *Lancet* 1990; 336: 193–7.

● 5. Elte JW, Bussemaker JK, Haak A. The natural history of euthyroid multinodular goitre. *Post Graduate Medical Journal* 1990; 66: 186–90.

6. Daniels GH. Thyroid nodules and nodular thyroids. A clinical overview. *Comprehensive Therapy* 1996; 22: 239–50.

* 7. Tunbridge WM, Evered DC, Hall R *et al.* The spectrum of thyroid disease in a community: The Wickham survey. *Clinical Endocrinology* 1977; 7: 481–93.

● 8. Neumanns S, Willgerodt H, Ackermann F *et al.* Linkage of the familial euthyroid goitre to the multinodular goitre-1 locus and exclusion of the candidate genes thyroglobulin thyroperoxidase and Na+/I– symporter. *Journal of Clinical Endocrinology and Metabolism* 1999; 84: 3750–6.

● 9. Gabriel EM, Bergert ER, Grant CS *et al.* Germline polymorphism of codon 727 of human thyroid stimulating hormone receptor is associated with toxic multinodular goitre. *Journal of Clinical Endocrinology and Metabolism* 1999; 84: 3328–35.

10. Huins CT, Georgalas C, Mehrzad H, Tolley NS. A new classification system for retrosternal goitre based on a systematic review of its complications and management. *International Journal of Surgery* 2008; 6: 71–6.

11. deSouza FM, Smith PE. Retrosternal goitre. *Journal of Otolaryngology* 1983; 12: 393–6.

◆ 12. Hollowell JG, Staehling NW, Hannon WH *et al.* Iodine nutrition in the United States. Trends and public health implications: iodine excretion data from National Health and Nutrition Examination Surveys 1 and 111 (1971–1974 and 1988–1994). *Journal of Clinical Endocrinology and Metabolism* 1998; 83: 3401–8.

* 13. Anglem TJ, Bradford ML. Nodular goitre and thyroid cancer. *New England Journal of Medicine* 1948; 239: 217–20.

14. Tan GH, Gharib H, Reading CC. Solitary thyroid nodule; comparison betweem palpation and ultrasonography. *Archives of Internal Medicine* 1995; 155: 2418–23.

● 15. Koh KB, Chang KW. Carcinoma in multinodular goitre. *British Journal of Surgery* 1992; 79: 266–7.

16. Berghout A, Wiersinga WM, Smits NJ *et al.* Interrelationship between age, thyroid volume, thyroid nodularity and thyroid function in patients with sporadic non-toxic goiter. *American Journal of Medicine* 1990; 89: 602–8.

17. Stoffer RP, Welch JW, Hellwig CA *et al.* Nodular goitre. *Archives of Internal Medicine* 1960; 106: 10–14.

18. Har-El G, Sundaram K. Powered instrumentation for transcervical removal of gigantic intrathoracic thyroid. *Head and Neck* 2001; 23: 322–5.

● 19. Thomusch O, Machers A, Sekulla C *et al.* Multivariate analysis of risk factors for post operative complications in benign goitre surgery surgery: prospective multicenter study in Germany. *World Journal of Surgery* 2000; 24: 1335–41.

20. Kraimps JL, Bouin-Pineau MH, Mathonnet M *et al.* Multicentre study of thyroid nodules in patients with Graves' disease. *British Journal of Surgery* 2000; 87: 1111–13.

21. Wagner HE, Seiler CA. Indications for and results of recurrent surgery of the thyroid gland. *Schweizerische Medizinischrift. Journal Suisse de Medicine* 1994; 124: 1222–6.

22. Wilson DB, Staren ED, Prinz RA. Thyroid reexploration; indications and risks. *American Surgeon* 1998; 64: 674–8.

23. Reeve TS, Delbridge L, Brady P *et al.* Secondary thyroidectomy: a twenty-year experience. *World Journal of Surgery* 1988; 12: 449–53.

* 24. Parry CH. Collections from the unpublished papers of the late Caleb Hilliel Parry. *Diseases of the Heart* 1825; 2: 111–65.

◆ 25. Gough S. The genetics of Graves' disease. *Endocrinology and Metabolism Clinics of North America* 2000; 29: 255–60.

26. Dabon-Almirante CLM, Surks MI. Clinical and laboratory diagnosis of thyrotoxicosis. *Endocrinology and Metabolism Clinics of North America* 1998; 27: 25–35.

27. Fatourechi V. Medical treatment of Graves' ophthalmopathy. *Ophthalmology Clinics of North America* 2000; 13: 683–91.

28. Bransom CJ, Talbot CH, Henry L, Elemenoglou J. Solitary toxic adenoma of the thyroid gland. *British Journal of Surgery* 1979; 66: 592–5.

◆ 29. Cooper DS. Antithyroid drugs for the treatment of hyperthyroidism caused by Graves' disease. *Endocrinology and Metabolism Clinics of North America* 1998; 27: 225–47.

◆ 30. Kaplan MM, Meier DA, Dworkin HJ. Treatment of hyperthyroidism with radioactive iodine. *Endocrinology and Metabolism Clinics of North America* 1998; 27: 205–23.

31. Van Isselt JW, Van Dongen AJ. The current status of radioiodine therapy for benign thyroid disorders. *Hellenic Journal of Nuclear Medicine* 2004; **7**: 104–10.

32. Alsenea O, Clark OH. Treatment of Grave's disease: the advantage of surgery. *Endocrinology and Metabolism Clinics of North America* 2000; **30**: 321–37.

◆ 33. Zimmerman D, Lteif AN. Thyrotoxicosis in children. *Endocrinology and Metabolism Clinics of North America* 1998; **27**: 109–26.

34. Mestman JH. Hyperthyroidism in pregnancy. *Clinical Obstetrics and Gynecology* 1997; **40**: 45–64.

● 35. Frilling A, Goretzki PE, Grussendorf M *et al.* The influence of surgery on endocrine ophthalmopathy. *World Journal of Surgery* 1990; **14**: 442–5.

36. Bartley GB, Fatourechi V, Kadrmas EF *et al.* Chronology of Graves' ophthalmopathy in an incidence cohort. *American Journal of Ophthalmology* 1996; **121**: 426–34.

37. Livraghi T, Paracchi MA, Ferrari C *et al.* Treatment of autonomous thyroid nodules with percutaneous ethanol injection – 4 year experience. *Radiology* 1994; **190**: 529–33.

38. Lippi F, Ferrari C, Manetta L *et al.* Treatment of solitary autonomous thyroid nodules by percutaneous ethanol injection; results of an Italian multicenter study. *Journal of Clinical Endocrinology and Metabolism* 1996; **81**: 3261–4.

39. Monzani F, Caraccio N, Goletti O *et al.* Five year follow up of percutaneous injection for the treatment of hyperfunctioning thyroid nodules: a study of 117 patients. *Clinical Endocrinology* 1997; **46**: 9–15.

40. Papini E, Pacella CM, Verdi G. Percutaneous ethanol injection (PEI): what is its role in the treatment of benign thyroid nodules? *Thyroid* 1995; **5**: 147–50.

41. Bennedback FN, Karstrup S, Hegedus L. Percutaneous ethanol injection therapy in the treatment of thyroid and parathyroid diseases. *European Journal of Endocrinology* 1997; **136**: 240–50.

42. Monzani F, Lippi F, Goletti O *et al.* Percutaneous aspiration and ethanol sclerotherapy for thyroid cysts. *Journal of Clinical Endocrinology and Metabolism* 1994; **78**: 800–2.

43. Zingrillo M, Torlontano M, Ghiggi MR *et al.* Percutaneous ethanol injection in large thyroid cystic nodules. *Thyroid* 1996; **6**: 403–8.

44. Chiang FY, Wang LF, Huang YF *et al.* Recurrent laryngeal nerve palsy after thyroidectomy with routine identification of the recurrent laryngeal nerve. *Surgery* 2005; **137**: 342–7.

45. Bergfelt G. Preoperative treatment of thyrotoxicosis with antithyroid drugs and thyroxine. *Journal of Clinical Endocrinology* 1961; **21**: 72–9.

46. Zonszein J, Santangelo RP, Mackin JF *et al.* Propanolol therapy in thyrotoxicosis: a review of 84 patients undergoing surgery. *American Journal of Medicine* 1979; **66**: 411–16.

47. Podrid PJ. Amiodarone reevaluation of an old drug. *Annals of Internal Medicine* 1995; **122**: 689–700.

● 48. Faarwell AP, Abend SL, Huang SK *et al.* Thyroidectomy for amiodarone-induced thyrotoxicosis. *Journal of the American Medical Association* 1990; **263**: 1526–8.

49. Goichot B. Amiodarone-induced hyperthyroidism. *Archives of Internal Medicine* 2001; **161**: 295.

50. Cardenas GA, Cabral JM, Leslie CA. Amiodarone induced thyrotoxicosis: diagnostic and therapeutic strategies. *Cleveland Clinic Journal of Medicine* 2003; **70**: 624–6.

● 51. Palit TK, Miller CC 3rd, Miltenburg DM. The efficacy of thyroidectomy for Graves' disease. A meta-analysis. *Journal of Surgical Research* 2000; **90**: 161–5.

52. Cakir M, Arici C, Alakus H *et al.* Incidental thyroid carcinoma in thyrotoxic patients treated by surgery. *Hormone Research* 2007; **67**: 96–9.

53. Pacini F, Elisei R, Di Coscio GC *et al.* Thyroid carcinoma in thyrotoxic patients treated by surgery. *Journal of Endocrinological Investigation* 1988; **11**: 107–12.

54. Mazzaferri EL. Thyroid cancer and Graves' disease. *Journal of Clinical Endocrinology and Metabolism* 1990; **70**: 826–9.

55. Wahl RA, Goretzki P, Meybier H *et al.* Coexistence of hyperthyroidism and thyroid cancer. *World Journal of Surgery* 1982; **6**: 385–90.

56. Lamade W, Renz K, Willeke F. Effect of training on the incidence of nerve damage in thyroid surgery. *British Journal of Surgery* 1999; **86**: 388–91.

57. Manolidis S, Takashima M, Kirby M *et al.* Thyroid surgery: a comparison of outcomes between experts and surgeons in training. *Otolaryngology – Head and Neck Surgery* 2001; **125**: 30–3.

● 58. Hermann M, Alk G, Roka R *et al.* Laryngeal recurrent nerve injury in surgery for benign thyroid diseases: effect of nerve dissection and impact of individual surgeons in more then 27,000 nerves at risk. *Annals of Surgery* 2002; **235**: 261–8.

59. Chiang FW, Wang LF, Huang YF *et al.* Recurrent laryngeal nerve palsy after thyroidectomy with routine identification of the recurrent laryngeal nerve. *Surgery* 2005; **137**: 342–7.

60. Martensson H, Terms J. Recurrent laryngeal nerve palsy in thyroid gland surgery related to operations and nerves at risk. *Archives of Surgery* 1985; **120**: 475–7.

61. Eisele DW. Intraoperative electrophysiologic monitoring of the recurrent laryngeal nerve. *Laryngoscope* 1996; **106**: 443–9.

62. Falk SA, Birken EA, Baran DT. Temporary post thyroidectomy hypocalcemia. *Archives of Otolaryngology – Head and Neck Surgery* 1988; **114**: 168–74.

63. Luu Q, Andersen PE, Adams J *et al.* The predictive value of perioperative calcium levels after thyroid/parathyroid surgery. *Head and Neck* 2002; **24**: 63–7.

64. Moore C, Lampe H, Agrawal S. Predictability of hypocalcaemia using early postoperative serum calcium levels. *Journal of Otolaryngology* 2001; **30**: 266–70.

65. De Pasquale L, Schubert L, Bastagli A. A post-thyroidectomy hypocalcaemia and feasibility of short stay thyroid surgery. *Chirurgia Italiana* 2000; **52**: 549–54.

66. Netterville JL, Aly A, Ossoff RH. Evaluation and treatment of complications of thyroid and parathyroid surgery. *Otolaryngologic Clinics of North America* 1990; **23**: 529–52.

67. Patel NN, Abkaham P, Buscombe J, Vanderpump MPJ. The cost effectiveness of treatment modalities for thyrotoxicosis in a UK centre. *Thyroid* 2006; **16**: 593–8.

68. Coyle PJ, Mitchell JE. Thyroidectomy: is Lugol's iodine necessary? *Annals of the Royal College of Surgeons* 1982; **64**: 334–5.

69. Marigold JH, Morgan AK, Earle DJ et al. Lugol's iodine: its effect on thyroid blood flow in patients with thyrotoxicosis. *British Journal of Surgery* 1985; **72**: 45–7.

70. Huscher CS, Recher A, Napolitano G, Chiodini S. Endoscopic right thyroid lobectomy. *Surgical Endoscopy* 1997; **11**: 877.

71. Yeung HC, Ng WT, Kong CK. Endoscopic thyroid and parathyroid surgery. *Surgical Endoscopy* 1997; **11**: 1135.

72. Shimizu K, Akira S, Tanaka S. Video-assisted neck surgery: endoscopic resection of benign thyroid tumor aiming at scarless surgery on the neck. *Journal of Surgical Oncology* 1998; **69**: 178–80.

73. Shimizu K. Minimally invasive thyroid surgery. *Best Practice and Research. Clinical Endocrinology and Metabolism* 2001; **15**: 123–37.

74. Ikeda Y, Takami H, Sasaki Y et al. Endoscopic resection of thyroid tumors by the axillary approach. *Journal of Cardiovascular Surgery* 2000; **41**: 791–2.

75. Ohgami M, Ishii S, Arisawa Y et al. Scarless endoscopic thyroidectomy; breast approach for better cosmesis. *Surgical Laparoscopy, Endoscopy and Percutaneous Techniques* 2000; **10**: 1–4.

76. Maeda S, Uga T, Hayashida N et al. Video-assisted subtotal or near-total thyroidectomy for Graves' disease. *British Journal of Surgery* 2006; **93**: 61–6.

77. Miccoli P, Berti P, Conte M et al. Minimally invasive surgery for thyroid small nodules: preliminary report. *Journal of Endocrinological Investigation* 1999; **22**: 849–51.

● 78. Miccoli P, Berti P, Raffaelli M et al. Comparison between minimally invasive video-assisted thyroidectomy and conventional thyroidectomy: a prospective randomized study. *Surgery* 2001; **130**: 1039–43.

79. Miccoli P, Berti P, Materazzi G et al. Minimally invasive video-assisted thryoidectomy. Five years of experience. *Journal of the American College of Surgeons* 2004; **199**: 243–8.

80. Miccoli P, Berti P, Frustaci GL et al. Video-assisted thyroidectomy; indications and results. *Archives of Surgery* 2006; **391**: 68–71.

* 81. Gagner M. Endoscopic subtotal parathyroidectomy in patients with primary hyperparathyroidism. *British Journal of Surgery* 1996; **83**: 875.

82. Gagner M. Endoscopic thyroidectomy for solitary thyroid nodules. *Thyroid* 2001; **11**: 161–3.

◆ 83. Ruggieri M, Straniero A, Maiuolo A et al. The minimally invasive surgical approach in thyroid diseases. *Minerva Chirurgica* 2007; **62**: 309–14.

23

Surgical management of differentiated thyroid cancer

JOHN M CHAPLIN, NEIL SHARMA AND JOHN C WATKINSON

There are in fact two things, science and opinion. The former begets knowledge, the latter ignorance.

Hippocrates (460–377 BC)

INTRODUCTION

Differentiated thyroid cancer (DTC) consists of a group of malignant tumours derived from the thyroid follicular cell.[1] Thyroid cancer is uncommon, making up around 1 per cent of all cancers[1,2] and DTCs (including papillary and follicular adenocarcinomas) make up around 90 per cent of all thyroid malignancy.[3] In the United Kingdom, there are about 1200 newly diagnosed thyroid cancers a year (3.5 per 100 000 women and 1.3 per 100 000 men per year) compared with an increasing US incidence of 37 000 new cases per year in 2009.[4,5] The incidence of DTC is higher in women, older patients and those with a family history or previous radiation exposure. There is evidence that the incidence of DTC,

particularly papillary thyroid carcinoma (PTC), is increasing,[4,6] especially in the USA and Canada although death rates in the UK and North America remain the same. Possible reasons for this are discussed later. Despite this, DTC remains an indolent disease with an excellent prognosis.

Interpreting the literature on DTC can be difficult as the disease is both uncommon, indolent and results in few deaths. The data are largely retrospective, often with inadequate follow up, and there are multiple variables and a definite outcome of any prospective trial is unlikely in any one clinician's working lifetime. By far the most common presentation of DTC is as a solitary thyroid nodule. However, papillary and follicular thyroid cancers may present with locally invasive symptoms and signs such as a laryngeal nerve palsy, dysphagia or airway compromise, evidence of metastatic disease with palpable lymph nodes or distant spread to the bones producing a pathological fracture.

Thyroid nodules are common and occur in approximately 5 per cent of women and 1 per cent of men living in iodine-sufficient areas.[7] Rates of up to 70 per cent can be shown by high resolution ultrasound in randomly selected individuals[8] although only 5–10 per cent of thyroid nodules represent malignancy.[9] The most appropriate initial investigation of a solitary or dominant thyroid nodule is fine needle aspiration cytology (FNAC). This investigation, combined with high resolution ultrasound, has allowed the design of surgical algorithms that have been incorporated in the recently published American and British Thyroid Association Guidelines.[4, 5]

These guidelines advocate a multidisciplinary approach to the management of DTC with teams which include surgeons, endocrinologists, oncologists as well as nuclear medicine physicians. This allows combined, coordinated and standardized treatment that results in the best possible prognosis for the disease.

PATHOLOGY AND CLASSIFICATION OF DTC

Differentiated carcinomas derived from the thyroid follicular cell can be separated into two main categories. The most common type is PTC, which makes up 75–80 per cent of all thyroid malignancies. Presentation ranges from intrathyroid lesions measuring less than 1 cm in diameter called papillary microcarcinomas, through to large tumour masses with extension beyond the thyroid capsule. There are three growth patterns: pure papillary, follicular and mixed. PTC, however, is defined pathologically by the cell type rather than the growth pattern. The PTC cell is oval shaped due to nuclear changes and shows chromatin margination along the nuclear membrane giving a clear nuclear appearance known as 'Orphan Annie' nuclei. Similar changes in the nuclear membrane cause the other characteristic nuclear features of longitudinal grooves and inclusions that appear in PTC cells (**Figure 23.1**). Psammoma bodies are also present in these tumours, particularly in tumours with a papillary growth pattern. These are concentric, lamellated, calcifications caused by repeated deposition of calcium onto necrotic cells at the tips of papillae. PTC is multifocal in up to 80 per cent of cases with up to 50 per cent of these foci being in the contralateral lobe.[10] These tumours tend to metastasize by lymphatic routes and positive nodes can be detected in up to 90 per cent of patients, although the presence of metastatic nodes is not felt to be prognostically significant. Vascular invasion is present in up to 7 per cent and distant metastases present in 5–7 per cent of cases.[10]

In addition to the standard patterns of PTC there are a number of variants, some of which have more aggressive behaviour with respect to distant metastases and death (**Box 23.1**).

The second most common type of DTC is follicular thyroid carcinoma (FTC), which accounts for approximately 10 per cent of all thyroid cancers. They are more common in women and usually present in an older age group. Again, the most common presentation is with a solitary thyroid nodule. These tumours are slow growing and metastasize via the blood stream. Distant metastases in lung and bone are therefore more common than in PTC, and can be the first signs of the disease. They are not multifocal, do not invade lymphatic channels and lymph node metastases are rare. There are two main types of follicular carcinoma: (1) Encapsulated or minimally invasive follicular carcinoma

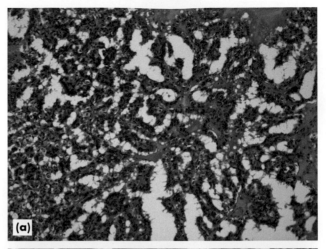

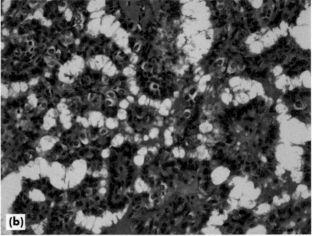

Figure 23.1   (a, b) Histological features of papillary thyroid carcinoma. Well-formed papillae with fibrovascular cores. Scalloping of darkly staining colloid is seen. H&E stain × 10 magnification. Papillae are lined by crowded cells with longitudinal nuclear grooves, intranuclear pseudo-inclusions, and optically clear nuclei. H&E stain × 40 magnification.

Box 23.1   Classification of papillary thyroid carcinoma

- PTC (papillary/follicular/mixed pattern)
- Follicular variant PTC
- Tall cell variant PTC
- Cribriform PTC
- Columnar cell variant PTC
- Papillary microcarcinoma
- Solid variant PTC
- Diffuse sclerosing variant PTC

(MIFC), which essentially looks like an adenoma and is classified as a malignancy because capsular and/or vascular invasion are demonstrated histologically (**Figure 23.2**); (2) Widely invasive follicular carcinoma (WIFC), where the tumour diffusely infiltrates the gland (**Figure 23.3**).[10] WIFC

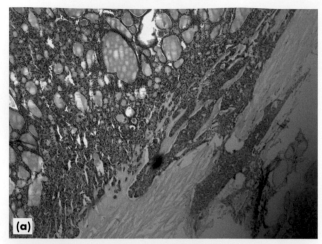

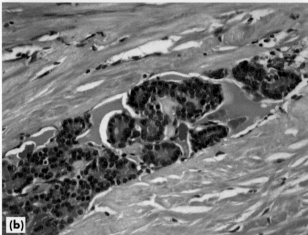

Figure 23.2 (a, b) Minimally invasive follicular carcinoma. Minimally invasive follicular carcinomas have limited (focal) capsular and/or vascular invasion. Capsular invasion (a) is defined as tumour penetration through the capsule (not associated with the site of previous fine needle aspiration biopsy). H&E stain × 10 magnification. Vascular invasion (b) is defined as the presence of intravascular tumour cells attached to the wall of the vessel, and either covered by endothelium or associated with thrombus.

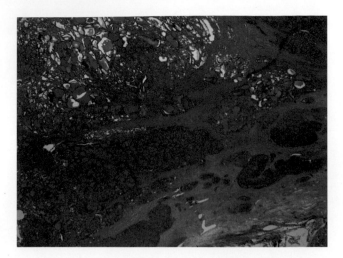

Figure 23.3 Widely invasive follicular carcinoma. Widely invasive follicular carcinomas have widespread infiltration of adjacent thyroid tissue and/or vessels. H&E stain × 20 magnification.

Table 23.1 Outcomes of 172 patients divided into two groups based on the invasiveness of follicular thyroid carcinoma.

Invasiveness	Minimal	Extensive
Patients at risk	98	72
End of follow up		
Alive	90	54
Dead (from tumour)	0	10
Metastases at diagnosis		
Regional	2	5
Distant	4	21
Metastases during follow up		
Regional	4	15
Distant	4	18

Reproduced with permission from Lang et al.[11]

can be subclassified into unencapsulated or encapsulated type, the latter showing extensive capsular and vascular invasion. WIFC tends to have poorer survival than MIFC (**Table 23.1**).

The difficulty with these tumours is differentiating MIFCs from adenomas and therein lies one of the great controversies of thyroid pathology and surgery. There is a lack of consensus among pathologists regarding the diagnostic criteria for MIFC.[10] A number of criteria have been cited in the literature, including tumour invasion into/through the capsule and into the capsular vessels. Some authors feel that the diagnosis of follicular carcinoma should be made on the basis of angioinvasion and that tumours that demonstrate capsular invasion only should be referred to as 'follicular tumours of unknown malignant potential'. These tumours have been shown to have metastatic potential.[12] Other authors have demonstrated disease-specific mortality and distant metastatic recurrence rates of 0 per cent for MIFC with capsular invasion only.[13] The reality probably is that

those with capsular invasion only have a very small chance of metastasizing.

THE THYROID NODULE

Determining which of the many thyroid nodules that a head and neck surgeon assesses are actually or potentially malignant and which require surgical excision is a complex and multifaceted task. It involves gathering as much information as possible about the nodule and then using a logical, well-defined decision-making process.

Clinical assessment

HISTORY

The majority of patients with thyroid tumours will present with a solitary thyroid nodule (**Figure 23.4**). The patient's

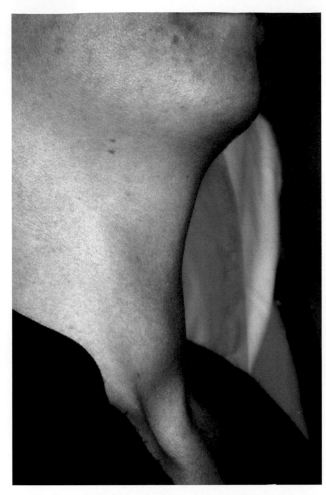

Figure 23.4   The solitary thyroid nodule. The most common way for thyroid cancer to present is as a solitary thyroid nodule in a young female euthyroid patient when the incidence of malignancy is between 10 and 20 per cent.

age is very important in determining the likelihood of a solitary nodule being malignant. A truly solitary thyroid nodule in a patient under 20 years old has a 25 per cent chance of malignancy.[14] The risk lessens in middle age to around 7–10 per cent[8] and increases again after the age of 50 when in men the likelihood of a solitary thyroid mass being malignant is 20–40 per cent. Solitary nodules that occur at either extreme of life are more likely to be malignant. Around 10 per cent of patients with DTC will present with palpable neck node metastases[15, 16] and 3–5 per cent will have hoarseness or obstructive symptoms.[17]

The other important historical risk factors in the development of thyroid cancer are radiation exposure, particularly in childhood,[18] and a family history of thyroid disease[19] (**Box 23.2**).

EXAMINATION

Distinguishing accurately between benign and malignant thyroid nodules can be difficult although certain clinical features of a thyroid nodule are typical of DTC. Papillary cancers tend to be harder than follicular tumours and have a

Box 23.2   Factors that increase the likelihood of malignancy in a thyroid nodule

A nodule is more likely to be malignant if:

- History of neck irradiation in childhood
- Endemic goitre
- Hashimoto's thyroiditis (risk of lymphoma)
- Prolonged stimulation by elevated TSH
- Solitary thyroid nodule
- Family or personal history of thyroid adenoma
- There is a history of previous thyroid cancer
- Genetic factors –
  - Familial thyroid cancer
  - Cowden's syndrome
  - Familial adenomatous polyposis
- There is an enlarging nodule (particularly on suppressive doses of thyroxine)
- The nodule develops in a person under 14 or over 65 years of age
- The patient is male

Table 23.2   Classification of thyroid nodule cytology.

Thy1	Inadequate for diagnosis
Thy2	Benign disease
Thy3	Suspicious for neoplasia
Thy4	Suspicious for malignancy
Thy5	Positive for malignant disease

higher rate of nodal metastases. A degree of fixation to surrounding structures may be associated with extrathyroid extension.

The neck must be palpated carefully for lymph nodes; levels of involvement are VI, III, II, IV, V and I in decreasing order of frequency.[20] Even with this knowledge, clinically involved lymph nodes can be difficult to palpate and a high degree of suspicion must be maintained.

Finally, the pharynx, larynx (and upper trachea if indicated) should be examined by direct fibreoptic endoscopy to look for vocal cord paralysis or invasion by tumour.

Investigations

CYTOLOGY

The interpretation of FNAC by an experienced cytopathologist has had a major impact in the management of nodular thyroid disease. FNAC is a safe, cheap and reliable investigation and, along with FT4, thyroid stimulating hormone (TSH), serum calcium and thyroid antibody levels together with an ultrasound scan should encompass the primary investigations in the management of thyroid nodules.[8] The classification of thyroid cytopathology is shown in **Table 23.2**. A Thy5 result is only possible in papillary and medullary thyroid carcinoma where a constellation of the expected cytological features are present.[10] Although lymphoma and anaplastic carcinoma can be occasionally diagnosed with confidence on FNAC, a firm diagnosis is usually only made on Trucut or open biopsy. The features of PTC are listed in **Table 23.3** and seen in **Figure 23.5**.

In follicular variant papillary tumours, there is significantly more difficulty in interpreting the cytological

findings because many features overlap with those of hyperplastic nodules or follicular neoplasms (**Figure 23.6**).[21] The aspirate from a lesion such as this is likely to be classified as Thy4. There are often some nuclear features suspicious for PTC, such as elongation and membrane thickening, but grooves and inclusions are frequently not seen. A lesion that has these features in the background of a mainly follicular pattern cytology is the only lesion that would justify a request for intraoperative frozen section.

The Thy3 category essentially represents lesions that have features that pathologists can only call a 'follicular neoplasm'. This reflects the fact that the diagnosis of follicular carcinoma is made only by observing capsular or vascular invasion and this cannot be determined by FNAC. The cytological features of a follicular neoplasm demonstrate a cellular aspirate with scant colloid. The cells are arranged in groups that often have a microfollicular pattern. There is frequently nuclear overlapping and although nuclear atypia can be present this does not indicate malignancy as this feature is also seen in benign follicular lesions (**Figure 23.7**).

Cytology representing a benign pattern (Thy2) would contain more colloid and a sparse cellular population with no repetitive microfollicular pattern and no atypical cellular features (**Figure 23.8**). In this situation there is still a small risk of the lesion being a follicular carcinoma.[22] Non-diagnostic cytology (Thy1) has been shown to be malignant in up to 9 per cent of cases on permanent histological examination.[8] The recommendation is to initially repeat the FNAC in this situation.

Table 23.3 Cytological features of classical papillary thyroid carcinoma.

Cells	Cellular aspirate in papillary groups, clusters or single cells
Background	Bubble gum colloid, stromal fragments, calcific debris (psammoma bodies), macrophages
Nuclear features	Elongation, membrane thickening, chromatin clearing, nuclear grooves and inclusions.

LABORATORY INVESTIGATIONS

Investigation of a thyroid nodule should include TSH, T3, T4 and thyroid antibodies. An elevated TSH is associated with an increased risk of malignancy.[4, 5, 23] Antibodies are useful in the interpretation of the thyroid function tests, the prediction

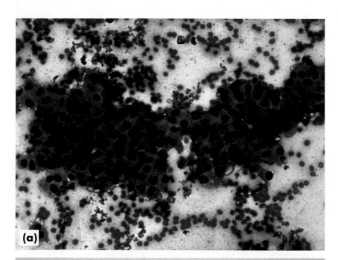

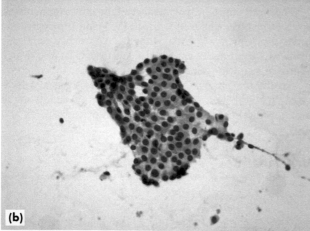

Figure 23.5 (a, b) FNAC cytological features of papillary thyroid carcinoma. (a) Neoplastic cells arranged in angulated sheets or papillae. Note the dense squamoid cytoplasm and nuclear enlargement. Diff-Quik stain™ × 40 magnification. (b) The diagnosis of papillary thyroid carcinoma rests on the identification of nuclear features which include crowding, longitudinal nuclear grooves, intranuclear pseudo-inclusions, and pale powdery chromatin. Papanicolaou stain × 40 magnification.

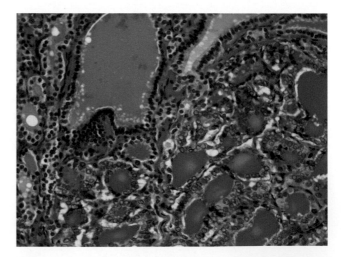

Figure 23.6 Follicular variant of papillary carcinoma. The follicular variant of papillary carcinoma may be difficult to distinguish from follicular adenoma or carcinoma. The diagnosis rests on identification of the nuclear features of papillary thyroid carcinoma. Contrast with benign follicular epithelium at the top left of the photograph. H&E stain × 20 magnification.

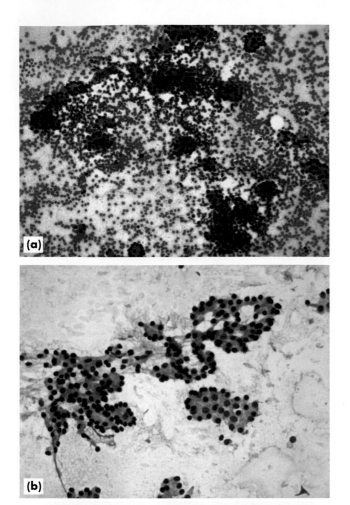

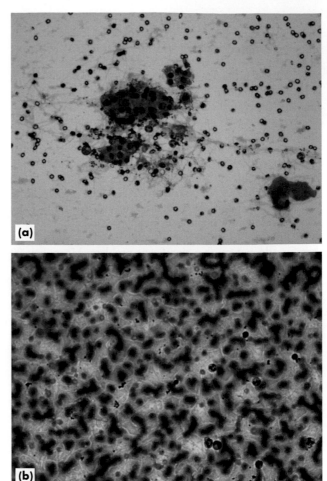

Figure 23.7 (a, b) Features suggestive of a follicular neoplasm. (a) Increased cellularity, scanty or absent colloid, and a recurring microfollicular pattern are suspicious for follicular neoplasia. Diff-Quik stain × 20 magnification. (b) Follicular cells with regular round to oval nuclei and dense chromatin, arranged in a recurring microfollicular pattern. Papanicolaou stain × 40 magnification.

Figure 23.8 (a, b) Colloid nodule. (a) Groups of evenly spaced follicular cells. Irregular amorphous dense colloid is seen in the lower right of the photograph. Diff-Quik stain × 40 magnification. (b) Abundant thin colloid showing 'cracking' artefact. Diff-Quik stain × 40 magnification.

of postoperative subclinical hypothyroidism and in the assessment of the serum thyroglobulin.[4] Preoperative measurement of thyroglobulin is not usually helpful unless the patient has had previous treatment. Serum calcium can also be considered to exclude hyperparathyroidism and to provide a baseline pre-surgery.

Radiology

ULTRASOUND

Ultrasound is useful in measuring tumour size, diagnosing multinodular goitres and excluding contralateral disease. Ultrasonography can also be used to evaluate complex cysts and can distinguish purely cystic nodules (only rarely is a cystic nodule associated with thyroid cancer). Calcification may be detected and although it occurs in both benign and malignant disease, it tends to have different features.

Microcalcification within a nodule has a high specificity for malignancy although its sensitivity is low.[24, 25] Colour flow Doppler sonography (CFDS), in addition to conventional scanning ultrasound, has been recently used to identify different types of blood flow within solid thyroid nodules,[26] with type III (marked intranodular) flow being a statistically significant criterion to suggest malignant disease ($p < 0.005$). Ultrasound is also useful for assessment of central and lateral neck lymph nodes and to detect metastases which can be difficult to assess clinically. Features suggesting malignancy in lymph nodes include increased size, rounded and bulging shape and loss of hilar echoes as the structure becomes disrupted.[27]

Authors recognize that there are limitations to the ability of ultrasound to detect malignancy and that biopsy is still a superior modality;[28] ultrasound can have an important role in guiding the pathologist's needle into a suspicious node.

Scintigraphy

Scintigraphy, which has been available for longer than both computed tomography (CT) and magnetic resonance imaging (MRI), was previously routinely used for investigation of the solitary thyroid nodule. Iodine-123 (^{123}I) is probably the optimal radionuclide for thyroid imaging because of its physiological properties but, as it is cyclotron generated, cost and availability limit its use. The radionuclide technetium-99m (^{99m}Tc), in the chemical form of pertechnetate (TcO$_4^-$), is trapped (but not organified) by the thyroid gland in a similar manner to the iodide ion. It has a 6-hour half-life and is cheap and readily available with a low radiation dose; it is therefore now used in thyroid imaging. Pertechnetate uptake, however, is low (0.4–4 per cent) and does not always match the physiological uptake of iodide which leads to a high background activity. Nonetheless, with careful attention to scanning technique the majority of nodules greater than 5 mm diameter can be visualized on scintigraphy. False negative results are often associated with smaller lesions in the isthmus, but these are usually easy to palpate and therefore do not cause a significant problem. More than 90 per cent of lesions identified will not concentrate the radio-nuclide ('cold' nodules). These clinically solitary non-functional nodules may be an adenoma, a carcinoma or a cystic or dominant nodule in a non-palpable multinodular goitre. Truly functioning nodules (also called 'hot' or 'toxic' nodules) are highly unlikely to be malignant so this investigation is probably not cost-effective for cancer assessment. Scintigraphy is now only used to identify hot nodules in a patient with elevated thyroxine or suppressed TSH levels. A diagnostic protocol is shown in **Figure 23.9**.

CT of the neck and thorax is of help in assessing the extent and relationship of larger thyroid tumours, particularly those involving the larynx, trachea, pharynx, oesophagus and major vessels (**Figure 23.10**). It is also used to demonstrate nodal deposits in the neck and mediastinum, direct retrosternal extension and pulmonary metastases (**Box 23.3**).

MRI allows multiplanar imaging of the neck and has good inherent soft tissue contrast. Vessel involvement can be assessed with MR angiography. Additional advantages over CT include the fact that iodine containing contrast is not required and there is no radiation exposure. Both MRI and CT may be difficult investigations for patients with a compromised airway for whom lying flat is uncomfortable.

Prognostic factors

There are a number of prognostic factors associated with DTC and these can be divided into those related to patient, tumour and management factors. They are listed in **Table 23.4**.

Box 23.3　Features of thyroid cancer identified on anatomical imaging

- Extracapsular extension
- Contralateral lobe
- Vascular invasion
- Mediastinal involvement
- Pharyngeal and oesophageal involvement
- Laryngeal and tracheal involvement
- Nodal disease (levels I–VII)
- Distant metastatic spread

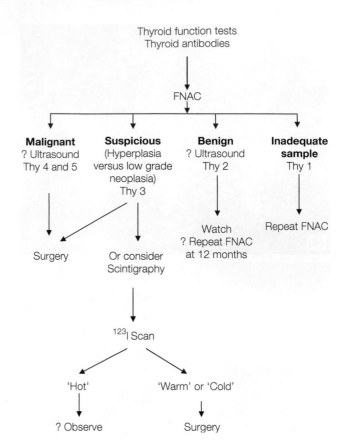

Figure 23.9　Investigations of a 'solitary' or 'dominant' thyroid nodule.

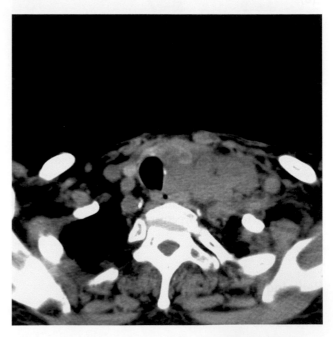

Figure 23.10　Computed tomography scan showing invasive thyroid carcinoma.

Patients under 45 years have a better prognosis and women in general do better than men. Tumours that present at advanced age generally have a poorer prognosis.[29] There is a linear relationship between the size of the tumour and prognosis[30] (**Figure 23.11**) and the grade of tumour is also important. The tall cell variant of PTC is particularly aggressive as are those follicular tumours which exhibit extensive vascular invasion (WIFC).[31] Patients with PTC fare better than those with follicular tumours. The presence of either local invasion or distant spread is associated with a worse prognosis, as are nodal metastases, particularly in elderly patients.[15, 31]

Staging

The staging system that is most widely used for DTC is the TNM classification for malignant tumours.[33] This classification is based on some of the prognostic factors listed above. There should be histological confirmation of the disease and division of cases by histological type. The current TNM (tumour, node, metastases) classification for carcinoma of the thyroid is set out in **Table 23.5** and **23.6**.

Table 23.4 Prognostic factors in differentiated thyroid cancer.

Patient factors	Tumour factors	Management factors
Age	Tumour size	Delay in therapy
Sex	Tumour histology	Extent of surgery
	Nodal metastases (in elderly patients)	Experience of the surgeon
	Local invasion	Thyroid hormone therapy
	Distant metastases	Treatment with postoperative radioiodine
No control	Control	Control

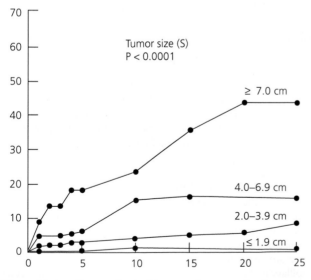

Figure 23.11 Prognostic significance of tumour size in papillary thyroid carcinoma. Reproduced with permission from Hay et al.[32]

Although the current thyroid staging systems in use around the world correctly stratify mortality rates among various subsets of patients, they have their limitations. Some patients in the lowest risk groups do die of cancer, particularly if the risk groups are only stratified into either low or high. In one study, 10 per cent of patients dying of DTC had been staged as either TNM stage I or II.[34] In addition, the systems that use age to stratify risk are often inaccurate in predicting the relationship between recurrence and survival since younger patients often have higher recurrence rates but lower death rates than older ones. Most staging systems have been derived from multivariant analysis and have survival as their end point. They frequently fail to consider recurrence or the effect of treatment and rely solely on information available postoperatively. Finally, recurrence free status and survival cannot be assured by low stage.

The first staging system was suggested by the European Organisation for Research and Treatment of Cancer (EORTC) in 1975 and incorporated a scoring system based on male gender, histology, 'T' stage and distant metastases.[35] In 1987, the Mayo clinic described the AGES classification system[32] for PTC which was based on age, tumour grade, extrathyroid invasion and tumour size. The main problem with this system was that reporting of tumour grade for PTC was variable among pathologists and was available only after surgery had been performed. The following year, Cady and Rossi from the Lahey clinic introduced the AMES classification for DTC (age, distant metastases, extrathyroid invasion and tumour size).[36] This system seemed user-friendly, however there still were some shortcomings: the data was retrospective, the earlier cases were incomplete with regard to tumour size and it included both papillary and follicular thyroid cancers. The Memorial Sloan Kettering (MSK) Hospital introduced the GAMES classification which is based on the size and extent of the tumour as well as its grade, the presence of distant metastases and patient gender.[37] In 1992, workers at the Karolinska Institute in Stockholm added the prognostic risk factor of DNA ploidy to the AMES system and came up with the DAMES classification for PTC.[38]

The Mayo clinic brought out a more elaborate staging system for PTC called the MACIS system[30] (**Table 23.7**). This system placed patients into four groups based on their scores. Patients with a MACIS score of less than 6 had a 99 per cent chance of living 20 years. In this system there was consideration of the impact of treatment; patients who had incomplete resection of tumour could be placed in a poorer prognostic group.

The problem with many of these classification systems is that they are based on retrospective data from single institutions and have no proven advantages over the universally used and widely accepted TNM system,[39] which can accurately predict survival based on a variety of prognostic factors (**Table 23.8**).

MOLECULAR GENETICS OF THYROID CANCER

The development of molecular technology over the last two decades has allowed insight into the genetic abnormalities associated with the molecular biology of thyroid cancer, although the development of novel diagnostic and therapeutic modalities is still awaited. Malignant thyroid tumours generally

Table 23.5 TNM staging for thyroid carcinoma from AJCC cancer staging manual, 7th edn, 2009.[33]

Stage	
TX	Primary tumour cannot be assessed
T0	No evidence of primary tumour
T1a	Tumour 1 cm or less in greatest dimension, limited to the thyroid
T1b	Tumour 1–2 cm in greatest dimension, limited to the thyroid
T2	Tumour more than 2 cm but not more than 4 cm in greatest dimension, limited to the thyroid
T3	Tumour more than 4 cm in greatest dimension, limited to the thyroid or any tumour with minimal extrathyroid extension (e.g. extension to sternothyroid muscle or perithyroid soft tissues)
T4a	Tumour of any size extending beyond the thyroid capsule and invades any of the following: subcutaneous soft tissues, larynx, trachea, oesophagus, recurrent laryngeal nerve
T4b	Tumour invades prevertebral fascia, mediastinal vessels, or encases carotid artery
NX	Regional lymph nodes cannot be assessed
N0	No regional lymph node metastasis
N1	Regional lymph node metastasis
N1a	Metastasis in level VI (pretracheal and paratracheal, including prelaryngeal and Delphian lymph nodes)
N1b	Metastasis in other unilateral, bilateral or contralateral cervical or upper/superior mediastinal lymph nodes.
cM0	Clinically no distant metastasis
cM1	Distant metastasis clinically
pTNM	Pathological classification
pN0	Histological examination of a selective neck dissection specimen will ordinarily include six or more lymph nodes. If the lymph nodes are negative, but the number ordinarily examined is not met, classify as pN0
pM1	Distant metastasis proven microscopically

Table 23.6 Stage grouping for papillary and follicular carcinoma from AJCC cancer staging manual, 7th edn, 2009.[33]

Stage			
Papillary or follicular under 45 years			
I	Any T	Any N	M0
II	Any T	Any N	M1
Papillary or follicular 45 years and older			
I	T1	N0	M0
II	T2	N0	M0
III	T3	N0	M0
	T1,T2,T3	N1a	M0
IVA	T1,T2,T3	N1b	M0
	T4a	N0, N1	M0
IVB	T4b	Any N	M0
Stage IVC	Any T	Any N	M1

Table 23.7 Prognostic variables for papillary thyroid carcinoma. The MACIS staging system.

Stage	
M	Distant 'M'etastases (3)
A	'A'ge (3.1 or 0.08 × age)
C	'C'ompleteness of excision (1)
I	extrathyroid 'I'nvasion (1)
S	'S'ize (cm)
Score =	$3.1 + (0.3 \times size) + 1 + 1 + 3.1$ ($0.08 \times age$ if <40 years)

Reproduced with permission from Hay et al.[30]

have a monoclonal origin, suggesting that genetic events in a single cell account for their development. These events may involve the activation of oncogenes or the inactivation of tumour suppressor genes. *In vivo* mechanisms of action of known oncogenic pathways have been identified in transgenic mice. Several oncogenes are known to play an important role in thyroid carcinogenesis and development, for example the RET and TRK rearrangements and BRAF and RAS mutations in PTC and PAX8-PPARγ translocations and RAS mutations in FTC.

RET/PTC

RET is a proto-oncogene located at chromosome 10q11.2 which encodes a transmembrane tyrosine kinase receptor.

The ligand for RET has recently been identified as glial cell-line neutrophilic factor (GDNF). RET has been identified principally in PTC and several mutations have been identified. These are all due to specific oncogenic rearrangements of the tyrosine kinase domain of the RET gene. More than 10 RET/PTC rearrangements have been identified, many of which are seen in radiation-induced tumours. The most common rearranged forms of RET are RET/PTC1 and RET/PTC3 occurring in 60–70 and 20–30 per cent of PTCs respectively.[40]

The role of the RET mutation has been demonstrated in transgenic mice with targeted overexpression of RET/PTC1 and RET/PTC3. The mice develop tumours similar to human PTC. RET rearrangements are found frequently in tumours from paediatric patients and those exposed to radiation in childhood. They are more frequent in papillary microcarcinomas, classic papillary and diffuse sclerosing variant and rare in the follicular variant. RET/PTC can transform transfected follicular cells *in vitro*, which then demonstrate the nuclear features of PTC. The RET/PTC mutation was found in 60 per cent of Ukrainian

Table 23.8 TNM staging system and mortality rates for differentiated thyroid cancer. BTA guidelines 2007.[4]

Stage		Ten-year cancer-specific mortality (%)
I	<45 years, tumour <1 cm, no metastases (any T, any N, M0)	1.7
	>45 years, tumour <1 cm, no distant metastases (T1, N0, M0)	
II	>45 years any tumour size including distant metastases (any T, any N, M1)	15.8
	>45 years tumour 1–4 cm and no metastases (T2, N0, M0 and T3, N0 M0)	30
III	>45 years with tumour extending beyond the thyroid capsule with or without lymph node metastases (T4, N0, M0 and any T, N1, M0)	
IV	>45 years with distant metastases (any T, any N, M1)	60.9

thyroid cancers after the Chernobyl accident, and RET/PTC3 was present in 19/25 of the unusual solid/follicular subset of papillary cancers seen in affected children.[41]

RAS

The RAS genes encode signal transducing proteins involved in the transduction of intracellular signalling from the cell surface to the nucleus in a similar way to G proteins. RAS activation stimulates mitosis and reduced differentiation. There are three separate RAS genes, Ki-RAS, N-RAS and Ha-RAS, and point mutations have been identified in thyroid cancers. These point mutations (usually codons 12, 13 or 61) can produce activated RAS, which is potently oncogenic. RAS mutations are uncommon in conventional papillary thyroid cancer (less than 10 per cent) but are frequently present in follicular variant PTC. RAS mutations are equally prevalent (around 50 per cent) in follicular adenomas and carcinomas. These mutations seem to predispose to development of poorly or undifferentiated carcinomas, such as anaplastic tumours. Activated RAS transfected into normal human follicular cells *in vitro* leads to an increase in cell proliferation, which is a key step in tumour formation.

TRK

TRK is an oncogene, located on chromosome 1q22, which codes for a transmembrane tyrosine kinase receptor, whose ligand is nerve growth factor. It is mutated in 10–25 per cent of papillary carcinomas. Similar to RET, the TRK gene undergoes oncogenic activation by rearrangement of chromosomes. They are less common than RET rearrangements in PTC and the incidence in post-Chernobyl PTC is around 3 per cent.

BRAF

The RAF proteins are serine/threonine protein kinases that are critically involved in cell proliferation, differentiation and apoptosis by signalling along the mitogen-activated protein kinase (MAPK) pathway. There are three forms: ARAF, BRAF and CRAF. BRAF is the prominent form in thyroid follicular cells and of the three it is the most potent activator of the MAPK pathway. BRAF mutations have been demonstrated in 40–70 per cent of PTC of most types, except follicular variant PTC. There is also evidence that BRAF mutations are associated with poor clinical outcome in PTC.[42] They are also frequently seen in poorly differentiated or anaplastic carcinomas, particularly those with a papillary component, implying these tumours may develop from BRAF-positive PTC that dedifferentiate.[43] BRAF mutations are, however, not commonly seen in radiation-induced thyroid cancers.

PPPAX8–PPARγ

This gene rearrangement is the result of a recurrent translocation seen in follicular lesions of the thyroid. The consequence of the translocation is fusion of the DNA of the thyroid transcription factor PAX8 to domains A–F of the peroxisome proliferation-activated receptor (PPAR). PAX8-PPARγ rearrangements are seen more commonly in follicular carcinomas compared to adenomas (53 versus 8 per cent)[44] and are more frequent in patients with a history of radiation exposure. PAX8-PPARγ-positive follicular carcinomas are likely to be widely invasive while tumours negative for this rearrangement are for the most part minimally invasive.

TREATMENT OF DTC

There are many historical controversies regarding the optimal treatment of DTC, which mainly relate to the type of operation and the extent of thyroid surgery. Few dispute that the mainstay of treatment for DTC is surgery with radioactive iodine remnant ablation and thyroxine suppression. External beam radiation (and even chemotherapy) is also occasionally offered as adjuvant therapy. However, the extent of surgery is a widely debated issue and relates to lobectomy versus near-total or total thyroidectomy, particularly in low risk disease based on the prognostic indicators discussed earlier. The arguments for and against total thyroidectomy are shown in **Table 23.9**.[45]

The arguments for and against lobectomy versus total thyroidectomy also vary with the tumour type. It is recognized that PTC can be multifocal in up to 80 per cent of cases and that 50 per cent of the foci can be in the contralateral lobe.[46] Despite this, local recurrence rates in patients with PTC have been shown to be only around 5 per cent.[47] The group at the MSK Cancer Centre argue strongly for conservative surgery in the form of lobectomy alone in low risk DTC, including PTC, because of the low mortality rates

Table 23.9 The arguments for and against total thyroidectomy.[45]

'Total' thyroidectomy	'Less than total' thyroidectomy
Radioactive iodine can be used to detect and treat residual normal thyroid or local or distant metastases	Fewer complications develop
Serum thyroglobulin is a more sensitive marker of recurrence when all normal thyroid is removed	One half of local recurrences can be cured with surgery
The microscopic foci of cancer present in up to 30–70% of patients are eliminated as sites of recurrence	Less than 5% of recurrences occur in the thyroid bed
Recurrent cancer develops in the remaining contralateral lobe in approximately 5–15% of patients and one half of these may die of thyroid cancer	Little clinical significance is given to multicentricity
Recurrence is lower in patients who have undergone total thyroidectomy	Prognosis is good with lesser procedures
Facilitates accurate follow up and staging	
Improved survival rates	
Is the treatment of choice for multinodular goitre and thyrotoxicosis	
Minimal complications of total thyroidectomy in experienced hands	

(1 per cent at 20 years).[48] However, little mention is made of the rates of local and regional recurrence which although may not influence survival, certainly contribute to the morbidity of the disease with respect to reoperation, further adjuvant therapy and potential complications. Analysis of a large series of patients with low risk PTC treated at the Mayo clinic over 50 years demonstrated a significant difference in local recurrence rates between those treated with bilateral lobar resection and unilateral lobectomy (2 and 14 per cent respectively ($p = 0.0001$)).[49] This paper also showed a significant difference in regional recurrence rates favouring bilateral resection but no difference between the two approaches with respect to distant recurrence rates or cause-specific mortality.[49] Total or near-total thyroidectomy is usually recommended because of the probable reduction in local and regional recurrence, even though there is probably no influence on survival.[50]

Postoperative radioactive iodine may obscure the effect of surgery, although it would seem that surgery and ^{131}I therapy have independent effects on recurrence and cancer mortality.[51]

In FTC, multifocality and lymph node recurrence are not common and the arguments for total thyroidectomy versus lobectomy surround detection of recurrence with thyroglobulin levels and risks of distant disease and mortality. Usually the decision to perform completion thyroidectomy at a second operation is made once formal analysis of the ipsilateral tumour has been performed following original lobectomy.[52] Data from the Mayo clinic showed that in low risk FTC where vascular invasion is absent there were no distant metastatic recurrences and no cause-specific deaths.[13] The authors in this series and others argue for conservative surgery in minimally invasive FTC because of the low recurrence and mortality rates.[11]

It is well recognized that there are difficulties with making evidence-based decisions in the management of DTC. The vast majority of patients are in the low risk category and the disease is indolent with low recurrence and mortality rates. For these reasons there are no large prospective series with adequate follow-up periods. The data available are therefore based on retrospective analysis of large groups of patients treated in single institutions over long periods of time. The data are often incomplete, and treatment strategies and quality can vary over the time the analysis occurs. Nevertheless, these data are the best that we have and surgeons treating patients with DTC must have a rational and consistent therapeutic strategy based on this evidence. In an attempt to standardize treatment, both the British Thyroid Association (BTA) in association with the Royal College of Physicians and the American Thyroid Association (ATA) have developed guidelines for the management of thyroid cancer. The BTA first published guidelines in 2002[53] and updated them in 2007.[4] The American guidelines were first published in 1996[54] and last updated in 2009.[5]

Although there are some recognized differences between these guidelines,[55] they both offer an up-to-date review of the current evidence available in the management of this complex disease. There is agreement in principle about methods of treatment, with recommendations including more use of ultrasound as both an initial investigation and at follow up, more total thyroidectomies, increased use of central neck dissection and less radioiodine. The UK guidelines[4] will form the basis of the recommendations for treatment made in this chapter.

SURGICAL TREATMENT OF DTC

Surgery is the mainstay of treatment in DTC and the main aim of initial therapy is to remove the primary tumour disease and that which has spread beyond the thyroid capsule and involved cervical lymph nodes. Other goals are to minimize treatment- and disease-related morbidity and to permit accurate staging of the disease. Thyroidectomy facilitates postoperative treatment with radioactive iodine and appropriate treatment minimizes the risk of disease recurrence and metastatic spread and caters for long-term accurate surveillance.[4] Surgical options for treatment of the thyroid gland should be limited to a lobectomy (the complete removal of one thyroid lobe including the isthmus), near-total lobectomy (a total lobectomy leaving behind the smallest amount of thyroid tissue (less than 1 g) to protect the recurrent laryngeal nerve), a near-total thyroidectomy (either a complete lobectomy on one side and near-total on the other or a bilateral near-total lobectomy or a total thyroidectomy (complete removal of both lobes of the gland, the isthmus and the pyramidal lobe). These operations are illustrated in **Figure 23.12**.

Traditionally, lymph node metastases have not been thought to be a significant prognostic indicator in DTC, but recent studies have demonstrated that this is not the case in high risk patients (particularly those over 45 years).[56] In addition, lymph node involvement has been shown to increase the risk of local and particularly regional recurrence.[56] Traditional methods of selective nodal excision (berry picking) have been shown to result in higher rates of recurrence than systematic compartment orientated nodal dissection such as a selective neck dissection[57] and most

institutions recommend selective or comprehensive dissection for previously untreated neck disease.

Surgical management of involved cervical lymph nodes requires an understanding of the lymph node anatomy of the neck and likely patterns of spread of disease to the lymph nodes. The neck is divided into lateral and central compartments. Each compartment is further divided into levels as outlined in **Table 23.10** and as seen in **Figure 23.13**. There are two main categories of neck dissection; a comprehensive neck dissection involves resecting levels I–V and is subclassified based on the type and amount of other structures excised; a selective neck dissection involves removing some, but not all, of levels I–V and preservation of the internal jugular vein, spinal accessory nerve and sternocleidomastoid muscle. The types of neck dissection are described in detail in Chapter 36, Neck dissection. It is well recognized that regional metastases from PTC are most commonly found in level VI.[58] These nodes are often very difficult to palpate and may therefore only be found at surgery or preoperatively with imaging and possibly ultrasound guided FNAC. In the lateral neck, in patients with palpable nodal disease, the most frequently involved levels are II, III and IV and of these level III is most common.[20] Level II is next most frequently involved and level IIb above the nerve is recognized to harbour positive lymph nodes in a significant number of patients.[59]

Levels V and I are usually only affected when there is involvement of multiple neck levels.[60] In addition, multiple levels are more frequently involved than single levels in this group of patients.[20] Recently, clinically node-negative high risk patients (more than 45 years) have been demonstrated to have higher rates of occult nodal involvement than low risk patients and that even rates in patients less than 45 years are around 30 per cent.[61] There is also an increase in the incidence of recurrence in the central compartment. Repeat surgery in the central area is associated with a higher risk of permanent hypoparathyroidism and recurrent laryngeal nerve injury than central neck dissection performed at the time of total thyroidectomy.[62, 63] It is advised that level VI node dissection should be performed at the same time as total thyroidectomy,[4] and that there is no increased morbidity associated with this procedure.[64] It is argued that microscopic nodal disease in the central compartment can be effectively treated by radioactive iodine. However, some papillary carcinomas do not concentrate iodine and this has been demonstrated particularly in the cells of older

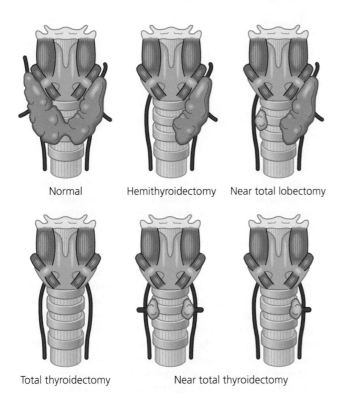

Normal   Hemithyroidectomy   Near total lobectomy

Total thyroidectomy   Near total thyroidectomy

Figure 23.12 Surgical options for management of the thyroid gland.

Table 23.10 Cervical lymph node levels.

Lateral compartment	I	Submental and submandibular nodes further divided by anterior belly of digastric muscle into Ia and Ib
	II	Deep cervical nodes from the skull base to the level of the hyoid. Further divided by the relationship to the accessory nerve (level 2a being medial and 2b lateral)
	III	Deep cervical nodes from the level of the hyoid to the cricoid
	IV	Deep cervical nodes from the level of the cricoid to the suprasternal notch
	V	Posterior triangle nodes can be divided by their relationship to a plane drawn through the level of the cricoid cartilage. (Va is above and Vb is below the accessory nerve)
Central compartment	VI	Pre- and paratracheal nodes from the level of the hyoid bone above to the sternal notch below and the carotid artery laterally
Mediastinal compartment	VII	Superior mediastinal nodes as far as the superior aspect of the brachiocephalic vein

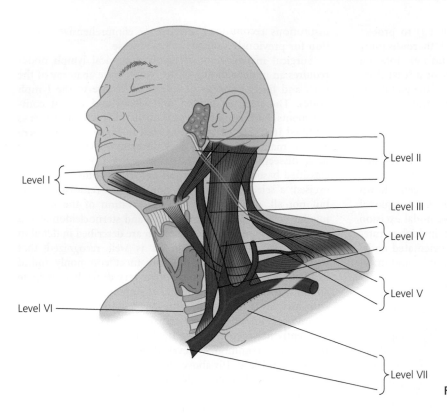

Level I

Level II

Level III

Level IV

Level V

Level VI

Level VII

Figure 23.13 Cervical lymph node levels.

patients' tumours, potentially reducing the efficacy of this treatment.[65]

SURGICAL MANAGEMENT OF THE THYROID GLAND IN PAPILLARY THYROID CANCER

Patients with cancers 1 cm in diameter or less without evidence of lymph node metastases can be adequately treated by lobectomy and thyroxine suppressive therapy. In the majority of patients with tumours greater than 1 cm, multifocal disease, familial disease, extrathyroid extension and positive lymph node involvement or distant metastases, total thyroidectomy is indicated. Total or near-total thyroidectomy is also indicated in those with a history of previous radiation exposure in childhood.[4] If the diagnosis of PTC is made after lobectomy and completion thyroidectomy is required, the operation should be offered within 8 weeks of histological diagnosis. In this situation, if the risk of recurrence is judged to be low, lobectomy alone may be appropriate in tumours larger than 1 cm in diameter.[4]

SURGICAL MANAGEMENT OF THE THYROID IN FTC

FNAC cannot differentiate between hyperplasia, a benign colloid nodule, a follicular adenoma or carcinoma and Thy3 cytology mandates at least a lobectomy and subsequent histological examination. Frozen section is not helpful when FNAC demonstrates a follicular lesion[66] and should not be used in lobectomy for Thy3 lesions. The UK guidelines for the management of thyroid cancer make the following grade B and

C recommendations based on level III and IV evidence.[4] A follicular carcinoma less than 1 cm in diameter with no capsular invasion should be treated by lobectomy only. Patients with follicular carcinoma showing evidence of vascular invasion should undergo total thyroidectomy. Patients with follicular carcinomas greater than 4 cm in diameter should be treated with a total or near-total thyroidectomy. Low risk patients (females, age less than 45 years) with tumours less than 2 cm in diameter may be managed by lobectomy and thyroxine therapy following multidisciplinary team (MDT) discussion and informed consent. Clear recommendations for low risk patients with tumours 2–4 cm in diameter cannot be made and treatment should be at the recommendation of the MDT. If the diagnosis of thyroid cancer is made and completion thyroidectomy is indicated, the guidelines recommend performing the surgery within 8 weeks of histological diagnosis.[4]

SURGICAL MANAGEMENT OF THE NECK IN DTC

The BTA 2007 guidelines make the following grade C recommendations based on level IV data. In PTC, nodal disease in level VI discovered at surgery is treated with a central (level VI) neck dissection. If suspicious or clinically involved nodes are identified in the lateral neck and are confirmed by FNAC or by intraoperative frozen section, then a selective neck dissection incorporating levels IIa–Vb with preservation of the spinal accessory nerve (SAN), internal jugular vein (IJV) and sternocleidomastoid muscle (SCM) should be performed. The guidelines also state that node-positive FTC should be managed in a similar way. In patients with PTC and clinically uninvolved nodes but who are deemed high-risk (i.e. any of the following features: male, age greater than 45 years, tumours greater than 4 cm diameter, presence of extracapsular or extrathyroidal disease), then total thyroidectomy and level VI node dissection should be performed.[4, 5]

If the neck disease involves surrounding structures such as the IJV, SCM or skin, then these structures, should also be excised as part of the lateral neck dissection. Level IIb may also be addressed as there is evidence of moderate risk of these nodes being involved and recurrent disease is difficult to treat at this site.[59]

The options for surgery on a solitary thyroid nodule based on Thy3, Thy4 or Thy5 findings are shown in **Table 23.11**.

MANAGEMENT OF EXTRATHYROID EXTENSION

Although DTC is usually an indolent disease with a good prognosis, 8–26 per cent of patients can present with locally advanced cancer with invasion of surrounding structures, leading to increased morbidity and mortality.[67, 68, 69] The presence of extrathyroidal extension (ETE) is associated with higher rates of overall recurrence and mortality than tumours confined to the thyroid,[68] with local airway invasion being the cause of death in up to 50 per cent of deaths due to DTC.[70]

Although ETE occurs in both papillary and follicular carcinomas with equal frequency, it is seen more frequently in PTC due to its higher incidence. The prognostic risk factors significantly associated with ETE in PTC include age greater than 50 years, tumour size greater than 4 cm, non-encapsulated tumours and aggressive histological variants (diffuse sclerosing, solid, tall cell and poorly differentiated).[68] The strap muscles, recurrent nerve and trachea are the most common extrathyroid structures involved in the central neck compartment; the oesophagus is less so but is usually associated with laryngotracheal invasion. In the lateral neck the SCM, IJV, carotid artery, cranial nerves X, XI, phrenic and cervical sympathetic chain can all be involved either from direct thyroid tumour extension or from extranodal extension from cervical metastatic nodes.[71] ETE is associated with higher rates of lymph node metastases and distant metastases than tumours without ETE[68] and it is also seen more commonly in patients who present with recurrent DTC. The MACIS and AMES prognostic scoring systems include ETE as an indicator of poorer prognosis and higher risk.

Surgery is widely recognized to be the most effective management of ETE in DTC and it is felt that complete excision of tumour results in lower recurrence rates and mortality.[67] This is, however, controversial and many papers present conflicting evidence. If the invaded structure is easily resected with minimal morbidity (e.g. strap muscles or recurrent laryngeal nerve), then there is generally no argument and most authors recommend excision to obtain clear histological margins. The more difficult decision is whether to perform radical excision when there is invasion of the laryngopharynx, trachea and oesophagus, or both recurrent laryngeal nerves. Some authors recommend preservation of a functional nerve even if it is clinically invaded by tumour because complete excision of papillary carcinoma with resection of the recurrent laryngeal nerve does not improve survival over incomplete excision.[72] The UK guidelines recommend incomplete excision of tumour, preservation of one or both recurrent laryngeal nerves and treatment with postoperative ^{131}I and thyroxine suppression, plus or minus external beam radiation if both recurrent laryngeal nerves are threatened.[4] Where there is superficial invasion of the laryngotracheal tree and where limited resection such as shaving leaves behind only microscopic disease, it appears that local recurrence and survival results are comparable with patients treated with completely excised invasive tumour. However, if gross disease is left behind, recurrence rates are significantly higher and survival is significantly reduced.[69, 73] If there is gross invasion of the trachea or larynx, and particularly if there is intraluminal involvement, then radical resection including circumferential or partial resection of the tracheal wall and partial or total laryngectomy will reduce local recurrence rates and improve survival. An alternative to surgery is external beam radiotherapy plus or minus radioactive iodine. In patients where there is ETE, it has been shown that the addition of external beam radiation therapy offers improved locoregional control even where gross macroscopic disease has been completely excised.[74] The UK guidelines recommend this treatment particularly in patients where the residual tumour fails to concentrate sufficient amounts of radioactive iodine.[4]

MANAGEMENT OF DIFFERENTIATED THYROID CANCER IN PREGNANCY

As DTC is three times more common in women and the majority is low risk disease occurring in younger people, it is

Table 23.11   Solitary thyroid nodule – options for surgery.

Follicular lesion (Thy3)	Suspicious for carcinoma (Thy4)	Papillary carcinoma (Thy5)	Medullary carcinoma (Thy5)
↓	↓	↓	↓
Diagnostic hemi-thyroidectomy	Diagnostic hemi-thyroidectomy ± complete Frozen section and proceed ?Total thyroidectomy	Total thyroidectomy ± neck dissection Central neck dissection in high risk patients	Total thyroidectomy and level 6+7 dissection Lateral neck dissection in high risk patients

inevitable that the head and neck surgeon will be faced with patients being diagnosed during pregnancy at some time during their career. Women presenting with a thyroid nodule during pregnancy have a higher chance of the nodule proving to be malignant than non-pregnant women.[75] A diagnosis of DTC during pregnancy creates added anxiety with uncertainty regarding the optimal timing of treatment delivery and the impact on maternal and neonatal morbidity. Human pregnancy has been shown to accelerate the growth of thyroid cancers,[76] but despite an increase in size of the tumours it seems that there is no impact on prognosis if treatment is delayed until after delivery compared to patients treated during their pregnancy.[77, 78, 79] If a woman is diagnosed early in her pregnancy there will obviously be greater delay to treatment time if surgery is postponed until after delivery than if she is diagnosed later on. There are reports suggesting that delays greater than one year can lead to poorer prognosis.[51, 80]

There is significant risk to the fetus if an operation is performed during the first trimester and a higher risk for maternal vascular complications if elective surgery is performed in the third trimester. Another consideration is that postponing surgery until the postpartum period can interfere with infant care and breastfeeding protocols and can lead to further delays in treatment. Clearly, if there is symptomatic compression with airway compromise caused by the thyroid disease at any time during pregnancy early intervention is necessary.[81] There is controversy regarding the optimal timing of surgery and authors generally recommend either performing surgery during the second trimester[4, 82] or to delay treatment until after delivery.[77, 78, 79] Adjuvant treatment with radioiodine should be delayed until after delivery and breastfeeding is completed but suppressive doses of thyroxine are safe to use during pregnancy.

MANAGEMENT OF DTC IN CHILDHOOD

Although uncommon, thyroid nodules presenting in children are more likely to be malignant than in their adult counterparts.[83] DTC frequently presents at a more advanced stage in children and young people than in adults, with a higher rate of lymph node and distant metastases and higher postoperative rates of lymph node recurrence, particularly if they are younger than 10 years old.[84, 85] Recurrences are also more common in patients who have positive lymph nodes and who have multifocal thyroid carcinoma.[86] Despite these seemingly poor features, DTC in children tends to be less fatal than in adults and overall survival is significantly better even if they have distant metastatic disease.[84, 87] Children with a history of radiation exposure are at particular risk of developing thyroid cancer and should be followed up closely. Any nodular thyroid disease should be regarded with a high index of suspicion and treated aggressively.[88]

The general principles of treatment are the same as in adults. A total thyroidectomy is usually recommended as management for the primary tumour site within the gland, and selective neck dissection performed for positive nodal disease. Radioactive iodine treatment is advised, particularly for patients under 10 years old, followed by vigilant follow up with thyroxine suppression and lifelong serial serum thyroglobulin levels.[4]

ADJUVANT THERAPIES

The relevant adjunctive treatment modalities in DTC include radioactive iodine treatment, TSH suppression using thyroxine and external beam radiotherapy in selected cases. Details of these therapies are covered in Chapter 26, Non-surgical management of thyroid cancer, but a summary is appropriate here.

Radioactive iodine

A recent systematic review and meta-analysis of studies investigating the effectiveness of radioactive iodine remnant ablation in DTC suggested a statistically significant reduction in locoregional recurrence, and that ten-year distant metastatic rates were lower in patients treated with radioactive iodine remnant ablation following bilateral surgery for DTC. The data from this analysis did not allow the formulation of an optimal dose of radioactive iodine, nor could they confirm the decrease in recurrence and possible mortality in low risk patients with DTC.[89] The BTA guidelines state that there is no indication for radioactive iodine ablation if patients have all of the following features: all tumours measuring 1 cm or less in diameter; N0, M0 tumours or MIFC without vascular invasion smaller than 2 cm in diameter; favourable histology; complete surgery and no extension beyond the thyroid capsule. Also included are absolute and relative indications for ablation, dose and safety recommendations.[4]

External beam radiotherapy

As discussed above under Management of extrathyroid extension, external beam radiotherapy is indicated where there is high risk of locoregional recurrence. This includes patients with extensive extrathyroid invasion and extranodal extension even where the disease has been completely resected. Also included are older patients in whom the tumour may fail to concentrate sufficient amounts of radioiodine.[5, 74] It may also be used as primary treatment in selected cases.[4]

Thyroxine suppressive therapy

There is evidence that doses of thyroxine adequate to suppress TSH can increase recurrence-free survival in patients with DTC and that TSH suppression is an independent predictor of recurrence-free survival.[90, 91] Not all studies confirm this and the evidence is certainly not as clear in low risk patients.[92] Because of this, and the long-term risk of osteoporosis and cardiac complications, most authors now recommend that TSH is maintained at the lower limit of normal with the T4 as close to the normal range as possible.[4]

FOLLOW UP

Recurrence rates in DTC are around 30 per cent over long periods and around 60 per cent of these recurrences occur in the first 10 years.[51] Early detection of both locoregional and distant recurrences can lead to cure or at least favourable long-term survival if the disease is surgically resectable or takes up radioactive iodine.[93] It is imperative, therefore, that the treating team has a surveillance strategy for patients treated for DTC.

A patient with low risk DTC is considered disease free after total thyroidectomy and ^{131}I remnant ablation if the following criteria are fulfilled: all identifiable tumour has been resected, there is no clinical evidence of tumour, post-radioiodine scanning shows no uptake outside the thyroid bed, neck ultrasound results are negative, serum Tg anti-bodies are negative and Tg is undetectable (less than 1 µg/L) during TSH suppression and stimulation.[94, 95]

It is highly likely based on recent observations with increasingly sensitive tools that these so-called recurrences are in fact cases of persistent tumour that have fallen below the threshold of detection offered by the tests available to treating surgeons and physicians.[4]

THYROGLOBULIN LEVELS

Thyroglobulin (Tg) is a 660 kDa, dimeric protein produced by and used entirely within the thyroid gland. Tg is produced by thyroid follicular cells and is secreted and stored in the follicular lumen. It is also produced by DTC cells and can be used to detect residual or recurrent carcinomas following total thyroidectomy and radioactive iodine ablation of thyroid remnants. Thyroglobulin levels are less sensitive in patients who have had lobectomy or in patients who have antithyroglobulin antibodies.[51, 96]

It is recognized that measurement of serum Tg levels during TSH suppression with thyroxine often leads to failure to identify persistent tumour. TSH-stimulated Tg measurements with either thyroxine withdrawal or recombinant human TSH (rhTSH) are required to accurately identify recurrences.[95, 97] It has been demonstrated that a combination of stimulated TSH measurements and ultrasound scan has the highest sensitivity and negative predictive value for monitoring patients with DTC.[98] In addition, it is recommended that serial stimulated TSH measurement should be the principal test in the follow-up management of low risk DTC. Serial measurements of TSH are more useful than one off measurements and recurrence in DTC is indicated by a gradual rise in the serum Tg levels which reflects a change in the tumour mass.[99]

RADIOLOGICAL IMAGING STUDIES IN PATIENTS WITH ELEVATED SERUM TG LEVELS

Of the 30 per cent of DTC patients that recur, around 70 per cent do so locoregionally and the remainder recur at distant sites, most frequently the lungs.[51] Imaging studies in patients with elevated serum Tg levels then should be primarily targeted to examining the central and lateral neck structures and secondarily to distant sites. The approach to detecting metastases should be the least disruptive to the patient and the most cost effective. Neck ultrasound is followed by low-dose radioiodine whole body scanning if no locoregional recurrence is detected. Other imaging modalities, such as CT or MRI should only be used to plan for surgical resection of macroscopic recurrence. F[18]-fluorodeoxyglucose positron emission tomography (FDG-PET) CT scans are expensive but may be useful in patients where neck ultrasound is negative, in patients who are whole body iodine image negative and Tg positive, or when there is poor uptake of radioactive iodine precluding the use of radioiodine whole body scanning.

Neck ultrasound

Scanning of the central and lateral neck in patients who have been treated for thyroid cancer and have an elevated Tg will demonstrate recurrence in the central or lateral nodes or in neck soft tissues in around two-thirds of cases.[96, 100] It is a much more sensitive investigation in detecting disease recurrence than palpation. Ultrasound is useful in differentiating malignant from benign lymph nodes as malignant nodes tend to be larger, rounder and lose their hilar characteristics.[27] Ultrasound can also be used to guide FNAC of radiologically suspicious lymph nodes or thyroid remnants to provide a tissue diagnosis and the needle washings can be analysed for thyroglobulin to increase the sensitivity of this test.[101] Ultrasound is a useful imaging modality in children who have a high rate of regional recurrence and require regular surveillance because it is less invasive than other imaging modalities and is well tolerated.[102]

Whole body radioactive iodine scanning

Following total thyroidectomy and radioactive iodine ablation, whole body scanning with low dose ^{131}I is a relatively insensitive test for disease recurrence when compared to serial thyroglobulin measurement.[95, 96] It has the potential to miss large numbers of foci of recurrent disease in all risk groups but there is a particular concern in older patients in whom DTC has a lower avidity for radioactive iodine[65] and in whom there is a higher risk of nodal disease and recurrence and a worse prognosis.[56] More and more, routine ^{131}I whole body scanning post-ablation is being abandoned in low risk patients since the majority will have negative scans and serum thyroglobulin is a more sensitive, accurate investigative and monitoring tool.[5] Post-treatment whole body scanning following ablative radioactive iodine treatment is more sensitive because of the higher doses used. It will reveal new foci of tumour in up to 50 per cent of patients who were negative on diagnostic scanning with a substantial number of these being distant metastases.[96] This has led to the empirical treatment of patients with elevated serum thyroglobulin levels with ablative doses of [131]I. The argument against this is that patients may be more effectively treated with targeted therapy and also that patients may be over-treated and cumulative high dose radioactive iodine treatment has some associated long-term risks.[96] However, there may be a role for empirical treatment in patients who have particularly high Tg levels or rising stimulated Tg levels on serial testing.[96]

FDG–PET CT scanning

Of the variety of imaging studies used to investigate patients with elevated or rising Tg levels following treatment for DTC, FDG-PET CT scanning appears to be the most sensitive test.[103] The sensitivity in detecting metastases in DTC increases with increasing thyroglobulin levels.[56] Studies have shown that in patients with elevated serum Tg levels and a negative diagnostic radioactive iodine whole body scan, FDG-PET CT scans can demonstrate disease that is amenable to surgery and can lead to disease-free status in a significant number of patients.[104] In addition, FDG-PET CT scanning appears particularly useful in tumours that do not concentrate radioactive iodine where radioiodine scanning is not at all useful and where metastases have a poorer prognosis.[96] One group of authors demonstrated the poor prognostic significance of a positive PET scan with a significant survival difference between patients that were PET positive and those that were negative. The avidity and volume of FDG uptake was also predictive of survival.[105] F[18]-FDG-PET scans are usually now performed with simultaneous CT scan to give accurate anatomical information in addition to the biological information offered by PET. PET-CT is the investigation of choice in this scenario.

A surveillance programme for patients treated for DTC therefore should include serial stimulated Tg levels either off thyroxine or after the use of intramuscular RhTSH. If the levels increase, a neck ultrasound should be performed and this can be combined with FNAC and Tg estimation on the needle washout if cytology is equivocal. If the ultrasound does not show adequate disease to explain the elevated Tg level, a diagnostic radioactive iodine scan is appropriate and if this is negative then progression to a F[18]-FDG-PET CT scan is appropriate.

SURGICAL MANAGEMENT OF RECURRENT DTC

It is likely that many of the recurrences seen in DTC are in fact progression of persistent initial disease that was not detected prior to primary treatment. There are a number of factors that predict for higher rates of recurrence. These can be split into patient (age greater than 60 or less than 20), tumour (size greater than 4 cm, multifocality, postoperative residual disease and lymph node involvement) and treatment (less than near-total thyroidectomy and the lack of use of radioiodine).[106] The experience of the surgeon should also be taken into account.[4] The majority of recurrences occur in the neck,[51] either in the thyroid bed or in the regional lymph node basins, and the prognosis is better for these patients than it is for patients who develop distant metastases.[107] This is mainly because locoregional disease can be treated in a multimodal fashion and treatment of distant disease is more limited. Recurrence of any sort has been shown to have a negative impact on survival and patients who develop multiple recurrences have a poorer prognosis.[108]

Management of locoregional recurrence includes accurate detection of the site, volume and invasiveness of disease, and determination of whether the disease takes up radioactive iodine. Surgery is again the mainstay of management of local and regional recurrence, particularly with palpable disease,

however there is evidence that disease detected by scintigraphy can be adequately treated using ablative doses of [131]I.[108] The issues in repeat central compartment surgery are whether the recurrence is in residual thyroid gland, nodes or invading surrounding tissues and the risk of re-operation to the recurrent and external laryngeal nerves and parathyroid glands. There are reports that demonstrate increased rates of nerve injury and hypoparathyroidism with revision central compartment surgery[62, 63] but there are also data that show with a systematic approach and careful technique complications can be minimized.[109, 110] A comprehensive compartment orientated clearance of level VI should be performed with skeletonization of the recurrent laryngeal nerves and careful preservation of the parathyroids on vascular pedicles. Recurrent nodal disease in the lateral neck is more frequent in the very young and in those who have had positive nodes previously treated, particularly those with large numbers of involved nodes.[86, 111] In a neck that has been previously dissected, a single focus or multiple separate foci of nodal recurrence may be treated by local lymphadenectomy, however if there has been only a 'berry pick' approach used then a compartment orientated selective neck dissection should be used to treat neck recurrence.

If the recurrence is not in the thyroid bed or cervical lymph nodes, then it is likely to involve one or more of the sites listed in **Box 23.4**.[4]

Details of how to manage these are covered in Chapter 26, Non-surgical management of thyroid cancer, as well as the BTA Guidelines.[4] Metastatic disease involving lung and other soft tissue areas are not usually amenable to surgery and should be treated with ^{131}I therapy. There is no maximum limit to the cumulative ^{131}I dose that can be given to patients with persistent recurrent disease.[4] Extensive bony metastases are generally not curable by ^{131}I therapy alone. For solitary or limited number of bony metastases that are not cured by ^{131}I therapy, external beam radiotherapy, with or without resection and/or embolization should be considered in selected cases.[4]

SURGICAL ANATOMY

It is vitally important for the head and neck surgeon to have a thorough understanding of thyroid anatomy as well as the pathology and natural history of thyroid nodules in order to be able to treat them with minimal morbidity since the majority are either usually benign or of low grade malignancy, all with an excellent prognosis. It is also important

---

Box 23.4   Likely metastatic sites of DTC (excluding cervical and mediastinal lymph nodes)

- Metastatic disease involving lung and other soft tissue areas
- Bone metastases
- Cerebral metastases
- Other metastatic sites
- Unknown metastatic sites

to note that the outcome of a poorly performed operation could be worse than the outcome from an untreated thyroid nodule.

The thyroid gland is made of up two lateral lobes, which extend from the sides of the thyroid cartilage down to the sixth tracheal ring. These are joined together in the midline by the isthmus, which overlies the second to fourth tracheal rings. In addition, there is often a pyramidal lobe which projects up from the isthmus, usually on the left-hand side. The gland is enclosed in the pretracheal fascia, covered by the strap muscles and overlapped laterally by the sternomastoid muscles. Superficial to the sternohyoid muscle, the anterior jugular veins cross over the central neck. On the deep aspect of the gland lie the larynx and the trachea with the pharynx and oesophagus behind and the carotid sheath laterally. On either side, there are two important nerves: the external branch of the superior laryngeal nerve and the recurrent laryngeal nerve; both lie in close proximity to the gland and its blood supply. In addition, the cutaneous nerves C2 and C3 run superficial to the deep investing layer of cervical fascia and can be damaged at the time of surgery when the flaps are elevated. This results in anaesthesia of the anterior neck skin, which can be particularly troublesome to men when shaving.

The external branch of the superior laryngeal nerve lies deep to the upper pole of the gland as it passes superficial to the cricothyroid muscle in the sternothyrolaryngeal (Joll's) triangle (**Figure 23.14**). This triangle is formed laterally by the upper pole of the gland and the superior thyroid vessels, superiorly by the attachment of the strap muscles and deep investing layer of fascia to the hyoid and medially by the midline. Its floor is the cricothyroid muscle and its roof is made up of the strap muscles, it usually contains the external laryngeal nerve running on cricothyroid. There are three anatomical variations of the nerve described.[112] A type I nerve (17 per cent) crosses the superior thyroid pedicle more than 1 cm above the superior thyroid pole and enters the cricothyroid muscle. In a type IIa configuration (the most common variant (56 per cent)), the nerve passes within 1 cm of the superior pole while in a type IIb variation, the external branch of the superior laryngeal nerve passes onto the cricothyroid muscle below the level of the superior thyroid pole. The type IIb nerve is the most commonly injured and the frequency of damage increases with the size of the goitre.[112]

The recurrent laryngeal nerves run in, or lateral to, the tracheo-oesophageal groove and have a variable relationship with the branches of the inferior thyroid artery. They can run either in front of, behind or indeed between these branches. It is common for the nerve to divide into several branches before entering the larynx and there may be extralaryngeal branches as far as 3–4 cm below the inferior border of the cricoid cartilage. On the left side, the nerve ascends from the chest having circumnavigated the aortic arch. However, on the right side the nerve is more superficial, being 45° to the tracheo-oesophageal groove since it only has to pass around the artery of the 4th arch (the subclavian). On the right, it is important to remember that in approximately 2 per cent of patients the nerve may be non-recurrent and is then found more superiorly in the paracarotid tunnel where it runs with the inferior thyroid vessels en route to the larynx.

The inferior thyroid artery arises from the thyrocervical trunk, a branch of the first part of the subclavian artery. It passes medially behind the carotid artery and then pierces the prevertebral fascia medial to the carotid sheath to enter the posterior part of the thyroid gland. Additional blood supply sometimes comes from an inconstant vessel, the thyroid ima artery, which occurs in around 15 per cent of patients and arises from either the aortic arch or innominate artery (**Figure 23.15**).

The venous drainage of the thyroid is into the internal jugular vein via the superior thyroid vein which drains the upper pole. The middle thyroid vein drains the lateral part of the gland and there are multiple inferior thyroid veins which drain the lower pole of the gland into the brachiocephalic vein.

The parathyroid glands lie outside the thyroid capsule beneath the pretracheal fascia. In approximately 90 per cent of patients the blood supply to both superior and inferior glands is from the inferior thyroid artery and in a third of these cases there is also a significant supply through the thyroid capsule. In the remainder, both glands are supplied either by an anastomotic arch from the superior and inferior thyroid vessels or from the superior thyroid artery alone via posterior branches. The superior glands are more constant in their location and usually lie near the cricothyroid joint close to the recurrent laryngeal nerve, cephalic to the inferior thyroid artery (which is probably the best initial marker to locate them). The inferior glands are often more variable in their location, being caudal to where the recurrent laryngeal nerve and the inferior thyroid artery cross at the apex of Beahr's triangle. In half of the cases the inferior parathyroid glands are found in and around the lower pole of the thyroid gland and a quarter may be close to, or within, residual thymus tissue. As a general rule, parathyroid glands are located symmetrically (for embryological reasons) on either side of the neck, and this is often helpful

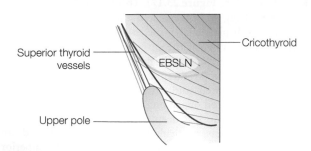

Figure 23.14 Joll's triangle.

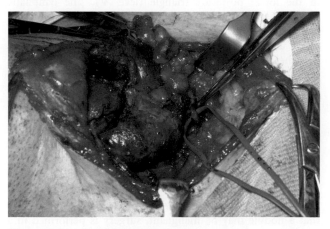

Figure 23.15 Thyroid Ima artery.

when looking for a missing gland. Most people have four parathyroids but approximately 10 per cent have more than four glands, while only 3 per cent have fewer than four glands. A healthy parathyroid usually measures on average just under 1 cm³ and is usually oval, varying in colour from light yellow in older patients to a reddish brownish colour in younger people, mainly because the fat content increases with age. It is useful to remember that in normal saline fat floats and parathyroid tissue sinks, although this is not a 100 per cent reliable test for parathyroid tissue and if there is doubt a frozen section should be performed on a small amount of gland. Parathyroid tissue can be found anywhere in the neck, including within the thyroid gland, as well as in the mediastinum where the location is usually intrathymic. Further detailed parathyroid anatomy is described in Chapter 27, Parathyroid tumours.

The primary lymphatic drainage from the thyroid is in a superior, lateral and inferior direction and follows the vascular pedicles of both the superior and inferior thyroid vessels, as well as the middle thyroid vein. The upper poles of the gland together with the isthmus and the pyramidal lobe drain superiorly, terminating in the lateral neck in levels II/III while the lateral aspect of each lobe drains into levels III and IV. The lower pole of the gland drains into the peri- and paratracheal nodes in level VI, and then onto both level IV and level VII nodes. Lymphatic drainage may also pass to nodes within the parapharyngeal and retropharyngeal spaces, but this usually tends to occur when other nodes are involved and shunting occurs, or when there has been previous treatment with either surgery or irradiation. It is very uncommon for differentiated thyroid malignancy to present initially with an isolated metastasis in the parapharyngeal space. There are also extensive communications between the lateral cervical lymph nodes in levels II, III and IV and the superior mediastinum via level VI. Subsequently, tumours in the upper pole tend to metastasize to levels II and III along the superior thyroid pedicle, in the middle third of the gland tumours spread to the perithyroid and paratracheal nodes (level VI) while those in the lower third spread predominately to the paratracheal nodes (level VI). Isthmus tumours spread most often to the pretracheal nodes (level VI). These drainage patterns are shown in **Box 23.5** and **Figure 23.16**.

From the primary echelon nodes in the central compartment, the major lymphatic drainage is to the middle and lower deep jugular nodes (level III and IV) and to the nodes in the lower posterior triangle (level V). The lymphatic pathways to these particular nodes follow the route of the inferior thyroid artery and frequently pass deep to the carotid artery and on the left can be intimately related to terminal branches of the thoracic duct. The inferior level VI nodes then drain to the mediastinal nodes (level VII).

SURGICAL TECHNIQUE IN DTC

Thyroidectomy

When a tumour is confined to the thyroid gland without any extrathyroidal extension, or when there is simply a suspicion that a nodule may be malignant, surgery is performed in a similar manner as for benign disease. A skin incision is made

---

> **Box 23.5 Lymphatic drainage of the thyroid gland**
>
> Major
>
> - Middle jugular nodes – level III
> - Lower jugular nodes – level IV
> - Posterior triangle nodes – level Vb
>
> Minor
>
> - Pretracheal and paratracheal nodes – level VI
> - Superior mediastinal nodes – level VII
>
> The lymph node groups at the highest risk of metastases from differentiated thyroid cancer are in the central compartment (level VI), lower jugular chain (levels III and VI) and the posterior triangle (level Vb).

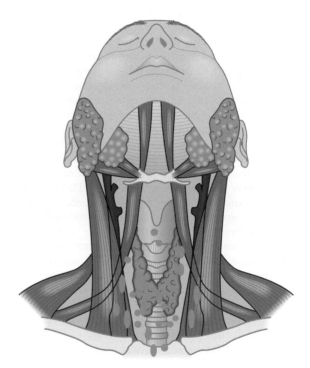

Figure 23.16   First echelon lymph node levels involved in thyroid cancer.

in, or closely paralleling, a low anterior neck skin crease (Kocher's incision; **Figure 23.17**). This is usually marked with the patient sitting up in the anaesthetic room.[113, 114] Flaps are raised in a sub-platysmal plane, or in a plane deep to the anterior jugular veins if the surgeon prefers to ligate these. The flaps are then sutured back, or kept open with a self-retaining Joll's retractor. Strap muscles are either separated in the midline, elevated and retracted laterally or they are divided and retracted depending on the surgeon's preference. One tip is to divide just deep to the sternothyroid muscle. This facilitates access, particularly to the upper pole, and can help minimize damage to the external branch of the superior laryngeal nerve. The muscle may be resutured back into position, or simply left which seems to have little effect on postoperative voice function. The thyroid gland is then exposed, the paracarotid tunnel entered and the middle thyroid vein divided. Dissection usually begins at the superior thyroid pole (particularly in the larger glands). The superior thyroid vessels are individually ligated and divided, and the superior pole is incrementally mobilized. Gentle downward and lateral retraction on the thyroid can be helpful during this procedure. As the mobilization proceeds, Joll's triangle is explored and the external branch of the superior laryngeal nerve may be seen at this point and identified and preserved although it is not necessary to find it in every case. Stimulation with an electrical nerve stimulator can help with identification. The posterior branches of the superior thyroid artery are often not dissected at this point because of their importance in the blood supply to the superior parathyroid glands. At this point, a superior parathyroid gland may be found medial to the upper pole in Joll's triangle although in 80 per cent of cases it is in its usual position, posterosuperiorly situated above the inferior thyroid artery (**Figure 23.18**).[113, 114] Attention then turns to the lower pole. Once the muscle and fascia have been elevated away from the inferior pole, the inferior thyroid veins are individually ligated and divided (**Figure 23.19**) and the anterior surface of the trachea exposed. It is important to realize that the recurrent laryngeal nerve can be damaged at this

point. The gland is mobilized medially, both parathyroids identified together with the recurrent laryngeal nerve. The lower parathyroid is usually found below and medial to the inferior thyroid artery close to or actually within the thyrothymic ligament (**Figure 23.20**).[113, 114] The recurrent laryngeal nerve is identified (with minimal disturbance) in the thyroid bed where it makes up the third side of Beahr's triangle,[113, 114] the other two sides being the inferior thyroid artery and the common carotid artery (**Figure 23.21**). An extracapsular dissection technique is then used on the gland across a broad front preserving the recurrent laryngeal nerve and two parathyroid glands. The assistant applies gentle but firm gradual sequential upward and medial traction using a swab (a technique known as 'creeping'), taking care to keep out of the surgeon's line of vision, to elevate the lobe from the thyroid bed as the capsule is being exposed. Vessels are ligated directly on the surface of the thyroid gland capsule and as dissection proceeds medially the parathyroids are noted to peel away within the fascia maintaining their blood supply (**Figure 23.22**). As the capsular dissection continues medially and the ligament of Berry is approached, the recurrent laryngeal nerve is seen and preserved within the fascia. At this

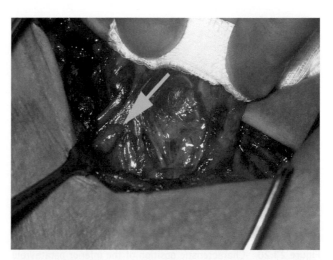

Figure 23.18   Position of the superior parathyroid (arrowed).

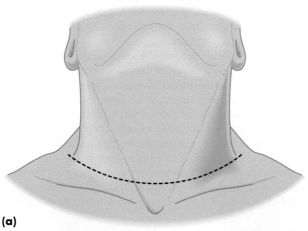

(a)

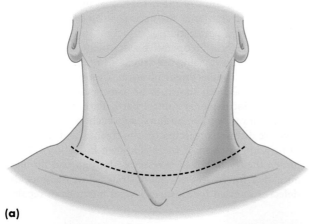

(b)

Figure 23.17   Low Kocher's incision.

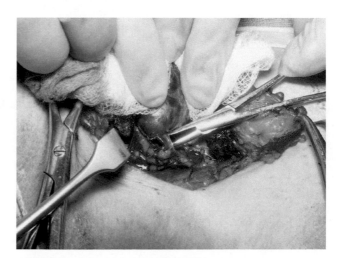

Figure 23.19   Ligation of the inferior thyroid veins.

point, and not before, the nerve may be gently exposed and then dissected up to where its various divisions enter the larynx. At the ligament of Berry, once the nerve is clear of the thyroid gland, sharp dissection on the trachea allows reflection of the lobe off the trachea to the point where the isthmus joins the contralateral lobe. This dissection of the ligament of Berry may be facilitated by the use of loupes. A Roberts clamp is placed across the gland and the lobe and isthmus excised if a lobectomy is being performed; a similar dissection is performed on the contralateral lobe for a total thyroidectomy. The parathyroids are carefully inspected and if one is particularly congested or devascularized it should be resected, morselized and placed into pockets in either the sternomastoid muscle or the brachioradialis muscle in the forearm. Some writers recommend routine reimplantation of parathyroid glands during total thyroidectomy, but there is little conclusive evidence for this. Haemostasis is established using a Valsalva manoeuvre and particular attention paid to the 'triangle of concern', which is where small blood vessels have been ligated medial to the recurrent laryngeal nerve.[113] The triangle consists of the recurrent laryngeal nerve, the trachea and the root of the neck (**Figure 23.23**).

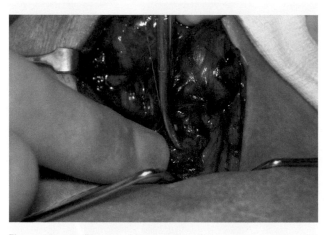

Figure 23.20 Characteristic position of the inferior parathyroid (indicated with forceps).

Techniques in managing extrathyroid extension

The approach here depends on the structures involved and note that more than one may be invaded.

Strap muscles: Most frequently the strap muscles are involved, and in this situation the muscles should be divided above and below the area of invasion and left attached to the gland. The approach to the gland itself is similar to above with access to the vessels and other extrathyroid structures around the attached individual strap muscles.

Recurrent laryngeal nerve: Involvement of the recurrent laryngeal nerve is not uncommon. If the nerve is non-functional prior to surgery, it can be resected without concern. If, however, it is functioning prior to surgery, all attempts should be made to preserve it. Frequently, the nerve itself will not be invaded and tumour is merely attached to the perineurium and can be carefully dissected off using sharp dissection under magnification with loupes or an operating microscope. If the nerve is clearly invaded then, functional or not, it should be resected.

Oesophagus: Although oesophageal muscle may be invaded, the lumen is only rarely involved. If oesophageal invasion is suspected clinically or radiologically, endoscopic examination of the lumen with a rigid oesophagoscope immediately prior to the surgery is essential. Placement of an oesophageal bougie or ET tube to aid identification of the oesophageal lumen while the surgeon is operating in the neck is also very helpful and can help avoid perforation.

Larynx and trachea: Preoperative assessment and endoscopy combined with imaging are crucial in managing tracheal or laryngeal compartment invasion. Complete resection of disease has been shown to be associated with improved locoregional control particularly where there is luminal invasion. The authors' approach is as follows: Invasive disease is resected off the trachea and the extent of invasion assessed. If there is known invasion of the lumen the tracheal wall is resected through and through and, after frozen section demonstrates clear margins, the defect is assessed for closure. Several methods of repair

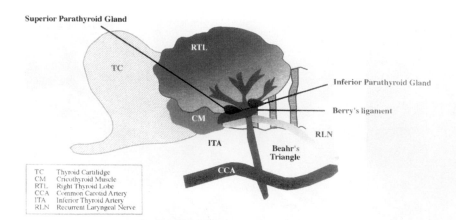

Superior Parathyroid Gland

RTL

TC

Inferior Parathyroid Gland

Berry's ligament

CM

RLN

ITA

Beahr's Triangle

CCA

TC	Thyroid Cartilidge
CM	Cricothyroid Muscle
RTL	Right Thyroid Lobe
CCA	Common Carotid Artery
ITA	Inferior Thyroid Artery
RLN	Recurrent Laryngeal Nerve

Diagram to show the relationships of the Recurrent Laryngeal Nerve

Note: The RLN may pass in front, behind or between the branches of the ITA. Such relationships should not be relied upon when searching for the nerve.

Figure 23.21 Beahr's triangle.

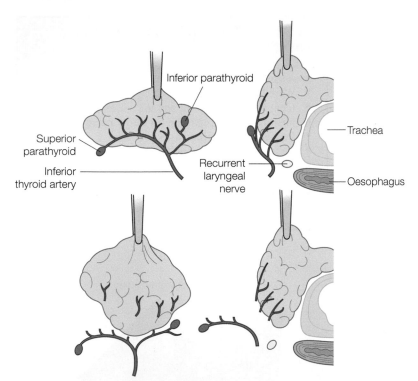

Figure 23.22 Extracapsular dissection of the thyroid gland preserving the parathyroid glands with their blood supply.

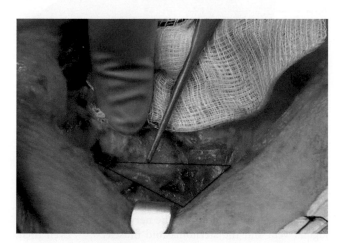

Figure 23.23 The triangle of concern.

are available including a patch of fascia or dermis, wedge excision and closure and segmental resection with end to end anastomosis. In the authors' opinion, unless the defect is very small, segmental resection and end to end anastomotic repair is the most reliable method and up to 4–5 cm of trachea can be resected and closed without difficulty. Only occasionally is a suprahyoid release required.[114] Laryngeal framework can be resected extensively with minimal impact on function, but once the laryngeal lumen is invaded, partial or total laryngectomy is required with the indications for the most appropriate procedure similar to those for mucosal based carcinomas. If a pharyngolaryngectomy is required, then reconstruction is usually either with free jejunum or anterolateral cutaneous thigh flap.

Large vessels: The jugular vein is not infrequently invaded by nodal disease and should be resected in this circumstance. The carotid artery may be encroached upon by metastatic nodal disease within the carotid sheath in levels III and IV but the artery is rarely involved and disease can usually be easily dissected away from the adventitia without damaging the vessel wall.

Central neck dissection (levels VI and VII)

Nodes in level VI can lie superficial and deep to the recurrent laryngeal nerve (RLN) and tend to be more frequent in the inferior part of the central compartment. Either electively or therapeutically, a central neck dissection is usually performed with a total thyroidectomy and involves an extension of extracapsular dissection (**Figure 23.24**). Initially, the RLN is skeletonized from the cricothyroid joint to the level of the sternal notch with the overlying tissue laid lateral and medial. Once the nerve can be seen along its length, it is carefully elevated off the underlying tissues. Vessel loops can be used but care should be taken not to apply any traction to the nerve. The node bearing tissue is then dissected as a compartment from lateral at the IJV passing it deep to the nerve and finally resecting it off the trachea. At the lower end, the thymic remnants and associated fatty tissue and lymph nodes are dissected and removed via the neck and the trachea is then completely skeletonized. The key to preserving parathyroid function is to retain the vascular supply to the superior parathyroids while resecting and reimplanting the inferior ones. Traditionally, a central neck dissection incorporates all node-bearing tissue from the hyoid bone to the sternal notch and laterally to the carotid sheath. However, the dissection in the superior compartment does not need to be as aggressive and this allows preservation of the superior glands which have a supply either wholly from the inferior thyroid artery (ITA) or partly from the ITA and partly from

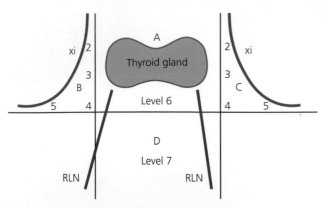

Figure 23.24   Extent of total thyroidectomy with either level VI (A) or level VII (D) neck dissection. A unilateral (C) or bilateral (C)+(B) selective neck dissection levels II–V can also be performed dissecting the accessory triangle below the accessory nerve.

the superior thyroid artery. Evidence suggests that this operation is associated with increased morbidity, including higher rates of recurrent laryngeal nerve damage and temporary and permanent hypoparathyroidism.[4] One technique that reduces this risk is to divide level VI into two parts, VIa and VIb, separated by the recurrent laryngeal nerve.[115] For small cancers in low risk patients, dissection could be confined to level VIa, greatly reducing the risks to the RLN and parathyroid glands. For high risk patients and those with large tumours, a full level VI dissection may be undertaken.

Lateral neck dissection

There is little role for elective lateral neck dissection in DTC. Therapeutic neck dissection will be discussed in detail in Chapter 36, Neck dissection. However, there are some particular points that should be raised in lateral neck dissection for thyroid carcinoma (**Box 23.6**). The incision may be either an extended conventional thyroid approach utilizing a lateral incision, or a superior extended thyroid excision overlying the cricoid cartilage. The inferior portion of level V is involved more frequently in metastatic DTC than in the more aggressive head and neck cancers. This is because, as previously mentioned, the nodal disease follows the inferior thyroid artery behind the common carotid and the internal jugular vein (Chassaignac's triangle) and it is here that scalene nodes may be missed (**Figure 23.25**).[114] On the left, the thoracic duct arches forward to enter the confluence of the IJV and innominate vein in the base of the triangle, and the sympathetic trunk is also close by. During a level Vb dissection (i.e. the region of level V below and anterior to the accessory nerve), the area must be carefully and thoroughly dissected in all cases of metastatic DTC. Level IIa (i.e. that area of level II anterior and inferior to the accessory nerve) must be cleared in every neck dissection, but if there is massive involvement of several levels, IIb may become involved and should also be cleared. Therefore a lateral neck dissection in DTC should incorporate a selective level IIa–level Vb dissection, unless there is massive multilevel disease and then a complete level II–V clearance should be

Box 23.6   Key points in selective neck dissection for DTC

- Adequate incision
- Work lateral to medial
- Identify levels II, III, IV and V
- Identify and preserve the accessory nerve
- Deal with the sternomastoid muscle
- Dissect corners one and two
- Preserve the internal jugular vein, phrenic nerve and brachial plexus
- Access Chassaignac's triangle
- Finally dissect levels IIa to Vb

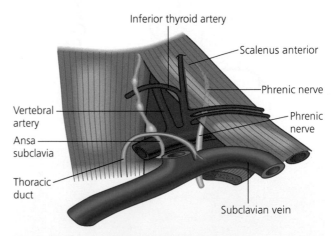

Figure 23.25   Chassaignac's triangle.

performed. Access to level IV, the carotid sheath and Chassaignac's triangle can be facilitated if needed by dividing the lower end of the sternomastoid muscle and peeling it upwards. The accessory nerve is then identified and level V below the accessory nerve along with levels IV, III and II are dissected, preserving not only the nerve but also the internal jugular vein and the sternomastoid muscle.[57, 114] Even then, level I does not usually need to be cleared. If there is extranodal extension and invasion of structures such as SCM or IJV, they should be excised in continuity such as in a modified radical neck dissection but again level I rarely needs to be dissected.[114]

COMPLICATIONS AND OUTCOME MEASUREMENTS

Thyroidectomy is a common surgical procedure that can be associated with significant complications, including haemorrhage, infection and both temporary and permanent recurrent laryngeal nerve palsy and hypoparathyroidism. The Third National Audit Report by the British Association of Endocrine and Thyroid Surgeons confirmed that complication rates are reduced in experienced hands, and that 25 per cent of thyroid surgery in the UK was consultant led.[116]

A complication is an unexpected adverse effect caused by thyroidectomy and this must be differentiated from natural sequelae (either temporary or permanent) which are inevitable following the operation (i.e. permanent hypothyroidism and temporary hypoparathyroidism following total thyroidectomy). Complications can be divided into early, intermediate and late, local and general and those specific to the operation.[113, 114]

Complications following thyroidectomy:

- early, intermediate and late;
- local and general;
- those specific to the operation.

Early complications following thyroidectomy include haemorrhage, voice change, airway obstruction and temporary hypoparathyroidism. The intermediate ones include seroma formation, infection and temporary palsy of the recurrent laryngeal nerve and the external branch of the superior laryngeal nerve. Late complications include subclinical hypothyroidism, permanent hypoparathyroidism, permanent injury to the recurrent laryngeal nerve, the external branch of the superior laryngeal nerve, the cutaneous nerves C2 and C3 and the accessory nerve and a poor scar. Techniques employed to avoid complications are summarized in **Table 23.12** and **Box 23.7** and discussed in detail in Chapter 25, Avoiding complications in thyroid and parathyroid surgery.

There are a number of important outcome measurements that can be used in the assessment of treatment for thyroid cancer (**Box 23.8**). These data are collected prospectively by the British Association of Endocrine and Thyroid Surgeons and form part of their National Audit Report,[116] allowing better quality of data for reporting results and taking informed consent. The importance of adequate low morbidity primary surgery has already being discussed along with the provision of radioiodine ablation and/or therapy, and treatment with long-term TSH suppression with regular monitoring of the serum thyroglobulin.

It is important to investigate an abnormal thyroglobulin promptly and to use local protocols which are approved by the multidisciplinary team. Because of a long natural history, the disease-free interval is important and although

recurrences have been reported up to 42 years following initial treatment, late recurrences are uncommon following

---

Box 23.7   Guidelines for difficult cases

- Make an adequate incision
- Do the easy side first
- Always consider cancer
- Consider total thyroidectomy for many benign and malignant cases; high-risk patients may need a level VI neck dissection
- Try to identify the recurrent laryngeal nerve and parathyroid glands
- Know the location of the external branch of the superior laryngeal nerve
- Consider using a nerve monitor
- Achieve good access in retrosternal goitre, do the easy side and the upper pole first, and divide the strap muscles at least on one side
- Do not hesitate to split the chest or sacrifice one recurrent laryngeal nerve if malignancy is present

---

Box 23.8   Outcome measurements following treatment for thyroid cancer[116]

- Adequate primary surgery
- Incidence of vocal cord paralysis
- Incidence of hypoparathyroidism (temporary and permanent)
- Achievement of TSH suppression
- Provision and treatment with radioiodine postoperatively when indicated
- Regular monitoring of serum thyroglobulin
- Abnormal thyroglobulin acted upon
- Disease-free interval
- Quality of life
- Survival

Table 23.12 Summary of important complications and avoidance measures.

Complication	Avoidance measures
RLN palsy	Identify the nerve early low down, use a meticulous surgical technique and consider using a nerve monitor
Damage to the EBSLN[13]	Know its course; if seen in Joll's triangle then confirm with a nerve stimulator, avoid and ligate superior thyroid vessels individually right on the gland
Temporary and permanent hypoparathyroidism	Identify all parathyroids, perform extracapsular dissection with preservation of blood supply and consider using loupes
Damage to the cutaneous nerves C2 and C3	Lift the upper and lower flaps by staying on the deep cervical fascia. Use bipolar diathermy
Haemorrhage	Meticulous surgical technique; doubly ligate or ligate and transfix the upper pole vessels, ligate the thyroid isthmus and close after a Valsalva. Consider using a drain
Poor scar	Mark correctly, ensure meticulous skin closure. Consider triamcinolone in patients with dark skin
Infection	Meticulous surgical technique. Consider prophylactic antibiotics in high risk cases

appropriate initial therapy. Common psychosocial issues relating to the anxiety of a cancer diagnosis, side effects of radioiodine treatment and the morbidity associated with major extirpative surgery are not uncommon, particularly in the young, and should be addressed by the multidisciplinary team which includes the appropriate counselling skills of a head and neck nurse and/or counsellor.

CONCLUSION

While thyroid nodules are common and cancer most commonly presents as a solitary thyroid nodule, thyroid malignancy still remains a rare entity. DTC is the most frequently seen of the thyroid cancers, and the incidence is increasing due to greater awareness and improved detection, together with an increase in surgery for benign disease and possibly greater environmental radiation exposure. Another important aetiological factor in DTC is a positive family history and although the genetics and molecular biology of these diseases are better understood than ever, effective novel therapies remain elusive.

Nevertheless, in the vast majority of cases DTC is an indolent disease with an excellent prognosis and low rates of recurrence and mortality. Several prognostic factors are recognized and among the most important are patient age, tumour size, extrathyroid extension and the presence of distant metastases. A number of prognostic scoring systems have been developed over the past three decades and although detailed analysis does support their validity, we would recommend the use of the AJCC/UICC staging system for DTC since it incorporates well-recognized prognostic risk factors, is accurate in predicting outcomes and is friendly and familiar to users because of its use in other head and neck malignancies.

The important primary investigations to exclude malignancy in a patient presenting with a solitary thyroid nodule include FNAC, T4 and TSH levels, thyroid antibodies and an ultrasound scan. Ultrasound can also be used to increase the accuracy of FNAC. There are five possible cytological outcomes of FNAC ranging from non-diagnostic (Thy1) to a definite cytological diagnosis of malignancy (Thy5). Anatomical imaging, such as CT scanning is important in investigating the extent of primary and particularly nodal disease in an established diagnosis of malignancy.

A total or near-total thyroidectomy is the appropriate operation when PTC has been diagnosed on FNAC. Following diagnostic thyroid lobectomy a completion thyroidectomy should be considered when PTC or follicular thyroid carcinoma is diagnosed.

Positive central or lateral nodal disease should be treated with selective neck dissection and in high risk PTC, elective central neck dissection may be indicated. Recurrent metastatic neck disease in a previously dissected neck may be treated by selective lymphadenectomy including single node removal. Widely invasive disease is best treated with complete resection, but morbidity should be minimized and incomplete resection with adjuvant therapy usually equates with excellent disease-free status and survival. DTC diagnosed during pregnancy is not uncommon and the prognosis is excellent despite any delay in surgical treatment until a successful delivery has been completed.

Vigilant follow up is important for the early diagnosis and management of recurrent DTC as 70 per cent of recurrences will be in the neck and therefore resectable. Serial unstimulated and stimulated thyroglobulin measurements are the mainstay of surveillance along with neck ultrasound, radioactive iodine whole body scanning and anatomical imaging where appropriate. PET-CT scanning is proving useful for those with rising Tg levels and negative ^{131}I/anatomical scans. PET-CT scans are also proving to be valuable in those with less well-differentiated tumours that do not concentrate iodine well.

Surgery for local recurrence in the thyroid bed or central neck has increased risks of laryngeal nerve injury and hypoparathyroidism, although this is not so in the lateral neck. A comprehensive understanding of the structural and lymphatic anatomy of the thyroid gland is essential in order for safe and effective surgery to be performed. Audit of performance indicators and a multidisciplinary approach to the management of patients with DTC are required to improve outcomes in this fascinating and complex disease.

DIRECTIONS FOR FUTURE RESEARCH

Cancer is a disease of genes. Genes encoding molecules involved in regulating the growth, differentiation and function of cells are mutated, lost or deregulated in cancer. The recognition of genetic changes, and potential to correct them, are leading to exciting new modalities for the diagnosis and treatment of thyroid cancer. Many of these are in early clinical trials, and their eventual impact on mortality from thyroid cancer remains to be seen.

FNAC is an important diagnostic test in use today.[117] Molecular techniques including reverse transcription-polymerase chain reaction (RT-PCR) have been used in an attempt to improve the accuracy of FNAC. This would be especially useful to distinguish between follicular adenoma and carcinoma, currently impossible on conventional cytological methods. There is currently no molecular marker specific enough to distinguish these, but detection of several mutations (Ras, Galectin-3 and PTTG) shows some promise.[118, 119] Other techniques including mass spectrometry, proteomics and gene array technology may allow accurate detection of cancer and differentiation of tumour subtypes, although further research is required.

Disease progression is currently monitored by serum thyroglobulin as well as ^{131}I scans and clinical examination. Up to 25 per cent of patients have antibodies which interfere with the thyroglobulin assays, and make interpretation difficult. Detection of serum thyroglobulin mRNA using quantitative RT-PCR may allow this subset of patients to be analysed more accurately, although preliminary studies require further clinical validation.[120]

Angiogenesis is the growth of new blood vessels by sprouting of existing capillaries and is essential for all tumour growth. Numerous angiogenic growth factors are elevated in thyroid cancers including vascular endothelial growth factor (VEGF), fibroblast growth factor (FGF) and the angiopoietins[12]. Bevacizumab is an anti-VEGF monoclonal antibody that already has FDA approval for use in several human malignancies including head and neck and colorectal cancers. There are several other anti-angiogenic agents in development (for example sorafenib which is a VEGF receptor inhibitor) that are entering clinical trials in other solid tumours. Many of these agents may soon be applied to thyroid cancers. Indeed, there is growing *in vitro* and preclinical evidence for use in thyroid cancer.[121] Several endogenous anti-angiogenic factors, including endostatin and angiostatin, have been effective at reducing or preventing tumour growth in an animal model of thyroid cancer, and may prove useful in human thyroid cancer.[122]

Further elucidation of thyroid cancer biology has led to the development of several other therapeutic targets, and many of these are in advanced stages of clinical development. More recently, targeted therapy against tyrosine kinase receptors has gained importance in the search for novel cancer treatments.[121] Cetuximab, a monoclonal antibody to epidermal growth factor receptor (EGFR – frequently overexpressed in many tumour types), has been thoroughly validated and is licensed for use in several human cancers including head and neck squamous carcinomas.[123] In thyroid cancer, RET, BRAF and PI(3)K kinases appear to be rational targets for the treatment of advanced thyroid cancer. RET is involved in the formation of both medullary and papillary thyroid cancers. BRAF mutations are highly prevalent in PTC. Two small molecular compounds ZD6474 (zactima) and BAY43-9006 (sorafenib) obstruct RET and BRAF signalling and are currently undergoing clinical evaluation (http://www.cancer.gov/clinical trials). Both compounds also inhibit VEGF receptors. The phosphoinositide-3-OH kinase (PI(3)K) pathway regulates cell proliferation and survival and has been shown to be hyper-activated in a high proportion of thyroid cancers. Two agents effective in inhibiting this pathway are CCI-770 (temsirolimus) and RAD001 (everolimus). Both compounds, derivatives of the macrolide antibiotic rapamycin, have been shown to have broad antitumour activity and are under advanced clinical study.[124]

Gene therapy is the treatment of disease by the transfer of genetic material. Several vector strategies may be employed, either viral such as retroviruses, adenoviruses and lentivirus which have relatively high transfer efficiency but may have unwanted effects due to the inherent properties of the virus, or physical methods such as liposomes or injection of naked DNA, which are safer, but less potent vectors. Approaches used include introduction of p53 into p53 deficient anaplastic carcinomas, transfer of suicide genes such as thymidine kinase into cancer cells, overexpression of interleukin-2 to increase immunological antitumour activity, and increased expression of the sodium iodide symporter into thyroid cancers that have become ^{131}I-resistant.[125] Despite the relatively modest results of gene therapy hitherto, it is likely that these approaches will prove to be clinically useful in the medium to long term, and have the potential to transform the treatment of many cancers, including thyroid cancer.

KEY EVIDENCE

- Essential preoperative investigations for thyroid surgery include clinical examination, thyroid function tests, thyroid antibodies, serum calcium, FNAC (plus or minus ultrasound) and voice assessment, and for established malignancy anatomical imaging is usually required.[4, 5]
- For differentiated thyroid cancer, the mainstay of treatment is near-total or total thyroidectomy, subsequent radioiodine ablation and lifelong follow up with TSH suppression and serum thyroglobulin measurement. There is a role for lobectomy alone in small cancers (<1 cm) in low risk patients.[4, 5]

KEY LEARNING POINTS

- Physicians and surgeons need to be aware that the most common way for thyroid cancer to present is as a solitary thyroid nodule in the euthyroid patient when the incidence of malignancy is approximately 10 per cent.
- Essential preoperative investigations include clinical examination, thyroid function tests, thyroid antibodies, serum calcium, FNAC (plus or minus ultrasound) and voice assessment.
- Anatomical imaging is usually required for established malignancy.
- For differentiated thyroid cancer, the mainstay of treatment is near-total or total thyroidectomy, subsequent radioiodine ablation and lifelong follow up with TSH suppression and serum thyroglobulin measurement.
- Neck disease is usually treatable by selective neck surgery.
- Major extirpative surgery may be required for advanced disease in selected cases
- Lymphoma and anaplastic carcinoma should be treated by the appropriate specialist team according to protocol. Surgery has little place to play apart from biopsy.
- Thyroid cancer is rare in children and those aged 10 years or less tend to have more aggressive disease. Total thyroidectomy is usually recommended for all patients.
- Quantitative outcome measurements are available and include adequacy of the primary surgery, incidence of complications, achievement of TSH suppression, regular monitoring of serum thyroglobulin together with quality of life, disease-free interval and survival.
- Working in multidisciplinary teams and further molecular biology research can only improve the way we diagnose, stage and treat thyroid cancer.

62. Hisham AN, Azlina AF, Harjit K. Reoperative thyroid surgery: analysis of outcomes. *ANZ Journal of Surgery* 2003; **73**: A30.

63. Tisell LE, Nilsson B, Molne J *et al.* Improved survival of patients with papillary thyroid cancer after surgical microdissection. *World Journal of Surgery* 1996; **20**: 854–9.

64. Grodski S, Cornford L, Sywak M *et al.* Routine level VI lymph node dissection for papillary thyroid cancer: surgical technique. *ANZ Journal of Surgery* 2007; **77**: 203–8.

65. Schlumberger M, Challeton C, De VF *et al.* Radioactive iodine treatment and external radiotherapy for lung and bone metastases from thyroid carcinoma. *Journal of Nuclear Medicine* 1996; **37**: 598–605.

66. Mulcahy MM, Cohen JI, Anderson PE *et al.* Relative accuracy of fine-needle aspiration and frozen section in the diagnosis of well-differentiated thyroid cancer. *Laryngoscope* 1998; **108**(4 Pt 1): 494–6.

67. Andersen PE, Kinsella J, Loree TR *et al.* Differentiated carcinoma of the thyroid with extrathyroidal extension. *American Journal of Surgery* 1995; **170**: 467–70.

68. Ortiz S, Rodriguez JM, Soria T *et al.* Extrathyroid spread in papillary carcinoma of the thyroid: clinicopathological and prognostic study. *Otolaryngology and Head and Neck Surgery* 2001; **124**: 261–5.

69. Nishida T, Nakao K, Hamaji M. Differentiated thyroid carcinoma with airway invasion: indication for tracheal resection based on the extent of cancer invasion. *Journal of Thoracic and Cardiovascular Surgery* 1997; **114**: 84–92.

70. McConahey WM, Hay ID, Woolner LB *et al.* Papillary thyroid cancer treated at the Mayo Clinic, 1946 through 1970: initial manifestations, pathologic findings, therapy, and outcome. *Mayo Clinic Proceedings* 1986; **61**: 978–96.

71. Kebebew E, Clark OH. Locally advanced differentiated thyroid cancer. *Surgical Oncology* 2003; **12**: 91–9.

72. Falk SA, McCaffrey TV. Management of the recurrent laryngeal nerve in suspected and proven thyroid cancer. *Otolaryngology and Head and Neck Surgery* 1995; **113**: 42–8.

73. McCaffrey JC. Aerodigestive tract invasion by well-differentiated thyroid carcinoma: diagnosis, management, prognosis, and biology. *Laryngoscope* 2006; **116**: 1–11.

74. Keum KC, Suh YG, Koom WS *et al.* The role of postoperative external-beam radiotherapy in the management of patients with papillary thyroid cancer invading the trachea. *International Journal of Radiation Oncology, Biology, Physics* 2006; **65**: 474–80.

75. Doherty CM, Shindo ML, Rice DH *et al.* Management of thyroid nodules during pregnancy. *Laryngoscope* 1995; **105**: 251–5.

76. Rosen IB, Walfish PG. Pregnancy as a predisposing factor in thyroid neoplasia. *Archives of Surgery* 1986; **121**: 1287–90.

77. Moosa M, Mazzaferri EL. Outcome of differentiated thyroid cancer diagnosed in pregnant women. *Journal of Clinical Endocrinology and Metabolism* 1997; **82**: 2862–6.

78. Nam KH, Yoon JH, Chang HS, Park CS. Optimal timing of surgery in well-differentiated thyroid carcinoma detected during pregnancy. *Journal of Surgical Oncology* 2005; **91**: 199–203.

79. Yasmeen S, Cress R, Romano PS *et al.* Thyroid cancer in pregnancy. *International Journal of Gynaecology and Obstetrics* 2005; **91**: 15–20.

80. Vini L, Hyer S, Pratt B, Harmer C. Management of differentiated thyroid cancer diagnosed during pregnancy. *European Journal of Endocrinology* 1999; **140**: 404–6.

81. Shaha A, Alfonso A, Jaffe BM. Acute airway distress due to thyroid pathology. *Surgery* 1987; **102**: 1068–74.

82. Rosen IB, Korman M, Walfish PG. Thyroid nodular disease in pregnancy: current diagnosis and management. *Clinical Obstetrics and Gynecology* 1997; **40**: 81–9.

83. Yip FW, Reeve TS, Poole AG, Delbridge L. Thyroid nodules in childhood and adolescence. *Australian and New Zealand Journal of Surgery* 1994; **64**: 676–8.

84. Zimmerman D, Hay ID, Gough IR *et al.* Papillary thyroid carcinoma in children and adults: long-term follow-up of 1039 patients conservatively treated at one institution during three decades. *Surgery* 1988; **104**: 1157–66.

85. Landau D, Vini L, A'Hern R, Harmer C. Thyroid cancer in children: the Royal Marsden Hospital experience. *European Journal of Cancer* 2000; **36**: 214–20.

86. Palmer BA, Zarroug AE, Poley RN *et al.* Papillary thyroid carcinoma in children: risk factors and complications of disease recurrence. *Journal of Pediatric Surgery* 2005; **40**: 1284–8.

87. Vassilopoulou-Sellin R, Goepfert H, Raney B, Schultz PN. Differentiated thyroid cancer in children and adolescents: clinical outcome and mortality after long-term follow-up. *Head and Neck* 1998; **20**: 549–55.

88. Rybakov SJ, Komissarenko IV, Tronko ND *et al.* Thyroid cancer in children of Ukraine after the Chernobyl accident. *World Journal of Surgery* 2000; **24**: 1446–9.

♦ 89. Sawka AM, Thephamongkhol K, Brouwers M *et al.* Clinical review 170: A systematic review and metaanalysis of the effectiveness of radioactive iodine remnant ablation for well-differentiated thyroid cancer. *Journal of Clinical Endocrinology and Metabolism* 2004; **89**: 3668–76.

90. Pujol P, Daures JP, Nsakala N *et al.* Degree of thyrotropin suppression as a prognostic determinant in differentiated thyroid cancer. *Journal of Clinical Endocrinology and Metabolism* 1996; **81**: 4318–23.

91. Hovens GC, Stokkel MP, Kievit J *et al.* Associations of serum thyrotropin concentrations with recurrence and death in differentiated thyroid cancer. *Journal of Clinical Endocrinology and Metabolism* 2007; **92**: 2610–15.

92. Cooper DS, Specker B, Ho M *et al.* Thyrotropin suppression and disease progression in patients with differentiated

thyroid cancer: results from the National Thyroid Cancer Treatment Cooperative Registry. *Thyroid* 1998; **8**: 737–44.

93. Hamby LS, McGrath PC, Schwartz RW *et al.* Management of local recurrence in well-differentiated thyroid carcinoma. *Journal of Surgical Research* 1992; **52**: 113–7.

94. Schlumberger M, Pacini F, Wiersinga WM *et al.* Follow-up and management of differentiated thyroid carcinoma: a European perspective in clinical practice. *European Journal of Endocrinology* 2004; **151**: 539–48.

◆ 95. Mazzaferri EL, Robbins RJ, Spencer CA *et al.* A consensus report of the role of serum thyroglobulin as a monitoring method for low-risk patients with papillary thyroid carcinoma. *Journal of Clinical Endocrinology and Metabolism* 2003; **88**: 1433–41.

96. Mazzaferri EL. Empirically treating high serum thyroglobulin levels. *Journal of Nuclear Medicine* 2005; **46**: 1079–88.

97. Haugen BR, Pacini F, Reiners C *et al.* A comparison of recombinant human thyrotropin and thyroid hormone withdrawal for the detection of thyroid remnant or cancer. *Journal of Clinical Endocrinology and Metabolism* 1999; **84**: 3877–85.

98. Pacini F, Molinaro E, Castagna MG *et al.* Recombinant human thyrotropin-stimulated serum thyroglobulin combined with neck ultrasonography has the highest sensitivity in monitoring differentiated thyroid carcinoma. *Journal of Clinical Endocrinology and Metabolism* 2003; **88**: 3668–73.

99. Bachelot A, Cailleux AF, Klain M *et al.* Relationship between tumor burden and serum thyroglobulin level in patients with papillary and follicular thyroid carcinoma. *Thyroid* 2002; **12**: 707–11.

100. Torlontano M, Attard M, Crocetti U *et al.* Follow-up of low risk patients with papillary thyroid cancer: role of neck ultrasonography in detecting lymph node metastases. *Journal of Clinical Endocrinology and Metabolism* 2004; **89**: 3402–7.

101. Baskin HJ. Detection of recurrent papillary thyroid carcinoma by thyroglobulin assessment in the needle washout after fine-needle aspiration of suspicious lymph nodes. *Thyroid* 2004; **14**: 959–63.

102. Antonelli A, Miccoli P, Fallahi P *et al.* Role of neck ultrasonography in the follow-up of children operated on for thyroid papillary cancer. *Thyroid* 2003; **13**: 479–84.

103. Lind P, Kohlfurst S. Respective roles of thyroglobulin, radioiodine imaging, and positron emission tomography in the assessment of thyroid cancer. *Seminars in Nuclear Medicine* 2006; **36**: 194–205.

104. Helal BO, Merlet P, Toubert ME *et al.* Clinical impact of (18)F-FDG PET in thyroid carcinoma patients with elevated thyroglobulin levels and negative ^{131}I scanning results after therapy. *Journal of Nuclear Medicine* 2001; **42**: 1464–9.

105. Wang W, Larson SM, Fazzari M *et al.* Prognostic value of [18F]fluorodeoxyglucose positron emission tomographic scanning in patients with thyroid cancer. *Journal of Clinical Endocrinology and Metabolism* 2000; **85**: 1107–13.

106. Tsang RW, Brierley JD, Simpson WJ *et al.* The effects of surgery, radioiodine, and external radiation therapy on the clinical outcome of patients with differentiated thyroid carcinoma. *Cancer* 1998; **82**: 375–88.

107. Waseem Z, Palme CE, Walfish P, Freeman JL. Prognostic implications of site of recurrence in patients with recurrent well-differentiated thyroid cancer. *Journal of Otolaryngology* 2004; **33**: 339–44.

108. Coburn M, Teates D, Wanebo HJ. Recurrent thyroid cancer. Role of surgery versus radioactive iodine (^{131}I). *Annals of Surgery* 1994; **219**: 587–93.

109. Kim MK, Mandel SH, Baloch Z *et al.* Morbidity following central compartment reoperation for recurrent or persistent thyroid cancer. *Archives of Otolaryngology – Head and Neck Surgery* 2004; **130**: 1214–16.

110. Palme CE, Freeman JL. Surgical strategy for thyroid bed recurrence in patients with well-differentiated thyroid carcinoma. *Journal of Otolaryngology* 2005; **34**: 7–12.

111. Pereira JA, Jimeno J, Miquel J *et al.* Nodal yield, morbidity, and recurrence after central neck dissection for papillary thyroid carcinoma. *Surgery* 2005; **138**: 1095–100, discussion.

112. Aina EN, Hisham AN. External laryngeal nerve in thyroid surgery: recognition and surgical implications. *Australian and New Zealand Journal of Surgery* 2001; **71**: 212–14.

113. Watkinson JC, Hobbs CGL. Thyroidectomy. *Surgery* 2007; **25**: 474–8.

114. Watkinson JC, Ramsden J. Thyroid cancer. In: Gleeson M, Browning GG, Burton MJ *et al.* (eds). *Otolaryngology – head and neck surgery*, 7th edn. London: Hodder Arnold, 2008.

115. Sharma N *et al.* Who should treat thyroid cancer? A UK surgical perspective. *Clinical Oncology* 2010; **22**: 413–18.

116. Scott-Combes D, Kinsman R, Walton P. British Association of Endocrine and Thyroid Surgeons. Third national audit report. London, 2009.

117. Boelaert K, Horacek RL, Holder JC *et al.* Serum thyrotropin concentration as a novel predictor of malignancy in thyroid nodules investigated by fine-needle aspiration. *Journal of Clinical Endocrinology and Metabolism* 2006; **91**: 4295–301.

118. Sciacchitano S, Paliotta D, Nardi F *et al.* PCR amplification and analysis of ras oncogenes from thyroid cytologic smears. *Diagnostic Molecular Pathology* 1994; **3**: 114–21.

119. Kim DS, McCabe CJ, Buchanan MA, Watkinson JC. Oncogenes in thyroid cancer. *Clinical Otolaryngology* 2003; **28**: 386–95.

120. Eszlinger M, Neumann S, Otto L, Paschke R. Thyroglobulin mRNA quantification in the peripheral blood is not a reliable marker for the follow-up of patients with differentiated thyroid cancer. *European Journal of Endocrinology* 2002; **147**: 575–82.

121. Santoro M, Fusco A. New drugs in thyroid cancer. *Arquivos Brasileiros de Endocrinologia e Metabologia* 2007; **51**: 857–61.

122. Ye C, Feng C, Wang S *et al.* Antiangiogenic and antitumour effects of endostatin on follicular thyroid carcinoma. *Endocrinology* 2002; **143**: 3522–9.

123. Grandis RJ, Melhem MF, Gooding WE *et al.* Levels of TGF-alpha and EGFR protein in head and neck squamous cell carcinoma and patient survival. *Journal of the National Cancer Institute* 1998; **90**: 824–32.

124. Bjornsti MA, Houghton PJ. The TOR pathway: a target for cancer therapy. *Nature Reviews. Cancer* 2004; **4**: 335–48.

125. DeGroot LJ, Zhang R. Gene therapy for thyroid cancer: where do we stand? *Journal of Clinical Endocrinology and Metabolism* 2001; **86**: 2923–8.

Medullary thyroid cancer

BARNEY HARRISON

I will not cut ... but will leave this to be done by men who are practitioners of this work ...

Extract from the Hippocratic Oath, fourth century BCE

INTRODUCTION

Medullary thyroid cancer (MTC) is uncommon and with the exception of those who work in tertiary referral centres will rarely be diagnosed or treated by individual surgeons. MTC is unique in that it occurs as genetically determined disease in 25 per cent of cases; it occurs in the paediatric and adult setting and is associated with other endocrine tumours. MTC merits a more aggressive surgical approach than differentiated thyroid cancer. Patients with MTC require care from an experienced multidisciplinary team that includes specialist surgeons, an endocrinologist, oncologist and pathologist who meet and discuss cases regularly with a radiologist, nuclear medicine physician and biochemist, all interested in the management of thyroid cancer. Close links and involvement with personnel from a Clinical Genetics Service are essential. National thyroid cancer guidelines in the UK recommend that patients with MTC should be referred for treatment to a cancer centre.

HISTORY

Medullary thyroid cancer was first described by Hazard et al.[1] in 1959. The recognition of calcitonin as a calcium lowering hormone in 1962 and its origin from the thyroid parafollicular cells, so named by Nonidez in 1932, was reported by Foster et al.[2] Pearse and Polak adopted the term C cells and first described their origin from neural crest tissue.[3]

A child with thyroid cancer containing amyloid stroma and bilateral phaeochromocytomas was reported in 1960.[4] The following year, a patient was described by Sipple with bilateral phaeochromocytomas, thyroid cancer and enlarged parathyroid gland (MEN type 2A, Sipple syndrome).[5] In a series of reports Dillwyn Williams linked medullary thyroid cancer, its origin in C cells,[6] association with diarrhoea,[7] phaeochromocytoma[8] and multiple mucosal neuromata.[9] In 1968, Schimke described three patients with MTC, multiple tumours involving the buccal mucosa; two of the patients had bilateral phaeochromocytomas and abnormal facies (MEN type 2B).[10]

Tashjian and Melvin[11] first described the production of calcitonin by MTC. MTC in three generations of a single family was reported by Cushman in 1962[12] in association with phaeochromocytoma and parathyroid disease.

The RET gene was first identified as a proto-oncogene in 1985[13] and cloned three years later.[14] RET was mapped to chromosome 10 in 1987[15, 16] and the mutations associated with MEN2A,[17] FMTC[18, 19] and MEN2B[20, 21] described in 1993 and 1994.

INCIDENCE OF MEDULLARY THYROID CANCER

In the United States, about 1000 people are diagnosed with MTC each year.[22] The disease accounts for approximately

3 per cent of all thyroid cancer in the USA[23, 24] and 5–10 per cent of paediatric thyroid cancers. SEER (Surveillance, Epidemiology and End Results) data from the USA from 1975 to 2000 indicates the maximum incidence of MTC as 4.4 per million per year in the 70–75-year-old age group, and in adolescents and young adults an incidence of less than one case/million per year.[25] The estimated incidence of MTC in the UK is 20–25 new cases per year among a population of 55 million.[26] In patients with nodular thyroid disease screened for MTC, the prevalence of MTC is reported as 0.4–1.8 per cent (see below under Diagnosis of medullary thyroid cancer).

PATHOLOGY

C cells and calcitonin

Medullary thyroid cancer arises from C cells that are found in the middle and upper third of the thyroid gland. These cells, of neural crest origin, will have migrated through the ultimobranchial body (branchial clefts 5 or 6). C cells produce calcitonin, a 32 amino acid peptide and calcitonin gene-related peptide (CGRP). C cells (parafollicular cells) are found adjacent to or within thyroid follicles (**Figure 24.1a**), between the follicular cell basement membrane and the

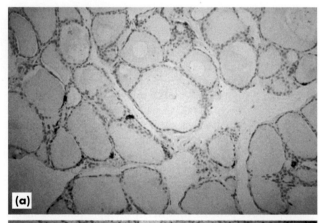

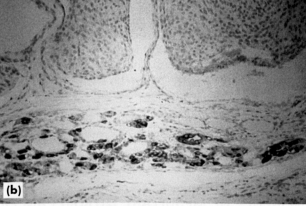

Figure 24.1 Histological sections of thyroid stained for calcitonin. (a) Normal C cells; (b) C cell hyperplasia in MEN2A patient.

surface epithelium. Typically, they have a polygonal or spindle shape, central nuclei and pale, granular cytoplasm. On immunohistochemical staining, C cells demonstrate marked staining for calcitonin, chromogranin, cytokeratin and carcinoembryonic antigen. Calcitonin is stored in dense cored secretory granules and released into the circulation. Circulating secretory products of MTC are listed in **Box 24.1**.

Calcitonin inhibits osteoclastic bone resorption and promotes calcium excretion by the kidney. Its physiological role is unclear in patients with medullary thyroid cancer, in whom calcitonin levels may be grossly elevated, and after total thyroidectomy, when levels are low, no derangement of calcium homeostasis is apparent. Calcium and pentagastrin are potent secretagogues of calcitonin. CGRP is a potent peripheral vasodilator.

C cell hyperplasia

C cell hyperplasia (CCH) is defined as a multifocal (diffuse or nodular) quantitative increase in C cells (**Figure 24.1b**). It can be found in post-mortem thyroid samples of men and women with no evidence of thyroid disease.[27] CCH occurs as a neoplastic precursor within the setting of MEN2-associated MTC, but can also accompany sporadic MTC. Two types of CCH are described that differ in morphological characteristics:[28, 29] (1) neoplastic – typically nodular and diffuse and indistinguishable from invasive MTC cells and (2) reactive (also called physiological) – typically diffuse associated with hypercalcaemia, hyperparathyroidism, chronic lymphocytic thyroiditis and follicular tumours. However, in terms of clinical decision making, a purely morphological distinction between 'physiological' and 'neoplastic' CCH, independent of *RET* status is unwise.[30]

Box 24.1 Circulating secretory products of medullary thyroid cancer

- Calcitonin
- Carcinoembryonic antigen
- Neuron-specific enolase
- Calcitonin gene-related peptide
- Katacalcin
- DOPA-decarboxylase
- Nerve growth factor
- ACTH
- Synaptophysin
- Somatostatin
- Neurotensin
- Serotonin
- Substance P
- Corticotrophin-releasing hormone
- Vasoactive intestinal peptide
- Bombesin
- Gastric-releasing peptide

Medullary thyroid cancer

MACROSCOPIC

Sporadic tumours are usually solitary and unilateral. In patients with familial disease, tumour foci are usually bilateral and multifocal. MTC on sectioning varies in colour from grey/white to pink with varied consistency. Calcification may be present.

CYTOLOGY

Tumour cell morphology is variable; oval/round/spindle-shaped cells may be seen in clusters or as single cells with pleomorphic nuclei and eosinophilic cytoplasm (**Figure 24.2a**). Eosinophilic extracellular material is amyloid.

HISTOPATHOLOGY

MTC may be encapsulated or unencapsulated with extension of the tumour into adjacent parenchyma. Nuclei may be eccentric, pleomorphic with a coarse chromatin pattern, and typically there is a low mitotic rate. A wide variety of histological variants and growth patterns are seen that include papillary, follicular, squamous and oncocytic subtypes.[31]

Amyloid is seen in 80 per cent of tumours, it may be focal or diffuse. On immunohistochemistry tumour cells stain positive for calcitonin (**Figure 24.2b**), CGRP, carcinoembryonic antigen (CEA) and chromogranin A. Thyroglobulin staining is negative. Other peptides that may be identified include adrenocorticotropic hormone (ACTH), somatostatin, serotonin and gut hormones.

MTC is staged as described in the American Joint Committee on Cancer (AJCC) Staging Manual (**Table 24.1**).[32]

HEREDITARY MEDULLARY THYROID CANCER

Genetically determined disease accounts for approximately 25 per cent of MTC cases. Three main clinical variants are recognized that include multiple endocrine neoplasia type 2A (MEN2A), multiple endocrine neoplasia type 2B (MEN2B) and familial medullary thyroid cancer (FMTC). All are inherited as autosomal dominant disorders (**Table 24.2**) with age-related penetrance and variable expression. The prevalence is estimated at one in 30 000. MTC is expressed in almost all patients with MEN2 and FMTC, and is usually the first manifestation of the syndrome; the age at onset is related to specific genotypes.

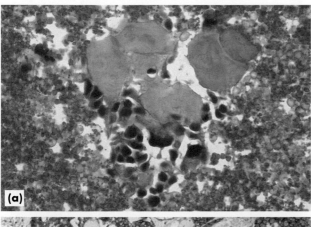

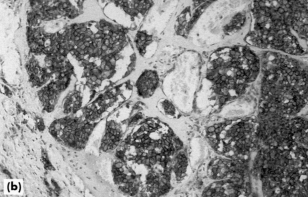

Figure 24.2 (a) MTC cytology obtained from fine needle aspiration of thyroid mass; (b) MTC histology showing strongly positive immunohistochemical staining for calcitonin.

Table 24.1 TNM clinical staging of medullary thyroid cancer.[32]

Clinical stage	
T0	Clinically occult disease
T1	Tumour 2 cm or less in greatest dimension, limited to the thyroid T1a, tumour 1 cm or less in greatest dimension, limited to the thyroid T1b, tumour more than 1 cm, but not more than 2 cm in greatest dimension, limited to the thyroid
T2	Tumour more than 2 cm, but not more than 4 cm in greatest dimension, limited to the thyroid
T3	Tumour more than 4 cm in greatest dimension, limited to the thyroid or any tumour with minimal extrathyroid extension (e.g. extension to sternothyroid muscle or perithyroid soft tissues)
T4a	Tumour extends beyond the thyroid capsule and invades any of the following: subcutaneous soft tissues, larynx, trachea, oesophagus, recurrent laryngeal nerve
T4b	Tumour invades prevertebral fascia, mediastinal vessels, or encases carotid artery

Stage			
I	T1a, T1b	N0	M0
II	T2, T3	N0	M0
III	T1, T2, T3	N1a	M0
IVA	T1, T2, T3	N1b	M0
	T4a	Any N	M0
IVB	T4b	Any N	M0
IVC	Any T	Any N	M1

Table 24.2   Clinical features of multiple endocrine neoplasia type 2.

		%
MEN2A	Medullary thyroid cancer	100
	Phaeochromocytoma	50
	Hyperparathyroidism	10–20
	Cutaneous lichen amyloidosis (rare)	
	Hirschsprung disease	Very rare
FMTC	Medullary thyroid cancer	100
MEN2B	Medullary thyroid cancer	100
	Phaeochromocytoma	50
	Marfanoid habitus	>95
	Mucosal neuromas and intestinal ganglioneuromatosis	>95

Germline and somatic mutations of the *RET* (*RE*arranged during *T*ransfection) proto-oncogene located on chromosome 10q11.2 are implicated in the pathogenesis of MTC. Gain of function germline mutations associated with MEN2/FMTC are found in seven of the *RET* gene's 21 exons. MEN2A accounts for approximately 85 per cent of genetically determined MTC and is associated with a mutation of codon 634 in 85 per cent of cases. At least 95 per cent of families with MEN2A have a *RET* mutation in exon 10 or exon 11. FMTC accounts for 5–15 per cent of hereditary cases, MEN2B accounts for 5 per cent of MEN2 cases.

RET encodes a plasma membrane bound receptor tyrosine kinase (**Figure 24.3**) that is expressed by thyroid C cells, cells of the adrenal medulla, autonomic nerve ganglia, colonic ganglia and parathyroid cells. The receptor consists of an *N*-terminal peptide, an extracellular domain important for cell-to-cell signalling (cadherin-like region) and receptor dimerization (cysteine-rich region), a transmembrane domain and two intracellular tyrosine kinase domains.

The C-terminal of RET protein has three splice variants; their various protein products have organ-specific physiological roles. Ligands of RET include glial cell line-derived neurotrophic factor (GDNF) in conjunction with a ligand-specific coreceptor (GFRα1-4), neurturin, artemin and persephin. Activation of the receptor leads to activation of various intracellular signalling pathways including c-JUN, Ras/ERK, MAPK, p38 that are involved in cell proliferation and survival, and the responses of cells to cytotoxic agents.

RET codon mutations correlate with the MTC phenotype (**Table 24.3**). The extracellular MEN2A 634 activating mutation induces a ligand-independent constitutive dimerization of the RET receptor which leads to abnormal cell growth, differentiation defects and cellular transformation. The intracellular 918 MEN2B mutation is associated with receptor activation in the absence of receptor dimerization by alteration of kinase substrate specificity.[21, 33]

Somatic mutations of *RET*, usually at codon 918, are found in approximately 25 per cent of sporadic MTC and linked with poorer prognosis.

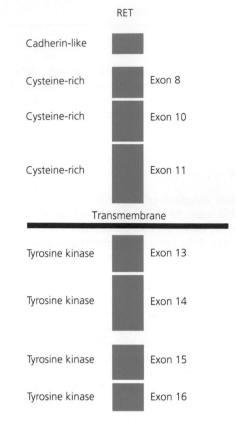

Figure 24.3   Schematic of membrane bound tyrosine kinase receptor encoded by *RET*.

CLINICAL FEATURES OF SPORADIC AND HEREDITARY MTC

The average age at presentation of sporadic MTC is in the fourth and fifth decade,[34, 35] while MEN2A typically presents in the second or third decades, MEN2B in the first and second decades, FMTC in the fourth and fifth decades.[36] The sex ratio is almost equal.

Local tumour growth, i.e. a thyroid mass, is normally the first indication of disease (>75 per cent), usually a non-tender thyroid nodule or diffuse thyroid enlargement. MTC metastasizes early to the locoregional lymph nodes. Cervical lymphadenopathy is seen as the first presenting feature in approximately 40–50 per cent of patients.[34, 37] Other MTC symptoms of either local mass effect or tumour invasion include airway compromise (10 per cent), neck sensitivity (9 per cent) and dysphagia (4 per cent). Recurrent laryngeal nerve palsy is rare as a presenting feature in MTC. Diarrhoea (the specific cause of which is unknown), flushing and bone pain are reported in 20–30 per cent of MTC and reflect tumour bulk; they are signs of disseminated disease. Blood-borne metastases are evident at presentation in the liver, lungs and bone of 12–28 per cent of patients. ACTH production by MTC in rare cases will cause Cushing syndrome.

Even patients with micro-MTC have a significant incidence of extrathyroidal manifestation of the disease at presentation, lymph node metastasis in 10 per cent, distant metastases in 6.3 per cent, diarrhoea and/or flushing in 7.5 per cent.[38]

Table 24.3 *RET* mutations associated with hereditary medullary thyroid cancer.

Exon	Codon	Syndrome	Frequency of mutation
	Cysteine–rich domain		
8	532	FMTC	
	533	FMTC	
10	609	MEN2A/ FMTC	<1%
	611	MEN2A/ FMTC	2–3%
	618	MEN2A/ FMTC	3–5%
	620	MEN2A/ FMTC	6–8%
11	630	MEN2A/ FMTC	<1%
	634	MEN2A	80–90%
	634, 635	MEN2A	
	635	MEN2A	
	637	MEN2A	
	Tyrosine kinase domain		
13	768	FMTC	
	790	MEN2A/ FMTC	
	791	FMTC	
14	804	MEN2A/ FMTC	
	804.806	MEN2B	
	844	FMTC	
15	883	MEN2B	
	891	FMTC	
16	912	FMTC	
	918	MEN2B	3–5%

When the same codon appears twice, the amino acid/nucleotide sequence is different.

Phaeochromocytoma will occur in up to 55 per cent of MEN2 patients. It is most commonly associated with codon mutations at 634 and 918, but found in association with nearly all MEN2 genotypes.[39] Phaeochromocytoma may be the first manifestation of the MEN2 syndrome in up to 25 per cent of cases; it is associated with adrenomedullary hyperplasia, sometimes bilateral phaeochromocytoma, but rarely extra-adrenal or malignant disease. Annual screening for phaeochromocytoma is warranted from the age of ten years in carriers of RET mutations in codons 918, 634 and 630, and from the age of 20 years in the remainder.[40] The average age at the time of diagnosis is the fourth decade.

In patients with MEN2A, hyperparathyroidism is reported to occur in 20–30 per cent of individuals, almost exclusively in those with mutations of codon 634 and 618.[41] Mean age at diagnosis is 38 years.[42] Patients are generally asymptomatic and the hypercalcaemia is often mild. Asymmetric parathyroid gland enlargement is the norm and resection of only the enlarged glands is recommended.[43, 44]

Rare forms of MEN2A with specific *RET* mutations are associated with Hirschsprung's disease[45] and cutaneous lichen amyloidosis (brownish plaques of multiple tiny papules, usually in the interscapular area).[46]

Four or more MTC-affected members of a kindred without other endocrine tumours are required for the clear diagnosis of FMTC. The age at onset of MTC in this syndrome is older than seen in MEN2A and MEN2B and the phenotype is less aggressive.

MEN2B has a specific phenotype that may be apparent in infancy. The facies are typical with enlarged lips (**Figure 24.4**). Mucosal ganglioneuromas arise in the digestive tract and are associated with abdominal distension, megacolon, constipation and diarrhoea. In infants, the colonic manifestations of MEN2B may be confused with Hirschsprung's disease, but the true diagnosis will be revealed on rectal biopsy.[47] Such presentation seems to be associated with early onset of MTC.[48] Ganglioneuromas can also be seen on the conjunctivae, lips and tongue (**Figure 24.5**). Other manifestations include skeletal abnormalities – marfanoid habitus, joint laxity, pes cavus, pectus cavatum, and markedly thickened corneal nerves. Patients with MEN2B will most likely (95 per cent) have a mutation at codon 918, 50 per cent of patients have a *de novo RET* mutation. Early diagnosis is essential in individuals with MEN2B because the onset of MTC occurs at a very early age. Those who have not undergone thyroidectomy within the first year of life are likely to develop metastatic disease.

DIAGNOSIS OF MEDULLARY THYROID CANCER

The diagnosis of MTC in most cases will result from the investigation of patients who present with a thyroid or lymph node mass. Fine needle aspiration biopsy, alone or in combination with immunocytochemistry, electron microscopy and serum calcitonin, will result in an accurate diagnosis in most cases.[49, 50, 51, 52] When cytology is not adequate, core needle biopsy, with or without ultrasound guidance avoids the need for open biopsy in nearly all cases. A preoperative diagnosis allows for a planned surgical intervention and reduces the need for completion thyroid and/or completion lymphadenectomy.

Routine measurement of basal calcitonin in patients presenting with nodular thyroid disease is recommended by some to identify otherwise undetected MTC (**Tables 24.4 and 24.5**) and lead to the potential benefit of better outcome.[56, 68] The prevalence of MTC in this group of patients varies from 0.4 to 1.8 per cent. Basal hypercalcitonaemia will be evident in at least 1.5 per cent of screened patients. In one study, approximately 60 per cent of patients with a high basal calcitonin did not have MTC, 57 per cent of hypercalcitonaemic patients without MTC had C-cell hyperplasia.[54] The positive predictive value of an abnormal basal calcitonin varies between studies, but for levels ≥20 pg/mL is reported as 23.1 per cent, for values >100 pg/mL as 100 per cent.[53] Pentagastrin stimulation testing (see below under Preoperative investigations) is required to confirm true positives. A positive test correlates with CCH and MTC, but false positives occur in up to 25 per cent of subjects.[55]

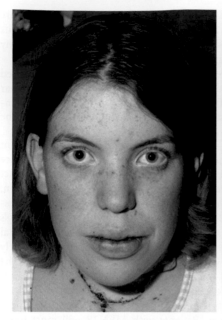
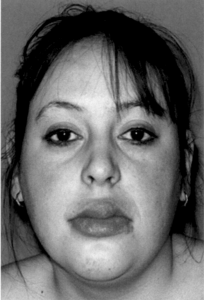
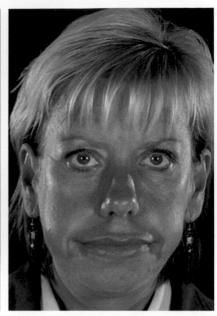

Figure 24.4   Typical facial phenotype of three unrelated MEN2B patients.

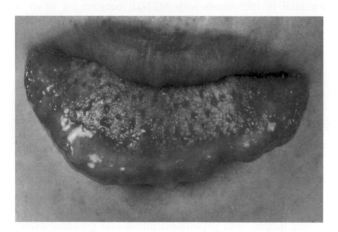

Figure 24.5   Tongue of 11-year-old MEN2B patient showing typical ganglioneuromas.

PREOPERATIVE INVESTIGATIONS

Calcitonin

Serum calcitonin (CT) is a sensitive and accurate marker of MTC; an elevated basal calcitonin level confirms the cytological or histological diagnosis of MTC in a symptomatic patient. False-positive serum calcitonin levels are recorded in patients with autoimmune thyroid disease, hypercalcaemia, foregut-derived neuroendocrine tumours, and renal failure. Conversely, MTC cases with normal basal serum calcitonin are recognized.[69]

Basal calcitonin should be measured in all patients with MTC prior to surgery. The level of calcitonin is a good indicator of disease extent: lymph node involvement may be found in patients with calcitonin as low as 10–40 pg/mL, distant metastasis and extrathyroidal growth can occur with calcitonin levels of 150–400 pg/mL.[70]

Table 24.4   Results of routine calcitonin screening in patients with nodular thyroid disease.

Author	No. patients screened	MTC detected
Costante et al.[53]	5817	15
Papi et al.[54]	1425	9
Vierhapper et al.[55]	14 000	32
Elisei et al.[56]	10 864	44
Niccoli et al.[57]	1167	16
Rink et al.[58]	21 900	28

In patients with potentially false-positive basal calcitonin levels, or when there is uncertainty about the histological diagnosis, a pentagastrin or pentagastrin/calcium stimulation test should be performed. The slow intravenous injection of 0.5 µg/kg pentagastrin and/or calcium gluconate 2 mg/kg is followed by venous sampling at 0, 1, 2, 3, 5 and 10 minutes. Peak calcitonin values are found at 1–2 minutes. The protocols for these tests and the definition of a positive test (two- or three-fold increase) or peak values >100–300 pg/mL are not standardized. Patients who have false-positive elevations of basal calcitonin will show a negative response to pentagastrin. Some patients with early MTC will have peak calcitonin values less than 100 pg/mL.[71] Side effects of the test include nausea, chest or abdominal pain, flushing and headache. The test has a further role, particularly in the setting of clinical research, to confirm biochemical cure of MTC after surgery.

Historically, patients at risk of genetically determined MTC were screened annually using pentagastrin/calcium stimulation in order to confirm the diagnosis of CCH or MTC. The requirement to subject patients to these tests is now superseded by the combination of RET mutation analysis, basal calcitonin estimation and a better understanding of genotype–phenotype correlation and the timing of surgery.

Table 24.5 Survival of patients with sporadic/hereditary MTC.

Author	Year	No.	Age (years)	5 year (%)	10 year (%)
Bergholm et al.[59]	1997	247[b]	11–85	69	65
Modigliani et al.[60]	1998	899[b]	–	85[a]	78[a]
Hyer et al.[61]	2000	162[c]	–	72	56
Kebebew et al.[62]	2000	104[c]	–	89[a]	87[a]
Bhattacharya et al.[24]	2003	499[b]	–	–	74
Clark et al.[63]	2005	30[c]	–	97[a]	74[a]
De Groot et al.[64]	2006	120[c]	1–35	–	73[a]
Pelizzo et al.[65]	2006	157[c]	6–79	–	72
Machens et al.[66]	2007	128[c]	–	89[a]	–
Ito et al.[67]	2009	118[c]	–	–	96[a]

[a]Cause-specific survival.
[b]National database.
[c]Single centre.
In Kebebew et al.,[62] 44 per cent of patients with familial disease, a third detected by screening.

Kindred of *RET* mutation-negative patients with apparent syndromic MTC and negative linkage studies will still require to undergo annual pentagastrin stimulation tests. Surgery is then proposed when the test is positive.

Urinary or plasma catecholamines/metanephrines

Phaeochromocytoma must be excluded prior to surgery in all patients with a diagnosis of MTC. Biochemical testing is mandatory. The absence of symptoms or hypertension does not indicate the absence of a catecholamine-secreting tumour. The absence of a family history does not preclude genetically determined disease; the patient may represent the index case of an MEN2 kindred. A 24-hour urine collection should be assayed for fractionated catecholamines, metanephrines and normetanephrines. Plasma-free normet/metanephrines can be assayed and have high sensitivity for the detection of familial phaeochromocytoma.[72]

Calcium

A serum calcium level should be obtained in all MTC patients prior to surgery. The results of *RET* mutation analysis may not be available before operation; a high serum calcium level may indicate previously undiagnosed MEN2A in the patient. A high or inappropriate level of serum parathyroid hormone (PTH) will indicate the need for careful assessment of the parathyroid glands at the time of thyroidectomy and, when necessary, excision of enlarged glands.

RET mutation analysis

Even in the absence of a positive family history, MEN2 should be suspected when MTC occurs at an early age or is multifocal/bilateral. In patients with apparently sporadic MTC, the prevalence of germline *RET* mutation is reported as high as 7.3 per cent.[73] All patients with a diagnosis of sporadic MTC should therefore undergo *RET* mutation

analysis because they may represent the index case of a previously undiagnosed MEN kindred. Predictive DNA tests should be carried out under the auspices of a clinical genetics service.

DNA-based testing will identify mutations in more than 95 per cent of individuals with MEN2A and MEN2B and in about 85 per cent of individuals with FMTC. When a patient with MTC is identified as carrying a *RET* mutation, genetic screening should then be offered to first-degree relatives of the proband. Family members identified as gene positive may then be offered therapeutic or risk reduction surgery for MTC (see below under Surgery for MTC) depending upon their age, genotype and disease extent.

Ultrasound

Ultrasound imaging of the thyroid and lymph nodes may have been performed prior to diagnosis as a part of non-specific thyroid work up or to guide fine needle aspiration (FNA). It is not mandatory prior to first time surgery, although it may provide a 'road map' of clinically undetectable disease. Ultrasound appearances of MTC in thyroid or lymph nodes are not specific, hypoechoic tumours less than 5 mm in diameter may be discovered. Ultrasound may identify bilateral and/or multiple thyroid lesions, suggestive of genetically determined disease, enlarged and abnormal lymph nodes. Microcalcification seen in lymph nodes is probably due to amyloid.[74]

CT/MRI

Preoperative assessment of the neck and mediastinum with computed tomography (CT) or magnetic resonance imaging (MRI) may alert the surgeon to the presence of extrathyroidal disease that involves the airway or oesophagus, and of lymph node enlargement outside the neck (**Figure 24.6**). Positive findings may result in an alteration in the surgical strategy to include planned resection of involved viscera or mediastinal lymphadenectomy requiring sternotomy. Cross-sectional imaging of the lungs and liver may reveal unsuspected distant

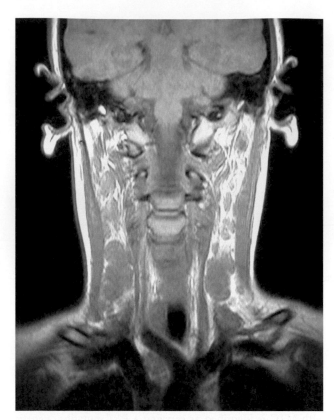

Figure 24.6   Magnetic resonance image showing bilateral cervical and infrabrachiocephalic lymphadenopathy in 17-year-old MEN2B patient following previous thyroidectomy.

disease that may result in planned restriction of the extent of neck surgery. A negative examination of the lungs and liver does not preclude pulmonary or hepatic spread as small MTC metastases are often below the lower limit of resolution of the scan.

An assessment of vocal cord function should be made prior to surgery in patients with proven or suspected MTC.

Invasive staging (laparoscopy, hepatic angiography) and radio-isotope scanning (^{131}I-MIBG, ^{99m}Tc-(V)-DMSA, ^{111}In-octreotide, ^{18}FDG-PET) are not routinely indicated prior to first time surgery. Their use is outlined below under Localization of persistent/recurrent MTC in the investigation of patients with residual or recurrent disease. If no metastases are identified on cross-sectional imaging, and there is a high index of suspicion of liver disease, laparoscopy is indicated.

SURGERY FOR MTC

The aim of surgery in patients with MTC is to remove all disease in the neck, to produce biochemical and clinical cure and minimize risk of locoregional relapse. This requires meticulous total thyroidectomy and lymph node dissection in most patients. ('Biochemical cure' is a term frequently misused as 'normalization' of basal calcitonin levels after surgery. It should probably be used only when pentagastrin stimulation does not result in a significant rise in hormone levels.) Surgery should be performed with the intention to preserve recurrent laryngeal nerves, superior laryngeal nerves and parathyroid function. There is little evidence other than non-randomized retrospective studies on which to base firm recommendations for surgical treatment.[75]

Rationale for lymph node dissection in MTC

Nodal metastases are common (>75 per cent) in patients with palpable MTC[76] and occur early in the disease. Spread of MTC to lymph nodes occurs in a characteristic pattern – ipsilateral central, ipsilateral lateral, then contralateral central neck. Further spread occurs to contralateral lateral and the upper mediastinal lymph nodes.[77] Lymph node involvement may be found when the basal calcitonin level is only minimally above the normal range.[70] The frequency can be predicted by tumour size and ranges from 17 (pT1) to 100 per cent (pT4).[78] Node metastases are uncommon in sporadic medullary microcarcinoma (1 cm diameter or less),[79, 80] but have been reported to occur in 30 per cent of patients.[38] The pattern of metastatic node distribution in the neck is not related to tumour size.[81] Historically, it has been considered that patients with familial MTC are more at risk of bilateral cervical node involvement because the frequency of multifocal, bilateral disease is high compared with sporadic MTC. However, central compartment node involvement is found in up to 80 per cent of patients with sporadic or hereditary disease. Ipsilateral lateral nodes are involved in 34->80 per cent and contralateral lateral nodes in 19->50 per cent of cases.[76, 81, 82, 83] The frequency of ipsilateral and contralateral lateral compartment node involvement reflects the degree of central compartment node positivity.[83] Skip metastases (negative central and positive lateral or mediastinal compartments) are found in approximately 20 per cent of patients.[84] Mediastinal node disease is more likely to occur in patients with positive cervical nodes and extrathyroidal extension;[85] contralateral cervical or mediastinal lymph node involvement predicts an increased risk of distant metastases.[86]

Standard texts describe the locoregional lymph nodes groups of the thyroid according to Robbins et al.[87] and UICC classifications. There is, however, a lack of clarity, accuracy and confusion in the anatomical terminology of lymph node groups and the surgical procedures described in the treatment of MTC that do not allow direct comparison of outcomes or easy understanding of surgical recommendations for treatment. This may partly explain the lack of compliance with guidelines for 'best surgical practice' which result in undertreatment of many patients with MTC.[88, 89, 90]

To this end, the following terms are defined:

- **Selective neck dissection**. Selective neck dissection preserves one or more of the lymph node groups removed by radical neck dissection.
- **Central compartment**. The area between the carotid arteries, the superior limit is the hyoid bone and inferiorly the suprasternal notch.
- **Central neck dissection**. Removal of lymph nodes in level 6 that include the pre- and paratracheal, pre-cricoid (Delphian) and perithyroidal nodes. The lower limit of a level 6 node dissection, often described as the 'suprasternal notch' and the definition of level 7 nodes

often described as 'superior mediastinal nodes' is unclear.

- **Lateral neck dissection.** Removal of lymph nodes in levels II, III and IV.
- **Posterolateral neck dissection.** Removal of lymph nodes in levels II, III, IV and V.

The compartment classification of Dralle et al.[91] (**Figure 24.7**) avoids much of the above confusion. The central compartment – C1a right and C1b left – (Robbins levels VI and VII) includes the pre- and paratracheal, pre-cricoid, perithyroidal, paraoesophageal nodes extending from the level of the submandibular glands superiorly, the brachiocephalic vein inferiorly and laterally to the carotid arteries. The cervical lateral compartments (C2, right; C3, left) include cervical lymph nodes (Robbins levels II, III, IV, V) from the carotid sheath to the trapezius muscle laterally, and inferiorly from the subclavian vein to the hypoglossal nerve superiorly. The mediastinal compartment (C4) includes all lymph nodes between the left brachiocephalic (inominate) vein and tracheal bifurcation within the upper anterior and posterior mediastinum. This classification is based on surgical anatomy, is of prognostic significance in MTC and includes the mediastinal nodes below the brachiocephalic vein.

The normal recommendation for the treatment of MTC is total thyroidectomy, although sporadic disease is usually unilateral and unifocal (80 per cent). A single prospective study reported the outcome following unilateral thyroidectomy (in addition to central and ipsilateral modified radical neck dissection) in gene-negative patients with MTC and compared this with historical controls who had undergone total thyroidectomy. The extent of thyroid resection in the 37 patients studied did not influence the rate of biochemical cure.[92]

Total thyroidectomy and compartment orientated node dissection is associated with improved survival[91] and a reduced risk of recurrence.[93] Biochemical cure can be obtained in up to 95–100 per cent of patients without lymph node metastases, and in 32–45 per cent of patients with lymph node metastases.[67, 77, 81] When fewer than ten lymph nodes are involved, an undetectable calcitonin level is observed in 57 per cent of patients.[81]

A rational approach to the primary surgical treatment of MTC without distant metastases includes:

- For the uncommon scenarios:
  - Micro-MTC when the basal and stimulated calcitonin is normal: <5 mm sporadic disease, hemithroidectomy,[94] otherwise total thyroidectomy.[79, 80]
  - MTC <1 cm or >1 cm in diameter when the basal calcitonin is normal and stimulated calcitonin levels are elevated – total thyroidectomy and central neck dissection (C1) (**Figure 24.8**).[78] Patients with stimulated calcitonin levels >560 pg/mL should be treated as having palpable disease[95] and considered for lateral neck dissection (C2/C3).
- For the common scenarios,
  - MTC with elevated basal calcitonin level and/or lymph node involvement – total thyroidectomy, central and lateral neck dissection (C1–C3).[78]
  - When preoperative imaging identifies mediastinal nodal disease or when there is a high risk of node involvement (patients with T4 tumours) mediastinal lymphadenectomy (C4) (via a trans-sternal approach) should be performed (**Figure 24.9**).

The addition of lymph node dissection to total thyroidectomy increases the likelihood of recurrent laryngeal nerve and parathyroid morbidity.[78, 88, 96] In all patients with MTC who undergo surgery, an attempt should be made to preserve parathyroid tissue *in situ* or by autotransplantation. Transient hypocalcaemia may occur in up to 60 per cent of patients who undergo central compartment neck dissection.[97] Permanent hypoparathyroidism after thyroidectomy and central compartment neck dissection is reported in 0.7–4.6 per cent of patients.[96, 97, 98] In expert hands,

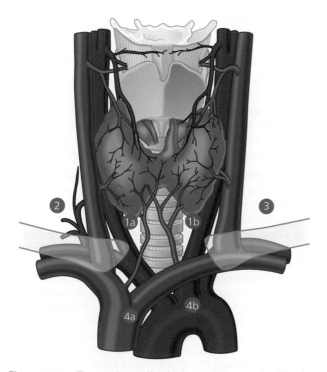

Figure 24.7 The cervicomediastinal compartment classification of Dralle et al.[91] Compartment: 1a/b, right/left central neck compartment; 2, right lateral neck; 3, left lateral neck; 4a/b, right/left mediastinal.

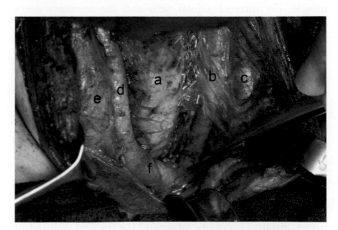

Figure 24.8 Central compartment of neck following C1–C3 lymph node dissection: (a) trachea; (b) left common carotid artery; (c) left internal jugular vein; (d) right common carotid artery; (e) right internal jugular vein; (f) brachiocephalic artery.

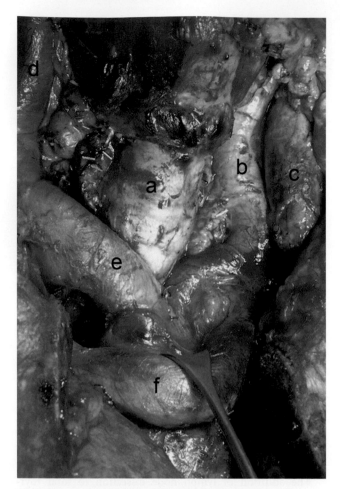

Figure 24.9 Central compartment of neck and anterior mediastinum following C1 and C4 lymph node dissection: (a) trachea; (b) left common carotid artery; (c) left internal jugular vein; (d) right common carotid artery; (e) brachiocephalic artery; (f) left inominate vein.

permanent recurrent laryngeal nerve palsy after neck dissection can be a very rare occurrence.[96, 99]

In the absence of direct invasion, the sternomastoid muscle, the internal jugular vein and the accessory nerve should be conserved. Routine dissection of levels I and IIb is not required unless there are palpable/suspicious nodes at these sites. In patients with locally advanced disease, when preoperative vocal cord examination has revealed no sign of recurrent laryngeal nerve involvement every attempt should be made to dissect the tumour from the nerve/s. In patients with unilateral nerve involvement associated with extensive extrathyroidal disease, the nerve may have to be sacrificed to achieve a 'curative' procedure. It may not be possible to remove the entire tumour without damaging both recurrent laryngeal nerves, in which case a small residue of tumour may be left behind to protect the nerve/s.

When locally advanced disease involves the upper aerodigestive tract and/or one or both recurrent laryngeal nerves, curative excisional surgery of the tracheal wall and/or oesophagus should be considered. Although pT4 tumours have an approximately 80 per cent risk of distant metastases,[78] survival may be prolonged. For this reason, most patients with confirmed distant metastases should undergo

total thyroidectomy and central neck dissection (C1) and should be considered for resection of bulky/symptomatic lymph node disease in the lateral neck (C2 and C3) and/or mediastinum (C4).

Follow up

Thyroid hormone replacement is required and monitored and all patients with MTC require life-long review. The most useful markers of disease status are calcitonin and CEA.[100] In some patients, the expected postoperative fall in calcitonin levels may be delayed.[101, 102] At each visit, a clinical and biochemical assessment should be performed as apparent biochemical cure of MTC after surgery may not be sustained.[60, 103] Patients with MEN2 require multidisciplinary follow up to diagnose, treat and monitor the other components of their syndrome.

PERSISTENT/RECURRENT HYPERCALCITONAEMIA AND RECURRENT MTC

The diagnosis of residual/recurrent disease is made on the basis of clinical symptoms, or signs, or an elevated/rising calcitonin. Locoregional and distant metastases from MTC occur preferentially within the first five years.[104] Approximately 50 per cent of patients who present with palpable MTC without lymphadenopathy will develop locoregional disease even after total thyroidectomy and lymph node dissection.[105] In contrast, a zero locoregional recurrence rate at five years is described in patients with histologically node-negative disease after compartment orientated node dissection.[66]

When a patient presents with persistent or recurrent hypercalcitonaemia, the key issues for the surgeon are:

- Was the initial surgery less that that recommended according to best practice?
- Is the source of calcitonin in the neck (residual thyroid or lymph nodes) or mediastinum and amenable to further surgery?
- Will further surgery result in cure or improved survival?

Many patients will be found to have undergone less than optimal initial surgery: SEER data indicate that between 1994 and 2000, 15 per cent of patients with MTC had less than total or near total thyroidectomy,[106] and between 1973 and 2002, 41 per cent had no cervical lymph node dissection and 51 per cent of patients had less than currently recommended treatment guidelines for MTC.[89]

A conservative surgical approach has been advised by some authors for patients with persistent hypercalcitonaemia because of five- and ten-year survival rates of 90 and 86 per cent, respectively.[107] The key issue is whether or not residual disease lies within the neck and is remediable by surgery. Reoperation in selected patients can result in normalization of calcitonin levels in 22–38 per cent of cases[77, 108] that persist up to ten years from surgery.[109] Biochemical cure is most likely to occur in those patients who have previously undergone inadequate first time surgery.[110] Reoperation may limit MTC progression. In one retrospective study, patients who had a greater than 50 per cent decrease in calcitonin levels after reoperation were less likely to develop distant metastases compared with patients who did not have a greater than 50 per cent decrease.[111]

In practical terms, patients with persistent or recurrent disease, as identified by elevated calcitonin levels, should undergo cross-sectional imaging studies to include the neck, mediastinum, chest and abdomen. Radiographic evidence of recurrent disease is unlikely when the calcitonin level is at or below 250 pg/mL.[93] In the absence of metastases and when first time neck surgery was less than adequate, reoperation should be performed for what is best considered persistent disease. This will usually require compartment orientated cervical node dissection. Mediastinal lymph node dissection should be considered in patients undergoing reoperation for node-positive medullary thyroid carcinoma who have extrathyroidal extension and cervical lymph node metastases.[85] When localization studies identify recurrent locoregional disease after appropriate first time surgery, reoperative surgery should also be performed. The presence of distant disease should not in isolation preclude surgery because even with distant metastases, bulky locoregional disease can cause significant morbidity and deterioration in quality of life,[112] survival may be prolonged. The aim of surgery is not only to cure or significantly reduce disease bulk or symptoms, but relieve or prevent future compression of the airway and oesophagus, as well as involvement of the brachial plexus or recurrent laryngeal nerves.

Localization of persistent/recurrent MTC

The purpose of diagnostic imaging studies in patients with persistent/recurrent hypercalcitonaemia is the identification of surgically remediable locoregional disease that may put the patient at risk of airway or oesophageal compression. In all other cases, in the current absence of effective/proven systemic therapy and with a clinical trial, the imaging technique will only serve to identify incurable and often untreatable metastases.

In patients with medullary thyroid cancer and elevated calcitonin levels following thyroidectomy, metastases are best detected when serum calcitonin levels are greater than 500–800 pg/mL.[113, 114] The most efficient detection of metastatic MTC consists of neck ultrasound, chest CT, liver MRI, bone scintigraphy and axial skeleton MRI.[115] ^{111}In-octreotide (Octreoscan) is superior to ^{99m}Tc-(V) DMSA and has a similar sensitivity rate to CT and MRI for the diagnosis of recurrent or metastatic MTC,[116, 117] and as with ^{68}Ga DOTA-TATE PET/CT may identify patients suitable for targeted radionuclide analogue therapy.[118] ^{18}F-FDG-PET has a sensitivity of up to 85 per cent for localizing metastatic disease[119] and is superior to conventional nuclear imaging.[120, 121] The sensitivity of ^{18}F-FDG-PET is limited when disease bulk is small, as indicated by calcitonin levels of less than 500 pg/mL.[122] ^{18}F-DOPA PET/CT, although not widely available, seems to provide better results than Octreoscan and ^{18}FDG-PET,[113, 123, 124] although FDG-PET positivity is associated with more aggressive disease and shorter calcitonin doubling times.[113, 125, 126] Laparoscopy can detect liver metastases not seen on cross-sectional imaging;[127] liver angiography (**Figure 24.10**), albeit invasive, is a sensitive technique to

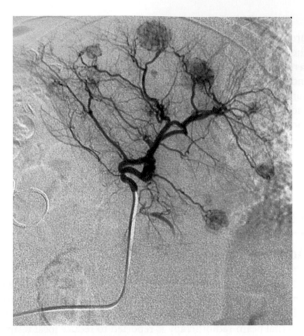

Figure 24.10 Selective hepatic artery angiogram showing metastases from a patient with long-standing medullary thyroid cancer. Patient asymptomatic ten years after diagnosis of these lesions.

confirm hepatic metastases as a source of hypercalcitonaemia.[128, 129] Selective venous sampling for calcitonin gradients may be useful to localize difficult to image residual, recurrent or metastatic MTC.[130, 131, 132]

OUTCOME AND PROGNOSIS

MTC is responsible for 10–15 per cent of deaths due to thyroid cancer;[23, 133] published survival rates at five and ten years range from 69 to 97 per cent and 56 to 96 per cent, respectively (**Table 24.5**). More than 50 per cent of patients with sporadic MTC will die of their disease. Biochemical cure following surgery is associated with 97.7 per cent survival at ten years,[60] survival for patients with micro-MTC is reported as 94 per cent at ten years.[38] Combined data from 61 European Cancer Registries indicate children with medullary carcinoma thyroid have five-year survival rates of 95 per cent.[134] Patients with advanced disease have a median survival of eight years[112] and a third of patients with systemic symptoms die within five years.[62]

On multivariate analysis, retrospective follow-up studies from single centres[61, 62, 65] and Swedish,[59] US National Cancer[23] and SEER databases[24, 89] indicate that younger age at diagnosis confers a survival advantage. A recent, single centre retrospective cohort study in which survival was adjusted for baseline population mortality did not confirm these findings.[135]

Preoperative basal calcitonin levels of less than 50 pg/mL (normal <10 pg/mL)[136] or more than 500 pg/mL[70] may predict the likelihood or failure of surgery to achieve biochemical cure, respectively. Post-treatment calcitonin doubling time of less than six months,[137] one year[135] and two years[114] indicates a worse prognosis. High preoperative CEA levels may indicate advanced disease.[138]

Histological features that are reported to indicate worse prognosis include the presence of lymphovascular invasion,[104] the number of positive lymph nodes, capsule invasion,[139] disseminated tumour cells in connective tissue.[140] Those that indicate a better prognosis include amyloid, DNA euploidy,[59] somatostatin expression in tumour cells,[141] absence of desmoplastic stromal reaction.[142] A somatic *RET* mutation,[143, 144] increased disease stage,[62] tumour size,[59, 65, 78] extent of local disease,[24, 104] extent of lymph node involvement,[61, 81] distant metastases, less extensive surgery[61, 65] and the presence of extrathyroidal disease[135] confer an adverse outcome.

NON-SURGICAL TREATMENT OF MTC

Adjuvant radiotherapy

Adjuvant radiation therapy has been found to be independently associated with a decreased survival,[89] although its use is inevitably confined to those patients with a worse prognosis. External beam radiotherapy is reported to reduce local relapse in patients with limited nodal disease,[61] in high risk patients[145] and in those presenting with more advanced disease.[146, 147] It has not been shown to produce a survival benefit.

Systemic therapy

Therapeutic ^{131}I-MIBG may provide transient, partial objective response or symptom palliation.[148] The somatostatin analogue octreotide (DOTATOC) labelled with ^{90}Y administered to patients with metastatic MTC that expresses somatostatin receptors can result in partial response, stable disease and survival benefit.[149, 150]

Combination regimes of chemotherapeutic agents that include doxirubicin, streptozotocin, 5 FU and dacarbazine have been studied in small series with minimal partial response and disease stabilization in approximately 50 per cent of patients.[151, 152, 153]

In vivo and *in vitro* studies using inhibitors of RET and FGFR4,[154] the P13K pathway,[155] tyrosine kinase,[156, 157] topoisomerase,[158] proteasome,[159] tumour suppressor gene activation,[160] targeted anti-CEA radioimmunotherapy[161] and somatostatin analogue therapy[162] provide a background for trials for patients with recurrent medullary thyroid carcinoma that include open and randomized phase II studies of ZD6474 (Zactima®; Astra Zeneca), Vandetanib®,[163, 164] Motesanib®,[165] Cabozantinib[166] and a phase II trial of pretargeted radioimmunotherapy using anti-CEA DTPA bispecific antibody and di-DTPA-^{131}I peptide of molecular targeted therapy. The subject is well covered in two recent reviews.[167, 168]

Table 24.6 Case history 1: 27-year-old male with apparently sporadic medullary thyroid cancer.

			Comments and learning points
	1999	Thyroid nodule. Referred to surgeon	
	2002	Subtotal thyroid lobectomy. Diagnosis: medullary thyroid cancer	2 year delay/inappropriate procedure
		Referred '… please advise as to further treatment …'	Young patient with MTC = ?MEN2A
Investigations			
	November 2002	Calcitonin 320 ng/L (NR, 0–11.5)	Calcitonin level indicating at least node metastases
		Urinary metanephrines and catecholamines – increased	
		Abdominal CT – bilateral adrenal masses (**Figure 24.11**)	'Asymptomatic' phaeochromocytomas
		RET 634 mutation, i.e. MEN2A	Index case in gene negative family
Treatment			
	February 2005	Bilateral laparoscopic adrenalectomy – cortical sparing	
	March 2005	Completion bilateral thyroidectomy and C1–C3 neck dissection	
Histology			
		Bilateral phaeochromocytomas MTC pT2N1aMx	
Follow up			
	November 2003	Calcitonin 5.1 ng/L (NR, 0–11.5)	
	April 2009	Calcitonin 14.2 ng/L (NR, 0–18.9)	Despite late presentation of hereditary disease
		Normal adrenal function. No recurrence of phaeochromocytoma	Good outcome with 'stable' calcitonin at 4 years
	September 2010	Calcitonin 6 ng/L (NR, 0–11.8)	

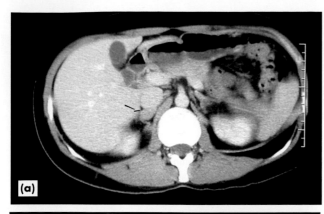

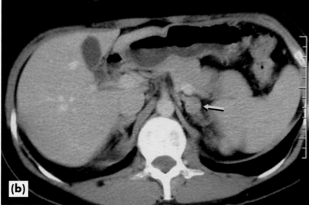

Figure 24.11 Abdominal CT scan showing asymptomatic (a) right and (b) left asymptomatic phaeochromocytoma in MEN2A patient who had undergone recent thyroid surgery without cardiovascular crisis!

PROPHYLACTIC SURGERY FOR HEREDITARY MTC

Children and adolescents identified by *RET* screening to be at risk for the development of medullary thyroid cancer can be treated with prophylactic thyroidectomy before developing the disease. The timing of the intervention is modified according to genotype and the age at presentation.

Age at onset of CCH and MTC and timing of thyroidectomy

The progression of C-cell hyperplasia to MTC and subsequent lymph node metastasis occurs in an age-related, codon-specific manner:

* Children with *RET* codon 883, 918 mutations (MEN2B), classified as level 3, have the highest risk from aggressive MTC. Neoplastic transformation of C cells occurs in the first year of life.
* Children with *RET* codon 609, 611, 618, 620, 630 or 634 mutations classified as level 2 have a high risk for MTC. Neoplastic transformation of C cells occurs in the first decade.
* Children with *RET* codon 768, 790, 791 804 and 891 mutations are classified as level 1 or as having the least high risk.

Cohort studies that include asymptomatic carriers with no malignancy or T1 N0 tumours[169] and index patients/carriers with various stages of disease[170] form the basis of recommendations as to at what age prophylactic/risk reduction total thyroidectomy should be performed:

* highest risk carriers within the first year of life, preferably in the first six months;
* high risk carriers before the age of five years;
* least high risk carriers before ten years of age.

The earliest manifestation of node-negative MTC, node-positive and metastatic disease for specific *RET* genotypes[171, 172] reveals that node-negative MTC can occur, albeit rarely, at an age earlier than that recommended for 'prophylactic' surgery. On that basis, decisions as to the timing and the extent of surgery should be based not only on the affected codon, but in addition the age of the patient, and the calcitonin level.

Timing of lymph node surgery

In ideal circumstances, risk reduction surgery (total thyroidectomy) should be performed before the onset of MTC, thereby reducing the need for lymph node dissection, which is associated with an increased risk of hypoparathyroidism and recurrent laryngeal nerve injury; it would be preferable to avoid this. In reality, cases often manifest when it is likely or evident that MTC is already present and occult lymph node metastasis may have occurred.

Current recommendations suggest that children with highest risk mutations (883, 918) should undergo routine lymph node dissection at the time of thyroidectomy in the first year of life. The evidence base for recommendations regarding lymph node dissection in children with high risk mutations is less clear. Although node metastasis has been identified in a child with MEN2A of five years 11 months,[172] the multicentre EUROMEN study did not find node involvement prior to the age of 14 years in individuals with a 634 codon mutation.[169] An evidenced-based review suggests that children with a 634 mutation should undergo lymph node dissection from the age of five years and those with mutations at codon 609, 611, 618, 620 and 630 from the ages of ten years.[171] Recommendations for those with least-high risk suggest node dissection should be performed from the age of 20 years. Recent studies suggest that in the absence of clinical features to the contrary, lymph node surgery can be avoided in *RET* carriers with a normal basal calcitonin.[173]

Results of 'prophylactic' surgery

Previously reported outcomes of 'prophylactic' surgery should be interpreted with the knowledge that MTC was often present at the time of surgery; the intervention would have been better termed 'risk reduction' or indeed therapeutic. By 2005, only 15 per cent of the 275 reported 'prophylactic' thyroidectomies performed on *RET* 634 children were carried out before the age of five years.[174] Studies of outcome from risk reduction surgery in young patients up to the age of 21 years confirm that biochemical cure is possible and sustained at follow up in the majority of individuals. In the landmark study, at a mean

Table 24.7 Case history 2: 42-year-old woman with sporadic medullary thyroid cancer.

			Comments and learning points
	2005	Thyroid nodule. Referred to surgeon	
		Subtotal thyroid lobectomy. Diagnosis: medullary thyroid cancer	
		Referred '... please advise as to further treatment...'	
Investigations			
	May 2005	Calcitonin 337 ng/L (NR, 0–4.6)	Calcitonin level indicating at least node metastases
		Urinary metanephrines and catecholamines – normal	
		RET mutation analysis – negative	Sporadic MTC
Treatment			
	October 2005	Completion thyroidectomy and C1–C3 neck dissection	
Histology			
		MTC. pT2 pN1b single unilateral positive node	
Follow up			
	November 2005	Calcitonin 362 ng/L (NR, 0–4.6)	Calcitonin level indicates distant metastasis
	April 2006	Calcitonin 553 ng/L (NR, 0–5.5)	
	August 2006	Calcitonin 1005 ng/L (NR, 0–5.5)	Rapid calcitonin doubling time – poor prognosis
		Extensive imaging chest/neck/abdomen CT/MRI/DOPA-PET – negative	
	June 2007	Calcitonin 5060 ng/L (NR, 0–5.5)	
	June 2007	Multiple liver metastases on MRI	
	February 2009	Calcitonin 3300 ng/L	Clinical trial of tyrosine kinase inhibitor
	May 2011	Calcitonin 5020 ng/L (NR, 0–4.8)	

of seven years from surgery (total thyroidectomy, central neck node dissection) 88 per cent of 50 patients who had undergone surgery between the ages of three and 19 years had undetectable basal and stimulated calcitonin levels.[175] A further report details outcome in 46 *RET* gene carriers (11 level 1 mutations and 35 level 2 mutations) who had undergone surgery at ages ranging from four to 21 years with a mean follow up of 6.4 years. All level 1 patients were cured. Of the level 2 patients, 24 patients had invasive disease (all pN0) at the time of surgery, five patients were not cured.[176]

CASE HISTORIES

Illustrative case histories of two patients with MTC are given in **Tables 24.6** and **24.7**.

KEY EVIDENCE

- Reoperation in patients with residual or recurrent MTC in the neck results in normalization of calcitonin in approximately a third of selected patients.[75]

- Genotype–phenotype correlations in genetically determined MTC provide a solid foundation on which to base recommendations for the timing of prophylactic surgery.[171, 177]
- Patients with MTC with suspected local metastatic disease to regional lymph nodes in the central compartment should undergo a total thyroidectomy and level VI compartmental dissection. When lymph node metastases are present in the paratracheal central compartment, the issue of lateral compartment node dissection is controversial.[178]

KEY LEARNING POINTS

- The care of patients with medullary thyroid cancer requires involvement of a specialist and an experienced multidisciplinary team that includes a clinical geneticist.
- All patients with MTC must undergo genetic testing for *RET* mutations to identify those with hereditary disease. When a patient is confirmed

as carrying a *RET* mutation, family members should be screened for the mutation. Prophylactic thyroidectomy should be offered to young gene-positive family members prior to the onset of malignancy.
- In patients with proven or suspected medullary thyroid cancer, phaeochromocytoma must be excluded prior to surgery by biochemical testing. An uneventful first operation does not preclude an 'eventful' reoperative procedure in a patient with a previously undiagnosed phaeochromocytoma.
- Meticulous surgery can result in biochemical cure of MTC.
- In patients with MTC, an elevated basal calcitonin, and/or involved nodes and no distant metastases – total thyroidectomy and node dissection of the central and lateral neck compartments (C1–C3) should be performed.

REFERENCES

1. Hazard JB, Hawk WA, Crile G Jr. Medullary (solid) carcinoma of the thyroid; a clinicopathologic entity. *Journal of Clinical Endocrinology and Metabolism* 1959; **19**: 152–61.
2. Foster GV, MacIntyre I, Pearse AG. Calcitonin production and the mitochondrion-rich cells of the dog thyroid. *Nature* 1964; **203**: 1029–30.
3. Pearse AG, Polak JM. Cytochemical evidence for the neural crest origin of mammalian ultimobranchial C cells. *Histochemie* 1971; **27**: 96–102.
4. Hayles AB, Kennedy RL, Beahrs OH, Woolner LB. Management of the child with thyroidal carcinoma. *Journal of the American Medical Association* 1960; **173**: 21–8.
5. Sipple J. The association of pheochromocytoma with carcinoma of the thyroid gland. *American Journal of Medicine* 1961; **31**: 163–6.
6. Williams ED. Histogenesis of medullary carcinoma of the thyroid. *Journal of Clinical Pathology* 1966; **19**: 114–18.
7. Williams ED. Diarrhoea and thyroid carcinoma. *Proceedings of the Royal Society of Medicine* 1966; **59**: 602–3.
8. Williams ED. A review of 17 cases of carcinoma of the thyroid and phaeochromocytoma. *Journal of Clinical Pathology* 1965; **18**: 288–92.
9. Williams ED, Pollock DJ. Multiple mucosal neuromata with endocrine tumours: a syndrome allied to von Recklinghausen's disease. *Journal of Pathology and Bacteriology* 1966; **91**: 71–80.
10. Schimke RN, Hartmann WH, Prout TE, Rimoin DL. Syndrome of bilateral pheochromocytoma, medullary thyroid carcinoma and multiple neuromas. A possible regulatory defect in the differentiation of chromaffin tissue. *New England Journal of Medicine* 1968; **279**: 1–7.
11. Tashjian AH Jr, Melvin EW. Medullary carcinoma of the thyroid gland. Studies of thyrocalcitonin in plasma and tumor extracts. *New England Journal of Medicine* 1968; **279**: 279–83.
12. Cushman P Jr. Familial endocrine tumors; report of two unrelated kindred affected with pheochromocytomas, one also with multiple thyroid carcinomas. *American Journal of Medicine* 1962; **32**: 352–60.
13. Takahashi M, Ritz J, Cooper GM. Activation of a novel human transforming gene, ret, by DNA rearrangement. *Cell* 1985; **42**: 581–8.
14. Takahashi M, Buma Y, Iwamoto T et al. Cloning and expression of the ret proto-oncogene encoding a tyrosine kinase with two potential transmembrane domains. *Oncogene* 1988; **3**: 571–8.
15. Simpson NE, Kidd KK, Goodfellow PJ et al. Assignment of multiple endocrine neoplasia type 2A to chromosome 10 by linkage. *Nature* 1987; **328**: 528–30.
16. Mathew CG, Chin KS, Easton DF et al. A linked genetic marker for multiple endocrine neoplasia type 2A on chromosome 10. *Nature* 1987; **328**: 527–8.
17. Mulligan LM, Kwok JB, Healey CS et al. Germ-line mutations of the RET proto-oncogene in multiple endocrine neoplasia type 2A. *Nature* 1993; **363**: 458–60.
18. Donis-Keller H, Dou S, Chi D et al. Mutations in the RET proto-oncogene are associated with MEN 2A and FMTC. *Human Molecular Genetics* 1993; **2**: 851–6.
19. Mulligan LM, Eng C, Attie T et al. Diverse phenotypes associated with exon 10 mutations of the RET proto-oncogene. *Human Molecular Genetics* 1994; **3**: 2163–7.
20. Carlson KM, Dou S, Chi D et al. Single missense mutation in the tyrosine kinase catalytic domain of the RET protooncogene is associated with multiple endocrine neoplasia type 2B. *Proceedings of the National Academy of Sciences of the United States of America* 1994; **91**: 1579–83.
21. Hofstra RM, Landsvater RM, Ceccherini I et al. A mutation in the RET proto-oncogene associated with multiple endocrine neoplasia type 2B and sporadic medullary thyroid carcinoma. *Nature* 1994; **367**: 375–6.
22. Gimm O. Thyroid cancer. *Cancer Letters* 2001; **163**: 143–56.
23. Hundahl SA, Fleming ID, Fremgen AM, Menck HR. A National Cancer Data Base report on 53,856 cases of thyroid carcinoma treated in the US, 1985–1995. *Cancer* 1998; **83**: 2638–48.
24. Bhattacharya N. A population-based analysis of survival factors in differentiated and medullary thyroid carcinoma. *Otolaryngology – Head and Neck Surgery* 2003; **128**: 115–23.
25. Waguespack S, Wells SA Jr, Ross J, Bleyer A. Thyroid cancer. In: Bleyer A, O'Leary M, Barr R, Ries LAG (eds). *Cancer epidemiology in older adolescents and young adults 15 to 29 years of age, including SEER incidence and survival: 1975–2000*. NIH Publication. No. 06-5767. Bethesda, MD: National Cancer Institute, 2006: 144–54.

26. Ponder B. Multiple endocrine neoplasia type 2. In: Vogelstein B, Kinzler K (eds). *The genetic basis of human cancer*. New York: McGraw-Hill, 2002: 501–13.

27. Guyetant S, Rousselet MC, Durigon M *et al.* Sex-related C cell hyperplasia in the normal human thyroid: a quantitative autopsy study. *Journal of Clinical Endocrinology and Metabolism* 1997; **82**: 42–7.

28. Perry A, Molberg K, Albores-Saavedra J. Physiologic versus neoplastic C-cell hyperplasia of the thyroid: separation of distinct histologic and biologic entities. *Cancer* 1996; **77**: 750–6.

29. Guyetant S, Blechet C, Saint-Andre JP. C-cell hyperplasia. *Annales d'Endocrinologie* 2006; **67**: 190–7.

30. Hinze R, Gimm O, Brauckhoff M *et al.* ['Physiological' and 'neoplastic' C-cell hyperplasia of the thyroid. Morphologically and biologically distinct entities?]. *Pathologe* 2001; **22**: 259–65.

31. Wenig BH, Heffess CS, Adair CF. Thyroid neoplasms. In: *Atlas of endocrine pathology*. Philadelphia, PA: WB Saunders, 1997: 83–159.

32. Edge S. American Joint Committee on Cancer. American Cancer Society. *AJCC cancer staging handbook: from the AJCC cancer staging manual*, 7th edn. New York: Springer, 2010.

33. Akhand AA, Ikeyama T, Akazawa S *et al.* Evidence of both extra- and intracellular cysteine targets of protein modification for activation of RET kinase. *Biochemical and Biophysical Research Communications* 2002; **292**: 826–31.

34. Saad MF, Ordonez NG, Rashid RK *et al.* Medullary carcinoma of the thyroid. A study of the clinical features and prognostic factors in 161 patients. *Medicine* 1984; **63**: 319–42.

35. Rosenberg-Bourgin M, Gardet P, de Sahb R *et al.* Comparison of sporadic and hereditary forms of medullary thyroid carcinoma. *Henry Ford Hospital Medical Journal* 1989; **37**: 141–3.

36. Farndon JR, Leight GS, Dilley WG *et al.* Familial medullary thyroid carcinoma without associated endocrinopathies: a distinct clinical entity. *British Journal of Surgery* 1986; **73**: 278–81.

37. Bergholm U, Adami HO, Bergstrom R *et al.* Clinical characteristics in sporadic and familial medullary thyroid carcinoma. A nationwide study of 249 patients in Sweden from 1959 through 1981. *Cancer* 1989; **63**: 1196–204.

38. Beressi N, Campos JM, Beressi JP *et al.* Sporadic medullary microcarcinoma of the thyroid: a retrospective analysis of eighty cases. *Thyroid* 1998; **8**: 1039–44.

39. Brandi ML, Gagel RF, Angeli A *et al.* Guidelines for diagnosis and therapy of MEN type 1 and type 2. *Journal of Clinical Endocrinology and Metabolism* 2001; **86**: 5658–71.

40. Machens A, Brauckhoff M, Holzhausen HJ *et al.* Codon-specific development of pheochromocytoma in multiple endocrine neoplasia type 2. *Journal of Clinical Endocrinology and Metabolism* 2005; **90**: 3999–4003.

41. Herfarth KK, Bartsch D, Doherty GM *et al.* Surgical management of hyperparathyroidism in patients with multiple endocrine neoplasia type 2A. *Surgery* 1996; **120**: 966–73; discussion 973–4.

42. Raue F, Kraimps JL, Dralle H *et al.* Primary hyperparathyroidism in multiple endocrine neoplasia type 2A. *Journal of Internal Medicine* 1995; **238**: 369–73.

43. O'Riordain DS, O'Brien T, Grant CS *et al.* Surgical management of primary hyperparathyroidism in multiple endocrine neoplasia types 1 and 2. *Surgery* 1993; **114**: 1031–7; discussion 1037–9.

44. Kraimps JL, Denizot A, Carnaille B *et al.* Primary hyperparathyroidism in multiple endocrine neoplasia type IIa: retrospective French multicentric study. Groupe d'Etude des Tumeurs a Calcitonine (GETC, French Calcitonin Tumors Study Group), French Association of Endocrine Surgeons. *World Journal of Surgery* 1996; **20**: 808–12; discussion 812–13.

45. Decker RA, Peacock ML. Occurrence of MEN 2a in familial Hirschsprung's disease: a new indication for genetic testing of the RET proto-oncogene. *Journal of Pediatric Surgery* 1998; **33**: 207–14.

46. Gagel RF, Levy ML, Donovan DT *et al.* Multiple endocrine neoplasia type 2a associated with cutaneous lichen amyloidosis. *Annals of Internal Medicine* 1989; **111**: 802–6.

47. Yin M, King SK, Hutson JM, Chow CW. Multiple endocrine neoplasia type 2B diagnosed on suction rectal biopsy in infancy: a report of 2 cases. *Pediatric and Developmental Pathology* 2006; **9**: 56–60.

48. Brauckhoff M, Gimm O, Weiss CL *et al.* Multiple endocrine neoplasia 2B syndrome due to codon 918 mutation: clinical manifestation and course in early and late onset disease. *World Journal of Surgery* 2004; **28**: 1305–11.

49. Lee MJ, Ross DS, Mueller PR *et al.* Fine-needle biopsy of cervical lymph nodes in patients with thyroid cancer: a prospective comparison of cytopathologic and tissue marker analysis. *Radiology* 1993; **187**: 851–4.

50. Collins BT, Cramer HM, Tabatowski K *et al.* Fine needle aspiration of medullary carcinoma of the thyroid. Cytomorphology, immunocytochemistry and electron microscopy. *Acta Cytologica* 1995; **39**: 920–30.

51. Forrest CH, Frost FA, de Boer WB *et al.* Medullary carcinoma of the thyroid: accuracy of diagnosis of fine-needle aspiration cytology. *Cancer* 1998; **84**: 295–302.

52. Bugalho MJ, Santos JR, Sobrinho L. Preoperative diagnosis of medullary thyroid carcinoma: fine needle aspiration cytology as compared with serum calcitonin measurement. *Journal of Surgical Oncology* 2005; **91**: 56–60.

53. Costante G, Meringolo D, Durante C *et al.* Predictive value of serum calcitonin levels for preoperative diagnosis of medullary thyroid carcinoma in a cohort of 5817 consecutive patients with thyroid nodules. *Journal of Clinical Endocrinology and Metabolism* 2007; **92**: 450–5.

54. Papi G, Corsello SM, Cioni K et al. Value of routine measurement of serum calcitonin concentrations in patients with nodular thyroid disease: A multicenter study. *Journal of Endocrinological Investigation* 2006; **29**: 427–37.

55. Vierhapper H, Niederle B, Bieglmayer C et al. Early diagnosis and curative therapy of medullary thyroid carcinoma by routine measurement of serum calcitonin in patients with thyroid disorders. *Thyroid* 2005; **15**: 1267–72.

56. Elisei R, Bottici V, Luchetti F et al. Impact of routine measurement of serum calcitonin on the diagnosis and outcome of medullary thyroid cancer: experience in 10,864 patients with nodular thyroid disorders. *Journal of Clinical Endocrinology and Metabolism* 2004; **89**: 163–8.

57. Niccoli P, Wion-Barbot N, Caron P et al. Interest of routine measurement of serum calcitonin: study in a large series of thyroidectomized patients. The French Medullary Study Group. *Journal of Clinical Endocrinology and Metabolism* 1997; **82**: 338–41.

58. Rink T, Truong PN, Schroth HJ et al. Calculation and validation of a plasma calcitonin limit for early detection of medullary thyroid carcinoma in nodular thyroid disease. *Thyroid* 2009; **19**: 327–32.

59. Bergholm U, Bergstrom R, Ekbom A. Long-term follow-up of patients with medullary carcinoma of the thyroid. *Cancer* 1997; **79**: 132–8.

60. Modigliani E, Cohen R, Campos JM et al. Prognostic factors for survival and for biochemical cure in medullary thyroid carcinoma: results in 899 patients, The GETC Study Group. Groupe d'etude des tumeurs a calcitonine. *Clinical Endocrinology* 1998; **48**: 265–73.

61. Hyer SL, Vini L, A'Hern R, Harmer C. Medullary thyroid cancer: multivariate analysis of prognostic factors influencing survival. *European Journal of Surgical Oncology* 2000; **26**: 686–90.

62. Kebebew E, Ituarte PH, Siperstein AE et al. Medullary thyroid carcinoma: clinical characteristics, treatment, prognostic factors, and a comparison of staging systems. *Cancer* 2000; **88**: 1139–48.

63. Clark JR, Fridman TR, Odell MJ et al. Prognostic variables and calcitonin in medullary thyroid cancer. *Laryngoscope* 2005; **115**: 1445–50.

64. de Groot JW, Links T, Plukker J. Disseminated medullary thyroid cancer after early thyroid surgery in multiple endocrine neoplasia type2A. *Thyroid* 2005; **15**: 1205–6; author's reply, 1206, 7.

65. Pelizzo MR, Boschin IM, Bernante P et al. Natural history, diagnosis, treatment and outcome of medullary thyroid cancer: 37 years experience on 157 patients. *European Journal of Surgical Oncology* 2007; **33**: 493–7.

66. Machens A, Hofmann C, Hauptmann S, Dralle H. Locoregional recurrence and death from medullary thyroid carcinoma in a contemporaneous series: 5-year results. *European Journal of Endocrinology* 2007; **157**: 85–93.

67. Ito Y, Miyauchi A, Yabuta T et al. Alternative surgical strategies and favorable outcomes in patients with medullary thyroid carcinoma in Japan: experience of a single institution. *World Journal of Surgery* 2009; **33**: 58–66.

68. Henry JF, Denizot A, Puccini M et al. Latent subclinical medullary thyroid carcinoma: diagnosis and treatment. *World Journal of Surgery* 1998; **22**: 752–6; discussion 756–7.

69. Dora JM, Canalli MH, Capp C et al. Normal perioperative serum calcitonin levels in patients with advanced medullary thyroid carcinoma: case report and review of the literature. *Thyroid* 2008; **18**: 895–9.

70. Machens A, Schneyer U, Holzhausen HJ, Dralle H. Prospects of remission in medullary thyroid carcinoma according to basal calcitonin level. *Journal of Clinical Endocrinology and Metabolism* 2005; **90**: 2029–34.

71. Barbot N, Calmettes C, Schuffenecker I et al. Pentagastrin stimulation test and early diagnosis of medullary thyroid carcinoma using an immunoradiometric assay of calcitonin: comparison with genetic screening in hereditary medullary thyroid carcinoma. *Journal of Clinical Endocrinology and Metabolism* 1994; **78**: 114–20.

72. Sawka AM, Jaeschke R, Singh RJ, Young WF Jr. A comparison of biochemical tests for pheochromocytoma: measurement of fractionated plasma metanephrines compared with the combination of 24-hour urinary metanephrines and catecholamines. *Journal of Clinical Endocrinology and Metabolism* 2003; **88**: 553–8.

73. Elisei R, Romei C, Cosci B et al. RET genetic screening in patients with medullary thyroid cancer and their relatives: experience with 807 individuals at one center. *Journal of Clinical Endocrinology and Metabolism* 2007; **92**: 4725–9.

74. Gorman B, Charboneau JW, James EM et al. Medullary thyroid carcinoma: role of high-resolution US. *Radiology* 1987; **162**: 147–50.

♦ 75. Moley JF, Fialkowski EA. Evidence-based approach to the management of sporadic medullary thyroid carcinoma. *World Journal of Surgery* 2007; **31**: 946–56.

76. Moley JF, DeBenedetti MK. Patterns of nodal metastases in palpable medullary thyroid carcinoma: recommendations for extent of node dissection. *Annals of Surgery* 1999; **229**: 880–7; discussion 887–8.

77. Gimm O, Ukkat J, Dralle H. Determinative factors of biochemical cure after primary and reoperative surgery for sporadic medullary thyroid carcinoma. *World Journal of Surgery* 1998; **22**: 562–7; discussion 567–8.

78. Ukkat J, Gimm O, Brauckhoff M et al. Single center experience in primary surgery for medullary thyroid carcinoma. *World Journal of Surgery* 2004; **28**: 1271–4.

79. Raffel A, Cupisti K, Krausch M et al. Incidentally found medullary thyroid cancer: treatment rationale for small tumors. *World Journal of Surgery* 2004; **28**: 397–401.

80. Hamy A, Pessaux P, Mirallie E *et al.* Central neck dissection in the management of sporadic medullary thyroid microcarcinoma. *European Journal of Surgical Oncology* 2005; **31**: 774–7.

81. Scollo C, Baudin E, Travagli JP *et al.* Rationale for central and bilateral lymph node dissection in sporadic and hereditary medullary thyroid cancer. *Journal of Clinical Endocrinology and Metabolism* 2003; **88**: 2070–5.

82. Machens A, Hinze R, Thomusch O, Dralle H. Pattern of nodal metastasis for primary and reoperative thyroid cancer. *World Journal of Surgery* 2002; **26**: 22–8.

83. Machens A, Hauptmann S, Dralle H. Prediction of lateral lymph node metastases in medullary thyroid cancer. *British Journal of Surgery* 2008; **95**: 586–91.

84. Machens A, Holzhausen HJ, Dralle H. Skip metastases in thyroid cancer leaping the central lymph node compartment. *Archives of Surgery* 2004; **139**: 43–5.

85. Machens A, Holzhausen HJ, Dralle H. Prediction of mediastinal lymph node metastasis in medullary thyroid carcinoma. *British Journal of Surgery* 2004; **91**: 709–12.

86. Machens A, Holzhausen HJ, Dralle H. Contralateral cervical and mediastinal lymph node metastasis in medullary thyroid cancer: systemic disease? *Surgery* 2006; **139**: 28–32.

87. Robbins KT, Medina JE, Wolfe GT *et al.* Standardizing neck dissection terminology. Official report of the Academy's Committee for Head and Neck Surgery and Oncology. *Archives of Otolaryngology – Head and Neck Surgery* 1991; **117**: 601–5.

88. Hundahl SA, Cady B, Cunningham MP *et al.* Initial results from a prospective cohort study of 5583 cases of thyroid carcinoma treated in the united states during, 1996, U.S. and German Thyroid Cancer Study Group. An American College of Surgeons Commission on Cancer Patient Care Evaluation study. *Cancer* 2000; **89**: 202–17.

89. Roman S, Lin R, Sosa JA. Prognosis of medullary thyroid carcinoma: demographic, clinical, and pathologic predictors of survival in 1252 cases. *Cancer* 2006; **107**: 2134–42.

90. Dotzenrath C, Goretzki PE, Cupisti K *et al.* Is there any consensus in diagnostic and operative strategy with respect to medullary thyroid cancer? A questionnaire answered by 73 endocrine surgical units. *Langenbecks Archives of Surgery* 2001; **386**: 47–52.

91. Dralle H, Damm I, Scheumann GF *et al.* Compartment-oriented microdissection of regional lymph nodes in medullary thyroid carcinoma. *Surgery Today* 1994; **24**: 112–21.

92. Miyauchi A, Matsuzuka F, Hirai K *et al.* Prospective trial of unilateral surgery for nonhereditary medullary thyroid carcinoma in patients without germline RET mutations. *World Journal of Surgery* 2002; **26**: 1023–8.

93. Yen TW, Shapiro SE, Gagel RF *et al.* Medullary thyroid carcinoma: results of a standardized surgical approach in a contemporary series of 80 consecutive patients. *Surgery* 2003; **134**: 890–9; discussion 899–901.

94. Pillarisetty VG, Katz SC, Ghossein RA *et al.* Micromedullary thyroid cancer: how micro is truly micro? *Annals of Surgical Oncology* 2009; **16**: 2875–81.

95. Scheuba C, Kaserer K, Bieglmayer C *et al.* Medullary thyroid microcarcinoma recommendations for treatment – a single-center experience. *Surgery* 2007; **142**: 1003–10.

96. Henry JF, Gramatica L, Denizot A *et al.* Morbidity of prophylactic lymph node dissection in the central neck area in patients with papillary thyroid carcinoma. *Langenbecks Archives of Surgery* 1998; **383**: 167–9.

97. Pereira JA, Jimeno J, Miquel J *et al.* Nodal yield, morbidity, and recurrence after central neck dissection for papillary thyroid carcinoma. *Surgery* 2005; **138**: 1095–100; discussion 1100–91.

98. Steinmuller T, Klupp J, Wenking S, Neuhaus P. Complications associated with different surgical approaches to differentiated thyroid carcinoma. *Langenbecks Archives of Surgery* 1999; **384**: 50–3.

99. Cheah WK, Arici C, Ituarte PH *et al.* Complications of neck dissection for thyroid cancer. *World Journal of Surgery* 2002; **26**: 1013–16.

100. Groot JW, Kema IP, Breukelman H *et al.* Biochemical markers in the follow-up of medullary thyroid cancer. *Thyroid* 2006; **16**: 1163–70.

101. Fugazzola L, Pinchera A, Luchetti F *et al.* Disappearance rate of serum calcitonin after total thyroidectomy for medullary thyroid carcinoma. *International Journal of Biological Markers* 1994; **9**: 21–4.

102. Brauckhoff M, Gimm O, Brauckhoff K *et al.* Calcitonin kinetics in the early postoperative period of medullary thyroid carcinoma. *Langenbecks Archives of Surgery* 2001; **386**: 434–9.

103. Franc S, Niccoli-Sire P, Cohen R *et al.* Complete surgical lymph node resection does not prevent authentic recurrences of medullary thyroid carcinoma. *Clinical Endocrinology* 2001; **55**: 403–9.

104. Peixoto Callejo I, Americo Brito J, Zagalo CM, Rosa Santos J. Medullary thyroid carcinoma: multivariate analysis of prognostic factors influencing survival. *Clinical and Translational Oncology* 2006; **8**: 435–43.

105. de Groot JW, Links TP, Sluiter WJ *et al.* Locoregional control in patients with palpable medullary thyroid cancer: Results of standardized compartment-oriented surgery. *Head and Neck* 2007; **29**: 857–63.

106. Kebebew E, Greenspan FS, Clark OH *et al.* Extent of disease and practice patterns for medullary thyroid cancer. *Journal of the American College of Surgeons* 2005; **200**: 890–6.

107. van Heerden JA, Grant CS, Gharib H *et al.* Long-term course of patients with persistent hypercalcitoninemia after apparent curative primary surgery for medullary thyroid carcinoma. *Annals of Surgery* 1990; **212**: 395–400.

108. Moley JF, Debenedetti MK, Dilley WG *et al.* Surgical management of patients with persistent or recurrent

medullary thyroid cancer. *Journal of Internal Medicine* 1998; **243**: 521–6.

109. Fialkowski E, DeBenedetti M, Moley J. Long-term outcome of reoperations for medullary thyroid carcinoma. *World Journal of Surgery* 2008; **32**: 754–65.

110. Fernandez Vila JM, Peix JL, Mandry AC *et al.* Biochemical results of reoperations for medullary thyroid carcinoma. *Laryngoscope* 2007; **117**: 886–9.

111. Kebebew E, Kikuchi S, Duh QY, Clark OH. Long-term results of reoperation and localizing studies in patients with persistent or recurrent medullary thyroid cancer. *Archives of Surgery* 2000; **135**: 895–901.

112. Chen H, Roberts JR, Ball DW *et al.* Effective long-term palliation of symptomatic, incurable metastatic medullary thyroid cancer by operative resection. *Annals of Surgery* 1998; **227**: 887–95.

113. Koopmans KP, de Groot JWB, Plukker JTM *et al.* 18F-Dihydroxyphenylalanine PET in patients with biochemical evidence of medullary thyroid cancer: relation to tumor differentiation. *Journal of Nuclear Medicine* 2008; **49**: 524–31.

114. Laure Giraudet A, Al Ghulzan A, Auperin A *et al.* Progression of medullary thyroid carcinoma: assessment with calcitonin and carcinoembryonic antigen doubling times. *European Journal of Endocrinology* 2008; **158**: 239–46.

115. Giraudet AL, Vanel D, Leboulleux S *et al.* Imaging medullary thyroid carcinoma with persistent elevated calcitonin levels. *Journal of Clinical Endocrinology and Metabolism* 2007; **92**: 4185–90.

116. Arslan N, Ilgan S, Yuksel D *et al.* Comparison of In-111 octreotide and Tc-99m (V) DMSA scintigraphy in the detection of medullary thyroid tumor foci in patients with elevated levels of tumor markers after surgery. *Clinical Nuclear Medicine* 2001; **26**: 683–8.

117. Faggiano A, Grimaldi F, Pezzullo L *et al.* Secretive and proliferative tumor profile helps to select the best imaging technique to identify postoperative persistent or relapsing medullary thyroid cancer. *Endocrine-Related Cancer* 2009; **16**: 225–31.

118. Conry BG, Papathanasiou ND, Prakash V *et al.* Comparison of (68)Ga-DOTATATE and (18)F-fluorodeoxyglucose PET/CT in the detection of recurrent medullary thyroid carcinoma. *European Journal of Nuclear Medicine and Molecular Imaging* 2010; **37**: 49–57.

119. Iagaru A, Masamed R, Singer PA, Conti PS. Detection of occult medullary thyroid cancer recurrence with 2-deoxy-2-[F-18]fluoro-D-glucose-PET and PET/CT. *Molecular Imaging and Biology* 2007; **9**: 72–7.

120. Diehl M, Risse JH, Brandt-Mainz K *et al.* Fluorine-18 fluorodeoxyglucose positron emission tomography in medullary thyroid cancer: results of a multicentre study. *European Journal of Nuclear Medicine* 2001; **28**: 1671–6.

121. de Groot JW, Links TP, Jager PL *et al.* Impact of 18F-fluoro-2-deoxy-D-glucose positron emission tomography (FDG-PET) in patients with biochemical evidence of recurrent or residual medullary thyroid cancer. *Annals of Surgical Oncology* 2004; **11**: 786–94.

122. Ong SC, Schoder H, Patel SG *et al.* Diagnostic accuracy of 18F-FDG PET in restaging patients with medullary thyroid carcinoma and elevated calcitonin levels. *Journal of Nuclear Medicine* 2007; **48**: 501–7.

123. Beuthien-Baumann B, Strumpf A, Zessin J *et al.* Diagnostic impact of PET with (18)F-FDG, (18)F-DOPA and 3-O-methyl-6-[(18)F]fluoro-DOPA in recurrent or metastatic medullary thyroid carcinoma. *European Journal of Nuclear Medicine and Molecular Imaging* 2007; **34**: 1604–9.

124. Beheshti M, Pocher S, Vali R *et al.* The value of 18F-DOPA PET-CT in patients with medullary thyroid carcinoma: comparison with 18F-FDG PET-CT. *European Radiology* 2009; **19**: 1425–34.

125. Marzola MC, Pelizzo MR, Ferdeghini M *et al.* Dual PET/CT with (18)F-DOPA and (18)F-FDG in metastatic medullary thyroid carcinoma and rapidly increasing calcitonin levels: Comparison with conventional imaging. *European Journal of Surgical Oncology* 2010; **36**: 414–21.

126. Bogsrud TV, Karantanis D, Nathan MA *et al.* The prognostic value of 2-deoxy-2-[18f]fluoro-D-glucose positron emission tomography in patients with suspected residual or recurrent medullary thyroid carcinoma. *Molecular Imaging and Biology* 2010; **12**: 547–53.

127. Tung WS, Vesely TM, Moley JF. Laparoscopic detection of hepatic metastases in patients with residual or recurrent medullary thyroid cancer. *Surgery* 1995; **118**: 1024–9; discussion 1029–30.

128. Esik O, Szavcsur P, Szakall S Jr *et al.* Angiography effectively supports the diagnosis of hepatic metastases in medullary thyroid carcinoma. *Cancer* 2001; **91**: 2084–95.

129. Szavcsur P, Godeny M, Bajzik G *et al.* Angiography-proven liver metastases explain low efficacy of lymph node dissections in medullary thyroid cancer patients. *European Journal of Surgical Oncology* 2005; **31**: 183–90.

130. Ben Mrad MD, Gardet P, Roche A *et al.* Value of venous catheterization and calcitonin studies in the treatment and management of clinically inapparent medullary thyroid carcinoma. *Cancer* 1989; **63**: 133–8.

131. Medina-Franco H, Herrera MF, Lopez G *et al.* Persistent hypercalcitoninemia in patients with medullary thyroid cancer: a therapeutic approach based on selective venous sampling for calcitonin. *Revista de Investigación Clínica* 2001; **53**: 212–17.

132. Frank-Raue K, Raue F, Buhr HJ *et al.* Localization of occult persisting medullary thyroid carcinoma before microsurgical reoperation: high sensitivity of selective venous catheterization. *Thyroid* 1992; **2**: 113–17.

133. Gilliland FD, Hunt WC, Morris DM, Key CR. Prognostic factors for thyroid carcinoma. A population-based study of 15,698 cases from the Surveillance, Epidemiology and End Results (SEER) program 1973–1991. *Cancer* 1997; **79**: 564–73.

25

Avoiding complications in thyroid and parathyroid surgery

MARCO RAFFAELLI, CELESTINO PIO LOMBARDI, ROCCO BELLANTONE, CARMELA DE CREA, DAVID LESNIK, ANDRE POTENZA AND GREGORY RANDOLPH

No sensible man will, on slight consideration, attempt to extirpate a goitrous thyroid gland. If a surgeon should be so adventurous or foolhardy as to undertake the enterprise … every stroke of his knife will be followed by a torrent of blood and lucky will it be for him if his victim lives long enough to enable him to finish his horrid butchery.

Samuel Gross, 1805–84

The extirpation of the thyroid gland for goitre typifies, perhaps better than any operation, the supreme triumph of the surgeon's art. A feat which today can be accomplished by any really competent operator without danger of mishap and which was conceived more than a thousand years ago.

William S Halsted, 1852–1922

INTRODUCTION

Although thyroidectomy is one of the most frequently performed surgical procedures worldwide, it was during the last century that it became an accepted operation. In fact, in the middle of the nineteenth century, the French Academy of Medicine banned thyroid surgery because of its high mortality rate.[1] Similarly in 1871, one of the pioneers of thyroid surgery, Greene, while reporting his three successful thyroidectomies, warned that the operation should be used 'never for the relief of deformity or discomfort merely; only to save life'.[2]

So it was that the risk of life-threatening complications forestalled the evolution of thyroid surgery until the end of the nineteenth century. It was only after T Kocher refined and described his meticulous technique and reported his excellent results, with a mortality rate of 0.5 per cent in 5000 thyroidectomies, that thyroidectomy became an accepted procedure. It is remarkable that he was the first surgeon to receive the Nobel Prize for this accomplishment in 1909.[3, 4] The history of parathyroid surgery is far more recent, with the first procedure performed by Felix Mandl in 1925.[5]

There is no doubt that competence in thyroid and parathyroid surgery requires a mastery of basic surgical techniques and thorough understanding of normal neck anatomy, as well as the possible anatomical variations one might encounter while performing these procedures.[6] It is currently performed with a low complication rate (<3 per cent) by experienced endocrine surgeons.[7] Several recent reports have demonstrated that these procedures may safely be performed by residents operating under supervision[8, 9] and the newly established surgical consultant.[10] However, in general, there is a significant inverse relationship between the number of procedures performed and the rate of complication.[11] In other words, surgical skill acquired through experience plays an important role in reducing one's complication rate. This has also been proven true in other fields of surgery.[6]

Indeed, lower complication rates are obtained in tertiary care referral centres where these procedures are regularly performed by dedicated endocrine surgical teams.[12]

Nonetheless, despite skill and experience, complications may occur, either as a result of surgical error or due to the extent of patient disease. The most effective way to avoid complications in endocrine surgery is to recognize how and why they occur. Thus, the aim of this chapter is to furnish the reader not only with a list of the possible complications, but more importantly with a description of common surgical errors and techniques that will help to avoid them.

PREOPERATIVE EVALUATION

When meticulous surgical technique is employed, the occurrence of complications may be attributed, at least in part, to factors related to patient disease or comorbidity. For this reason, thorough and accurate patient evaluation is necessary at the first consultation.

A careful history that emphasizes symptoms of endocrine disease, general physical status, cardiopulmonary status, genetic abnormalities, drug intake (particularly aspirin or other anticoagulants), response to previous anaesthesia and surgery, and any previous bleeding problems are important factors to consider in any preoperative evaluation. A thorough physical examination focusing on the stigmata of mass effect on the upper aerodigestive tract and signs of thyroid and parathyroid dysfunction must always be performed. Examination of the larynx by indirect laryngoscopy provides knowledge of the integrity of laryngeal function. Although it is frequently recommended, some surgeons question its utility in patients without previous operation and no change in voice quality.[13] However, occasionally, a paralyzed cord is found preoperatively in a patient who has achieved full vocal cord compensation and a normal voice. This preoperative finding might clearly have some value with respect to surgical treatment planning, not to mention possible medicolegal implications (see below under Recurrent laryngeal nerve, p. 478).

Standard blood chemistry, including thyroid functions and a serum calcium assay, should always be performed. Documenting euthyroidism is essential, lest one risk perioperative thyroid storm in thyrotoxic patients. If concomitant primary hyperparathyroidism is detected, which is not a rarity, a complete evaluation and possible exploration of all four parathyroid glands is clearly discussed with the patient. In summary, these and other findings may inform both patient and surgeon and may also reveal the need for further preoperative medical evaluation and management.

Infection and wound healing disorders

WOUND INFECTIONS

Thyroidectomy is associated with a low risk for wound infections (0.02–0.5 per cent).[14, 15] Apart from normal surgical disinfection prior to incision and accurate surgical field draping, no further preventive measures are usually required. As in other operations, polivinilpirrolidone (Betadine®) is the preferred disinfecting solution. In patients with known differentiated thyroid carcinoma, a non-iodinated disinfecting solution should be used so as not to interfere with a postsurgical radioiodine scintiscan and ablation. No difference in frequency of postoperative wound infections has been shown with antibiotic prophylaxis.[15] In spite of this evidence, others

still recommend routine intravenous prophylactic antibiotic administration at the induction of the anaesthesia.[16] In summary, antibiotic prophylaxis is not routinely advocated in the absence of well-known risk factors, such as diabetes, valvular heart diseases, immunodeficiency, etc. Another issue possibly related to wound infection is that of wound drainage. Some authors report that the utilization of closed suction drains reduces the amount of fluid collection in the operative bed and thus minimizes the risk of infection and abscess formation.[17] Others do not confirm a relationship between use of a drain and the risk of wound infection.[18] As the overall incidence of wound infection is so low, it is thought that most wound infections after endocrine neck surgery are endogenous.[18] For this reason, surgery should be avoided in patients with acute infectious illness. Minor cellulitis usually responds well to oral antibiotics. Frank abscesses are extremely rare and require incision and drainage in addition to intravenous antibiotics.

SCAR DISORDERS

Cosmesis after thyroid and parathyroid surgery is important given the prominent location of the surgical incision, as well as the fact that the patients are frequently young females. For the best cosmetic results, a well-positioned collar incision should be made in a normal skin crease approximately 1 cm below the cricoid cartilage.[18] Lower incisions are indeed more prone to hypertrophic scar and keloid formation because there is a higher degree of tension on the wound. This placement has another important advantage. It facilitates control and ligation of the superior pole vasculature. Over the last decade, the development of minimally invasive techniques, which are performed through small (1.5–4 cm) skin incisions, with or without endoscope utilization, has yielded even better cosmetic results compared to conventional approaches.[19, 20, 21, 22]

SEROMA

The seroma is a serum collection often associated with neck dissection during thyroid surgery. Its incidence has been reported to be between 0 and 6 per cent.[14, 15, 23, 24] When this occurs, it may be treated with repeated fine needle aspiration. However, this is associated with increased risk of infection. Drain utilization is usually suggested for its prevention, especially in cases of substernal goitre, Graves' disease or large multinodular goitre. In case of infection, open drainage is often necessary.

POSTOPERATIVE HAEMATOMA

Postoperative haematoma remains a fortunately uncommon, but potentially serious, complication of thyroid surgery. Postthyroidectomy haematoma is variably reported in the literature in 0.3–4.3 per cent of patients[23, 25, 26] and in about 0.3 per cent of patients after parathyroidectomy.[16, 27, 28]

A postoperative haematoma can lead to devastating consequences with tracheal compression and subsequent hypoxia, which may then lead to brain injury and even death.[29] The term 'compressive haematoma' has become well known in the medical literature, indicating potential airway compromise. The exact mechanism of airway obstruction is a matter of some debate. Some authors have questioned the ability of clots to cause compression of the rigid cartilaginous trachea. They have attributed airflow compromise to impairment of venous and lymphatic drainage within the laryngopharynx resulting in oedema and obstruction.[25] Whatever the cause, the patient may present with respiratory distress, pain or pressure sensation in the neck or dysphagia. Signs include progressive neck swelling, suture line bleeding, dyspnoea and/or stridor and possibly significant blood loss.

Intraoperative and postoperative haemorrhage may be venous or arterial in origin. It may be caused by dislodgment of ligatures, reopening of cauterized vessels, or bleeding from residual thyroid parenchyma. In some series, most of the haemorrhagic events occur early after surgery, with the patient still in the operating theatre or in the recovery room, or within the first 6 hours after the operation.[30, 31] However, in other series, more than 50 per cent of patients presented with haematoma beyond 6 hours after the operation, with up to 20 per cent of patients presenting beyond 24 hours after thyroidectomy.[14, 32, 33] This suggests that early discharge after thyroidectomy (<24 hours) bears the potential risk of missing some late haematomas that would require emergency evacuation. Using a decision analysis, it has been demonstrated that 94 deaths per 100 000 due to haemorrhage after thyroid operation could be prevented with 24 hours, rather than 6 hours hospital stay.[34]

Although it has been widely investigated, most published series have failed to definitively identify risk factors for this complication.[32] Patient risk factors include a history of coagulation disorder such as haemophilia, von Willebrand's disease, chronic renal failure and haemodialysis, use of anticoagulant or antiplatelet medications, etc. Preoperative optimization of these conditions prior to surgery is mandatory to avoid postoperative bleeding. Particular risk of haemorrhage associated with the underlying thyroid pathology has been postulated, but there is little evidence to support this. Toxic goitre and Graves' disease have been associated with increased risk of postoperative haematoma.[30, 35] Since Lugol's iodine solution has been proven efficacious in decreasing thyroid blood flow in toxic goitre, its utilization should be recommended in these conditions to reduce the risk of intra- and postoperative bleeding.[25] Substernal and intrathoracic goitres, as well as reoperative procedures, have been considered risks for postoperative bleeding.[35, 36] Other studies failed to identify these conditions as significant risk factors.[14, 32]

Surgeon-related risk factors obviously include experience and surgical technique. Despite this, in most studies, high surgical volume failed to reduce the rate of postoperative haemorrhage.[14, 32] Moreover, operations performed by supervised residents[37] and newly established consultants[38] do not seem to entail a higher risk of bleeding.

Another surgeon-related factor is the surgical access. If the strap muscles are sectioned, they may represent an additional source of bleeding.[25] Incomplete closure of the strap muscles, leaving a marginal 'weep hole', is widely proposed as a measure allowing early haematoma to spontaneously decompress.[12, 32] Care should also be taken to avoid injury to the anterior jugular veins during preparation of the flap or closure of the midline at the end of the operation. Another potential source of postoperative bleeding is residual thyroid tissue in partial resection. Recent reports showed a higher incidence of postoperative haemorrhage in patients who underwent bilateral subtotal thyroid resection.[15, 30]

In recent years, minimally invasive procedures for thyroid and parathyroid surgery have gained in popularity, particularly in specialized centres. Data from the literature demonstrate that the rate of major postoperative bleeding requiring surgical revision after video-assisted and endoscopic thyroid and parathyroid procedures approaches 0 per cent and only a few cases have been reported.[32, 39, 40, 41, 42] It could be inferred that the limited dissection which characterizes these techniques may reduce the risk of this complication.[25, 32] These results could be biased by the strict selection criteria for these procedures. For example, patients with large goitres, thyroiditis, aggressive and infiltrating tumours, node metastases, and those requiring reoperative surgery or bilateral exploration are generally not candidates for these procedures.

Postoperative bleeding is preventable in the majority of patients. A meticulous surgical technique with careful haemostasis is the best means of reducing the likelihood of haemorrhage. There are several manoeuvres that can assist the surgeon in the recognition of potential bleeding sources before wound closure. Neck hyperextension should be reduced so that bleeding vessels controlled under tension may be identified prior to closure. A Valsalva manoeuvre, which increases the venous pressure and reveals potential venous bleeding sources, is also of great value. Similarly, some authors suggest briefly tilting the head of the patient down about 30° in the Trendelenburg position at the end of the operation before wound closure.[43]

The traditional clamp and tie technique is clearly very effective for haemostasis. Additional methods include the application of surgical clips, as well as monopolar and bipolar electrocautery. Ligature and clips may become dislodged. For this reason, double ligature of prominent vessels is usually recommended.[32] In recent years, several new technologies for haemostasis have been developed for endocrine and other head and neck operations, initially for the minimally invasive approaches. These new technological devices for haemostasis include both ultrasonic shears (Harmonic scalpel, Ethicon endosurgery) and a computer-controlled bipolar electrothermal sealing system (Ligasure™; Valley Laboratory Corporation, a division of Tyco Healthcare, Boulder, CO, USA). Several comparative studies have evaluated their efficacy in thyroid surgery and have demonstrated that both instruments are safe alternatives to standard vessel ligation, with significant advantages in terms of shorter operative time.[44, 45, 46, 47, 48, 49, 50, 51] Whether these tools are effective in reducing blood loss remains to be determined.[25]

The use of haemostatic agents (i.e. oxidized cellulose, fibrin sealant, etc.) may be useful in selected cases to facilitate haemostasis by mechanical pressure and promoting coagulum formation, thus resulting in reduced capillary ooze.[12, 25, 32, 52] However, these agents increase the overall cost of the procedure and do no replace the need for meticulous haemostasis.

Many studies, including prospective, randomized investigations, have failed to demonstrate significant advantages in preventing postoperative haematoma with drain utilization.[53, 54, 55] Other studies have suggested that neither gland size, diagnosis, type of surgery, nor intraoperative bleeding were valid justifications for the use of an external drain.[30] Based on this, it would appear that drains should not routinely be used as a preventive measure. However, if used, they may signal the onset of bleeding and be particularly useful in alerting the nursing staff to the existence of postoperative haemorrhage. After wound closure, a smooth extubation without significant coughing or retching and adequate control of both postoperative pain and vomiting may help to avoid a sudden increase in venous and/or arterial pressure, and reduce the risk of postoperative bleeding.[18, 25] Pressure should be applied to the neck dressing if the patient struggles and coughs at the conclusion of the case or upon extubation. This manoeuvre could help to avoid the rise in the venous pressure at the wound site.[12] Conversely, pressure dressings can delay identification of a developing haematoma and should be avoided. After extubation, patients should be kept with the head and the shoulders elevated (10–20°) in order to maintain a negative venous pressure in the neck.

Beyond prevention, early recognition with immediate intervention is the key for the management of this potentially lethal post-thyroidectomy complication. It is important to ensure that a member of the surgical team remains with the patient during the extubation and transit to the recovery room. Furthermore, it is important for experienced personnel to closely monitor the patient upon return to the ward in order to detect signs of significant bleeding early. One recent review stressed the importance of recognizing early signs of hypoxia, such as tachycardia, diaphoresis, irritability and confusion, in order to avoid delays in reoperation.[56] In the event of significant airway compromise developing rapidly, bedside evacuation of the haematoma may be necessary. In such a circumstance, one must remove the superficial skin sutures and those closing the platysma to evacuate formed clots. If the patient is experiencing respiratory difficulty, it should be remembered that the supine position can exacerbate respiratory distress by increasing laryngeal oedema and may also complicate attempts at reintubation. For these reasons, intubation should be performed by experienced personnel. Inability to secure an adequate airway via intubation may result in the need for tracheotomy. Similarly, persistent laryngeal oedema after haematoma evacuation may indicate the need for prolonged intubation and systemic steroid administration and, in rare cases, tracheotomy. In a recent report from a high volume referral centre, tracheotomy was required in approximately a quarter of the patients who underwent re-exploration for haematoma (0.3 per cent of all thyroidectomies performed), although this percentage has diminished over recent years.[12]

A liberal attitude towards re-exploration in the case of symptomatic haematoma is mandatory. Patients are best served by early definitive intervention with evacuation of the clot rather than prolonged observation. Only a small subgroup of patients with minimal swelling, lack of symptoms and no progression of their haematoma should be considered for conservative management. However, even in these cases, conservative management would prolong hospitalization time, may require weeks to months of observation until complete reabsorption, and might also impair wound healing.[23]

At the time of re-exploration as always, protection of the structures at risk (i.e. laryngeal nerves, parathyroid glands) is paramount. Gentle irrigation and clot evacuation are mandatory. Saline solution is useful in cleaning the operative field and identifying any source of bleeding. Blind clamping of vessels is to be avoided. If no active source of bleeding is identifiable at reoperation, after all the potential sources have been adequately explored, drainage should be employed and closure should ensue.

Superior laryngeal nerve

Lesion of the external branch of the superior laryngeal nerve (EBSLN) may occur during thyroid surgery and may cause important voice changes, especially in professional voice users (singers, public speakers). Knowledge of its anatomy and its function is of utmost importance for thyroid surgeons. The superior laryngeal nerve (SLN) arises from the vagus nerve close to the caudal end of the nodose ganglion and descends in the neck behind the external carotid artery to the carotid bifurcation. At the level of the hyoid bone, it divides into an internal (sensory) branch and an external (motor) branch. The internal branch perforates the thyrohyoid membrane, providing sensory innervation of the pharyngeal and laryngeal mucosa from the base of the tongue to the glottis and the subglottic region. Lesions of the internal branch result in loss of sensation of the ipsilateral mucosa, determining defective sensory motor coordination of the glottis and subsequent aspiration on swallowing, but it is usually not at risk during thyroid and parathyroid procedures.

On the other hand, the course of the EBSLN is more caudal and near the superior thyroid vessels and thus it is at risk of lesion during thyroidectomy. After emerging from the SLN, the EBSLN runs in close proximity to the medial aspect of the superior thyroid artery and curves medially to provide motor innervation of the cricothyroid muscle. The function of this muscle is to lengthen and tense the ipsilateral true vocal cord.[57, 58] As a consequence, lesion of the EBSLN results in voice changes characterized by loss of high tone and pitch volume and fatigue after extensive use.[23, 59] Such changes are usually well tolerated by most patients, but may be career-threatening in voice professionals, such as singers and public speakers. The importance of this nerve for professional singers is underscored by the story of the famous opera soprano Amelita Galli-Curci whose professional career ended after undergoing a thyroidectomy for multinodular toxic goitre in 1935 performed by Dr Arnold Kegel. Indeed, after the operation she never sang well again due presumably to injury of the EBSLN.[60]

In most patients (about two-thirds of the cases), the nerve crosses medially into the cricothyroid muscle more than 1 cm cranially to the upper pole (Cernea's type 1). In the remaining one-third, the EBSLN runs within a distance of less than 1 cm from the upper pole of the thyroid gland (Cernea's type 2). In one half of these patients, the nerve remains cranial to the upper pole of the thyroid lobe (type 2a). In the remaining cases, the EBSLN has a more caudal course and lies below the superior thyroid pole (type 2b). This last position involves an increased risk of inadvertent nerve injury during dissection and ligation of the vessels of the superior pole (high-risk nerves).[61, 62]

Several technical methods have been proposed to reduce the risk of EBSLN injury, including skeletonization and individual ligation of the vessels of the superior thyroid pole adjacent to the capsule and visual identification of the nerve before ligation of the superior pole. However, at present, although the importance of preservation of the EBSLN is well recognized, the need for routine visualization is still controversial, because in 12–20 per cent of the cases, the nerve cannot be visualized since it is located within the cricothyroid muscle. A recently published prospective, randomized study comparing routine identification of the nerve versus individual ligation of the vessels of the superior pole close to the thyroid capsule, failed to demonstrate a significant difference in terms of EBSLN injury between the two techniques; no definitive EBSLN palsy was found in either group.[59] However, in absence of EBSLN identification, a meticulous surgical technique should be used to avoid injury. After careful division of the anterior suspensory ligament, the potential space between the medial portion of the superior pole and the cricothyroid muscle can be entered. The upper pole is then grabbed with a clamp or with a finger and retracted downward and outward. The connective tissue medial to the upper pole is completely opened. This allows good exposure of the vessels of the upper pole which are then individually ligated as distally as possible. Lateral and downward traction of the superior pole should put some tension on the EBSLN since it crosses the superior thyroid artery. This should aid in identification of the nerve if it is in a high-risk position. It is important to reduce the risk of EBSLN injury by avoiding en masse ligation of the superior pole. Moreover, dissection should be performed from medial to lateral.

Intraoperative utilization of a nerve stimulator has been demonstrated to be beneficial for the identification and preservation of the EBSLN. However, its utilization is not yet routine.[62, 63] EBSLN stimulation results in cricothyroid muscle contraction. This can help to identify the nerve during dissection of the superior pole and confirm its functional integrity at the end of the operation. It has been reported that the use of a nerve stimulator reduces the rate of EBSLN injury from 12 to 0 per cent, when compared with unaided visual identification.[62] Nerve detection technology may be especially useful in difficult cases, such as reoperative cases and large goitres which may alter normal anatomy as a result of cephalad growth of thyroid tissue behind the vascular pedicle.[64]

Identification and preservation of the EBSLN has been aided by video-assisted endoscopic techniques, largely due to the magnification provided by the endoscope.[39, 40] A recent randomized prospective study comparing voice after video-assisted versus conventional thyroid surgery has proposed a reduction in injury to the EBSLN using the former technique.[65]

Other factors may play a role in EBSLN injury. It has been reported that inappropriate use of diathermy close to the EBSLN or to the quite thin cricothyroid muscle itself can cause damage and it should be avoided.[66] In the same way, inappropriate utilization of novel technical devices for haemostasis (Ligasure and Harmonic scalpel) close to this nerve could result in thermal injury. Cautious use of these devices is recommended when sectioning the vessels of the upper pole. When using the Harmonic scalpel, it is necessary to have the active blade far from the nerve. Moreover, one should remember that small vessels run from the superior thyroid artery into the pharyngeal constrictor and the

cricothyroid muscles. As the EBSLN slips under these muscles, there is a risk of injury during cauterization of these little vascular branches. Clearly, this should be avoided.

Finally, every attempt should be made to avoid injury of the cricothyroid muscle itself. This may occur due to electrocautery or manual retraction. Indeed, lesions of the muscles may cause functional impairments similar to those related to EBSLN injury.

The reported incidence of injury to the EBSLN ranges from 0 to 20 per cent in the literature with most studies quoting a rate of <5 per cent.[17, 18, 23, 26, 59] The true incidence is hard to quantify because formal laryngeal evaluation is usually not performed as part of routine postoperative follow up in the absence of symptoms. In the case of unilateral paralysis, flexible laryngoscopy usually shows symmetry of the larynx at rest. During phonation, the cord on the affected side will appear shorter and bowed when compared with the normal. Inferior displacement of the affected vocal process may be seen, or, more commonly, sluggish vocal fold motion with an asymmetrical mucosal wave. This type of injury can result in rotation of the posterior glottis towards the affected side. This asymmetry will not be seen in patients with bilateral paralysis. The patients with EBSLN injury will not be able to produce high-pitch phonation because the vocal cords will not fully elongate.

Many of the symptoms or physical findings of injury to the EBSLN are subtle, especially in patients who are not professional voice users. The clinician must have a high degree of suspicion and be able to differentiate this injury from other voice disorders using indirect laryngoscopy, videostroboscopy and laryngeal electromyogram (EMG) to confirm the diagnosis. After the diagnosis is made, therapy by a speech and language pathologist should be promptly started to improve phonatory outcomes and avoid compensatory vocal abuses.

Recurrent laryngeal nerve

Recurrent laryngeal nerve palsy (RLNP) is the most feared and potentially serious complication following thyroid surgery as it may cause significant voice and airway problems. Although not all post-thyroidectomy voice and swallowing disturbances are related to laryngeal nerve injuries,[67, 68, 69, 70, 71] symptomatic RLNP has been proved to be a major cause of impaired quality of life and to have a negative impact on job performance.[72, 73] It accounts for most of the medicolegal claims that are related to complications of thyroidectomy.[74] A review of endocrine malpractice litigation, found that about 54 per cent of the adverse outcomes involved thyroid and parathyroid surgery and that about 79 per cent of these claims involved recurrent laryngeal nerve injury.[29]

The reported rates of recurrent nerve injury range from 0 to 6 per cent, or even more frequently in some studies.[15, 75, 76] About 50–88 per cent of all RLNPs are transient. Many series report an incidence of RLNP of 1–2 per cent with an incidence of permanent palsy of less than 1 per cent of cases performed by experienced surgeons.[23] However, these are likely underestimates since only patients with significant and persistent symptoms underwent postoperative laryngeal examination in many of these studies.

Symptoms are variable, since laryngeal nerve injury is not an all-or-none problem and partial injury is more common than complete transection.[77] Unilateral RLNP (URLNP) can sometimes be completely asymptomatic. However, most patients with URLNP do have some vocal impairment, ranging from mild vocal fatigue to severe hoarseness. In a significant percentage of patients, dysphagia for liquids and aspiration are also present.[77,78,79] Intermittent coughing paroxysms are frequently reported and are secondary to spontaneous saliva aspiration.[80] Dyspnoea may be apparent during exertion. URLNP is usually well tolerated, but in some patients it can be life-threatening, since aspiration pneumonia can be fatal, especially in older patients or those with impaired pulmonary function preoperatively.[78]

Bilateral vocal cord paralysis obviously represents a potential life-threatening condition and a 'real surgical calamity'.[81] Indeed, it is always associated with some degree of airway impairment, ranging from acute and severe upper airway obstruction, requiring emergent reintubation or tracheotomy, to marginal dyspnoea at rest. Respiratory problems are usually more troublesome than voice changes.

Prevention of RLNP begins in the preoperative period. In all the patients who are to undergo thyroid and parathyroid procedures, examination of the larynx by indirect or direct laryngoscopy should be performed. Indeed, since about 30–40 per cent of patients with URLNP are asymptomatic,[13,80] and since many patients with hoarseness may not have vocal cord paralysis,[68,69,70,71] this is a reliable way to preoperatively demonstrate laryngeal function. Preoperative recognition of impaired laryngeal function and RLNP is essential for the surgeon to reduce the risk of bilateral vocal cord paralysis.[12,13] Moreover, vocal cord paralysis has been demonstrated to be the most accurate marker of invasive thyroid malignancy. Therefore, detecting this finding on preoperative evaluation will allow thorough patient counselling and preparation for future intraoperative management of the potentially invaded RLN at surgery.

With regard to the invaded RLN, there is general agreement that in cases of preoperative vocal cord paralysis with macroscopic nerve infiltration by differentiated thyroid carcinoma, the nerve should be resected with the tumour. If preoperative vocal cord function is normal, the nerve should be left intact since microscopic residuum can be safely ablated with radioiodine.[13,79,82] On the other hand, some surgeons still question the utility of routine preoperative laryngoscopy in the absence of symptoms and recommend selective laryngoscopy in symptomatic patients. Recently published guidelines make no mention of laryngeal examination in patients with thyroid nodules and carcinoma.[83]

The risk of lesion of the recurrent laryngeal nerve exists in all neck dissections. Individual mechanisms of injury include stretch or traction, compression or crush (i.e. ligature entrapment, haematoma formation), and thermal, electrical and severing injuries (complete or partial transection).[77,82] Moreover, some conditions put the nerve at a higher risk of injury (e.g. lack of identification of RLN during surgery, bilateral surgery, surgery for malignant diseases, lymph node dissection, Graves' disease and thyroiditis, previous neck surgery, substernal goitre, longer operative times or greater blood loss, reoperation for bleeding).[80] The knowledge of the mechanism of injury and risk factors of RLNP should thus help in its prevention.

Positive identification of the recurrent laryngeal nerve is essential for preservation of its integrity and function. Until recently, some authors have questioned routine identification of RLN. Many recent studies have validated the importance of visual identification during any thyroid surgery.[75,82,84,85] Hermann et al.[86] in their review of more than 27 000 nerves at risk, demonstrated that the incidence of temporary and permanent RLNP is significantly reduced if the nerve is identified during thyroidectomy. Moreover, they demonstrated that routine complete nerve exposure is characterized by a lower incidence of RLNP when compared with simple nerve localization and partial exposure. Indeed, they reported an average permanent RLNP rate of 0.9 per cent for localization only, 0.3 per cent for partial dissection and 0.1 per cent for extensive dissection.[86]

One must bear in mind the possible anatomic variations in branching pattern that exist. In addition to the difference in origin and course between the left and the right side, numerous anatomic variations are well known with respect to its relationship with the inferior thyroid artery, the tracheo-oesophageal groove, the thyroid gland, and Berry's ligament.[26,87,88,89,90,91] Moreover, in addition to the well-described normal patterns of extralaryngeal and intralaryngeal ramifications, the inferior laryngeal nerve (ILN) may give off branches that do not enter the larynx at all but instead connect it with other structures within the neck (sympathetic system, superior laryngeal nerve, thyroid, trachea and oesophagus).[92] Furthermore, on rare occasions (0.3–0.8 per cent), the right ILN does not recur.[87,90,91] In these cases, it originates from the cervical portion of the vagus nerve. Non-recurrence of the ILN results from a vascular anomaly during the embryonic development of the aortic arches, determined by the absence of the innominate artery and the formation of an aberrant right subclavian artery that arises directly from the aorta left of the midline and crosses posterior to the oesophagus.[87,91] This anatomic variant is exceptionally rare on the left side.[87,91] A non-recurrent inferior laryngeal nerve has also been reported in association with an ipsilateral recurrent laryngeal nerve, in some cases even in the absence of any vascular anomaly.[90,91,93] The surgeon should also be aware that enlarged anastomotic branches between the RLN and the cervical sympathetic chain may mimic a non-recurrent laryngeal nerve in up to 7.5 per cent of cases.[91,94] Finally, another confounding condition is represented by small branches connecting a non-recurrent ILN and the stellate sympathetic ganglion with a course that is similar to that of a normally recurring ILN.[91,94]

Because of the broad spectrum of anatomical variations, identification of the RLN can be difficult in some cases. The most important rule to follow during thyroid and parathyroid surgery is that no structure should be cut until the RLN is identified.[80] Following this rule, RLN injury, and in particular transection injury, will be rare.

Several approaches have been proposed to identify the nerve. Palpation has been proposed by some as a valuable technique for nerve identification.[95] The nerve feels like a cord or a violin string that can be rolled against the trachea. To increase tension on the RLN, this approach involves upward and medial retraction of the partially mobilized thyroid lobe.[95] This could result in excessive stretching and consequent traction injury of the nerve,[80] if not performed with great care.

The RLN may be identified inferiorly at the thoracic inlet using the RLN triangle,[80] as described by Lore *et al.*[96] The RLN triangle has it apex inferior in the thoracic inlet. The medial wall is formed by the trachea. The lateral wall is formed by the medial edge of the retracted strap muscles and the superior base by the lower edge of the retracted thyroid's inferior pole.[80] After identifying the nerve, the surgeon should trace it along its entire course. The advantage of this technique resides first of all in the fact that the RLN is identified before it branches. Thus, all branches are easily identified and preserved. Moreover, at this level, the RLN lies in soft areolar tissue, that facilitates dissection, unlike the strong, fibrous tissue of Berry's ligament. This is of particular relevance in the reoperative cases, where the nerve should be identified out of the previous scar. Its principal disadvantage is that a long segment of the nerve is dissected, with potential risk of nerve injury by neuropraxia not to mention potential of devascularization of the inferior parathyroid glands.

Most endocrine surgeons nowadays rely on the more limited dissection of the nerve which characterizes the so-called capsular dissection.[12, 97] This implies division of the tertiary branches of the inferior thyroid artery, close to the thyroid capsule in order to preserve vascularization of the inferior parathyroid glands.[97] After dividing the superior pole, the lobe is retracted medially and the posterolateral aspects of the thyroid lobe are exposed. The RLN is thus encountered at a high level in the neck, usually close to the ligament of Berry.[97] Various landmarks have been proposed, including crossing of the inferior thyroid artery and the inferior edge of the thyroid cartilage's inferior cornu. Actually, it is current practice to identify the nerve where it crosses the inferior thyroid artery.[87, 91] This approach has the potential benefits of limiting the length of the RLN dissection and focusing attention on the real 'dangerous area' for the RLN, i.e. the area of Berry's ligament, and reducing the risk of jeopardizing inferior parathyroid vascular supply.[80] On the other hand, this approach is not suitable in cases with large masses with lateral displacement of the RLN, as well as in cases with dense scar tissue as in revision thyroidectomy.

Some surgeons have called attention to the Zuckerkandl's tubercle, a nodular thickening of the lateral edge of the thyroid lobe that is present in most patients. It usually enlarges lateral to the RLN, with the nerve appearing to pass into a cleft medial to it. Early elevation and medial displacement of the tubercle of Zuckerkandl usually allows identification of the RLN close to its entrance into the larynx. For this reason, this tubercle has been described as an 'arrow pointed toward the nerve'.[98] Moreover, the normal superior parathyroid glands, derived from the fourth brachial pouch, are commonly found in close association and cephalad to the tubercle of Zuckerkandl. On the other hand, in some cases, the RLN runs lateral to an enlarged tubercle of Zuckerkandl, which has been enlarging medially. In these cases, the RLN is at high risk if it is identified lower than this level.

In some situations (e.g. large substernal goitre), the RLN should be identified first at its entry point. The laryngeal entry point represents the most constant site for the RLN. The nerve can be found after superior pole reflection within or deep to the ligament of Berry, extending under the lower edge of the inferior constrictor. After its identification, the nerve should be followed downward before goitre delivery. Indeed, in case of large intrathoracic or meditational goitres,

the RLN can be significantly displaced by the thyroid mass, in a lateral, posterior, medial or even anterior position. This last position is especially dangerous as it makes the nerve vulnerable during delivery of the thyroid lobe. It is obvious that blind finger delivery could represent a manoeuvre that risks injury to the displaced RLN. This could explain the higher RLNP rate reported for mediastinal goitre operations. Conversely, RLN identification at the level of its entrance and subsequent tracing, with progressive dissection and delivery of the thyroid lobe (the so-called 'toboggan technique') reduces the risk of nerve injury.[99]

The main disadvantage of this superior approach resides in the fact that identification of the nerve occurs within the fibrous and dense ligament of Berry, which can easily bleed. Moreover, the surgeon should be aware that at this level, the nerve may already have branched. Additional challenges derive from the possible existence of a low-riding EBSL, potentially displaced by large upper poles, and from the need to avoid devascularization of the superior parathyroid, whose blood supply may depend upon the superior thyroid vessels. From a technical point of view, in such difficult cases, section of the strap muscles, and in particular of the sternothyroid muscle, can allow for a better preparation of the superior pole and easier and safer identification of the RLN at its entrance to the larynx.

It is clear that careful complete exposure allows the surgeon to prevent permanent injury. There are also some important points that should be kept in mind when performing a neck operation. The first is that the ligament of Berry represents the site of highest risk of nerve injury for several reasons. Usually, the RLN passes through this dense condensation of the thyroid capsule and is consequently fixed at this level. Excessive traction over the thyroid and the trachea during nerve dissection may result in stretching lesions of the nerve fibres. During thyroidectomy under local anaesthesia, we have observed immediate voice changes related to medial retraction of the thyroid lobe and stretching of the nerve. This underscores the particular susceptibility of the RLN to stretch injury.

Moreover, the ligament of Berry is both dense and well vascularized, along its inferior edge, from the inferior thyroid artery. These arterial branches are well known by thyroid surgeons and can cause troublesome haemorrhage during the final phase of the thyroid dissection. For this reason, meticulous dissection under direct visualization of the RLN, as well as individual ligation of small, fine arterial branches running in the ligament of Berry, are mandatory to avoid injury of the RLN in this area. If some bleeding does occur, blind coagulation should be avoided and direct ligature of the bleeding vessel should be accomplished with the nerve completely exposed. Application of small clips or small clamps and subsequent ligature with fine suture are essential. Monopolar cautery should be avoided in proximity to the RLN. Bipolar cautery is sometimes useful. To facilitate this step of the procedure, we suggest gentle downward (posterior) displacement of the RLN with atraumatic clamps or the back of scissors. This widens the space for ligature application. New technologies for haemostasis (Harmonic scalpel, Ligasure) should be avoided as well when dissecting the ligament of Berry, in order to avoid thermal injury of the RLN. Conventional ligature still represents the best approach during this step of the procedure.

The nerve itself may branch while passing through the ligament of Berry and thus surgeons should avoid clamping or cutting any portion of the ligament of Berry until he or she is completely sure that no nerve branch lies within the tissue involved.

Finally, one should remember that during less than total thyroid resection (i.e. subtotal thyroidectomy), the last portion of the RLN is not always completely visualized, regardless of whether or not its more proximal course is exposed. It is possible that the nerve runs medial to or within a crease on the surface of the thyroid remnant. As a consequence, haemostatic sutures on the remnant thyroid tissue could expose the nerve to injury. For this reason, we and other surgeons,[12] consider total resection a safer procedure in many cases since the RLN is completely exposed in its distal course.

On occasion, despite the best efforts of the surgeon, the RLN is not identified.[89] The rate of the unvisualized nerve is up to 12–18 per cent of the cases in recent large series.[14, 89] Obviously, these high rates could reflect lack of experience or technical mistakes during dissection, but some difficulties may rarely occur even in experienced hands.[100] Moreover, anatomic integrity does not imply functional integrity and the inability to intraoperatively visualize vocal cord movement implies uncertainty with respect to postoperative functional outcome.[101]

In recent years, several methods for RLN monitoring during neck dissection have been explored. Intraoperative nerve monitoring (IONM) has been described in the literature for nearly three decades,[102] but it has been advocated strongly only over the last several years as a means of assisting in nerve identification and mapping to reduce the risk of injury. Several methods of IONM have been evaluated. These include finger palpation of the posterior cricoarytenoid during RLN stimulation,[80, 103] observation of vocal cord movement during RLN stimulation by direct laryngoscopy or through fibreoptic nasopharyngoscopy by way of laryngeal mask airway,[104] glottic pressure/balloon transducers to detect vocal cord motion with stimulation,[105] and intramuscular vocal cord electrodes that are placed endoscopically[106, 107] or through the cricothyroid membrane.[108, 109, 110] Surface electrodes can be placed directly on the mucosa overlying the posterior cricoarytenoid muscle.[111, 112] At present, the most popular and preferred method for IONM is a technique employing endotracheal tube surface electrodes that are placed in contact with the mucosa of the vocal cord.[80, 82, 113] Surface electrodes are non-invasive and may theoretically represent better recording electrodes than needle electrodes in that they sample a greater region of evoked muscle action potentials.[80]

Some authors have described a significant reduction in both transient and permanent postoperative RLNP with the utilization of the IONM.[109] Also, it has been recently reported that IONM is associated with improved outcomes especially in selected high-risk procedures, such as reoperative surgery, malignant disease and substernal goitre.[113] Other studies, based on a large number of patients, failed to demonstrate significant improvement in rates of paralysis.[100, 113, 114]

In other words, from all the published experiences, it is clear that IONM adds to, but does not replace, meticulous surgical technique and knowledge of the anatomy of the nerve and its variations. It is true that in the hands of experienced and dedicated surgeons, information derived from IONM could expedite surgery and render safer nerve dissection, especially in difficult cases where nerve identification and preservation can be challenging (e.g. reoperative cases, malignancy).

This has led some authors to propose selective use of IONM, mainly because of the cost involved. However, since we cannot reliably predict preoperatively which cases will be challenging, its routine use should be common practice.

This is particularly true if one considers that the most important function of IONM is its ability to prognosticate regarding postoperative neural function. In other words, nerve monitoring provides the sole possibility to intraoperatively verify nerve function.[80] It is well known that even experienced surgeons usually underestimate actual RLNP.[113] Electrical testing is superior to visual inspection alone. EMG activity after stimulation of the vagus nerve at the end of lobectomy confirms functional integrity of RLN. The demonstration of impaired electrical activity at the end of the first lobectomy during bilateral resection, should lead the surgeon to postpone resection of the second side and avoid the risk of bilateral nerve palsy. Moreover, RLN monitoring should be strongly considered in the presence of a preoperative RLNP, as in malignancies or reoperative cases. These aspects obviously underscore the utility of routine intraoperative nerve monitoring in all cases.

Corticosteroids are extensively used to prevent the risk of postoperative RLNP related to oedema from manipulation or stretch injury,[115] in the case of an anatomically intact nerve. As in other operations,[116] some surgeons empirically administer steroids during thyroid surgery in an attempt to reduce postoperative neural oedema, as well as to promote recovery of nerve function when RLNP occurs. Some authors suggest that the rate of temporary RLNP can be reduced with the use of preoperative and/or intraoperative steroids.[96] Moreover, it has been recently demonstrated that the duration of RLNP can be significantly reduced with the use of a single dose of intraoperative steroids.[115] As a consequence, the utilization of intraoperative steroids should be recommended, if not routinely, at least in patients where difficult nerve dissection portends a higher risk of temporary RLNP[115] or in patients in whom intraoperative monitoring findings suggest a blunt non-transection injury.[80]

Management of inadvertent intraoperative division is still controversial. Primary reanastomosis can result in some functional recovery, but misdirected axonal regrowth is responsible for unintended synkinesis of the laryngeal musculature, due to reinnervation of both abductor and adductor musculature.[78, 117, 118] Anastomosis with an ansa cervicalis nerve graft can restore laryngeal tone and bulk, resulting in good voice.[118] Patients with URLNP should undergo a trial of speech therapy. This is appropriate whether or not the RLN is anatomically intact. On occasion, this alone may be an adequate treatment for RLNP.[23] However, vocal straining may lead to hyperactive compensatory mechanisms that can compromise vocal outcome after vocal cord medialization.[78] For minor aspiration in patients without underlying pulmonary disease, swallowing therapy can encourage compensation with the tongue base and supraglottic structures, although liquids may need to be thickened.[78]

An algorithm for the management of patients with URLNP should be based on the degree of associated symptoms: aspiration, increased vocal effort, altered voice quality, dyspnoea on exertion and decreased quality of life.[78] Vocal cord medialization is usually considered urgent if aspiration pneumonia occurs or if oral feeding is considered dangerous (patients with altered pulmonary function).[78] Endoscopic vocal fold injection of resorbable material (e.g. fat, collagen) does not compromise spontaneous functional recovery of the nerve and does not interfere with other subsequent medialization techniques.[17, 78] This is the technique of choice if spontaneous recovery is expected because of anatomic integrity of the RLN. On the other hand, if the URLNP is well tolerated, a waiting period combined with speech therapy is recommended. In the case of persistent unilateral RLNP after 12 months with poor voice quality, definitive vocal cord medialization by injection technique or thyroplasty is recommended.[17, 23, 78] The choice of technique is a matter of the surgeon's experience and depends on the glottic configuration upon phonation (the size of the glottic gap). Arytenoid adduction performed in conjunction with medialization thyroplasty has been shown to provide good results.[23, 119] All of these techniques provide a good voice, eliminate aspiration and improve quality of life.

Bilateral RLNP is far more evident in its clinical manifestations than URLNP. Although voice quality may be fairly good, because of paramedian vocal cord position, most cases are recognized immediately in the postoperative period because of severe respiratory distress. The first priority is to secure an adequate airway. Immediate reintubation is preferable to urgent tracheotomy in the acute setting. If the nerves are thought to be intact, the patient should remain intubated for several days and corticosteroid administered to reduce oedema.[17, 23, 76] After a few days, extubation can be safely performed in a controlled setting and, if airway compromise is still present, a tracheotomy should be performed. If laryngeal motility has recovered and the airway is adequate, no further manoeuvres are necessary and safe extubation is possible. Delaying performance of tracheotomy for several days has the two-fold advantage of allowing the nerves to recover their function in the case of transient injury and avoiding contamination of the fresh surgical field with a tracheotomy.[17, 23]

If recovery is anticipated, observation for up to 12 months is appropriate, and the airway is usually secured by tracheotomy or arytenoidopexy, which are reversible procedures.[17, 23] Recently, vocal cord laterofixation has been described as a solution for avoiding tracheotomy in the acute setting, when recovery is anticipated.[23] While multiple strategies have been used to rehabilitate the patient with bilateral vocal cord paralysis, ultimately each patient will present with a unique set of circumstances that mandate individualized care. In many cases, the simplest, most stable, and often overlooked option is the permanent tracheotomy. Patients are usually reluctant to accept such a solution. In these patients, lateralization of one cord by cordotomy or arytenoidectomy results in an improved airway and allows decannulation.[17, 23]

Voice and swallowing impairment in the absence of laryngeal nerve lesions

Most of the voice and swallowing alterations that occur following thyroidectomy are self-limited and not related to impaired laryngeal nerve function.[68, 69, 120, 121, 122] These symptoms are usually dismissed by the clinician or attributed to orotracheal intubation, because they cannot be translated into objective data by appropriate diagnostic tests. Nevertheless, their presence elicits anxiety among patients if they are uninformed about the risks. These symptoms should be regarded as true complications of thyroid surgery and treated appropriately by the consulted physicians.

Recent interest in these symptoms and their possible implications on patient quality of life after thyroidectomy, especially in voice professionals, has appeared in the world literature.[69, 70, 71, 76] Subjective voice and swallowing alterations after uncomplicated thyroidectomy include a broad spectrum of symptoms, and are usually temporary and resolve relatively quickly. However, in some cases symptoms tend to persist even years after thyroidectomy.[67, 71] Swallowing symptoms were reported more frequently and showed a tendency to persist longer than the voice changes.[67, 71]

In the absence of any videostrobolaryngoscopically demonstrable laryngeal nerve injury, the factors that could determine voice and swallowing disturbances seem related mainly to the normal healing process, or possibly to subclinical postoperative haematoma. After thyroid gland removal, the strap muscles become the sole support of the laryngotracheal unit, and these muscles often fuse through scar tissue formation.[67, 68, 121, 122] This results in laryngotracheal fixation with impairment of vertical movement. This problem seems more evident in the case of strap muscle division.[67, 71, 121, 122] However, a functional component related to local neck pain and an emotional or psychological reaction to the postoperative stress should also be considered as possible aetiologies. Nonetheless, in some cases, upper aerodigestive symptoms can persist for years after an 'uncomplicated' thyroidectomy. This can suggest that some symptoms may be due to an intraoperative injury of the fine anastomotic branches connecting the laryngeal nerves (RLN and the EBSLN) with the sympathetic cervical chain.[67, 71, 93] Some small branches of the laryngeal nerves, together with other cervical branches, participate in the autonomic, sensory and motor innervation of pharyngeal and laryngeal structures. Injury to this perivisceral nerve plexus during thyroidectomy could underlie at least some of the postoperative discomfort, which is variable in relation to the different anatomic pattern of nerve branches.[67, 71] These possible mechanisms underscore the importance of meticulous surgical technique to avoid this kind of post-thyroidectomy consequence. Strap muscle division should be avoided as far as possible. Accurate haemostasis and preservation of all fine nerve branches must be a primary goal. Less extensive neck dissection,[70] as performed in minimally invasive surgical techniques,[65] seems related to a lesser incidence of this kind of functional voice and swallowing alteration.

Regardless of the cause, these post-thyroidectomy vocal and swallowing changes are reported frequently, and we believe that surgeons should be aware of these subjective discomforts that commonly occur following thyroid surgery. Patients must also be informed and warned about these symptoms during the preoperative counselling session for ethical as well as legal reasons, especially in voice professionals.

Hypocalcaemia and hypoparathyroidism

Postoperative hypocalcaemia is one of the most common complications of thyroid and parathyroid surgery. Moreover, after RLN palsy, permanent hypoparathyroidism accounts for the largest number of thyroidectomy-related claims.[74]

Temporary hypocalcaemia has been reported to occur in 1.6–50 per cent of the patients undergoing bilateral thyroid resection and in 0–35 per cent of patients after parathyroidectomy. Permanent hypoparathyroidism results in 0–13 per cent of patients after bilateral thyroid surgery and in 0–2.2 per cent of patients after successful parathyroidectomy.[23]

Various factors account for these differences in the literature, such as the definition of hypocalcaemia, the type of disease, and the surgical technique. Moreover, hypocalcaemia following thyroid resection is somewhat different in origin versus that occurring after parathyroid surgery. Post-thyroidectomy hypocalcaemia is multifactorial in origin. Among the potential factors causing this decrease in serum calcium, there are postoperative hemodilution[123] and calcitonin release.[124] The so-called 'hungry bone syndrome' is also implicated in patients with hyperthyroidism or hyperparathyroidism and osteodystrophy.[125]

A moderate, asymptomatic hypocalcaemia is usually observed within 12 hours following unilateral or bilateral thyroidectomy, is associated with serum phosphorus decrease, and recovers spontaneously within 24 hours in most patients.[123, 126] Perioperative hemodilution may be responsible for this decrease and explains its occurrence with other extracervical operations.[123] This hypocalcaemia is self-limited, usually asymptomatic, and does not require supplementation.

Elevation of serum calcitonin (calcitonin leak), secondary to manipulation of the thyroid, was suspected to participate in this calcium decrease,[124] but this was not confirmed in further studies.[123, 125, 126, 127]

Preoperative hyperthyroid status is associated with decreased gastrointestinal calcium absorption and increased osteoclast activity, with increased bone resorption to maintain serum calcium levels.[128] The postoperative reversal of osteodystrophy and the accretion of calcium in bones may also contribute to the decreased serum calcium. The serum calcium generally reaches its nadir within 48 hours of surgery. The risk of hypocalcaemia is not alleviated by the correction of hyperthyroidism within a few weeks before thyroidectomy. It is correlated more closely with the pretreatment serum levels of free thyroxine[127] and with markers of bone turnover rate, such as serum alkaline phosphatase levels.[123] Similarly, hyperparathyroidism is associated with osteoclast activation and increased bone resorption. After thyroidectomy or parathyroidectomy, active calcium uptake by bone may result in postoperative hypocalcaemia. These possible mechanisms of postoperative hypocalcaemia underscore the need for adequate patient preparation before surgery for hyperthyroidism. Prophylactic supplementation should be considered to avoid severe hypocalcaemia in patients with significant osteodystrophy.[16]

Nonetheless, it is clear that impaired parathyroid function is the major contributing factor for clinically relevant hypocalcaemia. Proper surgical technique is of the utmost importance in preserving viable parathyroid glands and several factors have been associated with impaired postoperative function.

There is a risk of iatrogenic injury to the parathyroid glands during any operation in which both lobes are explored or resected. Bilateral neck exploration for hyperparathyroidism, with biopsy of all the glands necessarily involves the risk of parathyroid gland injury. Operation for known multiglandular disease (MEN1, MEN2A, familial hyperparathyroidism, parathyroid hyperplasia, and secondary and tertiary hyperparathyroidism) requires removal of most parathyroid tissue (subtotal or total parathyroidectomy with autotransplantation). In such cases, postoperative hypocalcaemia and hypoparathyroidism to some degree are consequences of the indicated operation itself.

Susceptibility of parathyroid glands to injury during neck dissection mainly resides in their widely variable anatomical position, their relationship with the thyroid gland, and in their very delicate vascular supply. Classically, there are four parathyroid glands in close association with the thyroid, although the number and positions of the glands may vary greatly among individuals. We know that there is an incidence of about 13 per cent of a supernumerary fifth parathyroid and, at most, a 3 per cent incidence of only three glands.[129]

The superior parathyroid glands are derived from the fourth branchial pouch and are relatively constant in their position since they have a short line of embryologic descent and remain close to the capsule on the posterolateral aspect of the superior third of the thyroid lobe near the cricothyroid junction. This is the level of Zuckerkandl's tubercle and is in close proximity to the RLN. The inferior parathyroid glands are derived from the third branchial pouch and descend along with the developing thymus. Therefore, they have a long line of descent and, consequently, their position is much more variable. An inferior parathyroid gland can be carried, with the thymus, into the anterior mediastinum, into the aortopulmonary window, or in the pericardium. It may also be left behind high in the carotid sheath, up to the carotid bifurcation, or even within the vagus nerve itself (undescended glands). Most inferior parathyroid glands, however, are found near the inferior pole of the thyroid in the vicinity of the thyrothymic tract. They frequently lie on the surface of the inferior pole of the thyroid, within the thyroid capsule. Despite the variability in the anatomy of the parathyroid glands, there is frequently a symmetric arrangement in the position of the glands on the two sides of the neck. Positional symmetry of the superior glands is found in about 80 per cent of cases and in 70 per cent of inferior glands.[129]

As first described by Halsted in 1907,[130] most of the parathyroid glands are supplied by a single, fine end-artery. There is a single arterial supply to 80 per cent of parathyroid glands, a dual arterial supply to 15 per cent, and multiple arteries to the remaining 5 per cent.[131] In most cases, these arteries originate from the inferior thyroid artery. However, in 15–20 per cent of cases the superior parathyroid is supplied by a branch from the superior thyroid artery, sometimes associated with an anastomotic branch running between the superior and inferior thyroid arteries.[132, 133]

The incidence of parathyroid gland injury is related to the extent of the operation and to the experience of the surgeon. A higher incidence is seen after total thyroidectomy versus subtotal thyroidectomy and after subtotal thyroidectomy versus excision of a single adenoma. Other factors associated with an increased incidence of postoperative hypocalcaemia are central compartment neck dissection, reoperative cases, surgery for substernal goitre, surgery for carcinoma, and surgery for Graves' disease.

A variety of strategies has been advocated to decrease the incidence of permanent hypoparathyroidism, including less than total thyroidectomy,[134] intracapsular dissection,[135] identification of the parathyroid glands with preservation of their vascular pedicle,[136] selective autotransplantation of inadvertently removed or nonviable parathyroid glands, and routine autotransplantation of at least one parathyroid gland if not all identified parathyroid glands.[137]

More limited thyroid resection (i.e. subtotal thyroidectomy) has been proposed to avoid inadvertent parathyroid injury.[137] Nonetheless, at present, total thyroidectomy is still considered the optimal procedure, even in cases of benign bilateral disease.[137]

It is now clear that the best way to avoid parathyroid damage is to clearly know the embryology and the surgical anatomy of the glands, including their blood supply, and to make every effort to preserve them *in situ* or to transplant one or more glands when this is not possible.

However, it should be stressed that despite the efforts of the surgeon, inadvertent parathyroid removal during thyroidectomy has been reported in 9–15 per cent of the cases, even in experienced centres according to recent reports.[133, 138, 139, 140] Even as incidental removal of one or two glands may not affect the incidence of postoperative hypocalcaemia,[133, 138, 140] it does demonstrate the difficulties surgeons encounter in preserving viable parathyroid glands during thyroidectomy. The incidence of intrathyroidal parathyroid glands is approximately 0.2 per cent according to autopsy studies,[129] but this incidence rises to between 2 and 5 per cent for patients with primary hyperparathyroidism[141, 142] and up to 11 per cent in those with persistent or recurrent hyperparathyroidism.[143, 144]

The surgeon should make every attempt to preserve viable parathyroid glands *in situ*. Some techniques play a crucial role in preserving parathyroid glands. First of all, a bloodless surgical field is essential, because any bleeding may stain the surface of the gland, obscuring its colour which is essential for parathyroid identification.[145] Although parathyroid glands can usually be identified based on their gross appearance, in some instances it may be difficult even for experienced surgeons to determine whether a structure represents a parathyroid gland, thyroid tissue, adipose tissue, or thymic tissue.[146, 147] In such cases, a liberal attitude toward biopsy and frozen section examination should be adopted.[146]

Because of the highly variable location of the inferior parathyroid glands, inability to identify one or both of the inferior parathyroids does not necessarily indicate inadvertent removal. The glands can be located cephalad or caudal (i.e. intrathymic) to the site of dissection. Conversely, not identifying a superior parathyroid gland more likely signifies inadvertent removal, since it is usually located on the posterior aspect of the thyroid lobe, close to the point where the RLN enters the larynx. In other words, the surgeon should make every effort to identify and preserve superior parathyroid glands, while this may not be possible with the inferior glands in all cases. If no inferior parathyroid gland is identified in close proximity to the thyroid, no further dissection of the thyrothymic tract or the thymus itself is necessary.[145] Extensive dissection may cause inadvertent devascularization of the inferior glands.

Once identified, the parathyroid gland should be preserved with its vascular pedicle intact as far as possible. This demands a very gentle, cautious and sometimes time-consuming dissection. The parathyroid itself should not be grasped, but gently detached from the thyroid capsule by retracting the surrounding fat which is usually present. Ligature of the most distal branches of the inferior thyroid artery usually allows for vascular pedicle preservation. Despite some reports demonstrating that truncal inferior artery ligation during subtotal thyroidectomy does not affect the incidence of postoperative hypocalcaemia and hypoparathyroidism,[128, 148] we (and most other authors) believe that it is necessary to ligate branches of the inferior thyroid artery in close proximity to the thyroid capsule to avoid devascularization of the parathyroid glands.

Excessive stretching of the vascular pedicle and the use of cautery should be avoided in close proximity to the parathyroid glands. Similarly, new devices for achieving haemostasis (i.e. Harmonic scalpel, Ligasure) should be avoided in close proximity to the parathyroid glands. In some cases, it may be very difficult to detach a parathyroid gland from the thyroid capsule, due to factors, such as inflammatory reaction (i.e. thyroiditis) or scarring after previous operation. In such cases, if dealing with benign disease, it is possible to perform an intracapsular dissection, with the aim of preserving the parathyroid gland *in situ*. Routine prophylactic central neck dissection in differentiated low-risk thyroid carcinoma is to be avoided in the absence of macroscopic involvement as it engenders a higher risk of postoperative hypoparathyroidism with arguably little patient benefit.[149]

Identifying and dissecting the parathyroid glands during thyroidectomy does not guarantee viability. Traditionally, judgement regarding the viability of a parathyroid gland has been made based on its colour. Unless a parathyroid is markedly discoloured (dark purple/black or pallid)), it is presumed to be viable.[145, 146] Vascular injury to the parathyroid pedicle may be arterial or venous. Arterial ischaemia (devascularization) implies a definitive parathyroid lesion. Macroscopically, the gland appears discoloured and pale, and should be transplanted when recognized intraoperatively. Impairment of venous drainage is usually characterized by venous congestion and it is indicated by dark purple or black discoloration of the parathyroid glands. In this case, incision of the parathyroid capsule may liberate excess venous blood and usually the gland will recover its normal appearance and colour. If this does not occur, the gland should be removed and autotransplanted.

Despite the adoption of this approach, some glands may be anatomically intact, but not physiologically viable.[137] Various methods of assessment have been adopted including the careful incision of the parathyroid capsule to assess for bleeding (knife test)[97, 146] and Doppler measurement of the parathyroid vessels.[150] This latter technique has not been reproducible and has not gained widespread acceptance. On the other hand, the knife test has been advocated by some, but may have the disadvantage of inducing iatrogenic injury to the already precarious blood supply of the parathyroid gland in question.[151]

Clearly, a reliable intraoperative method to identify patients with impaired parathyroid function could facilitate the decision to perform autotransplantation.[151] It has been suggested that intraoperative parathyroid hormone measurement may have a role in monitoring parathyroid function, but it is generally not employed in routine clinical practice currently.[137, 151] As a consequence, evaluation of the viability of parathyroid glands still relies mostly on macroscopic appearance.

Parathyroid autotransplantation during thyroidectomy was first described by Lahey in 1926.[81] However, only after the demonstration of the viability of the transplanted parathyroid tissue in humans,[152] was autotransplantation definitively included in the armamentarium of endocrine surgeons. Parathyroid autotransplantation is considered by most experts a useful technique for preserving parathyroid function, especially for non-viable parathyroid glands. However, strategies for parathyroid autotransplantation vary widely from a selective approach with transplantation of only non-viable or incidentally removed glands,[135, 147, 151] to routine autotransplantation of one gland[153] or even all the identified parathyroid glands.[154] Strategies that involve routine autotransplantation are obviously characterized by a higher incidence of early postoperative hypocalcaemia, but a low rate of permanent hypoparathyroidism. Nonetheless, in recent years groups that had previously proposed routine parathyroid autotransplantation have critically reviewed their experience and now propose a more selective approach to parathyroid autotransplantation.[137] In summary, there is no doubt that inadvertently removed or damaged parathyroid glands should undergo autotransplantation when they are recognized at operation. Intentional devascularization of all parathyroid glands should be avoided unless there is a reliable technique to ensure graft success after autotransplantation.[137, 151]

The technique of transplantation differs for different series. Thin sectioning (slicing),[152, 155] mincing[151, 154] and injection of a suspension of parathyroid tissue in buffered saline into muscle[97] have been described. Transplantation of thin sections in a muscular pocket closed and marked with a non-absorbable suture and titanium clips is the preferred option in transplantation of hyperplastic tissue, e.g. in parathyroid operations for multiglandular diseases. On the other hand, intramuscular injection of a suspension of parathyroid tissue in buffered saline seems an attractive, fast and easy option during thyroid operations.

There is also some variability in the site chosen for parathyroid transplantation. In most patients undergoing thyroid operations, parathyroid glands can be easily and safely transplanted into the sternocleidomastoid or strap muscles. In contrast, a remote site, such as the brachioradialis muscle, is more suitable for patients undergoing thyroidectomy for treatment of MEN2A (who are prone to development of hyperparathyroidism) or for aggressive malignancies such as poorly differentiated thyroid carcinoma or laryngeal cancer as these latter patients may need postoperative radiation therapy to the neck. The brachioradialis muscle is also a preferred site in patients with secondary hyperparathyroidism and multiglandular diseases (parathyroid hyperplasia, as observed in MEN1 and familial hyperparathyroidism), mainly because this facilitates evaluation of viable parathyroid tissue based on blood drawn from the forearm veins and facilitates localization and removal of parathyroid tissue in cases of recurrence. Irrespective of the site selected, it is important to histologically confirm the presence of parathyroid tissue before transplantation.

It is not clear in individual patients who have had a parathyroid transplantation and possible damage to the other parathyroid glands whether it is the transplant or possible supernumerary glands that are providing sufficient function for normocalcaemia.[12, 145]

In spite of all the efforts to avoid this complication, postoperative hypocalcaemia and hypoparathyroidism still occur. Temporary symptomatic hypocalcaemia is common after successful parathyroidectomy, despite the fact that minimally invasive and focused approaches have reduced its incidence when compared with bilateral neck exploration. Indeed, the targeted approaches to parathyroidectomy have the important advantage of avoiding manipulation of normal glands leading to normal parathyroid function postoperatively. In this setting, postoperative hypocalcaemia is usually self-limited and related to inhibition of normal glands by the hyperfunctioning one or to the existence of an underlying hungry bone syndrome. In any case, symptoms of hypocalcaemia are frequently observed, even in the absence of biochemical hypocalcaemia. These symptoms are usually mild to moderate and resolve spontaneously within weeks. With this phenomenon in mind, some authors propose prophylactic oral calcium administration in all patients undergoing parathyroidectomy. This is often done in order to relieve patient anxiety related to hypocalcaemic symptoms and also to allow the procedure to be performed on an ambulatory or same day basis.[156] On the contrary, permanent hypoparathyroidism is virtually impossible in the case of focused parathyroidectomy. On the other hand, bilateral neck exploration brings with it the possibility of injury to normal parathyroid glands, especially if biopsy is obtained to confirm parathyroid origin. In such situations, patients are at risk of clinically relevant hypocalcaemia and should not be selected for outpatient surgery.[157, 158] Operations for parathyroid hyperplasia (total parathyroidectomy plus autotransplantation, subtotal parathyroidectomy) are obviously characterized by a higher risk of postoperative hypocalcaemia and hypoparathyroidism.

Permanent hypoparathyroidism occurs in only 0–0.5 per cent of patients after initial exploration for sporadic primary hyperparathyroidism,[157, 159, 160] but is far more frequent after surgery for parathyroid hyperplasia, especially in patients undergoing total parathyroidectomy plus autotransplantation. The occurrence of permanent hypoparathyroidism is dependent on the viability of the parathyroid remnant or the parathyroid graft. Since its occurrence cannot be definitively predicted, cryopreservation of resected parathyroid tissue is usually recommended for all patients undergoing multigland parathyroid extirpation or reoperative parathyroid surgery. Cryopreserved tissue can be transplanted if permanent hypoparathyroidism occurs.

Although severe and symptomatic post-thyroidectomy hypocalcaemia is rare, it is of particular concern. Symptoms usually manifest 24–48 hours after operation and it is usually not easy to predict which patients will require oral calcium and/or vitamin D supplementation. In the absence of any reliable predictors of clinically relevant hypocalcaemia after bilateral thyroid resection, prolonged hospitalization to monitor serum calcium levels has been considered the standard of care. Conversely, current health-care practices encourage shorter and shorter hospitalizations to reduce costs.

For this reason, there has been a great deal of interest in identifying perioperative factors that can predict the development of post-thyroidectomy hypocalcaemia soon after surgery, allowing for early treatment of patients at risk and safe early discharge of patients not at risk.[127, 161] Calcium slopes monitoring in the early postoperative period has been demonstrated to be useful.[162, 163] More recently, parathyroid hormone measurement has been investigated. Several studies have demonstrated its usefulness in defining groups of patients at risk of postoperative hypocalcaemia. These patients should be treated early after surgery and are not candidates for early discharge, while those patients who are deemed not at risk can be discharged.[164] Encouraging initial results have not been uniformly confirmed by subsequent studies.[165] For this reason, postoperative monitoring of serum calcium levels still remains the standard of care. Another option to avoid symptomatic hypocalcaemia and to shorten hospital stay after thyroidectomy is routine prophylactic oral calcium/vitamin D supplementation.[166]

Despite uncertain utility of calcitriol administration in the early postoperative period, we believe that supplementation should include both vitamin D and oral calcium administration in all patients.[166] Vitamin D does not inhibit normal parathyroid gland function, but allows for a prompt recovery from hypocalcaemia.[166] Once started, supplementation should be tapered on the basis of serum calcium levels. Intravenous calcium gluconate administration should be reserved for patients who manifest symptoms or falling levels in spite of oral therapy.

Failed exploration – recurrent and persistent hyperparathyroidism

Parathyroid operations are among the most challenging in endocrine surgery because of the large variability in parathyroid anatomy. The enlarged parathyroid gland or glands can be almost anywhere; hence the term 'exploration'. To avoid unacceptably high failure rates, the surgeon should be familiar with normal parathyroid anatomy, but also with its variants. Moreover, he or she should be familiar with the common pathophysiology of the parathyroid diseases.

It has been demonstrated that low volume parathyroid surgeons report significantly higher rates of morbidity, most notably failed exploration.[167] Surgery performed by experienced surgeons would avoid complication in 95–98 per cent of the cases.[168, 169] However, the definition of the experienced parathyroid surgeon is not entirely clear. Based on the findings of published studies, demonstrating a lower complication rate among surgeons performing more than ten operations per year, this criterion has been used to support sufficient experience.[16, 170]

Operative failures can be grouped into persistent hyperparathyroidism, recurrent hyperparathyroidism, and errors in diagnosis. This last occurrence is a common cause of failed exploration. The surgeon must have a working understanding of basic endocrinology if this error is to be avoided and patients spared unnecessary surgery. It should be remembered that hypercalcaemia does not always indicate primary hyperparathyroidism and it should be correlated in all cases with serum parathyroid hormone (PTH) levels. One confounding condition the surgeon should remember is benign familial hypocalciuric hypercalcaemia (BFHH).

Persistent hyperparathyroidism is the most common result of operative failure and by convention is defined as postoperative hypercalcaemia occurring within six months after initial neck exploration. Causes of operative failure and persistent hyperparathyroidism include missed adenoma due to difficult anatomy or an ectopic or supernumerary gland, failure to recognize parathyroid hyperplasia, misinterpretation of localization data or intraoperative PTH monitoring results, and parathyromatosis. Parathyromatosis is a rare but feared complication in patients with hyperparathyroidism. Capsular rupture of the pathologic gland(s) may result in parathyroid seeding and consequent disseminated growth of the seeded hyperplastic cells.[171] This possibility underscores the importance of gentle handling of the affected glands, avoiding any capsular rupture. Grasping of the parathyroid capsule should be absolutely avoided in order to prevent this cause of persistent or recurrent hyperparathyroidism.

Recurrent hyperparathyroidism is characterized by at least six months of normocalcaemia after initial operation and typically indicates unrecognized, and therefore untreated, hyperplasia. It can also arise with parathyroid carcinoma, parathyromatosis, a missed synchronous or metachronous second adenoma, or recovery of a hyperfunctioning gland that was devascularized at initial dissection.

After successful operation for primary hyperparathyroidism, a significant percentage of patients show elevated levels of PTH with normal serum calcium levels (normocalcaemic hyperparathormonaemia). It generally resolves with six months' postoperative treatment with oral calcium and multivitamin supplementation.[27] In such patients, elevated parathormone seems to be a reflection of a dietary deficiency. Nonetheless, in about 1 per cent of the patients presumed to be successfully operated, this phenomenon predicts early operative failure due to unrecognized multiglandular disease.[16, 27] Patients with postoperative normocalcaemic hyperparathormonaemia should thus undergo close follow-up evaluation for recurrence.

Parathyroidectomy for primary hyperparathyroidism is associated with a success rate of 95–98 per cent.[16, 23] Primary hyperparathyroidism is caused by a single adenoma in most of the cases (85–95 per cent). Parathyroid hyperplasia has been reported in as many as 15 per cent of the cases, with most series reporting an incidence of 2–6 per cent. Double adenomas are present in 2–6 per cent of patients.[28, 142, 157, 159] Bilateral cervical exploration (without preoperative localization studies) with the removal of the suspected adenoma and biopsy of the normal appearing glands has long been considered the standard operation for primary hyperparathyroidism. Indeed, the requirement to clearly exclude multiglandular disease remains exploration with identification and assessment of all glands.[172] The only other way to exclude multiglandular disease is represented by intraoperative parathyroid hormone monitoring, which is based on measurement of serum intact PTH levels during surgery and analysed using a specially modified assay.[173, 174] After removal of a suspected adenoma, specific criteria indicate if further hyperfunctional glands exist. The criteria for interpretation vary somewhat between experts, but a PTH drop of more than 50 per cent of the highest pre-excision levels (and into the normal range) 5–10 minutes after parathyroid ablation are considered indicative of removal of all hyperfunctioning tissue by most.[173, 174, 175] It has been confirmed that PTH monitoring reliably predicts postoperative cure.[16, 157, 172, 173, 174, 175] Moreover, its introduction into clinical practice, along with improved preoperative localization studies (ultrasound and sestaMIBi scan) has allowed significant improvement in the surgical strategy in patients with primary hyperparathyroidism. If a single adenoma is suspected on the basis of preoperative localization studies, a minimally invasive, focused approach can be proposed with significant advantages for the patients not only in terms of cosmetic results, but more importantly in a lower incidence of postoperative complications (i.e. postoperative hypocalcaemia). At present, intraoperative PTH monitoring should be considered the new standard of care in patients undergoing parathyroidectomy for sporadic primary hyperparathyroidism.

Recurrence rates are higher (2–12 per cent) in patients undergoing parathyroidectomy for secondary hyperparathyroidism resulting from renal failure.[176, 177] This is usually the result of a missed gland in an unusual or ectopic location, supernumerary glands, or hyperplasia of remnant or grafted parathyroid tissue. These mechanisms highlight the need for an accurate and meticulous neck exploration in all cases and for the removal of a sufficient amount of parathyroid tissue. The decision between a subtotal and a total parathyroidectomy with autotransplantation is beyond the scope of this chapter. However, what is important in all cases of parathyroid hyperplasia is that the parathyroid remnant or graft should be carefully marked and the procedure well described in the operative report so that any possible re-exploration will have a higher chance of success, if it becomes necessary.

KEY LEARNING POINTS

- Complications associated with thyroid and parathyroid surgery may occur, either as a result of surgical error or due to the extent of patient disease. The aim of this chapter is to furnish the reader not only with a list of the possible complications, but more importantly with a description of common surgical errors and techniques that will help to avoid them.
- A post-operative hematoma is probably the most feared complication after thyroid and parathyroid surgery. It can lead to devastating consequences with tracheal compression and subsequent hypoxia, which may then lead to brain injury and death. The patient may present with respiratory distress, pain or pressure sensation in the neck or dysphagia. Signs include progressive neck swelling, suture line bleeding, dyspnoea and/or stridor. A liberal attitude towards re-exploration in the case of symptomatic hematoma is mandatory.
- Recurrent laryngeal nerve palsy is a potentially serious complication following thyroid and parathyroid surgery as it may cause significant voice and airway problems. Prior to thyroid and parathyroid procedures, examination of the larynx by indirect or direct laryngoscopy should be performed. About 30–40 per cent of patients with RLNP are asymptomatic, and many patients with hoarseness may not have vocal cord paralysis. Positive identification of the recurrent laryngeal nerve is essential for preservation of its integrity and function.
- Intraoperative nerve monitoring is a means of assisting in nerve identification and mapping to reduce the risk of injury. It also prognosticates nerve function postoperatively. Also, IONM is associated with improved outcomes especially in selected high-risk procedures, such as reoperative surgery, malignant disease and substernal goitre. IONM has a crucial role in the intraoperative decision-making process.
- Postoperative hypocalcaemia is one of the most common complications of thyroid and parathyroid surgery. Temporary hypocalcaemia has been reported to occur in 1.6–50 per cent of the patients undergoing bilateral thyroid resection and in 0–35 per cent of patients after parathyroidectomy. Permanent hypoparathyroidism results in 0–13 per cent of patients after bilateral thyroid surgery and in 0–2.2 per cent of patients after successful parathyroidectomy.
- Temporary symptomatic hypocalcaemia is common after successful parathyroidectomy, despite the fact that minimally invasive and focused approaches have reduced its incidence when compared with bilateral neck exploration. The targeted approaches to parathyroidectomy have the important advantage of avoiding manipulation of normal glands leading to normal parathyroid function postoperatively.
- Permanent hypoparathyroidism occurs in only 0–0.5 per cent of patients after initial exploration for sporadic primary hyperparathyroidism, but is far more frequent after surgery for parathyroid hyperplasia, especially in patients undergoing total parathyroidectomy plus autotransplantation. Cryopreserved tissue can be transplanted if permanent hypoparathyroidism occurs.
- Causes of operative failure and persistent hyperparathyroidism include missed adenoma due to difficult anatomy or an ectopic or supernumerary gland, failure to recognize parathyroid hyperplasia, misinterpretation of localization data or intraoperative PTH monitoring results, and parathyromatosis. After successful operation for primary hyperparathyroidism, a significant percentage of patients show elevated levels of PTH with normal serum calcium levels (normocalcaemic hyperparathormonaemia). It generally resolves with six months postoperative treatment with oral calcium and multivitamin supplementation. Intraoperative parathyroid hormone monitoring is a helpful tool to determine whether further hyperfunctional glands exist. It has been confirmed that PTH monitoring reliably predicts postoperative cure.

REFERENCES

♦ 1. Bliss RD, Gauger PG, Delbridge LW. Surgeon's approach to the thyroid gland: surgical anatomy and the importance of technique. *World Journal of Surgery* 2000; **24**: 891–7.

∗ 2. Greene WW. Three cases of bronchocele successfully removed. *American Journal of Medical Science* 1871; **121**: 80(cited in Ref. 1).

♦ 3. Becker WF. Presidential address: pioneer in thyroid surgery. *Annals of Surgery* 1977; **185**: 493–504.

● 4. Thompson N, Olsen WR, Hoffman GL. The continuing development of the technique of thyroidectomy. *Surgery* 1973; **73**: 913–27.

♦ 5. Slough CM, Johns R, Randolph GW *et al*. History of thyroid and parathyroid surgery. In: Randolph GW (ed.). *Surgery of the thyroid and parathyroid glands*. Philadelphia, PA: Saunders, 2003: 3–11.

♦ 6. McHenry CR. Patients volume and complications in thyroid surgery. *British Journal of Surgery* 2002; **89**: 821–3.

♦ 7. Soh EY, Clark OH. Surgical considerations and approach to thyroid cancer. *Endocrinology and Metabolism Clinics of North America* 1996; **25**: 115–39.

● 8. Manolidis S, Takashima M, Kirby M, Scarlett M. Thyroid surgery: a comparison of outcomes between experts and surgeons in training. *Otolaryngology – Head and Neck Surgery* 2001; **125**: 30–3.

● 9. Shindo ML, Sinha UK, Rice DH. Safety of thyroidectomy in residency: a review of 186 consecutive cases. *Laryngoscope* 1995; **105**: 1173–5.

● 10. Sywak MS, Yeh MW, Sidhu SB *et al*. New surgical consultant: is there a learning curve? *Australia and New Zealand Journal of Surgery* 2006; **76**: 1081–4.

● 11. Sosa JA, Bowman HM, Tielsch JM *et al*. The importance of surgeon experience for clinical and economic outcomes from thyroidectomy. *Annals of Surgery* 1998; **228**: 320–30.

♦ 12. Reeve T, Thompson NW. Complications of thyroid surgery: how to avoid them, how to manage them, and observations on their possible effect on the whole patient. *World Journal of Surgery* 2000; **24**: 971–5.

● 13. Randolph GW, Kamani D. The importance of preoperative laryngoscopy in patients undergoing thyroidectomy: voice, vocal cord function, and the preoperative detection of invasive thyroid malignancy. *Surgery* 2006; **139**: 357–62.

● 14. Bergamaschi R, Becouarn G, Ronceray J, Arnaud JP. Morbidity of thyroid surgery. *American Journal of Surgery* 1998; **176**: 71–5.

● 15. Rosato L, Avenia N, Bernante P *et al*. Complications of thyroid surgery: analysis of a multicentric study on 14934 patients operated on in Italy over 5 years. *World Journal of Surgery* 2004; **28**: 271–6.

♦ 16. Carty SE. Prevention and management of complications in parathyroid surgery. *Otolaryngologic Clinics of North America* 2004; **37**: 897–907.

♦ 17. Fewins J, Simpson B, Miller FR. Complications of thyroid and parathyroid surgery. *Otolaryngologic Clinics of North America* 2003; **36**: 189–206.

♦ 18. Zarnegar R, Brunaud L, Clark OH. Prevention, evaluation and management of complications following thyroidectomy for thyroid carcinoma. *Endocrinology and Metabolism Clinics of North America* 2003; **32**: 483–502.

● 19. Brunaud L, Zarnegar R, Wada N *et al*. Incision length for standard thyroidectomy and parathyroidectomy. When is it minimally invasive? *Archives of Surgery* 2003; **138**: 1140–3.

● 20. Bellantone R, Lombardi CP, Bossola M *et al*. Video-assisted vs conventional thyroid lobectomy – A randomized trial. *Archives of Surgery* 2002; **137**: 301–4.

● 21. Miccoli P, Berti P, Raffaelli M *et al*. Comparison between minimally invasive video-assisted thyroidectomy and conventional thyroidectomy: a prospective randomised study. *Surgery* 2001; **130**: 1039–43.

● 22. Lombardi CP, Raffaelli M, Princi P *et al*. Safety of video-assisted thyroidectomy versus conventional surgery. *Head and Neck* 2005; **27**: 58–64.

♦ 23. Gourin CG, Johnson JT. Postoperative complications. In: Randolph GW (ed.). *Surgery of the thyroid and parathyroid glands*. Philadelphia, PA: Saunders, 2003: 433–43.

● 24. Shaha AR, Jaffe BM. Selective use of drains in thyroid surgery. *Journal of Surgical Oncology* 1993; **52**: 241–3.

♦ 25. Harding J, Sebag F, Sierra M *et al*. Thyroid surgery: postoperative haematoma – prevention and treatment. *Langenbecks Archives of Surgery* 2006; **391**: 169–73.

♦ 26. Songun I, Kievit J, van de Velde CJH. Complication of thyroid surgery. In: Clark OH, Duh QY (eds). *Textbook of endocrine surgery*, 1st edn. Philadelphia, PA: WB Saunders, 1997: 167–74.

● 27. Carty SE, Roberts MM, Virij MA *et al*. Elevated serum parathormone level after concise parathyroidectomy for primary sporadic hyperparathyroidism. *Surgery* 2002; **132**: 1086–93.

● 28. Udelsman R. Six hundred and fifty-six consecutive explorations for primary hyperparathyroidism. *Annals of Surgery* 2002; **235**: 665–72.

● 29. Kern KA. Medical legal analysis in the diagnosis and treatment of surgical endocrine disease. *Surgery* 1993; **114**: 1167–74.

● 30. Hurtado-Lopez LM, Zaldivar-Ramirez FR, Basurto Kuba E *et al*. Causes for early re-intervention after thyroidectomy. *Medical Science Monitor* 2002; **8**: 247–50.

● 31. Shaha A, Jaffe B. Practical management of post-thyroidectomy haematoma. *Journal of Surgical Oncology* 1994; **57**: 235–8.

● 32. Burkey SH, van Heerden JA, Thompson GB *et al*. Reexploration for symptomatic haematomas after cervical exploration. *Surgery* 2001; **130**: 914–20.

33. Abbas G, Dubner S, Heller KS. Re-operation for bleeding after thyroidectomy and parathyroidectomy. *Head and Neck* 2001; **23**: 544-6.

34. Schwartz AE, Clark OH, Ituarte P. Thyroid surgery – the choice. *Journal of Clinical Endocrinology and Metabolism* 1998; **83**: 1097-105.

35. Palestini N, Tulletti V, Cestino L *et al.* Post-thyroidectomy cervical haematoma. *Minerva Chirurgica* 2005; **60**: 37-46.

36. Menegaux F, Turpin G, Dahman M *et al.* Secondary thyroidectomy in patients with prior thyroid surgery from benign disease: a study of 203 cases. *Surgery* 1999; **126**: 479-83.

37. Shaha A, Jaffe BM. Complications of thyroid surgery performed by residents. *Surgery* 1988; **104**: 1109-14.

38. Sywak MS, Yeh MW, Sidhu SB *et al.* New surgical consultants: is there a learning curve? *Australia and New Zealand Journal of Surgery* 2006; **76**: 1081-4.

39. Miccoli P, Berti P, Frustaci GL *et al.* Video-assisted thyroidectomy: indications and results. *Langenbecks Archives of Surgery* 2006; **391**: 68-71.

40. Lombardi CP, Raffaelli M, Princi P *et al.* Video-assisted thyroidectomy: report on the experience of a single center in more than four hundred cases. *World Journal of Surgery* 2006; **30**: 794-800.

41. Miccoli P, Berti P, Materazzi G *et al.* Results of video-assisted parathyroidectomy: single institution's six-year experience. *World Journal of Surgery* 2004; **28**: 1216-18.

42. Inabnet WB 3rd, Jacob BP, Gagner M. Minimally invasive endoscopic thyroidectomy by a cervical approach. *Surgical Endoscopy* 2003; **17**: 1808-11.

43. Farrar WB. Complications of thyroidectomy. *Surgical Clinics of North America* 1983; **63**: 1313-53.

44. Siperstein AE, Berber E, Morkoyun E. The use of the harmonic scalpel vs conventional knot tying for vessel ligation in thyroid surgery. *Archives of Surgery* 2002; **137**: 137-42.

45. Ortega J, Sala S, Flor B, Lledo S. Efficacy and cost-effectiveness of the Ultracision® harmonic scalpel in thyroid surgery: an analysis of 200 cases in a randomized trial. *Journal of Laparoendoscopic and Advanced Surgical Techniques* 2004; **14**: 9-12.

46. Cordon C, Fajardo R, Ramirez J, Herrera MF. A randomized, prospective, parallel group study comparing the harmonic scalpel to electrocautery in thyroidectomy. *Surgery* 2005; **137**: 337-41.

47. Petrakis I, Kogerakis NE, Lasithiotakis KG *et al.* Ligasure versus clamp-and-tie thyroidectomy for benign nodular disease. *Head and Neck* 2004; **26**: 903-9.

48. Franko J, Kish KJ, Pezzi CM *et al.* Safely increasing the efficiency of thyroidectomy using a new bipolar electrosealing device (Ligasure™) versus clamp-and-tie technique. *American Surgeon* 2006; **72**: 132-6.

49. Shen WT, Baumbusch MA, Kebebew E, Duh QY. Use of the electrothermal vessel sealing system versus standard vessel ligation in thyroidectomy. *Asian Journal of Surgery* 2005; **28**: 86-9.

50. Kiriakopoulos A, Dimitrios T, Dimitrios L. Use of a diathermy system in thyroid surgery. *Archives of Surgery* 2004; **139**: 997-1000.

51. Saint Marc O, Cogliandolo A, Piquard A *et al.* Ligasure vs clamp-and-tie technique to achieve the hemostasis in total thyroidectomy for benign multinodular goiter. *Archives of Surgery* 2007; **142**: 150-6.

52. Uwiera TC, Uwiera RRE, Seikaly H, Harris JR. Tisseel and its effect on wound drainage post-thyroidectomy: prospective, randomized, blinded, controlled study. *Journal of Otolaryngology* 2005; **34**: 374-8.

53. Defechereux T, Hamoir E, Nguyen D, Meurisse M. Drainage in thyroid surgery. Is it always a must? *Annales de Chirurgie* 1997; **51**: 647-52.

54. Khanna J, Mohil RS, Chintanami Bhatnagar D *et al.* Is the routine drainage after surgery for thyroid necessary? A prospective randomized clinical study. *BMC Surgery* 2005; **5**: 11.

55. Schoretsanitis G, Melissas J, Sanidas E *et al.* Does draining the neck affect morbidity following thyroid surgery? *American Surgeon* 1998; **64**: 778-80.

56. Agarwal A, Mishra SK. Post-thyroidectomy haemorrhage: an analysis of critical factors in successful management. *Journal of the Indian Medical Association* 1997; **95**: 418-19.

57. Friedman M, LoSavio P, Ibrahim H. Superior laryngeal nerve identification and preservation in thyroidectomy. *Archives of Otolaryngology, Head and Neck Surgery* 2002; **128**: 296-303.

58. Abelson TI, Tucker HM. Laryngeal findings in superior laryngeal nerve paralysis: a controversy. *Otolaryngology – Head and Neck Surgery* 1981; **89**: 463-70.

59. Bellantone R, Boscherini M, Lombardi CP *et al.* Is the identification of the external branch of the superior laryngeal nerve mandatory in thyroid operation? Results of a prospective randomised study. *Surgery* 2001; **130**: 1055-9.

60. Crookes PF, Recabaren JA. Injury to the superior laryngeal nerve branch of the vagus during thyroidectomy: lesson of myth? *Annals of Surgery* 2001; **233**: 588-93.

61. Cernea CR, Ferraz AR, Nishio S *et al.* Surgical anatomy of the external branch of the superior laryngeal nerve. *Head and Neck* 1992; **14**: 380-3.

62. Cernea CR, Ferraz AR, Furlani J *et al.* Identification of the external branch of the superior laryngeal nerve during thyroidectomy. *American Journal of Surgery* 1992; **164**: 634-9.

63. Eisele DW, Goldstone AC. Electrophysiologic identification and preservation of the superior laryngeal nerve during thyroid surgery. *Laryngoscope* 1991; **101**: 313-15.

64. Dackiw APB, Rotstein LE, Clark OH. Computer-assisted evoked electromyography with stimulating surgical instruments for recurrent/external laryngeal nerve

identification and preservation in thyroid and parathyroid operation. *Surgery* 2002; **132**: 1100–8.

● 65. Lombardi CP, Raffaelli M, D'Alatri L *et al.* Video-assisted thyroidectomy significantly reduces the risk of early postthyroidectomy voice and swallowing symptoms. *World Journal of Surgery* 2008; **32**: 693–700.

● 66. Lennquist S, Cahlin C, Smeds S. The superior laryngeal nerve in thyroid surgery. *Surgery* 1987; **102**: 999–1008.

● 67. Pereira JA, Girvent M, Sancho JJ *et al.* Prevalence of long-term upper aero-digestive symptoms after uncomplicated bilateral thyroidectomy. *Surgery* 2003; **133**: 318–22.

● 68. Stojadinovic A, Shaha AR, Orlikoff RF *et al.* Prospective functional voice assessment in patients undergoing thyroid surgery. *Annals of Surgery* 2002; **236**: 823–32.

● 69. Sinagra DL, Montesinos MR, Tacchi VA *et al.* Voice changes after thyroidectomy without recurrent laryngeal nerve injury. *Journal of the American College of Surgeons* 2004; **199**: 556–60.

● 70. Musholt TJ, Musholt PB, Garm J *et al.* Changes of the speaking and singing voice after thyroid or parathyroid surgery. *Surgery* 2006; **140**: 978–89.

● 71. Lombardi CP, Raffaelli M, D'Alatri L *et al.* Voice and swallowing changes after thyroidectomy in patients without inferior laryngeal nerve injuries. *Surgery* 2006; **140**: 1026–34.

● 72. Smith E, Verdolini K, Gray S *et al.* Effect of voice disorders on quality of life. *Journal of Medical Speech-Language Pathology* 1996; **4**: 223–44.

● 73. Smith E, Taylor M, Mendoza M *et al.* Spasmodic dysphonia and vocal cord paralysis: outcomes of voice problems on work-related functioning. *Journal of Voice* 1998; **12**: 223–32.

● 74. Ready AR, Barnes AD. Complications of thyroidectomy. *British Journal of Surgery* 1994; **81**: 1555–6.

● 75. Lo CY, Kwok KF, Yuen PO. A prospective evaluation of recurrent laryngeal nerve paralysis during thyroidectomy. *Archives of Surgery* 2000; **135**: 204–7.

● 76. Rosato L, Carlevato MT, De Toma G, Avenia N. Recurrent laryngeal nerve damage and phonetic modifications after total thyroidectomy: surgical malpractice only or predictable sequence? *World Journal of Surgery* 2005; **29**: 780–4.

● 77. Woodson GE. Pathophysiology of recurrent laryngeal nerve. In: Randolph GW (ed.). *Surgery of the thyroid and parathyroid glands.* Philadelphia, PA: Saunders, 2003: 366–73.

● 78. Hartl DM, Travagli JP, Leboulleux S *et al.* Current concepts in the management of unilateral recurrent laryngeal nerve paralysis after thyroid surgery. *Journal of Clinical Endocrinology and Metabolism* 2005; **90**: 3084–8.

● 79. Bou-Malhab F, Hans S, Perie S *et al.* Swallowing disorders in unilateral recurrent laryngeal nerve paralysis. *Annales d'Otolaryngologie et de Chirurgie Cervicofaciale* 2000; **117**: 26–33.

♦ 80. Randolph GW. Surgical anatomy of the recurrent laryngeal nerve. In: Randolph GW (ed.). *Surgery of the*

thyroid and parathyroid glands. Philadelphia, PA: Saunders, 2003: 300–42.

● 81. Lahey FH. Routine dissection and demonstration of the recurrent laryngeal nerve in subtotal thyroidectomy. *Surgery, Gynecology and Obstetrics* 1938; **66**: 775.

● 82. Affleck BD, Swartz K, Brennan J. Surgical considerations and controversies in thyroid and parathyroid surgery. *Otolaryngologic Clinics of North America* 2003; **36**: 159–87.

* 83. The American Thyroid Association Guidelines Taskforce. Management guidelines for patients with thyroid nodules and differentiated thyroid cancer. *Thyroid* 2006; **16**: 109–42.

● 84. Steurer M, Passler C, Denk D *et al.* Advantages of recurrent laryngeal nerve identification in thyroidectomy and parathyroidectomy and the importance of preoperative and postoperative laryngoscopic examination in more than 1000 nerves at risk. *Laryngoscope* 2002; **112**: 124–33.

● 85. Brauckhoff M, Walls G, Brauckhoff K. Identification of the non-recurrent inferior laryngeal nerve using intraoperative neurostimulation. *Langenbecks Archives of Surgery* 2002; **386**: 482–7.

● 86. Hermann M, Alk G, Roka R *et al.* Laryngeal recurrent nerve injury in surgery for benign thyroid diseases – Effect on nerve dissection and impact of individual surgeon in more than 27000 nerves at risk. *Annals of Surgery* 2002; **235**: 261–8.

● 87. Steinberg JL, Khane GJ, Fernandes CMC, Nel JP. Anatomy of the recurrent laryngeal nerve: a redescription. *Journal of Laryngology and Otology* 1986; **100**: 919–27.

♦ 88. Henry JF. Surgical anatomy and embryology of the thyroid and parathyroid glands and recurrent and external laryngeal nerves. In: Clark OH, Duh QY (eds). *Textbook of endocrine surgery.* Philadelphia, PA: Saunders, 1997: 8–14.

● 89. Sturniolo G, D'Alia C, Tonante A *et al.* The recurrent laryngeal nerve related to thyroid surgery. *American Journal of Surgery* 1999; **177**: 485–8.

● 90. Katz AD, Nemiroff P. Anastomoses and bifurcations of the recurrent laryngeal nerve: report of 1177 nerves visualized. *American Surgeon* 1993; **59**: 188–91.

♦ 91. Henry JF. Applied embryology of the thyroid and parathyroid glands. In: Randolph GW (ed.). *Surgery of the thyroid and parathyroid glands.* Philadelphia, PA: Saunders, 2003: 12–20.

● 92. Saudi RJ, Maranillo E, Léon X *et al.* An anatomic study of the anastomosis between laryngeal nerves. *Laryngoscope* 1999; **109**: 983–7.

● 93. Raffaelli M, Iacobone M, Henry JF. The false nonrecurrent inferior laryngeal nerve. *Surgery* 2000; **128**: 1082–7.

● 94. Proye CAG, Carnaille BM, Goropoulos A. Nonrecurrent and recurrent inferior laryngeal nerve: a surgical pitfall in cervical exploration. *American Journal of Surgery* 1991; **162**: 495–6.

95. Procacciante F, Picozzi P, Pacifici M et al. Palpatory method used to identify the recurrent laryngeal nerve during thyroidectomy. World Journal of Surgery 2000; 24: 571–3.

96. Lore JM Jr, Farrell M, Castillo NB. Endocrine surgery. In: Lore JM Jr, Medica JE (eds). An atlas of head and neck surgery, 4th edn. Philadelphia, PA: Elsevier, 2005: 963–5.

97. Delbridge L. Total thyroidectomy: the evolution of the surgical technique. Australia and New Zealand Journal of Surgery 2003; 73: 761–8.

98. Pelizzo MR, Toniato A, Gemo G. Zuckerkandl's tuberculum: an arrow pointing to the recurrent laryngeal nerve (constant anatomical landmark). Journal of the American College of Surgeons 1998; 187: 333–6.

99. Marescaux J. Thyroïde. In: Proye C, Dubost C (eds). Endocrinologie chirurgicale. Paris: McGraw-Hill, 1992: 13–54.

100. Wheeler MH. Thyroid surgery and the recurrent laryngeal nerve. British Journal of Surgery 1999; 86: 291–2.

101. Dralle H, Sekulla K, Haerting J et al. Risk factors of paralysis and functional outcome after recurrent laryngeal nerve monitoring in thyroid surgery. Surgery 2004; 136: 1310–22.

102. Flisberg K, Lindholm T. Electrical stimulation of the human recurrent laryngeal nerve during thyroid operation. Acta Otolaryngologica 1969; 263: 63–7.

103. Kratz RC. The identification and protection of the laryngeal motor nerves during thyroid and laryngeal surgery: a new microsurgical technique. Laryngoscope 1973; 83: 59–78.

104. Eltzschig HK, Posner M, Moore FD. The use of readily available equipment in a simple method for intraoperative monitoring of recurrent laryngeal nerve function during thyroid surgery. Archives of Surgery 2002; 137: 452–7.

105. Hvidegard T, Vase P, Jorgensen K, Blichert-Toft M. Identification and functional recording of the recurrent laryngeal nerve by electrical stimulation during neck surgery. Laryngoscope 1983; 93: 370–3.

106. Davis WE, Rea JL, Templer J. Recurrent laryngeal nerve localization using a microlaryngeal electrode. Otolaryngology – Head and Neck Surgery 1979; 87: 330–3.

107. Rice DH, Cone-Wesson B. Intraoperative recurrent laryngeal nerve monitoring. Otolaryngology, Head and Neck Surgery 1991; 105: 372–5.

108. Brauckhoff M, Walls G, Brauckhoff K et al. Identification of the non-recurrent inferior laryngeal nerve using intraoperative neurostimulation. Langenbecks Archives of Surgery 2002; 386: 482–7.

109. Thomusch O, Sekulla C, Walls G et al. Intraoperative neuromonitoring for benign goiter. American Journal of Surgery 2002; 183: 673–8.

110. Petro ML, Schweinfurth JM, Petro AB. Transcrithyroid intraoperative monitoring of the vagus nerve. Archives of Otolaryngology, Head and Neck Surgery 2006; 132: 624–8.

111. Rea LJ. Postcricoid surface laryngeal electrode. Ear, Nose and Throat 1992; 71: 267–9.

112. Rea JL, Khan A. Clinical evoked electromyography for recurrent laryngeal nerve preservation: use of an endotracheal tube electrode and a postcricoid surface electrode. Laryngoscope 1998; 108: 1418–20.

113. Chan WF, Lang BHH, Lo CY. The role of intraoperative neuromonitoring of recurrent laryngeal nerve during thyroidectomy: a comparative study of 1000 nerves at risk. Surgery 2006; 140: 866–73.

114. Yarbrough DE, Thompson GB, Kasperbauer JL et al. Intraoperative electromyographic monitoring of the recurrent laryngeal nerve in reoperative thyroid and parathyroid surgery. Surgery 2004; 136: 1107–15.

115. Wang LF, Lee KW, Kuo WR et al. The efficacy of intraoperative corticosteroids in recurrent laryngeal nerve palsy after thyroid surgery. World Journal of Surgery 2006; 30: 299–303.

116. Lee KJ, Fee WE, Terris DJ. The efficacy of corticosteroids in postparotidectomy facial nerve paresis. Laryngoscope 2002; 112: 1958–63.

117. Crumley RL. Laryngeal synkinesis and its significance to the laryngologist. Annals of Otology, Rhinology, and Laryngology 1989; 98: 87–92.

118. Crumley RL. Recurrent laryngeal nerve paralysis. Journal of Voice 1994; 8: 79–83.

119. McCulloch TM, Hoffman HT, Andrews BT, Karnell MP. Arytenoid adduction combined with Gore-Tex medialization thyroplasty. Laryngoscope 2000; 110: 1306–11.

120. Hong KH, Kim YK. Phonatory characteristics of patients undergoing thyroidectomy without laryngeal nerve injury. Otolaryngology – Head and Neck Surgery 1997; 117: 399–404.

121. Debruyne F, Ostyn F, Delaere P, Wellens W. Acoustic analysis of the speaking voice after thyroidectomy. Journal of Voice 1997; 11: 479–82.

122. McIvor NP, Flint DJ, Gillibrand J, Morton RP. Thyroid surgery and voice-related outcomes. Australia and New Zealand Journal of Surgery 2000; 70: 179–83.

123. Demeester-Mirkine N, Hooghe L, Van Geertruyden J, De Maertelaer V. Hypocalcemia after thyroidectomy. Archives of Surgery 1992; 127: 854–8.

124. Wilkin TJ, Paterson CR, Isles TE et al. Post-thyroidectomy hypocalcaemia: a feature of the operation or the thyroid disorder. Lancet 1977; 1: 621.

125. Michie W, Duncan T, Hamer-Hogdges DW et al. Mechanism of hypocalcemia after thyroidectomy for thyrotoxicosis. Lancet 1971; 1: 508–14.

126. Percival RC, Hargreaves AW, Kanis JA. The mechanism of hypocalcemia following thyroidectomy. Acta Endocrinologica 1985; 109: 220–6.

● 127. McHenry CR, Speroff T, Wentworth D, Murphy T. Risk factors for post-thyroidectomy hypocalcemia. *Surgery* 1994; **116**: 641–7.

● 128. See AC, Soo KC. Hypocalcemia following thyroidectomy for thyrotoxicosis. *British Journal of Surgery* 1997; **84**: 95–7.

∗ 129. Akerstrom G, Malmaeus J, Bergstrom R. Surgical anatomy of human parathyroid glands. *Surgery* 1984; **95**: 14–21.

∗ 130. Halsted WS, Evans HM. The parathyroid glandules, their blood supply and their preservation in operation upon the thyroid gland. *Annals of Surgery* 1907; **46**: 489.

● 131. Delattre JF, Flament JB, Palot JP, Pluot M. [Variations in the parathyroid glands. Number, situation and arterial vascularization. Anatomical study and surgical application]. *Journal de Chirurgie* 1982; **119**: 633–41.

♦ 132. Herrera MF, Gamboa-Dominguez A. Parathyroid embryology, anatomy and pathology. In: Clark OH, Duh QY (eds). *Textbook of endocrine surgery.* Philadelphia, PA: Saunders, 1997: 277–83.

● 133. Lin DT, Patel SG, Shaha AR et al. Incidence of inadvertent parathyroid removal during thyroidectomy. *Laryngoscope* 2002; **112**: 608–11.

● 134. Burnett HF, Mabry CD, Westbrook KC. Hypocalcemia after thyroidectomy: mechanism and management. *Southern Medical Journal* 1977; **70**: 1045–8.

● 135. Chamberlin JA, Fries JG, Allen HC. Thyroid carcinoma and the problem of potoperative tetany. *Surgery* 1964; **55**: 787–95.

● 136. Attie JN, Khafif RA. Preservation of parathyroid glands during thyroidectomy. *American Journal of Surgery* 1975; **130**: 399–404.

● 137. Palazzo FF, Sywak MS, Sidhu SB et al. Parathyroid autotransplantation during total thyroidectomy – Does the number of glands transplantated affect outcome? *World Journal of Surgery* 2005; **29**: 629–31.

● 138. Sippel RS, Ozgul O, Hartig GK et al. Risks and consequences of incidental parathyroidectomy during thyroid resection. *Australia and New Zealand Journal of Surgery* 2007; **77**: 33–6.

● 139. Lee NJ, Blakey JD, Bhuta S, Calcaterra TC. Unintentional parathyroidectomy during thyroidectomy. *Laryngoscope* 1999; **109**: 1238–40.

● 140. Sasson AR, Pingpank JFJr, Wetherington RW et al. Incidental parathyroidectomy during thyroid surgery does not cause transient symptomatic hypocalcemia. *Archives of Otolaryngology, Head and Neck Surgery* 2001; **127**: 304–8.

● 141. Bruining HA, van Houten H, Juttmann JR et al. Results of operative treatment of 615 patients with primary hyperparathyroidism. *World Journal of Surgery* 1981; **5**: 85–90.

∗ 142. Thompson NW, Eckhauser FE, Harness JK. The anatomy of primary hyperparathyroidism. *Surgery* 1982; **92**: 814–21.

● 143. Bruining HA, Birkenhager JC, Ong GL, Lamberts SW. Causes of failure in operations for hyperparathyroidism. *Surgery* 1987; **101**: 562–5.

● 144. Akerstrom G, Rudberg C, Grimelius L et al. Causes of failed primary exploration and technical aspect of re-operation in primary hyperparathyroidism. *World Journal of Surgery* 1992; **16**: 562–8.

● 145. Proye C, Carnaille B, Maynou C et al. Le risque parathyroidien en chirurgie thyroidienne. *Chirurgie* 1990; **116**: 493–500.

● 146. Kuhel WI, Carew JF. Parathyroid biopsy to facilitate the preservation of functional parathyroid tissue during thyroidectomy. *Head and Neck* 1999; **21**: 442–6.

● 147. Shaha AR, Burnett C, Jaffe BM. Parathyroid autotransplantation during thyroid surgery. *Journal of Surgical Oncology* 1991; **46**: 21–4.

● 148. Nies C, Sitter H, Zielke A et al. Parathyroid function following ligation of the inferior thyroid arteries during bilateral subtotal thyroidectomy. *British Journal of Surgery* 1994; **81**: 1757–9.

● 149. Hermann M, Hellebart C, Freissmuth M. Neuromonitoring in thyroid surgery. Prospective evaluation of intraoperative electrophysiological responses for prediction of recurrent laryngeal nerve injury. *Annals of Surgery* 2004; **240**: 9–17.

● 150. Henry JF, Gramatica L, Denizot A et al. Morbidity of prophylactic lymph node dissection in the central neck area in patients with papillary thyroid carcinoma. *Langenbecks Archives of Surgery* 1998; **383**: 167–9.

● 151. Ander S, Johansson K, Smeds S. *In situ* preservation of the parathyroid glands during operations on the thyroid. *European Journal of Surgery* 1997; **163**: 33–7.

♦ 152. Lo CY. Parathyroid autotransplantation during thyroidectomy. *Australia and New Zealand Journal of Surgery* 2002; **72**: 902–7.

∗ 153. Wells SA Jr, Gunnells JC, Shelburne JD et al. Transplantation of the parathyroid glands in man: clinical indications and results. *Surgery* 1975; **78**: 34–44.

● 154. Zedenius J, Wadstrom C, Delbridge L. Routine autotransplantation of at least one parathyroid gland during total thyroidectomy may reduce permanent hypoparathyroidism to zero. *Australia and New Zealand Journal of Surgery* 1999; **69**: 794–7.

● 155. Funahashi H, Satoh Y, Imai T et al. Our technique of parathyroid autotransplantation in operation for papillary thyroid carcinoma. *Surgery* 1993; **114**: 92–6.

● 156. Olson JA, DeBenedetti MK, Baumann DS, Wells SA. Parathyroid autotransplantation during thyroidectomy – Results of long-term follow-up. *Annals of Surgery* 1996; **223**: 472–80.

● 157. Carty SE, Worsey J, Virji MA et al. Concise prathyroidectomy: the impact of preoperative SPECT 99mTc sestaMIBI scanning and intraoperative quick parathormone assay. *Surgery* 1997; **122**: 1107–16.

● 158. Bergenfelz A, Lindblom P, Tibblin S, Westerdahl J. Unilateral versus bilateral neck exploration for primary hyperparathyroidism. *Annals of Surgery* 2002; **236**: 543–51.

159. Miura D, Wada N, Arici C *et al*. Does intraoperative quick parathyroid hormone assay improve the results of parathyroidectomy? *World Journal of Surgery* 2002; **26**: 926–30.

160. Monchik JM, Barellini L, Langer P, Kahya A. Minimally invasive parathyroid surgery in 103 patients with local/regional anaesthesia, without exclusion criteria. *Surgery* 2002; **131**: 502–8.

161. Pattou F, Combemale F, Fabre S *et al*. Hypocalcemia following thyroid surgery: incidence and prediction of outcome. *World Journal of Surgery* 1998; **22**: 718–24.

162. Adams J, Andersen P, Everts E, Cohen J. Early postoperative calcium levels as predictors of hypocalcemia. *Laryngoscope* 1998; **108**: 1829–31.

163. Husein M, Hier MP, Al-Abdulhadi K, Black M. Predicting calcium status post thyroidectomy with early calcium levels. *Otolaryngology – Head and Neck Surgery* 2002; **127**: 289–93.

164. Lombardi CP, Raffaelli M, Princi P *et al*. Early prediction of postthyroidectomy hypocalcemia by one single iPTH measurement. *Surgery* 2004; **136**: 1236–41.

165. Lombardi CP, Raffaelli M, Princi P *et al*. Parathyroid hormone levels 4 hours after surgery do not accurately predict post-thyroidectomy hypocalcemia. *Surgery* 2006; **140**: 1016–25.

166. Bellantone R, Lombardi CP, Raffaelli M *et al*. Is routine supplementation therapy (calcium and vitamin D) useful after total thyroidectomy? *Surgery* 2002; **132**: 1109–13.

167. Sosa JA, Powe NR, Levine MA *et al*. Thresholds for surgery and surgical outcomes for patients with primary hyperparathyroidism: a national survey of endocrine surgeons. *Journal of Clinical Endocrinology and Metabolism* 1998; **83**: 2658–65.

168. Shen W, Duren M, Morita E *et al*. Reoperation for persistent or recurrent primary hyperparaythyroidism. *Archives of Surgery* 1996; **131**: 861–7.

169. Doherty GM, Weber B, Norton JA. Cost of unsuccessful surgery for primary hyperparathyroidism. *Surgery* 1994; **116**: 954–8.

170. Malmaeus J, Granberg PO, Halvorsen J *et al*. Parathyroid surgery in Scandinavia. *Acta Chirurgica Scandinavica* 1988; **154**: 409–13.

171. Lee PC, Mateo RB, Clarke MR *et al*. Parathyromatosis: a cause for recurrent hyperparathyroidism. *World Journal of Surgery* 1991; **15**: 716–23.

172. Burkey SH, van Heerden JA, Farley DR *et al*. Will directed parathyroidectomy utilizing the gamma probe or intraoperative parathyroid hormone assay replace bilateral cervical exploration as the preferred operation for primary hyperparathyroidism? *World Journal of Surgery* 2002; **26**: 914–20.

173. Boggs JE, Irvin GL 3rd, Molinari AS, Deriso GT. Intraoperative parathyroid hormone monitoring as an adjunct to parathyroidectomy. *Surgery* 1996; **120**: 954–8.

174. Carneiro DM, Solorzano CC, Nader MC *et al*. Comparison of intraoperative iPTH assay (QPTH) criteria in guiding parathyroidectomy: which criterion is the most accurate? *Surgery* 2003; **134**: 973–9; discussion 9–81.

175. Di Stasio E, Carrozza C, Lombardi CP *et al*. Parathyroidectomy monitored by intra-operative PTH: the relevance of the 20 minutes end-point. *Clinical Biochemistry* 2007; **40**: 595–603.

176. Sancho JJ, Sitges-Serra A. Surgical approach to secondary hyperparathyroidism. In: Clark OH, Duh QY (eds). *Textbook of endocrine surgery*. Philadelphia, PA: WB Saunders, 1997: 403–9.

177. Akerstrom G, Juhlin C. Surgical management of multiglandular parathyroid diseases. In: Randolph GW (ed.). *Surgery of the thyroid and parathyroid glands*. Philadelphia, PA: Saunders, 2003: 529–48.

26

Non-surgical management of thyroid cancer

LAURA MOSS

Absence of evidence is not evidence of absence.

Carl Sagan, US astronomer (1934–96)

DIFFERENTIATED THYROID CANCER

There is a lack of prospective randomized controlled studies relating to the management of differentiated thyroid cancer as it is an uncommon disease with a long natural history. Many areas of thyroid cancer management remain controversial, including the indications for radioiodine ablation, the administered activity of radioiodine, timing and type of follow-up investigations, the degree and duration of thyroid-stimulating hormone (TSH) suppression, as well as indications and techniques for external beam radiotherapy. Evidence-based guidelines rely largely on retrospective and cohort studies, as well as consensus views. The recommendations in this chapter reflect common UK practice and advice from the British Thyroid Association, European Thyroid Association, the European Association of Nuclear Medicine and American Thyroid Association (ATA) guidelines.[1, 2, 3, 4]

^{131}I therapy

Normal thyroid gland tissue and differentiated thyroid cancer can concentrate iodine from the circulation and ^{131}I (an unsealed radionuclide of iodine) is taken up in the same way as stable iodine in the diet.

In practice, it is very difficult to achieve complete surgical ablation of the thyroid gland and some residual tissue is inevitably present and known as the thyroid remnant. As a rule, normal thyroid tissue within the remnant will preferentially take up the iodine compared to thyroid cancer tissue whether that is local or distant. Hence, if a large remnant is present postoperatively, the post-ablation full body radioiodine scan cannot be relied upon to exclude the presence of residual malignancy either locally in the neck or at distant sites as the iodine may be seen in the remnant only. Only when this remnant of normal thyroid tissue is ablated can you reliably expect to see any significant radioiodine uptake in sites of differentiated thyroid cancer.

INDICATIONS FOR ^{131}I

^{131}I aids the detection and earlier treatment of persistent/metastatic disease by destroying normal thyroid tissue; it may destroy microscopic foci of cancer in the thyroid remnant, and aids interpretation of serum thyroglobulin (Tg) measurements during follow up. It may be used for ablation of the thyroid remnant, or for treatment of residual or recurrent disease. Remnant ablation may reduce local recurrence and increase survival,[5, 6] although not all reported series support these findings.[7, 8, 9, 10]

In the absence of published randomized trials, recommendations on ^{131}I ablation have to be based on retrospective studies.[2, 11, 12, 13, 14, 15, 16, 17]

Postoperative radioactive iodine remnant ablation

This can be defined as the radioiodine uptake that is usually seen in the thyroid bed following a total or near total thyroidectomy. [131]I destruction of this residual tissue is called radioiodine remnant ablation.[1]

The following represents the British Thyroid Association's guidance on the indications for ^{131}I ablation.[1] It should be noted, however, that the recommendations for radioiodine remnant ablation vary slightly between the European, American and British guidelines.

- No indication for ^{131}I ablation (as low risk of recurrence or cancer-specific mortality):
  - complete surgery;
  - favourable histology;
  - unifocal tumour, ≤ 1 cm, N0 M0 or minimally invasive follicular thyroid carcinoma (FTC), without vascular invasion < 2 cm;
  - no extension beyond the thyroid capsule.
- Definite indications for radioiodine remnant ablation:
  - distant metastases;
  - incomplete resection;
  - tumour extension beyond capsule, > 10 involved lymph nodes, > 3 lymph nodes with extracapsular spread.
- Probable indications for radioiodine remnant ablation:
  - less than total thyroidectomy;
  - lymph node status not assessed at surgery;
  - tumour > 1 cm and < 4 cm;
  - < 1 cm with unfavourable histology (tall cell, columnar, diffuse sclerosing papillary thyroid carcinoma (PTC), widely invasive or poorly differentiated follicular thyroid cancers);
  - multifocal tumours < 1 cm.

Radioiodine therapy

This refers to administration of ^{131}I with the intention to treat recurrent or metastatic disease[1] and is indicated:

- if the primary tumour is inoperable;
- for postoperative residual neck disease;
- for distant metastases;
- for recurrent disease.

High versus low administered activity of [131]I

Administered activities of ^{131}I between 1.1 and 3.7 GBq show similar rates of successful remnant ablation,[18, 19, 20, 21] although there is a trend toward higher success rates with higher administered activities.

The American Thyroid Association[4] recommends that the minimum ^{131}I activity necessary to achieve successful remnant ablation should be chosen.

A recent systematic review has concluded that it is not possible to reliably determine whether ablation success rates using 1.1 GBq are similar to using 3.7 GBq and advocates large randomized trials to resolve the issue and guide clinical practice.[22]

In the UK in 2006, a multicentre randomized trial of high 'dose' versus low 'dose' radioiodine, with or without recombinant human thyroid-stimulating hormone, for thyroid remnant ablation following surgery for differentiated thyroid cancer was launched (HiLo Trial). The two aims are to (1) determine whether low-'dose' radioactive iodine (RAI) (1.1 GBq) is as effective as the standard 'high' dose (3.7 GBq) in ablating any remaining thyroid tissue after surgery and (2) determine whether patients given recombinant human TSH have a similar ablation success rate to those undergoing thyroid hormone withdrawal. Recruitment to this trial closed in 2010. Preliminary results suggest equivalent outcomes for all arms of the study and the final results are expected to be published in 2011.

[131]I administration procedure

Those prescribing radionuclide therapies in the UK must hold an appropriate Administration of Radioactive Substances Advisory Committee (ARSAC) certificate and the treatment must be given in appropriately designed areas.

Radioiodine is administered orally. Although it is available in liquid or capsule formulations, the latter is the preferred format as it is easier and safer to handle.

For successful remnant ablation to be achieved, the TSH level prior to the isotope administration must be elevated to > 25–30 mU/L in order to facilitate uptake of ^{131}I by thyroid tissue. If ^{131}I ablation can be performed approximately 4 weeks after surgery, there is no need for thyroid hormone supplementation to be commenced in the immediate postoperative period. If this is not possible, tri-iodothyronine (T3) 20 µg three times a day should be started postoperatively and then this is withdrawn 14 days before radioiodine use to allow sufficient time for the necessary rise in TSH. Elevated TSH level stimulates the sodium iodide symporter (membrane protein involved in active transport) and hence radioiodine uptake into thyrocytes. An alternative method is to administer recombinant human TSH (rhTSH, Thyrogen[TM]) as an exogenous source of TSH and allow the patient to continue with thyroid hormones throughout the radioisotope treatment period. The benefit with using rhTSH is the avoidance of potential significant physical and psychological symptoms of hypothyroidism resulting from thyroid hormone withdrawal.[23, 24]

If the patient is already established on thyroxine they will either need to discontinue this for 4 weeks or preferably commence T3 instead at 20 µg three times a day for 14 days and then discontinue this for a further 14 days prior to radioiodine. By swapping the thyroid hormones in this way, it is possible to reduce the length of time that the patient is rendered hypothyroid.

The decision whether a patient should receive ^{131}I remnant ablation after thyroid hormone withdrawal (THW) or after rhTSH injections depends on the current licensed indications of use, the patient's comorbidities and cost.

The current licensed indications for use are: (1) for pre-therapeutic stimulation in combination with radioactive iodine for ablation of thyroid tissue remnants in patients who have undergone a near total or total thyroidectomy for well-differentiated thyroid cancer and who do not have evidence of distant metastatic thyroid cancer; (2) for use with serum thyroglobulin testing with or without radioiodine imaging for the detection of thyroid remnants and well-differentiated thyroid cancer in post-thyroidectomy patients maintained on hormone suppression therapy; (3) for the follow-up assessment of patients with well-differentiated thyroid carcinoma who have undetectable serum Tg levels on hormone suppression therapy.

Patient factors that would warrant rhTSH use in preference to THW include hypopituitarism, functional metastases causing TSH suppression, severe ischaemic heart disease, previous history of psychiatric disturbance precipitated by hypothyroidism, advanced disease or frailty.

rhTSH injections (0.9 mg) are given by deep i.m. injection into the buttock on days 1 and 2 with radioiodine being administered on day 3. Thyroglobulin is measured on day 5 when it reaches its maximal response.

Possible side effects include flu-like myalgia, mild nausea and headache. There is also the possibility of stimulating thyroid remnant tissue and metastases resulting in local symptoms, and consideration should be given to prophylactic corticosteroids before use if residual neck disease or metastases are known to be present.

For diagnostic ^{131}I imaging, the method of TSH stimulation influences the optimal timing for the scan. If the patient has undergone THW the interval between administering the ^{131}I and scanning is usually 72 hours compared to 48 hours if the stimulation is provided by rhTSH

Serum Tg should be measured immediately prior to ^{131}I administration if THW preparation is undertaken or on day 5 if rhTSH is used.

The usual administered activity of ^{131}I used for remnant ablation is 3.7 GBq. However, the optimal administered activity is unknown as there are conflicting data between high and low ablation activities.[19, 25]

The administered activities of ^{131}I for therapy purposes are usually in the range 5.5–7.4 GBq. Whole body radioiodine scans are performed 2–10 days after giving radioiodine for ablation or therapy to determine the sites of radioiodine uptake and are more sensitive than diagnostic whole body scans due to the higher administered activity of radiation used.[26] The timing of the scan will depend on the administered activity of ^{131}I, the method of patient preparation (rhTSH versus thyroid hormone withdrawal) and the clinician's choice of the residual activity at which to image the patient.

Physiological ^{131}I uptake is seen in salivary tissue, genitourinary tract, gastrointestinal tract and sinuses.

Hürthle cell lesions are generally poorly responsive to radioiodine treatment and in particular distant metastases are often resistant to radioiodine therapy.

A preablation radioisotope scan is not routinely indicated, but it may be used to demonstrate the size of thyroid remnant. If a large remnant is seen, consideration of further surgery may be warranted. If further surgery is not appropriate it may influence the activity of radioiodine that is administered and prompt the prescription of premedication with corticosteroids prior to RAI to limit radiation thyroiditis symptoms.

If a preablation scan is performed, a low administered activity of ^{99m}Tc pertechnate or ^{123}I are preferred to ^{131}I as they reduce the risk of stunning.[27, 28] Stunning is the reduction in uptake of the ^{131}I therapy dose as a result of the pretreatment diagnostic dose.

Thyroid hormones are started 2–3 days after radioiodine administration if the patient has been withdrawn from hormones. If the patient has been given rhTSH, they can stay on thyroxine throughout the procedure.

Prior to radioiodine administration, the total body iodine pool should be reduced. A low daily intake of iodine can increase the effective radiation dose achieved with ^{131}I in the regions of interest.[29, 30, 31, 32] There is little consensus on the degree and the duration of dietary restriction required with each consensus guideline giving different advice, e.g. duration of the diet varies between 1 and 4 weeks with many centres using a 2-week period of restriction.[1]

Other sources of excess iodine should be eliminated before proceeding with ^{131}I administration, e.g. iodinated i.v. contrast and amiodarone.

^{131}I toxicity

- Neck discomfort and swelling due to an inflammatory response in the remnant, residual tumour or involved cervical lymph nodes. This is most likely to be seen when there is a large thyroid remnant present. If the swelling is significant or painful, corticosteroids can be helpful. If the patient has only had a debulking procedure and gross residual thyroid tissue is present, prophylactic corticosteroids are advisable to minimize the pain and swelling associated with the inflammatory response and can be started just prior to RAI administration.
- Altered sense of taste, nausea (vomiting is uncommon and prophylactic antiemetics are not routinely used).
- Sialadenitis arises due to physiological uptake of ^{131}I and subsequent excretion from salivary tissue. This can be reduced by encouraging patients to drink liberal quantities of fluids and possibly by encouraging salivary flow using sialogogues, such as lemon juice or sweets commencing 24 hours after ^{131}I administration.[33] In the long term, it is possible for tender parotid swelling to develop.
- Lacrimal gland dysfunction.
- Radiation cystitis. The risk may be reduced by maintaining a high fluid intake following radioiodine administration and during the isolation period.
- Gastritis.
- Bleeding/oedema in metastases.
- Bone marrow suppression. This reaches its peak 4–6 weeks after treatment. It is more likely in those patients who have extensive skeletal metastases or who have received prior external beam radiotherapy or chemotherapy.
- Gonadal tissue is exposed to radiation from radioiodine in the blood, urine and faeces.
  - **Male fertility**: a temporary rise in follicle-stimulating hormone (FSH) and a reduction in sperm count may be seen. High cumulative doses, e.g. >14 GBq may reduce fertility and consideration should be given to sperm storage in high-risk cases where multiple therapeutic doses of ^{131}I are expected.[34]
  - **Female fertility**: no significant difference in fertility rate, birth weights or prematurity rates. Temporary alterations in the menstrual cycle may last between four and ten months in about a quarter of female patients. Increased risk of miscarriage may

persist for up to one year following ^{131}I ablation/ therapy.[1,35,36,37,38,39] The risk of impaired fertility may be reduced by maintaining a high fluid intake following radioiodine administration and for the duration of the isolation period. This is in order to dilute the urine and therefore reduce concentration of radioactive iodine in the bladder and hence exposure of gonadal tissues.

- If the patient has undergone thyroid hormone withdrawal, constipation is a common symptom of the hypothyroid state and therefore the use of laxatives may also help in reducing the gonadal tissue exposure.
- If miliary pulmonary metastases are present, the patient may be at risk of developing pulmonary fibrosis especially if a high cumulative activity of radioiodine is administered. Consideration of pulmonary function test monitoring and corticosteroids immediately before and during treatment may reduce this risk. The data available are, however, fairly limited.[40,41,42]
- An increased risk of leukaemia and second cancers in organs that concentrate [131]I (salivary gland, breast, bladder, colon) is seen with the risk being highest with high cumulative activities of radioiodine, i.e. greater than 18.5 GBq, and after external beam radiotherapy.[1] The risk of leukaemia is lower than reported in earlier series due to deliberate attempts to limit the total body dose and to increase the interval between radioiodine administrations, whereas the risk of second solid malignancy might be higher than previously thought. Rubino et al.[43] have reported a 27 per cent increase in overall risk of second malignancy with an absolute excess risk of 14.4 per cent for solid tumours and 0.8 per cent for leukaemias, whereas Sandeep et al.[44] reported a 30 per cent risk of second primary cancer in patients with a history of thyroid cancer.
- Good hydration, frequent micturition and regular bowel activity will help reduce the level of whole body radiation.

Consideration should be given to the use of high-dose corticosteroids before radioiodine if there is bulky neck disease or metastatic disease.

Radiation protection issues

Before the administration of ^{131}I, pregnancy and lactation must be excluded. Following the administration of ^{131}I, pregnancy/conception must be avoided for six months.[45]

During the patient's stay in the isolation room, visiting of family and friends must be restricted to non-pregnant adults. They must not directly enter the patient's room, but must stay in a designated area outside the room and communication is often facilitated by an intercom system.

The patient's clothing must be washed separately on their return home, unless it is heavily soiled, when storage on the hospital site or disposal may be needed. The method of transport home may be determined by the patient's residual activity. For example, short distance travel in a private family vehicle, unoccupied by children, may allow discharge home with a higher residual activity than a longer journey via public transport where exposure to other members of the public, particularly children, may occur. Once at home, the patient must double flush the toilet; use separate cutlery and crockery, sleep alone, and restrict the time and extend the distance with their contacts. The duration of the restrictions is individualized for each patient and are longer for prolonged and close contact with children and pregnant women than they are with non-pregnant adults. Timing of a patient's return to work will depend on the type of work undertaken, the work environment and the surrounding work personnel involved.

TSH level

Following total thyroidectomy, thyroxine is required to both replace thyroid hormones no longer produced endogenously, as well as to suppress TSH levels.

The initial aim is to use a thyroxine dose sufficient to suppress TSH to between <0.1 mU/L (in high-risk cases) and 0.5 mU/L (in low-risk cases). The dosage tends therefore to be larger than that used for replacement purposes following thyroidectomy for a benign aetiology.[1,46,47,48,49,50]

Thyroxine in these larger doses prevents the pituitary from being stimulated to produce TSH and hence prevents stimulation of any remaining thyroid tissue, whether it is normal or malignant, with the intention of reducing the risk of recurrence, tumour progression and death.

The degree of suppression has not been tested in prospective studies and, due to concerns regarding the effects of prolonged supraphysiological thyroxine doses in low-risk cases, there has been recent interest in trying to relax the degree of TSH suppression in low-risk cases, aiming for a TSH within the lower part of the normal range.[51,52] The European consensus statement from 2006 advocates that low-risk patients, once they have achieved apparent remission, can immediately have their dose of thyroxine reduced to achieve a serum TSH within the lower part of the normal range (0.5–1.0 mU/L), whereas high-risk patients should continue with full TSH suppression (<0.1 mU/L) for between three and five years. The American Thyroid Association[52] recommends the initial TSH suppression to be kept below 0.1 mU/L for high-risk and intermediate-risk thyroid cancer patients, while maintenance of the TSH at or slightly below the lower limit of normal (0.1–0.5 mU/L) is appropriate for low-risk patients. Similar recommendations apply to low-risk patients who have not undergone remnant ablation, i.e. serum TSH 0.1–0.5 mU/L.

When TSH is being suppressed, the free T4 (FT4) level is often seen to be above the upper limit of the normal range. Nevertheless, such moderate elevation does not commonly result in symptoms or signs of thyrotoxicosis.

The average dose of thyroxine required is in the range 150–200 µg with the dose varying depending on the patient's age and weight.

Thyroxine is taken once daily, in the morning on an empty stomach. A number of medications can interfere with the absorption of thyroxine, so it is advisable to leave a 2-hour gap between taking thyroxine and other medications, such as calcium supplements, antacids and iron.

Thyroglobulin

Thyroglobulin is a glycosylated protein, which is a key substrate for biosynthesis and storage of thyroid hormones. It is secreted by normal and cancerous thyroid cells and its release is TSH-dependent. The diagnostic sensitivity of Tg is increased when the TSH level is elevated (ideally TSH above 30 mIU/L).[1, 53, 54] The Tg level may be undetectable in 20 per cent of cases in the presence of isolated lymph node metastases if it is measured while the patient is on TSH suppression therapy.

The serum Tg level is more sensitive than ^{131}I whole body scan (WBS) in detecting recurrent or metastatic disease.

Thyroglobulin autoantibodies interfere with the ability to accurately measure and follow Tg trends. The prevalence of thyroglobulin antibodies is higher in patients with differentiated thyroid cancer (DTC) than in the general population (up to 25 per cent versus 10 per cent).[55] There is some evidence that measuring TgAb levels and trends may be of some value in monitoring patients with thyroid cancer if the Tg cannot be relied upon in the presence of the autoantibodies,[1, 55, 56] e.g. a rising trend in TgAb levels may indicate disease relapse in a patient.[57]

In order to interpret the serum Tg level, it is necessary to know the TSH level and Tg antibody level.

Serum Tg is not useful as a diagnostic test preoperatively because thyroglobulin is a product of normal thyroid tissue and can be markedly elevated by inflammatory thyroid diseases. It is therefore not specifically a serum tumour marker; however, if elevated in a patient who has previously been rendered athyroid by surgery and or by radioiodine ablation it may indicate recurrent or metastatic differentiated tumour.

Follow up

There is significant international variation in practice relating to the timing and modalities used for assessing successfulness of thyroid remnant ablation. Whole body radionuclide imaging has largely been superseded by neck ultrasound and stimulated Tg assessment in many centres.

Diagnostic ^{131}I or ^{123}I scans can provide useful information on the effectiveness of ablation and the need for further [131]I.[58]

A follow-up scan should not routinely be performed earlier than six months following ablation.[1] Recent data indicate that low-risk cases, after the first negative radioiodine whole body scan and cervical ultrasound, may be monitored with a stimulated Tg assessment (in the absence of interfering antibodies) without the need for a diagnostic radioiodine scan.[4, 51, 58, 59, 60, 61] A diagnostic whole body radioiodine scan should be performed in all other cases.[1, 58]

Cervical ultrasound is a sensitive method for detection of residual disease in the thyroid bed or cervical lymph nodes. In the United States and mainland Europe, it is common practice for endocrinologists to perform ultrasound in the follow-up clinic, whereas in the UK there is often a lack of access to and availability of expert cervical ultrasound in the routine follow-up clinic setting. It is essential for the ultrasound to be performed by a highly skilled operator with knowledge of thyroid cancer behaviour and not as a routine investigation by a general ultrasonographer.[57] It is important to realize that low-risk intrathyroidal follicular thyroid cancer is very unlikely to recur in cervical lymph nodes or the thyroid bed, and therefore routine ultrasound is unlikely to detect any abnormalities in the neck if successful remnant ablation has been achieved. A raised Tg in these circumstances is therefore more likely to represent distant relapse.

For low-risk cases, if initial follow-up serum Tg is undetectable under TSH stimulation conditions then subsequent long-term, follow-up Tg assessments can be performed under TSH suppression conditions.[1, 2, 51, 60]

If the follow-up ^{131}I scan and stimulated Tg are within normal limits the patient is kept on clinical follow up with Tg annually and there will be no need for routine radionuclide imaging unless symptoms or signs arise or Tg rises on follow up. If the scan or the Tg are abnormal the patient would be considered for ^{131}I therapy. The usual administered activity of ^{131}I is 3.7–5.5 GBq[1] and this too will be followed up with repeat imaging and Tg assessment to assess response.

The TSH stimulated Tg level may remain detectable at low levels after ^{131}I ablation. This could represent residual/recurrent cancer, but in the majority of cases represents thyroid remnant. An expectant policy in low-risk cases is recommended with repeat TSH-stimulated Tg assessment at 6–12-month intervals. In many cases, repeat assessments will reveal a gradual decline in stimulated Tg to the point of no detection, when routine follow up should then be commenced.

Thyroglobulin–positive, radioiodine scan–negative disease

This is a not uncommon scenario seen in the follow up of patients with differentiated thyroid cancer and there is controversy about optimal management.

Before assuming that the reason for the results is the presence of unidentified recurrent disease, first make sure the scan is truly negative and that there has not been any interference, e.g. iodinated intravenous contrast for computed tomography (CT) imaging, no amiodarone, no high iodine content diet. The European Consensus recommendation is that iodine containing contrast media should be avoided for two to three months prior to radioiodine administration; however, there is considerable variation in international practice relating to the optimal interval to be used between iodinated contrast-enhanced CT and the administration of radioiodine. If a patient with an elevated thyroglobulin is to be investigated with regards to localizing the site of relapse, it is important to consider this potential interference if further radioiodine treatment is being considered and alternative imaging modalities may be indicated such as ultrasound or magnetic resonance imaging (MRI).

There are two possible explanations for this situation, once a false-negative scan or false-positive Tg has been ruled out: (1) a small volume of thyroid cancer cells not taking up enough radioiodine to be shown on gamma camera images, i.e. volume of disease below the sensitivity level of the imaging modality or (2) thyroid cancer cells which are non-iodine avid, dedifferentiated or of Hürthle cell type and are unable to take up radioiodine.

There are three main approaches in this situation:

1. No action until the patient becomes symptomatic.
2. Additional investigations aiming to localize the disease recurrence and offer specific therapy (in particular surgical resection of the disease wherever

possible). Use cross-sectional imaging and radioisotope functional imaging studies to find sites of disease. If an isolated lesion amenable to surgery or external beam radiation therapy (EBRT) is found then this and RAI therapy can be considered. A possible imaging strategy is as follows:

a. Neck ultrasound/MRI of neck and mediastinum as the thyroid bed, cervical and mediastinal nodes are the most common sites of recurrence for papillary thyroid cancer. If negative:

b. CT lungs to look for micronodular lung metastases. Remember the potential for iodinated intravenous contrast to inhibit subsequent radioiodine uptake and the recommendation for delaying ^{131}I treatment for two months. If negative:

c. [99m]Tc isotope bone scan. If negative, consider proceeding with a

d. [18]FDG-PET/CT and consider TSH stimulation before positron emission tomography (PET) imaging as there is some evidence to suggest this increases the sensitivity.[62, 63] Other radioisotopes for imaging purposes can be used such as thallium, tetrofosmin and sestamibi, but they lack specificity for thyroid cancer.

e. ^{111}In-labelled octreotide imaging[64] may demonstrate significant uptake in sites of tumour in a small percentage of cases and these patients may then be considered suitable for radiolabelled somatostatin analogue therapy.

f. If imaging suggests surgically resectable disease, its removal should be undertaken prior to further radioiodine therapy.

3. Empirical ^{131}I therapy.[1, 65, 66, 67]

The decision on whether to proceed with an empirical dose of ^{131}I needs to be made, bearing in mind the risk category of the patient and the rate of Tg rise. Proponents argue that a high proportion of patients will have positive post-therapy scans and or thyroglobulin response and some may achieve cure. Opponents argue that some of these patients have minimal disease and hence radioiodine is unlikely to improve survival and that treatment is associated with acute toxicity. A meta-analysis states that 50 per cent of post-therapy scans will be positive and of these positive cases 60 per cent will also show a fall in Tg.[66]

Recurrent or metastatic disease

Between 5 and 20 per cent of patients with papillary thyroid cancer relapse in the thyroid bed or cervical nodes and surgery is the treatment of choice for such locoregional recurrence. Ideally, complete resection is recommended, but if this is not feasible, debulking is beneficial as this will facilitate greater radioiodine uptake in a smaller volume of disease.[11] Distant metastases develop in 10–20 per cent with pulmonary and bone accounting for the majority. If the patient has radioiodine-avid disease, then repeated doses of radioiodine are indicated provided there is evidence of symptomatic, radiological or biochemical response.

Remission can be achieved in about two-thirds of patients with neck recurrence and one-third of those with distant metastases. Remission is more likely when a limited tumour burden is present.[13, 68, 69]

Prognosis depends on distribution and number of metastatic sites, tumour burden (microscopic foci are more likely to respond) and age at the time of diagnosis of metastases.[70, 71] If tumour takes up ^{131}I, then long-term survival is possible. The preferred treatment is repeated doses of ^{131}I with administered activities ranging between 3.7 and 11.1 GBq at three to nine month intervals (usually 5.5–7.4 GBq at 6–12 month intervals).[1, 40, 72, 73] The ATA guidelines[52] recommend repeated radioiodine therapies every 6–12 months for those patients with pulmonary micrometastases, as long as there is continued evidence of response.

Empirical administered activities of ^{131}I are generally used, but dosimetrically calculated activities are used in some centres.[74] There is no maximum limit to the cumulative administered activity of ^{131}I that can be used in the treatment of a patient with persistent disease.[1, 40] Normal bone marrow function is needed and reductions in the administered activity are required in the presence of renal impairment.

Extensive bony metastases are generally not curable by ^{131}I alone. For solitary or a limited number of bone metastases, external beam radiotherapy, resection or embolization with or without postoperative external beam irradiation may be associated with increased survival.[69]

External beam radiotherapy

The use and role of radiotherapy in differentiated thyroid cancer is debated due to conflicting results in published series. There are no randomized controlled trials and the retrospective reviews often extend over several decades resulting in considerable variation in extent of surgery and accuracy of staging investigations. Problems with selection bias are also encountered, as well as inappropriately short follow up for a disease with a long natural history.

The published data are also often lacking with regards to the radiotherapy techniques and doses used, the acute and late toxicity and study end points. The long natural history of the disease means that drawing conclusions from any treatment intervention is difficult.[75, 76, 77]

External beam radiotherapy is infrequently used but the main indications are:

- unresectable disease;
- non-iodine avid disease;
- gross local invasion with macro- or microscopic residual;
- recurrent neck disease not amenable to surgery;
- palliation of inoperable metastatic disease.

The radiotherapy treatment volume usually includes the thyroid bed, cervical and supraclavicular nodes and superior mediastinum. Technical difficulties arise due to the irregular shape of the areas requiring treatment and their proximity to the spinal cord which is more sensitive to the effects of radiotherapy than tumour tissue and is therefore a dose-limiting structure. Without careful attention to radiotherapy planning and delivery, the patient is at risk of radiation myelopathy. The anatomical relationship between the target area and the spinal cord makes it difficult to deliver an homogeneous dose to the areas at risk with conventional radiotherapy techniques.[78]

It is possible that radiotherapy may reduce the uptake of radioiodine into residual thyroid tissue and therefore consideration should be given to administering radioiodine therapy before external beam radiotherapy. However, in practice, there may be a significant delay before the patient can be admitted to the isolation room for radioiodine remnant ablation and for some patients it may be advisable to proceed with external beam radiotherapy, rather than delay both treatment modalities.

Intensity-modulated radiotherapy (IMRT) allows a better radiation dose distribution to the tumour while reducing the dose to radiosensitive organs close to the target areas. This technique can also reduce the volume of non-target tissue that is irradiated to high dose and may even allow dose escalation to at-risk areas.

During radiotherapy the patient is treated supine. Due to the proximity of the area for treatment to critical structures and the need to deliver treatment accurately and precisely over a number of weeks, an immobilization shell is required to keep the patient in a reproducible position.

Radiotherapy is most often required for both the thyroid bed and the locoregional nodes, including the superior mediastinal nodes, rather than the thyroid bed alone. This results in a more complex shape and a larger volume of tissue being irradiated resulting in greater acute toxicities. The most common acute toxicities seen with external beam radiotherapy in this situation are mucositis with associated odynophagia, skin erythema, skin desquamation and laryngitis. If level I and II cervical lymph node areas need irradiating, taste changes, xerostomia and accelerated dental decay and a small risk of osteoradionecrosis of the mandible can arise.

Chemotherapy

There are no data to support the use of adjuvant chemotherapy in the management of differentiated thyroid cancer and it is also not routinely used at the onset of locally recurrent or metastatic disease. Its use is restricted to symptomatic progressive disease when surgery, radiotherapy and radioactive iodine therapy have failed. Published studies have usually only included small numbers of patients and have often had a mixture of histological tumour types within the study population.

Doxorubicin is the most extensively studied agent in advanced thyroid cancer and the most frequently used drug, with a partial response rate of approximately 20–30 per cent reported.[79] There is no clear evidence, however, that its use increases survival. The published studies, however, include patients with variable tumour types and disease burdens and were performed prior to the routine use of high quality imaging and often have limited outcome data.

Doxorubicin in combination with cisplatin has demonstrated a higher response rate but with additional toxicity and no improvement in outcome.[80, 81] It has been reported that response rates to chemotherapy may increase in the presence of an elevated TSH level.[82] However, this has been based on a small series of patients and no large studies have been conducted to address this issue more formally.

Biological agents

As radioisotope therapies and conventional chemotherapy are frequently ineffective in treating symptomatic locally advanced and metastatic thyroid cancer, new treatment strategies are being developed. These new small molecule therapies, such as tyrosine kinase inhibitors, are being targeted at problematic areas in the thyroid cancer cell growth and apoptotic pathways. The following are some of the abnormal pathogenetic mechanisms observed in thyroid cancers:[83]

- RET gene rearrangements are present in 13–43 per cent of PTCs and 30–100 per cent of medullary thyroid carcinomas (MTC) (depending on whether sporadic, FMTC or MEN 2 related).
- BRAF mutations are seen in 29–69 per cent of PTC tumours.

These molecular alterations are now being used as targets for therapeutic strategies. A number of new agents are being investigated including sorafenib (Nexavar®) an inhibitor of BRAF, VEGFR, PDGFR-B, Flt3 and cKIT,[84] sunitinib (Sutent®) a receptor tyrosine kinase inhibitor that targets PDGFR, VEGFR and KIT, axitinib (AG-013736) a selective inhibitor of VEGFRs,[85] lenalidomide (Revlimid®) a derivative of thalidomide with anti-angiogenesis properties and motesanib (AMG 706), another multiple-receptor tyrosine kinase inhibitor that selectively targets and inhibits VEGFR, PDGFR, kit and RET receptors, thereby inhibiting angiogenesis and cellular proliferation.[86]

These agents are administered orally and have a different toxicity profile compared to conventional chemotherapy. The common toxicities are:

- hypertension;
- rash;
- diarrhoea;
- prolonged QT_C interval.

Other potential agents include PPARγ activators, COX 2 inhibitors, heat shock protein inhibitors, demethylating agents, histone deacetylase inhibitors, protease inhibitors and gene therapy. This is a rapidly evolving area and information on current clinical trial activity can be found at the following websites: www.clinicaltrials.gov, www.nci.nih.gov, www.centerwatch.com and www.thyroid.org.

Other radiolabelled therapies

Differentiated thyroid cancers express somatostatin receptors (mainly types 3 and 5) and a small proportion of patients may express the receptors to a significant degree thereby opening the possibility of using radiolabelled somatostatin analogues as a therapy in the metastatic setting.[64]

Childhood

Thyroid nodules are more likely to be malignant in children. Papillary carcinoma is the most common differentiated thyroid cancer seen, with 30–40 per cent being multifocal; 40–90 per cent of patients are found to have involved cervical nodes at initial surgery (compared with 20 per cent of adults).

Differentiated thyroid cancer tends to behave more aggressively in children younger than ten years of age and the chance of recurrence is also higher.[87, 88] [131]I ablation is indicated for all children and adolescents with differentiated thyroid cancers >1 cm following total thyroidectomy[88, 89, 90] and selective neck dissection is recommended for children with positive nodes.[91]

At presentation, 10–20 per cent have lung metastases, while bone metastases are rare (<1 per cent). Fewer than 10 per cent will die as a result of their disease.

Management of differentiated thyroid cancer during pregnancy

If differentiated thyroid cancer is diagnosed during pregnancy, it is essential to consider the risk to both mother and fetus of both the treatment options and the continuation of the pregnancy. Thyroidectomy in the first trimester of pregnancy is associated with a very high risk of miscarriage, but it may be performed safely in the second trimester.[1] Alternatively, surgery can be deferred until after the baby is delivered provided the thyroid tumour is monitored by ultrasound and found to be stable. Suppressive doses of thyroxine are safe in pregnancy and may be considered until surgery is possible. The dosage of thyroxine may need to be increased during pregnancy.[92] Termination of pregnancy is rarely indicated.

It is necessary to avoid pregnancy for six months after radioactive iodine.[44] There may be an increased risk of miscarriage in the first year following radioactive iodine.[35, 36, 37, 93] It is advisable to stop breast feeding at least 4 weeks and preferably 8 weeks prior to [131]I.[1]

Pretreatment sperm banking should be considered in male patients likely to have more than two high-dose ^{131}I therapy treatments (see above under ^{131}I toxicity).[1, 34, 94] Adequate hydration at the time of treatment and several days afterwards helps prevent a decrease in sperm count. Male patients should avoid fathering a child for a minimum of four months, and ideally six months, following [131]I.

Follow up

Frequency and type of follow up depends on an individual's risk of recurrence.[51, 60, 95] The aims of follow up are to detect tumour recurrence early, to monitor TSH suppression and to detect and manage hypocalcaemia. Protocols vary considerably between centres, but as an example the British Thyroid Association (BTA)[1] suggest that following the achievement of thyroid remnant ablation, the frequency of follow up in the first two years is three to six monthly, decreasing to six to eight monthly for three years and then annually thereafter.

The recommended duration of follow up is lifelong due to the long natural history, the possibility of late recurrences, to monitor for late side effects of radioactive iodine and the consequences of supraphysiological thyroxine replacement.

Clinical trials

Information on current clinical trials can be found at the following websites: www.clinicaltrials.gov, www.nci.nih.gov, www.centerwatch.com and www.thyroid.org.

MEDULLARY THYROID CARCINOMA

Surgery is the main modality of treatment for this disease and monitoring of serum calcitonin postoperatively is important in establishing whether biochemical control has been achieved. The calcitonin level of many patients remains elevated after surgery and it is frequently difficult to locate the site of residual disease whether it be local or at a distant site. Blood samples taken for calcitonin must be immediately stored in ice since rapid degradation occurs at room temperature and may give falsely low results. CEA is also commonly raised and can similarly be used to monitor progress and response to therapeutic intervention.

It is presumed that by rendering a patient calcitonin negative that they will have an improved chance of long-term survival and cure; however, long-term follow up of several patient series has lead to conflicting results. Tisel et al.[96] failed to demonstrate a survival advantage when meticulous attention to cervical lymph node dissection achieved normalization of calcitonin and many therefore advocate close clinical follow up and reserve surgery for when clinical relapse can be demonstrated.[97, 98]

Many patients with a raised calcitonin level remain well with an excellent performance status for many years, whereas others become symptomatic over a much shorter interval. In a retrospective review of 65 patients by Barbet et al.,[99] calcitonin doubling time during follow up was a significant predictor of survival in both univariate and multivariate analyses. A calcitonin doubling time greater than two years was associated with long-term survival, whereas patients with a doubling time of less than six months all died as a result of their medullary thyroid cancer.

External beam radiotherapy

Due to a lack of prospective studies, the role of radiotherapy remains uncertain. It is difficult to compare reported series due to considerable differences in radiotherapy dose fractionation, eligibility criteria and often due to the relative rarity of the disease, recruitment has been over very long periods of time. Reported series also often fail to report the associated toxicity and impact on quality of life of any treatment intervention.[100]

Radiotherapy may be indicated in the following situations:[101, 102]

- postoperatively, when the disease was locally advanced at presentation;
- multiple involved lymph nodes;
- persistently high calcitonin/CEA postoperatively;
- bulky inoperable tumours;
- palliation of distant metastases, e.g. bone.

Routine adjuvant radiotherapy in the postoperative setting has not been shown to improve survival.[1, 103, 104]

METASTATIC MEDULLARY THYROID CANCER

Many patients' survival can be measured in years and, even in the presence of significant disease bulk, quality of life can often be good.

Distant metastases frequently involve the liver, lungs and the skeleton and may first come to light when the serum calcitonin level rises significantly. Occasionally, the first sign of the development of distant metastases may be when the patient starts to experience diarrhoea as a result of excess peptide release or symptoms related to excess hormone production. As well as experiencing frequent loose bowel actions, wheezing and flushing are also possible. Cushing syndrome may also occur. These symptoms may respond to somatostatin analogue therapy (e.g. octreotide). Chemotherapy is rarely helpful unless there is rapidly progressive symptomatic disease.

There is no curative treatment option and therefore treatment interventions are usually reserved until the patient becomes symptomatic rather than at first presentation of asymptomatic radiologically diagnosed metastases.

When assessing response to treatment, it is often difficult to demonstrate an objective radiological response even in patients who have symptomatically responded or shown a biochemical response with falling calcitonin levels, by the conventional method of measuring a decrease in the size of tumour lesions. This phenomenon is characteristically seen in MTC and is possibly due to the inclusion of amyloid and calcification within the tumour.

Unlabelled somatostatin analogue therapy for diarrhoea

Somatostatin receptors can be found on medullary thyroid cancer cells and therefore blocking these receptors can result in a decrease in the amount of peptide and calcitonin released. However, a significant decrease in tumour mass is not seen and the aim of treatment is an improvement in symptoms – diarrhoea and flushing and quality of life. Unfortunately, any recorded benefits often seem to be short lived.

If a patient responds favourably to daily subcutaneous administration of octreotide, a synthetic somatostatin analogue (starting at 50–100 μg two or three times per day and escalating according to response up to a maximum of 1500 μg daily) with a reduction in diarrhoea frequency or severity, then they can be commenced on a depot preparation. However, with prolonged use, there is a risk of tachyphylaxis developing with loss of symptomatic benefit. However, if symptom control deteriorates it is important to consider if disease progression is the cause before attributing the change to tachyphylaxis.[105] Octreotide and lanreotide have a different spectrum of somatostatin receptor blockade. Side effects of the somatostatin analogues include gastrointestinal disturbances, such as anorexia, nausea, vomiting, abdominal pain, flatulence, diarrhoea and steatorrhoea, and rarely with long-term use gallstones may occur. Abnormalities of glucose metabolism may also occur. Local reactions at the site of administration may be seen and rotation of the injection site is recommended.

Targeted radiolabelled therapies

Once metastatic disease has been established, imaging with ^{123}I metaiodobenzylguanidine (mIBG) or ^{111}In octreotide may demonstrate selective uptake at sites of known tumour relapse, thereby opening up the possibility of using similar agents as targeted radiolabelled therapies.

As medullary thyroid cancer is not derived from follicular cells, it does not accumulate radioiodine.

METAIODOBENZYLGUANIDINE

Metaiodobenzylguanidine is a guanethidine derivative, structurally similar to noradrenaline. It is transported into neuroendocrine tumour cells by monoamine transport proteins and may be useful as a therapy in a small number of cases.[1, 106, 107]

Approximately 30–40 per cent of medullary thyroid cancers concentrate ^{131}I-mIBG,[108, 109, 110] but to date histological tumour characteristics that reliably predict isotope uptake and hence suitability for therapy have not yet been defined.

Prior to treatment, care must be taken to prevent the use of drugs that may interfere with the uptake and retention of mIBG. The following are some examples, but not an exhaustive list: tricyclic antidepressants, phenothiazines, calcium channel blockers, salbutamol and opioids.

The treatment is given in an isotope isolation room by intravenous infusion usually over a 1–2-hour period through a lead-shielded infusion system. Continuous blood pressure monitoring is required during the infusion and for a period of time afterwards, as unstable blood pressure can result. In practice, this is usually managed by slowing or interrupting the infusion, but in the case of a hypertensive crisis, intravenous phentolamine and propranolol may be required. These drugs should be immediately available during the infusion.

Prophylactic antiemetics, such as ondansetron, are indicated prior to the infusion and should be continued for 72 hours afterwards. It is advisable to insert two cannulae to allow simultaneous i.v. fluids to be given to ensure good hydration in case the patient is unable to take adequate fluids orally as a result of nausea. It is possible that the patient may experience diarrhoea, wheezing and flushing related to peptide and hormone release from the tumour. The patient remains in the isolation room for several days and will follow similar radiation protection procedures as described above under Differentiated thyroid cancer, p. 494.

Whole body gamma camera imaging is performed just before the patient is discharged home to demonstrate the distribution and intensity of isotope uptake.

A full blood count (FBC) should be checked weekly for 6 weeks afterwards as myelosuppression, particularly thrombocytopenia, can occur. This is more likely if there is widespread bone marrow involvement or if the patient has received chemotherapy.

mIBG treatment can be repeated. There are many regimes including three courses at 8–12-week intervals.

Response to treatment can be assessed in terms of symptom improvement, decreasing calcitonin levels or tumour regression on imaging. It is the former, however, which tends to dictate management decisions. Up to 60 per cent of patients may derive symptom benefit and 30–80 per cent may achieve disease stabilization. However, these data are derived from small series.[111, 112, 113] mIBG is traditionally reserved until patients become symptomatic from metastatic disease and it is unknown whether its use earlier in the natural history of the disease may be beneficial, for example when there is asymptomatic elevated serum calcitonin.

Radiolabelled somatostatin analogue therapy

Somatostatin receptor imaging is reported to have a sensitivity of 50–70 per cent in localizing medullary thyroid tumour.[114, 115]

Somatostatin analogues bound to ^{90}yttrium or ^{177}lutetium can therefore be used as therapy in those patients who demonstrate sufficient somatostatin analogue uptake within sites of tumour when compared to background physiological uptake. A subjective benefit may be seen after one to two treatments and this may be associated with a reduction in calcitonin/CEA and tumour stabilization. It is important to realize that a formal radiological assessment of response can be misleading. Often, overall tumour size remains static on cross-sectional imaging, even in the presence of significant radioisotope uptake, symptomatic response and biochemical response. Toxicity includes myelosuppression and nephrotoxicity. Pretreatment with an amino acid infusion can reduce binding of the somatostatin analogue to the renal tubules and hence reduce renal damage.

Chemotherapy

This is reserved for progressive and symptomatic metastatic disease.[1, 80, 81, 116]

There are no randomized controlled trials. The most commonly used drug is doxorubicin, with a response rate of 20–30 per cent that is usually short-lived.

Combination chemotherapy regimens (e.g. doxorubicin with cisplatin) are no more clinically effective and can add significant toxicity.

As medullary thyroid cancer is a neuroendocrine tumour (NET), chemotherapy regimens with activity in other NETs, such as carcinoids, have been suggested, e.g. 5-fluorouracil and streptozocin.

No significant survival benefit has ever been demonstrated and therefore this treatment modality is reserved until progressive symptomatic disease develops that is difficult to palliate with other less toxic modalities.

Biological agents

Preclinical studies have shown that RET inhibition can lead to growth restraint or apoptosis in medullary thyroid cancer cell lines. As a result, there has been significant recent interest in utilizing multikinase inhibitors with activity against RET, VEGF, EGFR, PDGF and KIT in locally advanced and metastatic thyroid cancer of all histological types. They may therefore have a dual mechanism of action with a direct action on tumour cells themselves and also an anti-angiogenic effect.

The toxicity profiles of these agents are different to those of cytotoxic chemotherapy agents. Common adverse events include diarrhoea, hypertension, skin rash, fatigue, headache and nausea. The side-effect profile needs to be balanced against potential improvement in disease-related symptoms, such as diarrhoea or flushing, as MTC is a slowly growing tumour in many cases.

Radiological evidence of significant disease progression along with the calcitonin doubling time, the patient's symptoms and their performance status should all be considered before deciding if systemic therapy is appropriate and likely to provide clinical benefit.

The first TKI to get Food and Drug Administration (FDA) approval for use in unresectable locally advanced or metastatic medullary thyroid cancer was vandetanib (Zactima^{TM}) in April 2011. This decision was based on the phase 3, double-blind placebo-controlled ZETA study that showed an increase in progression-free survival.[117]

Other oral TKIs currently being investigated include cabozantinib (XL184) and lenvatinib (E7080).

There is some evidence emerging that different RET mutations may have different drug sensitivities. For example, the codon 804 mutation seen in hereditary MTC shows *in vitro* resistance to vandetanib/ZD6474, but sensitivity to sorafenib.[118]

Clinical trials

Information on current clinical trials can be found at the following websites: www.clinicaltrials.gov, www.nci.nih.gov, www.centerwatch.com and www.thyroid.org.

ANAPLASTIC THYROID CANCER

Patients with this tumour have a very poor prognosis, with the median survival being six months from symptom onset.[119, 120]

External beam radiotherapy

This tumour is the least radiosensitive of the thyroid tumours. Tumour response tends to be partial even with high doses and the majority of patients still die as a result of locally progressive disease. It is also very important to appreciate that patients may spend a very significant proportion of their remaining lives undergoing treatment and recovering from its significant toxicity.

Attempts have been made to improve response to treatment by intensifying the radiotherapy regime by hyperfractionation (delivering more than the standard one fraction of radiotherapy per day) or by shortening the time period over which it is delivered (accelerated radiotherapy) and combining this with chemotherapy and in some cases surgery.[121, 122, 123, 124] This intensification has in some series resulted in improved response rates, but at the cost of increased toxicity.[125]

Chemotherapy

The response rate for doxorubicin is in the region of 20 per cent. The responses are often partial and of short duration.[79] Other agents are being investigated including the chemotherapy drugs paclitaxel[126] and combretastatin and biological agents, such as sorafenib.

Clinical trials

Information on current clinical trials can be found at the following websites: www.clinicaltrials.gov, www.nci.nih.gov, www.centerwatch.com and www.thyroid.org.

PRIMARY THYROID LYMPHOMA

Thyroid lymphomas constitute only 3 per cent of all non-Hodgkin lymphomas (NHL) and approximately 5 per cent of all thyroid neoplasms.[127] They are more frequently seen in patients with a history of Hashimoto thyroiditis. The majority of thyroid lymphomas are of B-cell origin. Diffuse large B-cell lymphoma accounts for up to 70 per cent of cases, while mucosa-associated lymphoid tissue (MALT)-positive lymphoma accounts for between 6 and 27 per cent.[128] If a diagnosis of thyroid MALT lymphoma is made, consideration should be given to performing a gastroscopy to check for involvement of the stomach as MALT lymphomas have a tendency to migrate to other areas with MALT.

The majority of patients present with cervical or mediastinal node involvement and are managed with a combination of external beam radiotherapy and systemic chemotherapy as both overall and distant relapse rates are lower in those patients receiving combined modality therapy compared to chemotherapy or radiotherapy alone.[129] Presentation with B symptoms is uncommon.

Six cycles of CHOP (cyclophosphamide, doxorubicin, vincristine and prednisolone) chemotherapy followed by radiotherapy increases survival when compared with radiotherapy alone (35 versus 65–90 per cent).[130] In general, the addition of rituximab, a chimeric monoclonal antibody against CD20, to CHOP chemotherapy in the management of NHL provides further benefit in survival and disease-free survival and it is therefore assumed that this also applies to primary thyroid lymphoma.

As lymphoma is a relatively radiosensitive tumour, the radiation dose required is appreciably lower than that used in the management of differentiated thyroid cancers.

Radiation therapy is most commonly given after between three and six courses of chemotherapy. The usual radiation fields either cover the areas involved at presentation only or they may be extended to include the thyroid, bilateral neck, supraclavicular regions and the mediastinum.

Radiotherapy alone may be indicated for stage I$_{AE}$ mucosa-associated lymphoid tissue-positive lymphoma as it tends to follow a more indolent course and a complete response of >90 per cent can be achieved with this single treatment modality. Laing et al.[131] report 100 per cent complete response with radiotherapy, a relapse rate of 30 per cent

and salvage rate >50 per cent with a 90 per cent overall cause-specific survival at five years.

KEY EVIDENCE

- I would really only recommend that practitioners are familiar with current international consensus documents/guidelines, e.g. American Thyroid Association (ATA) guidelines on management of differentiated thyroid cancer (DTC) and medullary thyroid carcinomas (MTC).

KEY LEARNING POINTS

- Differentiated thyroid cancer:
  - importance of risk stratification
  - degree of thyroid-stimulating hormone (TSH) suppression in long-term follow up
  - possibility of moving towards lower activity of radioactive iodine (RAI).
- Medullary thyroid carcinoma:
  - importance of calcitonin doubling time
- Progressive locally advanced/metastatic disease:
  - potential role of systemic treatment in the form of tyrosine kinase inhibitors (TKI).

REFERENCES

1. Perros P (ed.). British Thyroid Association, Royal College of Physicians. Guidelines for the management of thyroid cancer, 2nd edn. Report of the Thyroid Cancer Guidelines Update Group. London: Royal College of Physicians, 2007.
2. Pacini F, Schlumberger M, Dralle H et al. European Thyroid Cancer Taskforce. European consensus for the management of patients with differentiated thyroid carcinoma of the follicular epithelium. European Journal of Endocrinology 2006; 154: 787–803.
3. Luster M, Clarke S, Dietlein M et al. Guidelines for radioiodine therapy of differentiated thyroid cancer. European Journal of Nuclear Medicine and Molecular Imaging 2008; 35: 1941–59.
4. The American Thyroid Association Guidelines Taskforce. Management guidelines for patients with thyroid nodules and differentiated thyroid cancer. Thyroid 2006; 16: 109–44.
5. Sawka A, Thephamongkhol K, Brouwers M et al. Clinical review 170: A systematic review and metaanalysis of the effectiveness of radioactive iodine remnant ablation for well differentiated thyroid cancer. Journal of Clinical Endocrinology and Metabolism 2004; 89: 3668–76.

6. Samaan N, Schultz P, Hickey R et al. The results of various modalities of treatment of well differentiated thyroid carcinomas: a retrospective review of 1599 patients. *Journal of Clinical Endocrinology and Metabolism* 1992; **75**: 714–20.

7. Hay I, Thompson G, Grant C et al. Papillary thyroid carcinoma managed at the Mayo Clinic during six decades (1940–1999): Temporal trends in initial therapy and long term outcome in 2444 consecutively treated patients. *World Journal of Surgery* 2002; **26**: 879–85.

8. Sanders L, Cady B. Differentiated thyroid cancer: Reexamination of risk groups and outcome of treatment. *Archives of Surgery* 1998; **133**: 419–25.

9. Kim S, Wei J, Braverman J, Brams D. Predicting outcome and directing therapy for papillary thyroid carcinoma. *Archives of Surgery* 2004; **139**: 390–4.

10. Sugitani I, Fujimoto Y. Symptomatic versus asymptomatic papillary thyroid microcarcinoma: A retrospective analysis of surgical outcome and prognostic factors. *Endocrine Journal* 1999; **46**: 209–16.

11. Mazzaferri E, Jjhiang SM. Long term impact of initial surgical and medical therapy on papillary and follicular thyroid cancer. *American Journal of Medicine* 1994; **97**: 418–28.

12. Yamashita HNS, Murakami N, Kawamoto H, Watanabe S. Extracapsular invasion of lymph node metastatis is an indicator of distant metastasis and poor prognosis in patients with thyroid papillary carcinoma. *Cancer* 1997; **80**: 2268–72.

13. Pacini F, Cetani F, Miccoli P et al. Outcome of 309 patients with metastatic differentiated thyroid carcinoma treated with radioiodine. *World Journal of Surgery* 1994; **18**: 600–4.

14. Tsang R, Brierley J, Simpson W et al. The effects of surgery, radioiodine and external radiation therapy in the clinical outcome of patients with differentiated thyroid carcinoma. *Cancer* 1998; **82**: 375–88.

15. Brierley J, Tsang R, Panzarella T et al. Prognostic factors and the effect of treatment with radioactive iodine and external beam radiation on patients with differentiated thyroid cancer seen at a single institution over 40 years. *Clinical Endocrinology* 2005; **63**: 418–27.

16. Ringel M, Ladenson P. Controversies in the follow up and management of well differentiated thyroid cancer. *Endocrine-Related Cancer* 2004; **11**: 97–116.

17. Pacini F, Schlumberger M, Harmer C et al. Post surgical use of radioiodine (I^{131}) in patients with papillary and follicular thyroid cancer and the issue of remnant ablation: a consensus report. *European Journal of Endocrinology* 2005; **153**: 651–9.

18. Rosario P, Reis J, Barroso A et al. Efficacy of low and high I^{131} doses for thyroid remnant ablation in patients with differentiated thyroid carcinoma based on post operative cervical uptake. *Nuclear Medicine Communications* 2004; **25**: 1077–81.

19. Bal C, Padhy A, Jana S et al. Prospective randomized clinical trial to evaluate the optimal dose of I^{131} for remnant ablation in patients with differentiated thyroid carcinoma. *Cancer* 1996; **77**: 2574–80.

20. Creutzig H. High or low dose radioiodine ablation of thyroid remnants? *European Journal of Nuclear Medicine* 1987; **12**: 500–2.

21. Johansen K, Woodhouse N, Odugbesan O. Comparison of 1073 MBq and 3700 MBq iodine 131 in postoperative ablation of residual thyroid tissue in patients with differentiated thyroid cancer. *Journal of Nuclear Medicine* 1991; **32**: 252–4.

22. Hackshaw A, Harmer C, Mallick U et al. ^{131}I activity for remnant ablation in patients with differentiated thyroid cancer: A systematic review. *Journal of Clinical Endocrinology and Metabolism* 2007; **92**: 28–38.

23. Robbins R, Larson S, Sinha N et al. A retrospective review of the effectiveness of recombinant human TSH as a preparation for radioiodine thyroid remnant ablation. *Journal of Nuclear Medicine* 2002; **43**: 1482–8.

24. Pacini F, Ladenson P, Schlumberger M et al. Radioiodine ablation of thyroid remnants after preparation with recombinant human thyrotropin in differentiated thyroid carcinoma: results of an international, randomized, controlled study. *Journal of Clinical Endocrinology and Metabolism* 2006; **91**: 926–32.

25. Sirisalipoch S, Buachum V, Passawang P, Tepmongkol S. Prospective randomized trial for the evaluation of the efficacy of low vs high dose I^{131} for post-operative remnant ablation in differentiated thyroid cancer. *World Journal of Nuclear Medicine* **S36** (Suppl. 1) 2004; 36.

26. Fatourechi V, Hay I, Mullan B et al. Are post therapy radioiodine scans informative and do they influence subsequent therapy of patients with differentiated thyroid cancer? *Thyroid* 2000; **10**: 573–7.

27. Leger FA, Izembart M, Dagousset F et al. Decreased uptake of therapeutic doses of iodine 131 after 185 MBq iodine 131 diagnostic imaging for thyroid remnants in differentiated thyroid carcinoma. *European Journal of Nuclear Medicine* 1998; **25**: 242–6.

28. Park H, Park Y, Jhow X. Detection of thyroid remnant/metastases with stunning – an ongoing dilemma. *Thyroid* 1997; **7**: 277–80.

29. Maxon H, Boehringer T, Drilling J. Low iodine diet in I 131 ablation of thyroid remnants. *Clinical Nuclear Medicine* 1983; **8**: 123–6.

30. Pluijmen M, Eustatia-Rutten C, Goslings B et al. Effects of low-iodide diet on postsurgical radioiodide ablation therapy in patients with differentiated thyroid carcinoma. *Clinical Endocrinology* 2003; **58**: 428–35.

31. Maxon H. Quantitative radioiodine therapy in the treatment of differentiated thyroid cancer. *Quarterly Journal of Nuclear Medicine* 1999; **43**: 313–23.

32. Maxon H, Smith H. Radioiodine-131 in the diagnosis and treatment of metastatic well differentiated thyroid

cancer. *Endocrinology and Metabolism Clinics of North America* 1990; **19**: 685–718.

33. Nakada K, Ishibashi T, Takei T *et al.* Does lemon candy decrease salivary gland damage after radioiodine therapy for thyroid cancer? *Journal of Nuclear Medicine* 2005; **46**: 261–6.

34. Krassas G, Pontikides N. Gonadal effect of radiation from ^{131}I in male patients with thyroid carcinoma. *Archives of Andrology* 2005; **51**: 171–5.

35. Schlumberger M, De Vathaire F, Ceccarelli C *et al.* Exposure to radioiodine (I[131]) for scintigraphy or therapy does not preclude pregnancy in thyroid cancer patients. *Journal of Nuclear Medicine* 1996; **37**: 606–12.

36. Ayala C, Navarro E, Rodriguez J *et al.* Conception after I[131] therapy for differentiated thyroid cancer. *Thyroid* 1998; **8**: 1009–11.

37. Dottorinin M, Lomuscio G, Mazzucchelli L *et al.* Assessment of female fertility and carcinogenesis after iodine I[131] therapy for differentiated thyroid carcinoma. *Journal of Nuclear Medicine* 1995; **36**: 21–7.

38. Bal C, Kumar A, Tripathi M *et al.* High dose radioiodine treatment for differentiated thyroid carcinoma is not associated with changes in female fertility or any genetic risk to the offspring. *International Journal of Radiation Oncology, Biology, Physics* 2005; **63**: 449–55.

39. Vini L, Hyer S, Al-Saadi A *et al.* Prognosis for fertility and ovarian function after treatment with radioiodine for thyroid cancer. *Postgraduate Medical Journal* 2002; **78**: 92–3.

40. Brown A, Greening W, McCready V *et al.* Radioiodine treatment of metastatic thyroid cancer. Royal Marsden Experience. *British Journal of Radiology* 1984; **57**: 323–7.

41. Maheshwari Y, Hill C, Haynie G *et al.* I[131] therapy in differentiated thyroid carcinoma: MD Anderson Hospital Experience. *Cancer* 1981; **47**: 664–71.

42. Rall J, Alpers J, Lewallen C *et al.* Radiation pneumonitis and fibrosis: a complication of radioiodine treatment of pulmonary metastases from cancer of the thyroid. *Journal of Clinical Endocrinology and Metabolism* 1957; **17**: 1263–76.

43. Rubino C, de Vathaire F, Dottorinin M *et al.* Second primary malignancies in thyroid cancer patients. *British Journal of Cancer* 2003; **89**: 1638–44.

44. Sandeep T, Strachan M, Reynolds R *et al.* Second primary cancers in thyroid cancer patients: a multinational record linkage study. *Journal of Clinical Endocrinology and Metabolism* 2006; **91**: 1819–25.

45. Administration of Radioactive Substances Advisory Committee. *ARSAC notes for guidance on the clinical administration of radiopharmaceuticals and use of sealed radioactive sources.* Didcot, UK: ARSAC, 2006.

46. Biondi B, Filetti S, Schlumberger M. Thyroid hormone therapy and thyroid cancer: a reassessment. *Nature Clinical Practice. Endocrinology and Metabolism* 2005; **1**: 32–40.

47. Wang P, Wang S, Liu R. Levothyroxine suppression of thyroglobulin in patients with differentiated thyroid carcinoma. *Journal of Clinical Endocrinology and Metabolism* 1999; **84**: 4549–553.

48. Kamel N, Gullu S, Dagci I. Degree of thyrotropin suppression in differentiated thyroid cancer without recurrence or metastases. *Thyroid* 1999; **9**: 1245–8.

49. Pujol P, Daures J, Nsakala N *et al.* Degree of thyrotropin suppression as a prognostic determinant in differentiated thyroid cancer. *Journal of Clinical Endocrinology and Metabolism* 1996; **81**: 4318–23.

50. Cooper D, Specker B, Ho M *et al.* Thyrotropin suppression and disease progression in patients with differentiated thyroid cancer: results from the National Thyroid Cancer Treatment Cooperative Registry. *Thyroid* 1998; **8**: 737–44.

51. Schlumberger M, Berg G, Cohen O *et al.* Follow up of low risk patients with differentiated thyroid carcinoma: a European perspective. *European Journal of Endocrinology* 2004; **150**: 105–12.

52. Cooper DS, Doherty GM, Haugen BR *et al.* on behalf of the American Thyroid Association (ATA). Revised American Thyroid Association management guidelines for patients with thyroid nodules and differentiated thyroid cancer. *Thyroid* 2009; **19**: 1167–1214.

53. Demers LM, Spencer CA (eds) Laboratory support for the diagnosis and monitoring of thyroid disease. Laboratory Medicine Practice Guidelines prepared by the National Academy of Clinical Biochemistry. Franklin, TN: Durik Advertising, Inc. Available from the American Association of Clinical Chemistry at www.AACC.org. Monograph originally published in *Thyroid* 2003; **13**: 1–126.

54. Spencer C, Bergoglio L, Kazarosyan M *et al.* Clinical impact of thyroglobulin (Tg) and Tg autoantibody method differences on the management of patients with differentiated thyroid carcinomas. *Journal of Clinical Endocrinology and Metabolism* 2005; **90**: 5566–75.

55. Spencer C, Takeuchi M, Kazarosyan M *et al.* Serum thyroglobulin autoantibodies: Prevalence, influence on serum thyroglobulin measurement, and prognostic significance in patients with differentiated thyroid carcinoma. *Journal of Clinical Endocrinology and Metabolism* 1998; **83**: 1121–7.

56. Chiovato L, Latrofa F, Braverman L *et al.* Disappearance of humoral thyroid autoimmunity after complete removal of thyroid antigens. *Annals of Internal Medicine* 2003; **139**: 346–51.

57. Bal C, Padhy AK, Jana S *et al.* Prospective randomized clinical trial to evaluate the optimal dose of I[131] for remnant ablation in patients with differentiated thyroid carcinoma cancer. *Cancer* 1996; **77**: 2574–80.

58. Cailleux A, Baudin E, Travagli J *et al.* Is diagnostic I[131] scanning useful after total thyroid ablation for differentiated thyroid cancer. *Journal of Clinical Endocrinology and Metabolism* 2000; **85**: 175–8.

59. Haugen B, Pacini F, Reiners C *et al.* A comparison of recombinant human thyrotropin and thyroid hormone

withdrawal for the detection of thyroid remnant or cancer. *Journal of Clinical Endocrinology and Metabolism* 1999; **84**: 3877–85.

60. Mazzaferri E, Robbins R, Spencer C *et al.* A consensus report of the role of serum thyroglobulin as a monitoring method for low risk patients with papillary thyroid carcinoma. *Journal of Clinical Endocrinology and Metabolism* 2003; **88**: 1433–41.

61. Pacini F, Capezzone M, Elisei R *et al.* A diagnostic I[131] iodine whole body scan may be avoided in thyroid cancer patients who have undetectable stimulated serum thyroglobulin levels after initial treatment. *Journal of Clinical Endocrinology and Metabolism* 2002; **87**: 1499–501.

62. van Tol K, Jager P, Piers D *et al.* Better yield of 18 fluorodeoxyglucose positron emission tomography in patients with metastatic differentiated thyroid cancer during thyrotropin stimulation. *Thyroid* 2002; **12**: 381–7.

63. Petrich T, Börner AR, Otto D *et al.* Influence of rhTSH on 18 fluorodeoxyglucose uptake by differentiated thyroid cancer. *Journal of Nuclear Medicine and Molecular Imaging* 2002; **29**: 641–7.

64. Stokkel M, Reigman H, Verkooijen R, Smit J. Indium 111 octreotide scintigraphy in differentiated thyroid carcinoma metastases that do not respond to treatment with high dose I[131]. *Journal of Cancer Research and Clinical Oncology* 2003; **129**: 287–94.

65. McDougal I. Managament of thyroglobulin positive/whole body scan negative: is Tg positive/I[131] therapy useful? *Journal of Endocrinological Investigation* 2001; **24**: 194–8.

66. Ma C, Xie J, Kuang A. Is empiric I[131] therapy justified for patients with positive Tg and negative I[131] whole body scanning results? *Journal of Nuclear Medicine* 2005; **46**: 1164–70.

67. van Tol K, Jager P, de Vries E *et al.* Outcome in patents with differentiated thyroid cancer with negative diagnostic whole body scanning and detectable stimulated thyroglobulin. *European Journal of Endocrinology* 2003; **148**: 589–96.

68. Leeper R. The effect of I[131] therapy on survival of patients with metastatic papillary or follicular thyroid carcinoma. *Journal of Clinical Endocrinology and Metabolism* 1973; **36**: 1143–52.

69. Bernier M, Leenhardt L, Hoang C *et al.* Survival and therapeutic modalities in patients with bone metastases of differentiated thyroid carcinomas. *Journal of Clinical Endocrinology and Metabolism* 2001; **86**: 1568–73.

70. Schlumberger M, Mancusi F, De Vathaire F *et al.* Radioactive iodine treatment and external radiotherapy for lung and bone metastases from thyroid carcinoma. *Journal of Nuclear Medicine* 1996; **37**: 598–605.

71. Maxon H, Thomas S, Samaratunga R. Dosimetric considerations in the radioiodine treatment of macrometastases and micrometastases from differentiated thyroid cancer. *Thyroid* 1997; **7**: 183–7.

72. Harmer C, McCready V. Thyroid cancer: differentiated carcinoma. *Cancer Treatment Reviews* 1996; **22**: 161–77.

73. Wilson P, Millar B, Brierley J. The management of advanced thyroid cancer. *Clinical Oncology* 2004; **16**: 561–8.

74. Van Nostrand D, Atkins F, Yeganeh F *et al.* Dosimetrically determined doses of radioiodine for the treatment of metastatic thyroid carcinoma. *Thyroid* 2002; **12**: 121–34.

75. Meadows K, Amdur R, Morris C *et al.* External beam radiotherapy for differentiated thyroid cancer. *American Journal of Otolaryngology* 2006; **27**: 24–8.

76. Tubiana M, Haddad E, Schlumberger M *et al.* External radiotherapy in thyroid cancers. *Cancer* 1985; **55**(Suppl.): 2062–71.

77. Harmer C, Bidmead M, Shepherd S *et al.* Radiotherapy planning techniques for thyroid cancer. *British Journal of Radiology* 1998; **71**: 1069–75.

78. Ford D, Giridharan S, McConkey C *et al.* External beam radiotherapy in the management of differentiated thyroid cancer. *Clinical Oncology* 2003; **15**: 337–41.

79. Ahuja S, Ernst H. Chemotherapy of thyroid carcinoma. *Journal of Endocrinological Investigation* 1987; **10**: 303–10.

80. Shimaoka K, Schoenfeld D, Dewys W *et al.* A randomized trial of doxorubicin versus doxorubicin plus cisplatin in patients with advanced thyroid cancer. *Cancer* 1985; **56**: 2155–60.

81. Williams S, Birch R, Einhorn L. Phase II evaluation of doxorubicin plus cisplatin in advance thyroid cancer: a Southeastern Cancer Study Group Trial. *Cancer Treatment Reports* 1986; **70**: 405–7.

82. Santini F, Bottici V, Elisei R *et al.* Cytotoxic effects of carboplatinum and epirubicin in the setting of an elevated serum thyroglobulin for advanced poorly differentiated thyroid cancer. *Journal of Clinical Endocrinology and Metabolism* 2002; **87**: 4160–5.

83. Kondo T, Ezzat S, Asa S. Pathogenetic mechanisms in thyroid follicular-cell neoplasia. *Nature Reviews. Cancer* 2006; **6**: 292–306.

84. Gupta-Abramson V, Troxel AB, Nellore A *et al.* Phase II trial of sorafenib in advanced thyroid cancer. *Journal Clinical Oncology* 2008; **26**: 4714–19.

85. Cohen E, Rosen L, Vokes E *et al.* Axitinib is an active treatment for all histologic subtypes of advanced thyroid cancer: results from a phase II study. *Journal of Clinical Oncology* 2008; **26**: 3543.

86. Sherman S, Wirth L, Droz J *et al.* Motesanib diphosphate in progressive differentiated thyroid cancer. *New England Journal of Medicine* 2008; **359**: 31–42.

87. Schlumberger M, De Vathaire F, Travagli JP *et al.* Differentiated thyroid carcinoma in childhood: long term follow up of 72 patients. *Clinics in Endocrinology and Metabolism* 1987; **65**: 1088–94.

88. Jarzab B, Handkiewicz-Junak D, Wloch J *et al.* Multivariate analysis of prognostic factors for

27

Parathyroid tumours

R JAMES A ENGLAND AND NICK P MCIVOR

From there to here, from here to there, funny things are everywhere.

Dr Seuss: *One Fish, Two Fish, Red Fish, Blue Fish*

INTRODUCTION

Parathyroid tumours are benign in 99 per cent of cases. They usually present with primary hyperparathyroidism (HPT), normally characterized by hypercalcaemia in the presence of an inappropriate (i.e. unsuppressed) level of parathyroid hormone (PTH). Until the introduction of the automated serum autoanalyser in the 1970s, patients with these tumours typically presented late with severe symptoms or signs. Now, the majority are diagnosed in apparently asymptomatic patients with the discovery of incidental hypercalcaemia during biochemical analysis. Although making the diagnosis of HPT is normally straightforward, other causes for hypercalcaemia must always be considered and excluded.

In HPT, excess PTH is produced by the neoplastic or hyperplastic growth of parathyroid parenchymal cells. HPT is usually primarily due to a parathyroid abnormality and therefore unassociated with other biochemical influences – primary HPT. In some cases, it is due to other biochemical influences stimulating the parathyroid glands – secondary HPT. In chronic secondary hyperparathyroidism, the growth of a hyperplastic gland may become autonomous due to the resetting of the calcium receptor on individual parathyroid cells, such that the glands remain hyperplastic after the chronic stimulus has been removed. This situation is known as 'tertiary hyperparathyroidism'. Finally, HPT may be inherited as part of a MEN syndrome or less frequently in isolated form.

The vast majority of parathyroid surgery is carried out for primary HPT. The decision to operate is sometimes difficult as a significant proportion of these patients can be treated conservatively by regular monitoring and in some, symptomatic and biochemical improvement can be achieved with drugs. However, the only definitive treatment for hyperparathyroidism remains surgery and with the newer technique of targeted minimally invasive parathyroidectomy (MIP), many authors would argue that surgery should be considered in every case.

Surgery for familial hyperparathyroid syndromes is challenging because of the high incidence of multigland disease. Surgery is seldom required for secondary HPT, but those that persist after correction of the initiating stimulus, i.e. tertiary HPT, require specialized management.

THE CALCIUM–PTH RELATIONSHIP AND THE CALCIUM–SENSING RECEPTOR

There are usually four parathyroid glands in the neck (two on each side) that are responsible for maintaining the normal level of calcium in the blood specifically, and the body in general.

Normal parathyroid glands are regulated by a feedback mechanism. As the level of calcium in the blood increases, the stimulation to secrete PTH decreases and vice versa. This relationship between serum calcium and PTH is best represented by a sigmoidal curve: the PTH-Ca^{2+} curve. It is regulated via the parathyroid cell calcium-sensing receptor (CSR) which in turn is regulated by its coding gene and also by the 'set-point' which reflects sensitivity of the receptor. Various conditions shift the curve to the right (reduced sensitivity), e.g. lithium and chronic renal failure, while others shift it to the left (increased sensitivity), e.g. early renal failure.[1]

The CSR lies on the surface of parathyroid cells and responds to the ambient calcium of the pericellular fluid. Aberrations in the CSR gene which regulates the expression of this receptor, influence calcium homeostasis (see Familial hyperparathyroidism, p. 512). Also, there is a receptor 'set-point' which reflects the sensitivity of the CSR to calcium. The set-point is defined as the calcium level at half of the maximal inhibition of PTH release, i.e. 50 per cent of maximal PTH secretion.[2] There is always some basal PTH secretion, even in severe hypercalcaemia, whereas below the set-point there is an increasing stimulation of PTH production, PTH release, and parathyroid cell replication. Various conditions influence the set-point, e.g. lithium and renal failure cause a resetting of the set-point leading to states of persisting hypercalcaemia (see Secondary hyperparathyroidism, p. 512).

PRIMARY HYPERPARATHYROIDISM

Clinical presentation

The symptoms of primary HPT are due to hypercalcaemia and are listed in **Box 27.1**. These can be summarized by the aphorism 'bones, stones, groans and psychic moans'. However, 80 per cent of patients present incidentally with the finding of hypercalcaemia on routine blood testing.[3] Their condition is often labelled 'asymptomatic hyperparathyroidism', but as many of the symptoms of HPT may be attributed to the ageing process, the label 'asymptomatic' can be hard to validate. Patients may also be diagnosed while screening for osteopenia, osteoporosis or nephrolithiasis. Very rarely, patients may present with significant bone disease (osteitis fibrosa cystica) most clearly seen on x-rays of the middle phalanges showing subperiosteal bone resorption. This presentation tends to occur more frequently in severe long-standing disease, parathyroid cancer or secondary and tertiary hyperparathyroidism.

Box 27.1   Manifestations of hypercalcaemia

- Muscle weakness
- Muscle and bone aches and pains
- Depression
- Constipation
- Tiredness
- Peptic ulceration
- Pancreatitis
- Renal impairment
- Nephrogenic diabetes insipidus
- Nephrolithiasis
- Shortened QT interval
- Band keratopathy
- Thirst and polyuria

Diagnosis of primary hyperparathyroidism

PTH hypersecretion occurring as a primary event occurs at any age, but more commonly in older patients. By the sixth decade, the incidence has risen to approximately one in 1000 in men, and one in 500 in women.[4]

The diagnosis is usually first suspected by the finding of hypercalcaemia, although 10–20 per cent of hyperparathyroid patients may be normocalcaemic. This may be due to concomitant vitamin D insufficiency which must be screened for, or the fact that the parathyroid glands are intermittent secretors, and repeat Ca^{2+} monitoring or vitamin D replacement therapy in appropriate patients will normally unmask the diagnosis.[5]

In the presence of hypercalcaemia, an 'inappropriately' normal or elevated PTH level is indicative of HPT. Patients with nonparathyroid hypercalcaemia virtually always have PTH values below 25 pg/mL.[6] However, if the diagnosis is unclear, other causes of hypercalcaemia must be excluded.

The second most common cause of hypercalcaemia is cancer. There is secretion of parathyroid hormone-related peptide (PTHrP) causing the osteoclastic release of calcium and suppressing PTH. This diagnosis is normally easy to make as the tumour will be in an advanced state. However, in a clinically well, hypercalcaemic patient with a suppressed PTH, the diagnoses of malignant lymphoma and multiple myeloma must still be ruled out. PTH can be differentiated from PTHrP by a chemiluminescent assay so that primary HPT is not confused with the hypercalcaemia of malignancy.[7] Other causes of hypercalcaemia to be borne in mind are listed in **Box 27.2**.

Further useful tests in the diagnosis of primary hyperparathyroidism include serum phosphate, which is normally at the lower end of the normal range and serum creatinine, as renal impairment may occur as a result of chronic hypercalcaemia. In addition, a 24-hour urine collection is useful because 40 per cent of hyperparathyroid patients at diagnosis have hypercalciuria, the remainder having normal values.[8] Significant hypercalciuria is one of the criteria for advising surgery in asymptomatic primary hyperparathyroidism because of the increased risk of developing nephrocalcinosis or nephrolithiasis. If the urinary calcium is low, however, the diagnosis of familial hypercalcaemic hypocalciuria (FHH) must be considered (see Familial hyperparathyroidism).

that these patients are predisposed to persistent and recurrent HPT because of the persistence of parathyroid cell rests despite an apparently total (four gland) parathyroidectomy. The aims of surgery, therefore, include achieving and maintaining normocalcaemia for the longest time possible, avoiding iatrogenic hypocalcaemia and operative complications, and facilitating future surgery for recurrent disease.

MEN1

In this syndrome, the decision on timing of surgery can be difficult. While early intervention may avoid the long-term effects of hyperparathyroidism, it does expose the patient to the risk of recurrent HPT and of increasingly difficult revision surgeries at a younger age. Delaying surgery can allow the glands to become larger, thus facilitating the original surgery. Clearly, however, surgery is required when the effects of the disease are evident (osteoporosis, Zollinger–Ellison syndrome).

The initial surgical procedure should be either a subtotal procedure, leaving a remnant the size of a normal parathyroid gland (20–30 mg) or a total parathyroidectomy with autotransplantation of 20–30 mg of tissue. Both procedures require a meticulous search for ectopic parathyroid tissue and also a bilateral thymectomy not only to minimize the risk of persistence or recurrence of HPT, but also of thymic carcinoid tumours.[20] Because of the fallibility of preserved and transplanted tissue and when the facilities allow, parathyroid tissue should also be cryopreserved for later transplantation if required.

MEN2A

The management of this condition is typically dominated by the management of medullary thyroid carcinoma. The HPT tends to be mild and occurs in only 20–30 per cent. It is usually diagnosed at the same time or after the thyroid malignancy. All grossly abnormal glands should be removed.

Decision-making in secondary and tertiary hyperparathyroidism

RENAL

Secondary HPT patients are more symptomatic than both primary and tertiary HPT, but most can be treated medically with phosphate binders, calcitriol and calcium supplementation. Medical treatment fails in about 5 per cent of patients and they become unsuppressible or autonomous requiring parathyroidectomy.[26, 27]

The decision for parathyroid surgery in a renal failure patient with HPT is generally made by the renal physician to correct the biochemical abnormalities or the clinical symptoms or both. Bone pain and pruritus are likely to improve after surgery.[26] Pruritus is one the most disabling symptoms of secondary HPT and, although the pathophysiology is unclear, the reduction in PTH and the calcium/phosphate product must play a role.[26, 28] Vague symptoms, such as general muscle weakness[29] and irritability,[26] are improved after surgery for secondary HPT. Parathyroidectomy can also

be effective treatment in the life-threatening situation of calciphylaxis.[30] However, other vague symptoms, such as mood swings, depression, forgetfulness and fatigue, which can be expected to improve after surgery for primary HPT are variably ameliorated in patients with secondary HPT, presumably due to the continuing stimulation from chronic renal failure. Although these patients tend to improve with time, they remain symptomatic in some way, thus lowering quality of life.[31] In tertiary HPT, where the renal failure has been corrected by transplantation, the symptomatic improvement is similar to that in the primary HPT patient.[26]

The decision for surgery is based not only on symptoms, but also on the likelihood of calcium deposition in tissues. Deposition is likely to occur when the calcium/phosphate product exceeds 5 or when PTH reaches 100 pmol/L (normal, 1.7–7.3 pmol/L). Thus, uraemic patients in this situation are generally not put forward for renal transplantation until these parameters are improved, as the transplanted kidney is likely to fail. If oral or intravenous calcitriol is unsuccessful, then the patient is considered for parathyroidectomy. Similar parameters are used in post-transplant patients to avoid calcium deposition in the transplant.

The authors advocate total parathyroidectomy with autotransplantation of tissue into the forearm muscle or subcutaneous fat and with the cryopreservation of parathyroid tissue for subsequent grafting if the initial transplant fails. They argue that subtotal procedures may have higher rates of persistence and recurrence in a population in whom any parathyroid remnants retain an altered set-point and are therefore programmed to expand and hypersecrete. When the facilities are available, cryopreservation of surplus parathyroid tissue should proceed.

Others experienced in subtotal parathyroidectomy argue that the risk of recurrence is small and that permanent hypoparathyroidism and the long-term requirement for calcium and calcitriol should be avoided in the haemodialysis patient who is subject to potentially sudden changes in serum calcium without any functioning parathyroid reserve.[27] The vascularized parathyroid remnant resulting from subtotal parathyroidectomy is variably defined. Some advocate leaving half of the most normal gland[27]. However, Milas and Weber[30] comment that 'even leaving half' of a typically large parathyroid gland found in patients with renal disease 'preserves abnormal amounts of hyperfunctioning tissue'. They aim to leave a segment equal to approximately two normal parathyroid glands or approximately a $10 \times 5 \times 3$ mm segment which they define as 'near-total parathyroidectomy'.[30] With this approach, these authors report a 4 per cent rate of persistent HPT and 4 per cent recurrence.

LITHIUM

In a study of 15 patients undergoing parathyroidectomy for lithium-induced HPT, 14 (92 per cent) had adenomas (11 single, 3 double), and one (8 per cent) had four-gland hyperplasia.[32] In contrast, another study using intraoperative PTH (ioPTH) measurement to assess adequacy of resection in 12 patients, found that half had multiglandular disease. Mean ioPTH decrease from baseline following gland resection was 74 ± 4 per cent. Although 10 of 12 patients met criteria for curative resection, only eight remained normocalcaemic. The other two patients, who did not meet criteria, remained normocalcaemic. Of the ten normo-calcaemic patients, four had persistent elevation of PTH. The authors concluded that the incidence of multiglandular disease in lithium-induced HPT is higher than with standard HPT. They also concluded that ioPTH had a limited role in predicting durable normocalcaemia, and that bilateral neck exploration should be considered for these patients.[33]

In a group of 11 patients operated on by a Sydney group, a single adenoma was identified in six patients and multi-glandular disease in five. All subsequently resumed lithium with one developing recurrent HPT at three years, while another after one year had increased PTH, but was normo-calcaemic. They concluded that bilateral neck exploration should be performed routinely because of a relatively high frequency of multiglandular involvement, but that para-thyroid resection should be limited to evident disease.[34]

PARATHYROID LOCALIZATION

Preoperative localization techniques

Until recently, preoperative parathyroid localization techni-ques were employed predominantly when an initial exploration had failed to identify a parathyroid adenoma. However, with the increasing popularity of day-case parathyroidectomy, minimally invasive parathyroidectomy (MIP), targeted resection and parathyroidectomy under local anaesthesia, preoperative localization techniques are more commonly used prior to initial neck exploration. Their routine role still remains controversial as they add both time and expense to overall patient management and many point out that an experienced parathyroid surgeon will cure 95 per cent of patients without the benefit of preoperative localiza-tion, while the most accurate localization techniques will only identify 80 per cent of parathyroid tumours at best. Propo-nents of localization argue that reoperative parathyroid sur-gery can result in recurrent laryngeal nerve palsy rates of up to 7 per cent, and successful preoperative localization brings surgical success rates at initial exploration close to 100 per cent.[35]

SCINTIGRAPHY

Many imaging techniques have been tried in an attempt to improve parathyroid localization. Currently, nuclear scinti-graphy is seen as the most accurate localization technique. Although subtraction scanning with thallium chloride and pertechnetate was first proposed, technetium Tc99m sesta-mibi with either a subtraction technique using for example radioiodine I^{123} or used alone in a 'double-phase scan' where the scan is repeated at 2–3 hours gives the best results (**Figure 27.1**).[36, 37] The double-phase method relies on the differential washout rate of sestamibi from parathyroid tissue compared to thyroid tissue, due to the high metabolic rate of the parathyroids, particularly when adenomatous. Of the two technetium techniques, the subtraction technique is currently superior localizing solitary adenomata in 95 per cent of cases, and multigland disease in 80 per cent.[38]

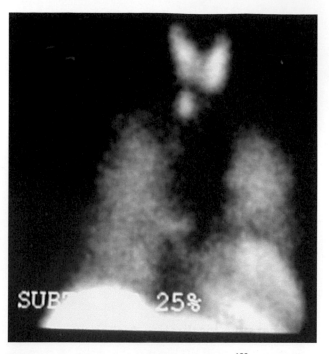

Figure 27.1 Technetium sestamibi scan with I^{123} subtraction demonstrating a large right inferior parathyroid adenoma.

ULTRASONOGRAPHY

Ultrasonography is also a frequently employed imaging modality when localizing parathyroid glands. Results are operator dependent, but in the best hands, solitary adenomas can be identified in 93 per cent of cases using colour Dop-pler.[39] Ultrasound is of limited value when glands are ectopic, particularly when they are located in the mediastinum. In ectopia, nuclear scintigraphy may also be less effective as it provides a planar image and the localization of abnormal glands may be hampered by overlying structures, particularly when the lesion is below the clavicles. Under these circum-stances, three-dimensional imaging techniques, such as single photon emission computed tomography (SPECT) or posi-tron emission tomography (PET) with either (^{18}F)-fluoro-2-deoxy-D-glucose or (^{11}C)-methionine are useful.

COMPUTED TOMOGRAPHY/MAGNETIC RESONANCE IMAGING

T_2-weighted magnetic resonance imaging (MRI) with gado-linium is a useful investigative tool, particularly when other tests have failed or following unsuccessful exploration. It has been shown to be more sensitive than contrast-enhanced computed tomography (CT).

VENOUS SAMPLING

Rarely, when planning revision surgery and when less inva-sive imaging and localization techniques have failed, venous sampling is employed. This involves femoral vein catheter-ization and the collection of blood samples from the draining veins of the thyroid plexus (high internal jugular, low internal jugular, brachiocephalic and subclavian from each side) and the superior vena cava. Intact PTH assays are measured from each sample and a plot of venous PTH:peripheral blood (control) PTH is tabulated. A ratio of two or greater is seen as significant. Using this technique, hyperfunctioning gland position can be predicted with 86 per cent specificity and 95 per cent sensitivity.[40] Interpretation of results is hampered somewhat by the knowledge that the middle and inferior thyroid veins may have been ligated during the previous procedure(s). Nevertheless, it can be useful in lateralizing the rogue gland(s) and determining whether it is higher or lower in the neck or likely to be in the superior mediastinum.

When planning targeted parathyroidectomy, the surgeon will normally only proceed if a technetium Tc99m sestamibi scan is concordant with a high resolution ultrasound scan in localizing the parathyroid tumour.[41] A successful resection can be effectively confirmed with the use of ioPTH, although if preoperative concordant double imaging suggests a solitary adenoma some would argue that this test is unnecessary.[42]

Intraoperative localization techniques

Parathyroid localization may be further enhanced intraoperatively by the use of the gamma probe. First described as a technique useful in both gland ectopia and hyperplasia in 1995, it depends on the identification by a gamma probe of a radioisotope injected preoperatively and selectively concentrated within parathyroid tissue.[43] Technetium 99m sestamibi tends to be the isotope of choice. The procedure depends on strict timing between radioisotope injection and time of surgery, and although not in widespread use has certainly gained some acceptance in MIP.[44]

METHYLENE BLUE

The other intraoperative localization technique employed by some parathyroid surgeons is the use of intravenous methylene blue.[45] This involves the preoperative intravenous administration of 5 mg/kg methylene blue in saline. The dye is preferentially taken up by the parathyroids particularly when adenomatous or hyperplastic, hence making their identification easier. Again, timing of infusion to surgery is crucial. The patient's skin will have a blue hue for a few days following surgery, and there may be some nausea.

SURGICAL ANATOMY

Parathyroid glands are simply called 'parathyroid', because they are 'next to' the thyroid gland (Greek, *para* beside). They develop at weeks 5 to 6 *in utero* from the endoderm of the third and fourth pharyngeal pouches. There are usually two parathyroid glands on each side, a superior and an inferior, although in a series of 547 autopsies Gilmour demonstrated that 87 per cent of patients have four parathyroid glands, 6 per cent three and 6 per cent five.[46]

The superior glands develop from the fourth pouch with the ultimobranchial bodies which form part of the lateral thyroid. Their descent in the neck is more limited and their

position therefore more constant than their inferior counterparts. The superior glands lie in a plane deep to the recurrent laryngeal nerve, but during exploration their position will generally be effectively inverted by retracting the thyroid lobe medially and 'out' of the neck, so that it lies on top of the trachea and its dorsal aspect can be properly inspected. In 80 per cent of cases, therefore, the superior gland is visualized on or just above the recurrent laryngeal nerve at the junction of the middle third and upper third of the thyroid lobe. It is extremely unusual for a normally situated superior gland to lie below the main branch of the inferior thyroid artery, a fact useful in preoperative parathyroid localization. In ectopia, the superior gland may lie in the retro-oesophageal or retropharyngeal gutter having descended posteriomedial to the nerve. This is purely a pulsion effect due to deglutition forcing the enlarging tumour in the direction of least resistance and, in extreme cases, a superior adenoma may be found in the posterior mediastinum.

Due to their joint origin with the ultimobranchial bodies, the superior glands are more likely to become truly intrathyroidal, although inferior parathyroids have certainly been reported within the thyroid parenchyma.[47] In addition, because of the variability in superior and inferior parathyroid development and descent, the relative positions of the parathyroid glands are occasionally reversed, i.e. the superior gland (parathyroid IV) may be more caudal than the inferior gland (parathyroid III). It is probably for this reason that some authors claim that intrathyroidal parathyroids represent ectopic superior glands, while others consider them to represent aberrant inferior glands.

The inferior parathyroids develop together with the thymus from the third pouch. Therefore, during the embryonic descent of the thymus, the inferior parathyroid is usually carried more caudal than the superior gland. The vast majority settle in the neck along this line of descent and separate somewhat from the thymus which continues into the chest leaving a thyrothymic tract in the neck in which the parathyroid is frequently situated. Most frequently located in a position caudal to the inferior aspect of the thyroid lobe, the inferior parathyroids lie in a plane superficial to the recurrent laryngeal nerve. In ectopia, their position is far more variable than the superior glands. They may be discovered as high as the carotid bifurcation and be associated with failure of thymic descent, or they may be more caudal than normal either lying within the substance of the normally situated thymus or more inferior, in the anterior or, more rarely, the posterior mediastinum. They may also be found within the carotid sheath. In 80 per cent of cases, the position of both the superior and inferior glands on each side is symmetrical, a fact that can be useful when a gland is proving hard to locate.

Finally, as the inferior parathyroids normally cross the position of the superior parathyroids during their developmental descent, both sets of glands may be extremely closely related. Therefore, a bilobed gland may be mistaken for two glands and vice versa.

The weight of a normal parathyroid gland may be 10–100 g with an average of 35–40 mg[48, 49] and the combined weight of parathyroid tissue averages 118 mg in men and 131 mg in women. They tend to be larger in those of AfroCaribbean origin, and increase in size with age up to the third and fourth decade. Fat content is highly variable and unevenly distributed throughout the gland.[48] When stimulated, parathyroid glands enlarge and their fat content decreases.

SURGICAL PATHOLOGY

The most common parathyroid tumour, the benign solitary adenoma, occurs with equal frequency in the superior and the inferior glands. A parathyroid adenoma macroscopically appears as an encapsulated tumour which is brown in colour, and normally of a darker shade than the other macroscopically normal glands. During exploration, a parathyroid gland is normally easily differentiated from surrounding structures as it is palpably much softer then thyroid tissue or lymph nodes. It is normally approximately 5–7 mm in its maximal dimension, elliptical in shape, brownish in colour and with fine tortuous vessels on its surface. The normal parathyroid is often within, or surrounded by, a layer of fatty tissue which tends to disappear if the gland becomes adenomatous. When traumatized, a parathyroid gland will bleed freely.

Microscopically, the adenomatous portion of an affected gland is normally made up predominantly of chief cells, although rarely the tumour may consist entirely of water-clear cells. There is a suppressed rim of normal parathyroid tissue around part of the periphery of the tumour, and this is often helpful in differentiating an adenomatous gland from a hyperplastic gland, a distinction that is not always clear cut. For the diagnosis of adenoma to be reliably made and hyperplasia excluded, a biopsy of a second histologically normal gland is generally required.[50]

Chief cell hyperplasia causes approximately 15 per cent of all primary hyperparathyroidism. This condition is a polyclonal cellular expansion resulting in proliferation of chief cells, oncocytes and transitional oncocytes in all glands, hence differing from the monoclonal expansion typical of parathyroid adenoma. Eighty per cent of hyperplasia is sporadic and 20 per cent familial, related to either familial hyperparathyroidism or a multiple endocrine neoplasia syndrome. In extremely rare instances, primary clear cell hyperplasia, which is never familial, may occur.

INTRAOPERATIVE PTH MONITORING

In 1987, the development of a two-site immunochemiluminescent assay for human PTH paved the way for intraoperative PTH monitoring (ioPTH) as a reliable indicator of success during parathyroidectomy.[51] The half-life of PTH is approximately 3–5 minutes and the assay measures the intact PTH molecule with no reaction to PTH fragments, hence avoiding erroneously elevated results of earlier assays. Modifications to the assay procedure have resulted in an approximate turnaround time of 10 minutes, making intraoperative PTH monitoring a realistically useful tool, particularly in minimal access, localized and day-case resections.[52]

The procedure of ioPTH varies slightly from centre to centre depending on the specifics of the immunoassay employed and local experience. An initial baseline blood sample is taken. This ideally is prior to the commencement of surgery (T-0), because it is recognized that manipulation of parathyroid glands intraoperatively can lead to spikes in PTH.[53] Further samples are then taken at 5 (T-5) and 10 (T-10) minutes after removal of each gland. Operative success is predicted if either the T-5 or T-10 sample demonstrates a PTH level 50 per cent or greater below the T-0 level.[54] The procedure indicates long-term operative success with about 95 per cent accuracy in single gland disease.[55] However, the results in multigland disease are less reliable with false-positive decreases occurring in as many as 75 per cent of patients.[56] In addition, recent work suggests that false-positive results, when followed up in the long term, may indicate germline mutations in the gene for multiple endocrine neoplasia, and genetic analysis of these patients is important.[57]

The role of ioPTH in secondary and tertiary HPT is less clear cut. In renal disease, the half-life of PTH is lengthened and there is very little long-term evidence of the predictive capabilities of ioPTH. However, short-term studies suggest that using ioPTH in a similar manner to how it is used in primary HPT is useful.[29] In addition, most work focuses on near total parathyroidectomy, or total parathyroidectomy with reimplantation. This, added to the fact that rests of parathyroid tissue when chronically stimulated by, in most instances, renal failure, can become autonomous, makes it impossible to accurately predict the completeness of the parathyroidectomy. However, recent work suggests that in total parathyroidectomy ioPTH predicts control of hyperparathyroidism, but fails to predict persistent hypoparathyroidism.[58]

Although ioPTH has many advantages, the procedure is expensive. In many institutions, therefore, its use remains controversial and without significant cost decreases is unlikely to become uniform.[59]

SURGICAL TREATMENT OF PRIMARY HYPERPARATHYROIDISM

Once the decision to operate has been made, the type of operation should be determined. In primary HPT, this decision will depend upon both the wishes of the patient and the abilities of the operating surgeon. In 80 per cent of cases, the causative lesion is a solitary parathyroid adenoma, and successful preoperative localization of such a lesion enables the surgeon to offer minimally invasive parathyroidectomy using a targeted approach. In this circumstance, parathyroidectomy under local anaesthesia is possible. The other option is the traditional four-gland exploration involving a bilateral dissection and ideally visualization of all four parathyroid glands. During this operation, the glands judged macroscopically normal are generally marked with a liga clip, and the macroscopically abnormal gland(s) removed and sent for histology. The procedure is often enhanced by intraoperative frozen section and ioPTH, the latter procedure to confirm cure following a successful dissection, or to point to the need for further exploration. Both the targeted approach and the four-gland exploration are performed endoscopically in some centres.

In 15–20 per cent of cases, HPT is caused by parathyroid hyperplasia which may be genetically predetermined. Here, preoperative imaging is far less effective at localizing the causative pathology[60, 61] and a four-gland exploration is generally appropriate. In 80 per cent of hyperplastic patients, the condition is non-familial. In this situation, a subtotal resection removing three and a half glands and leaving approximately 30–50 mg of functional tissue is the best approach as this minimizes the risk of recurrence and the need for reoperation, while preserving parathyroid function.[62]

The technique of parathyroidectomy

FOUR-GLAND EXPLORATION

Although we have mentioned other options, the open four-gland exploration remains the most common parathyroidectomy technique.

In this 'search and destroy' mission, the surgeon requires an orderly and thorough approach and an understanding of the unusual positions of enlarged parathyroids.

The principles

- Dissection should be as bloodless as possible.
- The superior gland is more constant and should be identified first.
- An enlarged parathyroid is easier to identify than a suppressed normal gland.
- Variability in development means that the relative positions of the parathyroids may be reversed, i.e. a missing superior parathyroid may be caudal to an already identified inferior gland and a missing inferior parathyroid more cephalad to the superior gland.
- If an adenoma is identified and not all parathyroids found, thymic delivery can be selective and it is not necessary to remove thyroid tissue.

With the patient in a supine position, and with approximately 30° of reverse Trendelenberg to decrease venous engorgement in the neck, the neck is extended where possible by appropriate placement of a head ring and sandbag. The approach is via a standard Kocher incision that is designed to lie within Langers lines, and is situated midway between the cricoid cartilage and the jugular notch. The incision level is best marked preoperatively with the conscious patient sat in a neutral position. The incision need only be 5 cm in length in most instances. The incision continues through the platysma to the level of the superficial layer of strap muscles and the superior myocutaneous flap is then raised to a level at least 2 cm above the cricoid cartilage. The inferior flap rarely requires raising. The linea alba is then identified and the strap muscles separated. Whether the surgeon goes medial or lateral to the straps is determined by preference, but the lateral approach requires less dissection and is preferred by some.

THE MEDIAL APPROACH

The linea alba is more easily identified caudally as the central straps tend to separate to some extent inferiorly. The procedure then involves peeling the straps off the ventral surface of one of the thyroid lobes, a relatively bloodless procedure which is kept dry by medial retraction on the thyroid lobe and lateral retraction on the straps minimizing the need for sharp dissection. The middle thyroid vein, when present, is then identified and ligated/divided. It is important at this stage to visualize the ventrocaudal surface of the thyroid for the rare ventrally placed parathyroid. The procedure then involves the separation of the thyroid lobe from the many fine fibrous bands that maintain it in its anatomical position. This process is greatly facilitated by medial digital retraction of the thyroid lobe, attempting to mobilize the lobe both medially and upwards out of the tracheo-oesophageal groove and on to the trachea. Simultaneously, the strap muscles are retracted laterally to keep the fibrous bands under tension. Fibrous tissue should divide easily in a previously unexplored neck, and when this does not happen this is because the structure is in fact a small blood vessel under tension and these must be diathermized rather than cut, as the maintenance of a bloodless field is vitally important for successful parathyroid identification. Once the thyroid lobe has been mobilized on to the trachea, it is often held in place by retracting a stay suture placed through it. With simultaneous lateral retraction of the strap muscles, the search for the parathyroid glands can begin.

THE LATERAL APPROACH

A subplatysmal plane is elevated from the thyroid notch above to the sternal notch below and to the medial border of sternomastoid on each side. The lateral approach involves separating the fascia between the sternomastoid and the strap muscles and identification of the carotid sheath more deeply. The omohyoid may require division for optimal exposure. The sternomastoid is retracted laterally and the medial border of the carotid sheath is then easily dissected from the level of the superior pole inferiorly to the level of the inferior thyroid artery. This gives an excellent view of the posterior aspect of the thyroid and the tracheo-oesophageal groove. During the subsequent parathyroid search, if greater exposure is required, it is a simple matter to divide the overlying sternothyroid muscle which gives the same exposure as the medial approach (**Figure 27.2**).

BASIC SEARCH FOR THE SUPERIOR GLAND

The inferior thyroid artery is readily identified deep to the carotid sheath usually around the mid-part of the thyroid lobe and followed bluntly to the thyroid lobe. The recurrent laryngeal nerve is identified (see Thyroidectomy chapter). An enlarged superior gland often descends in the space behind the thyroid lobe and oesophagus and deep to the recurrent laryngeal nerve and inferior thyroid artery. Therefore, the initial inspection of this potential space (retrothyroid/oesophageal) will frequently expose the adenoma. Should this space be empty then a more thorough dissection is employed on the posterior surface of the superior pole with the knowledge that the vast majority of superior parathyroids are within 1 cm of the cricothyroid joint. The next step is further exploration of the recurrent laryngeal nerve which is gently explored including deeply up to the cricothyroid joint. Not only does this decrease the risk to the nerve, but also the

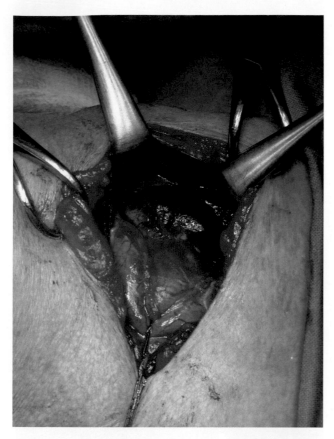

Figure 27.2 Delivering a large adenoma may be facilitated by dividing the strap muscles.

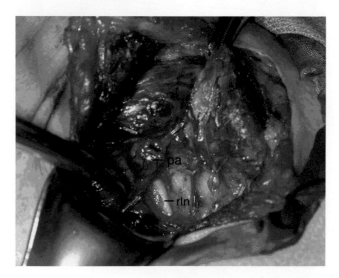

Figure 27.3 Right superior parathyroid adenoma (pa) overlying the recurrent laryngeal nerve (rln).

nerve is a good constant landmark for identification of the superior parathyroid position, and the plane of both superior and inferior glands (**Figure 27.3**). In most instances, the superior gland will be within a fat lobule in the position described. This position is often nicely demonstrated by palpating the area with a pledget and demonstrating differential movement of a subtly darker body within the fat, often with a small vessel on its surface. Blunt dissection is

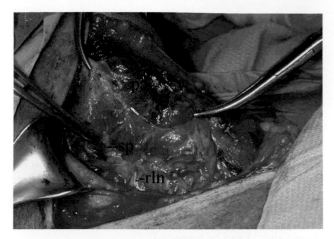

Figure 27.4 Right inferior parathyroid adenoma (pa) lying on the caudal end of the thyroid lobe as it is retracted 'out' of the neck. A normal superior parathyroid in fat (sp) and the recurrent laryngeal nerve (rln) are also highlighted.

employed with pledgets, mosquito forceps and bipolar diathermy division of fine vessels. Usually at this stage the surgeon will have either discovered the adenoma or a normal parathyroid gland, and a liga clip is applied. If not, the inferior gland is then sought.

BASIC SEARCH FOR THE INFERIOR GLAND

Inferior dissection proceeds with mobilization of the inferior pole and inspection particularly in the region of the thyrothymic tract. The inferior gland normally lies on or just below the inferior pole of the thyroid lobe as described, although it is ventral to the coronal plane of the recurrent nerve (**Figure 27.4**). For this reason, excision of an inferior adenoma can often be safely achieved without recurrent nerve identification, as long as the dissection, often with bipolar diathermy forceps, proceeds directly on the surface of the gland.

As the search continues, the tracheo-oesophageal groove is explored deep to the nerve. The examination of this area continues down to the sternal notch. Usually at this stage, both parathyroids will have been exposed, but not always. A small suppressed gland in a normal location may not be obvious, and a normal gland or an adenoma may be present in the thymus, mediastinum, thyroid or an unusual neck location. Rather than continue with further dissection that may devascularize a normal parathyroid, the surgeon proceeds to the opposite side employing the same orderly sequence of dissection and inspection.

FURTHER SEARCH STRATEGIES

After this initial bilateral exploration, in the vast majority of cases an adenoma will have been discovered and no further dissection is considered necessary even if one or more parathyroids remain hidden. The rationale for this is that a thorough exploration has been performed in all areas bar the thymus, the thyroid gland and unusual locations, such as lateral to the carotid sheath, the wall of the pyriform fossa, elsewhere in the neck and mediastinum. The return from further dissection is likely to be small with the added risk of devascularizing a small normal parathyroid. On the other hand, if this initial exploration fails to yield an adenoma, further ordered exploration is necessary, stopping when the adenoma is found. The direction of dissection is determined by what has been found already, but the surgeon must remember that the relative positions of the glands may be reversed.

A missing superior gland is sought around the cricothyroid joint, in the retropharyngeal space down into the posterior mediastinum, on the pharyngeal musculature which is easily separated from underlying mucosa by forceps dissection, and posteromedial to the superior thyroid pedicle back to the carotid sheath and carotid bifurcation. The thyroid should also be suspected.

A missing inferior gland is sought in the thymus, the thyroid and the carotid sheath.

THYMIC EXPLORATION

The thyrothymic tract is followed inferiorly on one side and the thymus gently teased into the neck by dividing the fascial capsule, clamping forceps to the thymic tissue and applying gentle traction. Small gains are accepted before the forceps are reapplied to the thymus more inferiorly. This in turn is put under tension, further fascia divided, small vessels liga-clipped, and the thymus gently lifted further into the neck. The sequence of small gains and reapplication of forceps is continued until the thymic remnant on that side of the neck is delivered (**Figures 27.5** and **27.6**). If the adenoma is found on one side of the thymic remnant and the opposite inferior parathyroid has not been identified, the opposite side of the thymus should be explored (80 per cent rule).

THYROID EXPLORATION

Exploration of the thyroid lobe includes first a reassessment to determine that all fascia has been cleared from the posterior aspect of the thyroid gland. Often a parathyroid may be subcapsular, but not truly intraglandular. Such glands may not be readily identifiable, but the bruising consequent to the initial dissection may highlight the colour and textural differences between thyroid and parathyroid tissue. The parathyroid gland may appear more brownish, reddish, blue or black (from venous congestion). Before proceeding to remove thyroid tissue, if possible the respective internal jugular veins (IJV) should be sampled for ioPTH to give an indication of which side of the neck the adenoma resides. While awaiting the assay, the surgeon should re-examine the retropharyngo-oesophageal region from the hyoid level to the superior mediastinum and similarly, the carotid sheaths. The entire cervical course of the recurrent laryngeal nerve, and tissue deep to it, must be gently exposed bilaterally.

The ioPTH determines which side of the thyroid to explore and if none is available, it is the surgeon's choice. An intra-thyroidal parathyroid is typically in the lower pole and excision of either the entire lobe or the lower two-thirds suffices. The excised thyroid tissue is then finely diced on a side table to determine whether a parathyroid adenoma is present.

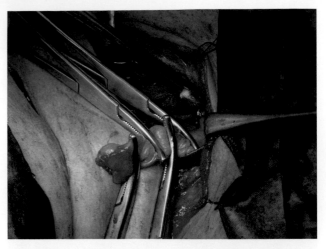

Figure 27.5 Delivery of the thymus during a neck dissection for medullary carcinoma thyroid (using a McFee incision).

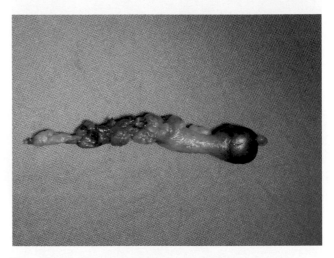

Figure 27.6 Parathyroid adenoma at the caudal end of a thymic remnant.

ACCEPTING FAILURE

In the event of no adenoma being found after the initial bilateral exploration, bilateral thymic delivery and a unilateral total or subtotal lobectomy, the authors do not advocate contralateral lobectomy without definite evidence of a hidden adenoma. The wound is washed and closed with the expectation that the rogue gland is hidden deeper in the mediastinum. Imaging studies and a targeted revision procedure are likely required.

MINIMAL ACCESS PARATHYROIDECTOMY/ VIDEO–ASSISTED/LAPAROSCOPIC PARATHYROIDECTOMY

Although the first parathyroidectomy, carried out in 1925, was under local anaesthesia, until recently the majority of procedures have been formal four-gland explorations under general anaesthesia. However, the development of ioPTH, the gamma probe and preoperative localization techniques have paved the way for novel surgical approaches aimed at minimizing inpatient stay and patient discomfort. This is particularly so as the predominant pathological cause of primary HPT is the solitary adenoma, and hyperplasia is being recognized as an increasingly rarer entity than was first believed.

Minimal access techniques which may be laporoscopic, video-assisted or without endoscopic enhancement normally depend on accurate preoperative localization with technetium 99m sestamibi with or without the additional use of ultrasound to localize the solitary parathyroid tumour. With accurate localization, unilateral explorations and single-gland targeted excisions through incisions of 1.5 cm become realistic options. In some institutions, minimal access video-assisted parathyroidectomy enables a bilateral four-gland exploration through a single medial horizontal 1.5 cm incision.[63] These advances have paved the way to local anaesthetic outpatient procedures producing comparable results to the traditional four-gland technique,[64] although patient selection criteria must be firmly established for such cases and patient suitability varies from 96 to 60 per cent depending on the reporting institution.[41, 65]

AUTOTRANSPLANTATION OF PARATHYROID TISSUE

To avoid the long-term consequences of hypoparathyroidism, whenever aparathyroidism is considered possible after the operation, immediate parathyroid autotransplantation should occur. Some authors will routinely cryopreserve parathyroid tissue, for subsequent autotransplantation if necessary, in all patients who undergo initial neck surgery for multigland hyperplasia and those who undergo reoperation for persistent or recurrent disease.[66]

Normal parathyroid

One intact parathyroid gland is all that is required to maintain calcium homeostasis. It follows that normocalcaemia can be achieved by the presence of an equivalent volume of parathyroid tissue even if in separate locations. Because the autotransplantation of a diced normal parathyroid into a vascular bed of connective tissue leads to a variable survival rate, to maximize the number of surviving parathyroid cells, any normal but devascularized parathyroid gland should be reimplanted.

The implanted cells are then under the same feedback mechanisms as they were in an intact gland. If there is initially a reduced take, one could expect that the resultant hypocalcaemia would lead to increased parathyroid cell growth, increased PTH production and increased secretion. However, in the postoperative setting, patients are not left to become hypocalcaemic. The best approach would seem to be to keep the serum calcium in the low–normal range so that there is a continuing stimulation.

Hyperplastic tissue

Autotransplantation of parathyroid cells in this situation differs from the above in that these cells are genetically altered

to have fewer CSRs and generally also have elevated set-points. They are therefore predetermined to proliferate and to secrete a greater than normal amount of PTH for a given calcium level. They are well suited for autotransplantation.

It is recommended that approximately 60 mg of diced hyperplastic parathyroid (15–20 1-mm^3 cubes) be implanted into muscle.[66] Others advocate 30 fragments, aiming to approximate two to three normal parathyroid glands.[30] Transplantation may be into the non-dominant brachioradialis for ease of access and facilitation of postoperative monitoring, or into the sternomastoid or deltoid. The transplantation site is marked with three liga clips orientated at 90° to one another.

Success rates are in the order of 30 per cent complete, 20 per cent partial, 40 per cent failure, 7 per cent hypercalcaemia, regardless of whether the autotransplantation is done immediately or subsequently with cryopreserved tissue. These rates remain unchanged with subsequent autotransplantation of cryopreserved tissue after an initial failure and appear to be independent of operator experience.[66]

Recent studies suggest that implantation into subcutaneous fat is as reliable and is certainly easier to do.[29]

CRYOPRESERVATION

Cryopreservation must be determined prior to surgery and scheduled with the regional tissue bank which will have a strict protocol.

As the parathyroid will be stored in a freezer along with other quarantined tissue, the tissue bank will require notification of any infectious disease (AIDS, hepatitis B, hepatitis C) and the risk profile for such diseases, for example, intravenous drug user, clotting disorder, risk profile for Creutzfeldt–Jakob disease (CJD). Prior to the surgery, a questionnaire must be completed by the patient concerning the risk profile and also consent for the disposal of unwanted tissue.

The tissue bank provides small vials on ice, containing cold parathyroid medium to transport the tissue.

Prior to removal of the gland for autotransplantation, the surgeon may wish to confirm that it is indeed parathyroid tissue with frozen section. If not, a small piece should still be sent in formalin to confirm its nature.

Once removed, the gland is cut it into approximately 1-mm^3 pieces and separated into a small number of the containers. Two 10 mL clotted blood samples for routine infectious screening are required, again because the tissue will be alongside other quarantined tissue. The containers are transferred to the tissue bank where they are placed in a controlled rate freezer, dropping the temperature 1 °C per minute down to −140 °C. Thereafter they are stored at −180 °C in liquid nitrogen for a determined period (usually three months). If stored beyond six months, a follow-up blood sample for infectious screening is required, again to assess infectious risk.

Should the tissue be required, it is thawed by the tissue bank by placing the containers in a 37 °C waterbath and gently agitating till thawed. The tissue is then washed repeatedly with a specific medium, resuspended in saline and transported to the surgeon for reimplantation.

POSTOPERATIVE HYPOCALCAEMIA

Symptoms of postoperative hypocalcaemia may develop due to a number of factors, as follows.

Temporary threshold shift

Patients with long-standing HPT, particularly with severe hypercalcaemia, may develop symptoms of hypocalcaemia even when the postoperative calcium is within the normal range presumably due to a temporary shift in what is perceived to be an optimal calcium level by nerves and muscles.

Hungry bone syndrome

Long-standing HPT causes a chronic stimulation of osteoclastic release of calcium from the skeleton. Removal of the source of elevated PTH brings about a sudden change in bone metabolism with increased calcium uptake into the skeleton leading to serum hypocalcaemia, but normal to high normal PTH levels.

Temporary hypoparathyroidism

Temporary hypoparathyroidism occurs due to manipulation and subsequent hypofunction of already suppressed parathyroid tissue leading to hypocalcaemia. In this era of miniparathyroid operations for primary HPT where dissection is confined to the adenomatous gland, injury to the other parathyroids and subsequent temporary HPT is much less frequent.

Permanent hypoparathyroidism

This can occur where a bilateral operation (single or staged) has removed or destroyed more than three parathyroid glands. In primary HPT, it is obviously more common in revision procedures where the adenoma may be the sole parathyroid remnant following earlier unsuccessful procedures. In tertiary HPT, permanent hypoparathyroidism is the aim of total parathyroidectomy (but not of subtotal).

MANAGEMENT OF POSTOPERATIVE CALCIUM LEVELS

Generally speaking, only symptomatic hypocalcaemia is treated. For those patients with an apparent threshold shift, the symptoms tend to resolve after a day or so. Either no treatment or oral calcium supplements for a week will suffice.

Hypocalcaemia whether from hungry bone syndrome or temporary hypoparathyroidism usually only lasts for days or weeks. In mild cases, calcium supplementation alone resolves symptoms, although more severe cases require calcitriol in addition.

The most complex patients to manage are those following parathyroidectomy for tertiary HPT. These cases have a threshold shift, hungry bones, permanent hypoparathyroidism and frequently autotransplanted tissue with an altered set-point.

Hypoparathyroidism is considered permanent to some degree when calcium and/or vitamin D supplementation is still required at three months.

PROTOCOL

Miniparathyroid surgery

A baseline calcium and PTH level is taken at the completion of parathyroid surgery. Further blood samples are taken according to patient symptoms. Generally, a further sample is taken the following morning either as an outpatient or inpatient.

Bilateral exploration or revision parathyroidectomy

Where there is the possibility of permanent hypoparathyroidism, serum calcium and perhaps also PTH is checked again approximately 12-hourly or twice daily. It is the trend in serum calcium that indicates the likely course of action. An initial low postoperative result may be due to dilutional effects and a further sample 6 hours later will determine whether there is a trend downwards or not. In the modern climate of day-stay and short-stay surgery, a downward trend is best managed with supplementation for a week or longer with twice weekly calcium checks. Treatment can be with oral calcium alone (1 g three times a day or 2 g twice a day) if the calcium level hovers around 2 mmol/L and above, otherwise calcitriol is added. Typically calcitriol 0.25 µg twice a day will control most, but some patients require 0.5 µg twice a day (occasionally, even more frequently).

Surgery for tertiary HPT

These complex patients are best managed on a renal ward in the perioperative period with regular input by the surgical team. On the night prior to surgery, to minimize the expected drop in serum calcium, these patients are admitted and given oral calcitriol 2 µg.

At the completion of surgery, blood should be taken for serum calcium and PTH with treatment dictated by the former. In this situation, intraoperative PTH is less reliable in assessing whether there has been complete removal of parathyroid tissue primarily because of the high initial PTH values. These are often in excess of 100 pmol/L (normal, 1.1–6.8) meaning that five half-lives or approximately 25 minutes is required before the second sample can be taken. Then there is the wait for the assay, meaning a total waiting time of 45–60 minutes. While tempting, a second sample taken after just one half-life may yield a halving of the initial PTH value yet the PTH fail to normalize due to a persisting hyperplastic parathyroid.

Following surgery and after confirmation of an aparathyroid patient, oral calcitriol 2 µg twice a day and calcium

1 g twice a day is continued. Serum calcium is checked 6 hours after surgery. A calcium infusion is required if serum calcium is less than 1.9 mmol/L and the oral doses may also require an increase. Regular serum checks continue.

Where autotransplantation has occurred and following discharge, serum calcium and PTH is checked twice weekly with the expectation that transplanted tissue will resume function 3–4 weeks post-surgery. Approximately 30 per cent of these patients will ultimately maintain a normal calcium level without supplementation, 20 per cent will continue to require some supplementation and 7 per cent will overproduce.

MANAGEMENT OF ACUTE HYPERCALCAEMIA

Severe hypercalcaemia is a rare but life-threatening complication of hyperparathyroidism. As the calcium level rises, the patient complains of thirst and polyuria with general malaise. However, as the condition worsens, the patient becomes gradually more confused and the conscious level decreases, finally resulting in coma. In this rare situation, acute medical intervention is necessary to prevent death and enable the underlying diagnosis to be confirmed and treated. As a rule of thumb, a patient with an adjusted serum calcium of 3.50 mmol/L or greater should be considered a metabolic emergency.[67]

The first treatment step should be to rehydrate the patient with isotonic saline. This will increase glomerular filtration rate and reduce sodium and hence calcium reabsorption. Serum calcium levels will also reduce due to the dilutional effect. Patients will symptomatically improve, but the effect will be short-lived. The addition of loop diuretics once rehydration has occurred can increase the rate of urinary calcium excretion, however, this must be done with care so as not to exacerbate dehydration.

Second-line therapy includes the use of calcitonin due to its inhibitory effect on osteoclasts. An initial rapid decrease in serum calcium may be achieved, but this is only maintained for up to 72 hours.[68] Glucocorticoids are also used as they inhibit vitamin D conversion to calcitriol. In rare instances, mithramycin, which is cytotoxic to osteoclasts and gallium nitrate, which inhibits osteoclast action, are used.[69] However, bisphosphonates provide the mainstay drug therapy for the management of severe hypercalcaemia. They decrease osteoclastic bone resorption and, although their speed of onset is slower than some other therapies, their duration of action is longer, the effect of pamidronate lasting a mean 28 days.[70] Because of their relatively slower speed of action, many advocate simultaneous bisphosphonate and calcitonin therapy.

SURGICAL FAILURE AND REOPERATIVE PARATHYROID SURGERY

The reasons for surgical failure in order of frequency are: inadequate cervical exploration, failure to diagnose or adequately resect multigland disease, gland ectopia and wrong diagnosis. It is vitally important to maximize surgical success rates at first operation, because surgical risks increase with further surgery. In addition, revision parathyroidectomy is less successful than first surgery with success rates ranging from 65 to 98 per cent.[71, 72, 73]

When failure occurs, the first step is to reconfirm the diagnosis. Other potential diagnoses, in particular FHH, pseudohyperparathyroidism and sarcoidosis must be excluded. Second, the requirement for curative surgery must be re-evaluated and its necessity reconfirmed. Patients without bony or renal complications, or normocalcaemic patients with an elevated PTH, for example, may opt to be observed rather than to undergo further surgery with increased complication rates and decreased cure rates. If re-exploration is judged appropriate, the histological specimens and operative notes from the first exploration should be examined, as these will often help in pointing to the likely location of the missing gland.

Preoperatively in revision surgery, attempts at localization are mandatory. High resolution ultrasound and technetium sestamibi scanning are the most common modalities used. If a mediastinal location is suspected, contrast-enhanced CT with technetium sestamibi scanning demonstrate the best sensitivities at 92 and 85 per cent, respectively.[74] MRI and highly selective venous sampling are also sometimes employed, and when other imaging techniques have failed ^{11}C-methionine PET has proved useful, however, this modality is not readily available.[75]

The operative procedure is often via a lateral approach dissecting in a plane between sternomastoid and the straps, and identifying the carotid sheath first. This avoids an approach through a densely scarred midline and enables the surgeon to localize normal landmarks early. The position and pathology of parathyroid disease varies at reoperation from centre to centre, but the overall percentage of hyperplastic glands is increased. The majority of reoperative pathologies are accessible by the transcervical approach. Akerstrom and Juhlin[76] pooled data from eight series and the positions of glands found at reoperation are demonstrated in **Table 27.1**. In the event of failure to find the pathological gland(s) at reoperation, all the likely ectopic sites should be explored and if the gland is still not evident, thyroid lobectomy on the side of the missing gland is justified as is transcervical thymectomy, if not previously performed. Ideally, ioPTH will be available and if the levels remain high, then intraoperative ultrasound and selective venous sampling are sometimes used.

Prior to reoperative surgery, the patient must be made aware of the increased risks to the recurrent laryngeal nerve, of failure and of permanent hypoparathyroidism.

Table 27.1 Percentage of parathyroid glands found in each anatomical position at reoperation.

Superior glands (%)	Inferior glands (%)
Normal position (40)	Normal position (39)
Retro/tracheo-oesophageal groove (17)	Intrathymic (46)
Posterior superior mediastinum (40)	Mediastinal (not in thymus) (3)
Intrathyroidal (1.5)	Intrathyroidal (7)
Carotid sheath (1.5)	Undescended (4)
	Carotid sheath (1)

PARATHYROID CARCINOMA

Parathyroid carcinoma (PC) is extremely rare, comprising less than 1 per cent of all hyperparathyroid presentations. Its incidence in Italy and Japan, however, seems to be higher (approximately 5 per cent).[77] Unlike benign hyperparathyroidism where there is a female predominance, its sex ratio is the same with a median age of occurrence of between 45 and 51 years.[78] Although rare, suspicion should be raised if calcium and parathyroid hormone levels are particularly high. The tumour is also often palpable (in 45 per cent of cases in the Mayo series[79]), which is not the case with benign parathyroid adenomata. In addition, patients with parathyroid carcinoma tend to be more symptomatic, having a high incidence of renal dysfunction, osteoporosis and gastrointestinal symptoms.[80] It seems that most cases of parathyroid carcinoma are idiopathic, although there are some reports suggesting that its incidence is raised in those who have undergone neck irradiation in the distant past. Molecular studies suggest that several genetic mutations are necessary in the pathogenesis of parathyroid carcinoma involving cyclin D1 on chromosome 13, the retinoblastoma and the p53 tumour suppressor genes.[77] More recently, the HRPT2 gene has been implicated in its pathogenesis and may provide a future genetic target.[81]

As with benign primary HPT, the only curative treatment modality for this condition is surgery. However, it is usually not possible to obtain a preoperative diagnosis of parathyroid carcinoma, and therefore for optimal outcome, intraoperative recognition is of the utmost importance.

The standard surgical treatment for this condition involves the en bloc resection of the tumour mass, together with the ipsilateral thyroid lobe and all other involved structures therefore avoiding transgression of the tumour capsule (**Figure 27.7**). Because of the difficulty of preoperative diagnosis, many patients require revision surgeries (60 per cent in the Mayo series). The usefulness of postoperative radiotherapy is debatable. Traditionally, PC is seen as radioresistant, but some retrospective data appear to suggest it is an effective treatment modality.[82] Ajuvant chemotherapy seems to confer short-lived, if any, benefit.[83]

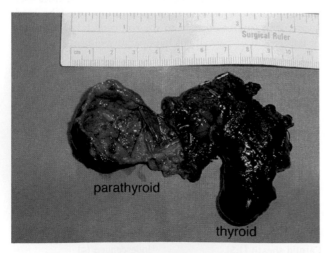

Figure 27.7 En bloc resection of malignant parathyroid tumour with ipsilateral thyroid lobe.

Ultimately, patients who die of PC do so from the effects of hypercalcaemia. Local recurrences should therefore be treated by further surgical resection, and bisphosphonates and calcimimetics are useful for symptom control.

KEY EVIDENCE

- In the presence of hypercalcaemia, an 'inappropriately' normal or elevated parathyroid hormone (PTH) level is indicative of hyperparathyroidism (HPT). Patients with nonparathyroid hypercalcaemia virtually always have PTH values below 25 pg/mL.[6]
- As many as 27 per cent of patients judged asymptomatic deteriorate over a ten-year period and eventually require surgery.[24]

KEY LEARNING POINTS

- Parathyroid tumours are benign in 99 per cent of cases or more.
- Parathyroid tumours are the most common cause of hypercalcaemia. The second most common cause is disseminated malignancy which should always be remembered.
- Primary hyperparathyroidism is diagnosed in relatively asymptomatic patients in 75 per cent of cases; there are well-recognized guidelines for when to advise surgery in these patients.
- Primary hyperparathyroidism is common in the over 60s, but occurs in all age groups.
- Renal failure is the most common, but not the only, cause of secondary hyperparathyroidism.
- Tertiary hyperparathyroidism is the continuation of hyperparathyroidism, once the extraneous stimulus causing secondary hyperparathyroidism has been removed.

REFERENCES

1. Bas S, Aguilera-Tejero E, Bas A et al. The influence of the progression of secondary hyperparathyroidism on the set-point of the parathyroid hormone-calcium curve. *Journal of Endocrinology* 2005; **184**: 241–7.
2. Kinugasa E, Akizawa T, Koshikawa S. Parathyroid function in end-stage renal failure. *Journal of Bone and Mineral Metabolism* 1993; **2**: S53–S58.
3. Silverberg SJ, Bilezikian JP. Evaluation and management of primary hyperparathyroidism. *Journal of Clinical Endocrinology and Metabolism* 1996; **81**: 2036–40.
4. Heath H, Hodgson SF, Kennedy M. Primary hyperparathyroidism: Incidence, morbidity, and potential

economic impact in a community. *New England Journal of Medicine* 1980; **302**: 189–93.

5. LoCascio V, Adami S, Galvanini G *et al*. Substrate-product relation of 1-hydroxylase activity in primary hyperparathyroidism. *New England Journal of Medicine* 1985; **313**: 1123–5.

6. Grant FD, Conlin PR, Brown EM. Complete rate and concentration dependence of parathyroid hormone dynamics during stepwise changes in serum ionized calcium in normal humans. *Journal of Clinical Endocrinology and Metabolism* 1990; **71**: 370–8.

7. Ratcliffe WA, Hutchesson CJ, Bundred NJ, Ratcliffe JG. Role of assays of parathyroid-hormone-related protein in investigation of hypercalcaemia. *Lancet* 1992; **339**: 164–7.

8. Silverberg SJ, Shane E, Jacobs TP *et al*. Nephrolithiasis and bone involvement in primary hyperparathyroidism. *American Journal of Medicine* 1990; **89**: 327–34.

9. Marx SJ, Stock JL, Attie MF *et al*. Familial hypocalciuric hypercalcemia: recognition among patients referred after unsuccessful parathyroid exploration. *Annals of Internal Medicine* 1980; **92**: 351–6.

10. Garfinkel PE, Ezrin C, Stancer HC. Hypothyroidism and hyperparathyroidism associated with lithium. *Lancet* 1973; **11**: 331–2.

11. Goodman WG, Misra S, Veldhuis JD *et al*. Altered diurnal regulation of blood ionized calcium and serum parathyroid hormone concentrations during parenteral nutrition. *American Journal of Clinical Nutrition* 2000; **71**: 560–8.

12. Rodriguez M, Almaden Y, Hernandez A, Torres A. Effect of phosphate on the parathyroid gland: direct and indirect? *Current Opinion in Nephrology and Hypertension* 1996; **5**: 321–8.

13. Chattopadhyay N. Biochemistry, physiology and pathophysiology of the extracellular calcium-sensing receptor. *International Journal of Biochemistry and Cellular Biology* 2000; **32**: 789–804.

14. Bendz H, Sjodin I, Aurell M. Renal function on and off lithium in patients treated with lithium for 15 years or more. A controlled, prospective lithium-withdrawal study. *Nephrology, Dialysis, Transplantation* 1996; **11**: 457–60.

15. Haden ST, Stoll AL, McCormick S *et al*. Alterations in parathyroid dynamics in lithium-treated subjects. *Journal of Clinical Endocrinology and Metabolism* 1997; **82**: 2844–8.

16. Brochier T, Adnet-Kessous J, Barillot M, Pascalis JG. Hyperparathyroidism with lithium. *Encephale* 1994; **20**: 339–49.

17. Nielsen JL, Pedersen EB, Amdisen A, Darling S. Reduced renal calcium exretion during lithium therapy. *Psychopharmacology* 1977; **54**: 101–3.

18. Tahara H, Arnold A. Molecular basis of hyperparathyroidism. *Journal of Bone and Mineral Metabolism* 1997; **15**: 173–8.

19. Carling T, Udelsman R. Parathyroid surgery in familial hyperparathyroid disorders. *Journal of Internal Medicine* 2005; **257**: 27–37.

20. Marx SJ, Simonds WF, Agarwal SK *et al*. Hyperparathyroidism in hereditary syndromes: special expressions and special managements. *Journal of Bone and Mineral Research* 2002; **17**: N37–43.

21. Brass EP. Effects of antihypertensive drugs on endocrine function. *Drugs* 1984; **27**: 447–58.

22. Locker FG, Silverberg SJ, Bilezikian JP. Optimal dietary calcium intake in primary hyperparathyroidism. *American Journal of Medicine* 1997; **102**: 543–50.

23. Orr-Walker B, Evans M, Clearwater J *et al*. Effects of hormone replacement therapy on bone mineral density in postmenopausal women with primary hyperparathyroidism. *Archives of Internal Medicine* 2000; **160**: 2161–6.

● 24. Silverberg SJ, Shane E, Jacobs TP *et al*. A 10-year prospective study of primary hyperparathyroidism with or without parathyroid surgery. *New England Journal of Medicine* 1999; **341**: 1249–55.

25. Bilezikian JP, Potts JT Jr. Asymptomatic primary hyperparathyroidism: new issues and new questions – bridging the past with the future. *Journal of Bone and Mineral Research* 2002; **17**: N57–N67.

26. Pasieka JL, Parsons LL. A prospective surgical outcome study assessing the impact of parathyroidectomy on symptoms in patients with secondary and tertiary hyperparathyroidism. *Surgery* 2000; **128**: 531–9.

27. Yu I, DeVita M, Komisar A. Long-term follow-up after subtotal parathyroidectomy in patients with renal failure. *Laryngoscope* 1998; **108**: 1824–8.

28. Chou FF, Ho JC, Huang SC, Sheen-Chen SM. A study of pruritus after parathyroidectomy for secondary hyperparathyroidism. *Journal of the American College of Surgeons* 2000; **190**: 65–70.

29. Chou FF, Lee CH, Chen JB *et al*. Intraoperative parathyroid hormone measurement in patients with secondary hyperparathyroidism. *Archives of Surgery* 2002; **137**: 341–4.

30. Milas M, Weber C. Near-total parathyroidectomy is beneficial for patients with secondary and teriary hyperparathyroidism. *Surgery* 2004; **136**: 1252–60.

● 31. Quiros RM, Alef MJ, Wilhelm SM *et al*. Health-related quality of life in hyperparathyroidism measurably improves after parathyroidectomy. *Surgery* 2003; **134**: 675–83.

32. Awad SS, Miskulin J, Thompson N. Parathyroid adenomas versus four-gland hyperplasia as the cause of primary hyperparathyroidism in patients with prolonged lithium therapy. *World Journal of Surgery* 2003; **27**: 486–8.

33. Hundley JC, Woodrum DT, Saunders BD *et al*. Revisiting lithium associated hyperparathyroidism in the era of intraoperative parathyroid hormone monitoring. *Surgery* 2005; **138**: 1027–32.

34. Abdullah H, Bliss R, Guinea AI, Delbridge L. Pathology and outcome of surgical treatment for lithium-associated hyperparathyroidsim. *British Journal of Surgery* 1999; **86**: 91–3.

35. Patow CA, Norton JA, Brennan MF. Vocal cord paralysis and reoperative parathyroidectomy. *Annals of Surgery* 1986; **203**: 282–5.

36. Thule P, Thakore K, Vansant J *et al.* Preoperative localization of parathyroid tissue with technetium-99m sestamibi-123-I subtraction scanning. *Journal of Clinical Endocrinology and Metabolism* 1994; **78**: 77–82.

37. Taillefer R, Boucher Y, Potvin C, Lambert R. Detection and localization of parathyroid adenomas in patients with hyperparathyroidism using a single radionuclide imaging procedure with technetium-99m-sestamibi (double phase study). *Journal of Nuclear Medicine* 1992; **33**: 1801–7.

38. Hindie E, Melliere D, Perlemuter L *et al.* Primary hyperparathyroidism: Higher success rate of first surgery after preoperative Tc-99m sestamibi-I-123 subtraction scanning. *Radiology* 1997; **204**: 221–8.

39. Reeder SB, Desser TS, Weigel RJ *et al.* Sonography in primary hyperparathyroidism. Review with emphasis on scanning technique. *Journal of Ultrasound in Medicine* 2002; **21**: 539–52.

40. Chaffanjon CJ, Voirin D, Vasdev A *et al.* Selective venous sampling in recurrent and persistent hyperparathyroidism: indication, technique, and results. *World Journal of Surgery* 2004; **28**: 958–61.

● 41. Inabnet WB, Fulla Y, Luton LP *et al.* Unilateral neck exploration under local anaesthesia: the approach of choice for asymptomatic primary hyperparathyroidism. *Surgery* 1999; **126**: 1004–9.

42. Stalberg P, Sidhu S, Sywak M *et al.* Intraoperative parathyroid hormone measurement during minimally invasive parathyroidectomy: does it 'value-add' to decision making? *Journal of the American College of Surgeons* 2006; **203**: 1–6.

43. Martinez DA, King DR, Romshe C *et al.* Intraoperative identification of parathyroid gland pathology: a new approach. *Journal of Pediatric Surgery* 1995; **30**: 1306–9.

44. Martinez DA, King DR, Romshe C *et al.* Experienced radio-guided surgery teams can successfully perform minimally invasive radio-guided parathyroidectomy without intraoperative parathyroid hormone assays. *American Surgeon* 2006; **72**: 785–9.

● 45. Dudley NE. Methylene blue for rapid identification of parathyroids. *British Medical Journal* 1971; **3**: 680–1.

● 46. Gilmour JR. The normal histology of the parathyroid glands. *Journal of Pathology and Bacteriology* 1937; **45**: 507–22 and **48**: 187–222.

47. Thompson NW, Eckhauser FE. Harness JK. The anatomy of primary hyperparathyroidism. *Surgery* 1982; **92**: 814–21.

48. Ghandur-Mnaymneh L, Cassady J, Hajianpour MA *et al.* The parathyroid gland in health and disease. *American Journal of Pathology* 1986; **125**: 292–9.

49. Wang CA. Parathyroid re-exploration: A clinical and pathological study of 112 cases. *Annals of Surgery* 1977; **186**: 140–5.

♦ 50. Lewis PD. Surgical pathology of the parathyroids in primary and secondary hyperparathyroidism. *Surgical Endocrinology* 1993; **31**: 370–9.

● 51. Brown RC, Aston JP, Weeks I *et al.* Circulating intact parathyroid hormone measured by a two-site immunochemiluminometric assay. *Journal of Clinical Endocrinology and Metabolism* 1987; **65**: 407–14.

52. Vignale E, Picone A, Materazzi G *et al.* A quick intraoperative parathyroid hormone assay in the surgical management of patients with primary hyperparathyroidism: a study of 206 consecutive cases. *European Journal of Endocrinology* 2002; **146**: 783–8.

● 53. Irvin GL, Molinari AS, Figueroa C. Improved success rate in reoperative parathyroidectomy with intraoperative PTH assay. *Annals of Surgery* 1999; **229**: 874–8.

54. Irvin GL, Dembrow VD, Prudhomme DL. Operative monitoring of parathyroid gland hyperfunction. *American Journal of Surgery* 1991; **162**: 299–302.

55. Westerdahl J, Lindblom P, Bergenfelz A. Measurement of intraoperative parathyroid hormone predicts long-term operative success. *Archives of Surgery* 2002; **137**: 186–90.

56. Clerici T, Brandle M, Lange J. Impact of intraoperative parathyroid hormone monitoring on the prediction of multiglandular parathyroid disease. *World Journal of Surgery* 2004; **28**: 187–92.

57. Westerdahl J, Bergenfelz A. Parathyroid surgical failures with sufficient decline of intraoperative parathyroid hormone levels: unobserved multiple endocrine neoplasia as an explanation. *Archives of Surgery* 2006; **141**: 589–94.

58. Roshan A, Kamath B, Roberts S *et al.* Intra-operative parathyroid hormone monitoring in secondary hyperparathyroidism: is it useful? *Clinical Otology* 2006; **31**: 198–203.

59. Ferzli G, Patel S, Graham A *et al.* Three new tools for parathyroid surgery: expensive and unnecessary? *Journal of the American College of Surgeons* 2004; **18**: 526–8.

60. Nguyen BD. Parathyroid imaging with Tc-99m sestamibi planar and SPECT scintigraphy. *Radiographics* 1999; **19**: 601–14.

61. Palestro CJ, Tomas MB, Tronco GG. Radionuclide imaging of the parathyroid glands. *Seminars in Nuclear Medicine* 2005; **35**: 266–76.

62. Wang CA, Castleman B, Cope O. Surgical management of hyperparathyroidism due to primary hyperplasia. *Annals of Surgery* 1982; **195**: 384–92.

● 63. Miccoli P, Berti P, Materazzi G *et al.* Results of video-assisted parathyroidectomy: single institution's six-year experience. *World Journal of Surgery* 2004; **28**: 1216–18.

64. Udelsman R. Six hundred and fifty-six consecutive explorations for primary hyperparathyroidism. *Annals of Surgery* 2002; **235**: 665–70.

65. Rubello G, Giannini S, De Carlo E *et al.* Minimally invasive (99m) Tc-sestamibi radioguided surgery of parathyroid adenomas. *Panminerva Medica* 2005; **47**: 99–107.

66. Feldman AL, Sharaf RN, Skarulis MC *et al.* Results of heterotopic parathyroid autotransplantation: A 13 year experience. *Surgery* 1999; **126**: 1042–7.

67. Swan JW, Stevenson JC. The medical management of hypercalcaemia. In: Lynn J, Bloom SR (ed.). *Surgical endocrinology.* Oxford: Butterworth Heinemann, 1993: 341–50.

68. Binstock ML, Mundy GR. Effect of calcitonin and glucocorticoids in combination on the hypercalcaemia of malignancy. *Annals of Internal Medicine* 1980; **93**: 269–72.

69. Carroll MF, Schade DS. A practical approach to hypercalcaemia. *American Family Physician* 2003; **67**: 1959–66.

70. Clines GA, Guise TA. Hypercalcaemia of malignanacy and basic research on mechanisms responsible for osteolytic and osteoblastic metastasis to bone. *Endocrine-Related Cancer* 2005; **12**: 549–83.

● 71. Low RA, Katz AD. Parathyroidectomy via bilateral cervical exploration: a retrospective review of 866 cases. *Head and Neck* 1998; **20**: 583–7.

72. Shen W, Duren M, Morita E *et al.* Reoperation for persistent or recurrent primary hyperparathyroidism. *Archives of Surgery* 1996; **131**: 861–7.

73. Järhult J, Nordenström J, Perbeck L. Reoperation for suspected primary hyperparathyroidism. *British Journal of Surgery* 1993; **80**: 453–6.

74. Nwariaku FE, Snyder WH, Burkey SH *et al.* Inframanubrial parathyroid glands in patients with primary hyperparathyroidism: alternatives to sternotomy. *World Journal of Surgery* 2005; **29**: 491–4.

75. Beggs AD, Hain SF. Localization of parathyroid adenomas using 11C-methionine positron emission tomography. *Nuclear Medicine Communications* 2005; **26**: 133–6.

76. Akerstrom G, Juhlin C. Reoperation in primary hyperparathyroidism. In: Akerstrom G (ed.). *Current controversy in parathyroid operation and reoperation.* Austin, TX: RG Landes, 1994: 131–65.

♦ 77. Lumachi F, Basso SM, Basso U. Parathyroid cancer: etiology, clinical presentation and treatment. *Anticancer Research* 2006; **26**: 4803–7.

78. Fraker DL. Parathyroid tumors. In: DeVita VT Jr, Hellmann S, Rosenberg SA (eds). *Cancer: principles and practice of oncology.* Philadelphia: Lippincott Williams & Wilkins, 2005: 1521–7.

79. Wynne AG, van Heerden J, Carney JA, Fitzpatrick LA. Parathyroid carcinoma: clinical and pathologic features in 43 patients. *Medicine* 1992; **71**: 197–205.

80. Chiofalo MG, Scognamiglio F, Losito S *et al.* Huge parathyroid carcinoma: clinical considerations and literature review. *World Journal of Surgical Oncology* 2005; **3**: 39.

81. Rawat N, Khetan N, Williams DW, Baxter JN. Parathyroid carcinoma. *British Journal of Surgery* 2005; **92**: 1345–53.

82. Busaidy NL, Jimenez C, Habra MA *et al.* Parathyroid carcinoma: a 22-year experience. *Head and Neck* 2004; **26**: 716–26.

83. Rodgers SE, Perrier ND. Parathyroid carcinoma. *Current Opinion in Oncology* 2006; **18**: 16–22.

28

Pituitary tumours

ALAN JOHNSON AND SHAHZADA AHMED

INTRODUCTION

Here in this well-concealed spot, almost to be covered by a thumb nail, lies the very mainspring of primitive existence – vegetative, emotional, reproductive – on which, with more or less success, man has come to superimpose a cortex of inhibitions.

Harvey Cushing, 1912

The pituitary gland is often known as the conductor of the endocrine orchestra because of its widespread effects on endocrine function. It consists of an anterior part, the 'adenohypophysis', and a posterior part, the 'neurohypophysis'. The gland is attached to the hypothalamus by the pituitary stalk. It is situated in a midline bony recess, the sella turcica, at the posterior superior corner of the sphenoid bone, a position which is in the middle of the head.

The adenohypophysis secretes a range of hormones with critical effects. Adrenocorticotrophic hormone (ACTH) acts on the adrenal cortex which secretes glucocorticoids, mineralocorticoids and androgens; thyroid-stimulating hormone (TSH) acts on the thyroid gland to stimulate thyroid hormone release; prolactin stimulates lactation; follicle-stimulating hormone (FSH) and luteinizing hormone (LH) control sexual and reproductive function; and growth hormone (GH) regulates growth before the epiphyses close and may have an effect on well-being throughout life.

The hypothalamus controls most anterior pituitary function by releasing hormones into a portal circulation which originates there and carries regulating hormones down the stalk to the cells of the adenohypophysis.

The neurohypophysis is made up of axons from the supraoptic and paraventricular nuclei of the hypothalamus which run through the stalk to the posterior pituitary. This part secretes oxytocin (causing milk ejection during lactation and uterine contraction during labour) and vasopressin or antidiuretic hormone (ADH), which stimulates the distal convoluted tubules and medullary collecting ducts in the kidney to reabsorb water.

The great majority of pituitary tumours arise within the adenohypophysis, but some arise within adjacent structures. Because most arise within the gland, this chapter concentrates on these tumours, their effects and their management.

ANATOMY OF THE PITUITARY GLAND

The gland lies in the sella turcica, a midline saddle-shaped bony recess in the posterior superior corner of the sphenoid sinuses (**Figure 28.1**). The anterior lobe, made up of the pars

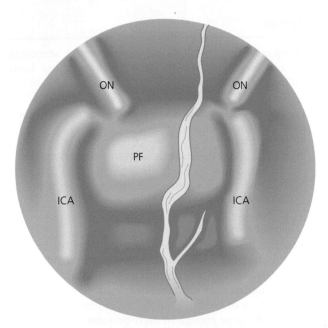

Figure 28.1 Diagram of endoscopic view of the interior of the sphenoid sinus with the intersinus septum taken down, showing the pituitary fossa (PF), optic nerves (ON) and internal carotid arteries (ICA).

anterior (80 per cent), pars intermedia and pars tuberalis, is quite firm yellow tissue. The neurohypophysis is adherent to its posterior aspect.

The arterial blood supply is from the superior and inferior hypophyseal arteries, which arise from the internal carotid. The anterior lobe also has its portal circulation from the medial eminence of the hypothalamus.

Bone of the sphenoid forms the anterior, inferior and posterior walls of the pituitary fossa. The lateral walls are formed by the cavernous sinuses, venous lakes which have dura mater and vein wall on their medial and lateral aspects and which contain the last part of the internal carotid arteries, the oculomotor (III), trochlear (IV) and abducent (VI) nerves, and the ophthalmic and maxillary divisions of the trigeminal (V) nerve. These sinuses are linked by connecting veins running within the anterior and inferior capsule of the gland. These connectors are important to the surgeon as they are easily opened when approaching the gland through the sphenoid and can cause troublesome bleeding. Blood from the opthalmic veins and pterygoid plexus of veins drains into the cavernous sinuses and flows from the cavernous sinuses into the superior and inferior petrosal sinuses.

The optic nerves, chiasm and tracts are closely associated with the gland. The nerves come from the orbital apices, between the anterior and middle clinoid processes on each side, just above the carotids and merge as the chiasm just anterior to the stalk. The chiasm then divides into the optic tracts, which pass either side of the stalk to head posterolaterally around the cerebral peduncles. The relevance of this anatomy is that a superiorly expanding pituitary lesion will come into contact with these structures, causing the typical clinical presentation of visual field loss.

The anatomy of sphenoid sinus is critical for pituitary surgery. The sphenoid is occasionally not aerated at all, in which case the sella sits in the top of a solid clivus. Normally, there are two sphenoid sinuses, which open into the nose in the sphenoethmoidal recesses on each side of the posterior septum. Aeration may range from minimal to highly aerated with large lateral extensions into the greater wings of the sphenoid bones. In addition to a septum separating the two sinuses, there are often additional septae within each sinus. These are valuable anatomical landmarks which can be noted on scans and used during surgery to navigate within the sinuses.

PHYSIOLOGY OF THE PITUITARY GLAND

This is a highly complex topic, and only a brief outline is given below, in order to allow an understanding of the pathology described in relation to the management of pituitary tumours.

Anterior pituitary function

PROLACTIN

Prolactin is a 199 amino acid protein. It has a 30 minute half-life in the circulation. It has similarities to GH and serum prolactin levels are a reliable measure of the amount of circulating hormone. The normal range of circulating hormone is 60–620 mU/L and it is higher in women than men. Its main action is to stimulate and maintain secretion of milk. It is regulated mainly by inhibition from the hypothalamus by prolactin inhibitory factor (PIF) and the main PIF is dopamine. Between 12 and 28 per cent of anterior pituitary cells secrete prolactin in a normal gland. Control of secretion is complex, but raised prolactin levels, caused by a prolactin secreting adenoma (prolactinoma), may suppress the release of gonadotrophins, as well as stimulating milk secretion, and so females often present with galactorrhoea and amenorrhoea. In men, there may be no obvious effect, although suppression of gonadotrophin secretion may cause low testosterone levels and loss of libido. It is important to be aware that stalk compression, whatever its cause, can cause a mild rise in prolactin levels by preventing PIF reaching the anterior gland.

Dopamine agonists are effective in treating prolactinomas. Cabergoline is the first-line treatment for prolactinoma in most cases in most centres. It can control prolactin levels and shrink tumours.

GROWTH HORMONE

Between 70 and 80 per cent of GH is a single chain 191 amino acid protein. About 50 per cent of the hormone-producing cells in the anterior pituitary secrete GH. It either acts directly on cells, binding to GH receptors, or it acts indirectly by triggering production of insulin-like growth factors (IGF) which are mainly synthesized in the liver. IGF1 is the most important and unlike GH, which has a very short half-life in the circulation, IGF1 levels do not fluctuate quickly and relate well to average GH levels. For this reason, IGF1 levels are useful when assessing acromegaly and its treatment. GH regulation is complex, but the hypothalamus produces both GH-releasing hormone (GHRH), which stimulates GH secretion and somatostatin, which inhibits it.

ADRENOCORTICOTROPHIC HORMONE

Adrenocorticotrophic hormone (ACTH) is a 39 amino acid peptide and it is regulated directly by circulating glucocorticoid levels and by the effect of corticotrophin-releasing hormone (CRH) and vasopressin from the hypothalamus. Glucocorticoid levels fluctuate on a diurnal rhythm, with levels being highest in the morning and lowest at night. ACTH levels fluctuate in a similar way and it is the major stimulus to the adrenal cortex, which secretes glucocorticoids, mineralocorticoids and adrenal androgens. Corticotropic cells constitute about 6–10 per cent of the cells in the normal anterior pituitary.

LUTEINIZING HORMONE, FOLLICLE-STIMULATING HORMONE AND THYROID-STIMULATING HORMONE

LH, FSH and TSH are all glycoproteins with a common alpha subunit (92 amino acids) and characteristic beta subunits (115 or 112 amino acid proteins). LH and FSH control sexual function and TSH regulates thyroid function. Functioning adenomas secreting these hormones are rare.

Posterior pituitary function

Antidiuretic hormone (ADH) and oxytocin are the hormones secreted by the posterior or neurohypophysis. ADH is the same as vasopressin. Both ADH and oxytocin are nine amino acid peptides. They are synthesized in the cells of the supraoptic and paraventricular nuclei of the hypothalamus, but individual cells in these nuclei secrete one or the other, not both. ADH acts on various receptors in the central nervous system (CNS), blood vessels, liver, adrenal cortex, uterus and platelets. Via different receptors, it acts on the anterior pituitary where it affects ACTH release, and via yet another type of receptor it affects the renal function by stimulating water reabsorption from the distal convoluted tubules and collecting ducts, hence the name 'antidiuretic hormone'. Oxytocin acts via receptors in the uterus to cause contraction of uterine smooth muscle and via receptors in the breast to cause contraction of myoepithelial cells resulting in ejection of milk. Receptors for oxytocin have been identified at other sites, including CNS, kidney, testis and thymus.

CLASSIFICATION OF PITUITARY TUMOURS

Pituitary adenomas can be classified in terms of function, size or histology.

Function

The great majority of pituitary tumours are benign adenomas which can broadly be divided into functioning and non-functioning adenomas.

- **Functioning adenomas**, from the most common to the most rare are as follows:
  - prolactinoma
  - growth hormone-secreting adenoma – acromegaly and gigantism
  - ACTH-secreting adenoma – Cushing disease and Nelson syndrome
  - TSHoma
  - Gonadotrophinoma.
- **Non-functioning adenomas**. These are more common than functioning adenomas and they present either by being large enough to compress adjacent structures or by causing pituitary hormone deficiency, or a combination of these. Of course, functioning adenomas can also be large enough to exert pressure on adjacent structures.
- **Incidental lesions** found on imaging for another indication. 'Incidentaloma' is a term used to describe the increasing number of adenomas identified in patients who have a head scan for other reasons. These imaging abnormalities may or may not prove to be significant, but depending on the size and imaging characteristics of the lesion, may merit investigation to exclude a functioning adenoma and at least continued surveillance (see below under Epidemiology and incidence).

TUMOUR SIZE

Tumour size is important when considering treatment. Pituitary adenomas are often described in terms of size:

- microadenomas, up to 10 mm in their largest dimension;
- macroadenomas, larger than 10 mm.
- the term 'mesoadenoma' is sometimes used to describe tumours of intermediate size (10 mm).

Of greater importance in larger tumours is their extent. Hardy and Somma[1] graded pituitary tumours on a scale of 0 to 4, where 1 and 2 are adenomas confined to the fossa, 3 has localized invasion and destruction of the sella and 4 has more extensive invasion and expansion beyond the sella. Extrasellar extension is described by further grades A to E. This classification is relevant to the surgical strategy as larger tumours require more extensive surgery to cure them and this is discussed below under Surgical approaches.

HISTOLOGY

Tumours used to be defined by the staining characteristics of the granules in the cells on haematoxylin and eosin staining into chromophobe, eosinophil (prolactin and GH) and basophil (ACTH, TSH, LH, FSH) tumours. However, with modern immunohistochemistry, histology can define type of hormone in the adenoma – for instance, a tumour may be described as corticotrophinoma (containing ACTH granules) or a somatotrophinoma (containing GH granules). It is interesting to note that adenomas may contain more than one hormone and positive immunohistochemistry does not always coincide with tumour function.

OTHER LESIONS ARISING IN AND ADJACENT TO THE PITUITARY

A range of other lesions can arise at this site. Below is a list of some of these, and this illustrates the diversity and the need for expert imaging and investigation in such cases. Many have particular characteristics on magnetic resonance imaging (MRI) and computed tomography (CT) which can be identified by an expert radiologist. Pituitary function may not be disturbed by these lesions, but if it is, function tends to be impaired:

- Rathke's pouch cyst
- Craniopharyngioma
- Chordoma
- Meningioma
- Carotid aneurysm
- Plasmacytoma
- Glioma
- Epidermoid cyst
- Dermoid cyst
- Nasopharyngeal carcinoma
- Metastatic cancer
- Granulomas.

EPIDEMIOLOGY AND INCIDENCE

Pituitary adenomas account for about 12 per cent of primary brain tumours and the incidence in various studies ranges from 0.6 to 2.8 tumours/100 000 population per annum.[2] Some studies show females to be more frequently affected than males, but this is not consistent. Non-functioning adenomas and prolactinomas are most common, with GH adenomas and ACTH adenomas third and fourth.

Post-mortem studies show a much higher incidence of adenomas – between 1.5 and 25 per cent, with an overall figure of 9.4 per cent.[2] Ten per cent of these were found to be multiple. This puts the finding of an incidental adenoma on a head scan into context.

Primary malignant tumours of the pituitary are extremely rare.

CLINICAL PRESENTATION OF PITUITARY LESIONS

As stated above, pituitary tumours present in one or more of three ways:

- Endocrine disturbance, caused by the effects of excess or deficient pituitary hormone secretion.

- As a space-occupying lesion spreading out of the pituitary fossa and compressing or invading adjacent structures.
- As an incidental finding on imaging of the brain.

The presentation of each type of pituitary tumour will be described in more detail under the individual tumour types.

INVESTIGATIONS

Pituitary imaging

MRI and CT scanning have made enormous advances over the last few decades. Modern MRI gives a wealth of information about the soft tissues in and around the pituitary gland at little risk to the patient. T_1-weighted images with and without contrast and T_2-imaging are most valuable. CT scanning obviously exposes the patient to significant doses of x-rays, but provides a wealth of detail about the bony anatomy when this is needed. Imaging of the pituitary is used to demonstrate the following:

- **Normality.** MRI gives details of the size, shape and intensity of the gland. On T_1-weighted imaging without contrast, the normal posterior pituitary is hyperintense in 90 per cent of children, but is less reliably so in adults. This is because the neurosecretory granules contain phospholipids which are bright on T_1. MRI also demonstrates the sphenoid sinus (air filled and so black on all weightings) and bone marrow (bright on T_1) within the clivus very well. CT defines the bony margins of the fossa and identifies bone asymmetry, expansion or erosion if present.
- **Abnormality within the gland.** MRI is best for identifying an abnormality within the gland. On this modality, the intensity of an adenoma is either iso- or hypointense. On T_1-weighted imaging with gadolinium, an adenoma will usually appear darker than the adjacent gland initially, because circulation is swifter to the normal gland than to the adenoma, but this may reverse in a delayed scan, where the adenoma may be bright after the contrast has moved out of the normal gland. T_2-weighted imaging will demonstrate cerebrospinal fluid (CSF) in the suprasellar cistern, a cyst in the gland if its contents have the appropriate signal characteristics, or a partially empty sella. CT is not likely to be useful in microadenomas. The presence of an abnormality in the gland must be treated with caution in light of the following:
  - A 10 per cent incidence of asymptomatic pituitary adenomas in the general population.
  - Small functioning adenomas may not be visible on standard MRI (about 25 per cent of Cushing adenomas cannot be seen on MRI). There is evidence that with improving techniques, imaging will become more accurate.[3]
- **Abnormality adjacent to the gland or extending beyond it.** Once again, MRI is likely to show most detail. Extension into the suprasellar cistern, chiasmal compression and cavernous sinus invasion will all be

seen on T_1-weighted imaging with contrast. The carotid arteries in the cavernous sinuses are seen clearly as flow voids. The optic nerves are easily seen after they have left the orbital apices, as is the optic chiasm. Invasion of the sphenoid sinus will be visible on all modalities of MRI and CT will show bone thinning or destruction when a tumour invades the sphenoid bone or sinuses.

The availability and quality of MRI means that this may be the only imaging needed, but some surgeons prefer to have imaging to demonstrate cortical bone detail clearly. Cortical bone is not seen clearly on MRI and so CT can be used to acquire this information. Both types of imaging can then be used by image guidance systems during surgery. This is helpful to guide the surgeon in the nose and sinuses. Angiography of any type is seldom required for pituitary adenomas because the carotids are seen clearly as flow voids on MRI and it is extremely unusual for a pituitary adenoma to affect the carotid arteries. If the signal characteristics of a lesion in or adjacent to the pituitary are in any way atypical of adenoma, an experienced neuroradiologist will advise on the differential diagnosis and any further types of imaging which should be used to define the nature of such a lesion. In many instances, MRI alone or MRI and CT are sufficient to make the diagnosis of whichever lesion is arising in this area (see the list of 'other lesions', above under Other lesions arising in and adjacent to the pituitary).

Endocrine investigations

The detail of the endocrine investigations needed to diagnose and assess pituitary function and abnormality will vary, dependent on the clinical diagnosis. The standard endocrine tests for pituitary function will measure plasma cortisol, urinary free cortisol, prolactin, growth hormone (GH), IGF1, LH, FSH, TSH, thyroid hormone levels, and plasma testosterone levels.

VISUAL FIELD TESTING

This is essential if there is suprasellar extension and the tumour reaches the optic nerves or chiasm. Documentation of the visual fields will demonstrate if the tumour is causing visual impairment, and provides a record which can be used to show the effect of surgery on the loss. Intrasellar tumours do not give rise to visual field problems but if any patient complains about visual disturbance, it is wise to document their visual fields preoperatively.

TREATMENT OPTIONS

If a pituitary tumour is suspected, it is important to investigate it as described above. The options for treatment will depend on the type of tumour, the overall health of the patient and how the tumour is affecting the patient. Treatment options vary for each type of tumour, as described below, but in general the options are:

- watchful waiting, with serial MRI;
- surgery;

- radiotherapy;
- medical treatment;
- combinations of these options.

NON-FUNCTIONING ADENOMA

Presentation

A non-functioning adenoma (NFA) can come to light for the following reasons:

1. Symptoms due to compression of the optic nerves and chiasm. If this is the presentation, the patient will usually be referred with the results of visual field testing showing the visual field loss. If the patient comes from an ophthalmologist, they may well have had MRI as well.
2. Symptoms of pituitary hypofunction, being investigated with a scan which demonstrates a pituitary adenoma.
3. An incidental finding when a patient has a scan for another reason (incidentaloma).

Investigation

VISUAL FIELD ASSESSMENT

If the patient has not had formal assessment of the visual fields, this will need to be accurately documented.

IMAGING

This will provide a great deal of valuable information for the surgeon about the adenoma.

- **Size and extent**. MRI will define the extent of the tumour and what structures are compressed or invaded by it. Obviously, if the tumour is causing visual disturbance, it will have grown upwards out of the fossa, but it may have invaded one or both cavernous sinuses or the sphenoid sinuses, or all of these structures. Its extent has important implications for planning the surgery and the more extensive the tumour, the more difficult it is to clear it completely at operation. Bone destruction may be evident on MRI, but CT will give more detail. This can be very important, for example it is valuable to know if the posterior clinoid processes and posterior wall of the pituitary fossa have been eroded by the adenoma, because if they have, there is nothing hard between the posterior capsule of the gland and the brain stem and basilar artery.
- **Shape**. A tumour may be a concentric enlargement, it may have a 'cottage loaf' shape or it may invade laterally or inferiorly. The waist in the cottage loaf is usually caused by the superior extent of the tumour pouting out through the diaphragma sellae. The superior part of a concentric tumour may descend into the fossa more readily during surgery than the upper part of a 'cottage loaf'.

- **Consistency.** MRI will often give some indication as to the consistency of the tumour. This is useful, because it is easier to remove cystic or 'soft-centred' tumours. If the tumour is tough and fibrous or proves to be adherent to the cavernous sinus during surgery, it is more difficult to remove completely. 'Soft-centred' tumours are often homogeneous or even have a slightly enhancing rim on T_1-weighted imaging with gadolinium with a homogeneous, hypointense centre. A heterogeneous signal on MRI may give the surgeon an indication that the tumour is going to be more fibrous and 'tough', making dissection and good clearance more difficult.

ENDOCRINE FUNCTION

It is essential to investigate pituitary endocrine function in the presence of a pituitary adenoma. A significant proportion of these patients are partially or totally deficient in anterior pituitary function. Any deficiencies identified can be treated prior to surgery if appropriate. If the presentation is as an emergency, the surgeon should be aware that the patient may be cortisol deficient and it is essential that this deficiency is treated urgently.

Prolactinomas may present as NFAs, particularly in men, and so a serum prolactin should be measured and a diagnosis of prolactinoma considered if the prolactin is greater than 2000 mU/L. If the patient has a prolactinoma, urgent treatment with a dopamine agonist should be considered because this is highly effective.

Treatment

Surgery is effective if needed to relieve the local pressure. This is described below under Surgical approaches, p. 537. If the adenoma is truly non-functioning, there is no medical treatment. Radiotherapy is effective but slow to act and is subject to its own complications.[4] Recurrence post-surgery can be treated by further surgery with a good prospect of controlling the tumour.[5]

Follow up

When a non-functioning adenoma is treated surgically, tumour removal may be partial or total. Most of these tumours are large and benign, and total removal may be unachievable or excessively risky. In that event and even with apparently complete removal, they can recur.

Routine follow up should include the following.

POSTOPERATIVE ENDOCRINE ASSESSMENT

The recovery of endocrine function that was deficient preoperatively is unpredictable, but on occasions recovery occurs. Surgery may also cause further loss of endocrine function and so full assessment of pituitary function should be undertaken postoperatively. Sometimes postoperative symptoms will give a good indication of lost or returning function. For instance, persistent diuresis occurs if the patient has developed diabetes insipidus, and if a woman's periods return, it is likely that LH and FSH secretion has recovered. It is important to assume that a patient is glucocorticoid deficient postoperatively until they have passed a short synacthen test which confirms a normal adrenocortical response to ACTH.

HISTOLOGY

Clearly, histological examination of the removed tissue is essential to confirm the diagnosis. It may also give some indication of the growth rate of the tumour, if there is a high mitotic rate and the Ki67 index is high.[6]

IMAGING

Recurrence of NFAs will depend on the degree of clearance obtained at surgery and the nature of the tumour. In view of this, it is recommended that all NFA patients should be rescanned. The timing of the first postoperative scan is at the surgeon's discretion. The authors rescan at about four to six months post-surgery, when healing is complete, and then serially at intervals of months or years to assess for evidence of recurrence. If there is persistent tumour on the scan and it starts to grow and if further treatment is considered necessary, the treatment options are further surgery or radiotherapy or both. This management avoids radiation for the majority of patients in whom the NFA never recurs.

FUNCTIONING ADENOMAS

These include the following:

- Prolactin-secreting adenoma – prolactinoma
- Growth hormone-secreting adenoma – acromegaly
- ACTH-secreting adenoma – Cushing disease
- TSHoma
- Gonadotrophinoma.

Prolactinoma

PRESENTATION

In women of reproductive age, a prolactinoma is most likely to present with secondary amenorrhoea and galactorrhoea. This is because high prolactin levels suppress gonadotrophin release and stimulate milk secretion. In men, they may cause no obvious symptoms, but gonadotrophin suppression may cause loss of libido or impotence. Prolactinomas are the most common functioning pituitary adenomas. They can vary from microadenomas to large macroadenomas which may even be invasive and very rarely truly malignant. The larger tumours can give rise to the same symptoms as a NFA.

INVESTIGATION

Serum prolactin levels will be elevated to over 2000 mU/L. In larger tumours, the levels may well be > 10 000 mU/L.

Gonadotrophin and testosterone levels may be low. Full endocrine assessment is important. Occasionally, tumours secrete both prolactin and GH.

TREATMENT

Medical treatment is effective to treat prolactinoma. Dopamine agonists lower the prolactin levels and shrink the tumour in most cases. Cabergoline is the drug of choice and is usually commenced at a low dose twice weekly and increased until a suitable response occurs. The effect on prolactin levels can be measured in the blood and tumour size can be monitored with serial MRI and serial visual field testing if there is visual field loss initially. Surgery is only indicated if one or more of the following applies:

- The tumour does not respond to medical treatment, either with a failure of prolactin levels to drop, or the tumour to shrink or both. Typically, the levels drop quite rapidly, but tumour shrinkage occurs over a longer period.
- The patient cannot tolerate medical treatment.
- The tumour expands, causing sudden loss of vision or other intracranial complications. This may be sudden, due to haemorrhage into an adenoma.
- Occasionally, a large tumour may shrink so much that a CSF leak develops and needs closure.

Should surgery prove necessary, it is important to screen the patient for cardiac valve disease, because this can arise from dopamine agonist treatment.[7]

It is important to check the serum prolactin in all patients presenting with what is thought to be a non-functioning adenoma, because some of these may be prolactinomas. In the event that the serum prolactin is significantly elevated, unless there is an immediate indication for surgery, such as sudden loss of vision, giving a dopamine agonist may well be effective in shrinking the tumour avoiding unnecessary surgery.

Acromegaly

PRESENTATION

The clinical picture in acromegaly is of enlargement of the hands, feet, soft tissues and bones of the face. Patients note these features, but the onset is typically insidious, and so it is often someone other than the patient who notices the change and triggers medical interest. Headaches, excessive sweating, snoring, nasal symptoms (an association with nasal polyposis), tight rings, enlarging feet, the onset of diabetes, hypertension and muscle and joint pains are all features of the condition. Family photographs can often help in identifying the onset of this disorder. Excessive secretion in childhood results in gigantism and following fusion of the epiphyses, acromegaly.

INVESTIGATIONS

Growth hormone is a protein with a half-life of a few minutes. There is a diurnal variation in the secretion, but in addition to this, the hormone is secreted in pulses. GH antagonizes insulin and its secretion is suppressed by a high blood sugar. If this condition is suspected, growth hormone levels should be measured during an oral glucose tolerance test (OGTT), because in normal people high glucose levels suppress GH levels below $0.6\,\mu g/L$ and if GH levels remain persistently high during this test, it is diagnostic. IGF1 (insulin-like growth factor 1) is produced in the liver in response to circulating GH and this is useful because it has a long half-life. Elevated IGF1 levels are strongly supportive of a diagnosis of acromegaly.

MRI of the pituitary fossa will usually demonstrate an adenoma, which may be anything from a microadenoma to a tumour spreading well beyond the limits of the gland.

TREATMENT

It is important to treat acromegaly. This condition is associated with a significantly increased risk of premature death if left untreated, due to a variety of causes, but mainly due to vascular disease and cancer.

Surgical

In this condition, surgery remains the treatment of choice in most centres. If the tumour is fully surgically accessible and there is normal gland in the fossa, it is possible to cure the disease and retain normal function. In microadenomas, surgical cure is obtainable in more than 85 per cent of tumours. Where tumours are larger or more invasive, the cure rate drops.

Medical

Somatostatin suppresses the secretion of GH, and somatostatin analogues are now available. These are quite short-acting drugs which have to be administered by injection, but once the treatment has been established and proved effective in controlling symptoms, depot preparations requiring just one injection every few weeks can be used. Tumour regression is variable and not very reliable, but somatostatin analogues are effective in lowering GH levels and will often rapidly relieve the patient's symptoms.

Radiotherapy

Radiotherapy has a role, as in other pituitary tumours, but given the slow-growing and benign nature of these tumours, the action on tumour size and hormone secretion is slow, taking years to show its full effect.

FOLLOW UP

Endocrine assessment is essential to assess the effect of treatment on growth hormone and IGF1 levels. These should fall following surgery. As with preoperative assessment, growth hormone levels should be measured during an oral glucose tolerance test, and should be low at rest and suppress to less than $0.6\,\mu g/L$ on the OGTT. Surgery ideally cures the disease and preserves other normal pituitary function, but this does not always happen, and so all anterior pituitary function should be assessed postoperatively and any deficiencies treated as appropriate.

Postoperative imaging is of value in assessing the removal of the adenoma and the presence of tissue within the fossa, but it is of secondary importance from the point of view of the patient, because restoring normal GH levels and maintaining this state of affairs is the goal of treatment. Life-long follow up is essential, because there is an incidence of a late recurrence in acromegaly.

Cushing disease and Nelson syndrome

PRESENTATION

'Cushing syndrome' is the term used to describe the clinical features of this condition whatever the source of glucocorticoid excess. This may be from an adrenal tumour, a pituitary tumour, an ectopic tumour secreting ACTH or due to medication with glucocorticoids. 'Cushing disease' is the term used when this is due to an ACTH-secreting adenoma in the pituitary. Whatever the cause of hypercortisolaemia, the presentation is similar. The effects of glucocorticoids on the body are wide ranging and the typical clinical picture is of increasing central obesity with a moon face and a buffalo hump, peripheral wasting with associated muscle weakness, skin changes which may include acne, hirsuitism, striae, easy bruising and easily damaged skin, bone demineralization which may cause pathological fractures, hypertension and diabetes. Untreated, this is a lethal disease, but once again the onset is usually insidious and the diagnosis is often missed early in the disease.

Nelson syndrome is included here because this arises in some patients who have adrenalectomy for Cushing disease without the pituitary adenoma being treated. The effect of adrenalectomy under these circumstances is to remove the inhibitory effect of high circulating levels of glucocorticoids on the adenoma, so it may undergo rapid growth giving rise to a larger more invasive ACTH-producing adenoma. The clinical features of Nelson's are hyperpigmentation (due to high levels of ACTH and associated hormones) in the presence of a rapidly expanding pituitary tumour in a patient who has had an adrenalectomy. The treatment is hypophysectomy in combination with radiotherapy if this has not already been used, but the cure rate is low.

INVESTIGATIONS

Adrenocorticotrophic hormone regulates glucocorticoid secretion and glucocorticoids are essential for life. Pituitary ACTH secretion is partially regulated by direct feedback of circulating glucocorticoid levels and partially by CRH and vasopressin. However, the diagnosis of Cushing disease may be complicated by ectopic secretion of ACTH, typically from a neuroendocrine tumour. Normally, glucocorticoid levels have a characteristic diurnal rhythm, with levels being highest in the morning and lowest at night. ACTH levels regulate this and fluctuate in a similar way.

Endocrine assessment

Because ACTH is a 39 amino acid protein with a short half-life, it is easier to measure plasma cortisol and 24-hour urinary-free cortisol levels when assessing pituitary/adrenal function.

- The loss of diurnal rhythm can be detected by measuring plasma cortisol levels at 9 a.m. (normal 180–550 nmol/L) and midnight (normal <130 nmol/L). In normal people, an overnight dexamethasone suppression test – a low dose of dexamethasone (2 mg) at night – will suppress plasma cortisol levels the next morning and this can be used to exclude a diagnosis of Cushing syndrome.
- Because ACTH may also be secreted by ectopic sources, such as neuroendocrine tumours, and such tumours give rise to a similar clinical picture, the diagnostic pathway needs to include a method of distinguishing between Cushing disease and syndrome. The behaviour of tumours secreting ectopic ACTH differs from that of pituitary adenomas because most ectopic tumours do not suppress in the presence of high circulation levels of glucocorticoids. Because the management is obviously radically different, it is essential to distinguish between ACTH arising from a pituitary adenoma and from an ectopic source. The dexamethasone suppression test has traditionally been used to distinguish between normal, where suppression occurs with a low dose of dexamethasone, pituitary adenomas, which suppress with high-dose dexamathasone and most ectopic adenomas which do not suppress at all. However, this is not infallible.
- If there is doubt remaining, giving the patient a dose of corticotrophin-releasing factor (CRF) will cause a rapid rise in ACTH in Cushing disease, but does not usually make any difference if the ACTH is from an ectopic source.
- Finally, the current preferred technique is to do inferior petrosal sinus sampling (IPSS) for ACTH during a CRF test. If there is a significantly greater rise in ACTH in the inferior petrosal sinuses than in peripheral blood, this indicates a pituitary source of ACTH.

This is a complex field and any surgeon treating this condition needs to work in close collaboration with a specialist endocrine team.

Imaging

These adenomas are usually small and may be undetectable on imaging. MRI is most useful and most adenomas are less than 1 cm. As stated above, a significant proportion cannot be clearly identified on MRI. This leaves the surgeon dependent on the endocrine results to make the diagnosis, but the presence of an abnormality on MRI does not guarantee that the ACTH secretion is arising from that abnormality, for the reasons stated above under Epidemiology and incidence.

TREATMENT

As stated, this is a dangerous condition with a high mortality rate if left untreated. The treatment options are surgery, medication and radiation, but in Cushing disease, pituitary surgery is the main option. Medication, using Metyrapone®, suppresses the symptoms by blocking the peripheral effects of glucocorticoids, but this is not a definitive treatment. Radiation is not used alone, as the onset of effect is too slow and unpredictable.

FOLLOW UP

The ideal outcome is a cure for the disease with maintenance of normal pituitary function. This requires excision of the adenoma with preservation of sufficient normal gland to function adequately. Even if this is achieved, recovery of normal ACTH secretion in the pituitary remnant takes months because in Cushing's this will have been suppressed by the disease. For this reason, patients should be given replacement hydrocortisone at physiological doses postoperatively and this should not be stopped until there is evidence of recovery of adequate ACTH secretion. Follow up will always include a full endocrine assessment in case there has been collateral damage to pituitary function.

Imaging is of secondary significance in the follow up of Cushing disease, but is essential if further surgery is being considered.

In our hospital, the optimal indicators for a good outcome are:

* an identified adenoma on preoperative imaging;
* histological confirmation that the tumour has been excised;
* a plasma cortisol which is undetectable on blood testing in the early postoperative period when the patient is off all steroids. This is measured on the 4th postoperative day.

Even if all these criteria are satisfied, we have had three patients whose Cushing's recurred. This once again emphasizes the fact that these patients all need life-long follow up from an endocrine service.

Other pituitary adenomas

TSHomas are rare functioning adenomas which present with hyperthyroidism. In a hyperthyroid patient who does not have suppression of TSH, this diagnosis should be considered. Treatment may be surgical or medical, because somatostatin analogues are useful in this condition.

Gonadotrophinoma is a diagnosis which is usually made on immunohistochemistry, so most patients with this diagnosis present as if they had non-functioning adenomas.

Other lesions in and around the pituitary

These have been listed above under Other lesions arising in and adjacent to the pituitary. Such lesions may present in a similar way to a non-functioning adenoma, as a space-occupying lesion in or near the pituitary fossa. Imaging may suggest the diagnosis, and often the neuroradiologist reporting the scan will identify features atypical of a pituitary adenoma and characteristic of an alternative diagnosis, such as calcification in a craniopharyngioma or a meningeal tail in meningioma. The presence of clinical signs, such as an ophthalmoplegia, should alert the clinician to the possibility

of a diagnosis other than pituitary adenoma, because pituitary adenomas very seldom give rise to symptoms or signs caused by invasion or destruction of adjacent structures. The treatment of such lesions may be surgical, but this is a decision which should only be made when the diagnosis is clear.

HYPOPHYSECTOMY

Contraindications for surgery

GENERAL CONTRAINDICATIONS

General contraindications include:

* **Uncontrolled disease**, for example severe Cushing disease where the patient's condition could be improved by controlling their hypertension or diabetes.
* **Poor general health** where the patient is at significantly increased risk from the anaesthetic or surgery. Coexisting medical conditions should be optimally treated.
* **Risk of haemorrhage** is an important consideration. Any anticoagulant, including aspirin, should be stopped. If the patient is on warfarin and this cannot be stopped, hypophysectomy is contraindicated.

LOCAL CONTRAINDICATIONS

* **Abnormal anatomy**, such as a solid sphenoid, needs to be considered, but it is not a contraindication. Abnormal position of the carotid arteries can occur and needs careful consideration. Image guidance is valuable in these situations.
* **Local infection**, such as sinusitis or nasal vestibulitis, needs to be eliminated or optimally treated before surgery to minimize the risk of meningitis.

PATIENT INFORMATION AND CONSENT

All pituitary surgery is performed in specialist centres and often patients are aware of the diagnosis and treatment options by the time they are first seen in a specialist clinic. Patients may have information on their condition or have searched the internet. However, a detailed individual explanation is always necessary, whatever the patient's state of knowledge. It should include the following:

* A careful explanation of the treatment options, with the benefits and shortcomings of each, including the consequences of no treatment.
* For surgical consent, the surgeon needs to explain:
  - the reason why surgery is the preferred option;
  - the nature of the operation;
  - the risks;
  - the likely outcomes and chances of these being achieved;

- the complications and their consequences;
- the likely time off work;
- what follow up is required and why, how and by whom the patient will be followed up and for how long.

Supporting literature is valuable and is available from the Pituitary Foundation (www.pituitary.org.uk).

PREOPERATIVE INVESTIGATIONS

The patient should be as fit as possible preoperatively. The preoperative assessment for each condition is described above, but the patient should be fully assessed with regard to their medical history and any abnormal physical findings and any pre-existing conditions should be treated to avoid or minimize the risk of problems in the perioperative period. Both Cushing's and acromegalic patients have significant increased risk of cardiac problems, hypertension and diabetes mellitus and this should be assessed and optimally treated before surgery. Dopamine agonists are also recognized to be associated with a risk of cardiac valve anomalies and so patients on these drugs should be assessed for this possibility.[7]

Preparation for surgery

- **Nasal preparation**. Bleeding can be minimized by using vasoconstrictors to reduce bleeding and improve access. Topical vasoconstriction (e.g. xylomatazoline 0.1 per cent spray) to the nasal mucosa and injection of local anaesthetic with adrenaline (lignocaine 2 per cent with 1:80 000 adrenaline) achieves this.
- **General anaesthesia** is obviously essential. It is useful if the anaesthetist is able to raise the CSF pressure when requested, to push the upper part of the gland into the fossa during the dissection of a macroadenoma.
- **Positioning**. The patient's head must be stable, but does not need to be fixed. If image guidance is being used, this needs to be set up appropriately.

SURGICAL APPROACHES

The pituitary has been approached from many different routes over the history of this surgery, but the basic requirements of any approach are the following:

- There must be adequate access to the gland and tumour.
- Intraoperative complications – the surgeon must be able to control bleeding and CSF leak.
- The approach must minimize complications intraoperatively and postoperatively.

The two main routes to the pituitary gland are trans-sphenoidal and transcranial. The first is now the method of choice in the vast majority of cases. Morbidity is significantly lower in trans-sphenoidal surgery and recent technical developments particularly in imaging, video technology, image guidance and instrumentation such as surgical debriders have resulted in the endoscopic trans-sphenoidal approach being the preferred technique. A transcranial approach is still indicated if there is an intracranial portion of tumour which is inaccessible from below.

Endoscopic transnasal route to the sphenoid sinus

ENDOSCOPIC TRANSNASAL ROUTE

This approach is particularly applicable since the introduction of Hopkin's rod endoscopes to nasal surgery. These instruments come in various angles of vision, but for this surgery 0° and 45° are ideal. The advantage of using this system is that the surgeons' vision is the view at the tip of the endoscope. Perspective is altered, but the angle of vision is dramatically wider than down a microscope. Ideally, two surgeons work together, one holding the endoscope and another instrument such as a sucker, the other using one or two other instruments as required. Both surgeons work from a television screen, and so it is essential to have a high quality video system attached to the endoscope and an efficient means of keeping the tip of the endoscope clean to maintain illumination and visibility. This is very much a team activity.

- The middle turbinate is lateralized.
- The spheno-ethmoidal recess and the sphenoid ostium are then identified.
- The anterior wall of the sphenoid sinus is removed inferiorly, widening the ostium. The same is done in the other nostril.
- The surgeon makes an incision in the posterior septum about 1 cm anterior to the rostrum of the vomer, does a subperiosteal dissection of the rostrum, which is then removed. Septal bone is useful if the surgeon wishes to repair the defect in the anterior wall of the pituitary fossa with bone. A long-shafted drill is important to get good access where the bone is thick.
- Bone and mucosa are then removed to obtain a clear view of the interior of the sphenoid sinuses. A surgical debrider is very useful for this purpose.

Advantages

- This is a simple rapid approach with minimal bleeding in a well-prepared nose.
- This provides a very similar approach angle as the trans-septal approach without the dissection involved – it can be used through both nostrils.
- There is no risk of damage to nasal skeleton and so no risk of postoperative nasal deformity.

Disadvantages

- This technique requires two people who are familiar with the technique and the equipment.

THE TRADITIONAL TRANS-SPHENOIDAL APPROACHES

1. **Trans-septal route**. This route follows the subperichondrial and subperiosteal plane to the

rostrum of the vomer, which is removed to gain entry to the sphenoid sinuses. This plane can be entered through an SMR (submucous resection) incision in the nasal septum or through a sublabial incision in the mouth. It is an excellent approach, but requires careful dissection. When using retractors in the wound and a microscope, this approach is useful, but it has been superseded by the endoscopic approach, which provides much better visibility in the sphenoid and pituitary fossa.

2. **Transethmoidal route.** This approach requires an incision from the medial end of the eyebrow, curved round the medial aspect of the orbit, inferiorly to the level of the upper edge of the piriform aperture of the nose. Care must be taken to make this incision well anteriorly, away from the medial canthus to avoid webbing of the scar. The approach is then through a window in the medial wall of the orbit, through the ethmoid complex to the sphenoid to gain an excellent view of the pituitary fossa. This view is maintained using a Talbot retractor (the same orbital blades as the Ferris Smith, but the self-retaining system is as for a mastoid retractor). This is the shortest route to the pituitary gland. It allows vision through the ethmoids and instrumentation through the nose and there is a wider view of the operative field than with a trans-septal approach. This is particularly advantageous if there is extensive disease in the sphenoid sinus or clivus. There is no risk of destruction of the anterior nasal septum or deformity of the external nose. The disadvantages of this approach are a facial scar, however minimal, more bleeding during the approach, and a poorer superior view within the pituitary.

With extensive experience of all these approaches, the authors' preference is for the endoscopic approach. This requires two surgeons, and painstaking attention to maintaining illumination and visibility, but the benefit for the surgeons is a much better view of the operative field. The benefit for the patient is a technique with the lowest morbidity and a shorter hospital stay. The other approaches have some specific advantages and are available if indicated. For instance, the transethmoid approach can be useful for extensive lesions within the sphenoid sinus and clivus.

Given that most pituitary surgery has a low morbidity, it is increasingly important that the surgeon takes care of the nasal structures. Nasal septal perforations, postoperative crusting, collapse of the nasal skeleton with the associated nasal deformity and unsightly facial scarring are now all avoidable complications of this surgery.

INDICATIONS FOR TRANSCRANIAL APPROACH TO THE PITUITARY GLAND

- If there is a large intracranial element of the tumour which is unlikely to be accessible by a trans-sphenoidal approach, then this approach should be considered. Tumours with a 'cottage loaf' or 'hour glass' shape are theoretically more difficult to remove from below, but normally they are amenable and so this appearance is not a contraindication to trans-sphenoidal surgery.

- If the surgeon suspects that the tumour is not an adenoma, but some other pathology such as a craniopharyngioma or meningioma, trans-sphenoidal surgery may well be inappropriate. However, the scope of the endoscopic skull base surgery is advancing so fast that many lesions previously considered inappropriate for this technique are becoming part of the normal repertoire.

Occasionally, a dual approach, either simultaneously or as a staged procedure, is necessary. Obviously, any approach to the pituitary from above is strictly a neurosurgical procedure.

TRANS-SPHENOIDAL HYPOPHYSECTOMY

The structures are described as the surgeon encounters them in this approach.

- **The sphenoid sinuses** are very variable in size and shape, and are normally asymmetrical. MRI and CT allow the surgeon to have a map of the route to the gland. Poor aeration of the sphenoid sinus has been quoted as a contraindication to surgery by this route, but with modern imaging, even unaerated sphenoid sinuses seldom pose a problem. Image guidance systems provide further assistance in this situation, but intraoperative x-rays are of value in the absence of image guidance.

- The **optic nerves** and the **internal carotid arteries** usually create indentations in the roof and lateral walls of the sphenoid sinuses. These are visible to the surgeons using the endoscope. Seldom does either cause a problem, but the surgeon should know their location from the MRI prior to starting surgery, and the images should be on display in theatre during surgery. If they or the pituitary adenoma are in an abnormal location and the bone over these structures is thought to be dehiscent, a CT scan is valuable. The optic nerves and chiasm are at some risk when the surgeon is operating above the pituitary fossa, although they lie outside the gland. They are seldom visible to the surgeon using a microscope, but they may well be visible with the endoscope and can be avoided.

- The thickness of the **anterior bony wall of the pituitary fossa** is inversely related to the degree of aeration of the sphenoid sinuses. In a well-aerated sphenoid or an expanded fossa, it may be dehiscent or paper thin so that it will crack with gentle pressure, allowing it to be dissected off the dura and removed. With thicker bone, the preferred techniques are a drill or a bone-penetrating laser. Once the pituitary fossa is open, its posterior limit (the dorsum sellae) is palpable with a pituitary dissector. This provides useful guidance on the anatomy of the fossa during surgery, but occasionally large tumours erode the dorsum sellae, in which case such a manoeuvre is inappropriate.

- The **dura mater** lines the pituitary fossa and forms a tough fibrous layer which is encountered as soon as the bone of the anterior bulge of the gland is removed. This has to be cut to enter the gland. Sharp dissection, diathermy or a laser can be used. Deep to this is a thinner layer of pituitary capsule, which can also be opened or the surgeon may choose to develop a plane between normal gland and the tumour capsule. It is important to be through the dura, or the surgeon may find that the dissection is in the plane of the intercavernous connecting veins which may result in brisk venous bleeding.

- The **cavernous sinuses** lie lateral to the pituitary gland, but their **interconnecting veins** are directly in the way of the surgeon. These may be visible in the dura, in which case the surgeon may be able to avoid them. Bleeding can be controlled with gentle pressure and haemostatic sponge (Lyostypt®) or similar material. If the tumour extends laterally into one or both cavernous sinuses, it can be removed, at least partially, with blunt ring dissectors such as Hardy's dissectors, angled suction or a combination. More caution is required if the internal carotid artery is surrounded by tumour. Given the nature and contents of cavernous sinuses, great caution is advisable when dissecting laterally. It is wise to refer to the scans, to check the relationship between the tumour, the internal carotid artery and the cavernous sinus. The III, IV, V and VI cranial nerves can also be damaged at this point, although this is uncommon.
- The normal **anterior pituitary gland** is quite firm, pale yellow tissue with a lobular structure. **Adenomas** are very variable in macroscopic appearance. Occasionally, they pop out as a discrete nodule, but more often there is an area of softer, sometimes discoloured gland. Macroadenomas are often bulky pinkish grey soft tumours (much of which will go up the sucker to leave a cavity), the walls of which consist of soft adenoma. This can be removed by gentle blunt dissection in all directions using purpose designed dissectors. The common varieties are the Angel-James and Hardy dissectors. If there is a large superior extension of adenoma, raising the intracranial pressure will push the tumour down into the fossa from where the surgeon can remove it. The anaesthetist can do this by raising the intrathoracic pressure. Using 0° and 45° endoscopes passed into the pituitary fossa, angled suction and angled dissectors, tumour that is not visible from outside the fossa may become visible and can be removed, particularly if it is soft. Some surgeons use a lumbar canula and infuse an appropriate solution to raise CSF pressure.
- The **pars posterior of the pituitary**, lying at the back of the gland, is often well seen on T_1-weighted MRI because of its fat content. It can be displaced by an adenoma. It is seldom involved in the disease process and care should be taken to leave it intact to avoid diabetes insipidus.
- When operating at the upper edge of the gland, **the diaphragma sellae**, the pia arachnoid attached to the upper surface of the gland, is a very delicate bluish membrane which has a venous pulsation in it. This is very easy to perforate and may be dehiscent. When dissecting in this plane, it is usual to see CSF seeping from it. If torn, a free flow of CSF occurs. As the dissection is taken posteriorly, the stalk of the gland can be seen penetrating the diaphragma.

- Once the surgeon has removed all or part of the gland and considers the operation within the fossa is complete, the means of closure depends on the presence or absence of a CSF leak. When there is no leak, the surgical defect used for the approach is closed gently, using synthetic material such as a gelatin sponge (Gelfoam® or similar) or collagen sponge (Lyostypt). Surgical practice varies at this stage of the operation, but the authors' preference is to use collagen foam in the fossa, a piece of bone from the nasal septum to repair the fossa itself and sphenoid mucosa on the outer aspect of the fossa. The opening in the fossa is covered with more Lyostypt, then the sinus is filled with Nasopore impregnated with bismuth and iodoform paraffin paste (BIPP). This avoids the need for a nasal pack, which is a great benefit to the patient.

In the event of an obvious CSF leak, a more comprehensive repair is required. The authors have two methods, the first is a patch of material such as Surgisis (Cook Medical, Bloomington, IN, USA) and bone flake repair of the anterior wall, with a Lyostypt (B Braun Biosurgicals, Tuttlingen, Germany) and DuraSeal (Covidien, Basingstoke, UK) or Tisseal (Baxter Healthcare, Compton, UK), covered with Nasopore (Polyganics, Groningen, The Netherlands), as described above. The second is a vascularized septal flap to cover the front of the pituitary fossa. In the presence of a persistent leak, the vascularized septal flap is now the preferred closure technique.[8]

POSTOPERATIVE MANAGEMENT

A protocol for the management of patients in the perioperative period is very valuable. This needs to cover the hormonal requirements of the patient, prevention of infection, fluid balance, the prevention of complications and their early detection and treatment. The protocol should be agreed with the involved endocrinologist and microbiologist. It should cover the following.

Steroid replacement

Our standard policy is to cover all patients for the perioperative period with hydrocortisone, giving 150 mg in divided doses on the day of surgery, reducing to 15 mg in the morning and 5 mg in the afternoon by the 5th day. Patients are all discharged on a maintenance dose of hydrocortisone 15 and 5 mg, as above, and instructed to stay on this all the time until they are reassessed at 4 weeks. A short synachthen test is performed at about 4 weeks and, if this indicates sufficient adrenal function, hydrocortisone is stopped. Patients treated for Cushing disease need a higher replacement dose and are reduced to and discharged on 20 mg at 9 a.m., 10 mg at noon and 10 mg at 4 p.m.

Antibiotic cover

Perioperative use of antibiotics is important in this surgery because the approach is through a contaminated field.

Prophylactic antibiotic use should be agreed with the local microbiologist and be part of the hospital antibiotic policy. CSF penetration is useful, and the first dose must be given early enough to ensure that there is an effective circulating level of antibiotic at the time the gland is opened and dissected. The duration of antibiotic cover is the perioperative period only, unless there is an indication to continue it for longer, such as a persistent CSF leak through the pack.

Neurological observations

All patients should be fully alert and orientated as soon as they have recovered from the general anaesthetic. The neurological status of the patient should be observed and recorded regularly for the first 12–24 hours to detect any developing intracranial complications as soon as they occur.

Fluid balance and the management of diabetes insipidus

An accurate fluid balance record must be maintained from the time of surgery. Diabetes insipidus (DI) is likely to occur when the pars posterior or pituitary stalk has been traumatized during surgery and may be transient in up to a third of patients, but is persistent in up to 9 per cent.[9] The diuresis normally begins on the first postoperative day, but a diuresis can occur for reasons other than DI, and so it is essential to monitor the serum electrolyte levels daily and ensure that the serum sodium level is greater than 140 mmol/L before treating a diuresis with synthetic ADH (DDAVP). If the patient is passing high volumes of dilute urine, DDAVP 1 µg subcutaneously will control this rapidly. Regular doses are seldom required. DI is usually transient, but if it persists and continues to require treatment, DDAVP injections can be replaced with ADH analogues given either orally or as a nasal spray. If it is necessary to confirm that the diuresis is indeed DI, urinary and plasma osmolality should be measured. The other problem of fluid balance which may arise in the postoperative period is the syndrome of inappropriate ADH secretion (SIADH). This causes water retention and a fall in plasma sodium levels. The patient may develop a range of symptoms including confusion and convulsions. Treatment is by strict fluid restriction.

Management of postoperative CSF leakage

The purpose of the absorbable nasal dressing is to hold the repair to the pituitary fossa in place while the pituitary fossa heals and becomes sealed from the nose. Although healing takes months to complete, there is usually an effective seal within days of surgery.

If there was no CSF leak on the table, this is very unlikely to occur during the postoperative period. If there was a leak during surgery, the surgeon will have repaired it, but in a proportion of patients the leak may persist, or start during the postoperative period. It may resolve spontaneously, but if it persists for more that a few days, it is wise to repair it to avoid the risk of meningitis. The approach is simple because it has already been done at the first operation. The techniques are described above.

DISCHARGE FROM HOSPITAL

The patient is discharged home when well enough and when any diuresis has settled or been controlled. Serum urea and electrolytes should be normal. If there was a visual field defect before surgery, postoperative visual fields may be measured prior to discharge. In Cushing disease, a plasma cortisol level of less that 20 nmol/L (undetectable) in the early postoperative period is a significant indicator of surgical cure. This needs to be measured with the patient off all hydrocortisone for 12 hours. Discharge medication should include hydrocortisone or the equivalent in physiological doses unless the surgeon is certain that the patient has sufficient ACTH. The patient must remain on hydrocortisone until adequate adrenal function has been confirmed, must understand the importance of this medication and must carry a Steroid Card, in the event of accident or hospital admission.

COMPLICATIONS OF SURGERY

Intraoperative complications

HAEMORRHAGE

The most common source of troublesome bleeding is the intercavernous connecting veins in the anterior capsule of the gland, which are easily controlled by packing. Haemorrhage from an internal carotid artery is a rare but potentially lethal complication if the artery is torn. This must be avoided by knowing where the arteries are from the scans and using only gentle blunt dissection when working in the gland. Should this complication occur, immediate packing to control the bleeding and transfer to an interventional neuroradiological facility are vital, to use endovascular techniques to identify and control the bleeding vessel.

CEREBROSPINAL FLUID LEAK

If a CSF leak arises during surgery, it is repaired at the time. If it persists or recurs postoperatively, it needs to be repaired before discharge, as described above.

Early postoperative complications

- Diabetes insipidus is discussed above under Fluid balance and the management of diabetes insipidus.
- Meningitis is rare, but serious. Antibiotic prophylaxis is always used, but neurological observations are done to enable early detection and prompt treatment of this complication.
- Significant intracranial haemorrhage is very rare. If it is suspected from the clinical signs, it constitutes a neurosurgical emergency and should be investigated with early scans and intervention to stop the bleeding.

- Pneumocephalus. Air may enter the CSF space if there is a connection into the nose. If suspected, it can be seen on a plain x-ray or CT scan. Nurse the patient flat, and if it persists, early repair of the defect is necessary.

Late postoperative complications

- Anterior pituitary deficiency. This is detected on postoperative endocrine assessment and needs to be adequately treated with replacement therapy.
- Persistent diabetes insipidus is a recognized complication. It needs to be treated with replacement antidiuretic hormone. It presents in the early postoperative period and often it settles, but in some cases it persists and necessitates life-long replacement therapy.
- Failure to cure the endocrine disorder. Pituitary surgery has a failure rate. In most cases, the abnormal levels of hormone will fall, but may not reach the criteria for cure. There is often a corresponding improvement in symptoms. The decisions on the need for and nature of further treatment are best made within the multidisciplinary team.
- Nasal and sinus complications are increasingly rare with endoscopic surgery, but sinusitis can arise. Trans-septal surgery can damage the nose and septum. Transethmoidal surgery causes a scar, which may be unsightly, and it can also result in a frontal sinus mucocele.
- Recurrence of the tumour can occur many years later. The postoperative protocol for these patients includes long-term follow up.

Treated **functioning adenomas** can be monitored by measuring the relevant hormone levels. In most cases, a good early response to surgery is a strong indication of cure, but this is not invariable.

Non-functioning adenomas are followed up by repeated MRI. They may regrow very slowly, hence the need for life-long follow up. Further treatment may be indicated with surgery or radiotherapy or both. The role of radiotherapy to these lesions is discussed below.

SURGICAL OUTCOMES

In functioning adenomas, success or failure can be categorized into four categories:

1. **Cure with normal pituitary function.** In this case, the patient's symptoms resolve and their biochemistry returns to normal, with normal pituitary function. If the patient had partial or complete hypopituitarism preoperatively, return of normal function may occur, but is unpredictable.
2. **Cure with partial or complete hypopituitarism** and requirement for replacement therapy. Once again, the patient's symptoms resolve, but they will be on life-long replacement medication for the persistent deficiencies. One of the current debates in the postoperative period is growth hormone deficiency.

Some patients are symptomatic from GH deficiency and improve if they are given a replacement dose of GH.
3. **Failure to cure, but otherwise normal pituitary function.** Further treatment will be required for the relevant hormone excess.
4. **Failure to cure, but with partial or complete hypopituitarism.** Further treatment and replacement therapy are required.

For non-functioning adenomas causing symptoms due to compression of adjacent structures, cure can be defined as:

- resolution of the clinical features – return of normal visual fields, subjective improvement in vision, resolution of headache.
- reduction in size or complete removal of the tumour on imaging, and no regrowth of the tumour on serial imaging over time.

Revision hypophysectomy

The best chance of curing a pituitary adenoma is at the first operation. However, if cure is not achieved and the surgeon and endocrinologist feel that revision surgery is the best option, this should be done. If the first operation was a microadenectomy, removal of all the remaining gland is likely to be appropriate unless the surgeon can easily identify an adenoma in the gland remnant, excise it and leave some normal anterior pituitary tissue. All series quote substantially lower cure rates and higher rates of hypopituitarism and increased complication rates in revision surgery.[10, 11]

ROLE OF RADIOTHERAPY IN PITUITARY ADENOMAS

Radiotherapy can be delivered by external beam, gamma knife, cyber knife and stereotactic conformal radiotherapy to treat pituitary tumours. Radiotherapy is seldom used as first-line treatment, but it is effective and can be used as the sole or main treatment to cure pituitary adenomas, as well as an adjunct to surgery if indicated. It is mainly used where the alternatives are contraindicated (too unfit for surgery) or as an additional therapy where the tumour is not amenable to total surgical removal, where biochemistry or imaging indicate recurrence, or in special situations such as following adrenalectomy for Cushing disease, where radiotherapy to the pituitary reduces the risk of Nelson syndrome.

The effect is gradual over a period of years and so if it is used as the primary treatment, symptomatic control may be needed while the effect of treatment develops. It has potential side effects too.[4] Important among these are:

- a long-term incidence of hypopituitarism (13–56 per cent);
- a risk of optic neuropathy or rarely, brain necrosis;
- a secondary risk of tumours arising in the irradiated field;
- an increased risk of cerebrovascular accident.

For these reasons, radiotherapy is reserved for the following patients:

- Those with postoperative regrowth of non-functioning adenomas showing signs of further growth on serial imaging. Fifty per cent of NFAs will regrow after surgery if there is residual tumour on imaging, and about 20 per cent will regrow even if there is no evidence of tumour on postoperative imaging.[11] Long-term follow up and serial imaging will identify those patients who need further treatment. Radiotherapy is effective in controlling NFAs following surgery.
- Those with functioning adenomas which have not been cured by surgery or show evidence of relapse, either on biochemical assessment or imaging or both. Here the options may include medical therapy, revision surgery, radiotherapy or combined treatment.
- Patients who have had adrenalectomy for Cushing disease. This may prevent them from developing Nelson syndrome.
- Patients who need treatment but are unfit for surgery.

THE FUTURE FOR THE SURGICAL MANAGEMENT OF PITUITARY TUMOURS

- Improved preoperative imaging of adenomas. This particularly applies to Cushing disease and it may be that MET-PET and high resolution MRI will prove successful here.[3]
- Intraoperative MRI is becoming available and does allow assessment of the tumour during surgery. This will hopefully become less expensive, more available and accurate over time.[12, 13]
- Improved instrumentation for surgery. Rigid endoscopes allow the surgeon to see round corners within the pituitary fossa. The next advance will be the generation of instruments which allow the surgeon to see and operate round these corners to remove parts of large adenomas which are currently inaccessible through the sphenoid.

KEY EVIDENCE

- Endoscopic surgery offers significant advantages over traditional approaches and should be considered in all patients undergoing pituitary surgery.[14]

KEY LEARNING POINTS

- Pituitary surgery is only one facet of the management of diseases of the pituitary gland. It requires a multidisciplinary approach

including endocrinologists, radiologists, surgeons, pathologists and radiation oncologists.
- Imaging has made enormous strides in the last two decades and improved accuracy in preoperative imaging has contributed significantly to improved outcomes. Intraoperative imaging is likely to improve outcomes in the next decade.
- Endoscopic surgery offers significant advantages over traditional approaches and the use of the operating microscope, for the following reasons:
  - reduced surgical morbidity
  - extended scope of surgery
  - improved surgical outcomes.

REFERENCES

1. Hardy J, Somma M. Acromegaly. Surgical treatment by transsphenoidal microsurgical removal of the pituitary adenoma. In: Collins WF, Tindall GT (eds). *Clinical management of pituitary disorders*. New York: Raven Press, 1979: 209–17.
2. Yamada S. Epidemiology of pituitary tumours. In: Tharpar K, Kovacs K, Scheithauer BW, Lloyd RV (eds). *Diagnosis and management of pituitary tumors*. New York: Humana Press, 2001: 57–69.
3. Ikeda H, Abe T, Watanabe K. Usefulness of composite methionine-positron emission tomography/3.0-tesla magnetic resonance imaging to detect the localisation and extent of early stage Cushing adenoma. *Journal of Neurosurgery* 2010; **112**: 750–5.
4. Erridge SC, Conkey DS, Strachan MW *et al*. Radiotherapy for pituitary adenomas: long term efficacy and toxicity. *Radiotherapy and Oncology* 2009; **93**: 597–601.
5. Chang EF, Sughrue ME, Zada G *et al*. Long term outcome following repeat transsphenoidal surgery for recurrent endocrine-inactive pituitary adenomas. *Pituitary* 2010; **13**: 223–9.
6. Chacko G, Chacko AG, Kovacs K *et al*. The clinical significance of MIB-1 labeling index in pituitary adenomas. *Pituitary* 2010; **13**: 337–44.
7. Schade R, Andersohn F, Suissa S *et al*. Dopamine agonists and the risk of cardiac-valve regurgitation. *New England Journal of Medicine* 2007; **356**: 29–38.
8. Hadad G, Bassagasteguy L, Carrau RL *et al*. A novel reconstructive technique after endoscopic expanded endonasal approaches: vascular pedicle nasoseptal flap. *Laryngoscope* 2006; **116**: 1882–6.
9. Kristof RA, Rother M, Neuloh G, Klingmuller D. The incidence, clinical manifestations and course of water and electrolyte metabolism disturbances following transsphenoidal pituitary adenoma surgery: a prospective observational study. *Journal of Neurosurgery* 2009; **111**: 555–62.

10. Chee GH, Mathias DB, James RA, Kendall-Taylor P. Transsphenoidal pituitary surgery in Cushing's disease: can we predict the outcome. *Clinical Endocrinology* 2001; **54**: 617–26.

11. Greenman Y, Ouaknine G, Veshchev I *et al*. Postoperative surveillance of clinically nonfunctioning pituitary macroadenomas: markers of tumour quiescence and regrowth. *Clinical Endocrinology* 2003; **58**: 763–9.

12. Netuka D, Masopust V, Belsan T *et al*. One year experience with 3.0 T intraoperative MRI in pituitary surgery. *Acta Neurochirurgica* 2011; **109**(Suppl.): 157–9.

13. Gerlach R, de Rochement Rdu M, Gasser T *et al*. Implementation of the ultra low field intraoperative MRI Polestar N20 during resection control of pituitary adenomas. *Acta Neurochirurgica* 2011; **109**(Suppl.): 73–9.

14. National Institute for Health and Clinical Excellence. Endoscopic transsphenoidal pituitary adenoma resection. Available from: www.nice.org.uk/guidance/IPG32.

PART FOUR

MALIGNANT DISEASE

Surgery by primary site

Section editors: Ken MacKenzie and Gerald McGarry

29

Lip and oral cavity

TIM MARTIN AND KEITH WEBSTER

> Make accurate incisions surrounding the whole tumour, so as to not leave a single root.
>
> Galen (129–200 AD)

INTRODUCTION

The oral cavity is the uppermost part of the digestive tract. It starts at the mucocutaneous junction of the lips (the vermilion border) extending posteriorly to the junction of the hard and soft palate superiorly, anterior fauces laterally and the junction of the anterior two-thirds and posterior third of the tongue inferiorly.

The oral cavity is lined by stratified squamous epithelium of varying degrees of keratinization. Primary tumours of the oral cavity may be derived from the mucosa, salivary glands, neurovascular tissues, bone or dental tissues. Over 90 per cent of tumours of the oral cavity are squamous cell carcinomas.

Globally over 300 000 people are diagnosed with oral cancer each year and it is the eighth most common malignancy.[1] There is considerable geographic variation, oral cancer being the third most common cancer in South East Asia. The incidence of oral cancer in males in England approximates six per 100 000 per annum compared to four per 100 000 per annum for females. The age-standardized incidence rate for oral cancer in South East Asia is as high as 25 per 100 000 per annum (**Figure 29.1**).

The registration rate for oral cancer has risen by over 20 per cent in the last 30 years in England and Wales, particularly in those under 65 years of age.[2, 3] The increasing incidence of oral cancer has been noted in other populations[4] and may be as a consequence of increasing alcohol consumption. Oral cancer is more common in males, patients usually presenting in their sixth and seventh decade of life (**Figure 29.2**), although the incidence of oral cancer in young people seems to be increasing.[5, 6]

Smoking and alcohol consumption are the major aetiological factors in the development of oral cancer,[7] oral cancer being considered largely preventable (**Figure 29.3**).

If oral cancer is detected when it is confined to the oral mucosa five-year survival rates exceed 80 per cent, decreasing to 40 per cent for those with regional disease at presentation and 20 per cent if distant metastasis has occurred (**Figure 29.4**).

Early presentation with oral cancer is associated with an improved prognosis and less extensive treatment in attempt to cure the patient. Research is required regarding selected or opportunistic screening for oral cancer, but at present there is insufficient evidence to support screening.[8]

The management of patients with oral cancer requires a concentration of medical expertise and resources. For the patient to receive optimal management, a truly multidisciplinary approach is required.

PATIENT WORK UP

History

The work up of a patient with suspected oral cancer starts with a detailed accurate history. The patient's symptoms

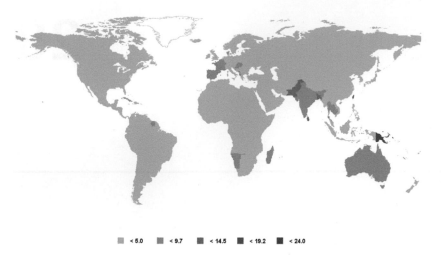

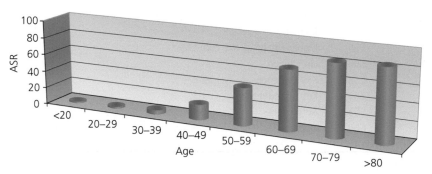

■ < 5.0   ■ < 9.7   ■ < 14.5   ■ < 19.2   ■ < 24.0

Figure 29.1   Age-standardized incidence rate per 100 000 for lip and oral cancer, 2008. Reproduced with permission from Ferlay J, Shin HR, Bray F *et al.* GLOBOCAN 2008, *Cancer incidence and mortality worldwide*: IARC CancerBase No. 10. Lyon: International Agency for Research on Cancer, 2010. Available from: http://globocan.iarc.fr.

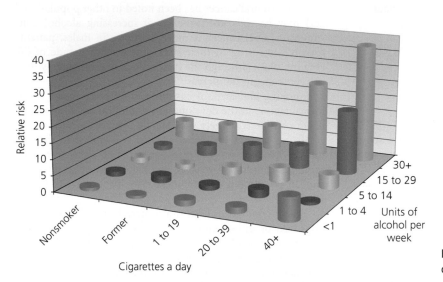

Figure 29.2   Age-standardized incidence rate per 100 000 (SEER data, 1992–2005).

Figure 29.3   Relative risk of developing oral cancer associated with drinking and smoking.

should be documented and a thorough history of each symptom clarified. A short systematic review should be included, asking specifically for symptoms suggestive of metastatic disease or synchronous aerodigestive tract tumour.

The patient's medical history, including medications and allergies, should be recorded. A frequently neglected aspect of history taking is the patient's social history. Patients with oral cancer are likely to face the prospect of major surgery, radiotherapy or chemoradiotherapy. The social circumstances of a patient will significantly influence management decisions. Support packages instituted early in the patient's management may help with timely delivery of care and

increased patient compliance. If it is anticipated that free flap reconstruction may form part of the treatment plan, then direct questions regarding proposed donor sites should be asked, such as hand dominance, intermittent claudication or chronic chest disease.

Examination

While taking a history from a patient, the clinician should make note of such things as the patient's mobility when they

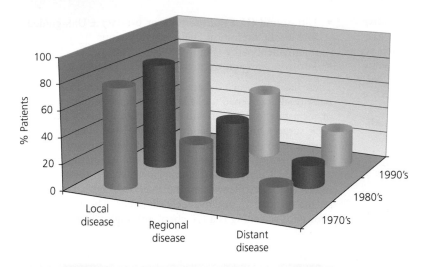

Figure 29.4 Five-year survival related to stage at presentation (SEER data).

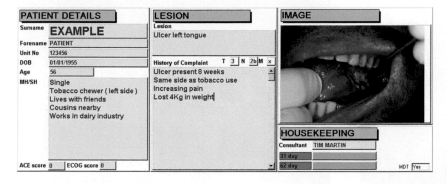

Figure 29.5 Patient information and photograph projected at multidisciplinary meeting to facilitate discussion.

enter the room, the patient's affect, dysarthria or clues to smoking and drinking habits.

The formal examination should ideally be conducted in a dental chair with good lighting. The neck should be systematically palpated for cervical lymphadenopathy. Using two dental mirrors to help with retraction and visualization, the oral cavity and oropharynx should be examined in their entirety in a systematic manner. All patients should undergo nasendoscopy if there is a high index of suspicion that they have oral cancer. A dental examination should form part of the initial consultation so that dental treatment may be started early in anticipation of surgery or radiotherapy.

Occasionally, pain or trismus may limit the examination; in these circumstances an examination under anaesthetic should be conducted.

Investigations

Investigations conducted at the initial consultation will depend on the clinician's suspicion that the patient may have oral cancer. Simple investigations that may be conducted at the first appointment include:

- photographs (**Figure 29.5**);
- incisional biopsy of mucosal lesions;
- fine needle aspiration cytology (FNAC) of suspicious lymphadenopathy;
- orthopantomogram (**Figure 29.6**);
- chest radiograph;
- electrocardiogram;

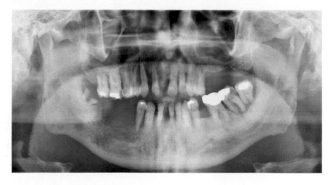

Figure 29.6 Orthopantomogram demonstrating bone loss of the right mandible associated with a T4 squamous cell carcinoma and poor dental status.

- routine bloods – full blood count, urea and electrolytes, liver function tests and clotting.

Biopsy should always be conducted prior to definitive treatment, preferably by a senior member of the team. The biopsy site should be at the periphery of the lesion to include a sample of normal mucosa. A large, deep biopsy may give information regarding depth of invasion and hence the potential necessity to conduct a neck dissection. It has been demonstrated that if tumour thickness on biopsy is > 2 mm, then the final tumour thickness is usually greater than 3.5 mm,[9] suggesting an elective neck dissection may need to be considered. Unfavourable tumour factors, such as perineural spread, vascular permeation and a noncohesive invasive front are indicators to the probability of positive margins and long-term prognosis. Unfavourable features may lead one to consider wider surgical margins where feasible so as to reduce local recurrence (accepting that these same features suggest a poorer long-term prognosis), while balancing the quality of life issues raised by conducting such a resection.

Once oral malignancy is confirmed histologically, additional investigations may be conducted.

STAGING OF THE DISEASE

- Computed tomography (CT) $\pm$ CT of the chest (**Figures 29.7** and **29.8**)
- Magnetic resonance imaging (MRI) (**Figure 29.9**)

- Ultrasound (USS) of the neck or primary $\pm$ USS-guided fine needle aspiration (FNA) of suspicious lymphadenopathy (**Figure 29.10**)
- Positron emission tomography (PET) (**Figure 29.11**).

There has been much debate regarding the extent to which an individual is screened for second aerodigestive tract tumours or metastatic disease. To subject a patient to major head and neck surgery and an extended hospital stay is clearly inappropriate in the presence of established distant disease, however extensive surgery may be an excellent mode of palliation. Currently, screening for distant metastases is indicated in patients with multiple cervical nodes, recurrence, second primary[10] or advanced disease.[11] The modality of choice for screening is a CT chest, although [18]FDG-PET may

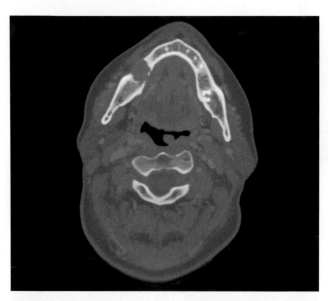

Figure 29.7 Computed tomographic scan demonstrating squamous cell carcinoma invading the right mandible.

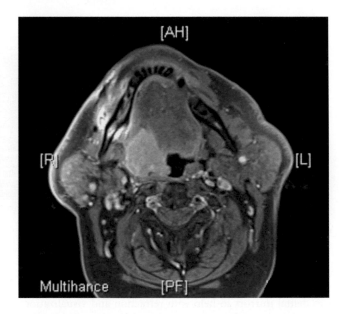

Figure 29.9 Magnetic resonance image of the tongue demonstrating squamous cell carcinoma of oropharynx and base of tongue.

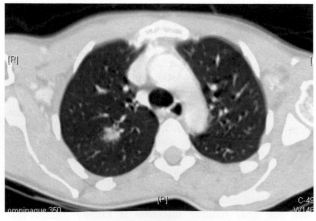

Figure 29.8 Computed tomographic scan of the chest demonstrating metastasis of oral squamous cell carcinoma to the right lung.

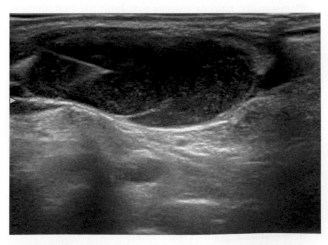

Figure 29.10 Ultrasound-guided fine needle aspiration sampling of an abnormal cervical node.

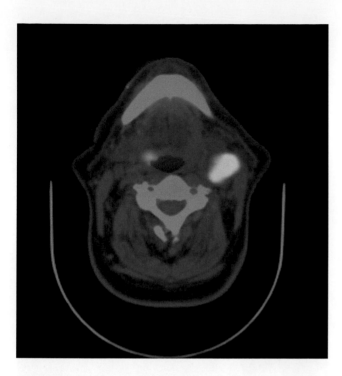

Figure 29.11 Positron emission tomographic scan demonstrating squamous cell carcinoma of the right oropharynx and left cervical nodes.

have an increasing role.[10] The routine use of panendoscopy in the work up of the patient with oral cancer is not warranted.[12] Once the patient has had appropriate investigations, the tumour may be staged using the TNM (tumour, node, metastasis) system (**Tables 29.1** and **29.2**).[13]

PLANNING OF RECONSTRUCTION

The most appropriate reconstruction will be determined by multiple factors, notably characteristics of the primary site and the anticipated defect, the medical and social history of the patient and donor site characteristics. The reconstructive surgeon should have the ability to raise or harvest many different types of local, regional or distant flaps when dealing with head and neck malignancy. Focused examination or investigations regarding proposed reconstruction include:

- Allen's test of the vascular supply to the hand if a radial free forearm flap is anticipated (**Figure 29.12**).
- Magnetic resonance angiography (MRA)/angiography of the leg vessels, if composite fibula reconstruction is anticipated (**Figure 29.13**).
- Thorough examination of the chest and abdomen if a DCIA (deep circumflex iliac artery) free flap is anticipated.
- Doppler ultrasound of potential perforator flap donor sites (**Figure 29.14**).
- CAD/CAM (computer-aided design/computer-aided modelling) models, if complex composite reconstruction is anticipated (**Figure 29.15**).
- Dental impressions for all maxillary tumours.

Table 29.1 TNM staging of oral tumours: AJCC Cancer Staging Manual.[13]

Stage		
T stage	Tx	Primary tumour cannot be assessed
	T0	No evidence of primary tumour
	T1	Tumour 2 cm or less in greatest dimension
	T2	Tumour more than 2 cm, but no more than 4 cm in greatest dimension
	T3	Tumour more than 4 cm in greatest dimension
	T4a	Tumour invades through cortical bone, into deep (extrinsic) muscle of tongue (genioglossus, hyoglossus, palatoglossus or styloglossus), maxillary sinus or skin of face
	T4b	Tumour involves masticator space, pterygoid plates or skull base and/or encases internal carotid artery
N stage	Nx	Regional lymph nodes cannot be assessed
	N0	No regional lymph node metastasis
	N1	Metastasis in a single ipsilateral lymph node, 3 cm or less in greatest dimension
	N2a	Metastasis in a single ipsilateral lymph node more than 3 cm, but not more than 6 cm in greatest dimension
	N2b	Metastasis in multiple ipsilateral lymph nodes, none more than 6 cm in greatest dimension
	N2c	Metastasis in bilateral or contralateral lymph nodes, none more than 6 cm in greatest dimension
	N3	Metastasis in a lymph node more than 6 cm in greatest dimension
M stage	Mx	Distant metastasis cannot be assessed
	M0	No distant metastasis
	M1	Distant metastasis

Table 29.2 Stage grouping of oral tumours: AJCC Cancer Staging Manual.[13]

Stage	T stage	N stage	M stage
I	T1	N0	M0
II	T2	N0	M0
III	T3	N0	M0
	T1	N1	M0
	T2	N1	M0
	T3	N1	M0
IVA	T4a	N0	M0
	T4a	N1	M0
	T1	N2	M0
	T2	N2	M0
	T3	N2	M0
	T4a	N2	M0
IVB	T4b	Any N	M0
	Any T	N3	M0
IVC	Any T	Any N	M1

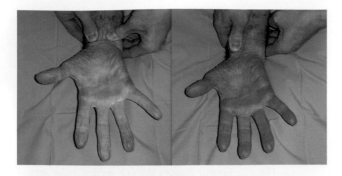

Figure 29.12 Allens test demonstrating good vascular return to the hand following release of digital occlusion of the ulnar artery.

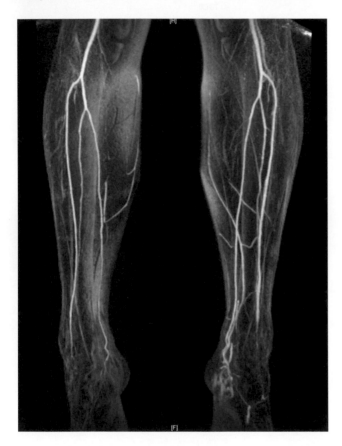

Figure 29.13 Magnetic resonance angiography of the lower limbs demonstrating vascular anatomy prior to fibula free flap harvest.

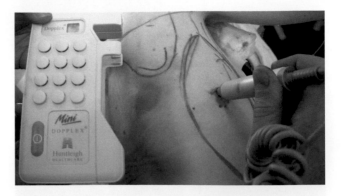

Figure 29.14 Doppler ultrasound of perforators prior to harvest of a scapula-thoracodorsal artery perforator flap.

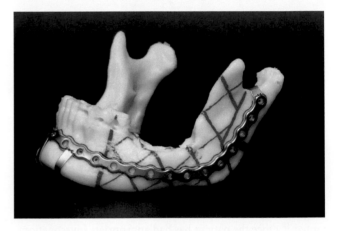

Figure 29.15 CAD-CAM model of mandible demonstrating planned resection and precontoured, prelocalized reconstruction plate.

ANAESTHETIC ASSESSMENT OF THE PATIENT

It is advisable to liaise with the anaesthetist early in the patient's treatment plan. Investigations that may help assess the patient's fitness for anaesthetic include:

- echocardiography;
- exercise tolerance test;
- nuclear cardiac perfusion scan;
- lung function tests.

The patient should be seen by the dietician early in management for dietary advice. Early consideration should be given to a percutaneous endoscopic gastrostomy[14] or a radiologically inserted gastrostomy to supplement feeding, particularly if radiotherapy is anticipated. Nasogastric feeding may be more appropriate if the surgery anticipated is not complex and the need for postoperative radiotherapy unlikely. It is beneficial if the patient meets the speech and language therapist, and counsellor prior to definitive treatment starting.

Once the patient has been thoroughly worked up, a discussion should occur with the whole head and neck team to formulate an appropriate treatment plan. The proposed treatment should then be discussed with the patient and informed consent gained. Informed consent should be tailored to the individual and results achieved in the operating unit. The general success rate of microvascular free flap surgery is greater than 95 per cent, however 5–15 per cent of patients may require return to theatre for complications such as flap compromise, haematoma or infection. It should be remembered that the perioperative mortality rate for major head and neck surgery is 1–3 per cent. Patient's age alone should not rule out major surgery and microvascular reconstruction,[15] as it is the patient's comorbidity that primarily influences the incidence of postoperative complications[16, 17] and prognosis.[18] The benefit of major microvascular surgery in patients with an Adult Comorbidity Evaluation Index 27 of grade 3, unstable angina, respiratory disease with breathlessness at rest, etc., should be carefully considered.

SURGICAL ACCESS

The ultimate aim of surgical resection is removal of the tumour with adequate margins. For the majority of oral tumours, this may be achieved via a peroral route with good retraction and lighting.

Patients with trismus, microstomia, large or posteriorly based oral tumours may require additional access procedures to ensure adequate clearance of the tumour.

Mandibulotmomy

Bone resection is no longer an acceptable method of improving access to oral tumours. A mandibulotomy gives good access to large or posteriorly located tumours. An orthopantomograph (OPG) is required prior to conducting this procedure to demonstrate the dental anatomy of the area. Typically, the procedure is accompanied with a lip split. Mandibulotomy without lip split has been described,[19] however access is not as great as when a lip split is conducted.

The neck dissection incision is extended anteriorly to split the lip. Multiple incision designs have been proposed for the lip split.[20] An incision around the chin prominence tends to make the prominence more pronounced, a vertical incision over the chin point producing a more cosmetic result. Incorporation of a chevron between the chin prominence and vermilion aids closure and breaks up the scar. The intended incision should be marked and temporary tattoos created with needle and ink at the vermilion to ensure accurate reapproximation at the end of the procedure.

The osteotomy should be conducted anterior to the mental foramen so as to preserve labial sensation. The preferred site for the osteotomy is the paramidline area (between the lateral incisor and canine) since the distance between the tooth roots is greater[21] and an osteotomy in this area preserves the attachments of geniohyoid, genioglossus and digastric, only mylohyoid requiring division. If the distance between the lateral incisor and canine roots is insufficient to accept a saw blade, then the lateral incisor should be removed and the osteotomy conducted through the socket to minimize the possibility of osteoradionecrosis should a tooth be damaged. Once the site of osteotomy is established, miniplates are adapted and applied to the mandible bridging the proposed osteotomy site. The plates are then removed and the osteotomy conducted using a fine reciprocating saw blade.[22] The mandible and cheek flap may now be retracted laterally and superiorly giving excellent access to the posterior oral cavity and oropharynx (**Figure 29.16**).

The nonanatomical position adopted by the temporomandibular joint (TMJ) during this procedure does not give rise to long-term TMJ dysfunction.[23] The osteotomy is plated with the preadapted and drilled plates at the end of the procedure, ensuring the occlusion is accurately preserved (**Figure 29.17**).

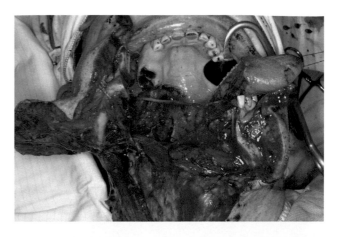

Figure 29.16 Lip split mandibulotomy to facilitate access to posterior tumours.

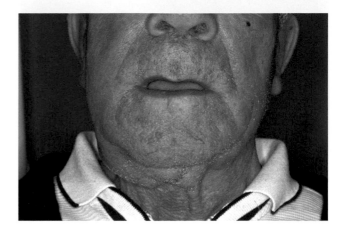

Figure 29.17 Cosmetic appearance of healed lip split mandibulotomy at six months.

Visor approach and lingual release

This approach is generally reserved for when bilateral neck dissections are to be performed. The visor approach may also be appropriate for recurrence or second primary tumours in patients who have received previous radiotherapy to the mandible. The visor approach avoids facial incisions, the incision being located in a cervical skin crease. A mastoid to mastoid visor flap is elevated in the subplatysmal plane to the lower border of the mandible. An intraoral mucosal incision is made in the lingual gingival sulcus from the posterior molar on one side to the posterior molar of the other. In edentulous patients, the incision is made on the alveolar crest. The mylohyoid, geniohyoid, genioglossus and digastrics are detached from the lingual aspect of the mandible allowing the floor of the mouth and tongue to be dropped into the neck (**Figure 29.18**).

Care should be taken to ensure the lingual and hypoglossal nerves are not injured during the dissection. The reattachment of geniohyoid and genioglossus muscles at the end of the procedure is important to reconstitute the floor of the mouth. This may be facilitated by drilling holes in the

Invariably, it is the deep margin that is close or positive,[34] however close deep margins do not necessarily require adjunctive treatment.[35] The use of ultrasonography to aid in determining deep margin resection has been described.[36]

Frozen sections are not routinely used by many surgeons,[25, 26] reasons cited being potential cost,[37] inability to reliably prevent positive final margins[37, 38] and poor relocation of biopsy site should the result be positive.[39] Ninety-nine percent of American head and neck surgeons routinely use frozen section intraoperatively, however overreliance on frozen section may result in undertreatment of tumours.[29]

When conducting a bony resection, a 1 cm margin should be achieved. It has been demonstrated that it is unusual for extension of tumour in bone to exceed the overlying soft tissue extension.

BUCCAL CARCINOMA

Surgical anatomy

The buccal mucosa is the mucosal lining of the inner surface of the cheek. The area extends from the oral commisure anteriorly to the retromolar trigone posteriorly. The junction between the buccal mucosa and retromolar trigone is an arbitrary line drawn from the maxillary tuberosity to the distobuccal aspect of the mandibular third molar (or its anticipated position if not present).

The inferior and superior boundaries of the area are delineated by the mandibular and maxillary gingivobuccal sulci, respectively.

The buccal mucosa is not exposed to masticatory loads and so is covered by a lining mucosa with nonkeratinizing stratified squamous epithelium. The mucosa is firmly attached to the underlying buccinator muscle. Minor salivary glands are located within the cheek. The parotid duct pierces the buccinator muscle to enter the oral cavity adjacent to the first maxillary molar tooth.

Sensory innervation to the area is via the buccal branch of the mandibular division of the trigeminal nerve. Lymphatic drainage of the site is via the ipsilateral facial and submandibular nodes to the deep cervical chain. The thickness of the cheek, from mucosal lining to external skin, is 1–3 cm.

Epidemiology

The buccal mucosa is the most common site for oral cancer in South East Asia, up to 40 per cent of oral cancers arising at this site. This contrasts with North America and Western Europe where buccal carcinoma only accounts for 2–10 per cent of oral carcinomas.[26, 40] The consumption of betel quid is socially and culturally embedded in the countries of South East Asia and is responsible for the difference in site predilection. The ingredients of betel quid (paan/paan masala) varies throughout South East Asia. The main ingredients include the Piper betel leaf, slaked lime, spices, tobacco and areca nut. For many years, the tobacco content alone was credited as being the carcinogenic agent in betel quid, however it is now recognized that the areca nut is also carcinogenic, as well as being the main aetiological agent in oral

submucous fibrosis. Individuals who consume betel quid frequently have a preference regarding which side they chew betel, this corresponding to the side of tumour development. There is a strong association with smoking and alcohol consumption in populations where betel chewing is not prevalent.[40, 41, 42]

The male-to-female ratio in Western countries approximates 1:1, however in South East Asia the ratio reflects the consumption of betel quid. In India, the male-to-female ratio is approximately 4:1, however in the Taiwanese population, where betel quid use occurs primarily in the male population, the ratio may be as high as 27:1.[43]

Buccal carcinoma typically occurs over the age of 40 years, although it may occur in younger patients,[44] particularly when associated with the habit of betel chewing.[45]

Presentation

Buccal carcinoma may be described as verrucous, exophytic or ulceroinfiltrative in character (**Figures 29.23** and **29.24**).

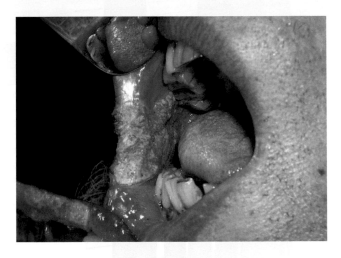

Figure 29.23 Squamous cell carcinoma buccal mucosa of verrucous appearance.

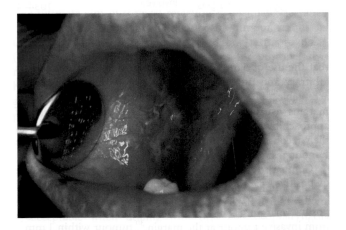

Figure 29.24 Squamous cell carcinoma buccal mucosa of ulceroinfiltrative appearance.

Patients may present with pain, an intraoral mass, ulceration or trismus. Patients who chew betel often have areas of erythroleukoplakia of the buccal mucosa or submucous fibrosis and consequent trismus, making the detection of invasive squamous cell carcinoma difficult. Advanced buccal carcinomas may extend into adjacent sites to include external skin, mandible or maxilla.

It is not unusual for patients to present with advanced disease, 40 per cent or more presenting with stage III/IV disease.[40, 41, 46] Palpable lymphadenopathy on presentation may be as high as 57 per cent for T3/4 lesions. Occult nodal metastasis may be present in 26 per cent of those who are clinically N0 at presentation.[40, 41, 46, 47] Tumours greater than T2, are poorly differentiated, have a poor lymphocytic response[47] or are thicker than 5 mm[47, 48] are more likely to demonstrate cervical metastasis. Tumours are usually well differentiated.[40, 49]

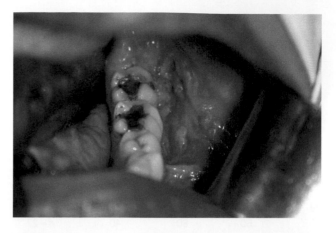

Figure 29.25 Case 1: Squamous cell carcinoma buccal mucosa.

Work up

Biopsies of buccal carcinomas should be of sufficient depth to help the pathologist give an indication of depth of invasion, since this will help decide on management of the neck. Buccal carcinoma may rapidly extend to adjacent sites, thus accurate imaging is required. Most patients will require MRI/CT imaging, augmented with ultrasound scan if necessary to help in the assessment of depth of primary and cervical lymphadenopathy.

Treatment

PRIMARY SITE

Traditional treatment of buccal carcinoma is surgery with PORT for selected patients.[41, 43] T1/2 disease can typically be resected perorally, however T3/4 disease may require facial access incisions and bony resection of the maxilla and/or mandible.

The primary tumour should be resected with a 1 cm margin[26] and up to 2 cm if skin is involved.[50] The buccinator muscle should be included as the deep margin at the very least.[50] The parotid duct may need to be repositioned or ligated.[49] External skin should be taken with the specimen if there is any evidence clinically or on imaging that it is involved. Partial maxillectomy or mandibular resection (rim or segmental) may be required.

Small T1 tumours may be resected and reconstructed by primary closure. Healing by secondary intention may be considered, however postoperative trismus may be anticipated unless vigorous mouth opening exercises are conducted. Split thickness skin grafts may be used, the use of silicone sheets to stabilize the graft being useful.[51] The use of a skin graft to reconstruct deeper resections may leave a very thin cheek with potentially poor aesthetics. Local flaps such as the buccal fat pad or temporoparietal fascial flap may be used for reconstruction if tumour extension does not compromise their use. Microvascular free flap reconstruction with a radial free forearm flap or anterolateral thigh flap[52] restores the thickness of the cheek and if external skin is involved, the flaps can be bipaddled to provide

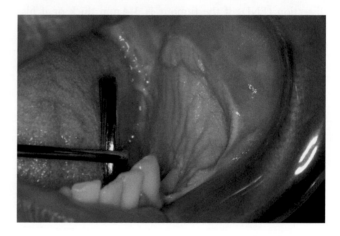

Figure 29.26 Case 1: Radial free forearm flap reconstruction.

reconstruction of mucosal and skin surfaces. T4 tumours requiring segmental resection of the mandible may require composite free flap reconstruction. Reconstruction with a radial free forearm flap has been shown to give better postoperative mouth opening than reconstruction with a split skin graft or buccal fat pad (**Figures 29.25** and **29.26**).[53]

Radiotherapy as a single treatment modality for T1/2 tumours has been advocated,[54, 55] however, a change of practice from radiotherapy to surgery at Memorial Sloan Kettering was associated with improved prognosis.[56] Brachytherapy or external beam irradiation may be considered.

NECK

Regional spread of disease in buccal carcinoma is usually to the ipsilateral level I and II lymph nodes.[57, 58] Patients with palpable lymphadenopathy or pathological nodes on imaging should have a comprehensive neck dissection, although if pathological nodes are only located in level I, a level I–III selective neck dissection (SND) may be considered.[59] Nodes in the region of the facial artery as it crosses the mandible should be removed with the neck dissection specimen.

Patients with T2 or greater primary tumours or tumours with a thickness >5 mm should have an elective neck dissection.[41, 60] Some institutions will conduct an elective neck

Table 29.3 Recurrence of buccal carcinoma.

Local (%)	Regional (%)	Locoregional (%)	
46	28	26	n = 147 (all N0 primaries)[49]
53	28	22	n = 119[41]

Table 29.4 Five-year survival for stage I–IV buccal carcinoma.

I (%)	II (%)	III (%)	IV (%)	
78	66	62	50	n = 119[41]
71	60	60	40	n = 27[40]
83	71	57	42	n = 280[45]

dissection (END) if the tumour is 3–4 mm thick or if histological examination of the tumour demonstrates lymphatic infiltration.[41]

PORT

The indications for postoperative radiotherapy to the locoregional area are similar to other sites, notably two or more nodes in the neck, extracapsular spread (ECS), positive margins or stage III/IV disease.[46] The beneficial role of PORT in selected patients with buccal carcinoma has been demonstrated by several authors.[61, 62] Some authors suggest that PORT should be considered even in stage I and II disease,[40, 46] or tumours greater than 10 mm thick.[61]

Recurrence

Recurrence rates for buccal carcinoma are 26–80 per cent,[40, 41, 43, 46, 47, 49] usually occurring within two years (**Table 29.3**).[41, 43, 49]

Involvement of the parotid duct and buccinator have not been found to be significant indicators of recurrence.[40] Factors that influence recurrence include tumour thickness[47, 48, 63] and tumour differentiation.[49]

Prognosis

Buccal carcinoma is considered by many to be particularly aggressive. Five-year survival figures vary depending on population studied and treatment modality (**Table 29.4**).[41, 46]

Factors that potentially influence survival include regional metastasis,[41, 64] extracapsular spread,[41] tumour thickness >5–6 mm,[47, 48] skin involvement,[43] positive margins,[65] stage[45] and recurrent disease.[47]

FLOOR OF MOUTH CARCINOMA

Surgical anatomy

The floor of mouth is the mucosal lining of the anterior and lateral floor of the mouth. The area is bound anteriorly and laterally by the attached mucoperiosteum of the mandibular alveolus. The lateral floor of mouth is bound posteriorly by the anterior tonsillar pillars. Medially, the floor of mouth merges with the ventral and lateral aspects of the tongue.

The floor of mouth is lined by nonkeratinizing stratified squamous epithelium similar to the buccal mucosa, but with a less dense submucosa. Underlying the mucosa lie minor salivary glands, the sublingual glands, submandibular ducts, hypoglossal nerves, lingual nerves and genioglossus muscles. These structures are located in an area bound by the mylohyoid muscle laterally and hypoglossal muscle medially. The submandibular ducts enter the mouth anteriorly either side of the lingual frenum.

Sensory innervation to the area is by the lingual branch of the mandibular division of the trigeminal nerve. Lymphatic drainage of the lateral floor of the mouth is via the ipsilateral submandibular nodes to the deep cervical chain. Lymphatic drainage of the anterior floor of mouth is via the submental nodes to both the left and right deep cervical chains.[66] Lingual lymph nodes in the floor of mouth, above the mylohyoid, may have implications regarding the management of tumours of the floor of mouth.[58, 67]

Epidemiology

The floor of mouth is a common site for oral cancer, 18–33 per cent of oral cancers developing at this site.[26, 68, 69, 70, 71] It is thought that the high incidence of cancer at this site may be due to pooling of saliva with dissolved carcinogens or lack of keratinized epithelium.[72] Within the anatomical site, tumours are more likely to occur anteriorly.[73, 74, 75]

Floor of mouth carcinoma occurs more frequently in men,[70, 71, 74, 76, 77] the age at diagnosis usually being in the sixth to seventh decade.[70, 76, 77] Floor of mouth cancer, as does oral cancer at all sites, has a strong association with smoking[72] and the consumption of alcohol.[76]

Presentation

Since the floor of mouth is a relatively small anatomical area, tumours frequently extend into adjacent sites notably the tongue or mandible.[78] Patients may present with a sore lesion, ulceration or obstructive submandibular gland symptoms.[79] Leukoplakia of the floor of mouth may be considered a premalignant condition with an annual transformation rate of 1–2.9 per cent,[80, 81] the demonstration of carcinoma within an excised leukoplakia not being uncommon.

Stage at presentation varies considerably between institutions, although approximately 50 per cent present with advanced disease (**Table 29.5**).

Cervical lymphadenopathy is present in 17–45 per cent of patients on presentation,[70, 71, 74, 82] up to 22 per cent of those clinically N0 at presentation having occult metastasis.[70, 77, 82, 83] Depending on the location of the tumour, up to 28.6 per cent of patients may have bilateral nodal involvement.[71, 82] Many tumours of the floor of mouth are well or moderately differentiated.[74]

Work up

Work up of patients with floor of mouth tumours should follow that of any patient with oral cancer. Particularly important in larger floor of mouth tumours is assessment of invasion of the base of tongue or mandible. The loose connective tissue of the floor of mouth presents a poor barrier to local spread.

Treatment

PRIMARY SITE

The need for aggressive treatment of floor of mouth carcinomas is well recognized.[84]

Surgical resection with a 1 cm margin should be achieved if surgery is the preferred treatment modality. Even in the best surgeon's hands, positive or close margins may be seen in up to 47 per cent of resections,[70, 78] despite the use of intraoperative frozen section.[71] Many floor of mouth tumours are infiltrative with indistinct edges, possibly explaining the high incidence of positive margins.[71] Further resection is advocated if margins are positive.[71] Although 1 cm margins are considered by most surgeons to be adequate, extended 2 cm margins have been advocated by some.[85]

The early extension of floor of mouth tumours into the tongue or mandible is demonstrated by the fact that many patients require rim or segmental resection of the mandible.[70] Surgical resection of the floor of mouth in the majority of circumstances will involve resection of part of the submandibular ducts. Typically, the ducts will be resected at the resection margin, well away from their orifice, however in smaller resections at least 3 mm length of duct proximal to the orifice should be taken to ensure surgical clearance of carcinoma or dysplasia that may extend along the duct.[86] Management of the submandibular ducts is of great importance if a neck dissection is not being conducted with consequent removal of the submandibular gland. Stricture of the duct in the presence of a functioning gland may give rise to obstructive symptoms of the gland and difficulty in differentiating the potential submandibular gland swelling from cervical disease. The ducts should be transected obliquely to minimize stricture formation and repositioned at the margin of resection, ideally being stented.[87] Alternatively, the ducts

may be found proximal to the resection margin, a longitudinal incision made and the duct 'marsupialized' to the floor of mouth mucosa. Uninvolved branches of the lingual nerve should be identified and preserved.

Small resections may be left to heal by secondary intention or a split thickness skin graft applied (**Figures 29.27, 29.28** and **29.29**). A more substantial reconstruction may be achieved using local nasolabial[88] or facial artery musculomucosal flaps,[89] however an edentulous segment is required when using both of these flaps to accommodate their pedicle. If a neck dissection is required and surgical facilities allow, microvascular reconstruction provides a far more flexible reconstructive option, without necessarily prolonging operative time if a two team approach is adopted (**Figures 29.30 and 29.31**).

The radial free forearm flap is an ideal reconstructive option for floor of mouth defects, easily being converted to a composite flap if segmental resection of an edentulous mandible is required. Prefabricated fasciomucosal free flaps have been described in oral reconstruction,[90] however their role in oncological reconstruction is questioned. The fibula osteocutaneous flap provides superior reconstruction if a

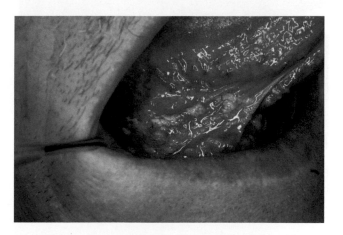

Figure 29.27 Case 2: Squamous cell carcinoma floor of mouth.

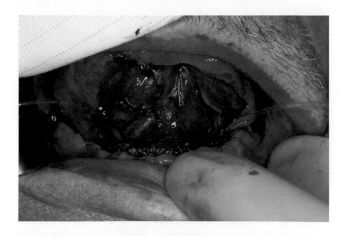

Figure 29.28 Case 2: Laser resection of tumour and stenting of submandibular ducts.

Table 29.5 Floor of mouth carcinoma stage at presentation.

Stage I/II (%)	Stage III/IV (%)		
43	57	$n = 99$[70]	United States
50	50	$n = 280$[71]	United States
15	85	$n = 144$[76]	United States (tertiary referral centre, 45 previously treated elsewhere)
76	24	$n = 207$[74]	France
49	51	$n = 320$[77]	United States
64	35	$n = 248$[82]	United States

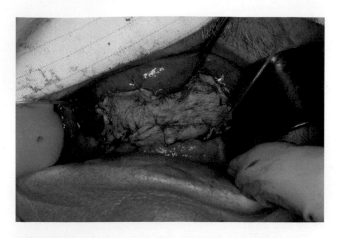

Figure 29.29 Case 2: Reconstruction with split skin graft.

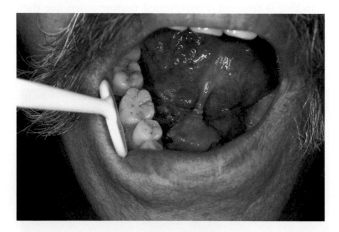

Figure 29.30 Case 3: Squamous cell carcinoma floor of mouth involving alveolar bone.

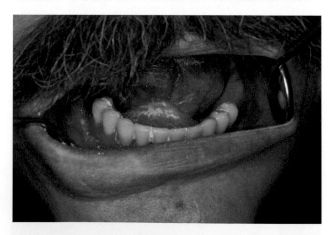

Figure 29.31 Case 3: Reconstruction with anterolateral thigh free flap and implant retained denture.

segmental resection is anticipated in a dentate patient, although like the composite radial free flap, flexibility of the skin paddle is limited. The scapula osteocutaneous flap with two skin paddles, or one skin paddle and muscle left to

mucosalize, provides an excellent reconstruction of large defects involving mucosa, bone and external skin.

Radiotherapy techniques (brachytherapy or external beam) for T1/2 primaries have been shown to provide results similar to surgery.[74, 75, 91] The proximity of the floor of the mouth to the mandible is of concern when using brachytherapy, since up to 8.5 per cent of patients treated with this modality require segmental resection of the mandible due to osteoradionecrosis within 10 years.[74, 75]

Several units have described a change in practice from brachytherapy to surgery as the primary treatment modality due to the risk of complications.[71, 77, 92] T3/4 lesions are best treated with surgery and postoperative radiotherapy.

NECK

Regional spread of disease in floor of mouth carcinomas is usually to the ipsilateral level I to III lymph nodes,[58, 77] involvement of multiple levels not being unusual. Lesions towards the midline may spread to both sides of the neck, hence bilateral neck dissections should be considered. The presence of lingual lymph nodes has raised the concept of in-continuity neck dissection[93] in an attempt to reduce local recurrence and improve survival. Resection of the tumour accompanied with the complete clearance of the floor of the mouth, preserving mylohyoid, hyoglossus and genioglossus if possible, so clearing the lingual lymph nodes would seem an acceptable method of managing lingual lymph nodes.[67]

The decision to conduct an elective neck dissection has been related to tumour size or depth of invasion. Lesions that are T2 or greater should have an elective I–III/IV selective neck dissection,[70, 94] although elective neck dissections have been advocated for T1 lesions.[74, 95]

Tumour thickness of 4 mm is often used as a 'generic' critical thickness, greater than which an elective neck dissection is indicated, since the risk of occult metastasis is greater than 20 per cent.[96] It has been demonstrated that the risk of cervical metastasis of floor of mouth tumours exceeds 20 per cent in tumours as thin as 1.5–2 mm.[94, 97] Using a thickness of 1.5 mm may result in up to 32 per cent of patients requiring END based on thickness criteria.[97]

PORT

The indications for postoperative radiotherapy to the loco-regional area are similar to other sites, notably two or more involved nodes in the neck, extracapsular spread, positive margins or stage III/IV disease.

The beneficial role of PORT in selected patients with floor of mouth carcinoma has been demonstrated.[70, 78, 82]

Recurrence

Recurrence rates for floor of mouth carcinoma are 26–55 per cent,[70, 77, 84] usually within the first two years.

Factors that influence recurrence include tumour size,[70, 77] margin status[70, 71] and tumour thickness,[94] and advanced nodal disease.[77]

Table 29.6 Prognosis for floor of mouth carcinoma.

I (%)	II (%)	III (%)	IV (%)		
89	73	65	30	5-year DSS[93]	United States
95	86	82	52	5-year DSS[70]	S+PORT
88	80	66	32	$n = 320$[77]	

DSS, disease-specific survival; PORT, postoperative radiotherapy.

Prognosis

Overall five-year survival for floor of mouth carcinoma is 52–76 per cent (**Table 29.6**).[70, 71, 77, 82] Factors that potentially influence survival include nodal status,[71, 82] thickness,[94] margin status and recurrence.[71]

TONGUE CARCINOMA

Surgical anatomy

The oral tongue is the freely mobile anterior two-thirds of the tongue. The oral tongue is demarcated from the base of tongue by the circumvallate papillae posteriorly. The tongue may be subdivided into the tip, dorsum, lateral borders and ventral surface. The ventral and lateral surfaces are in continuity with the floor of mouth, having a lining mucosa with nonkeratinizing stratified squamous epithelium. The dorsum and tip of tongue are lined by specialized gustatory mucosa, with a thick, primarily keratinized epithelium. The mucosa of the tongue overlies the intrinsic muscles of the tongue, in addition to the four paired extrinsic muscles of the tongue – genioglossus, hyoglossus, styloglossus and palatoglossus.

Motor innervation to muscles of the tongue is via the hypoglossal nerve, except palatoglossus which is supplied by the vagus nerve. Sensation of the tongue is supplied by the lingual nerve, a branch of the mandibular division of the trigeminal nerve. Taste sensation of the oral tongue is supplied by fibres of the facial nerve that run with the lingual nerve before passing to the chorda tympanic branch of the facial nerve.

Lymphatic drainage of the lateral borders of the tongue is to the ipsilateral cervical nodes; however, drainage of the midline, tip and base of tongue occurs bilaterally. The blood supply to the tongue is provided by the paired lingual arteries, the third branches of the external carotid artery. During resection of posterior tongue lesions, the contralateral vascular pedicle should be preserved if the tongue tip is to be maintained.

The tongue is a complex structure with an important role in mastication, deglutition and speech.

Epidemiology

In populations where tobacco chewing is not endemic, the oral tongue is one of the most common sites for oral cancer, 22–39 per cent of oral cancers developing at this site.[26, 69, 98]

Within the site, most tumours occur in the middle third of the tongue,[99, 100] commonly on the lateral aspect, followed by the ventral aspect of the tongue. Only 4–5 per cent of tongue carcinomas occur on the dorsum of the tongue.[101]

Tongue cancer occurs slightly more frequently in males,[99, 102, 103, 104, 105] the age at diagnosis usually being in the sixth to eighth decades,[99, 103, 104] 90 per cent of patients being greater than 40 years of age.[102] The male-to-female ratio has decreased in recent years, possibly due to increased alcohol consumption by females.

Smoking and alcohol consumption is common among patients with tongue cancer,[102] up to 70 per cent describing significant tobacco and alcohol use.[99]

Presentation

Patients with oral cancer may present with several symptoms notably pain, ulceration or a lump on the tongue.[99, 102, 104, 106] Lesions of the oral tongue are more likely to be symptomatic than lesions of the base of the tongue, although despite this many patients still present with a four- to six-month history of symptoms prior to seeking medical advice.[102, 104, 107] The majority of patients with cancer of the oral tongue present with stage I/II disease,[99, 102, 103, 106] which contrasts significantly with cancers of the base of the tongue that are usually stage III/IV at presentation.[102] Clinically positive cervical lymphadenopathy at presentation is in the region of 21–34 per cent.[99, 103, 105] Occult cervical metastasis has been demonstrated in up to 53 per cent of patients with tongue cancer,[99, 104, 107, 108] being related to tumour thickness.[109] Tumours arising on the lateral aspect of the tongue tend to be thicker than those of the ventral aspect of the tongue.[105] Up to 4.5 per cent may have occult cervical disease in the contralateral neck.[104] Clinical examination, CT and MRI have relatively poor sensitivity at determining cervical lymphadenopathy.[105, 110]

The majority of tongue tumours are well to moderately differentiated on histological examination.[99, 102, 103, 106]

Work up

As with many sites, management of the neck is frequently determined by tumour thickness. Tumour thickness can be assessed accurately with intraoral sonography, or immediate sonography of the resected tumour[39] prior to proceeding to a neck dissection if access to the neck is not required for reconstructive purposes.

Biopsies should endeavour to include the deep margin of the tumour in addition to mucosa at the periphery of the tumour. Deep biopsies may give an indication of tumour depth, but also multifactorial histological malignancy grading of the most dysplastic areas of the invasive front may help in assessing the risk of cervical metastasis.[105]

Treatment

PRIMARY

Resection of the tumour with a 1 cm margin in three dimensions should be conducted if surgery is the treatment of choice. The use of ultrasonography to aid in assessment of surgical clearance had been advocated,[39, 111] particularly for the deep margin. Frozen section is not routinely used in many units. Even with apparently adequate margins during surgery, 10 per cent of resections may demonstrate histologically positive margins.[99]

The aim of reconstruction of the oral tongue following resection is to ensure maximum function of the residual tongue tissue, since the complex function of the tongue cannot be replicated with current reconstructive techniques.[112] Preservation of the tip of the tongue, while maintaining oncologically sound resection margins, helps maximize postoperative function.[113]

The use of monopolar electrocautery, 'cutting' through mucosa changing to 'coagulation' when in muscle, or the harmonic scalpel helps reduce bleeding during the resection, however this is at the cost of lack of feel afforded by the use of scalpel or scissors. If both lingual vessels are resected, then the viability of the tip of tongue remnant should be carefully assessed. Sacrifice of both hypoglossal nerves results in a nonfunctioning tongue tip.

Small lesions may be removed with a laser and allowed to heal by secondary intention (**Figures 29.32** and **29.33**).

T1 and small T2 primary tumours may be excised with a vertical wedge and the defect closed primarily, if the defect does not extend to significantly include the floor of mouth. Many larger lesions benefit from free flap reconstruction of the defect, usually with a radial free forearm flap, although the anterolateral thigh free flap is being used more frequently (**Figures 29.34** and **29.35**).

The skin paddle of the chosen free flap should be fashioned so as not to restrict residual tongue function and should hopefully augment swallowing. Typically, the reconstruction should be of the same size, or slightly smaller than the defect created by the resection. Care should be taken in the design of the flap when the defect extends to include

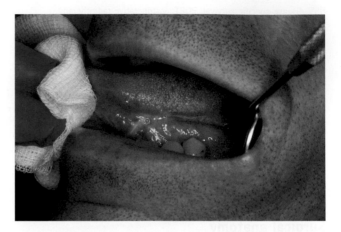

Figure 29.33　Case 4: Appearance following laser resection.

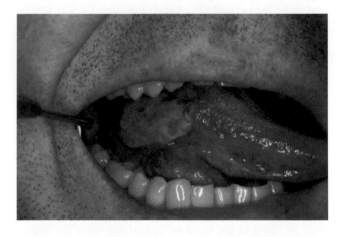

Figure 29.34　Case 5: Squamous cell carcinoma right tongue.

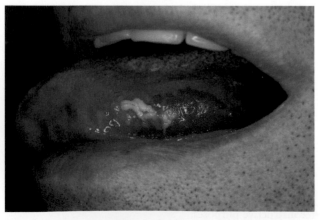

Figure 29.32　Case 4: Squamous cell carcinoma left lateral tongue.

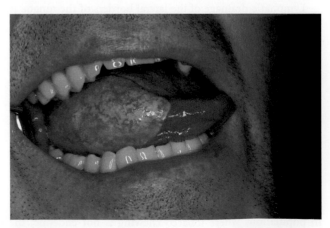

Figure 29.35　Case 5: Reconstruction with radial free forearm flap.

adjacent sites, such as the soft palate or floor of mouth. The mobile tongue and floor of mouth should be 'separated' in the reconstruction to minimize restriction of movement of the residual tongue.[112] Thin radial free flaps may have their bulk increased by extending fascial flaps beyond the skin island, the fascial flaps then being folded and buried underneath the epithelial reconstruction.[112]

Reconstruction of large resections may be accompanied by measures aimed to improve postoperative function, such as static laryngeal suspension to the mandible and cricopharyngeal myotomy.[112]

Once the specimen is removed, it is examined for clearance and orientated for the pathologist, a digital photograph being useful.

Radiotherapy as the primary treatment modality has been advocated since it conserves tongue volume and morphology, brachytherapy being considered preferable to external beam radiotherapy.[114] Osteoradionecrosis of the mandible is a recognized complication of brachytherapy of the tongue, up to 9 per cent developing some form of osseous complication.[103] The use of brachytherapy to the primary site requires either surgery or external beam radiotherapy to the neck in an elective or therapeutic manner. When surgery is not conducted as the primary treatment valuable prognostic information is lost, since the primary tumour is not examined histologically. This makes the decision as to whether to conduct an END more difficult. It has been suggested that surgery is superior to brachytherapy in the management of stage I/II tongue cancer.[115] By conducting surgery as the primary treatment modality, radiotherapy is kept in reserve for either poor prognostic indicators of the resected specimen, for management of recurrence or management of second primaries which commonly occur at a later date.

NECK

Tumours of the tongue initially metastasize to levels I and II, lateral tongue tumours frequently metastasizing directly to level II nodes.[58] Involvement of level V nodes, in the absence of positive nodes in levels I–IV is rare, however it is not unusual for nodes in level IV to be involved,[105, 116] hence even in elective neck dissections levels I–IV should be dissected.

Like floor of mouth tumours, the presence of lingual lymph nodes should be considered and either an in-continuity resection with the neck specimen or clearance of tissue above the mylohyoid conducted.

Bilateral neck dissections should be considered in tumours that extend to or beyond the midline.

The management of the neck in larger primary tumours is usually straightforward since the neck is accessed for microvascular or pedicled flap reconstruction of the primary site. Management difficulties arise with smaller tumours amenable to peroral resection and local closure.[109]

It has been proposed that the increased incidence of nodal metastasis associated with tongue carcinoma may be due to contraction of tongue muscles promoting entry of cancer cells into the lymphatics.[117] It is thought that mechanism by which tumour thickness is related to cervical metastasis is that thicker tumours have access to wider lymphatics in which tumour emboli can form more readily.

Although tumours arising on the lateral aspect of the tongue tend to be thicker than those of the ventral aspect of the tongue,[105] this may not manifest as a greater risk of cervical metastasis, since the 'critical thickness' for tumours of the floor of mouth is less than other oral sites.

Elective neck dissection or elective neck radiotherapy should be considered for tumours thicker than 3–4 mm,[109, 118, 119] T2 or greater in dimension and T1 tumours that demonstrate poor histological features (poor differentiation, double DNA aneuploidy or degree of differentiation at the advancing front).[100, 119]

Elective neck dissection significantly improves locoregional control.[118] It has been demonstrated that conducting an END reduces regional recurrence from 47 per cent in 'watch and wait' patients to 9 per cent if END is conducted.[108]

END has been shown by some to improve five-year survival,[108] the five-year survival of patients undergoing therapeutic neck dissection following a 'watch and wait' policy being 35 per cent, as opposed to 69 per cent when an elective neck dissection is conducted.[107] Others, however, have not demonstrated a survival advantage.[99, 118]

PORT

PORT has been advocated for positive margins,[99, 100] multiple cervical nodes,[100] extracapsular spread in the neck,[100] stage III/IV disease,[99, 100] perineural spread[100] or tumours thicker than 9–10 mm even in the absence of other features.[109, 117, 120] Based on involved margins, ECS of cervical nodes or multiple positive nodes, 62 per cent of patients receiving surgery as the primary treatment modality may require PORT.[105]

Local failure following PORT to tongue tumours has been demonstrated to be higher than comparable floor of mouth tumours, leading some to suggest higher doses of PORT should be considered for tongue tumours.[78]

Recurrence

Recurrence rates for oral tongue carcinoma are 10–50 per cent,[104, 109] usually being locoregional.[99, 105]

Similar to other sites, recurrence usually occurs within the first two years.[99, 106]

Factors that influence local recurrence include tumour thickness and the presence of perineural spread.[109, 121] It has been proposed that recurrence of thicker tumours is related to difficulty in assessing deep clearance intraoperatively compared to assessing mucosal clearance.[117]

Patients younger than 40 years have been demonstrated to be significantly more likely to develop locoregional failure, although this does not influence survival.[122] Ten per cent of patients who have developed a tongue tumour will develop metachronous second tumours of the oral cavity.[104]

Prognosis

Tumour thickness,[95, 105, 118, 119, 121] the presence of perineural invasion,[109, 121] cervical metastasis[99, 104] or dysplasia at the

Table 29.7 Tongue prognosis.

I	II	III	IV		
82%	65%	54%	22%	n = 322 (mainly radiotherapy)[2]	Overall 5-year 56%
90	72	54	34	n = 297 (mainly surgery)[99]	Overall 65%
				n = 448 (brachytherapy only)[3]	45% 5-year DSS

DSS, disease-specific survival.

resection margins[119] have all been demonstrated to influence prognosis. Patients with tumours greater than 9 mm thick have been shown to have a five-year survival of 66 per cent compared to 100 per cent survival for tumours less than 3 mm thick (**Table 29.7**).[109]

RETROMOLAR CARCINOMA

Surgical anatomy

The retromolar trigone is a triangular area of mucosa that overlies the ascending ramus of the mandible. The base of the triangle is in the region of the mandibular third molar inferiorly, the apex being adjacent to the maxillary tuberosity superiorly. The area is bound by the buccal mucosa laterally and the anterior tonsillar pillar medially. The retromolar mucosa is not exposed to masticatory loads and so is covered by a lining mucosa with nonkeratinizing stratified squamous epithelium, similar to the buccal mucosa. Sensory innervation to the area is by the buccal branch of the mandibular division of the trigeminal nerve. Lymphatic drainage is to the ipsilateral submandibular and deep cervical nodes.

Epidemiology

The retromolar trigone is a relatively unusual site for carcinoma of the oral cavity, only 6–7 per cent of oral carcinomas arising at this site.[26, 123] The disease is more common in males and like other sites is typically a disease of older individuals.[123, 124, 125] In common with other oral sites, there is a strong association with smoking[125, 126] and alcohol consumption.

Presentation

Patients typically present late with pain, trismus, otalgia and lingual paraethesia.[123, 126, 127]

Since the retromolar trigone is an anatomically small site, tumours often extend to involve adjacent subsites: buccal mucosa (84 per cent), oropharynx (14 per cent), masticator space, involving the medial pterygoid, masseter, temporalis, mandibular branch of the trigeminal nerve (22 per cent). Bone involvement of the mandible and/or maxilla is present in 12–34 per cent of retromolar tumours,[123, 125, 126, 127, 128] although a higher incidence of up to 75 per cent has been reported.[129] The posterior maxilla is more frequently involved than the mandible when bone invasion occurs.[123]

Retromolar carcinoma usually presents as advanced disease, 55–73 per cent having stage III/IV disease at presentation.[123, 124, 125] Spread to regional lymph nodes occurs in 26–56 per cent of patients at presentation,[123, 125, 130] 8–15 per cent having occult cervical node involvement.[123, 130]

Tumours of the retromolar trigone are usually well or moderately differentiated.[125]

Work up

The complex anatomy of the retromolar region and the frequent extension of retromolar carcinoma make accurate preoperative imaging essential. CT has been demonstrated to have a high specificity, but low sensitivity for predicting mandibular bone invasion of retromolar carcinomas.[129, 131] MRI is considered the imaging modality of choice for retromolar tumours due to its ability to accurately stage the disease and demonstrate accurately anatomical relationships of the tumour,[132] although mandibular invasion may still be hard to define.

Treatment

PRIMARY

The treatment of choice for retromolar tumours is surgical resection with pre/postoperative radiotherapy or chemoradiotherapy dependent on the stage of the tumour and histological findings.[123, 124, 125, 127, 128] Radiotherapy as a sole treatment modality for retromolar carcinoma has been demonstrated to be associated with significantly worse recurrence rates and disease-free survival,[124, 125] although others have been unable to demonstrate this significance.[126, 133] The debate regarding the use of surgery or radiotherapy as the primary treatment modality is hampered by the lack of data regarding tumour thickness in this anatomical site. It is recognized that tumours in this site may be T3 in size, but superficial in nature.[134]

Resection should be achieved with a 1 cm margin in all planes. It is recognized that the incidence of positive margins following resection of retromolar tumours is higher than other oral sites.[25]

Small tumours of the retromolar trigone may be resected via a transoral route, however the posterior location of retromolar tumours and frequent extension of disease into adjacent anatomical sites often necessitates a mandibulotomy to facilitate access.[123, 127] Extensive tumours extending into the masticator space may require a cervicofacial incision, parotidectomy, ± zygomatic osteotomy and preservation of the facial nerve for access, or an anterior approach including maxillectomy.[135]

Defects following the resection of small mucosal tumours may be left to heal by secondary intention, however larger lesions require reconstruction to prevent trismus. Simple reconstructive methods include use of a split skin graft or buccal fat pad reconstruction (**Figures 29.36** and **29.37**).

Tongue flaps and masseteric flaps have been described,[128] however they lack flexibility and may be compromised in anything but the smallest of tumours.

Given the low negative predictive value of CT for bone involvement and the high incidence of bone involvement demonstrated in retrospective series, a low threshold for bone resection should be adopted. A posterior marginal mandibulectomy (including coronoid) conducted via a visor or lip split soft tissue flap is oncologically safe in patients with no history of previous radiotherapy and no radiological signs of cortical bone involvement.[127, 136] Patients demonstrating cortical bone involvement on imaging, or who have previously received radiotherapy should have a segmental mandibular resection. A posterior maxillectomy should be conducted when indicated.

The combination of mandibulotomy and posterior marginal mandibulectomy for large soft tissue lesions should be avoided in view of the increased risk of osteoradionecrosis, a segmental resection being warranted in these circumstances.[137]

Pedicled myocutaneous flaps, such as the pectoralis major flap, are stretched to their limit at this anatomical site, often resulting in delayed healing.[127] The use of the radial free forearm flap or anterolateral thigh flap provides excellent reconstruction of larger soft tissue defects in the retromolar region, it being important to pay particular attention to flap design in this area. Where the resection involves the soft palate, the combination of free flap and superiorly based pharyngeal wall flap should be considered to minimize nasopharyngeal reflux.

Reconstruction following segmental resection should ideally be with free tissue transfer, such as the fibula, scapula or DCIA flaps. Since radiotherapy will almost certainly be indicated following segmental resection, the use of vascularized bone flaps results in more predictable healing with lower risk of nonunion/resorption.[127] The use of reconstruction plates and purely soft tissue cover is particularly prone to failure in the retromolar region.[138]

Large tumours extending into mandible, maxilla, soft palate, tongue base and buccal mucosa require careful consideration regarding reconstructive options. Dual free flaps may provide ideal soft tissue and bony reconstruction, but at the increased risk of complications. The scapula flap is versatile enough in thin individuals to be able to reconstruct these extensive defects (**Figures 29.38, 29.39** and **29.40**).

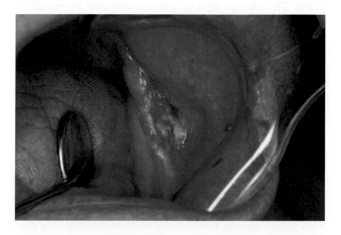

Figure 29.36 Case 6: T1 Squamous cell carcinoma left retromolar area.

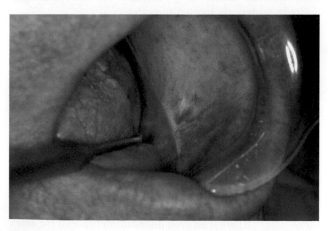

Figure 29.37 Case 6: Healing following buccal fat pad reconstruction.

NECK

Lymphatic spread to the neck is usually to levels I and II in the absence of detectable lymphadenopathy, however involved nodes in levels III–V may occur in the presence of nodes in levels I and/or II.[130]

Unlike tumours at other sites, there are few data correlating tumour thickness to incidence of cervical metastasis.

An END (levels I–III/IV) is indicated for any tumour bigger than T1,[123, 127, 130, 136] or where access to vessels in the neck is required for reconstruction.

PORT

Up to 58 per cent of patients may require postoperative radiotherapy/chemoradiotherapy,[123] an indication of the typically advanced nature of retromolar carcinomas.

Recurrence

Local and/or regional recurrence may occur in 20–37 per cent,[123, 124, 125] depending on primary treatment modality and stage of disease on presentation. Recurrence usually occurs in the first two years.[130]

Prognosis

Factors influencing survival are stage, involvement of the masticator space[123] and cervical metastasis,[123, 125, 130] mean

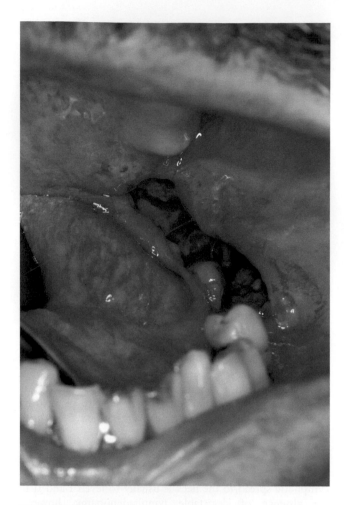

Figure 29.38 Case 7: T4 squamous cell carcinoma left retromolar region.

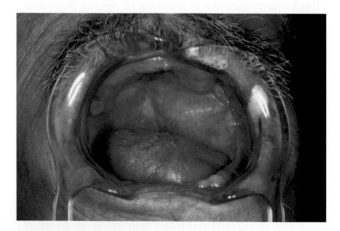

Figure 29.39 Case 7: Composite osseomyocutaneous scapula free flap reconstruction.

survival in patients with masticator space involvement being 38 months.[123] Patients receiving surgery combined with radiotherapy have been demonstrated to have a significant survival advantage over patients receiving radiotherapy alone (**Table 29.8**).[124]

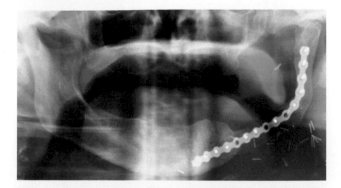

Figure 29.40 Case 7: Orthopantomogram of composite reconstruction of mandible.

MAXILLARY ALVEOLUS AND HARD PALATE

Surgical anatomy

The maxilla comprises the maxillary alveolus and the hard palate. The osseous alveolar process supports the maxillary dentition, being covered by a mucoperiosteum with a stratified squamous epithelium. The maxillary alveolus merges laterally with the buccal mucosa and lips at the gingival sulcus and medially with the hard palate. The alveolar process extends to the upper end of the pterygopalatine arches posteriorly. The hard palate lies within the horseshoe shape of the maxillary alveolus, merging imperceptibly with the alveolar mucosa. The hard palate has minor salivary glands located in the submucosa, 33 per cent of palatal tumours being derived from salivary epithelium.[139] Posteriorly, the hard palate merges with the soft palate at the posterior edge of the palatine bone. Sensory innervation to the maxillary mucosa is by branches of the maxillary division of the trigeminal nerve. The nasopalatine nerve supplies the anterior hard palate, passing through the incisive foramen, the posterior palate being supplied by the paired greater palatine nerves that pass through the greater palatine foraminae. Lymphatic drainage is to the ipsilateral cervical nodes via the submandibular nodes or potentially the retropharyngeal nodes in posteriorly located tumours.

Epidemiology

Squamous cell carcinoma of the maxillary alveolus represents 3.5–6.5 per cent[34, 69] of oral cancers, being approximately one-third as common as mandibular alveolar carcinoma. Carcinoma of the hard palate is very unusual representing only 1–3 per cent[140, 141] of oral cancers. Aetiological factors include tobacco use and alcohol consumption. Palatal carcinoma is particularly associated with reverse smoking, a habit practised in parts of India by women.[142, 143, 144]

Patients tend to present in their sixth to seventh decade of life.[140, 143, 145] There is an even distribution between the sexes, except where reverse smoking is practised when there is a greater frequency in females.[143]

Table 29.8   Retromolar prognosis.

I (%)	II (%)	III (%)	IV (%)		
100	74	75	43.6	Surgery and PORT $(n = 50)^{23}$	Overall 5 year 60%
	I–III, 83		IV, 61	Surgery and radiotherapy[24]	Overall 5 year 69% (DSS)

DSS, disease-specific survival.

Presentation

Patients may present with pain, ulceration, loose teeth or poorly fitting dentures. Symptoms of advanced disease may include infraorbital paraethesia, trismus or nasal obstruction. Most patients present with stage I or II disease.[140, 145]

Eight per cent of patients with carcinoma of the hard palate or maxillary alveolus present with cervical lymphadenopathy, a further 27 per cent having occult metastasis.[145]

Work up

The surface extent of a maxillary carcinoma may be relatively easy to determine from clinical examination alone, however extension into the maxillary antrum and beyond requires additional imaging. Extension of tumour through the pterygoid plates into the masticator space may render a tumour inoperable. CT scans and MRI are complementary in the assessment of maxillary tumours.[146]

Intranasal examination with a nasendoscope should be conducted to determine the extent of the tumour through the floor of the nose or medial antral wall.

All patients should have impressions taken for the provision of a temporary obturator, even if free flap reconstruction is anticipated. In the unfortunate situation of free flap failure, the presence of presurgical models will make prosthetic salvage considerably easier. If prosthetic reconstruction is to be considered from the outset, then early consultation with a prosthodontist is required.

Treatment

PRIMARY

Anaesthesia is usually accomplished with an oral tube, a tracheostomy only being considered for larger resections or free flap reconstruction. Patients requiring an upper cheek flap for access should have their eyes protected with corneal shields or temporary tarsorraphies.

The surgical goals that apply to hard palate and maxillary alveolar tumours are the same as those at other sites, notably surgical clearance of 1 cm in three dimensions. Small tumours may be approached perorally, however larger tumours may require an upper cheek flap or midfacial degloving to augment access.

Once the mucosal incisions have been completed, the soft tissues are elevated in a subperiosteal plane away from the tumour to allow access for bone cuts. Teeth may need to be extracted to allow osteotomy cuts and minimize postoperative complications. The use of a fine reciprocating or saggital saw allows accurate bony resection. Care should be

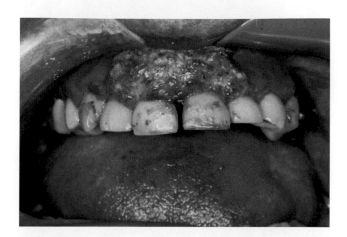

Figure 29.41   Case 8: Alveolar squamous cell carcinoma anterior maxilla.

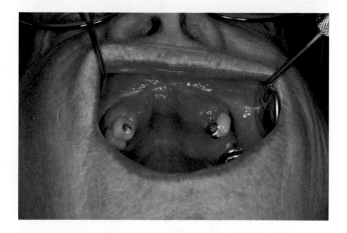

Figure 29.42   Case 8: Surgical defect following resection.

taken to avoid tooth roots. If the margins of resection extend posteriorly, the specimen may be disarticulated from the pterygoid plates with a curved osteotome. Posterior dissection may be completed with large curved scissors. The posterior dissection in the region of the pterygoids should be the last part of the resection due to the bleeding that occurs in this area. An ipsilateral coronoidectomy should be conducted to minimize impingement of the coronoid on the prosthesis or flap reconstruction. Defects that are to be reconstructed with a prosthesis should be lined with a split skin graft (**Figures 29.41, 29.42** and **29.43**).

Surgical closure of small maxillectomy defects may be achieved with local flaps, such as buccal fat pad, temporalis flaps or facial artery musculomucosal flaps. Large defects may require soft tissue[147] or composite free tissue transfer (**Figures 29.44, 29.45** and **29.46**).[148]

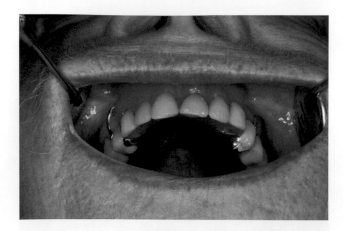

Figure 29.43 Case 8: Dental obturator to reconstruct defect.

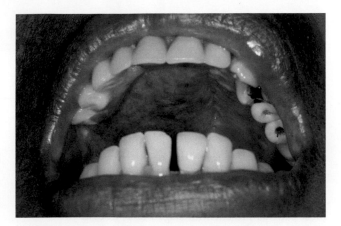

Figure 29.45 Case 9: Fibula osseocutaneous reconstruction of maxillary defect with implant retained prosthesis.

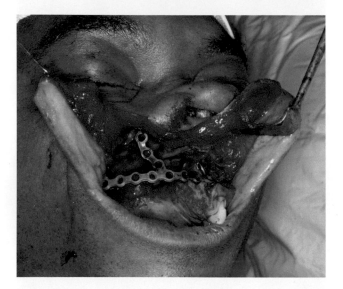

Figure 29.44 Case 9: Resection of squamous cell carcinoma right maxilla.

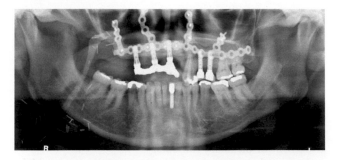

Figure 29.46 Case 9: Orthopantomogram of fibula free flap reconstruction of maxilla (note ossified pedicle).

The use of an appropriate defect classification system[149] allows for planning of reconstruction and communication with colleagues.

NECK

Historically, regional spread from maxillary tumours has been considered low, however this may be due to coregistration of hard palate and alveolar tumours such as sinonasal tumours.[139] Cervical metastasis has been demonstrated in 35 per cent of patients with hard palate or maxillary alveolar carcinomas,[145] an elective I–III neck dissection being considered appropriate for lesions of T2 size or greater.[139] Consideration should be given to clearing the facial lymph nodes when conducting a neck dissection for maxillary tumours.

PORT

Postoperative radiotherapy has been suggested for T3 or greater disease, positive margins, perineural or perivascular invasion or multiple cervical nodes, particularly if they demonstrate extracapsular spread.[139]

Recurrence

Locoregional control of hard palate and alveolar tumours following initial therapy is in the region of 40–45 per cent,[140, 145] increasing to 68 per cent following secondary intervention.[140] Salvage of local recurrence may be achieved in 33 per cent and regional recurrence in 71 per cent.[145] Over 90 per cent of recurrence occurs within the first two years, similar to other sites.

Prognosis

Five-year absolute survival for hard palate carcinoma is 57 per cent, five-year survival for alveolar carcinoma being 49 per cent.[140] Tumour stage and presence of cervical metastasis influence long-term survival.[140]

MANDIBULAR ALVEOLUS

Surgical anatomy

The mandibular alveolus represents that part of the mandible that is 'intraoral'. The osseous alveolar process of the mandible supports the dentition and is covered by a mucoperiosteum. The mandibular alveolus merges laterally with the buccal mucosa/lips at the gingival sulcus and medially with the floor of mouth. The alveolar process extends to the retromolar trigones posteriorly. Sensory innervation to the mandibular alveolus is by the mandibular division of the trigeminal nerve. Lymphatic drainage is to the ipsilateral submandibular and submental nodes to the deep cervical chain. Lymphatic drainage towards the midline may be bilateral. Following loss of the dentition, there is considerable resorption of the alveolar process, leaving only a thin strip of attached mucoperiosteum on the crest of the mandible between the floor of mouth and buccal mucosa.

Epidemiology

Squamous cell carcinoma of the mandibular alveolus represents 7.5–17.5 per cent[34, 69, 141] of oral cancers, although it represents up to 30 per cent of oral cancers in the Japanese population.[150] Mandibular alveolar carcinoma is three times more common than maxillary alveolar carcinoma.[151] Rarely, primary intraosseous carcinomas may occur, being derived from residues of odontogenic epithelium within the mandible.[152] The use of tobacco, particularly chewing tobacco, and alcohol is associated with alveolar carcinoma.

Patients tend to present later in life in their seventh decade, the disease being slightly more common in males.[150, 151, 153]

Presentation

The most common presenting symptom is pain, occurring in 54–86 per cent of patients.[150, 151, 153] Patients who are dentate may note loosening of teeth while edentulous patients may note a change of fit of their dentures. Labial paraesthesia may be a presenting feature in up to 14 per cent of patients. Unfortunately, patients still present with a history of delayed healing of an extraction socket in up to 28 per cent of cases.[150] The majority of lesions of the mandibular alveolus are located posterior to the canines, extension to the floor of mouth or buccal mucosa being common (**Table 29.9**).[151]

Alveolar tumours are staged by their size until there is invasion of tumour through cortical bone into marrow space when the tumour becomes T4. Cervical lymphadenopathy is present in 24–32 per cent of patients at presentation, usually to levels I and II,[150, 151, 153] 15 per cent of patients having occult metastasis.[151] Up to 94 per cent of patients have evidence of bone involvement clinically.[150] Most tumours at this site are usually well or moderately differentiated.[150, 153]

Work up

The most important aspect of working up mandibular alveolar tumours is to determine the degree of bone involvement since this determines the extent of tumour resection.

Treatment

PRIMARY

Mandibular alveolar carcinoma is considered a surgical disease.[153] Invariably, some degree of bone resection is required, 6–7 per cent requiring soft tissue resection only.[150, 153, 154] Small alveolar carcinomas with no clinical evidence of significant bone involvement may be resected via a peroral approach and a marginal mandibulectomy, aiming for a 1 cm soft tissue and bony margin. Larger tumours with obvious bone involvement require segmental resection and extraoral access incisions. Segmental resection should also be considered for small tumours abutting a mandible previously treated with radiotherapy, massive soft tissue tumours adjacent to the mandible, involvement of the inferior dental nerve or intraosseous tumours (primary or secondary). Marginal mandibulectomy is preferable to segmental resection whenever oncologically acceptable. If a marginal resection is conducted, then reconstruction may usually be achieved by primary closure (**Figures 29.47, 29.48** and **29.49**).

More extensive mucosal defects may require reconstruction with a skin graft; local flaps such as the FAMM (facial artery muscular mucosal) flap, nasolabial flap or buccal fat pad; or microvascular free tissue transfer to achieve acceptable soft tissue closure. Segmental mandibular resection should be accompanied with composite microvascular free flap reconstruction whenever feasible (**Figures 29.50, 29.51, 29.52** and **29.53**).

The use of a recognized mandibular defect classification helps surgeons plan appropriate reconstruction and communicate effectively with colleagues. The H, C, L, o, m, s classification system[155] accurately describes mandibular surgical defects.

NECK

Regional spread of mandibular alveolar tumours is usually to the ipsilateral level I–III nodes. Elective neck dissection is

Table 29.9 Mandibular alveolus presentation.

Stage I/II (%)	Stage III/IV (%)	
60	40	United States ($n = 155$)[51]
40	60	Japan ($n = 50$)[50]

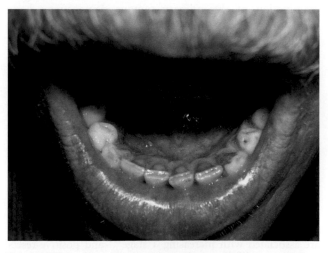

Figure 29.47 Case 10: Alveolar carcinoma anterior mandible.

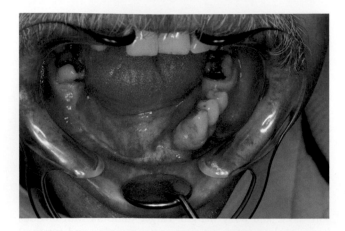

Figure 29.48 Case 10: Surgical defect following rim resection.

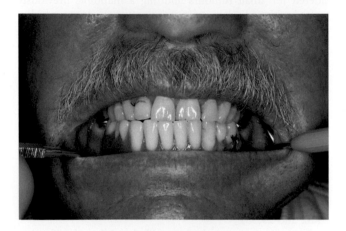

Figure 29.49 Case 10: Tooth supported denture reconstruction.

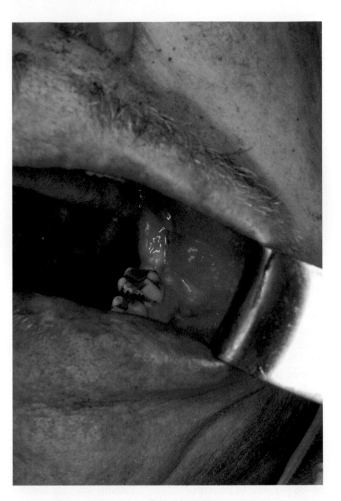

Figure 29.50 Case 11: Deeply invasive T4 carcinoma of left mandible.

indicated in tumours T2 in size or greater or any tumour with demonstrable bone invasion, clearance of levels I–III being adequate.[156] Lesions overlying the symphysis are thought to be associated with a higher risk of cervical metastasis and may require bilateral neck dissections. It has been argued that a staged neck dissection should be considered if histological examination of the primary tumour demonstrates bone involvement.[156] A more extensive neck dissection should be conducted in the presence of confirmed cervical metastasis, level V requiring treatment.[156]

PORT

Indications for postoperative radiotherapy include positive margins (soft tissue or bone), multiple positive nodes or extracapsular spread.[151]

Recurrence

Recurrence rates for mandibular alveolar carcinoma at two years are 13–25 per cent.[150, 151, 153] Higher recurrence rates are associated with increasing T stage[151] and positive resection margins.[150, 151]

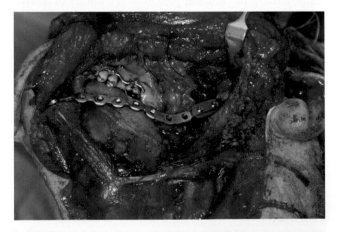

Figure 29.51 Case 11: Hemimandibulectomy, including condyle and application of precontoured reconstruction plate to facilitate accurate location of fibula free flap reconstruction.

Prognosis

Overall five-year survival for lower alveolus carcinoma is 50–60 per cent, disease-specific survival being 73–80 per cent.[150, 151]

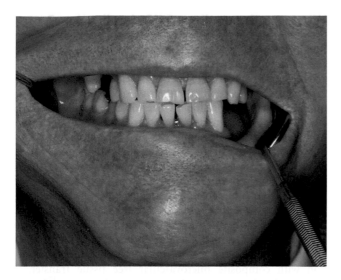

Figure 29.52 Case 11: Postoperative occlusion and intraoral fibula skin paddle.

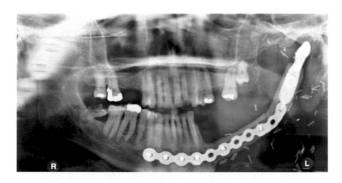

Figure 29.53 Case 11: Postoperative orthopantomogram demonstrating fibula flap *in situ*.

Cervical metastasis has been demonstrated to significantly reduce prognosis for lower gingival carcinoma.[156] Increasing T stage (and particularly tumours greater than 3 cm),[151] bone involvement (cortical or cancellous)[151] and positive resection margins[150, 151] are associated with decreased prognosis.

Tooth extraction at the site of primary tumour does not influence prognosis.[150, 151]

MANAGEMENT OF THE MANDIBLE

Tumours of the mandibular alveolus, the floor of mouth, buccal mucosa or retromolar trigone may involve the bone of the mandible. Involvement of the mandible has significant consequences regarding management of the patient.

Several questions need to be answered when managing a patient with potential mandibular involvement.

How does squamous cell carcinoma invade the mandible?

Squamous cell carcinoma (SCC) invades the mandible either in an invasive or erosive manner.[154, 157] Invasive tumours

Table 29.10 Mandible imaging.

	Sensitivity (%)	Specificity (%)
Clinical examination	82	61
Plain films	76	81
Computed tomography[61]	75	86
Magnetic resonance imaging	85	72
Single photoemission computed tomography	97	65
Bone scintigraphy	93	74

demonstrate fingers or islands of tumour advancing deeply into bone with no obvious osteoclastic activity. Erosive tumours have a broad advancing front with osteoclast activity and connective tissue between the tumour and bone, although as the depth of invasion increases, they may become more invasive in character. Large, deeply invading tumours are more likely to demonstrate an invasive pattern of spread and involve the mandible.[154, 158]

Tumours enter the mandible at the point of contact,[154, 159] usually the junction of the attached and reflected mucosa, whether the patient is edentulous or dentate. The mandible should be considered at risk at any point where tumour is in contact and this is taken into account when planning resection. Clinical fixation of the tumour to bone is not necessary for bone invasion to occur.

It has been demonstrated that it is primarily the size and extent of the tumour that dictates the pattern of spread once in bone rather than anatomical features, such as the inferior alveolar nerve or periodontal ligament. Preferential spread within the mandible via the inferior alveolar nerve or medullary space is rare,[154, 160] justifying 1 cm margins.

Tumours demonstrating an invasive pattern of spread are more likely to give rise to cervical metastasis with extracapsular extension,[154] an indication of their more aggressive nature.

How do we detect bony invasion?

Preoperative imaging of the mandible is necessary to determine if bone resection is required, and if so the appropriate type of resection.[161]

At present, there is no single investigation that can reliably predict bone invasion (**Table 29.10**). An OPG radiograph should be requested for all cancer patients. This plain radiograph is not only useful for demonstrating bony invasion, but also for assessing mandibular height, dental anatomy and dental pathology. It should be remembered that plain radiographs do not detect initial invasion until 30 per cent demineralization has occurred, giving rise to reduced sensitivity.[162] Clinical examination and OPG alone are probably inadequate for accurate assessment of mandibular invasion.[162]

Axial MRI views with T1 and STIR fat suppression are very sensitive for imaging the primary site of oral cancer with an adequate specificity.[163] Bone scintigraphy or

Lower lip defect

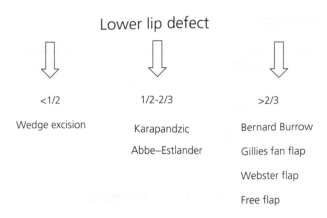

<1/2	1/2-2/3	>2/3
Wedge excision	Karapandzic	Bernard Burrow
	Abbe–Estlander	Gillies fan flap
		Webster flap
		Free flap

Figure 29.56 Lower lip reconstruction.

course of a few months. Following treatment, advice on the use of sun block to the lip to prevent recurrence of the original problem is given.

LOWER LIP

The techniques for treating defects of the lower lip are summarized in **Figure 29.56**, and described in detail below.

Infiltrating lesions of the lower lip affecting less than one third

Small lesions invading into the adjacent muscle are amenable to a wedge excision. A through and through surgical defect is thus created. In closing the defect, the vermilion is temporarily approximated with a resorbable suture. This allows the underlying muscle to be closed in two layers. The external skin is closed with an interrupted monofilament and the labial and intraoral wound is closed with a resorbable suture. The excision can also be completed using a W-plasty or half W-plasty to avoid the bottom of the excision encroaching on the crease line of the chin (**Figure 29.57**).

Lower lip defects one-third to two-thirds

Defects of the lower lip over one-third require a different surgical approach. The dimensions of the lip resection require the introduction of tissue from the other lip by means of an Abbe or an Abbe-Estlander flap or rotation of tissue from the adjacent lip via a Karapandzic.[181, 182, 183, 184]

Abbe-Estlander flap

The Abbe-Estlander staged reconstruction requires the development of a triangular full thickness flap from the upper lip. The width of the flap is one-half to two-thirds the horizontal length of the lower lip defect, with the vertical dimension of the flap being the same as the surgical defect. The flap is pedicled on the labial artery with the full thickness incision extending within 2–3 mm of the vermilion border. With the flap mobilized, initial inset into the defect is completed in a layered fashion flap (**Figure 29.58**). Two to three weeks after the harvest of the flap, the pedicle is divided and the final insetting of the flap is completed. Care is taken to reconstruct accurately the white line. The Estlander modification of the cross-lip flap is used to reconstruct the oral commissure. (An Estlander flap is a laterally based Abbe

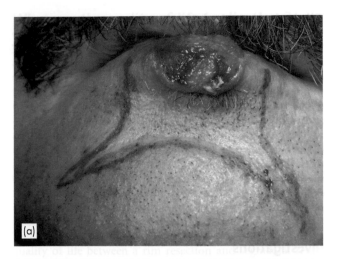

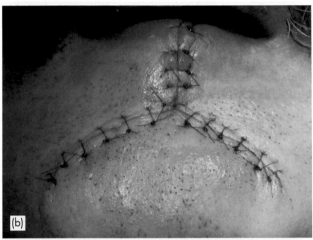

Figure 29.57 Lower lip cancer W excision.

flap that is used when defects affect the commissure.) The commissure is thus rotated when the tissue is transferred to the defect in the lower lip. The patient needs to be placed on a soft diet while the transposed flap takes. Venous compromise of the flap is usually due to leaving too thin a bridging pedicle or too tight a closure. A few sutures should be removed in the early stages to see if this reverses the venous compromise, or consideration to the use of medicinal leeches to deal with the venous stasis needs to be undertaken. The bridging pedicle is divided under local anaesthetic after 2–3 weeks.

Karapandzic flap

The Karapandzic flap is useful for defects involving more than two-thirds of the lower lip where the defect is in the midline.[185] The main advantage of the Karapandzic flap is that the nerve and blood supply to the underlying orbicularis oris muscle is retained and the underlying orbicularis muscle is rotated so that a sensate functional lip reconstruction occurs. The tissue is rotated from the nasolabial region and this tissue is shifted medially and rotated into the lower lip. The lateral incisions of the Karapandzic flap follow the nasolabial skin creases. Resection of the tumour on the lower lip is performed in the usual manner and then the skin

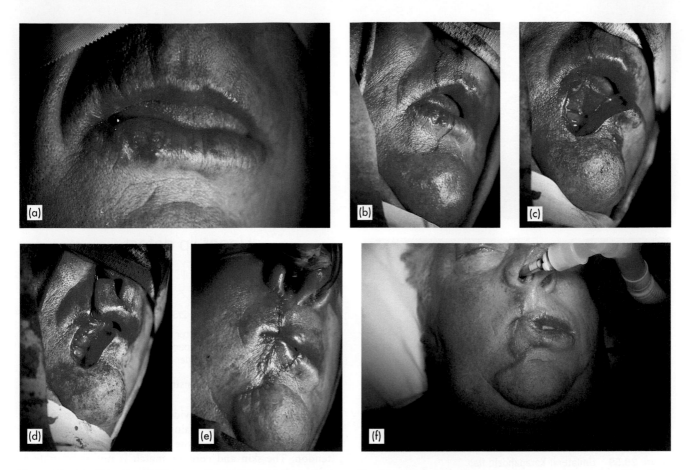

Figure 29.58 Abbe flap. (a) T1 squamous cell carcinoma, right lower lip; (b) outline of excision marked on lower lip and rotation flap on upper lip; (c) the tumour has been excised; (d) the upper lip rotation flap has been raised. Note the anterior limit of the incision at the vermilion border; (e) the upper lip rotation has been inserted into the lower lip and the donor site repaired; (f) three weeks later, just prior to incising the pedicle.

incisions for elevation of the Karapandzic flap are made. It is important to avoid division of the muscle fibres containing the neuromuscular control of the orbicularis under the skin. To aid mobilization, mucosal incisions are placed in the gingival labial and gingival buccal sulcus on each side. The flap is elevated in a subcutaneous plane remaining superficial to the orbicularis oris muscle. Sufficient length in the mucosal incisions must be performed to permit medial mobilization of both flaps for a midline closure. The repair of the defect begins with the vertical midline closure of the lower lip with approximation of the vermilion border by a temporary nylon suture. The advanced muscle in the orbicularis oris is closed in the midline followed by external skin closure. Following this, reapproximation of the suture line between the advanced cutaneous margin of the flap and the residual cutaneous margin of the chin and nasolabial region is undertaken (**Figure 29.59**). The larger the defect, the tighter the reconstructed lip will be, and thus a certain amount of microstomia can be present following Karapandzic flap reconstruction. This is more easily accommodated in the elderly edentulous patient where there is a certain amount of skin laxity. The restricted oral aperture will stretch gradually over the course of a few months and the stretching can be augmented by physiotherapy.

Lower lip defects greater than two-thirds

With larger defects of the lower lip, reconstruction requires either large cheek flaps to be advanced to repair the defect or the use of free tissue transfer. The common forms of cheek flap include the bilateral Gillies fan flaps or the Bernard–Webster cheek flap reconstruction.[186]

In the Gillies fan flap, a full thickness incision is made around the commissure extending on to the upper lip at the nasolabial fold. The incision is cut and advanced almost to the vermilion border of the upper lip. The flap is now pedicled on labial vessels and can be advanced unilaterally or bilaterally and closed in layers. The modified fan flap differs from a classical fan flap in that the flap rotates around the angle of the mouth to fill in the defect. The vermilion is reconstructed by mucosal advancement of a tongue mucosal flap which is divided at 10–14 days (**Figure 29.60**). In the Webster cheek advancement flap, horizontal incisions are extended laterally from the base of the defect and the commissure. The resulting four Burrows triangles are excised above and below the lateral aspect of the flaps. The flaps are advanced bilaterally and closed in layers, and the resulting triangles are closed. The vermilion is reconstructed by mucosal advancement or a tongue flap.

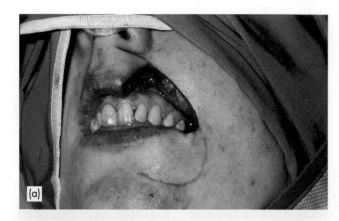

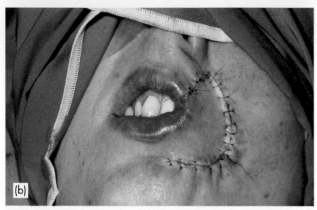

Figure 29.59   Unilateral Karapandzic flap.

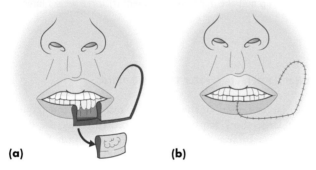

Figure 29.60   Gillies fan flap.

In the Bernard–Webster flap, Burrows triangles are formed at the edge of the lower lip excision. Incisions are extended laterally from the base of the defect. The buccal mucosa from the base of the excised Burrows triangles are rotated inferiorly over the free margin of the triangle and used to reconstruct the lateral vermilion of the lip. The two flaps are advanced medially, the triangles closed and the flaps are approximated in layers (**Figure 29.61**).

Free tissue transfer is required for lip reconstruction when the total remaining lip or adjacent rotated tissue is insufficient to create a reasonable circular and symmetrical mouth. Often these defects include cheek, skin and underlying mandible. In this case, a radial artery free forearm flap using the palmaris longus tendon to suspend the lower lip is used. This reconstruction technique, however, is insensate and

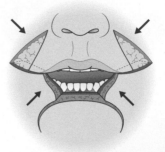

Figure 29.61   Webster–Bernard reconstruction.

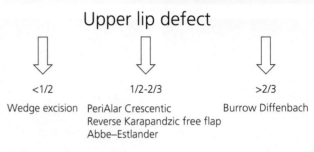

Figure 29.62   Upper lip reconstruction.

immobile and merely provides a static platform for the mobile upper lip to close against. The flap is used as a double paddled flap rotated on the underlying palmaris longus tendon. The skin and contour match is not as accurate as when using adjacent rotated tissue. The lip can remain ptotic and may require wedge excisions a few months following reconstruction to improve the lip tone, allowing the formation of an adequate seal with the upper lip. Similarly, fascial slings may be required to maintain lip closure.

UPPER LIP

In the upper lip, defects again can be divided into: less than a third, one-third to two-thirds and greater than two-thirds to complete defects. The techniques for treating them are summarized in **Figure 29.62**.

Defect involving up to a third of upper lip

Similar to lower lip defects, wedge excisions and advancement flaps can address upper lip defects which involve up to one-half of the width of the upper lip. Care is taken to respect the relevant aesthetic subunits. Defects of less than a third in the midline can be closed primarily.

Defects between one-third and two-thirds

These can be reconstructed with cross lip flaps from the lower lip. Perialar crescentic advancement flaps can be used to disguise the advancement of the upper lip when the advancement encroaches on the medial part of the nose.

Defects greater than two-thirds of the upper lip

A Burrow-Diffenbach reconstruction can be performed. The Burrow-Diffenbach flap replaces upper lip defects by utilization

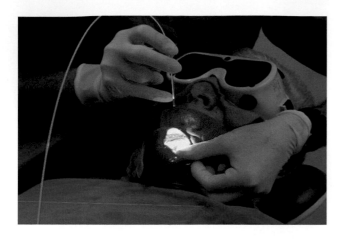

Figure 29.63 Photodynamic therapy for lip cancer.

of laterally based advancement flaps. Bilateral perialar crescentic excisions are required to provide adequate advancement.

NECK DISSECTION IN LIP CANCER

Squamous cell carcinoma of the lip does not appear to be as lethal as squamous cell carcinoma at other sites in the oral cavity. The favourable survival rate of lip cancer is often due to the early stage of the presentation of tumours[187] and most large series in the literature show that the majority of patients have small lesions without palpable cervical metastases. The local recurrence rate is low due to the relative ease of surgical excision and even re-excision because of local failure leads to salvage in 75–80 per cent of patients.[183] The incidence of synchronous cervical metastases increases as the size of the primary tumour increases. The primary lymphatic drainage of the lower lip is to the submental and submandibular level Ia and Ib cervical lymph nodes. Neck dissection is generally not performed in the absence of clinically suspicious cervical lymph nodes as less than 5 per cent of patients are likely to develop recurrence in the neck following treatment of the primary lesion.[187]

RADIOTHERAPY TECHNIQUES

Various studies have shown that for small tumours, radiation therapy can achieve a cure rate equivalent to that obtained surgically.[188, 189] However, the cosmetic results of radiation therapy to the lip may not be as satisfactory as surgical excision and repair. Surgical excision of small lip tumours involves relatively minor surgery, often under local anaesthetic and may be therefore less burdensome for the patient than a course of radiotherapy.

EXTERNAL BEAM THERAPY

The lower lip is one of the few ideal sites for orthovoltage x-ray therapy. Using a single anterior field a fractionated course of 50 Gy in 15 fractions over 3 weeks is given.

Table 29.12 Tumour thickness and survival rate in lip cancer.

Tumour size (cm)	Five-year survival (%)
1	94
<2	84
<3	58
<4	67
>4	62

Presence of nodal disease and five-year survival: N+ 61%; N0 89%.

BRACHYTHERAPY

192-iridium brachytherapy can be used in the treatment of lip cancer. Patients can be treated twice a day for 4–5 days with a total radiation dose between 40 and 45 Gy in eight to ten fractions. The Paris system is often used, where needles are placed horizontally and parallel to the mucosa of the lip with 9 mm spacing between them.[188]

PHOTODYNAMIC THERAPY

Photodynamic therapy can also be used to treat primary cancer of the lip.[190] The light sensitizing drug, such as photofrin, is given intravenously followed 4 days later by a single nonthermal illumination of the tumour using a light dose of 20 J/cm with an irradiance of 100 mW/cm^2 (**Figure 29.63**).

This form of treatment yields complete response rates comparable to those published for surgery or radiotherapy.[191] As this treatment works by a cold photochemical process producing apoptosis and vascular shut down, less scarring should occur compared to radiotherapy and surgery. However, clinical experience suggests that some scarring does occur with larger lesions and the problems of light sensitivity and pain following treatment may limit its general application. However, the lack of tissue memory for photodynamic therapy means that, unlike radiotherapy, this treatment can be given on a number of occasions.

Survival rates for lip cancer

The survival rates for lip cancer are shown in **Table 29.12**.[192]

KEY EVIDENCE

- Although screening for cancer has proved effective for some major cancers there is no evidence to support screening for oral cancer.[193]
- The routine use of panendoscopy in the work up of patients with oral cancer is not warranted,[12] however a computed tomography (CT) scan of the chest is indicated in most patients.
- Management of the primary tumour involves surgical resection and appropriate reconstruction. Radiotherapy (brachytherapy) may be considered for accessible, well-

demarcated lesions not adjacent to the mandible.
- Patients should be offered elective neck treatment if characteristics of the primary tumour suggest there is a greater than 20 per cent risk of occult nodal metastasis,[194] althugh entry into appropriate clinical trials should be offered.

KEY LEARNING POINTS

Buccal carcinoma

- The most common site for oral cancer in South East Asia.
- Associated with betal/paan consumption.
- Good surgical reconstruction is required to prevent postoperative trismus.
- Up to 26 per cent have occult nodal metastasis at presentation.
- Consider elective neck dissection if tumour >4 mm thick.

Floor of mouth carcinoma

- One of the most common sites for oral cancer.
- Leukoplakia of the floor of mouth has a 1–2.9 per cent annual malignant transformation rate.
- Careful consideration should be given to management of the submandibular ducts.
- Anterior lesions may require treatment of both necks.
- Tendency for cervical metastasis to occur in thinner tumours than other sites.

Tongue carcinoma

- One of the most common sites for oral cancer.
- Usually presents as stage I/II disease.
- Elective neck dissections should include levels I–IV because of skip metastases.
- Reconstruction should maximize function of the residual tongue.

Retromolar carcinoma

- Represents 6–7 per cent of oral carcinomas.
- Frequently presents as stage III/IV disease with extension into adjacent sites.
- Accurate preoperative imaging is required to determine the extent of disease.

Maxillary alveolus and hard palate

- Carcinoma of the maxillary alveolus is three times less common than the mandibular alveolus.
- Carcinoma of the hard palate represents only 1–3 per cent of oral cancers.

- Palatal carcinoma is associated with reverse smoking.
- All patients should have dental impressions as part of their work up.
- Some degree of bone removal is nearly always required.

Mandibular alveolus

- Represents approximately 10 per cent of oral cancers, although it represents up to 30 per cent in the Japanese population.
- Ninety-four per cent of tumours involve bone.
- Alveolar carcinoma is a surgical disease requiring a rim or segmental resection of the mandible.

Management of the mandible

- Bone involvement may be by erosion or invasion.
- Bone involvement occurs at any point where tumour contacts bone.
- Magnetic resonance imaging, computed tomography, single-photon emission computed tomography and periosteal stripping are complimentary in assessing bone involvement.
- Bone margins should be dictated by overlying soft tissue margins.
- Rim resection should be conducted when oncologically acceptable.

Lip cancer

- Lip cancer arises mainly as a result of solar radiation.
- Surgical reconstruction usually involves local rotation flaps.
- Neck metastases are unusual.
- Radiotherapy is reserved for elderly and medically unfit patients.

REFERENCES

1. Ferlay J, Bray F, Pisani P, Parkin DM. GLOBOCAN. *Cancer incidence, mortality and prevalence worldwide.* IARC CancerBase No. 5, version 2.0. Lyon: IARC Press, 2004.
2. Quinn MJ. Cancer trends in England and Wales 1950–1999. *Studies on medical and population subjects No. 66.* London: The Stationery Office, 2001.
3. Conway DI, Stockton DL, Warnakulasuriya KA *et al.* Incidence of oral and oropharyngeal cancer in United Kingdom (1990–1999) – recent trends and regional variation. *Oral Oncology* 2006; **42**: 586–92.
4. Shiboski CH, Schmidt BL, Jordan RC. Tongue and tonsil carcinoma: increasing trends in the US population ages 20–44 years. *Cancer* 2005; **103**: 1843–9.

5. Franceschi S, Levi F, Lucchini F *et al.* Trends in cancer mortality in young adults in Europe, 1955–1989. *European Journal of Cancer* 1994; **30**: 2096–118.

6. Shiboski CH, Shiboski SC, Silverman S Jr. Trends in oral cancer rates in the United States, 1973–1996. *Community Dentistry and Oral Epidemiology* 2000; **28**: 249–56.

7. Blot WJ, McLaughlin JK, Winn DM *et al.* Smoking and drinking in relation to oral and pharyngeal cancer. *Cancer Research* 1988; **48**: 3282–7.

◆ 8. Kujan O, Glenny AM, Oliver RJ *et al.* Screening programmes for the early detection and prevention of oral cancer. *Cochrane Database of Systematic Reviews*; 2006; **(3)**: CD004150.

9. Karas DE, Baredes S, Chen TS, Karas SF. Relationship of biopsy and final specimens in evaluation of tumor thickness in floor of mouth carcinoma. *Laryngoscope* 1995; **105**: 491–3.

10. Brouwer J, Senft A, de Bree R *et al.* Screening for distant metastases in patients with head and neck cancer: is there a role for (18)FDG-PET? *Oral Oncology* 2006; **42**: 275–80.

11. Loh KS, Brown DH, Baker JT *et al.* A rational approach to pulmonary screening in newly diagnosed head and neck cancer. *Head and Neck* 2005; **27**: 990–4.

12. Davidson J, Gilbert R, Irish J *et al.* The role of panendoscopy in the management of mucosal head and neck malignancy – a prospective evaluation. *Head and Neck* 2000; **22**: 449–54.

13. Edge SB, Byrd DR, Compton CC *et al.* (eds). Lip and oral cavity. In: *AJCC cancer staging manual*, 7th edn. New York: Springer 2010: 29–40.

14. Chandu A, Smith AC, Douglas M. Percutaneous endoscopic gastrostomy in patients undergoing resection for oral tumors: a retrospective review of complications and outcomes. *Journal of Oral and Maxillofacial Surgery* 2003; **61**: 1279–84.

15. Beausang ES, Ang EE, Lipa JE *et al.* Microvascular free tissue transfer in elderly patients: the Toronto experience. *Head and Neck* 2003; **25**: 549–53.

16. Borggreven PA, Kuik DJ, Quak JJ *et al.* Comorbid condition as a prognostic factor for complications in major surgery of the oral cavity and oropharynx with microvascular soft tissue reconstruction. *Head and Neck* 2003; **25**: 808–15.

17. Ferrier MB, Spuesens EB, Le Cessie S *et al.* Comorbidity as a major risk factor for mortality and complications in head and neck surgery. *Archives of Otolaryngology – Head and Neck Surgery* 2005; **131**: 27–32.

18. Borggreven PA, Kuik DJ, Langendijk JA *et al.* Severe comorbidity negatively influences prognosis in patients with oral and oropharyngeal cancer after surgical treatment with microvascular reconstruction. *Oral Oncology* 2005; **41**: 358–64.

19. Baek CH, Lee SW, Jeong HS. New modification of the mandibulotomy approach without lip splitting. *Head and Neck* 2006; **28**: 580–6.

20. Hayter JP, Vaughan ED, Brown JS. Aesthetic lip splits. *British Journal of Oral and Maxillofacial Surgery* 1996; **34**: 432–5.

21. Shohat I, Yahalom R, Bedrin L *et al.* Midline versus paramidline mandibulotomy: a radiological study. *International Journal of Oral and Maxillofacial Surgery* 2005; **34**: 639–41.

22. Nam W, Kim HJ, Choi EC *et al.* Contributing factors to mandibulotomy complications: a retrospective study. *Oral Surgery, Oral Medicine, Oral Pathology, Oral Radiology, and Endodontics* 2006; **101**: e65–70.

23. Devine JC, Rogers SN, McNally D *et al.* A comparison of aesthetic, functional and patient subjective outcomes following lip-split mandibulotomy and mandibular lingual releasing access procedures. *International Journal of Oral and Maxillofacial Surgery* 2001; **30**: 199–204.

24. Loree TR, Strong EW. Significance of positive margins in oral cavity squamous carcinoma. *American Journal of Surgery* 1990; **160**: 410–14.

25. Sutton DN, Brown JS, Rogers SN *et al.* The prognostic implications of the surgical margin in oral squamous cell carcinoma. *International Journal of Oral and Maxillofacial Surgery* 2003; **32**: 30–4.

26. McMahon J, O'Brien CJ, Pathak I *et al.* Influence of condition of surgical margins on local recurrence and disease-specific survival in oral and oropharyngeal cancer. *British Journal of Oral and Maxillofacial Surgery* 2003; **41**: 224–31.

27. Mistry RC, Qureshi SS, Kumaran C. Post-resection mucosal margin shrinkage in oral cancer: quantification and significance. *Journal of Surgical Oncology* 2005; **91**: 131–3.

28. Batsakis JG. Surgical excision margins: a pathologist's perspective. *Advances in Anatomic Pathology* 1999; **6**: 140–8.

29. Meier JD, Oliver DA, Varvares MA. Surgical margin determination in head and neck oncology: current clinical practice. The results of an International American Head and Neck Society Member Survey. *Head and Neck* 2005; **27**: 952–8.

30. Jacobs JR, Ahmad K, Casiano R *et al.* Implications of positive surgical margins. *Laryngoscope* 1993; **103**: 64–8.

31. Helliwell T, Woolgar JA. *Standards and minimum datasets for reporting common cancers. Minimum dataset for head and neck carcinoma histopathology reports.* London: The Royal College of Pathologists, 1988.

32. Lee JG. Detection of residual carcinoma of the oral cavity, oropharynx, hypopharynx, and larynx: a study of surgical margins. *Transactions of the American Academy of Ophthalmology and Otolaryngology* 1974; **78**: 49–53.

33. Leemans CR, Tiwari R, Nauta JJ *et al.* Recurrence at the primary site in head and neck cancer and the significance of neck lymph node metastases as a prognostic factor. *Cancer* 1994; **73**: 187–90.

34. Woolgar JA, Triantafyllou A. A histopathological appraisal of surgical margins in oral and oropharyngeal cancer resection specimens. *Oral Oncology* 2005; **41**: 1034–43.

35. Weijers M, Snow GB, Bezemer DP *et al.* The status of the deep surgical margins in tongue and floor of mouth squamous cell carcinoma and risk of local recurrence; an analysis of 68 patients. *International Journal of Oral and Maxillofacial Surgery* 2004; **33**: 146–9.

36. Helbig M, Flechtenmacher C, Hansmann J *et al.* Intraoperative B-mode endosonography of tongue carcinoma. *Head and Neck* 2001; **23**: 233–7.

37. DiNardo LJ, Lin J, Karageorge LS, Powers CN. Accuracy, utility, and cost of frozen section margins in head and neck cancer surgery. *Laryngoscope* 2000; **110**: 1773–6.

38. Ord RA, Aisner S. Accuracy of frozen sections in assessing margins in oral cancer resection. *Journal of Oral and Maxillofacial Surgery* 1997; **55**: 663–9.

39. Kerawala CJ, Ong TK. Relocating the site of frozen sections – is there room for improvement? *Head and Neck* 2001; **23**: 230–2.

40. Sieczka E, Datta R, Singh A *et al.* Cancer of the buccal mucosa: are margins and T-stage accurate predictors of local control? *American Journal of Otolaryngology* 2001; **22**: 395–9.

41. Diaz EM Jr, Holsinger FC, Zuniga ER *et al.* Squamous cell carcinoma of the buccal mucosa: one institution's experience with 119 previously untreated patients. *Head and Neck* 2003; **25**: 267–73.

42. Chhetri DK, Rawnsley JD, Calcaterra TC. Carcinoma of the buccal mucosa. *Otolaryngology – Head and Neck Surgery* 2000; **123**: 566–71.

43. Fang FM, Leung SW, Huang CC *et al.* Combined-modality therapy for squamous carcinoma of the buccal mucosa: treatment results and prognostic factors. *Head and Neck* 1997; **19**: 506–12.

44. Iype EM, Pandey M, Mathew A *et al.* Squamous cell cancer of the buccal mucosa in young adults. *British Journal of Oral and Maxillofacial Surgery* 2004; **42**: 185–9.

45. Lee JJ, Jeng JH, Wang HM *et al.* Univariate and multivariate analysis of prognostic significance of betel quid chewing in squamous cell carcinoma of buccal mucosa in Taiwan. *Journal of Surgical Oncology* 2005; **91**: 41–7.

46. Lin CS, Jen YM, Cheng MF *et al.* Squamous cell carcinoma of the buccal mucosa: an aggressive cancer requiring multimodality treatment. *Head and Neck* 2006; **28**: 150–7.

47. Jing J, Li L, He W, Sun G. Prognostic predictors of squamous cell carcinoma of the buccal mucosa with negative surgical margins. *Journal of Oral and Maxillofacial Surgery* 2006; **64**: 896–901.

48. Urist MM, O'Brien CJ, Soong SJ *et al.* Squamous cell carcinoma of the buccal mucosa: analysis of prognostic factors. *American Journal of Surgery* 1987; **154**: 411–14.

49. Iyer SG, Pradhan SA, Pai PS, Patil S. Surgical treatment outcomes of localized squamous carcinoma of buccal mucosa. *Head and Neck* 2004; **26**: 897–902.

50. Hao SP, Cheng MH. Cancer of the buccal mucosa and retromolar trigone. *Operative Techniques in Otolaryngology* 2004; **15**: 239–51.

51. Robiony M, Forte M, Toro C *et al.* Silicone sandwich technique for securing intraoral skin grafts to the cheek. *British Journal of Oral and Maxillofacial Surgery* 2007; **45**: 166–7.

52. Ozkan O, Mardini S, Chen HC *et al.* Repair of buccal defects with anterolateral thigh flaps. *Microsurgery* 2006; **26**: 182–9.

53. Chien CY, Hwang CF, Chuang HC *et al.* Comparison of radial forearm free flap, pedicled buccal fat pad flap and split-thickness skin graft in reconstruction of buccal mucosal defect. *Oral Oncology* 2005; **41**: 694–7.

54. Nair MK, Sankaranarayanan R, Padmanabhan TK. Evaluation of the role of radiotherapy in the management of carcinoma of the buccal mucosa. *Cancer* 1988; **61**: 1326–31.

55. Chaudhary AJ, Pande SC, Sharma V *et al.* Radiotherapy of carcinoma of the buccal mucosa. *Seminars in Surgical Oncology* 1989; **5**: 322–6.

56. O'Brien PH. Cancer of the cheek (mucosa). *Cancer* 1965; **18**: 1392–8.

57. Gray L, Woolgar J, Brown J. A functional map of cervical metastases from oral squamous cell carcinoma. *Acta Oto-Laryngologica* 2000; **120**: 885–90.

58. Woolgar JA. Histological distribution of cervical lymph node metastases from intraoral/oropharyngeal squamous cell carcinomas. *British Journal of Oral and Maxillofacial Surgery* 1999; **37**: 175–80.

59. Pradhan SA, D'Cruz AK, Gulla RI. What is optimum neck dissection for T3/4 buccal-gingival cancers? *European Archives of Oto-Rhino-Laryngology* 1995; **252**: 143–5.

60. Rodgers GK, Myers EN. Surgical management of the mass in the buccal space. *Laryngoscope* 1988; **98**: 749–53.

61. Dixit S, Vyas RK, Toparani RB *et al.* Surgery versus surgery and postoperative radiotherapy in squamous cell carcinoma of the buccal mucosa: a comparative study. *Annals of Surgical Oncology* 1998; **5**: 502–10.

62. Mishra RC, Singh DN, Mishra TK. Post-operative radiotherapy in carcinoma of buccal mucosa, a prospective randomized trial. *European Journal of Surgical Oncology* 1996; **22**: 502–4.

63. Mishra RC, Parida G, Mishra TK, Mohanty S. Tumour thickness and relationship to locoregional failure in cancer of the buccal mucosa. *European Journal of Surgical Oncology* 1999; **25**: 186–9.

64. Bloom ND, Spiro RH. Carcinoma of the cheek mucosa. A retrospective analysis. *American Journal of Surgery* 1980; **140**: 556–9.

65. Badakh DK, Grover AH. The efficacy of postoperative radiation therapy in patients with carcinoma of the

buccal mucosa and lower alveolus with positive surgical margins. *Indian Journal of Cancer* 2005; **42**: 51–6.

66. DiNardo LJ. Lymphatics of the submandibular space: an anatomic, clinical, and pathologic study with applications to floor-of-mouth carcinoma. *Laryngoscope* 1998; **108**: 206–14.

67. Dutton JM, Graham SM, Hoffman HT. Metastatic cancer to the floor of mouth: the lingual lymph nodes. *Head and Neck* 2002; **24**: 401–5.

68. Shah JP, Candela FC, Poddar AK. The patterns of cervical lymph node metastases from squamous carcinoma of the oral cavity. *Cancer* 1990; **66**: 109–13.

69. Garzino-Demo P, Dell'Acqua A, Dalmasso P *et al.* Clinicopathological parameters and outcome of 245 patients operated for oral squamous cell carcinoma. *Journal of Cranio-Maxillo-Facial Surgery* 2006; **34**: 344–50.

70. Hicks WL Jr, Loree TR, Garcia RI *et al.* Squamous cell carcinoma of the floor of mouth: a 20-year review. *Head and Neck* 1997; **19**: 400–5.

71. Sessions DG, Spector GJ, Lenox J *et al.* Analysis of treatment results for floor-of-mouth cancer. *Laryngoscope* 2000; **110**: 1764–72.

72. Schmidt BL, Dierks EJ, Homer L, Potter B. Tobacco smoking history and presentation of oral squamous cell carcinoma. *Journal of Oral and Maxillofacial Surgery* 2004; **62**: 1055–8.

73. Aygun C, Salazar OM, Sewchand W *et al.* Carcinoma of the floor of the mouth: a 20-year experience. *International Journal of Radiation Oncology, Biology, Physics* 1984; **10**: 619–26.

74. Pernot M, Hoffstetter S, Peiffert D *et al.* Epidermoid carcinomas of the floor of mouth treated by exclusive irradiation: statistical study of a series of 207 cases. *Radiotherapy and Oncology* 1995; **35**: 177–85.

75. Marsiglia H, Haie-Meder C, Sasso G *et al.* Brachytherapy for T1–T2 floor-of-the-mouth cancers: the Gustave-Roussy Institute experience. *International Journal of Radiation Oncology, Biology, Physics* 2002; **52**: 1257–63.

76. Klotch DW, Muro-Cacho C, Gal TJ. Factors affecting survival for floor-of-mouth carcinoma. *Otolaryngology – Head and Neck Surgery* 2000; **122**: 495–8.

77. Shaha AR, Spiro RH, Shah JP, Strong EW. Squamous carcinoma of the floor of the mouth. *American Journal of Surgery* 1984; **148**: 455–9.

78. Zelefsky MJ, Harrison LB, Fass DE *et al.* Postoperative radiotherapy for oral cavity cancers: impact of anatomic subsite on treatment outcome. *Head and Neck* 1990; **12**: 470–5.

79. Mashberg A, Meyers H. Anatomical site and size of 222 early asymptomatic oral squamous cell carcinomas: a continuing prospective study of oral cancer. II. *Cancer* 1976; **37**: 2149–57.

80. Schepman KP, van der Meij EH, Smeele LE, van der Waal I. Malignant transformation of oral leukoplakia: a follow-up study of a hospital-based population of 166 patients with oral leukoplakia from The Netherlands. *Oral Oncology* 1998; **34**: 270–5.

81. Scheifele C, Reichart PA. Is there a natural limit of the transformation rate of oral leukoplakia? *Oral Oncology* 2003; **39**: 470–5.

82. Zupi A, Califano L, Mangone GM *et al.* Surgical management of the neck in squamous cell carcinoma of the floor of the mouth. *Oral Oncology* 1998; **34**: 472–5.

83. McGuirt WF Jr, Johnson JT, Myers EN *et al.* Floor of mouth carcinoma. The management of the clinically negative neck. *Archives of Otolaryngology – Head and Neck Surgery* 1995; **121**: 278–82.

84. McColl HA Jr, Horwood J. 'Localized' carcinoma of the mobile tongue and floor of the mouth – a lesion frequently misjudged and undertreated. *Journal of Surgical Oncology* 1978; **10**: 337–45.

85. Yco MS, Cruickshank JC. Treatment of stage I carcinoma of the anterior floor of the mouth. *Archives of Otolaryngology – Head and Neck Surgery* 1986; **112**: 1085–9.

86. Daley TD, Lovas JG, Peters E *et al.* Salivary gland duct involvement in oral epithelial dysplasia and squamous cell carcinoma. *Oral Surgery, Oral Medicine, Oral Pathology, Oral Radiology, and Endodontics* 1996; **81**: 186–92.

87. Ord RA, Lee VE. Submandibular duct repositioning after excision of floor of mouth cancer. *Journal of Oral and Maxillofacial Surgery* 1996; **54**: 1075–8.

88. Maurer P, Eckert AW, Schubert J. Functional rehabilitation following resection of the floor of the mouth: the nasolabial flap revisited. *Journal of Cranio-Maxillo-Facial Surgery* 2002; **30**: 369–72.

89. Joshi A, Rajendraprasad JS, Shetty K. Reconstruction of intraoral defects using facial artery musculomucosal flap. *British Journal of Plastic Surgery* 2005; **58**: 1061–6.

90. Chiarini L, De Santis G, Bedogni A, Nocini PF. Lining the mouth floor with prelaminated fascio-mucosal free flaps: clinical experience. *Microsurgery* 2002; **22**: 177–86.

91. Panje WR, Smith B, McCabe BF. Epidermoid carcinoma of the floor of the mouth: surgical therapy vs combined therapy vs radiation therapy. *Otolaryngology – Head and Neck Surgery* 1980; **88**: 714–20.

92. Rodgers LW Jr, Stringer SP, Mendenhall WM *et al.* Management of squamous cell carcinoma of the floor of mouth. *Head and Neck* 1993; **15**: 16–19.

93. Leemans CR, Tiwari R, Nauta JJ, Snow GB. Discontinuous vs in-continuity neck dissection in carcinoma of the oral cavity. *Archives of Otolaryngology – Head and Neck Surgery* 1991; **117**: 1003–6.

94. Spiro RH, Huvos AG, Wong GY *et al.* Predictive value of tumor thickness in squamous carcinoma confined to the tongue and floor of the mouth. *American Journal of Surgery* 1986; **152**: 345–50.

95. Dias FL, Kligerman J, Matos de Sa G *et al.* Elective neck dissection versus observation in stage I squamous cell carcinomas of the tongue and floor of the mouth.

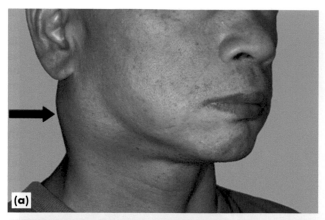

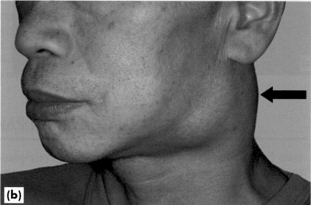

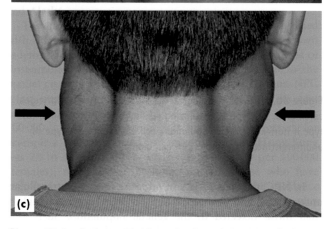

Figure 30.2 Patient with bilateral enlarged upper cervical lymph nodes (arrow).

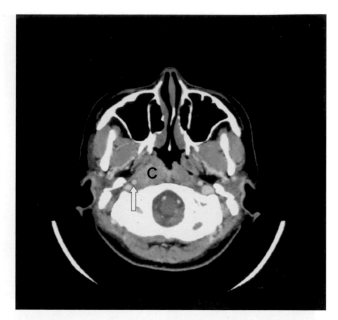

Figure 30.3 Computed tomography (axial view) showing an extensive left nasopharyngeal carcinoma (C) encasing the internal carotid artery (arrow).

The increasing trend of both the antibody levels or copies of EBV DNA on serial testing in any individual is an indication for further investigation.

Imaging studies

The development of cross-sectional computed tomography (CT) and magnetic resonance (MR) imaging have revolutionized the diagnosis, evaluation and treatment of NPC. The extent of the primary tumour and its involvement of adjacent structures can be clearly determined (**Figure 30.3**). The presence of cervical metastasis can also be determined (**Figure 30.4**). These imaging studies have improved the accuracy of staging and have also allowed radiotherapy planning and treatment.[20]

It has been shown recently that better treatment results, especially the reduction of side effects, can be achieved with intensity modulated radiotherapy (IMRT). This therapeutic modality employs composite CT-MR images,[21] and enables radiotherapy to be targeted even more accurately onto the tumour while at the same time sparing adjacent tissue.

MAGNETIC RESONANCE IMAGING

MRI is superior to CT in displaying both superficial and deep nasopharyngeal soft tissues and differentiating tumour from normal tissue. Its multiplanar capability also gives a three-dimensional impression of the tumour (**Figures 30.5, 30.6, 30.7**). MRI can demonstrate the infiltration of muscle by tumour laterally (**Figure 30.8**) and superiorly to affect the cavernous sinus (**Figure 30.9**). It is also useful in the detection of the presence, location and extent of paranasopharyngeal and cervical nodal metastases (**Figure 30.10**).[22] MRI, however, is of

measured by real time quantitative PCR and this is related to the stage of disease with high copies more commonly detected in advanced stage,[17] however its value in the early detection of recurrent locoregional NPC is limited.

The quantity of EBV DNA measured before and after treatment is also an important predictive factor of outcome. One study reported patients with post-treatment EBV DNA above 500 copies/mL had a higher chance of developing relapse and death.[18] Another study reported pre-treatment EBV DBA above 4000 copies/mL in stage I–II patients was associated with a higher risk of distant failure.[19] These results suggested that pre- and post-therapy EBV DNA may provide important prognostic information which allows clinicians to define a high risk patient group that warrants more aggressive treatment.

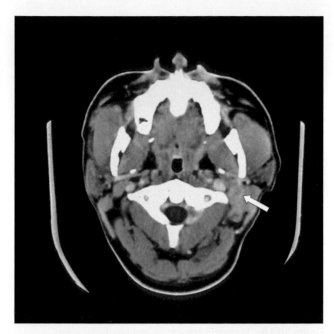

Figure 30.4 Computed tomography showing a metastatic cervical lymph node with central necrosis (arrow).

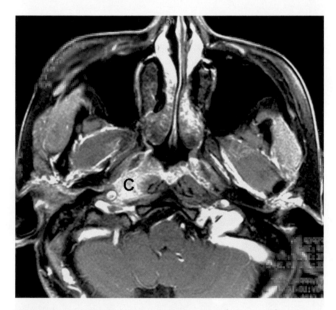

Figure 30.5 Magnetic resonance imaging (axial view) showing nasopharyngeal carcinoma (C).

limited effectiveness in evaluating the extent of bone involvement.

COMPUTED TOMOGRAPHY

CT is useful for detecting bone skull base erosion by tumour (**Figure 30.11**). CT can also identify the paranasopharyngeal extension of the tumour which is one of the most common modes of extension of NPC,[23] and perineural spread through the foramen ovale as an important route of intracranial extension. Perineural spread through the foramen ovale is the explanation for cavernous sinus involvement without skull base erosion.[24]

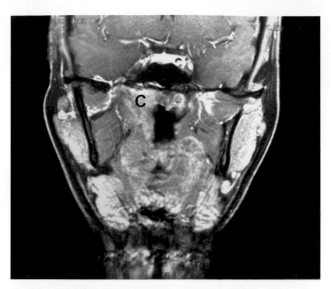

Figure 30.6 Magnetic resonance imaging (direct coronal view) showing nasopharyngeal carcinoma (C).

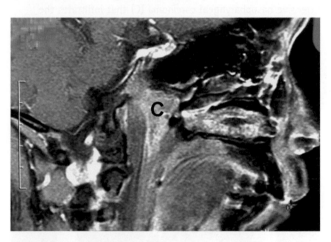

Figure 30.7 Magnetic resonance imaging (sagittal view) showing nasopharyngeal carcinoma (C).

OTHER IMAGING STUDIES

Imaging studies to detect distant metastases at diagnosis are less successful in early disease (scale 1) in patients with advanced disease (N3); staging with chest x-ray, bone scan and liver ultrasonography is indicated.[25] The reactive policy of imaging only when patients have symptoms of distant metastasis is the best policy.

Both CT and MRI are not sensitive in detecting residual or recurrent disease following radiation or chemoradiation.[26] Positron emission tomography (PET) is more sensitive than CT and MRI in detecting persistent and recurrent tumours in the nasopharynx[27] (**Figure 30.12**).

Endoscopic examination and biopsy

Endoscopic examination provides valuable information on mucosal involvement and tumour extent and allows guided biopsy. The endoscopic examination, however, cannot

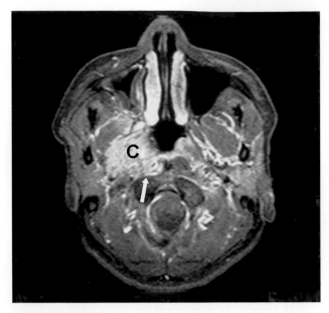

Figure 30.8   Magnetic resonance imaging (axial view) showing extensive nasopharyngeal carcinoma (C) that infiltrates the prevertebral muscle (arrow).

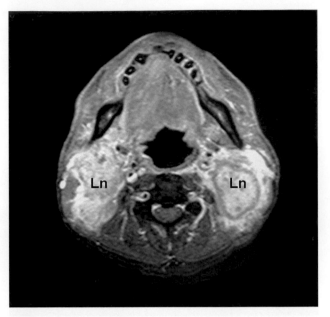

Figure 30.10   Magnetic resonance imaging (axial view) showing bilateral metastatic nasopharyngeal carcinoma in the cervical lymph nodes (Ln).

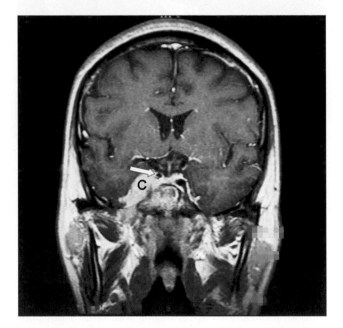

Figure 30.9   Magnetic resonance imaging (direct coronal view) showing nasopharyngeal carcinoma (C) that has extended upwards to affect the cavernous sinus involving the internal carotid artery (arrow).

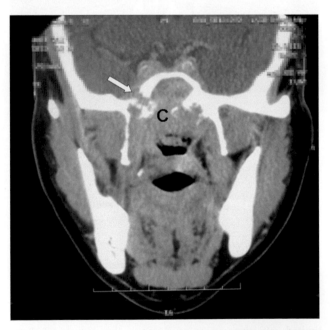

Figure 30.11   Computed tomography (direct coronal view) showing an extensive nasopharyngeal carcinoma (C) eroding the skull base (arrow).

determine deep extension or skull base involvement of the tumour. The endoscopic examination and biopsy can be carried out under local anaesthesia using both flexible and rigid endoscopes.

FIBREOPTIC FLEXIBLE ENDOSCOPE

A fibreoptic flexible endoscope with a suction and biopsy forcep channel should be used. Flexible biopsy forceps are

small however, and this limits the amount of tissue obtained. As the carcinoma cells may lie submucosally, the biopsy forceps should pierce the nasopharyngeal mucosa and be inserted deep to ensure a good biopsy.[28] The optical image obtained with the flexible endoscope is slightly inferior to that of the rigid endoscope. The flexibility of the scope and its incorporated biopsy forceps channel are the main advantages (**Figure 30.13**).

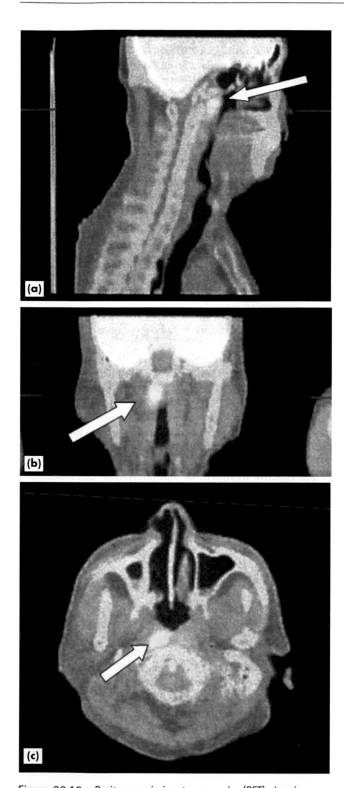

Figure 30.12   Positron emission tomography (PET) showing residual tumour in the nasopharynx after chemoradiation (arrows).

RIGID ENDOSCOPE

A 4 mm Hopkins rod rigid endoscope provides a better optical image. Endoscopes with different visual angles can be used for inspection of different regions in the nasopharynx. The rigid endoscopes that are frequently used include

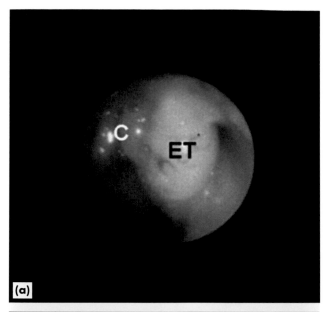

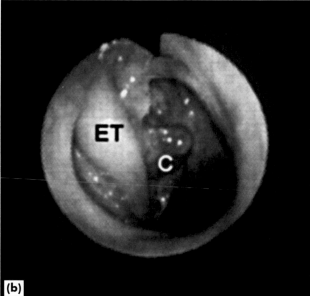

Figure 30.13   Flexible endoscopic view of nasopharynx. (a) Scope through the left nasal cavity, showing a tumour (C) in the left fossa encroaching onto the medial crura of the Eustachian tube (ET). (b) Scope through the right nasal cavity, showing a polypoid tumour (C) arising from the right fossa, attaching to the medial crura of the Eustachian tube (ET).

the 0° and 30° lens scopes (**Figure 30.14**). The rigid endoscope can be inserted through either nasal passage to reach the pathology in the nasopharynx, a biopsy forceps can be introduced either alongside the endoscope or via the opposite nostril so that biopsy is taken under direct vision.

Staging of nasopharyngeal carcinoma

There are a few staging systems for NPC. The American Joint Committee on Cancer Staging and/or UICC system is used in

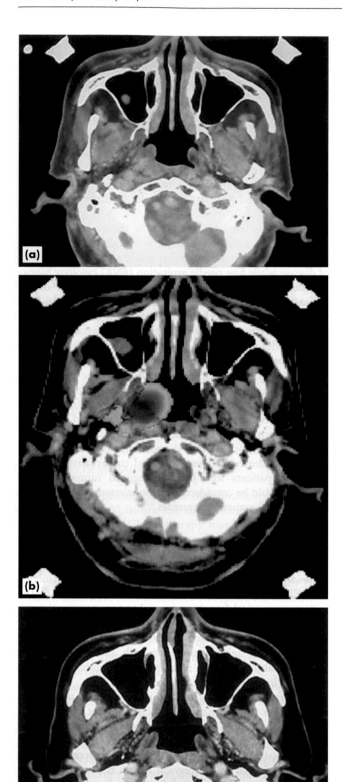

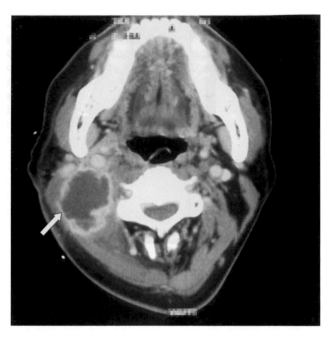

Figure 30.20 Computed tomography (axial view) showing that an enlarged right neck node with central necrosis showing extensive infiltration (arrow).

clinically evident; (2) over 70 per cent of the nodes exhibited extracapular spread; (3) 30 per cent of positive nodes were lying close to the spinal accessory nerve.[79]

In some cases cervical lymph nodes at presentation are already of a significant size to suggest extensive extracapsular spread (**Figure 30.19**). The extension beyond the confines of the lymph nodes can involve surrounding neck structures such as the overlying skin (**Figure 30.20**) and muscle carotid sheath. For these patients, even after radical neck dissection, removing all macroscopic tumour, the resection margins would be close and there might be microscopic residual disease. After-loading brachytherapy delivered to the tumour bed following radical neck dissection has been shown to be useful. In this situation, nylon tubes are placed on the tumour bed accurately at the time of the neck dissection (**Figure 30.21**). The overlying skin has to be removed as it will not survive further radiation from the brachytherapy. A skin flap is used to cover the tumour bed and bring in new blood supply and thus decrease the risk of necrosis. Adjuvant brachytherapy in extensive neck diseases allows a similar tumour control rate to that achieved when radical neck dissection alone was performed in less extensive neck disease.[86]

DISEASE IN THE NASOPHARYNX

Reirradiation

External reirradiation of NPC with curative intent is often undesirable given the large numbers of critical structures in the vicinity of the primary radiotherapy field. Whenever possible, brachytherapy or stereotactic radiosurgery should be considered for reirradiation of treatments. Reported five-year survival rates after external reirradiation using the conventional technique range from 8 to 36 per cent.[85, 87, 88] A high incidence of late complications, mostly neurological

Figure 30.19 Stereotactic radiosurgery as salvage treatment for nasopharyngeal carcinoma. (a) CT showing recurrent lesion at right lateral wall of nasopharynx. (b) Isodose distribution of target covered by radiosurgery with single isocentre with a dose of 12.5 Gy to target periphery. (c) CT taken 12 months after radiosurgery showing complete regression of tumour.

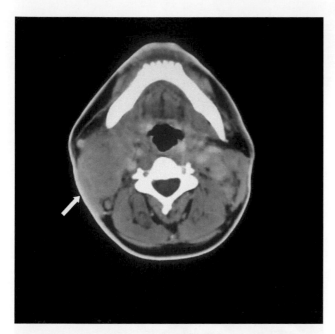

Figure 30.21 Computed tomography (axial view) showing that the enlarged right neck node has infiltrated the overlying neck skin (arrow).

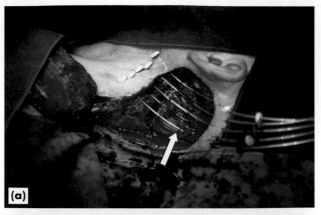

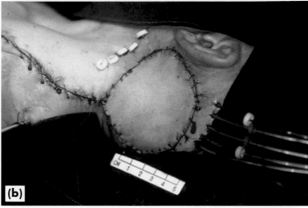

Figure 30.22 (a) Clinical photograph showing the placement of hollow nylon tube (arrow) over the tumour bed after radical neck dissection. The overlying skin was removed with the radical neck dissection. (b) The cutaneous defect in the neck was covered with the pectoralis major myocutaneous flap.

damage and soft tissue fibrosis, is commonly seen after external reirradiation. The use of three-dimensional conformal radiotherapy and more recently IMRT has improved the outlook of patients receiving external reirradiation. In one study using three-dimensional conformal radiotherapy for retreatment of nasopharyngeal carcinoma, the five-year local control rate was 71 per cent but the actuarial incidence of major late toxicities was still high with at least grade 3 toxicities in 100 per cent and grade 4 in 49 per cent at five years.[89] Several preliminary reports using IMRT for re-irradiation of nasopharyngeal carcinoma also reported good short-term control with a relatively low incidence of severe late toxicities.[90, 91]

Chemoradiotherapy may also improve treatment outcome in locally recurrent nasopharyngeal carcinoma. One study employed induction chemotherapy to shrink the tumour volume followed by reirradiation using IMRT and reported 75 per cent local control rate at one year.[92] Another study employed concurrent chemoradiotherapy and reported a one-year progression-free rate of 42 per cent.[93] In patients with advanced local recurrence in which treatment planning for reirradiation is difficult, induction rather than concurrent chemotherapy is preferred as the former may allow tumour shrinkage to take place and thus facilitate subsequent radiotherapy planning and whole target coverage.

Stereotactic radiosurgery

The technique of stereotactic radiosurgery involves the localization of a small target which is irradiated by multiple convergent beams providing a large single dose of radiation. The technique was originally developed for the treatment of functional neurological disorders, but was later found to be useful for vascular malformations, benign intracranial/skull base neoplasms and cerebral metastases. Stereotactic

radiosurgery has also been used in nasopharyngeal carcinoma to deliver a boost dose after a second course of radiotherapy or as a salvage treatment for local recurrence (**Figure 30.22**). Stereotactic radiosurgery alone can achieve local control rates of 53–86 per cent for locally recurrent nasopharyngeal carcinoma.[94, 95] For recurrent disease confined to nasopharynx or adjacent soft tissues, the reported local control rate at two years was 72 per cent.[96] When stereotactic radiosurgery was administered as a boost dose after reirradiation, the three-year control rate ranged from 52 to 58 per cent.[92, 97, 98] Based on these results, there is strong evidence indicating that radiosurgery is an effective salvage treatment for local failures of nasopharyngeal carcinoma. There are, however, no data comparing the relative efficacy and complications of radiosurgery with other salvage treatments. In practice, the selection of treatment modalities depends mainly on the extent of disease and expertise available. For recurrent disease confined to the nasopharynx or adjacent soft tissues, results of radiosurgery appear to be comparable to brachytherapy or surgery, and can be considered as a treatment option. The advent of intensity-modulated radiotherapy appears to have improved the outcome of recurrent nasopharyngeal carcinoma. Reirradiation using IMRT is recommended for patients with extensive local recurrence while reserving radiosurgery as a boost treatment or for further recurrence. Although most series reported a relatively low risk of late complications following radiosurgery, massive potentially fatal haemorrhage remains the most severe form of complication.[99] Massive haemorrhage after radiosurgery is usually due to radiation damage to the carotid artery, often as a result of using a large fraction dose and high cumulative dose. To minimize the risk of haemorrhage, radiosurgery should only be used in the absence of direct tumour encasement of the carotid artery.

Brachytherapy

When brachytherapy is used, the radiation dosage is highest at the source and decreases rapidly towards the periphery. This enables a high dose of irradiation to be delivered to the residual or recurrent tumour while surrounding tissue receives a much smaller dose. Brachytherapy radiation also delivers radiation at a continuous low dose rate, which gives a further radiobiological advantage over fractionated external radiation.

Intracavitary brachytherapy has been used traditionally for nasopharyngeal carcinomas.[100] With this method, the radiation source is placed either in a tube or over a mould and then inserted into the nasopharynx (**Figure 30.23**). The irregular contour of the nasopharynx and the variable dimensions and location of persistent or recurrent tumours make it difficult to position radiation sources accurately in the nasopharynx. To circumvent this problem, radioactive interstitial implants have been used to treat small localized residual or recurrent tumour in the nasopharynx.

Radioactive gold grains (198Au) have been used as an interstitial radiation source. Gold grains can be implanted into the tumour either transnasally under endoscopic guidance[101] or using the split-palate approach.[102] The latter approach gives the surgeon a direct view of the tumour, its location and its extent in the nasopharynx. This enables the precise implanting of the gold grains permanently into the tumour.

Using a soft palate split in the midline and to one side of the uvula, the mucoperiosteum over the hard palate is lifted. The attachment of the soft palate to the posterior edge of the hard palate is detached and the tumour in the nasopharynx is exposed (**Figure 30.24**). The surgeon inserts the endoscope into the nasopharynx while the oncologist implants the gold grains into the tumour under direct vision with the introducer (**Figure 30.25**). The palatal wound is then closed in layers. During the closure, a thick lead shield is used to reduce the radiation dose to the body of the surgeon and the patient's eyes are protected with a lead glass (**Figure 30.26**).

As brachytherapy is effective over short distances it is used only for shallow tumours localized in the nasopharynx and without bone invasion. The split palate implantation of gold grains as a brachytherapy source has provided effective salvage with minimal morbidity (**Figure 30.27**).[103] Where gold grain implants were applied to treat persistent and recurrent tumours after radiotherapy, the five-year local tumour control rates were 87 and 63 per cent, respectively, and the corresponding five-year disease-free survival rates were 68 and 60 per cent, respectively.[104]

Nasopharyngectomy

When persistent or recurrent tumour in the nasopharynx is too extensive for brachytherapy or has extended to the

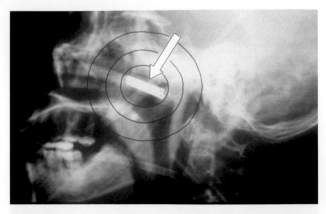

Figure 30.23   Radiation source is placed in a tube (arrow) and this is introduced into the nasopharynx.

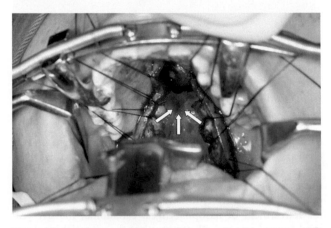

Figure 30.24   Intraoperative photography showing exposure of the oral cavity with the Dingman's mouth gag. The soft palate and the mucoperiosteum of the hard palate have been retracted laterally with stay sutures. The shallow tumour in the nasopharynx can be seen (arrows).

paranasopharyngeal space, then surgical salvage may be an option. Nasopharyngectomy can achieve salvage in selected patients.

Adequate surgical exposure to allow oncological extirpation of tumour in the nasopharynx region is a technical challenge. A number of approaches have been described including the infratemporal approach from the lateral aspect,[105] transpalatal, transmaxillary and transcervical approaches from the inferior aspect,[106, 107] and an anterolateral approach.[108] The overall mortality associated with all these salvage surgical procedures is low. As all patients have undergone previous radical radiotherapy, meticulous tissue handling during surgery is essential for satisfactory healing.

The choice of the surgical approach to carry out the nasopharyngectomy depends on the location and extent of the tumour in the nasopharynx. For localized tumour in the lower part of the posterior wall of the nasopharynx, the transpalatal approach is usually adequate. The disadvantage of this approach is that the lateral extent of resection is limited. When the main tumour bulk is located in the paranasopharyngeal space, lying close or lateral to the

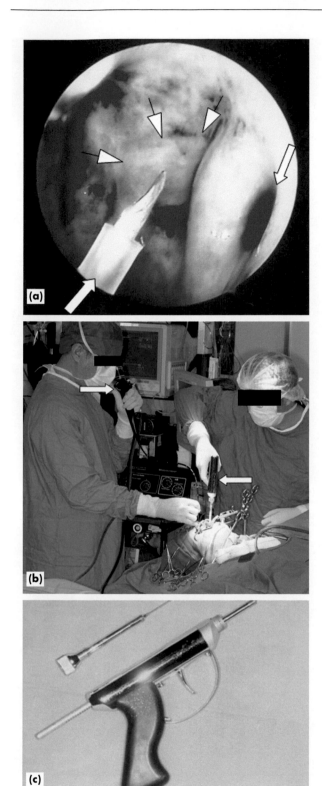

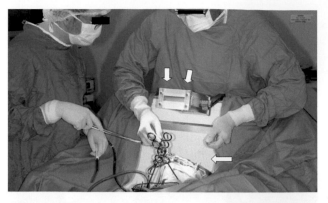

Figure 30.26   During closure of the palatal wound, the bodies of the surgeons are protected by a lead shield (arrow) and the eyes are protected by a thick lead glass mounted on the shield (arrows).

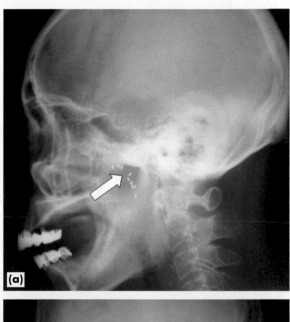

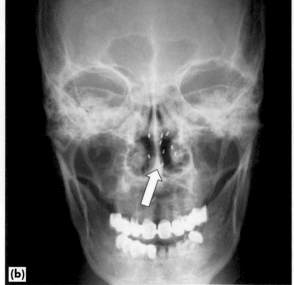

Figure 30.25   (a) Endoscopic view showing the Eustachian tube opening (arrow), the shallow tumour in the nasopharynx (arrow heads) and the tip of the gold grain introducer (solid arrow). (b) The surgeon on the left examines the tumour in the nasopharynx with the flexible endoscope (arrow) and the clinical oncologist standing on the right inserts the gold grains into the tumour with the introducer (arrow). (c) The cartridges of gold grains and the introducer.

Figure 30.27   Plain x-rays showing the implanted gold grains (arrow). (a) Lateral view; (b) anteroposterior view.

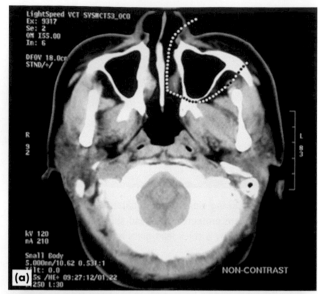

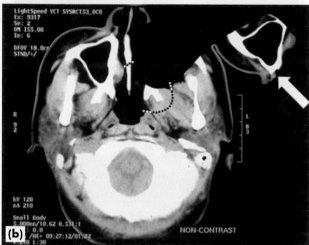

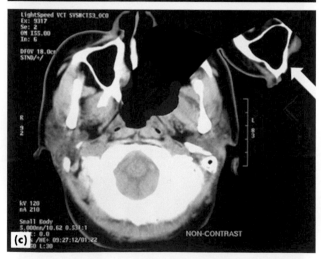

Figure 30.28 Schematic axial view computed tomography. (a) The dotted lines mark the osteotomies on the maxilla. (b) The maxilla is swung laterally but remains attached to the anterior cheek flap (arrow). Pterygoid plate and the posterior part of nasal septum can be removed. (c) Whole nasopharynx exposed after the maxilla is swung laterally and removing the pterygoid plates and posterior part of nasal septum.

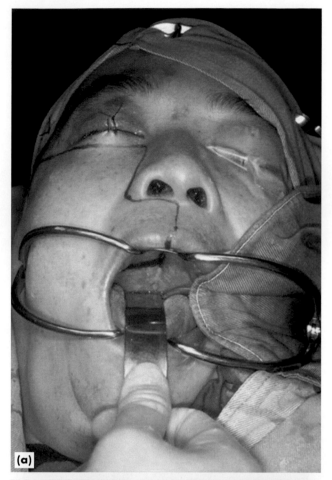

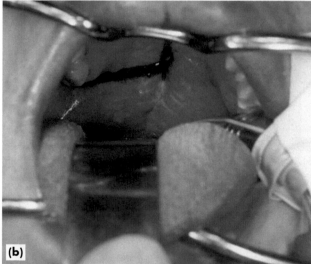

Figure 30.29 (a) Weber Ferguson facial incision extends between the central incisors onto the hard palate. (b) The midline palatal incision turns laterally behind the maxillary tuberosity.

internal carotid artery, then the lateral infratemporal fossa approach is applicable. The limitation of this approach is that many structures have to be mobilized in order to obtain an adequate exposure. The various other anterior and inferior approaches may give adequate visualization of the tumour but do not allow the resection of the tumour from all sides in

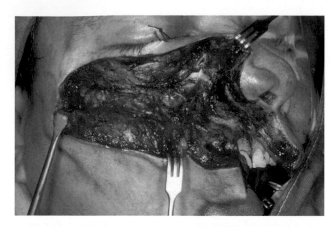

Figure 30.30 Soft tissue over the face was retracted to expose a narrow strip of anterior maxillary bone for osteotomy (purple marking).

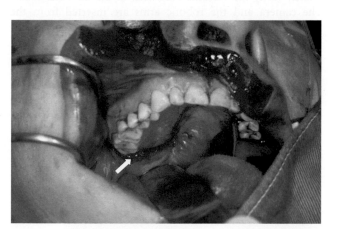

Figure 30.31 Clinical photograph showing the incision over the hard palate. A curved osteotome would be used to separate the maxillary tuberosity from the pterygoid plates (arrow).

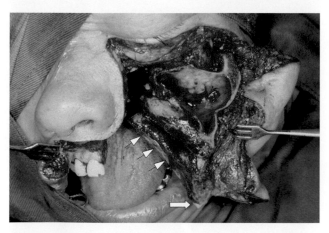

Figure 30.32 Another patient with the left triangular-shaped maxilla swung laterally. The retractor is on the anterior cheek flap. The hard palate (arrow heads) with the central incisor tooth (arrow) can be seen.

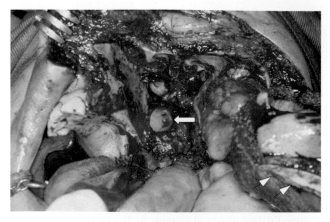

Figure 30.33 After nasopharyngectomy, the sphenoid sinus is opened (arrow). The posterior edge of the hard palate on the side of the swing is seen on the left side (arrow heads).

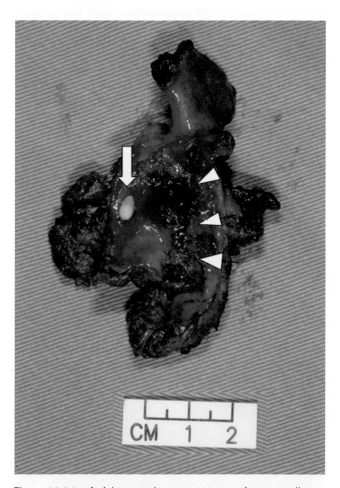

Figure 30.34 A right nasopharyngectomy specimen: a yellow tube is inserted in the Eustachian tube (arrow) opening. The tumour is marked (arrow heads).

an oncological fashion. As most nasopharyngeal carcinoma is closely associated with the crura at the opening of the Eustachian tube, a curative oncological resection should always include these structures. Serial sectioning of nasopharyngectomy specimens has shown that the persistent or recurrent nasopharyngeal carcinoma exhibits extensive submucosal extension and a wide resection of the nasopharynx is essential in order to achieve a favourable outcome.[109]

As most of the residual and recurrent nasopharyngeal carcinoma in the nasopharynx affects the fossa of

Rosenmüller and the crura of the Eustachian tube, the anterolateral or maxillary swing approach is a common route for surgical salvage. The procedure applied for salvage nasopharyngectomy was first reported in 1991 (**Figure 30.28**).[108] The facial incisions start with the Weber–Ferguson incision as for maxillectomy and this is continued between the central incisor teeth onto the hard palate in the midline and then turned laterally along the attachment of the soft palate to the hard palate (**Figure 30.29**). The soft tissue over the anterior wall of the maxilla is lifted to expose a small portion of the bone for osteotomy (**Figure 30.30**). The osteotomy goes through the anterior wall of the maxilla below the floor of the orbit and includes the lower part of the zygomatic arch. The hard palate is divided in the midline and a curved osteotome used to separate the maxillary tuberosity from the pterygoid plates (**Figure 30.31**). After the osteotomies, the maxilla is dropped down but remains attached to the anterior cheek flap (**Figure 30.32**). The maxilla can be swung laterally as an osteocutaneous complex to expose the nasopharynx and the paranasopharyngeal space (**Figure 30.33**). This wide exposure allows persistent or recurrent tumour in the region to be removed en bloc (**Figure 30.34**).

Patient selection is crucial as surgical salvage in the form of nasopharyngectomy is only indicated for tumours localized in the nasopharynx without infiltration of the skull base or internal carotid artery. As long as the residual or recurrent tumour can be removed adequately, i.e. when the surgical margins are negative, the long-term aesthetic and functional results are satisfactory (**Figure 30.35**). The five-year actuarial control of tumours in the nasopharynx has been reported to be 74 per cent and the five-year disease-free survival rate is around 56 per cent.[110] As all these patients have undergone radical radiotherapy, they develop morbidities such as trismus and occasionally palatal fistula. Palatal fistula risk can be minimized by avoiding placing the soft tissue incision in the same plane as the osteotomy over the hard palate (**Figure 30.36**).[111]

Recently, resection of a small tumour localized at the posterior wall of the nasopharynx has been reported using endoscope and instruments inserted through the nasal and oral cavities.[112] The rigid endoscopic instruments limit the en bloc removal of larger or laterally located tumour. For small tumours located over the lateral wall but not extending into the paranasopharyngeal space, they might be resected adequately using the versatile endowrist of the da Vinci robot. The camera and the robotic arms are inserted from the inferior aspect with a split palate approach.[113]

For a successful salvage of localized small tumour in the nasopharynx, brachytherapy or surgery could be considered. The choice of approaches of surgical salvage of recurrent nasopharyngeal carcinoma depends on the location and extent of the tumour. For those tumours involving skull base or those that are too extensive for surgery, stereotactic

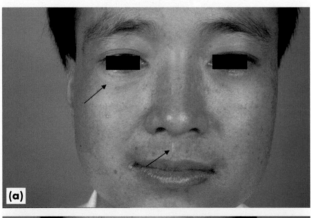

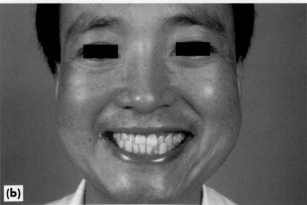

Figure 30.35 Postoperative photograph at 1.5 years after the operation. (a) The facial wound has healed and is nearly invisible (arrows). (b) All the teeth on the side of the swing have survived.

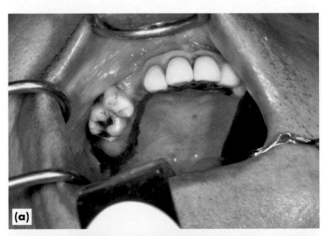

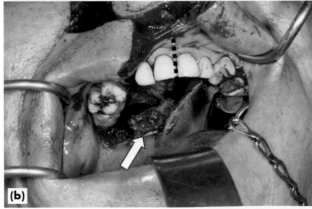

Figure 30.36 (a) The palatal incision is modified to go along the root of the upper alveolus. (b) The palatal flap (arrow) is raised so that the osteotomy (dotted line) of the hard palate is not in the same plane as the incision on the palate.

radiation or intensity modulated radiotherapy could be tried and this is sometimes combined with chemotherapy.[114]

KEY EVIDENCE

- Epstein–Barr viral DNA determination has been established as a diagnostic means for nasopharyngeal carcinoma, especially for early stage disease.
- Concurrent chemoradiation employed for the treatment of advanced stage nasopharyngeal carcinoma has improved survival outcome when compared with radiation alone.
- Salvage surgery for residual or recurrent disease either in the neck or in the nasopharynx gives satisfactory results with limited morbidity.

KEY LEARNING POINTS

- Nasopharynx is anatomically difficult to examine.
- In southern China the most common malignant pathology is nasopharyngeal carcinoma.
- Imaging studies determine the extent of the pathology while the diagnosis of nasopharyngeal carcinoma has to be confirmed with biopsy through endoscopic examination.
- The primary treatment modality for early stage nasopharyngeal carcinoma is radiotherapy and for advanced stage concurrent chemoradiation.
- For residual or recurrent nasopharyngeal carcinoma in the cervical lymph nodes, the optimal salvage is radical neck dissection.
- For residual or recurrent nasopharyngeal carcinoma in the nasopharynx, the optimal salvage is nasopharyngectomy.

REFERENCES

1. Harrison DF. The natural history, pathogenesis, and treatment of juvenile angiofibroma. Personal experience with 44 patients. *Archives of Otolaryngology – Head and Neck Surgery* 1987; **113**: 936–42.
2. Sham JS, Wei WI, Zong YS *et al.* Detection of subclinical nasopharyngeal carcinoma by fibreoptic endoscopy and multiple biopsy. *Lancet* 1990; **335**: 371–4.
3. Curado MP, Edwards B, Shin HR *et al.* (eds). *Cancer incidence in five continents*, vol. IX. IARC Scientific Publications No.160. Lyon: IARC, 2007: 141–3.
4. Buell P. The effect of migration on the risk of nasopharyngeal cancer among Chinese. *Cancer Research* 1974; **34**: 1189–91.
5. Prasad U. Cells of origin of nasopharyngeal carcinoma: an electron microscopical study. *Journal of Laryngology and Otology* 1974; **88**: 1087.
6. Shanmugaratnam K, Sobin LH. Histological typing of tumours of the upper respiratory tract and ear. International Histological Classification of Tumours: No 19. Geneva: World Health Organization, 1991: 32–33.
7. Nicholls JM. Nasopharyngeal carcinoma: Classification and histological appearances. *Advances in Anatomic Pathology* 1997; **4**: 71–84.
8. Reddy SP, Raslan WF, Gooneratne S *et al.* Prognostic significance of keratinization in nasopharygeal carcinoma. *American Journal of Otolaryngology* 1995; **16**: 103–8.
9. Marks JE, Philips JL, Menck HR. The National Cancer Data Base report on the relationship of race and national origin to the histology of nasopharyngeal carcinoma. *Cancer* 1998; **83**: 582–8.
10. Lee AW, Foo W, Law SC *et al.* Nasopharyngeal carcinoma: presenting symptoms and duration before diagnosis. *Hong Kong Medical Journal* 1997; **3**: 355–61.
11. Ozyar E, Atahan IL, Akyol FH *et al.* Cranial nerve involvement in nasopharyngeal carcinoma: its prognostic role and response to radiotherapy. *Radiation Medicine* 1994; **12**: 65–8.
12. Henle G, Henle W. Observations on childhood infections with the Epstein-Barr virus. *Journal of Infectious Diseases* 1970; **121**: 303–10.
13. Klein G, Giovanella BC, Lindahl T *et al.* Direct evidence for the presence of Epstein-Barr virus DNA and nuclear antigen in malignant epithelial cells from patients with poorly differentiated carcinoma of the nasopharynx. *Proceedings of the National Academy of Sciences of the United States of America* 1974; **71**: 4737–41.
14. Ho HC, Ng MH, Kwan HC, Chau JC. Epstein–Barr-virus-specific IgA and IgG serum antibodies in nasopharyngeal carcinoma. *British Journal of Cancer* 1976; **34**: 655–60.
15. Chien YC, Chen JY, Liu MY *et al.* Serologic markers of Epstein–Barr virus infection and nasopharyngeal carcinoma in Taiwanese men. *New England Journal of Medicine* 2001; **345**: 1877–82.
16. Lo DYM, Leung SF, Chan LYS *et al.* Kinetics of plasma Epstein–Barr virus DNA during radiation therapy for nasopharyngeal carcinoma. *Cancer Research* 2000; **60**: 2351–5.
17. Lin JC, Wang WY, Chen KY *et al.* Quantification of plasma Esptein–Barr virus DNA in patients with advanced stage nasopharyngeal carcinoma. *New England Journal of Medicine* 2004; **350**: 2461–70.
18. Chan AT, Ma BB, Lo YM *et al.* Phase II study of neoadjuvant carboplatin and paclitaxel followed by radiotherapy and concurrent cisplatin in patients with locoregionally advanced nasopharyngeal carcinoma: therapeutic monitoring with plasma Epstein-Barr virus DNA. *Journal of Clinical Oncology* 2004; **22**: 3053–60.

19. Leung SF, Chan AT, Zee B *et al.* Pretherapy quantitative measurement of circulating Epstein-Barr virus DNA is predictive of posttherapy distant failure in patients with early-stage nasopharyngeal carcinoma of undifferentiated type. *Cancer* 2003; **98**: 288–91.

20. Cellai E, Olmi P, Chiavacci A *et al.* Computed tomography in nasopharyngeal carcinoma: Part II: Impact on survival. *International Journal of Radiation Oncology, Biology, Physics* 1990; **19**: 1177–82.

21. Emami B, Sethi A, Petruzzelli GJ. Influence of MRI on target volume delineation and IMRT planning in nasopharyngeal carcinoma. *International Journal of Radiation Oncology, Biology, Physics* 2003; **57**: 481–8.

22. Dillon WP, Mills CM, Kjos B *et al.* Magnetic resonance imaging of the nasopharynx. *Radiology* 1984; **152**: 731–8.

23. Sham JS, Cheung YK, Choy D *et al.* Nasopharyngeal carcinoma: CT evaluation of patterns of tumor spread. *AJNR American Journal of Neuroradiology* 1991; **12**: 265–70.

24. Chong VF, Fan YF, Khoo JB. Nasopharyngeal carcinoma with intracranial spread: CT and MR characteristics. *Journal of Computer Assisted Tomography* 1996; **20**: 563–9.

25. Kumar MB, Lu JJ, Loh KS *et al.* Tailoring distant metastatic imaging for patients with clinically localized undifferentiated nasopharyngeal carcinoma. *International Journal of Radiation Oncology, Biology, Physics* 2004; **58**: 688–93.

● 26. Chong VF, Fan YF. Detection of recurrent nasopharyngeal carcinoma. MR imaging versus CT: *Radiology* 1997; **202**: 463–70.

27. Yen RF, Hung RL, Pan MH *et al.* 18-fluoro-2-deoxyglucose positron emission tomography in detecting residual/recurrent nasopharyngeal carcinomas and comparison with magnetic resonance imaging. *Cancer* 2003; **98**: 283–7.

28. Wei WI, Sham JS, Zong YS *et al.* The efficacy of fiberoptic endoscopic examination and biopsy in the detection of early nasopharyngeal carcinoma. *Cancer* 1991; **67**: 3127–30.

● 29. Sobin LH, Wittekind CH (eds). *TNM classification of malignant tumours*, 5th edn. New York: Wiley-Liss, 1997: 25–30.

● 30. Fleming ID, Cooper JS, Henson DE *et al.* (eds). *AJCC cancer staging manual*, 5th edn. Philadelphia: Lippincott-Raven, 1997: 33–5.

31. Ho JHC. An epidemiologic and clinical study of nasopharyngeal carcinoma. *International Journal of Radiation Oncology, Biology, Physics* 1978; **4**: 182–98.

◆ 32. Ho JH. Stage classification of nasopharyngeal carcinoma: a review. *International Agency for Research on Cancer* 1978; **20**: 99–113.

33. Edge SB, Byrd DR, Carducci MA *et al.* (eds). American Joint Committee on Cancer (AJCC). *Cancer staging manual*, 7th edn. New York: Springer, 2009.

34. Cooper JS, Cohen R, Stevens RE. A comparison of staging systems for nasopharyngeal carcinoma. *Cancer* 1998; **83**: 213–19.

35. Özyar E, Yildiz F, Akyol FH, Atahan IL. Comparison of AJCC 1988 and 1997 classifications for nasopharyngeal carcinoma. *International Journal of Radiation Oncology, Biology, Physics* 1999; **44**: 1079–87.

36. Moss WT. *Therapeutic radiology*, 2nd edn. St Louis: CV, Mosby, 1965: 142–180.

◆ 37. Lee AWM, Poon YF, Foo W *et al.* Retrospective analysis of 5037 patients with nasopharyngeal carcinoma treated during 1976–1985: overall survival and patterns of failure. *International Journal of Radiation Oncology, Biology, Physics* 1992; **23**: 261–70.

38. Lee AW, Sze WM, Au JS *et al.* Treatment results for nasopharyngeal carcinoma in the modern era: the Hong Kong experience. *International Journal of Radiation Oncology, Biology, Physics* 2005; **61**: 1107–16.

39. Lee AWM, Sham JS, Poon YF, Ho JH. Treatment of Stage I nasopharyngeal carcinoma: analysis of the patterns of relapse and the results of withholding elective neck irradiation. *International Journal of Radiation Oncology, Biology, Physics* 1989; **17**: 1183–90.

40. Kwong DL, Sham JS, Chua DT *et al.* The effect of interruptions and prolonged treatment time in radiotherapy for nasopharyngeal carcinoma. *International Journal of Radiation Oncology, Biology, Physics* 1997; **39**: 703–10.

41. Wu PM, Chua DT, Sham JS *et al.* Tumor control probability of nasopharyngeal carcinoma: a comparison of different mathematical models. *International Journal of Radiation Oncology, Biology, Physics* 1997; **37**: 913–20.

42. Levendag PC, Lagerwarrd FJ, de Pan C *et al.* High-dose, high-precision treatment options for boosting cancer of the nasopharynx. *Radiotherapy and Oncology* 2002; **63**: 67–74.

43. Teo PM, Leung SF, Fowler J *et al.* Improved local control for early T-stage nasopharyngeal carcinoma: a tale of two hospitals. *Radiotherapy and Oncology* 2000; **57**: 155–66.

44. Le QT, Tate D, Koong A *et al.* Improved local control with stereotactic radiosurgical boost in patients with nasopharyngeal carcinoma. *International Journal of Radiation Oncology, Biology, Physics* 2003; **56**: 1046–54.

45. Teo PM, Leung SF, Chan AT *et al.* Final report of a randomized trial on altered-fractionated radiotherapy in nasopharyngeal carcinoma prematurely terminated by significant increase in neurologic complications. *International Journal of Radiation Oncology, Biology, Physics* 2000; **48**: 1311–22.

46. Lee AW, Sze WM, Yau TK *et al.* Retrospective analysis on treating nasopharyngeal carcinoma with accelerated fractionation (6 fractions per week) in comparison with conventional fractionation (5 fractions per week): report on 3-year tumor control and normal tissue toxicity. *Radiotherapy and Oncology* 2001; **58**: 121–30.

47. Hsiung CY, Yorke ED, Chui CS et al. Intensity-modulated radiotherapy versus conventional three-dimensional conformal radiotherapy for boost or salvage treatment of nasopharyngeal carcinoma. International Journal of Radiation Oncology, Biology, Physics 2002; 53: 638–47.

∗ 48. Lee N, Xia P, Quivey JM et al. Intensity-modulated radiotherapy in the treatment of nasopharyngeal carcinoma: an update of the UCSF experience. International Journal of Radiation Oncology, Biology, Physics 2002; 53: 12–22.

49. Kam MK, Teo PM, Chau RM et al. Treatment of nasopharyngeal carcinoma with intensity-modulated radiotherapy: the Hong Kong experience. International Journal of Radiation Oncology, Biology, Physics 2004; 60: 1440–50.

● 50. Kwong DL, Pow EH, Sham JS et al. Intensity-modulated radiotherapy for early-stage nasopharyngeal carcinoma: a prosepective study on disease control and preservation of salivary function. Cancer 2004; 101: 1584–93.

51. International Nasopharynx Cancer Study Group: VUMCA I Trial: Preliminary results of a randomized trial comparing neoadjuvant chemotherapy (cisplatin, epirubicin, bleomycin) plus radiotherapy vs. radiotherapy alone in stage IV (≥ N2, M0) undifferentiated nasopharyngeal carcinoma: A positive effect on progression-free survival. International Journal of Radiation Oncology, Biology, Physics 1996; 35: 463–9.

52. Chua DTT, Sham JST, Choy D et al. Preliminary report of the Asian-Oceanian Clinical Oncology Association randomized trial comparing cisplatin and epirubicin followed by radiotherapy versus radiotherapy alone in the treatment of patients with locoregionally advanced nasopharyngeal carcinoma. Cancer 1998; 83: 2270–83.

53. Ma J, Mai H, Hong M et al. Results of a prospective randomized trial comparing neoadjuvant chemotherapy plus radiotherapy with radiotherapy alone in patients with locoregionally advanced nasopharyngeal carcinoma. Journal of Clinical Oncology 2001; 19: 1350–7.

54. Hareyama M, Sakata K, Shirato H et al. A prospective, randomized trial comparing neoadjuvant chemotherapy with radiotherapy alone in patients with advanced nasopharyngeal carcinoma. Cancer 2002; 94: 2217–23.

◆ 55. Chua DT, Ma J, Sham JS. Long-term survival after cisplatin-based induction chemotherapy and radiotherapy for nasopharyngeal carcinoma: A pooled data analysis of two phase III trials. Journal of Clinical Oncology 2005; 23: 1118–24.

56. Rossi A, Molinari R, Boracchi P et al. Adjuvant chemotherapy with vincristine, cyclophosphamoide, and doxorubicin after radiotherapy in local-regional nasopharyngeal cancer: Results of a 4-year multicenter randomized study. Journal of Clinical Oncology 1988; 6: 1401–10.

57. Chi KH, Chang YC, Guo WY et al. A phase III study of adjuvant chemotherapy in advanced nasopharyngeal carcinoma patients. International Journal of Radiation Oncology, Biology, Physics 2002; 52: 1238–44.

∗ 58. Al-Sarraf M, LeBlanc M, Shanker Giri PG et al. Chemoradiotherapy versus radiotherapy in patients with advanced nasopharyngeal cancer: Phase III randomized intergroup study 0099. Journal of Clinical Oncology 1998; 16: 1310–17.

∗ 59. Lin JC, Jan JS, Hsu CY et al. Phase III study of concurrent chemoradiotherapy versus radiotherapy alone for advanced nasopharyngeal carcinoma: Positive effect on overall and progression-free survival. Journal of Clinical Oncology 2003; 21: 631–7.

◆ 60. Chan AT, Leung SF, Ngan RK et al. Overall survival after concurrent cisplatin-radiotherapy compared with radiotherapy alone in locoregionally advanced nasopharyngeal carcinoma. Journal of the National Cancer Institute 2005; 97: 536–9.

● 61. Wee J, Tan EH, Tai BC et al. Randomized trial of radiotherapy versus concurrent chemoradiotherapy followed by adjuvant chemotherapy in patients with American Joint Committee on Cancer/International Union Against Cancer Stage III and IV nasopharyngeal cancer of the endemic variety. Journal of Clinical Oncology 2005; 23: 6730–8.

62. Kwong DL, Sham JS, Au GK et al. Concurrent and adjuvant chemotherapy for nasopharyngeal carcinoma: a factorial study. Journal of Clinical Oncology 2004; 22: 2643–53.

◆ 63. Lee AW, Lau WH, Tung SY et al. Preliminary results of a randomized study on therapeutic gain by concurrent chemotherapy for regionally-advanced nasopharyngeal carcinoma: NPC-9901 trial by the Hong Kong Nasopharyngeal Cancer Study Group. Journal of Clinical Oncology 2005; 23: 6966–75.

64. Rischin D, Corry J, Smith J et al. Excellent disease control and survival in patients with advanced nasopharyngeal cancer treated with chemoradiation. Journal of Clinical Oncology 2002; 20: 1845–52.

65. Pow EH, McMillan AS, Leung WK et al. Salivary gland function and xerostomia in southern Chinese following radiotherapy for nasopharyngeal carcinoma. Clinical Oral Investigations 2003; 7: 230–4.

● 66. Ho WK, Wei WI, Kwong DL et al. Long-term sensorineural hearing deficit following radiotherapy in patients suffering from nasopharyngeal carcinoma: a prospective study. Head and Neck 1999; 21: 547–53.

67. Leung SF, Zheng Y, Choi CY et al. Quantitative measurements of post-radiation neck fibrosis based on the Young modulus: description of a new method and clinical results. Cancer 2002; 95: 656–62.

68. Lin YS, Jen YM, Lin JC. Radiation-related cranial nerve palsy in patients with nasopharyngeal carcinoma. Cancer 2002; 95: 404–9.

69. Chang YC, Chen SY, Lui LT et al. Dysphagia in patients with nasopharyngeal cancer after radiation therapy: a videofluoroscopic swallowing study. Dysphagia 2003; 18: 135–43.

70. Fang FM, Chiu HC, Kuo WR et al. Health-related quality of life for nasopharyngeal carcinoma patients with cancer-free survival after treatment. *International Journal of Radiation Oncology, Biology, Physics* 2002; **53**: 959–68.

71. Cheng SW, Ting AC, Lam LK, Wei WI. Carotid stenosis after radiotherapy for nasopharyngeal carcinoma. *Archives of Otolaryngology – Head and Neck Surgery* 2000; **126**: 517–21.

72. Lam LC, Leung SF, Chan YL. Progress of memory function after radiation therapy in patients with nasopharyngeal carcinoma. *Journal of Neuropsychiatry and Clinical Neurosciences* 2003; **15**: 90–7.

73. Cheung M, Chan AS, Law SC et al. Cognitive function of patients with nasopharyngeal carcinoma with and without temporal lobe radionecrosis. *Archives of Neurology* 2000; **57**: 1347–52.

74. Lee PW, Hung BK, Woo EK et al. Effects of radiation therapy on neuropsychological functioning in patients with nasopharyngeal carcinoma. *Journal of Neurology, Neurosurgery, and Psychiatry* 1989; **52**: 488–92.

* 75. Jen YM, Shih R, Lin YS et al. Parotid gland-sparing 3-dimensional conformal radiotherapy results in less severe dry mouth in nasopharyngeal cancer patients: a dosimetric and clinical comparison with conventional radiotherapy. *Radiotherapy and Oncology* 2005; **75**: 204–9.

76. Kwong DL, Nicholls J, Wei WI et al. The time course of histologic remission after treatment of patients with nasopharyngeal carcinoma. *Cancer* 1999; **85**: 1446–53.

77. Hong RL, Lin CY, Ting LL et al. Comparison of clinical and molecular surveillance in patients with advanced nasopharyngeal carcinoma after primary therapy: the potential role of quantitative analysis of circulating Epstein–Barr virus DNA. *Cancer* 2004; **100**: 1429–37.

78. Lee AW, Foo W, Law SC et al. Recurrent nasopharyngeal carcinoma: the puzzles of long latency. *International Journal of Radiation Oncology, Biology, Physics* 1999; **44**: 149–56.

● 79. Wei WI, Ho CM, Wong MP et al. Pathological basis of surgery in the management of postradiotherapy cervical metastasis in nasopharyngeal carcinoma. *Archives of Otolaryngology – Head and Neck Surgery* 1992; **118**: 923–9.

80. Kao CH, Tsai SC, Wang JJ et al. Comparing 18-fluoro-2-deoxyglucose positron emission tomography with a combination of technetium 99m tetrofosmin single photon emission computed tomography and computed tomography to detect recurrent or persistent nasopharyngeal carcinomas after radiotherapy. *Cancer* 2001; **92**: 434–9.

81. Chua DT, Sham JS, Kwong DL et al. Locally recurrent nasopharyngeal carcinoma: treatment results for patients with computed tomography assessment. *International Journal of Radiation Oncology, Biology, Physics* 1998; **41**: 379–86.

◆ 82. Wei WI, Sham JS. Nasopharyngeal carcinoma. *Lancet* 2005; **365**: 2041–54.

● 83. Huang SC, Lui LT, Lynn TC. Nasopharyngeal cancer: study III. A review of 1206 patients treated with combined modalities. *International Journal of Radiation Oncology, Biology, Physics* 1985; **11**: 1789–93.

84. Sham JS, Choy D. Nasopharyngeal carcinoma: treatment of neck node recurrence by radiotherapy. *Australasian Radiology* 1991; **35**: 370–3.

* 85. Wei WI, Lam KH, Ho CM et al. Efficacy of radical neck dissection for the control of cervical metastasis after radiotherapy for nasopharyngeal carcinoma. *American Journal of Surgery* 1990; **160**: 439–42.

● 86. Wei WI, Ho WK, Cheng AC et al. Management of extensive cervical nodal metastasis in nasopharyngeal carcinoma after radiotherapy: a clinicopathological study. *Archives of Otolaryngology – Head and Neck Surgery* 2001; **127**: 1457–62.

87. Öksüz DÇ, Meral G, Uzel Ö et al. Reirradiation for locally recurrent nasopharyngeal carcinoma: treatment results and prognostic factors. *International Journal of Radiation Oncology, Biology, Physics* 2004; **60**: 388–94.

88. Chang JT, See LC, Liao CT et al. Locally recurrent nasopharyngeal carcinoma. *Radiotherapy and Oncology* 2000; **54**: 135–42.

* 89. Zheng XK, Ma J, Chen LH et al. Dosimetric and clinical results of three-dimensional conformal radiotherapy for locally recurrent nasopharyngeal carcinoma. *Radiotherapy and Oncology* 2005; **75**: 197–203.

* 90. Lu TX, Mai WY, The BS et al. Initial experience using intensity-modulated radiotherapy for recurrent nasopharyngeal carcinoma. *International Journal of Radiation Oncology, Biology, Physics* 2004; **58**: 682–7.

91. Chua DT, Sham JS, Leung LT, Au GK. Reirradiation of nasopharyngeal carcinoma with intensity-modulated radiotherapy. *Radiotherapy and Oncology* 2005; **77**: 290–4.

92. Chua DT, Sham JS, Au GK. Induction chemotherapy with cisplatin and gemcitabine followed by reirradiation for locally recurrent nasopharyngeal carcinoma. *American Journal of Clinical Oncology* 2005; **28**: 464–71.

◆ 93. Poon D, Yap SP, Wong ZW et al. Concurrent chemoradiotherapy in locoregionally recurrent nasopharyngeal carcinoma. *International Journal of Radiation Oncology, Biology, Physics* 2004; **59**: 1312–18.

94. Cmelak AJ, Cox RS, Adler JR et al. Radiosurgery for skull base malignancies and nasopharyngeal carcinoma. *International Journal of Radiation Oncology, Biology, Physics* 1997; **37**: 997–1003.

95. Chua DT, Sham JS, Hung KN et al. Stereotactic radiosurgery as a salvage treatment for locally persistent and recurrent nasopharyngeal carcinoma. *Head and Neck* 1999; **21**: 620–6.

* 96. Chua DT, Sham JS, Kwong PW et al. Linear accelerator-based stereotactic radiosurgery for limited, locally persistent, and recurrent nasopharyngeal carcinoma:

efficacy and complications. *International Journal of Radiation Oncology, Biology, Physics* 2003; **56**: 177–83.

97. Chen HJ, Leung SW, Su CY. Linear accelerator based radiosurgery as a salvage treatment for skull base and intracranial invasion of recurrent nasopharyngeal carcinoma. *American Journal of Clinical Oncology* 2001; **24**: 255–8.

98. Pai P, Chuang C, Wei K *et al.* Stereotactic radiosurgery for locally recurrent nasopharyngeal carcinoma. *Head and Neck* 2002; **24**: 748–53.

99. Xiao JP, Xu GZ, Miao YJ. Fractionated stereotactic radiosurgery for 50 patients with recurrent or residual nasopharyngeal carcinoma. *International Journal of Radiation Oncology, Biology, Physics* 2001; **51**: 164–70.

100. Wang CC, Busse J, Gitterman M. A simple afterloading applicator for intracavitary irradiation of carcinoma of the nasopharynx. *Radiology* 1975; **115**: 737–8.

101. Harrison LB, Weissberg JB. A technique for interstitial nasopharyngeal brachytherapy. *International Journal of Radiation Oncology, Biology, Physics* 1987; **13**: 451–3.

∗ 102. Wei WI, Sham JS, Choy D *et al.* Split-palate approach for gold grain implantation in nasopharyngeal carcinoma. *Archives of Otolaryngology – Head and Neck Surgery* 1990; **116**: 578–82.

103. Choy D, Sham JS, Wei WI *et al.* Transpalatal insertion of radioactive gold grain for the treatment of persistent and recurrent nasopharyngeal carcinoma. *International Journal of Radiation Oncology, Biology, Physics* 1993; **25**: 505–12.

104. Kwong DL, Wei WI, Cheng AC *et al.* Long term results of radioactive gold grain implantation for the treatment of persistent and recurrent nasopharyngeal carcinoma. *Cancer* 2001; **91**: 1105–13.

105. Fisch U. The infratemporal fossa approach for nasopharyngeal tumors. *Laryngoscope* 1983; **93**: 36–44.

106. Fee WE Jr, Roberson JB Jr, Goffinet DR. Long-term survival after surgical resection for recurrent nasopharyngeal cancer after radiotherapy failure. *Archives of Otolaryngology – Head and Neck Surgery* 1991; **117**: 1233–6.

107. Morton RP, Liavaag PG, McLean M, Freeman JL. Transcervico-mandibulo-palatal approach for surgical salvage of recurrent nasopharyngeal cancer. *Head and Neck* 1996; **18**: 352–8.

∗ 108. Wei WI, Lam KH, Sham JS. New approach to the nasopharynx: the maxillary swing approach. *Head and Neck* 1991; **13**: 200–7.

109. Wei WI. Carcinoma of the nasopharynx. *Advances in Otolaryngology Head and Neck Surgery* 1998; **12**: 119–32.

● 110. Wei WI, Chan JY, Ng RW, Ho WK. Surgical salvage of persistent or recurrent nasopharyngeal carcinoma with maxillary swing approach – Critical appraisal after 2 decades. *Head and Neck* 2011; **33**: 969–75.

111. Ng RW, Wei WI. Elimination of palatal fistula after the maxillary swing procedure. *Head and Neck* 2005; **27**: 608–12.

∗ 112. Chen MK, Lai JC, Chang CC, Liu MT. Minimally invasive endoscopic nasopharyngectomy in the treatment of recurrent T1 – 2a nasopharyngeal carcinoma. *Laryngoscope* 2007; **117**: 894–6.

∗ 113. Wei WI, Ho WK. Transoral robotic resection of recurrent nasopharyngeal carcinoma. *Laryngoscope* 2010; **120**: 2011–14.

◆ 114. Wei, WI, Kwong DL. Recurrent nasopharyngeal carcinoma: surgical salvage vs. additional chemoradiation. *Current Opinion in Otolaryngology and Head and Neck Surgery* 2011; **19**: 82–6.

Pharynx: oropharynx

JARROD HOMER AND GUY REES

The art of medicine is long and life is short; opportunity fleeting; the experiment perilons; judgment flawed.

Hippocrates

INTRODUCTION

Arguably, patterns of incidence and treatment have changed the management of oropharyngeal cancer more than any other site of the head and neck in the last decade. The incidence of squamous cell carcinoma (SCC) in the oropharynx has increased greatly over this period of time, more than other sites of the upper aerodigestive tract (UADT). This has mainly been due to the rise in non-smokers with human papilloma virus (HPV)-induced tumours, something that has been described as an 'epidemic'. At the same time, there has been an increase in the practice of chemoradiotherapy, with a decrease in radical surgery and postoperative radiotherapy (RT). HPV-induced tumours are particularly radiosensitive. These issues, together with the introduction of transoral laser resection techniques, means that decision-making in oropharyngeal cancer is complex and a significant challenge to the multidisciplinary team.

SURGICAL ANATOMY

The oropharynx includes the soft palate, tonsillar fossae, tongue base and the pharyngeal walls from the level of the soft palate to the level of the epiglottis caudally. The most distinguishing anatomical characteristic is the location for most of Waldeyer's lymphatic ring, including the palatine and lingual tonsils. Other pertinent features include a complex muscular structure that is critical to speech, mastication and swallowing and a rich blood supply.

The oropharynx extends from the level of the hard palate superiorly to the level of the hyoid bone inferiorly. Its anterior limit is the anterior faucal pillar, but this is contiguous with the retromolar trigone. It is divided into the following components:

- The anterior wall, which is made up of the base of the tongue posterior to the foramen caecum, the vallecula and the lingual surface of the epiglottis; it is bounded by the pharyngoepiglottic folds.
- The lateral wall, which is made up of the anterior pillar (palatoglossus), posterior pillar (palatopharyngeus) and the pharyngeal palatine tonsil.
- The roof, which is formed by the soft palate containing the two heads of palatopharyngeus, the levator palati, the tensor palati and the palatoglossus. The oral surface of the soft palate is in the oropharynx and the nasopharyngeal surface is part of the nasopharynx.

- The posterior wall, which extends from the level of the hard palate to the level of the hyoid and is anterior to the second and third cervical vertebrae. This consists of the superior and middle constrictors and the buccopharyngeal fascia, which separates it from the prevertebral fascia.
- The tongue base, or posterior tongue. This is made up of the genioglossus muscle, which is attached to the hyoid. The base of the tongue is contiguous with the vallecula, which is the roof of the pre-epiglottic space.

Like the rest of the UADT, the oropharynx is lined with squamous epithelium. However, there is abundant lymphoid tissue particularly in the palatine tonsil and also lingual tonsil of the tongue base. These can be affected in head and neck lymphoma. The soft palate is especially rich in minor salivary glands and is a site of minor salivary gland tumours.

FUNCTION

The oropharynx plays a central role in speech and swallowing. Movement of the soft palate modifies the size and shape of the resonating cavities, influencing vowel production. Closure of the soft palate prevents food regurgitating into the nose. The base of tongue modulates the production of vowels and consonants because of its obstruction of the vocal tract. Movement and the bulk of the base of the tongue forces the food bolus into the oropharynx, powering this phase of swallowing and helping protection against aspiration.

PATHOLOGY

Oropharyngeal tumour histological types

SCC is the most common malignancy and forms 90 per cent of the tumours in this region. Non-Hodgkin's lymphomas account for 8 per cent and minor salivary gland tumours for 2 per cent. With regard to squamous cell carcinoma, the frequency of affected sites is tonsil/lateral wall (60 per cent), tongue base (25 per cent), soft palate (10 per cent) and posterior wall (5 per cent).

Lymphoma

These consist almost entirely of non-Hodgkin's lymphoma. The histological classification, staging and relative site incidence of these lymphomas are described in Chapter 4, Assessment and staging (**Table 31.1**). Lymphomas particularly affect younger patients, and usually occur in the tonsil or tongue base.

Minor salivary gland tumours

On the soft palate, most minor salivary gland tumours are benign pleomorphic adenomas. Elsewhere in the oropharynx, however, malignant tumours are the rule, with adenoid cystic and mucoepidermoid tumours being the most common. Adenoid cystic tumours invade perineural lymphatics and there is a rich source of tumour spread in this area along the greater and lesser palatine nerves and the inferior alveolar nerves.

Table 31.1   TNM and overall staging of oropharyngeal tumours.

TNM and staging			
T: Primary tumour			
T_X	Primary tumour cannot be assessed		
T_0	No evidence of primary tumour		
T_{is}	Carcinoma *in situ*		
T_1	Tumour 2 cm or less in greatest dimension		
T_2	Tumour more than 2 cm but not more than 4 cm in greatest dimension		
T_3	Tumour more than 4 cm in greatest dimension		
T_4	Tumour invades adjacent structures, e.g. pterygoid muscles, mandible, hard palate, deep muscle of the tongue, larynx		
Stage grouping			
0	T_{is}	N_0	M_0
I	T_1	N_0	M_0
II	T_2	N_0	M_0
III	T_1	N1	M_0
	T_2	N1	M_0
	T_3	N0, T_1	M_0
IVA[a]	T_4	N_0, T_1	M_0
	Any $T_{1,2,3}$	N_2	M_0
IVB[a]	Any $T_{1,2,3}$	N_3	M_0
IVC[a]	Any T	Any N	M

Edge SB, Byrd DR, Compton CC *et al. American Joint Committee on Cancer (AJCC): Cancer staging manual,* 7th edn. New York: Springer, 2009.
[a]New inclusion.

TREATMENT

Minor salivary gland tumours of the oropharynx are treated with primary surgery. Small benign and low grade tumours of the soft palate can often be treated by narrow margin transoral laser excision. Elsewhere in the oropharynx, minor salivary gland tumours are more likely to be high grade malignant and are generally treated with primary surgery, in the same manner as a squamous cell carcinoma in the same location, as described later in this chapter. Postoperative radiotherapy tends to be the rule due to high grade features.

These tumours are discussed in more detail in Chapter 37, Salivary gland tumours.

SQUAMOUS CELL CARCINOMA

Epidemiology and HPV

The true incidence of oropharyngeal cancer is difficult to determine because the term oropharyngeal cancer is often used to include oral cavity cancer. Most true oropharyngeal cancers are captured in the ICD-10 codes, C01 (base of tongue), C09 (tonsil) and C10 (oropharynx). The crude incidence rates of these groups combined in the UK in 2006 were 3.6 (males) and 1.2 (females)/100 000/year and have steadily increased in the previous decade.[1] This is similar to the incidence in the US.[2] There is consistent evidence of increasing incidence of oropharyngeal squamous cell carcinoma (OPSCC) in many different countries, and the rate of increase is itself increasing.

Like other UADT squamous cell carcinoma, the most significant aetiological factor is tobacco, alcohol to a lesser degree but with significant synergy between the two.[3] The effect, however, of HPV-16 has been profound on OPSCC. It is this effect that is responsible for the increase in incidence of OPSCC over the last decade or more, so much so that now as

much as 50 per cent of OPSCC is thought to be HPV-induced.[4] Recent rises in the incidence of tonsillar cancer have paralleled the rise in the proportion of HPV-positive cancers. This has led to claims of a developing 'epidemic' of HPV-induced OPSCC with most cancers in the near future being HPV-induced, in the same way as cervical carcinoma.[5] Moreover, this increase is particularly marked in younger patients (typically 40–60 years) and in non-smokers.[2, 6]

HPV-16 infection is spread by orogenital sex and typically presents earlier than smoking/alcohol-induced tumours. There is much to suggest that HPV-induced SCC is distinct from its smoking-induced counterpart at every level. This is summarized in **Table 31.2**.

There is a lack of consensus as to how to define an OPSCC as HPV-induced. The different definitions and biomarkers used reflect the variability in the exact frequency of HPV-induced tumours from series to series. The most robust biomarker is arguably a combination of proof of HPV infection and integration into the host genome (e.g. *in situ* hybridization) AND proof of downstream activity of HPV E7 protein overexpression of p16.

A summary of the issues around HPV and OPSCC can be found in a Adelstein's monograph.[7] While it remains unclear as to how exactly treatment should be modified according to HPV status, there has been much progress in integrating HPV status together with stage and smoking history to define low, intermediate and high risk groups.[8] This is shown in **Figure 31.1**

TUMOUR PROGRESSION

Local progression

Local progression is discussed below under Patterns of presentation.

Table 31.2   Characteristics of HPV-induced OPSCC.

Characteristic	Comments
Epidemiology	HPV-induced SCC affects generally younger patients and relatively more females. This reflects the population groups at risk of sexually transmitted disease, albeit with long latency
Aetiology	HPV-16 infection through orogenital sex. No relationship with tobacco and alcohol usage[9]
Histopathologic morphology	HPV-induced SCC typically displays non/poorly-keratinizing basaloid morphology[9, 10]
Genomic profile and gene expression	HPV-induced cancers have distinct and different patterns of chromosomal loss and deletions, e.g. loss at 13q and gain at 20q, and do not demonstrate common patterns seen in non-HPV cancers, such as allelic loss on 3p, 9p and 17p.[11] HPV-induced tumours tend not to have disruptive p53 mutations
Clinical behaviour and prognosis	There is overwhelming evidence that HPV-induced tumours have a substantially improved prognosis, especially with radiotherapy/chemoradiotherapy,[9] with survival rates approaching 90–95 per cent overall survival at 3 years.[8, 12] This has led many to call for less aggressive and less toxic treatments for this group of patients.[13] Data from Sydney Cancer Institute show that while HPV status has a significant impact on outcome when radiotherapy is all or part of the treatment, it has no effect on outcome in patients treated with surgery only

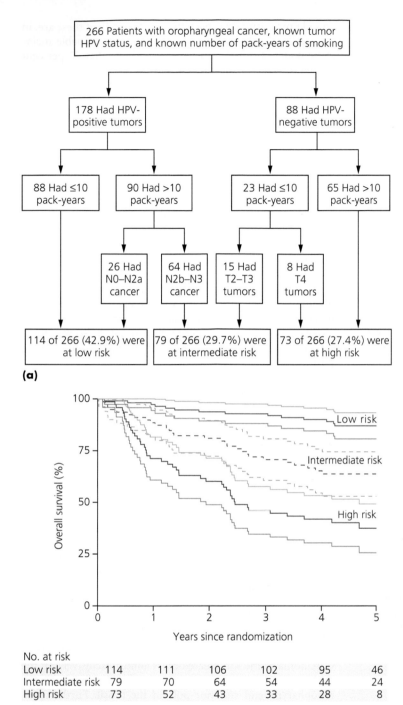

(a)

(b)

No. at risk						
Low risk	114	111	106	102	95	46
Intermediate risk	79	70	64	54	44	24
High risk	73	52	43	33	28	8

Figure 31.1 Classification of stage III and IV OPSCC into risk groups with chemoradiotherapy treatment. Reproduced with permission from Bonner JA, Harari PM, Giralt J *et al.* Radiotherapy plus cetuximab for squamous-cell carcinoma of the head and neck. *New England Journal of Medicine* 2006; **354**: 567–78.

Lymphatic metastasis

Lymph node metastases at presentation are common in OPSCC, with over half of patients having clinical or radiological evidence of cervical metastasis, and around a third of patients diagnosed as cN0 having pathologic evidence of lymph node metastasis.[14, 15]

The lymphatic drainage from the oropharynx is mainly to levels II, III and IV.[15, 16] Frequencies of involvement of different levels are shown in **Table 31.3**. It should be borne in mind that, by virtue of such data coming from patients undergoing neck dissection, there will be a bias towards patients with cN+ necks, and these are therefore not representative of patients staged with cN0 necks.

It also drains into the retropharyngeal (RP) nodes, which need to be considered in the assessment of disease in this area.[17] The risk of metastasis to RP lymph nodes depends on subsite, a meta-analysis of papers suggests risk of RP lymphadenopathy being 19 per cent for soft palate; 12 per cent for tonsil; 6 per cent for base of tongue and 21–57 per cent for posterior pharyngeal wall tumours (including hypopharynx).[18] The prognostic impact of positive RP lymph node metastasis is disputed, some authors showing an adverse impact[19, 20] and others not.[14, 21]

Table 31.3 Frequency of lymph node level involvement in patients with OPSCC (adapted from Buckley and Feber[15] and Shimizu et al.[13]).

Lymph node level	N (from 6 series)	Total number of neck dissections	Frequency of cervical metastases (%)
1	48	406	12
2	222	406	55
3	134	406	33
4	77	406	19
5	26	406	6

A particular feature of OPSCC is the propensity to metastasis to the contralateral neck, this occurring in up to 30 per cent of patients overall in one series.[14, 15] The subsites in which this is mostly likely to occur are the soft palate, base of tongue and posterior pharyngeal wall. However, even tonsil cancers have an approximate rate of contralateral nodal spread of 10 per cent.[22]

Distant metastasis

As distinct from other head and neck tumours, as many as 8 per cent of patients will have distant metastases which are apparent at presentation. This is probably due to the rich lymphatic drainage of the oropharynx, which leads to a higher incidence of local and hence distant metastases. Distant metastasis will occur at some stage of the disease in 15–20 per cent, with 80 per cent of such cases being apparent within two years of diagnosis, and is most commonly to the lungs (around 50 per cent) followed by bone and liver, these being relatively common for this site compared to other head and neck sites. Patients who present with advanced disease, particularly more advanced cervical lymph node metastasis, are at increased risk of distant metastasis (DM), as are patients who recur locally.[23, 24, 25, 26] However, of those patients who achieve locoregional control, only around 5 per cent will go on to develop DM.[26]

Second primary

One in three patients with oropharyngeal tumours will, at some time, develop a second primary, so it is important to consider the presence of a synchronous second primary, especially if contralateral nodes are found.

PATTERNS OF PRESENTATION

OPSCC tends to present in one of three ways: (1) symptoms from primary disease with or without lymph node metastases; (2) lymph node metastasis with clinically detectable OPSCC primary; (3) lymph node metastasis with unknown primary. With the introduction of PET-CT in patients with an unknown primary cancer, the vast majority of these are, in fact, OPSCC. Fifty per cent of patients have palpable metastatic nodes at initial presentation, with another 25 per cent having occult disease in a clinically N0 neck.

Lateral wall tumours

These are the most common tumours (50 per cent) and usually involve the tonsil. They may spread anteriorly and upwards to the retromolar trigone and on to the buccal mucosa, as well as into the tongue base. If they erode deeply, they involve the pterygoid muscles producing trismus and pain. Further posterolateral invasion will involve the parapharyngeal space and structures including the carotid sheath (carotid artery, internal jugular vein and vagus nerve), the symphathetic chain, the styloglossus, the stylopharyngeus. Disease here is usually contiguous with lymph node metastases. Anterolateral extension can involve the angle of the mandible and the inferior alveolar nerve, especially in elderly patients, since in the edentulous mandible the inferior alveolar nerve is more superior than usual. Inferiorly, these tumours can extend down the lateral pharyngeal wall into the piriform sinus.

Tonsil primaries, especially in the inferior pole, are often submucosal and difficult to detect on examination.

Tongue base

These are the next most common oropharyngeal tumours (40 per cent). As above, early tumours are often submucosal and difficult to detect. Symptoms frequently do not appear until the lesions are at an advanced stage, by which time tumours often have crossed the midline and through the genioglossus. In doing so, the oral tongue and floor of the mouth can be involved. Spread can also be posterior and inferiorly into the vallecula, the epiglottis and hence into the supraglottis and the pre-epiglottic space.

Soft-palate tumours

Carcinoma of the soft palate occurs almost exclusively on the anterior surface. As the tumour progresses, it will involve the nasopharynx and superior pole of the tonsil. Further progression may involve the palatine nerves and the back of the maxillary antrum. A particular feature of these tumours is aggressive, not uncommonly bilateral lymph node metastases, in association with very little primary tumour volume.

Posterior wall tumours

These are relatively unusual and often are associated with contiguous submucosal spread in a superior and inferior direction to involve the nasopharyngeal or hypopharyngeal posterior wall. In the untreated patient, the prevertebral fascia often acts as a barrier to spread. The majority of patients present late and usually complain of a sore throat, otalgia or dysphagia.

EXAMINATION

Key considerations when examining a patient with possible OPSCC are that: (1) a systematic upper aerodigestive tract examination, including fibre-optic endoscopy should be performed; and (2) the tongue base should be additionally palpated (as many tumours here are submucosal).

INVESTIGATION

Radiology

The role of radiology in the assessment of oropharyngeal tumours is discussed in Chapter 42, Principles of radiotherapy. In general, MR imaging is preferred to CT, particularly for assessing tongue base and parapharyngeal spread. Mandible invasion can be assessed by CT or MR with high sensitivity (combined with clinical examination).[27]

As with all UADT cancers, it is mandatory to image the thorax with CT to ascertain distant metastasis and/or second primary cancers.

Cytology

Patients who present with a neck mass will have fine needle aspiration cytology at initial assessment. This can be carried out under ultrasound guidance for increased diagnostic accuracy, as well as for staging information.

Biopsy

This is generally performed under general anaesthetic, as part of a systematic panendoscopy, the latter to exclude any UADT second primary tumours. As well as a means of obtaining definitive histology, the primary tumour is accurately staged and an assessment of whether it is surgically resectable can be made (and by what means). If the diagnostic biopsy/endoscopy is not carried out by a surgical oncologist, this may need to be repeated in order to make a decision about treatment with regards to surgery.

With regard to tonsil tumours, the preferred means of biopsy is a deep incisional biopsy, rather than tonsillectomy. Performing a tonsillectomy at diagnostic stage often means that it is difficult to judge the margins of any remaining tumour for later definitive surgical resection, either open or transoral. Therefore, a well intentioned tonsillectomy as a debulking procedure might exclude the possibility of definitive primary surgery while achieving nothing oncologically. Nevertheless, if there is not an obvious tumour, then tonsillectomy will be necessary. This applies to the context of evaluating an unknown primary, when 'blind' biopsies will also be carried out of the tongue base, and there is a strong argument for bilateral tonsillectomy also. This is discussed in more detail in Chapter 35, Management of an unknown primary carcinoma.

TREATMENT POLICY

General comments

The treatment of OPSCC has changed considerably over the last two decades. In the 1980s, surgical resection and reconstruction for patients with advanced tumours was the rule, with postoperative radiotherapy, on the basis that this approach offered the best chance of disease-specific cure, particularly for more advanced disease.[28] Patients with early disease or those not suitable for this were given RT.

The 1990s saw the introduction and increasing use of definitive concomitant chemoradiotherapy (CRT), which offers better survival compared to RT.[29] Initially, this was seen as a better way of treating patients who would otherwise simply have RT. However, even before the popularization of CRT, there was some suggestion that definitive RT offered comparable survival with better function.[30, 31, 32] For example, results from definitive RT (twice daily in some), with planned post-RT neck dissection in a series of 490 patients, yielded the following oncologic results: local control T1 87 per cent, T2 82 per cent, T3 70 per cent, T4 43 per cent; disease-free survival I 89 per cent, II 89 per cent, III 87 per cent, IVa 69 per cent, IVb 61 per cent.[33]

With the additional advantage of concomitant CRT, the balance has fallen to CRT over surgery and this has now become the standard of care for most patients with OPSCC.[34]

While the results of CRT for early OPSCC seem to be excellent, the results for more advanced OPSCC are disappointing. The overall survival in a series of 48 patients was 84 per cent for T1–2 OPSCC and 27 per cent for T3–4, treated with concomitant CRT.[35]

Intensive modulated radiotherapy (IMRT) may reduce morbidity without oncologic compromise.[36]

CRT has evolved to be generally in the form of induction chemotherapy, with three cycles of TPF (docetaxel–cisplatin–5-fluorouracil) and then concurrent chemoradiotherapy with platinum.[37, 38]

However, some have questioned the major toxicity of this treatment approach and the encouraging oncologic results may, in part, reflect the increasing influence of HPV-induced OPSCC. The acute toxicity and late effects of chemotherapy and RT are significant in terms of mucositis, haematological toxicity, long-term dysphagia and dependence of feeding tubes.

In Bonner et al.'s trial of radiotherapy versus radiotherapy and cetuximab, the effect of cetuximab was most pronounced in OPSCC.[39] This observation, coupled with the possible overtreatment of HPV OPSCC with conventional chemoradiotherapy, has led to proposals for using cetuximab with radiotherapy for OPSCC, especially HPV-induced tumours.

In the last decade, transoral microsurgery has gained popularity as a means of carrying out effective oncologic resection with much less morbidity. This has been in the form of CO_2 laser transoral microsurgery, but recently, transoral robotic surgery (TORS) has attracted interest, particularly for oropharyngeal resections. Most patients treated by transoral microsurgery have postoperative RT or CRT. The oncologic results appear promising, with a disease-free survival of 94 per cent in one series of 71 tongue base OPSCC (18 per cent T1; 51 per cent T2; 21 per cent T3), as do the functional results with no patients requiring tube feeding.[40]

With regard to neck disease, there has been a parallel evolution. In the 1980s, most patients with clinically evident neck disease (certainly >N1) would be treated with a comprehensive neck dissection, whether the primary was treated with surgery or not.[41] The introduction of CRT saw this being used for definitive treatment of N2 and even N3 disease, if the primary was being treated in the same fashion. Initially, this would generally be followed by planned post-CRT neck dissection, for N2 and N3 disease.[42] This has given way to an increasingly acceptable policy of definitive CRT with neck dissection only if there is clinical or radiological evidence of residual disease.[43] Thus, it has become routine practice to perform a positron emission tomography-computed tomography (PET-CT) scan after CRT to guide the need for neck dissection.

Options for definitive treatment of OPSCC are shown in **Table 31.4**.

Treatment of the neck

Patients with clinical and/or radiologic evidence of neck metastases (cN+) should have a comprehensive neck dissection or CRT. As alluded to above, if CRT is used for definitive treatment of the N+ neck, it is increasing practice for that to be followed by PET-CT and only neck dissection if there is clinical or radiologic evidence of residual disease.

A comprehensive neck dissection can be done as part of primary tumour surgery, or before definitive RT/CRT.[44] The role of selective neck dissection for N+ disease is more controversial. However, there is growing evidence to suggest that level 5 can be spared, if there is no preoperative evidence

of involvement and there is no multiple lymphadenopathy (i.e. N1 or N2a).[46] Quality of life studies indicate improved pain scores if level 5 is not dissected.[47, 48, 49] Similarly, in cases staged below cN2b, level 1 can be modified so as not to include perifacial lymph nodes.[50]

Treatment of N0 neck

It is the rule that all N0 necks in OPSCC have elective treatment, either by selective neck dissection or RT. If primary surgery is being carried out, selective neck dissection (SND) should be performed, dissecting levels 2/3/4.[15] When studies began to show that level 2b does not routinely need to be dissected for N0 neck, it was thought that this should not apply to OPSCC.[51] However, more recent work has suggested that this does indeed apply to OPSCC, as long as there is no finding preoperatively of level 2a disease.[52] With primary treatment with CRT or RT, it would be routine to include levels 2–4 in the RT fields.

Treatment of the contralateral N0 neck

Contralateral metastases are a feature of all OPSCC subsites to a degree and clinicians should be alert to this. The contralateral neck should be treated as for the ipsilateral N0 neck for tumours arising in the soft palate, posterior pharyngeal wall and/or near midline, large tumours (T>2) and advanced ipsilateral nodal involvement (N2b, N3) due to the high frequency of lymph node metastases.[53, 54] For other tumours, in most cases it will remain untreated (by surgery

Table 31.4 Overview of treatment options for OPSCC.

Primary	Neck	Comment/arguments for
RT	RT	There is growing opinion that such a less toxic treatment may be suitable for HPV-induced tumours. Some patients will be unsuitable for cytotoxic chemotherapy. Targeted therapy could be considered with RT (EGFR inhibitor or monocloncal antibody)
RT/CRT	ND followed by RT	Initial ND may be preferred if safe to perform more function-sparing ND, particularly if the primary tumour is small. The results from this treatment approach for T1–2 N+ OPSCC have been shown to be excellent (93.5 per cent disease-free survival, median follow up 33 months)[42]
CRT	CRT followed by PET-CT ± ND	PET-CT is sensitive and specific for residual disease and spares ND in many patients. CRT in this context is usually induction+concurrent and is very toxic
CRT	CRT followed by planned ND	See comments above. Planned ND after CRT is becoming unusual if there is access to PET-CT
Trans-oral surgery ± RT/CRT	ND ± RT/CRT	It is unusual for tumours treated with transoral surgery NOT to have postoperative RT.[44] Postoperative RT (or CRT) may also be required on neck metastatic criteria regardless
Open surgery ± RT/CRT	ND ± RT/CRT	More morbidity than transoral surgery but some tumours will not be suitable for transoral approach. It does offer more definitive histologic analysis of tumour clearance and margins and, in some cases, may offer more chance of single modality treatment[45] (no RT)

CRT, chemoradiotherapy; EGFR, epidermal growth factor receptor; HPV, human papillomavirus; ND, neck dissection; OPSCC, oropharyngeal squamous cell carcinoma; PET-CT, positron emission tomography-computed tomography; RT, radiotherapy.

or RT) in the absence of clinical or radiologic suspicion of involvement. In a series of 642 patients treated with ipsilateral RT (mostly T1–2), only 3.5 per cent failed in the contralateral neck.[54]

Functional considerations

Percentage tongue base resected and total volume resected are most often correlated with swallowing function.[55] In patients closed with a flap, the excess bulk of the flap compared to the size of the defect is related to a poorer outcome with swallowing. The best outcomes are for patients with no flap closure. The use of postoperative radiotherapy worsened swallow, on a dose-related level.

Twenty patients with stage III/IV oropharyngeal cancer were treated by surgical extirpation, free flap and postoperative radiotherapy.[56] Average time to decannulation was 15 days. Thirteen of 20 started oral intake before RT (average 19.5 days); by four months after surgery 10/20 took all food orally and ten were tube fed (6/10 managing some oral intake).

There is a tendency to worse swallowing outcomes in patients with advanced T stage and with base of tongue rather than tonsil subsite of disease.

SURGICAL RESECTION

Open techniques

There are three technical considerations in open surgery for the oropharynx: access technique (generally via mandibulotomy or transcervical); reconstruction; and mandibulectomy (see **Table 31.5**).

Mandibulectomy

Advanced tumours of the lateral oropharynx, particularly when extending into the retromolar trigone of the oral cavity, may require segmental or rim mandibulectomy. This should be anticipated on clinical or radiological grounds. The operative technique, including reconstructive issues, are discussed in Chapter 51, Defect-based reconstruction: mandible and oral cavity.

Access techniques

The two main access techniques are via paramedian mandibulotomy or transcervical/pharyngotomy. Lateral mandibulotomy should not be used mainly because the inferior alveolar nerve is divided, which renders the lower lip insensate and leads to drooling.

Paramedial mandibulotomy is used for access for lateral oropharyngeal wall (± lateral tongue) tumours, or tongue base cancers extending laterally. For small tongue base tumours, an elegant posterior approach is via a lateral pharyngotomy. This can be extended by removing the ipsilateral hyoid bone. The functional results from this approach are superior to mandibulotomy.[57]

Any incisions which relate to access must consider the levels required for neck dissection, which will usually be at least level II, III and IV for the N_0 neck, or otherwise a modified radical or radical neck resection. Such an operation

Table 31.5 Open techniques.

Technique	Comment
Access	
Paramedian mandibulotomy	Standard access technique for most oropharyngeal tumours
Lateral mandibulotomy	Rarely used. Sacrifices inferior alveolar nerve and places osteotomy in radiotherapy field
Lingual release	Unusual approach for oropharyngeal resections. Offers little extra compared to transoral approach
Lateral pharyngotomy	Very useful technique for tongue base tumours without significant lateral extension, with good functional results[57]
Midline suprahyoid pharyngotomy	Unusual approach
Reconstructive	
Radial artery free flap	Generally the flap of choice, as it is pliable enough to reconstruct the three-dimensional nature of the oropharynx, and can be modified to optimize palatal closure[56]
Anterolateral thigh free flap	Reduced donor site morbidity. Increased bulk compared to RAFF may be preferable when there is significant tongue base resection
Pectoralis major myocutaneous flap	Not ideal for the oropharynx, as it is generally at the limits of the arc of rotation, and the weight tends to make it pull inferiorly
Other pedicled flaps	Several local pedicled flaps can be used and have been described. For a tumour to be large enough to warrant an open resection and reconstruction rather than CRT or a transoral approach, these will often be inadequate. Examples include sternomastoid myofascial flap, buccal mucosal transposition flap, lingual flap, temporalis flap
None	Many defects can be primarily closed or left to heal by secondary intention

CRT, chemoradiotherapy; RAFF, rectus abdominus free flap.

facilitates exposure of the major vessels, which will provide the facility for microvascular free transfer. The oropharynx is a difficult area to reconstruct, given its three-dimensional complexity and the need for sensation. The principles for reconstruction are discussed in Chapter 51, Defect-based reconstruction: pharynx.

Paramedian mandibulotomy

- Tracheostomy – it is standard to perform tracheostomy as part of any open OPSCC resection, in order to protect the airway from postoperative obstruction at the resection/reconstruction site and from aspiration. This is generally performed at the beginning of the operation through a separate small incision.
- Incision – usually involves a lip split with paramedian mandibulotomy and access via a mandibular swing (**Figure 31.2**). It is important to preserve the mental nerve to ensure that lower lip sensation remains intact. The incision can be extended into the neck as either a modified Schobinger or a 'T' on its side.
- Neck dissection is carried out, the type and selectivity depending on individual circumstances. It is important to preserve all candidate vessels, where possible, for microvascular anastomosis, assuming that a free flap reconstruction will be employed. This includes the lingual-facial trunk, superior thyroid artery, (occasionally) transverse cervical artery, internal jugular vein and facial vein. The neck dissection may be left pedicled on the parapharyngeal space adjacent to the primary tumour to allow for a primary neck dissection single specimen, or can be taken separately.
- Mandibulotomy – the periosteum of the mandible is cleared either side of the mandibulotomy site, usually at or around the lateral incisor or canine tooth. The mental nerve is identified and preserved. The mandibulomy can be either between tooth roots or through one. The exact location depends on the OPG XR assessment (i.e. through an appropriate socket after extraction or between two roots that diverge, allowing enough room). The inner periosteum is also cleared but only immediately around the mandibulotomy site. The mandibulotomy is planned as a stepped incision and is pre-plated with titanium plates and screws beforehand. The bone cuts can be done with a reciprocating or an oscillating saw.
- Tumour access and resection. The mandible is then swung laterally, as the mylohyoid and anterior belly of digastric are cut, whilst making a mucosal incision in the gingival mucosa towards the retromolar trigone (it is important to leave enough mucosa on the mandible-side for later closure). The lingual and hypoglossal nerves are identified and preserved. At this point, the access depends on the exact location of the tumour. Generally, dissection will be performed around the tumour medially via glossotomy, while lateral dissection will extend from the retromolar trigone, around the anterior faucal pillar to the soft palate. The external carotid artery and internal carotid artery can be followed superiorly in the parapharyngeal space, as this marks the deep aspect of the tumour dissection. The

pterygoid muscles can be resected at the deep margin also.
- Reconstruction is performed, usually with a radial artery free flap for most OPSCC.
- Closure.

Lateral pharyngotomy approach

A neck dissection incision (as above) with a selective or modified radical neck dissection is performed as required. In dissection of level 1, the lingual artery is dissected, ligating any posterior branches feeding the inferior tonsil or tongue base, clipping branches to posterior tongue. Following this, the hypoglossal nerve is dissected from the anterior edge of the carotid artery to the hyoglossus muscle. Elevation of the nerve away from the tongue base area akin to a clothes line and elevation away from posterior tongue over hyoglossus allows access to the tongue base without compromise to motor innervation of the mid and anterior tongue. Inferior to the hypoglossal nerve, and above the superior thyroid artery, the internal branch of the superior laryngeal nerve is encountered. Careful dissection of this nerve is essential to reduce the risk of denervation and loss of sensation of the ipsilateral supraglottic larynx.

At this stage, attention passess to the hyoid bone. Periosteal dissection of bone from midline to greater cornua is performed with separation of digastric, mylohyoid and hyoglossus from hyoid. The ipsilateral hyoid is resected from the lesser cornua to the apex of the greater cornua. More extensive tumours will require resection of the entire ipsilateral hyoid. Incision through the base of hyoid into ipsilateral vallecula with a hockey-stick extension posterosuperiorly allows exposure of the lower pole of tonsil, and base of tongue. Transoral digital palpation of the tumour allows approach to the tumour without trangression of the lesion directly and maintenance of tissue margins.

Once the pharyngotomy is made, direct view of the tumour with controlled margin resection is made in three dimensions.

Dependent upon the volume of tissue resected, the pharyngotomy can be closed and the defect left to heal by secondary intention. In larger defects, local mucosal flaps can be developed from the tongue base and pharyngeal wall to close the defect. Some defects may require free flap closure – most probably a radial forearm free flap, with vascular access to the superior thyroid artery and internal jugular vein close by for anastomosis.

Midline vallecula approach

In the case of midline tongue base, following bilateral level I and II anatomical dissection and bilateral dissection of the lingual arteries and hypoglossal nerves, a suprahyoid release of geniohyoid, mylohyoid and hyoglossus muscles with transoral digital palpation allows incision into the apex of the vallecula from one tonsillolingual sulcus to the opposite sulcus. Retraction of the tongue base into the neck allows direct resection of the tumour with three-dimensional marginal control. Tissue closure may occur primarily with small defects, or with tongue/pharyngeal flaps from larger defects.

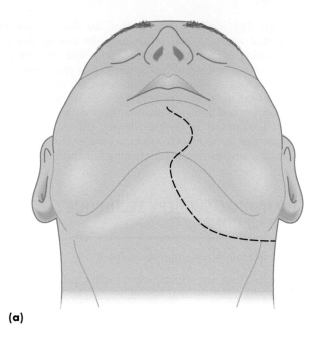

(a)

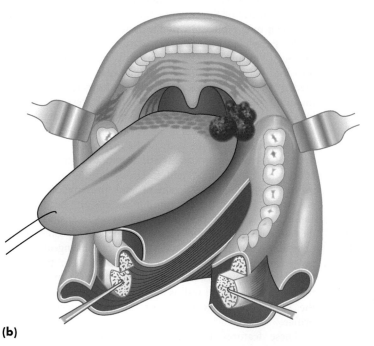

(b)

Figure 31.2 Lip split incision (a) with paramedian mandibulotomy and a mandibular swing (b). Panel (b) reproduced with permission from Aug KK, Harris J, Wheeler R *et al*. Human papillomavirus and survival of patients with oropharyngeal cancer. *New England Journal of Medicine* 2010; **363**: 24–35.

The use of a free flap to repair a defect in the entire tongue base is associated with significant loss of swallowing function requiring a PEG tube and persistent swelling requiring prolonged tracheostomy tube dependence.

Lingual release approach

In the case of large tonsillar or tongue base tumours, especially those requiring a free flap closure, a lingual release allows excellent tumour exposure, direct margin control in three dimensions of the primary tumour and more straightforward free flap insertion and vascular anastomosis.

The release commences with transoral exposure of the tumour using plastic cheek/lip retractors and a bite block with silk suture retraction of the tongue. Incision of oral mucosa allowing a cuff of mucosa and mylohyoid muscle to remain on the inner surface of the mandible is made. This allows maintenance of vascular supply to the mandible and eases muscle and mucosal repair with a watertight seal at the end of the procedure. Following myomucosal incisions laterally, the genial tubercle muscles and the anterior attachment of the anterior bellies of the digastric muscles are divided, again leaving a cuff of muscle/tendon attached to the inner surface of the mandible to allow postresection repair. At this point, there should be a through and through defect from the oral cavity from one retromolar space to the other and the entire tongue will be dropped out into the neck. Pulling forward on the tongue allows the entire oropharynx to be visualized for controlled tumour resection. In the case of tonsillar extension of the tumour, transoral release of the tonsil from the soft palate and resection lateral to the superior constrictor muscle, anterior to the buccopharyngeal raphe and inferior to the retromolar trigone, allows the tonsil to drop out into the neck in continuity with the tongue base. Resection of the inferior-medial extension of the tumour is now performed with three-dimensional marginal control.

One benefit of this approach is that the ipsilateral hypoglossal and lingual nerves may be preserved if not invaded by tumour, and vascular control of external carotid vessel branches can be achieved. Second, insertion of a free flap is straightforward with closure of inferior and posterior mucosal surfaces with the tongue in the neck and then with the tongue returned to the oral cavity, repair of the flap to soft palate and superior pharynx can be achieved under direct view. Muscle and mucosal closure allows a watertight seal and avoids the possibility of postoperative fistula formation. In addition, muscle closure returns the normal diaphragm function of mylohyoid supporting tongue movement and returns the geniohyoid anatomy to normality with stability of the airway and larynx.

RECONSTRUCTION

Tissue reconstruction in oropharyngeal defects follows the standard 'ladder' approach, as with other tissue sites.

Generally speaking, the simplest closure which achieves watertight closure without tension and maximal retention of organ function directs the technique used.

Small lesions may be closed primarily, following the principles above. Medium-sized defects of the tonsil and tongue base which do not expose major vessels may be left to heal by secondary intention. A combination of fibrotic scar contracture and re-epithelialization of the defect allows excellent functional recovery in most cases. There is a small risk of secondary bleeding, which may require return to theatre, and the patient should be alert to this possibility.

Larger defects, and especially those associated with major vessel exposure or direct communication with the neck as a through and through defect, will require myomucosal closure. This may be achieved in some cases by use of local myomucosal flaps, such as the buccinator flap, posterior tongue flap, lateral pharyngeal flap or superior constrictor advancement flap. In these situations, a palatopharyngoplasty may reduce the risk of velopharyngeal incompetence. Larger defects where these local approaches are insufficient for tissue coverage will be repaired with free flaps.[58] In general, lateral pharyngeal defects may be commonly closed with a radial forearm flap or, in thin patients, an anterolateral thigh flap. In general, it is helpful not to design the flap to completely replace three dimensionally the tissue resected, but to slightly reduce the flap size, allowing a slightly more constricted

closure. The ideology here is that the flap is insensate, immobile and stiff, and minimizing the size of this non-functioning portion of the oropharynx will improve postoperative oropharyngeal functionality. It is vitally important not to leave the pharynx overly constricted, or to make the closure too tight, increasing the risk of impaired mucosal breakdown and fistula formation. Flap design needs to be three-dimensional in design, allowing palate, pharynx and tongue base to be maintained in normal anatomical configuration after flap repair, maintaining functionality.

TRANSORAL SURGERY TECHNIQUE DESCRIPTIONS

The two main access approaches are:

1. Boyle Davis gag – mainly for tonsillar, palatal and limited tonsillolingual tumours.
2. FK retractor system – useful for base of tongue tumours, inferiorly extending lateral pharyngeal tumours.

At the time of initial tumour evaluation at panendoscopy, a trial of exposure of the tumour with the above systems is made. Biopsies of the primary tumour and marginal tissues are taken and evaluation of the mobility of the tumour is made. Particular note is taken of deep invasion of tonsil tumours through the superior constrictor and anterior invasion behind the pterygomandibular raphe into the medial pterygoid muscle and ascending ramus of the mandible. Invasion anterior to the medial pterygoid muscle inferiorly brings the tumour into contact with the lingual nerve, inferior alveolar nerve, nerve branch to mylohyoid and to the periosteum of the body of the mandible. Examination of the tongue base to assess the extent of tumour spread across the tongue base and inferiorly to the apex of the vallecula, hyoepiglottic ligament and pre-epiglottic space is made. Palpation for tumour extension deeply into genioglossus, and inferolaterally into styloglossus, as well as palpation of the carotid vessels through the posterolateral oropharyngeal mucosa and for retropharyngeal nodes posteriorly, is made. Elevation and inspection or transnasal rigid endoscopic assessment of the superior portion of the lateral pharyngeal wall is made to look for extension into the salpingopharyngeus and up to the Eustachian tubal orifice.

These features are critical to achieve a clear margin resection and avoiding untoward neural and vascular injury and to identify areas of extended resection including marginal mandibulectomy. In addition, the requirement for reconstruction is made – none, mucosal advancement, buccinator myomucocutaneous flap or free flap.

At the time of resection surgery, tracheostomy may be electively planned for large transoral resection with associated modified radical neck dissections and free flap reconstruction. Patients with smaller tumours requiring no or local flap closure may be managed by extubation on the table with a covering nasopharyngeal airway or remain intubated in ICU overnight and electively extubated the following day.

During the neck dissection, elective ligation of the posterior lingual artery branch(es) to the tongue base and ascending pharyngeal artery may be associated with reduced risk of primary and secondary bleeding.

The use of dilute adrenaline (1:200 k) to the tissue surrounding the tumour acts to maintain a clear surgical field and a heat sink to reduce thermal injury to non-resected tissue during electrocautery or laser resection.

The tumour may be resected with a CO_2 laser, set at 10–15 watts superpulse continuous mode via a microslad on an operating microscope or a hand-held attachment using operating loupes (2.5–3 × magnification). The use of electrocautery using a switching pen with a guarded tip or Colorado needle, set at 20 joules cautery and 40 joules cutting, allows an extended and malleable attachment to be used, reaching margins tangential to the line of sight. Bipolar cautery and ligaclips are used to seal small and larger vascular structures.

Commonly, tumours may require alteration of the angle of view, requiring replacement of retraction systems to access the three-dimensional nature of the tumour. At all times the operator must be clear as to the volume of the tumour and surrounding structures. It is commonplace to dissect immediately along the adventitia of the carotid artery, and to dissect across the tongue base to identify the lingual artery and ligate it.

For superiorly based tumours (palate and tonsil), a superior to inferior approach is used, maintaining a view of the depth of the tumour and allowing the field to be kept clear of blood. For tongue base lesions, the medial and inferior edges of the tumour may be exposed using the FK retractor, resecting perpendicular to the epithelial surface. Following replacement of the retractor, the lateral and anterior margins are exposed and the other two sides of the box cut are made with resection of the tumour, taking care of the third dimension margin.

In the case of tonsillar tumours, an incision at the level of the buccopharyngeal raphe in the vertical plane, extending superiorly across the soft palate with an adequate mucosal margin, and across the tonsillolingual sulcus with a similar margin, is made.

At this point, deepening the incision through the superior constrictor muscle allows entry to the space. In this area, loose areolar tissue and fat is encountered with vessels crossing the space from lateral to medial. These may be ligaclipped, harmonic scissor coagulated or bipolar diathermied appropriate to the size of the vessel. Continual assessment of the deep margin of tumour resection is made, and dissection of the space posteriorly with scissors or an artery clip allows exposure of the internal carotid artery. Dissection medial to the artery allows the tumour flap to be elevated to the posterolateral pharyngeal wall and the posterior mucosal incision can be made, again with appropriate margins. It is the author's preference to take frozen section tissue of superficial and deep margins to allow confidence in clear tumour resections. It is noted that other centres may take the primary tumour directly to the pathologist at this stage, and with coloured inking of the specimen, allow frozen section margins to be taken of the resected tumour with a similar outcome.

In the case of tongue base tumours, the use of the FK retractor system allows access to the apex of the vallecula and lateral pharyngeal wall. It is critical to have a clear idea of the depth of invasion of the tumour to plan an adequate depth to tumour resection. This is achieved by a combination of radiologic review and palpation of the tumour on the table. The asymmetric blade is positioned to allow complete visualization of the ipsilateral hemitongue base. The author uses electrocautery to release the tumour from the base of the tonsil, with a clear margin, extending across the level of the ipsilateral circumvallate papillae to the midline, and then inferiorly to the apex of the vallecula. The anterolateral quadrant of the dissection is the critical point of exposure as this is where the lingual artery and two medially directed transverse tongue base branches are encountered. Knowledge of the anatomy of this area through cadaveric dissection practice and training in a centre with a regular approach to this area is vital at this time to avoid transgression of the arterial branches. Inferomedial retraction of the tumour with dissection in the line of the pedicle allows the lingual artery to be identified and ligated with ligaclips if required for tumour resection. Similarly, the two medially directed tongue base branches are similarly ligated. Once vascular control is achieved, the mucosal incision laterally is taken down to the pharyngo-epiglottic fold and across the apex of the tongue base to the midline. At the pharyngo-epiglottic fold, there is a constant arterial vessel passing in the fold medially towards the apex of the vallecula. This will also require ligaclipping. At this point, the quadrantic resection of the tongue base tissue is achieved and the marked and orientated specimen sent to the pathologist. As indicated above, frozen section of the margins can be taken from the patient in superficial and deep areas or from the tumour resected. As appropriate, further tissue may be resected to achieve a clear margin.

Currently, one of the authors is using Da Vinci Transoral Robotic Surgery (TORS) to resect tongue base tumours. In comparison to standard transoral resection, there are three benefits. First, binocular magnification at the surface of the resection allows clearer visualization of tumour boundaries, vascular tissue and aids accurate assessment of tumour margins. Second, the use of 'wristed' three-dimensionally mobile grasping and cutting instruments allows better resection of the tumour in a plane tangential to the view achieved with direct transoral view. This improves the accuracy of tumour resection and manipulation of the specimen and vessels, making the surgery easier to perform. Third, the 'robotic surgeon' operating through two hand controls allows the 'manual assistant' to grasp, cut, ligate and suction in the field simultaneously. It would be very difficult for a standard transoral procedure to take place with four surgeons' hands working on the tongue base!

Whatever way the tumour is resected, haemostasis with intraoperative vasalva is checked and titanium clips are used adequately to seal all major vessels. Following tumour resection of the tonsil or tongue base, and establishment of haemostasis, Surgi-Flo or Surgicell Fibrillar may be placed over the deep resection surfaces to allow small vessels' coagulation to occur and minimize surface oozing.

The requirement for tissue repair is now made. Essentially, extended tonsil tumour resections may not require any closure, behaving like a normal tonsillectomy with healing by secondary intention. Resection involving the soft palate at risk of developing velopharyngeal incompetence should be closed using a posteriorly based buccinator artery myomucosal flap (BAMMF) or palatal island flap (PIF). Tumours involving exposure of mandibular bone should always be covered, usually using a BAMMF to avoid issues of osteoradionecrosis following the planned postoperative radiotherapy. Lesions of the tonsil extending into tongue base will benefit from a BAMMF to reduce tethering and tongue mobility issues. Because this flap is neurotized, sensation of this important area is maintained. It is not critical to close small tongue base lesion resections (less than 30 per cent surface) as these will also mucosalize similar to tonsil lesions.

Tumours extending widely onto the lateral pharyngeal wall whose resection exposes carotid vessels or where oral secretions may contaminate the neck around the great vessels should be repaired. Small defects may be covered with the BAMFF, but larger lesions will require a radial forearm free flap.

It should be noted that these larger lateral pharyngeal resections will probably be through and through resections with contact to the neck dissection. This situation will commonly occur if high level IIa or lateral retropharyngeal nodes are resected at the time of the neck dissection. In some centres, staging of the surgery with primary resection is followed by a neck dissection at a 1-week interval, allowing tissue healing to start to close the primary defect prior to the neck dissection. It is the author's preference to close pharyngeal defects which expose the carotid artery as indicated above, however. At the time of neck dissection, the use of the posterior belly of digastric muscle and stylohyoid muscle to close the defect will reduce neck contamination.

When tumour invasion extends into the mandible and is visible radiologically preoperatively, or evident at the time of surgical resection, it should be treated by segmental mandibulectomy. This will usually require a fibula or deep circumflex iliac artery osseomyocutaneous flap repair.

As can be seen from the above, most lesions will not require free flap closure, and those that will should be predicted from preoperative imaging and panendoscopic tumour assessment.

Most patients will require a period of at least 4 days nil by mouth with NET feeding, and then assessment by a speech pathologist to commence liquid diet intake. Patients with mandibulectomy and free flap closure often will require a prolonged period of nutritional support, especially as they will have significant deterioration of swallowing with adjuvant radiotherapy. These patients should be planned to have a PEG tube insertion prior to the resection surgery, as there will be a deterioration in swallowing related to radiotherapy and planned PEG insertion will avoid delays and interruptions in delivery of radiotherapy.

Those patients who require a tracheostomy will commonly have staged decannulation starting at day 4–5 postoperatively.

The surgical approach indicated above would be expected to allow one modality (surgery) treatment to be definitive in approximately 10 per cent of patients, and to avoid the need for chemotherapy in postsurgical treatment in 30–40 per cent of patients. The subsequent de-escalation of treatment in a planned, histologically directed manner allows tumour control and minimizes treatment-related morbidity.

POSTOPERATIVE RADIOTHERAPY AND CHEMORADIOTHERAPY

The principles and indications for postoperative radiotherapy and chemoradiotherpy are discussed in Chapter 44, Postoperative radiotherapy in head and neck cancer and Chapter 45, Chemoradiation in head and neck cancer. The indications after OPSCC resection are no different from other primary tumours. Most pN+ and T>2 OPSCC are treated with postoperative radiotherapy, with specific adverse features being treated with postoperative CRT, these being extracapsular invasion and positive surgical margins,[59, 60, 61] although many would also include other adverse features, such as perineural or lymphovascular invasion. After transoral resections of the oropharynx, most patients have postoperative RT or CRT, with results that appear to be comparable to open surgery and postoperative radiotherapy.[62]

RADIOTHERAPY AND CHEMORADIOTHERAPY TECHNIQUES

The radiotherapeutic technique chosen depends on whether or not the tumour is well lateralized. If there is a central tumour, or a large, lateral one which either crosses or even encroaches on the midline, there is a high probability of bilateral nodal involvement. In such cases, the whole width of the neck must be irradiated, whereas for small, laterally placed tumours, treatment of a limited volume can be effective. Such a set-up enables the contralateral mucosa and parotid gland to be spared, and therefore it causes much less morbidity.

Carcinomas of the tonsil or lateral wall

SMALL TUMOURS WITHOUT NODES

Before considering small-volume treatment for a lateral oropharyngeal tumour, it is essential that its limits have been precisely identified at examination under anaesthesia, and that any clinically occult extension has been excluded by a CT scan. As in the case of oral cavity tumours, it can be helpful for treatment planning if the tumour margins are marked by the insertion of inert metal seeds, which are used to indicate the position of the tumour on radiographs. For T1 or T2 squamous carcinoma of the tonsil or fauces which do not extend significantly into the base of tongue or parapharyngeal area, and where there is no lymphatic spread, small-volume treatment is appropriate. Two ipsilateral fields are used (**Figure 31.3**), a posterior oblique and an anterior oblique. Wedges are used to ensure that a homogeneous dose distribution is achieved (**Figure 31.4**).

The fields extend from the level of the hard palate superiorly down to the hyoid. Their anterior border is through the central part of the tongue and their posterior limit is through the vertebral bodies. The volume encompassed therefore includes the primary tumour with an adequate margin and the jugulodigastric and parapharyngeal nodes, and extends to the midline. For T1–2N0 tumours it is not necessary to irradiate the lower neck prophylactically. The patient is planned lying supine in a shell with the mouth closed. A simulator check film is taken as a permanent record of the intended treatment, and portal verification films are taken or megavoltage imaging is performed to ensure that treatment is executed as planned. A dose of 55 Gy in 20 fractions over 4 weeks or its equivalent is given, using 4–6 MV x-rays from a linear accelerator.

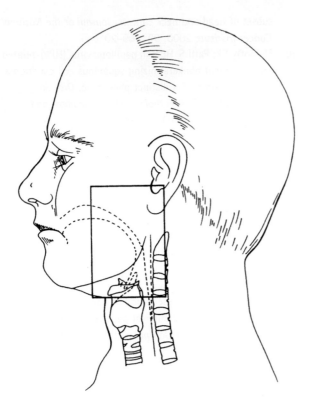

Figure 31.3 Volume to be irradiated in a patient with a small carcinoma of the lateral oropharynx without nodal involvement.

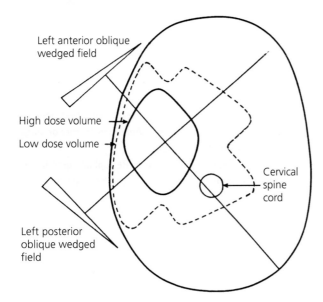

Left anterior oblique wedged field

High dose volume

Low dose volume

Cervical spine cord

Left posterior oblique wedged field

Figure 31.4 Plan of the radiotherapy field arrangement for a small lateral oropharyngeal tumour without nodal metastases.

EXTENSIVE LATERAL TUMOURS AND SMALLER ONES WITH NODES

To embrace the primary tumour adequately and upper deep cervical nodes bilaterally a pair of lateral parallel opposed fields is used. Their margins are essentially the same as described for more limited tumours. Care is taken to ensure that these are extended if necessary to cover any direct

tumour extension or nodal involvement. Although in most circumstances radiotherapists attach great importance to achieving a homogeneous dose distribution, the oropharynx provides an exception. If the tumour is confined to the tonsillar region and does not infiltrate the base of tongue or extend on to the palate, it is possible to weight the treatment, giving a greater dose to the affected side and an adequate prophylactic dose to the contralateral nodes. If there is palpable nodal enlargement, the lower neck is also treated. An anterior field is used, the upper border of which matches the lower border of the parallel opposed fields. If the lymphadenopathy is bilateral, then both sides of the lower neck are treated. A single anterior field covering the width of the neck is used and a midline block is required to shield the cervical cord. If there is extensive or bulky nodal disease, primary surgery with postoperative radiotherapy is usually preferred. Nonetheless, primary radical radiotherapy is sometimes appropriate, in which case it may not be possible to achieve adequate coverage without including the spinal cord in the high-dose volume. A two-phase technique, similar to that described for piriform fossa carcinoma (Chapter 42, Principles of radiotherapy), enables the dose to the cord to be kept within safe limits. In such circumstances the likelihood of cure is slim, but radical treatment may be attempted as it is sometimes successful. A dose of 55 Gy in 20 fractions over 4 weeks is often given, but for the reasons set out in the section on supraglottic carcinoma (Chapter 42, Principles of radiotherapy), many radiotherapists prefer a more protracted fractionation schedule.

Carcinoma of the base of tongue

The technique here is similar to that described above for bulky lateral wall tumours, or those with nodes. The inferior margin of the lateral fields should, however, be lower to cover actual or potential spread into the supraglottis. In addition, if the tumour is confined to the tongue base, the upper margin is placed below the level of the hard palate and the patient is treated with the mouth open and the tongue depressed. This enables the mucosa of the roof of the mouth to be spared to some extent. Treatment of nodal disease and selection of a fractionation schedule are as indicated above.

Sometimes, a brachytherapy boost can be given to the primary tumour using looped iridium wires, as described in Chapter 42, Principles of radiotherapy.

Carcinoma of the soft palate

In most cases this is treated by evenly weighted parallel opposed lateral fields, as described for extensive lateral wall tumours. In the rare event of finding a small T1 squamous carcinoma, interstitial therapy alone may be chosen. The principal advantage of this approach is that because the treatment volume is small, the reaction will be minimized. Implantation is a particularly valuable treatment method when irradiation of a previous primary tumour has limited the scope for further external beam radiotherapy.

KEY LEARNING POINTS

- The incidence of oropharyngeal squamous cell carcinoma (OPSCC) has dramatically increased over the last decade.
- This is due to HPV-16-induced cancers, which comprise the majority of cases.
- HPV-induced OPSCC is distinct from smoking-induced OPSCC.
- HPV-induced cancers have significantly better prognosis.
- There are many different treatment options, and combinations thereof, which provide a challenge to multidisciplinary teams (MDTs).

REFERENCES

1. Office of National Statistics. Cancer statistics registrations 2006. Registrations of cancer diagnosed in 2006, England. Series MB1 No. 37, 2008. Available from: www.statistics.gov.uk/downloads/theme_health/MB1_37_2006.pdf.
2. Ryerson AB, Peters ES, Coughlin SS et al. Burden of potentially human papillomavirus-associated cancers of the oropharynx and oral cavity in the US, 1998–2003. Cancer 2008; 113: 2901–9.
3. Hashibe M, Brennan P, Chuang SC et al. Interaction between tobacco and alcohol use and the risk of head and neck cancer: pooled analysis in the International Head and Neck Cancer Epidemiology Consortium. Cancer Epidemiology, Biomarkers and Prevention 2009; 18: 541–50.
4. Romanitan M, Nasman A, Ramqvist T et al. Human papillomavirus frequency in oral and oropharyngeal cancer in Greece. Anticancer Research 2008; 28: 2077–80.
5. Nasman A, Attner P, Hammarstedt L et al. Incidence of human papillomavirus (HPV) positive tonsillar carcinoma in Stockholm, Sweden: an epidemic of viral-induced carcinoma? International Journal of Cancer 2009; 125: 362–6.
6. Golas SM. Trends in palatine tonsillar cancer incidence and mortality rates in the United States. Community Dentistry and Oral Epidemiology 2007; 35: 98–108.
7. Adelstein DJ, Ridge JA, Gillison ML et al. Head and neck squamous cell cancer and the human papillomavirus: summary of a National Cancer Institute State of the Science Meeting, November 9–10, 2008, Washington, DC. Head and Neck 2009; 31: 1393–422.
8. Ang KK, Harris J, Wheeler R et al. Human papillomavirus and survival of patients with oropharyngeal cancer. New England Journal of Medicine 2010; 363: 24–35.
9. Gillison ML, Koch WM, Capone RB et al. Evidence for a causal association between human papillomavirus and a subset of head and neck cancers. Journal of the National Cancer Institute 2000; 92: 709–20.
10. El-Mofty SK, Patil S. Human papillomavirus (HPV)-related oropharyngeal nonkeratinizing squamous cell carcinoma: characterization of a distinct phenotype. Oral Surgery, Oral Medicine, Oral Pathology, Oral Radiology, and Endodontics 2006; 101: 339–45.
11. Smeets SJ, Braakhuis BJ, Abbas S et al. Genome-wide DNA copy number alterations in head and neck squamous cell carcinomas with or without oncogene-expressing human papillomavirus. Oncogene 2006; 25: 2558–64.
12. Fakhry C, Westra WH, Li S et al. Improved survival of patients with human papillomavirus-positive head and neck squamous cell carcinoma in a prospective clinical trial. Journal of the National Cancer Institute 2008; 100: 261–9.
13. Worden FP, Kumar B, Lee JS et al. Chemoselection as a strategy for organ preservation in advanced oropharynx cancer: response and survival positively associated with HPV16 copy number. Journal of Clinical Oncology 2008; 26: 3138–46.
14. Shimizu K, Inoue H, Saitoh M et al. Distribution and impact of lymph node metastases in oropharyngeal cancer. Acta Oto-laryngologica 2006; 126: 872–7.
15. Lim YC, Koo BS, Lee JS et al. Distributions of cervical lymph node metastases in oropharyngeal carcinoma: therapeutic implications for the N0 neck. Laryngoscope 2006; 116: 1148–52.
16. Buckley JG, Feber T. Surgical treatment of cervical node metastases from squamous carcinoma of the upper aerodigestive tract: evaluation of the evidence for modifications of neck dissection. Head and Neck 2001; 23: 907–15.
17. Ballantyne AJ. Significance of retropharyngeal nodes in cancer of the head and neck. American Journal of Surgery 1964; 108: 500–4.
18. Ferlito A, Shaha AR, Rinaldo A. Retropharyngeal lymph node metastasis from cancer of the head and neck. Acta Oto-laryngologica 2002; 122: 556–60.
19. Dirix P, Nuyts S, Bussels B et al. Prognostic influence of retropharyngeal lymph node metastasis in squamous cell carcinoma of the oropharynx. International Journal of Radiation Oncology, Biology, Physics 2006; 65: 739–44.
20. McLaughlin MP, Mendenhall WM, Mancuso AA et al. Retropharyngeal adenopathy as a predictor of outcome in squamous cell carcinoma of the head and neck. Head and Neck 1995; 17: 190–8.
21. Gross ND, Ellingson TW, Wax MK et al. Impact of retropharyngeal lymph node metastasis in head and neck squamous cell carcinoma. Archives of Otolaryngology – Head and Neck Surgery 2004; 130: 169–73.
22. Northrop M, Fletcher GH, Jesse RH, Lindberg RD. Evolution of neck disease in patients with primary squamous cell carcinoma of the oral tongue, floor of mouth, and palatine arch, and clinically positive neck

nodes neither fixed nor bilateral. *Cancer* 1972; **29**: 23–30.

23. Kowalski LP, Carvalho AL, Martins Priante AV, Magrin J. Predictive factors for distant metastasis from oral and oropharyngeal squamous cell carcinoma. *Oral Oncology* 2005; **41**: 534–41.

24. Merino OR, Lindberg RD, Fletcher GH. An analysis of distant metastases from squamous cell carcinoma of the upper respiratory and digestive tracts. *Cancer* 1977; **40**: 145–51.

25. Goodwin WJ. Distant metastases from oropharyngeal cancer. *ORL; Journal for Oto-rhino-laryngology and its Related Specialties* 2001; **63**: 222–3.

26. Beer KT, Greiner RH, Aebersold DM, Zbaren P. Carcinoma of the oropharynx: local failure as the decisive parameter for distant metastases and survival. *Strahlentherapie und Onkologie* 2000; **176**: 16–21.

27. Jones AS, England J, Hamilton J *et al.* Mandibular invasion in patients with oral and oropharyngeal squamous carcinoma. *Clinical Otolaryngology and Allied Sciences* 1997; **22**: 239–45.

28. Carvalho AL, Magrin J, Kowalski LP. Sites of recurrence in oral and oropharyngeal cancers according to the treatment approach. *Oral Diseases* 2003; **9**: 112–18.

29. Calais G, Alfonsi M, Bardet E *et al.* Randomized trial of radiation therapy versus concomitant chemotherapy and radiation therapy for advanced-stage oropharynx carcinoma. *Journal of the National Cancer Institute* 1999; **91**: 2081–6.

30. Parsons JT, Mendenhall WM, Stringer SP *et al.* Squamous cell carcinoma of the oropharynx: surgery, radiation therapy, or both. *Cancer* 2002; **94**: 2967–80.

31. Mendenhall WM, Amdur RJ, Stringer SP *et al.* Radiation therapy for squamous cell carcinoma of the tonsillar region: a preferred alternative to surgery? *Journal of Clinical Oncology* 2000; **18**: 2219–25.

32. Mendenhall WM, Stringer SP, Amdur RJ *et al.* Is radiation therapy a preferred alternative to surgery for squamous cell carcinoma of the base of tongue? *Journal of Clinical Oncology* 2000; **18**: 35–42.

33. Fein DA, Lee WR, Amos WR *et al.* Oropharyngeal carcinoma treated with radiotherapy: a 30-year experience. *International Journal of Radiation Oncology, Biology, Physics* 1996; **34**: 289–96.

34. Chen AY, Schrag N, Hao Y *et al.* Changes in treatment of advanced oropharyngeal cancer, 1985–2001. *Laryngoscope* 2007; **117**: 16–21.

35. Nguyen NP, Vos P, Smith HJ *et al.* Concurrent chemoradiation for locally advanced oropharyngeal cancer. *American Journal of Otolaryngology* 2007; **28**: 3–8.

36. Lee NY, de Arruda FF, Puri DR *et al.* A comparison of intensity-modulated radiation therapy and concomitant boost radiotherapy in the setting of concurrent chemotherapy for locally advanced oropharyngeal

carcinoma. *International Journal of Radiation Oncology, Biology, Physics* 2006; **66**: 966–74.

37. Pignon JP, Syz N, Posner M *et al.* Adjusting for patient selection suggests the addition of docetaxel to 5-fluorouracil-cisplatin induction therapy may offer survival benefit in squamous cell cancer of the head and neck. *Anticancer Drugs* 2004; **15**: 331–40.

38. Posner MR, Hershock DM, Blajman CR *et al.* Cisplatin and fluorouracil alone or with docetaxel in head and neck cancer. *New England Journal of Medicine* 2007; **357**: 1705–15.

39. Bonner JA, Harari PM, Giralt J *et al.* Radiotherapy plus cetuximab for squamous-cell carcinoma of the head and neck. *New England Journal of Medicine* 2006; **354**: 567–78.

40. Camp AA, Fundakowski C, Petruzzelli GJ, Emami B. Functional and oncologic results following transoral laser microsurgical excision of base of tongue carcinoma. *Otolaryngology – Head and Neck Surgery* 2009; **141**: 66–9.

41. Jones AS, Fenton JE, Husband DJ. The treatment of squamous cell carcinoma of the tonsil with neck node metastases. *Head and Neck* 2003; **25**: 24–31.

42. Frank DK, Hu KS, Culliney BE *et al.* Planned neck dissection after concomitant radiochemotherapy for advanced head and neck cancer. *Laryngoscope* 2005; **115**: 1015–20.

43. Clayman GL, Johnson CJ 2nd, Morrison W *et al.* The role of neck dissection after chemoradiotherapy for oropharyngeal cancer with advanced nodal disease. *Archives of Otolaryngology – Head and Neck Surgery* 2001; **127**: 135–9.

44. Reddy AN, Eisele DW, Forastiere AA *et al.* Neck dissection followed by radiotherapy or chemoradiotherapy for small primary oropharynx carcinoma with cervical metastasis. *Laryngoscope* 2005; **115**: 1196–200.

45. Hicks WLJr, Kuriakose MA, Loree TR *et al.* Surgery versus radiation therapy as single-modality treatment of tonsillar fossa carcinoma: the Roswell Park Cancer Institute experience (1971–1991). *Laryngoscope* 1998; **108**: 1014–19.

46. Lim YC, Koo BS, Lee JS, Choi EC. Level V lymph node dissection in oral and oropharyngeal carcinoma patients with clinically node-positive neck: is it absolutely necessary? *Laryngoscope* 2006; **116**: 1232–5.

47. Terrell JE, Welsh DE, Bradford CR *et al.* Pain, quality of life, and spinal accessory nerve status after neck dissection. *Laryngoscope* 2000; **110**: 620–6.

48. Chepeha DB, Taylor RJ, Chepeha JC *et al.* Functional assessment using Constant's Shoulder Scale after modified radical and selective neck dissection. *Head and Neck* 2002; **24**: 432–6.

49. Bradford CR. Selective neck dissection is an option for early node-positive disease. *Archives of Otolaryngology – Head and Neck Surgery* 2004; **130**: 1436.

50. Lim YC, Lee JS, Choi EC. Perifacial lymph node metastasis in the submandibular triangle of patients with oral and oropharyngeal squamous cell carcinoma with clinically node-positive neck. *Laryngoscope* 2006; **116**: 2187–90.

51. Corlette TH, Cole IE, Albsoul N, Ayyash M. Neck dissection of level IIb: is it really necessary? *Laryngoscope* 2005; **115**: 1624–6.

52. Lee SY, Lim YC, Song MH *et al.* Level IIb lymph node metastasis in elective neck dissection of oropharyngeal squamous cell carcinoma. *Oral Oncology* 2006; **42**: 1017–21.

53. Lim YC, Lee SY, Lim JY *et al.* Management of contralateral N0 neck in tonsillar squamous cell carcinoma. *Laryngoscope* 2005; **115**: 1672–5.

54. O'Sullivan B, Warde P, Grice B *et al.* The benefits and pitfalls of ipsilateral radiotherapy in carcinoma of the tonsillar region. *International Journal of Radiation Oncology, Biology, Physics* 2001; **51**: 332–43.

55. Pauloski BR, Rademaker AW, Logemann JA *et al.* Surgical variables affecting swallowing in patients treated for oral/oropharyngeal cancer. *Head and Neck* 2004; **26**: 625–36.

56. Skoner JM, Andersen PE, Cohen JI *et al.* Swallowing function and tracheotomy dependence after combined modality treatment including free tissue transfer for advanced stage oropharyngeal cancer. *Laryngoscope* 2003; **113**: 1294–8.

57. Klozar J, Lischkeova B, Betka J. Subjective functional results 1 year after surgery and postoperative radiation for oropharyngeal carcinoma. *European Archives of Oto-rhino-laryngology* 2001; **258**: 546–51.

58. Pradier O, Christiansen H, Schmidberger H *et al.* Adjuvant radiotherapy after transoral laser microsurgery for advanced squamous carcinoma of the head and neck. *International Journal of Radiation Oncology, Biology, Physics* 2005; **63**: 1368–77.

59. Moerman M, Vermeersch H, Van Lierde K *et al.* Refinement of the free radial forearm flap reconstructive technique after resection of large oropharyngeal malignancies with excellent functional results. *Head and Neck* 2003; **25**: 772–7.

60. Bernier J, Cooper JS, Pajak TF *et al.* Defining risk levels in locally advanced head and neck cancers: a comparative analysis of concurrent postoperative radiation plus chemotherapy trials of the EORTC (#22931) and RTOG (# 9501). *Head and Neck* 2005; **27**: 843–50.

61. Allal AS, Nicoucar K, Mach D, Dulgueroy P. Quality of life in patients with oropharynx carcinomas: assessment after accelerated radiotherapy with or without chemotherapy versus surgery and post operative radiotherapy. *Head and Neck* 2003; **25**: 833–40.

62. Spiro RH. Less can mean more. The Hayes Martin Lecture. *American Journal of Surgery* 1993; **166**: 322–55.

Hypopharyngeal cancer

PATRICK J BRADLEY AND NIGEL BEASLEY

Cancer of the hypopharynx remains a dismal disease that poses a therapeutic challenge to the treating physician, with an extremely high incidence of morbidity and distant metastases.

Ferlito (2001)

INTRODUCTION

Hypopharyngeal cancer is uncommon in the United Kingdom, 10 per million per year, with the majority of patients presenting with advanced primary and metastatic disease. Patients with hypopharyngeal cancers usually present with significant comorbidities: respiratory, cardiac and nutritional, which may restrict the therapeutic options. The selection of treatment is dependent on the stage of disease and a thorough understanding of cancer spread and its natural history. Frequently, the relief of symptoms may be the best therapeutic intent allowable, and maintenance of nutrition and airway, with relief of pain is all that can be realistically achievable. However, in selected patients aggressive treatment will result in cure of disease, but may result in significant life-long morbidity, particularly voice and swallowing, which will require support and rehabilitation.

ANATOMY

The hypopharynx is interposed between the oropharynx superiorly and the upper oesophagus inferiorly, with the larynx located anteriorly. In the adult, the hypopharynx extends from the hyoid bone (fourth cervical vertebrae) above to below the cricopharyngeus muscle, lower border of the cricoid cartilage (sixth cervical vertebrae). The cervical oesophagus extends from the lower border of the cricoid cartilage into the thorax. The hypopharynx includes the posterior pharyngeal wall, the piriform fossae or sinuses, and the postcricoid area or space (**Figure 32.1a,b** and **Table 32.1**).

The wall of the hypopharynx is composed of four layers:

1. An inner mucosal lining of stratified squamous epithelium over a loose stroma.
2. A fibrous layer of pharyngeal aponeurosis.
3. A muscular layer formed by the inferior constrictor muscle and, in the upper part by the distal portion of the middle constrictor. The most distal fibres of the inferior constrictor condense into the cricopharyngeus muscle; just proximal to this muscle on the posterior wall is an area of relative weakness known as Killian's dehiscence.
4. An outer layer of fascia that derives from the buccopharyngeal fascia.

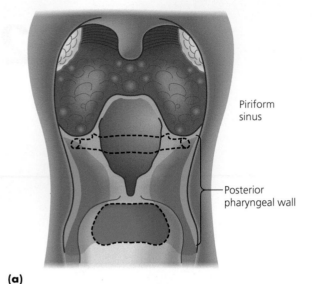

Piriform
sinus

Posterior
pharyngeal wall

(a)

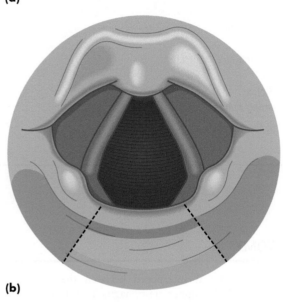

(b)

Figure 32.1 (a,b) Subsites of the hypopharynx: piriform sinus, posterior pharyngeal wall and postcricoid space.

The piriform sinus is divided into a superior or membranous part, and an inferior or cartilaginous part. The thyrohyoid membrane bounds the superior aspect of the piriform sinus laterally, through which passes the internal branch of the superior laryngeal nerve. Sensory innervation of this area synapses with the jugular ganglion, along with sensory nerves of the external auditory canal (Arnold's nerve), which accounts for the referred otalgia frequently encountered with the patient presenting with tumours of the piriform sinus. The lower portion of the piriform sinus is bounded by the ala of the thyroid cartilage. The terminal branches of the recurrent laryngeal nerve pass through the fibres of the cricopharyngeus muscle and the posterior cricoarytenoid muscle and the posterior cricoarytenoid muscles of the larynx. Motor and sensory innervation of the hypopharynx occurs via the pharyngeal plexus, which is formed by branches of the cranial nerves IX and X. The arterial supply arises from branches of the superior thyroid arteries along

Table 32.1 Hypopharynx – UICC anatomical descriptions (C12, C13).

	Anatomical description
C13.0	Pharyngo-oesophageal junction (postcricoid area) extends from the level of the arytenoid cartilages and connecting folds to the inferior border of the cricoid cartilage, thus forming the anterior wall of the hypopharynx
C12.9	Piriform sinus extends from the pharyngoepiglottic fold to the upper end of the oesophagus. It is bounded laterally by the thyroid cartilage and medially by the hypopharyngeal surface of the aryepiglottic fold, the hypopharyngeal surface of the aryepiglottic fold (C13.1) and the arytenoid and cricoid cartilages
C13.2	Posterior pharyngeal wall extends from the superior level of the hyoid bone (or floor of the valleculae) to the level of the inferior border of the cricoid cartilage and from the apex of the piriform sinus to the other

with collateral vessels from the lingual and ascending pharyngeal arteries.

Lymphatic drainage of the hypopharynx terminate in lymph nodes along the jugular vein (levels II, III and IV) and appear to a lesser extent in the nodes along the spinal accessory nerve (level V) and even less frequently in the submandibular area (level Ib). Significant lymphatic drainage occurs from the posterior pharyngeal wall and drains to the retropharyngeal lymph nodes. Lymphatics from the inferior part of the piriform sinus, the postcricoid area and the upper oesophagus often drain to the nodes along the recurrent laryngeal nerves to the paratracheal lymph nodes (level VI).

PATHOLOGY AND CLASSIFICATION

Macroscopic pathology

The majority of tumours present as ulcers and are widely infiltrative. They have a tendency to extend submucosally and also to metastasize to the local lymph nodes.

Histopathologic types

The most common (90 per cent) histologic type of cancer is squamous cell carcinoma. Other malignant tumours present in a similar manner either with ulceration or as a non-ulcerative swelling: malignant minor salivary gland tumours, lymphomas and sarcomas.

Epidemiology

The hypopharynx is an uncommon site of tumours, the majority being malignant, and accounts for less than

Table 32.2 Geographical distribution of hypopharyngeal cancers.

	United States	Europe	Northern Europe
Piriform sinus	66–75%	75–80%	60%
Posterior pharyngeal wall	20–25%	20–25%	10%
Postcricoid space	>10%	>15%	30%

10 per cent of all squamous cell carcinomas overall. The overall incidence in the Western world is one per 100 000 per year. There is a high incidence in Northern France of 14.8 per 100 000 per year, which accounts for 18 per cent of head and neck cancer seen. The distribution macroscopically of hypopharyngeal cancer varies geographically, with tumours of the piriform sinus being the most common subsite in North America and Europe, and postcricoid lesions more common in Northern Europe and the UK (**Table 32.2**).

The mean age at presentation is 60 years. Piriform sinus and posterior pharyngeal wall carcinomas demonstrate a male dominance, 5–20:1. Postcricoid lesions unlike other sites, shows a moderate female preponderance 1.5:1.

Aetiology

As with all head and neck cancers, there is a significant association with alcohol and smoking, acting synergistically. Postcricoid carcinoma is associated with previous irradiation exposure, and sideropenic dysphagia, with up to 10 per cent having a history of Plummer–Vinson, Kelly–Patterson Brown syndrome.

SECOND PRIMARY CANCER

Hypopharyngeal cancer patients are at risk of having a synchronous or metachronous cancer. Little work has been reported on this topic. In a series of 38 patients treated surgically[1] who had a cancer in their upper oesophagus or hypopharynx, 14 had multiple primaries in addition to their main primary cancer. They reported that synchronous, previous metachronous and subsequent metachronous carcinomas occurred in 26, 17 and 8.5 per cent of instances, respectively. Twenty of the 25 (80 per cent) multicentric carcinomas were invasive. This finding lends weight to the concept of total pharyngolaryngectomy as the treatment of choice for hypopharyngeal cancer because it includes all the condemned upper pharyngolaryngeal mucosa. A similar study in the UK,[2] has shown that patients with a hypopharyngeal cancer have a greater than 20 per cent chance of developing a second primary cancer. Half of all will present within two years of the index tumour diagnosis. Another publication[3] reports that there is an excess risk for the development of a second primary cancer in the upper aerodigestive tract and lung following initial hypopharyngeal cancer, but no excess risk was observed in organs outside the respiratory tract and/or the upper aerodigestive tract.

They recommend that stopping smoking and alcohol consumption, as well as increased consumption of citrus fruits should be recommended as a means to reduce the risk of second primary cancer.

Routes of primary tumour spread

Cancer of the medial wall of the piriform sinus may spread superficially towards the aryepiglottic folds and arytenoids. It also may infiltrate deeply into the larynx, to include the cricoarytenoid joint area. Involvement of the paraglottic and pre-epiglottic spaces frequently explains the frequency of early vocal cord fixation.[4] Involvement of the recurrent laryngeal nerve beneath the mucosa of the piriform sinus may also fix the hemilarynx. Tumours of the lateral wall spread rapidly to the ala of the thyroid cartilage and thereafter to involve the lobe of the thyroid gland.

Cancers of the postcricoid space frequently invade the posterior cricoarytenoid muscles and the cricoid and arytenoid cartilages. The apex of the piriform sinus terminates in the postcricoid area and is often invaded early. Advanced tumours may totally encircle the hypopharyngeal lumen.

Cancer of the posterior pharyngeal wall usually presents as an ulcer that infiltrates the whole of the posterior wall both superficially and deeply, and may involve from the nasopharynx down to the upper oesophagus. Tumours may spread to involve the prevertebral muscles and the retropharyngeal space, and may spread laterally to involve both piriform sinuses.

Regional metastases

In more than 80 per cent of patients, tumours spread to involve the local lymph nodes are detected on physical examination or by imaging at first presentation. The lymphatics fluid flows mostly via collectors into the lymph nodes of levels II and III. A direct relationship to level I has not been detected. Drainage to involve level IV occurs frequently. The lymphatic drainage of the posterior pharyngeal wall occurs mainly first into the retropharyngeal lymph nodes, and accounts for over 40 per cent of cases.[5]

In hypopharyngeal cancers, because of its advanced stage at presentation and its involvement or extension to cross the midline, the risk of contralateral metastases is high, with histological identification of tumour in more than 20 per cent of cases treated surgically[3, 4, 5, 6, 7] and supports the therapeutic decision to treat both sides of the neck, either by surgery or by radiotherapy in the N0 neck.[8] Other areas of lymph node drainage that require specific attention, when evaluating and considering the treatment of patients with hypopharyngeal cancers include retropharyngeal and parapharyngeal nodes,[9, 10] paratracheal nodes[11] and mediastinal nodes.[12]

Distant metastases

Distant spread has been reported in up to 3 per cent of patients who present for treatment of a hypopharyngeal cancer, and related to site – piriform sinus, advanced T stage, as well as the presence of nodal metastases. The most frequent sites involve the lungs, liver, bones and brain. However, as the cancer progresses, distant metastases are a common feature of hypopharyngeal malignancy. The majority of patients at presentation have advanced disease when diagnosed.[13, 14]

CLASSIFICATION

- **T1**, Tumour limited to one subsite of hypopharynx and 2 cm or less in greatest diameter.
- **T2**, Tumour invades more than one subsite of hypopharynx or an adjacent site, or measures more than 2 cm, but not more than 4 cm in greatest dimension, without fixation of hemilarynx.
- **T3**, Tumour more than 4 cm in greatest dimension, or with fixation of hemilarynx.
- **T4a**, Tumour invades any of the following: thyroid/cricoid cartilage, hyoid bone, thyroid gland, oesophagus, central compartment soft tissue (prelaryngeal strap muscles and subcutaneous fat).
- **T4b**, Tumour invades prevertebral fascia, encases carotid artery, or invades mediastinal structures.

The nodal classification for the hypopharynx is the same as for other regions in the head and neck, resulting in similar stage groupings of disease into early and late stage, depending on T and N stage.

PATIENT EVALUATION

Presenting symptoms

Patients with cancer of the hypopharynx commonly present with a history of sore throat, dysphagia, referred otalgia, hoarseness and/or a neck mass. Dysphagia, while common, commences with a vague pain or discomfort in the throat, and may be associated with problems with swallowing of saliva initially, then food (usually solids), then followed by difficulty with fluids. Severe dysphagia and otalgia are signs of advanced-staged disease that involve the lower regions of the piriform sinus/postcricoid area and the upper oesophagus. Hoarseness is not uncommon with cancer of the hypopharynx and may be due to invasion of the larynx or paralysis of the recurrent laryngeal nerve. Dyspnoea is uncommon in the early stage, but when present suggests that the larynx is extensively involved or may be due to bilateral recurrent nerve involvement, resulting in bilateral vocal cord fixity. This progressive difficulty with swallowing results in weight loss and hyponatraemia – adding to the associated comorbidity of patients who present with advanced head and neck cancers.

Cervical adenopathy is frequent at the time of presentation and is most often detected at level IIa and III. Thus, in patients who present with palpable cervical adenopathy, who may have a sore throat, otalgia and with known risk factors (smoking and drinking), a tumour located in the hypopharynx needs to be excluded.

Clinical assessment

The assessment of patients with a hypopharyngeal cancer begins with a global evaluation of their general health – nutritional status and anaemia. Also, requiring assessment are their social habits, such as chronic smoking and excessive alcohol intake, which may have an effect on their respiratory and hepatorenal systems. Evaluation of the airway for patency and possible dyspnoea and hoarseness may suggest a large tumour involving the supraglottis or even the subglottis or the trachea.

Evaluation of the primary tumour can be performed by indirect and direct examination of the hypopharynx recording the subsites involved, whether the vocal cords are mobile or paralysed. Next is palpation of the neck, to determine the presence of enlarged lymph nodes, and record their number, size and distribution. Also, during neck palpation, it is possible to assess laryngopharyngeal mobility on the cervical vertebrae. Extension of the tumour to the prevertebral muscles when early causes loss of laryngeal crepitus indicating significant oedema or swelling around the hypopharynx, usually associated with a large tumour.

Endoscopic assessment

Almost every clinic has a flexible fibreoptic nasolaryngoscope which is used widely to evaluate patients who have head and neck pain, as well as throat symptoms. Frequently, a tumour of the hypopharynx is first diagnosed in this way, and the extent of the lesion can be assessed. Movements of the vocal cords can be noted, together with any distortion, swelling or ulceration suggesting involvement of the larynx, as well as narrowing of the laryngeal or upper tracheal airway. The transverse extent of hypopharyngeal cancers can usually be determined by flexible endoscopic examination, whereas evaluation of the vertical extent is difficult if not impossible with any degree of accuracy. This is particularly challenging when the tumour is located in the postcricoid region. One useful tip, is to get the patient to swallow the endoscope into the oesophagus and during gentle withdrawal of the viewing end, the lower end of the tumour can be evaluated.

The vertical extent of the tumour is best evaluated by the use of the rigid endoscope, however, this procedure requires the use of a general anaesthetic. The larynx can be lifted forward opening the lower end of the hypopharynx for inspection and facilitates biopsy to be performed. Sometimes, the use of bougies to dilate the stenosed tumour segment may be required to evaluate the lower extent, as well as estimating the vertical length. This procedure is traumatic and bleeding can occur, obstructing the view, and may increase the possibility of perforation.

Imaging studies

The aim of imaging studies is to determine the exact three-dimensional extent of tumour involvement, to detect the presence of locoregional neck metastases, to detect pulmonary metastases or synchronous second primary, so as to allow the patient's therapy or treatment to be optimized. The lateral soft tissue radiograph may be a good screener in a busy clinic, to determine the urgency of patients' investigation, in that patients with hypopharyngeal upper oesophageal cancers will have expansion of the prevertebral soft tissue, the space between the tracheal air column and the cervical vertebral bodies. In some large tumours, involvement of the trachea or vertebral bodies themselves may be visible.

CONTRAST STUDIES OR BARIUM SWALLOW

Performing a barium study may not be appropriate because of the potential risk of aspiration and also may not with any degree of accuracy identify any mucosal irregularities, so it may need to be modified by the radiologist. By using a modified Valsalva or Toynbee manoeuvre, it is possible to distend the hypopharynx and allow the barium to coat the mucosa, thus increasing the surface area covered by the barium suspension. The longitudinal extent of the hypopharyngeal cancer has been shown to be a significant prognostic indicator, however, the lower end of the tumour is notoriously difficult to predict with accuracy on contrast studies. Should a perforation or a pharyngotracheal fistula be suspected, then a non-ionic and low osmolar water-soluble contrast agent should be used to minimize the resultant chemical pneumonitis and pulmonary oedema.

COMPUTED TOMOGRAPHY

Computed tomography (CT) is currently the most frequently employed imaging study used to evaluate the extent of hypopharyngeal cancers (**Table 32.3**). Its use can identify the tumour itself, the surrounding structure (larynx, thyroid) and assessment of the likely involvement of the cervical nodes. The primary tumour may extend or invade in all directions; a piriform sinus tumour may invade medially into the larynx or laterally to or through the thyrohyoid membrane. Also, in all subsites whether the tumour has crossed the midline, it is imperative to evaluate the upper and lower extent of the tumour, which may involve the oropharynx above or below the oesophagus. One of the limitations of CT is that it is difficult to differentiate between tumour and soft tissue oedema.

MAGNETIC RESONANCE IMAGING

Magnetic resonance imaging (MRI) is superior to CT scanning at demonstrating soft tissue abnormalities such as prevertebral fascia invasion. The limitations of MRI in the

Table 32.3 Advantages and disadvantages of computed tomography (CT) and magnetic resonance imaging (MRI) in the evaluation of hypopharyngeal tumours.

	CT scan	MRI
Planes of investigation	Two	Three
Assessment bone/cartilage	Good	Poor
Differentiate tumour from oedema	Poor	Good
Radiation hazard	Mild	None

hypopharyngeal imaging are that it is time consuming and images can be blurred because patients have a tendency to swallow excessive saliva. Also, metallic implants, such as cardiac pacemakers and intracerebral aneurysm clips, are a contraindication to the use of MRI as an imaging technique.

POSITRON EMISSION TOMOGRAPHY

Positron emission tomography (PET) when used with the contrast fluorine-18-fluoro-deoxy-glucose (FDG) has a high sensitivity in the detection of occult, residual and recurrent tumours, but has a low specificity. While contrast CT and MRI remain the mainstay of initial radiological evaluation, imaging usually upstages the tumour at presentation. After treatment, including surgery and/or chemoradiotherapy, using CT and MRI to differentiate residual and recurrent tumour from oedema and scarring may be impossible. The combination of PET and CT increases the specificity and is increasingly being used to image post-treatment cases. Other newer imaging modalities, such as diffusion-weighted imaging (DWI), MR spectroscopy and MRI with superparamagnetic iron oxide (SPIO) contrast agent are reported to be useful and should be employed more widely in difficult cases.[15, 16]

CURRENT MANAGEMENT PHILOSOPHY

The optimal treatment for hypopharyngeal cancer depends on the stage at presentation. For early disease, radiotherapy and surgery achieve similar results.[17] For advanced disease, radical surgery followed by radiotherapy may be applicable when the tumour stage is operable in selected patients. Many hypopharyngeal cancer patients present with significant comorbidity, thus limiting the choices of available treatment. The functional outcome following treatment is important and the appropriate therapeutic measure chosen should be 'cost-effective' in that the treatment duration should be short and the associated morbidity minimal.[17] In a review of treatment of hypopharyngeal cancer as practised in the United States in the 1980s and 1990s,[18] survival was best for surgery only (50.4 per cent), similar with combined surgery and irradiation (48 per cent), and worst for irradiation only (25.8 per cent). However, the appearance of active chemotherapy regimens has shifted many paradigms in head and neck oncology, and no more so than in the treatment of hypopharyngeal cancer (**Box 32.1**). The tendency to avoid removal of the larynx has led many clinicians to assess preservation strategies using up-front or concurrent chemotherapy with irradiation as an alternative for candidates for surgery.[19] The evidence-based management of hypopharyngeal cancer in the UK has been summarized as of practice in 2001.[20] It was suggested that early disease be managed by organ-sparing techniques – both surgical and non-surgical. Radical surgery in early cancer is not justified on available evidence.

A retrospective review of whether radiotherapy or surgery alone as primary treatment results in any survival advantage when applied to a retrospective population-based study of 595 patients from Ontario, Canada, treated between 1990 and

Box 32.1 Options for treatment

Early hypopharyngeal carcinoma

- Surgical excision ± neck dissection(s) (endoscopic (CO_2) or open surgery)
- Conservation surgery ± bilateral selective neck dissection ± postoperative radiotherapy ± chemotherapy
- Concurrent chemoradiotherapy to primary site and both necks
- Radiotherapy alone – where significant comorbidity prevents the above options

Locally advanced hypopharyngeal carcinoma

- Concurrent chemo ± bioradiotherapy to primary and neck
- Radical surgery; pharyngolaryngectomy ± reconstruction ± bilateral selective or modified neck dissection, with postoperative chemoradiotherapy.

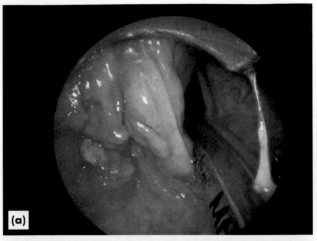

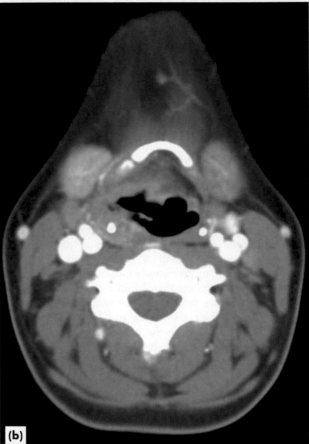

Figure 32.2 (a) Clinical picture of T2 left piriform sinus tumour demonstrating lateral wall involvement of hypopharynx. (b) Computed tomography scan of the same patient demonstrating a more extensive tumour than clinically apparent.

1999, has been reported.[21] Three different methodological approaches were used for the survival analysis, including a restricted cohort study, a matched case–control study, and natural experiment study across defined geographical regions. The authors report that there was no survival advantage for either radiotherapy ± salvage surgery or surgery ± postoperative radiotherapy. It must be commented that there has been no analysis of the modern inclusion of chemotherapy to the treatment regimen. However, a more recent commentary on the widespread use of primary chemoradiotherapy as a laryngeal organ-preserving protocol when applied to hypopharyngeal cancer (extralaryngeal sites) lacks a paucity of randomized controlled trials comparing non-operative treatments to the gold standard of surgery followed by postoperative radiation for adverse pathological features, as the likelihood of a successful surgical salvage does not translate to extralaryngeal sites compared to that of larynx cancer.[22]

Useful and practical guidance has recently been developed by the Scottish Intercollegiate Guidelines Network (SIGN). These are clear, comprehensive and well referenced.[23]

Early hypopharyngeal carcinoma is relatively unusual (**Figure 32.2a,b**). Treatment options include radical surgery, conservation surgery and radiotherapy with or without induction or concurrent platinum-based chemotherapy. At present, there are no randomized controlled trials comparing these treatment modalities. It is noted that surgery and radiotherapy are equal modalities for cure with equal morbidity for early hypopharyngeal cancers. However, there is a paucity of well-designed prospective clinical trials to support this statement because early hypopharyngeal cancer occurs infrequently and, therefore, does not frequently appear in the reported large series.[24, 25]

Cancer of the hypopharynx is known to invade insidiously, and the presence of submucosal spread is considered an indication for wide resection, well beyond gross clinical margins. If practised in small tumours, this will result in an extensive surgical procedure. As a result, the frequent reporting of pathologic specimens with incomplete excisions has resulted so that when advocating surgical treatment for larger tumours, it is considered best that radiotherapy is given postoperatively. Thus, currently, because of the likely risk of complications and loss of laryngeal function when treating advanced surgically curable disease, patients are now recommended to consider treatment with concurrent chemoradiotherapy. Should the hypopharyngeal cancer recur or persist after such treatment, then salvage surgery consisting of total pharyngolaryngectomy with neck dissections may be feasible. This programme is generally associated with a poor prognosis. When one reviews large patient series of consecutive patients with hypopharyngeal cancer, up to 25 per cent of patients are considered untreatable for a variety of reasons, such as comorbidity, inoperability, second primary cancer, and refusal to consent to treatment.[26]

SURGICAL PATHOLOGY

The results of radical surgery for hypopharyngeal cancer have remained poor with a five-year survival rate with postoperative radiotherapy in the range of 25–40 per cent. The main cause of failure is thought to be due to submucosal extension of the primary tumour. Poor survival is associated with the high rate of involvement of the cervical nodes, as well as the resection margins and usually presents within two years of treatment, the overall five-year survival rates being in the region of 30 per cent in stage III/IV.[27, 28]

In a series from Hong Kong,[29] using whole organ serial sections, submucosal tumour extension was found in 58 per cent (33 of 57) and most (67 per cent) could be detected grossly at the time of surgery. These investigators recommend that surgical resection margins should be 3 cm inferiorly and 2 cm both superiorly and laterally. However, it is agreed that the extent of invasion into the laryngeal framework and the surrounding tissues after radiotherapy is unpredictable. Thus, conservative surgery is considered unsafe.

In another study,[30] they looked at radial clearance in resected hypopharyngeal cancer. It was considered important to be aware that tumours can infiltrate into the muscular wall of the pharynx and the laryngeal cartilage. A total of 56 per cent of patients had a radial clearance of <1 mm, but the incidence of local recurrence was only 19 per cent, and occurred usually in the upper and lower margins of resection. This narrow margin would appear sufficient as long as the patients were treated with postoperative radiotherapy. Naturally as wide a margin as possible is to be recommended.

Treatment of the thyroid gland in hypopharyngeal cancer is dependent on the clinical and radiologic findings at tumour assessment. However, in certain circumstances, total thyroidectomy has been advocated in resection of postcricoid and upper oesophageal cancer. It is recommended that resection of the thyroid isthmus and lobe ipsilateral to the tumour be removed in cancers of the piriform sinus. Because many of these patients currently are treated in addition by chemoradiotherapy, the possibility of hypothyroidism and hypocalcaemia needs to be considered during each and every visit for the duration of the patient's life.[31]

SURGERY FOR HYPOPHARYNGEAL CANCER

A classification for surgery of the hypopharynx is important (**Table 32.4**) to discuss the specific procedures available when treating patients with a tumour involving specific sites or areas within the hypopharynx.[32] It is recognized that in many patients with advanced disease, the site of origin of the tumour is impossible to determine because frequently all

Table 32.4 Classification of surgery on the hypopharynx.

Classification	
Internal excision	CO$_2$ laser or 'cold steel'
External excision (with or without flap repair)	Partial pharyngectomy
	Partial pharyngectomy/partial laryngectomy
	Partial pharyngectomy/total laryngectomy
	Total pharyngolaryngectomy
	Extended pharyngolaryngectomy

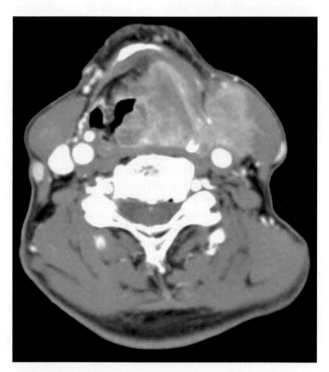

Figure 32.3 Computed tomography scan demonstrating an extensive hypopharyngeal primary with cervical nodal involvement.

three subsites are involved with tumour (**Figure 32.3**). A classification of defect repair has been suggested, but does not consider preservation of the larynx, and is best used by surgeons when describing repair of pharyngeal defects.[33]

A review of the reconstructive options used in the UK found that the use of the stomach pull up was the most commonly used method, but the jejunal free flap was becoming increasingly more popular because of its associated lower morbidity and mortality.[34]

SURGICAL TECHNIQUES

Internal excision

The operative technique of transoral partial hypopharyngectomy is well established, and current preference is to use the endoscopic technique with the carbon dioxide laser.[35, 36]

A spreadable supraglottoscope is used for exposure of the hypopharynx in the orally intubated patient. In patients whose tumour has spread caudally to involve the oropharynx or even nasopharynx, a mouth gag is also used. In lesions involving the posterior wall of the hypopharynx, a resection line is drawn around the tumour with the laser at the beginning of the procedure, followed by performing a deeper incision made using the laser approximately 1 cm cranial to the superior border of the tumour, until the prevertebral fascia is reached. Using this incision, the complete or total tumour volume along with all of the layers of the pharyngeal wall is dissected off the prevertebral fascia using the CO_2 laser, exactly like a scalpel or scissors, while remaining inside the excision borders marked initially. Because grafts do not cover the wounds adequately, healing is by most usually by secondary intent, taking about 3–4 weeks to granulate and heal. In such cases, the need for a tracheostomy and nasogastric tube feeding is seldom required.

The lateral and medial hypopharyngeal walls of the piriform sinus can be treated in a similar manner. If blood vessels of more than 0.5 mm are encountered, they are grasped with an alligator clamp, which is insulated except for the jaws, coagulated, and then divided by the laser. Postcricoid tumours are only resected, if the tumour is limited to one arytenoid and the cricoid cartilage is not infiltrated. Also if the apex of the piriform sinus is involved or low postcricoid cancer, access may be difficult or impossible to view, and if resected with safe margins, patients are at high risk of developing pharyngeal stenosis, which may require further surgery. Complications reported with the use of laser excision include local infection, emphysema, pharyngocutaneous fistula, postoperative bleeding, dyspnoea due to oedema or stenosis, swallowing difficulties and aspiration problems, including pneumonia.[37]

External excision

PARTIAL PHARYNGECTOMY ± PARTIAL LARYNGECTOMY ± FLAP REPAIR

Cancer of the posterior pharyngeal wall and some cancers of the lateral wall of the piriform sinus may be small enough to employ local excision via a lateral pharyngotomy approach and primary repair with skin, free tissue or allowed to heal by secondary intent. However, these patients need to be carefully selected so that the larynx can be preserved, with minimal morbidity. The types of tissue described which have been used in such defects have included radial forearm, platysma muscle flap and pectoralis myocutaneous flap.[38, 39]

Many investigators have advocated the use of partial laryngeal surgery with partial pharyngectomy. Ogura and Mallen[40] described select patients who had cancer of the medial wall of the piriform sinus without involvement of the apex, who were suitable for treatment with partial laryngopharyngectomy. They advocated entering the hypopharynx away from the clinically evident tumour, permitting surgical exposure of the lesion, while preserving as much pharyngeal wall as possible for subsequent reconstruction. The extent of the laryngeal resection depends upon the degree of involvement by the piriform sinus primary and may

range from subglottic laryngectomy to resection of the arytenoid.

The use of the supracricoid hemilaryngopharyngectomy was popularized in the mid-1960s and was indicated for tumours of the supracricoid upper part of the piriform sinus and carcinomas of the lateral wall with normal mobility of the vocal cord.[41, 42]

The use of near-total laryngectomy has also been advocated for more advanced cancer of the piriform sinus, which includes both the lateral and medial wall sites, with or without fixation of a vocal cord. This procedure, recently reported has resulted in preservation of speech and aspiration-free swallowing in the majority, thus many patients may avoid a permanent tracheostoma.[43]

TOTAL LARYNGECTOMY AND PARTIAL PHARYNGECTOMY – PRIMARY WITH AND WITHOUT FLAP CLOSURE

In the vast majority of patients worldwide who have cancer of the hypopharynx, the prime subsite location is the piriform sinus. Surgical treatment of these cancers requires total laryngectomy and partial pharyngectomy. Indications for this procedure include involvement of the apex of the sinus, partial involvement of the postcricoid mucosa, and invasion of the thyroid cartilage or the presence of a paralysed hemilarynx.

After total laryngectomy with partial pharyngectomy, it is possible to close the pharynx primarily if the narrowest width of the pharyngeal remnant is 1.5 cm relaxed or 2.5 cm stretched in the absence of tumour. This amount of residual pharyngeal tissue is sufficient to restore swallowing function.[44]

When there is less than 50 per cent or <2.5 cm of mucosa stretched after removal of a hypopharyngeal tumour, then the remaining mucosa needs to be supplemented by a 'patch technique' using either a free tissue flap, such as a radial forearm or a pectoralis myocutaneous flap; this will minimize the possibility of a fistula and subsequent pharyngeal stenosis.[45, 46] It is considered that using a 'patch technique' in such circumstances results in better swallowing function than repair of a full circumferential defect, the use of residual pharyngeal tissue will maintain accurate length and better physiology (**Figure 32.4**).

The concept of hypopharyngeal reconstruction must deal with restoration of not a simple tubed conduit but a complex arrangement of constrictive and propulsive forces with fine sensory circuits.[46] The chosen surgical approach should aim to achieve both complete removal of tumour and re-establishment of two primary functions: swallowing and phonation. To date, the use of free flaps represents the first choice for both partial and total oncologic hypopharyngeal reconstruction, and pedicled flaps should be considered only when free flaps are contraindicated by general and vascular conditions.

TOTAL PHARYNGOLARYNGECTOMY AND FLAP REPAIR

The need for complete excision of the hypopharynx, in addition to a total laryngectomy, is based on the circumferential extent of the tumour and the presence of

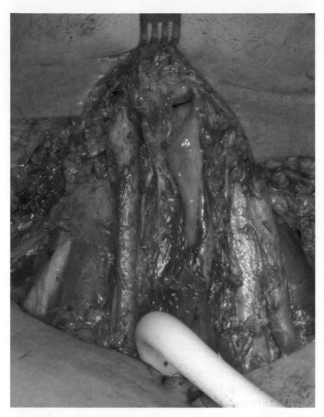

Figure 32.4 Resected hypopharyngeal cancer, with bilateral neck dissection, preservation of the posterior pharyngeal mucosal strip, suitable for pharyngeal repair by the 'on lay patch technique'.

tumour inferiorly in the postcricoid area, extending towards or involving the cervical oesophagus. The hypopharynx is a funnel-shaped tube, with a larger upper circumference that narrows down towards the pharyngo-oesophageal junction. Hence, cancer at the lower end of the hypopharynx and upper oesophagus requires a complete circumferential resection and repair. The surgical defect thus created requires a tubular replacement which can be skin, skin and muscle (a myocutaneous or free tissue), viscus (either free jejunum, caecum, greater curve of stomach with omentum or a pedicled stomach) or colon graft.[47, 48, 49, 50, 51, 52, 53, 54, 55, 56, 57]

The problems or difficulties associated with primary and secondary (salvage) hypopharyngectomy are different and the surgical defects require differing management and realistic expectations, not only by clinicians but by the patients and their carers. Patients considered for salvage are a high-risk group in terms of both operative morbidity and survival. It has been proposed that the use of the gastro-omental flap because of its anatomical, physiological and immunological properties is the ideal reconstructive technique in repair of surgical defects, especially for hypopharyngeal cancers, when considered after failed primary treatment having used chemoradiotherapy.[58] Patients with nodal metastases, extracapsular spread and poorly differentiated tumours are likely to succumb to their disease and should be selected for adjuvant therapy when possible.[59]

The ideal reconstructive technique for circumferential defects of the hypopharynx and upper oesophagus should have as many of the following attributes as possible: adequate surgical margins, especially the inferior margin; low rate of stenosis or fistula formation; short time to swallowing; normal sounding of conversational speech; ability of tissue to withstand postoperative radiotherapy with or without chemotherapy; simultaneous harvesting at the same time as the excisional surgery to reduce time 'on the table'; short hospitalization; and surgeon team experienced with the procedure and handling of complications.[60]

CERVICAL LYMPH NODES

In view of the high propensity of metastases to cervical lymph nodes in patients suffering from hypopharyngeal cancer, attention to these is as important as resecting and repairing the primary defect. The method of treating the likely cervical nodal metastases will depend on the method of primary treatment whether it is surgery, or radiotherapy ± chemotherapy.

For patients with no palpable cervical lymph nodes, then selective neck dissection removing the lymph nodes at levels II, III and IV should be performed with resection of the primary tumour. When cervical nodal disease is palpable, then a modified neck dissection should be considered. Nodal disease along the paratracheal gutter should be sought for when the primary tumour is located low in the piriform sinus or postcricoid space.[11] Occasionally, the upper mediastinum will need to be approached and a mediastinal neck dissection performed.[12, 61]

THE THYROID GLAND

Involvement of the thyroid gland in hypopharyngeal carcinoma is difficult to predict preoperatively, unless there is gross invasion seen on imaging studies. In early disease confined to one side, e.g. piriform fossa carcinoma, a hemithyroidectomy can be performed on the involved side preserving the contralateral thyroid. If the patient receives postoperative radiotherapy, hypothyroidism may still result and thyroid function should be monitored.

In more advanced disease, total thyroidectomy is usually required. The indications for total thyroidectomy have been summarized when surgically managing laryngeal and hypopharyngeal cancers including the presence of subglottic extension of more than 2 cm, cricoid cartilage invasion and perithyroidal soft tissue involvement.[62] The significant morbidity from this does not usually arise from removal of the thyroid whose function can be simply replaced with thyroid hormone supplements, but from resection of the parathyroid glands and the resulting hypocalcaemia. In these cases, careful titration of 1-alpha calcidol against calcium levels should result in normal calcium levels, but can be difficult to achieve and may be disturbed by comorbidity or intercurrent illness. In all cases, the aim should be to preserve one of the parathyroid glands, which may be difficult with extensive neck disease. If possible, the parathyroid gland should be left *in situ*, but if removed can be reimplanted into the sternomastoid muscle.

COMPLICATIONS

Complications associated with surgery for hypopharyngeal cancer may occur either during or after the operation. The problems may be grouped in relation to the procedure of resection or reconstruction.[62] Early recognition of these is mandatory if successful discharge from hospital is to be anticipated.[63, 64]

Resection-related problems

BLEEDING

Intraoperative bleeding during the resection can be controlled easily by pressure, as the neck is wide open! Bleeding from the carotid artery requires prompt attention and appropriate suturing of the defect in the wall, or ligation of a branch as appropriate. More extensive defects may require a venous patch, or even a bypass temporarily to maintain blood flow while the defect is controlled. Consideration to repairing an arterial defect by use of a vein bypass may be occasionally required to excise tumour adherent to the carotid system.

Bleeding intrathoracically during blunt dissection of the oesophagus may be profuse and sometimes may even be fatal, if the aorta or a large branch is avulsed. Bleeding from the azygos vein if injured can be torrential, and direct visualization of the bleeding area or vessel may be very difficult to view and additional access may be required with appropriate use of suction and light, as a matter of urgency. The anaesthetist should be advised should bleeding occur, as it is important that the patient's blood pressure is maintained, either by giving blood or plasma expander. A torn azygos vein can be approached by extending the abdominal incision into a right anterior thoracotomy incision, by retracting the right lung, allowing identification of the azygos vein and ligation. With experience, this vein can be dissected under direct vision, using thorascopic techniques and the vein ligated, so avoiding this complication.

Bleeding from the jugular vein in the neck can be controlled by pressure and, with appropriate assistance, the defect can be ligated, avoiding the possibility of air embolism.

DAMAGE TO THE POSTERIOR WALL OF THE TRACHEA

Injury to the posterior wall of the trachea may occur during separation of the posterior wall from the upper part of the oesophagus. This is likely when the tumour of the hypopharynx indents the oesophageal wall and has invaded the wall of the oesophagus, or in the clinical situation when the patient is being salvaged from previous treatment, such as radiotherapy. During the separation, the cuff of the endotracheal tube or the tracheostomy should be deflated to reduce the distension of the posterior tracheal wall. When the posterior tracheal wall is damaged in the upper portion of the trachea, it can be repaired from the neck wound. When the tear is more distal and cannot be repaired from the neck, then the repair procedure requires better access.

Injury at a lower level above the carina, can occur when mediastinal dissection is being performed. When the damage is through the lower trachea, the anaesthetist may notice that they are unable to maintain ventilation pressures, and gas will leak through the tear. An upper midline sternotomy, sometimes with retraction of the trachea with paratracheal traction sutures, may allow for the trachea to be presented into the neck, so that the tear can be sutured. Occasionally, a thoracotomy may be required to gain access. The endotracheal tube may be pushed further down to the level of the carina, to bypass the damaged area and maintain ventilation. Should a ventilation leak persist, then it may be necessary to insert a pneumonectomy double ventilation tube into each main bronchus to maintain ventilation. The damaged tracheal wall can be repaired directly, but usually involves drawing the cartilaginous rings posteriorly together to gain an air seal, or a partial pleural or pericardial flap can be sutured into the defect to reinforce the weakened area. Also, bringing the stomach into the neck will provide additional support to the repaired posterior tracheal wall.[61]

Intraoperative problems

TENSION AT THE ANASTOMOSIS

This problem occurs and depends on the type of tissue used for repair and the technique and size of the surgical defect.

When a patch technique is being used, the current preferred flaps available include the myocutaneous flap, free jejunal graft, free gastro-omental or stomach. When a pedicled flap is used, tension of the muscle pedicle must be avoided so as to minimize tension on the anastomosis. With jejunum, an adequate length is essential and should be sutured under adequate tension so there is minimal redundant tissue. The jejunal lumen is usually too small to fill the defect at the oropharynx, so additional diameter can be achieved by making an incision on the anti-mesenteric border to increase the lumen size.

When the stomach is used, it is usually brought up through the posterior mediastinum as this is the shortest route and will allow for maximum length of stomach to be achieved. Other ways to increase length are to reduce the tension at the pharyngogastric anastomosis by mobilizing the pharynx, or increasing the length of the stomach. Also, if the opening into the fundus of the stomach extends anteriorly about 1–1.5 cm distal from the free border, this will give additional length posteriorly, the tongue will always be mobile enough to be sutured more caudal, or alternatively a lingual flap can give additional length. If the stomach will not reach the oropharyngeal defect, then it is recommended that a gastrostomy be created in the neck as high as is possible, the orostome closed and then wait for 2–3 weeks and re-explore the wounds and see if further mobilization is possible. Alternatively, an additional graft may need to be piggy-backed to repair the short segment.

LEAKAGE FROM THE PHARYNGEAL RECONSTRUCTION

Leakage may manifest during the early and the late recovery phase. The causes associated with other fistulae apply here, such as previous radiotherapy, poor nutrition and techniques of closure (**Figure 32.5**).[63, 64]

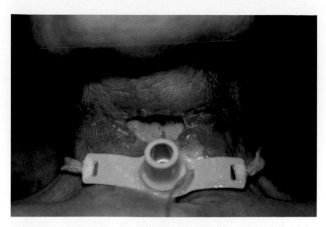

Figure 32.5 A pharyngocutaneous fistula, following an attempt at primary partial pharyngeal closure.

Minor leaks may be detected at the time of imaging with barium contrast. The general condition of the patient and the timing of the leak detection will dictate the form of intervention required. For minor leaks with no systemic upset, continue nil per oral, feeding via a nasogastric tube, or through a percutaneous endoscopic gastrostomy (PEG) and continue antibiotics for another week or so. The majority will settle.

When the anastomosis dehiscence or flap failure manifests in the early postoperative period (i.e. the first few days), the leakage should be identified, and the discharge exteriorized onto healthy skin to divert saliva, food, pus and gastric contents from the local tissue including blood vessels, in particular the carotid artery. Should tissue necrosis be evident, then the dead tissue should be debrided and no attempt to be made in performing further surgery until the infection and oedema has subsided, which may take some weeks.

WHAT ABOUT CARCINOMA IN A HYPOPHARYNGEAL DIVERTICULUM?

Carcinoma arising in a pharyngeal pouch is rare. There have been reports in the literature of carcinoma developing in long-standing, untreated pouches and also in pouches that have been treated by surgical methods.[65] A UK community study from the estimates an annual incidence of pharyngeal pouches at two per 100 000 per year.[66] Endoscopic stapling is currently the procedure of choice for the surgical treatment of pharyngeal pouches.[67] In a consecutive series of 50 patients treated surgically,[68] with excision of the pouch and a cricopharyngeal myotomy, all tissue was subjected to histopathologic examination – two cases of carcinoma in situ and two cases of squamous cell carcinoma were detected. In one case, the squamous carcinoma was suspected at the time of endosocopy. The authors advocate discussion of theoretical possibility of cancer in patients who present under the age of 65 years, and recommend excision and histological examination, as the pouch is likely to get bigger with time. Does endoscopic stapling eradicate symptoms and prevent increase in size of the remaining pouch stump? There has been no long-term follow up of such a patient group. Recently, there has been a report[69] of a male patient who had previously had his pouch endoscopically stapled, at the age of 65 years, who developed recurrence of his symptoms six years later, and was found to have cancer in the residual pouch. Treatment was by excision of the pouch with the carcinoma followed by external beam radiotherapy.

Use of radiotherapy with or without chemotherapy

Although radiotherapy alone is effective,[70, 71] concurrent chemoradiotherapy has become the treatment of choice for those patients able to tolerate treatment, as a survival benefit of around 16 per cent has been demonstrated on meta-analysis.[72] Neck node metastases to levels II, III and IV are common in hypopharyngeal carcinoma and the N0 neck is usually treated either by selective neck dissection, if surgery is the primary modality of treatment, or radiotherapy. The N+ neck is considered below.

Treatment of advanced hypopharyngeal carcinoma is challenging. Options include radical surgery or non-surgical organ preservation strategies. Radiotherapy alone has little chance of controlling advanced disease and the outcomes are poor. Induction chemotherapy with cisplatin and 5FU followed by radical radiotherapy, for those with a complete response, gives similar survival figures to historical controls having radical surgery and post-operative radiotherapy.[73] More recently, the concurrent administration of chemotherapy and radiotherapy has increased in popularity for those patients able to tolerate the treatment.[74] Subsequent publication of a number of randomized studies and meta-analyses indicates increased laryngeal preservation rates after concurrent platinum chemotherapy and radiation.[75, 76] This regimen has also resulted in improved survival in non-resectable disease. Novel agents, such as the monoclonal antibody cetuximab and its analogues, have shown significant improvement in locoregional control and disease-free survival when added to conventional radiotherapy in randomized studies.[77, 78] Altered fractionation radiotherapy, either hyperfractionation or acceleration, can improve locoregional control when an increased overall dose of treatment is given, but this may result in an increase in early and late side effects.[79, 80]

As indicated above, nodal metastases to levels II, III and IV are common in hypopharyngeal carcinoma and the N0 neck is usually treated actively. Patients with low volume neck disease (N1), particularly those with nodes <2 cm in diameter and no evidence of necrosis on imaging studies can be treated in the same way as the N0 neck, with selective neck dissection if the primary treatment is surgery or extension of the radiotherapy treatment fields to include the neck. Advanced neck disease (N2 or N3) is usually resected. The extent of surgery should be tailored to the extent of disease, preserving the accessory nerve and internal jugular vein if possible, but not at the risk of leaving disease in the neck. This strategy can be used with early or advanced disease at the primary site and irrespective of the treatment of the primary site.[81]

Assessment of the primary site and the neck after organ preservation strategies is vital to determine whether surgical salvage is required. Clinical examination and outpatient endoscopy should be carried out on all patients at regular intervals following treatment to assess tumour response.

Persistent pain or dysphagia should alert the clinician to the possibility of residual disease. Much of the hypopharynx is hidden and endoscopy under general anaesthetic may be required. Imaging modalities, such as CT and MRI can give an indication of response to treatment, but are a crude indicator of disease eradication. PET scanning has increased in popularity over the last decade as it measures glucose uptake in metabolically active residual carcinoma cells. It must be carried out at least 8 weeks after the completion of treatment and has a higher specificity than CT alone for residual disease.[82, 83] If positive, a concerted effort can be made to locate the residual disease and treat appropriately.

MORBIDITY AND QUALITY OF LIFE

Two major problems for patients treated for hypopharyngeal cancer are breathing and swallowing.[84] As commented above, early hypopharyngeal cancers are uncommon, with the majority of patients having advanced stage disease at presentation. Patients treated surgically will result in a pharyngolaryngectomy and result in a tracheostoma and difficulty with their swallow. Minimal problems with swallowing in patients who have had a gastric transposition are reported. As a consequence of laryngectomy, they will require altered voicing techniques such as electrolarynx or tracheo-esophageal (TEP) puncture. Much has been written about TEP voice restoration in laryngectomy patients, but a lesser quality of voice and increased risks of complications are associated with patients who have extensive replacement of their hypopharynx by free tissue or viscus flaps.[85, 86, 87] Swallowing is also a major problem either in the early phase with fistulae or in the late period with stricture formation.[88, 89, 90]

Patients who are treated by radiation or chemoradiation have associated complications, including mucositis and swallowing problems. The incidence of mucositis and, as a consequence, swallowing problems, is high, but varies depending on tumour location, radiation dose and schedule, and the use of concomitant chemotherapy.[91, 92] Problems with swallowing may interfere with all three phases of swallowing, and the following have been observed in studies using a modified barium swallow: reduction of posterior tongue base movement, reduced tongue strength, impairment of laryngeal elevation, pharyngeal stasis, piriform and vallecular residue, and aspiration. Interestingly, pre-treatment swallowing abnormalities became severe following treatment, suggesting that chemoradiotherapy did not produce any new swallowing abnormalities, but exacerbated pre-existing ones.[93] Dysphagic patients tend to be isolated and depressed as they cannot comfortably participate in social activities, such as going out to dinner, because of fear of embarrassment. In a retrospective survey of patients who had a modified barium study and responded to quality of life (QoL) questionnaires, the degree of anxiety and depression was correlated with dysphagia severity. Patients who required prolonged tube feeding because of aspiration had the worst QoL.[94] Once chronic dysphagia occurred, it rarely returned to normal in studies with sequential modified barium studies for monitoring long-term dysphagia.[95] In addition, pharyngeal or oesophageal stenosis occurred late (more than one

year) after chemoradiation, and required repeated dilatations, thereby increasing treatment morbidities.[96] Thus, the management of patients following treatment of hypopharyngeal cancers requires the care of a multidisciplinary team, involving not only doctors but physicians, speech and language therapists, dieticians and psychologists.[97]

Salvage after initial curative treatment

Relapse-free survival of patients who have a cancer located in the hypopharynx is strongly related to the localization and initial tumour stage; 25 per cent of relapses remain undetected by patients themselves. To detect relapse at an early stage, oncologic follow up should be performed at close intervals during the first three years. The use of PET-FDG has helped to increase likely detection of persistent and/or recurrent disease, and should be performed 12 weeks after completion of treatment, but beware of the possible confusion with chondronecrosis. Sadly, most of these relapses are already incurable at the time of diagnosis. In a recent analysis of treated cases of hypopharyngeal cancer, the median relapse-free survival was 45 months.[98] Another analysis of the 'natural history' of hypopharyngeal cancer from Canada,[99] reports that up to 20 per cent of patients after curative treatment had residual disease, recurrences tended to appear in the first year and 50 per cent of first recurrences included distant metastases. Overall, 47 per cent of patients were disease free at three years, but eventually 64 per cent of patients died of their cancer.

SUMMARY

The treatment of hypopharyngeal carcinoma remains one of the most challenging areas of head and neck cancer management. Patients often present late with advanced disease and significant co-morbidity. Appropriate decision-making is helped by careful clinical and radiological assessment of the patient and tumour, and discussion with colleagues in a multidisciplinary team environment. There is little hard evidence to guide treatment decisions due to the paucity of well-conducted randomized trials, but the addition of chemotherapy to organ-preservation strategies has improved survival. One of the hardest decisions to make with a patient is to follow a non-curative pathway and institute active palliation with symptom support, but for many with advanced disease this is the appropriate course of action.

KEY EVIDENCE

- The majority of patients when diagnosed with hypopharyngeal cancer have advanced stage disease with evidence of advanced local disease T3/T4,[80] regional involvement of level II, III, IV, paratracheal and retropharyngeal lymph nodes (>80 per cent)[5, 9, 11] and involvement of contralateral lymph nodes (>20 per cent)[6] and distant metastases (3 per cent),[14] thus restricting the options for curative treatment.[17, 26]

- Those few patients who present with early primary site (T stage) disease should be considered for treatment by surgical excision (endoscopic (CO_2) or open surgery) when possible, so that organ function (voice and swallowing) can be preserved.[24]
- In the recent past, treatment for operable patients was surgery with post-operative chemoradiotherapy. However, because of the morbidity of the procedure and the likely risk of local recurrence and/or distant metastases manifesting within two years, the option of 'organ preservation' treatment has been explored.[76]
- Patients with advanced inoperable disease should be treated by chemo ± biotherapy + radiotherapy regimens with possible surgery for persisting neck disease, aiming to maximize symptom relief, with minimal treatment toxicity while maintaining good quality of life for the remainder of such patients' life.[78, 80]

KEY LEARNING POINTS

- There is a high risk of synchronous and metachronous second primary tumours.
- Treat the neck in all cases – 80 per cent are N+ at the time of presentation.
- Submucosal spread is common – surgical margins should be 3 cm inferiorly and 2 cm both superiorly and laterally.
- Prevent tracheal tears by deflating the cuff of the endotracheal tube when dissecting the trachea from the oesophagus during gastric transposition.
- Consider the addition of chemotherapy to organ-preservation treatment strategies and post-operative radiotherapy.

REFERENCES

1. Martins AS. Multicentricity in pharyngoesophageal tumours: Argument for total pharyngo-laryngo-esophogectomy and gastric transposition. *Head and Neck* 2000; 22: 156–63.
2. Raghavan U, Quraishi Q, Bradley PJ. Multiple primary tumours in patients diagnosed with hypopharyngeal cancer. *Otolaryngology and Head and Neck Surgery* 2003; 128: 419–25.
3. Dikshit RP, Boffetta P, Bouchardy C *et al.* Risk factors for the development of second primary tumours among men

4. Deleyiannis FW, Piccirillo JF, Kirchner JA. Relative importance of histologic invasion of the laryngeal framework by hypopharyngeal cancer. *Annals of Otology, Rhinology and Laryngology* 1996; 105: 101–8.
5. Buckley JG, MacLennan K. Cervical node metastases in laryngeal and hypopharyngeal carcinoma. *Clinical Otolaryngology* 1999; 22: 380–5.
6. Aluffi P, Pisani P, Policarpo M, Pia F. Contralateral cervical lymph node metastases in piriform sinus carcinoma. *Otolaryngology and Head and Neck Surgery* 2006; 134: 650–3.
7. Koo BS, Lim YC, Lee JS *et al.* Management of contralateral N0 neck in piriform sinus carcinoma. *Laryngoscope* 2006; 116: 1268–72.
8. Ferlito A, Shaha AR, Buckley JG, Rinaldo A. Selective neck dissection for hypopharyngeal cancer in the clinically negative neck: should it be bilateral? *Acta Otolaryngologica* 2001; 121: 329–35.
9. Kamiyama R, Saikawa M, Kishimoto S. Significance of retropharyngeal node dissection in hypopharyngeal cancer. *Japanese Journal of Clinical Oncology* 2009; 39: 632–7.
10. Sakata K, Aoki Y, Nakagawa K *et al.* Analysis of treatment results of hypopharyngeal cancer. *Radiation Medicine* 1998; 16: 31–6.
11. Timon CV, Toner M, Conlon BJ. Paratracheal lymph node involvement in advanced cancer of the larynx, hypopharynx, and cervical oesophagus. *Laryngoscope* 2003; 113: 1595–9.
12. Martins AS. Neck and mediastinal dissection in pharyngolaryngoesophageal tumors. *Head and Neck* 2001; 23: 772–9.
13. Lefebvre JL. What is the role of primary surgery in the treatment of laryngeal and hypopharyngeal cancer? *Archives of Otolaryngology – Head and Neck Surgery* 2000; 126: 285–8.
14. Spector GJ. Distant metastases from laryngeal and hypopharyngeal cancer. *ORL, Journal for Otorhinolaryngology and its Related Specialties* 2001; 63: 224–8.
15. Wycliffe ND, Grover RS, Kim PD, Simental A Jr. Hypopharyngeal cancer. *Topics in Magnetic Resonance Imaging* 2007; 18: 243–58.
16. Zbaren P, Weidner S, Thoeny HC. Laryngeal and hypopharyngeal carcinomas after (chemo) radiotherapy: a diagnostic dilemma. *Current Opinion in Otolaryngology and Head and Neck Surgery* 2008; 16: 147–53.
17. Lefebvre JL, Lartigau E. Preservation of form and function during management of cancer of the larynx and hypopharynx. *World Journal of Medicine* 2003; 27: 811–16.
18. Hoffman HT, Karnell LH, Shah JP *et al.* Hypopharyngeal cancer patient care evaluation. *Laryngoscope* 1997; 107: 1005–17.

after laryngeal and hypopharyngeal carcinoma. *Cancer* 2005; 103: 2326–33.

♦ 19. Wei HI. The dilemma of treating hypopharyngeal carcinoma: more or less. *Archives of Otolaryngology – Head and Neck Surgery* 2002; **128**: 229–32.

20. Robson A. Evidence based management of hypopharyngeal cancer. *Clinical Otolaryngology* 2002; **27**: 413–20.

♦ 21. Hall SF, Groome PA, Irish J, O'Sullivan B. Radiotherapy or surgery for head and neck squamous cell cancer: establishing the baseline for hypopharyngeal carcinoma? *Cancer* 2009; **115**: 5711–22.

22. Gourin CG, Johnson JT. A contemporary review of indications for primary surgical care of patients with squamous cell carcinoma of the head and neck. *Laryngoscope* 2009; **119**: 2124–34.

23. Scottish Intercollegiate Guidelines Network (SIGN). Diagnosis and management of head and neck cancer 90: A national clinical guideline, 2006. *Clinical Otolaryngology* 2007; **32**: 111–18. Available from: www.sign.ac.uk.

● 24. Martin A, Jackel MC, Christiansen H *et al.* Organ preservation transoral laser microsurgery for cancer of the hypopharynx. *Laryngoscope* 2008; **118**: 398–402.

● 25. Karatzanis AD, Psychogios G, Waldfahrer F *et al.* T1 and T2 hypopharyngeal cancer treatment with laser microsurgery. *Journal of Surgical Oncology* 2010; **102**: 27–33.

26. Eckel HE, Staar S, Volling P *et al.* Surgical treatment for hypopharyngeal carcinoma: feasibility, mortality and results. *Otolaryngology and Head and Neck Surgery* 2001; **124**: 561–9.

27. Johansen LV, Grau C, Overgaard J. Hypopharyngeal squamous cell carcinoma: treatment results in 138 consecutively admitted patients. *Acta Oncologica* 2000; **39**: 529–36.

● 28. Sewaik A, Hoorweg JJ, Knegt PP *et al.* Treatment of hypopharyngeal carcinoma: analysis of nation-wide study in the Netherlands over a 10 year period. *Clinical Otolaryngology* 2005; **30**: 52–7.

● 29. Ho CH, Ng WF, Lam KH *et al.* Submucosal tumour extension in hypopharyngeal cancer. *Archives of Otolaryngology and Head and Neck Surgery* 1997; **123**: 959–65.

● 30. Ho CH, Ng WF, Lam KH *et al.* Radial clearance in resection of hypopharyngeal cancer. *Head and Neck* 2002; **24**: 181–90.

31. Price JC, Ridley MB. Hypocalcaemia following pharyngoesophageal ablation and gastric pull-up reconstruction: pathophysiology and management. *Annals of Otology, Rhinology and Laryngology* 1988; **97**: 521–6.

♦ 32. Bradley PJ. Cancer of the hypopharynx. *Operative Techniques in Otolaryngology* 2005; **16**: 55–66.

♦ 33. Disa JJ, Pusic AL, Hidalgo DA *et al.* Microvascular reconstruction of the hypopharynx; defect classification, treatment algorithm and functional outcome based on 165 consecutive cases. *Plastic and Reconstructive Surgery* 2003; **111**: 652–63.

34. Ayshford CA, Walsh RM, Watkinson JC. Reconstructive techniques currently used following resection of hypopharyngeal carcinoma. *Journal of Laryngology and Otology* 1999; **113**: 145–8.

35. Martin A, Jackel MC, Christiansen H *et al.* Organ preserving trans-oral laser microsurgery for cancer of the hyopharynx. *Laryngoscope* 2008; **118**: 398–402.

36. Eckel HE, Schroder U, Jungehulsing M *et al.* Surgical treatment options in laryngeal and hypopharyngeal cancer. *Wiener Medizinische Wochenschrift* 2008; **158**: 255–63.

37. Vilaseca-Gonzalez I, Bernal-Sprekelsen M, Blanch-Alejandro J-L *et al.* Complications in trans-oral CO_2 laser surgery for carcinoma of the larynx and hypopharynx. *Head and Neck* 2003; **25**: 382–8.

38. Julieron M, Kolb F, Schwaab G *et al.* Surgical management of posterior pharyngeal wall carcinoma: functional and oncologic results. *Head and Neck* 2001; **23**: 80–6.

39. Lydiatt WM, Kraus DH, Cordeiro PG *et al.* Posterior pharyngeal carcinoma resection with laryngeal preservation and radial forearm free flap reconstruction: a preliminary report. *Head and Neck* 1996; **18**: 501–5.

40. Ogura JH, Mallen RW. Partial laryngopharyngectomy for supraglottic and pharyngeal carcinoma. *Transactions of the American Academy of Ophthalmology and Otolaryngology* 1965; **69**: 832–45.

41. Chevalier D, Watelet J-B, Darras J-A, Piquet J-J. Supraglottic hemilaryngopharyngectomy plus radiation for the treatment of early lateral margin and piriform sinus carcinoma. *Head and Neck* 1997; **19**: 1–5.

42. Papacharalampous GX, Kotsis GP, Vlastarakos PV *et al.* Supracricoid hemilaryngectomy for selected pyriform sinus carcinoma patients – a retrospective chart review. *World Journal of Surgical Oncology* 2009; **7**: 65.

43. Shenoy AM, Sridharan S, Srihariprasad AV *et al.* Near-total laryngectomy in advanced cancers of the larynx and pyriform sinus: a comparative study of the morbidity and functional and oncological outcomes. *Annals of Otology, Rhinology and Laryngology* 2002; **111**: 50–6.

● 44. Hui Y, Wei WK, Yuen PW *et al.* Primary closure of pharyngeal remnant after total laryngectomy and partial pharyngectomy: how much residual mucosa is sufficient? *Laryngoscope* 1996; **106**: 490–4.

45. Azizzadeh B, Yafai S, Rawnsley JD *et al.* Radial forearm free flap pharyngo-oesophageal reconstruction. *Laryngoscope* 2001; **111**: 807–10.

♦ 46. Benazzo M, Bertino G, Spasiano R *et al.* Decisional algorithm in extended neoplasms of the hypopharynx and the cervical oesophagus. *Supplementi di Tumori* 2005; **4**: S190–2.

47. Couch ME. Laryngopharyngectomy with reconstruction. *Otolaryngologic Clinics of North America* 2002; **35**: 1097–114.

48. Gender EM, Kaufman MR, Katz B *et al.* Tubed gastro-omental free flap for pharyngo-oesophageal reconstruction. *Archives of Otolaryngology – Head and Neck Surgery* 2001; **127**: 847–53.

♦ 49. Hartley BEJ, Botterill ID, Howard DJ. A third decade's experience with the gastric pull-up operation for hypopharyngeal carcinoma: changing patterns of use. *Journal of Laryngology and Otology* 1999; **113**: 241–3.

50. Kim A, Wu H-G, Heo D-S *et al.* Advanced hypopharyngeal carcinoma treatment results according to treatment modalities. *Head and Neck* 2001; **23**: 713–17.

♦ 51. Lorenz RR, Alam DS. The increasing use of enteral flaps in reconstruction for the upper aerodigestive tract. *Current Opinion in Otolaryngology and Head and Neck Surgery* 2003; **11**: 230–5.

52. Makitie AA, Beasley NJ, Neligan PC *et al.* Head and neck reconstruction with anterolateral thigh flap. *Otolaryngology and Head and Neck Surgery* 2003; **129**: 547–55.

53. Martins AS. Gastric tansposition for pharyngo-laryngo-oesophogeal cancer: the Unicamp Experience. *Journal of Laryngology and Otology* 2000; **114**: 682–9.

54. Scharpf J, Esclamado RM. Reconstruction with radial forearm flaps after ablative surgery for hypopharyngeal cancer. *Head and Neck* 2003; **25**: 261–6.

55. Schilling WK, Eichenberger M, Maurer CA *et al.* Long-term survival of patients with stage IV hypopharyngeal cancer: impact of fundus rotation gastroplasty. *World Journal of Surgery* 2002; **26**: 561–5.

56. Wei WI, Lam LK, Yuen PW, Wong J. Current status of pharyngo-laryngo-esophogectomy and pharyngo-gastric anastomosis. *Head and Neck* 1998; **20**: 240–4.

57. Yamamoto Y, Sugihara T. Reconstruction following total laryngo-pharyngo-oesophogectomy and extensive resection of the superior mediastinum: an update. *Plastic and Reconstructive Surgery* 2003; **111**: 828–30.

♦ 58. Patel RS, Gilbert RW. Utility of the gastro-omental free flap in head and neck reconstruction. *Current Opinion in Otolaryngology and Head and Neck Surgery* 2009; **17**: 258–62.

♦ 59. Clark JR, de Almeida J, Gilbert R *et al.* Primary and salvage (hypo) pharyngectomy: analysis and outcome. *Head and Neck* 2006; **28**: 671–7.

60. Chu P-Y, Chang S-Y. Reconstruction after resection of hypopharyngeal carcinoma: comparison of the postoperative complications and oncologic results of different methods. *Head and Neck* 2005; **27**: 901–8.

61. Wei WI, Lam KH, Lau WF *et al.* Salvagable mediastinal problems in pharyngo-laryngo-esophagectomy and pharyngo-gastric anastemosis. *Head and Neck Surgery* 1988; **10**: S60–8.

62. Gurunathan RK, Panda NK, Das A, Karuppiah S. Thyroid gland in carcinoma of the larynx and hypopharynx: analysis of factors indicating thyroidectomy. *Journal of Otolaryngology and Head and Neck Surgery* 2008; **37**: 435–9.

63. Chang DW, Hussussian C, Lewin JS *et al.* Analysis of pharyngocutaneous fistula following free jejunal transfer for total laryngopharyngectomy. *Plastic and Reconstructive Surgery* 2002; **109**: 1522–7.

♦ 64. Gender EM, Rinaldo A, Shaha AR *et al.* Pharyngocutaneous fistula following laryngectomy. *Acta Otolaryngologica* 2004; **124**: 117–20.

65. Saunders MW, Murty GE, Bradley PJ. Pharyngeal pouch carcinoma. *ENT Journal* 1993; **72**: 149–50.

66. Laing MR, Murthy P, Ah-See KW, Cockburn JS. Surgery for pharyngeal pouch: audit of management with short and long-term follow up. *Journal of the Royal College of Surgeons of Edinburgh* 1995; **40**: 315–18.

67. Siddiq MA, Sood S. Current management in pharyngeal pouch surgery by UK otorhinolaryngologists. *Annals of the Royal College of Surgeons of England* 2004; **86**: 247–52.

♦ 68. Bradley PJ, Kochaar A, Quraishi MS. Pharyngeal pouch carcinoma: real or imaginary risks? *Annals of Otology, Rhinology and Laryngology* 1999; **108**: 1027–32.

● 69. Acharya A, Jennings S, Douglas S *et al.* Carcinoma arising in a pharyngeal pouch previously treated by endoscopic stapling. *Laryngoscope* 2006; **116**: 1043–5.

70. Garden AS, Morrison WH, Clayman GL *et al.* Early squamous cell carcinoma of the hypopharynx: outcomes of treatment with radiation alone to the primary disease. *Head and Neck* 1996; **18**: 317–22.

71. Godballe C, Jorgensen K, Hansen O, Bastholt L. Hypopharyngeal cancer: results of treatment based on radiation therapy and salvage therapy. *Laryngoscope* 2002; **112**: 834–8.

♦ 72. Pignon JP, Bourhis J, Domenge C, Designe L. Chemotherapy added to locoregional treatment for head and neck squamous-cell carcinoma: three meta-analyses of updated individual data. MACH-NC Collaborative Group. Meta-analysis of Chemotherapy on Head and Neck Cancer. *Lancet* 2000; **355**: 949–55.

73. Lefebvre JL, Chevalier D, Luboinski B *et al.* Larynx preservation in pyriform sinus cancer: preliminary results of a European Organization for Research and Treatment of Cancer phase III trial. EORTC Head and Neck Cancer Cooperative Group. *Journal of the National Cancer Institute* 1996; **88**: 890–9.

74. Forastiere AA, Goepfert H, Maor M *et al.* Concurrent chemotherapy and radiotherapy for organ preservation in advanced laryngeal cancer. *New England Journal of Medicine* 2003; **349**: 2091–8.

75. Winiquist E, Oliver T, Gilbert R. Postoperative chemoradiotherapy for advanced squamous cell carcinoma of the head and neck: a systematic review with meta-analysis. *Head and Neck* 2007; **29**: 38–46.

● 76. Takes RP, Strojan P, Silver CE *et al.* Current trends in initial management of hypopharyngeal cancer: the declining use of open surgery. *Head and Neck* 2010 Nov 10 [Epub ahead of print].

77. Bonner JA, Harari PM, Giralt J et al. Radiotherapy plus cetuximab for squamous-cell carcinoma of the head and neck. New England Journal of Medicine 2006; 354: 567–78.

● 78. Wang CJ, Kneckt R. Current concepts of organ preservation in head and neck cancer. European Archives of Otorhinolaryngology 2011; 268: 481–7.

79. Cancer Care Ontario Initiative, Practice Guidelines. Accelerated radiotherapy for locally advanced squamous cell carcinoma of the head and neck. Toronto: Cancer Care Ontario, 2002. Available from: www.cancercare.on.ca.

80. Pracy P, Laughran S, Parmar S et al. Hypopharyngeal cancer. In: Roland NJ, Palerie V (eds). Head and neck cancer: multidisciplinary management guidelines, 4th edn. London: ENTUK, 2011.

81. Byers RM, Clayman GL, Guillamondequi OM et al. Resection of advanced cervical metastasis prior to definitive radiotherapy for primary squamous carcinomas of the upper aerodigestive tract. Head and Neck 1992; 14: 133–8.

82. Andrade RS, Heron DE, Degirmenci B et al. Post-treatment assessment of response using FDG-PET/CT for patients treated with definitive radiation therapy for head and neck cancers. International Journal of Radiation Oncology, Biology, Physics 2006; 65: 1315–22.

83. Kutler DI, Wong RJ, Schoder H, Kraus DH. The current status of positron-emission tomography scanning in the evaluation and follow-up of patients with head and neck cancer. Current Opinion in Otolaryngology and Head and Neck Surgery 2006; 14: 73–81.

◆ 84. Malik T, Bruce I, Cherry J. Surgical complications of treacheo-oesophageal puncture and speech valves. Current Opinion in Otolaryngology and Head and Neck Surgery 2007; 15: 117–22.

85. Ahmad I, Kumar BN, Radford K et al. Surgical voice restoration following ablative surgery for laryngeal and hypopharyngeal carcinoma. Journal of Laryngology and Otology 2000; 114: 522–5.

86. Lewin JS, Barringer DA, May AH et al. Functional outcomes after circumferential pharyngoesophageal reconstruction. Laryngoscope 2005; 115: 1266–71.

87. Benazzo M, Occhini A, Rossi V et al. Jejunum free flap in hypopharynx reconstruction: case series. BMC Cancer 2002; 2: 13.

88. Temam S, Janot F, Germain M et al. Functional results with advanced hypopharyngeal carcinoma treated with circular near total pharyngolaryngectomy and jejunal free-flap repair. Head and Neck 2006; 28: 8–14.

89. Clark JR, Gilbert R, Irish J et al. Morbidity after flap reconstruction of hypopharyngeal defects. Laryngoscope 2006; 116: 173–81.

90. Andrades P, Pehier SF, Baranano CF et al. Fistula analysis after radial forearm free flap reconstruction of hypopharyngeal defects. Laryngoscope 2008; 118: 1157–63.

● 91. Treister N, Sonis S. Mucositis: biology and management. Current Opinion in Otolaryngology and Head and Neck Surgery 2007; 15: 123–9.

92. Trotti A, Bell LA, Epstein JB et al. Mucositis, incidence, severity and associated outcomes in patients with head and neck cancers receiving radiotherapy with or without chemotherapy: a systematic literature review. Radiotherapy and Oncology 2003; 66: 253–62.

93. Logermann JA, Rademaker AW, Pauloski BR et al. Site of disease and treatment protocol as correlates of swallowing function in patients with head and neck cancer treated with chemoradiation. Head and Neck 2006; 28: 64–73.

94. Nguyen NP, Frank C, Moltz CC et al. Impact of dysphagia on quality of life after treatment of head and neck cancer. International Journal of Radiation Oncology, Biology, Physics 2005; 61: 772–8.

95. Nguyen NP, Moltz CC, Frank C et al. Severity and duration of chronic dysphagia following treatment of head and neck cancer. Anticancer Research 2005; 25: 2929–34.

96. Nguyen NP, Moltz CC, Frank C et al. Evolution of chronic dysphagia following treatment for head and neck cancer. Oral Oncology 2006; 42: 374–80.

◆ 97. Nguyen NP, Smith HJ, Sallah S. Evaluation and management of swallowing dysfunction following chemoradiation for head and neck cancer. Current Opinion in Otolaryngology and Head and Neck Surgery 2007; 15: 130–3.

98. Sesterhenn AM, Muller HH, Weigand S et al. Cancer of the oro- and hypopharynx – when to expect recurrences? Acta Otolaryngologica 2008; 128: 925–9.

99. Hall SF, Groome PA, Irish J, O'Sullivan B. The natural history of patients with squamous cell carcinoma of the hypopharynx. Laryngoscope 2008; 118: 1362–71.

FURTHER READING

Delaere P. Reconstruction of the cervical aerodigestive tract. Brussels: Leuven University Press, 2006.

Wei WI, Sham J. Cancer of the larynx and hypopharynx. Oxford: Isis Medical Media, 2000.

Larynx

KENNETH MACKENZIE AND HISHAM MEHANNA

It is not the years in your life but the life in your years that counts.

Adlai Stevenson

INTRODUCTION

Laryngeal cancer is the eighteenth most common cancer in the UK. It has an incidence of 6.2 per 100 000 males and 1.3 per 100 000 females, resulting in approximately 1800 cases a year.[1] In recent years, there has been a small decrease in incidence, seen in males only. Incidence is strongly related to age, and is rare before 40 years of age. Laryngeal cancer incidence also has a strong socioeconomic association, being twice as common in the more deprived groups compared to the more affluent groups. There is also a wide geographic variation, being highest in Scotland and the north of England, mirroring the socioeconomic profiles. A recent comparison of head and neck audits involving more than 4000 patients in Scotland and south and west England found that there was significantly more laryngeal cancer presenting at an advanced stage in Scotland than south and west England.[2]

Tobacco smoking and alcohol are the main risk factors for laryngeal cancer, and their effects are synergistic.[3] Smoking is the main risk factor for glottic cancers, whereas alcohol appears to be the bigger risk factor for supraglottic tumours. Recently, a large study has shown the relative contributions of smoking and alcohol to the risk of head and neck cancer in the population. This shows that the population attributable risk is multiplicative and is 89 per cent for laryngeal cancer; being almost half due to tobacco alone and half due to tobacco and alcohol combined, and a small percentage due to alcohol alone.[4]

Within the larynx, tumours may arise from the vocal cords (glottic), superior to the vocal cords (supraglottic), or from below the vocal cords (subglottic). This subclassification of site of origin is historical but serves to allow comparison of tumours between individuals as part of the 'TNM' classification (see **Table 33.1**). In practical terms, however, in all but the very early stage tumours the allocation of a tumour to a subsite is highly subjective. Tumours do not adhere to subsites and indeed the definition of most T2 stages and beyond involve two subsites or more. Definition of the site of origin is subjective and is generally concluded at initial examination without the benefit of detailed imaging. Despite this, it is of value to allocate an index primary site to allow relevant discussion in the patient's management.

The most common site is glottis (approximately 49 per cent) followed by supraglottis (16 per cent). Eighty-five per cent of tumours are squamous carcinomas.

In recent years, there has been a significant change in the philosophy behind the treatment of laryngeal cancer. Previously, radiotherapy was the mainstay of treatment for most early and low volume tumours, and total laryngectomy for advanced disease. Partial laryngectomy was performed in a few selected cases in a few specialist centres. Increasing application and popularization of endoscopic resection techniques and organ preservation strategies, coupled with improvement and increased availability of imaging techniques, such as PET scanning, has resulted in a considerable

Table 33.1 T categories for laryngeal cancers from UICC: TNM classification of malignant tumours.[34]

Larynx	
Supraglottis	
T1	One subsite, normal mobility
T2	Mucosa of more than one adjacent subsite of supraglottis or glottis or adjacent region outside the supraglottis; without fixation
T3	Cord fixation or invades postcricoid area, pre-epiglottic tissues, paraglottic space, thyroid cartilage erosion
T4a	Through thyroid cartilage; trachea, soft tissues of neck: deep/extrinsic muscle of tongue, strap muscles, thyroid, oesophagus
T4b	Prevertebral space, mediastinal structures, carotid artery
Glottis	
T1	Limited to vocal cord(s), normal mobility
T1a	One cord
T1b	Both cords
T2	Supraglottis, subglottis, impaired cord mobility
T3	Cord fixation, paraglottis space, thyroid cartilage erosion
T4a	Through thyroid cartilage; trachea, soft tissues of neck: deep/extrinsic muscle of tongue, strap muscles, thyroid, oesophagus
T4b	Prevertebral space, mediastinal structures, carotid artery
Subglottis	
T1	Limited to subglottis
T2	Extends to vocal cord(s) with normal/impaired mobility
T3	Cord fixation
T4a	Through cricoid or thyroid cartilage; trachea, soft tissues of neck: deep/extrinsic muscle of tongue, strap muscles, thyroid, oesophagus
T4b	Prevertebral space, mediastinal structures, carotid artery

change in approach to management considerations by head and neck multidisciplinary teams.

Previous treatment strategies resulted in overall survival of approximately 84 per cent at one year, 64 per cent at five years and 54 per cent at 10 years.[5] This is an increase of 3.3 per cent every five years since the 1980s, and is mainly due to improvement in survival of affluent groups.

SURGICAL ANATOMY

The principal bony and cartilaginous structures in the larynx are the hyoid bone, thyroid cartilage, the cricoid cartilage and the trachea, each being attached to the surrounding structures. Within the larynx are the arytenoids, positioned on the cricoid, and the epiglottis. The cartilages, with the exception of the epiglottis, may have degrees of differential ossification. These structures are further interconnected by a series of membranes, ligaments and muscles with whole assembly being covered by an overlying epithelium (**Figures 33.1, 33.2 and 33.3**).

It is from this epithelium that dedifferentiation may occur and result in an invasive tumour. The epithelium within the

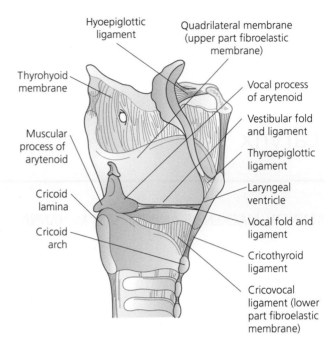

Figure 33.1 Sagittal section across the larynx looking laterally.

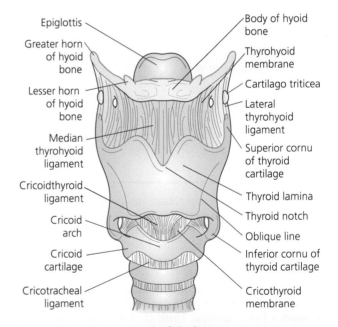

Figure 33.2 The framework of the larynx.

larynx is respiratory in nature, pseudostratified columnar epithelium, and squamous in other regions. The areas within the larynx most susceptible to change are the glottic and supraglottic structures, as these are the areas most likely to be exposed to the aetiological co-carcinogens of smoking and, to a lesser extent, alcohol.

The larynx develops from the respiratory and upper digestive tracts. The supraglottic region is derived from arches II and IV (buccopharyngeal anlage) and the glottic and subglottic regions from the VIth arch (respiratory). Effectively, the division between the respiratory and digestive tracts occurs

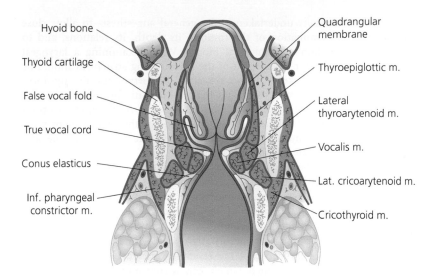

Hyoid bone

Thyoid cartilage

False vocal fold

True vocal cord

Conus elasticus

Inf. pharyngeal constrictor m.

Quadrangular membrane

Thyroepiglottic m.

Lateral thyroarytenoid m.

Vocalis m.

Lat. cricoarytenoid m.

Cricothyroid m.

Figure 33.3 Coronal section through the larynx looking anteriorly.

laterally in the ventricle. It is widely regarded that the vocal folds anteriorly and laterally act as the point of division of lymphatic drainage and as such have very little lymphatic drainage themselves. With such a clear division of origin, regional lymphatic drainage is clearly demarcated, namely:

- supraglottis – via superior laryngeal vessels to levels II and III;
- anterior glottis and subglottis – through cricothyroid ligament anteriorly to level VI and laterally to level IV;
- posterior glottis and subglottis – through cricotracheal membrane to the paratracheal nodes in level VI and laterally to level IV.

Chijiwa *et al.*[6] describe the importance of paraglottic or cricoid involvement in patients with glottic carcinoma and the significantly increased occurrence of lymph node metastases in this group.

PRESENTATION

The cardinal symptom of laryngeal cancer presentation is hoarseness. There is not any particular type of hoarseness which is more indicative of cancer than a benign aetiology. However, the hoarseness is frequently persistent with resumption of a normal voice occurring extremely rarely. With increasing size of an intralaryngeal lesion, vocal cord mobility may be reduced with a subsequent breathy component to the voice. As the volume of the tumour increases, less of the laryngeal airway remains patent. This increases turbulence, and stridor ensues. Associated symptoms may include dysphagia, choking attacks, odynophagia, otalgia and weight loss.

DIAGNOSIS

Clinical examination

In a patient presenting with hoarseness, visualization and assessment of their larynx while they are awake is essential.

This is generally carried out in the outpatient setting, traditionally by indirect laryngoscopy using a mirror. Although this technique has almost universally been replaced by fibreoptic naso-laryngoscopy as the standard for laryngeal assessment, it may still be of value in assessing the tongue base or in those patients who cannot comply with nasal instrumentation.

Fibreoptic nasolaryngoscopy can be carried out following installation of topical local anaesthesia, such as co-phenylcaine, or without any anaesthesia using a lubricating gel. The advantage of fibreoptic nasolaryngoscopy is that the tongue base and posterior and lateral pharyngeal walls can be visualized and an impression of the pyriform fossa obtained, in addition to a detailed examination of the larynx. It is important to conclude the most likely subsite of origin of the index tumour. Thereafter, the extent of the tumour should be described in detail with particular regard to the laryngeal subsites. The tumour area is effectively a surrogate for a volume assessment, which is confirmed by subsequent computed tomography (CT) scanning or magnetic resonance imaging (MRI). An accurate commentary on the macroscopic appearance of tumour involvement of the subsites allows provisional T stage categorization, although this will be confirmed later at examination under general anaesthesia.

The main advantage, however, is in the assessment of the mobility of the vocal cord, which is pivotal in the determining T staging. It is important that this is carried out in a fully awake patient, as it is inaccurate if carried out in a sedated patient, for example when awakening from general anaesthesia. Mobility is categorized into fully mobile, reduced mobility, or fixed. This assessment can sometimes be difficult due to the vocal cord being obscured by the tumour mass.

Videostroboscopy is not an essential part of examination, but it may have a role in early stage lesions. The detail of the vocal cords can be highlighted with the use of the rigid endoscope. Subtle movement deficits within the vocal cords may then be elucidated by using the videostroboscopic function. The theory is that as the malignancy involves more structures of the larynx, the dysfunction of the vocal cord will increase, culminating in complete involvement of the intralaryngeal musculature with marked reduction in the movement, or fixation, of the vocal cord. The advantage of this instrumentation is that intralaryngeal detail can be recorded, and is of specific relevance when contemplating partial laryngeal surgery either by an endoscopic or external approach.

Imaging

The main imaging modality for staging the larynx is CT scanning. Usually, it is used to complement direct examination of the larynx when staging laryngeal cancers. Fine slice CT scanning provides a detailed impression of the extent of the tumour, in particular the inferior extension, invasion of the paraglottic and pre-epiglottic spaces and/or extension through the thyroid cartilage to the paralaryngeal soft tissues. It can also identify possible nodal metastases. Extending scanning down to the chest will also identify abnormalities in the lung, the most common site of distant metastases and second primary tumours in this patient group.

It should be noted that MRI has a better sensitivity, but less specificity, for laryngeal cartilage invasion.[7] Therefore, when there is concern about invasion of the laryngeal cartilages, an MRI scan may provide additional useful information. A further indication for the use of MRI is concern about involvement of the tongue base.

Ideally, scanning should be performed before examination under anaesthesia as the manipulation of the tumour and the larynx by direct laryngoscopy may result in inflammatory changes around the tumour, with the possibility of upstaging of the tumour.

When assessing imaging of a laryngeal tumour, consideration should be given to the following:

- the subsites involved, including extension across the mid line, and the approximate volume;
- paraglottic and pre-epiglottic space extension, as this can upstage the tumour;
- laryngeal cartilage invasion – especially the outer cartilage invasion, which upstages the tumour to T4. It can sometimes be difficult to be certain if this has occurred, because of differential ossification of the thyroid cartilage. In general, the only way of concluding that there is unequivocal invasion is if there is tumour lateral to, i.e. 'outside', the thyroid cartilage;
- the subglottis and anterior subglottic wedge which can be particularly involved in anterior commissure tumours, and may result in upstaging the tumour significantly;
- an examination of pyriform fossae and postcricoid region should also be made;
- tongue base involvement;
- assessment of the neck, including the central compartment (level 6), for nodal metastases.

If there is any suspicion of lymph node involvement then this can be confirmed, or refuted, by ultrasound scanning with sampling by fine needle aspiration cytology or core biopsy as appropriate.

Examination by microlaryngoscopy

Once a laryngeal lesion is identified, a full examination of the larynx and surrounding sites is necessary for staging. This is usually undertaken under general anaesthesia to allow close examination of the tumour, its depth, its relations, and to obtain a histological biopsy. When examining a laryngeal tumour, assessment of the surrounding structures should be undertaken. This is especially important for the pyriform fossae and postcricoid region. Tumour can extend through the aryepiglottic folds into these sites, resulting in an upstaging of the tumour and a change of the management plan. Assessment of the extension into the base of tongue and vallecula should also be made.

The ideal form of anaesthesia allows examination of each of the subsites while at the same time maintaining the delivery of the anaesthetic gaseous agents. When examining all aspects of the larynx, including the subglottis, it is best to use a Venturi type of delivery of entrained air and an appropriate microlaryngoscope. There are many types of microlaryngoscope but essentially they are of a design with a proximal lumen which can accommodate the many and varied microlaryngeal instruments and with a distal lumen which sits in the supraglottic larynx displaying the appropriate mucosal surfaces of the larynx. The illumination is fibreoptic and delivered distally. One such laryngoscope is the 'Dedo' laryngoscope (Pilling) which satisfies the above criteria very well and is currently in regular clinical use.

Due to patient anatomical issues such as the length of their neck, and upper dentition, it is not always possible to visualize all areas of each of the subsites of the larynx. It is mandatory to achieve this in patients in whom there is a clinically obvious lesion or in whom there is a high level of suspicion. To obtain this, an anterior commissure laryngoscope is used. This scope must be available for all microlaryngoscopy cases, as it may be the only method of intubating a patient with a large laryngeal lesion, and can often obviate the need for a surgical tracheostomy, especially in the emergency situation. The key features of this type of laryngoscope are that it is smaller in each of the main dimensions of the laryngoscope. Namely, it is shorter and narrower but of a similar shape. This allows the laryngoscope to be positioned through a gap in the upper dentition, or gain access to the supraglottis in prominent dentition. The difficulty with it is the diameter of the proximal end, which does not allow ease of use of the microlaryngeal instruments. This is even more problematic when trying to use the CO_2 laser through it, the difficulty on this occasion being the alignment of the laser beam onto the target area. A further problem is the use of the Venturi system with this laryngoscope as it is not possible to fix it to the laryngoscope as the surgical access is then obscured. To allow access in the non-laser cases, fine bore laryngeal intubation can be used with a system attached to the insufflator. The tube sits in the posterior commissure and allows near total access to all parts of the larynx. An example of this type of tube is a Hunsakker tube, which has the added advantage of having a portal through which to measure the patient's CO_2 levels. It is imperative, however, that a CO_2 laser is not used if there is any kind of endotracheal tube in the airway other than a specified laser tube.

Irrespective of the instrument used, each laryngeal subsite must be inspected thoroughly. It is best to start by identifying if there is an obvious lesion. The ventricle, false cords and the remainder of the supraglottis must be examined, and may present difficulties for examination. This may require retraction of the false cords with examination of all aspects of the ventricle. The most difficult area to obtain a complete assessment is the laryngeal surface of the epiglottis, and in particular the petiole. The reason for this is the introduction of the endoscope which obscures the area. To overcome this difficulty, the endoscope should be introduced to the level of the anterior commissure and then withdrawn slowly, gradually exposing the mucosal surface of the petiole and laryngeal surface of the epiglottis.

When a tumour is present, it is necessary to map it out carefully in relation to all of the areas of the larynx and surrounding structures. It is best to start by deciding (estimating) from where the tumour has originated. This is known as the index primary site. Although it is of importance for reference for treatment and epidemiological reasons, in high volume tumours it can be difficult to determine the epicentre of the tumour. On some occasions, this is not possible and the tumour is registered as 'indeterminate'.

Having established the index site, the involvement of all the surrounding structures is noted in detail. This should be considered in all directions within the larynx with attention paid to the subglottis, particularly anteriorly, the anterior commissure, the ventricles, and the petiole and all areas of the supraglottis. The tumour extension out with the larynx is then described – the most commonly involved areas being the aryepiglottic fold into the pyriform fossa, the epiglottis into the vallecula, and the subglottis into the trachea.

To examine these areas comprehensively, telescopes should be used. Hopkins rods are a form of telescope which can be coupled to a video camera system to allow accurate recording of the tumour. The optical system uses angles of 0, 30 and 70 degrees to allow differing perspectives of the laryngeal subsites. They are of particular value in the glottis, subglottis and ventricle. The 70 degree telescope is invaluable in early laryngeal malignancy, particularly if endoscopic resection, with or without, the CO_2 laser, is planned. It allows accurate assessment of the volume of the lesion and its position on the glottis, thereby allowing accurate planning and resection of the tumour while preserving as much of the laryngeal structures as possible.

Using the camera, linked to the telescope, the lesion can be digitally recorded and reproduced for informed discussion at clinicopathological and multidisciplinary team meetings. This ensures that all health care professionals in the MDT are able to appreciate the extent of the tumour, and acts as a focus when discussing further management. It is advisable to attach a 'hard copy' of the photo of the lesion as a permanent record in the patient's case notes. Photos can also be attached to the pathology request form.

PRINCIPLES OF MANAGEMENT OF LARYNGEAL CANCER

The management of laryngeal cancer depends in the first instance on the stage at presentation. However, a variety of other factors are also involved in the decision-making, including the patient's age, comorbidities, surgical access issues, the skills and preferences of the treating multidisciplinary team and, importantly, the wishes of the patient.

Early laryngeal cancer

For T1 N0 and T2 N0 lesions, the options for treatment are mainly radiotherapy or transoral endolaryngeal surgery. For a small number of patients, there is the option, or need, for open partial laryngeal surgery. This is now undertaken infrequently following the introduction of transoral endolaryngeal laser surgery.

It should be noted that there have been no direct comparisons of the efficacy of the two main treatment modalities, radiotherapy and endoscopic laryngeal surgery. However, on examining the literature, including cohort studies, they appear to have very similar cure rates. For example, Moreau[8] reported on a review of the literature on CO_2 laser surgery for T1 and T2 glottic squamous cell carcinomas (SCCs). They found a 6.5 per cent recurrence rate in the series of 400 cases; 10 out of the 26 recurrences required total laryngectomy with an overall survival rate of 99 per cent. Ambrosh et al.[9] reported on a series of 48 cases of supraglottic stage 1 and stage 2 SCCs, demonstrating a five-year control rate of 100 per cent for T1 tumours, and 89 per cent for T2 tumours, and a five-year recurrence-free survival of 86 per cent. Similarly, many radiotherapy cohort studies report excellent success rates for early laryngeal cancer.[10]

There are relative advantages and disadvantages for each of the modalities. For endolaryngeal surgery, advantages include treatment in a single sitting, minimal absence from employment, certainty of removal of the specimen and the ability to assess margins surgically. Importantly, it also allows further laryngeal surgery or radiotherapy in case of recurrence. The disadvantage of transoral laser surgery is that it can affect the voice quality and access is sometimes difficult. It is also requires a general anaesthetic, and may need repeated operations, for which patients may not be fit.

The main advantage of radiotherapy is that it is potentially achievable in patients with poor reserve. In addition, it has been thought to have better voice outcomes. This hypothesis is based on the principle that the laryngeal structures are being 'preserved'. The flaw to this is that at the time of presentation the laryngeal structures will already have been destroyed to a certain extent by the malignant process. In addition, radiotherapy is in itself a radical treatment so it will have a deleterious effect on the structures. To date, definitive comparison of voice outcomes between the two treatment methods has not yet been possible. However, a study has shown that quality of life outcomes for the two modalities appear to be similar.[11]

While reported control rates after open partial laryngeal surgery for small tumours are probably as good as the other modalities, there is only a very limited role for open partial surgery for T1 and small T2 tumours. This is because the approach carries more morbidity with poorer outcomes than transoral laser surgery. Its only conceivable role would be for a patient whose access transorally is not possible, and who has refused radiotherapy. In addition, there may also be a limited role in low volume recurrences following radiotherapy.[12] Due to the small numbers of cases being performed, these operations should be undertaken by someone with specialized interest in open partial surgery.

Advanced laryngeal cancer

The main options for the treatment of advanced laryngeal cancer currently are total laryngectomy or chemoradiotherapy. Other options used less commonly include partial open laryngectomy, near total laryngectomy and laser CO_2 transoral surgery.

LARYNGECTOMY

The first total laryngectomy was reportedly carried out in 1873 by Billroth. Since then, it has been the standard by which other treatments are compared. This is because it results in excellent local and regional control of the cancer. However, it results in considerable effects on voice production and communication, as well as resulting in psychological effects due to disfigurement and the production of an end stoma. This has led to the development of organ preservation treatments. Interestingly however, some cross-sectional studies have shown no difference in the quality of life between patients who have had total laryngectomy and those who have had radiotherapy or conservation surgery.[13, 14] This suggests that any treatment of advanced laryngeal surgery considerably affects the function and overall quality of life of patients.

OPEN PARTIAL LARYNGECTOMY AND TRANSORAL LASER SURGERY

Other surgical options for the treatments of advanced laryngeal cancer include open partial laryngectomy, near total laryngectomy and laser CO_2 transoral surgery. These techniques are not suitable for the majority of advanced laryngeal patients. However, they do have an important role in selected patients with selected pathologies such as liposarcomas or neuroendocrine tumours.

Options include partial and supracricoid laryngectomy for certain moderately sized (T2 and small T3) primary or recurrent tumours involving one half of the larynx or for those limited to the supraglottis, with no paraglottic space involvement respectively. Laccourreye et al. reported on 21 T2–T4 laryngeal SCCs treated with supracricoid partial laryngectomy, with a local control rate of 95 per cent and a laryngeal function preservation rate of 90 per cent over five years.[15] In addition, CO_2 laser transoral surgery has also been used for advanced laryngeal and hypopharyngeal squamous cell carcinomas. For example, Iro et al.[16] reported a series of 141 supraglottic carcinomas, eight of which were T3 and T4 – over 50 per cent of whom also received postoperative radiotherapy. He reported a five-year disease-free survival of 75 per cent for stage 3 and 45 per cent for stage 4.[16] Steiner et al. reported on 96 stage 3 and 4 hypopharyngeal SCCs with five-year overall survival of 37 per cent.[17]

However, it should be noted that the above management options are not standard treatment options, and that they need to be recommended within the context of a multidisciplinary team discussion. Furthermore, these operations should only be carried out by surgeons experienced in conservation laryngeal surgery. Such cases should be referred to regional centres and nominated surgeons to ensure that there are surgeons who are performing adequate numbers of such operations.

LARYNGEAL PRESERVATION CHEMORADIOTHERAPY

The first generation of larynx preservation chemotherapy trials appeared in the 1990s, and randomized patients into surgery and radiotherapy or to induction chemotherapy cycles of cisplatin/5FU. Patients who responded to chemotherapy then received radiotherapy, with possible salvage surgery. If they did not respond to the chemotherapy, they received surgery and postoperative radiotherapy. Generally, the results of these studies showed no significant difference in survival between the two treatment arms. The larynx was preserved in 56 per cent of patients undergoing the experimental chemoradiotherapy arm.[18]

In 2000, Pignon et al.[19] published a meta-analysis of the first generation of laryngeal preservation chemoradiotherapy trials. In the main, they included T3 laryngeal and hypopharyngeal cancers. There was no statistically significant difference in overall survival. However, it is important to note that there was a trend to benefit from surgery (hazard ratio 1.19 intervals 0.97–1.46). Surgery $\pm$ radiotherapy resulted in overall survival of 45 per cent compared to an overall survival from chemoradiotherapy of 39 per cent. On the other hand, 56 per cent of those who survived with chemoradiotherapy managed to avoid laryngectomy, giving an overall laryngectomy survival rate of 23 per cent at five years. Patients treated with chemoradiotherapy had almost double the local recurrence rate, but less distant metastases than the patients treated with surgery. Analysis of laryngeal cancer patients separately from hypopharyngeal cancer patients showed that laryngeal cancer patients in the surgical arm demonstrated a risk reduction of 32 per cent. This suggests that advanced laryngeal tumours would be better treated with surgery than chemoradiotherapy. On the other hand, hypopharyngeal cancer patients showed no difference in survival between the two modalities of treatment.

Furthermore, the meta-analysis showed that the overall survival benefit from chemotherapy in addition to radiotherapy was 4 per cent at five years. Concomitant chemotherapy resulted in an 8 per cent overall survival benefit, compared to a 4 per cent overall survival benefit from neoadjuvant chemoradiotherapy. Adjuvant chemoradiotherapy resulted in no overall survival benefit. These findings have resulted in the adoption of concomitant chemoradiotherapy as the standard regimen for delivery of chemotherapy when treating laryngeal and pharyngeal cancers. Recently, an update of this meta-analysis confirmed an overall survival effect of 6.5 per cent for concomitant chemoradiotherapy.[20]

The second generation of laryngeal preservation trials were published in 2003.[21] The RTOG 91-11 trials showed that both concomitant and neo-adjuvant chemoradiotherapy with cisplatin resulted in no statistically significant differences in survival compared to radiotherapy alone. However, laryngeal preservation was highest with concomitant chemoradiotherapy (84 per cent) compared to neo-adjuvant chemoradiotherapy (72 per cent) and radiotherapy alone (67 per cent). On the other hand, concomitant chemoradiotherapy resulted in significantly worse acute toxicity compared to induction and chemotherapy and radiotherapy alone.

Third generation organ preservation trials have now started reporting. They show that the addition of doxitacel to standard induction chemoradiotherapy with cisplatin and 5-fluorouracil results in significantly higher survival rates.

More studies are required to prove the superiority of these enhanced induction regimens compared to standard concomitant cisplatin regimens.[22, 23]

It should also be noted that oncological alternatives to chemoradiotherapy also exist. A meta-analysis by Bourhis et al.[24] in the Lancet in 2006 showed that hyper-fractionation and accelerated fractionation without total dose reduction results in better local regional control compared to radiotherapy alone. These altered regimens can be used in patients who would not tolerate chemotherapy.

Laryngeal preservation strategies are clearly an attractive option. However, the concept of organ preservation is not clearly defined. There has been little research into what constitutes a preserved larynx. From an oncological perspective, the effects of the therapy are generally reported by assessing the local toxic effects, such as mucositis and xerostomia. Although this level of toxicity is used to compare various therapeutic regimes, it should not be regarded as the sole assessment of organ preservation. Organ preservation is not merely the presence of the organ in situ, but it also has to have useful function, however that might be defined. As such, an assessment of end organ function would be appropriate. This can be achieved relatively easily by using patient-centred, patient report questionnaires, addressing voice (VoiSS, VHI), swallowing (MD Anderson Dysphagia Inventory) and quality of life (University of Washington or FACT). This is of considerable importance and is an area of clinical research which needs to be addressed.

MANAGEMENT OF NODAL METASTASES

For early laryngeal cancer, the risk of metastases, especially for glottic cancer, is negligible. Therefore, the nodal basins are not treated electively, unless there is clinical evidence of metastases.

In advanced laryngeal tumours, there is a high risk of occult nodal metastases, of up to 60 per cent, especially when the supraglottis is involved. Therefore, in the N0 neck, the primary echelon nodes are treated electively either by radiotherapy or surgery. The risk of occult metastasis in a lesion confined to the glottis is only 10 per cent. Therefore, elective treatment for a N0 neck is not indicated for this subsite.

For the N1 neck, if treatment of the primary is by surgery, then treatment is by selective 2–4 neck dissection, followed by chemoradiotherapy where appropriate. If the primary is being treated by chemoradiotherapy, then treatment of the nodal metastases can also be performed by chemoradiotherapy followed by assessment of the neck.[25]

In advanced nodal disease (N2 and N3 disease), if the primary is being treated by surgery then a modified radical neck dissection should be performed with consideration of postoperative radiotherapy or chemoradiotherapy. Increasingly, some are carrying out selective neck dissections instead. If the primary is being treated by chemoradiotherapy, further treatment is controversial. The options are a neck dissection or treatment followed by assessment with a PET CT scan. Currently, a multicentre PET Neck trial is taking place in the UK examining this question.

DECISION-MAKING IN THE MANAGEMENT OF LARYNGEAL TUMOURS

It should be noted that there are multiple factors involved in decision-making process for treatment. These include:

- Tumour stage and characteristics: the presence of laryngeal cartilage invasion suggests the need for a laryngectomy. Nodal metastasis also affects the type of treatment required.
- Patient's comorbidity: patient comorbidity affects the degree to which they can be treated. Cardiac disease precludes the use of cisplatin and may mandate carboplatin or fractionated radiotherapy.
- Patient's lifestyle and social support network may also strongly affect the choice of treatment modality. Patients who require the use of their voice, e.g. for teaching or in meetings, may wish to have organ preservation treatment. Self-employed patients may choose laryngeal conservation surgery over radiotherapy for early laryngeal tumours due to the convenience of a shorter treatment course with less absence from work.
- The expertise of the treating centre can also affect the treatment that is offered. Some of the alternative surgical treatment options should not be offered by occasional operators.
- Finally, the patient's preference is of utmost importance. It should be noted that there may be up to a 70 per cent discordance between patients' and clinicians' preference in the decision on treatment modality, as demonstrated by List et al.[26]

SURGICAL TECHNIQUES

Principles of surgical treatment of an early suspicious laryngeal lesion

Diagnosis of the cause of an abnormality in the larynx, most frequently arising in the glottis, requires the acquisition of representative tissue while ensuring minimal damage to the underlying and surrounding structures of the larynx. This is a frequent challenge to the laryngologist.

In **Figure 33.4**, a lesion, suspicious of being malignant can be seen to be arising from the right vocal cord. Ideally, the surgical procedure would not only treat the lesion but would also ensure that there is a representative specimen for histological examination. The key considerations in this situation are the position and the volume of the tumour. Extreme care must be taken when the excision might involve the anterior commissure. Webbing can occur even when there has been very little damage to the contralateral mucosa. Such a result can affect voice quality considerably, as any significant degree of webbing will result in dysphonia. If the lesion is in the anterior two-thirds of the vocal cord, then once again care must be taken as excessive damage will result in deficiency in the vocal cord structure or scarring, with subsequent abnormality in its vibration.

The key is to carry out a dissection which will preserve the integrity of the vocal ligament. Furthermore, it must be possible to visualize the lateral margin and thereby achieve a

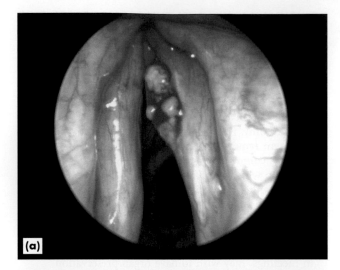

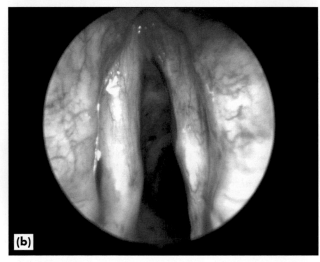

Figure 33.4 (a) T1A right vocal cord; (b) right vocal cord following excision of T1A.

dissection margin. If each of these criteria can be satisfied, then the lesion in its entirety can be excised with care. To achieve this is, it is necessary to use fine instrumentation, such as that produced by Bouchayeur (Microfrance). Some laryngologists use the technique of hydrodissection to delineate and facilitate the plane of dissection by injection of saline into the submucosal space, Reinke's space, thereby allowing the dissection to remain superficial to the vocal ligament.

In the majority of appropriate cases, however, dissection proceeds by incision of the mucosa either posteriorly or laterally to the lesion. This allows entry into Reinke's space, with microdissection of the lesion by freeing the tissue gently from the vocal ligament. Dissection is best achieved by anteromedial retraction of the lesion and extension of the lateral incision anteriorly, leaving a macroscopic 1 mm margin. Removal of the lesion is completed by excision of the mucosa anteriorly and in the inferomedial or subglottic aspect of the vocal cord. Haemostasis is achieved by placing one in 1000 adrenaline on a neurosurgical pattie on the excised area. Although there is very little absorption of adrenaline from this technique, unlike when it is in the

trachea, it is imperative that the anaesthetist is informed prior to its application.

Although initially used in these situations, the CO_2 laser has fallen from favour for excision of these suspicious lesions. This is mainly because it results in a large amount of 'diathermy artefact', which affects the histological examination. Furthermore, there is a risk of potential thermal damage to the residual vocal cord.

If it is not possible to carry out a definitive diagnostic and therapeutic excisional biopsy of the suspicious area, then representative tissue should be obtained from the lesion. The same principles apply in that the biopsy has to be taken from the specimen at an area which should have a minimal effect on the voice. The biopsies are taken from the most abnormal area(s) which may have been highlighted by its friability on contact bleeding. The most appropriate instrument to achieve this is usually cupped biopsy forceps. Crushing should be avoided by using a needle to manipulate the specimen when transferring the specimen to the histopathology container. Drying of the tissue should also be avoided so placement in formalin should not be delayed. An acceptable alternative to the cupped biopsy forceps would be 'cold steel' excision of part of the lesion.

Technique of endoscopic resection of an early laryngeal malignancy

The microlaryngeal assessment of the laryngeal lesion is carried out in a similar fashion to that described above for any suspicious laryngeal lesion. Once SCC is confirmed on biopsy, the approach for resection is planned. The key assessment is the extension of the lesion into the various subsites as determined using a combination of microlaryngoscopic and telescopic techniques described previously and by imaging, generally CT scanning.

The lesion can be excised either by a conventional approach where it is removed by creating an excision margin around the circumference (**Figure 33.5a**) Alternatively, if this type of excision is not possible then it can be divided into sections (**Figure 33.5b**) and removed sequentially. The advantage of the first technique is that the specimen is removed en bloc and as such is easier to orientate in relation to the excision margins. The second technique tends to be used in bigger lesions or those that extend into various subsites and has the advantage of being able to assess the tumour depth during the procedure, thereby increasing the chance of achieving macroscopic margins. Sequential subdivision of the lesion into multiple sections can be carried out until excision is complete. The disadvantage is that there has to be accurate orientation and assessment of the tumour 'segments' which can be challenging even when the clinico-pathological team is experienced.

The technique will be described in relation to glottic lesions, although a very similar technique applies to supraglottic and subglottic lesions.

The patient is placed in a supine position, the general anaesthesia being delivered via an intravenous infusion, with muscle relaxant, and the patient being maintained oxygenated using a Venturi entrainment system. The most frequently used laryngoscope is the 'Dedo' laryngoscope, the

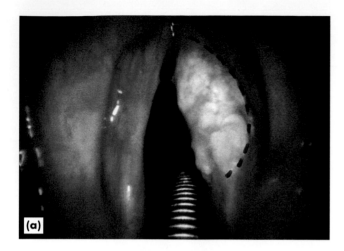

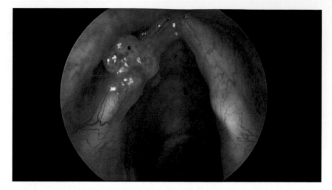

Figure 33.6 T1A left vocal cord viewed through 30° endoscope.

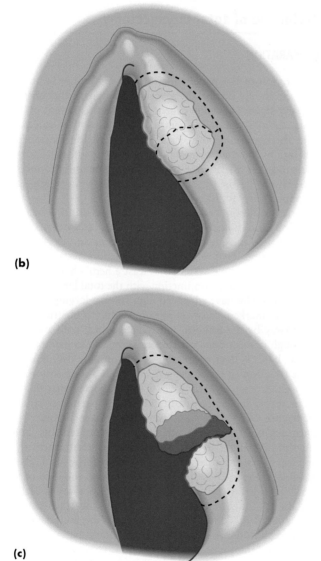

Figure 33.5 (a–c) T1A right vocal cord showing transtumour method of resection.

design of which is suitable because of the shape of the distal end in conjunction with the distal fibreoptic illumination. In patients who need repeated microlaryngoscopies, as in this

clinical situation, an individually manufactured laser mouth guard, which is laser resistant, should be used if possible. The laryngoscope is placed in the supraglottis, displaying all areas of the glottis. The laryngoscope is suspended with the larynx view maximized by applying pressure to the cricoid or fixing it with some adhesive tape. Updated photography with digital capture is carried out using 0, 30 and 70 degree Hopkins rods (**Figure 33.6**).

Having tested that the CO_2 laser system is functioning correctly, it is set at the optimal setting. This is often dot size of 1 mm, exposure time of 0.1 second, and a power of 5–10 watts, in a repeated mode. This can be modified by reducing the power or putting it onto single fire. The tumour is held using aspirating forceps and retracted medially. The laser incision commences posteriorly, or posterolaterally, the laser plume being aspirated through the aspirating forceps or through the aspirating portal on the laryngoscope. The dissection proceeds while maintaining at least a 1 mm margin. On occasion, it may not be possible to visualize the entire lesion and so to achieve this it may be necessary to remove the ipsilateral false cord, known as a ventriculotomy. This can be simply achieved by vapourizing the false cord, but care should be taken not to disrupt the surface appearances of the glottic lesion so that an accurate macroscopic resection can take place. Dissection proceeds from posterior to anterior, although one must be constantly aware of the three-dimensional perspective of the resection. The mucosal margin is relatively obvious and so therefore should be the maintenance of a 1 mm excision margin. Resection of the deep margin is more difficult. It can be judged by the appearance of the submucosal structures, which in the case of the true vocal cord, are the vocal ligament and the vocalis muscle. If there is any significant bleeding, this can be arrested by use of one of the bipolar systems. A disposable variety is that designed for intranasal use. Its end is fine enough for most bleeding points and is used in conjunction with a separate microlaryngeal metal suction. Alternatively, a combined suction monopolar diathermy, such as that produced by Steiner, could be used.

The problematic area during the dissection of the lesion is the anterior commissure. It is well recognized that there is a significant effect on the quality of voice if the endoscopic resection involves the anterior commissure. It is necessary to ensure that the anterior subglottis is resected adequately while ensuring that there is no unnecessary sacrifice of the anterior commissure mucosa.

Having completed the resection, it is useful to view the resection site by once again using the 0, 30 and 70 degree Hopkins rods. This ensures that the operator is satisfied with the macroscopic clearance and that there is no gross disease remaining. Furthermore, the photograph of the resection site facilitates discussion at the multidisciplinary team meeting.

Previously, 'standard' practice involved taking a series of samples for frozen section examination at selected areas around the resection site to ensure that the excision is complete. A useful way of recording the sites of these is to annotate a stylized larynx diagram and photograph it, with the clinical images, for clinicopathological discussion. However, there are difficulties using a frozen section strategy. First, there can be considerable difficulty with the histopathological processing of frozen section samples, not only because of the size but also with the difficulty in interpreting the cellular appearance following the thermal effects of the laser. Second, there is reluctance by surgeons to remove a large specimen for frozen section as it may compromise the quality of the postoperative voice. It is highly debatable as to whether there is significant value from frozen section assessment or whether it is a case of 'treating the surgeon'. At the UK consensus meeting on the endoscopic management of early laryngeal cancer it was concluded that the use of frozen sections was not required routinely.[27]

The resected specimen requires a detailed and accurate pathological assessment. The standard approach would be to 'pin the specimen' using a cork base and pins around the edge of the specimen. Unfortunately, this destroys the accuracy of the assessment of the margins. If no base is used, orientation is extremely difficult. This can be overcome by mounting the specimen on an organic mount which can be subsequently sectioned. A good example of this is to use dehydrated cucumber as the organic mount.[28]

The cucumber is prepared by removing the skin and cutting the cucumber into 5 mm thick transverse sections. The seeds are removed from the centre, leaving a triangular appearance with the sides of the 'triangle' being of the approximate dimensions of the vocal cords. The cucumber is then dehydrated by placing it in absolute alcohol for 24 hours and repeating the process for two further 24-hour periods. The cucumber is stored in absolute alcohol and can be removed as required. The specimen is mounted onto the cucumber using histoacryl tissue glue. To ensure correct histological orientation, the lateral border of the specimen is marked using black ink. Having been allowed to dry for a few minutes, the mounted specimen is placed in a container with standard formalin solution. Gross pathological assessment starts by photographing the gross specimen and mount and printing an A4 copy. This allows an accurate recording of where the transverse sections are made. The histopathological sections are examined sequentially and so an accurate map of the tumour and its margins can be made. By using the diagram, it is possible to delineate where there are 'near' or 'involved' margins. This allows targeted further resection to be carried out if necessary, achieving adequate margins while at the same time minimizing the amount of tissue resected and thus minimizing the effect on the patient's voice.

Once the patient has been discharged from hospital, voice therapy by speech and language therapists should be carried out. Close monitoring of the larynx is necessary and should be carried out every month for the first 12 months, looking for any recurrent, or persistent, intralaryngeal pathology or any change in the vocal cord mobility. Electively, there should be repeat microlaryngoscopy with detailed examination of the larynx under general anaesthesia, paying particular attention to any area or subsite which was of concern at the initial resection. There are no accepted guidelines about the frequency or timing of check microlaryngoscopy. It will depend on confidence of a clear margin at the initial histological examination and the level of suspicion in individual cases. If routine monitoring is to be carried out, then it should probably be approximately 2–4 months post-endoscopic resection. Should there be a recurrence, then a decision has to be made regarding further treatment, namely further surgical excision or radical radiotherapy. This decision is based on the definitive histopathology and the volume, site and stage of recurrence.

Technique of total laryngectomy

PREPARATION

Preparation of the patient for total laryngectomy is important and should involve the speech and language therapists at an early stage. This allows them to advise the patient on the sequence of events postoperatively and how they can cope with the communication issues, ultimately advising on the self care of the tracheo-oesophageal voice prosthesis. Part of this process is offering the patient the opportunity to meet a patient who has had a laryngectomy to allow an insight and an opportunity to ask questions.

Prior to the procedure being performed, routine haematological and biochemical investigations are carried out. These should include full blood count, urea and electrolytes, liver function tests and thyroid function tests. Thyroid function should be assessed as at least a hemi-thyroidectomy will be performed in conjunction with the total laryngectomy.

Patients who have advanced high volume laryngeal cancer may have marked airway compromise due to obstruction of the airway by the tumour and reduced vocal cord mobility. Although in most circumstances it is possible to maintain the airway by CO_2 laser or microdebrider tumour debulking, in some situations it is necessary to carry out a tracheostomy to ensure a safe airway. Some series have reported that there is an increased incidence of tumour, and in particular stomal, recurrence in those patients who have required a tracheostomy.[29] However, others have discounted this. In an attempt to minimize the risk of stomal recurrence, it is necessary first to carry out the tracheostomy as high as possible in the trachea and should be around the level of the first tracheal ring. Second, when the laryngectomy is carried out the specimen is excised by including the tracheostomy with a 'cuff' of skin of the tracheostomy site included in it. Third, a thorough level six dissection should be carried out. This should minimize the risk of tumour recurrence as one of the main reasons for stomal recurrence is the deposit of tumour in paratracheal lymph nodes in level six.

ANAESTHESIA

The patient is anaesthetized using a reinforced endotracheal tube, the tube fixed in the midline and connected to the ventilator by taking the connecting tubing over the patient's head. This allows the dissection to proceed and the tube to be changed during the procedure. In general, the endotracheal tube is removed at the point of larynx removal and replaced by a preformed tube, such as a Montandon tube. The timing of this tube change is dependent on the progress of the procedure but is generally once the trachea has been entered and just prior to larynx removal.

SURGICAL APPROACH

The horizontal skin incision is made in the midcervical region at around the level of the cricoid cartilage, extended over the anterior border of sternocleidomastoid bilaterally and curved gently superolaterally. It should be positioned so that the tracheostome can be placed in the inferior flap with a sufficient bridge of skin between the superior edge of the tracheostome and the incision, this being of the order of 2 cm.

The use of the eponymously named 'Gluck–Sorenson incision' is an alternative approach. Once again midcervical, but this time lower, more 'U' shaped, and running into the proposed tracheostome. This incision is convenient to close but care has to be taken as there is a three-point junction at either side of the stoma. Such an incision is of value when a tracheostomy has been carried out to relieve obstruction preoperatively. The aim is to excise the skin around the tracheostomy and the tract to the trachea in these patients. This tracheostome resection, combined with a superolateral extension, effectively produces a Gluck–Sorenson incision.

If a neck dissection is to be carried out at the same time as the laryngectomy, the extent and the direction of the incision will depend on the levels of lymph nodes being cleared. However, most of the time, the neck dissections can be performed through the same incision as the laryngectomy.

MOBILIZATION

Following an appropriate incision, the skin flaps are elevated with the platysma in continuity, so maintaining the vascularity of the flap. As there is little platysma in the midline the subplatysmal flap is best elevated by commencing it laterally. This flap is elevated easily by sharp dissection using a scalpel, probably best with a number 10 blade, and by dissecting directly onto the deep aspect of the platysma muscle. This is best achieved by traction on the flap by the assistant using initially a cat's paw and thereafter a rake retractor, and with countertraction of the soft tissues by the principal operator. When in the correct surgical plane, as might be expected, the flap elevation is relatively bloodless. Involvement of the platysma by tumour occurring unexpectedly should be relatively rare as detailed pre-operative imaging is mandatory. It is sensible, however, to elevate the flaps with particular care when overlying the index primary site as extralaryngeal spread may have occurred. The elevated flaps can be retracted by either sewing them in a retracted position or using some kind of elasticated retractor.

Having exposed the larynx, the aim of surgical removal is to resect the tumour while maintaining the maximum amount of residual mucosa and, to a lesser extent, muscle. To achieve this, it is necessary to mobilize the larynx and disconnect it from its blood supply, the pharynx, the tongue base and the trachea. When considering this, it is also necessary to decide if a total thyroidectomy will be performed; for example, when there is extensive tumour around the anterior commissure, the petiole or anterior subglottis. In other words when there is a high chance of 'escape' of the tumour out of the larynx through the cricothyroid membrane. In the majority of patients, there will be a preponderance of tumour to one side of the midline and it is the hemi-thyroid of this side which will be resected, with preservation of the contralateral lobe on its inferior vascular pedicle.

Mobilization will be discussed without reference to any form of neck dissection being performed. The most appropriate plane to establish first is in the paralaryngeal, parapharyngeal space between the carotid sheath (containing the internal jugular vein, the carotid arterial systems and the vagus nerve) and the constrictor muscles attached to the pharynx and larynx.

This space is entered by sharp dissection in a direction parallel to the constrictors and with division of omohyoid in the tendinous mid-portion. Dissection proceeds superiorly and inferiorly to the level of the thyroid. Superiorly, the pedicle is identified as a branch of the external carotid artery, the superior thyroid artery and is divided as it enters the larynx as it pierces the thyrohyoid membrane. The artery is best transfixed and divided. The superior thyroid vein is taken separately as are any other remaining vessels.

If the hemi-thyroid is to be resected with the tumour specimen on this side, then dissection proceeds inferiorly with division of the inferior thyroid pedicle. Prior to identifying the pedicle, the inferior strap muscles are divided inferiorly. These are sternohyoid and sternothyroid muscles. The inferior thyroid artery is easily identified as a branch of the thyrocervical trunk. Once again, this is divided and transfixed. The inferior venous drainage from the hemi-thyroid is present around the lateral and inferior aspects of the thyroid and is divided with the vessels being tied or clipped with stainless steel clips. Dissection proceeds onto the trachea with clearance of soft tissue from it, thus clearing the level six lymph nodes.

On the contralateral side, mobilization takes place in a similar fashion. There are no hard and fast rules about which order mobilization should occur. This is dependent on the presence of concurrent neck dissection and the extent of the index tumour.

The technique is then repeated on the contralateral side. The paralaryngeal, parapharyngeal space is identified and entered by sharp dissection, with division of omohyoid with this space being opened posteriorly down to the level of the prevertebral muscles. The superior vascular pedicle is divided in a similar fashion to the contralateral side.

Inferiorly, the strap muscles, sterno-hyoid and sterno-thyroid muscles are divided as inferiorly as possible and reflected by sharp dissection from the anterior surface of the capsule of the thyroid gland until the hemi-thyroid has been exposed completely. The thyroid gland is transfixed and divided in the midline. The hemi-thyroid is elevated from the trachea by sharp dissection and bipolar diathermy, this ensures that the thyroid gland and the ipsilateral parathyroid glands are preserved on their vascular pedicle.

Any lymph nodes from level six should be included with the laryngeal resection.

RESECTION

At this stage, it is timely to enter into the trachea to establish a secure airway before proceeding to the laryngeal resection.

Having ensured that the soft tissue has been cleared from the trachea, the anaesthetist frees the taped fixation of the endotracheal tube prior to removal. The trachea is entered by sharp incision anteriorly, probably at the space between the second and third tracheal ring. The exact level will depend on the extent, and in particular the subglottic extent of the index tumour. Clearly, if there is any significant extension into the subglottis an appropriate margin will be needed. If following resection inspection of the larynx reveals a close margin, another tracheal ring can be excised to ensure an adequate margin. Prior to tracheal entry a stay suture, using a relatively heavy suture such as 2/0 suture, is placed in the lateral wall of the trachea at the level of the proposed incision. As the trachea is entered, the endotracheal tube is retracted by the anaesthetist to a level just proximal to the tracheostomy and can be watched by the operator. This allows the patient's ventilation to be maintained throughout. An appropriate endotracheal tube is inserted with a pre-formed tube probably being the most appropriate. A good example of this is a Montandon tube. With this in place, anaesthesia is continued through this tube.

The larynx has had the external infrahyoid muscles divided and has been mobilized from its vascular supply. The areas of connection which remain are at the trachea and tongue base.

Dissection proceeds by removing the larynx from the tongue base by using the monopolar diathermy or scalpel dissection of the suprahyoid muscles in the midline. It is important to 'stay on the hyoid' during this dissection until all of the muscle has been divided. By so doing, any damage to the hypoglossal nerve on either side should be avoided as the nerve lies superomedial to the hyoid. It is extremely important to maintain the integrity and function of the hypoglossal nerve as paralysis significantly compromises voice and swallowing rehabilitation post-laryngectomy.

The muscles are removed from the greater and lesser horns of the hyoid until the superolateral aspect of the hyoid has been exposed. The medial aspect of the hyoid is mobilized by using curved Mayo scissors.

The pharynx has to be entered, bearing in mind at all time that the tumour has to be resected with an appropriate margin, at least 1 cm macroscopically, while at the same time maximizing the amount of mucosa which remains. This is of importance to ensure there is minimal tension in the pharyngeal repair and voice and swallowing rehabilitation is maximized.

The pharynx is entered by continuing the dissection at the level of the hyoid in the midline at the genioglossus and proceeds until the vallecula is entered. An alternative is to enter the pharynx from a lateral approach. The epiglottis edge is palpated and dissecting scissors are aimed just posterior to the edge and directed medially and the mucosa opened. The advantage of the lateral to midline approach is that the mucosa can be seen clearly, of particular importance

when the lesion arises from the supraglottis or there is involvement of the pyriform fossa. The mucosa is divided in the vallecula and the pharynx opened fully thus maintaining symmetry of dissection.

Before proceeding further, it is necessary to divide the constrictors from the thyroid cartilage, approximately 1 cm anterior to the posterior edge of the thyroid cartilage, using a scalpel or monopolar diathermy. The muscle is elevated from the cartilage and around its posterior edge.

Removal of the larynx proceeds from superiorly and by retracting the epiglottis anteriorly, holding it with tissue holding forceps such as 'Alices' or 'Babcocks'. This places the pharyngeal mucosa on a stretch. If the lesion is intralaryngeal then the mucosa is divided along the lateral border of the epiglottis parallel to the aryepiglottic folds, aiming towards the superior horn of the thyroid cartilage. This proceeds into the pyriform fossa bilaterally by taking the larynx forward and dividing the mucosa, bearing in mind to preserve as much mucosa as possible on the contralateral side to the lesion, while carrying out an effective mucosal resection ipsilaterally. Maintaining symmetry, mucosal division is carried out immediately post-cricoid. By completing the incision, mobilization of the larynx from the cervical oesophagus is carried out by retracting the larynx and dissecting the cervical oesophagus from it, by scissors or blunt dissection. It is facilitated by pulling the larynx superiorly and maximizing the amount of trachea mobilized by blunt dissection of the soft tissues. The larynx is disconnected from the trachea by dividing the trachea at the level of the tracheostomy and bevelling the incision posterosuperiorly.

Cricopharyngeal myotomy can be carried out at this stage by vertical incision through the muscle down to the mucosa, leaving the mucosa intact. Whether this is necessary or not is dependent on the experience, and preference, of the head and neck team and the benefit of the procedure to the voice rehabilitation outcomes.

STOMA CREATION

At this point, it is worthwhile creating the end stoma for the trachea. An appropriate incision has to be made for the stoma between the horizontal incision for the laryngectomy and the sternal notch, approximately half way between, leaving an appropriate bridge of skin superiorly, 15–20 mm in breadth. The opening for the stoma should be an ellipse/oval in shape, with the larger axis horizontal. The crucial aspect is that the skin to mucosa has to be aligned in such a fashion that the stoma remains open and there is no concentric scarring and subsequent closure of the stoma. To achieve this, the tracheal mucosa is positioned at least 5 mm above the skin edge. This should maintain it in an everted position. To prevent the concentric scarring, a bilateral 'v' plasty can be used as a primary procedure. When designing the ellipse of skin excision two small triangles of skin are preserved at the lateral edge of the oval (**Figure 33.7**). These are then inserted into the two lateral incision in the trachea of similar 'height' to the skin triangles. This is an extremely effective method of ensuring the stoma size and shape and facilitates tracheo-oesophageal voice prosthesis use.

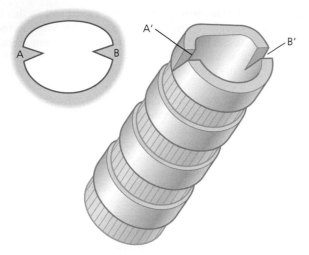

Figure 33.7 Stomaplasty technique.

TRACHEO–OESOPHAGEAL TRACT CREATION

Once the stoma has been created the set up for the tracheo-oeaophageal voice prosthesis should be considered. It is only in rare circumstances that a voice prosthesis would be inserted via a secondary tracheo-oesophageal puncture. Mostly the debate is whether to create a tracheo-oesophageal puncture at the time of laryngectomy and fit a voice prosthesis at a later date or to insert a tracheo-oesophageal prosthesis during the laryngectomy. The former strategy is carried out by taking a pair of curved forceps, such as a 'Cushing Cairns', passing them into the cervical oesophagus, position anteriorly, and then cut down onto them. The forceps are advanced and tent up the posterior tracheal mucosa, approximately 5 mm inferior to the mucosal edge and cut down onto it. A size 14 nasogastric tube is grasped by the forceps and delivered posteriorly into the oesophagus and advanced inferiorly into the distal oesophagus.

Postoperatively feeding can be commenced through this tracheogastric tube. This will act as the final conduit for the tracheo-oesophageal voice prosthesis. The advantage of this strategy is that it allows the tracheo-oesophageal fistula to heal fully and so the fitting of the voice prosthesis can be carried out accurately. Alternatively, a voice prosthesis can be inserted at the time of laryngectomy and feeding carried out through a nasogastric tube placed through it. This has the advantage of not needing a valve inserted at a later date. However, the disadvantage is that the inserted valve may not be the most appropriate size and could potentially be damaged by the insertion of the tracheogastric tube. The choice of which strategy to adopt is dependent on the local expertise and preference.

CLOSURE

Closure of the pharynx is an extremely important issue and should be carried out meticulously. The aim is to ensure that the mucosal edges are inverted throughout the length of the closure. The amount of residual mucosa will clearly depend on the extent of the pharyngeal resection and so the line of mucosal closure may vary. Individual surgeons have personal preferences on the optimal way of closing, ranging from horizontal to 'T' shaped to vertical. Rather than adhering to a standard shape of closure, it is probably more rational to close as it most naturally wishes to come together while doing so with no tension in the surrounding tissues. Closure should be with an absorbable suture and is probably best as interrupted for the first layer. This allows the mucosal edges to be accurately approximated with appropriate tension. The second layer can be continuous, by picking up the serosa and ensuring that the suture line is inverted. Finally, the cut edges of the constrictors are approximated, without excess tension, using the same absorbable suture.

Drains are inserted bilaterally, size 18 gauge, fixed and attached to continuous suction once the skin has been closed. The skin and subcutaneous tissues are closed in two layers. The first layer is the apposition of the platysma layer. This is achieved by using an absorbable suture in a continuous format. The skin is closed using staples.

The stoma is fashioned by using subcutaneous suture and a nylon-based suture for skin. The 'triangle' of the stoma-plasty is inserted and placed *in situ* with no suture within them.

The question of whether to have a tracheostomy tube in place is dependent on the local arrangement with the postoperative care team. Ideally, there would be no tube *in situ* as it would allow the healing to take place without any local pressure on the skin around the stoma and the mucosa of the trachea. The advantage of a tracheostomy tube is that a gentle pressure in the cuff prevents blood tracking down the trachea and also means that the postoperative humidified oxygen can be delivered and bronchial toilet can be carried out with relative ease.

Postoperative care following laryngectomy

Routine postoperative measures should be instituted. These should include the following:

1. Adequate fluid replacement until tracheogastric feeding has been established.
2. Monitoring urine output by use of a urinary catheter.
3. Intravenous antibiotic cover. There has been considerable debate about the type, dosage and frequency of the antibiotics which are used. SIGN guideline review[30] recommends antibiotic prophylaxis, covering aerobic and anaerobic organisms, for 24 hours.
4. Tracheostomy tube should be left *in situ*, with the endotracheal cuff deflated, and oxygen delivered in a humidified format. This should be removed as soon as possible.
5. The patient should be nil by mouth. Enteral feeding is commenced via the stomagastric tube when the gastrointestinal tract is receptive. This generally starts in the first or second postoperative days, when any pharmacologically induced ileus has settled.
6. Routine blood tests should be carried out, initially full blood count, calcium levels and later thyroid function tests. It is unlikely that the calcium levels will be affected significantly in those cases where only a hemi-thyroidectomy has been carried out. Patients may have insidious onset of hypothyroidism

after a few months, especially if they receive postoperative radiotherapy. It is imperative to monitor thyroid levels as significant proportions are having a salvage laryngectomy post-radiotherapy or chemoradiotherapy.

7. Fitting of a tracheo-oesophageal voice prosthesis occurs at approximately 2–4 weeks once the stoma has healed and the interparty wall has settled to it its near final size. Some fit the voice prosthesis 7–10 days after surgery.

PATHOLOGICAL ASSESSMENT

At the time of the operation, most surgeons would want to assess the macroscopic clearance of the total laryngectomy procedure in relation to the extent of the laryngeal tumour. It is imperative that the 'formal' excision margins are not compromised by any per-operative examination. To achieve this, the most effective way of assessing the endolaryngeal extent is to 'split' the larynx posteriorly between the arytenoids and through the cricoid cartilage. This allows the tumour to be visualized and the main margin, i.e. that in the trachea, to be assessed.

The excised larynx, with or without an attached neck dissection, is placed in a container with formalin. In general, it is preferable to 'pin out' the specimen so that the larynx can be examined in relation to the associated levels of lymph nodes. The neck specimen should be annotated either by marking the cork onto which the specimen has been pinned or by attaching 'dog tag' number labels. When requesting pathological assessment, key elements of the history should be stated. These include previous radiotherapy ± chemotherapy, smoking status, clinical staging including vocal cord mobility and specific areas of concern such as areas of potentially close excision margins.

At pathological assessment, the specimen should be photographed macroscopically prior to sectioning. Essentially, the larynx can be sectioned in the sagittal, coronal or axial planes, or a combination of them depending on the area being examined. From an ideal surgical anatomical perspective, the most effective method would be to section the larynx from the glottis inferiorly in the axial plane and superior to this in the sagittal plane. This would allow the most appropriate examination of the laryngeal spaces, but most of all the pre-epiglottic space. In general, however, most larynges are sectioned throughout in an axial plane. To allow sectioning to take place, the laryngeal specimen has to be decalcified and this, in conjunction with the definitive histological examination, can take several weeks. This is not only important when considering the potential requirement for postoperative radiotherapy but also in advising the patient that it may be some time before this is known. Radiotherapy is considered when there is concern about the excision margins or the metastatic tumour volume in the cervical lymph nodes. In general, if the excision margins are less than 5 mm, then radiotherapy is considered.

Excision margins have to be interpreted with care. During the orientation of the excised specimen, there is only a certain amount of margin which is possible as a result of the anatomical structures. For example, anteriorly the skin or subplatysmal layers must be the anterior extent and so this is the anterior margin. Equally the margins, or free edge, in the pyriform fossa can be difficult to orientate. It is essential that following full assessment, preferably in conjunction with the clinician, that the full extent of the tumour, including detailed assessment of lymph nodes, numbers of nodes, their appropriate levels and the presence, or otherwise, of extracapsular spread, are stated. These various aspects when combined must be noted as a pTNM staging. Such a staging is regarded as the 'gold standard' with which to compare all aspects of management, for example determining the sensitivity and specificity of key investigations such as CT or MR scanning, or evolving techniques such as PET CT. It is imperative that there is regular audit of the validity of the pathological assessments and staging conclusions. It is incumbent on each head and neck multidisciplinary team to ensure that they are satisfied with their clinicopathological processes.

SALVAGE SURGERY

As part of an effective organ preservation strategy, it is mandatory to have surgical resection as the main salvage treatment modality. There are effectively two forms of index primary treatment which may need surgery should there be persistence or recurrence.

Post-endoscopic resection

As part of the endoscopic resection strategy it is necessary to reexamine or reoperate on individuals depending on the certainty and security of the initial resection. Separate from this, however, is the small group of patients in whom there is recurrence of the disease following a period of the patient having been disease free. If there is a recurrence, great care has to be taken in restaging the recurrence, with this effectively meaning that the original assessments are repeated. If there is low volume recurrence, then it may be possible to carry out endoscopic resection.[31] If not, then radiotherapy, total laryngectomy, or in rare circumstances, partial laryngectomy, are carried out.[32]

Post-radiotherapy or chemoradiotherapy

With the increased use of 'organ preservation' strategies using radiotherapy, and ever increasing chemoradiotherapy regimes, surgical resection needs to be employed should there be recurrence or persistence at the index site, the neck, or both. These situations may be challenging, not only during the surgical resection but also in the healing process.

The principal procedure employed is total laryngectomy. There are no specific issues which need to be addressed except to maintain a meticulous surgical technique and be aware of potential areas where the healing may be compromised. Particular attention needs to be paid to the skin, where on occasions new tissue is needed in the form of a myocutaneous flap or free tissue transfer. Care also needs to be taken with pharyngeal repair and closure. Use of a muscle-only pectoralis major pedicled flap, laid over the pharyngeal repair, improves healing of both the pharynx and the overlying skin.

There has been increasing use of endoscopic resection techniques when there is 'low volume' recurrence following radiotherapy or chemoradiotherapy. There are questions surrounding the applicability of the technique for curative intent in radio recurrent situations. However, it is of value when there is a palliative intent or where the patient is unfit or unwilling to undergo total laryngectomy.

STOMAL RECURRENCE

Recurrence of malignant tumours in or around the stoma following total laryngectomy is a specific and difficult problem to manage. There has been a long held belief that this can be associated with a pre-laryngectomy tracheostomy. This would appear to be the case and hence the requirement for excision of the tracheal cuff of skin and soft tissues during laryngectomy.

The principal cause of stomal recurrence is the persistence of disease in lymph nodes in the central compartment or paratracheal region. If it occurs then the most effective way of managing it is by surgical excision with appropriate reconstruction, and postoperative radiotherapy if possible. This should only be undertaken for limited, small volume disease, mainly situated above the '3 to 9 o'clock' line. Large recurrences, and those below this line, have a very poor prognosis despite resection. Resection will involve the trachea, levels six and seven, and possibly part of the manubrium.

Horizon scanning

Transoral robotic surgery of the larynx: transoral robotic surgery has recently been performed for oropharyngeal lesions. There is also some preliminary work on glottic surgery using the robot in dogs. There have been early reports regarding using this technique in humans.[33] This may become an established procedure in due course.

KEY EVIDENCE

- Laser microsurgery is an effective treatment option for early laryngeal cancer.[9]
- The addition of chemotherapy to radiotherapy improves survival of advanced head and neck cancer by approximately 6 per cent.[19]
- Supracricoid laryngectomy is an effective treatment for a small selected number of patients with laryngeal cancer.[15]

KEY LEARNING POINTS

- Laryngeal anatomy is complex.

- Thorough assessment using a combination of imaging and examination under anaesthetic is essential for planning and treatment.
- Early laryngeal cancer can be treated with single modality treatment: either transoral surgery or radiotherapy.
- Advanced laryngeal cancer can be treated with combined modality: either surgery and postoperative chemoradiotherpay or primary chemoradiotherapy.
- Laryngeal cartilage invasion is usually an indication for laryngectomy.
- Partial laryngectomy techniques can be used for a few selected primary and recurrent laryngeal cancers, and should be undertaken in specialist centres.
- Elective treatment of neck nodes is usually indicated in advanced supraglottic or transglottic laryngeal cancer.

REFERENCES

1. Cancer Research UK website, 2009. http://info.cancerresearchuk.org/cancerstats/types/larynx/ accessed October 5, 2009.
2. MacKenzie K, Savage SA, Birchall MA. Processes and outcomes of head and neck cancer patients from geographically disparate regions of the UK. A comparison of Scottish and English cohorts. *European Journal of Surgical Oncology* 2009; **35**: 1113–18.
3. Tuyns AJ, Audigier JC. Double wave cohort increase for oesophageal and laryngeal cancer in France in relation to reduced alcohol consumption during the second world war. *Digestion* 1976; **14**: 197–208.
◆ 4. Hashibe M, Brennan P, Chuang SC et al. Interaction between tobacco and alcohol use and the risk of head and neck cancer: pooled analysis in the International Head and Neck Cancer Epidemiology Consortium. *Cancer Epidemiology, Biomarkers and Prevention* 2009; **18**: 541–50.
5. Nutting CM, Robinson M, Birchall M. Survival from laryngeal cancer in England and Wales up to 2001. *British Journal of Cancer* 2008; **99**(Suppl 1): S38–9.
6. Chijiwa H, Sato K, Umeno H, Nakashima T. Histopathological study of correlation between laryngeal space invasion and lymph node metastasis in glottic carcinoma. *Journal of Laryngology and Otology* 2009; **123**(Suppl 31): 48–5.
7. Kaanders JH, Hordijk GJ. Dutch Cooperative Head and Neck Oncology Group. Carcinoma of the larynx: the Dutch national guideline for diagnostics, treatment, supportive care and rehabilitation. *Radiotherapy and Oncology* 2002; **63**: 299–307.
8. Moreau PR. Treatment of laryngeal carcinomas by laser endoscopic microsurgery. *Laryngoscope* 2000; **110**: 1000–6.

◆ 9. Ambrosch P, Kron M, Steiner W. Carbon dioxide laser microsurgery for early supraglottic carcinoma. *Annals of Otology, Rhinology, and Laryngology* 1998; **107**: 680–8.

10. Inoue T, Inoue T, Ikeda H *et al.* Comparison of early glottic and supraglottic carcinoma treated with conventional fractionation of radiotherapy. *Strahlentherapie und Onkologie* 1993; **169**: 584–9.

11. Loughran S, Calder N, MacGregor FB *et al.* Quality of life and voice following endoscopic resection or radiotherapy for early glottic cancer. *Clinical Otolaryngology* 2005; **30**: 42–7.

12. Yiotakis J, Stavroulaki P, Nikolopoulos T *et al.* Partial laryngectomy after irradiation failure. *Otolaryngology – Head and Neck Surgery* 2003; **128**: 200–9.

13. List MA, Ritter-Sterr CA, Baker TM *et al.* Longitudinal assessment of quality of life in laryngeal cancer patients. *Head and Neck* 1996; **18**: 1–10.

14. El-Deiry M, Funk GF, Nalwa S *et al.* Long-term quality of life for surgical and nonsurgical treatment of head and neck cancer. *Archives of Otolaryngology – Head and Neck Surgery* 2005; **131**: 879–85.

◆ 15. Laccourreye O, Brasnu D, Jouffre V *et al.* Supra-cricoid partial laryngectomy extended to the anterior arch of the cricoid with tracheo-crico-hyoido-epiglottopexy. Oncologic and functional results. *Annales d'Oto-laryngologie et de Chirurgie Cervico Faciale* 1996; **113**: 15–19.

16. Iro H, Waldfahrer F, Altendorf-Hofmann A *et al.* Transoral laser surgery of supraglottic cancer: follow-up of 141 patients. *Archives of Otolaryngology – Head and Neck Surgery* 1998; **124**: 1245–50.

17. Steiner W, Ambrosch P, Hess CF, Kron M. Organ preservation by transoral laser microsurgery in piriform sinus carcinoma. *Otolaryngology – Head and Neck Surgery* 2001; **124**: 58–67.

● 18. The Department of Veterans Affairs Laryngeal Cancer Study Group. Induction chemotherapy plus radiation compared with surgery plus radiation in patients with advanced laryngeal cancer. *New England Journal of Medicine* 1991; **324**: 1685–90.

● 19. Pignon JP, Bourhis J, Domenge C, Designé L. Chemotherapy added to locoregional treatment for head and neck squamous-cell carcinoma: three meta-analyses of updated individual data. MACH-NC Collaborative Group. Meta-Analysis of Chemotherapy on Head and Neck Cancer. *Lancet* 2000; **355**: 949–55.

20. Pignon JP, le Maître A, Maillard E *et al.* Meta-analysis of chemotherapy in head and neck cancer (MACH-NC): an update on 93 randomised trials and 17,346 patients. *Radiotherapy and Oncology* 2009; **92**: 4–14.

● 21. Forastiere AA, Goepfert H, Maor M *et al.* Concurrent chemotherapy and radiotherapy for organ preservation in advanced laryngeal cancer. *New England Journal of Medicine* 2003; **349**: 2091–8.

22. Posner MR, Hershock DM, Blajman CR *et al.* Cisplatin and fluorouracil alone or with docetaxel in head and neck cancer. *New England Journal of Medicine* 2007; **357**: 1705–15.

◆ 23. Vermorken JB, Remenar E, van Herpen C *et al.* Cisplatin, fluorouracil, and docetaxel in unresectable head and neck cancer. *New England Journal of Medicine* 2007; **357**: 1695–704.

◆ 24. Bourhis J, Overgaard J, Audry H *et al.* Meta-Analysis of Radiotherapy in Carcinomas of Head and neck (MARCH) Collaborative Group. Hyperfractionated or accelerated radiotherapy in head and neck cancer: a meta-analysis. *Lancet* 2006; **368**: 843–54.

25. Brizel DM, Prosnitz RG, Hunter S *et al.* Necessity for adjuvant neck dissection in setting of concurrent chemoradiation for advanced head-and-neck cancer. *International Journal of Radiation Oncology, Biology, Physics* 2004; **58**: 1418–23.

26. List MA, Stracks J, Colangelo L *et al.* How do head and neck cancer patients prioritize treatment outcomes before initiating treatment? *Journal of Clinical Oncology* 2000; **18**: 877–84.

27. Bradley P, MacKenzie K, Wight R *et al.* Consensus statement on management in the UK: Transoral laser assisted microsurgical resection of early glottic cancer. *Clinical Otolaryngology* 2009; **34**: 367–73.

28. Murray CE, Cooper L, Handa KK *et al.* A technique for the orientation of endoscopically resected laryngeal lesions. *Clinical Otolaryngology and Allied Sciences* 2007; **32**: 201–3.

29. Halfpenny W, McGurk M. Stomal recurrence following temporary tracheostomy. *Journal of Laryngology and Otology* 2001; **115**: 202–4.

30. Scottish Intercollegiate Guidelines Network. Diagnosis and management of head and neck cancer. Available from: www.sign.ac.uk/guidelines/fulltext/90/index.html.

31. Grant DG, Salassa JR, Hinni ML *et al.* Transoral laser microsurgery for recurrent laryngeal and pharyngeal cancer. *Otolaryngology – Head and Neck Surgery* 2008; **138**: 606–13.

32. Marioni G, Marchese-Ragona R, Lucioni M, Staffieri A. Organ-preservation surgery following failed radiotherapy for laryngeal cancer. Evaluation, patient selection, functional outcome and survival. *Current Opinion in Otolaryngology and Head and Neck Surgery* 2008; **16**: 141–6.

33. O'Malley BW Jr, Weinstein GS, Hockstein NG. Transoral robotic surgery (TORS): glottic microsurgery in a canine model. *Journal of Voice* 2006; **20**: 263–8.

34. Sobin L, Gospodarowicz M, Wittekind C (eds). *TNM classification of malignant tumours*, 7th edn. Oxford: Blackwell.

34

Metastatic neck disease

VINIDH PALERI AND JOHN C WATKINSON

Subclinical disease is not early cancer.

Helmuth Goepfurt

INTRODUCTION

One of the most important prognostic factors in head and neck cancer is the presence or absence, level and size of metastatic neck disease. Many tumours of the head and neck will at some stage metastasize to lymph nodes and a number of factors control the natural history and spread of disease.

Several controversies exist about the management of malignant neck disease, with varying practices on choice, timing and combination of treatment modalities. This is primarily due to the paucity of high level evidence to many treatment paradigms, but this trend may be reversing with some randomized controlled trials and systematic reviews published in the last decade and a few more in progress. However, many organizations have generated guidelines following rigorous evidence-gathering exercises, suggesting best management practices based on available evidence in many countries.

This chapter identifies the evidence base and discusses the principles of management of metastatic head and neck squamous cell carcinoma (HNSCC) at initial presentation, residual disease following treatment and recurrent neck disease. It also outlines major clinical controversies regarding the management of the neck in relation to when to treat, how much to treat and which modality to use. It reviews tumour biology behind metastatic disease, the various rationales for assessment, as well as methods for elective and therapeutic treatment and focuses on quality-of-life issues. The management of tumours other than HNSCC (i.e. salivary gland and thyroid tumours) are not covered in this chapter.

TUMOUR BIOLOGY AS RELATED TO METASTASES

Significant progress has been made in understanding at the molecular level the processes that trigger the metastatic cascade. Tumours do not have primary lymphatics and cancer cells were thought to gain access to the lymphatic system through pre-existing lymphatic vessels near the tumour. Recent studies on animal models have shown that solid tumours can induce lymphangiogenesis. In the context of HNSCC, intratumoral and peritumoral lymphangiogenesis has been correlated with lymph node metastases.[1, 2, 3] Vascular endothelial growth factor (VEGF)-C and VEGF-D, secreted by the tumour, have been shown to play an active role in lymphangiogenesis by binding to VEGF receptor-3, a tyrosine kinase receptor, expressed on the surface of lymphatic endothelial cells (**Figure 34.1**). This pathway is also the focus for research into antilymphangiogenetic therapeutics.

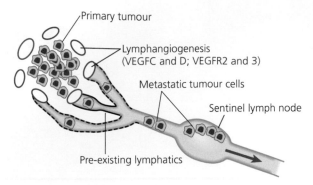

Figure 34.1 Mechanisms of lymphatic invasion.

The metastatic potential of primary tumours varies considerably, even among tumours of the same site and extent. One factor that affects the metastatic potential is the genetic make up of the tumour. Metastatic primary tumours have been shown to express distinct signature genes that set them apart from non-metastatic tumours.[4, 5] This metastatic profile includes genes related to the extracellular matrix, adhesion, motility and protease inhibition. The products of these genes help local invasion and spread into the intra- and peritumoral lymphatics, which is the next essential step in the metastatic cascade. This is facilitated by three molecular events: (1) Cellular adhesion molecules, such as E cadherin, responsible for tissue architecture and differentiation, are downregulated, making the cancer cells free to migrate. (2) Integrins are adhesion receptors that provide a linkage between the cell cytoskeleton and the extracellular matrix. Overexpression of integrins is associated with increased cellular motility and the production of matrix metalloproteinases (MMP 1, 2, 3, 9 and 14) that act upon the matrix to enhance migration. The MMPs are produced both by tumour and stromal cells, lending credence to the important role that the 'soil' plays in the metastatic cascade.[6] A meta-analysis pooling data from 710 patients indicated that MMPs played a significant role in metastatic behaviour.[7] Cathepsins are lysosomal endopeptidases with a similar role in promoting metastases. (3) Active migration of cancer cells into lymphatics is driven by the production of autocrine and paracrine cytokines, mediated by integrin receptors. Tumour cell homing to lymph nodes is probably mediated by L-selectin, a migratory cell–cell interaction molecule. In summary, a variety of genotypic (e.g. p53 and MET oncogene mutation), phenotypic (e.g. E cadherin downregulation) and microenvironmental (e.g. expression of VEGF-C) processes conspire to facilitate what is probably an inefficient process.

The milieu in the node is hostile to the cancer cells, with the preponderance of immune effector cells and cytokines. The immunoresistant clones are thus selected out for establishing metastases. Once adapted to the lymphatic nodal environment, these cells can invade the rest of the lymphatic system with little need for further adaptation.

The exact role of the regional lymph node system in the spread of HNSCC has yet to be fully defined, although it is established that they are not simple mechanical barriers, but are involved in conferring anti-tumour immunity, primarily through cytotoxic T lymphocytes. However, defects in the antigen-presenting machinery of the cancer cells and reduced expression of HLA class I antigens are the mechanisms that have evolved to avoid detection by immune effector cells.[8]

Behaviour of disease within the cervical lymph nodes

Multiple afferent lymph vessels bring lymph into the lymph node, branching extensively in the capsule of the node. Several variations exist in the way afferent vessels interface with the node, and this is important in understanding patterns of lymph nodal infiltration and why extracapsular spread (ECS) can occur earlier in the natural history. While the afferent channels may penetrate the capsule and discharge the lymph into the subcapsular sinus, many run obliquely into the capsule, while others travel along the capsule for considerable distances before penetrating it. Valves are often found in these afferent channels that run on the capsule, forming a network of capsular lymphatics.

Toker[9] described four distinct growth patterns of squamous cell carcinoma (SCC) within cervical lymph nodes:

1. Following initial cancerous deposits in the subcapsular sinus, growth within the affected node takes place, replacing the architecture of the node before ECS occurs. Ultimately, ECS occurs by the direct penetration and destruction of the capsule, or by the arrest of further underlying capsular or juxtacapsular lymphatics.
2. Metastatic deposits extensively infiltrate the lymphatic sinuses, leaving the germinal centres and trabeculae intact. ECS occurs by the direct penetration and destruction of the capsule, or by the arrest of tumour emboli in underlying capsular or juxtacapsular lymphatics.
3. A less common pattern involves the deposition of a malignant embolus within the subcapsular sinus together with the simultaneous arrest of tumour within capsular or juxtacapsular lymphatics. This results in the coincident and equivalent proliferation of cancer both within and outside the node.
4. Another uncommon metastatic pattern is where capsular or juxtacapsular emboli grow with no intranodal cancer. In these instances, ECS can occur much earlier in the natural history of the disease process.

Metastatic involvement of various lymph node regions usually progresses from superior to inferior in an orderly fashion, but it has been shown that in some situations lymph node groups can be bypassed, leading to 'skip metastases'. Once tumour cells arrive at a draining lymph node, they can proliferate, die, remain dormant or enter the circulation.

Haematogenous spread

From the node, efferent channels leave the hilum to join the terminal collecting trunks (the right and left lymphatic ducts) and then drainage is into the venous system. However, there are other routes whereby cancer cells can access the bloodstream and these include entering directly from a node. Vascularization of tumours usually occurs when growths are greater than 0.1–1 mm in size and following this, rapid rates of neoplastic growth and increased rates of vessel invasion can occur. These may be released as single cells, cell clumps or a thrombus fragment containing tumour cells. The success of implantation is determined by both tumour and host factors. In the context of HNSCC, disseminated and circulating tumour cells in the bone marrow and venous blood occur at a low frequency compared to other tumour sites (one to five cells per 6×10^7 leukocytes).[10, 11] Owing to very small numbers of cells in the circulation, low levels of tumour-specific markers and heterogeneity of marker gene expression transcripts, work in this field has been hampered. However, using highly sensitive and specific techniques and a panel of tumour markers, circulating tumour cells have been demonstrated in the setting of HNSCC and shown to predict disease-free survival.[10, 12]

CLINICAL IMPLICATIONS OF METASTASES

The presence of regional lymph node metastases acts as an indicator of the ability of the primary tumour to metastasize locally and to distant sites, rather than acting as an instigator of distant metastases on their own. This is because lymph node involvement indicates a host response which is permissive for the development of metastases, not only in the regional lymph nodes, but also to distant sites. Therefore, the degree of lymph node involvement should be regarded as an indirect index of the systemic tumour burden. Therefore, elective removal of regional lymph nodes serves as a biopsy staging procedure to ascertain whether or not metastatic disease is present and to identify high risk patients who might benefit from systemic adjuvant therapy, but is not expected to diminish the metastatic potential. This means that, like breast cancer, tumour-free survival depends more on the biology of the tumour present at the operation rather that the extent of surgery. This explains why patients with metastatic lymph nodes in HNSCC have a significantly reduced chance of survival when compared with those who are disease free.[13]

It has long been recognized that systemic spread can occur early in many solid tumours and this includes HNSCC. The question that one must ask is, 'If cancer is a systemic disease, how can cure ever be effected?' Traditional teaching has been to offer wide margin radical surgery to the neck, with the premise that patients who have a large number of occult positive nodes fare better since these nodes are discovered earlier. This philosophy is now being questioned with regard to locoregional disease being cured with locoregional treatments, since recent advances mean patients are now living longer only to die more frequently of second primaries or distant metastases. Overall survival has not changed significantly.

It becomes clear from the above discussion that the spread of HNSCC to the regional lymph nodes indicates an aggressive tumour where the tumour–host balance has swung in favour of the tumour. While there are structural and immunobiological mechanisms that may affect tumour lysis within the lymph node itself, in a certain proportion of cases, systemic spread occurs early on. This can take place by lymphaticovenous or haematological routes. These processes of spread and tumour arrest can be affected by previous treatment. As the systemic immunosuppressive effects of multimodality head and neck cancer therapy are taken into consideration, both the number and the complexity of modalities that are used become ever more important.

NECK LEVELS

It is useful to introduce the concept of neck levels here. In 1981, the Memorial Sloan-Kettering Hospital published a number of levels or regions within the neck which contain groups of lymph nodes representing the first echelon sites for metastases from head and neck primary sites.[14] These levels have been widely accepted and currently six neck levels are recognized, with level VII being outside the neck and referring to the chain of paratracheal nodes below the suprasternal notch to the level of the innominate artery. These neck node levels (**Figure 34.2**) along with their respective boundaries are described in **Table 34.1**.[15] Levels I, II and V can be further subdivided into (a) and (b). These subdivisions were introduced to recognize certain areas in the neck that have a biological significance independent of the

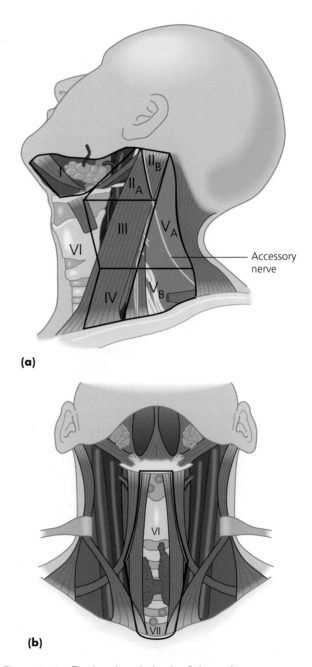

(a)

(b)

Figure 34.2 The lymph node levels of the neck.

Table 34.1 Neck levels as defined by the American Academy of Otolaryngology-Head and Neck Surgery.

Level	Clinical location	Surgical boundaries	Radiological boundaries
Ia	Submental triangle	S, Symphysis of mandible I, Hyoid bone A (M), Left anterior belly of digastric P (L), Right anterior belly of digastric	Nodes above the level of lower body of hyoid bone, below mylohyoid muscles and anterior to a transverse line drawn through the posterior edge of submandibular gland on an axial image
Ib	Submandibular triangle	S, Body of mandible I, Posterior belly of digastric A (M), Anterior belly of digastric P (L), Stylohyoid muscle	
IIa	Upper jugular	S, Lower level of bony margin of jugular fossa I, Level of lower body of hyoid bone A (M), Stylohyoid muscle P (L), Vertical plane defined by accessory nerve	Superior and inferior limits as described under surgical boundaries. Nodes posterior to a transverse plane defined by the posterior surface of submandibular gland and anterior to a transverse line drawn along the posterior border of the sternomastoid. Note: Nodes lying medial to the carotids are retropharyngeal and not level II
IIb	Upper jugular	S, Lower level of bony margin of jugular fossa I, Level of lower body of hyoid bone A (M), Vertical plane defined by accessory nerve P (L), Posterior border of sternomastoid muscle	
III	Mid jugular	S, Level of lower body of hyoid bone I, Horizontal plane along inferior border of anterior cricoid arch A (M), Lateral border of sternohyoid muscle P (L), Posterior border of sternocleidomastoid muscle or sensory branches of the cervical plexus	Superior and inferior limits as described under surgical boundaries. Nodes anterior to a transverse line drawn on each axial scan through the posterior edge of the SCM and lateral to the medial margin of the common carotid arteries
IV	Lower jugular	S, Horizontal plane along inferior border of anterior cricoid arch I, Clavicle A (M), Lateral border of sternohyoid muscle P (L), Posterior border of sternocleidomastoid muscle or sensory branches of the cervical plexus	Superior and inferior limits as described under surgical boundaries. Nodes anterior to a transverse line drawn on each axial scan through the posterior edge of the SCM and lateral to the medial margin of the common carotid arteries
Va	Posterior triangle	S, Convergence of SCM and trapezius muscles I, Horizontal plane along inferior border of anterior cricoid arch A (M), Posterior border of sternocleidomastoid muscle or sensory branches of the cervical plexus P (L), Anterior border of trapezius muscle	
Vb	Posterior triangle (supraclavicular)	S, Horizontal plane along inferior border of anterior cricoid arch I, Clavicle A (M), Posterior border of sternocleidomastoid muscle or sensory branches of the cervical plexus P (L), Anterior border of trapezius muscle	Nodes posterior to a transverse line drawn on each axial scan through the posterior edge of the SCM
VI	Anterior compartment	S, hyoid bone I, sternal notch A (M), common carotid artery P (L), common carotid artery	
VII	Superior mediastinum	S, sternal notch I, innominate artery A (M), common carotid artery P (L), common carotid artery	

A, anterior; I, inferior; L, lateral; M, medial; P, posterior; SCM, sternocleidomastoid; S, superior.

larger zone that they lie in. For instance, level Ia is rarely involved in malignant processes excluding the lip, anterior floor of mouth and midface. The prognostic significance of level Vb involvement is grave and thus merits the subdivision. The rationale behind subdivision of level II is discussed below under Elective neck treatment.

NECK DISSECTION TERMINOLOGY

Standardized neck dissection terminology that was first produced by the American Academy of Otolaryngology and Head and Neck Surgery in 1991 has been updated by the Committee for Neck Dissection Classification of the American Head and Neck Society in 2002 and is widely used (**Table 34.2**). There is an increasing trend to divide neck dissections into two broad types with subdivisions: (1) comprehensive (removal of levels I–V) and (2) selective neck dissection (SND) (less than five levels).

The previous division of SND into named subtypes has been superseded by recommendations that the levels or sublevels removed during SND be precisely stated in the operation notes.[16] There is an even greater need for this in the chemoradiation era, where specific levels may need to be cleared along with some non-lymphatic structures, leading to calls for further modification of the terminology.[17] The term 'elective neck dissection' (END) is used to describe any type of neck dissection that is performed on the neck that is clinically and radiologically free of disease.

REGION-SPECIFIC LYMPHATIC DRAINAGE

There are approximately 150 lymph nodes on either side of the neck. The normal range in size is from 3 mm to 3 cm, but most nodes are less than a centimetre. Within the upper deep cervical

Table 34.2 Classification of neck dissection techniques.

Classification	
Radical neck dissection (RND)	Removal of levels I–V, accessory nerve, internal jugular vein and sternomastoid muscle
Modified radical neck dissection (MRND)	Removal of levels I–V dissected; preservation of one or more of the accessory nerve, internal jugular vein or sternomastoid muscle (types I, II and III, respectively)
Selective neck dissection (SND)	Preservation of one or more levels of lymph nodes
Extended radical neck dissection (ERND)	Removal of one or more additional lymphatic and/or non-lymphatic structures(s) relative to a radical neck dissection, e.g. level VII, retropharyngeal lymph nodes, hypoglossal nerve

nodes in level II, the largest node is often called the jugulodigastric node and is situated within the triangle formed by the internal jugular vein, facial vein and posterior belly of the digastric muscle. It is important because it receives lymph from a wide area which includes the submandibular region, the oropharynx and oral cavity. The jugulo-omohyoid nodes are situated at the junction between the middle and lower cervical group (low level III/high level IV) where the omohyoid muscle crosses the internal jugular vein and receives lymph from a wide area which includes the anterior floor of mouth, oropharynx and larynx. It is important to realize that contralateral neck spread may occur early in those tumours situated in or near the midline.

- The nasopharynx, nasal cavities and sinuses drain via the junctional nodes into the upper deep cervical nodes (levels II and III) having passed through retropharyngeal or submandibular lymph nodes.
- The oropharynx similarly drains into the upper, middle and lower deep cervical nodes (levels II, III and IV) again either directly or via the retropharyngeal nodes. Within these areas of deep lymph node collections in the neck, certain nodes can reach quite large proportions.
- The oral cavity has a wide area of drainage and this is important because there is often free communication between the two sides of the tongue. This means that the normal acts of mastication and swallowing facilitate tongue massage and can promote both early and rapid lymphatic spread directly to low in the neck. The posterior parts of the oral cavity either drain directly into the upper deep cervical nodes (level II/III) or indirectly via the submandibular nodes (level Ib). More anterior parts of the oral cavity and tongue also drain to these nodes but, in addition, may drain to the submental nodes (level Ia) or directly to the jugular nodal chain (levels II–IV). The tongue especially is known to cause 'skip metastases' to level IV.
- The larynx drainage is separated into upper and lower systems based on its embryological origins, with a division that occurs at the level of the true vocal cord. The supraglottis drains through vessels which accompany the superior laryngeal pedicle via the thyroid membrane to reach the upper deep cervical nodes (levels II/III), with a greater tendency for bilateral nodal drainage. The lower system drains directly into the deep cervical nodes (levels III/IV) through vessels which pass through or behind the cricothyroid membrane and also into the prelaryngeal, pretracheal or paratracheal nodes (level VI), before reaching the deep cervical nodes. Because the vocal cords are relatively avascular, they have an extremely sparse lymphatic drainage, hence lymph node metastases from small carcinomas at this site are uncommon.
- The hypopharynx is similar to the supraglottic larynx, and both may have contralateral spread, particularly in those areas that are either close to the midline or have significant communications across the midline, such as the epiglottis, posterior pharyngeal wall and postcricoid region. Drainage is to levels III, IV, VI and VII.

The region-specific drainage translates well into clinical practice and it is possible to predict the site of a primary tumour based upon the distribution of cervical metastases and vice versa. In a landmark study of 1155 patients with previously untreated HNSCC published by Lindberg in 1972,[18] the topographical distribution of clinically evident cervical metastases was set out. This identified distinct patterns of spread to the neck based on the primary site. Histological proof of this concept was produced in 1990 by Shah,[19] in a series of 1119 neck dissections.

It is widely accepted that patterns of subclinical microscopic metastases follow a similar distribution. The high incidence of occult metastases in tumours of the oral cavity, pharynx and the supraglottic larynx forms the basis for SND and removal of the echelon lymph nodes which are the most likely sites of initial metastatic deposits. The echelon nodes for each site are as follows: levels I, II and III for the oral cavity, levels II, III, IV for the larynx and pharynx, and levels IV, VI and VII for the thyroid gland. For the parotid gland, the first echelon lymph nodes are the pre-auricular, periparotid and intraparotid lymph nodes along with those in levels II, III and the upper accessory chain (level Va). For the submandibular and sublingual gland, the echelon lymph nodes lie in levels I, II and III.

METASTATIC BEHAVIOUR IN THE PREVIOUSLY TREATED NECK

Treatment modalities can affect tumour–host equilibrium in unpredictable ways and these include surgery, radiotherapy and chemotherapy.

Surgery can undoubtedly mechanically alter the locoregional tumour environment. Considerable gaps between lymphatics mean that collateral channels form, and the ability to do this relates to the nature of connective tissue through which the lymphatics must grow. These mechanical effects can alter patterns of lymphatic metastatic spread and divert lymph flow to the contralateral neck and sometimes even cause retrograde spread. Surgical scarring can trap tumour cells, although this may not always ultimately lead to established local recurrence.[20] It seems sensible to suggest that gentle handling of cancer tissues may decrease the amount of exposure that a surgical wound gets to free cancer cells and as such minimize the potential for any growth.

Lymphoid tissue and circulating small lymphocytes are sensitive and very small doses of radiotherapy (as low as 2.5 Gy) may produce a detectable decrease in the peripheral lymphocyte count. Suppressor T cells are also thought to be particularly radiosensitive. There is evidence in the literature that the systemic cellular immune response is significantly compromised following locoregional radiation therapy (RT) in head and neck cancer patients. Radiation is associated with changes in the regional lymph nodes and lymphatics in general. Thus, within a few days of starting RT, there is a decrease in the numbers of lymphocytes within lymph nodes and thickening of the walls of both lymph nodes and blood vessels can be noted. Some of these changes explain why previous RT can cause lymphatic obstruction and shunting of lymph both into the subdermal vessels and also to the contralateral neck. All of the above lead to unpredictable changes in the pattern of lymphatic drainage, and thus, the echelon levels described above for the various sites will not be applicable to disease recurrence following treatment.

OCCULT NODAL DISEASE

The term 'occult disease' is used to describe the presence of metastases in the neck nodes that cannot be clinically or radiologically identified. This falls into two categories: (1) occult metastases that can be identified on light microscopy and (2) micrometastases measuring less than 2 mm that need special histological techniques (immunohistochemistry, step serial sectioning and molecular analysis) - for identification. The incidence of occult disease as assessed by routine histological examination varies by the site and stage of tumour (**Table 34.3**), but use of molecular techniques to look for metastatic disease will increase the incidence rates.

The natural history and the clinical significance of occult metastases is an important, yet largely unanswered question.

Table 34.3 The probability of cervical metastases (N) related to primary (T) staging in patients with head and neck squamous carcinoma.

Primary site	T-stage	N0%	N1 %	N2–N3%
Floor of mouth	T_1	89	9	2
	T_2	71	18	10
	T_3	56	20	24
	T_4	46	10	43
Oral tongue	T_1	86	10	4
	T_2	70	19	11
	T_3	52	16	31
	T_4	24	10	66
Retromolar trigone anterior faucial pillar	T_1	88	2	9
	T_2	62	18	20
	T_3	46	21	33
	T_4	32	18	50
Nasopharynx	T_1	8	11	82
	T_2	16	12	72
	T_3	12	9	80
	T_4	17	6	78
Soft palate	T_1	92	0	8
	T_2	64	12	24
	T_3	35	26	39
	T_4	33	11	56
Base of tongue	T_1	30	15	55
	T_2	29	14	56
	T_3	26	23	52
	T_4	16	8	76
Tonsillar fossa	T_1	30	41	30
	T_2	32	14	54
	T_3	30	18	52
	T_4	10	13	76
Supraglottic larynx	T_1	61	10	29
	T_2	58	16	26
	T_3	36	25	40
	T_4	41	18	41
Hypopharynx	T_1	37	21	42
	T_2	30	20	49
	T_3	21	26	54
	T_4	26	15	58

Table adapted from Lindberg[17] and Shah.[19]

Neck dissection may arrest progress of some cancer cells. However, a lymph node may be negative on examination because either cancer never reached it or if it did, it was not retained or indeed was destroyed. This has led to several controversies in the management of the occult neck. It is important to address this question because this affects whether or not the disease needs to be treated and by what method. Observational data suggest that the conversion rate from the N0 to the N+ neck without neck treatment is similar to the incidence of pathological positive nodes in END specimens (around 30 per cent).[20] There is no doubt that occult neck disease does have the potential to manifest itself, but it is impossible to predict with reasonable certainty in individual patients. This is one of several arguments that justify the elective treatment of the occult neck. The clinical significance is discussed in depth below under The N0 neck.

MICROMETASTASES AND ISOLATED TUMOUR CELLS

Micrometastases are deposits of cancer cells between 0.2 and 2 mm in size. Presence of micrometastases upstages the neck status (pN1mi). One of the many goals of translational research in cancer has been to refine disease prediction by detecting tumour-specific molecular alterations in histological normal tissues either at resection margins or identifying 'subpathological' metastases in regional lymph nodes. Specific clonal genetic changes seen in tumour cells can be used as molecular markers for their detection in lymph nodes. However, the heterogeneity seen in HNSCC, like other solid cancers, precludes the use of a single tumour specific marker. Thus, these studies are dependent on the amplification of less specific epithelial genes or a panel of their transcripts.

Several molecular markers have been used to identify the presence of 'subpathological' metastases in lymph nodes. Using immunohistochemistry, micrometastases can be detected in between 5 and 25 per cent of tumour-positive elective neck dissections of clinically N0 necks,[21, 22] with upstaging occurring in up to 12 per cent of patients.[23, 24] Results using techniques such as quantitative reverse transcriptase-polymerase chain reaction (QRT-PCR) can be obtained within 2 hours of tissue harvesting.

The clinical significance of micrometastases is undetermined. Prospective studies have used different markers and techniques to assess micrometastases and have arrived at diametrically opposite conclusions. In the absence of a universally acceptable marker or a battery of markers, it will be difficult to design clinical trials. Because of the unknown prognostic significance of micrometastases or indeed implications for additional postoperative treatment, the extra work involved in discovering it on a routine basis is not currently justified.

Isolated tumour cells (ITC) are defined as malignant deposits within lymph nodes that measure ≤0.2 mm in greatest extent or appear as single cells or small clusters of <200 cells, detectable on standard processing or immunohistochemistry, that show no evidence of metastatic activity. Unlike micrometastases, the presence of ITCs does not upstage the pathological stage, with their presence being denoted as pN0[i+].

CYSTIC NECK METASTASES/BRANCHIOGENIC CARCINOMA

Cystic neck metastases are usually of oropharyngeal origin, with the most common site being the tonsil. Human papilloma virus-related tumours are usually associated with cystic metastases.[25] These patients tend to have a better prognosis than their non-cystic counterparts. This has been reported as branchiogenic carcinoma in the past. Any diagnosis of branchiogenic carcinomas should be viewed with scepticism.[26, 27] The majority of branchiogenic carcinomas are in fact cystic metastases from oropharyngeal carcinoma, most commonly originating in the tonsils, and not true carcinomas arising in a branchial cleft cyst.

A diagnosis of branchiogenic carcinoma arising from the branchial system can only be made if the criteria in **Box 34.1**, are fulfilled. One could add to this list that the tumour should be human papilloma virus (HPV)-negative, as identification of HPV would point to an oropharyngeal origin.

PROGNOSTIC NODAL FEATURES

There are a number of features of metastatic cervical nodal disease which indicate a poor prognosis (**Box 34.2**). However, much of the data used to arrive at these conclusions are retrospective. Lefebvre et al.[28] looked at the impact of various regional factors on regional recurrence and distant metastases. This study with 1330 patients showed that irrespective of T staging, ECS, three or more positive nodes and positive level IV nodes doubled the risk of regional recurrence and trebled the risk of distant metastases.

Box 34.1 Criteria for the diagnosis of branchiogenic carcinoma

- The carcinoma should be demonstrated as arising in the wall of the branchial cyst.
- The tumour should occur in line running from a point just anterior to the tragus along the anterior border of sternomastoid muscle to the clavicle.
- The histology should be compatible with an origin from tissue found in branchial vestiges.
- No evidence of high risk human papilloma virus should be identified in the tumour tissue.
- No other primary should become evident within a five-year follow up.

Box 34.2 Prognostic nodal features

- Site, size and number
- Low neck nodes
- Extracapsular spread
- Morphology
- Bilateral and contralateral spread

Extracapsular spread

There is a general consensus that the presence of ECS in a lymph node is associated with a poor prognosis.[20, 29, 30, 31, 32, 33] Both prospective and retrospective evidence suggests that ECS decreases survival rates by approximately half compared to those patients whose tumour was confined to the nodes. Also, patients who have occult involvement of nodes and ECS statistically do worse.[20, 34] A meta-analysis concluded that perinodal spread adversely affected five-year survival, with a summarized odds ratio of 2.7.[35] Some workers have noted that invasion of the soft tissues of the neck by tumour lowers treatment success rates by 80 per cent. Other studies show that patients with ECS are at increased risk of local recurrence, distant metastases and that the time to recurrence is shorter. It is likely that ECS may have a differential impact depending on the primary sites. For instance, Oosterkamp et al.[36] showed that ECS adversely affected survival in laryngeal cancer by increasing the risk of metastases nine times, compared to a three times greater risk in patients without this finding.

Currently, it is not clear whether or not ECS represents an increase in tumour burden or an increase in tumour aggressiveness. As previously discussed, Toker[9] demonstrated that a primary deposit of tumour emboli within the node capsule may lead to ECS occurring quite early in the metastatic process and as such may represent an anatomical variation rather than an aggressive tumour. In addition, not all nodes within a neck dissection specimen show ECS and there may be a threshold volume of ECS above which the prognosis is poor.

The literature almost universally recommends that the standard treatment if ECS is detected following surgery is to add postoperative radiotherapy or chemoradiation, even for those who have only one node involved.[20, 37] Currently, based on level 1 evidence, many centres recommend adjuvant chemoradiation in the presence of extracapsular spread.[38]

Retropharyngeal nodes

Tumours that are associated with these nodes include primary disease of the oropharynx, paranasal sinuses and pyriform sinus, as well as advanced primary tumours at any site together with massive unilateral or bilateral neck disease, which presumably involves retropharyngeal nodes due to shunting from obstructed lymphatic ducts or channels. Retropharyngeal node invasion is almost always a radiologic diagnosis. There are a number of reports in the head and neck literature that associate the presence of retropharyngeal nodes with a very poor prognosis,[20, 39, 40] but a recent study of 51 patients concluded otherwise.[41]

CLINICAL STAGING

The joint UICC/AJCC classification for regional cervical lymphadenopathy, published in 2009 is the current system used for staging (**Table 34.4**).[42]

A classification system is essential for documentation of disease extent, comparisons of results between centres and stratifying patients for inclusion into trials. This is based not

Table 34.4 TNM classification of regional nodes.

N_x	Regional lymph nodes cannot be assessed
N_0	No regional lymph node metastases
N_1	Metastasis in a single ipsilateral lymph node 3 cm or less in greatest dimension
N_2	Metastasis in a single ipsilateral lymph node, more than 3 cm, but not more than 6 cm in greatest dimension or in multiple ipsilateral lymph nodes none more than 6 cm in greatest dimension, or in bilateral or contralateral lymph nodes, none more than 6 cm in greatest dimension
N_{2a}	Metastasis in a single ipsilateral lymph node, more than 3 cm, but not more than 6 cm in greatest dimension
N_{2b}	Metastasis in multiple ipsilateral lymph nodes, none more than 6 cm in greatest dimension
N_{2c}	Metastasis in bilateral or contralateral lymph nodes, none more than 6 cm in greatest dimension
N_3	Metastasis in a lymph node more than 6 cm in greatest dimension

UICC, 2009. Adapted from Sobin et al.[42]
Note: Midline nodes are considered ipsilateral nodes.

only on the presence or absence of cervical lymphadenopathy, but also the size, number and laterality of the lymph nodes. It applies to all head and neck tumours apart from those arising from primaries of the nasopharynx, thyroid gland and mucosal melanomas.

Limitations of the current staging system

The staging system is primarily anatomical and does not take into account very important prognostic factors such as concurrent comorbidity, HPV status in oropharyngeal cancers, the presence of vascular invasion and ECS in lymph nodes. It also does not take into account the level of the lymph nodes, and the worse prognosis conferred by some nodal groups, e.g. retropharyngeal nodes.

Furthermore, clinical staging gives great weight to laterality whereas pathological studies have shown that bilateral nodes, particularly if they are small (<3 cm), do not carry any worse prognosis than N1 nodes at certain sites, i.e. supraglottis. For other sites, contralateral and bilateral nodes carry a dismal prognosis and, as such, probably deserve an N3 grouping. This scheme does not allow independent classification of massive nodes on both sides of the neck which are often fixed and almost universally fatal.

CLINICAL PRESENTATION OF NECK DISEASE

The pattern of spread of malignant disease to the neck depends upon both patient and tumour factors. These are identified in **Box 34.3**. The site of the primary tumour is important with some sites having a higher incidence of

Box 34.3 Factors implicated in pattern of metastatic nodal disease

- Tumour site
- Tumour size
- Tumour thickness
- Previous treatment
- Tumour recurrence

metastases, both palpable and otherwise, at presentation (**Table 34.3**). Neck metastases usually present as neck masses, usually firm to hard on palpation. They may be mobile or fixed to surrounding structures, usually determined by the degree of ECS.

ASSESSMENT OF CERVICAL LYMPHADENOPATHY

Any patient with a head and neck primary tumour requires careful assessment of the neck. This begins with a full clinical examination which may be supplemented by an examination under anaesthetic. Further assessment of the neck with fine needle aspiration cytology and radiological imaging can help confirm or refute the diagnosis. Occasionally, an open biopsy may be required.

Clinical examination

Clinical examination remains an important initial method of assessing regional lymph nodes. Clinical examination of the neck has a variable diagnostic accuracy.[43, 44] Based on a systematic review,[45] physical examination has a sensitivity of 74 per cent, specificity of 81 per cent and an overall accuracy of 77 per cent. This can be particularly difficult in necks that are difficult to examine, i.e. for restaging or in short, stocky necks. In these instances, nodes may go unnoticed until they reach a considerable size. In addition, some regions are inaccessible, such as the retropharyngeal area.

Fine needle aspiration cytology

In the presence of palpable disease and a proven primary, treatment will usually be directed towards the assessment of the neck disease rather than confirming that a metastasis is present by fine needle aspiration cytology (FNAC). However, in many cases it is beneficial to perform an FNAC on a palpable node since a positive result is often back before assessment under anaesthesia can be performed. Few surgeons would ignore a clinically palpable node in the presence of proven primary disease, even if the FNAC shows no evidence of malignancy. The technique is particularly useful in the assessment of a palpable node when searching for an unknown primary as the cytological aspirate can be subjected to tests that may help in the search for the primary tumour. For example, evidence of human papilloma virus or

Epstein–Barr virus transcripts (or their surrogate markers) will point to a primary site in the oropharynx or nasopharynx, respectively. The possibility of anaplastic carcinoma or lymphoma usually makes a core biopsy or open biopsy mandatory. The technique is easy to perform, can be reported immediately (particularly if a cytopathologist is present in the outpatient clinic) and has overall accuracy rates exceeding 90 per cent.[46] There is, however, a well-recognized learning curve associated with the technique.

Ultrasound scan

This technique can detect the presence of malignant cervical lymph nodes with sensitivity rates between 70 and 90 per cent. When combined with FNAC, this figure increases to 90 per cent. The technique may require an ultrasonographer to be present in the outpatient clinic, is operator dependent and labour intensive. However, more clinicians are integrating portable ultrasound machines into the outpatient practice, and perform the procedure themselves. The addition of power Doppler to assess vascular flow[47] and molecular analysis of the aspirate[48] does improve on these figures. It should be noted that there are no absolute criteria for differentiating benign from malignant disease, but absent hilar echoes and increases in short axis length are generally considered to be features of metastatic neck nodes. Sonoelastography is a new imaging technique where low-amplitude, low-frequency shear waves are propagated through internal organs, while real-time Doppler techniques are used to image the resulting vibration pattern.

The decrease in vibration amplitude caused by the presence of non-homogeneity, such as a tumour within a region of soft tissue, is measured. This has shown promise in the evaluation of neck nodes.[49] There is also an increasing vogue for adding ultrasound with or without guided FNAC to follow up neck disease in patients after chemoradiation.[50]

Computed tomography

The diagnostic accuracy of computed tomography (CT) scanning in detecting malignant cervical lymphadenopathy is higher than clinical examination. The range of non-malignant cervical lymphadenopathy is 3 mm up to 3 cm, but most authors recognize that nodes greater than 1 cm in size on CT may contain metastatic disease. The criteria used for categorizing metastatic deposits include lymph nodes with short axis diameter larger than 1 cm, cluster of three or more borderline enlarged nodes larger than 0.8 cm, and nodal necrosis or patchy enhancement within the nodes.[51, 52, 53]

A meta-analysis of CT versus physical examination with 647 neck dissections showed CT to have a sensitivity of 83 per cent with a specificity and overall accuracy of 83 per cent.[45] This figure has remained stable in a more recent meta-analysis.[54] The detection of malignant disease is based on the fact that as cancer invades the lymph node, its size, shape and characteristics change so that as it enlarges, its centre dies and appears necrotic, and there is a thin rim of inflammation around the edge which shows up on scanning as rim enhancement.

It is important to realize that the two most difficult areas in imaging head and neck cancer are the detection of low volume neck disease and residual and recurrent disease following surgery and irradiation. Based on the above imaging criteria, it is possible to miss metastatic deposit in an 8 mm cervical lymph node, at which stage, the lymph node would contain 10^8 malignant cells. With increasing use of organ-preservation modalities, conventional imaging (CT and magnetic resonance imaging (MRI)) has assumed an important role in the assessment of treatment response after chemoradiation. In this setting, CT has been demonstrated to have negative predictive values in excess of 90 per cent.[55, 56, 57, 58, 59]

However, it is important not to rely on imaging alone and management decisions must be made after correlating with the clinical findings. Indications for neck imaging are set out in **Box 34.4**.

Magnetic resonance imaging

Meta-analyses suggest that this technique can detect cervical lymphadenopathy with overall similar accuracy rates to CT.[54, 60] However, MRI may be better in evaluating the N0 neck and in the presence of deep invasion. Similar criteria for malignancy are used in both techniques. Initial experience with ultrasmall paramagnetic iron oxide-enhanced MRI has shown this modality to have superior diagnostic efficacy compared to conventional imaging.[61, 62]

Computed tomography–positron emission tomography fusion imaging

Positron emission tomography (PET) using ^{18}F-2-fluoro-2-deoxy-D-glucose (^{18}FDG) as a radioactive tracer has proven efficacy in the functional imaging of solid tumours. Tumour cells metabolize more glucose compared to normal tissue and the increased uptake of the glucose analogue FDG can be imaged. However, the major drawback of this technique is the limited morphological information, making the exact anatomical localization of an area of increased glucose metabolism difficult. On its own, ^{18}FDG-PET has inferior sensitivity and specificity compared to conventional imaging,[63] but has been shown to have the ability to change the management in up to 15 per cent of patients when used prior to commencing treatment.[64, 65]

Coregistered anatomic and functional imaging techniques using dual modality CT-PET scanners lead to accurate image fusion, thus harvesting the advantages of both techniques. With relevance to metastatic neck disease, CT-PET has been investigated in the following settings: initial staging, radiotherapy planning and evaluation of response to radiation or chemoradiation.

There are calls for using this modality in routine practice to stage patients prior to treatment planning, as apart from diagnosis, this may have an impact on the treatment; for example, the presence of distant metastases, otherwise not detected on conventional scanning may be picked up on PET imaging, leading to a more palliative approach. This can help more treatment resources to be directed to those who are more likely to do well following locoregional treatment.[66, 67] High sensitivity (90–95 per cent) and specificity (95–99 per cent) rates have been observed in the pretreatment setting.[60, 67, 68, 69] However, lack of high quality prospective evidence about the impact the imaging has on the outcome and cost–benefit has delayed widespread use. CT-PET detection rate for nodes less than 1 cm is reported at 71 per cent.[70] Thus, this modality has poor detection rate (0–30 per cent) in the setting of the N0 neck.[67, 71, 72, 73]

Currently, the widespread role of CT-PET is confined to detecting the occult primary and for assessment of residual and recurrent disease following surgery and irradiation. If a primary site is not immediately apparent on clinical examination, all efforts must be taken to identify the primary site. Where the primary site remains undiscovered, a larger mucosal field may need to be radiated to cover all possible sites, thus increasing the morbidity. This is best done in a manner that maximizes the diagnostic efficacy of all modalities. Prospective and retrospective studies have shown that CT-PET scans will detect a primary site in between 25 and 60 per cent of patients in whom no primary is evident on clinical examination and using conventional radiology[74, 75] and combined with panendoscopy and biopsy, a primary will be identified in about 50 per cent of patients. CT-PET scans are best done prior to the panendoscopy to reduce false-positive rates. Our suggested algorithm for investigating an unknown primary is set out in **Figure 34.3**.

It is worth noting that false-positive results are common in the first few weeks after treatment and scans should be deferred until at least 8–12 weeks after completion of treatment. The scan has a high sensitivity (100 per cent) and negative predictive value (98–100 per cent)[76, 77] in the evaluation of the post-treatment neck, and these figures also hold good on meta-analyses.[78] Based on this finding, its use has been recommended to avoid salvage neck surgery following chemoradiation (see below under The chemoradiated neck). A prospective randomized controlled trial to evaluate the role of CT-PET in the post-treatment setting, to compare the outcomes of a watchful waiting policy based on a negative CT-PET scan to planned neck dissection is currently in progress. The Scottish Intercollegiate Network Guidelines recommend that FDG-PET be performed where neck recurrence is suspected and conventional imaging is non-confirmatory.[79] However, when this modality is used to assess the primary tumour status following treatment or for suspected recurrence, the results are much inferior.

Open biopsy

In general, this diagnostic procedure is best avoided as an initial diagnostic modality. However, in situations where

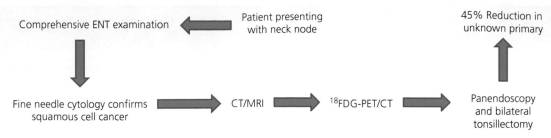

Figure 34.3   Algorithm for investigating an unknown primary with neck metastases.

FNAC is not available, equivocal or non-diagnostic, or when the results suggest either a lymphoma or an anaplastic carcinoma, or when a primary site is occult, it may be necessary. There is no evidence in the literature that an open biopsy alters the prognosis, as long as correct treatment is instigated within 6 weeks.[37] Any incision should be made to facilitate the removal of the scar via a subsequent standard neck dissection incision and previous surgery may mean that vital structures, such as the sternomastoid muscle, may have to be sacrificed due to scar tissue.

Sentinel node biopsy

The sentinel node biopsy (SNB) is a diagnostic technique used to assess the presence of occult metastatic disease in the N0 neck. The SNB concept is based on the principle that identification of the echelon nodes and assessing them for metastatic spread will provide information regarding the status of the rest of the neck. Using radioactive probes and/or blue dye around the tumour site, the first to third echelon nodes are identified with the help of gamma cameras and peri-operative hand-held probes; these nodes are subsequently harvested and analysed for tumour deposits. From a pathological point of view, these nodes undergo a much more comprehensive analysis (step-serial sectioning, immunohistochemistry) as missing a small deposit in the node could result in a wrong decision to not treat the neck. The assumption here is that if these echelon nodes are negative for secondary deposit, it is unlikely for the rest of the neck to have metastases, thus avoiding further treatment to the neck.

It has been shown in patients with early-stage malignant melanoma that selective lymphatic dissection performed after confirmation of positive sentinel node(s) is therapeutically equivalent to elective lymphatic dissection. Although the technique is considered standard for melanoma in non-head and neck sites as well as breast cancer, in the head and neck the technique suffers from a number of inherent problems. The head and neck lymphatic drainage can be variable with skip metastases, collateral channels are often present and the technique potentially involves the violation of oncologic principles. In addition, the technique is operator dependent with a recognized learning curve[80] and there is an inherent risk of facial nerve damage when assessing parotid nodes. Its role would only be mainly in the treatment of disease within the oral cavity and oropharynx as injection of the tracer around laryngeal and hypopharyngeal tumours is very cumbersome and satisfactory injection all around the tumour

is difficult, if not impossible, to perform. A multicentre trial showed that SNB procedure is reproducible in early oral cavity and oropharynx tumours with good sensitivity rates.[81] A diagnostic meta-analysis incorporating a decision analysis model[82] demonstrated pooled sensitivity rates for the SNB procedure using radionuclides from all published studies to be 92 per cent. When compared to elective neck dissection, the decision analysis model showed that the cumulative outcomes (including recurrence and mortality) for SNB were poor by about 1 per cent. The outcomes did not take into account the morbidity caused by the procedures. Within the head and neck, its use remains to be established outside trial settings. A Europe-wide multicentre trial is now underway to establish the role and efficacy of this modality in oral cancer. Other prospective trials are also in progress in the United States.

Pathology

The head and neck pathologist has the final say in the assessment and staging of cervical lymphadenopathy. Following neck dissection, the specimen should be pinned out on a board and orientated as to the levels, or the specimen separated into respective levels before presenting it to the pathologist. It will then be examined to assess the total number of lymph nodes in the specimen, the number that are positive, the levels that are involved along with the presence or absence of ECS, vascular and lymphatic permeation. Within the current UICC/AJCC classification, histological examination of a selective neck dissection will ordinarily include six or more lymph nodes and examination of a radical neck dissection will include ten or more lymph nodes. Standardization of pathological reporting is essential in order to compare data across centres and to facilitate comparative audit and there is currently a standardized reporting form, which has recently been produced by the Royal College of Pathologists.[83]

DRAWBACKS IN THE LITERATURE WHEN ASSESSING TREATMENT OUTCOME

The majority of papers published in the literature which relate to HNSCC are retrospective, and because of this many of the controversies that existed 50 years ago have yet to be resolved.

Retrospective data suffer from several biases. These include variation in treatment protocols caused by factors relating to the patient, the tumour and treating physician. Diagnostic and treatment expertise varies between centres and therapeutic schedules applied in various ways and at various times. Data collection may require perusal of the notes, which are often incomplete and studies that report different end points are not strictly comparable. For example, survival is the usual end point reported by head and neck surgeons, but when studying the efficacy of any type of neck treatment, locoregional control is more important.

When assessing any single or combination treatment with regards to the control of neck disease, it is important that the study meets the requirements set out in **Box 34.5**. Prospective randomized therapeutic trials control for all these variables, but unfortunately there is a paucity of surgical trials in the current head and neck literature, although this situation may be remedied by several trials that are currently in progress.

TREATMENT OF METASTATIC NECK DISEASE

After controlling for patient and tumour factors, the treatment of metastatic neck disease is usually decided by the stage of neck disease as identified by the joint UICC/AJCC classification for regional cervical lymphadenopathy.[42] The following section discusses treatment of neck disease for each N stage. It is worthwhile identifying the broad areas where there is a lack of high level evidence and controversy exists (**Box 34.6**). Most of these topics are being actively investigated and the treatment paradigms are evolving.

It is worth reiterating a few important general principles regarding neck spread when discussing the surgical management of metastatic neck disease. (1) In the untreated neck, patterns of spread may be predictable. (2) In the N0 neck, occult disease is usually found within the first echelon lymph node drainage basin. This permits the principle of selective neck dissection. (3) Previous treatment alters drainage patterns significantly. (4) Patients with palpable neck disease are more likely to have non-palpable spread in other levels.

The N0 neck

Historically, evaluation and treatment for the N0 neck has been one of the great dilemmas in head and neck surgery and its treatment today is still controversial. The problem that faces the head and neck oncologist is whether or not to treat the neck electively. The reason why elective treatment to the N0 neck has been proposed is that retrospective evidence from elective radical neck dissection (RND) specimens suggests there is a high incidence of subclinical disease for SCC affecting the oral cavity, pharynx and supraglottic larynx. As shown in **Table 34.3**, the likelihood of there being involved nodes depends not only on the site of the primary disease, but also on tumour size and histological differentiation. The controversy extends to when and how the N0 neck should be treated.

There are a number of treatment options for the N0 neck. These include the following:

- elective surgery;
- elective radiotherapy;
- adopting a policy of 'wait and see';
- elective neck investigation.

Elective neck treatment

Proponents of elective neck treatment maintain it prevents some cancer-related deaths because untreated neck disease can shed tumour into the vascular or lymphatic system and produce distant metastases. Unfortunately, only distant metastases which are seeded from developing nodal disease can be prevented by elective neck treatment and since spread can occur by other routes, or at inception of tumour, then quite clearly the argument for elective treatment is weakened.

EVIDENCE FOR ELECTIVE NECK TREATMENT VERSUS OBSERVATION

Five randomized prospective trials that have examined the issue of elective neck treatment are summarized in **Table 34.5**. Four compared surgical clearance of the neck,[84, 85, 86, 87] and one elective neck irradiation,[88] with observation. The bulk of this level 1 evidence is based on cohorts with oral cavity primaries.

As can be seen, only one trial,[85] favoured elective neck treatment. Careful five-year follow up detected no difference in survival between the two groups in the French trial,[84] but in the delayed treatment group, tumour problems or the patient's general condition precluded an operation when nodes were palpable in two patients, one of the objections to adopting a policy of 'wait and see' for N0 disease. In addition, more than 50 per cent of patients in both arms received radiation, which may have contributed to the lack of difference. Although the trial by Fakih et al.[86] showed no difference in control rates between the arms, it must be noted that the results reported were one-year survival data, despite a median follow-up period of 20 months. Chi-square tests were used to compare the proportion who were disease free at one year and no actuarial methods were used. Careful perusal of this trial shows that patients who underwent elective treatment did well in all comparisons, without achieving statistical significance. A recent randomised trial from Hong Kong by Yuen et al.[87] with 71 patients showed no difference in disease free survival between the groups. However, the observed group had a significantly higher incidence of regional recurrences, which were picked up on close surveillance and successfully salvaged. This group had earlier published significantly better five-year disease-free survival in a retrospective cohort who had been compared to observation alone.[89] The major difference is close follow up in the observation arm, leading to earlier identification of neck metastases. It must also be noted that all these studies are not adequately powered.

In addition to the trials by Vandenbrouck et al,[84] Yuen et al.[87] and Pointon and Gleave,[88] other studies support a wait and watch policy for the N0 neck. D'Cruz et al.[90] found no differences in the three- and five-year disease-free survival in a retrospective cohort of 359 patients (200 observed versus 159 treated with END) who had early tongue cancer. Leyland et al.[91] looked at the influence of neck disease on the outcome in a large retrospective cohort of 3887 patients with SCC at all subsites in the head and neck. The results suggested that close observation with subsequent salvage in the event of recurrence produced statistically similar disease-specific survival to elective treatment, be it radiation, surgery or combined modality. This approach can be complemented by meticulous follow up using ultrasound-guided cytology and salvage when appropriate.[50, 92] These studies seem to support the contention that elective treatment of the neck is not prophylactic in that it does not prevent cancer-related deaths or improve survival. Currently, multicentre prospective randomized trials designed to address this question in oral cavity cancer are in progress in the United Kingdom and in India.

However, many retrospective studies and recently, other prospective non-randomized studies, including an evidence-based review,[37] that have looked at the treatment of the N0 neck in oral cavity carcinomas[93, 94] suggested improved outcome when the neck was electively treated. A 'wait and watch' policy will result in 25–35 per cent of patients presenting with overt disease, needing therapeutic neck treatment, although the results from the randomized trials quoted above suggest a much higher conversion rate. Control rates in this scenario approximate 30–50 per cent, leading to around 15 per cent of patients who have progressive disease. This figure is still higher than the widely accepted 5–7 per cent failure rate where the neck is electively treated. In the presence of only limited high-level evidence for a watch and wait policy, the general consensus in the literature is to err on the side of caution and it is prudent to treat the neck when the risk of occult spread is more than 15–20 per cent. The latter figure is derived from a rather simplistic decision analysis model performed in the 1990s,[95] which showed that at a threshold occult metastatic rate of 20 per cent, the morbidity of treatment is offset by its benefit, and is widely accepted. It must be noted that the surgical treatment considered in the model was radical neck dissection. Many surgeons and oncologists would perform elective neck treatment for lesser probability (5–15 per cent) of occult metastases.[96] The Scottish Intercollegiate Guidelines Network also espouses elective treatment of the neck in this scenario.[79]

Currently, both elective neck dissection and irradiation are viewed as prophylactic treatments, but if one recognizes the significance of occult neck disease as a marker of the ability of

Table 34.5 Randomized controlled studies in management of the N0 neck.

Study	Treatment arms	No. patients	Primary site	Positive necks	Disease-free survival (%)	Follow up (years)	Difference
Pointon and Gleave[88]	ENI	100	–	–	80	2	NS
	OBS	105		–	65		
Vandenbrouck et al.[84]	END	39	Oral tongue and	19	NA	5	NS
	OBS	36	floor of mouth	19	NA		
Kligerman et al.[85]	END	34	Oral tongue and	7	72	3	$p = 0.04$
	OBS	33	floor of mouth	13	49		
Fakih et al.[86]	END	30	Oral tongue	10	63	1	NS
	OBS	40		23	52		
Yuen et al.[87]	END	36	Oral tongue	2	89%	5	NS
	OBS	35		11	87%		

END, elective neck dissection; ENI, elective neck irradiation; NA, not available; NS, not significant; OBS, observation.

any individual tumour to metastasize thereby providing a significant prognostic indicator of eventual distant metastases and the possible need for systemic adjuvant chemotherapy, then only surgery can provide the histological data to give this information (**Box 34.7**).

Choice of treatment modality for the N0 neck

Although there are no prospective trials, retrospective data from studies with large numbers suggest that elective neck dissection and irradiation are equally effective in controlling subclinical disease.[97] The choice of treatment modality is dictated by numerous factors, including physician and patient choices, quality-of-life issues and how the primary site is managed. When the primary tumour is being treated with radiotherapy, then elective treatment should be with radiotherapy to at least the first echelon lymph nodes (or the whole neck) and where midline extension occurs, treatment should be bilateral. If the primary tumour is being treated with interstitial brachytherapy then the neck may be treated electively with either surgery or irradiation. When the primary tumour is treated with surgery, then elective neck surgery should be carried out since it provides further information for clinical staging, lymph nodes in the area are cleared to give access to vessels for reconstructive purposes, local recurrence rates may be reduced and survival enhanced. The appropriate levels to be dissected out in an SND are based on the site of the primary tumour and this is discussed under Elective surgery below. **Figure 34.4**, summarizes our recommendations for management of the ipsilateral N0 neck.

ELECTIVE SURGERY

The pros and cons of elective neck surgery are set out in **Boxes 34.8** and **34.9** below.

The concept of therapeutic equivalence of selective neck dissection and comprehensive neck dissection for elective treatment of the neck is widely accepted[98] and based on prospective studies, there is little justification for a comprehensive neck dissection in this setting.[99, 100] Levels II–IV need to be cleared for laryngeal and hypopharyngeal cancer.[100] For patients with oral cavity cancer, SND of at least levels I–III should be carried out, with the addition of level IV for tongue cancers.[99] Levels II–IV are recommended for oropharyngeal cancers.[101] There appears to be little advantage in dissecting level V for any of the mucosal primaries electively.[102, 103, 104] Excellent local control rates can be obtained with SND, with

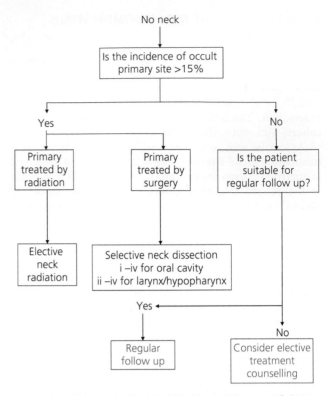

Figure 34.4 Recommendations for the management of the ipsilateral N0 neck.

recurrence rates of around 5 per cent with the primary controlled.

Current work focuses on selecting the levels that need to be dissected in the elective setting. For example, clearance of level IIb during SND involves dissection in a relatively narrow field

- Control rates are no lower when a 'wait and see' policy is followed and therapeutic neck dissection is performed.
- Careful clinical follow up combined with imaging has the potential to detect early conversion from N0 to N1.
- Radiation is as effective as neck dissection for non-palpable disease.
- Elective neck dissection results in a large number of unnecessary surgical procedures associated with inevitable morbidity.
- Elective neck dissection removes the barrier to the spread of disease and may have a detrimental immunological effect.
- Elective neck dissection can cause a scarred, hypoxic field that can reduce radiation kill.

and significant retraction of the sternomastoid muscle is needed. It is likely that the accessory nerve can be subjected to traction injury and segmental devascularization, causing shoulder dysfunction. Prospective studies[105] have shown that SND causes a small, but significant impairment to the shoulder function. The incidence of isolated metastases in this level is very low at 0.3 per cent.[106] Prospective studies have shown little oncologic benefit in clearing this level in laryngeal cancer as the occult metastatic rate is low at 0.4 per cent,[106, 107] but higher incidence rates are seen in oral cavity (3.9 per cent) and oropharyngeal (5.2 per cent) cancer, needing clearance of this level. Whether preservation of level IIb necessarily leads to improved shoulder outcomes needs to be verified in prospective studies. Other reviews have promoted evidence to suggest that level IV need not be dissected in patients with N0 supraglottic and glottic squamous carcinoma.[108]

END can undoubtedly serve as a biopsy and a subsequent indicator of the risk of systemic disease since local neck and distant metastases are manifestations of the same process and represent the ability of the tumour to metastasize in an individual host.

ELECTIVE NECK IRRADIATION

Retrospective evidence suggests that external beam radiation of approximately 40–50 Gy to the clinically N0 neck will control occult metastases in more than 90–95 per cent of cases.[109] In addition to the prospective study identified,[88] other retrospective studies evaluating its role in the treatment of patients with SCC of the oral cavity and tongue[110] did show that elective neck irradiation improves locoregional control and may prolong survival in some cases. This is based on the observed rate of conversion of N0 to N+ necks after elective neck irradiation (3–15 per cent) and the expected rate of appearance of nodes when the neck is observed, based on a 20–40 per cent histological incidence of occult neck disease. However, this assumes that all occult lymph node cancer deposits are clinically significant and evidence from other studies suggests this is not necessarily the case.

ELECTIVE NECK INVESTIGATION

Another option in the N0 neck is to consider elective neck investigation. Could a radiological investigation such as CT, MRI or ultrasound demonstrate malignant cervical lymphadenopathy at the subclinical stage and if so, could a treatment plan be adopted on the basis of these scans?

It would seem that many of the arguments levelled against neck dissection could be levelled against elective neck imaging.[111] If false-positive results are inevitable in the presence of inflammatory neck nodes and false negatives do occur, then imaging could play no role in the routine evaluation of the N0 neck. Treatment should be based upon the understanding of the natural history in question and currently it is probably cheaper and as effective to offer elective treatment to those high-risk patients who need it and 'wait and see' in the others. This will avoid large numbers of unnecessary CT scans and subsequent inevitable inappropriate surgery. It is perfectly reasonable to adopt a policy of 'wait and see' in low-risk necks, i.e. carcinoma of the glottis or the gingiva, but for those who are high risk, waiting for the neck to develop from N0 to N1 may have a detrimental effect on the patient unless scrupulous follow-up policies are instituted.

The follow-up protocol for the observation arm in the randomized trial by Yuen et al.[87] included three-monthly ultrasonograms of the neck for the first three years. This policy led to earlier diagnosis of neck recurrences and prompt salvage with no decrease in disease-specific survival. Van den Brekel et al.[112] evaluated the outcome of observing the clinically N0 neck in high-risk patients (mainly oral carcinoma) using ultrasonographic-guided (US) FNAC for follow up after transoral excision. Patients were followed up for between one and four years using palpation and US-FNAC. The high salvage rate (71 per cent) was attributed to a strict follow-up policy using US-FNAC and concluded that a policy of 'wait and see' was justified. Other studies and reviews have come to similar conclusions.[113, 114]

The contralateral N0 neck

In the setting of a unilateral primary and ipsilateral metastases, data suggest that the contralateral neck has a very high incidence of occult metastases, between 30 and 70 per cent, especially in supraglottic[115, 116, 117] hypopharyngeal[118, 119, 120, 121] and oropharyngeal tumours.[122, 123] In the presence of advanced primaries at high risk of occult spread, contralateral neck treatment is warranted. Recurrence in the untreated contralateral neck has been shown to be the most common cause of failure in supraglottic cancer, with improved local control and two-year survival when dissected.[124, 125, 126, 127] There is no benefit in clearing level IIb in the contralateral N0 neck for any primary site.[106, 128]

The N+ neck

Management of the N+ neck is continuously evolving as more and more data are accrued. Traditionally, advanced neck disease has needed a combination of surgery and radiation therapy for control of disease. The treatment offered to the neck often depends on the modality used to treat the primary site, as seen in the suggested algorithms for patients undergoing primary surgery (**Figure 34.5**) and primary chemoradiation (**Figure 34.6**).

SINGLE PALPABLE METASTASIS IN THE IPSILATERAL NECK LESS THAN 3 CM IN DIAMETER (N1)

Similar to the N0 neck, the choice of modality is usually dictated by the treatment to the primary site. Where the primary is treated with irradiation, the neck is also covered in the field. ECS is uncommon in this stage and since the survival figures are good, conservation neck surgery is feasible. It is important to remember that in palpable neck disease, all five levels may be involved and should usually be dissected. In the majority of cases, the accessory nerve can be preserved, enabling modified radical neck dissection (MRND). Based on assessment of the best available evidence,[37] there is no evidence that RND achieves better survival figures than MRND.

It is widely accepted that single treatment modality gives good control rates for N1 neck disease,[129] although review of large databases suggests that there may be survival advantage to adding RT even for N1 necks.[130] As approximately 50 per cent of clinically N1 necks are upstaged after pathological assessment, many patients subsequently require postoperative radiation. Single modality usually suffices to control N1 neck disease, with both radiation and surgery having equivalent control rates.

SELECTIVE NECK DISSECTION IN THE N1 NECK AS PRIMARY TREATMENT

The role of SND in the N+ neck is less controversial today than it was two decades ago. There is no doubt that the morbidity of a neck dissection arises largely from level V dissection and there is a low incidence of nodal involvement at this level unless two or more levels (especially level IV) are involved.[37, 102] There is a clear pathological basis for SND in N1 and N2a disease. The proponents for a 'less than five level'

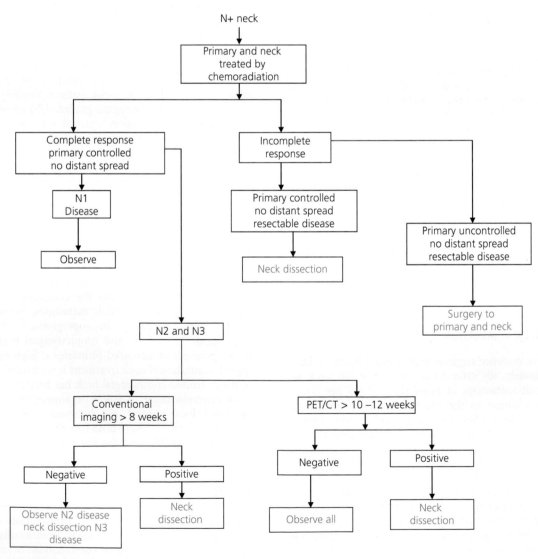

Figure 34.5 Algorithm for patients undergoing primary surgery.

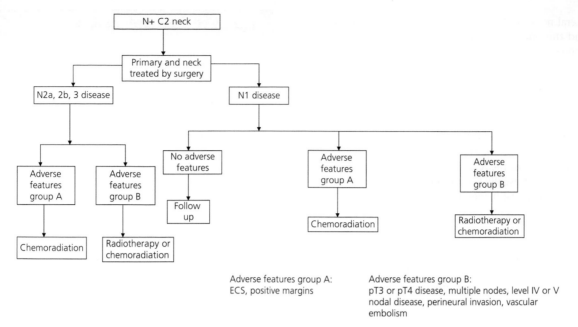

Figure 34.6 Algorithm for patients undergoing primary chemoradiation.

Adverse features group A:
ECS, positive margins

Adverse features group B:
pT3 or pT4 disease, multiple nodes, level IV or V nodal disease, perineural invasion, vascular embolism

neck dissection for N1 disease argue that the distribution of metastases within first echelon lymph nodes in non-palpable disease can be applied to early palpable disease. However, this sort of surgery requires considerable expertise and is not recommended for the trainee surgeon.

Byers *et al.*[131] looked at the outcomes of SNDs in 517 patients. They found that recurrence rates in patients with N1 disease were 5.6 and 35.6 per cent with and without postoperative radiation, respectively. Other retrospective studies also vouch for the efficacy of the SND alone in the N1 neck, as long as adjuvant treatment is provided if the disease is upstaged following surgery or other adverse factors exist.[132, 133, 134, 135, 136, 137]

Prospective studies are yet to be performed to evaluate this further, but on the basis of a large body of retrospective evidence, it can be concluded that SND may be sufficient treatment for N1 disease confirmed on pathological examination. We recommend that where there is doubt regarding the spread and extent of disease, it is better to perform a comprehensive procedure the first time around.

CONCURRENT CHEMORADIATION THERAPY FOR THE N1 NECK

Concurrent chemoradiation (given for treating the primary site) offers excellent control rates.[138, 139] No treatment is required in the event of a complete response, but partial responders merit a neck dissection. The type of neck dissection for partial responders is discussed below.

IPSILATERAL LARGE NODE (>3–6 CM, N2A) OR MULTIPLE UNILATERAL NODES (N2B)

The treatment depends on the management of the primary and if deemed operable, the neck should be treated with comprehensive neck dissection. If possible, a MRND sparing

---

Box 34.10 Indications for postoperative adjuvant treatment

- Extracapsular spread
- Two or more positive nodes
- N2–3 stages
- Residual disease

---

the accessory nerve gives equivalent control rates to a RND.[37, 140, 141] Larger neck nodes are at a greater risk of ECS, and following primary surgery are best treated by postoperative adjuvant treatment (**Box 34.10**). Analysis of large databases show that adjuvant radiotherapy confers a 10 per cent absolute increase in five-year cancer-specific survival and overall survival for patients with lymph node-positive HNSCC compared with surgery alone.[142] Recent randomized controlled trials performed in Europe and the United States confirm the clear benefit provided by adjuvant chemoradiation in the presence of ECS.[38, 143, 144] If the primary site is being irradiated, and incomplete response ensues, a neck dissection is warranted. Patients who achieve a complete response may not need surgical salvage and the rationale behind this is discussed in more detail below under The chemoradiated neck. This group represents advanced disease and retrospective and prospective studies clearly show that if primary surgery is performed, postoperative adjuvant therapy is required to achieve good regional control rates.

BILATERAL AND CONTRALATERAL NODES (N2C)

Patients with bilateral neck nodes are uncommon and occur overall in about 5 per cent of head and neck cancers. The common primary sites involved are the tongue base, supraglottic larynx and hypopharynx. Conventionally, the presence of bilateral neck disease was thought to be a grave prognostic sign and this was indicated historically in its staging. However, subsequent careful pathological studies have shown that, in certain instances, this is not so. The prognosis is determined more by the size, number of nodes and by the presence or absence of ECS within the neck rather than by pure laterality. This is particularly true for the supraglottic larynx and in those patients where the bilateral nodes do not feature massive and multiple nodes, treatment can be worthwhile using conventional surgery.[145] Conservation neck surgery may be possible on the less involved side and postoperative radiotherapy will usually be administered.[13, 146] The decision to treat will often be helped by the location and size of the primary site. Laryngeal tumours with extralaryngeal spread and bilateral nodes are often eminently treatable with laryngectomy and appropriate neck dissection, but patients with an extensive tongue base tumour and bilateral cervical lymphadenopathy will usually be inoperable at presentation. Patients with bilateral nodes when one side is fixed are usually incurable.

MASSIVE NODES (> 6 CM, N3)

The presence of massive nodes is again an uncommon event occurring in patients with head and neck cancer. Only 5 per cent of all patients will present with N3 neck disease in the United Kingdom. It is important to realize that many nodes that do reach 6 cm in size are often fixed to the skin and/or underlying structures. The decision whether or not to operate depends upon the stage and site of the primary site, presence or absence of fixation, what the node is fixed to, the experience of the surgeon and the needs of the patient. The incidence of true fixation of neck masses is often difficult to determine from the literature with reported figures up to 30 per cent. Fixation to the mandible, sternomastoid muscle or muscles in the midline may not represent as much a problem as fixation to the brachial plexus or carotid artery. These patients are at high risk of distant metastases and may present a special group where CT-PET scans may be warranted to fully evaluate this problem.

Long-term control rates are poor and the benefit of treatment must be carefully weighed against the morbidity caused by it, including the chances of control at the primary site. Radical treatment is warranted in patients who have less advanced disease at the primary site, and has been shown to achieve long-term control.[147] Combined modality therapy leads to better control rates,[148] although recent studies report similar control rates by reserving surgical salvage for clinical or radiologic evidence of residual disease.[149] In many patients, palliation will be the best option.

The unknown primary

There is no consensus on the management of squamous cancer arising from occult primaries. Options include primary surgery (comprehensive neck dissection) followed by radiotherapy (plus chemotherapy where indicated) to either the ipsilateral involved neck alone or to the bilateral neck and mucosa of the upper aerodigestive tract. Alternatively, primary chemoradiation to the neck or to the neck and all mucosal sites can be delivered, with

---

> **Box 34.11   The difficult neck**
>
> - Difficult to assess
> - Short stocky neck
> - Retropharyngeal nodes
> - Recurrent disease
> - Involvement of vital structures

surgical salvage as discussed above. Extending the radiation field to encompass all possible mucosal primary sites results in lower locoregional failure at five years (27 versus 51 per cent for ipsilateral irradiation), but has no advantage in terms of disease-free survival and emergence of primary cancer, but is associated with increased toxicity.[150] This entity is discussed in further detail in Chapter 35, Management of an unknown primary carcinoma.

The difficult neck

The scenarios that present a difficult neck are set out in **Box 34.11**.

Careful clinical assessment with mandatory radiological imaging will help to assess operability and some of these patients will be helped by extended radical neck dissection. Fixation to the skull base and brachial plexus is certainly a contraindication to surgical treatment, but fixation to the skin may be treated by wide resection and flap repair.

CAROTID INVASION

In current day practice, most tumours that present with clinical and radiological signs of invasion are likely to be radiorecurrent.[151] Indications for considering carotid resection include clinical evidence of fixation of the tumour to the carotid, invasion confirmed on imaging, and encroachment of tumour which encompasses more than 270 degrees of the vessel wall. Luminal invasion is rare and pathological evidence of invasion, limited to the adventitia, is seen in only 40–50 per cent of resected arteries.[152, 153, 154]

The plan to resect the carotid should always be a preoperative decision and almost never should a situation arise where this is contemplated for the first time peri-operatively. Preoperative work up is essential to plan the resection. Balloon occlusion of the artery with single photon emission computed tomography (SPECT) is performed to prognosticate the possibility of neurological deficit following resection. If the test shows adequate crossflow and does not cause symptoms, permanent occlusion can be performed with coils pre-operatively, with resection being performed 2 weeks later. Intraoperative ligation without reconstruction is fraught with a high risk of complications owing to the haemodynamic instability that can occur. This is likely even in those patients who demonstrate good crossflow and a stump pressure of more than 70 mmHg. If the crossflow is inadequate, reconstruction is necessary to reduce chances of neurologic complications. Most studies report using the saphenous vein graft.

A high operative morbidity (33 per cent hemiplegia) and mortality (12 per cent) has been quoted from work undertaken in the 1980s, but recent studies where resection and reconstruction of the carotid artery is performed have shown much lower figures.[155, 156] A review of 148 patients published between 1987 and 1998 demonstrated combined major neurological morbidity and mortality rates of 10 per cent.[157]

It is well recognized that in untreated patients with HNSCC, the carotid artery may not often be involved even when massive disease is present in the neck and that neck dissection may be possible. However, in the presence of radiological evidence of invasion, surgeons have traditionally opted to resect the carotid. In a review of 90 patients with documented radiological evidence of invasion, Ozer et al.[151] showed that this need not be the case and in over 70 per cent of cases dissection of the carotid is feasible and the tumour can be removed without recourse to carotid resection.

Traditionally, carotid resections were regarded to be unrewarding in HNSCC from the point of either achieving locoregional control or improving survival. A review of the literature in 1992[154] reported a two-year survival rate of 22 per cent following carotid artery resection. This study has been criticized for failing to identify those patients who had been treated previously, for not distinguishing between the treatment of isolated neck recurrence compared with recurrent disease at the primary site, as well as the neck. Aggressive disease in a radiated neck may be associated with residual tumour following resection and there is high risk of systemic disease; thus resection of the carotid artery was thought not to affect the natural history of the disease. Papers published in the last decade suggest that poor outcomes are especially seen in patients who have had previous radiation. Those patients with demonstrable carotid invasion who undergo primary surgical resection with or without reconstruction of the carotid may have a much superior outcome, with control rates between 30 and 50 per cent at five years.[151, 156, 157, 158] There may be a subgroup of patients who present with bulky neck disease and carotid invasion, who are best managed by primary resection and reconstruction with adjuvant radiation.

This is often a difficult scenario and decisions should be made after careful consideration of the morbidity and mortality of the procedure, patient expectations and the expertise of the treating team.

THE IRRADIATED N0 NECK WITH RECURRENCE AT THE PRIMARY SITE

Very few studies[159, 160, 161] have addressed this question, but have happily arrived at the same conclusion. There appears to be no increased risk of occult metastases in this setting and SND is oncologically adequate to clear the neck.

THE CHEMORADIATED NECK

Organ-preservation protocols have established a firm place in head and neck oncologic practice. Using concurrent chemoradiation, they aim to avoid resection and thus sacrifice of the organ where the primary is sited, even for advanced primaries. The following discussion assumes that the primary site has been controlled in all instances.

Although histological evidence of residual disease has been demonstrated in only 40–45 per cent of partial responders, few centres would argue against salvage neck surgery in this setting. The extent of the procedure remains a point of controversy as it is rare to find viable disease in levels that are clinically negative.[162, 163]

However, there is no universal agreement on how the advanced neck should be dealt with following chemoradiation when a complete response is obtained. Pathologic examination of the neck dissection specimen reveals residual disease in up to 25 per cent of patients who have achieved a complete response,[138, 164] but the presence of tumour cells does not indicate that they are viable. Some studies show a clear benefit in regional control when planned neck dissection is undertaken even in the presence of complete response.[138] However, prospective studies of patients with a complete response as assessed radiologically have mature long-term clinical follow up and show very low regional relapse rates that are comparable to the regional failure rates reported in planned neck dissection series.

Several studies have demonstrated the high sensitivity and negative predictive value of CT-PET imaging to assess residual disease in complete[76, 165, 166] and partial responders,[76, 77] performed at least 8 weeks after treatment. Earlier scanning increases false-positive results and is not recommended. A recent meta-analysis showed that highest sensitivity results are seen in studies performing CT-PET 10 weeks after treatment.[78] This has been used as a decision-making tool in recommending neck dissection after chemoradiation, with surgery being limited to cases where there is evidence of uptake. The literature has slowly shifted towards a non-surgical management for patients who experience a complete response[167, 168, 169] with some international groups endorsing this in consensus statements.[170] Emerging data suggest some role for an SND or even a lesser procedure (superselective neck dissection) in this setting when a complete response is obtained.[171, 172, 173, 174]

We recommend that necks staged N2 undergo conventional imaging between 8 and 12 weeks and that the decision is made for the surgical salvage in partial responders. Complete responders can be observed. Where there is access for CT-PET imaging, this can be used to decide if neck salvage is required, assuming all quality control assurances are met. For N3 necks, as the incidence of residual disease is high, we would recommend neck salvage irrespective of the response (see Massive nodes (>6 cm N3) above). In the absence of sufficiently sensitive diagnostic techniques, it is prudent to perform a comprehensive neck dissection in N2–3 necks, regardless of the response.[138, 162, 164, 175] Metastases from nasopharyngeal carcinomas are excluded from this recommendation, and observation alone will suffice when a complete response is obtained even with N3 disease.

The timing of neck dissection after chemoradiation has not been systematically assessed. Nodes tend to regress at variable rates after irradiation. Bataini et al.[176] suggested an interval of at least 8 weeks for nodes 6 cm and less and longer periods (16–20 weeks) for those greater than 6 cm. Pathological studies have shown that metastatic disease can be demonstrated in 30 per cent of necks after chemoradiation, despite clinical and radiological evidence of complete response, but this does not correlate with the clinical outcome of low (5 per cent) recurrence.[177, 178, 179, 180]

This may be due to non-viable cells and the fact that many of the dissections were done 4–6 weeks after treatment. The neck is best assessed between 8 and 12 weeks as discussed above and salvage offered following this. Surgical procedures on necks after chemoradiation are fraught with more complications.

TREATMENT OUTCOMES

Regional recurrence rates in the pN0 neck are consistently good between 3 and 7 per cent, largely irrespective of the modality of treatment. Recurrence rates following therapeutic neck treatment will vary depending on other factors, such as control of the primary site, ECS and the stage. Where the primary tumour has been controlled, overall recurrence rates range from approximately 10 per cent for N1 disease without ECS, 20–30 per cent for N2 disease and up to 85 per cent for N3 disease, although some series quote better results.[13, 148, 149, 181] In many cases of N3 disease, the primary site remains uncontrolled.[20, 147]

RECURRENT NECK DISEASE

Recurrence in the neck following previous treatment carries a gloomy prognosis. In accordance with the natural history of HNSCC, the majority of recurrences occur within the first two years of treatment. Various considerations including status of the primary site, extent and nature of recurrence, distant metastases and comorbidity dictate the treatment. Thus, a comprehensive investigation of the general status of the patient and distant metastases should be performed. Many of these masses will be fixed to vital structures which will negate extensive surgery. In patients who present with unresectable disease, reirradiation with or without chemotherapy should be considered, particularly in those who present more than two years since their previous treatment. Evidence of partial repair of radiotherapy-induced spinal cord subclinical damage and newer radiotherapy delivery techniques (intensity-modulated radiotherapy (IMRT), tomotherapy, protons) that allow better sparing of neurological structures at risk make this a realistic option in a larger number of patients. If surgery is possible, wide resections should be undertaken and postoperative radiotherapy given. If the patient has already received postoperative irradiation, then further radiotherapy using brachytherapy may be given when margins are close or when complete resection was not possible. About one-third of patients will be untreatable at presentation.

Recurrence in the ipsilateral untreated neck

In this situation, neck dissection is usually the preferred treatment with or without postoperative radiotherapy based on the histology. This group of patients do relatively well and local control rates between 50 and 60 per cent can be expected. Alternatively, irradiation with surgical salvage may be used along the principles described above.

Recurrence in the contralateral untreated neck

A proportion of patients in whom metastases occur on the untreated contralateral side of the neck some time after a dissection on the other side may be salvaged, provided there is no recurrence at the primary site. In a retrospective review of 2550 patients, Spector et al.[182] concluded that delayed metastases occurring on the untreated contralateral side were associated with significantly better salvage rates (42.5 per cent) than the ipsilateral previously treated neck (17 per cent).

Recurrence in the previously treated neck

Radical radiotherapy can be used if there is recurrent disease in the neck developing after previous surgery, which was not followed by postoperative irradiation. Owing to scarring from previous treatment, the neck stage is often N2a or more at presentation and ECS occurs in the vast majority of patients.

A multi-institutional review[183] studied 77 patients with cervical recurrence on the treated side, in the setting of a controlled primary. The review found that attempting salvage was useful in selected patients, giving a 33 per cent control rate at three years. Results were better when surgical salvage was performed, but this probably reflects the low disease volume. Salvage rates were significantly better in the previously radiated neck rather than the neck treated by previous surgery, with disease-free intervals being 46 months and eight months, respectively.

Nodal recurrence after combination treatment

The prognosis is extremely poor in those patients who suffer a neck recurrence following previous surgery and radiotherapy, with median disease-free intervals of four months.[183] This clinical situation is often associated with distant metastases. However, the presence of such disease in the neck causes distressing symptoms, such as pain or bleeding, together with offensive fungation and in selected cases further treatment may be appropriate. This includes wide excision of the tumour and the overlaying skin, flap reconstruction and brachytherapy. In very selected cases, reirradiation may be an option. Evidence of partial repair of radiotherapy-induced spinal cord subclinical damage and newer radiotherapy delivery techniques (IMRT, tomotherapy, protons) that allow better sparing of neurological structures at risk make this a realistic option in a larger number of patients.

IMPACT OF NECK TREATMENT ON QUALITY OF LIFE

The issues that relate to quality of life and the treatment of metastatic neck disease are discussed below.

Elective surgery versus irradiation of the N0 neck

There are no studies comparing quality of life between these two treatments and there is very little morbidity associated with a well-executed SND. This is because vital structures are preserved and level V is not usually dissected. In contrast, a strategy of uniformly irradiating both sides of the neck to try and decrease the likelihood of occult cancer growth may be associated with numerous problems since radiation does not always control occult neck cancer. The fate of recurrent cancer in an electively irradiated neck is much more difficult to salvage and isolated recurrence in the contralateral neck is extremely unlikely.[20] In addition, treatment options for second primary tumours are diminished when wide field radiotherapy has been applied to both sides of the neck and there are no prospective randomized studies which demonstrate a survival disadvantage when the N0 neck is observed. In summary, the quality-of-life issues relating to elective irradiation appear less transparent than those for elective surgery and should not be underestimated when prescribing its use. Further studies are awaited.

Impact of neck treatment on the shoulder

Neck surgery for node-positive disease usually involves a five level dissection and there are quality-of-life issues that relate both to the extent of the dissection and which tissues are sacrificed (i.e. accessory nerve, sternomastoid muscle and the internal jugular vein). Shoulder problems are greater in patients undergoing a RND as opposed to a MRND.[184, 185] Despite preserving the accessory nerve in MRND, dysfunction occurs due to the nerve being devascularized and stretched. The fewest problems are seen in patients undergoing an SND.[105] It is noteworthy that SNDs that clear levels II to IV can also affect the shoulder by stretching the accessory nerve during dissection of the submuscular recess (level IIb).[186] Quite clearly, if level V is not dissected, this may improve quality of life. However, it must be noted that the trade-off for not dissecting all five levels may be the subsequent morbidity of postoperative radiotherapy, which does contribute to shoulder dysfunction.[135]

The use and extent of radiotherapy to the neck

While the effects of neck surgery are confined to the neck, radiotherapy fields often include the salivary glands and some of the viscera, leading to side effects such as mucositis and xerostomia. Use of IMRT has allowed parotid sparing techniques. Results from randomized controlled trials indicate that IMRT does improve quality of life, at least in the early years.[187] In addition, the evidence that both sides of the neck need to be irradiated in well-lateralized primaries postoperatively is flimsy since the incidence of contralateral neck disease is relatively uncommon.[20] Unfortunately, many oncologists continue to routinely prescribe bilateral postoperative radiotherapy to the neck.

In our efforts to improve quality of life and reduce the traumatic psychosocial impact, a number of specialist centres are now in the process of balancing science with ethics and the human experience with a surge of quality of life (QoL) research and, hopefully, an evidence-based rationale to guide us in the future. Until a major therapeutic breakthrough takes place, reducing physical treatment morbidity, improving patients, overall quality of life and minimizing the psychosocial impact of therapy will continue to present our greatest challenge in the practice of head and neck surgery.

FUTURE RESEARCH

The quality and quantity of randomized trials of surgical techniques for metastatic neck disease are acknowledged to be limited. There are several problems that make running surgical trials a difficult prospect. Further research should involve the integration of modified randomized trials with prospective audit and quality control studies.[188] The following are areas where further work needs to be addressed:

- Imaging of low volume disease
- Significance of occult cancer in the neck
- Molecular detection of occult neck disease and its significance
- Sentinel node biopsy for occult neck cancer
- Selective neck dissection for palpable disease
- Assessment of the chemoradiated neck
- Superselective neck dissection for residual disease after chemoradiation
- Management of the contralateral neck
- Quality of life should be investigated following various treatment modalities
- Centralization with specialization and appropriate data collection should improve research, audit and quality control.

KEY EVIDENCE

- Where rigorous, close and frequent clinical and radiologic follow up can be assured with the resources for rapid intervention when necessary, it appears that observation of the N0 neck for early oral tongue squamous cell carcinoma offers equivalent regional control rates to elective neck dissection. Where this management policy cannot be ensured, selective neck dissection is more appropriate.
- Selective neck dissection alone offers equivalent control rates to modified radical neck dissection in histologically confirmed N0 and N1 neck disease.
- Following neck dissection, adjuvant radiation is necessary to enhance regional control rates in the presence of adverse histological findings.
- In the presence of extracapsular spread, the use of concomitant cisplatin during adjuvant radiation increases tumour control and overall survival.

- Prospective uncontrolled evidence from several centres suggests that demonstration of radiological complete response after chemoradiation, especially on computed tomography–positron emission tomography imaging, is an excellent indicator of the absence of viable tumour in the neck and needs no further treatment.

KEY LEARNING POINTS

- Head and neck squamous cell cancer is a systemic disease.
- Tumour–host interaction has a major role to play in the outcomes of treatment.
- Metastatic cervical lymphadenopathy is the most important prognostic factor in head and neck squamous cell carcinoma.
- Patterns of neck metastases are altered by previous treatment.
- Subclinical neck disease is not early cancer.
- A key determinant in the choice of modality to manage neck disease is the treatment given to the primary site.
- Elective neck dissection is as effective as elective irradiation in controlling regional disease.
- Selective neck dissection is adequate in the management of N0 necks.
- Modified radical neck dissection is as good as radical neck dissection in regional control.
- Adjuvant radiotherapy or chemoradiotherapy is indicated for surgically managed N2 and N3 disease, and for N1 disease with poor prognostic features.
- Management of the neck following chemoradiation continues to evolve. Neck salvage for complete and partial responders should be based on availability of local imaging expertise.
- In selecting treatment options, quality of life issues are important considerations.

REFERENCES

1. Beasley NJ, Prevo R, Banerji S et al. Intratumoral lymphangiogenesis and lymph node metastasis in head and neck cancer. Cancer Research 2002; 62: 1315–20.
2. Franchi A, Gallo O, Massi D et al. Tumor lymphangiogenesis in head and neck squamous cell carcinoma: a morphometric study with clinical correlations. Cancer 2004; 101: 973–8.
3. Audet N, Beasley NJ, MacMillan C et al. Lymphatic vessel density, nodal metastases, and prognosis in patients with head and neck cancer. Archives of Otolaryngology, Head and Neck Surgery 2005; 131: 1065–70.
4. Akervall J. Gene profiling in squamous cell carcinoma of the head and neck. Cancer Metastasis Reviews 2005; 24: 87–94.
5. Roepman P, de Jager A, Marian JA et al. Maintenance of head and neck tumor gene expression profiles upon lymph node metastasis. Cancer Research 2006; 66: 11110–14.
6. Jodele S, Blavier L, Yoon JM et al. Modifying the soil to affect the seed: role of stromal-derived matrix metalloproteinases in cancer progression. Cancer Metastasis Reviews 2006; 25: 35–43.
7. Wiegand S, Dunne AA, Muller HH et al. Metaanalysis of the significance of matrix metalloproteinases for lymph node disease in patients with head and neck squamous cell carcinoma. Cancer 2005; 104: 94–100.
8. Whiteside TL. Immunobiology of head and neck cancer. Cancer Metastasis Reviews 2005; 24: 95–105.
9. Toker C. Some observations on the deposition of metastatic carcinoma within cervical lymph nodes. Cancer 1963; 16: 364–74.
10. Partridge M, Brakenhoff R, Phillips E et al. Detection of rare disseminated tumor cells identifies head and neck cancer patients at risk of treatment failure. Clinical Cancer Research 2003; 9: 5287–94.
11. Pantel K, Cote RJ, Fodsyod O. Detection and clinical importance of micrometastatic disease. Journal of the National Cancer Institute 1999; 91: 1113–24.
12. Winter SC, Stephenson SA, Subramaniam SK et al. Long term survival following the detection of circulating tumour cells in head and neck squamous cell carcinoma. BMC Cancer 2009; 9: 424.
13. Mastronikolis NS, Fitzgerald D, Owen C et al. The management of squamous cell carcinoma of the neck. The Birmingham UK experience. European Journal of Surgical Oncology 2005; 31: 461–6.
14. Shah JP, Strong E, Spiro RH, Vikram B. Surgical grand rounds. Neck dissection: current status and future possibilities. Clinical Bulletin 1981; 11: 25–33.
15. Robbins KT, Clayman G, Levine PA et al. Neck dissection classification update: revisions proposed by the American Head and Neck Society and the American Academy of Otolaryngology-Head and Neck Surgery. Archives of Otolaryngology, Head and Neck Surgery 2002; 128: 751–8.
16. Robbins KT, Shaha AR, Medina JE et al. Consensus statement on the classification and terminology of neck dissection. Archives of Otolaryngology, Head and Neck Surgery 2008; 134: 536–8.
17. Ferlito A, Robbins KT, Shah JP et al. Proposal for a rational classification of neck dissections. Head and Neck 2011; 33: 445–50.
18. Lindberg R. Distribution of cervical lymph node metastases from squamous cell carcinoma of the upper

respiratory and digestive tracts. *Cancer* 1972; **29**: 1446–9.

19. Shah JP. Patterns of cervical lymph node metastasis from squamous carcinomas of the upper aerodigestive tract. *American Journal of Surgery* 1990; **160**: 405–9.

20. Collins SL. Controversies in management of cancer of the neck. In: Thawley SE, Panje WR, Batsakis JG, Lindberg RD (eds). *Comprehensive management of head and neck tumours*. Philadelphia: WB Saunders, 1999: 1479–563.

21. Ambrosch P, Brinck U. Detection of nodal micrometastases in head and neck cancer by serial sectioning and immunostaining. *Oncology* 1996; **10**: 1221–6; discussion 1226, 1229.

22. van den Brekel MW, van der Waal I, Meijer CJ *et al.* The incidence of micrometastases in neck dissection specimens obtained from elective neck dissections. *Laryngoscope* 1996; **106**: 987–91.

23. Enepekides DJ, Sultanem K, Nguyen C *et al.* Occult cervical metastases: immunoperoxidase analysis of the pathologically negative neck. *Otolaryngology – Head and Neck Surgery* 1999; **120**: 713–17.

24. Hamakawa H, Takemura K, Sumida T *et al.* Histological study on pN upgrading of oral cancer. *Virchows Archiv* 2000; **437**: 116–21.

25. Goldenberg D, Begum S, Westra WH *et al.* Cystic lymph node metastasis in patients with head and neck cancer: an HPV-associated phenomenon. *Head and Neck* 2008; **30**: 898–903.

26. Jereczek-Fossa BA, Casadio C, Jassem J *et al.* Branchiogenic carcinoma – conceptual or true clinico-pathological entity? *Cancer Treatment Reviews* 2005; **31**: 106–14.

27. Devaney KO, Rinaldo A, Ferlito A *et al.* Squamous carcinoma arising in a branchial cleft cyst: have you ever treated one? Will you? *Journal of Laryngology and Otology* 2008; **122**: 547–50.

28. Lefebvre JL. *Oral cavity, pharynx, and larynx cancer. Prognostic factors in cancer*. New York: Wiley-Liss, 2001.

29. Johnson JT, Barnes EL, Myers EN *et al.* The extracapsular spread of tumors in cervical node metastasis. *Archives of Otolaryngology* 1981; **107**: 725–9.

30. Ferlito A, Rinaldo A, Devaney KO *et al.* Prognostic significance of microscopic and macroscopic extracapsular spread from metastatic tumor in the cervical lymph nodes. *Oral Oncology* 2002; **38**: 747–51.

31. Jose J, Coatesworth AP, Johnston C, MacLennan K. Cervical node metastases in squamous cell carcinoma of the upper aerodigestive tract: the significance of extracapsular spread and soft tissue deposits. *Head and Neck* 2003; **25**: 451–6.

32. Woolgar JA, Rogers SN, Lowe D *et al.* Cervical lymph node metastasis in oral cancer: the importance of even microscopic extracapsular spread. *Oral Oncology* 2003; **39**: 130–7.

33. Gourin CG, Conger BT, Porubsky ES *et al.* The effect of occult nodal metastases on survival and regional control in patients with head and neck squamous cell carcinoma. *Laryngoscope* 2008; **118**: 1191–4.

34. Alvi A, Johnson JT. Extracapsular spread in the clinically negative neck (N0): implications and outcome. *Otolaryngology – Head and Neck Surgery* 1996; **114**: 65–70.

35. Dunne AA, Muller HH, Eisele DW *et al.* Meta-analysis of the prognostic significance of perinodal spread in head and neck squamous cell carcinomas (HNSCC) patients. *European Journal of Cancer* 2006; **42**: 1863–8.

36. Oosterkamp S, de Jong JM, van den Ende PL *et al.* Predictive value of lymph node metastases and extracapsular extension for the risk of distant metastases in laryngeal carcinoma. *Laryngoscope* 2006; **116**: 2067–70.

37. Robson A. The management of the neck in squamous head and neck cancer. *Clinical Otolaryngology and Allied Sciences* 2001; **26**: 157–61.

38. Bernier J, Cooper JS, Pajak TF *et al.* Defining risk levels in locally advanced head and neck cancers: a comparative analysis of concurrent postoperative radiation plus chemotherapy trials of the EORTC (#22931) and RTOG (#9501). *Head and Neck* 2005; **27**: 843–50.

39. Dirix P, Nuyts S, Bussels B *et al.* Prognostic influence of retropharyngeal lymph node metastasis in squamous cell carcinoma of the oropharynx. *International Journal of Radiation Oncology, Biology, Physics* 2006; **65**: 739–44.

40. McLaughlin MP, Mendenhall WM, Mancuso AA *et al.* Retropharyngeal adenopathy as a predictor of outcome in squamous cell carcinoma of the head and neck. *Head and Neck* 1995; **17**: 190–8.

41. Gross ND, Ellingson TW, Wax MK *et al.* Impact of retropharyngeal lymph node metastasis in head and neck squamous cell carcinoma. *Archives of Otolaryngology, Head and Neck Surgery* 2004; **130**: 169–73.

42. Sobin LH, Gospodarowicz MK, Wittekind C (eds). *TNM classification of malignant tumours*, 7th edn. Oxford: Wiley-Blackwell, 2009.

43. Haberal I, Celik H, Gocmen H *et al.* Which is important in the evaluation of metastatic lymph nodes in head and neck cancer: palpation, ultrasonography, or computed tomography? *Otolaryngology – Head and Neck Surgery* 2004; **130**: 197–201.

44. Rottey S, Petrovic M, Bauters W *et al.* Evaluation of metastatic lymph nodes in head and neck cancer: a comparative study between palpation, ultrasonography, ultrasound-guided fine needle aspiration cytology and computed tomography. *Acta Clinica Belgica* 2006; **61**: 236–41.

45. Merritt RM, Williams MF, James TH, Porubsky ES. Detection of cervical metastasis. A meta-analysis comparing computed tomography with physical examination. *Archives of Otolaryngology, Head and Neck Surgery* 1997; **123**: 149–52.

46. Amedee RG, Dhurandhar NR. Fine-needle aspiration biopsy. *Laryngoscope* 2001; **111**: 1551–7.

47. Ahuja AT, Ying M, Ho SS et al. Distribution of intranodal vessels in differentiating benign from metastatic neck nodes. Clinical Radiology 2001; 56: 197–201.

48. Nieuwenhuis EJ, Jaspars LH, Castelijns JA et al. Quantitative molecular detection of minimal residual head and neck cancer in lymph node aspirates. Clinical Cancer Research 2003; 9: 755–61.

49. Lyshchik A, Higashi T, Asato R et al. Cervical lymph node metastases: diagnosis at sonoelastography – initial experience. Radiology 2007; 243: 258–67.

50. van der Putten L, van den Broek GB, de Bree R et al. Effectiveness of salvage selective and modified radical neck dissection for regional pathologic lymphadenopathy after chemoradiation. Head and Neck 2009; 31: 593–603.

51. Moreau P, Goffart Y, Collignon J. Computed tomography of metastatic cervical lymph nodes. A clinical, computed tomographic, pathologic correlative study. Archives of Otolaryngology, Head and Neck Surgery 1990; 116: 1190–3.

52. van den Brekel MW, Stel HV, Castelijns JA et al. Cervical lymph node metastasis: assessment of radiologic criteria. Radiology 1990; 177: 379–84.

53. Som PM. Detection of metastasis in cervical lymph nodes, CT and MR criteria and differential diagnosis. American Journal of Roentgenology 1992; 158: 961–9.

54. de Bondt RB, Nelemans PJ, Hofman PA et al. Detection of lymph node metastases in head and neck cancer: a meta-analysis comparing US, USgFNAC, CT and MR imaging. European Journal of Radiology 2007; 64: 266–72.

55. Liauw SL, Mancuso AA, Amdur RJ. Postradiotherapy neck dissection for lymph node-positive head and neck cancer: the use of computed tomography to manage the neck. Journal of Clinical Oncology 2006; 24: 1421–7.

56. Corry J, Peters L, Fisher R et al. N2–N3 neck nodal control without planned neck dissection for clinical/radiologic complete responders-results of Trans Tasman Radiation Oncology Group Study 98.02. Head and Neck 2008; 30: 737–42.

57. Lau H, Phan T, Mackinnon J et al. Absence of planned neck dissection for the N2–N3 neck after chemoradiation for locally advanced squamous cell carcinoma of the head and neck. Archives of Otolaryngology, Head and Neck Surgery 2008; 134: 257–61.

58. Lopez Rodriguez M, Cerezo Padellano L, Martin Martin M et al. Neck dissection after radiochemotherapy in patients with locoregionally advanced head and neck cancer. Clinical and Translational Oncology 2008; 10: 812–16.

59. Vedrine PO, Thariat J, Hitier N et al. Need for neck dissection after radiochemotherapy? A study of the French GETTEC Group. Laryngoscope 2008; 118: 1775–80.

60. Choi HJ, Ju W, Myung SK et al. Diagnostic performance of computer tomography, magnetic resonance imaging, and positron emission tomography or positron emission tomography/computer tomography for detection of metastatic lymph nodes in patients with cervical cancer: meta-analysis. Cancer Science 2010; 101: 1471–9.

61. Sigal R, Vogl T, Casselmann J et al. Lymph node metastases from head and neck squamous cell carcinoma: MR imaging with ultrasmall superparamagnetic iron oxide particles (Sinerem MR) – results of a phase-III multicenter clinical trial. European Radiology 2002; 12: 1104–13.

62. Baghi M, Mack MG, Hambek M et al. Iron oxide particle-enhanced magnetic resonance imaging for detection of benign lymph nodes in the head and neck: how reliable are the results? Anticancer Research 2007; 27: 3571–5.

63. Dammann F, Horger M, Mueller-Berg H et al. Rational diagnosis of squamous cell carcinoma of the head and neck region: comparative evaluation of CT, MRI, and 18FDG PET. American Journal of Roentgenology 2005; 184: 1326–31.

64. Lonneux M, Hamoir M, Reychler H et al. Positron emission tomography with [18F]fluorodeoxyglucose improves staging and patient management in patients with head and neck squamous cell carcinoma: a multicenter prospective study. Journal of Clinical Oncology 2010; 28: 1190–5.

65. Goerres GW, Schmid DT, Gratz KW et al. Impact of whole body positron emission tomography on initial staging and therapy in patients with squamous cell carcinoma of the oral cavity. Oral Oncology 2003; 39: 547–51.

66. MacManus M, Peters L, Duchesne G et al. How should we introduce clinical positron emission tomography in the UK? Oncologists need to have a (clearer) view. Clinical Oncology 2004; 16: 492–3.

67. Fleming AJ Jr, Smith SP Jr, Paul CM et al. Impact of [18F]-2-fluorodeoxyglucose-positron emission tomography/computed tomography on previously untreated head and neck cancer patients. Laryngoscope 2007; 117: 1173–9.

68. Menda Y, Graham MM. Update on 18F-fluorodeoxyglucose/positron emission tomography and positron emission tomography/computed tomography imaging of squamous head and neck cancers. Seminars in Nuclear Medicine 2005; 35: 214–19.

69. Schwartz DL, Ford E, Rajendran J. FDG-PET/CT imaging for preradiotherapy staging of head-and-neck squamous cell carcinoma. International Journal of Radiation Oncology, Biology, Physics 2005; 61: 129–36.

70. Brink I, Klenzner T, Krause T et al. Lymph node staging in extracranial head and neck cancer with FDG PET – appropriate uptake period and size-dependence of the results. Nuklearmedizin 2002; 41: 108–13.

71. Stoeckli SJ, Steinert H, Pfaltz M, Schmid S. Is there a role for positron emission tomography with 18F-fluorodeoxyglucose in the initial staging of nodal negative oral and oropharyngeal squamous cell carcinoma. Head and Neck 2002; 24: 345–9.

72. Civantos FJ, Gomez C, Duque C et al. Sentinel node biopsy in oral cavity cancer: correlation with PET scan and immunohistochemistry. Head and Neck 2003; 25: 1–9.

73. Hyde NC, Prvulovich E, Newman L et al. A new approach to pre-treatment assessment of the N0 neck in oral

squamous cell carcinoma: the role of sentinel node biopsy and positron emission tomography. *Oral Oncology* 2003; **39**: 350–60.

74. Johansen J, Buus S, Loft A *et al*. Prospective study of 18FDG-PET in the detection and management of patients with lymph node metastases to the neck from an unknown primary tumor. Results from the DAHANCA-13 study. *Head and Neck* 2008; **30**: 471–8.

75. Waltonen JD, Ozer E, Hall NC *et al*. Metastatic carcinoma of the neck of unknown primary origin: evolution and efficacy of the modern workup. *Archives of Otolaryngology, Head and Neck Surgery* 2009; **135**: 1024–9.

76. Yao M, Graham MM, Hoffman HT *et al*. The role of post-radiation therapy FDG PET in prediction of necessity for post-radiation therapy neck dissection in locally advanced head-and-neck squamous cell carcinoma. *International Journal of Radiation Oncology, Biology, Physics* 2004; **59**: 1001–10.

77. Porceddu SV, Jarmolowski E, Hicks RJ *et al*. Utility of positron emission tomography for the detection of disease in residual neck nodes after (chemo)radiotherapy in head and neck cancer. *Head and Neck* 2005; **27**: 175–81.

78. Isles MG, McConkey C, Mehanna HM. A systematic review and meta-analysis of the role of positron emission tomography in the follow up of head and neck squamous cell carcinoma following radiotherapy or chemoradiotherapy. *Clinical Otolaryngology* 2008; **33**: 210–22.

79. Scottish Intercollegiate Guidelines Network. Diagnosis and management of head and neck cancer: A national clinical guideline. February 7, 2007. Available from www.sign.ac.uk/pdf/sign90.pdf.

80. Alkureishi LW, Burak Z, Alvarez JA *et al*. European Association of Nuclear Medicine Oncology Committee; European Sentinel Node Biopsy Trial Committee. Joint practice guidelines for radionuclide lymphoscintigraphy for sentinel node localization in oral/oropharyngeal squamous cell carcinoma. *Annals of Surgical Oncology* 2009; **16**: 3190–210.

81. Alkureishi LW, Ross GL, Shoaib T *et al*. Sentinel node biopsy in head and neck squamous cell cancer: 5-year follow-up of a European multicenter trial. *Annals of Surgical Oncology* 2010; **17**: 2459–64.

82. Paleri V, Rees G, Arullendran P *et al*. Sentinel node biopsy in squamous cell cancer of the oral cavity and oral pharynx: a diagnostic meta-analysis. *Head and Neck* 2005; **27**: 739–47.

83. Helliwell TR, Woolgar JA. *Histopathology reports on head and neck carcinomas and salivary neoplasms*. London: Royal College of Pathologists, 2005.

84. Vandenbrouck C, Sancho-Garnier H, Chassagne D *et al*. Elective versus therapeutic radical neck dissection in epidermoid carcinoma of the oral cavity: results of a randomized clinical trial. *Cancer* 1980; **46**: 386–90.

85. Kligerman J, Lima RA, Soares JR *et al*. Supraomohyoid neck dissection in the treatment of T1/T2 squamous cell carcinoma of oral cavity. *American Journal of Surgery* 1994; **168**: 391–4.

86. Fakih AR, Rao RS, Borges AM *et al*. Elective versus therapeutic neck dissection in early carcinoma of the oral tongue. *American Journal of Surgery* 1989; **158**: 309–13.

87. Yuen AP, Ho CM, Chow TL *et al*. Prospective randomized study of selective neck dissection versus observation for N0 neck of early tongue carcinoma. *Head and Neck* 2009; **31**: 765–72.

88. Pointon RC, Gleave EN. Lymphatic spread. In: Sikora K, Halnan KE (eds). *Treatment of cancer*. London: Chapman and Hall, 1990.

89. Yuen AP, Wei WI, Wong Y *et al*. Elective neck dissection versus observation in the treatment of early oral tongue carcinoma. *Head and Neck* 1997; **19**: 583–8.

90. D'Cruz AK, Siddachari RC, Walvekar RR *et al*. Elective neck dissection for the management of the N0 neck in early cancer of the oral tongue: need for a randomized controlled trial. *Head and Neck* 2009; **31**: 618–24.

91. Leyland MK, Sessions DG, Lenox C. The influence of lymph node metastasis in the treatment of squamous cell carcinoma of the oral cavity, oropharynx, larynx, and hypopharynx: N0 versus N+. *Laryngoscope* 2005; **115**: 629–39.

92. Nieuwenhuis EJ, Castelijns JA, Pijpers R *et al*. Wait-and-see policy for the N0 neck in early-stage oral and oropharyngeal squamous cell carcinoma using ultrasonography-guided cytology: is there a role for identification of the sentinel node? *Head and Neck* 2002; **24**: 282–9.

93. Wolfensberger M, Zbaeren P, Dulguerov P *et al*. Surgical treatment of early oral carcinoma – results of a prospective controlled multicenter study. *Head and Neck* 2001; **23**: 525–30.

94. Haddadin KJ, Soutar DS, Oliver RJ *et al*. Improved survival for patients with clinically T1/T2, N0 tongue tumors undergoing a prophylactic neck dissection. *Head and Neck* 1999; **21**: 517–25.

95. Weiss MH, Harrison LB, Isaacs RS. Use of decision analysis in planning a management strategy for the stage N0 neck. *Archives of Otolaryngology, Head and Neck Surgery* 1994; **120**: 699–702.

96. Ferlito A, Rinaldo A, Silver CE *et al*. Elective and therapeutic selective neck dissection. *Oral Oncology* 2006; **42**: 14–25.

97. Chow JM, Levin BC, Krivit JS *et al*. Radiotherapy or surgery for subclinical cervical node metastases. *Archives of Otolaryngology, Head and Neck Surgery* 1989; **115**: 981–4.

98. Clayman GL, Frank DK. Selective neck dissection of anatomically appropriate levels is as efficacious as modified radical neck dissection for elective treatment of the clinically negatice neck in patients with squamous cell carcinoma of the upper respiratory and digestive

tracts. *Archives of Otolaryngology, Head and Neck Surgery* 1998; **124**: 348–52.

99. Brazilian Head and Neck Cancer Study Group. Results of a prospective trial on elective modified radical classical versus supraomohyoid neck dissection in the management of oral squamous carcinoma. *American Journal of Surgery* 1998; **176**: 422–7.

100. Brazilian Head and Neck Cancer Study Group. End results of a prospective trial on elective lateral neck dissection vs type III modified radical neck dissection in the management of supraglottic and transglottic carcinomas. *Head and Neck* 1999; **21**: 694–702.

101. Lim YC, Koo BS, Lee JS, Choi EC. Level V lymph node dissection in oral and oropharyngeal carcinoma patients with clinically node-positive neck: is it absolutely necessary? *Laryngoscope* 2006; **116**: 1232–5.

102. Davidson BJ, Kulkarny V, Delacure MD, Shah JP. Posterior triangle metastases of squamous cell carcinoma of the upper aerodigestive tract. *American Journal of Surgery* 1993; **166**: 395–8.

103. Cole I, Hughes L. The relationship of cervical lymph node metastases to primary sites of carcinoma of the upper aerodigestive tract: a pathological study. *Australia and New Zealand Journal of Surgery* 1997; **67**: 860–5.

104. Leon X, Quer M, Orus C *et al*. Selective dissection of levels II–III with intraoperative control of the upper and middle jugular nodes: a therapeutic option for the N0 neck. *Head and Neck* 2001; **23**: 441–6.

105. Laverick S, Lowe D, Brown JS *et al*. The impact of neck dissection on health-related quality of life. *Archives of Otolaryngology, Head and Neck Surgery* 2004; **130**: 149–54.

106. Paleri V, Subramaniam SK, Oozeer N *et al*. Dissection of the submuscular recess (level IIb) in squamous cell cancer of the upper aerodigestive tract: prospective study and systematic review of the literature. *Head and Neck* 2008; **30**: 194–200.

107. Rinaldo A, Elsheikh MN, Ferlito A *et al*. Prospective studies of neck dissection specimens support preservation of sublevel IIB for laryngeal squamous carcinoma with clinically negative neck. *Journal of the American College of Surgeons* 2006; **202**: 967–70.

108. Ferlito A, Silver CE, Rinaldo A. Selective neck dissection (IIA, III): a rational replacement for complete functional neck dissection in patients with N0 supraglottic and glottic squamous carcinoma. *Laryngoscope* 2008; **118**: 676–9.

109. Bar Ad V, Chalian A. Management of clinically negative neck for the patients with head and neck squamous cell carcinomas in the modern era. *Oral Oncology* 2008; **4**: 817–22.

110. Dearnaley DP, Dardoufas C, A'Hearn RP, Henk JM. Interstitial irradiation for carcinoma of the tongue and floor of mouth, Royal Marsden Hospital Experience 1970–1986. *Radiotherapy and Oncology* 1991; **21**: 183–92.

111. Watkinson JC. The Clinically N0 neck: investigation and treatment. *Clinical Otolaryngology and Allied Sciences* 1993; **18**: 443–5.

112. van den Brekel MW, Castelijns JA, Reitsma LC *et al*. Outcome of observing the N0 neck using ultrasonographic-guided cytology for follow-up. *Archives of Otolaryngology, Head and Neck Surgery* 1999; **125**: 153–6.

113. Hodder SC, Evans RM, Patton DW *et al*. Ultrasound and fine needle aspiration cytology in the staging of neck lymph nodes in oral squamous cell carcinoma. *British Journal of Oral and Maxillofacial Surgery* 2000; **38**: 430–6.

114. Richards PS, Peacock TE. The role of ultrasound in the detection of cervical lymph node metastases in clinically N0 squamous cell carcinoma of the head and neck. *Cancer Imaging* 2007; **7**: 167–78.

115. Hicks WL Jr, Kollmorgen DR, Kuriase MA *et al*. Patterns of nodal metastasis and surgical management of the neck in supraglottic laryngeal carcinoma. *Otolaryngology – Head and Neck Surgery* 1999; **121**: 57–61.

116. Gallo O, Fini-Storchi I, Napolitano L. Treatment of the contralateral negative neck in supraglottic cancer patients with unilateral node metastases (N1–3). *Head and Neck* 2000; **22**: 386–92.

117. Redaelli de Zinis LO, Nicolai P, Tomenzoli D *et al*. The distribution of lymph node metastases in supraglottic squamous cell carcinoma: therapeutic implications. *Head and Neck* 2002; **24**: 913–20.

118. Byers RM, Wolf PF, Ballantyne AJ *et al*. Rationale for elective modified neck dissection. *Head and Neck Surgery* 1988; **10**: 160–7.

119. Buckley JG, MacLennan K. Cervical node metastases in laryngeal and hypopharyngeal cancer: a prospective analysis of prevalence and distribution. *Head and Neck* 2000; **22**: 380–5.

120. Aluffi P, Pisani P, Policarpo M, Pia F. Contralateral cervical lymph node metastases in pyriform sinus carcinoma. *Otolaryngology – Head and Neck Surgery* 2006; **134**: 650–3.

121. Koo BS, Lim YC, Lee JS *et al*. Management of contralateral N0 neck in pyriform sinus carcinoma. *Laryngoscope* 2006; **116**: 1268–72.

122. Lim YC, Lee SY, Lim J-Y *et al*. Management of contralateral N0 neck in tonsillar squamous cell carcinoma. *Laryngoscope* 2005; **115**: 1672–5.

123. Lim YC, Koo BS, Lee JS *et al*. Distributions of cervical lymph node metastases in oropharyngeal carcinoma: therapeutic implications for the N0 neck. *Laryngoscope* 2006; **116**: 1148–52.

124. Lutz CK, Johnson JT, Wagner RL *et al*. Supraglottic carcinoma: patterns of recurrence. *Annals of Otology, Rhinology and Laryngology* 1990; **99**: 12–17.

125. Weber PC, Johnson JT, Myers EN. The impact of bilateral neck dissection on pattern of recurrence and survival in

supraglottic carcinoma. *Archives of Otolaryngology, Head and Neck Surgery* 1994; **120**: 703–6.

126. Scola B, Fernandez-Vega M, Fernandez-Vega S, Ramirez C. Management of cancer of the supraglottis. *Otolaryngology – Head and Neck Surgery* 2001; **124**: 195–8.

127. Chiu RJ, Myers EN, Johnson JT. Efficacy of routine bilateral neck dissection in the management of supraglottic cancer. *Otolaryngology – Head and Neck Surgery* 2004; **131**: 485–8.

128. Lee SY, Lim YC, Song MH *et al.* Level IIb lymph node metastasis in elective neck dissection of oropharyngeal squamous cell carcinoma. *Oral Oncology* 2006; **42**: 1017–21.

129. Mendenhall WM, Cassisi NJ, Stringer SP, Tannehill SP. Therapeutic principles in the management of head and neck tumours. In: Souhami RL, Tannock I, Hohenberger P, Horiot JC (eds). *Oxford textbook of oncology*. New York: Oxford University Press, 2002: 1322–43.

130. Kao J, Lavaf A, Teng MS *et al.* Adjuvant radiotherapy and survival for patients with node-positive head and neck cancer: an analysis by primary site and nodal stage. *International Journal of Radiation Oncology, Biology, Physics* 2008; **71**: 362–70.

131. Byers RM, Clayman GL, McGill D *et al.* Selective neck dissections for squamous carcinoma of the upper aerodigestive tract: patterns of regional failure. *Head and Neck* 1999; **21**: 499–505.

132. Kolli VR, Datta RV, Orner JB *et al.* The role of supraomohyoid neck dissection in patients with positive nodes. *Archives of Otolaryngology, Head and Neck Surgery* 2000; **126**: 413–16.

133. Ambrosch P, Kron M, Pradier O *et al.* Efficacy of selective neck dissection: a review of 503 cases of elective and therapeutic treatment of the neck in squamous cell carcinoma of the upper aerodigestive tract. *Otolaryngology – Head and Neck Surgery* 2001; **124**: 180–7.

134. Andersen PE, Warren F, Spiro J *et al.* Results of selective neck dissection in management of the node-positive neck. *Archives of Otolaryngology, Head and Neck Surgery* 2002; **128**: 1180–4.

135. Chepeha DB, Hoff PT, Taylor RJ *et al.* Selective neck dissection for the treatment of neck metastasis from squamous cell carcinoma of the head and neck. *Laryngoscope* 2002; **112**: 434–8.

136. Muzaffar K. Therapeutic selective neck dissection: a 25-year review. *Laryngoscope* 2003; **113**: 1460–5.

137. Simental AA Jr, Duvvuri U, Johnson JT, Myers EN. Selective neck dissection in patients with upper aerodigestive tract cancer with clinically positive nodal disease. *Annals of Otology, Rhinology and Laryngology* 2006; **115**: 846–9.

138. Brizel DM, Prosnitz RG, Hunter S *et al.* Necessity for adjuvant neck dissection in setting of concurrent chemoradiation for advanced head-and-neck cancer. *International Journal of Radiation Oncology, Biology, Physics* 2004; **58**: 1418–23.

139. Moore MG, Bhattacharyya N. Effectiveness of chemotherapy and radiotherapy in sterilizing cervical nodal disease in squamous cell carcinoma of the head and neck. *Laryngoscope* 2005; **115**: 570–3.

140. Andersen PE, Shah JP, Cambronero E *et al.* The role of comprehensive neck dissection with preservation of the spinal accessory nerve in the clinically positive neck. *American Journal of Surgery* 1994; **168**: 499–502.

141. Richards BL, Spiro JD. Controlling advanced neck disease: efficacy of neck dissection and radiotherapy. *Laryngoscope* 2000; **110**: 1124–7.

142. Lavaf A, Genden EM, Cesaretti JA *et al.* Adjuvant radiotherapy improves overall survival for patients with lymph node-positive head and neck squamous cell carcinoma. *Cancer* 2008; **112**: 535–43.

143. Bernier J, Domenge C, Ozsahin M *et al.* Postoperative irradiation with or without concomitant chemotherapy for locally advanced head and neck cancer. *New England Journal of Medicine* 2004; **350**: 1945–52.

144. Cooper JS, Pajak TF, Forastiere A *et al.* Postoperative concurrent radiotherapy and chemotherapy for high-risk squamous-cell carcinoma of the head and neck. *New England Journal of Medicine* 2004; **350**: 1937–44.

145. Cagli S, Yuce I, Yigitbasi OG *et al.* Is routine bilateral neck dissection absolutely necessary in the management of N0 neck in patients with supraglottic carcinoma? *European Archives of Otorhinolaryngology* 2007; **264**: 1453–7.

146. Watkinson JC, Owen C, Thompson S *et al.* Conservation surgery in the management of T1 and T2 oropharyngeal squamous cell carcinoma: the Birmingham UK experience. *Clinical Otolaryngology and Allied Sciences* 2002; **27**: 541–8.

147. Jones AS, Goodyear PW, Ghosh S *et al.* Extensive neck node metastases (n3) in head and neck squamous carcinoma: is radical treatment warranted? *Otolaryngology – Head and Neck Surgery* 2011; **144**: 29–35.

148. Chan SW, Mukesh BN, Sizeland A *et al.* Treatment outcome of N3 nodal head and neck squamous cell carcinoma. *Otolaryngology – Head and Neck Surgery* 2003; **129**: 55–60.

149. Moukarbel RV, Fung K, Venkatesan V *et al.* The N3 neck: outcomes following primary chemoradiotherapy. *Journal of Otolaryngology, Head and Neck Surgery* 2011; **40**: 137–42.

150. Grau C, Johansen LV, Jakobsen J *et al.* Cervical lymph node metastases from unknown primary tumours. Results from a national survey by the Danish Society for Head and Neck Oncology. *Radiotherapy and Oncology* 2000; **55**: 121–9.

151. Ozer E, Agrawal A, Ozer HG *et al.* The impact of surgery in the management of the head and neck carcinoma involving the carotid artery. *Laryngoscope* 2008; **118**: 1771–4.

152. Huvos AG, Leaming RH, Moore OS et al. Clinicopathologic study of the resected carotid artery. Analysis of sixty-four cases. *American Journal of Surgery* 1973; **126**: 570–4.

153. McCready RA, Miller SK, Hamaker RC et al. What is the role of carotid arterial resection in the management of advanced cervical cancer? *Journal of Vascular Surgery* 1989; **10**: 274–80.

154. Snyderman CH, D'Amico F. Outcome of carotid artery resection for neoplastic disease: a meta-analysis. *American Journal of Otolaryngology* 1992; **13**: 373–80.

155. Jacobs JR, Korkmaz H, Marks SC et al. One stage carotid artery resection: reconstruction in radiated head and neck carcinoma. *American Journal of Otolaryngology* 2001; **22**: 167–71.

156. Roh JL, Kim MR, Choi SH et al. Can patients with head and neck cancers invading carotid artery gain survival benefit from surgery? *Acta Otolaryngologica* 2008; **128**: 1370–4.

157. Katsuno S, Takemae T, Ishiyama T et al. Is carotid reconstruction for advanced cancer in the neck a safe procedure? *Otolaryngology – Head and Neck Surgery* 2001; **124**: 222–4.

158. Muhm M, Grasl MCh, Burian M et al. Carotid resection and reconstruction for locally advanced head and neck tumors. *Acta Otolaryngologica* 2002; **122**: 561–4.

159. Solares CA, Fritz MA, Esclamado RM. Oncologic effectiveness of selective neck dissection in the N0 irradiated neck. *Head and Neck* 2005; **27**: 415–20.

160. Temam S, Koka V, Mamelle G et al. Treatment of the N0 neck during salvage surgery after radiotherapy of head and neck squamous cell carcinoma. *Head and Neck* 2005; **27**: 653–8.

161. Farrag TY, Lin FR, Cummings CW et al. Neck management in patients undergoing postradiotherapy salvage laryngeal surgery for recurrent/persistent laryngeal cancer. *Laryngoscope* 2006; **116**: 1864–6.

162. Stenson KM, Haraf DJ, Pelzer H et al. The role of cervical lymphadenectomy after aggressive concomitant chemoradiotherapy: the feasibility of selective neck dissection. *Archives of Otolaryngology, Head and Neck Surgery* 2000; **126**: 950–6.

163. Frank DK, Hu KS, Culliney BE et al. Planned neck dissection after concomitant radiochemotherapy for advanced head and neck cancer. *Laryngoscope* 2005; **115**: 1015–20.

164. Lavertu P, Adelstein DJ, Saxton JP et al. Management of the neck in a randomized trial comparing concurrent chemotherapy and radiotherapy with radiotherapy alone in resectable stage III and IV squamous cell head and neck cancer. *Head and Neck* 1997; **19**: 559–66.

165. Andrade RS, Heron DE, Degirmenci B et al. Posttreatment assessment of response using FDG-PET/CT for patients treated with definitive radiation therapy for head and neck cancers. *International Journal of Radiation Oncology, Biology, Physics* 2006; **65**: 1315–22.

166. Chen AY, Vilaseca I, Hudgins PA et al. PET-CT vs contrast-enhanced CT: what is the role for each after chemoradiation for advanced oropharyngeal cancer? *Head and Neck* 2006; **28**: 487–95.

167. Ferlito A, Corry J, Silver CE et al. Planned neck dissection for patients with complete response to chemoradiotherapy: a concept approaching obsolescence. *Head and Neck* 2010; **32**: 253–61.

168. Corry J, Smith JG, Peters LJ. The concept of a planned neck dissection is obsolete. *Cancer Journal* 2001; **7**: 472–4.

169. Grabenbauer GG, Rodel C, Ernst-Stecken A et al. Neck dissection following radiochemotherapy of advanced head and neck cancer – for selected cases only? *Radiotherapy and Oncology* 2003; **66**: 57–63.

170. Wee JT, Anderson BO, Corry J et al. Management of the neck after chemoradiotherapy for head and neck cancers in Asia: consensus statement from the Asian Oncology Summit 2009. *Lancet Oncology* 2009; **10**: 1086–92.

171. Clayman GL, Johnson CJ 2nd, Morrison W et al. The role of neck dissection after chemoradiotherapy for oropharyngeal cancer with advanced nodal disease. *Archives of Otolaryngology, Head and Neck Surgery* 2001; **127**: 135–9.

172. Robbins KT, Doweck I, Samant S, Vieira F. Effectiveness of superselective and selective neck dissection for advanced nodal metastases after chemoradiation. *Archives of Otolaryngology, Head and Neck Surgery* 2005; **131**: 965–9.

173. Robbins KT, Shannon K, Vieira F. Superselective neck dissection after chemoradiation: feasibility based on clinical and pathologic comparisons. *Archives of Otolaryngology, Head and Neck Surgery* 2007; **133**: 486–9.

174. Mukhija V, Gupta S, Jacobson AS et al. Selective neck dissection following adjuvant therapy for advanced head and neck cancer. *Head and Neck* 2009; **31**: 183–8.

175. McHam SA, Adelstein DJ, Rybicki LA et al. Who merits a neck dissection after definitive chemoradiotherapy for N2-N3 squamous cell head and neck cancer? *Head and Neck* 2003; **25**: 791–8.

176. Bataini JP, Bernier J, Jaulerry C et al. Impact of neck node radioresponsiveness on the regional control probability in patients with oropharynx and pharyngolarynx cancers managed by definitive radiotherapy. *International Journal of Radiation Oncology, Biology, Physics* 1987; **13**: 817–24.

177. Roy S, Tibesar RJ, Daly K et al. Role of planned neck dissection for advanced metastatic disease in tongue base or tonsil squamous cell carcinoma treated with radiotherapy. *Head and Neck* 2002; **24**: 474–81.

178. Velazquez RA, McGuff HS, Sycamore D, Miller FR. The role of computed tomographic scans in the management of the N-positive neck in head and neck squamous cell carcinoma after chemoradiotherapy. *Archives of Otolaryngology, Head and Neck Surgery* 2004; **130**: 74–7.

179. Stenson KM, Huo D, Blair E *et al.* Planned post-chemoradiation neck dissection: significance of radiation dose. *Laryngoscope* 2006; **116**: 33–6.

180. Sewall GK, Palazzi-Churas KL, Richards GM. Planned postradiotherapy neck dissection: Rationale and clinical outcomes. *Laryngoscope* 2007; **117**: 121–8.

181. Medina JE, Byers RM. Supraomohyoid neck dissection: rationale, indications, and surgical technique. *Head and Neck* 1989; **11**: 111–22.

182. Spector JG, Sessions DG, Emami B *et al.* Delayed regional metastases, distant metastases, and second primary malignancies in squamous cell carcinomas of the larynx and hypopharynx. *Laryngoscope* 2001; **111**: 1079–87.

183. Krol BJ, Righi PD, Weisberger EC *et al.* Factors related to outcome of salvage therapy for isolated cervical recurrence of squamous cell carcinoma in the previously treated neck: a multi-institutional study. *Otolaryngology – Head and Neck Surgery* 2000; **123**: 368–76.

184. Kuntz AL, Weymuller EAJr. Impact of neck dissection on quality of life. *Laryngoscope* 1999; **109**: 1334–8.

185. Talmi YP, Horowitz Z, Pfeffer MR *et al.* Pain in the neck after neck dissection. *Otolaryngology – Head and Neck Surgery* 2000; **123**: 302–6.

186. Cappiello J, Piazza C, Giudice M *et al.* Shoulder disability after different selective neck dissections (levels II–IV versus levels II–V): a comparative study. *Laryngoscope* 2005; **115**: 259–63.

187. Pow EH, Kwong DL, McMillan AC *et al.* Xerostomia and quality of life after intensity-modulated radiotherapy vs. conventional radiotherapy for early-stage nasopharyngeal carcinoma: Initial report on a randomized controlled clinical trial. *International Journal of Radiation Oncology, Biology, Physics* 2006; **66**: 981–91.

188. McCulloch P, Taylor I, Sasako M *et al.* Randomised trials in surgery: problems and possible solutions. *British Medical Journal* 2002; **324**: 1448–51.

35

Management of an unknown primary carcinoma

JAWAHER ANSARI AND JOHN GLAHOLM

Seek, and ye shall find.

Matthew 7:7

INTRODUCTION

The definition of an unknown or occult primary carcinoma is the presentation of metastatic neck lymphadenopathy without the development of a primary lesion within a subsequent five-year period. The diagnosis is, however, one of exclusion and consequently depends upon the diligence exercised in the search for a primary tumour. Failure to identify an occult primary has been attributed to spontaneous regression of the primary tumour possibly as a result of autoimmune destruction, although the exact reason is unknown. The term 'carcinoma of unknown primary origin' (UPC or CUP) should be used if no evidence of primary tumour is found after adequate clinical examination, fibreoptic endoscopy, imaging investigations which include fluorine 18-labelled deoxyglucose positron emission tomography (FDG-PET) ideally with CT fusion imaging (FDG) PET-CT and biopsy of putative mucosal sites.

The presentation of metastatic carcinoma involving neck nodes without clinical evidence of a primary tumour is an unusual scenario and accounts for only 2–3 per cent of patients with head and neck malignancy.[1] Metastasis most commonly occurs to nodal levels II and III with less frequent involvement of levels I, IV, V and VI.[2] Squamous carcinoma is the most common histological tumour type and poses the greatest diagnostic dilemma because of the large number of primary upper aoerodigestive sites from which nodal metastases may arise. The prognosis for these patients is relatively good with five-year survival rates exceeding 50 per cent, irrespective of the management strategy.[3] Isolated supraclavicular nodal involvement is almost invariably related to malignant disease arising below the clavicles, with the most likely origin of squamous carcinoma being from lung and oesophagus and adenocarcinoma from thyroid, breast, gastrointestinal and gynaecological tracts. Such tumours have discrete histological and immunohistochemical characteristics and are outwith the remit of this discussion.

DIAGNOSIS

When a patient presents with an isolated neck mass, a thorough clinical history with emphasis on smoking and drinking habits and clinical examination are essential, including a full ear, nose and throat (ENT) assessment with nasendoscopic examination of the upper aerodigestive tract.

Metastatic nodal disease in level I is most commonly associated with a primary tumour of the lip, anterior tongue, anterior floor of mouth and buccal mucosa and, in patients from the Indian subcontinent, there may be a history of betel nut or paan chewing. The majority of patients presenting with a level II/III mass will have a primary tumour of the tonsil or tongue base and so particular attention must be paid to the examination of these areas. It must be emphasized that bulky neck nodes can present in conjunction with a very small primary tumour of the tonsil or a submucosal tumour of the tongue base. Additionally, the skin in the head and neck region including scalp should be carefully assessed together with the external ear and auditory canal. Disease in level IV is most commonly associated with tumours of the hypopharynx and larynx, whereas isolated level V nodal metastasis is a typical feature of nasopharyngeal carcinoma. Isolated level VI disease is unusual, most will be carcinoma of thyroid origin, although subglottic squamous carcinoma may occasionally present with metastasis to this nodal level.

Fine needle aspirate cytology (FNAC), ideally using ultrasound guidance, from the abnormal neck node should then be performed and will often afford a clear indication of the pathological nature of the lesion. In cases of uncertainty, ultrasound-guided core biopsy or open biopsy will be necessary. Excision biopsy is no longer considered to compromise outcome in metastatic squamous carcinoma provided definitive treatment, such as neck dissection and/or radiotherapy is undertaken soon afterwards.[4, 5] A chest x-ray will exclude primary bronchial carcinoma in the majority of patients with squamous histology and must not be overlooked.

Traditionally, anatomical imaging with computed tomography (CT) and magnetic resonance imaging (MRI) of the head and neck, was the next diagnostic stage of the process and while they remain important techniques for the staging of established disease, (FDG) PET-CT, which will be discussed in detail later in this chapter, should now be considered to be the optimal diagnostic investigation. This must be undertaken before examination under general anaesthesia and biopsy of putative mucosal sites, because if scanning is performed after biopsy, subsequent swelling and inflammation may result in FDG uptake and confound interpretation.

Examination under general anaesthesia should then be performed. This consists of pharyngolaryngo-oesophagoscopy and careful palpation of the tongue base. PET-CT may assist in targeting a specific structure for biopsy. However if PET-CT is negative and there is no obvious primary on endoscopy, tonsillectomy, tongue base biopsy and biopsies of the postnasal space and pyriform fossa should be performed. The nasopharynx is of particular importance in patients whose nodal metastasis lies in level V and in those with an undifferentiated histology. Tonsillectomy is recommended because up to 25 per cent of tumours are found at this site.[6, 7, 8] Traditionally, tonsillectomy ipsilateral to the nodal metastasis has been recommended, however contralateral spread from occult tonsilar lesions may be as high as 10 per cent, consequently bilateral tonsillectomy will offer a higher diagnostic yield.[9] Tongue base biopsy will subsequently reveal an additional 10–15 per cent of occult primaries. Biopsy of the tongue base can be difficult and many occult carcinomas are submucosal. Consideration should be given to performing a wedge biopsy, cutting deeply into the tongue base rather than just using cupped forceps.

A note of caution is warranted in a patient presenting with a presumed branchial cyst over the age of 40, particularly if they smoke and drink alcohol. The diagnosis must be treated with considerable suspicion even if FNAC is reported as being benign. If subsequent histological examination reveals squamous carcinoma, the diagnosis will most likely be metastatic squamous carcinoma from the upper aerodigestive tract most commonly from the tongue base or tonsil. Malignant transformation in a branchial cyst is extremely unusual and should never be assumed as the definitive diagnosis. Therefore, branchial cyst in the >40-year-old group should be considered as a patient presenting with an unknown primary.

Conventional processes of clinical examination, panendoscopy, CT and/or MRI followed by panendoscopy with biopsy have been shown to reveal the primary site in over 40 per cent of patients initially diagnosed with neck node metastatic squamous carcinoma of unknown primary origin[10] and is further improved with (FDG) PET and more recently (FDG) PET-CT. Diagnostic accuracy may also be enhanced using laser-induced fluorescence endoscopy in parallel with conventional panendoscopy and biopsy. In a study of 13 patients reported by Kulapaditharom et al.[11] the identification rate of an occult primary was increased from 15.4 to 38.5 per cent.

GENETICS AND MOLECULAR ANALYSIS

Undifferentiated carcinoma is a special example in which the diagnosis of nasopharyngeal carcinoma can be strengthened by the detection of Epstein–Barr virus in the lymph node metastasis either by polymerase chain reaction (PCR) or in-situ hybridization, techniques which have sufficient sensitivity to detect the virus in FNAC[12] or in core biopsy. Serology combining IgA with early antigen serology will also provide a high degree of sensitivity and specificity when type III nasopharyngeal carcinoma is suspected.

Genetic alterations in apparently normal tissue from putative primary sites should be identical to those from a metastatic lymph node and can be defined by microsatellite identification. This technique has been used successfully by Califano et al.[13] where 10 of 18 patients demonstrated identical molecular abnormalities in apparently benign mucosa from surveillance biopsies. The technique may prove clinically useful in patients with an unknown primary squamous cell carcinoma and warrants further assessment. Cytomorphological characteristics, such as monolayered papillary fronds with intranuclear cytoplasmic inclusions in thyroid papillary carcinoma; large, polygonal, keratinized cells with a low nuclear/cytoplasmic ratio in perioral cancers; and numerous naked nuclei with marked lymphocytic infiltrates in nasopharyngeal cancer could possibly be utilized for presumption of primary site in cases of UPC. In a retrospective review of 133 cytologically diagnosed carcinomas, the accuracy rate of presumption of primary sites was 100 per cent in thyroid papillary carcinoma (6/6), 83 per cent in perioral cancer (24/29) and 77 per cent in nasopharyngeal cancer (26/34), but low in other malignancies.[14]

Positron emission tomography

Positron emission tomography using 18-fluorodeoxyglucose (FDG) PET is a promising disease detection modality because of its ability to differentiate between tissue with a high rate of metabolism, such as tumour, inflammation or infection, and tissue with a low metabolic rate, for example scar tissue. The technique is being increasingly used to detect occult primary lesions which other conventional methods have failed to identify.

Historically, the data have been somewhat heterogeneous with results which have been misleading and frequently contradictory. Detection rates for single modality FDG-PET following conventional procedures, including anatomical imaging have been variable with reports ranging from 14 to almost 50 per cent.[15, 16] This wide range can also be attributed to small sample sizes and varied definitions of UPC.

Fogarty et al.[17] have reported a series of 21 patients with UPC who underwent FDG-PET. A potential primary tumour was detected by the procedure in eight patients, although none was considered unequivocally PET-positive. Only one case was pathologically confirmed, in five this could not be confirmed, of which three had no evidence of primary disease within a subsequent two-year period. The authors concluded that FDG-PET did not add significantly to conventional comprehensive investigations as previously discussed. In contrast, a similar-sized prospective study performed at Christie Hospital, Manchester, drew differing conclusions recommending routine use of FDG-PET scans in the management of patients with unknown head and neck primary carcinoma. In this study, a primary site was identified in nine out of 25 patients with UPC on the basis of positive FDG-PET scans. Although 42 per cent of patients had a positive PET scan, only 33 per cent had a true positive PET scan confirmed by histopathology (three out of nine patients). The rate of true negative scans was very high at 88 per cent (14 out of 16 patients). Although, an occult primary was detected only in a small number of patients, nearly a third of the patients studied had abnormalities on PET scans in terms of locoregional disease and distant metastases in 23 and 6 per cent, respectively.[18] Similar conclusions were drawn by Bohuslavizki et al.[19] in a study of 28 patients with UPC. Sixteen out of 28 patients showed increased tracer uptake corresponding to potential primary tumour sites. Of these, nine tumours were found suggesting that approximately a third of patients may benefit from the procedure. Wong et al.[20] reported treatment-related benefits of FDG-PET scans in nine out of 17 patients (53 per cent) with UPC. Of concern, in one series reported by Greven et al.,[21] the apparent false-positive rate was as high as 46 per cent which could have significant implication should the technique be used to select treatment options. Higher false-positive rates in some studies could be attributed to the fact that the PET scans may have been performed after the biopsy.[18] FDG-PET has been summarized as having a positive predictive value of 56 per cent, a negative predictive value of 86 per cent and an overall accuracy of 69 per cent.[22] However, the benefit of FDG-PET scans is not only limited to identifying a primary carcinoma, as the detection of advanced locoregional disease or distant metastases can significantly alter management in terms of modifying radiotherapy fields from unilateral to contralateral neck or changing treatment intent from radical to palliative.[18, 20]

The more recent advance using CT cross-sectional image co-registration with (FDG) PET specifically using a single scanning device termed 'PET-CT' has provided more detailed anatomical localization of FDG avid tissue and together with improved scanning technology may prove to offer greater sensitivity, selectivity and specificity (**Figure 35.1**). Fakhry et al.[23] reported a prospective study of 20 patients with UPC who underwent PET-CT scan, and concluded the sensitivity and specificity of PET/CT to be 70 per cent. Additionally, the use of PET-CT fusion imaging has also significantly reduced the number of false-positive results.[24]

A recent meta-analysis of (FDG) PET-CT from the Netherlands has reported data from 11 studies comprising 433 patients with unknown primary carcinoma. Overall primary detection rate was 37 per cent, with sensitivity of 84 per cent and specificity of 84 per cent, however there was considerable heterogeneity of results between individual studies.[25] A negative PET/PET-CT result clearly does not preclude the requirement for panendoscopy under anaesthesia and biopsy of putative sites, including deep biopsy of the tongue base.[26]

It is important to emphasize that if biopsies have been undertaken prior to PET scanning, false-positive uptake will occur at the biopsy sites and PET-CT scanning will need to be delayed for up to 6 weeks thereafter. Such delay is unacceptable in the time course of the patient's treatment.

CLINICAL MANAGEMENT

Despite extensive investigations, a primary tumour will nevertheless remain elusive in approximately 60 per cent of cases. Management of patients with UPC presents a clinical dilemma due to the lack of evidence-based treatment, exclusion of most patients from randomized clinical trials and rarity of the disease. Controversies in the management of patients with UPC, range from types of neck dissection to be performed, fields of radiotherapy (whether ipsilateral neck only, whole neck or additional panmucosal fields), role of chemotherapy, to sequencing of radiotherapy and neck dissection. The optimal management strategy for patients with UPC is yet to be defined. Therapeutic options include excision biopsy of involved lymph nodes, neck dissection, radiotherapy, chemoradiotherapy or radiotherapy with salvage neck dissection. The only randomized phase III study (EORTC-24001-22005) looking into the selection of the target volume for postoperative radiotherapy in patients with cervical lymph node metastases from UPC closed in July 2004 with very poor accrual.

Surgical management of the neck

Modified radical neck dissection is the most commonly used technique for management of nodal metastatic disease. The procedure can be considered definitive if the histological specimen reveals no more than two involved nodes without evidence of extracapsular spread. Postoperative radiotherapy will then be unnecessary and an active surveillance policy for the occult primary carcinoma can be safely adopted avoiding definitive treatment to putative mucosal sites and consequent treatment-related morbidity.

There is evidence to support the use of radiotherapy alone for management of the neck following the excision of a single metastatic node without recourse to neck dissection, with 88–100 per cent control rates quoted in the literature.[27, 28] A Canadian retrospective study of 61 patients with UPC compared outcomes after panmucosal radiotherapy, preceded by either biopsy (67 per cent) or neck dissection (23 per cent). There was no statistically significant difference in eight-year overall survival between patients who had biopsy (FNAC or

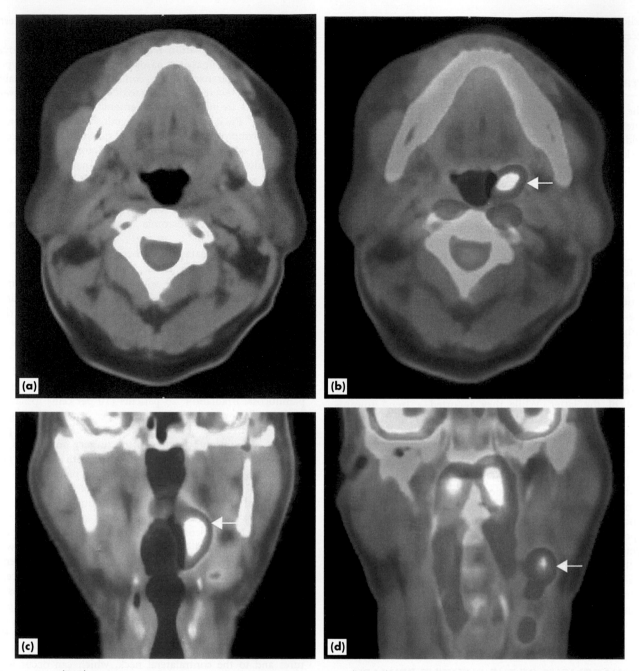

Figure 35.1 (FDG) positron emission tomography–computed tomography (PET-CT) images showing 'occult' carcinoma of left tonsillar fossa subsequently confirmed by biopsy and level II lymphadenopathy.

excision biopsy) or neck dissection (64.8 and 67.6 per cent, respectively). They concluded that definitive radiotherapy to the neck and potential mucosal sites is effective in achieving good local control rates, whether preceded by neck dissection or not.[29] A retrospective review of 106 patients with UPC demonstrated a reduction in mucosal and neck recurrences with the addition of radiotherapy, but failed to show a survival improvement.[3] Coster *et al.*[30] reviewed records of 117 patients with UPC and concluded that patients with N1 neck disease with no extracapsular extension can be managed by surgery alone. However, they recommended postoperative radiotherapy for patients with a pathologic

stage N2 or higher or with evidence of extracapsular extension.

However, the present authors would advise definitive modified neck dissection following excision biopsy in all cases, because recurrent disease in the irradiated neck usually presents as a diffuse tumour infiltrate for which successful salvage rates are low. An exception to this would be where the nodes are small (<2 cm) and where there is no evidence of extracapsular spread. For N2 and N3 disease, the consensus at the present time is for dual modality therapy, involving both neck dissection and radiotherapy. Both neck dissection followed by postoperative irradiation to the neck, and radiotherapy followed by an interval neck dissection are acceptable.

Irradiation limited to the involved neck

The most commonly used techniques employ either an anterior radiation field or anterior–posterior parallel opposed fields to encompass the clinical target volume of the lateral neck nodal compartments and to exclude the midline structures, thereby reducing mucosal toxicity. Sinnathamby et al.[31] reported their series of 69 patients treated between 1983 and 1992. Sixty-three patients were treated with radical radiotherapy, 23 by radiotherapy alone and 40 with surgery and postoperative radiotherapy, with only four patients having surgery alone. The actuarial incidence of primary mucosal occurrence at ten years was 30 per cent and appeared unrelated to whether or not the mucosa was irradiated. This value is equivalent to the ten-year risk of second primaries in patients with successfully treated head and neck cancer. Their five-year overall survival was 36 per cent, which is consistent with most other series. A retrospective study of 144 patients by Wier et al.[28] compared 85 patients receiving radiotherapy to the neck only, with 59 patients who were treated with irradiation to both neck and mucosa. Primary tumours developed in only 8 per cent of the former group and in 2 per cent of the latter. While they reported a trend towards improved survival in those receiving neck and mucosal irradiation, the difference was no longer evident once the extent of nodal involvement was taken into account. Their overall five-year survival rate was reported as 41% with no significant difference between the two groups. The authors cautiously suggest that radiation to the involved nodal region alone may be adequate.[28] These data corroborate the earlier much quoted work from the Middlesex Hospital, London reported in 1990 in which 83 unselected patients at that centre over a 30-year period were treated with radiotherapy to the neck alone, 58 with radical intent for which the overall five-year survival was 40%. Only 7% subsequently developed a primary tumour above the clavicles, supporting the argument for avoidance of routine panmucosal irradiation in this circumstance.[32]

MANAGEMENT OF THE PUTATIVE PRIMARY SITE

When there is a clear indication for postoperative irradiation to the neck, the choice of management strategy becomes considerably more challenging. Irradiation of lateral neck structures will largely preclude irradiation of subsequently occurring primary sites, particularly those which lie in the midline because there will be considerable overlap with radiation fields required to treat a primary site. The management choice will be either to treat putative mucosal sites by panmucosal irradiation, or alternatively by selective mucosal irradiation, using techniques which will also include the involved neck, or alternatively to irradiate the involved neck alone. Postoperative neck irradiation requires a dose of 60–63 Gy over 6–6.5 weeks, or biological equivalent,[33] is well tolerated with mild acute toxicity primarily short-term skin erythema and confers a low risk of associated long-term toxicity.

Panmucosal irradiation requires doses of 50–60 Gy over 5–6 weeks encompassing nasopharynx, oropharynx, hypopharynx and larynx, and in contrast causes considerable morbidity.[34] Acute mucosal toxicity is usually severe and patients frequently require enteral support with nasogastric or PEG (percutaneous endoscopic gastrostomy) feeding. Symptomatic xerostomia is unavoidable with conventional two- or three-dimensional CT treatment planning and results from irradiation of both major and minor, mucosal, salivary glands. When the probability of an occult nasopharyngeal tumour is low, selective mucosal irradiation avoiding this site can be employed and reduces mucosal dryness, although xerostomia may nevertheless remain significant.

At present, all data are retrospective and there are no completed randomized trials. Published reports can be broadly divided into those which propose elective panmucosal irradiation and into those which suggest that avoidance of irradiation to mucosal sites is a safe alternative incurring significantly less morbidity.

The Danish Society for Head and Neck Oncology reported their series of 277 patients from five oncology centres with unknown primary carcinoma treated radically between 1975 and 1995. The majority, 224 patients (81 per cent), received panmucosal irradiation, 26 patients (10 per cent) ipsilateral neck irradiation and 23 patients (9 per cent) neck surgery alone. The five-year actuarial risk of emergence of the primary was significantly higher in the surgery only group, 54 per cent, compared to those treated with surgery and radiotherapy, 15 per cent. When comparing panmucosal with 'neck only' irradiation, the five-year actuarial control rates were 51 and 27 per cent, respectively, although the number of patients was small in the latter group.[2] A smaller study from Reddy and Marks[35] compared 36 patients treated with panmucosal and bilateral neck irradiation to 16 patients who received irradiation to the ipsilateral neck alone. Occurrence of a primary tumour at five years was 8 versus 44 per cent, respectively, and contralateral neck node control 86 versus 56 per cent suggesting superior control rates for more comprehensive irradiation. Patient numbers are small, however, the study is noteworthy because electrons were used to treat the neck only, avoiding incidental irradiation of midline structures and to the contralateral neck, which can occur with photon (x-ray) beam techniques. Earlier reports from the University of Florida and from Institut Curie, Paris, have also alluded to the efficacy of mucosal radiotherapy for eradicating occult primary tumours, although neither included data from nonirradiated patients.[34, 36]

RECENT ADVANCES

Intensity-modulated radiotherapy

Intensity-modulated radiotherapy (IMRT), a new technique for delivering tumoricidal radiation doses to mucosal sites, yet permitting a reduction in dose to sensitive structures including major salivary glands, is still in the early stages of implementation in the UK.

A comparison of IMRT versus conventional radiotherapy treatment plans for six patients undertaken by Bhide *et al.*[37] at the Royal Marsden Hospital has shown improved radiation coverage of the mucosa including nasopharynx with a significant reduction of dose to the parotid gland contralateral to the involved neck, thereby reducing the risk of severe xerostomia.

Results with IMRT in patients with unknown primary carcinoma have been encouraging as recently reported by Memorial Sloane-Kettering Cancer Center for a series of 21 patients. Two-year regional progression-free survival, distant metastasis-free survival and overall survival were 90, 90 and 85 per cent, respectively. The incidence of acute grade 1 xerostomia was 57 and 43 per cent for grade 2 xerostomia. Salivary function improved over time, however dysphagia as a result of oesophageal stricture occurred in three patients all of whom improved following oesophageal dilatation.[38] A group in Ghent has reported similar results using IMRT compared to their historical controls treated with conventional radiotherapy. Grade 3 acute dysphagia was 4.5 compared to 50 per cent. By six months, grade 3 xerostomia was 11.8 per cent in the IMRT group and 53 per cent in the historical controls. There were no cases of late grade 3 dysphagia in the IMRT patients. Control rates and the emergence of a subsequent primary tumour were equivalent.[39]

Inclusion of the nasopharynx in nasopharyngeal carcinoma (NPC)-endemic China has resulted in high control rates and a low risk of development of a primary.[40] Nevertheless, inclusion of the nasopharynx increases the dose to the parotid gland even using IMRT[37] and selective mucosal irradiation should still be considered in patients with a low risk of NPC.

Chemoradiotherapy

Concurrent chemoradiotherapy is now a standard nonsurgical management option for patients with locally advanced head and neck cancers. The role of chemoradiotherapy for patients with UPC has not been fully established. Shehadeh *et al.*[41] reported a benefit in locoregional disease control with postoperative radiotherapy with concurrent cisplatin (100 mg/ m^2 given 3 weekly) in 37 patients with UPC. The majority of patients in this cohort had greater than N2b disease (71 per cent) and extracapsular spread (68 per cent). After a median follow up of 42 months, regional and distant recurrences were noted in 5 and 11 per cent of patients, respectively. Substantial acute and late morbidities were seen, particularly incidence of grade 3/4 mucositis in 46 per cent and xerostomia in a third of patients.[41]

CONCLUSIONS

- All patients with suspected UPC should be thoroughly examined and investigated with panendoscopy, CT or MRI of head and neck, and (FDG) CT-PET.
- Biopsies from putative mucosal sites should only be undertaken after PET-CT scanning targeting sites of increased uptake, the tongue base, postnasal space and pyriform fossa, along with bilateral tonsillectomy.

- Modified neck dissection is recommended for all patients with UPC with cervical lymphadenopathy outside the context of a clinical trial.
- Postoperative selective or panmucosal radiotherapy is indicated for most patients with advanced operable neck disease.
- IMRT should be considered to be the optimal radiotherapy technique in order to maximize coverage of putative mucosal sites and to spare major salivary gland tissue.

FUTURE RESEARCH AND DEVELOPMENT

Issues in the management of patients with UPC continue to remain unresolved. With the current lack of randomized clinical trials for UPC along with a reduced incidence of these tumours, the clinical management of these patients remains challenging. The majority of evidence used to guide investigations and management of these tumours is limited to small retrospective case series.

- Is definitive neck dissection sufficient for patients with N1 and N2a disease, avoiding the need for elective mucosal irradiation (EMI) and its associated morbidity?
- The optimal field for elective irradiation is yet to be defined – whether selective irradiation of the ipsilateral neck is adequate, or is panmucosal or selective mucosal irradiation required for an improvement in disease-free survival and overall survival?

KEY EVIDENCE

- There is no level I evidence for guidance in managing the UPC patient. Data are at best level II.
- PET-CT has been shown to have a key role in the management of patients presenting with UPC, and should precede putative biopsy.
- Postoperative selective or panmucosal radiotherapy is indicated for most patients with advanced operable neck disease.
- Strategies for the use of new treatment technologies, IMRT and modified radiation fractionation, are largely based upon extrapolation of data accumulated for the treatment of known sites of head and neck squamous carcinoma.

KEY LEARNING POINTS

- Unknown primary carcinoma is an unusual clinical scenario and accounts for only 2–3 per cent of patients with head and neck malignancy.

- Involvement of nodal levels I–IV is almost exclusively associated with occult upper aerodigestive tract primary squamous carcinoma, with level II being the most common site.
- CT, MRI or (FDG) CT-PET scans should be performed prior to biopsy in order to guide subsequent biopsy and to avoid imaging artefacts or false-positive results with PET scans.
- The only tumour marker of clinical value is Epstein–Barr virus serology. Positive EBV serology should be followed on by multiple biopsies of the nasopharynx in the search for an occult primary.
- The usefulness of FDG-PET scans in the diagnostic pathway of patients with UPC has been reported with varying degrees of success. Careful analysis of all available data reveals that FDG-PET can alter management in up to a third of patients with UPC. Simultaneous image coregistration PET-CT should be considered optimal.
- There is good evidence to recommend tonsillectomy, but the evidence for tongue base and nasopharyngeal biopsy is less compelling.
- Definitive modified neck dissection should be performed in all patients with UPC after either FNAC or biopsy.
- Panmucosal radiotherapy has demonstrated a reduction in primary site occurrence without any improvement in overall survival. Associated morbidity is high, in particular grade 3/4 mucositis and xerostomia.
- Radiotherapy-related morbidity may be reduced if selective mucosal irradiation is undertaken, most commonly by exclusion of the postnasal space within the clinical target volume in patients who present with nodal involvement of levels I–IV.
- IMRT should be considered to be the optimal technique for radiation dose delivery.
- For panmucosal radiotherapy, a dose of 50 Gy in 25 daily fractions, five fractions per week is sufficient for control of occult primary disease.
- Nodal stage is the most important risk factor for local relapse.
- Chemoradiotherapy in patients with UPC should be considered when neck nodes have extracapsular spread or when resection margins are positive.

REFERENCES

◆ 1. Million RR, Cassisi NJ, Mancuso AA (eds). The unknown primary. In: *Management of head and neck cancer: a multidiscliplinary approach*, 2nd edn. Philadelphia: JB Lippincott, 1994; 311–21.

2. Grau C, Johansen LV, Jakobsen J *et al*. Cervical lymph node metastases from unknown primary tumours. Results from a national survey by the Danish Society for Head and Neck Oncology. *Radiotherapy and Oncology* 2000; **55**: 121–9.

3. Iganej S, Kagan R, Anderson P *et al*. Metastatic squamous cell carcinoma of the neck from an unknown primary: management options and patterns of relapse. *Head and Neck* 2002; **24**: 236–46.

* 4. Mack Y, Parsons JT, Mendenhall WM. Squamous cell carcinoma of the head and neck: management after excisional biopsy. *International Journal of Radiation, Oncology, Biology, Physics* 1993; **25**: 619–22.

5. Ellis ER, Mendehall WM, Rao PV *et al*. Incisional or excisional biopsy before definitive radiotherapy alone or followed by neck dissection. *Head and Neck* 1991; **13**: 177–83.

6. Randall DA, Johnstone PA, Foss RD, Martin PJ. Tonsillectomy in the diagnosis of the unknown primary tumor of the head and neck. *Otolaryngology – Head and Neck Surgery* 2000; **122**: 52–5.

7. Lapyere M, Malissard L, Peiffert D. Cervical lymph node metastasis from an unknown primary: is a tonsillectomy necessary? *International Journal of Radiation, Oncology, Biology, Physics* 1997; **39**: 291–6.

8. Kothari P, Randhawa PS, Farrell R. Role of tonsillectomy in the search for a squamous carcinoma from an unknown primary of the head and neck. *British Journal of Oral and Maxillofacial Surgery* 2008; **46**: 283–7.

9. Koch WM, Bhatti N, Williams MF, Eisele DW. Oncologic rationale for bilateral tonsillectomy in head and neck squamous carcinoma of unknown primary source. *Otolaryngology – Head and Neck Surgery* 2001; **124**: 331–3.

10. Mendenhall WM, Mancuso AA, Parsons JT *et al*. Diagnostic evaluation of squamous cell carcinoma metastatic to cervical lymph nodes from an unknown head and neck primary site. *Head and Neck* 1998; **20**: 739–44.

* 11. Kulapaditharom B, Boonkitticharoen V, Kunachak S. Fluorescence-guided biopsy in the diagnosis of an unknown primary cancer in patients with metastatic cervical lymph nodes. *Annals of Otology, Rhinology and Laryngology* 1999; **108**: 700–4.

* 12. Lee WY, Hsaio JR, Tsai ST. Epstein–Barr virus detection in neck metastases by in situ hybridization in fine-needle aspiration cytologic studies: an aid for differentiating the primary site. *Head and Neck* 2000; **22**: 336–40.

* 13. Califano J, Westra WH, Koch W *et al*. Unknown primary head and neck squamous cell carcinoma: molecular identification of the site of origin. *Journal of the National Cancer Institute* 1999; **91**: 599–604.

14. Liu YJ, Lee YT, Hsieh SW, Kuo SH. Presumption of primary sites of neck lymph node metastases on fine needle aspiration cytology. *Acta Cytologica* 1997; **41**: 1477–82.

● 15. Safa AA, Tran LM, Rege S *et al*. The role of positron emission tomography in occult primary head and neck cancers. *Cancer Journal from Scientific American* 1999; **5**: 214–18.

16. Aassar OS, Fischbein NJ, Caputo GR *et al.* Metastatic head and neck cancer: role and usefulness of FDG PET in locating occult primary tumors. *Radiology* 1999; **210**: 177–81.

17. Fogarty GB, Peters LJ, Stewart J *et al.* The usefulness of fluorine 18-labelled deoxyglucose positron emission tomography in the investigation of patients with cervical lymphadenopathy from an unknown primary tumour. *Head and Neck* 2003; **25**: 138–45.

18. Silva P, Hulse P, Sykes AJ *et al.* Should FDG-PET scanning be routinely used for patients with an unknown head and neck squamous primary? *Journal of Laryngology and Otology* 2007; **121**: 149–53.

19. Bohuslavizki KH, Klutmann S, Sonnemann U *et al.* FDG PET for detection of occult primary tumor in patients with lymphatic metastases of the head and neck. *Laryngorhinootology* 1999; **78**: 445–9.

20. Wong WL, Saunders M. The impact of FDG PET on the management of occult primary head and neck tumours. *Clinical Oncology* 2003; **15**: 461–6.

21. Greven KM, Keyes JW, Williams DW *et al.* Occult primary tumors of the head and neck: lack of benefit from positron emission tomography imaging with 2-[F-18] fluoro-2-deoxy-D-glucose. *Cancer* 1999; **86**: 114–18.

22. Nieder C, Gregoire V, Kian Ang K. Cervical lymph node metastases from an occult squamous cell carcinoma: cut down a tree to get an apple. *International Journal of Radiation, Oncology, Biology, Physics* 2001; **50**: 727–33.

23. Fakhry N, Jacob T, Paris J *et al.* Contribution of 18 F-FDG PET for detection of head and neck carcinomas with an unknown primary tumor. *Annales d'Oto-laryngologie et de Chirurgie Cervico Faciale* 2006; **123**: 17–25.

24. Gutzeit A, Antoch G, Kuhl H *et al.* Unknown primary tumors: detection with dual-modality PET/CT – initial experience. *Radiology* 2005; **234**: 227–34.

25. Kwee TC, Kwee RM. Combined FDG-PET/CT for the detection of unknown primary tumours: systematic review and meta-analysis. *European Radiology* 2009; **19**: 731–44.

26. Miller FR, Karnad AB, Eng T *et al.* Management of the unknown primary carcinoma: long-term follow-up on a negative PET scan and negative panendoscopy. *Head and Neck* 2008; **30**: 28–34.

27. Colletier PJ, Garden AS, Morrison WH *et al.* Postoperative radiation for squamous cell carcinoma metastatic to cervical lymph nodes from an unknown primary site: outcomes and patterns of failure. *Head and Neck* 1998; **20**: 674–81.

28. Wier L, Keane T, Cummings B *et al.* Radiation treatment of cervical lymph node metastases from an unknown primary: an analysis of outcome by treatment volume and other prognostic factors. *Radiotherapy and Oncology* 1995; **35**: 206–11.

29. Aslani M, Sultanem K, Voung T *et al.* Metastatic carcinoma to the cervical nodes from an unknown head and neck primary site: is there a need for neck dissection? *Head and Neck* 2007; **29**: 585–90.

30. Coster, Foote RL, Olsen KD *et al.* Cervical nodal metastasis of squamous cell carcinoma of unknown origin: indication for withholding radiation therapy. *International Journal of Radiation, Oncology, Biology, Physics* 1992; **23**: 743–9.

31. Sinnathamby K, Peters LJ, Laidlaw C, Hughs PG. The occult head and neck primary: to treat or not to treat? *Clinical Oncology* 1997; **9**: 322–9.

32. Glynne-Jones RG, Anand AK, Young TE, Berry RJ. Metastatic carcinoma in the cervical lymph nodes from an occult primary: a conservative approach to the role of radiotherapy. *International Journal of Radiation, Oncology, Biology, Physics* 1990; **18**: 289–94.

33. Peters LJ, Goepfert H, Ang KK *et al.* Evaluation of the dose for postoperative radiation therapy of head and neck cancer: first report of a prospective randomised trial. *International Journal of Radiation, Oncology, Biology, Physics* 1993; **26**: 3–11.

34. Harper CS, Mendenhall WM, Parsons JT *et al.* Cancer in neck nodes with unknown primary site: role of mucosal radiotherapy. *Head and Neck* 1990; **12**: 463–9.

35. Reddy SP, Marks JE. Metastatic carcinoma in the cervical lymph nodes from an unknown primary site: results of bilateral neck plus mucosal irradiation. *International Journal of Radiation, Oncology, Biology, Physics* 1997; **37**: 797–802.

36. Bataini JP, Rodriguez J, Jaulerry C *et al.* Treatment of metastatic neck nodes secondary to an occult epidermoid carcinoma of the head and neck. *Laryngoscope* 1987; **97**: 1080–4.

37. Bhide S, Clarke C, Harrington K, Nutting CM. Intensity modulated radiotherapy improves target coverage and parotid sparing when delivering total mucosalirradiation in patients with squamous cell carcinoma of the head and neck of unknown primary site. *Medical Dosimetry* 2007; **32**: 188–95.

38. Klem ML, Mechalakos JG, Wolden SL, Zelefsky MJ *et al.* Intensity-modulated radiotherapy for head and neck cancer of unknown primary: toxicity and preliminary efficacy. *International Journal of Radiation, Oncology, Biology, Physics* 2008; **70**: 1100–7.

39. Madani I, Vakaet L, Bonte K *et al.* Intensity-modulated radiotherapy for cervical lymph node metastasis from unknown primary cancer. *International Journal of Radiation, Oncology, Biology, Physics* 2008; **71**: 1158–66.

40. Lu H, Yao M, Tan H. Unknown primary head and neck cancer treated with intensity-modulated radiation therapy: to what extent the volume should be irradiated. *Oral Oncology* 2009; **45**: 474–9.

41. Shehadeh NJ, Ensley JF, Kucuk O *et al.* Benefit of postoperative chemoradiotherapy for patients with unknown primary squamous cell carcinoma of the head and neck. *Head and Neck* 2006; **28**: 1090–8.

primary tumour is dissected in continuity with the neck, especially in instances where the mandible is split for access. It may also be advisable to perform an elective tracheostomy in patients who are undergoing a bilateral neck dissection.

Prophylactic antibiotic regimes of 24 hours', duration, covering aerobic, anaerobic and Gram-negative bacteria, based on local sensitivities, are mandatory for clean-contaminated surgery. Their use is advised in clean major oncological head and neck surgery. A urinary catheter can be eschewed if the sole procedure to be performed is a neck dissection.

The following description of neck procedures assumes that several conditions are met: patients are fit for a major surgical endeavour and fully understand the risks of the procedure, the metastatic lesion is resectable, and the primary tumour is controlled or will be addressed concurrently, unless there are over-riding palliative indications for the procedure that have been discussed with the patient and preferably in a multidisciplinary setting. Distant metastases are not necessarily a contraindication for surgery if it is judged that locoregional control will be obtained by the surgical procedure and the benefits outweigh the risks.

Position of the patient during surgery

The patient is laid supine on the operating table and intubated. The authors prefer for the patient not to be paralysed in case a need arises to use nerve stimulators during the procedure. The head is turned to the opposite side and is hyperextended, resting on a head ring. A sandbag, or a towel, pillow or inflatable rubber bag, is placed under the shoulders in order to obtain the desired surgical position of the neck. The upper end of the operating table is elevated to approximately 30°, which decreases the amount of blood loss during surgery and further extends the neck.

A disinfectant surgical solution is applied, with ample margins, to prepare the operative field before draping the patient. Draping may vary according to hospital custom. In general, two horizontal drapes and two vertical drapes are fixed to the skin. Basically, when draping the surgical field the following ipsilateral landmarks should remain visible: mastoid tip, ear lobe, body of the mandible, midline of the chin, suprasternal notch, clavicle and region of trapezius muscle insertion.

A scrub nurse as well as two surgical assistants, one in front of the surgeon and one at the patient's head, is usually present. Few general instruments are used for the operation.

Type of incision

A number of eponymous incisions have been described (**Figure 36.1**). The choice for a specific incision is based on a variety of factors, including personal preference, previous radiotherapy or surgery, the site of the primary tumour and its resection.

The following are the main goals that should be achieved by the skin incision:

- assure adequate vascularization of the skin flaps;
- adequate exposure of the surgical field;
- consider the localization of the primary tumour;
- adequate protection of the major vessels if the sternocleidomastoid muscle is resected;

- consider preoperative factors, such as previous radiotherapy;
- consider as well as facilitate reconstructive surgery, if needed;
- include previous surgical fields (scars, incisions for biopsies, etc.);
- produce acceptable cosmetic results.

Variations of the classical Y-incision (Crile), such as the Gluck, Schobinger, Conley or Martin incision, were used commonly for the excellent exposure they provide, but have the drawback of a trifurcation point or narrow flaps which are prone to breakdown, especially in previously radiated necks. Other alternatives such as the utility incision, hockey stick incision and the apron flap also give good exposure, while avoiding trifurcation points. The McFee incision with two horizontal limbs limits exposure, but has a low incidence of wound dehiscence.

When a neck dissection is performed on a planned basis or for salvage after radiation, it is very unlikely for all five levels to be dissected, thus limiting the need for extensive exposure. A smaller vertical, hockey stick or horizontal incision, based on the levels that need extirpation, will suffice in some selected cases.

When an extensive neck dissection is performed for salvage after chemoradiation, it is advised that myofacial flaps are used to prevent wound breakdown and further complications.

Generic steps for all neck dissections

After positioning and draping of the patient, the desired incision is drawn using a marking pen or ink. The incision should provide adequate exposure and therefore suitable access to the complete operative field. There are four areas of special attention that define the limits of the dissection, and adequate exposure of these areas may constitute the difference between failure and success (**Box 36.1** and **Figure 36.2**). The goal of surgery is to resect both visible and occult disease, and it is in these corners that further occult disease may lurk. Also, when marking the desired incision, care should be taken not to place three-point junctions over the carotid artery.

Before making the incision, slight scratch marks can be made at right angles across to the incision or matching dots can be made/tattooed at three or four points with the tip of an intramuscular green needle dipped in ink, in order to facilitate placement of critical sutures.

The incision is made with a blade No. 10 through the skin down to and through the fibres of the platysma muscle. During the incision, the assistant helps apply adequate traction and countertraction to the skin. The skin flaps are elevated using the platysma muscle as identification of the correct dissection plane. Keeping the platysma muscle into the elevated skin flap ensures appropriate blood supply to the skin flaps and also increases the strength of the wound in the postoperative period. In certain situations, it may be necessary to keep the platysma in the dissection specimen due to tumour invasion, and in these cases it is often wiser to resect the overlying skin as well. In the cranioposterior part of the neck, the fibres of the sternocleidomastoid muscle insert

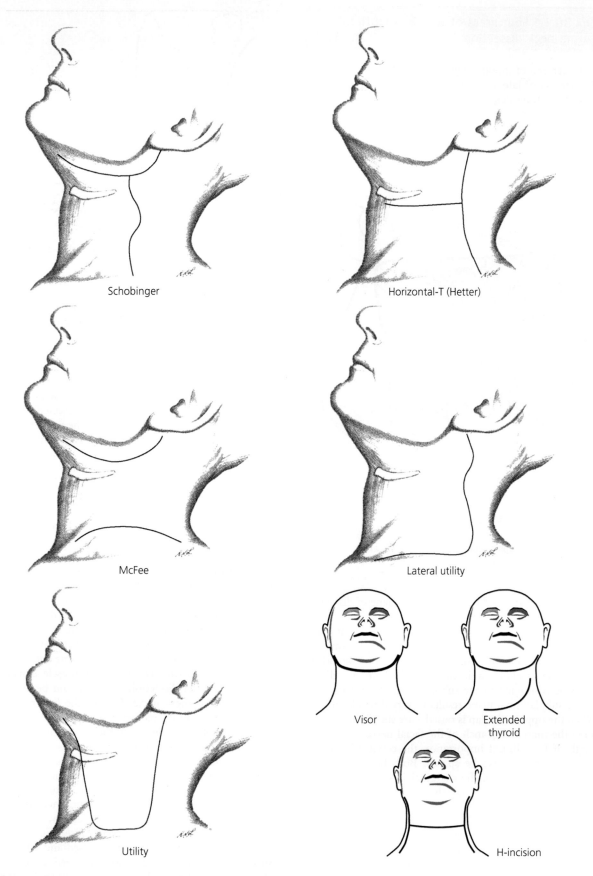

Figure 36.1   Various incisions for neck dissection.

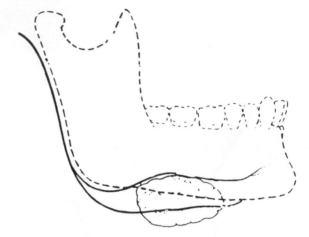

Figure 36.3   Cervical and marginal branches of the facial nerve.

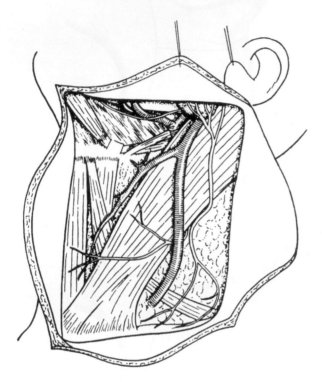

Figure 36.2   Skin flaps raised showing the four areas of special attention.

directly into the skin, and the appropriate plane of dissection is less easily found.

Raising the skin flaps is made easier if the assistant places double skin hooks or a rake retractor under the platysma and applies upward traction. Also, countertraction should be applied to the specimen and, still using the knife, the dissection can be continued in the subplatysmal plane. Dissection along the subplatysmal plane results in very little bleeding.

When the upper skin flap is raised, care should be taken to preserve the marginal branch of the facial nerve. If possible, although of less clinical importance, the cervical branch of the facial nerve can also be spared. Both branches supply tension to the lower lip; the marginal branch supplies the muscles of the corner of the mouth, while the cervical branch supplies the platysma muscle that crosses the mandible and is inserted into the corner of the mouth. Both branches emerge from the lower pole of the parotid gland, curve around the angle of the mandible, cross the facial vessels and then run parallel – approximately at a finger breadth – to the body of the mandible. At the level of the submandibular gland, the marginal mandibular branch is found immediately superior and the cervical branch lateral to the gland. Next, the

branches both curve upwards and cross the mandible (**Figure 36.3**).

One should always bear in mind that neck dissection is an oncological procedure with the goal of cancer cure and this should not be compromised by preserving the nerve. Specifically, if nodal disease is present in the close proximity of the nerve branches, then they should be dissected.

If a McFee incision is being used, the next step is to make the lower skin incision and the lower and middle skin flaps are elevated. Following the subplatysmal plane, the lower flap is easily elevated, and the middle skin flap (also referred to as the bridge) is elevated by dissecting both from the caudal as well as from the cranial field of dissection.

If a trifurcate incision is being used, then the anterior and posterior skin flaps are next to be elevated. Care should specifically be taken when the posterior flap is elevated as it is the most difficult of the three flaps to be raised. This is due to the insertion into the skin of the cranial fibres of the sternocleidomastoid muscle, as well as absence of the platysma muscle over part of its extent, causing the appropriate plane of dissection to be less easily found. The flap is easily made too thick or too thin, and it is easiest to achieve uniform thickness by holding the flap both between retractor and fingers. The posterior flap is elevated to the anterior border of the trapezius muscle. The trapezius muscle constitutes the posterior limit of dissection and it should be exposed from mastoid tip to the clavicle. Due to the hyperextended and rotated position of the patient, the trapezius muscle is lax and it can therefore be more difficult to find. One should remember that the accessory nerve runs through the posterior triangle at a superficial level and is therefore close to the plane of dissection and it is sometimes injured at this point in modified neck dissection procedures. Even though the accessory nerve is resected in a radical neck dissection, the surgeon should be aware of its trajectory, and it is a safe custom to identify the nerve before resecting it.

Once the skin flaps have been raised and adequate exposure is obtained to the aforementioned corners of consternation, the flaps, if desired, can be sutured to the drapes. The flaps should be preferably protected with a moist gauze or sponge to keep them in good condition.

RADICAL NECK DISSECTION

Despite the diminished role of RND in head and neck surgical practice, this is discussed first as a description of radical neck dissection provides greater insight into the neck levels and regional anatomy.

Surgical boundaries and indications

The surgical field has the following boundaries: superior, the inferior border of the mandible; anterior, the contralateral anterior belly of the digastric muscle, the hyoid bone and the sternohyoid muscle; inferior, the clavicle; and posterior, the anterior border of the trapezius muscle.

The indications and contraindications for radical neck dissection are set out in **Box 36.2**.

FIRST AREA OF SPECIAL ATTENTION: THE LOWER END OF THE INTERNAL JUGULAR VEIN

According to personal preference and institution, the dissection can be started at any chosen point, some surgeons like to locate the accessory nerve first, but usually dissection is started at the lower end in the first (lower end of internal jugular vein) or second area (junction of the lateral border of the clavicle with the trapezius muscle) of special attention.

Opinions differ as to whether the lower end or upper end of the main draining vein from the operative field should be ligated first; ligation of the lower end prevents transport of possible tumour emboli into the bloodstream by manipulation of the tumour, but ligation of the lower end of the internal jugular vein causes distension above the ligature rendering dissection more difficult.

Usually, the lower end of the internal jugular vein is approached first by continuing the dissection along the upper border of the clavicle from trapezius muscle to the suprasternal notch. The supraclavicular nerves and vessels (such as the

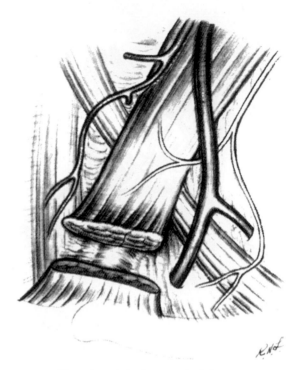

Figure 36.4 Dissection of the lower end of the sternocleidomastoid muscle.

external jugular vein) are divided as well as the sternocleidomastoid muscle. The internal jugular vein lies between the sternal and clavicular heads of the sternomastoid muscle, and dividing the muscle fibres just above the clavicle reveals the vein. This can be done by using blunt-tipped scissors, isolating the muscle by pushing the scissors under the muscle and then keeping the scissors in place to protect the underlying vein, the muscle can be cut (**Figure 36.4**). After dividing the sternocleidomastoid muscle, the blueness of the internal jugular vein can be seen as the vein lies encompassed within the carotid sheath. The carotid sheath contains the internal carotid artery, the internal jugular vein, the vagus nerve and usually also branches of the ansa cervicalis.

The carotid sheath is opened and the internal jugular vein is exposed for at least a few centimetres in order to allow for adequate access for ligation. The position of the vagus nerve is verified before ligation of the internal jugular vein. Three ligating sutures, i.e. vicryl 0/0, are placed around the vein: a ligature and an additional transfixion at the lower end and a ligature at the upper end of the vein remaining within the dissection specimen (**Figure 36.5**).

The vein can be easily damaged during dissection, either when dividing the overlying sternocleidomastoid muscle or when the vein itself is manipulated for its dissection. Damage to the internal jugular vein, but also to small contributing vessels in its proximity, can lead to alarming bleeding during which it is of the utmost importance to remain calm and instruct the assistant not to grab the bleeding vessel with artery forceps or use diathermy as this will enlarge the hole in the vessel. The trick in stopping the bleeding is to apply pressure with a finger or apply arterial clamps and then ligate the vessel. If a large hole occurs or the vein is torn, adequate finger pressure should be applied and the patient should ideally be placed in the Trendelenburg position before

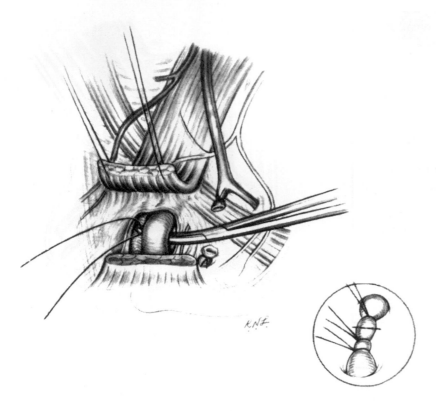

Figure 36.5 Ligation of the internal jugular vein.

clamping and ligating the vein, as the main danger of a torn internal jugular vein is not the blood loss but the possibility of an air embolism.

When performing neck dissection on the left side, one should be alert in the angle between the internal jugular vein, subclavian vein and the clavicle because of the thoracic duct. The thoracic duct passes medial to the jugular vein, then posterior to it and finally curves around to enter the junction of the internal jugular and subclavian vein (**Figure 36.6**). One should note that when performing dissection on the right side, a similar but much smaller duct (accessory duct) is encountered.

After ligation of the vein, the carotid artery and vagus nerve are carefully retracted medially allowing for dissection of the internal jugular vein and its associated lymph nodes. It is of great importance to bear the position of the sympathetic chain in mind – deep to the carotid artery – and it should be preserved.

Once the internal jugular vein has been tied, the dissection extends laterally towards Chaissaignac's triangle, which is defined as the triangle between where the longus colli and scalenus anterior attach to the tubercle of C6 (Chaissaignac's or carotid tubercle) with the subclavian artery as the base (**Figure 36.6**). Here are found the scalene nodes (which should be removed) and the main jugular lymph duct that terminates here on the left side with the thoracic duct, and it is at risk of being damaged. If the duct is damaged, noticeable by extra clear fluid welling up into the dissection area, the source should be found and transfixed. At the end of the operation, it is important to return to this point and check that there are no further leaks. Occasionally, not one large duct but a convolute of lymphatic vessels is found in this area and the utmost care should be taken to prevent chyle leakage.

SECOND AREA OF SPECIAL ATTENTION: JUNCTION OF CLAVICLE AND ANTERIOR BORDER OF TRAPEZIUS

Next, the dissection proceeds towards the second area of special attention formed by the junction of the trapezius muscle and the clavicle (**Box 36.3**). One way to do this is, having tied off the internal jugular vein (**Figure 36.7**), move directly towards the second area and begin the dissection at the lower end of the trapezius muscle. The fatty tissues in the supraclavicular region are divided and care should be taken not to pull these tissues from behind the clavicle into the neck. While the fat is retracted upwards, the inferior belly of the omohyoid muscle is encountered and, according to institutional preference, it is either cut or ligated and it can then be retracted upwards.

Deeper to the omohyoid, the transverse cervical artery and vein are found as they run laterally across the floor of the posterior triangle. They are normally ligated, and in some instances the artery is spared as a possible anastomosis for free flap reconstruction purposes. Both the artery and particularly the vein have small branches across the anterior border of the trapezius muscle. These vessels can often be the source of bleeding during dissection of the posterior triangle, particularly in the short thick neck if they retract into the fat below the trapezius muscle.

Dissection is then continued further, either sharp or blunt with a swab, on to the underlying level of the prevertebral fascia overlying the scalene muscles. Directly beneath the prevertebral fascia, the phrenic nerve and the brachial plexus are seen and, as long as the fascia is not breached, these structures are protected. The phrenic nerve descends from lateral to medial through the neck over the anterior scalenus muscle and the brachial plexus emerges from between the

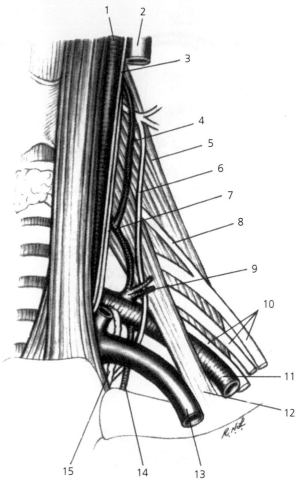

Figure 36.6 Anatomy of the root of the neck. 1, common carotid artery; 2, internal jugular vein; 3, vagus nerve; 4, ascending cervical artery; 5, scalenus medius muscle; 6, phrenic nerve; 7, inferior thyroid artery; 8, C5 nerve; 9, thyrocervical trunk; 10, plexus brachialis; 11, subclavian artery; 12, anterior scalene muscle; 13, subclavian vein; 14, internal thoracic artery; 15, thoracic duct.

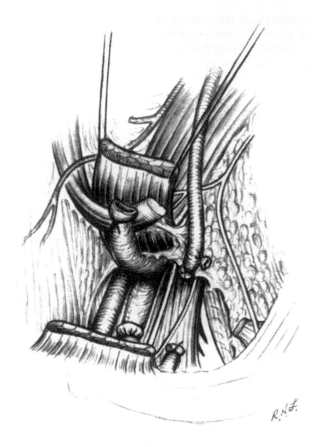

Figure 36.7 Ligation and dissection of the lower end of the internal jugular vein and dissection from the carotid sheath.

Box 36.3 Critical steps in radical neck dissection: the lower neck

- Divide the lower end of the sternocleidomastoid muscle in the first area
- Isolate and ligate the internal jugular vein
- Look for and avoid damage to the thoracic duct and branches of the jugular lymphatic duct in Chaissaignac's triangle
- Remove scalene nodes
- Divide and retract the omohyoid muscle upwards
- Mobilize the fat pad overlying the prevertebral fascia
- Identify and preserve the brachial plexus
- Identify and preserve the phrenic nerve
- Deal with the second area

medial and anterior scalenus muscles. If bleeding occurs in this part of the dissection, bipolar diathermy should be used because of the proximity of the nerves. The supraclavicular dissection is continued to the anterior border of the trapezius muscle and here the dissection proceeds in an upward direction, thus dissecting the posterior triangle of the neck. A note of caution should be made not to exert excessive traction when dividing the supraclavicular tissue as it is possible to inadvertently pull the subclavian vein out of the upper chest with obvious consequences.

Dissection of the posterior triangle

The dissection continues upwards following the anterior border of the trapezius muscle to the uppermost point of the triangle at the mastoid tip where the trapezius and sterno-cleidomastoid meet. By following the anterior border of the trapezius, but dissecting on to the prevertebral fascia the posterior triangle can be cleared. Particularly in patients with a short thick neck, the volume of fatty tissue dissected increases and the clearance of the posterior triangle can be a major problem area for the inexperienced surgeon.

It is however, often thought easiest to dissect the posterior triangle working from the mastoid tip downwards to the clavicle; at the tip of the dissected triangle, the layer of tissue is still thin and it is easier to identify the desired dissection plane. The anterior border of the trapezius muscle constitutes the lateral border of the dissection and the floor of the posterior triangle is formed by the prevertebral fascia overlying the deeper muscles of the neck: the splenius capitis (cranially) and the levator scapulae. The prevertebral fascia is left intact. The method of dissection used is one of personal preference, varying from scissors to sharp scalpel dissection, or in some instances blunt, with the aid of dry gauze.

As a matter of routine, the accessory nerve should be identified before dissection of the posterior triangle. As the nerve runs in the roof of the posterior triangle, it is often identified by the surgeon early during neck dissection when the skin flaps are raised.

Several methods can be used to identify the accessory nerve, based on its anatomical trajectory and surgical landmarks. The accessory nerve innervates the trapezius muscle and the nerve exits from its trajectory through the sternocleidomastoid muscle, approximately at the junction of the upper and lower two-thirds of the sternocleidomastoid and runs in a caudolateral direction to the anterior border of the trapezius. The exit point of the nerve from within the sternocleidomastoid muscle can be predicted by the rule of thumb that it is located approximately 1 cm above Erb's point, the point where the great auricular nerve winds from behind the muscle on its route to supply the skin over the parotid gland. Another way to identify the accessory nerve, but often thought more difficult, is to locate it at its entry point into the anterior border of the trapezius muscle a few centimetres above the clavicle. The dissected tissues are retracted forward and the retraction is hindered by branches of the cervical plexus (C2, C3 and C4). These branches emerge immediately posterolateral to the carotid artery and internal jugular vein and enter the dissection specimen. To enable further retraction, the branches are cut; however, some surgeons prefer to spare the branches of C3 and C4 contributing to shoulder function if the accessory nerve is divided.

The dissected tissue now hinges on the mastoid and skin insertions of the sternocleidomastoid muscle; these are dissected as well as the lower lobe of parotid gland at the level of the angle of the mandible. The mass of the sternocleidomastoid muscle varies considerably; it can be particularly bulky in patients with a short, thick neck. It is of great reassurance for any surgeon to remember that no structures run between the sternocleidomastoid muscle and the posterior belly of the digastric muscle and if these landmarks are defined, the muscle can be divided safely.

THIRD AREA OF SPECIAL ATTENTION: THE UPPER END OF THE INTERNAL JUGULAR VEIN

The posterior belly of the digastric muscle – often referred to as the resident's friend – is cleared and, using a Langenbeck retractor, it can be retracted superiorly exposing the internal jugular vein and the accessory nerve (**Figure 36.8**). The accessory nerve runs along with the internal jugular vein from the jugular foramen and crosses the jugular vein from medially to laterally as the nerve enters the sternocleidomastoid muscle at approximately the junction of the upper and middle third of the muscle. The transverse process of the atlas serves as a useful anatomical landmark. As the muscle has been divided from its cranial insertion into the skin and the mastoid process, and the muscle is retracted caudally, the accessory nerve can be transposed in a craniolateral direction. The dissection plane across the jugular vein lies close to the

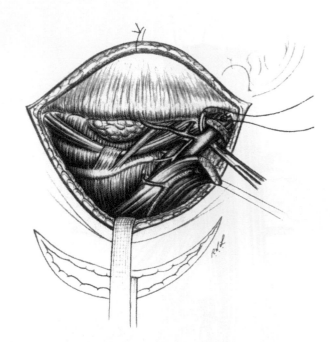

Figure 36.8 Dissection of the upper end of the internal jugular vein.

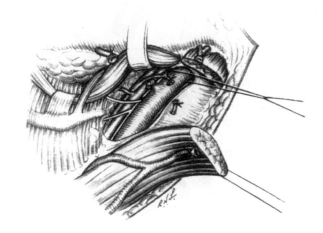

Figure 36.9 Retraction of the posterior belly of the digastric muscle to show the upper end of the internal jugular vein (third area of special attention).

vessel wall and the vein is cleared and mobilized over a few centimetres. The vein is divided after ligation and transfixion with sutures, e.g. Vicryl 0/0 (**Figure 36.9**).

Two important structures should be identified before ligating the internal jugular vein: the vagus and hypoglossal nerves. The vagus nerve runs along with the internal and common carotid artery and its position is verified during dissection. The hypoglossal nerve is a very useful landmark during dissection, specifically if the tumour is fixed near or to the carotid bifurcation. The hypoglossal nerve runs across the carotid bifurcation, the lingual and occipital arteries and forms a rather convenient tunnel along which the dissection can be continued. The occipital artery is usually encountered when the internal jugular vein is cleared as the artery crosses the vein and is often the source of bleeding.

Dissection across the carotid bifurcation may cause bradycardia and changes in blood pressure due to triggering of the carotid sinus lying within the bifurcation. Usually, these symptoms disappear when manipulation ceases and if necessary lidocaine can be applied locally.

Once the internal jugular vein has been ligated and dissected at the upper end, the surgical specimen is mobilized by working both from a cranial and a caudal direction. It is useful to remember that usually all branches of the internal jugular vein arise from its anteromedial surface, but of course there are exceptions to this rule, and the branches are ligated. Working from a caudal to cranial direction, the dissection is completed by following the anterior belly of the omohyoid muscle – which is the anterior border of the dissection – to its insertion at the hyoid bone from which it is divided (**Box 36.4**).

FOURTH AREA OF SPECIAL ATTENTION: THE SUBMANDIBULAR TRIANGLE

It is important to recognize that clearance of level I for oncologic purposes is not synonymous with removal of the submandibular salivary gland. The contents of the triangle, including lymph nodes and fatty tissue must be removed, leaving behind clean muscles that form the boundaries. Dissection of the submandibular triangle (**Figure 36.10**) is usually begun in the midline, by dividing the fatty tissue on to the dissection plane of the anterior belly of the contralateral digastric muscle. The fatty tissue in the submental triangle between the anterior bellies of digastric muscles is included in the dissection specimen and the dissection continues over the anterior belly of the ipsilateral digastric muscle and the mylohyoid muscle, which are cleared of their covering tissues.

The fascia, including the submandibular gland, is dissected from its attachments across the lower border of the mandible and from its insertion directly behind the digastric muscle to the mandibular angle. The facial artery and vein are encountered and ligated as they cross the corpus of the mandible towards the masseter muscle. It is important to include the tissue in close continuity to the facial artery and vein as this may include a small lymph node regularly found at this site.

By retracting the mylohyoid muscle medially and at the same time retracting the submandibular gland inferolaterally, the floor of the submandibular triangle becomes visible with the lingual and hypoglossal nerve overlying the deep plane formed by the genioglossus and hyoglossus muscles.

Because of the downward traction of the submandibular gland, the lingual nerve is extended slightly. This allows for placement of a ligature around its ganglion – supplying secretomotor innervation – as well as the small accompanying blood vessel which can be the source of bleeding if severed. After dissecting the ganglion and connecting tissues, the lingual nerve retracts upwards to its original position behind the body of the mandible, out of the surgical field.

The hypoglossal nerve is identified on its anterosuperior anatomical trajectory, medial to the anterior belly of the digastric muscle. While keeping the hypoglossal nerve under direct vision, the submandibular duct is ligated or divided according to the surgeon's preference and the entire gland is

---

Box 36.4   Critical steps in radical neck dissection: upper neck

- Divide the upper end of the sternocleidomastoid muscle in the third area
- Retract the posterior belly of the digastric muscle upwards
- Identify and ligate the internal jugular vein
- Identify and preserve the hypoglossal nerve

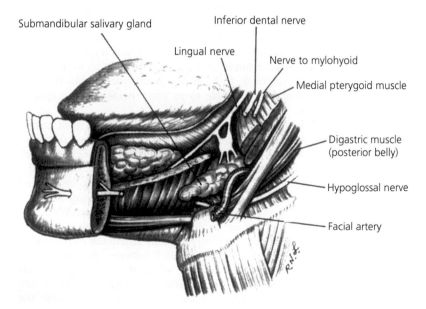

Submandibular salivary gland

Inferior dental nerve

Lingual nerve

Nerve to mylohyoid

Medial pterygoid muscle

Digastric muscle (posterior belly)

Hypoglossal nerve

Facial artery

Figure 36.10 Anatomy of the submandibular triangle.

mobilized with the specimen. One of the last steps before removing the entire specimen is formed by ligating the facial artery. The facial artery is encountered (again) at the posterior inferior border of the submandibular gland as it rounds the posterior belly of the digastric muscle; it can be ligated at its point of origin (external carotid) or directly near the submandibular gland. The latter preserves a large part of the artery and forms a suitable microvascular anastomosis site for free flaps if the neck dissection is part of major ablative and reconstructive surgery.

Complications of radical neck dissection

An extensive overview of the possible complications of radical neck dissection has been given in Chapter 11, Complications and their management. The most troublesome and crippling long-term complication of radical neck dissection is the shoulder syndrome. It is a direct consequence of the denervation of the shoulder musculature, specifically the trapezius muscle, caused by cutting the spinal accessory nerve and possibly its cervical plexus branches. Due to denervation of the trapezius muscle, several changes within the shoulder girdle and arm movements occur: complete abduction of the arm is impeded at 75°, the shoulder girdle is tilted downwards, rotation is impeded and flexion of the arm can only be performed by the deltoid muscle, resulting in maximal flexion of 45°. Furthermore, the shoulder syndrome is extremely troublesome because of the accompanying long-term pain and it is of the utmost importance that all patients are referred to a physiotherapist postoperatively.

Extended radical neck dissection

In addition to all structures resected during radical neck dissection, it may be necessary to extend the surgical procedure including other adjacent structures due to tumour involvement or lymph node metastasis into additional lymph node groups, such as retropharyngeal lymph nodes or nodes in the parotid gland, and nodes in levels VI (prelaryngeal) or VII. In these cases, the dissection is performed as described for the radical neck dissection procedure with inclusion of the additional levels or structures.

Modified radical neck dissection

SURGICAL BOUNDARIES AND INDICATIONS

The surgical field for an MRND shares the same boundaries as an RND. It is difficult to be certain preoperatively which structures can be spared based on the clinical and radiological findings. In a clinical N1 or N2a, N2b neck in which the accessory nerve is free from the lymph node metastases, it is safe to preserve the nerve. It is often safe to preserve both the nerve and internal jugular vein, specifically if the contralateral neck is also dissected at the same time and in those cases where there is need for a microvascular anastomosis site. Preservation of all three major non-lymphatic structures

Box 36.5 Preservation of all three major non-lymphatic structures
Modified radical neck dissection with:
• Preservation of accessory nerve • Preservation of accessory nerve and internal jugular vein • Preservation of accessory nerve, internal jugular vein and sternocleidomastoid

is specifically advocated for the treatment of cancer of the thyroid gland with lymph node metastases (**Box 36.5**).

Sparing of the accessory nerve

If the accessory nerve is to be spared, extra care should be taken when the skin flap of the posterior triangle is developed, as the nerve runs at a superficial level and is therefore close to the plane of dissection. It is at this point that the nerve is often damaged during modified radical neck dissection procedures, and it is a safe practice for many surgeons to identify the nerve at an early stage of the dissection, often during the elevation of the skin flaps. Several methods to identify and locate the nerve can be used. These methods are based on the anatomical trajectory of the nerve and on the use of surgical landmarks.

The accessory nerve supplies the innervation of the trapezius muscle and the nerve exits from its trajectory through the sternocleidomastoid muscle, approximately at the junction of the upper third and lower two-thirds of the sternocleidomastoid and runs in a caudolateral direction to the anterior border of the trapezius. The exit point of the nerve from within the sternocleidomastoid muscle can be predicted by the rule of thumb that it is located approximately 1 cm above Erb's point, the point where the great auricular nerve winds from behind the muscle on its trajectory to supply the skin of the face. Another way, but often thought more difficult, to identify the accessory nerve is to locate it at its entry point into the anterior border of the trapezius muscle a few centimetres above the clavicle. The accessory nerve is then dissected free from its surrounding tissues in its lower course through the neck, from its exit point from within the sternocleidomastoid muscle to its entry point at the trapezius muscle.

It is safe to locate the accessory nerve in its most cranial part as it enters the neck together with the internal jugular vein from within the jugular foramen. Through superior retraction of the posterior belly of the digastric muscle, the accessory nerve and the internal jugular vein can be exposed and the nerve can be identified as it runs along with the internal jugular vein and crosses it medially to laterally across its anterior surface to innervate the sternocleidomastoid muscle. The accessory nerve usually enters the sternocleidomastoid muscle at the junction between the upper and middle third of the muscle, where the transverse process of the atlas serves as a useful landmark. The nerve can safely be dissected from within its trajectory through the sternocleidomastoid muscle by placing Ellis clamps or clips on the edge of the sternocleidomastoid muscle at either side of the nerve and lifting the muscle up, thus creating a tunnel and the nerve can be followed while dissecting the overlying muscle fibres. During the dissection of the accessory nerve through the sternocleidomastoid, its branch supplying this muscle is cut. The dissection of the nerve involves manipulation as well as devascularization of the nerve possibly leading to unpredictable postoperative loss of function.

Sparing of the sternocleidomastoid muscle

Preservation of the sternocleidomastoid muscle requires mobilization of the deep inserting fascia from the anterior border of the sternocleidomastoid muscle and dissection of the muscle from the fascia below allowing for upward retraction of the muscle using loops or retractors. The neck dissection is more difficult to perform if the sternocleidomastoid muscle is preserved and it is often wise for the surgeon to consider the merit of its preservation. The dissection itself is continued under the sternocleidomastoid muscle in the same way as one would proceed as in a radical neck dissection. Sometimes, surgeons opt for division of the sternocleidomastoid muscle in its caudal end, pulling the muscle up during surgery and resuturing it into place at the end of the procedure.

Sparing of the internal jugular vein

Preservation of the internal jugular vein requires careful dissection along the surface of the vein over its complete course through the neck. As in radical neck dissection, the vein is located preferably first in the lower neck, after having completed the dissection across the clavicle from trapezius to suprasternal notch. The supraclavicular nerves and vessels (such as the external jugular vein) are divided as well as the sternocleidomastoid muscle. The sternocleidomastoid lies directly over the internal jugular vein and the muscle fibres are divided – if the sternocleidomastoid is to be sacrificed – just above the clavicle. This can be done by using blunt-tipped scissors, isolating the muscle by pushing the scissors under the muscle and then, keeping the scissors in place to protect the underlying vein, the muscle can be cut. After dividing the sternocleidomastoid muscle, the blueness of the internal jugular vein can be seen as the vein lies encompassed within the carotid sheath.

The carotid sheath is opened and the internal jugular vein is exposed. The vein can be easily damaged during dissection, either when dividing the overlying sternocleidomastoid muscle or when the vein itself is manipulated for its dissection. The upper part of the internal jugular vein is also identified by superior retraction of the posterior belly of the digastric muscle and by dissection along the internal jugular vein the vein can be dissected from the surrounding tissues over its entire course through the neck. Of course, all relevant branches of the vein are encountered during dissection, usually branching from the anterior surface of the vein, and ligated.

Postoperative management and complications of modified radical neck dissection

The postoperative care of modified radical neck dissection does not differ from the radical neck dissections. Complications have been described in Chapter 11, Complications and their management.

SELECTIVE NECK DISSECTION

Surgical boundaries and indications

The boundaries of the surgical field are defined by the lymph node levels that are dissected and are thus less extensive than in modified or radical neck dissection.

SND is commonly used for a clinically disease-free neck in which the lymph node levels at the highest risk of containing possible micrometastatic disease are dissected. There is increasing support for the use of SND in N1 neck disease. One should bear in mind that if peroperative positive lymph nodes are found, especially at multiple levels, it may be necessary to convert the dissection to a modified radical neck dissection. However, when postoperative irradiation is planned for favourable N2 disease, SND may still be appropriate in very selected cases. The lymph node levels/groups dissected are determined by the patterns of metastatic spread for specific tumour locations.

Based on these patterns of metastatic spread the following indications and corresponding SND can be defined.[11, 12, 19, 20, 21]

SELECTIVE NECK DISSECTION FOR ORAL CANCER: SND (I–III) AND SND (I–IV)

The SND (I–III) is indicated for oral cancer, T1 to T4 with clinical N0 neck, in which levels I–III are the node groups/levels at risk (**Figure 36.11**). It is also indicated for the contralateral neck in midline lesions of the floor of mouth or ventral tongue. Other indications include extension of parotid surgery in cases of malignancy or facial skin malignancies in a line anterior to the tragus. The SND (I–IV) is indicated for oral cancer of the anterolateral part of the tongue in which lymph node level IV is also considered to be at risk (**Figure 36.11**).

SELECTIVE NECK DISSECTION FOR OROPHARYNGEAL, HYPOPHARYNGEAL AND LARYNGEAL CANCER: SND (II–IV) AND SND (II–IV AND VI)

The SND (II–IV) is indicated in oropharyngeal, hypopharyngeal and laryngeal tumours in which levels II–IV are the most at risk (**Figure 36.11**). Furthermore, tumours at these sites often cross the midline and thus a bilateral SND (II–IV) is often the case if the neck is managed surgically.

There is good prospective evidence to suggest that dissection of level IIb may be unnecessary for some N0 necks.[17] Patients with laryngeal primaries and contralateral N0 necks are ideal scenarios for preservation of sublevel IIb. In laryngeal cancer with subglottic extension, hypopharyngeal

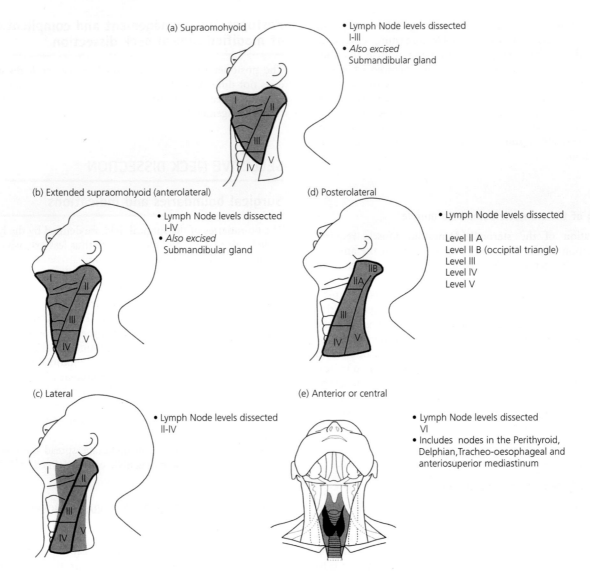

Figure 36.11 Types of selective neck dissection. (a) Levels I–III (supraomohyoid); (b) levels I–IV (extended supraomohyoid); (c) levels II–IV (lateral); (d) levels II–V (posterolateral); (e) level VI–VII (anterior/paratracheal).

cancer and medullary thyroid cancer level VI is also included in the dissection, as well as in some instances level VII.

SELECTIVE NECK DISSECTION FOR METASTASES OF CUTANEOUS CANCER: SND (II–V, POSTAURICULAR AND SUBOCCIPITAL/POSTEROLATERAL DISSECTION)

Selective neck dissection for lymph node metastases of skin tumours of the scalp and neck (posterior to the tragus) should include the suboccipital and postauricular levels in addition to levels II–V (**Figure 36.11**).

Operative techniques for selective neck dissection

Positioning, preparation of the surgical field and draping of the patient are largely comparable to radical neck dissection, but in accordance with the levels included in the dissection,

variations in position, incision, as well as surgical preference, may occur.

SND (I–III) AND (I–IV)

Once adequate exposure is obtained, the investing fascia of the sternomastoid muscle is mobilized anteriorly and the muscle is retracted laterally. Care should be taken not to injure the greater auricular nerve as most of the sensory branches from the cervical plexus can be preserved for selective neck dissections not involving level V. The investing fascia is then dissected off the undersurface of the sternomastoid muscle to its posterior border, along its entire length. The accessory nerve comes into view when the upper third of the sternomastoid is being mobilized. Mobilizing the muscle laterally will lead the surgeon on to the fat and lymphatic tissue in the posterior triangle. The posterior boundary of the dissected specimen usually corresponds to the posterior border of the sternomastoid and the branches of the cervical plexus. Dissection should now proceed deeper, cutting though the fatty tissue, leading the surgeon to the prevertebral fascia overlying the paraspinal muscles. The specimen is mobilized working from inferior to superior, staying superficial to the cervical plexus branches, which are preserved.

The dissection is taken up to the level of the posterior belly of the digastric muscle where the internal jugular vein is identified along with the accessory nerve as it enters the neck, usually crossing the anterior surface of the IJV to enter the sternomastoid muscle. Here, a decision will need to be made whether to dissect level IIb, which lies posterosuperior to the accessory nerve. If level IIb is to be dissected, the fibrofatty tissue needs to be mobilized off the underlying splenius capitis and levator scapulae and the accessory nerve gently lifted off it, before being passed under the nerve to maintain continuity with the rest of the specimen. Working along the inferior belly of omohyoid muscle that is left in place to form the inferior border of the dissection (levels I–III), the lymph nodal tissue is mobilized further anteriorly in a plane superficial to the prevertebral fascia along a broad front. The IJV is encountered and meticulous sharp dissection helps swing the specimen towards the superior belly of omohyoid. The omohyoid can now be followed to the hyoid, which is skeletonized, and this leads to the contralateral anterior belly of digastric muscle. The fatty contents of the submental and submandibular triangles are cleared as described in earlier sections.

If level IV also has to be dissected, the dissection is extended inferiorly to include this lymph node level. The omohyoid muscle is left in place, but does not constitute the inferior border of the dissection.

SND (II–IV) AND (VI)

The dissection of levels II–IV is performed as described above. If level VI is also dissected, as in laryngeal cancer and total thyroidectomy, the pre- and paratracheal nodes in this level are also included. Level VI dissection is discussed in Chapter 23, Surgical management of differentiated thyroid cancer.

SND (II–V, POSTAURICULAR AND SUBOCCIPITAL/ POSTEROLATERAL DISSECTION)

This procedure needs greater exposure than required for the other SND types described, with skin flap elevation to ensure the trapezius is identified. The procedure commences with mobilization of the sternomastoid, as discussed above under Operative techniques for selective neck dissection. Following this, the dissection and mobilization of the fatty tissue is started in the posterior triangle, identifying the accessory early in the dissection. Levels Va and Vb are cleared with anterior retraction of the sternomastoid. The dissected fibrofatty tissue in level Va usually will merge with the tissue in level IIb, which will need to be passed under the accessory nerve. This will enable the specimen to be delivered anteriorly under the sternomastoid and the rest of the dissection will proceed as described under SND (II–IV). For cutaneous primaries, this will include clearance of the suboccipital and postauricular lymph node levels. It should be noted that the

cervical plexus branches may need to be sacrificed in this type of neck dissection.

SUPERSELECTIVE NECK DISSECTION AND OTHER UNCLASSIFIED VARIANTS

These entities are not currently included in the neck dissection classification update published in 2002, but are practised more widely than is recognized. The indications are exclusively in the setting of residual disease following chemoradiation, where appropriate investigations have revealed the absence of active disease in the primary site or at multiple neck levels. It should be noted that these procedures are not yet backed by high level evidence and are best confined to trial settings at present.

The incision is based on the exposure needed, and given the indications for primary chemoradiation in practice today, it is very likely that the lymph node will be in levels II, III or IV. These can be easily accessed through a horizontal incision. The same principles as for the other neck dissections hold, but it must be noted that normal anatomy may be difficult to recognize, with scarred fibrotic tissue making dissection challenging. In most circumstances, the residual lump with adjacent fibrofatty tissue in the same or adjacent level is removed. Sometimes, based on the extent of scarring, the residual node may be adherent to non-lymphatic structures (sternomastoid muscle, accessory nerve or internal jugular vein), making it impossible to safely remove the nidus without their sacrifice. The extent of sternomastoid to be removed in such an instance is only a segment that covers one or two levels as the case may be.

Haemostasis, closure and postoperative care

Haemostasis is checked and irrigation of the wound is performed according to the surgeon's or institutional custom. One or two drains are placed, taking care that they are not placed in proximity to microvascular anastomosis sites and that they do not cross the carotid. Before closing the wound in two layers, subcutis with Vicryl and cutis with staples or Ethilon sutures, a last inspection of the wound is made checking for possible chylous leak and haemostasis.

No dressings are applied to the wound and specific postoperative care is given along individual institutional custom.

Orientating specimen for pathological examination

To maximize the yield from pathology services, the authors recommend three important strategies: ensure high quality clinical information about the patient is communicated, identify if any special information is required from the pathological examination and orientate the resection specimen for the pathologist. Broadly, two techniques are used for orientation. The specimen can be pinned on to a cork or polystyrene blocks, with coloured pins used to identify the levels (**Figure 36.12**). An alternative recommended for SNDs is for the surgeon to separate the node groups, mark the

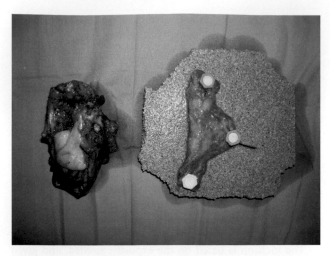

Figure 36.12 Total laryngectomy with selective neck dissection (II–IV) specimen. Note how the specimen has been mounted and orientated using different coloured pins.

superior margin of each group with a suture and place each group in a separately labelled container.[22] Surgically important margins may be marked with Indian ink or an appropriate dye. Where feasible, it is desirable to supplement this with a photograph of the specimen.

Postoperative management and complications of SND

The postoperative care of selective neck dissections does not differ from radical neck dissections. Complications are described in Chapter 11, Complications and their management.

Neck dissection as part of a combined surgical procedure: site of desired continuity between the specimens

A neck dissection is often part of a combined surgical procedure in which the primary tumour is also resected. It is preferable, but not mandatory, that continuity is preserved between the two specimens. Despite the widespread practice of not preserving continuity, there exists no evidence of adverse effect.

- **Oral cancer.** Oral lymphatic drainage is to the submental, submandibular and upper deep cervical lymph nodes of levels I, II and III. Continuity between the dissection specimens can be maintained along the lower border of the mandible, ensuring that the inner layer of periosteum is included.
- **Oropharyngeal cancer.** Oropharyngeal lymphatic drainage is primarily to the upper cervical lymph nodes of levels II, II and IV. Continuity between the dissection specimens can be maintained with the tissue lying medial to the corner of the mandible and oropharynx.
- **Laryngeal cancer.** The neck dissection specimen is left attached to the whole length of the larynx in a total

laryngectomy, thus including the superior and inferior laryngeal lymphatic pedicles, and including lymphatic drainage regions of levels II, III, IV and VI. In a supraglottic laryngectomy, the neck dissection specimen is left attached at the thyrohyoid membrane.

- Neck dissection following chemoradiation, especially performed well after fibrosis has set in, can prove to be a challenging operation.

REFERENCES

1. Crile GW. Excision of cancer in the head and neck. With special reference to the plan of dissection based on one hundred and thirty-two operations. *Journal of the American Medical Association* 1906; **47**: 1780-6.
2. Chelius JM. *A system of surgery*, vol. III. Philadelphia: Lea and Blanchard, 1847: 515.
3. Kocher T. Ueber Radicalheilung des Krebses. *Deutsche Zeitschrift für Chirurgie* 1880; **13**: 134-66.
4. Butlin HT. *Diseases of the tongue*. London: Cassell, 1885.
5. Jawdyński F. Przypadek raka pierwotnego szyi. t.z. raka skrzelowego Volkmann'a.Wycięcie nowotworu wraz z rezekcyją tętnicy szyjowej wspólnej i żyly szyjowej wewnętreznej. *Wyzdrowienie Gaz Lek* 1888; **8**: 530-7.
6. Crile GW. On the surgical treatment of cancer of the head and neck. With a summary of one hundred and twenty-one operations performed upon one hundred and five patients. *Transactions of the Southern Surgical and Gynecological Association* 1905; **18**: 108-27.
7. Martin H, Del Valle B, Ehrlich H, Cahan WG. Neck dissection. *Cancer* 1951; **4**: 441-99.
8. Suárez O. El problema de las metastasis linfáticas y alejadas del cáncer de laringe e hipofaringe. *Revue de Otorrinolaringologia* 1963; **23**: 83-99.
9. Bocca E. Evidement 'fonctionel' du cou dans la thérapiede principedes metastases ganglionnaires du cancer du larynx (introduction a la presentation d'un film). *Journal Français d'Oto-rhino-laryngologie* 1964; **13**: 721-3.
10. Ferlito A, Rinaldo A. Osvaldo Suárez: often forgotten father of functional neck dissection (in the non-Spanish-speaking literature). *Laryngoscope* 2004; **114**: 1177-8.
11. Lindberg R. Distribution of cervical lymph node metastases from squamous cell carcinoma of the upper aerodigestive tracts. *Cancer* 1972; **29**: 1446-9.
12. Shah JP, Anderson PE. The impact of patterns of neck metastasis on modifications of neck dissection. *Annals of Surgery and Oncology* 1994; **1**: 521-32.
13. Jesse RH, Ballantyne AJ, Larson D. Radical or modified neck dissection: a therapeutic dilemma. *American Journal of Surgery* 1978; **136**: 516-19.
14. Robbins KT, Medina JE, Wolfe GT *et al.* Standardizing neck dissection terminology. Official report of the Academy's Committee for Head and Neck Surgery and Oncology. *Archives of Otolaryngology – Head and Neck Surgery* 1991; **117**: 601-5.
15. Robbins KT, Clayman G, Levine PA *et al.* Neck dissection classification update. Revisions proposed by the American Head and Neck Society and the American Academy of Otolaryngology-Head and Neck Surgery. *Archives of Otolaryngology – Head and Neck Surgery* 2002; **128**: 751-8.
16. Lim YC, Choi EC, Lee JS *et al.* Is dissection of level IV absolutely necessary in elective lateral neck dissection for clinically N0 laryngeal carcinoma? *Oral Oncology* 2006; **42**: 102-7.
17. Paleri V, Kumar Subramaniam S, Oozeer N *et al.* Dissection of the submuscular recess (sublevel IIb) in squamous cell cancer of the upper aerodigestive tract: prospective study and systematic review of the literature. *Head and Neck* 2008; **30**: 194-200.
18. Robbins KT, Shannon K, Vieira F. Superselective neck dissection after chemoradiation: feasibility based on clinical and pathologic comparisons. *Archives of Otolaryngology, Head and Neck Surgery* 2007; **133**: 486-9.
19. Ferlito A, Robbins KT, Shah JP *et al.* Proposal for a rational classification of neck dissections. *Head and Neck* 2011; **33**: 445-50.
20. Patel KN, Shah JP. Neck dissection: past, present, future. *Surgical Oncology Clinics of North America* 2005; **14**: 461-77.
21. Ferlito A, Rinaldo A, Silver CE *et al.* Changing concepts in the surgical management of the cervical node metastasis. *Oral Oncology* 2003; **39**: 429-35.
22. Helliwell TR, Woolgar JA, Dataset for histopathology reports on head and neck and salivary cancers. London: Royal College of Pathologists, 2005. Last accessed June 19, 2011. Available from: www.rcpath.org/publications.

37

Salivary gland tumours

PATRICK SHEAHAN AND ASHOK R SHAHA

Don't just do something ... stand there and think.

Ron Hoille, 1999

INTRODUCTION

Salivary glands are a common source of benign pathology. In contrast, salivary carcinoma is uncommon. However, salivary neoplasms possess some features which make them unlike any other head and neck neoplasm. In the first instance, there is a multiplicity of tumour types, many of which are characterized by a variable and diverse histological appearance. Thus, distinction between tumour types, including the distinction between benign and malignant, may be very difficult on the basis of fine needle aspiration (FNA) or small biopsies. Second, the most common benign tumour (pleomorphic adenoma) has a premalignant potential, which is unique in the head and neck. Third, many salivary malignancies are characterized by an indolent growth pattern, but with a high tendency to recur locally or give rise to distant metastases. Such recurrences may appear after many years of apparent disease-free survival. Thus, a thorough understanding of the nature of salivary neoplasms is essential to the head and neck surgeon.

SURGICAL ANATOMY

Parotid glands

The parotid glands are paired glands situated on either side of the face, between the ear and the ramus of the mandible.

Superiorly, the gland extends above the level of the external auditory canal, up to the temporomandibular joint. Anteriorly, it extends superficial to the masseter muscle. In around 20 per cent of individuals, a portion of the gland (the 'accessory' lobe) may be separate from the main gland, over the masseter muscle, in proximity to the parotid duct. The bulk of the gland (the 'tail') extends inferiorly, between the mandible and the upper part of the sternomastoid muscle. A lump in the tail of the parotid gland may easily be confused with an upper deep cervical node. There may be an extension of the gland deep to the mandible (the 'pterygoid' process) (**Figure 37.1**).

The parotid gland is surrounded by a thick capsule derived from the investing layer of deep cervical fascia. Histologically, it is composed of serous secretory units (acini), which drain into intercalated (terminal) ducts. The intercalated ducts converge to form striated (intralobular) ducts, which in turn converge to form secretory (interlobular) ducts, found within connective tissue septae. Secretory ducts empty into the main parotid duct.

The main trunk of the facial nerve enters the posterior surface of the gland and quickly bifurcates into upper and lower divisions. These in turn split into further branches. The pattern of branches is variable. As a general rule, the upper division gives rise to frontal, zygomatic and upper buccal branches; and the lower division gives rise to lower buccal, marginal mandibular and cervical branches. The upper division branches tend to be thicker and more resilient than the lower division branches, and take a more superficial course through the gland before exiting. The lower division branches are thinner and more delicate, and take a deeper course. Neuropraxia after surgical manipulation is seen particularly with the lower division branches. The most

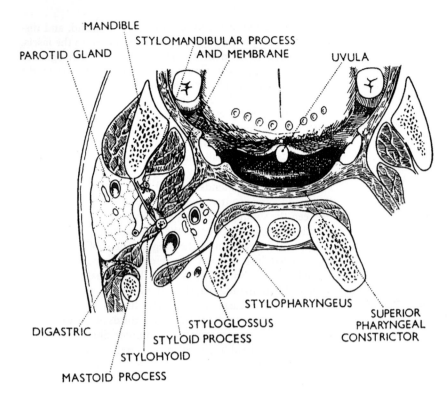

MANDIBLE

STYLOMANDIBULAR PROCESS
AND MEMBRANE

PAROTID GLAND

UVULA

STYLOPHARYNGEUS

SUPERIOR
PHARYNGEAL
CONSTRICTOR

STYLOGLOSSUS

STYLOID PROCESS

DIGASTRIC

STYLOHYOID

MASTOID PROCESS

Figure 37.1   Cross-sectional/transverse diagram showing relationships of the parotid gland.

important branches of the facial nerve are the zygomatic and marginal mandibular branches, injury to which leads to considerable functional and cosmetic problems. The facial nerve and its branches arbitrarily define the superficial and deep lobes and of the parotid gland; however, it should be stressed that there is no histological demarcation between these two 'lobes' (**Figure 37.2**).

The facial nerve exits the skull base at the stylomastoid foramen. Several landmarks may help the surgeon identify the nerve at this point, prior to tracing its course through the gland. The posterior belly of the digastric arises from the digastric ridge just below the stylomastoid foramen, and at the same depth, and is probably the most useful landmark. The surgeon can safely deepen the plane of dissection until the level of the digastric muscle is reached, before looking for the nerve just superior to the muscle's upper border. The tragal pointer is a deep cartilaginous landmark which is 1 cm superior to and 1 cm superficial to the nerve. The tympanomastoid suture line is easily palpable as a hard ridge deep to the cartilaginous portion of the external auditory canal. The facial nerve emerges a few millimeters deep to its outer edge. The styloid process lies deep to the nerve and so should not be used as a landmark. It should be noted that tumours of the parotid gland may displace the facial nerve inwards, outwards, superiorly, or inferiorly, depending on their location (**Figure 37.3**).

The greater auricular nerve courses superiorly over from the posterior border of the sternomastoid muscle towards the parotid gland. It is usually necessary to sacrifice this nerve when performing parotid surgery, leading to sensory deficit which is most noticeable over the earlobe. The posterior branch of the greater auricular nerve, which supplies the earlobe, may occasionally be preserved.

The tissues superficial to the parotid gland include skin, subcutaneous tissue and the greater auricular nerve. Occasional lymph nodes are also present. Lymph nodes are

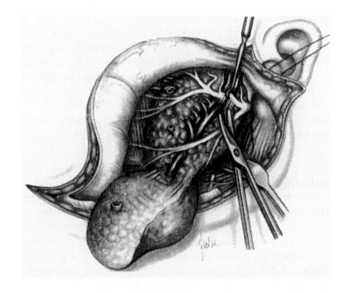

Figure 37.2   Diagram with superficial lobe of parotid gland removed, showing division of facial nerve into terminal branches.

also found deep to the parotid fascia within the parotid parenchyma.

The retromandibular vein traverses the parotid gland deep to the facial nerve branches. It is frequently encountered in the inferior part of the gland, where, classically, the marginal mandibular and cervical branches cross directly over it. The terminal branches of the external carotid artery are deep to the retromandibular vein and are much less commonly encountered.

The deep lobe of the parotid gland extends medial to the level of the ramus of the mandible. The presence of the mandibular ramus constricts the gland at this point. Deep

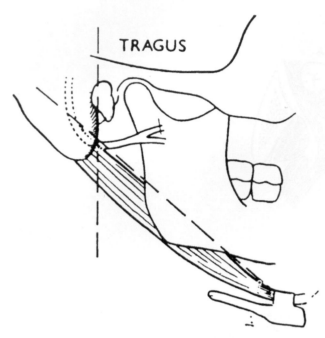

Figure 37.3 Location of main trunk of the facial nerve having traced the posterior belly of digastric backward.

to the deep lobe, minor salivary glands are present in the parapharyngeal space.

The parotid duct (Stenson's duct) extends forward from the superficial part of the parotid gland, superficial to the masseter muscle, a fingerbreadth inferior to the zygomatic arch. At the anterior border of the masseter muscle, it pierces the buccal fat pad and the buccinator muscle. It then courses between the buccinator and buccal mucosa before opening opposite the upper second molar tooth. The intraoral course provides a valve-like mechanism preventing reflux.

Submandibular/sublingual glands

The submandibular glands are paired structures situated medial to the posterior part of the body of the mandible. Each gland is composed of a large superficial and small deep part, which are continuous posteriorly around the posterior border of the mylohyoid muscle. The posterior belly of the digastric lies posterior to the gland. The facial artery enters the submandibular triangle deep to the posterior belly of the digastric, is related to the posterior and then superior surfaces of the gland, before emerging at the lower border of the mandible at the anterior border of the masseter.

Superficial to the submandibular gland is skin, subcutaneous tissue, platysma muscle and submandibular fascia (derived from the investing layer of cervical fascia). The facial vein courses superficial to the gland and digastric muscle on its way from the face to the internal jugular vein. The marginal mandibular and cervical branches of the facial nerve lie superficial to the submandibular fascia overlying the gland, also crossing superficial to the facial vein. The marginal mandibular nerve curves superiorly and crosses the lower border of the mandible close to the facial artery and the supramandibular lymph node. In order to avoid injury to the branches of the facial nerve, the submandibular fascia

should be incised at the lower border of the gland, and dissection should proceed right on the gland, deep to the fascia.

The deep portion of the gland lies on the hyoglossus muscle. The lingual nerve passes anteriorly superior to the gland. The submandibular ganglion is connected to the lingual nerve and is related to the superior surface of the gland. Blood vessels are present between the gland and ganglion which require division during submandibular gland removal. The hypoglossal nerve, which is inferior to the deep portion of the gland, is usually not encountered during simple submandibular gland surgery. The submandibular duct (Wharton's duct) extends forward from the deep portion of the gland, and courses beneath the floor of the mouth between the sublingual glands laterally, and the genioglossus muscle medially, to open at the submandibular papilla just lateral to the frenulum of the tongue. The sublingual glands are situated just beneath the floor of the mouth, closely related to the submandibular duct. The lingual nerve winds around the submandibular duct, lying first on its lateral, then inferior, then medial surfaces. The lingual nerve supplies somatic sensation to the anterior two-thirds of the tongue. In addition, this nerve supplies secretomotor fibres to the submandibular and sublingual glands, as well as taste sensation from the tongue. The secretomotor and special sensory fibres derive from the facial nerve, and reach the lingual nerve via the chorda tympani nerve.

Minor salivary glands, numbering approximately 600–800 in any individual, are spread throughout the upper aerodigestive tract. The greatest concentration is in the hard palate.

SURGICAL PATHOLOGY

Salivary gland tumours are relatively rare, with an overall incidence of between 2.5 and 3.0 per 100 000 per year. About 80 per cent are benign. Salivary malignancies account for around 5 per cent of malignancies of the head and neck.[1, 2]

Salivary tumours present a significant pathological challenge. The reasons for this are as follows: (1) the present classification includes a large number of different types of tumours, with the latest World Health Organization (WHO) classification including over 40 types; (2) many types of salivary tumours are characterized by marked morphological diversity, and thus can have overlapping morphological features, making these tumours very prone to diagnostic confusion; (3) salivary tumours are rare, with some of the subtypes extremely rare, so that most pathologists are likely to have limited experience with the rarer types; (4) rapid changes in nomenclature and classification of the various pathologies have occurred in recent years. Reclassification of tumours according to updated classifications may change the diagnosis in nearly one in three cases.[3]

Approximately 70–90 per cent of salivary tumours are located in the parotid gland.[1, 2, 4, 5] The vast majority (85 per cent) of these are benign.[1] Pleomorphic adenoma comprises 60–80 per cent of parotid neoplasms. Warthin's tumour (adenolymphoma) is the next most common benign lesion. The most common malignant parotid tumour is mucoepidermoid carcinoma (21–26 per cent), followed by carcinoma ex pleomorphic adenoma (5–18 per cent) and acinic cell carcinoma (9–24 per cent), and adenocarcinoma not otherwise specified (NOS) (11–15 per cent).[6, 7, 8] Adenoid cystic carcinoma and polymorphous low-grade adenocarcinoma are rare in the parotid gland. Of note, the parotid gland is a common site for metastases from squamous cell carcinomas and malignant melanomas arising in the skin of the head and neck, particularly from the region of the temple. In Australia, such metastases typically outnumber primary parotid cancers.[7]

Submandibular gland tumours are much less common than parotid tumours (4–11 per cent of total).[1, 2, 5] Roughly half are benign pleomorphic adenomas. Most of the remainder are malignant.[1] Adenoid cystic carcinoma is the most common malignancy. Carcinoma ex pleomorphic adenoma, mucoepidermoid carcinoma, non-Hodgkin's lymphoma and squamous cell carcinoma are also reported.[1, 9]

Just over half (56–58 per cent) of intraoral salivary tumours are benign, most of these being pleomorphic adenomas (59–71 per cent).[1, 10, 11, 12, 13] Canalicular adenoma is the next most common benign tumour.[10, 13] The most common malignant tumours are mucoepidermoid carcinoma (47–52 per cent), followed by adenoid cystic carcinoma (14–23 per cent) and polymorphous low-grade adenocarcinoma (12–19 per cent).[10, 13] The most common site for intraoral minor salivary tumours is the palate (33 per cent),[11, 12, 13] followed by the upper lip (20 per cent) and buccal mucosa (17 per cent).[11] Most neoplasms of the upper lip are benign; in contrast, those on the lower lip, floor of mouth, lower gingiva, retromolar area and tongue are more likely to be malignant.[1, 10, 11, 13] Minor salivary tumours are more common in females,[10, 11, 12] except for adenoid cystic carcinoma, which has an equal sex predilection.[10, 13]

Tumours of the sublingual gland are rare. Most are malignant with adenoid cystic carcinoma being the most commonly reported.[1, 14]

BENIGN TUMOURS

Pleomorphic adenoma

Pleomorphic adenoma is by far the most common salivary tumour. It occurs in patients of all ages, with the highest incidence reported in the fourth to fifth decades. Both sexes are affected equally. Of those arising in the parotid gland, 80 per cent are located in the superficial lobe in the tail of the gland; however they are also seen in the deep lobe, the pre-auricular area, and anteriorly over the masseter muscle.

Histologically, the tumour is characterized by marked morphological diversity, with glandular areas, myxomatous areas, and solid areas seen. Seifert et al.[15] classified these tumours into cellular types (27–35 per cent), myxoid (stroma-rich) type (35–51 per cent) and the classic type (14–37 per cent), where there is a balanced amount of epithelial and myoepithelial cells and stroma component.[16, 17] A capsule is usually present around the tumour, however, this capsule is usually focally thin or absent, particularly with the myxoid subtype[16, 17, 18] and with larger tumours.[18] In 24–28 per cent of cases, projections of tumour through dehiscences in the capsule are present which are in continuity with the main tumour.[16, 17, 19, 20] It is because of these projections that the recurrence rate after enucleation (21–45 per cent over 30

years[21, 22, 23, 24, 25, 26]) is so high.[20, 27] On the other hand, when the tumour removal includes a cuff of surrounding parotid tissue, recurrence rates are typically less than 2 per cent.[5, 28, 29, 30] Incomplete capsules with tumour cells immediately next to the mucosa are also reported in intraoral pleomorphic adenomas, suggesting that the overlying mucosa should always be removed during complete excision of these tumours.[13]

Parotid pleomorphic adenomas usually present as slow-growing, painless tumours. Facial nerve palsy is never seen in benign cases. However, left untreated, up to 5 per cent may become malignant (carcinoma ex pleomorphic adenomas, also known as malignant mixed tumour). For this reason, surgical excision is always to be advised.

Warthin's tumour (adenolymphoma)

Warthin's tumour (adenolymphoma) is the second most common benign parotid tumour. It occurs almost exclusively in the tail of the parotid gland. Multifocal (20–23 per cent) or bilateral (6–10 per cent) tumours are often seen.[31, 32] It is far more common in males than females (M:F ratio, 7:1), with an average age at presentation of 70 years. It is reported to be more common in smokers.[33]

Histologically, it is composed of tall columnar epithelium with glands and papillae with a stroma of abundant lymphoid tissue with germinal centres. Cysts containing mucoid fluid are typically present.

Warthin's tumours are generally slow-growing, however, the abundant lymphoid tissue in these tumours is susceptible to acute inflammation. Such inflammation may be precipitated by an upper respiratory infection. This may lead to marked swelling, tenderness and even ulceration of the tumour(s). On palpation, they generally have a soft or fluctuant consistency, but may also be firm depending on the extent of previous inflammation. The presence of multilobulated or multifocal tumours on palpation or imaging is suggestive of Warthin's tumour.

The usual treatment of Warthin's tumours is simple excision via partial superficial parotidectomy.[31] Unlike pleomorphic adenoma, Warthin's tumours do not have any premalignant potential. Thus, in elderly males with significant medical comorbidities presenting with parotid lumps, with a cytological diagnosis of Warthin's tumour on fine needle aspiration, observation alone is reasonable management.

Other benign tumours

Oncocytomas are benign tumours composed of large eosinophilic cells with mitochondria. They are usually found in the superficial lobe of the parotid gland. Males and females are equally affected with most patients aged over 50 years.

Monomorphic adenoma is a term which was used in the past to lump all apparently benign lesions which were morphologically homogenous, but that did not meet the criteria for pleomorphic adenoma. These lesions are now reclassified into such entities as canalicular adenoma, basal cell adenoma and myoepithelioma.[3] The term 'monomorphic adenoma' is not used in the most recent WHO classification.

MALIGNANT TUMOURS

Mucoepidermoid carcinoma

Mucoepidermoid carcinoma is the most common salivary malignancy in most series, accounting for roughly 45 per cent of cases. Between 50 and 70 per cent arise in the parotid gland, 15–35 per cent in oral cavity minor salivary glands and 6–11 per cent in the submandibular glands.[34] Patients of all ages and both sexes are affected. Mucoepidermoid carcinomas account for the vast majority of salivary carcinomas in children.[35, 36]

Histologically, the tumour is composed of three cell types: epidermoid cells, mucous cells and intermediate cells. Mucus secreted by the mucous cells accounts for the tumour's partly cystic structure. On the basis of the histological features, these tumours may be divided into high, intermediate and low grade. This grading is based loosely on the prevalence of cell types and cystic areas, and on features of aggressiveness or cytological atypia, but has mostly been subjective.[4, 37] Recently, numerical scoring systems have been devised in an effort to make the grading more objective, however, these schemes are still prone to interobserver error. There is good evidence that grading of mucoepidermoid carcinoma does have prognostic significance. Brandwein et al.[38] reported that low-grade tumours never metastasized, and that 100 per cent of patients were disease-free at ten years, compared to 70 per cent of patients with intermediate-grade, and less than 40 per cent of patients with high-grade tumours. Other series have reported metastasis and death to occur in a higher proportion of patients with low-grade tumours;[37] it is possible that much of this variance is due to differences in the criteria used to grade the tumours. On the other hand, Spiro et al.[39, 40] believed tumour stage to be a much better indicator of prognosis than grade. Other authors also report tumour size and stage to be an important prognostic factor.[37, 38, 41] At ten years, over 90 per cent of patients with stage I and II disease are tumour-free, compared to less than 30 per cent with stage III or IV disease.[38]

Mucoepidermoid carcinoma generally has an indolent natural history, however, high-grade tumours may grow rapidly and give rise to pain and local symptoms. It shows a propensity to metastasize to regional lymph nodes; this occurs in 30–50 per cent of patients with high-grade tumours.

Adenoid cystic carcinoma

Adenoid cystic carcinoma comprises around 30 per cent of salivary malignancies. Most (60 per cent) arise in minor salivary glands. Between 25 and 33 per cent arise in the parotid gland, however, it comprises a small proportion of parotid gland neoplasms.[42, 43, 44]

Three histological patterns of adenoid cystic carcinoma are recognized: (1) cribriform, or Swiss-cheese pattern, which is the most common; (2) tubular, the next most common; and (3) solid, which occurs in around 21 per cent of cases, and has the worst prognosis. Histological grading of adenoid cystic carcinoma has some prognostic value,[43] however, the significance of this has been contested.[45, 46] On the other hand, Spiro and others have shown clinical stage to be the most important prognostic factor.[43, 46, 47]

Adenoid cystic carcinoma generally presents as a slow-growing mass. This tumour has a marked propensity for neural invasion, which occurs in up to 50 per cent of cases.[44] Thus, symptoms of pain and facial palsy are common. Skip metastases may be seen along nerves. The presence of facial palsy or perineural invasion of large (named) nerves is a well-established adverse prognostic factor.[44, 48, 49, 50] Adenoid cystic carcinoma also has a propensity for spread along Haversian canals of bone, often with little apparent bony erosion. Lymph node metastases are rare.[43] Local recurrences are common (30–50 per cent of cases), even after clear surgical margins and many years of disease-free status. Distant metastases occur in around 24–39 per cent of patients within ten years, with the lung being the most common site.[43, 44, 49]

The usual treatment for adenoid cystic carcinoma is surgery with postoperative radiotherapy. This cancer has a very indolent natural history, and patients may survive with disease for many years, however, they are rarely cured. The five-year survival rate is around 72 per cent, with 15-year survival rate around 34 per cent. Even with pulmonary metastases, patients may live up to five years and even longer.[43]

Carcinoma ex pleomorphic adenoma (malignant mixed tumour)

Carcinoma ex pleomorphic adenoma, or malignant mixed tumour, is the second most common parotid malignancy. The risk of developing carcinoma ex pleomorphic adenoma is estimated at around 5–6 per cent over 20 years. Patients are typically 10–20 years older than those with benign pleomorphic adenoma.[51] Tumours are typically larger and of longer duration than their benign counterparts.[51, 52] Pain and facial nerve paresis may also be present.[53] It is an aggressive cancer.[53] Currently it is generally recognized that there is a progression of benign to malignant change in pleomorphic adenoma, however, to date, no histological features have been identified which are predictive of malignant transformation. The risk of malignant transformation would appear to be higher in tumours of the submandibular gland compared to the parotid gland.[51, 52]

Three variants are recognized:

1. Carcinoma in pleomorphic adenoma. This is the most common form. The malignant component is usually either a salivary duct carcinoma or adenocarcinoma, and the metastases contain only carcinoma.
2. True malignant mixed tumour (carcinosarcoma), in which the malignant components are both carcinoma and sarcoma, and the metastases contain both elements.
3. Metastasizing pleomorphic adenoma. The rarest variety, in which both the primary tumour and metastases consist only of structures typical of benign pleomorphic adenoma.

It has been suggested that the number of carcinoma ex pleomorphic adenomas encountered depends to a large extent on the diligence of the pathologist in searching for areas of residual pleomorphic adenoma in parotid cancers.

By the time of surgical removal, the carcinoma typically makes up more than half of the tumour mass.[53] The malignant component most commonly consists of adenocarcinoma NOS or salivary duct carcinoma. Epithelial-myoepithelial carcinoma, adenoid cystic carcinoma, adenosquamous carcinoma and undifferentiated carcinoma have also been reported.[53] The pathology is usually high grade.[53] Cervical metastases are common.[53, 54] The depth of invasion beyond the mixed tumour capsule is a valuable guide to prognosis.[53] Intracapsular and minimally invasive (<5–8 mm) tumours generally do well.[53, 54, 55] More invasive tumours have a poor prognosis, with high rates of local recurrence, distant metastases and death. Other adverse prognostic factors are large size, local extension, presence of cervical metastases, origin from major (as opposed to minor) salivary gland, high grade and carcinoma making up more than half of the tumour mass.[53, 56]

It has been suggested that pleomorphic adenoma recurrence and the use of postoperative radiotherapy to treat tumour spillage may be factors in malignant transformation, however, there is little evidence to support these notions.

Acinic cell carcinoma

Acinic cell carcinoma is the third most common cancer of the parotid gland. The vast majority arise in the parotid gland.[44, 57, 58] It is a slow-growing tumour, with a propensity for local recurrence and distant metastases, which may occur after many years of apparent disease-free survival. Like adenoid cystic carcinoma, patients may have prolonged survival even after the diagnosis of distant metastases.[44] Lymph node metastases are uncommon. Five- and 15-year survival rates of 76–96 and 50–55 per cent have been reported.[57, 59] Rarely, the tumour may be multifocal or bilateral.

Polymorphous low–grade adenocarcinoma

This is a more recently described entity which is increasingly recognized. Recent reports suggest that in fact it is more common than adenoid cystic carcinoma, and is the third most common salivary neoplasm after pleomorphic adenoma and mucoepidermoid carcinoma. It is almost predominantly a tumour of minor salivary glands, with 60 per cent arising on the palate, 20 per cent in the cheek, and 12 per cent in the upper lip. It is rare in the parotid gland.

Histologically, polymorphous low-grade adenocarcinoma shows marked morphological diversity, but a striking cytological uniformity and bland nuclear morphology. It is thus easily confused with pleomorphic adenoma or adenoid cystic carcinoma on small biopsies. Examination of the entire tumour shows the characteristic infiltrative growth pattern. Like adenoid cystic carcinoma, it has a propensity for perineural invasion. Most cases show an indolent natural course.

Although polymorphous low-grade carcinoma has traditionally been considered to be a low-grade tumour, it does not always behave in a low-grade fashion. In fact, this tumour would appear to have a very unpredictable behaviour, with up to 15 per cent of patients reported to develop cervical metastases and 12.5 per cent dying from disease. Local recurrences may develop as late as 15 years after treatment of the primary site with negative pathological margins.[60]

Salivary ductal carcinoma

Salivary ductal carcinoma is an aggressive malignancy which is believed to arise from the excretory duct. It most frequently arises in the parotid gland. Neural invasion and extraglandular extension are commonly seen. Most patients die within three years.

Epithelial–myoepithelial carcinoma

This a rare tumour composed of both epithelial and myoepithelial cells. It is found predominantly in the parotid (77 per cent) and submandibular (10 per cent) glands. It is generally considered to be a low-grade neoplasm, however, aggressive and lethal cases have been reported.[61]

Basal cell adenocarcinoma

This is a low-grade malignancy which is usually found in the parotid gland. It is generally considered to be low-grade with a good prognosis.

Papillary cystadenocarcinoma

This is a low-grade malignancy which may occur in either major (65 per cent) or minor (35 per cent) salivary glands. It has an indolent behaviour.[62]

Adenocarcinoma NOS

The term 'adenocarcinoma NOS' is used to encompass a variety of neoplasms recognized as being of salivary origin, but lacking sufficient histological features to place them into any of the named subcategories. Thus it represents a heterogenous group of tumours. The relative frequency of adenocarcinoma NOS varies between different series. They are generally considered to be aggressive tumours with a propensity for perineural invasion[44] and lymph node metastases.[44, 63, 64]

Squamous cell carcinoma

Most squamous cell carcinomas to the parotid are metastases from skin squamous cell carcinomas. Occasionally, no primary site may be found. It is unknown whether or not such cases represent true primary parotid squamous carcinomas. Concomitant cervical nodal disease and cervical nodal conversion are common, thus surgical therapy should always include a neck dissection, even in clinically N0 necks.[65]

Lymphoma

Non-Hodgkin's lymphomas may develop in intraparotid lymph nodes. The risk of lymphoma is increased in patients with Sjogren's syndrome. On fine needle aspiration cytology, parotid lymphomas are frequently confused with Warthin's tumour or benign reactive intraparotid lymph nodes. Flow cytometry immunophenotyping may be useful in distinguishing these lesions. In many cases, open or core biopsy is necessary to arrive at the correct diagnosis. Rarely, high-grade lymphomas may masquerade as parotid abscesses. Diagnosis in these cases can be extremely difficult due to the abundance of necrotic tissue and paucity of representative tumour cells.

STAGING

The T-staging for parotid carcinomas is given in **Table 37.1**.[66] The N-staging and stage grouping are identical to that for the larynx.

HISTORY AND EXAMINATION

The usual presentation of a parotid tumour is a painless mass within the parotid gland. Tumours in the tail of the parotid may appear quite low in the neck, particularly in older patients, and so may easily be confused with enlarged upper deep cervical lymph nodes. Benign tumours are usually slow-growing and so have a long history, however, rapid enlargement and even ulceration may occur in Warthin's tumours secondary to acute inflammation of the lymphoid tissue. Pain is unusual in benign tumours and usually indicates an acute inflammatory pathology or a malignant tumour.

Parotid swellings usually have limited mobility because of the dense fascia surrounding the gland, however, tumours low down in the tail of the parotid may be reasonably mobile. On the other hand, marked immobility suggests location in the deep lobe.

The overlying skin should be examined to rule out cellulitis (suggestive of an acute inflammatory process) or skin fixation (suggestive of malignancy). In addition, careful attention should be paid to the remainder of the parotid gland, as well as the contralateral parotid gland to rule out multiple or bilateral lesions. Bilateral parotid swellings most commonly occur in patients with Warthin's tumours, HIV-related lymphoepithelial cysts, Sjogren's syndrome or sarcoidosis. The remainder of the neck should be checked for lymphadenopathy. Examination of all five main branches

Table 37.1   T-staging of parotid carcinomas.[66]

Stage	
T1	Tumour 2 cm or less in greatest dimension with no extraparenchymal extension
T2	Tumour more than 2 cm, but no more than 4 cm in greatest dimension with no extraparenchymal extension
T3	Tumour more than 4 cm or having extraparenchymal extension
T4a	Tumour invades skin, mandible, ear canal and/or facial nerve
T4b	Tumour invades skull base, pterygoid plates and/or carotid artery

of the facial nerve is an integral part of the examination and should be performed in all cases. In addition, intraoral examination should be performed to check for swelling of the parapharyngeal space (usually manifest by medial deviation of the tonsil or a bulge in the lateral wall of the oropharynx) or any abnormality in the region of Stenson's duct (situated opposite the upper second molar). Of note, deep lobe parotid tumours may be completely asymptomatic and be an incidental finding on routine head and neck examination or imaging.

There are certain features that are highly suggestive of malignancy and so should be checked for in every patient with a parotid swelling. These are pain, rapid growth, facial palsy, skin fixation and cervical lymphadenopathy.

Occasionally, parotid tumours may present with facial weakness without any noticeable parotid swelling. It should be remembered that facial weakness which is insidious in onset, recurrent, associated with twitching or synkinesis, or isolated to only some branches of the facial nerve, is usually a sign of malignancy, and should prompt imaging of the parotid gland.

INVESTIGATIONS

Imaging

The use of routine imaging in the investigation of parotid lumps is controversial. In cases of small, mobile, well-circumscribed lumps within the tail of the parotid, it can be argued that imaging is unlikely to add any further information that will influence management. Imaging is obviously more useful in patients with fat necks where examination of the parotid is difficult. Imaging can help confirm that the lump is definitely located within the parotid gland. In addition, by demonstrating the relationship between the lump and the retromandibular vein, it can help determine whether the lump is located in the superficial or deep lobe. Imaging is definitely helpful in large tumours or with suspected malignancy, for better evaluation of the tumour's third dimension and relationship to the surrounding structures. Imaging may also detect other features suggestive of malignancy (e.g. central necrosis, infiltration of adjacent structures), as well as the presence of suspicious cervical lymphadenopathy. Imaging is also important in cases of deep lobe tumours.

Both computed tomography (CT) and magnetic resonance imaging (MRI) (**Figure 37.4**) may be used. MRI affords better definition between the tumour and surrounding parotid tissue.[67]

Fine needle aspiration cytology

Fine needle aspiration of parotid masses is a commonly performed procedure. It has been shown to be safe and does not cause tumour spread along the needle tract. However, cytological diagnosis of salivary aspirates is far from straightforward. The reasons for this are as follows: (1) There is an enormous number and diversity of salivary tumours. (2) Most salivary tumours are uncommon, thus most pathologists will have limited experience with the rarer types.

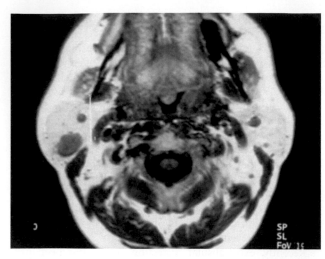

Figure 37.4 Magnetic resonance image of parotid tumour.

(3) Many of the salivary tumours display marked morphological diversity, and many very distinct tumours show overlapping morphological features. (4) Many salivary carcinomas are cytologically bland with little evidence of mitotic activity or cellular pleomorphism. Tumour invasion as a defining feature of malignancy is beyond the recognition of cytology. Because of this, distinguishing between different parotid tumours, including the distinction between benign and malignant, can be very difficult. In particular, such disparate tumours as pleomorphic adenoma, adenoid cystic carcinoma and polymorphous low-grade adenocarcinoma may display such markedly variable and similar features that differentiation in some cases may be near impossible.[68]

Proponents of fine needle aspiration cytology argue that it has a high accuracy rate (80–98 per cent). However, it should be borne in mind that reports of the accuracy of parotid aspirates may be misleading. This is because most parotid lumps are pleomorphic adenomas; hence, as long as most aspirates are reported as being consistent with this diagnosis, then the specificity and sensitivity for the diagnosis of pleomorphic adenoma is always going to be quite high. On the other hand, fine needle aspiration cytology may fail to diagnose a sizeable proportion of malignancies.[69, 70] A review of data from the College of American Pathologists Interlaboratory Comparison Program reported 32 per cent of malignant salivary lesions to be falsely reported as benign. The highest false-negative rates were for lymphoma (57 per cent), acinic cell carcinoma (49 per cent), low-grade mucoepidermoid carcinoma (43 per cent) and adenoid cystic carcinoma (33 per cent). For benign lesions, the 'true negative' rate (i.e. the proportion of cases correctly diagnosed as benign) was 91 per cent.[71]

A common scenario in practice is an aspirate being reported as consistent with pleomorphic adenoma, but 'suspicious' and/or not able to rule out adenoid cystic carcinoma or other malignancy. In reality, most of these cases will transpire to be pleomorphic adenomas, so this type of report does not necessarily help the surgeon greatly.

A further argument against the use of fine needle aspiration cytology is that, in the vast majority of cases, parotid lumps will require surgical excision, and fine needle aspiration will not change that management. Certainly, surgical excision should be recommended in all cases of malignant parotid tumours, as well as in pleomorphic adenomas, given the risk of carcinoma ex pleomorphic adenoma in untreated cases. However, there are exceptions to the above dictum. In elderly males, who have multiple medical problems and so are not good candidates for general anaesthesia, a cytological diagnosis of Warthin's tumour may obviate the need for surgery, as this pathology does not have any premalignant potential. Cytology may also obviate the need for surgery in granulomatous disorders. In clinically indeterminate salivary lesions, cytology may help in distinguishing between salivary and non-salivary pathology. Finally, a cytological report which is highly suggestive of malignancy may allow the patient to be counselled preoperatively on the possibility of sacrifice of a branch of the facial nerve.

It is important for the surgeon to be aware of the most commonly confused diagnoses. The confusion between pleomorphic adenoma, adenoid cystic carcinoma and polymorphous low-grade adenocarcinoma is well recognized.[71] In addition, Warthin's tumours, lymphomas and benign or reactive intraparotid lymph nodes are frequently confused because of the abundant lymphoid stroma.[71] Inflammatory and cystic conditions like chronic sialadenitis with squamous metaplasia, lymphoepithelial cysts and low-grade mucoepidermoid carcinoma may be difficult to distinguish cytologically. Acinic cell carcinoma, oncocytoma and Warthin's tumour may be easily confused with normal parotid tissue.[71]

Open biopsy

As a general rule, open incisional biopsy of parotid lesions should be avoided, due to the risk of causing tumour implantation, particularly if the lesion is a pleomorphic adenoma, which is what the vast majority of parotid tumours will turn out to be. If fine needle aspiration cytology fails to yield a diagnosis, then the surgeon should proceed to superficial parotidectomy with *in toto* removal of the tumour. On the other hand, open biopsy may be appropriate in very superficial tumours, where fine needle aspiration cytology suggests lymphoma, in order to obtain more tissue to rule out a reactive process, and for classification of the lymphoma type; or in the case of extensive tumours where cytology clearly shows malignancy. In such cases, biopsy may allow the tumour to be categorized, a metastatic process to be ruled out, and definitive treatment to be planned. In cases of diffuse salivary enlargement, incisional biopsy may be appropriate to diagnose Sjogren's syndrome, sarcoidosis, or other granulomatous disorder, and to rule out lymphoma or other malignant process.

Incisional biopsy is the usual initial diagnostic procedure of choice in minor salivary gland tumours located on the palate. However, the surgeon should be aware that, similar to the case with fine needle aspiration cytology, differentiation between the three most common lesions (pleomorphic adenoma, adenoid cystic carcinoma and polymorphous low-grade adenocarcinoma) can be very difficult on the basis of small biopsies.

Intraoperative frozen section

Intraoperative frozen section for salivary cancers as a diagnostic procedure is prone to the same difficulties as that encountered in fine needle aspiration cytology, on account of the small sample size submitted to the pathologist. Studies have shown a similar overall accuracy for FNA and frozen section,[72] however, it would appear that sensitivity of frozen section for malignancy (69–77 per cent) is slightly lower than that of FNA, while specificity (96–100 per cent)[72, 73, 74] is higher. Frozen section is useful in determining the extent of tumour spread, including the presence and extent of invasion of the facial nerve, and the assessment of surgical margins. Frozen section as a diagnostic procedure may be useful when preoperative FNA is non-diagnostic, or when the FNA diagnosis is at odds with the clinical and/or intraoperative findings. The results of frozen section may help in intraoperative decision-making. In cases where frozen section shows high-grade carcinoma, the surgeon may proceed to perform at least a limited neck dissection with the parotidectomy. It may also be helpful in deciding whether or not to proceed with facial nerve sacrifice in case of the unexpected finding of a tumour clinically infiltrating the facial nerve, as well as the extent of resection of other involved structures, e.g. skin or temporomandibular joint.

TREATMENT POLICY

Pleomorphic adenoma

The vast majority of parotid tumours are pleomorphic adenomas, and the bulk of these are located in the superficial lobe of the gland. Simple enucleation of pleomorphic adenomas is not appropriate treatment as this leads to recurrence in 21–45 per cent of cases.[21, 22, 23, 24, 25, 26] These recurrences occur because of projections of tumour through dehiscences in the tumour capsule which are sheared off and left behind when simple enucleation is performed.[16, 17, 19, 20]

Because of the high recurrence rates for simple enucleation, the traditional treatment for these tumours has been superficial parotidectomy, with removal of all the parotid gland superficial to the facial nerve. More recently, partial superficial parotidectomy, with dissection of less than the full facial nerve, but with removal of a generous cuff all around the tumour, except where the tumour abuts the facial nerve, has become standard of care. Initially, a 2 cm margin was considered the minimum allowable for partial surgery. More recently, a 1 cm margin has been shown to be adequate.[75] With the use of these techniques, when negative pathological margins are obtained, then recurrences should occur in less than 1 per cent of cases.[30, 76, 77, 78]

A common intraoperative finding with pleomorphic adenomas is that the deep surface of the tumour capsule directly abuts the branches of the facial nerve. Thus, in many cases, it is not possible to take a cuff of parotid tissue all around; rather, the surgeon has to dissect right on the tumour capsule in the vicinity of these branches. Thus, focal capsular exposure occurs in the vast majority of parotid operations, regardless of the technique used.[17, 27, 79] However, this practice does not appear to lead to any increased risk of recurrence.[80] Furthermore, in most cases of pleomorphic adenomas located in the deep lobe of the parotid gland, or in the parapharyngeal space, the operation performed to

remove them is little better than enucleation. However, again this does not appear to increase the likelihood of recurrence. The reasons for the low recurrence rate despite the high incidences of capsule exposure are unclear. Suggested reasons include: more meticulous surgical technique which prevents separation of pseudopodia[27] and the presence of pseudopodia predominantly on the superficial surface of the parotid gland.[81] In the case of deep lobe tumours, it has been suggested that they have a more complete capsule and less tumour projections through the capsule.[82, 83] Of note, it has been found that although a significant incidence of recurrences is seen when tumour is present histologically at the margin of excision (17.6 per cent), recurrences are rare (<2 per cent) in the case of close (<1 mm) margins. These findings suggest that a margin of a fraction of a millimetre is adequate to prevent recurrence.[78]

Recently, extracapsular dissection (ECD) has been proposed as a surgical treatment for pleomorphic adenoma. In this technique, a small cuff of normal parotid parenchyma just outside the tumour capsule is dissected. Careful attention is paid to the lobulations of the tumour and their relationship to the branches of the facial nerve. This is a technically demanding procedure which requires the tumour to be mobile and large enough to allow digital manipulation. The incidence of capsular exposure and positive margins is reported to be no different between ECD and superficial parotidectomy.[27, 78] Proponents of ECD have claimed reduced complication rates, particularly facial nerve neuropraxia and Frey's syndrome, with no increase in recurrence.[84, 85] On the other hand, others have reported this technique to be associated with an unacceptably high incidence of tumour spillage and tumour recurrence, despite short follow up and the use of postoperative radiotherapy in selected cases.[86]

Tumour spillage

Capsular rupture and tumour spillage has been associated with a two- to three-fold increased recurrence rate for pleomorphic adenoma,[27, 79, 87] however, other authors have disputed this.[20, 80] In any case, great care should be taken intraoperatively not to penetrate the tumour and cause tumour spillage. Cutting into the tumour should be absolutely avoided. In cases where inadvertent tumour spillage does occur, the most appropriate treatment is probably to remove as much parotid tissue as possible without jeopardizing the branches of the facial nerve. At the conclusion of the case, the wound should be meticulously washed out. The use of postoperative radiotherapy in such cases has been advocated, however, there is no evidence that this is either necessary or beneficial.[20, 80]

Recurrent pleomorphic adenoma

Recurrent pleomorphic adenoma is a difficult surgical challenge. Most patients (55–100 per cent) present with a multiplicity of nodules in the surgical bed,[88, 89, 90, 91] which are slow growing and often underestimated by palpation. The typical time lag after the initial surgery is between 5 and 12 years, but may be much longer.[20, 78, 80, 91, 92] Facial paresis may be due to previous surgery or scarring of the nerve, however, the possibility of carcinoma ex pleomorphic adenoma should always be considered in patients with new-onset facial weakness. Carcinoma has been reported in 6–17 per cent of such cases.[93, 94]

Revision surgery is difficult because of scarring and the multiplicity of nodules, the distorted anatomy, and the more superficial location of the facial nerve branches. In addition, tumour frequently involves the old scar, the facial subcutaneous tissues, the external auditory canal and middle ear, and may encase or involve the facial nerve.[90, 91]

In most cases, the treatment of recurrent pleomorphic adenoma is total parotidectomy with scar excision and preservation of the branches of facial nerve. It may be impossible to identify the main trunk of the facial nerve. In such cases, identification of the branches of the facial nerve in the neck and face with retrograde dissection may be necessary. Patients should be counselled regarding the significantly increased risk of transient or permanent facial weakness postoperatively. In cases with facial nerve involvement, frozen sections should be sent to check for carcinoma ex pleomorphic adenoma, and consideration should be given to nerve resection with or without nerve grafting.[90, 91]

An alternative approach in cases with multifocal recurrence, multiple previous recurrences and where there is little remaining normal parotid tissue is conservative 'cosmetic' enucleation, however, this is likely to lead to an increased recurrence rate.[90]

The incidence of re-recurrence after reoperation for recurrent pleomorphic adenoma varies from 8 to 52 per cent,[88, 90, 91, 93, 95] but is much higher (32–52 per cent) in studies with longer periods of follow up.[90, 93] The risk of re-recurrence has been suggested to be higher in cases of multinodular recurrence[95] and lower in cases where the initial surgery was an enucleation (as opposed to a formal parotidectomy),[88, 93] where the revision surgery is a total parotidectomy (as opposed to subtotal parotidectomy)[91] and after facial nerve resection.[91] The use of postoperative radiotherapy to decrease the probability of further recurrence has been suggested,[88, 92, 95] however, there is little strong evidence that this has any major impact on recurrence or the probability of later malignant change. Of note is that even in cases where the facial nerve is successfully preserved, a significant proportion of patients are likely to have long-term weakness.[90, 91, 93, 95]

Malignancies

The mainstay of treatment for salivary carcinomas is surgical resection with or without postoperative radiotherapy. In the case of parotid malignancies, every effort should be made to preserve the facial nerve, particularly in cases where it is functioning preoperatively. In most cases, it is possible to find a plane of cleavage between the nerve and the tumour.

The goal of surgical treatment is to achieve local control. For early stage cancers, this usually equates to cure. On the other hand, a significant proportion of patients with advanced stage cancers will represent with distant metastases. There may be a lengthy time lag between surgical treatment of the primary site and development of distant metastases. The development of distant metastases is not prevented by

either postoperative radiotherapy or by elective neck dissection. It may be that in some patients with advanced tumours, distant metastases are already present at a microscopic level at the time of initial treatment, but, because of the slow-growing nature of the tumour, they do not become clinically evident for many years. Indeed, in the case of adenoid cystic carcinoma, patients with established distant metastases may survive with disease for many years.[43]

This propensity to develop distant metastases, sometimes many years after apparently successful primary treatment, is a feature characteristic of nearly all salivary carcinomas. Failure in the neck, in contrast, is much less common. A propensity for cervical metastases is seen in some subtypes of salivary carcinoma (mucoepidermoid carcinoma, carcinoma ex pleomorphic adenoma, adenocarcinoma NOS); however, cervical metastases are uncommon with most of the other subtypes. Thus, although the presence of nodal metastases is a well-established adverse prognostic factor in salivary cancers, the benefits of elective treatment of the clinically negative neck are much more contentious.

Overall, most salivary carcinomas are slow growing and have an indolent natural history. However, they show a striking tendency for local recurrence and delayed development of distant metastases. Thus, reports of five-year survival may be misleading; and significant differences between five- and ten-year survival outcomes may be present. Furthermore, it has been suggested that patients with treated salivary cancer should undergo lifelong follow up.

Extent of surgery

The extent of surgery is dependent on the size and site of the tumour. The surgeon should endeavour to take a reasonable margin of normal tissue all around the tumour. In the case of tumours located in the superficial lobe, the deep surgical margin is determined by the plane of the branches of the facial nerve. Thus, most such cases will be treated by superficial parotidectomy with facial nerve preservation. Resecting part of the deep lobe for the sake of it in such cases does not make sense when the closest margin has been determined by the relationship of the tumour to the facial nerve. In addition, parotid malignancies are very rarely multifocal, and are very unlikely to metastasize to the deep lobe. In fact, for tumours less than 4 cm in size, it is likely that partial superficial parotidectomy is adequate treatment, provided that adequate horizontal margins are obtained.[96] More extensive surgery is likely to increase the risk of facial nerve paralysis without improving local control.[97]

It should be noted that in cases where the tumour abuts or is adherent to one or more of the branches of the facial nerve, the final pathology report will typically state that the margin is close or involved. In such cases, the adequacy of surgical clearance is best judged by the surgeon.

Management of the facial nerve

As a general rule, every effort should be made to preserve a nerve which was functioning normally preoperatively. Facial nerve sacrifice should be reserved for cases of preoperative paralysis, cases of recurrent malignancy or of gross encasement and infiltration of the nerve. Microscopic invasion of the facial nerve is generally not considered an indication for nerve sacrifice. Although this may improve local control, it will not improve survival.[98, 99, 100] Furthermore, it is likely that the addition of postoperative radiotherapy will negate any benefit of nerve sacrifice on local control.[101] An exception to this may be in cases of involvement of a single branch where sacrifice would not lead to unacceptable morbidity.

When facial nerve sacrifice is necessary, then the margins should be checked by frozen section. Immediate repair should be performed using the greater auricular nerve. This nerve is easily accessible, provides adequate length, diameter and arborization. Function may take up to two years to return. A reasonable objective is House-Brackman grade 3.[99, 102] In the case of the zygomatic branch, the optimum rehabilitation may be by means of a gold weight implant, as, unlike nerve repair, this allows for synchronized blinking.

Neck dissection

In cases of parotid carcinoma with clinically N+ necks, neck dissection should be performed at the time of parotidectomy. The management of the clinically N0 neck is more controversial. Arguments for performing an elective neck dissection include the following: (1) There is a high rate of occult metastases in high-grade mucoepidermoid carcinomas, carcinoma ex pleomorphic adenoma and adenocarcinoma.[44] (2) Pathological examination of the submitted neck specimen provides prognostic information. (3) The upper neck levels are readily accessible by making a small extension to the standard parotidectomy incision, so that adding a selective neck dissection to the parotidectomy is associated with only a small amount of extra operating time and surgical morbidity.

On the other hand, opponents of elective neck dissection make the following arguments: (1) Cervical metastases are uncommon in adenoid cystic carcinoma, acinic cell carcinoma and many other types of salivary carcinoma.[44] (2) Patients with locally advanced or high-grade cancers will require postoperative radiotherapy regardless, and the pathological information provided by a selective neck dissection will thus not change management, and that this should sterilize any occult disease in the clinically negative neck. (3) Patients with salivary carcinomas usually fail from distant metastases and not from regional disease.

Certain parotid tumours show a high nodal relapse rate in untreated necks. These tumours include T3+ mucoepidermoid carcinoma, carcinoma ex pleomorphic adenoma, adenocarcinoma NOS, squamous cell carcinoma and undifferentiated carcinoma.[44] Thus, if neck dissection is not performed, patients should receive postoperative neck irradiation.[103]

Radiotherapy and adjunctive treatment

In general, salivary gland carcinomas are not particularly radiosensitive, although this has been disputed.[104] In a large series of previously untreated patients with salivary carcinoma, all treated with curative intent, those who were treated by radiotherapy alone had a significantly lower ten-year local control rate (42 per cent) compared to those treated by surgery with postoperative radiotherapy (90 per cent).[105] Thus, the role of radiotherapy as primary treatment for salivary carcinomas is limited to unresectable tumours.

On the other hand, adjuvant radiotherapy in the postoperative setting may be useful in improving local control rates. Although there are no randomized data available which assess the efficacy of postoperative radiotherapy, several retrospective series have reported a higher local control rate in patients treated with postoperative radiotherapy compared to patients treated with surgery alone.[8, 44, 106, 107, 108, 109] Other series have not found any significant difference,[43, 110, 111] however, it should be remembered that in most single-institution retrospective series, patients are selected to undergo postoperative radiotherapy on the basis of uncertainty over the completeness of resection, the status of margins, or other poor prognostic factors. Other authors have found improvements in local control for postoperative radiotherapy only in patients with stage III/IV disease (i.e. tumours greater than 4 cm, and/or with extraparenchymal spread and/or with nodal disease).[112, 113]

The effect of postoperative radiotherapy on survival is more controversial. Koul et al.[6] found higher disease-specific survival in patients who received combined treatment. Other authors have failed to find any survival benefit,[44, 106, 111] although a trend towards improved survival in patients with advanced stage tumours has been reported by some.[8, 112] However, given that patients with salivary carcinoma may survive for many years before dying from distant metastases, the addition of postoperative radiotherapy to improve local control may reduce morbidity and increase quality of life.

In general, postoperative radiotherapy is indicated for tumours greater than 4 cm, in the presence of positive surgical margins or in cases where the branches of the facial nerve were preserved despite being adherent to the tumour, and in cases with lymph node metastases.[114] Other factors which may be relative indications for radiotherapy include histological grade, adenoid cystic carcinoma and perineural invasion. The histological grade of the tumour would appear to be less important than tumour stage in determining prognosis and need for postoperative radiotherapy; thus, it is controversial whether radiotherapy is indicated in cases of adenoid cystic carcinoma or high-grade mucoepidermoid carcinoma staged T1/T2,[112] although some authors have claimed a benefit.[115]

In patients with unresectable cancers, the use of neutron radiotherapy has been advocated. This modality has resulted in impressive local control rates.[116, 117] In a trial of 25 patients with unresectable salivary carcinomas randomized to receive either conventional or neutron radiotherapy, neutron radiotherapy was found to have superior ten-year locoregional control (56 versus 17 per cent), but no improvement in survival (15 versus 25 per cent). Most patients treated with neutron radiotherapy developed distant metastases, whereas most patients treated with conventional radiotherapy developed local recurrence. A much higher incidence of severe complications was also seen in the neutron treatment group.[117]

The key to improving long-term survival in patients with salivary cancer would appear to be systemic treatment aimed at reducing the incidence of distant disease. However, to date, salivary carcinomas have shown poor response rates to combination chemotherapy and molecular therapies.[118]

Unexpected report of malignancy

Occasionally, after having performed a superficial parotidectomy where the preoperative diagnosis was pleomorphic adenoma, the pathology is unexpectedly reported as showing parotid carcinoma. This presents the surgeon with a difficult dilemma. The options for the patient at this point are observation alone, referral for postoperative radiotherapy or reoperation with performance of subtotal parotidectomy with or without subsequent postoperative radiation. The correct option will vary from case to case. Factors to be considered include the type of cancer, the size of the cancer, the histological grade, the surgeon's confidence in having cleared the tumour during the original operation, and the pathological margin status. For tumours which are small, low-grade and where the surgeon feels confident with the clearance, then observation alone may be adequate. On the other hand, large, high-grade tumours will usually warrant a more aggressive approach. Adding to the dilemma is that margins are frequently reported as close or positive on account of having dissected right on the capsule of the tumour in the vicinity of the branches of the facial nerve.

Recurrent malignancies

Recurrent salivary cancers usually warrant aggressive surgical therapy, consisting of wide resection of the tumour. More often than not this involves radical parotidectomy with sacrifice of the facial nerve and resection of overlying skin.

SURGICAL TECHNIQUE

Surgical technique of superficial parotidectomy

PREPARATION

Many surgeons use intraoperative facial nerve monitoring. Intraoperative nerve monitoring may be particularly useful for patients with large and/or malignant tumours, patients undergoing revision surgery, cases where retrograde dissection of the facial nerve may be required, and for less experienced surgeons. The facial nerve monitor should be applied and testing prior to prepping and draping the patient.

INCISION

An incision should be carefully marked out extending from the preauricular region, around the lobule of the ear towards the mastoid tip, and then curving back down to join a neck crease, well below the angle of the mandible. If a preauricular crease is present, this should be used. Otherwise the incision may be hidden behind the tragus (**Figure 37.5**).

Prior to making the incision, it is very useful to make a single crosshatch in the region of the lobule. When making the

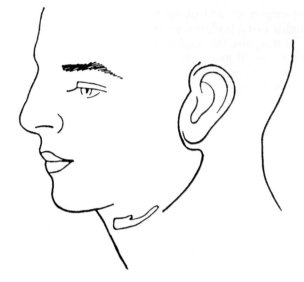

Figure 37.5   Incision for parotidectomy.

incision, it is important not to bevel the blade in the postauricular region, as this may compromise the skin in this region.

FLAPS

In the face, the anterior skin flap should be raised superficial to the parotid fascia, leaving subcutaneous fat on the flap. It is very easy to buttonhole this flap. If the surgeon sees hair follicles, he is probably getting too superficial. Strong traction and countertraction, with the countertraction being applied as far into the wound as possible, is very helpful in defining the plane. Alternatively, dissecting scissors may be used to open the plane and then cut the intervening fibres.

In the neck, the flap may be raised either superficial or immediately deep to the platysma. A 'white line' which defines the plane the surgeon needs to be in is usually apparent between these facial and neck planes.

When raising the flap, it is of utmost importance that the surgeon keeps palpating the tumour and does not inadvertently enter it.

Posteriorly, the neck part of the incision should be deepened to the sternomastoid muscle. The greater auricular nerve can be seen. This is usually sacrificed, leading to some permanent numbness of the ear lobe, although the posterior branch, which supplies the earlobe, may frequently be preserved. The anterior border of the sternomastoid should be defined and followed up to the mastoid tip. The fascia should be raised anteriorly off the sternomastoid muscle. In doing so, the surgeon should stay behind any posterior extension of the parotid gland or the tumour. The surgeon should also be aware of the proximity of the accessory nerve while dissecting on the medial surface of the sternomastoid muscle. The deep cervical fascia should then be incised to display the posterior belly of the digastric muscle, which is an important landmark.

In the region of the ear, the incision should be deepened along the cartilage of the external auditory canal, taking care not to damage this cartilage. As long as the surgeon stays right on the external auditory canal, the incision can be safely deepened all the way to the bony-cartilaginous junction.

The surgeon should look out for the 'tragal pointer', which is another useful landmark for the facial nerve.

At this point, the surgeon should divide the tissue anterior to the mastoid process in order to join the dissection in the region of the external auditory canal to that in the region of the sternomastoid muscle. The depth of this should remain superficial to the digastric muscle. There are many blood vessels around the mastoid which will require appropriate control.

LOCATING THE FACIAL NERVE

The facial nerve emerges from the stylomastoid foramen just superior to the posterior belly of the digastric muscle, at the same depth as this muscle. The tragal pointer is 1 cm superficial and above this point. The styloid process is medial to the facial nerve so is not a good landmark. The direction of the nerve is anterior, superficial and inferior (**Figure 37.3**).

Prior to looking for the facial nerve, the posterior belly of the digastric and tragal pointer should be well defined, and the surgeon should have opened a broad plane of dissection, so that he is not working down a narrow 'hole'. The surgeon should then proceed to look for the nerve using an Adson clamp or artery forceps. This may be opened gently in a direction parallel to the nerve to avoid causing inadvertent damage. Surgeons should thus note that from this standpoint, the nerve is coming towards them. There are usually many fibrous strands in the region of the nerve which will need to be divided in order to find the nerve. In addition, there are usually some blood vessels just superficial to the nerve which, if injured, will cause troublesome bleeding which will make identification of the nerve difficult. It is best to divide these blood vessels after cauterizing them using bipolar diathermy, however, the surgeon must be certain that the facial nerve is not cauterized.

When there is difficulty finding the nerve, the surgeon should look a little more anterior and/or inferior, as often the problem is that the surgeon is too close to the external auditory canal.

Once the facial nerve is found, it should be followed to its bifurcation, prior to division of any parotid tissue.

FOLLOWING THE BRANCHES

The branches should be followed in sequence, starting either superiorly or inferiorly. A clamp should be inserted along the nerve, then lifted away from the nerve and opened. The assistant should then divide the parotid tissue between the tines of the clamp (insert – lift – spread – cut). Once inserted and opened, the clamp should not be closed without first withdrawing it. The surgeon should try to divide some tissue with every manoeuvre, otherwise little progress will be made. The surgeon should remember that as the branches are traced distally, they become more superficial, particularly the upper branches.

The dissection should commence over a branch which is clear of the tumour, and then proceed to the successive branches. In so doing, parotid tissue should be divided clear of the tumour. Once two branches have been followed, the intervening tissue at the anterior part of the gland is divided so that the superficial part of the gland containing the tumour can be peeled up or downwards. The surgeon may

come towards the tumour both superiorly and inferiorly, so the superficial lobe is well mobilized by the time the tumour is approached.

For tumours located in either the upper or lower pole of the gland, it is not necessary to remove the whole of the superficial lobe. It may be possible to remove the tumour with an adequate cuff while following only either the upper or lower division branches.

Commonly, the deep part of the tumour capsule is applied directly onto the branches of the facial nerve. In this situation, the surgeon should carefully separate the tumour from the nerve, taking great care not to rupture the capsule. If this is done, there is no increased recurrence rate.

CLOSURE

Prior to closure, a drain should always be placed, as otherwise the wound will inevitably accumulate saliva and serous fluid. The drain should be ideally left for at least 48 hours. Closure is then performed according to surgeon's preference.

Difficult cases

DEEP LOBE TUMOURS

For tumours situated in the deep lobe, the operation begins with a standard superficial parotidectomy, as described above. Having completed this, the branches of the facial nerve overlying the tumour are now easily visible. The branches overlying the tumour are then separated from the tumour and mobilized. The underlying tumour is then mobilized and separated from the deep tissue. This is usually easily accomplished and, although it usually results in the operation leading to little more than an enucleation, there does not appear to be an increased recurrence rate, similar to that seen if enucleation is performed for superficial lobe tumours. The tumour is then removed between two of the mobilized facial nerve branches. Not uncommonly, particularly in the buccal region, extensive arborization and communicating branches are present. In such cases, it may be necessary to sacrifice some of the minor communicating branches, although this should, if possible, be avoided.

REVISION CASES

Revision parotid surgery is one of the most difficult surgeries in head and neck. Usually, it will be necessary to resect the previous scar. Occasionally, skin resection will also be necessary and the surgeon should be prepared to reconstruct the defect. If the previous surgery comprised a formal superficial parotidectomy, then the branches of the facial nerve will be just beneath the skin flap, without any intervening parotid fascia, and so will be vulnerable to injury while raising the skin flap. Extending the previous incision, and identifying the correct plane in virgin tissue, may be a useful manoeuvre. Identification of the main trunk of the facial nerve may be difficult or impossible due to scarring. In such cases, it may be necessary to identify the branches of the facial nerve in the neck and/or face and perform retrograde dissection. The retromandibular vein, if still present, is a useful landmark as the marginal mandibular and cervical branches pass directly over it. If this vein has been previously ligated, then the marginal mandibular nerve may be identified beneath the angle of the mandible, or crossing the facial artery at the mandibular notch on the inferior border of the mandible. The cervical branch is a variable distance below the marginal mandibular branch. There is variable arborization and anatomy of the remaining branches, but as a rough guide the temporal branch crosses the zygomatic arch 1 cm anterior to the ear, and courses superficial to the deep temporal fascia, coming to within 1.5 cm of the lateral border of the eye. The zygomatic branch crosses the zygomatic arch further forward. The upper buccal branch runs forward roughly 1 cm below the zygomatic arch; and the lower buccal branch runs towards the corner of the mouth. These nerves are superficial to the masseter muscle. It should be noted that retrograde dissection of the branches of the facial nerve may lead to a higher incidence of neuropraxia than traditional prograde dissection.

Complications of parotid surgery

FACIAL NERVE INJURY

Facial nerve injury is usually the biggest concern in parotid surgery. Postoperative weakness may be temporary, if the injury is a neuropraxia, or permanent, due to transection of, or cautery injury to, the main trunk of the facial nerve, or, more commonly, one of the terminal branches. Temporary weakness is much more common and is seen in between 10 and 50 per cent of parotidectomies.[28, 77] It occurs more commonly in difficult cases, i.e. large tumours, tumours located in the deep lobe, malignant cases and revision surgery. The precise cause of neuropraxia is not known, but probably results from a combination of trauma while dissecting right on the nerve, traction injury to the nerve, heat injury secondary to the use of cautery, and prolonged operating time. The lower division branches, in particular, the marginal mandibular branch, would appear to be particularly susceptible to neuropraxia. This is probably due to the thinner, more fragile nature of these branches. Neuropraxia usually recovers in a few weeks, but may take many months, particularly in elderly patients. The incidence of permanent facial nerve injury is generally reported as 0–5 per cent.[28, 30, 77]

HAEMATOMA

Haematoma is reported to occur in up to 5 per cent of parotidectomies. As a general rule, small haematomas should be evacuated promptly, as their presence leads to compromise of the skin flap with possible necrosis.

SEROMA/SALIVOMA/SALIVARY FISTULA

After superficial parotidectomy, leakage of serous fluid and saliva from the transected parotid tissue is an expected occurrence. This usually lasts for a few days. Thus, a drain should always be placed after parotid surgery and left in place for at least 2–3 days. At this stage, the skin flap should have begun to adhere to the parotid bed, so obliterating the dead space in which fluid can accumulate.

If, after removing the drain, patients develop swelling underneath the wound, this should be aspirated. Seromas usually resolve within a few days of serial aspiration. In the case of salivary collections, drainage of saliva out of the drain site or through the wound when the patient is eating is not uncommon. Any collection should be aspirated. A pressure dressing, similar to the type used after otoplasty, may also be useful to speed resolution.

FREY'S SYNDROME

Frey's syndrome, or gustatory sweating, is a phenomenon seen after parotid surgery where the patient develops sweating on the side of the face while eating. It is believed to be due to transection of cholinergic secretomotor fibres to the secretory units of the parotid gland, which subsequently sprout new axons and come to innervate sweat glands in the skin flap, which are also responsive to acetylcholine. It is reported that around 10 per cent of patients who undergo parotidectomy will complain of gustatory sweating, but that on questioning, 30–40 per cent will reply that they experience it, while it can be demonstrated objectively in 95 per cent of patients.[119] Objective demonstration is possible using Minor's starch-iodine test. This is performed by covering the affected skin with iodine solution. Once this has dried, it is dusted with starch powder, and the patient given a lemon sweet. As a result of absorption of the wet iodine by starch, the affected area will turn deep blue purple.[119]

Frey's syndrome usually develops within weeks or months of surgery, but its onset may be delayed for several years.[119, 120] It occurs more commonly with more extensive parotid surgeries. Several techniques for preventing Frey's syndrome have been described. These include raising a thick skin flap,[121] rotation of a superficial temporal artery-based temporoparietal vascular flap,[122] rotation of the superficial musculoaponeurotic system (SMAS),[123, 124, 125] and rotation of sternomastoid muscle flaps.[125, 126] However, there are disadvantages to most of these techniques.[119] In established cases, topical anticholinergics may be useful, but have variable efficacy and may lead to anticholinergic side effects.[119, 120] For persistent cases, the most effective treatment would appear to be injection of botulinum type A toxin. This inhibits neurotransmitter release and gives long-lasting relief, and may be repeated if recurrent symptoms develop.[127, 128]

OTHER

Ear numbness is an expected outcome from parotid surgery. It results from transection of the greater auricular nerve. Occasionally, the posterior branch of the nerve can be preserved, which minimizes the sensory deficit. Patients are usually very aware of sensory change immediately after the surgery. Over the course of several months, the area of numbness diminishes, but patients are usually left with an area of persistent numbness around the ear lobe. Patients

recurrence. *Archives of Pathology and Laboratory Medicine* 1976; **100**: 271–5.

19. Patey D, Thackeray AC. The treatment of parotid tumors in the light of a pathological study of parotidectomy material. *British Journal of Surgery* 1957; **45**: 477–87.

20. Henriksson G, Westrin KM, Carlsoo B, Silfversward C. Recurrent primary pleomorphic adenomas of salivary gland origin: intrasurgical rupture, histopathological features, and pseudopodia. *Cancer* 1998; **82**: 617–20.

21. Rawson AJ, Howard JM, Royster HP. Tumors of the salivary glands. A clinicopathological study of 160 cases. *Cancer* 1950; **3**: 445–8.

22. McFarland J. Three hundred mixed tumors of the salivary glands of which 69 recurred. *Surgery, Gynecology and Obstetrics* 1936; **88**: 457–68.

23. Stein I, Geschickter CF. Tumors of the parotid gland. *Archives of Surgery* 1934; **28**: 482–526.

24. Krolls SO, Boyers RC. Mixed tumors of salivary glands: long-term follow-up. *Cancer* 1972; **30**: 276–81.

25. Benedict EG, Meigs JV. Tumors of the parotid gland. A study of 225 cases with complete end-results in 80 cases. *Surgery, Gynecology and Obstetrics* 1930; **51**: 626–47.

26. Wood FC. Mixed tumors of the salivary glands. *Annals of Surgery* 1904; **39**: 57.

27. Witt RL. The significance of the margin in parotid surgery for pleomorphic adenoma. *Laryngoscope* 2002; **112**: 2141–54.

28. Leverstein H, van der Waal JE, Tiwari RM *et al.* Surgical management of 246 previously untreated pleomorphic adenomas of the parotid gland. *British Journal of Surgery* 1997; **84**: 399–403.

29. Debets JM, Munting JD. Parotidectomy for parotid tumors: 19-year experience from the Netherlands. *British Journal of Surgery* 1992; **79**: 1159–61.

30. Guntinas-Lichius O, Kick C, Klussman JP *et al.* Pleomorphic adenoma of the parotid gland: a 13-year experience of consequent management by lateral or total parotidectomy. *European Archives of Otorhinolaryngology* 2004; **261**: 143–6.

31. Leverstein H, van der Waal JE, Tiwari RM *et al.* Results of the surgical management and histopathological evaluation of 88 parotid gland Warthin's tumors. *Clinical Otolaryngology* 1997; **22**: 500–3.

32. Maiorano E, Lo Muzio L, Favia G, Piatelli A. Warthin's tumor: a study of 78 cases with emphasis on bilaterality, multifocality, and association with other malignancies. *Oral Oncology* 2002; **38**: 35–40.

33. Klussman PJ, Wittekindt C, Preuss FS *et al.* High risk for bilateral Warthin tumor in heavy smokers – review of 185 cases. *Acta Otolaryngologica* 2006; **126**: 1213–17.

34. Luna MA. Salivary mucoepidermoid carcinoma: revisited. *Advances in Anatomic Pathology* 2006; **13**: 293–307.

35. Callender DL, Frankenthaler RA, Luna MA *et al.* Salivary gland neoplasms in children. *Archives of Otolaryngology, Head and Neck Surgery* 1992; **118**: 472–6.

36. Guzzo M, Ferrari A, Marcon I *et al.* Salivary gland neoplasms in children: the experience of the Instituto Nazionale Tumori of Milan. *Pediatric Blood and Cancer* 2006; **47**: 806–10.

37. Goode RK, Auclair PL, Ellis GL. Mucoepidermoid carcinoma of the major salivary glands: clinical and histopathologic analysis of 234 cases with evaluation of grading criteria. *Cancer* 1998; **82**: 1217–24.

38. Brandwein MS, Ivanov K, Wallace DI *et al.* Mucoepidermoid carcinoma: a clinicopathological study of 80 patients with special reference to histological grading. *American Journal of Surgical Pathology* 2001; **25**: 835–45.

39. Spiro RH, Huvos AG, Berk R, Strong EW. Mucoepidermoid carcinoma of salivary gland origin. A clinicopathological study of 367 cases. *American Journal of Surgery* 1978; **136**: 461–8.

40. Spiro RH, Thaler HT, Hicks WF *et al.* The importance of clinical staging of minor salivary gland carcinoma. *American Journal of Surgery* 1991; **162**: 330–6.

41. Plambeck K, Friedrich RE, Hellner D *et al.* Mucoepidermoid carcinoma of the salivary glands: clinical data and follow-up of 52 cases. *Journal of Cancer Research and Clinical Oncology* 1996; **122**: 177–80.

42. Bradley PJ. Adenoid cystic carcinoma of the head and neck: a review. *Current Opinion in Otolaryngology and Head and Neck Surgery* 2004; **12**: 127–32.

43. Khan AJ, DiGiovanna MP, Ross DA *et al.* Adenoid cystic carcinoma: a retrospective clinical review. *International Journal of Cancer* 2001; **96**: 149–58.

44. Terhaard CH, Lubsen H, Van der Tweel I *et al.* Salivary gland carcinoma: independent prognostic factors for locoregional control, distant metastases, and overall survival: results of the Dutch Head and Neck Oncology Cooperative Group. *Head and Neck* 2004; **26**: 681–92.

45. Spiro RH, Huvos AG, Strong EW. Adenoid cystic carcinoma of salivary origin. A clinicopathologic study of 242 cases. *American Journal of Surgery* 1974; **128**: 512–20.

46. Spiro RH, Huvos AG. Stage means more than grade in adenoid cystic carcinoma. *American Journal of Surgery* 1992; **164**: 623–8.

47. Nascimento AG, Amaral AL, Prado LA *et al.* Adenoid cystic carcinoma of salivary glands: a review of 61 cases with clinicopathological correlation. *Cancer* 1986; **57**: 312–19.

48. Fordice J, Kershaw C, El-Nagger A, Goepfert H. Adenoid cystic carcinoma of the head and neck: predictors of morbidity and mortality. *Archives of Otolaryngology, Head and Neck Surgery* 1999; **125**: 149–52.

49. Garden AS, Weber RS, Morrison WH *et al.* The influence of positive margins and nerve invasion in adenoid cystic carcinoma of the head and neck treated with surgery and radiation. *International Journal of Radiation Oncology, Biology, Physics* 1995; **32**: 619–26.

50. Triantafillidou K, Dimitrakopoulos J, Iordanidis F, Koufogiannis D. Management of adenoid cystic

carcinoma of minor salivary glands. *Journal of Oral and Maxillofacial Surgery* 2006; **64**: 1114–20.

51. Auclair PL, Ellis GL. Atypical features in salivary gland mixed tumors: their relationship to malignant transformation. *Modern Pathology* 1996; **9**: 652–7.

52. Spiro RH, Huvos AG, Strong EW. Malignant mixed tumor of salivary origin: a clinicopathologic study of 146 cases. *Cancer* 1977; **39**: 388–96.

53. Olsen KD, Lewis JE. Carcinoma ex pleomorphic adenoma: a clinicopathologic review. *Head and Neck* 2001; **23**: 705–12.

54. Tortoledo ME, Luna MA, Batsakis JG. Carcinomas ex pleomorphic adenoma and malignant mixed tumors. Histomorphologic indexes. *Archives of Otolaryngology* 1984; **110**: 172–6.

55. Brandwein M, Huvos AG, Dardick I *et al.* Noninvasive and minimally invasive carcinoma ex mixed tumor: a clinicopathologic and ploidy study of 12 patients with major salivary tumors of low (or no?) malignant potential. *Oral Surgery, Oral Medicine, Oral Pathology, Oral Radiology, and Endodontics* 1996; **81**: 655–64.

56. LiVolsi VA, Perzin KH. Malignant mixed tumors arising in salivary glands. I. Carcinomas arising in benign mixed tumors: a clinicopathologic study. *Cancer* 1977; **39**: 2209–30.

57. Spiro RH, Huvos AG, Strong EW. Acinic cell carcinoma of salivary origin. A clinicopathologic study of 67 cases. *Cancer* 1978; **41**: 924–35.

58. Guimaraes DS, Amaral AP, Prado LF, Nascimento AG. Acinic cell carcinoma of salivary glands. 16 cases with clinicopathologic correlation. *Journal of Oral Pathology and Medicine* 1989; **18**: 396–9.

59. Luukkaa H, Klemi P, Leivo I *et al.* Salivary gland cancer in Finland 1991–1996. An evaluation of 237 cases. *Acta Otolaryngologica* 2005; **125**: 207–14.

60. Pogodzinski MS, Sabri AN, Lewis JE, Olsen KD. Retrospective study and review of polymorphous low-grade adenocarcinoma. *Laryngoscope* 2006; **116**: 2145–9.

61. Seethala RR, Barnes EL, Hunt JL. Epithelial-myoepithelial carcinoma: a review of the clinicopathological spectrum and immunophenotypic characteristics in 61 tumors of the salivary glands and upper aerodigestive tract. *American Journal of Surgical Pathology* 2007; **31**: 44–57.

62. Foss R, Ellis GL, Auclair PL. Salivary gland cystadenocarcinomas: a clinicopathologic study of 57 cases. *American Journal of Surgical Pathology* 1996; **20**: 1440–7.

63. Li J, Wang BY, Nelson M *et al.* Salivary adenocarcinoma, not otherwise specified. A collection of orphans. *Archives of Pathology and Laboratory Medicine* 2004; **128**: 1385–94.

64. Sheahan P, Byrne M, Hafidh M *et al.* Neck dissection findings in primary head and neck high-grade adenocarcinomas. *Journal of Laryngology and Otology* 2004; **118**: 532–6.

65. Ying YL, Johnson JT, Myers EN. Squamous cell carcinoma of the parotid gland. *Head and Neck* 2006; **28**: 626–32.

66. Sobin LH. *TNM classification of malignant tumours*, 7th edn. London: John Wiley & Sons, 2009.

67. Yousem DM, Kraut MA, Chalian AA. Major salivary gland imaging. *Radiology* 2000; **216**: 19–29.

68. Alphs HH, Eisele DW, Westra WH. The role of fine needle aspiration in the evaluation of parotid masses. *Current Opinion in Otolaryngology and Head and Neck Surgery* 2006; **14**: 62–6.

69. Balakrishnan K, Castling B, McMahon J *et al.* Fine needle aspiration cytology in the management of a parotid mass: a two centre retrospective study. *Surgeon* 32005: 67–72.

70. Das DK, Petkar MA, Al Mane NM *et al.* Role of fine needle aspiration cytology in the diagnosis of swellings in the salivary gland regions: a study of 712 cases. *Medical Principles and Practice* 2004; **13**: 95–106.

71. Hughes JH, Volk EE, Wilbur DC. Pitfalls in salivary gland fine-needle aspiration cytology. Lessons from the College of American Pathologists Interlaboratory Comparison Program in Nongynaecologic Cytology. *Archives of Pathology and Laboratory Medicine* 2005; **129**: 26–31.

72. Seethala RR, LiVolsi VA, Baloch ZW. Relative accuracy of fine needle aspiration and frozen section in the diagnosis of lesions of the parotid gland. *Head and Neck* 2005; **27**: 217–23.

73. Badoual C, Rousseau A, Heudes D *et al.* Evaluation of frozen section diagnosis in 721 parotid gland lesions. *Histopathology* 2006; **49**: 538–40.

74. Heller KS, Attie JN, Dubner S. Accuracy of frozen section in the diagnosis of salivary tumors. *American Journal of Surgery* 1993; **166**: 424–7.

75. Witt RL. Minimally invasive surgery for parotid pleomorphic adenoma. *Ear, Nose and Throat Journal* 2005; **84**: 308–11.

76. Bradley PJ. Pleomorphic salivary adenoma of the parotid gland: which operation to perform? *Current Opinion in Otolaryngology and Head and Neck Surgery* 2004; **12**: 69–70.

77. O'Brien CJ. Current management of benign parotid tumors: the role of limited superficial parotidectomy. *Head and Neck* 2003; **25**: 946–52.

78. Ghosh S, Panarese A, Bull PD, Lee JA. Marginally excised pleomorphic salivary adenomas: risk factors for recurrence and management: a 12.5 year mean follow-up study of histologically marginal excisions. *Clinical Otolaryngology and Allied Sciences* 2003; **28**: 262–6.

79. Donovan DT, Conley JJ. Capsular significance in parotid surgery: reality and myths of lateral lobectomy. *Laryngoscope* 1984; **94**: 324–9.

80. Natvig K, Soberg R. Relationship of intraoperative rupture of pleomorphic adenomas to recurrence: an 11–25 year follow-up study. *Head and Neck* 1994; **16**: 213–17.

81. Lawson HH. Capsular penetration and perforation in pleomorphic adenoma of the parotid salivary gland. *British Journal of Surgery* 1989; **76**: 594–6.

82. Harney MS, Murphy C, Hone S *et al.* A histological comparison of deep and superficial lobe pleomorphic adenomas of the parotid gland. *Head and Neck* 2003; **25**: 649–53.

83. Fliss DM, Rival R, Gullane P *et al.* Pleomorphic adenoma: a preliminary histopathological comparison between tumors occurring in the deep and superficial lobes of the parotid gland. *Ear, Nose and Throat Journal* 1992; **71**: 254–7.

84. McGurk M, Thomas BL, Renehan AG. Extracapsular dissection for clinically benign parotid lumps: reduced morbidity without oncological compromise. *British Journal of Cancer* 2003; **89**: 1610–13.

85. Hancock BD. Clinically benign parotid tumours: local dissection as an alternative to superficial parotidectomy in selected cases. *Annals of the Royal College of Surgeons of England* 1999; **81**: 299–301.

86. Piekarski J, Nejc D, Szymczak W *et al.* Results of extracapsular dissection of pleomorphic adenoma of parotid gland. *Journal of Oral and Maxillofacial Surgery* 2004; **62**: 1198–202.

87. Liu FF, Rotstein L, Davison AJ *et al.* Benign parotid adenomas: a review of the Princess Margaret Hospital experience. *Head and Neck* 1995; **17**: 177–83.

88. Carew JF, Spiro RH, Singh B *et al.* Treatment of recurrent pleomorphic adenomas of the parotid gland. *Otolaryngology, Head and Neck Surgery* 1999; **121**: 539–42.

89. Stennert E, Wittekindt C, Klussman JP *et al.* Recurrent pleomorphic adenoma of the parotid gland: a prospective histopathological and immunohistochemical study. *Laryngoscope* 2004; **114**: 158–63.

90. Wittekindt C, Streubel K, Arnold G *et al.* Recurrent pleomorphic adenoma of the parotid gland: analysis of 108 consecutive patients. *Head and Neck* 2007; **29**: 822–8.

91. Leonetti JP, Marzo SJ, Petruzzelli GJ, Herr B. Recurrent pleomorphic adenoma of the parotid gland. *Otolaryngology, Head and Neck Surgery* 2005; **133**: 319–22.

92. Dawson AK. Radiation therapy in recurrent pleomorphic adenoma of the parotid gland. *International Journal of Radiation Oncology, Biology, Physics* 1989; **16**: 819–21.

93. Phillips PP, Olsen KD. Recurrent pleomorphic adenomas of the parotid gland: report of 126 cases and a review of the literature. *Annals of Otology, Rhinology, and Laryngology* 1995; **104**: 100–4.

94. Chilla R, Schneider K, Droese M. Recurrence tendency and malignant transformation of pleomorphic adenomas. *HNO* 1986; **34**: 467–9.

95. Renehan A, Gleave EN, McGurk M. An analysis of the treatment of 114 patients with recurrent pleomorphic adenomas of the parotid gland. *American Journal of Surgery* 1996; **172**: 710–14.

96. Lim YC, Lee SY, Kim K *et al.* Conservative parotidectomy for treatment of parotid cancers. *Oral Oncology* 2005; **41**: 1021–7.

97. Bron LP, O'Brien CJ. Facial nerve function after parotidectomy. *Archives of Otolaryngology, Head and Neck Surgery* 1997; **123**: 1091–6.

98. O'Brien CJ, Adams JR. Surgical management of the facial nerve in the presence of malignancy about the face. *Current Opinion in Otolaryngology and Head and Neck Surgery* 2001; **9**: 90–4.

99. Vander Poorten VL, Balm AJ, Hilgers FJ. Management of cancer of the parotid gland. *Current Opinion in Otolaryngology and Head and Neck Surgery* 2002; **10**: 134–44.

100. Guntinas-Lichius O, Klussman JP, Schroeder U *et al.* Primary parotid malignoma surgery in patients with normal preoperative facial nerve function: outcome and long-term postoperative facial nerve function. *Laryngoscope* 2004; **114**: 949–56.

101. Leverstein H, van der Waal JE, Tiwari RM *et al.* Malignant epithelial parotid gland tumors: analysis and results in 65 previously untreated patients. *British Journal of Surgery* 1998; **85**: 1267–72.

102. Reddy PG, Arden RL, Mathog RH. Facial nerve rehabilitation after radical parotidectomy. *Laryngoscope* 1999; **109**: 894–9.

103. Chen AM, Garcia J, Lee NY *et al.* Patterns of nodal relapse after surgery and postoperative radiation therapy for carcinomas of major and minor salivary glands: what is the role of elective neck irradiation? *International Journal of Radiation Oncology, Biology, Physics* 2007; **67**: 988–94.

104. Chen AM, Kara Bucci M, Quivey JM *et al.* Long-term outcome of patients treated by radiation therapy alone for salivary gland carcinomas. *International Journal of Radiation Oncology, Biology, Physics* 2006; **66**: 1044–50.

105. Mendenhall WM, Morris CG, Amdur RJ *et al.* Radiotherapy alone or combined with surgery for salivary gland carcinoma. *Cancer* 2005; **103**: 2544–50.

106. Chen AM, Kara Bucci M, Weinberg V *et al.* Adenoid cystic carcinoma of the head and neck treated by surgery with or without postoperative radiation therapy: prognostic features of recurrence. *International Journal of Radiation Oncology, Biology, Physics* 2006; **66**: 152–9.

107. North CA, Lee DJ, Piantadosi S *et al.* Carcinoma of the major salivary glands treated by surgery or surgery plus postoperative radiotherapy. *International Journal of Radiation Oncology, Biology, Physics* 1990; **18**: 1319–26.

108. Miglianico L, Eschwege F, Marandas P *et al.* Cervico-facial adenoid cystic carcinoma: study of 102 cases. Influence of radiation therapy. *International Journal of Radiation Oncology, Biology, Physics* 1987; **13**: 673–8.

109. Simpson JR, Thawley SE, Matsuba HM. Adenoid cystic salivary carcinoma: treatment with irradiation and surgery. *Radiology* 1984; **151**: 509–12.

110. Kokemueller H, Eckardt A, Brachvogel P *et al.* Adenoid cystic carcinoma of the head and neck – a 20 year experience. *International Journal of Oral and Maxillofacial Surgery* 2004; **33**: 25–31.

111. Lima RA, Tavares MR, Dias FL *et al.* Clinical prognostic factors in malignant parotid gland tumors. *Otolaryngology, Head and Neck Surgery* 2005; **133**: 702–8.

112. Armstrong JG, Harrison LB, Spiro RH *et al.* Malignant tumors of major salivary gland origin: a matched-pair analysis of the role of combined surgery and postoperative radiotherapy. *Archives of Otolaryngology, Head and Neck Surgery* 1990; **116**: 290–3.

113. Silverman DA, Carlson TP, Khuntia D *et al.* Role for postoperative radiation therapy in adenoid cystic carcinoma of the head and neck. *Laryngoscope* 2004; **114**: 1194–9.

114. Chen AM, Granchi PJ, Garcia J *et al.* Local-regional recurrence after surgery without postoperative irradiation for carcinomas of the major salivary glands: implications for adjuvant therapy. *International Journal of Radiation Oncology, Biology, Physics* 2007; **67**: 982–7.

115. Zbaren P, Nuyens M, Caversaccio M *et al.* Postoperative radiation therapy for T1 and T2 primary parotid carcinoma: is it useful? *Otolaryngology, Head and Neck Surgery* 2006; **135**: 140–3.

116. Laramore GE, Krall JM, Griffin TW *et al.* Neutron versus photon irradiation for unresectable salivary gland tumors: final report of an RTOG-MRC randomized clinical trial. *International Journal of Radiation Oncology, Biology, Physics* 1993; **27**: 235–40.

117. Pommier P, Liebsch NJ, Deschler DG *et al.* Proton beam radiation therapy for skull base adenoid cystic carcinoma. *Archives of Otolaryngology, Head and Neck Surgery* 2006; **132**: 1242–9.

118. Dodd RL, Slevin NJ. Salivary gland adenoid cystic carcinoma: a review of chemotherapy and molecular therapies. *Oral Oncology* 2006; **42**: 759–69.

119. De Bree R, van der Waal I, Leemans CR. Management of Frey syndrome. *Head and Neck* 2007; **29**: 773–8.

120. Clayman MA, Clayman SM, Seagle MB. A review of the surgical and medical treatment of Frey syndrome. *Annals of Plastic Surgery* 2006; **57**: 581–4.

121. Singleton GT, Cassisi NJ. Frey's syndrome: incidence related to skin flap thickness in parotidectomy. *Laryngoscope* 1980; **90**: 1636–9.

122. Ahmed OA, Kolhe PS. Prevention of Frey's syndrome and volume deficit after parotidectomy using the superficial temporal artery fascial flap. *British Journal of Plastic Surgery* 1999; **52**: 256–60.

123. Allison GR, Rappaport I. Prevention of Frey's syndrome with superficial musculoaponeurotic system interposition. *American Journal of Surgery* 1993; **166**: 407–10.

124. Bonanno PC, Casson PR. Frey's syndrome: a preventable phenomenon. *Plastic Reconstructive Surgery* 1992; **89**: 452–6.

125. Casler JD, Conley J. Sternomastoid muscle transfer and superficial musculoaponeurotic system plication in the prevention of Frey's syndrome. *Laryngoscope* 1991; **101**: 95–100.

126. Sood S, Quraishi MS, Jennings CR, Bradley PJ. Frey's syndrome following parotidectomy: prevention using rotation sternocleidomastoid muscle flap. *Clinical Otolaryngology* 1999; **24**: 365–8.

127. Naumann M, Zellner M, Toyka KV, Reiners K. Treatment of gustatory sweating with botulinum toxin. *Annals of Neurology* 1997; **42**: 973–5.

128. Dulguerov P, Quinodoz D, Cosendal G *et al.* Frey syndrome treatment with botulinum toxin. *Otolaryngology, Head and Neck Surgery* 2000; **122**: 821–7.

129. Fee WEJr, Tran LE. Functional outcome after total parotidectomy reconstruction. *Laryngoscope* 2004; **114**: 223–6.

130. Filho WQ, Dedivitis RA, Rapoport A, Guimaraes AV. Sternocleidomastoid flap preventing Frey syndrome following parotidectomy. *World Journal of Surgery* 2004; **28**: 361–4.

131. Gooden EA, Gullane PJ, Irish J *et al.* Role of the sternocleidomastoid muscle flap preventing Frey's syndrome and maintaining facial contour following superficial parotidectomy. *Journal of Otolaryngology* 2001; **30**: 98–101.

132. Kerawala CJ, McAloney N, Stassen LF. Prospective randomized trial of the benefits of a sternocleidomastoid flap after superficial parotidectomy. *British Journal of Oral and Maxillofacial Surgery* 2002; **40**: 468–72.

133. Foustanos A, Zavrides H. Face-lift approach combined with a superficial musculoaponeurotic system advancement flap in parotidectomy. *British Journal of Oral and Maxillofacial Surgery* 2007; **45**: 652–5.

134. Meningaud JP, Bertolus C, Bertrand JC. Parotidectomy: assessment of a surgical technique including facelift incision and SMAS advancement. *Journal of Craniomaxillofacial Surgery* 2006; **34**: 34–7.

135. Honig JF. Omega-incision face-lift approach and SMAS rotation advancement flap in parotidectomy for prevention of contour deficiency and conspicuous scars affecting the neck. *International Journal of Oral and Maxillofacial Surgery* 2005; **34**: 612–18.

136. Taylor SM, Yoo J. Prospective cohort study comparing subcutaneous and sub-superficial musculoaponeurotic system flaps in superficial parotidectomy. *Journal of Otolaryngology* 2003; **32**: 71–6.

137. Boynton JF, Cohen BE, Barrera A. Rhytidectomy and parotidectomy combined in the same patient. *Aesthetic Plastic Surgery* 2006; **30**: 125–31.

138. Zenk J, Koch M, Bozzato A, Iro H. Sialoscopy – initial experiences with a new endoscope. *British Journal of Oral and Maxillofacial Surgery* 2004; **42**: 293–8.

139. Nahlieli O, Nakar LH, Nazarian Y, Turner MD. Sialoendoscopy: a new approach to salivary gland obstructive pathology. *Journal of the American Dental Association* 2006; **137**: 1394–400.

140. Nahlieli O, Nazarian Y. Sialadenitis following radioiodine therapy – a new diagnostic and treatment modality. *Oral Diseases* 2006; **12**: 476–9.

141. Meningaud JP, Pitak-Arnnop P, Bertrand JC. Endoscope-assisted submandibular sialadenectomy: a pilot study. *Journal of Oral and Maxillofacial Surgery* 2006; **64**: 1366–70.

38

Non-melanoma and melanoma skin cancer

RICHARD CW MARTIN AND JONATHAN CLARK

An expert is a man who has made all the mistakes which can be made, in a narrow field.

Niehls Bohr 1885–1962

INTRODUCTION

Skin cancer is the most common malignancy in the world. The highest rates are seen in countries with fair-skinned, Anglo-Celtic populations and high sun exposure. Australia and New Zealand lead the world in this regard, where the annual incidence of basal cell carcinoma (BCC) is 788 per 100 000, squamous cell carcinoma (SCC) is 321 per 100 000 and melanoma is 40 per 100 000 per year. The incidence in other fair-skinned nations such as the United States is considerably lower, where BCC is 146 per 100 000 and SCC is 100 per 100 000.[1] However, the incidence worldwide is increasing at a rate of 2–3 per cent per year, making this a global oncological problem. Cutaneous malignancy is divided into melanoma and non-melanoma skin cancer (NMSC) with BCC and SCC representing the vast majority (**Box 38.1**). In general, NMSC is a highly curable disease using basic surgical techniques. However, selected cases can challenge the surgical oncologist either due to patient self-neglect, immunosuppression, extensive superficial disease or aggressive variants with the propensity for local invasion and metastases, particularly in the head and neck. Neuroendocrine tumours, such as Merkel cell carcinoma (MCC) and melanoma, represent a completely different spectrum of disease that are characterized by locoregional and distant failure. The search continues, without success, for effective treatment strategies for patients with distant metastatic disease.

NON-MELANOMA SKIN CANCER

Epidemiology

The most common sites affected by NMSC are the sun-exposed areas of head and neck, as well as hands and fore-

---

Box 38.1 Types of non-melanoma skin cancer

- Basal cell carcinoma
- Squamous cell carcinoma
- Merkel cell carcinoma
- Other rare
  - Sarcoma
    - Fibrous tissue (malignant fibrous histiocytoma, dermatofibrosarcoma)
    - Vascular tissue (angiosarcoma, Kaposi's sarcoma, hemangiopericytoma)
  - Skin appendage carcinomas (e.g. sebaceous carcinoma)

arms. NMSC is a multifactorial disease and aetiology can be divided into individual, environmental and genetic factors.[1]

Individual

Individual risk factors include male gender and Anglo-Celtic ancestry. The typical patient has pale complexion, blue or green eyes, fair hair, skin freckles and poor tanning ability. The incidence rises with increasing age and with a history of precancerous (solar keratosis) or cancerous skin conditions.

Immunosuppression is a potent cause of both SCC and BCC and is seen most commonly in transplant patients who have been on long-term immunosuppressive medication such as cyclosporin. This often results in widespread multiple tumours that are locally aggressive and have increased metastatic potential. This can be challenging because of rapidly advancing disease, local recurrence and numerous lesions. The option of cessation of treatment and probably transplant loss needs to be discussed with these patients. This represents an important complication of immunosuppressive treatment. The cumulative incidence at five years in patients with heart transplants was reported at 24 per cent.[1] SCC may also occur in chronic inflammatory disorders and arise in scars of skin burns or chronic ulcers (Marjolin's ulcer).

Environmental

The main environmental risk factor is solar ultra-violet (UV) radiation, UVB is more carcinogenic than UVA. However, there are several other potent risk factors (**Table 38.1**) such as iatrogenic ionizing radiation and occupational exposure to arsenic and polycyclic hydrocarbons. The important role of viruses in many forms of cancer is emerging and human papilloma virus (HPV) is well established in cervical and tonsillar SCC. HPV is also implicated in cutaneous SCC, however its role is less well defined but appears to be important in the immunosuppressed.

Genetic

The genetic syndromes associated with NMSC (**Table 38.2**) are rare causes of skin cancer but are important in terms of early identification and genetic counselling. Furthermore, because tumours are usually multiple, minimizing the functional and aesthetic morbidity of surgery and timing of radiotherapy (where indicated) is an additional challenge.

Table 38.1 Risk factors for NMSC.

Basal cell carcinoma	Squamous cell carcinoma
Solar UV radiation	Solar UV radiation
Ionizing radiation	Ionizing radiation
Arsenic exposure	Tobacco
	HPV[2, 3, 4, 5]
	Polycyclic aromatic hydrocarbons
	Arsenic exposure
	Chronic ulcers/sinus tracts/scars

Xeroderma pigmentosum (SCC, BCC and melanoma) is caused by a defect in DNA repair and synthesis, clinical features include sun sensitivity, ocular involvement and severely damaged skin. Gorlin's syndrome is characterized by multiple BCCs, palmar pits, jaw cysts, rib abnormalities, calcification of falx cerebri, characteristic facies (frontal bossing, hypoplastic maxilla, broad nasal root, ocular hypertolerism). Bazex's syndrome (Acrokeratosis paraneoplastica) produces BCCs, SCCs, follicular atrophoderma, hypotrichosis and hypohidrosis or hyperhydrosis. Patients with albinism especially develop SCCs. Patients with dyskeratosis congenita have increased skin pigmentation, nail dysplasia and leukoplakia of mucous membranes and are prone to SCCs. Epidermolysis bullosa is characterized by atrophy of blistered areas, severe scarring and nail changes. It presents at birth or in early infancy and BCCs and SCCs develop early.

BASAL CELL CARCINOMA

BCC is the most common malignancy in humans. They typically occur in the head and neck region, most commonly on the nose, but can occur anywhere that is sun exposed. There are five histological subtypes (**Box 38.2**) which are important to recognize because their clinical behaviour is distinct (see **Figures 38.1, 38.2** and **38.3**).

Nodular BCC is the most common subtype and has the distinctive features of a small pearly dome-shaped nodule with surface telangiectasia and a raised rolled edge. As these increase in size they may ulcerate and become locally invasive and have been termed a 'rodent ulcer'. Superficial BCC is also common and the least aggressive subtype. Features include

Table 38.2 Genetic syndromes associated with skin cancer.

Syndrome	Inheritance
Xeroderma pigmentosum	Autosomal recessive
Gorlins syndrome (nevoid basal cell carcinoma syndrome)	Autosomal dominant
Bazex's syndrome	Autosomal dominant
Albinism	Autosomal recessive
Epidermodysplastic verruciformis	Autosomal recessive
Dyskeratosis congenita	X-linked recessive
Epidermolysis bullosa	Autosomal dominant and recessive

Box 38.2 Histological subtypes of BCC

- Types of BCC
  - Nodular
  - Superficial
  - Basosquamous
  - Pigmented
  - Morpheic

scaly, dry, erythematous plaques which are round or oval in shape and typically occur on the limbs and trunk. Baso-squamous BCC is a more aggressive tumour, often ulcerated with histologic features of SCC and BCC and has limited but definite metastatic potential. Pigmented BCC is seen in darker skinned individuals. The pigment is due to melanin and easily confused with melanoma. Morpheic (sclerosing) BCC characteristically appear as an indurated pale plaque with indistinct borders. These are locally aggressive tumours where margin control is particularly difficult and as such have a high propensity for local recurrence. Patients with these tumours need to be counselled in advance that the surgical defect may be much larger than the visible lesion and intraoperative frozen section is recommended to optimize initial disease control.

Most BCCs are low-grade malignant tumours, however massive or deeply infiltrative examples can be problematic in the head and neck, particularly in the peri-ophthalmic region and midface. Regional and distant metastases are very rare and most of these unusual cases will show some degree of squamous differentiation. In contrast with SCC, BCC does not express CD44, a cell adhesion molecule, and this may, in part, explain its low metastatic potential.

SQUAMOUS CELL CARCINOMA

SCCs classically occur in elderly males on sun-exposed sites, especially in the head and neck region (**Figures 38.4** and **38.5**). They may arise from precursor lesions such as actinic keratosis (solar keratosis). The transformation rate is estimated to be between 5 and 20 per cent over 10–25 years with an individual lesion risk of 0.24 per cent. Bowen's disease or SCC-*in situ*, surprisingly has a lower transformation rate of

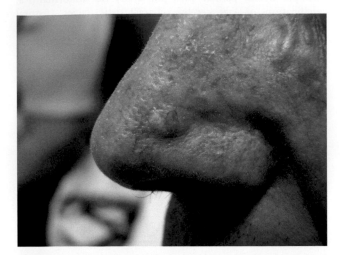

Figure 38.1   Early nodular basal cell carcinoma nose.

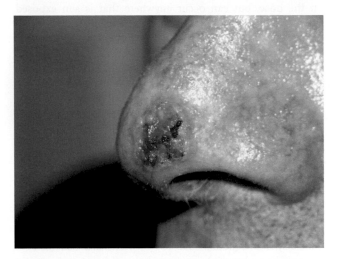

Figure 38.2   Ulcerated nodular basal cell carcinoma nose.

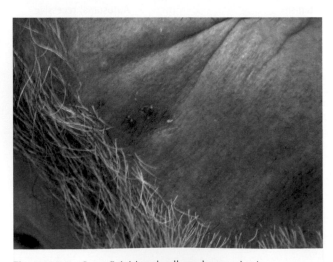

Figure 38.3   Superficial basal cell carcinoma cheek.

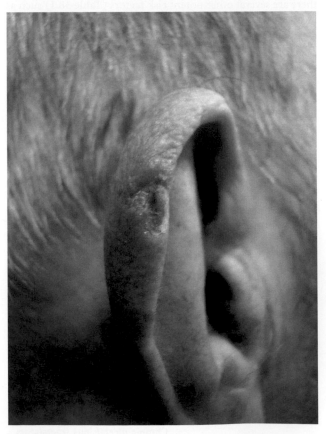

Figure 38.4   Squamous cell carcinoma pinna.

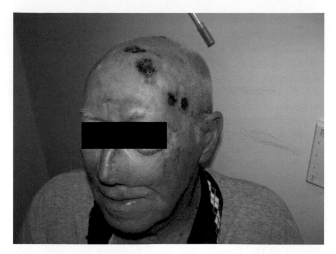

Figure 38.5 Multiple squamous cell carcinoma scalp.

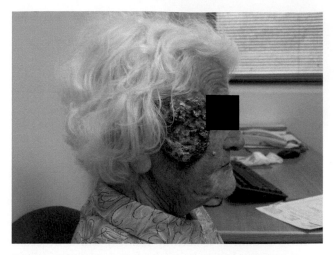

Figure 38.7 Advanced squamous cell carcinoma cheek.

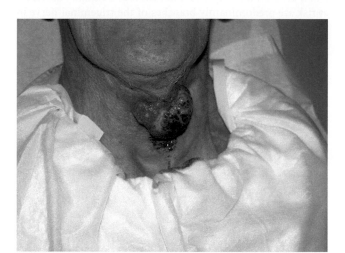

Figure 38.6 Advanced cutaneous squamous cell carcinoma neck.

Box 38.3   Clinicopathological features of high risk SCC

- Size > 2 cm
- Invasion into subcutaneous fat (depth > 4–5 mm)
- Poorly differentiated
- Perineural invasion
- Lymphovascular invasion
- Site: ear or lip
- Incomplete excision
- Local recurrence
- Immunosuppression

---

up to 5 per cent. Early lesions appear as an enlarging erythematous nodule or scaly plaque. Ulceration (volcano-like) and crusting occur later followed by invasion of deep structures (**Figures 38.6** and **38.7**).

Regional metastases are uncommon, occurring in 5 per cent overall. However, certain clinicopathological features increase the risk of lymphatic spread (**Box 38.3**) and these high risk SCCs metastasize in approximately 20 per cent of cases.[6,7] The parotid gland represents an important receptacle for regional disease in the head and neck (**Figure 38.8**).[8] Current evidence suggests that between 25 and 50 per cent of patients with parotid node metastases from SCC will have concurrent cervical nodal disease, either clinical or pathological.[9] Overall mortality for cutaneous SCC is only 3.4 per cent but increases substantially in patients with regional metastases.[10] In a multicentre study of patients with metastatic SCC to the parotid, overall survival was 72 per cent at five years and over 25 per cent of patients had concurrent neck disease.[11] Until recently, the AJCC staging system for cutaneous SCC was very limited in its description of nodal disease and several alternative staging systems have

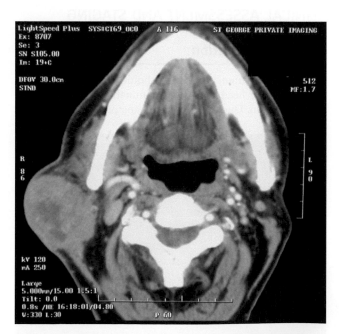

Figure 38.8 CT scan of metastatic cutaneous squamous cell carcinoma to the parotid gland.

been proposed to better stratify patients with metastatic cutaneous SCC.

MERKEL CELL CARCINOMA

MCC is a rare neuroendocrine tumour of skin with approximately 50 per cent of tumours occurring in the head and neck region. The annual incidence is 0.23 per 100 000 and mainly affects elderly males. MCC is thought to arise from mechanoreceptor (Merkel) cells, however the exact aetiology of MCC is unknown. Ultraviolet radiation exposure appears to be an important factor and implicated environmental agents include arsenic, methoxysalen and UVA treatment for psoriasis.

MCC is difficult to identify clinically and is frequently passed over as a benign lesion. It often presents as a solitary cutaneous papule or nodule, and may be purplish or pink in colour (see **Figure 38.9**). Multiple nodules or satellitosis is relatively common, demonstrating its potential for local recurrence. MCCs are very aggressive malignancies with a high metastatic potential. As such, a common initial presentation is a neck or parotid mass. Of those patients who present with primary disease, 30 per cent have lymph node metastases at diagnosis and 50 per cent develop distant metastases. Sites of distant disease include liver, bone, lung, brain and skin.[12]

The largest reported series of head and neck MCC reported pathological nodal metastases in 48 of 110 patients.[13] MCC is associated with a high mortality and behaves quite differently to cutaneous SCC and is much more akin to melanoma. Important predictors of disease-specific survival include increasing age (hazard ratio 6.19 for patients over 70 years of age) and primary tumour size (hazard ratio 7.55 for tumours greater than 1 cm in size).

CLINICAL ASSESSMENT AND STAGING

Patient examination

Assessment of cutaneous lesions should be combined with a comprehensive head and neck examination and generalized skin evaluation. Due to the complex anatomy in the head and neck, particular consideration needs to be given to the likely aesthetic and functional consequences of treatment. Areas that are prone to suboptimal surgical therapy include the periorbital region, periauricular region (temporal bone and facial nerve), nose and commissure of the lip. Inexperience or lack of preoperative planning may result in inadequate tissue margins or unacceptable morbidity that could have been avoided. Furthermore, the surgeon needs to consider whether resection alone will constitute comprehensive management or is adjuvant therapy likely to be necessary. Where adjuvant therapy is considered, the patient should be assessed in a multidisciplinary head and neck clinic, particularly as many lesions may be appropriately managed with radiotherapy as a single modality rather than combination therapy.

Cranial nerve examination to assess for perineural invasion should be performed for cutaneous SCC on the face (**Figure 38.10**). Despite this, many tumours with perineural invasion may not be clinically evident. Motor nerves at risk include peripheral branches of the facial nerve or the nerve trunk division for deeply invasive tumours. Cutaneous nerves at risk are predominantly branches of the trigeminal nerve in the face and less commonly branches of the cervical plexus in the neck, scalp and ear. In particular, the supraorbital and supratrochlear nerves in the forehead and infraorbital nerve in the mid face appear to be most susceptible.

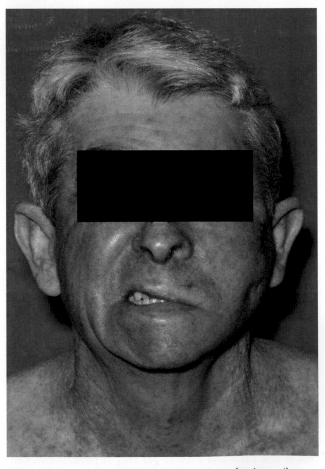

Figure 38.10 Facial paresis from facial nerve (perineural) invasion from metastatic squamous cell carcinoma to the parotid gland.

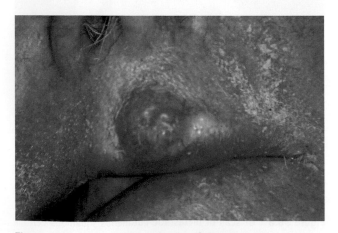

Figure 38.9 Merkel cell carcinoma of the upper lip.

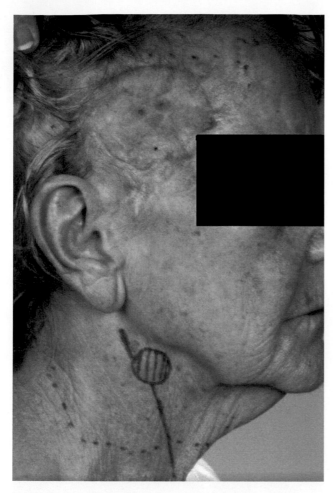

Figure 38.11 Metastatic squamous cell carcinoma to the external jugular lymph node from temple primary.

Examination of regional lymph nodes fields is essential for all head and neck pathology, however the distribution of nodal metastases in cutaneous malignancy has critical differences to mucosal cancer. Lymphoscintigraphy and sentinel node biopsy in melanoma have demonstrated that cutaneous lymphatic drainage is less predictable than expected.[14] Areas peculiar to cutaneous malignancy include the parotid gland (preauricular lymph nodes), postauricular nodes, the external jugular lymph node (**Figures 38.11** and **38.12**)[15] and suboccipital lymph nodes.

Biopsy

The majority of NMSC can be managed without biopsy, but if doubt exists histopathology should be obtained. Excision biopsy for suspicious lesions with 3–4 mm margins can be performed routinely for small tumours in non-critical regions without the need for further treatment. Where diagnosis is uncertain and excision is likely to be morbid, an incisional biopsy can be performed.

All patients with enlarged or suspicious lymph nodes should undergo fine needle aspiration biopsy (FNAB) prior to definitive therapy. Ultrasound-guided aspiration and immediate cytological assessment decreases non-diagnostic

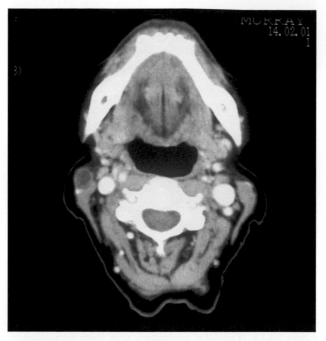

Figure 38.12 CT scan corresponding to **Figure 38.11**.

aspirates and should be performed routinely for lesions that are difficult to palpate.[16]

Imaging

While imaging is not routinely indicated for early stage disease, it is mandatory in advanced lesions and selected recurrent tumours. The technique of choice depends on institutional expertise and the primary concern that has warranted imaging. The standard choice in patients with advanced disease is high resolution multislice computed tomography (CT) scanning with intravenous contrast (see **Figure 38.13**). This allows assessment of the tumour and surrounding soft tissue structures. Bone windows are used to determine cranial or mandibular invasion. CT examines the parotid and neck for subclinical disease in patients with advanced primaries and extent in patients with palpable nodes. CT of the chest has a low yield for distant disease in cutaneous SCC but is a simple investigation in high risk SCC and MCC.

Magnetic resonance imaging (MRI) can substitute CT in all regards except cortical bone definition. It is the modality of choice for neurotropic cancers and in tumours with intracranial, orbital or parapharyngeal extension (**Figures 38.14, 38.15** and **38.16**). Cervical node assessment with MRI is equivalent to multislice CT and we reserve MRI for selected patients with nerve deficit or extensive disease. Ultrasound is highly specific and sensitive for cervical node disease in selected series and can be combined with ultrasound-guided fine needle aspiration, but has a limited role in structural definition of primary malignancies.

There are few data examining the role of positron emission tomography (PET) in NMSC. [18]FDG-PET and PET-CT is being used more frequently as a standard investigation in the assessment of regional and distant metastatic disease. Distant metastases are uncommon in cutaneous SCC,

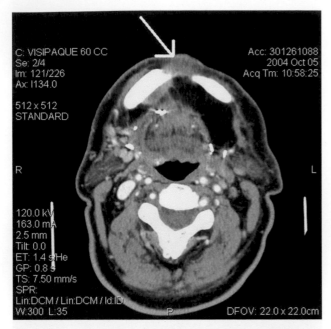

Figure 38.13 Computed tomography scan (with intravenous contrast) of basal cell carcinoma invading anterior mandible.

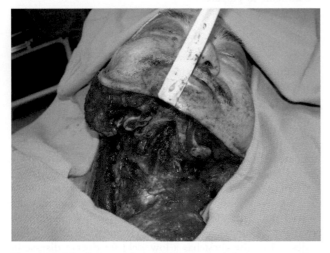

Figure 38.14 Segmental mandibulectomy defect corresponding to **Figure 38.13**.

including patients with nodal metastases, and our preference is to perform a chest CT with the head and neck scan. PET is more likely to be positive in patients with MCC where distant disease is common, although because of rarity there are no large series to establish its utility in this setting. Lymphoscintigraphy is also unproven in NMSC but may have a role in high risk SCC and is increasingly used in stage I MCC.

Staging for NMSC

The seventh American Joint Committee on Cancer (AJCC) TNM staging has seen major modifications in the renamed chapter of 'Cutaneous squamous cell carcinoma and other cutaneous carcinomas', and a new separate classification for

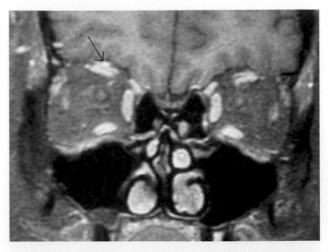

Figure 38.15 Magnetic resonance image demonstrating right supraorbital nerve perineural invasion from squamous cell carcinoma of the forehead (sequence T_1-weighted image with gadolinium and fat suppression).

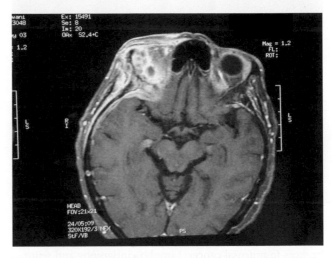

Figure 38.16 Magnetic resonance scan demonstrating orbital invasion by recurrent basal cell carcinoma (sequence T_1-weighted image with gadolinium and fat suppression).

MCC.[17] As the majority of cutaneous SCCs occur on the head and neck, the staging system has been made congruent with that for mucosal head and neck SCC (**Tables 38.3** and **38.4**). The 5 cm size cut-off for the T category in the previous edition has been abolished. Two centimetres continues to differentiate between T1 and T2 (<2 and >2 cm, respectively). T3 represents deep invasion into muscle, cartilage and bone, whereas T4 is reserved for involvement of skull base and axial skeleton.

Previously, the TNM staging system was not specific for cutaneous SCC of the head and neck (CSCCHN) and has had minimal clinical applicability and limited prognostic value. Excluding T4 disease, the only variable considered in T classification was horizontal dimension. N status did not discriminate between the number, size and location of the nodes. This has prompted a number of studies aimed at designing a staging system that could be applied in a similar manner to that of mucosal SCC. Fortunately, the latest

Table 38.3 AJCC staging system for cutaneous squamous cell carcinoma, 7th edn.[17]

Stage	
T1	≤2 cm
T2	>2 cm
T3	Deep: muscle, bone, cartilage, jaws, orbit
T4	Skull base, axial skeleton
N1	Single ipsilateral node ≤3 cm
N2a	Single ipsilateral node ≥3 cm, ≤6 cm in greatest dimension
N2b	Multiple ipsilateral nodes ≤6 cm in greatest dimension
N2c	Bilateral or contralateral nodes, ≤6 cm in greatest dimension
N3	Any node >6 cm

Anatomical stage groups

Stage I	T1 N0
Stage II	T2 N0
Stage III	T3 N0
	T1, 2, 3 N1
Stage IV	T1, 2, 3 N2
	T4 or N3 or M1

AJCC prognostic groups

Stage I[a]	T1 N0
Stage II	T2 N0
Stage III and IV	Same as anatomical above

[a]Stage I with >1 high risk factor = stage II.
High risk factors (AJCC): >4 mm thickness, Clark IV, perineural invasion, lymphovascular incasion, ear, nonglabrous lip, poorly or undifferentiated.

Table 38.4 AJCC staging system for Merkel cell carcinoma, 7th edn.[17]

Stage	
T1	≤2 cm
T2	>2–5 cm
T3	>5 cm
T4	Deep extradermal structures, e.g. bone and muscle
N1a	Microscopic metastasis
N1b	Macroscopic metastasis
N2	In-transit metastasis
M1a	Skin, subcutaneous, non-regional lymph node
M1b	Lung
M1c	Other sites
I	T1 N0
IA	T1 pN0
IB	T1 cN0
IIA	T2,3 pN0
IIB	T2,3 cN0
IIC	T4 N0
IIIA	Any T N1a
IIIB	Any T N1b,2
IV	Any T Any N M1

edition of the AJCC staging manual has taken a substantial amount of recent data into consideration.

O'BRIEN P/N SYSTEM

O'Brien proposed the P/N staging system to allow for better assessment of the prognostic factors and treatment outcomes. Initially, this system was applied to a cohort of 72 patients finding that increasing P stage, positive margins, and failure to give adjuvant radiotherapy was associated with decreased local control, and advanced neck disease had a negative impact on survival.[8] The P/N system was then applied to 322 patients with metastatic CSCCHN in a multi-institutional international trial, concluding that advanced P stage (P3) and neck disease (N1/2) were independently associated with reduced survival.[11] Although the staging system was a major step forward, the model was complex and did not stratify risk well within P and N groups. However, the discrimination between parotid and neck metastases is still important as it underlies our current treatment philosophies.

N1S3 SYSTEM

In an attempt to simplify the O'Brien P/N system and by incorporating the parotid as one of the regional nodal levels, we carried out a further analysis of clinical and pathological information from 215 patients treated with primary surgery for metastatic CSCCHN.[12] N1S3 refers to the number (one or more) and size of nodes (<3 or >3 cm), which were found to be significant predictors of survival along with extracapsular spread (ECS). The N1S3 system shown in **Table 38.5** is easily applied to both clinical and pathological data.

ITEM PROGNOSTIC SCORE

The ITEM prognostic score moves away from traditional models that can be applied clinically to include pathological information only available in the postoperative setting and separates patients into three (low, medium and high) risk groups.[18] It takes into account four variables (immunosuppression, treatment, extranodal spread and margin) that are significantly associated with survival to calculate the ITEM score. In the cohort of patients tested, the five-year risk of dying from disease for patients with high-risk (>3.0), moderate-risk (>2.6–3.0) and low-risk (2.6) ITEM scores was 56, 24 and 6 per cent, respectively. An inherent problem with the ITEM score is that untreated patients cannot be staged and the staging system cannot be used to select patients at low risk of recurrence who may be suitable for less intensive treatment regimens.

CURRENT TNM STAGING SYSTEM

The 7th edition of the AJCC staging manual for cutaneous SCC has incorporated current information available to make substantial changes to the T and N staging criteria.

Table 38.5 N1S3 staging system for metastatic SCC of the head and neck.[12]

Stage		Disease-specific survival at two years (%)	Disease-specific survival at five years (%)
I	Single node ≤3 cm	95	90
II	Single node >3 cm or multiple nodes ≤3 cm	88	75
III	Multiple nodes >3 cm	66	42

The T stage incorporates size, bone invasion and several pathological high-risk criteria (thickness, perineural invasion, site and differentiation). The N staging criteria is identical to that of mucosal head and neck SCC, thus using extent of disease (nodal size and number), but introduces criteria that have not been validated, such as laterality of nodes.

MANAGEMENT OF NON-MELANOMA SKIN CANCERS

Treatment for early stage NMSC

Surgery remains the mainstay of treatment after biopsy to confirm diagnosis. The recommended margins for SCC are 4 mm for lesions under 2 cm and 6 mm for greater than 2 cm. BCCs should be excised with a minimum 3 mm margin.[1] Moh's micrographic surgery or complete resection with comprehensive frozen section analysis of all margins can be utilized in difficult areas where wide excision is impractical.[19]

Radiotherapy may be preferred as primary treatment where surgical excision with reconstruction may produce significant cosmetic and/or functional sequelae.[2] Radiation techniques for small cutaneous tumours often differs from mucosal disease. Electrons may be used rather than photons due to their ability to distribute energy superficially without damage to deeper structures. Since regional metastases are unlikely in small NMSC, the fields are generally smaller and both early and late toxicity is less. Cure rates between 60 to 90 per cent are reported for both SCC and BCC.[1] Despite the apparent benefits of this approach, on average 4–6 weeks of daily therapy is necessary which may have a significant socioeconomic impact on patients. Early toxicity usually consists of erythema, desquamation, pain and crusting which resolves within 4 weeks of therapy. However, late radiation sequelae include pigmentation or depigmentation, tissue fibrosis, contracture and atrophy. This may develop over years and is generally irreversible. The theoretical risk of a second radiation-induced malignancy is generally very small when treating small volumes to moderate doses, but does need to be discussed with patients, particularly under the age of 40 years.

There are a number of topical drug therapies including 5 fluorouracil cream for treatment of SCC/BCC *in situ*[20] and imiquimod 5 per cent for SCC *in situ* and superficial BCCs.[3] Cryotherapy should be reserved for superficial, non-pigmented lesions only (SCC/BCC *in situ*, superficial BCCs, actinic keratoses).

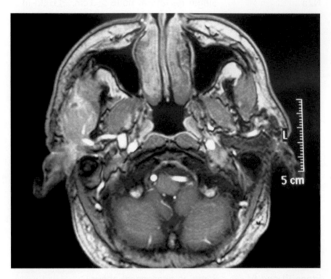

Figure 38.17 Magnetic resonance imaging demonstrating extensive perineural invasion of the facial nerve extending to the stylomastoid foramen (sequence T_1-weighted image with gadolinium and fat suppression).

TREATMENT FOR ADVANCED STAGE NMSC

Surgery

Advanced NMSC (T3/T4) require en-bloc resection of tumour incorporating invaded structures (fat, muscle, bone, orbit) (**Figures 38.17**, **38.18**, **38.19**, **38.20** and **38.21**). These patients should be assessed in a multidisciplinary clinic prior to surgery as many patients will require adjuvant post-operative radiotherapy. Furthermore, the option of definitive radiotherapy with or without concurrent chemotherapy should be considered in select patients where the morbidity of surgery is excessive. A number of reconstructive options are available for these patients, however direct closure is usually impossible. Skin graft (full thickness or split-skin) may be possible for large superficial lesions, but is unlikely to be a viable option alone for invasive tumours where bone or mucosal surfaces are involved. Generally, local and regional flaps are preferable over free tissue transfer in terms of contour and skin colour match which are important aesthetic factors in the head and neck. However, locoregional flaps are less reliable in terms of wound healing and if adjuvant therapy is planned the most reliable technique of tissue closure should be adopted to minimize time to radiotherapy with the aim of maximizing disease control. In using free tissue for reconstruction, a range of flaps is available and

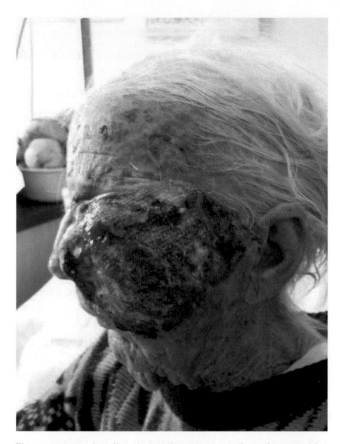

Figure 38.18   Locally advanced squamous cell carcinoma with orbital invasion.

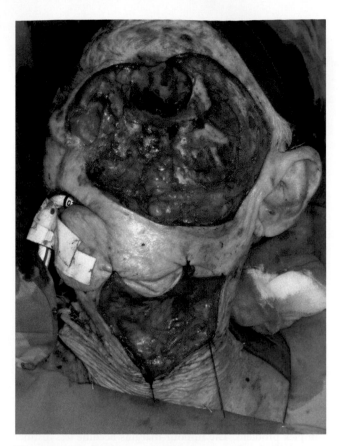

Figure 38.20   Orbital exenteration corresponding to **Figure 38.18**.

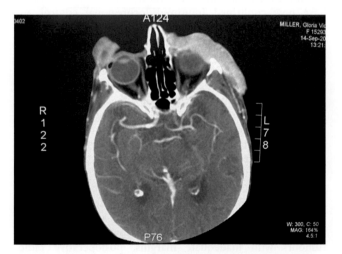

Figure 38.19   Computed tomography scan corresponding to **Figure 38.18**.

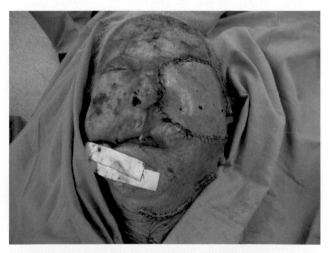

Figure 38.21   Reconstruction following exenteration corresponding to **Figure 38.18**.

depending on ethnicity and patient preference free flap choice should be aimed at achieving the optimal contour and colour match. Specifics regarding local, regional and free flap reconstruction is beyond the scope of this chapter and there are many excellent texts and articles discussing these options.[21, 22, 23, 24, 25]

Management of subclinical nodal disease in advanced NMSC is controversial and there is little high-level evidence

to guide surgeons. In many patients, the choice as to whether a neck dissection is indicated will be predetermined by the method of reconstruction. There is no doubt that patients with clinical disease should undergo neck dissection, however most selective dissections are based upon evidence for mucosal SCC rather than cutaneous SCC. We have adopted a selective technique in the majority of patients with the anticipation of adjuvant radiotherapy in patients who have pathological neck or parotid disease.

For anterior tumours of the face, nodal groups at risk include the parotid, external jugular nodes and levels I (including submental and peri-facial lymph nodes), II, III and IV. For posterior tumours of the scalp, nodal groups at risk include the retroauricular, external jugular, occipital nodes and levels II, III, IV and V. Hence a standard modified radical neck dissection for a patient with a cheek primary will not include some of the high risk groups, in particular the parotid. While location of the primary tumour predicts nodal fields at risk, recent evidence from the melanoma literature suggests a variance in clinically predicted drainage in one-third of patients.[15] Selective lymphadenectomy in melanoma is based on the lymphoscintogram and at risk second tier nodes. One of the most important nodes in head and neck cutaneous malignancy is the external jugular node[16] and this must be removed during lymphadenectomy. Patients with positive nodes in the parotid have approximately a 30 per cent chance of having metastatic disease in the neck.[16] Elective parotidectomy in patients with cervical disease is not generally employed.

Sentinel node biopsy remains a new technique to NMSC but is likely to become more widely applied for high risk SCC and MCC. In addition to providing information regarding the presence of nodal disease, lymphoscintigraphy allows a more selective approach to the removal of at-risk nodal groups.

Surgery following radiotherapy constitutes a particularly complex problem. The tumour margins become less distinct and often recurrence is multifocal. The tissue is indurated and oedematous and clinical judgement can be unreliable. In addition, the pathologist often finds distinguishing islands of tumour within fibrous tissue difficult on frozen (quick) section. Surgery should be preceded by adequate imaging with high resolution CT, MRI and PET-CT. Wide margins should be taken (1–2 cm) where feasible and because of the poor vascularity of surrounding tissue, a low threshold for free tissue reconstruction should be maintained, especially if retreatment with radiotherapy is contemplated.

Adjuvant therapy

The standard indications for postoperative radiotherapy for SCC are close or positive margins, perineural invasion, two or more positive nodes, extracapsular spread and nodes greater than 3 cm in size (see **Box 38.4**). Parotid nodal metastases and poorly differentiated tumours are also considered to be high risk groups. Recent data from the TransTasman Oncology Group Post-Operative Skin Trial (POST study)[26] has highlighted parotid metastasis in the high risk group for adjuvant therapy comparing surgery and radiotherapy with surgery and chemoradiotherapy.

Various radiation schedules have been used for regional metastases, however standard fractionation has been advocated as described below. Data from MD Anderson demonstrated that increasing the postoperative dose beyond a biologically effective dose of 60 Gy increased the risk of late complications, with no increased benefit in locoregional control.[27] Where metastases have occurred greater than 12 months following definitive treatment to the primary lesion, consideration should be given to including the primary site

---

> **Box 38.4 High risk nodal disease with any T-stage[25]**
>
> - Presence of extracapsular extension
> - Intraparotid nodal metastasis regardless of size or number
> - ≥2 cervical nodes
> - Cervical nodes >3 cm in size

> **Box 38.5 Radiotherapy treatment**
>
> - Clinical target volume (CTV)
> - The volume including the site of resected gross disease, surgical bed/scar and next echelon of draining lymph nodes with a minimum of a 0.5 cm margin in all dimensions
> - Planning target volume
> - Defined as CTV 1 with a minimum of a 1.0 cm margin in all dimensions
> - Radiation dose: 50–60 Gy in 25–30 fractions, 2 Gy per fraction, five fractions per week

---

and intervening dermal lymphatics in the treatment volume (see **Box 38.5**).[26]

Chemotherapy remains experimental and patients should be entered into appropriate clinical trials.[28] Several studies have now confirmed improved locoregional control and survival with concurrent chemoradiation in the postoperative setting for high risk mucosal cancer.[29] This is at the cost of a substantial increase in both early and late adverse effects. At present there is no compelling data to suggest that the same benefit is present in cutaneous SCC, however this question will be answered by the POST study.[26] Most studies examining mucosal SCC use cisplatin and fluorouracil in conjunction with radiotherapy. More recently, carboplatin has been used to minimize toxicity. This is important for elderly patients who are more likely to present with advanced disease and will not tolerate standard treatment protocols with concurrent cisplatin. For the POST study, carboplatin is given once per week for 6 weeks concurrently with radiotherapy.

BCCs with close or positive margins are best managed with repeat surgery where feasible. However, for advanced tumours with inadequate margins, postoperative radiotherapy should be considered, particularly if there is calvarial or orbital involvement. Most patients with dural or brain invasion will require adjuvant therapy and there should be a low threshold for treating recurrent BCCs with postoperative radiotherapy. Regional therapy is not indicated in BCC unless there is documented nodal disease, which is rare.

TREATMENT OF MERKEL CELL CARCINOMA

The treatment of MCC depends on its stage, see **Table 38.6**.[30] There is strong evidence from a large single institutional

Table 38.6 Suggested treatment for Merkel cell carcinoma.

Stage	Suggested treatment
I	Wide excision+SNB
	Radiotherapy to primary and neck if SNB positive. (May be definitive treatment in patients with poor performance status)
II	Wide excision+SNB (NO) or neck dissection (N1)
	Radiotherapy to primary and neck. (May be definitive treatment in patients with poor performance status)
III	Wide excision+neck dissection
	Radiotherapy to primary and neck. (May be definitive treatment in patients with poor performance status)
	Consider concurrent chemotherapy in patients with good performance status
IV	Palliative
	Consider radiotherapy to primary and neck
	Concurrent/adjuvant chemotherapy
	Consider clinical trial

series[31] that small volume primary disease (stage I MCC) can be managed by wide excision alone. Clark et al.[14] have demonstrated that disease-specific survival for patients with head and neck tumours less than 1 cm in size and no nodal metastases is approximately 95 per cent at five years. The ideal margin of excision is unknown and has not been shown to alter survival. MCC is exquisitely radiosensitive and adjuvant radiotherapy is recommended for patients with large primary tumours or nodal metastases (stage II and III). The dose and volume of radiotherapy is adjusted to the volume of nodal disease, but typically requires 60–70 Gy in 2 Gy daily fractions for clinical disease and 50 Gy for subclinical disease. The target volume should include the draining nodal basin, primary site and also the intervening dermal lymphatics due to the high relapse rate (up to 70 per cent).[5]

Sentinel node biopsy is increasingly being used in MCC[32] and is probably of greatest benefit in patients where comprehensive radiotherapy is not planned (stage I). There is no proven benefit for elective neck dissection in MCC.

The evidence for radiotherapy alone for MCC is increasing[5] and should be considered in patients who are poor surgical candidates due to either comorbidity or where the morbidity of resection is excessive. Despite aggressive treatment, prognosis remains poor due of the high rate locoregional failure and also the development of distant metastases. The search for effective chemotherapeutic agents and novel therapies has been disappointing thus far and there is limited evidence to suggest that adjuvant chemotherapy should be regarded as standard treatment.[33, 34, 35, 36, 37] Despite this, the authors advocate concurrent chemoradiation for patients with high risk disease. The most common chemotherapeutic agents used to date are carboplatin, etoposide and anthracyclines.[37] Patients with distant metastases are generally incurable (stage IV), and radiotherapy should be reserved for symptomatic disease, however chemotherapy may be appropriate as palliative therapy in selected patients.

CUTANEOUS MELANOMA OF THE HEAD AND NECK

Melanoma incidence has undergone an exponential increase in the past 30 years. Australia and New Zealand have the

Table 38.7 Melanoma risk factors.[41]

Risk factor	Relative risk
Strong family history	35–70
Atypical naevi	11
Previous melanoma	8.5
Immunosuppression	1.5–3
Skin type	1.7–2.5

highest rates (35–40/100 000), three times greater than that of the USA and Europe.[38] Ten to 20 per cent of cutaneous melanoma arises in the head and neck[39] and approximately 20 per cent of patients develop regional metastases.

Melanoma is predominantly a disease of fair-skinned individuals, typically of Celtic background. Sun exposure is the most important risk factor for melanoma, in particular intermittent sunburn during early life.[40] Other risk factors for melanoma are listed in **Table 38.7**.[41] While environmental factors feature strongly, certain genetic defects have been linked with melanoma and a strong family history increases the risk. Mutations of CDKN2A, which is located on chromosome 9, are associated with the development of melanoma in up to 90 per cent of affected individuals by the age of 80.[42]

Diagnosis

The majority of melanomas can be detected by the history of the lesion, and comparison with other pigmented lesions (**Figures 38.22** and **38.23**). Morphologically, melanomas are classified into six types, as shown in **Box 38.6**. The most difficult to diagnose and the most commonly missed melanoma is the amelanotic variant.

Early diagnosis is the key to the effective treatment of melanoma. The ABCD system:[43] Asymmetry, Border irregularity, Colour variation and Diameter greater than 6 mm is a useful tool. Recently 'E' was added for elevation or evolution. Surface microscopy with a hand-held dermatoscope is used by some clinicians to improve the clinical diagnosis of skin lesions. The technique uses application of oil to the cutaneous lesion and examination of the pigmented

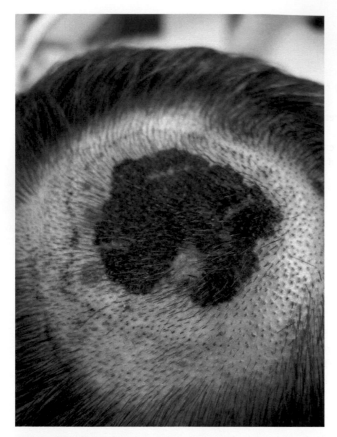

Figure 38.22 Primary cutaneous melanoma scalp.

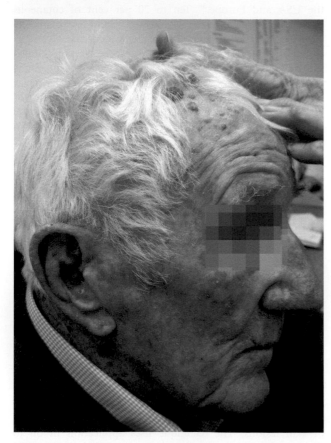

Figure 38.23 Primary cutaneous melanoma forehead.

structures of the epidermis and dermis via magnification and illumination. In expert hands, a sensitivity of 92 per cent and specificity of 71 per cent can be achieved.[44] Any suspicious lesion should be biopsied with a 2–3 mm margin of normal skin. The pathologist will then produce a synoptic report from which definitive management can be planned (**Box 38.7**).[45]

Staging of melanoma

The mortality for cutaneous melanoma of the head and neck is high, with overall survival being 66 per cent at ten years. This falls to 34 per cent for patients with proven nodal metastases and further decreases with an increasing number of positive nodes.[46] Clinicopathological features that predict for nodal disease and mortality are listed in **Box 38.8**.

A new AJCC staging system for melanoma was released in December 2009.[48] The new staging system found that in patients with localized melanoma, tumour thickness, mitotic rate (histologically defined as mitoses/mm^2), and ulceration were the most dominant prognostic factors. Mitotic rate replaces Clark's level of invasion in T1b melanoma. Nodal disease now incorporates immunohistochemically positive nodes and micrometastases less than 0.1 mm in staging (N+). See **Table 38.8** for the latest AJCC staging system for melanoma (2009).

The Breslow depth was devised in 1970,[49] and is measured from the granular layer of the epidermis or the base of an ulcer to the deepest contiguous melanoma cell with an ocular micrometer. Clark levels[50] are not as accurate as Breslow depth, but are important in sub-millimetre primaries when deciding on sentinel needle biopsy (SNB) (see **Table 38.9**).

Management of cutaneous melanoma

MARGINS

Excision margins for melanoma have changed over the years but are still primarily based on Breslow thickness. Numerous retrospective studies[51] and three prospective studies[52, 53, 54] provide evidence for the accepted margins of excision. More recently, the Clinical Practice Guidelines for the Management of Melanoma in Australia and New Zealand have made evidence based recommendations for margins of excision (**Table 38.10**).[55]

Melanoma in the head and neck region provides more of a challenge because wide excision is often not physically possible or may increase morbidity and disfigurement. A compromise on margins is thus considered acceptable in the region.[56]

SENTINEL NODE BIOPSY

SNB for melanoma was first reported by Morton in the early 1990s (see **Figures 38.24** and **38.25**).[57] Since then it has been used in numerous other malignancies.[58] Controversy reigns over the use of SNB, however the majority of surgical oncologists perform the procedure for melanomas greater than 1 mm thick. SNB is also offered for melanomas 0.75–1 mm thick that show Clark IV or V, ulceration, high mitotic count or in patients <45 years old. The only randomized control trial to date (Melanoma Sentinel Lymph Trial (MSLT) 1)

Table 38.8 AJCC staging system for melanoma, 7th edn (2009).

Stage	

Primary tumour (T)

TX	Primary tumour cannot be assessed (see comment)
T0	No evidence of primary tumour
Tis	Melanoma *in situ* (i.e. not an invasive tumour: level I)
T1a	Melanoma 1.0 mm or less in thickness and mitotic count $<1/mm^2$, no ulceration
T1b	Melanoma 1.0 mm or less in thickness and mitotic count $>1/mm^2$ or with ulceration
T2a	Melanoma 1.01–2.0 mm in thickness, no ulceration
T2b	Melanoma 1.01–2.0 mm in thickness, with ulceration
T3a	Melanoma 2.01–4.0 mm in thickness, no ulceration
T3b	Melanoma 2.01–4.0 mm in thickness, with ulceration
T4a	Melanoma greater than 4.0 mm in thickness, no ulceration
T4b	Melanoma greater than 4.0 mm in thickness, with ulceration

Regional lymph nodes (N)

NX	Regional lymph nodes cannot be assessed
N0	No regional lymph node metastasis
N1	Metastasis in one regional lymph node
N1a	Micrometastasis[a,b]
N1b	Macrometastasis[b]
N2	Metastasis in 2–3 regional nodes or intralymphatic regional metastasis without nodal metastasis
N2a	Micrometastasis[a,b]
N2b	Macrometastasis[b]
N2c	Satellite or in-transit metastasis without nodal metastasis
N3	Metastasis in four or more regional lymph nodes, or matted metastatic nodes, or in-transit metastasis or satellites(s) with metastasis in regional node(s)

Distant metastasis (M)

MX	Presence of distant metastasis cannot be assessed
M0	No distant metastases
M1a	Metastasis in skin, subcutaneous tissues, or distant lymph nodes
M1b	Metastasis to lung
M1c	Metastasis to all other visceral sites or distant metastasis at any site associated with an elevated serum lactic dehydrogenase (LDH)

[a]Micrometastases are diagnosed after sentinel node biopsy.
[b]Macrometastases are defined as clinically detectable nodal metastases confirmed pathologically.

Table 38.9 Clark levels.

Clark level	Definition
I	Epidermis only
II	Into papillary dermis
III	Into reticular dermis
IV	Into deep dermis
V	Into subcutaneous fat

Table 38.10 Recommended surgical margins for melanoma.

	Margin
Melanoma *in situ*	5 mm
<1 mm Breslow thickness	1 cm
>1 mm Breslow thickness	1-2 cm

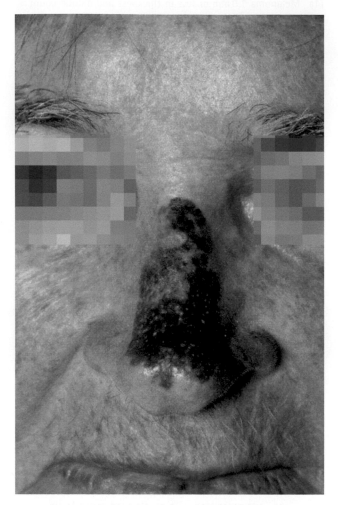

Figure 38.24 Primary cutaneous melanoma nose.

shows no overall survival benefit, but a 20 per cent survival benefit was seen on subset analysis for sentinel node positive patients who underwent immediate completion lymphadenectomy versus those on observation who develop clinical lymph node metastases.[59] Patients who are found to be sentinel node positive should undergo completion selective lymphadenectomy as predicted by the lymphoscintigram. The prognostic and staging information gained from SNB is vital for entry into adjuvant treatment trials and for survival prediction (**Table 38.11**). SNB is a minor surgical procedure with low reported complication rates of 10 per cent (seroma, haematoma, infection, nerve damage).[61]

TECHNIQUE OF SNB

SNB in the head and neck is often technically challenging due to complex anatomy, small nodes, close proximity of primary

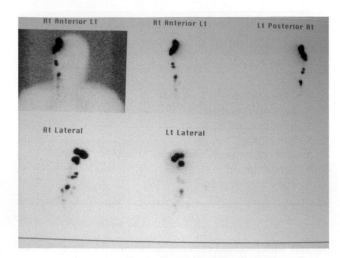

Figure 38.25 Lymphoscintigraphy for melanoma.

Table 38.11 Prognosis of sentinel node biopsy.[60]

	5 years (%)
Sentinel node positive	56
Sentinel node negative	90

melanoma and multiple drainage patterns.[15, 62, 63, 64, 65] Preoperative lymphoscintigraphy is essential to identify which draining lymph node fields contain the sentinel node(s). Technetium[99] antimony sulphur colloid is injected intradermally around the scar, and dynamic and static lymphoscintigrams obtained.[62] SNB should be performed within 18 hours of lymphoscintigraphy.

Incisions are marked out with consideration given to therapeutic neck dissection access should nodes be positive. Patent blue dye (1 mL) or isosulfan blue (USA only) is injected into the dermis around the primary scar. This should be performed once the patient is anaesthetized to allow the dye to move to the sentinel nodes (slow transit on the lymphoscintigraphy may require a small delay). Negative pressure on withdrawal of the needle is helpful to prevent inadvertent spraying of the dye (NB always wear gloves and a mask!). The primary site is widely excised first to avoid 'shine through' interference of isotope from the primary site. The sentinel nodes are then identified with the use of a gamma probe and blue dye. The blue dye is particularly important in the parotid where high radioactivity is found, making the gamma probe less accurate.

LYMPHADENECTOMY

Elective lymph node dissection has not demonstrated a survival benefit apart from a subgroup of intermediate thickness melanomas of the trunk.[66] However, this study did not use lymphoscintigraphy to predict the draining nodal field which is essential in truncal melanomas to avoid dissecting the wrong nodes. No randomized studies have examined head and neck melanoma. Therapeutic node dissection (TND) is considered standard treatment for patients who are sentinel node positive unless they are part of the MSLT II trial, or comorbidity precludes major surgery. Subset analysis of the MSLT 1 trial showed a 20 per cent survival benefit for sentinel node positive patients who underwent immediate completion lymphadenectomy versus those who develop clinical lymph node metastases.[59] The extent of the TND is guided by the lymphoscintogram so that all potential second tier nodes are removed. All patients who are found to be node positive should undergo a whole body staging CT scan or PET/CT scan prior to definitive lymphadenectomy.

Patients presenting with palpable metastatic nodes should undergo a comprehensive neck dissection after confirmation with fine needle aspiration biopsy (**Figures 38.26** and **38.27**). The recurrence rate is reported at 0 per cent for modified radical neck dissection but 23 per cent when a selective approach is taken.[67] However, the routine use of lymphoscintigraphy may enable more accurate prediction of at-risk nodal levels and a more selective approach. As with all cutaneous malignancies, the external jugular node should be removed with the specimen and other nodal groups not incorporated in standard comprehensive dissections may be at risk depending on the primary site (parotid, retro-auricular and occipital).[15] Consideration should be also given to adjuvant radiotherapy as discussed below under Adjuvant radiotherapy.

UNKNOWN PRIMARY

In patients who present with cervical melanoma metastases, approximately 10 per cent will not have an identifiable primary site. A thorough head and neck examination should be completed including mucosal membranes and opthalmoscopy, as well as potential non-head and neck draining sites (upper back/shoulders). Whole body CT should be used to complete staging prior to treatment.

There is little in the literature on the management of the unknown primary.[68, 69] A comprehensive neck dissection should be performed based on the site of the metastasis. Prognosis is dependent on the nodal status more than the type of dissection[68] and outcome is better than cases with known primaries.

ADJUVANT RADIOTHERAPY

Desmoplastic neurotropic melanomas have recurrence rates of up to 50 per cent,[70] postoperative adjuvant radiotherapy has been shown to improve local control.[71] Other indications for irradiation include microscopically involved or close surgical margins where further resection is impractical, perineural spread or tumour satellites.[72]

The current indications for postoperative radiotherapy after lymphadenectomy are listed in **Table 38.12**. To date, no study has shown a significant improvement in regional control with radiotherapy, but an answer should be found with the TROG adjuvant radiotherapy trial.[73]

ADJUVANT CHEMOTHERAPY/ IMMUNOTHERAPY

Dacarbazine, temozolamide and fotemustine are the most commonly used single agents for metastatic melanoma. They have a low toxicity profile and are easily administered, however response rates are only 18–24 per cent with complete response rates less than 5 per cent.[41, 74] Vaccines remain experimental and occasional dramatic responses have been reported. Unfortunately, overall, no survival benefit has been shown. Interferon alpha 2 B is approved for the treatment of metastatic melanoma, a meta-analysis showed a significant improvement in disease free survival but not overall survival.[75]

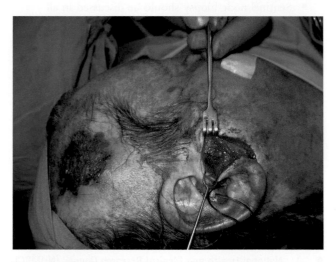

Figure 38.26 Sentinal node biopsy for melanoma.

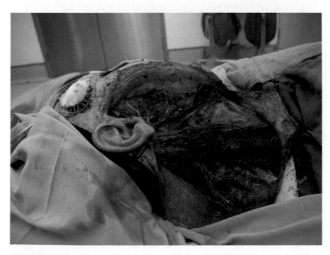

Figure 38.27 Comprehensive neck dissection (type III modified radical) and parotidectomy for metastatic melanoma.

Table 38.12 Indications for postoperative radiotherapy.

Palpable nodes	Parotid >1
	Neck >2
Extranodal spread	
Maximum metastatic node diameter	Neck >3 cm

Table 38.13 Suggested follow-up regime.

Melanoma *in situ*	Every 6 months for life
Melanoma <1 mm	Every 4 months for three years
	Every 6 months for life
Melanoma >1 mm	Every 3 months for three years
	Every 6 months for life
	plus CXR ± LDH

Recently, a monoclonal antibody (anti-CTLA-4) called ipiluminab has shown a survival benefit. The median survival was 10 versus 6.4 months, but there are significant side effects including skin rashes, gastrointestinal and hepatic toxicity. Grade III and IV toxicity was seen in 10–15 per cent.[76]

However, a major advance in melanoma treatment has recently been made with targeted therapy known as BRAF and MEK inhibitors. Only 60 per cent of melanomas have the V600 BRAF mutation required for treatment to work. Dramatic results are seen within days of starting this oral medication. The side effects are minimal but interesting, with 27 per cent of patients in one study developing cutaneous SCCs. This mode of therapy is likely to become available off trial in the near future.[77, 78]

FOLLOW UP

Patients are followed up for a variety of reasons: to identify recurrence or new primaries (melanoma or NMSC); for education and for psychosocial support plus reassurance. Eighty five per cent of recurrences occur in the first three years following diagnosis, and most are symptomatic or clinically detectable. Routine investigations (imaging and blood tests) are unreliable and not cost effective, except for a chest x-ray and a rising LDH.[41] See **Table 38.13** for recommended follow up, but this should be tailored to the individual patient and institution.

KEY EVIDENCE

- Understanding the differences in biological behaviour and metastatic potential of different cutaneous cancers is key to appropriate management.
- Aggressive and metastatic cutaneous cancers should be managed in a multidisciplinary setting.

KEY LEARNING POINTS

- Basal cell cancers have very limited metastatic potential, but less common subtypes may be difficult to treat on the face due to extensive local invasion and indistinct margins.
- Cutaneous squamous cell carcinoma metastasize in less than 5 per cent of cases, however particular high risk features may increase this risk to 20 per cent. High risk patients should be considered for sentinel nodes biopsy or close observation.
- Most patients with metastatic cutaneous squamous cell carcinoma should be managed with parotidectomy or neck dissection and adjuvant radiotherapy. Early identification of nodal metastases may allow single modality therapy.
- Merkel cell carcinoma is a rare but aggressive cutaneous cancer with high regional and distant metastatic potential. Merkel cell carcinoma is radiosensitive and optimal management depends on tumour size and the presence of nodal metastases.
- Early diagnosis is the key to the effective treatment of melanoma.
- Sentinel node biopsy should be discussed in all patients with melanoma greater than 1 mm.
- Targeted therapy with new oncology drugs is showing great promise in the future management of melanoma, however currently there are few chemotherapeutic agents with demonstrated benefit in any form of cutaneous malignancy. Several trials are underway to further define the role of systemic therapy in melanoma and non-melanoma skin cancer.

REFERENCES

◆ 1. National Health and Medical Research Council (NHMRC). Non-melanoma skin cancer. Guidelines for treatment and management in Australia. Available from www.nhmrc.gov.au/publications/_files/cp87.pdf.

2. Morrison WH, Garden AS, Ang KK. Radiation therapy for nonmelanoma skin carcinomas. *Clinics in Plastic Surgery* 1997; **24**: 719–29.

3. Chang YC, Madkan V, Tyring S *et al.* Current and potential uses of imiquimod. *Southern Medical Journal* 2005; **98**: 914–20.

4. Brizel D, Albers M, Fisher S *et al.* Hyperfractionated irradiation with or without concurrent chemotherapy for locally advanced head and neck cancer. *New England Journal of Medicine* 1998; **338**: 1798–804.

5. Veness MJ, Morgan GJ, Gebski V. Adjuvant locoregional radiotherapy as best practice in patients with Merkel cell carcinoma of the head and neck. *Head and Neck* 2005; **27**: 208–16.

◆ 6. Veness MJ. Defining patients with high-risk cutaneous squamous cell carcinoma. *Australasian Journal of Dermatology* 2006; **47**: 28–33.

7. Brian A, Moore BA, Weber RS *et al*. Lymph node metastases from cutaneous squamous cell carcinoma of the head and neck. *Laryngoscope* 2005; **115**: 1561–7.

8. O'Brien CJ. The parotid gland as a metastatic basin for cutaneous cancer. *Archives of Otolaryngology – Head and Neck Surgery* 2006; **131**: 551.

9. O'Brien CJ, McNeil E, McMahon J *et al*. Incidence of cervical node involvement in metastatic cutaneous malignancy involving the parotid gland. *Head and Neck* 2001; **23**: 744–8.

10. Joseph MG, Zulueta WP, Kennedy PJ. Squamous cell carcinoma of the skin of the trunk and limbs: the incidence of metastases and their outcome. *Australian and New Zealand Journal of Surgery* 1992; **62**: 697–701.

11. Andruchow J, Veness MJ, Morgan GL *et al*. Implications for clinical staging of metastatic cutaneous squamous carcinoma of the head and neck based on a multicentre study of treatment outcomes. *Cancer* 2006; **106**: 1078–83.

12. Forest VI, Clark JR, Veness MJ, Milross C. Veness N1S3: a revised staging system for head and neck cutaneous squamous cell carcinoma with nodal metastases – the results of two Australian Cancer Centres. *Cancer* 2010; **116**: 1298–304.

♦ 13. Poulsen M. Merkel-cell carcinoma of the skin. *Lancet Oncology* 2004; **5**: 595–9.

14. Clark JR, Veness MJ, Gilbert R *et al*. Merkel cell carcinoma of the head and neck: is adjuvant radiotherapy necessary? *Head and Neck* 2007; **29**: 249–57.

♦ 15. de Wilt JHW, Thompson JF, Uren RF *et al*. Correlation between preoperative lymphoscintography and metastatic nodal disease sites in 362 patients with cutaneous melanomas of the head and neck. *Annals of Surgery* 2004; **239**: 544–52.

16. O'Brien CJ, McNeil EB, McMahon JD *et al*. Incidence of cervical node involvement in metastatic cutaneous malignancy involving the parotid gland. *Head and Neck* 2001; **23**: 744–8.

17. International Union Against Cancer. Carcinoma of the skin (excluding eyelid, vulva and penis). *TNM – Classification of malignant tumours*, 5th edn. Geneva: UICC, 1997.

18. Oddone N, Morgan GJ, Palme CE *et al*. Metastatic cutaneous squamous cell carcinoma of the head and neck: the Immunosuppression, Treatment, Extranodal spread, and Margin status (ITEM) prognostic score to predict outcome and the need to improve survival. *Cancer* 2009; **115**: 1883–91.

19. Smeets NW, Kuijpers DI, Nelemans P *et al*. Mohs' micrographic surgery for treatment of basal cell carcinoma of the face – results of a retrospective study and review of the literature. *British Journal of Dermatology* 2004; **151**: 141–7.

20. Bargman H, Hochman J. Topical treatment of Bowen's disease with 5-fluorouracil. *Journal of Cutaneous Medicine and Surgery* 2003; **7**: 101–5.

21. Weerda H. *Reconstructive facial plastic surgery*. Stuttgart: Thieme, 2001.

♦ 22. Urken M. *Atlas of regional and free flaps for head and neck reconstruction*. Philadelphia: Lippincott Williams and Wilkins, 1995.

23. Disa JJ, Pusic AL, Hidalgo DH, Cordeiro PG. Simplifying microvascular reconstruction: a rational approach to donor site selection. *Annals of Plastic Surgery* 2001; **47**: 385–9.

24. Pistre V, Pelissier P, Martin D *et al*. Deep plane cervicofacial flap: a useful and versatile technique in head and neck surgery. *Head and Neck* 2006; **28**: 46–55.

25. Disa JJ, Pusic AL, Hidlago DH, Cordeiro PG. 10 years experience with the submental flap. *Plastic and Reconstructive Surgery* 2001; **108**: 1576–81.

26. Trans-Tasman Radiation Oncology Group. TROG 05.01. Post-operative concurrent chemo-radiotherapy versus post-operative radiotherapy in high-risk cutaneous squamous cell carcinoma of the head and neck. Version 1:11 March 2005.

27. Peters LJ, Goepfert H, Ang KK *et al*. Evaluation of the dose for post-operative radiation therapy of head and neck cancer: first report of a prospective randomized trial. *International Journal of Radiation Oncology, Biology, Physics* 1993; **26**: 3–11.

28. Martinez JC, Otley CC, Okuno SH *et al*. Chemotherapy in the management of advanced cutaneous squamous cell carcinoma in organ transplant recipients: theoretical and practical considerations. *Dermatologic Surgery* 2004; **30**: 679–86.

29. Cooper JS, Pajak TF, Forastiere AA *et al*. Postoperative concurrent radiotherapy and chemotherapy for high risk squamous cell carcinoma of the head and neck. *New England Journal of Medicine* 2004; **350**: 1937–944.

30. Yiengpruksawan A, Coit D, Thaler H *et al*. Merkel cell carcinoma: prognosis and management. *Archives of Surgery* 1991; **126**: 1514–19.

31. Allen PJ. Merkel cell carcinoma, prognosis and treatment of patients from a single institution. *Journal of Clinical Oncology* 2005; **23**: 2300–9.

32. Pan D, Narayan D, Ariyan S. Merkel cell carcinoma: five case reports using sentinel lymph node biopsy and a review of 110 new cases. *Plastic and Reconstructive Surgery* 2002; **110**: 1259–65.

33. Poulsen M, Harvey J. Is there a diminishing role for surgery for Merkel cell carcinoma of the skin? A review of current management. *Australia and New Zealand Journal of Surgery* 2003; **72**: 142–6.

34. Poulsen M, Risichen D, Walpole E *et al*. High risk Merkel cell carcinoma of the skin treated with synchronous carboplatin/etoposide and radiation. *Journal of Clinical Oncology* 2003; **21**: 4371–6.

35. Miller SJ, Andersen J, Beenken SW *et al*. Merkel cell carcinoma: clinical practice guidelines in oncology. *Journal of National Comprehensive Cancer Network* 2004; **2**: 80–7.

39

Nose and sinuses

VALERIE J LUND AND DAVID J HOWARD

To see what is in front of one's nose, needs a constant struggle

George Orwell (1903–50)

INTRODUCTION

Malignant tumours in the nose and paranasal sinuses present some of the most challenging problems in head and neck cancer. First, they are rare, making it difficult for any one person or institution to accrue large numbers and expertise in their management. They represent the area of greatest histological diversity in the body with every tissue type represented. This myriad of individual histologies with individual natural histories renders statistical analysis difficult. Patients initially develop relatively innocuous symptoms which are often ignored by them, their general practitioners and even ENT surgeons. As a consequence, patients more often present with extensive tumours with significant invasion of important adjacent structures, such as the intracranial cavity and orbit.

The combination of these factors means that optimum management can only really be offered in tertiary referral centres where expert imaging and histopathology underpin the medical and surgical oncology.

SURGICAL ANATOMY

The complex anatomy of the nose and paranasal sinuses and close proximity of the orbit and skull base can mask early presentation of tumours and compromise oncologic resection (**Figure 39.1**). The ethmoid bone can be viewed as a cross (perpendicular plate, crista galli and cribriform plate) with the two labyrinths hanging at either side composed of a number of individual cells (3–17). The cells are divided into an anterior and posterior group by the basal lamella of the middle turbinate. Both the lamina papyracea and skull base are intrinsically weak structures, with natural dehiscences where neurovascular structures cross. The roof of the ethmoids is largely composed of hard frontal bone, but the lateral lamella of the cribriform niche offers a route into the anterior cranial fossa as do the anterior and posterior ethmoidal foramina. Similarly, these provide a route into the orbit. The rule of 24-12-6 is well known, representing the average distance in millimetres from the anterior lacrimal crest to the anterior ethmoidal foramen (24), the anterior to posterior ethmoidal foramen (12) and the posterior ethmoid foramen to the optic canal (6), but there is considerable range in these distances and the optic canal can be very close to the posterior ethmoidal artery.[1] Furthermore, the ethmoidal vessels may be multiple or missing. The anterior ethmoidal artery is more vulnerable during endoscopic surgery, running across the anterior skull base posterior to the suprabullar cell and frontal recess, often in a mucosal fold or dehiscent canal.

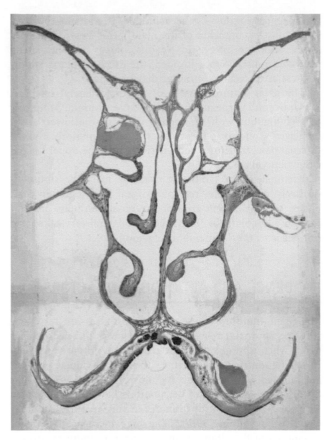

Figure 39.1 Coronal section through midfacial block (H and E staining) showing close proximity of orbit and anterior skull base to nasal cavity and sinuses.

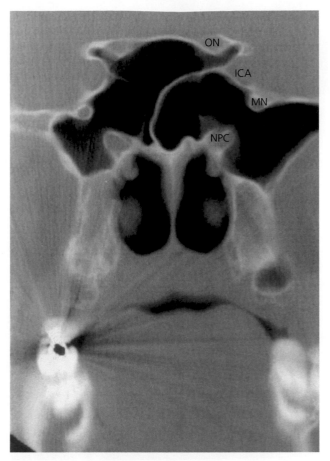

Figure 39.2 Coronal computed tomography scan showing a well-pneumatized sphenoid with optic nerves, carotid artery, maxillary nerve and nerve of the pterygoid canal in close proximity in the walls of the sinus. ON, optic nerve; ICA, internal carotid artery; MN, maxillary nerve; NPC, nerve pterygoid canal.

The posterior ethmoidal artery is usually more protected running within the bone of the roof.

The length and depth of the cribriform niche vary considerably (length 15.5–25.8 mm; depth 0–15.5 mm).[2] Anterior to the crista galli an emissary vein connects to the sagittal sinus, providing a route of spread as do the olfactory fibres passing with their dural prolongation through the cribriform plate. The dura is closely applied in this area and has to be sharply dissected during craniofacial resection.

Behind the cribriform plate lies the jugum of the sphenoid and posterior to this the optic chiasm (mean 21 mm).[2] Tumours invading the medial orbit may run subperiosteally to the apex and thence into the middle cranial fossa. The superior and inferior orbital fissures also offer routes of tumour exit and entry. The inferior fissure communicates with the pterygopalatine fossa medially and the infratemporal fossa laterally while the superior fissure leads to the cavernous sinus.

The sphenoid sinus is variable in size and shape and the optic nerve and internal carotid artery run in the lateral wall. The bone overlying these structures has been estimated to be clinically dehiscent in up to 20 per cent of cases and the opticocarotid recess is variable in depth. The cavernous sinus lies laterally and the foramen rotundum (V2) and pterygoid canal may impinge on the sinus cavity especially if well pneumatized (**Figure 39.2**). Superiorly sits the pituitary gland. The intersinus septum can be asymmetric and may attach to the lateral wall in the region of the carotid. When posterior ethmoid cells extend superiorly and lateral to the sphenoid (sphenoethmoidal or Onodi cells), the optic nerve and carotid are often exposed in the lateral wall of these cells (**Figure 39.3**).

The frontal sinus is variable in size and shape. It has asymmetric septations and may be impinged on by anterior ethmoidal cells pneumatizing from below. This makes drainage into the middle meatus more like an hourglass than a 'duct' and is referred to as the frontonasal recess.

The maxillary sinus is a bony box bounded by eye, nose, mouth, cheek, pterygoid space and nasopharynx. The palatine process of the maxilla forms the hard palate and floor of nasal cavity. Natural areas of weakness exist into the nose via the ostium and fontanelles, into the mouth via the premolar and molar teeth roots and into the eye and cheek via the infraorbital canal and foramen. The medial wall has a large opening, the maxillary hiatus, which in life is closed by inferior turbinate, uncinate and bulla of the ethmoid, lacrimal and perpendicular plate of the palatine. Areas without bone lying anterior and posterior to the uncinate are filled by mucosa and fibrous tissue and are referred to as 'fontanelles'. The lateral wall is thus easily breached by tumours which may arise in the middle meatus.

Attached to the posterior wall of the maxilla are the pterygoid plates, part of the sphenoid. The space between the plates and the sinus is the pterygomaxillary fissure, through which the maxillary artery runs. This, in turn, connects with the pterygopalatine fossa and the infratemporal fossa. The pterygopalatine fossa is divided into a neural component composed of pterygopalatine ganglion and maxillary nerve and a vascular component containing the terminal part of the maxillary artery and its branches. The infratemporal fossa lies beneath the skull base between the sidewall of the pharynx

and ascending ramus of the mandible. It contains the pterygoid muscles, branches of the mandibular nerve, maxillary artery and the pterygoid venous plexus in the lateral pterygoid muscle. Once invaded, the excellent blood supply of these areas facilitate tumour dissemination.

The nasal septum consists of the quadrilateral cartilage, the vomer and perpendicular plate of the ethmoid. Anteriorly it is contiguous with the medial crura of the lower lateral cartilages. Tumours in this area can escape superiorly into the external nasal structures and inferiorly into the upper lip and gingivobuccal sulcus.[3]

Fortunately, the lymphatic drainage from the sinuses is relatively poor to the retropharyngeal and jugulodigastric nodes, but this is not true of the nasal vestibule, anterior septum and columella from whence bilateral cervical spread can occur to the submandibular region.

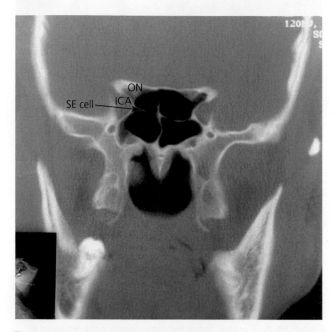

Figure 39.3 Coronal computed tomography showing sphenoethmoidal (SE) (Onodi) cells above sphenoid with optic nerve and carotid artery in close proximity. ON, optic nerve; ICA, internal carotid artery.

INCIDENCE AND AETIOLOGICAL FACTORS

Malignant tumours of the nose and sinuses are rare constituting approximately 3 per cent of head and neck malignancy when tumours of the external nasal skin are excluded. In most countries fewer than 1/100 000 individuals per year are affected but other factors, notably occupational, may distort this. A number of occupations have been associated with the development of tumours in this area most notably woodworking (**Table 39.1**).[4] The high incidence of adenocarcinoma of the ethmoids in the furniture industry around High Wycombe was first noted by Acherson and colleagues[5] and was subsequently shown to be due to hard wood exposure, such as mahogany. Only those jobs, such as lathing and sanding which create dust particles of greater than 5 μm diameter seem susceptible, increasing the relative risk as compared to the normal population by 70-fold, although it

Table 39.1 Occupational agents correlated with sinonasal cancer (after Roush[4]).

Occupation	Relative risk	Suspected carcinogen	Latent period (year)	Histology
Woodworkers	70	Dust 5 μm diameter Tar Aldehydes Aflatoxins Chromium Tannins	35	Adenocarcinoma (hardwood); squamous (softwood)
Leather/shoe manufacturers	87	Dust Tar Aldehydes Aflatoxins Tannins	55	Adenocarcinoma
Chrome pigment manufacturers	>21	Calcium chromate Zinc potassium chromate	–	Adenocarcinoma
Isopropyl alcohol manufacturers	>21	Isopropyl oil	<20	Adenocarcinoma
Textile and clothing	5–8	Wool dust and dyes	–	Adenocarcinoma Malignant melanoma

is not known which component of the dust is responsible. The duration of exposure and interval between exposure and development of the tumour was initially reported as over 20 years in both respects. However, it is clear that there are a number of individuals who develop the tumour with much shorter exposure and lag time.

Other occupations have also been implicated although exposure to cigarette smoke and alcohol appears less damaging in this area than in the rest of the upper aerodigestive tract.[4, 6, 7]

AGE AND SEX

Malignant tumours in this area can occur at any age though the majority present in the sixth and seventh decades with some tumours, such as malignant melanoma, having a propensity for the elderly. When occupational factors are excluded the male to female ratio is approximately 2:1.

HISTOLOGY

As previously stated, the nose and sinuses have one of the largest ranges of histopathologies in the body (**Table 39.2**). As a consequence, considerable histological expertise may be required to confirm the diagnosis utilizing a battery of immunohistochemistry.

The distinction between benign and malignant is less clear in this area where individuals may succumb to the local effects of a malignant tumour before manifesting the *sine qua non* of metastatic disease and, similarly, very large benign tumours may also lead to the demise of their host.

Squamous cell carcinoma remains the most common sinonasal malignancy but it can often be difficult to say exactly where the tumour arose as often the nasal cavity and antroethmoid regions are affected. The majority probably arise in the maxillary sinus (**Figure 39.4**). The degree of differentiation varies and may be getting poorer with time[8] though generally combined surgical and medical oncologic treatment is used. In poorly differentiated or undifferentiated sinonasal carcinomas however, chemoradiation alone may be curative. Rarely the nasal septum or columella are the primary site. These tumours have a particularly poor prognosis in part due to the possibility of bilateral metastatic spread to cervical nodes.

Adenocarcinoma is well recognized due to its association with occupation although <30 per cent of patients with this condition are woodworkers.[9] These tumours usually arise in the middle meatus and spread into the ethmoid (**Figure 39.5**). However, they can spread anteriorly to present with a mass in the glabella or posteriorly into the sphenoethmoidal recess and nasopharynx.[9] Differentiation ranges from high to low grade with a commensurate effect on outcome.[10] Adenocarcinoma is generally rather radioresistant but combined therapy is usually offered.[11] Many patients require a craniofacial but in selected cases have been treated successfully by an endoscopic resection.[12, 13, 14] The use of topical 5-fluorouracil and surgical debulking has been advocated by some.[15]

Table 39.2 Histology of malignant sinonasal neoplasia.

Epithelial epidermoid	Squamous cell carcinoma (+spindle cell, verrucous, transitional)
Epithelial non-epidermoid	Adenoid cystic carcinoma
	Adenocarcinoma
	Mucoepidermoid carcinoma
	Acinic cell carcinoma
Neuroectodermal	Malignant melanoma
	Olfactory neuroblastoma
	Neuroendocrine carcinoma
	Sinonasal undifferentiated carcinoma
	Ewing's sarcoma/primitive peripheral neuroectodermal tumour
Odontogenic tumours	Ameloblastoma
Mesenchymal	Fibrosarcoma
	Liposarcoma
	Malignant fibrous histiocytoma
	Alveolar soft-part sarcoma
Vascular	Angiosarcoma
	Kaposi's sarcoma
	Glomangiopericytoma (haemangiopericytoma)
Muscular	Leiomyosarcoma
	Rhabdomyosarcoma
Cartilaginous	Chondrosarcoma (+mesenchymal)
Osseous	Osteosarcoma
Lymphoreticular	Non-Hodgkin's lymphoma
	Burkitt's lymphoma
	Extramedullary plasmacytoma
	T/NK lymphoma
	Histiocytic/dendritic cell malignancies
Metastasis	

Adenoid cystic carcinoma is well known for its propensity to spread along perineural lymphatics which compromises attempts at excision. However, it can also embolize along these routes and is known to produce blood-borne metastases, classically to the lung while lymphatic spread is rare.[16] The natural history can be extensive, with good five-year figures, but there is progressive loss with time so that at 20 years survival is quoted at 5 per cent or less. Indeed, it is likely that all patients eventually die from this disease unless some other event intervenes. Treatment is generally combined surgery and radiotherapy though there is no evidence that radiotherapy adds any additional chance of cure, rather it delays recurrence.

Malignant melanoma is a rare mucosal neoplasm of neural crest origin usually affecting the elderly.[17] It typically affects the nasal mucosa and presents with nasal blockage and bleeding (**Figure 39.6**). Satellite lesions and areas of amelanotic tumour can make it difficult to determine tumour extent. However, the tumour exhibits an immunological symbiosis with its host which means that some patients may survive for extended periods with residual disease while

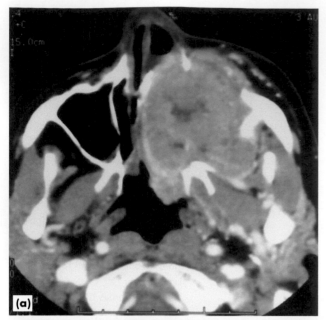

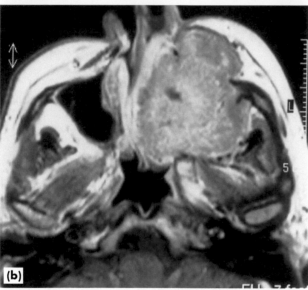

Figure 39.4 (a) Axial computed tomography showing extensive squamous cell carinoma of the right maxillary antrum; (b) axial magnetic resonance imaging T₁ with gadolinium in the same patient.

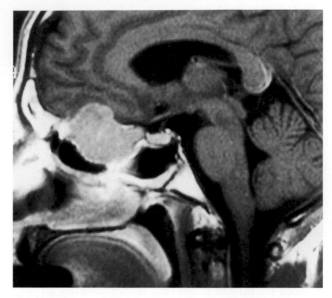

Figure 39.5 Sagittal magnetic resonance imaging T_1 with gadolinium showing adenocarcinoma arising in the middle meatus and spreading into the anterior cranial fossa.

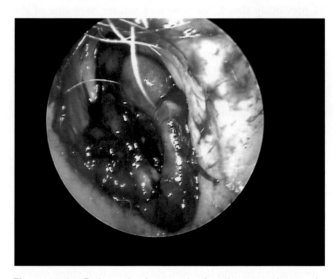

Figure 39.6 Endoscopic photograph of malignant melanoma in the nasal cavity.

others are overwhelmed by disease in a matter of weeks.[18] Consequently, an endoscopic resection is as effective as more radical procedures and craniofacial is contraindicated. The role of radiotherapy is debated but may confer a small advantage. However, this cannot be confirmed statistically, largely due to the poor prognosis and rarity of the condition. In a cohort of 58 patients, five-year actuarial survival was 28 per cent falling to 20 per cent at ten years.[19]

Olfactory neuroblastoma or esthesioneuroblastoma[20] classically arises from olfactory epithelium in the upper nasal vault although can originate elsewhere in the nose. Once considered very rare, with improved histologic techniques, it is more frequently diagnosed.[21, 22] Its symptoms of blockage (93 per cent), bleeding (53 per cent) and reduced olfaction

are not specific though the presence of a mass in the upper nasal cavity with associated skull base erosion is typical (**Figure 39.7**). Age ranged from 12 to 70 years (mean 46 years) in a cohort of 42 patients[23] (though 3–90 years has been described with a bimodal peak in the second/third and sixth/seventh decades[24]). As a neuroendocrine tumour, metabolites such as vanilylmandelic acid may be detected.[25] Cervical metastases have been described in up to 23 per cent.[26, 27] The craniofacial resection was designed to deal with this tumour, which can involve the olfactory bulbs and tracts microscopically at an early stage.[28] Consequently, these are routinely resected in craniofacial approaches.[29, 30] Outcome analysis showed a higher rate of recurrence when craniofacial resection was not combined with radiotherapy so

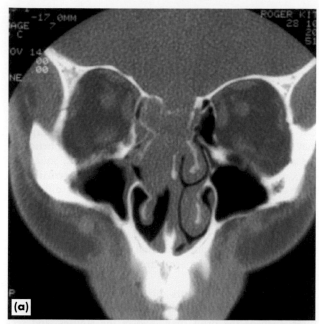

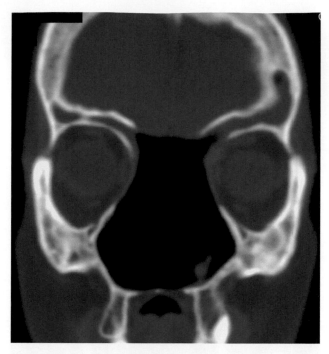

Figure 39.8 Coronal computed tomography showing effects of an NK T-cell lymphoma with massive midline destruction.

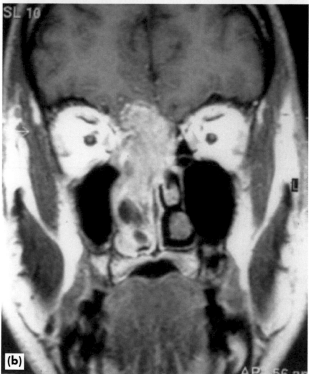

Figure 39.7 (a) Coronal computed tomography showing an olfactory neuroblastoma affecting the right nasal cavity; (b) coronal magnetic resonance imaging T₁ with gadolinium in the same patient showing intracranial extension above the cribriform plate.

this should be offered.[23] Endoscopic resection is being increasingly offered for this tumour particularly when it arises from the middle and superior turbinates.[13, 31, 32] However, this should always be combined with radiotherapy.[33] Adjuvant chemotherapy is also being offered in many protocols.[34] Late recurrence has been observed up to

14 years after initial treatment, sometimes in the contralateral eye or as disseminated dural plaques at some distance from the original lesion.[23]

Lymphoma. No area of histology has been subject to so many changes in classification as lymphoid lesions. In addition to plasmacytoma, extranodal lymphoma, such as sinonasal B cell and T/NK-cell lymphomas present specific problems. Lymphomas comprise approximately 6 per cent of malignant sinonasal tumours and less than 1 per cent of lymphomas occur in this area.[35] B-cell tumours present as an infiltrating indurated mass often affecting the external nose and soft tissues. T/NK-cell tumours are associated with Epstein–Barr exposure and are therefore more common in the Far East.[36] They produce aggressive destructive lesions of the midface (**Figure 39.8**), previously referred to as 'midline granuloma' and a host of other pseudonyms. The most important thing is to obtain representative tissue and alert the pathologist about your suspected diagnosis as this can be difficult in the presence of significant inflammation and necrosis. Once diagnosed, a full staging is undertaken and treatment is by established chemoradiotherapy regimes depending on the extent of spread.[37]

Chondrosarcomas arise in the nasal cavity, often from the septum or maxillary alveolus, and spread superiorly into the skull base and inferiorly into the palate (**Figure 39.9**).[38] They may be multifocal and often pursue an indolent course of frequent recurrence over many years.[12] They may be well differentiated resembling normal cartilage, but the term chondroma should not be used as these tumours are associated with a high morbidity as cranial nerves become involved, sometimes bilaterally, and death results from uncontrolled local intracranial disease. The age range includes both young and old and the tumour is generally more aggressive in younger patients. Craniofacial resection usually offers the best

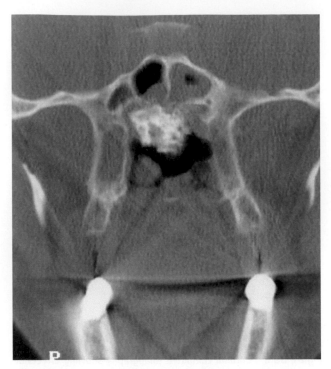

Figure 39.9 A coronal computed tomography scan showing chondrosarcoma of the posterior nasal septum and basisphenoid.

oncologic approach particularly as these tumours are not radiosensitive.[12]

A particularly aggressive and fortunately rare form, mesenchymal chondrosarcoma, can affect the nose and sinuses. It affects the young, metastasizes to nodes and bone and despite radical medical and surgical oncologic treatment, there are few survivors.

CLASSIFICATION AND STAGING

Although various classification systems have been devised for the nasal cavity and paranasal sinuses, these are of less prognostic use than elsewhere in the head and neck. The diversity of histology and associated natural histories undermines the value of five-year survival rates nor are modern imaging and management options taken into account by these systems.

The TNM classification (**Table 39.3**) may be of some value but most patients present with advanced local disease whereas lymphatic and haematogenous spread occurs relatively late, if at all, as patients often succumb before this becomes evident.[39]

There have been a number of attempts to classify according to extent, e.g. Kadish *et al.*'s staging for olfactory neuroblastoma,[40] but these are relatively crude. Histological classification based on degree of differentiation may be of some help in predicting prognosis, e.g. in adenocarcinoma. An interesting study compared the AJCC-UICC 1997, 2002 and their own classification system, perhaps not surprisingly, finding their own to be superior.[41]

SITE

It can be difficult to determine the exact site of origin in tumours which are often extensive at presentation. However, improvements in imaging and endoscopy have helped enormously in this respect with sometimes apparently extensive tumours having limited origin from the lateral wall of the nose. The different disciplines dealing with these tumours can also give a false impression as maxillofacial surgeons may deal with maxillary tumours leading to a reduction in the numbers seen by ENT colleagues. However, squamous cell carcinoma of the maxilla almost certainly remains the most common tumour in this area even if it is difficult to estimate the percentage of the whole group. Tumours arising in the middle meatus will involve the nasal cavity, ethmoid and antrum at an early stage. From there, disease may spread into the sphenoid and/or frontal sinus whereas primary tumours of these sinuses are extremely rare for reasons that are unclear.

While primary tumours predominate in this area, it should not be forgotten that tumours from adjacent structures, such as the orbit may involve the sinuses, and secondary deposits from other sites, such as kidney, bronchus, breast, thyroid and pancreas have all be described (**Figure 39.10**). However, these occur with sufficient rarity to render total body screening less than cost-effective except in the presence of a clear cell adenocarcinoma of the ethmoid (often from a hypernephroma of the kidney) or where there are suggestive symptoms and/or a previous history.

MANAGEMENT

Diagnosis

CLINICAL FEATURES

See also **Table 39.4** and **Figure 39.11**.

Nasal cavity

Tumours arising in the nasal cavity present with unilateral nasal obstruction, discharge which may be blood-stained, a reduction in the sense of smell and occasionally facial discomfort. These symptoms do not always arouse suspicion and it is only when the eye or external soft tissues are involved that the problem may be diagnosed. Rarely some tumours, such as malignant melanoma disseminate locally with multiple satellite lesions on the mucosa and may extend into the soft tissues of the midface.

Ethmoid

Ethmoidal tumours readily transgress the lamina papyracea and anterior skull base, but both dura and orbital periosteum are relatively resistant to spread. They produce nasal symptoms as before and may extend across the midline into the contralateral ethmoid to produce bilateral symptoms. Displacement of the eye anteriorly may produce double vision due to a mass effect or latterly by infiltration. The size of tumour required to produce clinical symptoms is greater here than in the posterior ethmoid where infiltration of the

Table 39.3   TMN classification.[39]

Classification Primary tumour (T)	

Maxillary sinus

TX	Primary tumour cannot be assessed
T0	No evidence of primary tumour
Tis	Carcinoma *in situ*
T1	Tumour limited to the maxillary sinus mucosa with no erosion or destruction of bone
T2	Tumour causing bone erosion or destruction including extension into the hard palate and/or middle nasal meatus, except extension to posterior wall of maxillary sinus and pterygoid plates
T3	Tumour invades any of the following: bone of the posterior wall of maxillary sinus, subcutaneous tissues, floor or medial wall of orbit, pterygoid fossa, ethmoid sinuses
T4a	Tumour invades anterior orbital contents, skin of cheek, pterygoid plates, infratemporal fossa, cribriform plate, sphenoid or frontal sinuses
T4b	Tumour invades any of the following: orbital apex, dura, brain, middle cranial fossa, cranial nerves other than maxillary division of trigeminal nerve V_2, nasopharynx or clivus

Nasal cavity and ethmoid sinus

TX	Primary tumour cannot be assessed
T0	No evidence of primary tumour
Tis	Carcinoma *in situ*
T1	Tumour restricted to any one subsite, with or without bony invasion
T2	Tumour invading two subsites in a single region within the nasoethmoidal complex, with our without bony invasion
T3	Tumour extends to invade the medial wall or floor of the orbit, maxillary sinus, palate or cribriform plate
T4a	Tumour invades any of the following: anterior orbital contents, skin of the nose or cheek, minimal extension to anterior cranial fossa, pterygoid plates, sphenoid or frontal sinuses
T4b	Tumour invades any of the following: orbital apex, dura, brain, middle cranial fossa, cranial nerves other than V_2, nasopharynx or clivus

Regional lymph nodes (N)

NX	Regional lymph nodes cannot be assessed
N0	No regional lymph node metastasis
N1	Metastasis in a single ipsilateral lymph node, 3 cm or less in greatest dimension
N2	Metastasis as described below:
N2a	Metastasis in a single ipsilateral lymph node, more than 3 cm but not more than 6 cm in greatest dimension
N2b	Metastasis in multiple ipsilateral lymph nodes, none more than 6 cm in greatest dimension
N2c	Metastasis in bilateral or contralateral lymph nodes, none more than 6 cm in greatest dimension
N3	Metastasis in a lymph node, more than 6 cm in greatest dimension

Distant metastasis (M)

MX	Distant metastasis cannot be assessed
M0	No distant metastasis
M1	Distant metastasis

orbital apex may affect vision, movement and the position of the eye at an early stage. The degree of diplopia varies with the speed of tumour growth and rapid displacement can be associated with exposure of the cornea, keratosis and ulceration. Involvement of the nasolacrimal apparatus will result in epiphora, again a relatively common symptom. From the orbital apex tumour can spread posteriorly either intra- or extraperiosteally to affect the cavernous sinus with its respective cranial nerves, the internal carotid artery and thence reach the middle cranial fossa. Superior extension of the tumour through the lateral lamella of the cribriform plate, along the anterior and posterior neurovascular bundles or directly through the fovea is usually asymptomatic. Cerebrospinal fluid leaks and meningitis are exceptionally rare and even when the dura has been breached and extensive frontal lobe infiltration occurs, any personality changes are usually too subtle to be noticed.

Tumours arising within the anterior ethmoids/middle meatus can spread into the maxillary sinus and/or into the frontal sinus via the frontal recess occasionally producing a mucocele, though this is a rare phenomenon in the presence of a malignant tumour.

Maxillary sinus

In addition to medial spread into the nasal cavity tumours may spread superiorly, particularly through the infraorbital canal.[42] This can produce paraesthesia of the cheek in addition to orbital symptoms. Tumour can also spread directly through bone or infraorbital foramen to produce a mass in the cheek which may ulcerate. Inferior spread produces a mass, loosening of teeth and/or an oroantral fistula. Posterior spread into the pterygoid region and infratemporal fossa is associated with trismus and pain.

Sphenoid and frontal sinuses

It is not known why these sinuses are rarely the site of primary malignant tumours and are generally only involved by local spread or due to involvement of the surrounding bone. A frontal sinus tumour is most likely to present with swelling of the forehead. Sphenoid tumours produce orbital symptoms, in particular visual loss. In certain tumours, such as chondrosarcoma, this can be bilateral.

Orbit

Over 50 per cent of patients with sinonasal tumours present with orbital symptoms, most commonly orbital displacement and periorbital swelling, followed by reduction in visual acuity in up to 20 per cent of patients.[43] Orbital symptoms are most frequently associated with ethmoidal tumours (62 per cent) but occur in just under half of nasal tumours. Orbital invasion occurs in 60–80 per cent of maxillary sinus malignancies.[44] Iannetti et al.[45] have identified three stages of orbital invasion: (1) erosion or destruction of the medial orbital wall; (2) extraconal invasion of periorbital fat; and (3) invasion of the medial rectus muscle, optic nerve, ocular bulb or eyelid skin.

Metastatic spread

The paucity of lymphatic drainage from the sinuses and the propensity for local spread results in a low cited incidence of cervical lymphadenopathy (approximately 10 per cent of epithelial malignancy). However, this varies from tumour to tumour and may occur at any time during the course of the disease. The submandibular, jugulodiagastric, prefacial and postfacial nodes are most commonly involved by tumours from the septum and in particular columellar region which

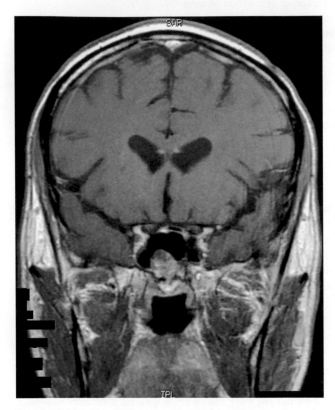

Figure 39.10 A secondary deposit of adenocarcinoma from the lung in the floor of sphenoid sinus.

Table 39.4 Site of origin and clinical features.

	Primary	Symptoms
Nasal cavity		Nasal blockage, bleeding, hyposmia
	Inferiorly into palate	Mass
	Posteriorly into nasopharynx and Eustachian orifice	Middle ear effusion
	Anterosuperiorly into the nasal bone	Glabellar mass
	Externally into skin	Mass/ulceration
	Superiorly into anterior cranial fossa	Minimal, personality change?, headache
Maxillary sinus		
	Medially into nasal cavity	As above
	Anteriorly into cheek directly or via infraorbital canal	Mass, ulceration of skin, paraesthesia
	Posteriorly into pterygoid region and infratemporal fossae	Trismus and pain
	Inferiorly into the palate or alveolar ridge	Mass, loosening of teeth, malignant oroantral fistula
	Superiorly into orbit	Proptosis, diplopia
Ethmoid sinuses		
	Medially into nasal cavity	As above, can cross to contralateral side
	Inferolaterally into maxilla	Mucus retention
	Medially into orbit	Proptosis, chemosis, diplopia, visual loss, epiphora
	Superiorly into the anterior cranial fossa	Minimal, personality change?

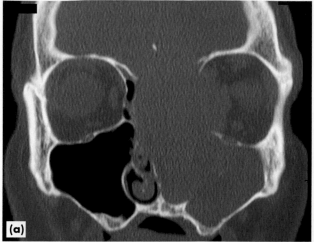

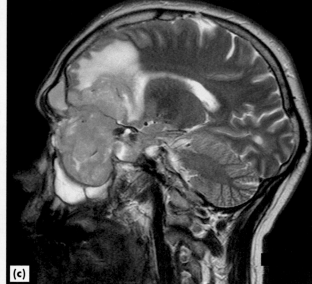

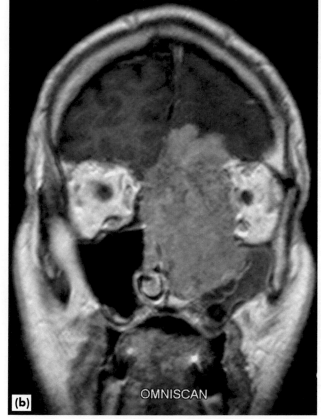

Figure 39.11   (a) A coronal computed tomography showing extensive undifferentiated sinonasal carcinoma eroding anterior skull base and laminae papyracea; (b) coronal magnetic resonance imaging (MRI) T_1 with gadolinium showing the same patient with the relationship of the tumours to the orbit and anterior cranial fossa better shown; (c) sagittal MRI T_1 with gadolinium showing intracranial extension with associated frontal lobe oedema and secretion in the frontal sinus and maxilla.

sometimes spread bilaterally. This is invariably associated with a poor prognosis.

Blood-borne metastases are relatively uncommon but with longer follow up and in the presence of uncontrolled local disease may be relatively common. This is particularly true of olfactory neuroblastoma and malignant melanoma. Adenoid cystic carcinoma is also known to spread along perineural lymphatics either directly or by embolization, often presenting at some distance from the original tumour though patients can survive for some time with disseminated disease.

Thus, although these problems are rare, particularly at presentation, complaints of an unresolving non-productive cough, bone pain or significant fatigue should prompt further investigation.

IMAGING

The availability of fine detail and rapidly performed computed tomography (CT) producing images in the coronal, axial and sagittal plane combined with magnetic resonance imaging (MRI) provides an accurate depiction of tumour extent and sometimes an indication of tumour type.[46, 47] The preoperative evaluation protocol developed at the Royal National Throat Nose and Ear Hospital is shown in **Table 39.5**.[48] Earlier studies suggest that a combination of these modalities produced an accuracy of 98 per cent in predicting extent of tumour, though the assessment of spread through the orbital periosteum and dura still requires macro- and microscopic confirmation.[46] MRI alone is not sufficient as

Table 39.5 Protocol for investigation of sinonasal malignancy.[48]

Preoperative: endoscopic examination under anaesthesia	Imaging	CT	Fine detail coronal, axial ± sagittal
			Contrast enhancement if skull base affected
		MRI	Coronal, axial and sagittal T_1 sequences, pre- and post-gadolinium–DTPA
			Axial T_2-weighted sequences
		± CXR/CT chest[a]	
		± CT abdomen[a]	
Postoperative follow-up protocol: endoscopic examination under anaesthesia	Imaging	MRI[b]	Coronal, axial and sagittal T_1 sequences, pre- and post-gadolinium–DTPA
			Axial T_2-weighted sequences

[a]Depending on histology.
[b]Every four months for first two years, then six-monthly thereafter depending on histology.
CT, computed tomography; CXR, chest x-ray; DTPA, diethylenetriamine penta-acetic acid; MRI, magnetic resonance imaging.

early erosion of the cribriform plate is still best shown on coronal CT.[46]

The extent to which imaging beyond the nose and sinuses is undertaken will depend to some extent upon the histology and patient symptoms. For most malignant tumours, it is not routinely undertaken but poorly differentiated tumours, such as sinonasal undifferentiated carcinoma, neuroendocrine carcinoma and lymphomas require more extensive staging. Similarly, adenoid cystic carcinoma which has a propensity to spread to the lung, requires a chest x-ray and/or chest CT.

BIOPSY

Although this can sometimes be performed under no or local anaesthesia in the outpatient setting, it is generally more appropriate to perform a biopsy under endoscopic control and general anaesthesia. This is most likely to produce representative tissue, without transgression of normal tissue planes in a controlled setting.

During the surgical procedure, frozen section facilities should be available to confirm complete resection.

ULTRASOUND AND FINE NEEDLE ASPIRATE

If ultrasound facilities are available, this is offered to selected patients combined with fine needle aspiration which offers an accurate staging and an important base line for subsequent follow up.[49]

ADDITIONAL TESTS

The accuracy and utility of positron electron transmission (PET) remain to be established in the nose and sinuses but may prove of value, particularly as it becomes more readily available.[50] In patients in whom bone metastases are suspected, a formal radionucleotide bone scan should be undertaken.

Haematological investigations including bone marrow aspirate may be appropriate in cases of chloroma (leukaemic deposits), lymphoma and in individuals where bone and liver secondaries are suspected.

ANAESTHESIA

All the following procedures are performed under general anaesthesia in the reversed Trendelenburg position with 15–20° of head elevation. Nasal mucosal vasoconstriction is achieved by instilling 2–4 mL of Moffat's solution (10 per cent cocaine, 2 mL, 1:1000 adrenaline 2 mL and 0.9 per cent sodium bicarbonate 1 mL) in the anaesthetic room with the patient head down for approximately 10 minutes. The incision line(s) is infiltrated with 2 per cent xylocaine and adrenaline 1:80 000 and during the procedure ribbon gauzes soaked in 1:1000 adrenaline are applied to the surgical field.

In the case of craniofacial resection, patients are started on phenytoin 200 mg/day 48 hours before surgery. During the surgery, manipulation of the blood pressure and pCO_2 are generally sufficient to reduce brain mass without resort to systemic diuretics.[51]

A broad-spectrum antibiotic, e.g. co-amoxicillin clavulanate or a cephalosporin and metronidazole, is generally administered with induction and continued while any packing is in place.

SURGERY

Craniofacial resection

Since its introduction in the 1970s, craniofacial resection has become the 'gold standard' for tumours affecting the anterior skull base.[52, 53, 54, 55] This approach in its many variations offers a genuine attempt at oncologic resection of the tumour.

INDICATIONS

- Malignant tumours which require surgical resection, involving the anterior skull base.

CONTRAINDICATIONS

- Extensive frontal lobe and/or middle cranial fossa involvement or bilateral orbital invasion/optic chiasm.

- Certain histologies, such as mucosal malignant melanoma where extent of surgery does not influence outcome and those where surgery is not appropriate, such as sinonasal undifferentiated carcinoma, lymphoma, plasmacytoma.
- Distant metastasis. However, craniofacial may be considered as a palliative procedure in certain circumstances such as lung metastases in adenoid cystic carcinoma.

INCISION

Following bilateral temporal tarsorrhaphies, an extended lateral rhinotomy is made on the side of maximal tumour involvement (**Figure 39.12**). Many variations on this theme have been described including a coronal flap combined with a midfacial degloving which is generally employed in young patients[56] and a subcranial approach.[57, 58, 59]

TECHNIQUE

The soft tissues of the face are mobilized by subperiostial elevation to expose the nasal bones, frontal processes of the maxilla and frontal bone up to the hairline via an extended lateral rhinotomy.[12] A self-retaining retractor is then placed superiorly. If a midfacial degloving approach is used, the middle third of the face is elevated as described while the forehead is elevated in the subperiosteal plane via a coronal scalp incision.

Through the lateral rhinotomy, the upper lateral cartilage is separated from the nasal bone to allow complete retraction of the nasal ala, and the incision may be carried on into the vestibule though wherever possible this attachment is preserved.

Usually the tumour is mobilized to define its relationship with the orbit. The orbital periosteum is elevated to expose the lacrimal fossa and the medial orbital wall. The nasolacrimal duct is often transected obliquely at this point. The trochlea is sharply detached and the anterior and posterior ethmoidal arteries are divided after bipolar coagulation. This allows lateral retraction of the orbital contents. If the lamina

has been eroded by tumour, the adjacent periorbita should be resected for frozen section assessment.

A shield-shaped craniotomy is performed above the level of the supraorbital rim to include the frontal sinus (**Figure 39.13**). The size and symmetry of the craniotomy will vary depending upon the extent of the tumour but is usually approximately $3 \times 3 \times 3.5$ cm. The bone cuts are made with a rosehead cutting burr or fissure burr until the dura is just visible. Mini-plates are then drilled and attached (**Figure 39.14**). The bone flap is then removed using straight and curved osteotomes and stored for subsequent reconstruction.

The frontal sinus which has been opened by this manoeuvre is cleared of its mucosa and the posterior wall removed combined with a wide dissection of the dura. It is important to extend this dissection as far laterally to allow the dura to fall back as the brain shrinks with the anaesthesia.

Dissection around the cribriform plate and crista galli is facilitated by the use of the operating microscope. The dural prolongations and olfactory fibres are cut using a No. 11 scalpel blade and the dissection continued using neurosurgical patties and a Freer's elevator. This dissection continues until the cribriform plate is exposed and continues on to the jugum of the sphenoid. Tumour may be encountered during the dissection and will necessitate adjacent dural

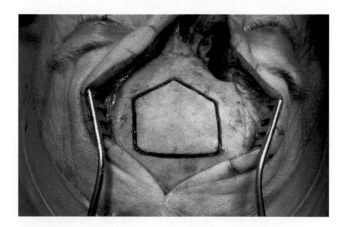

Figure 39.13 Clinical photograph showing shield-shaped frontal osteotomy.

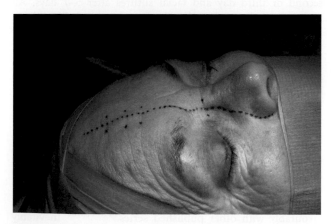

Figure 39.12 Clinical photograph showing extended lateral rhinotomy incision for craniofacial resection.

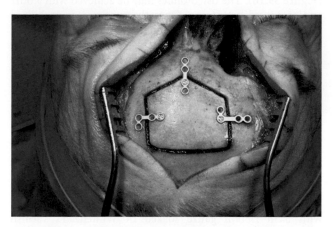

Figure 39.14 Attachment of miniplates to the frontal osteotomy.

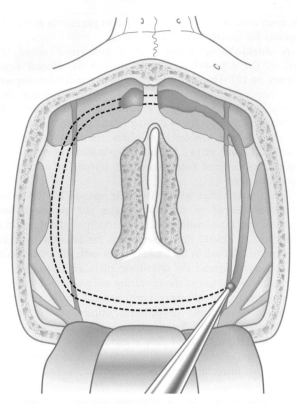

Figure 39.15 A diagram showing osteotomies in the anterior skull base around roof of ethmoids and cribriform plate.

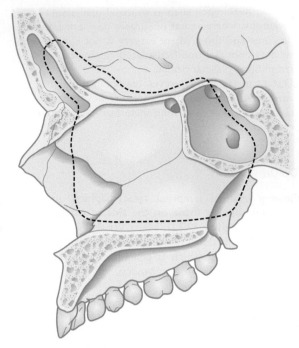

Figure 39.16 Sagittal diagram showing osteotomies through septum, sphenoid, anterior skull base and frontal sinus.

resection. The extent of the dural resection will depend upon the extent of the tumour, but in cases of olfactory neuroblastoma routinely the olfactory bulb and tracts are removed in continuity. The anterior and posterior ethmoidal arteries are coagulated with the bipolar diathermy although care must be exercised as the optic nerve is approached.

Osteotomies are performed around the cribriform plate through the ethmoidal and sphenoid roofs (**Figure 39.15**). These osteotomies are joined to those around the lamina papyracea and through the perpendicular plate/place of the ethmoid. The posterior osteotomy crosses the planum sphenoidale to include the anterior face of the sphenoid and the nasal septum is separated by quadrilateral cuts (**Figure 39.16**). The osteotomies may be achieved with a burr and/or curved osteotome. Once the specimen is mobilized this can be removed, haemostasis achieved and the cavity inspected for further resection. This can be done using the operating microscope or endoscope allowing complete exenteration of any residual ethmoidal cells, removal of mucosa of the sphenoid and maxillary antrum if required. It is advisable to fashion a large middle meatal antrostomy to prevent subsequent infection.

Occasionally, the dura has small defects which can be repaired primarily but more often a formal repair is required. Generally, this is undertaken with fascia lata held in place with fibrin glue to which a split-skin graft taken from the thigh is applied inferiorly. A layer of Sofradex® soaked gel foam is applied to the skin graft and the cavity is packed with 5 cm ribbon gauze soaked in Whitehead's varnish (compound iodoform paint: iodoform, benzoin prepared storax, tolu balsam and solvent ether).[60]

In common with the variations of the incision (subcranial, coronal), a variety of other repair techniques have been described including pericranial flaps and free flaps.

The frontal bone flap is replaced and secured with miniplates. The periosteum and subcutaneous layer is closed with absorbable sutures and the skin closed with clips or fine skin sutures. A pressure dressing is applied to both the head and leg.

POSTOPERATIVE CARE

Patients are kept in a neutral position of approximately 15° for the first 2 or 3 days and then gently elevated, usually getting out of bed on the fifth day. Neurological observations continue for at least 24 hours. Fluid intake is initially restricted to match the inevitable diuresis experienced in the first 24–36 hours. The urinary catheter is removed on the second or third day and facial sutures after 5–7 days. All patients experience some degree of cerebrospinal rhinorrhoea initially so broad-spectrum antibiotics are continued until the nasal packing is removed under a general anaesthetic at 10–12 days. The anticonvulsant is continued for 6 weeks following the operation and patients must douche the nose long term.

COMPLICATIONS

Complications using the extended lateral rhinotomy and fascia lata/skin graft repair are few. Duration of the entire operation is a mean of 3.3 hours and the hospital stay 14 days.[12] The number of serious complication compares favourably with other published series.[61, 62, 63, 64] Inevitably all patients lose their sense of smell as a result of this intervention which has quite an impact on quality of life.[65]

Complications are:

- immediate:
  - convulsions
  - haemorrhage
  - air embolism
- intermediate:
  - cerebrovascular accident
  - confusion
  - pulmonary embolism
  - meningitis
  - aerocele
- long term:
  - haemorrhage
  - frontal abscess/encephalitis
  - bone necrosis/fistula
  - cerebrospinal fluid leak
  - epilepsy
  - epiphora
  - diplopia
  - serous otitis media
  - sinusitis/mucocele
  - cellulitis
  - pituitary deficiency.

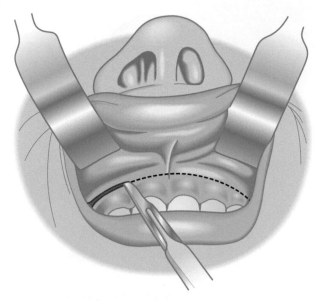

Figure 39.17 Midfacial degloving: a diagram showing a bilateral sublabial incision from maxillary tuberosity to tuberosity down to bone.

Midfacial degloving

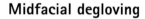

The degloving approach affords excellent access to the middle third of the face and can be used alone or combined with a coronal scalp incision for craniofacial resection or with an endoscope or even microscope for greater visualization. It was popularized by Casson et al.[66] in the 1970s and Price[67] in the 1980s.

INDICATIONS

- Selected malignant tumours affecting the nasal cavity, maxilla, ethmoids, sphenoid, pterygopalatine and infratemporal fossae.[56] A bilateral maxillectomy can be performed via this approach if required.

CONTRAINDICATIONS

- The limits of resection are posteriorly the posterior wall of the sphenoid, pterygoid plates and muscles, superiorly the skull base and laterally the coronoid process of the mandible.

INCISION

After temporary tarrsoraphies, a bilateral sublabial incision is made from maxillary tuberosity to tuberosity down to bone (**Figure 39.17**). Routine rhinoplasty intercartilaginous incisions are made extending into a transfixion incision along the dorsal and caudal borders of the cartilaginous septum, separating it from the medial crura of the lower lateral cartilages (**Figure 39.18**). The circumferential incisions are joined across the floor of the nose just anterior to the pryriform aperture.

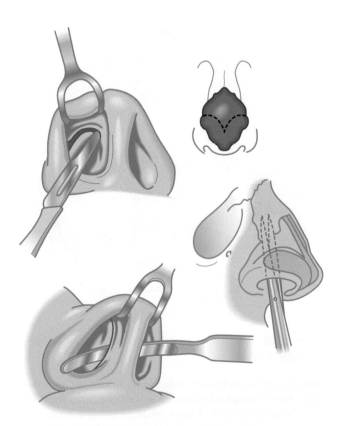

Figure 39.18 Rhinoplasty type intercartilaginous incisions, transfixion and complete mobilization.

TECHNIQUE

The soft tissues of the midface are elevated subperiosteally up to the infraorbital nerve on each side to display the pyriform aperture (**Figure 39.19**). The soft tissues over the nasal bridge are elevated as far as the root of the nose and laterally to

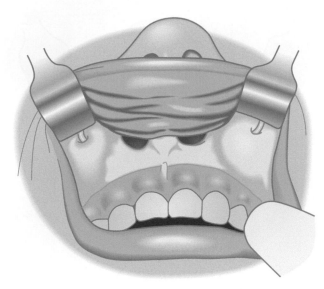

Figure 39.19 Elevation of periosteum from anterior face of maxilla as far as infraorbital nerves.

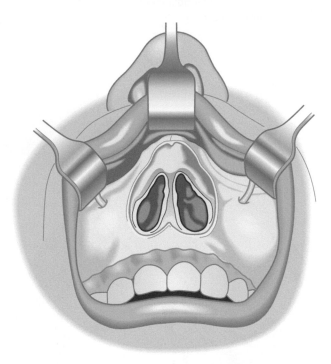

Figure 39.20 Exposure of midface after mobilization of tissues over nasal skeleton.

complete the mobilization from below so that the mid-third of the face is completely elevated and can be lifted superiorly over the nasal skeleton (**Figure 39.20**). Having achieved this, the nasal cavities and maxillary sinuses can be opened using drills, hammers and osteotomes and upcutting bone forceps and thence the maxillary and sphenopalatine arteries accessed and ligated.

Thence the ethmoids, sphenoid, nasopharynx and structures posterior and lateral to the maxillae are reached for further resection. A Whitehead's varnish pack[60] can be inserted if there is a significant ooze at the end of the procedure.

Closure of the incisions must be done with care to avoid complications, using absorbable suture material. The bridge of the nose may be taped or a rhinoplasty dressing applied for a few days.

Packing is usually removed under a short general anaesthetic and patients advised to use saline douching daily until crusting settles.

COMPLICATIONS

These are generally rare and are:[56]

- immediate/early:
  - haemorrhage
  - facial bruising
  - infraorbital paraesthesia
- late:
  - vestibular stenosis
  - oro-antral fistula
  - epiphora
  - septal perforation
  - upward tip rotation.

Lateral rhinotomy

This operation has been available since 1848 but is usually ascribed to Moure in 1902.[68] It is rapid and gives excellent access to the nasal cavity through which a medial maxillectomy can be undertaken. It can be extended both superiorly (and inferiorly) if required.

INDICATIONS

- Any malignant tumour affecting the nasal septum, lateral wall and extending into ethmoid, sphenoid, maxillary sinuses and up to the anterior skull base.

CONTRAINDICATIONS

- Malignant tumours which have spread beyond these areas when an extended procedure is required, i.e. craniofacial, maxillectomy.

INCISION

After a temporary tarrsoraphy, the incision runs from the level of the medial canthus, midway between the canthus and nasal bridge in the nasomaxillary groove, curving round the lower ala into the nasal cavity (**Figure 39.21**). The incision is made down to bone and a subperiosteal dissection undertaken over the anterior face of the maxilla. The nasal cavity is opened and the nasal flap lifted and also dissected off the nasal bones and cartilages (**Figure 39.22**). However, if possible, the incision should stop before the ala to avoid postoperative alar lift.

TECHNIQUE

Through this incision, the orbital periosteum can be dissected from the lamina and the nasolacrimal duct mobilized.

The duct can be transected obliquely adjacent to the sac with little risk of stenosis, although sometimes an O'Donoghue stent may be inserted or the sac opened as a formal rhinostomy. The anterior and posterior ethmoidal arteries can be ligated or bipolar diathermied (with care in the posterior ethmoid due to the proximity of the optic nerve). An en bloc or piecemeal removal of the lateral nasal wall can be undertaken including the pyriform aperture, nasal bones, frontal process of the maxilla and anterior maxillary wall, the medial orbital floor and rim, ethmoids, lamina papyracea and lacrimal fossa depending on the extent of the tumour. Then the sphenoid sinus can be opened and if the incision is extended superiorly, the frontal can be accessed. Orbital periosteum can be resected if required and grafted with skin or fascia.

As before, Whitehead's varnish packing[60] can be used if necessary and the incision closed with absorbable subcutaneous and skin sutures. Considerable care must be exercised at the alar margin to get good approximation and minimize the risk of contracture.

COMPLICATIONS

Complications are:

- early:
  - haemorrhage
  - orbital oedema
  - cerebrospinal fluid leak/meningitis
- late:
  - epiphora
  - diplopia
  - cosmetic – webbing, alar lift, vestibular stenosis
  - facial paraesthesia
  - frontal sinus obstruction, infection, mucocele.

Maxillectomy

A traditional total maxillectomy via a Weber-Fergusson or Weber-Dieffenbach incision (**Figures 39.23** and **39.24**) may still be employed but may be replaced by a midfacial degloving approach particularly in younger patients.

INDICATIONS

- Malignant tumours of the maxilla involving the inferior, superior, anterior or posterior walls. Extension through the orbital perisoteum superiorly will necessitate orbital clearance. Preoperatively, the patient should consult a prosthetic orthodontist to take an impression of the upper alveolus for future reconstruction.

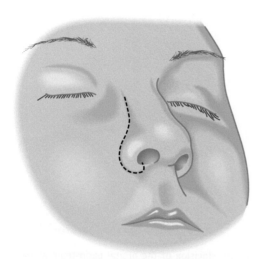

Figure 39.21   Diagram showing lateral rhinotomy incision.

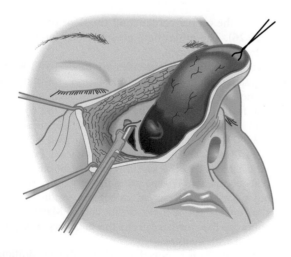

Figure 39.22   Diagram showing medial maxillectomy being performed through lateral rhinotomy.

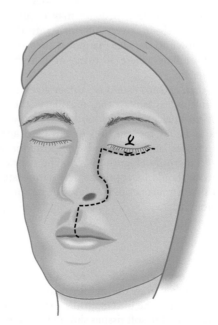

Figure 39.23   Total maxillectomy: classic Weber-Ferguson incision on face.

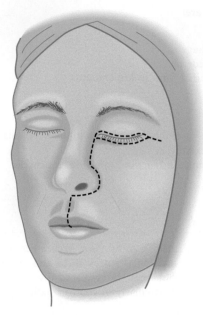

Figure 39.24 Maxillectomy with orbital clearance employing modified Weber-Dieffenbach incision skirting both lash margins.

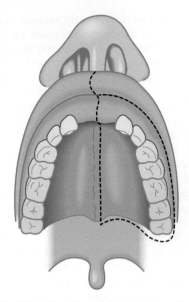

Figure 39.25 Palatal incisions during total maxillectomy.

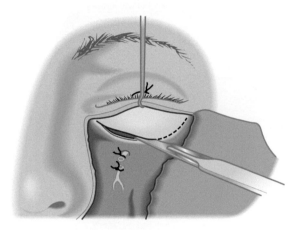

Figure 39.26 Incision of the orbital periosteum at the bony rim allowing dissection of the orbital contents off the floor of the socket.

CONTRAINDICATIONS

• Extension superiorly to the skull base will require an additional craniofacial approach.

INCISION

After temporary tarrsoraphy, the classic Weber-Fergusson incision extends 1 cm lateral to the lateral canthus and medially approximately 3 mm below the lower eyelash. The placement is important as if too close to the lashes, ectropion can result, whereas if too low, oedema may occur. At the medial canthus, the incision curves inferiorly into the naso-maxillary groove down to the alar margin. It then continues medially to the midline where it turns at a right angle dividing the upper lip.

The incision then extends round the upper alveolus in the gingivobuccal sulcus as far as the maxillary tuberosity. Medially the incision passes onto the hard palate between the central incisors as far as the junction of the hard and soft palate where it crosses laterally towards the posterior aspect of the maxillary tuberosity (**Figure 39.25**). The palatal incision in the mucosa should lie approximately 3 mm lateral to the midline so that a mucoperiosteal flap can be formed to cover the raw bony edge.

TECHNIQUE

The entire soft tissues of the cheek are raised subperiosteally off the anterior maxilla from the pyriform aperture to the zygomatic arch including the buccinator. If the anterior wall has been breached, a cuff of soft tissues should be left over the tumour. The orbicularis oculi is left intact around the eye but the orbital periosteum is incised at the bony rim allowing dissection of the orbital contents off the floor of the socket (**Figure 39.26**). The infraorbital neurovascular bundle is cut at the infraorbital foramen.

To free the maxilla, osteotomies are made (with a drill, oscillating saw, Gigli saw or osteotomes) through the zygoma, beneath the infraorbital rim if the eye is being preserved, across the frontal process of the maxilla, into the pyriform fossa, and inferiorly through the central upper alveolus (**Figure 39.27**). The lateral nasal wall is divided below the superior turbinate. The hard palate is transected from front to back, just medial to the septum and the mobilization of the maxilla completed by separating the tuberosity from the pterygoid plates with a curved osteotome. Additional soft tissue attachments can be divided with curved Mayo scissors. Once removed, haemorrhage from the maxillary artery can be controlled with ligatures.

Once the maxilla is removed, together with any additional surrounding tissues if involved, a variety of reconstructions are available. At its simplest, a split-skin graft can be applied to the

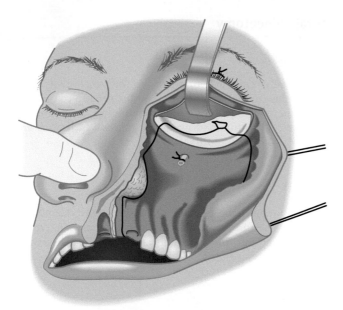

Figure 39.27 Osteotomies through zygoma, floor of orbit, frontal process of maxilla and cribriform aperture.

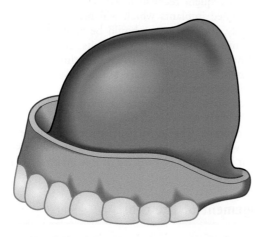

Figure 39.28 Temporary gutta percha prosthesis.

cavity walls held in place with quilting incisions, biological glues, a Whitehead's varnish pack[60] and a temporary gutta percha prosthesis (**Figure 39.28**). Alternatively, a free flap can be utilized, e.g. rectus abdominis, latissimus dorsi, radial or fibula osteocutaneous flaps with osseointegration.[69, 70, 71, 72] Other methods include vascularized calvarial bone flaps[73] and coronoid-temporalis pedicled rotation flaps.[74] Whatever is used, it is important that the patient can eat and speak in the immediate postoperative period. Closure of the flap can then be effected with absorbable subcutaneous and skin sutures, taking especial care at the vermillion border. A light pressure dressing is usually applied.

Repairing lost orbital support decreases the risk of globe malposition, diplopia and disturbance of extraocular muscle function.[75] Small defects in the floor can be left, larger ones can be repaired using a fascia lata sling secured to the margins of the bony defect. Subtotal or complete defects require some form of rigid reconstruction.

Initial refashioning of an artificial prosthesis is usually undertaken under general anaesthetic and thereafter a permanent prosthesis/denture is made once the cavity has healed complemented by osseointegration.

Extensive spread of the tumour anteriorly into the facial skin may necessitate sacrifice of this with repair using a local pedicled or free microvascular flap. More frequently, extension occurs posteriorly into the pterygoid region which adversely affects prognosis. Limited areas of pterygoid muscle can be removed, but a partial mandibulectomy may be required.[76] Further clearance of the pterygopalatine and infratemporal fossae can be undertaken, bearing in mind the close relationship of the internal carotid artery.

COMPLICATIONS

Complications are:

- early:
  - haemorrhage
  - infection
- late:
  - epiphora
  - paraesthesia
  - ectropion or lower lid oedema
  - facial contracture, notching of the lip
  - diplopia.

Endoscopic resection

Since its introduction, endoscopic sinus surgery has been extended to the skull base and orbit. The ability to repair skull base defects and resect orbital periosteum has facilitated the use of this approach alone or in combination with a craniotomy in the management of selected malignant sinonasal tumours.[77, 78] The principle of complete excision of the tumour must be observed and the options discussed with the patient, who should understand that a craniofacial may still be required if there is significant dural invasion and/or infiltration of the superior sagittal sinus. Endoscopic resection should not be employed or regarded as a 'smaller' operation but rather an equivalent resection via an endonasal route.

TECHNIQUE

A complete resection of the tumour is undertaken including a wide field clearance of adjacent mucosa, bone and cartilage. On the skull base, the bone and dural defects can be repaired using combinations of fascia, pinna cartilage and contralateral nasal mucosa dependent on the size of the defect.[79, 80] Ipsilateral septal mucosal flaps are less useful in malignant disease due to the possibility of field-change. Similarly, orbital periosteum can be resected and repaired with contralateral mucosa or a split skin graft held with fibrin glue, gelatin sponge and a Whitehead's varnish pack.[60] In practice, a complete fronto-ethmo-sphenoidectomy is generally undertaken (Draf III), combined with removal of the lateral nasal wall (at the least, including a middle meatal antrostomy) and/or septal resection as dictated by the tumour extent

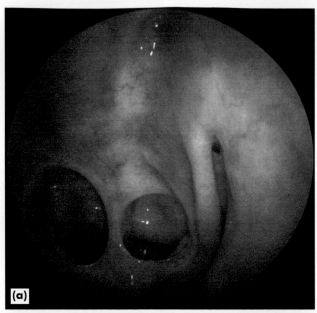

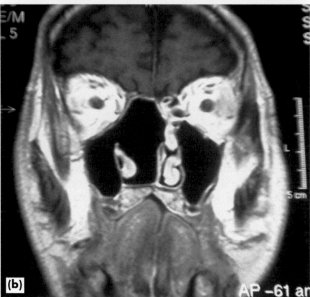

Figure 39.29 (a) Postoperative endoscopic view of cavity after endoscopic resection of an adenocarcinoma five years at follow up; (b) coronal magnetic resonance imaging T_1 with gadolinium in the same patient.

(**Figure 39.29**). It is technically possible to undertake an endoscopic craniofacial resection in selected cases. Image guidance is frequently employed. The advent of neuroendoscopic techniques is pushing the boundaries of what can be resected via an endonasal approach, though careful patient selection is paramount to maximize cure and minimize morbidity.[81]

COMPLICATIONS

Theoretically, these are the same as for craniofacial but in practice are negligible and the patients generally have a very low morbidity and short hospital stay.

Total rhinectomy

INDICATIONS

Occasionally, extensive tumours in the nasal cavity will involve the external nose resulting in the need to completely excise the nose. Squamous cell carcinoma of the columella, vestibule and septum and malignant mucosal melanoma are the most common culprits.

INCISION

A cut down to bone is made circumferentially around the pyriform aperture remembering that tumour can escape submucosally into the upper lip and premaxilla so a wide margin is recommended.

TECHNIQUE

The entire nasal mucosal cuff can be removed together with septum, lateral wall and floor as dictated by the tumour. If it is possible to retain any portion of the nasal bone, this will facilitate subsequent reconstruction and allow placement of osseointegrated implants which will need to be covered by skin. Ideally, the skin edge should be approximated to any residual mucosa and while skin grafts may be applied to exposed bone, this will mucosalize with time.

A Whitehead's pack[60] is placed in the cavity for a few days and can usually be removed under sedation.

Reconstruction may involve a palatal prosthesis if the premaxilla has been resected, often achieved by modifying an existing denture. The superstructure of the nose can be replaced with an artifical prosthesis secured by osseointegration or by a variety of pedicled or free microvascular flaps.

Management of the orbit

Involvement of the orbit is an important predictor of recurrence-free, disease-specific and overall survival. As a consequence, in the past if tumour had reached the orbital periosteum the patient was advised to have the eye removed. However, it is increasingly apparent that a more conservative strategy can be adopted without adversely affecting outcome. Therefore, in most instances if tumour has eroded the lamina, is abutting the perisoteum but has not penetrated into the orbital fat, the periosteum can be widely resected and repaired with split skin or fascia. The position of the eye can be maintained with a Whitehead's pack[60] while healing takes place and significant enophthalmos avoided. Frozen section is invaluable in making this assessment preoperatively as even the most accurate imaging cannot absolutely predict whether the periosteum has been breached (**Figure 39.30**).

In the presence of intraperiosteal spread, in cases where cure is possible, the eye should be sacrificed. In most cases, the eyelids can be spared as sinonasal tumours rarely spread pre-septally and there is no lymphatic drainage anteriorly. This constitutes orbital clearance as opposed to orbital exenteration where the lids are also sacrificed. The lids are incised leaving the lash margin on the specimen and the

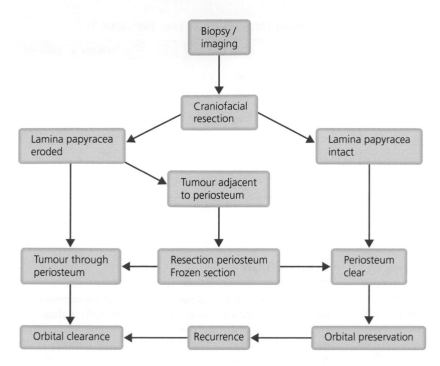

Figure 39.30 The management algorithm of the orbit.

skin and subcutaneous tissues of the lid are dissected free of the tarsal plates. A circumferential incision is made around the socket, down to bone and the canthal ligaments divided. The periosteum is then elevated using a Freer and ribbon gauze soaked in 1:1000 adrenaline. Care should be taken not to extend out through the fissures. Once the orbital contents are mobilized, the apex is divided with curved Mayo scissors. The anaesthetist should be warned as patients often develop a marked bradycardia as the optic nerve is cut. Significant bleeding is encountered from the ophthalmic artery though this quickly vasoconstricts. It is advisable to put a stay suture through the optic neurovascular bundle, not only for haemostasis but also to close the cerebrospinal fluid space around the nerve.

Primary osseointegrated implants may be placed in the orbital rim but may take up to a year to integrate, especially if radiotherapy is given. The socket is filled with a portion of the Whitehead's pack and the lids are sutured together using fine absorbable sutures. An orbital prosthesis can be applied once the lids have sunk back to form a skin-lined socket, initially held with adhesives or on a spectacle frame while integration takes place.

After orbital exenteration or if the lids fistularize, the socket may be filled with a temporalis muscle flap to which a split-skin graft can be applied or a variety of free microvascular flaps used.[82, 83]

FOLLOW UP

The lack of specific symptoms and involvement of silent areas combined with a natural history spanning a lifetime, makes careful long-term follow up mandatory. A protocol has been developed which may be modified depending on the histology and patient but involves regular endoscopic examination, initially performed as a formal examination under anaesthesia combined with biopsy and regular MRI (**Table 39.5**). It is not possible to determine the cost-effectiveness of this approach, suffice to say that patients have been diagnosed with recurrence and salvaged over ten years after their initial presentation.

Outcome and prognosis

While lateral rhinotomy, rhinectomy and midfacial degloving still have a role for selected malignancies, craniofacial resection has dramatically improved the outcome for those tumours affecting the anterior skull base. In a cohort of 308 patients undergoing craniofacial resection, the follow up ranged from 6 to 259 months (mean 63 months).[12] There were 259 patients with malignant tumours in whom the actuarial disease-free survival was 59 per cent at five years dropping to 40 per cent at ten years and 33 per cent at 15 years. Placing these results in context, the five-year survival figure for olfactory neuroblastoma prior to craniofacial was 35 per cent and is now 74 per cent. In other words, craniofacial resection has doubled the survival for many of these rare tumours. However, late recurrence can be seen in most tumours (**Table 39.6**) which emphasizes the fallibility of five-year actuarial survival in predicting cure.

Multivariant analysis unsurprisingly identifies brain involvement, type of malignancy and orbital involvement as the three most significant prognostic factors.[12, 61, 84, 85] This applies to the nasal cavity[86, 87] and maxillary sinus tumours[88, 89] as well as those in the ethmoid. However, survival is not affected when invasion is limited to orbital periosteum and this is resected, with orbital preservation.[12, 75, 90]

By contrast, involvement of the orbital apex significantly reduces survival even if orbital clearance is undertaken.[91] In 170 patients with orbital invasion by squamous cell carcinoma, five-year survival and local recurrence were 41 and 20 per cent when the eye was preserved compared to 37 and

Table 39.6 Craniofacial resection: actuarial survival for whole group and individual histologies comparing 1997–2004.[12]

Histology	5 Year (%)	10 Year (%)	15 Year (%)	Number of patients
Overall	65	47	41	308
Benign	92	82	76	49
Malignant	59	40	33	259
Adenocarcinoma	58	40	33	62
Olfactory neuroblastoma	74	50	40	56
Squamous cell carcinoma	53	35	35	34
Chondrosarcoma	94	56	37	24
Adenoid cystic carcinoma	61	31	31	19

36 per cent when the eye was removed.[44] The impact of orbital invasion on survival can also be related to tumour type. Nishino et al.[92] reported a five-year overall survival of 74 per cent for squamous cell carcinoma versus 40 per cent for non-squamous tumours where limited orbital invasion was treated with combined therapy but orbital preservation.

However, timing of radiotherapy does not seem to affect outcome with no statistical difference demonstrated between those receiving this preoperatively and those treated post-operatively ($p = 0.87$).[12]

The most frequent recurrence is local and was amenable to treatment with intention to cure in 14 per cent of our series, most of whom underwent surgery in the form of revision craniofacial resection.[12] This can be repeated, in some cases on numerous occasions, with minimal morbidity and emphasizes the palliative role of the procedure.

Fewer patients have undergone endoscopic resection, with limited follow up to date, so it is not possible to make meaningful comparisons with alternative approaches and statistically robust actuarial survival data are difficult to obtain. Patients are necessarily selected for their limited disease so one would anticipate similar if not better results and this appears to be the case in emerging series.[13, 14, 31, 32, 93, 94, 95] In addition, there are obvious advantages in terms of morbidity, hospital stay and the ability to start chemoradiation shortly after surgery. However, the principle of oncologic resection must be observed wherever possible and the full menu of surgical approaches available if the excellent results of recent years are to be maintained.

SPECIAL CONSIDERATIONS IN CHILDREN

Most malignant sinonasal tumours, albeit rarely, can affect children and should be excluded in any case of unilateral obstruction. Rhabdomyosarcoma is the most common and good results are now obtained using a protocol of chemor-adiation with surgery, though this is often reserved for sal-vage. Embryonal and botryoid subtypes are most common in the young. These represent a better prognosis than alveolar and undifferentiated types.[96]

If radical surgery is required, it may be undertaken without significant deleterious effects on facial development as long as the cartilaginous septum, upper lateral cartilages and palate are preserved.[97]

CONCLUSION

There have been tremendous strides in the management of malignant tumours in the sinonasal region, both in diagnosis and treatment with improvement in outcome while mini-mizing morbidity.[95, 98] The task is to identify patients at the earliest opportunity in order to give them the best chance of survival from these rare and distressing conditions.

KEY EVIDENCE

- Epidemiological studies confirm an association between adenocarcinoma of the ethmoids and the woodworking industry.[5]
- Prognosis in the anterior skull base relates to the spread into brain, orbit and the type of malignancy.[12]
- Craniofacial remains the gold standard by which other treatment strategies must be measured, but prospective data on endoscopic resection is increasing.[12, 95]

KEY LEARNING POINTS

- Malignant tumours of the nose and sinuses are rare and present late due to initially innocuous symptoms.
- These tumours have the greatest histological diversity with individual natural histories.
- Their management requires expertise in histopathology imaging, as well as surgical and medical oncology.
- Rehabilitation may require prostheses and a range of reconstructive techniques, as well psychological support for the patient.
- Survival has doubled for a number of tumours since the introduction of craniofacial resection.

- In selected patients, an endoscopic approach may be employed to perform surgical exenteration of the tumour.
- All patients require long-term follow up including endoscopic examination and imaging.

REFERENCES

1. Rontal E, Rontal M, Guildford FT. Surgical anatomy of the orbit. *Annals of Otology, Rhinology and Laryngology* 1979; **88**: 382–6.
2. Lang J. *Clinical anatomy of the nose, nasal cavity and paranasal sinuses.* New York: Thieme, 1989; 65, 82.
3. Gullane PJ, Conley J. Carcinoma of the maxillary sinus. A correlation of the clinical course with orbital involvement, pterygoid erosion or pterygopalatine invasion and cervical metastases. *Journal of Otolaryngology* 1983; **12**: 141–5.
♦ 4. Roush GC. Epidemiology of cancer of the nose and paranasal sinuses. Current concepts. *Head and Neck Surgery* 1979; **2**: 3–11.
● 5. Acherson E, Cowdell R, Rang E. Adenocarcinoma of the nasal cavity and sinuses in England and Wales. *British Journal of Industrial Medicine* 1972; **29**: 21–30.
6. Holmstrom M, Lund V. Malignant melanoma of the nasal cavity following occupational exposure to formaldehyde. *British Journal of Industrial Medicine* 1991; **48**: 9–11.
7. Lund VJ, Howard DJ, Battershill J. Olfactory neuroblastoma and occupation. In: Columbus F (ed.). *Focus on neuroblastoma research.* Hauppauge, NY: Nova Science Publishers, in press.
8. Norlander T, Frodin JE, Silfversward C, Anggard A. Decreasing incidence of malignant tumors of the paranasal sinuses in Sweden. An analysis of 141 consecutive cases at Karolinska Hospital from 1960–1980. *Annals of Otology, Rhinology, and Laryngology* 2003; **112**: 236–41.
9. Harrison DNF, Lund VJ (eds). Adenocarcinoma. In: *Tumours of the upper jaw.* New York: Churchill Livingstone 1993: 115–21.
10. Núñez F, Suárez C, Alvarez I *et al.* Nasosinusal adenocarcinoma. Clinicopathological and epidemiological study of 34 cases. *Journal of Otolaryngology* 1993; **22**: 86–90.
11. Cawte T, Taskin M, Kacker A, Wahl S. Low-grade adenocarcinoma of nasal passages. *Otolaryngology and Head and Neck Surgery* 1997; **117**: 116–19.
● 12. Howard DJ, Lund VJ, Wei WI. Craniofacial resection for sinonasal neoplasia – a twenty-five year experience. *Head and Neck* 2006; **28**: 867–73.
● 13. Lund VJ, Howard DJ, Wei WI. Endoscopic resection of malignant tumours of the nose and sinuses. *American Journal of Rhinology* 2007; **21**: 89–94.
14. Goffart Y, Jorissen M, Daele J *et al.* Minimally invasive endoscopic management of malignant sinonasal tumours. *Acta Oto-rhino-laryngologica Belgica* 2000; **54**: 221–32.
15. Knegt PP, de Jong PC, van Andel JG *et al.* Carcinoma of the paranasal sinuses. Results of a prospective pilot study. *Cancer* 1985; **56**: 57–62.
16. Howard DJ, Lund VJ. Reflections on the management of adenoid cystic carcinoma of the nose and paranasal sinuses. *Otolaryngology and Head and Neck Surgery* 1985; **93**: 338–41.
17. Chiu NT, Weinstock MA. Melanoma of oronasal mucosa. Population based analysis of occurrence and mortality. *Archives of Otolaryngology – Head and Neck Surgery* 1996; **122**: 985–8.
18. Peralta E, Yarrington C, Glenn M. Malignant melanoma of the head and neck: effects of treatment on survival. *Laryngoscope* 1998; **108**: 220–3.
19. Lund VJ, Howard DJ, Harding L, Wei W. Management options and survival in malignant melanoma of the sinonasal mucosa. *Laryngoscope* 1999; **109**: 208–11.
20. Berger L, Luc R, Richard D. L'estheioneuroepitheliome olfactif. *Bulletin de l'Association Française pour l'Etude du Cancer* 1924; **13**: 410–21.
21. Lund VJ, Milroy C. Olfactory neuroblastoma: clinical and pathological aspects. *Rhinology* 1993; **31**: 1–6.
22. Hirose T, Scheithauer BW, Lopes MB *et al.* Olfactory neuroblastoma: an immunohistochemical, ultrastructural, and flow cytometric study. *Cancer* 1995; **76**: 4–19.
23. Lund VJ, Howard D, Wei W, Spittle M. Olfactory neuroblastoma. *Laryngoscope* 2003; **113**: 502–7.
♦ 24. Dulguerov P, Abdelkarim SA, Calcaterra TC. Esthesioneuroblastoma: a meta-analysis and review. *Lancet Oncology* 2001; **2**: 683–8.
25. Singh W, Ramage C, Best P *et al.* Nasal neuroblastoma secreting vasopressin. *Cancer* 1980; **45**: 961–6.
26. Rinaldo A, Ferlito A, Shaha AR *et al.* Esthesioneuroblastoma and cervical lymph node metastases: clinical and therapeutic implications. *Acta Oto-Laryngologica* 2002; **122**: 215–21.
27. Ferlito A, Rinaldo A, Rhys-Evans PH. Contemporary clinical commentary: esthesioneuroblastoma: an update on management of the neck. *Laryngoscope* 2003; **113**: 1935–8.
28. Harrison D. Surgical pathology of olfactory neuroblastoma. *Archives of Otolaryngology* 1984; **7**: 60–4.
29. Eden BV, Debo RF, Larner JM. Esthesioneuroblastoma: long-term outcome and patterns of failure – the University of Virginia experience. *Cancer* 1994; **73**: 2556–62.
30. Levine PA, Gallagher R, Cantrell RW. Esthesioneuroblastoma: reflections of a 21-year experience. *Laryngoscope* 1999; **109**: 1539–43.
31. Walch C, Stammberger H, Anderhuber W *et al.* The minimally invasive approach to olfactory neuroblastoma:

combined endoscopic and stereotactic treatment. *Laryngoscope* 2000; **110**: 635–40.

32. Casiano RR, Numa WA, Falquez AM. Endoscopic resection of esthesioneuroblastoma. *American Journal of Rhinology* 2001; **15**: 271–9.

33. Foote RL, Morita A, Ebersold M *et al.* Esthesioneuroblastoma: the role of adjuvant radiation therapy. *International Journal of Radiation Oncology, Biology, Physics* 1993; **27**: 835–42.

34. Kim D, Jo Y, Heo D *et al.* Neoadjuvant etoposide, ifosfamide and cisplatin for the treatment of olfactory neuroblastoma. *Cancer* 2004; **101**: 2257–60.

35. Mills SE, Gaffey MJ, Frierson HF (eds). Lymphoid lesions. In: *Tumours of the upper respiratory tract and ear.* Washington DC: Armed Forces Institute of Pathology, 2000: 201–42.

36. Harabuchi Y, Yamanaka N, Kataura A. Epstein–Barr virus in nasal T-cell lymphomas in patients with lethal midline granuloma. *Lancet* 1990; **335**: 128–30.

37. Lodgson MD, Ha CS, Kavadi VS *et al.* Lymphoma of the nasal cavity and paranasal sinuses: improved outcome and altered prognostic factors with combined modality modality therapy. *Cancer* 1997; **80**: 477–88.

38. Rassekh CH, Nuss DW, Kapadia SB *et al.* Chondrosarcoma of the nasal septum: skull base imaging and clinicopathologic correlation. *Otolaryngology and Head and Neck Surgery* 1996; **115**: 29–37.

39. Sobin L, Gospodarowicz M, Wittekind C (eds). *UICC TNM classification of malignant tumours*, 7th edn. Oxford: Wiley Blackwell, 2009.

40. Kadish S, Goodman M, Wang C. Olfactory neuroblastoma: a clinical analysis of 17 cases. *Cancer* 1976; **37**: 1571–6.

41. Cantu G, Solero CL, Miceli R *et al.* Which classification for ethmoid malignant tumors involving the anterior skull base? *Head and Neck* 2005; **27**: 224–31.

42. Tiwari R, van der Wal J, van der Waal I, Snow G. Studies of the anatomy and pathology of the orbit in carcinoma of the maxillary sinus and their impact on preservation of the eye in maxillectomy. *Head and Neck* 1998; **20**: 193–6.

43. Lund VJ. Tumours of the nasal cavity and paranasal sinuses. *ORL; Journal for Oto-rhino-laryngology and Its Related Specialties* 1983; **45**: 1–12.

44. Carrau RL, Segas J, Nuss DW *et al.* Squamous cell carcinoma of the sinonasal tract invading the orbit. *Laryngoscope* 1999; **109**: 230–5.

45. Iannetti G, Valentini V, Rinna C *et al.* Ethmoido-orbital tumors: our experience. *Journal of Craniofacial Surgery* 2005; **16**: 1085–91.

● 46. Lund VJ, Howard DJ, Lloyd GA, Cheesman AD. Magnetic resonance imaging of paranasal sinus tumours for craniofacial resection. *Head and Neck Surgery* 1989; **11**: 279–83.

47. Phillips C. Current status and new developments in techniques for imaging the nose and sinuses.

Otolaryngologic Clinics of North America 1997; **30**: 371–87.

48. Lloyd GAS, Lund VJ, Howard DJ *et al.* Optimum imaging for sinonasal malignancy. *Journal of Laryngology and Otology* 2000; **114**: 557–62.

49. Collins B, Cramer H, Hearn S. Fine needle aspiration cytology of metastatic neuroblastoma. *Acta Cytologica* 1997; **41**: 802–10.

50. Koshy M, Paulino A, Howell R *et al.* F-18 FDG PET-CT fusion in radiotherapy treatment planning for head and neck cancer. *Head and Neck* 2005; **27**: 494–502.

51. Lund VJ, Howard DJ, Wei WI *et al.* Craniofacial resection for tumors of the nasal cavity and paranasal sinuses – a 17-year experience. *Head and Neck* 1998; **20**: 97–105.

52. Cheesman AD, Lund VJ, Howard DJ. Craniofacial resection for tumours of the nose and paranasal sinuses. *Head and Neck Surgery* 1986; **8**: 429–35.

53. Ketcham AS, Van Buren JM. Tumors of the paranasal sinuses: a therapeutic challenge. *American Journal of Surgery* 1985; **150**: 406–13.

54. Clifford P. Transcranial approach to cancer of the antroethmoidal area. *Clinical Otolaryngology and Allied Sciences* 1977; **2**: 115–30.

55. Terz JJ, Young HF, Lawrence W Jr. Combined craniofacial resection for locally advanced carcinoma of the head and neck. *American Journal of Surgery* 1980; **140**: 613–24.

● 56. Howard DJ, Lund VJ. The role of midfacial degloving in modern rhinological practice. *Journal of Laryngology and Otology* 1999; **113**: 885–7.

57. Shah JP, Kraus DH, Bilsky MH *et al.* Craniofacial resection for malignant tumors involving the anterior skull base. *Archives of Otolaryngology – Head and Neck Surgery* 1997; **123**: 1312–17.

58. Kellman RM, Marentette L. The transglabellar/subcranial approach to the anterior skull base. *Archives of Otolaryngology – Head and Neck Surgery* 2001; **127**: 687–90.

59. Raveh J, Laedrach K, Speiser M *et al.* The subcranial approach for fronto-orbital and anteroposterior skull-base tumors. *Archives of Otolaryngology – Head and Neck Surgery* 1993; **119**: 385–93.

60. Lim M, Lew-Gor S, Sandhu G *et al.* Whitehead's varnish nasal pack. *Journal of Laryngology and Otology* 2007; **121**: 592–4.

◆ 61. Ganly I, Patel SG, Singh B *et al.* Craniofacial resection for malignant paranasal sinus tumors: Report of an International Collaborative Study. *Head and Neck* 2005; **27**: 575–84.

62. Richtsmeier WJ, Briggs RJ, Koch WM *et al.* Complications and early outcome of anterior craniofacial resection. *Archives of Otolaryngology – Head and Neck Surgery* 1992; **118**: 913–17.

63. Kraus DH, Shah JP, Arbit E *et al.* Complications of craniofacial resection for tumors involving the anterior skull base. *Head and Neck Surgery* 1994; **16**: 307–12.

64. Deschler DG, Gutin PH, Mamelak AN et al. Complications of anterior skull base surgery. Skull Base Surgery 1996; 6: 113–18.

65. Lloyd S, Devesa-Martinez P, Howard DJ, Lund VJ. Quality of life of patients undergoing surgical treatment of head and neck malignancy. Clinical Otolaryngology 2003; 28: 524–32.

66. Casson PR, Bonnano PC, Converse JM. The midface degloving procedure. Plastic and Reconstructive Surgery 1974; 53: 102–3.

67. Price JC. The midfacial approach to the central skull base. Ear, Nose, and Throat Journal 1986; 65: 174–80.

68. Schram VL, Myers EN. Lateral rhinotomy. Laryngoscope 1978; 88: 1042–5.

69. Cordeiro PG, Santamaria E. A classification system and algorithm for reconstruction of maxillectomy and midfacial defects. Plastic and Reconstructive Surgery 2000; 105: 2331–46.

70. Triana RJJr, Uglesic V, Virag M et al. Microvascular free flap reconstructive options in patients with partial and total maxillectomy defects. Archives of Facial Plastic Surgery 2000; 2: 91–101.

71. Santamaria E, Cordeiro PG. Reconstruction of maxillectomy and midfacial defects with free tissue transfer. Journal of Surgical Oncology 2006; 94: 522–31.

72. Kakibuchi M, Fujikawa M, Hosokawa K et al. Functional reconstruction of maxilla with free latissimus dorsi-scapular osteomusculocutaneous flap. Plastic and Reconstructive Surgery 2002; 109: 1238–44.

73. Lee HB, Hong JP, Kim KT et al. Orbital floor and infraorbital rim reconstruction after total maxillectomy using a vascularized calvarial bone flap. Plastic and Reconstructive Surgery 1999; 104: 646–53.

74. Pryor SG, Moore EJ, Kasperbauer JL et al. Coronoid-temporalis pedicled rotation flap for orbital floor reconstruction of the total maxillectomy defect. Laryngoscope 2004; 114: 2051–5.

75. Imola MJ, Schramm VL Jr. Orbital preservation in surgical management of sinonasal malignancy. Laryngoscope 2002; 112: 1357–65.

76. Donald P. Management of sinus malignancy. Current Opinion in Otolaryngology and Head and Neck Surgery 1997; 5: 73–8.

77. Thaler ER, Kotapka M, Lanza D, Kennedy DW. Endoscopically assisted anterior cranial skull base resection of sinonasal tumors. American Journal of Rhinology 1999; 13: 303–10.

78. Batra PS, Citardi MJ, Worley S et al. Resection of anterior skull base tumors: comparison of combined traditional and endoscopic techniques. American Journal of Rhinology 2005; 19: 521–8.

79. Lund VJ. Endoscopic management of CSF leaks. American Journal of Rhinology 2002; 16: 17–23.

80. Zuckerman J, Stankiewicz JA, Chow JM. Long-term outcomes of endoscopic repair of cerebrospinal fluid leaks and meningoencephaloceles. American Journal of Rhinology 2005; 19: 582–7.

81. Kassam A, Horwitz M, Welch W. The role of endoscopic assisted microneurosurgery (image fusion technology) in the performance of neurosurgical procedures. Minimally Invasive Neurosurgery 2005; 48: 191–6.

82. Menderes A, Yilmaz M, Vayvada H et al. Reverse temporalis muscle flap for the reconstruction of orbital exenteration defects. Annals of Plastic Surgery 2002; 48: 521–26.

83. Pryor SG, Moore EJ, Kasperbauer JL. Orbital exenteration reconstruction with rectus abdominis microvascular free flap. Laryngoscope 2005; 115: 1912–16.

84. McCaffrey TM, Olsen KD, Yohanan JM et al. Factors affecting survival of patients with tumors of the anterior skull base. Laryngoscope 1994; 104: 940–5.

85. Suárez C, Llorente JL, Fernández de León R, Maseda E. Prognostic factors in sinonasal tumors involving the anterior skull base. Head and Neck 2004; 26: 136–44.

86. Diaz E, Johnigan R, Pero C. Olfactory neuroblastoma. The 22 year experience at one comprehensive cancer center. Head and Neck 2005; 27: 138–49.

87. Bhattacharyya N. Cancer of the nasal cavity: survival and factors influencing prognosis. Archives of Otolaryngology – Head and Neck Surgery 2002; 128: 1079–83.

88. Nazar G, Rodrigo JP, Llorente JL et al. Prognostic factors of maxillary sinus malignancies. American Journal of Rhinology 2004; 18: 233–8.

89. Carrillo JF, Guemes A, Ramirez-Ortega MC, Onate-Ocana LF. Prognostic factors in maxillary sinus and nasal cavity carcinoma. European Journal of Surgical Oncology 2005; 31: 1206–12.

90. McCary WS, Levine PA, Cantrell RW. Preservation of the eye in the treatment of sinonasal malignant neoplasms with orbital involvement. A confirmation of the original treatise. Archives of Otolaryngology – Head and Neck Surgery 1996; 122: 657–9.

91. Cantù G, Solero CL, Mariani L et al. Anterior craniofacial resection for malignant ethmoid tumors. A series of 91 patients. Head and Neck 1999; 21: 185–91.

92. Nishino H, Ichimura K, Tanaka H et al. Results of orbital preservation for advanced malignant maxillary sinus tumors. Laryngoscope 2003; 113: 1064–9.

93. Draf W, Schick B, Weber R et al. Endoscopic micro-endoscopic surgery of nasal and paranasal sinus tumours. In: Stamm AC, Draf W (eds). Micro-endoscopic surgery of the paranasal sinuses and the skull base. Berlin: Springer, 2000: 481–8.

94. Stamm AC, Watashi CH, Malheiros PF et al. Micro-endoscopic surgery of benign sino-nasal tumours. In: Stamm AC, Draf W (eds). Micro-endoscopic surgery of the paranasal sinuses and the skull base. Berlin: Springer, 2000: 489–514.

95. Lund V, Stammberger H, Nicolai P et al. European position paper on endoscopic management of tumours of the

nose, paranasal sinuses and skull base. *Rhinology* 2010;
22(suppl.): 1–144.

96. Newton W, Gehan E, Webber B. Classification of
rhabdomyosarcomas and related sarcomas. Pathologic
aspects and proposal for a new classification: an
Intergroup Rhabdomyosarcoma Study. *Cancer* 1995; **76**:
1073–85.

97. Lund VJ, Neijens HJ, Clement PA *et al.* The treatment of
chronic sinusitis: a controversial issue. *International Journal
of Pediatric Otorhinolaryngology* 1995; **32**: S21–35.

♦ 98. Dulguerov P, Jacobsen M, Allal A *et al.* Nasal and
paranasal sinus carcinoma: are we making progress? A
series of 220 patients and a systematic review. *Cancer*
2001; **92**: 3012–29.

40

Lateral skull base surgery

BENEDICT PANIZZA, C ARTURO SOLARES AND MICHAEL GLEESON

To live without hope is to cease to live.

Fyodor Dostoyevsky

INTRODUCTION

In this chapter, we will discuss temporal bone resections for primary malignant tumours of the temporal bone and malignant tumours extending to the temporal bone. The remaining aspects of lateral skull base surgery will be reviewed elsewhere in the text.

HISTORY

The first comprehensive description of carcinomas of the external auditory canal and middle ear is attributed to Politizer.[1] His report was followed by initial descriptions of piecemeal removal. Later, treatment for this condition included radical mastoidectomy and radiotherapy, which sometimes included radioactive implants.[2] During the 1950s, more radical surgical treatments for temporal bone carcinoma were proposed with the first report, in 1954, of a one-stage temporal bone resection.[3] Five-year survival rates of 25 per cent for squamous cell carcinoma were later reported.[4] In 1960, a less radical temporal bone resection, now known as 'lateral temporal bone resection', was described.[5]

In the 1980s, reports on improved survival appeared. Goodwin and Jesse,[6] in a report on 136 patients, demonstrated a 58 per cent overall five-year survival rate for squamous cell carcinoma of the temporal bone. This is, to our knowledge, the largest reported series on temporal bone resections. Importantly, it was demonstrated that deep temporal bone involvement resulted in a poor outcome due to difficulty in obtaining clear margins. This landmark study also demonstrated that postoperative radiotherapy was of no benefit when clear margins could not be achieved. A benefit in local control was observed when radiotherapy was used as an adjuvant in those patients with clear margins. No benefit on survival was observed.[6] This study is the basis for modern practice in the management of temporal bone malignancies. Also in the 1980s, there were various reports on temporal bone resections with carotid artery resections without significant impact on survival.[7, 8]

ANATOMY

A thorough understanding of the temporal bone anatomy is paramount during oncologic surgery of the temporal bone. The temporal bone anatomy is quite complex and an in-depth description is beyond the aims of this chapter. Briefly, the temporal bone has four components. The squamosa constitutes a vertical plate whose medial surface forms part of the middle cranial fossa. On the lateral surface, the zygomatic process projects from it, and the mandibular fossa is located

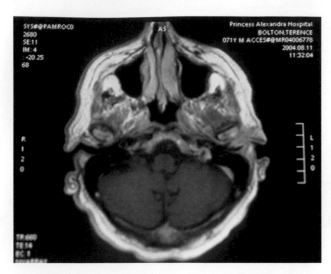

Figure 40.1 T_1-weighted magnetic resonance image with axial cuts demonstrating a tumour involving the anterior wall of the external auditory canal and the temporomandibular joint.

below its root. The mastoid process, which projects from the squamous and petrous parts, articulates with the occipital and parietal bones. The petrous bone is a pyramidal projection from the mastoid portion, the apex of which inserts in the angle between the occipital and sphenoid bones. It divides the middle and posterior cranial fossae. The tympanic bone is a ring opened superiorly which forms the anterior and inferior walls, as well as part of the posterior wall of the external auditory canal (EAC). The temporal bone occupies the inferolateral skull base. Although osseous, it also houses the epithelialized ear canal, mastoid and middle ear. In addition, cranial nerves VII–XI, the carotid artery, and the sigmoid sinus all traverse the temporal bone.

Several tissue types, from cartilaginous to glandular, can be found within the temporal bone. Any of these structures can potentially give rise to a malignancy. However, as already mentioned, most temporal bone cancers arise from the EAC, and of these, squamous cell carcinomas (SCC) is the most common. These tumours can spread (1) anteriorly, into the parotid gland, infratemporal fossa, glenoid fossa (**Figure 40.1**) or facial skin; (2) posteriorly, into the bony EAC, mastoid air cells and posterior fossa; (3) inferiorly, into the neck soft tissue, jugular foramen, foramen magnum or cervical spine, and (4) superiorly into the epitympanum, tegmen tympani and middle fossa. Tumour spread may dictate the need for additional procedures (i.e. parotidectomy, neck dissection, and mandibular condylectomy).[9]

Lymphatic drainage from the EAC is into the parotid and pre-auricular lymph nodes anteriorly; inferiorly, into the upper deep cervical and deep internal jugular nodes; and posteriorly into the post-auricular nodes. The middle ear and mastoid lymphatics drain into the Eustachian tube area and then into the deep upper jugular and retropharyngeal nodes.[9]

PATHOLOGY AND EPIDEMIOLOGY

Malignant tumours of the temporal bone are rare and therefore it is difficult to establish treatment protocols that are universally applicable. Primary tumours of the temporal bone are usually SCC of the external auditory canal or middle ear. SCC of the pinna is considered a cutaneous malignancy, with a different staging and prognosis. The prevalence of temporal bone carcinomas is approximately six cases per million in the general population.[10] The main risk factor is a long, often two or more decade history of chronic suppurative otitis media.[11] Other potential inciting factors include chronic dermatitis,[12] cholesteatoma[13] and history of previous radiation.[14, 15] Less commonly, adenocarcinomas and adenoid cystic carcinomas may be observed. In addition, the temporal bone may be affected by direct extension of parotid malignancies. Less commonly metastatic spread from the breast, prostate, lung or kidney to the marrow containing petrous apex can occur.[16, 17, 18, 19] In our practice, perineural spread through the facial nerve from skin SCC is a frequent indication for some form of temporal bone resection along with direct spread of cutaneous malignancy to the temporal bone.

CLINICAL EVALUATION AND STAGING

Otorrhoea, often blood stained, an external auditory canal mass and pain are usually the initial signs and symptoms. As the disease progresses, the pain becomes severe or excruciating. Facial and vagal palsies are late signs.[20, 21, 22] A high index of suspicion is necessary as the initial presentation may mimic more common otologic conditions. An ear examination under magnification, a complete head, neck and cranial nerve examination, and audiometry should be performed.

Because SCC of the temporal bone routinely invades bone and soft tissues, most patients should ideally undergo fine-cut computed tomography (CT) of the temporal bone with bone windows and magnetic resonance imaging (MRI) of the head and neck. We obtain a fine-cut high resolution CT scan to identify the tumour extent and degree of bone erosion. An MRI is performed on all cases unless the tumour is localized to the external auditory canal and there is no bone erosion on CT. If the carotid artery is suspected to be involved (rare with poor prognosis), angiography with trial ipsilateral balloon occlusion should be performed, followed by xenon diffusion test to assess the adequacy of cerebral blood flow from the contralateral carotid artery. Special attention is also given to the venous outflow phase to determine the adequacy of the torcula and contralateral drainage pathway, in case the surgery requires sacrifice of the sigmoid sinus or internal jugular vein. In a cadaveric study, up to 25 per cent of specimens did not have a patent torcula.[23] Despite this, in our experience, sacrifice of the sigmoid sinus/jugular bulb is feasible in a significant proportion of cases. Even after careful work up and state-of-the-art imaging, the extent of disease may be underestimated and, thus intraoperative clinical judgement is imperative.

No staging system for temporal bone malignancies is universally accepted. Many authors have proposed staging systems concurrent with a review of patient series from major institutions; however, the small number of patients per group, the disparity of staging criteria, the diversity in management protocols, and the use of non-standardized surgical nomenclature prohibits meaningful comparison of outcomes. In addition, some patients are reportedly classified into groups with variability in histology types and sites of tumour origin, which further confounds analysis of outcome by stage.

A staging system for squamous cell cancers of the EAC proposed by the University of Pittsburgh[24] has been shown to be useful and has gained support in the literature.[9, 25, 26] This staging system is based on clinical, radiologic and pathologic findings. In general, tumours that are limited to the EAC are defined as early disease, and those that extend beyond the external canal to invade the surrounding soft tissues, the middle ear, the mastoid, or cranial nerves are recognized as advanced disease.

The Pittsburgh staging system was modified by the authors after further review of patients from an extended series.[27] In the modified staging system, facial nerve weakness is considered a criterion for a T4 lesion. The authors observed that facial nerve paresis did not occur in lesions otherwise classified as limited T1, T2 or T3 lesions. Involvement of the facial nerve would be otherwise classified as T4 based on the anatomical area of involvement, including the medial wall of the middle ear (horizontal segment), extensive bony erosion within mastoid (vertical segment), or involvement of stylomastoid foramen. **Table 40.1** summarizes the University of Pittsburgh staging system for temporal bone SCC (most commonly used). Nodal and metastatic disease is staged according to the American Joint Committee System. Nodal metastasis is extremely important in temporal bone carcinoma as N1 disease in a T2 or higher lesion is considered stage IV. In addition to the Pittsburgh staging system, other staging systems include Clark/Stell and the Otology Group staging system.[10, 24, 28, 29, 30]

Table 40.1 The University of Pittsburgh staging system for temporal bone squamous cell carcinoma.

T1	Tumour limited to the EAC without bony erosion or evidence of soft tissue involvement
T2	Tumour with limited EAC bone erosion (not full thickness) with limited (<0.5 cm) soft tissue involvement
T3	Tumour eroding the osseous EAC (full thickness) with limited (<0.5 cm) soft tissue involvement or tumour involving the middle ear, mastoid, or both
T4	Tumour eroding the cochlea, petrous apex, medial wall of the middle ear, carotid canal, or jugular foramen of dura; or with extensive soft tissue involvement (>0.5 cm), such as involvement of the TMJ or stylomastoid foramen; or with evidence of facial paresis
Stage I	T1 N0 M0
Stage II	T2 N0 M0
Stage III	T3 N0 M0, T1 N1 M0
Stage IV	T4 N0 M0, T2–4 N1 M0, any T N2 M0, any T N3 M0, any T any N M1

EAC, external auditory canal; TMJ, temporomandibular joint.

TEMPORAL BONE RESECTIONS: RATIONALE

With the advent of modern skull base surgery techniques, our ability to remove temporal bone malignancies has been expanded. Nevertheless, the dilemma of defining resectability still persists. Although it is technically feasible to remove structures such as the petrous carotid artery, the morbidity associated with it is significant and surgical cure rates in these scenarios are not significantly improved. The rarity of the problem results in a small collective surgical experience which complicates matters further. Pensak *et al.*[21] consider that invasion of any of the following structures:

- cavernous sinus,
- carotid artery,
- infratemporal fossa,
- paraspinous musculature

make a patient unresectable.[21] All patients in their series of 46 individuals with SCC of the temporal bone with such invasion died within three years despite surgery and postoperative radiotherapy.[21] The difficulty hinges on the reliability of preoperative staging. This is a subject of significant controversy.[9]

In our practice, a temporal bone resection is performed for malignant tumours involving the temporal bone. We recommend en-bloc resection of the entire specimen by either a complete external auditory canal excision (i.e. lateral temporal bone resection (LTBR)), or a near total temporal bone excision (NTTBR) (**Figure 40.2**). Any potentially involved adjacent soft tissue is included en bloc with the specimen by means of additional ancillary procedures, commonly a parotidectomy and less so the temporomandibular joint (TMJ) and capsule. We perform a lateral temporal bone resection with preservation of the facial nerve in tumours located lateral to the tympanic membrane.

Tumours medial to the tympanic membrane are best treated with a NTTBR. The assessment of medial spread can

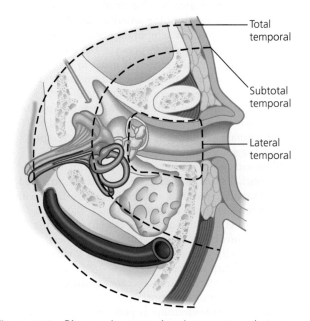

Total temporal

Subtotal temporal

Lateral temporal

Figure 40.2 Diagram demonstrating the structures that are removed with each of the temporal bone resection types.

be made preoperatively by clinical signs (facial nerve palsy) and radiological assessment. Intraoperative assessment is made by inspection of the middle ear cavity via a posterior tympanotomy. Soft tissue thickening in the middle ear may be due to a mucosal reaction to the tumour or frank tumour invasion. Thus, frozen section verification is recommended.

In essence, three types of temporal bone resections can be performed (i.e. LTBR, NTTBR and TTBR). In addition, sleeve resections of the EAC skin have been described. These are mentioned here briefly mainly to dissuade the reader from using this technique in the management of EAC carcinoma. Sleeve resections are simply striping of the EAC skin and thus are not an oncologically sound operation, but may be applicable in certain basal cell carcinomas limited to the lateral aspect of the EAC.

SURGICAL TECHNIQUE

Lateral temporal bone resection

This operation requires complete en bloc removal of the entire osseous and cartilaginous EAC with the intact tympanic membrane.[31, 32, 33] The surgical steps for this operation are outlined below.

1. A postauricular C-shaped incision approximately 1 cm behind the postauricular sulcus is performed. This incision may be extended inferiorly into the neck for a parotidectomy as required (**Figure 40.3**).
2. The skin flaps are elevated anteriorly above the parotidomasseteric and temporalis fascia. The posterior skin flap is elevated above the temporalis fascia, mastoid bone and sternocleidomastoid fascia. If it is required, the tragus and part of the conchal cartilage may be included in the resection. If the retromandibular area is to be involved in the resection, the depth of the anterior skin flap is extended deep to the temporalis fascia at the root of the zygoma in order to preserve the temporal branch of the facial nerve. It is usual to bring the pinna forward with the wide-based postauricular incision. However, where large amounts of the concha are involved with tumour, then the incision may have to extend in a preauricular fashion with the remnant pinna taken posteriorly to attempt to preserve some vascularity.
3. Blind sac closure of the canal is performed (tragal to conchal skin), if the lateral canal is not involved, after cartilage removal and reinforced medially with an anteriorly based musculoperiosteal flap. This situation is uncommon. If the lateral end of the canal is involved, it is resected and the defect repaired with a local rotation, such as a temporalis rotational flap or free flap.
4. The lateral external auditory canal is sutured closed if tumour spread is a concern.
5. A routine mastoidectomy is performed to expose the bony plate of the sigmoid sinus and the middle cranial fossa dura. A posterior

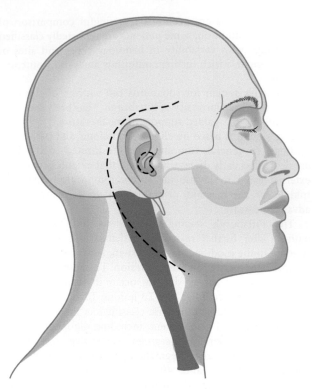

Figure 40.3 Postauricular C-shaped incision commonly utilized for lateral temporal bone resections. Extending the incision into the neck allows access for a parotidectomy and/or neck dissection.

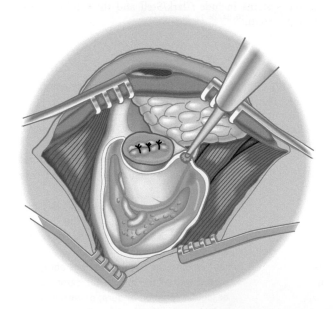

Figure 40.4 A cortical mastoidectomy has been performed and extended into the root of the zygoma.

tympanotomy is fashioned and the middle ear is inspected through it.
6. The incudostapedial joint is disarticulated.
7. The mastoidectomy is extended into the root of the zygoma and the epitympanum opened (**Figure 40.4**).

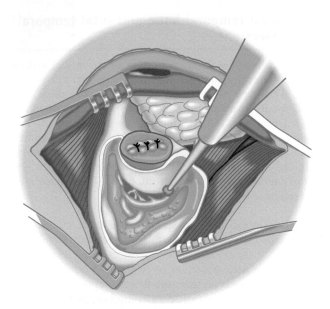

Figure 40.5 Diagram showing an extended posterior tympanotomy being performed.

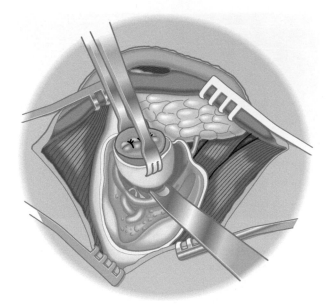

Figure 40.7 A 2 mm osteotome is being used via the posterior tympanotomy to liberate the anterior component of the tympanic plate. In a narrow posterior tympanotomy, this allows for extra space to complete the anterior drilling.

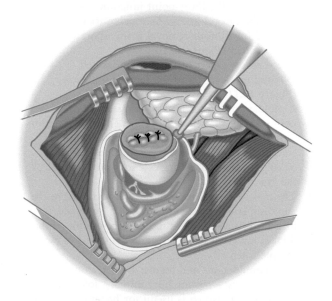

Figure 40.6 The hypotympanic opening is being extended anteriorly towards the inferior part of the temporomandibular joint.

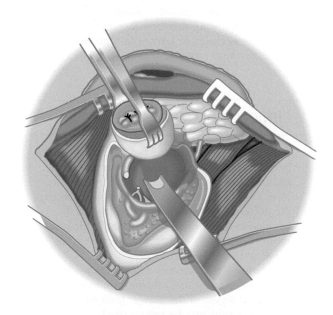

Figure 40.8 Specimen being removed en bloc.

8. The posterior tympanotomy is extended inferiorly into the hypotympanum, sacrificing the chorda tympani. Care must be taken to dissect the chorda tympani and transect it with a sharp instrument to avoid traction injury to the facial nerve (**Figure 40.5**).
9. The anterior epitympanic region is drilled extending anteroinferiorly and medially to reach the superior part of the TMJ.
10. The hypotympanic opening is extended anteriorly, lateral to the jugular bulb and internal carotid to reach the inferior part of the TMJ (**Figure 40.6**). Occasionally, it is necessary to raise the facial nerve

from the stylomastoid foramen to the second genu in order to drill the hypotympanic region.
11. The specimen is then removed en bloc by pushing forward on it. Should resistance be present, a 2 mm osteotome may be used via the posterior tympanotomy to liberate the anterior component of the tympanic plate. With a narrow posterior tymanotomy (facial nerve to tympanic annulus), once the temporal bone is fractured forward, the space opens a further couple of millimetres allowing completion of the anterior drilling and clean removal of the specimen (**Figures 40.7, 40.8 and 40.9**).

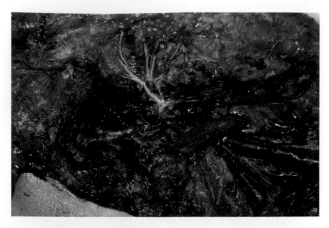

Figure 40.9 Resultant defect after a lateral temporal bone resection with resection of the temporomandibular joint and superficial parotidectomy.

12. The Eustachian tube is plugged with muscle and fascia.
13. The defect is filled with temporalis muscle rotated inferiorly. Free abdominal fat grafts are avoided if radiation therapy is planned. Obliteration of the mastoid cavity prevents osteoradionecrosis from developing following radiation therapy.[34]
14. The wound is closed in layers and a padded lightly compressive head bandage is then applied.

TECHNICAL NOTES

- The vertical portion of the facial nerve may drift lateral to the annulus in the inferior half of the annulus. Care must therefore be taken, in those cases with facial nerve preservation, in extending the posterior tympanotomy inferiorly. As the annulus in this area curves anteriorly, adequate room is present to allow drilling between the nerve and the annulus.
- In extending the posterior tympanotomy into the hypotympanum and forward on to the TMJ, the lateral aspect of the jugular bulb and internal carotid may be encountered.
- The middle cranial fossa descends in the anterior part of the epitympanum. On occasion, it may be necessary to elevate the dura to perform the superior part of the resection.
- The geniculate ganglion sits immediately medial to the medial wall of the anterior epitympanum. Extension of the mastoidectomy into the root of the zygoma and medially into the superoposterior aspect of the TMJ should be performed with care.
- In using the temporalis muscle to obliterate the defect, the anterior half is left *in situ* to prevent a cosmetic defect in the temporal fossa.

Near-total temporal bone and total temporal bone resections

A NTTBR describes en-bloc resection of the medial surfaces of the mesotympanum, leaving the air cells of the petrous apex. This type of resection is indicated for those with malignancies involving the middle ear without extension into the petrous apex. A TTBR involves an en-bloc resection of the entire temporal bone, including the petrous apex and the sigmoid sinus. The petrous internal carotid artery may be included in this resection. There is questionable added benefit of a total temporal bone resection.[21, 35] The surgical steps to perform a NTTBR are outlined below.

1. The skin incision must allow access to the middle cranial fossa, mastoid, parotid and retromandibular fossa. It should also allow extension of the incision should a neck dissection be required. A large C-shaped incision from the frontotemporal region 6–8 cm above the auricle, extending up to 4–5 cm behind the retroauricular sulcus, then running 4 cm below the horizontal aspect of the mandible and ending in the submental region may be used. A vertical limb can be made for a neck dissection, ensuring that the three-point junction does not overlie the carotid artery. As much auricle as is required for tumour removal is incorporated with the specimen (**Figure 40.10**).
2. The superior aspect of the flap is elevated followed by elevation of the temporal muscle (**Figure 40.11**).
3. A middle-posterior temporal craniotomy is performed. A drill hole is performed at the asterion to find the junction of the lateral and sigmoid sinuses. The craniotomy is commenced here and usually measures 6 × 4 cm extending to the root of the zygoma.
4. The middle cranial fossa dura is dissected from the anterosuperior aspect of the petrous bone and is inspected to ensure the tumour is resectable. If the dura is involved here, it is incised and left as part of the specimen.
5. The sigmoid sinus and jugular bulb regions are exposed using a cutting burr initially, followed by a diamond burr which is useful for haemostasis. The dura in front of the sigmoid is then sufficiently exposed so that it is possible to dissect the dura over the posterior aspect of the petrous bone toward the area of the internal auditory meatus and pars nervosa of the jugular foramen. The dura in this region is also inspected for tumour.
6. A total parotidectomy and, if necessary, a neck dissection are performed. Any resection required of tissue anterior to the external auditory canal may also be performed at this stage. If dural involvement and therefore resectability is not a concern, this step is performed prior to the craniotomy.
7. The sigmoid is opened and packed with haemostatic packing proximally and distally down towards the jugular bulb region. The jugular bulb is then opened and the inferior petrosal sinus

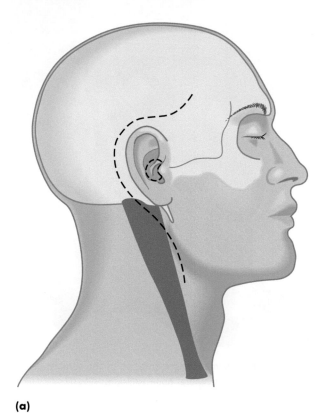

(a)

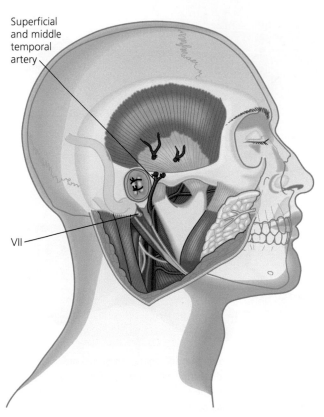

Superficial and middle temporal artery

VII

Figure 40.11 Schematic representation of the anatomy following flap elevation during a near total temporal bone excision.

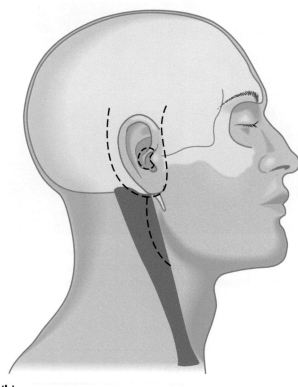

(b)

Figure 40.10 Incision options when performing a near total temporal bone excision. (a) A large C-shaped incision from the frontotemporal area, extending post-auricular and the running below the body of the mandible. (b) A Y-shaped incision.

openings are gently packed. A preoperative magnetic resonance venogram should be performed to assess the adequacy of the torcula.

8. A diamond drill is used to make a cut along the superomedial aspect of the jugular bulb into the hypotympanum and up to the posterior wall of the carotid canal.

9. The middle cranial fossa dura is dissected free to the posterior part of the foramen ovale coagulating and cutting the middle meningeal artery in the process. It is then continued to the connective tissue of the posterolateral margin of the foramen lacerum and along the petrous ridge. The roof and lateral wall of the internal carotid canal are removed using a diamond drill all the way to the level of the cochlea.

10. A diamond drill is used to create an osteotomy via the middle cranial fossa across the petrous bone just lateral to the porus acousticus to reach the carotid canal anteriorly and the posteromedial part of the preserved wall of the jugular fossa inferiorly. Care must be taken in performing this step so as to prevent injury to the lower cranial nerves.

11. The final cut is made medial to lateral joining the area of the glenoid fossa or root of the zygoma, across the floor of the middle cranial fossa, to run immediately behind the foramen ovale to the carotid canal.

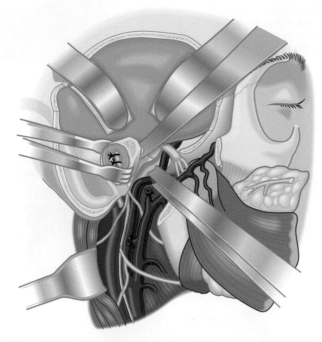

Figure 40.12 A total parotidectomy, temporomandibular joint resection and neck dissection have been performed, as well as a temporal craniotomy. The sigmoid sinus has been exposed and the carotid artery has been dissected. A cut along the middle fossa floor allows for removal of the specimen.

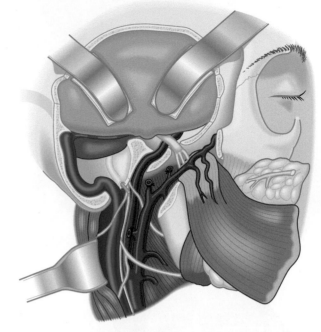

Figure 40.13 Schematic representation of the surgical defect following near total temporal bone excision.

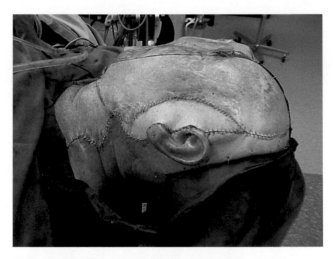

Figure 40.14 Post-operative result following near total temporal bone excision, radical parotidectomy and neck dissection, followed by an anterolateral thigh free-flap reconstruction.

12. The specimen is then cracked free by pushing anteroinferiorly from the posterior surface of the petrous bone using a rocking motion. There are usually some soft tissue attachments preventing liberation of the specimen, including the nerves of the internal auditory canal (IAC), which need to be cut. Bleeding from the inferior petrosal sinus is managed with haemostatic packing (**Figures 40.12, 40.13** and **40.14**).

13. Haemostasis is achieved and any dural defect is repaired. This may require primary closure with, or a fascial graft for, larger defects. We favour a 5-0 non-absorbable monofilament suture for dural suturing.

14. The facial nerve rehabilitated either by a crossface cable graft or by a split XII–VII neurorraphy. Experience at the Cleveland Clinic has been favourable with XII–VII anastomosis.[36] The split XII–VII neurorraphy can also be used as a babysitter graft in patients in whom a crossface anastomosis is performed to maintain the viability of the motor end plates.[37] Our practice is to perform static reanimation with facial slings and gold weight concurrently with cable grafting.

Our preference is to repair the defect with a free flap graft (**Figure 40.14**). We feel that free flaps are better at preventing leakage of cerebrospinal fluid and at protecting the carotid artery in large resections which is important because these patients will routinely receive post-operative radiotherapy or have already failed radiotherapy.

TECHNICAL NOTES

- Drilling anterior to the sigmoid to allow elevation of the dura is generally safe as this region is rarely involved with tumour. On the occasions where tumour is seen anterior to the sigmoid sinus or if the sinus is very anterior, drilling is commenced retrosigmoid and the sigmoid opened and packed from behind.

- Care must be taken in packing the inferior petrosal openings into the jugular bulb as excessive pressure may cause a palsy of the glossopharyngeal and possibly the vagal nerves.
- Exposure of the carotid via the middle cranial fossa should be adequate for the insertion of a small dissector to free the carotid artery from the wall of the carotid canal.
- In freeing the carotid from its canal, it may be necessary to bipolar coagulate the caroticotympanic or periosteal branches.
- The framework of the medial porus acousticus is preserved if possible to allow packing with bone wax and prevent a cerebrospinal fluid leak.
- A total resection of the petrous bone is almost never necessary; if it is required, closure is more difficult.
- In our experience, facial nerve grafting when followed with postoperative radiotherapy has lead to poor outcomes. We always perform static facial reanimation with a gold eyelid weight and static fascial slings concurrently with cable grafting.

Ancillary procedures

As mentioned above under Clinical evaluation and staging, p. 780, tumours of the temporal bone can extend outside the temporal bone necessitating ancillary procedures. More commonly, parotid tumours will extend to the temporal bone. In either case, the procedure planned should encompass a complete tumour resection. Thus, ancillary procedures commonly performed with a temporal bone resection include parotidectomy with or without facial nerve sacrifice, condyle/temporomadibular joint resection, auriculectomy and a neck dissection. A superficial parotidectomy is generally performed to obtain clear margins in tumours extending to the gland or in close contact with it. The decision to perform a total parotidectomy and/or facial nerve sacrifice is based on the extension of the tumour within the gland and the pre-operative nerve function. In addition, a neck dissection can be performed if there is evidence of neck lymphadenopathy. This is preferably removed en bloc with the temporal bone specimen. A routine neck dissection is not performed due to the low incidence (10–15 per cent) of occult involvement of the cervical lymphatics and the routine use of post-operative radiation therapy which includes treatment of the neck.

A unique circumstance in our practice is perineural spread from skin SCC. In these cases, we advocate for a radical resection of the disease. Thus, if the magnetic resonance neurography study demonstrates perineural spread up to the stylomastoid foramen, a cortical mastoidectomy with dissection of the facial nerve should be performed and the nerve is sacrificed at the second genu with intraoperative frozen section control. If the margins are positive at this stage, or if pre-operative magnetic resonance neurography suggested that the disease extends further, a NTTBR should be performed to achieve clear neural margins. If there is further extension, resection of the facial nerve up to the brainstem may be required. With gross involvement of the facial nerve,

it is common for the third branch of the trigeminal nerve to be involved as well. If the MRI suggests that the disease is resectable, the temporal bone is resected en bloc with a radical parotidectomy, ascending mandible and infra-temporal fossa contents up to the Gasserian ganglion.

RADIOTHERAPY

Radiotherapy as the sole modality for the treatment of temporal bone malignancies has a very limited role and is mostly historical. Before the development of modern skull base, surgery techniques radiotherapy was used because of the dismal surgical results. Birzgalis et al.[38] reported on 53 patients with radical radiotherapy. An overall 32 per cent five-year survival rate was noted. Unfortunately, an unspecified number of these patients also had radical mastoidectomy. Early (T1) cancers had excellent control, with eight of ten cases being alive at five years, but, as mentioned above, the contribution from surgery was unclear.[38] Zhang et al.[25] had a 29 per cent survival rate for radiotherapy alone, and a rate of 60 per cent for combined surgery and radiation. These and other authors have recommended combined therapy for advanced disease.[25, 39, 40] Similarly, Hahn et al.[41] noted that survival rates improved from 14 per cent with surgery alone to 50 per cent with surgery and radiotherapy. Importantly, none of three patients with advanced disease who received radiotherapy alone were alive at five years. The authors concluded that surgery or radiotherapy alone is not sufficient for most of the cases of carcinoma of the middle ear because of late presentation.[41] Only isolated reports of stereotactic radiotherapy are available.[21, 27] At this juncture, we can recommend radiotherapy has an adjuvant to surgical clearance of disease.

TREATMENT OUTCOMES

Fortunately, improved survivals have been observed over the last 50 years from a five-year survival rate of 25 per cent to a current rate of 50 per cent. The survival rates of T1 and T2 carcinomas are 80–100 per cent.[27] The main controversy is whether a larger operation gives better results for advanced disease (T3 and T4 lesions). As with smaller lesions, there are advocates of a limited surgical procedure coupled with postoperative radiation for advanced disease. Chao et al.[42] used a radical mastoidectomy and postoperative radiation in a series of 47 patients, 29 of whom had cancer originating in the middle ear with an overall survival rate of 53 per cent. With a similar approach, Zhang et al.[25] reported a 69 per cent survival rate in stage III patients and a 20 per cent survival rate in stage IV patients, whereas Liu et al.[43] had a 54 per cent survival rate with combined radiation and radical mastoidectomy.

On the other hand, Moffat et al.[44] reported on 15 patients with recurrent, extensive squamous cell carcinomas of the temporal bone. The primary site of origin in nine patients was the middle ear and mastoid, and all patients had undergone previous partial temporal bone resection, usually followed by radiotherapy. Five patients had T3 tumours, and ten patients had T4 tumours. The five-year survival rate in

suggested staging system. *Journal of Laryngology and Otology* 1985; **99**: 847–50.

31. Conley JJ, Novack AJ. The surgical treatment of malignant tumors of the ear and temporal bone. Part I. *Archives of Otolaryngology* 1960; **71**: 635–52.

32. Crabtree JA, Britton BH, Pierce MK. Carcinoma of the external auditory canal. *Laryngoscope* 1976; **86**: 405–15.

33. Kinney SE, Wood BG. Malignancies of the external ear canal and temporal bone: surgical techniques and results. *Laryngoscope* 1987; **97**: 158–64.

34. Nadol JB Jr, Schuknecht HF. Obliteration of the mastoid in the treatment of tumors of the temporal bone. *Annals of Otology, Rhinology and Laryngology* 1984; **93**: 6–12.

35. Pomeranz S, Sekhar LN, Janecka IP *et al.* Classification, technique, and results of surgical resection of petrous bone tumors. In: Sekhar LN, Janecka IP (eds). *Surgery of cranial base tumors*. New York: Raven Press, 1993: 317–35.

36. Shipchandler TZ, Alam D. *Split hypoglossal-facial nerve transfer for treatment of the paralyzed face*. Chicago, IL: American Academy of Facial Plastic and Reconstructive Surgery, 2008.

37. Kalantarian B, Rice DC, Tiangco DA, Terzis JK. Gains and losses of the XII-VII component of the 'babysitter' procedure: a morphometric analysis. *Journal of Reconstructive Microsurgery* 1998; **14**: 459–71.

38. Birzgalis AR, Keith AO, Farrington WT. Radiotherapy in the treatment of middle ear and mastoid carcinoma. *Clinical Otolaryngology and Allied Sciences* 1992; **17**: 113–16.

39. Korzeniowski S, Pszon J. The results of radiotherapy of cancer of the middle ear. *International Journal of Radiation, Oncology, Biology, Physics* 1990; **18**: 631–3.

40. Pfreundner L, Schwager K, Willner J *et al.* Carcinoma of the external auditory canal and middle ear. *International Journal of Radiation, Oncology, Biology, Physics* 1999; **44**: 777–88.

41. Hahn SS, Kim JA, Goodchild N, Constable WC. Carcinoma of the middle ear and external auditory canal. *International Journal of Radiation, Oncology, Biology, Physics* 1983; **9**: 1003–7.

42. Chao CK, Sheen TS, Shau WY *et al.* Treatment, outcomes, and prognostic factors of ear cancer. *Journal of the Formosan Medical Association* 1999; **98**: 314–18.

43. Liu FF, Keane TJ, Davidson J. Primary carcinoma involving the petrous temporal bone. *Head and Neck* 1993; **15**: 39–43.

44. Moffat DA, Wagstaff SA, Hardy DG. The outcome of radical surgery and postoperative radiotherapy for squamous carcinoma of the temporal bone. *Laryngoscope* 2005; **115**: 341–7.

♦ 45. Prasad S, Janecka IP. Efficacy of surgical treatments for squamous cell carcinoma of the temporal bone: a literature review. *Otolaryngology – Head and Neck Surgery* 1994; **110**: 270–80.

46. Arriaga M, Hirsch BE, Kamerer DB, Myers EN. Squamous cell carcinoma of the external auditory meatus (canal). *Otolaryngology – Head and Neck Surgery* 1989; **101**: 330–7.

47. Spector JG. Management of temporal bone carcinomas: a therapeutic analysis of two groups of patients and long-term followup. *Otolaryngology – Head and Neck Surgery* 1991; **104**: 58–66.

41

Rare cancers of the head and neck

ANDREW K CHAN, ANDREW HARTLEY, ROBERT J GRIMER, RABIN PRATAP SINGH AND PREM MAHENDRA

If you do not expect the unexpected, you will not find it; for it is hard to be sought out, and difficult

Heraclitus (c.535–475BC)

NEUROECTODERMAL MALIGNANCIES OF THE HEAD AND NECK

Introduction

Sinonasal undifferentiated carcinoma (SNUC), olfactory neuroblastoma (ONB) and neuroendocrine carcinoma (NEC) form a spectrum of rare malignancies of neuroectodermal origin. The rarity of these tumours precludes any prospective trials and reports in the literature of management have been limited to retrospective single institution series. These tumours are therefore best managed in specialized centres with treatment options largely dictated by local expertise and patient choice. SNUC and NEC are aggressive tumours which require a multimodality approach with surgery, radiotherapy and chemotherapy, whereas early stage ONB may be treated with local therapy.

Sinonasal undifferentiated carcinoma

Sinonasal undifferentiated carcinoma was first described by Frierson et al.[1] in 1986 as a clinicopathological entity arising from the Schneiderian epithelium or from the nasal ectoderm of the paranasal sinuses. Reports in the literature are emerging since its recognition as a distinct entity; however, the true incidence is not known with fewer than 100 reported cases.[2] The majority arise from the nasal cavity with the remaining cases originating from the maxillary and ethmoid sinuses. The age range is broad with a bimodal distribution affecting young adults and the elderly. A median age of presentation of 50 years (range 20–77 years) has been reported.[1, 3, 4, 5, 6, 7]

CLINICAL FEATURES

SNUC commonly presents with locally advanced features with its propensity to aggressively invade local structures, such as the orbit, cranial cavity, nasopharynx, and sphenoid and frontal sinuses. Symptoms and signs characteristically develop over a short period of weeks to a few months in keeping with its locally aggressive behaviour. These include nasal obstruction, epistaxis, propotosis, periorbital discomfort with swelling, diplopia, and other cranial nerve palsies.[1] Locoregional nodal involvement and distant metastases, particularly to the lung and bone, can also occur in up to 30 per cent.[8]

PATHOLOGY

Light microscopy can differentiate most cases of SNUC from other undifferentiated tumours but immunohistochemistry and electron microscopy can be helpful to confirm the diagnosis. Features seen on light microscopy include small to medium-sized undifferentiated cells showing significant pleomorphism, a high nuclear–cytoplasmic ratio and moderate eosinophilic cytoplasm. These cells are classically arranged in nests, trabeculae or sheets. Large ovoid nuclei with numerous mitotic figures, extensive vascular invasion and necrosis can also be prominent features.[9] SNUC stains positive for keratin and epithelial membrane antigen. Some cases show neuroendocrine differentiation. Neuron-specific enolase and CD99 are often expressed, but chromogranin, synaptophysin, S-100 and vimentin markers are usually negative.[1,3] SNUCs are typically negative for Epstein–Barr virus on immunohistochemistry.[3,5]

DIFFERENTIAL DIAGNOSIS

Given the lack of differentiation seen with SNUC, the differential diagnosis can be very broad and includes ONB, lymphoma, embryonal rhabdomyosarcoma, melanoma, nasopharyngeal carcinoma (lymphoepithelioma) and small cell carcinoma. It is crucial to differentiate SNUC from ONB because natural history, treatment and prognosis differ greatly. SNUC is characteristically locally aggressive associated with a poor prognosis, whereas ONB generally has a slower natural history.

INVESTIGATIONS

Initial assessment of a sinonasal mass routinely includes nasoendoscopy, examination under anaesthesia and biopsy. Initial imaging is often with a computed tomography (CT) scan which commonly shows a non-calcified mass arising either from the nasal cavity or paranasal sinuses with local bone destruction and invasion of adjacent structures, such as the orbit, anterior cranial cavity or nasopharynx. A magnetic resonance (MR) scan with gadolinium contrast is also frequently undertaken to complement the CT scan and complete local staging. It characteristically shows heterogenous gadolinium-enhancement of the tumour with a superior soft tissue resolution compared with a CT scan which, in contrast, provides superior bone delineation.

MANAGEMENT

SNUC is a locally destructive tumour and therefore is often found to be unresectable at presentation. A radical approach to treatment involves the combined modalities of surgery (craniofacial resection), radiotherapy and chemotherapy. Craniofacial resection entails an en bloc resection of the tumour, the cribriform plate and any intracranial extension. However, the aims of treatment are realistically to control disease.[4,10,11,12] Other approaches have been to give neoadjuvant radiotherapy followed by surgery, or concurrent chemoradiotherapy in those that are not resectable. The role of adjuvant chemotherapy is unclear. In view of its rarity, the optimal sequence of treatment has yet to be established.

Chen et al.[13] recently reported one of the largest series of SNUC (21 patients) treated in a single institution. The majority of patients had T4 disease. Seventeen patients were treated with surgery followed by postoperative radiotherapy with or without adjuvant chemotherapy. Two patients received neoadjuvant chemoradiotherapy followed by surgery and two patients received definitive chemoradiotherapy alone. Five-year overall survival was 43 per cent and two-year local control rate was 60 per cent. No difference

in local control was seen between the treatment approaches but it was observed, among the patients who underwent surgery, that local control was significantly better in those who had gross tumour resection compared to those with a subtotal resection (two-year local control 74 versus 24 per cent, respectively, $p = 0.001$). However, in view of the small study size, this did not translate to a survival difference between the groups. The median dose of radiotherapy given was 60 Gy in those treated with definitive chemoradiotherapy and 57 Gy in those given postoperative radiotherapy. Chemotherapy regimes used varied: cyclophosphamide, doxorubicin and vincristine given in five patients; cisplatin and etoposide in four patients; cisplatin and 5-fluorouracil in two patients; carboplatin and etoposide in one patient; and cisplatin alone in one patient. The investigators concluded that gross tumour resection was the only factor which demonstrated a significant benefit in local control and therefore aggressive surgical resection either up front or after neoadjuvant therapy, in those with initially unresectable tumours, should be the main objective of treating non-metastatic SNUC.

A further recent series reported that surgery combined with radiotherapy, either given preoperatively or postoperatively, demonstrated the highest locoregional control. Of the 15 patients, nine were treated with surgery and radiotherapy (two patients received preoperative radiotherapy with concurrent cisplatin, seven patients received postoperative radiotherapy) demonstrating a three-year locoregional control rate of 78 per cent.[14]

It has also been advocated that, in view of the poor prognosis associated with most cases of SNUC, induction chemotherapy followed by concurrent chemoradiotherapy should be considered primary treatment. A series of seven patients treated with three cycles of platinum and 5-fluorouracil followed by radiotherapy with concurrent platinum showed a two-year overall survival of 64 per cent.[15]

Olfactory neuroblastoma

Olfactory neuroblastoma is a tumour of neural crest origin arising from the olfactory neuroepithelium of the roof of the nasal cavity and paranasal sinuses. It was first described by Berger et al.[16] in 1924 and has also been known as esthesioneuroblastoma, esthesioneuroepithelioma, esthesioneurocytoma and neuroendocrine carcinoma.[17,18] ONB represents 5–10 per cent of sinonasal malignancy and has no sex predilection. It has a bimodal age distribution peaking at 15 years and 50 years of age.[18]

CLINICAL FEATURES

The symptoms of ONB include nasal obstruction, rhinorrhea, epistaxis, anosmia, facial pain and diplopia. However, patients often present with non-specific symptoms resembling chronic sinusitis and therefore many cases are diagnosed late with advanced disease.[19] It has been reported that up to 70 per cent of patients present at a locally advanced stage.[19,20,21] Nasoendoscopy usually confirms an exophytic polypoid or sessile mass arising from the superior portion of the nasal cavity. The risk of cervical lymph node involvement is approximately 8–25 per cent and tends to occur late in the natural history.[22, 23] A CT scan will assess local invasion into the adjacent bony structures, particularly the cribriform plate, and a MR scan will assess the extent of soft tissue invasion, particularly involvement into the anterior cranial cavity and orbit. A small unilateral mass in the nasal cavity with or without bony involvement is seen in the early stages. More advanced stages present with extensive bone destruction, involvement of the paranasal sinuses, and orbital and intracranial involvement (**Figure 41.1**).

PATHOLOGY

The hallmark of ONB is the formation of tumour cells into rosettes, pseudorosettes, or sheets and clusters separated by a fibrovascular stroma.[24] Tumour cells characteristically have round nuclei containing dense chromatin which are surrounded by pale eosinophilic cytoplasm with indistinct borders. Necrosis is infrequent and is generally associated with high mitotic rates.[25] However, most ONBs have a low mitotic rate with mild to moderate nuclear pleomorphism.[26] Homer Wright pseudorosettes are seen in a half of ONBs. These are composed of tumour cells surrounding a central pink fibrillar material. True rosettes (known as Flexner type), which are uncommon, are formed by tumour cells surrounding a central lumen.[27]

Electron microscopy and immunohistochemical studies are frequently needed to establish the diagnosis. ONB stains strongly positive for a variety of neuroendocrine markers, such as neuron-specific enolase, chromogranin and synaptophysin. The rosettes may be surrounded by several spindle or stellate cells which stain positive for S-100.[9]

It is well established that the degree of histopathological differentiation is strongly correlated with the biological behaviour and prognosis.[28] Hyams et al.[29] introduced four grades of differentiation based on growth, architecture, mitotic activity, necrosis, nuclear pleomorphism, rosette formation and fibrillary stroma. A higher grade in the Hyams classification is associated with a poorer prognosis.

HYAMS HISTOLOGICAL GRADING SYSTEM

The grading system is as follows:[29]

- Grade I tumours have a prominent fibrillary matrix, tumours cells which have uniform nuclei and lack nuclear pleomorphism, mitotic activity and necrosis.
- Grade II tumours have some fibrillary matrix, moderate nuclear pleomorphism and some mitotic activity. No necrosis is present.
- Grade III tumours are characterized by minimal fibrillary matrix and Flexner-type rosettes are seen. Prominent mitotic activity, nuclear pleomorphism and some necrosis may be present.
- Grade IV tumours have no fibrillary matrix or rosettes. Marked nuclear pleomorphism and increased mitotic activity with frequent mitoses are seen.

STAGING

Despite three staging classifications being devised over the past three decades to help predict prognosis and tailor treatment strategies, there is no established consensus on the staging system for ONB. Kadish et al.[20] first introduced a three-tier classification in 1976 based on local disease extent with Morita et al.[21] later adding a stage D in 1993 (**Table 41.1**).

A further staging system devised by Dulguerov et al.[30] was introduced in 1992 based on the TNM system (**Table 41.2**).

Some centres have found the TNM classification to be more accurate in correlating prognosis and in guiding treatment compared with the original Kadish system.[31] The TNM classification takes into consideration involvement of the cribriform plate and intracranial extension without dural invasion. Tumours arising below and not involving the cribriform plate can potentially be managed with a more conservative approach rather than extensive surgery. Similarly, intracranial involvement which is extradural carries a better

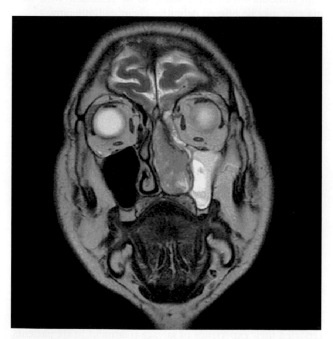

Figure 41.1 Coronal T_2-weighted magnetic resonance image of an olfactory neuroblastoma. A soft tissue mass is arising from the left nasal cavity causing deviation of the septum. No orbital invasion (courtesy of Gerald McGarry).

Table 41.1 Kadish stages of olfactory neuroblastoma,[20] modified by Morita.[21]

Stage	Features
A	Disease confined to the nasal cavity
B	Disease confined to the nasal cavity and paranasal sinuses
C	Disease beyond the nasal cavity and paranasal sinuses, including involvement of the cribriform plate, base of skull, orbit or intracranial cavity
D	With metastasis to cervical lymph nodes or distant metastases

Table 41.2 TNM staging of olfactory neuroblastoma.[30]

T/N/M	Characteristics
Primary tumour (T)	
T1	Tumour involving the nasal cavity and/or paranasal sinuses (excluding sphenoid), sparing the most superior ethmoidal cells
T2	Tumour involving the nasal cavity and/or paranasal sinuses (including the sphenoid), with extension to or erosion of the cribriform plate
T3	Tumour extending into the orbit or protruding into the anterior cranial fossa, without dural invasion
T4	Tumour involving the brain
Regional lymph nodes (N)	
N0	No cervical lymph node metastasis
N1	Any form of cervical lymph node metastasis
Distant metastasis (M1)	
M0	No metastasis
M1	Distant metastasis

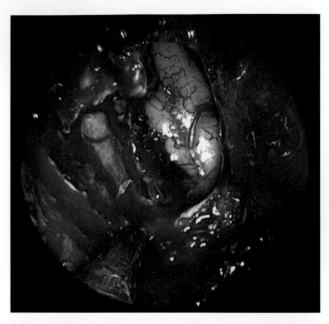

Figure 41.2 Transnasal endoscopic resection of an olfactory neuroblastoma (courtesy of Gerald McGarry).

prognosis than true invasion of the cerebral parenchyma and this is recognized in the TNM staging.

MANAGEMENT

There is no universally accepted optimal treatment for ONB in view of its rarity and the lack of randomized trials. Small tumours confined to the nasal or paranasal sinuses may be considered for an endoscopic resection providing appropriate expertise is available. However, a combined treatment modality approach with surgery and radiotherapy is needed for more advanced stage disease.[30, 31, 32, 33, 34, 35]

Endoscopic endonasal resection has been receiving attention recently in order to minimize surgical morbidity, such as cerebrospinal fluid leakage, intracranial haemorrhage and infection, as well as to reduce cosmetic complications associated with craniofacial resection (**Figure 41.2**). Tumours confined to the nasal or paranasal sinuses (Kadish A and B) and highly selected cases of Kadish C without deep infiltration of the orbit and pterygoplatine fossa or gross intracranial extension can be considered for this endoscopic approach. A few institutions have recently reported their experience showing good outcomes.[36, 37, 38]

Craniofacial resection is the standard surgical approach for most cases enabling en bloc resection with the cribriform plate. This has been shown to improve overall survival as well as disease-free survival.[22, 32, 33, 39, 40] Five-year survival has been shown to improve from 37.5 to 82 per cent with craniofacial resection.[33] However, despite macroscopic clearance, there is a relatively high risk of locoregional recurrence of 10–30 peer cent[19, 32] and therefore adjuvant therapies with radiotherapy with or without chemotherapy have been explored.[33, 41, 42]

A review of 390 cases published between 1990 and 2000 supports the addition of radiotherapy to surgery demonstrating a five-year survival of 65 per cent for those treated with surgery and radiotherapy compared with 48 per cent for

surgery alone.[43] This is consistent with a recent analysis from the Surveillance, Epidemiology, and End Results (SEER) database reporting a five-year survival of 66 per cent with surgery and radiotherapy compared to 51 per cent with surgery alone.[44]

Similar to SNUC, the timing of radiotherapy around surgery varies in practice. Some centres prefer using preoperative radiotherapy with concurrent chemotherapy,[33, 45, 46] whereas others prefer using postoperative radiotherapy.[21, 30, 47] Patients with tumours which are unlikely to be resectable with clear margins may be offered definitive chemoradiotherapy.

Levine et al.[33] reported their experience with surgery followed by postoperative radiotherapy demonstrating a five-year survival rate of close to 100 per cent for Kadish stage A and 75 per cent for Kadish stage B tumours. Kadish stage C tumours were associated with a relatively high incidence of local recurrence and distant metastases (10–20 per cent), and therefore adjuvant chemotherapy can be considered in this group.

Cisplatin-based chemotherapy has generally been used in the adjuvant or palliative setting. The Mayo Clinic reported a case series of ten Kadish stage C patients with recurrent disease who were treated with platinum chemotherapy.[42] The investigators concluded that cisplatin has activity in advanced ONB and that the Hyams grading is important at predicting response to chemotherapy with high-grade tumours having the most tumour regression. Non-platinum chemotherapy, such as irinotecan and docetaxel, have also been shown to have activity in advanced ONB.[48]

Locoregional recurrence can be salvaged with a radical neck dissection or radiotherapy depending on the site of recurrence and the original treatment modality. Kim et al.[49] reported their experience of salvage treatment in six patients. Nodal recurrence was generally managed with a radical neck dissection or a radical course of radiotherapy. Distant metastases, commonly to the central nervous system or bone, were associated with a dismal prognosis despite palliative chemotherapy with agents such as cisplatin, etoposide and ifosfamide.

The Hyams grading system is helpful for planning treatment. Surgical resection alone can be considered for small, low-grade tumours providing an R0 resection has been carried out. For high-grade tumours, which have a high risk of both local and distant recurrence, postoperative radiotherapy with or without chemotherapy is usually recommended.[17, 34]

Small cell undifferentiated (neuroendocrine) carcinoma

Neuroendocrine carcinomas can occur in any site of the head and neck region with a predilection to the larynx. They have been traditionally classified into three groups: carcinoid tumour, atypical carcinoid and small cell carcinoma. Those involving the sinonasal tract are usually small cell undifferentiated carcinoma; however, it is the least prevalent type of sinonasal carcinoma of neuroectodermal origin. It is believed to originate from the glandular epithelium of the exocrine glands of the olfactory mucosa.[50] The development and behaviour of NECs are distinct from those of ONB. NEC tends to arise more inferiorly in the nasal cavity, infrequently presents with regional nodal involvement, and has more potential for distant spread than ONB. It more frequently affects the elderly and has a poorer prognosis than ONB. In contrast, ONB can usually affect a younger age group, develops in the superior nasal cavity with a higher risk of regional nodal disease.

PATHOLOGY

Neuroendocrine carcinoma of the paranasal sinuses is microscopically indistinguishable from those of the bronchogenic origin. Light microscopy characteristically shows nests of poorly differentiated cells separated by thin branches of connective tissue. Nucleoli are often not prominent with nuclear chromatin having a fine granular appearance and the cytoplasm is scanty to moderate. NEC stains positive for the neuroendocrine markers (chromogranin, neuron-specific enolase, synaptophysin) and usually for cytokeratins.[51]

CLINICAL FEATURES

The presentation of NEC of the paranasal sinuses is similar to SNUC with nasal obstruction and epistaxis as common early symptoms, and cranial nerve palsies as more locally advanced features. Direct extension into the brain and multiple local recurrences are common. Distant metastases to the lungs, liver and bone are often relatively late events when compared to NEC arising from other anatomic sites. Furthermore, NEC may metastasize to the paranasal sinuses, and therefore a primary NEC of another site, such as the lungs, should always be sought and excluded.

MANAGEMENT

There is no recommended standard treatment for NEC of the nasal cavity or paranasal sinuses as a result of its rarity, and evidence to tailor treatment is extrapolated from data from small cell lung carcinoma. In view of its propensity to metastasize and its sensitivity to chemo-/radiotherapy, surgery is often considered not appropriate. The role of surgery is limited to very early stage disease which is uncommon. If surgery is used as primary treatment, craniofacial resection may not be necessary providing the cribriform plate, dura or brain are not involved. Locally advanced cases of NEC can be treated with induction chemotherapy, with regimens including a platinum, followed by a radical course of radiotherapy with consideration of concurrent chemotherapy in those who have responded and who are fit to receive this form of treatment. Metastatic NEC can be treated with chemotherapy, using a platinum plus etoposide, with consideration of radiotherapy to the primary or metastatic sites for palliation of local symptoms.

Outcome

SNUC and NEC are aggressive tumours with a high risk of locoregional and distant recurrence. Despite a radical treatment approach for SNUC, prognosis still remains very poor with median survival ranging from 10 to 18 months.[3, 5] NEC shares the same poor clinical outcome as SNUC with a reported median survival of 14.5 months.[52] Although prognosis of ONB is largely determined by the extent of disease at presentation, it can vary widely despite the Kadish staging and Hymans grading. ONB can show an indolent natural history with survival of more than 20 years in some cases. However, more aggressive cases of ONB which metastasize rapidly have survival often limited to a few months. Five-year survival rates have been reported as 57–88 per cent for Kadish stage A, 58–60 per cent for stage B and 0–50 per cent for stage C.[30, 53]

Follow up

Clinical follow up is determined by the aggressiveness of the tumour. However, this is often balanced by the potential for any salvageable treatment options which is largely influenced by the previous treatment and the patient's fitness. Follow up is usually a minimum of five years with a general ENT examination with locoregional nodal assessment and nasoendoscopy every two months for the first two years, then every six months for the third to fifth years, then annually as guided by local practice. ONB may need to be followed up for ten years or more as late recurrences can occur with indolent cases. Repeat imaging can be undertaken with either a CT or MR scan after six months, and then annually. Thyroid and pituitary function should both be monitored following radiotherapy.

BONE AND SOFT TISSUE SARCOMAS

Introduction

Both bone and soft tissue sarcomas are rare in the head and neck, but when encountered, treatment will follow the principles of managment of these tumours at their more usual sites, but modified to suit the anatomical constraints of the head and neck. Advice and shared care with a sarcoma specialist team will ensure appropriate diagnosis and treatment is achieved.[54, 55]

Bone sarcomas

Primary malignant bone sarcomas are very rare. There are approximately 400 each year in the UK (population 50 million) so the incidence is about 8/million population per year. The most common bone sarcoma is osteosarcoma, followed by Ewing's sarcoma and chondrosarcoma, while there are a smaller number of other primary malignant bone sarcomas which do not have typical features of any of the above three and are known as spindle cell sarcomas, including such diagnoses as a fibrosarcoma, leiomyosarcoma or MFH (malignant fibrous histiocytoma). The most common site for bone sarcomas to develop is in the long bones of the skeleton and about two-thirds of all primary bone sarcomas will arise around the knee. Less than 10 per cent of all bone sarcomas arise in the axial skeleton and of these only a few will arise in the head and neck.

This chapter gives details about the current management of primary malignant bone sarcomas, so that a head and neck surgeon encountering one of these will have an idea of their current management and outcome and can discuss the case with the appropriate bone sarcoma experts for advice on management.

OSTEOSARCOMA

Osteosarcoma is principally a disease of adolescents with the most common age being 15 years and is slightly more common in males than females. Most osteosarcomas are high-grade malignant tumours presenting with a short history of pain followed by swelling. In the peripheral skeleton, the classic radiological features include sunray spiculations and periosteal elevation known as Codman's triangle. These classical features may not be present in other sites and any patient presenting with an x-ray exhibiting any of the four following characteristics should be considered to have a potential bone tumour until proved otherwise:

- periosteal elevation;
- soft tissue swelling;
- bone destruction;
- new bone formation.

There are, however, a variety of other types of osteosarcoma:

- **Parosteal osteosarcoma.** This is a relatively low-grade variant of surface osteosarcoma typically arising at the back of the knee. It is densely calcified.[56, 57]
- **Periosteal osteosarcoma.** This arises within the periosteum and usually presents relatively early. It has a better prognosis than conventional osteosarcoma, but is treated similarly.[58, 59]
- **Low-grade central osteosarcoma.** This is a slowly progressive and difficult to diagnose condition. Histologically, it looks remarkably similar to fibrous dysplasia and there can be significant delays in diagnosis because of this. Treatment is surgical.[60]

- **Paget's osteosarcoma.** This is a highly malignant and rapidly progressive tumour arising in patients with pre-existing Paget's disease.[61, 62]
- **Radiation-induced osteosarcoma.** This is an osteosarcoma developing in bone which has previously been exposed to radiation, usually following treatment for a previous malignancy lying adjacent to the bone (e.g. thyroid cancer, orbital cancer). The sarcoma typically develops from five to 30 years later and should be treated like a conventional high-grade osteosarcoma.[63, 64]

A few patients with osteosarcoma will have the Li–Fraumeni syndrome (a familial cancer clustering of breast cancer, brain tumours, leukaemia and sarcomas). There is an increased incidence of osteosarcoma in patients with previous retinoblastoma because of the *RB1* gene. The risk is related to age of diagnosis and treatment of the retinoblastoma with a 25 per cent incidence for those treated prior to 12 months of age and 3 per cent for those treated after that age.[65]

In the head and neck region, osteosarcoma usually arises in young males who present with pain and swelling of the face. Radiological investigations will reveal abnormalities either involving the maxilla or mandible. The tumours are often relatively low grade, but careful histological analysis by a sarcoma expert is recommended in all cases to confirm the diagnosis and guide treatment.

Any patient with a bone sarcoma requires staging, which is the assessment of the extent of the disease, both locally and distantly.[66] Sarcomas spread by the bloodstream and metastases nearly always arise in the lungs, but occasionally another bone will be involved. Staging will thus consist of imaging of the chest (a computed tomography (CT) scan), a bone scan, and magnetic resonance imaging (MRI) or CT of the primary site.

The outcome for patients with osteosarcoma has been dramatically changed by the use of chemotherapy. For patients with high-grade osteosarcoma, survival rates of 65 per cent or greater would now be expected. Treatment consists of a combination of chemotherapy and surgical excision of the primary site with reconstruction if required. A raised alkaline phosphatase at diagnosis and the presence of metastases are both poor prognostic indicators, as are a poor response of the tumour to chemotherapy, axial site (including head and neck), large size of the tumour, as well as older age of the patient.[67, 68]

Chemotherapy is based on regimes using cisplatin, doxorubicin, methotrexate and ifosfamide. Most chemotherapy for osteosarcoma will be given in specialist centres where there is expertise in using these regimes. It is standard practice to give approximately ten weeks of chemotherapy before proceeding to surgery. Following resection of the tumour, the removed specimen is analysed to assess the amount of necrosis caused by the chemotherapy. If more than 90 per cent of the tumour is found to be necrotic, this is a very good prognostic indicator. For those patients with poor necrosis however, there is no evidence that changing the chemotherapy improves survival, although this is currently the subject of an international trial.[69, 70]

Surgical resection of the tumour remains essential for both local control and cure. The principle is to excise the tumour with a 'wide' margin of normal tissue around the tumour itself. Effective chemotherapy will help improve the margins of excision.

In the head and neck, obtaining wide margins will be extremely difficult, but every attempt must be made to achieve them. The narrower the margin of excision and the worse the response to chemotherapy, the greater the risk of local recurrence.[71] There is a natural tendency to consider the use of radiotherapy in cases where a wide margin cannot be achieved, but there is at the moment little evidence that this improves local control. Radiotherapy can be used for palliation in cases of extensive recurrence.[72]

There have been no large studies of osteosarcoma of the head and neck, but there are a number of case series. All these comment on the necessity for a multidisciplinary approach and the need for clear margins of excision to maximize local control.[73, 74, 75]

Patients with low-grade central osteosarcoma or low-grade parosteal osteosarcoma do not require chemotherapy and can be managed purely surgically.[76]

The techniques of reconstruction used in the head and neck will be very similar to those used for other tumour types arising in similar sites and will not be documented further.

CHONDROSARCOMA

Chondrosarcoma is the second most common type of bone tumour and is more common in older people from about 40 years onwards. It is slightly more common in males than females and on the whole it is a low-grade, slow-growing type of sarcoma. It frequently presents as a painless mass arising either within the bone (central) or on the surface (peripheral). Chondrosarcoma is graded from one to three based on the histological appearance and most will be grade one or two. Grade 3 chondrosarcoma is a highly malignant tumour with a poor prognosis. Rarely, a chondrosarcoma will dedifferentiate to a high-grade spindle cell sarcoma and again the prognosis is poor.[77]

Chondrosarcomas do not respond to chemotherapy or radiotherapy and treatment is by surgical excision and reconstruction if necessary. Clear margins of excision are absolutely essential for local control.[78, 79]

Chondrosarcoma of the head and neck is rare but a review by the National Cancer database in the United States identified 400 cases of head and neck chondrosarcoma in a ten-year period.[80] The authors reported a disease-specific survival of 87 per cent at five years dropping to 70 per cent at ten years. Complete surgical excision led to the best chance of local control and survival.

EWING'S SARCOMA

Ewing's sarcoma of bone arises in children and young adults and although common in the axial skeleton (25 per cent of cases arise in the pelvis), it is rare in the head and neck. The cell of origin remains uncertain, but the tumours are small blue round cell tumours characteristically demonstrating a t(11;22) translocation. The histological diagnosis can be extremely difficult, in particular differentiating these tumours from rhabdomyosarcoma or synovial sarcoma and the use of molecular genetic studies is essential to confirm the diagnosis prior to treatment starting.[81]

Ewing's sarcoma usually responds very well to chemotherapy using ifosfamide, doxorubicin, vincristine and etoposide. The tumour is also usually very sensitive to radiotherapy. In the past, treatment with chemotherapy and radiotherapy resulted in a high rate of local recurrence (20 per cent or more) and so now attempts are made in most cases to surgically remove the tumour once it has been downstaged by preoperative chemotherapy. Postoperative radiotherapy will still be used if there is a poor response of the tumour to chemotherapy or if the margins are not wide. If the surgical excision would not achieve clear margins or there would be a major functional deficit following the surgery, then consideration should still be given to definitive radiotherapy despite the increased risk of local recurrence. The overall prognosis for patients with Ewing's sarcoma is dependent upon the presence or absence of metastases at the time of diagnosis, the age of the patient and the size of the initial tumour, as well as the response to chemotherapy. Overall, survival rates of approximately 70 per cent at five years are to be expected.[82, 83]

SPINDLE CELL SARCOMAS

Spindle cell sarcomas of bone are treated in a very similar manner to osteosarcoma with chemotherapy and surgical excision and reconstruction. Because these patients tend to be older, it is often more difficult to give them a full course of chemotherapy and beyond the age of 60 years, chemotherapy proves very toxic and it may not be possible to use this. Survival rates are slightly better than for osteosarcoma in a similar age group.[84, 85]

There are a variety of other bone tumours which may affect the head and neck region, the most important of which is in giant cell tumour of bone (osteoclastoma). This is a benign but locally aggressive tumour where the bone is simply eaten away. The aetiology is unknown and treatment is by curettage of the giant cell tumour. The site and size of the tumour will depend on whether any form of reconstruction is needed. A bone graft or bone cement can both be used to fill the defect. Although some people use adjuvants, such as liquid nitrogen or phenol, to clean out the cavity, local recurrence rates vary between 10 and 25 per cent.[86, 87] In cases of very aggressive or recurrent tumours, complete surgical excision may be required for local control and radiotherapy can also be used if essential. The main differential diagnosis of a giant cell tumour both radiologically and histologically is a brown tumour of hyperparathyroidism and it is mandatory to check the serum calcium of any patient with a suspected giant cell tumour of bone.

CHORDOMAS

Chordomas are tumours arising from the primitive notochord. The most common site is in the sacrococcygeal area, but about 25 per cent will arise in the cervical spine or base of skull. They are slow growing, but locally aggressive malignant tumours with a low rate of metastasis. Surgical excision with clear margins is the treatment, but can be very difficult to achieve. Conventional radiotherapy seems to have little role in controlling progression of the tumour, but in very selective cases heavy particle proton beam radiotherapy may have a role.[88, 89, 90]

FOLLOW UP

Any patient who has been diagnosed and treated for a sarcoma should be regularly followed up to try and identify locally recurrent disease at a stage when it is still treatable. The other purpose of follow up is to identify early metastatic disease because surgical resection of metastases (usually in the lungs) can be worthwhile, providing long-term cure in up to 30 per cent of cases. It is usually recommended that patients should be seen clinically every three months for the first two years, six monthly the next three years and annually thereafter. They should have a routine x-ray of the primary site and a chest x-ray on each occasion. At the present time, there is no proof that regular follow up with either CT or MRI is beneficial or cost-effective.

Soft tissue sarcomas

Soft tissue sarcomas are malignant tumours originating from various soft components of the mesenchymal tissue anywhere in the body. They are rare in the head and neck accounting for less than 10 per cent of all soft tissue sarcomas and approximately 1 per cent of all head and neck tumours.[91, 92, 93, 94, 95] There is a variable male predominance with median age between 50 to 55 years.[92, 93] In children, head and neck soft tissue sarcomas are much more common comprising 35–40 per cent of all soft tissue sarcomas.[96, 97]

A variety of histological entities, some clearly defined, others more ambiguous, with varied biological behaviour are observed (**Box 41.1**). This heterogeneity makes individual subtypes of the disease even more rare, although the more commonly reported subtypes are fibrosarcoma, liposarcoma and malignant fibrous histiocytoma, each accounting for about 20 per cent in most studies.[93, 98] Rhabdomyosarcoma is rare in adults, but is the principal paediatric type.[98] It has a distinct natural history and is managed differently to other soft tissue sarcomas, and is thus discussed separately.

Box 41.1   Histological subtypes of soft tissue sarcomas

- Malignant fibrous histiocytoma
- Liposarcoma
- Fibrosarcoma
- Malignant peripheral nerve sheath tumour (MPNST)
- Spindle cell sarcoma
- Ewing's sarcoma
- Synovial sarcoma
- Dermatofibrosarcoma protuberans
- Leiomyosarcoma
- Myxoid chondrosarcoma
- Sclerosing epithelioid fibrosarcoma
- Angiosarcoma
- Epithelioid sarcoma
- Rhabdomyosarcoma
- Lymphangiosarcoma
- Unclassified sarcoma

The rarity of soft tissue sarcomas suggests that they are best treated at multidisciplinary specialist sarcoma units where the opportunity is available to gather knowledge and skills, and develop expertise.[98]

AETIOLOGY

The majority of patients do not have any obvious risk factors, however a number of genetic and environmental exposures have been associated with an increased risk of soft tissue sarcomas. The Li–Fraumeni syndrome is an autosomal dominant disorder involving a mutation of p53 tumour-suppressor gene and is associated with soft tissue sarcomas, as well as multiple other malignancies.[99] Neurofibromatosis type 1 is associated with rhabdomyosarcoma, liposarcoma and fibrosarcoma in children and MPNST (malignant peripheral nerve sheath tumor) in adults.[99, 100] Other conditions which have been implicated in the increased risk for soft tissue sarcomas include hereditary retinoblastoma and Gardner's syndrome.[97, 99] Previous radiotherapy to treat other conditions, especially breast cancer has been associated with increased risk of late development of soft tissue sarcomas in the head and neck.[93, 101, 102, 103, 104]

CLINICAL FEATURES

Soft tissue sarcomas may occur in any part of the head and neck, although the most commonly reported primary sites include scalp, face and neck.[93, 97] The clinical presentation is mostly related to the anatomical site of the lesion and presence or absence of compression of the surrounding structures by the lesion. The most common presenting feature of head and neck sarcomas is a painless mass which is reported in 80 per cent of cases.[105] A wide spectrum of other symptoms have been reported which include nasal blockage, epistaxis, proptosis, diplopia, otalgia, deafness, tinnitus, vertigo, dental pain, tooth mobility, dysphagia, alteration in voice quality and facial palsy. Most tumours are nonmetastatic at presentation. Occasionally, the patients may present with an enlarged neck node due to regional spread. It is extremely unlikely for the patients to present with symptoms related to spread to distant sites.

It is common to discover soft tissue sarcomas incidentally following excision of a lump, without prior suspicion of a sarcoma. The clinical signs are mostly nonspecific, however a submucosal or subcutaneous mass may be expected.[97] Angiosarcoma typically presents as a macule or plaque resembling dermatological entities on the forehead and scalp of elderly white males.[106, 107]

Current guidance issued by National Institute for Health and Clinical Excellence (NICE) recommends that a lump with any of the following features should be investigated for potential malignancy:

- larger than 5 cm;
- increasing in size;
- deep to the fascia;
- painful.

Similar guidance published about early diagnosis of head and neck cancer recommends urgent referral for any unexplained lump in the neck, of recent onset, or a previously undiagnosed lump that has changed over a period of 3–6 weeks.[108]

There should be clearcut pathways for referring patients in either of the above categories either to a head and neck or a sarcoma rapid diagnosis unit.

INVESTIGATIONS

Delay in diagnosis for soft tissue sarcomas is common as often the patients and clinicians do not perceive the symptoms and signs as sinister. The initial role of the head and neck surgeon includes assessment of the primary tumour and clinical investigations including nasendoscopy, examination under general anaesthesia and biopsy. Because soft tissue sarcomas are so rare, it is unlikely that the diagnosis will be initially considered, but it is important not to jeopardise subsequent management of a potential sarcoma by hasty treatment.

Any patient with a suspicious lump should undergo appropriate investigation, which, in the head and neck will usually follow the pathway recommended for the site of the lesion. While imaging to asses the anatomical location of the mass is essential, biopsy is mandatory in confirming the diagnosis of soft tissue sarcoma.

Very few pathologists, even in specialist centres, will be happy to diagnose a soft tissue sarcoma on a fine needle aspiration (FNA) cytology sample, although this is frequently the first procedure carried out in head and neck clinics. A needle core biopsy will however be diagnostic in most cases and should be the next step in investigation if FNA is not helpful.[93, 101] An incisional transmucosal biopsy is appropriate for lesions in the aerodigestive and sinonasal tracts. Complete resection of the tumour in the parotid, neck and parapharyngeal space is preferable to incisional biopsy to prevent iatrogenic seeding of tumour cells into a possible future operative site. An incisional biopsy on these sites may only be considered if unacceptable level of cosmetic or functional morbidity is expected if complete resection was undertaken.[97]

The patients should undergo imaging studies, such as MRI and/or CT, to enable accurate assessment of the lesion and to ascertain regional node status although the risk of regional spread is low.[93, 97] The most common site for distant metastases is the lungs and therefore the patients should have a CT scan of the chest before treatment to rule out the possibility of metastatic disease, especially in cases of high-grade tumours. In the absence of lung metastases, other distant metastases are highly unlikely and therefore further investigations are not essential.[93, 97]

PATHOLOGY

Most soft tissue sarcomas are high grade and are located deep to the superficial fascia.[93] Establishing accurate histological subtype of the tumour is unfortunately not straightforward as it requires complex immunohistochemical and cytogenetic studies by specialist pathologists, and all cases of suspected sarcoma should be referred to a specialist sarcoma pathologist for confirmation of diagnosis prior to treatment.[95, 97, 109] An accurate histological diagnosis will provide helpful information on the likely prognosis for the patients. Malignant fibrous histiocytoma, rhabdomyosarcoma,

angiosarcoma, synovial sarcoma, alveolar soft part sarcoma and Ewing's sarcoma are generally high-grade tumours with poorer prognosis, whereas dermatofibrosarcoma protuberans and desmoid tumours are low-grade tumours with better prognosis.[91, 97, 105, 110, 111, 112]

There is currently no universally accepted staging system for soft-tissue sarcomas. Several staging systems are used, of which the most commonly used are the TNM (tumour, node, metastasis) system developed by the American Joint Committee on Cancer and the Enneking system.[66, 113] Both of these staging systems take histological grade into account, as well as size and spread of the tumour.

MANAGEMENT

Soft tissue sarcomas are best managed by a multidisciplinary team which may include a sarcoma specialist, a site-specific head and neck surgeon and an oncologist, as well as the sarcoma pathologist and appropriate radiologists. The important features that determine management of soft tissue sarcomas are site, size and grade of the tumour, and presence or absence of nodal or distant metastases.[93, 97]

Complete surgical resection is the treatment of choice for all soft tissue sarcomas. Surgical excision with a wide margin of normal tissue around the lesion should be attempted in all cases unless contraindicated by the possibility of an unacceptable level of functional or cosmetic morbidity or in those tumours in close proximity to vital anatomical structures. Contemporary surgical advances, such as free tissue transfer with microvascular reconstruction, have made it possible for larger tumours to be resected and this may require a multidisciplinary surgical team consisting of a sarcoma surgeon, head and neck surgeon, and a maxillofacial or plastic surgeon. Locoregional lymph node dissection is rarely necessary for sarcomas, however it may be considered in certain tumours with a predilection for lymph node metastases (e.g. epithelioid sarcoma, clear cell sarcoma and occasionally synovial sarcoma).

Adjuvant radiotherapy is indicated for all high- or intermediate-grade tumours and also for marginally or incompletely resected low-grade tumours. Radiotherapy alone may be used in cases of unresectable tumours and may provide temporary local control in some patients.[93]

Chemotherapy is not usually used for soft tissue sarcomas as it has not been shown to produce an overall survival benefit. It does however have a role in the treatment of specific soft tissue sarcomas, such as Ewing's tumour, and soft tissue sarcomas in children.[73, 114] A meta-analysis published in the *Lancet* revealed a 10 per cent benefit of chemotherapy on recurrence-free survival which may support a case for considering adjuvant chemotherapy for patients with large, high-grade deep soft tissue sarcomas in an attempt to improve relapse-free survival (**Figure 41.3**).[114] The treatment is essentially palliative if metastatic disease is present.

OUTCOME

The most significant prognostic factors for overall survival of soft tissue sarcomas are grade, size and depth, while margin status of the excised tumours is the most important prognostic factor for local control.[115] High grade, tumour size

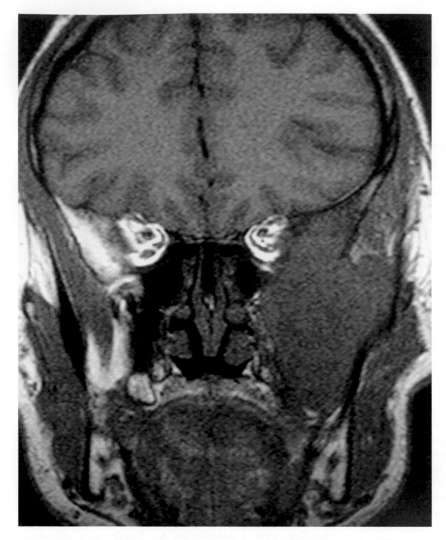

Figure 41.3 Magnetic resonance image (MRI) of the face of a 26-year-old male who presented with a painless swelling of the face. MRI revealed this soft tissue tumour (arrowed) extending from the base of skull to the hard palate. Biopsy confirmed synovial sarcoma. Treatment was with chemotherapy to downsize the tumour, followed by surgical excision and radiotherapy.

larger than 5 cm in diameter, tumours incompletely excised and location deep to the superficial fascia are all associated with poorer survival.[95, 97, 106, 110, 112, 116, 117, 118]

Head and neck soft tissue sarcomas are recognized to have a worse prognosis than similar sarcomas elsewhere in the body. The five-year overall survival and local control rates for soft tissue sarcomas of the head and neck ranges from 60 to 70 per cent.[93] This is much lower compared with local control rates of up to 90 per cent for sarcomas of the extremities.[93, 119] This is most likely related to the difficulty of obtaining wide surgical margins in many cases in the head and neck. Unlike limb soft tissue sarcomas, there is no option of undertaking an amputation if local recurrence occurs.

The local recurrence rates for high-grade soft tissue sarcomas after surgical excision is as high as 50 per cent and the risk is increased with intralesional or marginal surgical margins.[92, 93, 119, 120] It is therefore extremely important that every effort is made to maximize the margins at the time of the first surgical procedure. If the margins prove positive at the first attempt, performing a further and wider excision should always be considered. Patients who present after inadvertent excision of a lump which turns out to be a sarcoma should always be considered for a further wide excision as residual tumour cells will be found in up to 70 per cent of cases.[121] The risk of developing distant metastases is between 10 and 30 per cent and the risk is higher for large, intermediate or high-grade and deep lesions.[93] The majority of patients who develop metastatic disease do so within two to three years of receiving the treatment.[93, 122, 123]

A nomogram to predict survival of patients following excision of soft tissue sarcomas is available online (www.mskcc.org/mskcc/html/6181.cfm).[124]

FOLLOW UP

Following definitive treatment, patients should be followed up routinely in order to detect treatable local recurrence or metastatic disease at a stage when it can be dealt with. A minimum period of up to five years is recommended as it is uncommon for local recurrence to occur after this period and prolonged follow up may result in unnecessary distress to the patients and inappropriate use of resources. Clinical assessment and chest radiograph should be considered at each clinic visit. These would usually be four times a year for two years following diagnosis then twice a year for the next three years. Surgical excision of local recurrence or metastatic disease should be considered if possible. Palliative chemotherapy or radiotherapy may have a role.

Rhabdomyosarcoma

Rhabdomyosarcoma is a distinct clinicopathological entity and its management is significantly different from other types of soft tissue sarcomas. It accounts for about one-fourth of all head and neck sarcomas and 4–8 per cent of all paediatric cancers.[105, 118, 125, 126] Other than in the head and neck, it may arise in genitourinary organs, limbs and may also rarely occur elsewhere.

There are four different histological types of rhabdomyosarcoma-embryonic, alveolar (**Figure 41.4**), botryoidal and pleomorphic, of which the embryonic types are the most common and the alveolar tumours have the worst prognosis.[127] Rhabdomyosarcoma arises in three main head and neck primary sites with different prognostic significance – orbit, parameningeal sites (nasopharynx, nasal fossa, paranasal sinuses, infratemporal fossa, ptrygoid fossa, middle ear and mastoid) and non-parameningeal sites (scalp, face, parotid, oral cavity, oropharynx, larynx and neck).[127] Those arising at parameningeal sites have an affinity to invade the cranial cavity via basal skull foramina and are consequently associated with the worst prognosis.

Rhabdomyosarcoma has a propensity to metastasize early to regional lymph nodes[126, 127] and therefore radiological investigation of the neck with MRI should be undertaken routinely. In cases of parameningeal rhabdomyosarcoma, a MRI of the brain and cytological examination of cerebrospinal fluid (CSF) may be needed.[97]

The specific site of origin of rhabdomyosarcoma is incorporated into the TNM staging system as it correlates well with the outcome.[127] The Children's Oncology Group (COG) based in the United States and European Paediatric Soft Tissue Sarcoma Study Group (EPSTSSG) conduct studies and produce protocols for management of soft tissue sarcomas in children. They have used surgicopathologic criteria including local extension, regional and distant metastases, and amount of residual tumour after surgical resection of the tumour, to stage rhabdomyosarcoma.[127]

Complete surgical excision remains a critical component of treatment for rhabdomyosarcoma, however radical surgery is frequently not possible due to close proximity of the tumours to vital structures and also due to the possibility of significant postoperative cosmetic and functional morbidity.

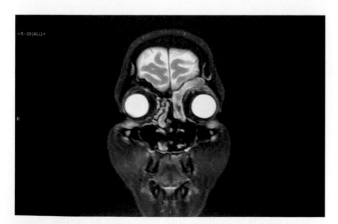

Figure 41.4 Coronal T$_2$-weighted magnetic resonance image showing an alveolar rhabdomyosarcoma of the left fronto-ethmoidal sinuses (figure courtesy of Gerald McGarry).

Combination chemotherapy with or without adjuvant surgery and/or radiotherapy is commonly used as primary treatment for rhabdomyosarcoma.[127, 128, 129]

The five-year overall survival for rhabdomyosarcoma in children ranges from 74 to 77 per cent, while the five-year disease-free survival ranges from 58 to 74 per cent. The outcome in adults is unclear due to lack of studies, however may be significantly worse.[127, 128, 129, 130, 131]

HEAD AND NECK LYMPHOMAS

Introduction

Lymphomas involving the head and neck broadly fall into four main categories:

1. Primary central nervous system lymphoma (PCNSL) is rare and accounts for 1–2 per cent of all lymphomas. It is defined as a non-Hodgkin's lymphoma (NHL) that is confined to the craniospinal axis without systemic involvement. Patients present with symptoms due to either ocular or involvement of the brain (in 50 per cent of cases the frontal lobes are involved). Patients with either congenital or acquired immunodeficiency (e.g. due to human immunodeficiency virus or immunosuppression secondary to solid organ transplantation) have a significantly greater risk of developing PCNSL. Patients with PCNSL usually present to neurologists, neurosurgeons or ophthalmologists and hence further information about this rare but complex lymphoma is not included in this chapter.

2. Primary extranodal lymphomas are defined as lymphomas occurring in tissue other than lymph nodes, spleen or bone marrow. Approximately 25 per cent of NHL occur in extranodal sites. Lymphoma involving Waldeyer's ring (tonsil, nasopharynx and base of tongue) accounts for approximately 10–15 per cent of extranodal lymphomas. NHL involving the sinuses accounts for approximately 4 per cent of all extranodal lymphomas. Thyroid lymphomas account for 5 per cent of thyroid cancers and 5 per cent of extranodal lymphomas.

3. Nasal T/NK-cell lymphoma is now considered to be a distinctive pathological entity and typically is a destructive tumour which affects the midline facial structure. It has an unusual epidemiological pattern and is seen predominantly in the Far East (China, Hong Kong, Japan, Malaysia and Korea), as well as Central and South America (Mexico and Peru). Sporadic cases in other parts of the world are only rarely seen. It is an exceedingly rare lymphoma and even in places where it is observed more frequently, such as the Far East, it accounts for only 5 per cent of all lymphomas.

4. Hodgkin's lymphoma is relatively rare and in the UK there are approximately 1500 new cases/year. The disease has a bimodal age distribution with one peak between 15 and 35 years, and a second peak in patients older than 50 years. Cure rates for patients

with Hodgkin's lymphoma are generally better than for NHL and are usually in excess of 50 per cent.

Primary extranodal lymphomas involving the head and neck

LYMPHATICS OF THE HEAD AND NECK

The lymphatics of the head and neck are arranged in deep and superficial chains. The deep jugular chain extends from the skull base to the clavicle and is formed into superior, middle and inferior groups of lymph nodes.

The superior deep jugular nodes receives primary drainage from the soft palate, tonsils, palatoglossal and palatopharyngeal arches, posterior and base of tongue, pyriform sinus and larynx above the vocal folds. The middle deep jugular nodes receive primary drainage from the larynx above the vocal folds, lower pyriform sinus and posterior cricoid. The inferior deep jugular nodes receive primary drainage from the thyroid, trachea and cervical oesophagus (see **Figure 41.5a,b**). The retropharyngeal and paratracheal nodes receive drainage from deep structures in the midline of the head, including the nasopharynx, posterior nasal cavity, paranasal sinuses and posterior oropharynx.

The superficial nodes are the submental, superficial cervical, submandibular, spinal accessory and anterior scalene. The submental nodes drain the chin, tip of the tongue, anterior mouth and middle of the lower lip. The submandibular nodes drain the upper lip, lateral lower lip, lower nasal cavity, anterior mouth and the skin of the cheek. The superficial cervical nodes receive drainage from around the parotid gland, behind the ear, parotid and occipital nodes. The nodes in the posterior triangle lie around the spinal accessory nerve and drain the parietal and occipital regions of the scalp. The anterior scalene (Virchow's) nodes are located at the junction of the thoracic duct and the left subclavian vein and receive drainage form the thoracic duct. They are usually the site for metastases from the stomach. The supraclavicular nodes receive drainage from the spinal accessory nodes and infraclavicular sources (see **Figure 41.6**).

All the lymphatics from the head and neck region eventually drain into the venous system either through the thoracic duct on the left or the right lymphatic duct.

Clinical presentation

Patients with head and neck lymphomas generally present with airway obstruction, difficulty in swallowing, mass lesion, blockage of the Eustachian tube or neck nodes. Frequently, the mass may be palpable. However, a flexible direct endoscopy is recommended in all patients since such an assessment may reveal multiple sites of involvement. Fine needle aspiration/cytology is inadequate to make a detailed pathological diagnosis and hence a tissue biopsy or excision biopsy is required in all patients. To allow for full molecular, cytogenetic and immunohistochemical analysis, the sample should be sent fresh to the pathology laboratory as a matter of urgency. Although surgery may debulk the tumour, surgical resection alone is not curative and hence full staging is required on all patients.

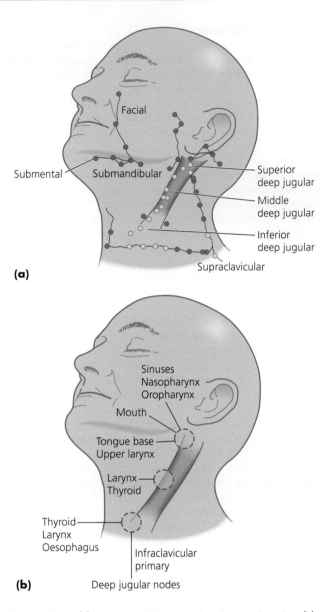

Figure 41.5 (a) Drainage of the deep jugular lymph nodes. (b) Drainage of the deep jugular nodes.

Staging investigations

The following investigations are recommended at diagnosis:

- Computed tomography (CT) or magnetic resonance imaging (MRI) scan of the head and neck
- Whole body CT/positron emission tomography (PET) scan or if not available, CT scan of the chest, abdomen and pelvis
- Bone marrow aspirate and trephine biopsy
- Full blood count
- Biochemistry profile, including lactate dehydrogenase (LDH)
- For patients presenting with lymphoma involving Waldeyer's ring, investigation of the gastrointestinal (GI) tract with either endoscopy or contrast imaging is required.

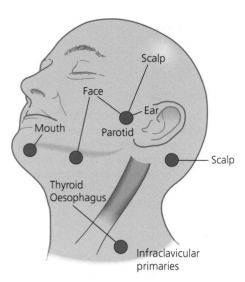

Figure 41.6 Drainage of superficial nodes.

Approximately 30 per cent of patients with tonsillar lymphoma have systemic disease. There is an association between Waldeyer's ring lymphoma and the GI tract. In a large randomized trial,[132] approximately a third of patients with relapsed Waldeyer's ring lymphoma, relapsed in the GI tract.

Diffuse large B-cell lymphoma (a type of high-grade or aggressive B-cell NHL) accounts for 60–80 per cent of non-Hodgkin's lymphoma occurring in the head and neck region, other histological types include follicular (14 per cent), mantle cell (12 per cent) and mucosa-associated lymphoid tissue (MALT)-lymphoma (9 per cent). Sixty per cent of patients present with localized disease.

Treatment

Limited stage

Surgical resection is rarely curative and treatment of patients with localized head and neck lymphomas generally consists of a combination of chemotherapy and radiotherapy. The chemotherapy schedule that is almost universally used for patients with high-grade B-cell NHL is R-CHOP.[133] This consists of a cocktail of five drugs: rituximab (a monoclonal antibody against CD20), cyclophosphamide, doxorubicin, vincristine and prednisolone. The chemotherapy schedule is given on a 3-weekly basis. For patients with limited stage disease, treatment generally consists of three cycles of chemotherapy followed by radiotherapy. A randomized trial of 316 patients with stage I Waldeyer's ring high-grade lymphoma showed a higher relapse rate for patients treated with CHOP or irradiation alone compared with combined modality treatment.[132] Twenty-three per cent of patients treated with chemotherapy alone relapsed compared to 5 per cent treated with a combination of chemotherapy plus radiotherapy. In a retrospective review of 130 adult patients with stage I and II NHL affecting the Waldeyer's ring, Ezzat et al.[134] found that 84 per cent had diffuse large B-cell NHL, 58 per cent had primary tonsillar, 35 per cent nasopharyngeal and 7 per cent base of the tongue lymphoma. Fifty-eight per cent received chemotherapy alone, 20 per cent received radiotherapy and 35 per cent were managed with a combination of chemotherapy and radiotherapy. The complete

remission rate of approximately 80 per cent was no different between the three treatment modalities. Most distant relapses were seen in non-gastrointestinal sites. Patients treated with combined modality treatment had a better event-free survival; this study did not show a difference in overall survival for the combined modality treatment when compared with single modality treatment. However, a further study from Italy[135] in 107 patients with localized extranodal head and neck lymphoma treated with either radiotherapy alone ($n = 59$) or chemotherapy plus radiotherapy ($n = 48$) showed a significant improvement in five-year overall survival for combined modality treatment; 63 versus 38 per cent for radiotherapy alone. In multivariate analysis, the only significant prognostic factor was age <60 years. Eighty per cent of the relapses occurred systemically and only 7.5 per cent of patients relapsed in-field.

Contrary to diffuse large B-cell or aggressive NHL, patients with indolent, localized lymphoma of the Waldeyer's ring can achieve long-term disease control with radiotherapy alone.

Advanced stage disease

Patients with stage III/IV diffuse large B-cell NHL, those with B-symptoms or bulky disease (>10 cm) should be treated with between six and eight cycles of R-CHOP chemotherapy, followed by radiotherapy to any residual sites of disease. Residual disease is best assessed by a PET scan.

Patients with extensive low-grade lymphoma can be treated with single agent (e.g. chlorambucil or fludarabine) or combination (R-CVP, rituximab in combination with cyclophosphamide, vincristine and prednisolone) chemotherapy.

Nasal T/NK–cell lymphoma

SINUS LYMPHOMA

Approximately 3 per cent of extranodal lymphomas involve the sinuses. The sinuses most commonly involved include the ethmoid, frontal, maxillary and sphenoid.

Presenting symptoms

Patients usually present with:

- Local pain and/or facial swelling.
- Nasal or airway obstruction.
- Rhinorrhoea.
- Epistaxis.
- If the tumour involves the periorbital area, patients may present with proptosis, loss of vision or diplopia.

In British Columbia, a retrospective survey was carried out of 44 patients with primary paranasal lymphoma presenting between 1980 and 1999.[135] Eighty-four per cent of patients had diffuse large B-cell lymphoma, 8 per cent had T/NK nasal type and 8 per cent had T-cell/not classified. Median age at presentation was 66 years (range, 27–97 years). All patients were treated with chemotherapy plus radiotherapy. In addition, from 1985, they received intrathecal chemotherapy. The addition of intrathecal chemotherapy reduced the risk of central nervous system (CNS) relapse and also improved overall and disease-free survival (from 20 to 51 per cent and 40 to 65 per cent, respectively).

Sinus lymphoma usually follows an aggressive course and has a tendency to cause bony destruction, break down natural anatomic barriers and systemically disseminate. Once the diagnosis is confirmed, patients should be commenced on chemotherapy (which will be R-CHOP in the majority of cases). Patients usually receive between six and eight cycles of chemotherapy followed by involved field radiotherapy. Given the anatomical proximity of the sinuses to the central nervous system, it is not surprising that this type of lymphoma has a tendency to spread to the central nervous system. The risk of spread has been estimated to be as high as between 20 and 40 per cent.[136] Administering prophylactic intrathecal chemotherapy may reduce the risk of CNS relapse to less than 10 per cent.

THYROID LYMPHOMA

Primary thyroid lymphoma is a lymphoma that arises from the thyroid. It is relatively rare and accounts for 5 per cent of all thyroid malignancies. It is more common in women and the median age of presentation is 60 years. Lymphomas affecting the thyroid are usually non-Hodgkin's lymphomas. The incidence of thyroid lymphoma in patients with Hashimoto thyroiditis is markedly increased and the incidence of pre-existing autoimmune thyroiditis in patients with thyroid lymphoma ranges from 27 to 100 per cent.[137, 138, 139] The risk of developing thyroid lymphoma in a patient with Hashimoto's thyroiditis is 40–80 times greater than that of the general population.[140]

Presenting symptoms

Patients most commonly present with:

- Patients with diffuse large B-cell NHL present with a rapidly enlarging thyroid mass. Patients with mucosa-associated lymphoid tissue (MALT-lymphoma) have an indolent histology and can present with a slowly growing mass which has been present for months or sometimes years.
- Hoarseness.
- Respiratory difficulty.
- Cough.

Diagnosis

Fine needle aspiration (FNA) is insufficient for diagnosis and for histological diagnosis to be made, an incisional biopsy is required. Over 80 per cent of thyroid lymphomas are diffuse large cell B-cell lymphoma (DLBCL) and most (80 per cent) present with stage I or II disease. The second most common histological variety is the indolent B-cell marginal cell lymphoma (also known as MALT-oma).

Staging

Before commencing treatment, the following are required to fully stage a patient:

- CT scan of neck, chest, abdomen and pelvis or CT/PET scan;

- bone marrow aspirate, immunophenotyping and trephine biopsy;
- serum LDH.

Treatment

Diffuse large B-cell lymphoma

All patients with DLBCL of the thyroid are treated with R-CHOP chemotherapy. For patients with stage I/II disease, three cycles of chemotherapy followed by involved field radiotherapy is usually given. For patients with stage III/IV disease, B symptoms or bulky disease more than 10 cm, more prolonged chemotherapy with between six and eight cycles of R-CHOP chemotherapy is indicated.

MALT-lymphoma of thyroid

Patients with localized MALT-lymphoma are treated with involved field radiotherapy and this can result in five-year survivals of 90 per cent. For more extensive disease, chemotherapy is indicated. Agents commonly used include chlorambucil, cyclophosphamide, rituximab and fludarabine. Combination regimens such as R-CVP may also be used.

Patients with treated thyroid lymphoma (especially those treated with radiotherapy) are usually rendered hypothyroid and hence lifelong monitoring of thyroid function tests is required.

Nasal T/NK cell lymphoma

Nasal natural killer cell/T-cell cell lymphoma typically affects the midline facial structures and has distinctive pathological and immunophenotypic characteristics.

It has a strong association with Epstein–Barr virus and is the most common extranodal lymphoma in Taiwan. It is seen predominantly in the Far East (China, Japan, Korea and Malaysia) and less commonly in Central and South America.[141] Median age of onset is 50 years and there is a slight male preponderance. Measurement of EBV DNA load by PCR (polymerase chain reaction) is used as a surrogate marker of tumour load.

Patients usually present with a nasal mass causing obstruction and bleeding. The tumour usually causes bony destruction to the maxillary sinuses and nasal passages. It frequently has an aggressive course with a poor outcome.

Treatment usually consists of a combination of chemotherapy and radiotherapy. CHOP chemotherapy is generally ineffective and hence regimens such as the SMILE (steroid = dexamethasone, methotrexate, ifosphamide, L-asparaginase and etoposide) are more commonly used. There is some evidence to suggest that radiotherapy doses ≥ 50 Gy may result in more favourable local control.[142]

Hodgkin's lymphoma

The vast majority of patients with Hodgkin's lymphoma present with lymphadenopathy. In about 75 per cent, the lymph nodes are enlarged in the neck.[143] The enlarged nodes may wax and wane over time. About a third of patients with Hodgkin's lymphoma present with B-symptoms (fevers, sweats or weight loss > 10 per cent). Alcohol-induced pain/

pruritus is rare, but is typically associated with Hodgkin's lymphoma. Histologically, the disease is characterized by the presence of Reed–Sternberg cells. The aetiology of Hodgkin's lymphoma is unknown, but there is an association with Epstein–Barr virus. Similar to non-Hodgkin's lymphoma, there is a higher incidence in patients who are HIV positive.

As with other lymphomas, diagnosis requires an incisional biopsy (FNA is inadequate). Once the diagnosis is confirmed, full staging as with a newly diagnosed patient with non-Hodgkin's lymphoma is required.

Treatment

Most patients will require combination chemotherapy. The most common regimen used is ABVD (adriamycin, bleomycin, vinblastine and dacarbazine).[144] Patients usually require between six and eight cycles of treatment. Patients with bulky disease at presentation or those with residual masses post-chemotherapy may benefit from adjuvant radiotherapy. Patients presenting with limited early stage disease (stage I/IIA) may be treated by two to four cycles of ABVD followed by radiotherapy. CT/PET scanning is particularly useful in assessing response to treatment.

KEY EVIDENCE

- The rarity of neuroectodermal malignancies of the head and neck precludes any randomized trials and evidence is from a collection of institutional experiences.
- Gross tumour resection either up front or after neoadjuvant therapy is the main aim of treating non-metastatic SNUC to maximize on local control.[66] Adjuvant radiotherapy is associated with improved locoregional control.[67]
- A combined treatment modality approach with surgery and radiotherapy has been associated with improved survival compared with surgery alone for ONB.[96, 97]

KEY LEARNING POINTS

Neuroectodermal malignancies of the head and neck

- In view of the rarity, these tumours are best managed in specialized centres with the appropriate histopathological, radiological, surgical and oncological expertise.
- The biological behaviour of sinonasal malignancies of neuroectodermal origin can be broadly divided into two main groups: ONB or non-ONB.
- ONB can be associated with a very good prognosis following local therapy, typically surgery and postoperative radiotherapy. Late locoregional recurrences can be seen with ONB

and long-term follow up is therefore needed. Salvage neck dissection can be considered for nodal recurrences.
- Endoscopic endonasal resection is emerging as a more conservative surgical approach to craniofacial resection in highly selected cases of early ONB providing appropriate surgical expertise is available.
- Non-ONB (such as SNUC and NEC) have high rates of locoregional and systemic failure, and therefore combined treatment modality approaches are necessary for disease control. However, prognosis of non-ONB generally remains poor and more effective therapies are needed for the future.

Bone sarcomas

- Bone sarcomas are difficult to diagnose and manage, and the opinion of a specialist sarcoma team should be considered in every case.
- Chemotherapy has dramatically improved survival for osteosarcoma and Ewing's sarcoma.
- Resection with clear margins remains essential for cure.

Soft tissue sarcomas

- Soft tissue sarcomas are rare in the head and neck.
- Diagnosis is frequently delayed.
- Wide surgical excision is the mainstay of treatment unless contraindicated.
- The overall five-year survival after treatment ranges from 60 to 70 per cent.
- There is high incidence of local recurrence and metastatic disease.
- Lungs are the most common distant site.
- They are best treated at specialist sarcoma units.

Rhabdomyosarcoma

- Rhabdomyosarcoma is a significant disease of children comprising 4–8 per cent of all paediatric cancers.
- The head and neck sites include orbit, parameningeal and nonparameningeal region.
- They are usually treated with combination chemotherapy and adjuvant radiotherapy, and/ or surgery.
- Five-year survival for children after treatment is around 75 per cent.

Head and neck lymphomas

For patients being investigated/diagnosed as having a head and neck lymphoma:

- Flexible direct endoscopy is recommended for all patients.
- Fine needle aspiration is insufficient to make a tissue diagnosis and all patients require an incisional biopsy.
- Lymph node biopsies need to be sent 'fresh' (i.e. not in formalin) as a matter of urgency to a designated lymphoma pathologist.

- Surgical resection is never curative and full staging is required in all patients.
- The most common histological type is diffuse large B-cell non-Hodgkin's lymphoma.
- Patients with diffuse large B-cell NHL will require chemotherapy with R-CHOP ± radiotherapy.
- Patients with sinus lymphoma benefit from administration of prophylactic intrathecal chemotherapy.
- Assessing response to treatment is best done by combined CT/PET scanning.

REFERENCES

● 1. Frierson HF Jr, Mills SE, Fechner RE *et al.* Sinonasal undifferentiated carcinoma. An aggressive neoplasm derived from schneiderian epithelium and distinct from olfactory neuroblastoma. *American Journal of Surgical Pathology* 1986; **10**: 771–9.

2. Wenig BM. Undifferentiated malignant neoplasms of the sinonasal tract. *Archives of Pathology and Laboratory Medicine* 2009; **133**: 699–712.

3. Cerilli LA, Holst VA, Brandwein MS *et al.* Sinonasal undifferentiated carcinoma: immunohistochemical profile and lack of EBV association. *American Journal of Surgical Pathology* 2001; **25**: 156–63.

4. Levine PA, Frierson HF Jr, Stewart FM *et al.* Sinonasal undifferentiated carcinoma: a distinctive and highly aggressive neoplasm. *Laryngoscope* 1987; **97**: 905–8.

5. Jeng YM, Sung MT, Fang CL *et al.* Sinonasal undifferentiated carcinoma and nasopharyngeal-type undifferentiated carcinoma: two clinically, biologically, and histopathologically distinct entities. *American Journal of Surgical Pathology* 2002; **26**: 371–6.

6. Smith SR, Som P, Fahmy A *et al.* A clinicopathological study of sinonasal neuroendocrine carcinoma and sinonasal undifferentiated carcinoma. *Laryngoscope* 2000; **110**: 1617–22.

7. Miyamoto RC, Gleich LL, Biddinger PW, Gluckman JL. Esthesioneuroblastoma and sinonasal undifferentiated carcinoma: impact of histological grading and clinical staging on survival and prognosis. *Laryngoscope* 2000; **110**: 1262–5.

◆ 8. Mendenhall WM, Mendenhall CM, Riggs CE *et al.* Sinonasal undifferentiated carcinoma. *American Journal of Clinical Oncology* 2006; **29**: 27–31.

9. Houston GD, Gillies E. Sinonasal undifferentiated carcinoma: a distinctive clinicopathologic entity. *Advances in Anatomic Pathology* 1999; **6**: 317–23.

10. Deutsch BD, Levine PA, Stewart FM *et al.* Sinonasal undifferentiated carcinoma: a ray of hope. *Otolaryngology and Head and Neck Surgery* 1993; **108**: 697–700.

11. Kerrebijn JD, Tietze L, Mock D, Freeman JL. Sinonasal undifferentiated carcinoma. *Journal of Otolaryngology* 1998; **27**: 40–2.

◆ 12. Gorelick J, Ross D, Marentette L, Blaivas M. Sinonasal undifferentiated carcinoma: case series and review of the literature. *Neurosurgery* 2000; **47**: 750–4.

13. Chen AM, Daly ME, El-Sayed I *et al.* Patterns of failure after combined-modality approaches incorporating radiotherapy for sinonasal undifferentiated carcinoma of the head and neck. *International Journal of Radiation Oncology, Biology, Physics* 2008; **70**: 338–43.

14. Tanzler ED, Morris CG, Orlando CA *et al.* Management of sinonasal undifferentiated carcinoma. *Head and Neck* 2008; **30**: 595–9.

15. Rischin D, Porceddu S, Peters L *et al.* Promising results with chemoradiation in patients with sinonasal undifferentiated carcinoma. *Head and Neck* 2004; **26**: 435–41.

● 16. Berger L, Luc G, Richard D. L'esthesioneuroepitheliome olfactif [in French]. *Bulletin de l'Association Française pour l'Etude du Cancer* 1924; **13**: 410–21.

17. Bhattacharyya N, Thornton AF, Joseph MP *et al.* Successful treatment of esthesioneuroblastoma and neuroendocrine carcinoma with combined chemotherapy and proton radiation. Results in 9 cases. *Archives of Otolaryngology – Head and Neck Surgery* 1997; **123**: 34–40.

18. Silva EG, Butler JJ, Mackay B, Goepfert H. Neuroblastomas and neuroendocrine carcinomas of the nasal cavity: a proposed new classification. *Cancer* 1982; **50**: 2388–405.

19. Levine PA, Gallagher R, Cantrell RW. Esthesioneuroblastoma: reflections of a 21-year experience. *Laryngoscope* 1999; **109**: 1539–43.

● 20. Kadish S, Goodman M, Wang CC. Olfactory neuroblastoma. A clinical analysis of 17 cases. *Cancer* 1976; **37**: 1571–6.

● 21. Morita A, Ebersold MJ, Olsen KD *et al.* Esthesioneuroblastoma: prognosis and management. *Neurosurgery* 1993; **32**: 706–14.

22. Constantinidis J, Steinhart H, Koch M *et al.* Olfactory neuroblastoma: the University of Erlangen-Nuremberg experience 1975–2000. *Otolaryngology and Head and Neck Surgery* 2004; **130**: 567–74.

23. Ferlito A, Rinaldo A, Rhys-Evans PH. Contemporary clinical commentary: esthesioneuroblastoma: an update on management of the neck. *Laryngoscope* 2003; **113**: 1935–8.

24. Barnes L. *Surgical pathology of the head and neck*, 2nd edn. New York: Marcel Dekker, 2001.

25. Ordóñez NG, Mackay B. Neuroendocrine tumors of the nasal cavity. *Pathology Annual* 1993; **28**: 77–111.

26. Hyams VJ, Batsakis JG, Michaels L (eds). Neuroectodermal lesions. In: *Tumours of the upper respiratory tract and ear*, 2nd edn. Washington DC: Armed Forces Institute of Pathology, 1988: 226–57.

27. Hirose T, Scheithauer BW, Lopes MB *et al.* Olfactory neuroblastoma. An immunohistochemical, ultrastructural, and flow cytometric study. *Cancer* 1995; **76**: 4–19.

28. Girod D, Hanna E, Marentette L. Esthesioneuroblastoma. *Head and Neck* 2001; **23**: 500–5.

29. Hyams VJ. Olfactory neuroblastomas (case 6). In: Batsakis JG, Hyams VJ, Morales AR (eds). *Special tumours of the head and neck.* Chicago, IL: American Society of Clinical Pathologists Press, 1992: 24–9.

● 30. Dulguerov P, Calcaterra T. Esthesioneuroblastoma: the UCLA experience 1970–1990. *Laryngoscope* 1992; **102**: 843–9.

31. Bachar G, Goldstein DP, Shah M *et al.* Esthesioneuroblastoma: The Princess Margaret Hospital experience. *Head and Neck* 2008; **30**: 1607–14.

32. Diaz EM Jr, Johnigan RH 3rd, Pero C *et al.* Olfactory neuroblastoma: the 22-year experience at one comprehensive cancer center. *Head and Neck* 2005; **27**: 138–49.

33. Levine PA, McLean WC, Cantrell RW. Esthesioneuroblastoma: the University of Virginia experience 1960–1985. *Laryngoscope* 1986; **96**: 742–6.

34. Eriksen JG, Bastholt L, Krogdahl AS *et al.* Esthesioneuroblastoma – what is the optimal treatment? *Acta Oncologica* 2000; **39**: 231–5.

35. Koka VN, Julieron M, Bourhis J *et al.* Aesthesioneuroblastoma. *Journal of Laryngology and Otology* 1998; **112**: 628–33.

36. Folbe A, Herzallah I, Duvvuri U *et al.* Endoscopic endonasal resection of esthesioneuroblastoma: a multicenter study. *American Journal of Rhinology and Allergy* 2009; **23**: 91–4.

37. Castelnuovo PG, Delu G, Sberze F *et al.* Esthesioneuroblastoma: endonasal endoscopic treatment. *Skull Base* 2006; **16**: 25–9.

38. Suriano M, De Vincentiis M, Colli A *et al.* Endoscopic treatment of esthesioneuroblastoma: a minimally invasive approach combined with radiation therapy. *Otolaryngology and Head and Neck Surgery* 2007; **136**: 104–7.

39. Resto VA, Eisele DW, Forastiere A *et al.* Esthesioneuroblastoma: the Johns Hopkins experience. *Head and Neck* 2000; **22**: 550–8.

40. Walch C, Stammberger H, Anderhuber W *et al.* The minimally invasive approach to olfactory neuroblastoma: combined endoscopic and stereotactic treatment. *Laryngoscope* 2000; **110**: 635–40.

41. Sakata K, Aoki Y, Karasawa K *et al.* Esthesioneuroblastoma. A report of seven cases. *Acta Oncologica* 1993; **32**: 399–402.

42. McElroy EA Jr, Buckner JC, Lewis JE. Chemotherapy for advanced esthesioneuroblastoma: the Mayo Clinic experience. *Neurosurgery* 1998; **42**: 1023–7.

◆ 43. Dulguerov P, Allal AS, Calcaterra TC. Esthesioneuroblastoma: a meta-analysis and review. *Lancet Oncology* 2001; **2**: 683–90.

◆ 44. Platek ME, Mashtare SR, Popat M *et al.* Improved survival following surgery and radiation for olfactory neuroblastoma: analysis of the SEER database. *International Journal of Radiation Oncology, Biology, Physics* 2009; **75**: S396.

45. Spaulding CA, Kranyak MS, Constable WC, Stewart FM. Esthesioneuroblastoma: a comparison of two treatment eras. *International Journal of Radiation Oncology, Biology, Physics* 1988; **15**: 581–90.

46. Loy AH, Reibel JF, Read PW *et al.* Esthesioneuroblastoma: continued follow-up of a single institution's experience. *Archives of Otolaryngology – Head and Neck Surgery* 2006; **132**: 134–8.

47. Zappia JJ, Carroll WR, Wolf GT *et al.* Olfactory neuroblastoma: the results of modern treatment approaches at the University of Michigan. *Head and Neck* 1993; **15**: 190–6.

48. Kiyota N, Tahara M, Fujii S *et al.* Nonplatinum-based chemotherapy with irinotecan plus docetaxel for advanced or metastatic olfactory neuroblastoma: a retrospective analysis of 12 cases. *Cancer* 2008; **112**: 885–91.

49. Kim HJ, Cho HJ, Kim KS *et al.* Results of salvage therapy after failure of initial treatment for advanced olfactory neuroblastoma. *Journal of Cranio-maxillo-facial Surgery* 2008; **36**: 47–52.

● 50. Silva EG, Butler JJ, Mackay B, Goepfert H. Neuroblastomas and neuroendocrine carcinomas of the nasal cavity: a proposed new classification. *Cancer* 1982; **50**: 2388–405.

51. Perez-Ordonez B, Caruana SM, Huvos AG, Shah JP. Small cell neuroendocrine carcinoma of the nasal cavity and paranasal sinuses. *Human Pathology* 1998; **29**: 826–32.

52. Galanis E, Frytak S, Lloyd RV. Extrapulmonary small cell carcinoma. *Cancer* 1997; **79**: 1729–36.

53. Appelblatt NH, McClatchey KD. Olfactory neuroblastoma: a retrospective clinicopathologic study. *Head and Neck Surgery* 1982; **5**: 108–13.

● 54. Wanebo HJ, Koness RJ, MacFarlane JK *et al.* Head and neck sarcoma: report of the Head and Neck Sarcoma Registry. *Society of Head and Neck Surgeons Committee on Research. Head and Neck* 1992; **14**: 1–7.

∗ 55. National Institute for Health and Clinical Excellence. Improving outcomes for people with sarcoma. NICE guidance. Available from www.nice.org.uk/guidance/csgsarcoma.

56. Campanacci M, Picci P, Gherlinzoni F *et al.* Parosteal osteosarcoma. *Journal of Bone and Joint Surgery* 1984; **66**: 313–21.

57. Vlychou M, Ostlere SJ, Kerr R, Athanasou NA. Low-grade osteosarcoma of the ethmoid sinus. *Skeletal Radiology* 2007; **36**: 459–62.

◆ 58. Grimer RJ, Bielack S, Flege S *et al.* Periosteal osteosarcoma – a European review of outcome. *European Journal of Cancer* 2005; **41**: 2806–11.

59. Yoon JH, Yook JI, Kim HJ *et al.* Periosteal osteosarcoma of the mandible. *Journal of Oral and Maxillofacial Surgery* 2005; **63**: 699–703.

60. Fukunaga M. Low-grade central osteosarcoma of the skull. *Pathology, Research and Practice* 2005; **201**: 131–5.

61. Mankin HJ, Hornicek FJ. Paget's sarcoma: a historical and outcome review. *Clinical Orthopaedics and Related Research* 2005; **438**: 97–102.

62. Gleich LL, Eberle RC, Shaha AR, Solomon M. Paget's sarcoma of the mandible. *Head and Neck* 1995; **17**: 425–30.

63. Shaheen M, Deheshi BM, Riad S *et al.* Prognosis of radiation-induced bone sarcoma is similar to primary osteosarcoma. *Clinical Orthopaedics and Related Research* 2006; **450**: 76–81.

64. Kasthoori JJ, Wastie ML. Radiation-induced osteosarcoma of the maxilla. *Singapore Medical Journal* 2006; **47**: 907–9.

65. Moll AC, Imhof SM, Bouter LM *et al.* Second primary tumours in patients with hereditary retinoblastoma: a register-based follow up study. *International Journal of Cancer* 1996; **67**: 515–19.

66. Enneking WF, Spanier SS, Goodman MA. Current Concepts Review. The surgical staging of musculoskeletal sarcoma. *Journal of Bone and Joint Surgery of America* 1980; **62A**: 1027–30.

● 67. Bielack SS, Kempf-Bielack B, Delling G *et al.* Prognostic factors in high-grade osteosarcoma of the extremities or trunk: an analysis of 1702 patients treated on Neoadjuvant Cooperative Osteosarcoma Study Group protocols. *Journal of Clinical Oncology* 2002; **20**: 776–90.

68. Wafa H, Grimer RJ. Surgical options and outcomes in bone sarcoma. *Expert Reviews of Anticancer Therapy* 2006; **6**: 239–48.

● 69. Lewis IJ, Nooij MA, Whelan J *et al.* MRC BO06 and EORTC 80931 collaborators, European Osteosarcoma Intergroup. Improvement in histologic response but not survival in osteosarcoma patients treated with intensified chemotherapy: a randomized phase III trial of the European Osteosarcoma Intergroup. *Journal of the National Cancer Institute* 2007; **99**: 112–28.

∗ 70. European and American Osteosarcoma Study Group. Euramos 1 trial. Available from www.ctu.mrc.ac.uk/euramos.

71. Picci P, Sangiorgi L, Rougraff BT *et al.* Relationship of chemotherapy-induced necrosis and surgical margins to local recurrence in osteosarcoma. *Journal of Clinical Oncology* 1994; **12**: 2699–705.

72. Nissanka E, Amaratunge E, Tilakaratne W. Clinicopathological analysis of osteosarcoma of jaw bones. *Oral Diseases* 2007; **13**: 82–7.

◆ 73. Ha PK, Eisele DW, Frassica FJ *et al.* Osteosarcoma of the head and neck: a review of the Johns Hopkins experience. *Laryngoscope* 1999; **109**: 964–9.

◆ 74. Patel SG, Meyers P, Huvos AG *et al.* Improved outcomes in patients with osteogenic sarcoma of the head and neck. *Cancer* 2002; **95**: 1495–503.

75. Gadwal SR, Gannon FH, Fanburg-Smith JC *et al.* Primary osteosarcoma of the head and neck in pediatric patients: a clinicopathologic study of 22 cases with a review of the literature. *Cancer* 2001; **91**: 598–605.

76. Rodriguez-Arias CA, Lobato RD, Millan JM *et al.* Parosteal osteosarcoma of the skull. *Neurocirugia* 2001; **12**: 521–4.

77. Staals EL, Bacchini P, Bertoni F. Dedifferentiated central chondrosarcoma. *Cancer* 2006; **106**: 2682–91.

78. Fiorenza F, Abudu A, Grimer RJ *et al.* Risk factors for survival and local control in chondrosarcoma of bone. *Journal of Bone and Joint Surgery* 2002; **84**: 93–9.

79. Lee FY, Mankin HJ, Fondren G *et al.* Chondrosarcoma of bone: an assessment of outcome. *Journal of Bone and Joint Surgery* 1999; **81**: 326–38.

80. Koch BB, Karnell LH, Hoffman HT *et al.* National cancer database report on chondrosarcoma of the head and neck. *Head and Neck* 2000; **22**: 408–25.

81. Bernstein M, Kovar H, Paulussen M *et al.* Ewing's sarcoma family of tumors: current management. *Oncologist* 2006; **11**: 503–19.

● 82. Cotterill SJ, Ahrens S, Paulussen M *et al.* Prognostic factors in Ewing's tumor of bone: analysis of 975 patients from the European Intergroup Cooperative Ewing's Sarcoma Study Group. *Journal of Clinical Oncology* 2000; **18**: 3108–14.

83. Wexler LH, Kacker A, Piro JD *et al.* Combined modality treatment of Ewing's sarcoma of the maxilla. *Head and Neck* 2003; **25**: 168–72.

84. Nooij MA, Whelan J, Bramwell VH *et al.* European Osteosarcoma Intergroup. Doxorubicin and cisplatin chemotherapy in high-grade spindle cell sarcomas of the bone, other than osteosarcoma or malignant fibrous histiocytoma: a European Osteosarcoma Intergroup Study. *European Journal of Cancer* 2005; **41**: 225–30.

85. Grimer RJ, Cannon SR, Taminiau AM *et al.* Osteosarcoma over the age of forty. *European Journal of Cancer* 2003; **39**: 157–63.

86. Prosser GH, Baloch KG, Tillman RM *et al.* Does curettage without adjuvant therapy provide low recurrence rates in giant-cell tumors of bone? *Clinical Orthopaedics and Related Research* 2005; **435**: 211–18.

87. Stolovitzky JP, Waldron CA, McConnel FM. Giant cell lesions of the maxilla and paranasal sinuses. *Head and Neck* 1994; **16**: 143–8.

88. Hulen CA, Temple HT, Fox WP *et al.* Oncologic and functional outcome following sacrectomy for sacral chordoma. *Journal of Bone and Joint Surgery* 2006; **88**: 1532–9.

89. Mendenhall WM, Mendenhall CM, Lewis SB *et al.* Skull base chordoma. *Head and Neck* 2005; **27**: 159–65.

90. Hug EB, Slater JD. Proton radiation therapy for chordomas and chondrosarcomas of the skull base. *Neurosurgical Clinics of North America* 2000; **11**: 627–38.

91. Farhood AI, Hajdu SI, Shiu MH, Strong EW. Soft tissue sarcomas of the head and neck in adults. *American Journal of Surgery* 1990; **160**: 365–9.

● 92. Chen SA, Morris CG, Amdur RJ *et al.* Adult head and neck soft tissue sarcomas. *American Journal of Clinical Oncology* 2005; **28**: 259–63.

◆ 93. Mendenhall WM, Mendenhall CM, Werning JW *et al.* Adult head and neck soft tissue sarcomas. *Head and Neck* 2005; **27**: 916–22.

94. Eeles RA, Fisher C, A'Hern RP *et al.* Head and neck sarcomas: prognostic factors and implications for treatment. *British Journal of Cancer* 1993; **68**: 201–7.

95. Huber GF, Matthews TW, Dort JC. Soft tissue sarcomas of the head and neck: a retrospective analysis of the Alberta experience 1974 to 1999. *Laryngoscope* 2006; **116**: 780–5.

96. Figueiredo MT, Marques LA, Campos-Filho N. Soft-tissue sarcomas of the head and neck in adults and children: Experience at a single institution with a review of literature. *International Journal of Cancer* 1988; **41**: 198–200.

◆ 97. Sturgis EM, Potter BO. Sarcomas of the head and neck region. *Current Opinion in Oncology* 2003; **15**: 239–52.

98. Watkinson JC, Gaze MN, Wilson JA. *Stell and Maran's head and neck surgery*, 4th edn. Oxford: Butterworth-Heinemann, 2000.

99. Zahm SH, Fraumeni JF Jr. The epidemiology of soft tissue sarcoma. *Seminars in Oncology* 1997; **24**: 504–14.

100. Viskochil D, White R, Cawthon R. The neurofibromatosis type 1 gene. *Annual Reviews of Neuroscience* 1993; **16**: 183–205.

● 101. Balm AJ, Vom Coevorden F, Bos KE *et al.* Report of a symposium on diagnosis and treatment of adult soft tissue sarcomas in the head and neck. *European Journal of Surgical Oncology* 1995; **21**: 287–9.

102. Pierce SM, Recht A, Lingos TI *et al.* Long term radiation complications following conservative surgery (CS) and radiation therapy (RT) in patients with early stage breast cancer. *International Journal of Radiation, Oncology, Biology, Physics* 1992; **23**: 915–23.

103. Taghian A, de Vathaire F, Terrier P *et al.* Long-term risk of sarcoma following radiation treatment for breast cancer. *International Journal of Radiation, Oncology, Biology, Physics* 1991; **21**: 361–7.

104. Mark RJ, Bailet JW, Poen J *et al.* Postirradiation sarcoma of the head and neck. *Cancer* 1993; **72**: 887–93.

105. Weber RS, Benjamin RS, Peters LJ *et al.* Soft tissue sarcomas of the head and neck in adolescents and adults. *American Journal of Surgery* 1986; **152**: 386–92.

106. Aust MR, Olsen KD, Lewis JE *et al.* Angiosarcomas of the head and neck: clinical and pathologic characteristics. *Annals of Otology, Rhinology and Laryngology* 1997; **106**: 943–51.

107. Lydiatt WM, Shaha AR, Shah JP. Angiosarcoma of the head and neck. *American Journal of Surgery* 1994; **168**: 451–4.

＊ 108. National Institute for Health and Clinical Excellence. Referral guidelines for suspected cancer, June 2005. Last accessed January 22, 2007. Available from www.nice.org.uk/page.aspx?o = cg027.

109. Arca MJ, Sondak VK, Chang AE. Diagnostic procedures and pretreatment evaluation of soft tissue sarcomas. *Seminars in Surgical Oncology* 1994; **10**: 323–31.

● 110. Bentz BG, Singh B, Woodruff J *et al.* Head and neck soft tissue sarcomas: a multivariate analysis of outcomes. *Annals of Surgical Oncology* 2004; **11**: 619–28.

111. Laskin WB. Dermatofibrosarcoma protuberans. *CA Cancer Journal for Clinicians* 1992; **42**: 116–25.

112. Dudhat SB, Mistry RC, Varughese T *et al.* Prognostic factors in head and neck soft tissue sarcomas. *Cancer* 2000; **89**: 868–72.

113. Enneking WF, Spanier SS, Goodman MA. A system for the surgical staging of musculoskeletal sarcoma. *Clinical Orthopaedics and Related Research* 2003; **415**: 4–18.

● 114. Sarcoma Meta-Analysis Collaboration. Adjuvant chemotherapy for localised resectable soft-tissue sarcoma of adults: meta-analysis of individual data. *Lancet* 1997; **350**: 1647–54.

115. Pisters PW, Leung DH, Woodruff J *et al.* Analysis of prognostic factors in 1041 patients with localized soft tissue sarcomas of the extremities. *Journal of Clinical Oncology* 1996; **14**: 1679–89.

116. Le QT, Fu KK, Kroll S *et al.* Prognostic factors in adult soft-tissue sarcomas of the head and neck. *International Journal of Radiation, Oncology, Biology, Physics* 1997; **37**: 975–84.

117. Willers H, Hug EB, Spiro IJ *et al.* Adult soft tissue sarcomas of the head and neck treated by radiation and surgery or radiation alone: patterns of failure and prognostic factors. *International Journal of Radiation, Oncology, Biology, Physics* 1995; **33**: 585–93.

118. Le Vay J, O'Sullivan B, Catton C. An assessment of prognostic factors in soft tissue sarcoma of the head and neck. *Archives of Otolaryngoogy – Head and Neck Surgery* 1994; **120**: 981–6.

119. Parsons JT, Zlotecki RA, Reddy KA *et al.* The role of radiotherapy and limb-conserving surgery in the management of soft-tissue sarcomas in adults. *Hematology-Oncology Clinics of North America* 2001; **15**: 377–88.

120. O'Sullivan B, Gullane P, Irish J *et al.* Preoperative radiotherapy for adult head and neck soft tissue sarcoma: assessment of wound complication rates and cancer outcome in a prospective series. *World Journal of Surgery* 2003; **27**: 875–83.

121. Goodlad JR, Fletcher CD, Smith MA. Surgical resection of primary soft tissue sarcoma. Incidence of residual tumour in 95 patients needing re-excision after local resection. *Journal of Bone and Joint Surgery* 1996; **78**: 658–61.

122. Kraus DH, Dubner S, Harrison LB *et al.* Prognostic factors for recurrence and survival in head and neck soft tissue sarcomas. *Cancer* 1994; **74**: 697–702.

123. Barker JL Jr, Paulino AC, Feeney S *et al.* Locoregional treatment for adult soft tissue sarcomas of the head and neck: an institutional review. *Cancer Journal* 2003; **9**: 49–57.

124. Grobmyer SR, Brennan MF. Predictive variables detailing the recurrence rate of soft tissue sarcomas. *Current Opinion in Oncology* 2003; **15**: 319–26.

125. Nayar RC, Prudhomme F, Parise O Jr *et al.* Rhabdomyosarcoma of the head and neck in adults: a study of 26 patients. *Laryngoscope* 1993; **103**: 1362–6.

● 126. Callender TA, Weber RS, Janjan N *et al.* Rhabdomyosarcoma of the nose and paranasal sinuses in adults and children. *Otolaryngology, Head and Neck Surgery* 1995; **112**: 252–7.

◆ 127. Dagher R, Helman L. Rhabdomyosarcoma: an overview. *Oncologist* 1999; **4**: 34–44.

● 128. Crist WM, Anderson JR, Meza JL *et al.* Intergroup rhabdomyosarcoma study-IV: results for patients with nonmetastatic disease. *Journal of Clinical Oncology* 2001; **19**: 3091–102.

● 129. Baker KS, Anderson JR, Link MP *et al.* Benefit of intensified therapy for patients with local or regional embryonal rhabdomyosarcoma: results from the Intergroup Rhabdomyosarcoma Study IV. *Journal of Clinical Oncology* 2000; **18**: 2427–34.

130. Kraus DH, Saenz NC, Gollamudi S *et al.* Pediatric rhabdomyosarcoma of the head and neck. *American Journal of Surgery* 1997; **174**: 556–60.

131. Anderson GJ, Tom LW, Womer RB *et al.* Rhabdomyosarcoma of the head and neck in children. *Archives of Otolaryngology – Head and Neck Surgery* 1990; **116**: 428–31.

132. Aviles A, Delgado S, Ruiz H *et al.* Treatment of non-Hodgkin's lymphoma of Waldeyer's ring: radiotherapy versus chemotherapy versus combined therapy. *European Journal of Cancer, B Oral Oncology* 1996; **32B**: 19–23.

● 133. Coiffier B, Lepage E, Briere J *et al.* CHOP chemotherapy plus rituximab compared with CHOP alone in elderly patients with diffuse large B-cell lymphoma. *New England Journal of Medicine* 2002; **346**: 235–42.

134. Ezzat AA, Ibrahim EM, El Weshi AN *et al.* Localized non-Hodgkin's lymphoma of Waldeyer's ring: clinical features, management and prognosis of 130 adult patients. *Head and Neck* 2001; **23**: 547–58.

● 135. Laskin J, Savage K, Voss N *et al.* Primary paranasal sinus lymphoma: natural history and improved outcome with central nervous system chemoprophylaxis. *Leukemia and Lymphoma* 2005; **46**: 1721–7.

◆ 136. Shenkier T, Connors J. Primary extranodal non-Hodgkin's lymphoma. In: Canellos GP, Lister TA, Young B (eds). *The lymphomas*. Philadelphia: Saunders Elsevier, 2006: 334.

137. Matsuzuka F, Miyauchi A, Katayama S *et al.* Clinical aspects of primary thyroid lymphoma: diagnosis and treatment based on our experience of 119 cases. *Thyroid* 1993; **3**: 93–9.

138. Limanova Z, Neuwirtova R, Smejkal V. Malignant lymphoma of the thyroid. *Experimental and Clinical Endocrinology* 1987; **90**: 113–19.

139. Anscombe AM, Wright DH. Primary malignant lymphoma of the thyroid – a tumour of mucosa-associated lymphoid tissue: review of seventy six cases. *Histopathology* 1985; **9**: 81–97.

● 140. Pedersen RK, Pedersen NT. Primary non-Hodgkin's lymphoma of the thyroid gland: a population based study. *Histopathology* 1996; **28**: 25–32.

141. Liang R. Nasal T/NK cell lymphoma. In: Canellos GP, Lister TA, Young B (eds). *The lymphomas*. Philadelphia: Saunders Elsevier, 2006: 451.

142. Isobe K, Uno T, Tamaru J *et al.* Extranodal natural killer/T-cell lymphoma, nasal type: the significance of radiotherapeutic parameters. *Cancer* 2006; **106**: 609–15.

143. Kennedy BJ, Loeb V Jr, Peterson VM *et al.* National survey of patterns of care for Hodgkin's disease. *Cancer* 1985; **56**: 2547–56.

● 144. Cannellos GP, Anderson JR, Propert KJ *et al.* Chemotherapy of advanced Hodgkin's disease with MOPP, ABVD or MOPP alternating with ABVD. *New England Journal of Medicine* 1992; **327**: 1478–84.

FURTHER READING

Mendenhall WM, Mendenhall CM, Werning JW *et al.* Adult head and neck soft tissue sarcomas. *Head and Neck* 2005; **27**: 916–22.

Sturgis EM, Potter BO. Sarcomas of the head and neck region. *Current Opinion in Oncology* 2003; **15**: 239–52.

SECTION B

Non-surgical treatments

Section editor: Nick Slevin

42

Principles of radiotherapy

NICK ROWELL

Let the wise listen and add to their learning and let the discerning get guidance.

Proverbs 1:5

INTRODUCTION

Radiotherapy is the application of radiation for the purpose of therapeutic gain. Most commonly, this is by means of external beam radiotherapy (sometimes known as teletherapy) where a radiation beam is directed from a machine placed outside the patient to a treatment volume located within. Alternatively, radioactive material can be introduced directly to within a tumour or tumour-bearing area (brachytherapy). Recent decades have seen considerable progress in technology, with more effective means of immobilizing patients, of defining the treatment volume and of limiting dose to normal tissues. With this, our understanding of tumour and normal tissue biology has steadily evolved as has our understanding of fractionation and, more recently, the consequences of adding chemotherapy (either sequentially, concurrently or both). There remain significant areas of uncertainty and many areas where further research is needed. The balance between delivering treatment of sufficient intensity to cure the highest proportion of patients and minimizing the risk of serious sequelae remains a challenge for oncologists, just as it remains a challenge for surgeons in the surgical arena.

RADIOTHERAPY EQUIPMENT AND PHYSICS

Treatment with photons (x-rays and gamma rays)

Historically, external beam radiotherapy began with low energy x-ray beams generated by modified diagnostic tubes. Beams with peak energies between 50 and 300 kV (known as orthovoltage) are still used in the treatment of superficial tumours, principally skin cancer. The van de Graff generator bridged the gap between orthovoltage and megavoltage (beams of $\geq 1\,MV$) but was quickly overtaken by the advent of the cobalt unit. This contained a cobalt-60 source within the head of the machine which would traverse from a shielded 'safe' position within the head of the machine to the treatment position for a specified time. Gamma rays (which arise from radioactive decay) have the same biological and physical properties as x-rays (which are produced artificially). The rate of decay of cobalt sources necessitated replacement approximately every five years. A small amount of radiation would still leak through the head of the machine so that treatment staff on cobalt units received greater radiation exposure than those on other units. Concerns about misuse of radioactive sources around the world has led to most cobalt units being replaced with linear accelerators, the standard megavoltage treatment unit in use today. A beam from a cobalt unit (1.1 MeV photons arising from the natural decay of cobalt-60) has similar tissue penetration properties as a 3 MV beam from a linear accelerator.

In a linear accelerator, a stream of electrons produced from a filament in an electrically charged field is accelerated through a series of wave guides in conjunction with a

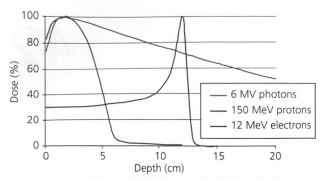

Figure 42.1 Comparison of depth dose characteristics of a 6 MV photon beam and a 12 MeV electron beam from a linear accelerator and a 150 MeV proton beam from a cyclotron. The photon beam shows a degree of skin sparing with the maximum dose apparent at 1.5 cm. The proton beam shows an initial plateau then a peak (the Bragg peak) followed by a rapid decline.

radiofrequency pulse to within a fraction of the speed of light. This electron beam can itself be used for treatment or can impact on a target to produce a photon beam of maximum energy between 4 and 20 MV according to the design and calibration of the machine. Beams of 10 MV or greater are mostly used in the treatment of abdominal or pelvic tumours, while beams of 4–6 MV are most appropriate for the treatment of head and neck cancer (**Figure 42.1**).

All photons interact with matter by producing secondary electrons, which have a finite range according to the amount of energy imparted to them, which in turn is determined by the energy of the photon beam. Secondary electrons cause a number of ionization events along their path and it is these events, together with oxygen, which are responsible for free radical formation and consequent tissue damage. This also means that it takes a finite depth in tissue (defined by the maximum path length of the secondary electrons) before the dose builds up to a maximum (the build-up depth). This accounts for the relative skin sparing of megavoltage photon beams – the maximum absorbed dose from a 6 MV photon beam is 1.5 cm beneath the skin surface. Mostly this is an advantage in reducing the severe skin reactions associated with earlier forms of irradiation.

Electron beams can treat to depths of up to 5 cm or so according to the beam energy used; a 4–6 MeV beam would be mostly used to treat skin tumours and a beam of approximately 12 MeV to treat neck nodes (**Figure 42.1**).

Brachytherapy

Radium needles were the first to be used for this purpose and resulted in significant radiation dose for the operator. Iridium (Ir-192) wire is the source of choice for modern head and neck brachytherapy. Radio-opaque hollow needles or tubes (applicators) can be inserted under general anaesthetic and then following return of the patient to a radiation-protected side-room, the sources are introduced (afterloaded). Nowadays, a remote afterloading device houses the sources within a lead chamber in the treatment room and is connected to each applicator within the implant. This then

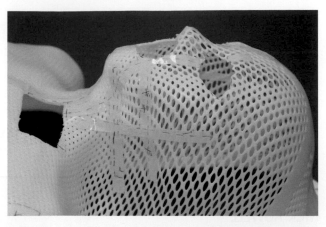

Figure 42.2 Individually moulded thermoplastic shell covering the head and neck area used for patient immobilization. Field centres and field borders are marked on the outside of the shell. The areas around the eyes and mouth are cut out for patient comfort and the part of the lower neck field to reduce the surface dose.

automatically loads each applicator with a predetermined length of active iridium wire when treatment and nursing staff have left the room, thereby minimizing radiation exposure to staff. In most cases, the volume at risk is implanted with either one or two planes of radioactive sources, where individual sources and planes of sources lie parallel to each other and evenly spaced (generally about 1 cm apart). The implant is imaged prior to afterloading to allow precise calculation of radiation dose, which is delivered over 2–5 days depending on the specific activity of the iridium wire and the dose to be delivered.

The advantage of brachytherapy is that it provides a means of delivering a high dose to a small area and as the radiation dose falls off rapidly outside the treatment volume, the dose to adjacent normal tissues can be kept within acceptable limits. On the other hand, a major limitation is the need for adequate radiation protection and that the technique is not appropriate where wider field irradiation is required, for example to cover adjacent nodal areas. Brachytherapy, both as primary and postoperative treatment for oral cancer, has largely been replaced by resection and repair with free flaps, but is still sometimes used for recurrent disease in the neck or nasopharynx.[1]

Immobilization

Accuracy of delivery of external beam radiotherapy is dependent on maintaining a stable target volume. Individually moulded thermoplastic shells covering the head and neck area are used to immobilize patients (**Figure 42.2**). These are located onto a fixed frame on the treatment couch. Reference marks are placed on the outside of the shell, avoiding the need for any skin marks or tattoos. Standard techniques allow treatment accuracy to within approximately 3 mm. More rigid frames providing accuracy closer to 1–2 mm have been developed for stereotactic radiotherapy (sometimes referred to as radiosurgery) and intensity modulated radiotherapy (IMRT) where movement can be more critical to dose delivery.

Target definition and coverage

The vast majority of radiotherapy planning is now done using computed tomography (CT) images obtained within the immobilization shell. According to the clinical situation, the gross tumour volume (GTV) and/or clinical target volume (CTV)[2, 3] is outlined on screen. This allows for inclusion of areas at risk, such as nodal areas, or potential routes of spread. A number of radiotherapy treatment plans include two consecutive phases of treatment, the first covering areas of known involvement together with areas at risk and the second solely the areas of known involvement. In this case, a phase 1 CTV and a phase 2 CTV are outlined separately. These volumes are 'grown' three-dimensionally to derive the planning target volume (PTV) for each phase by adding an additional margin. This margin allows for patient movement and normal set-up variation. In most cases, this margin is 1 cm although tighter margins may be used in circumstances where there is a need to minimize dose to adjacent normal tissues. Organs at risk, such as spinal cord, parotid and submandibular glands are also outlined (**Figure 42.3**). Radiotherapy planning technicians and physicists then devise a treatment plan which defines the positioning and weighting of two or more photon beams to provide adequate coverage of the PTV while not exceeding agreed maximum doses to adjacent normal tissues (see below under Treatment morbidity). Current convention[2] stipulates that the stated dose is the dose to the centre of the treatment volume and that all of the PTV receives at least 95 per cent of this dose and that there is no point which receives greater than 107 per cent.

All megavoltage units (i.e. cobalt units and linear accelerators) vary the size of the irradiated field by moving large lead blocks within the head of the machine (collimators) in and out of the beam thus generating square or rectangular fields of any size. Individual beams are shaped either by the introduction of custom-made lead or alloy blocks mounted onto a perspex plate and positioned just below the head of the machine or by multileaf collimators. Rather than using single large blocks, the collimators of modern linear accelerators are constructed with individual leaves of approximately 0.5 cm width. These multileaf collimators can be programmed to produce any shape of field allowing the 95 per cent isodose to conform closely to the PTV in three dimensions (**Figure 42.4**).

BIOLOGICAL EFFECTS OF RADIATION: DNA DAMAGE AND REPAIR

Photon beams interact with matter by producing secondary electrons. Ionization events along the path of secondary electrons result in very localized tissue damage. Although many events will occur in non-critical parts of the cell, some will occur within DNA. A wide range of types of damage are described and there is now a good understanding of repair mechanisms in response to each. While ionization events resulting in single strand breaks within DNA are generally repairable, double strand breaks frequently cannot be repaired faithfully so that cell death will occur within the next few cell divisions. Sublethal damage refers to DNA damage

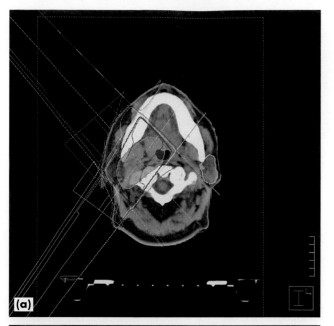

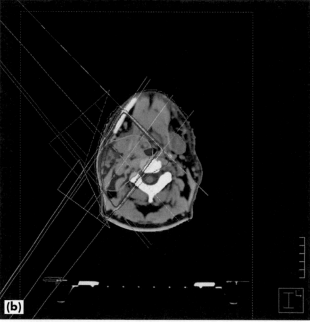

Figure 42.3 Treatment plan for irradiation of a T_2N_0 tonsillar carcinoma showing outlining of the contralateral parotid (a) and submandibular gland (b). Anterior and posterior oblique fields are used to cover the planning target volume (PTV, pale blue shading). The PTV is surrounded by the 95 per cent isodose (red line). The parotid and submandibular glands lie between the exit beams of the two fields thus ensuring minimal disruption to saliva production.

that can be repaired given the right cellular conditions and sufficient time. It is known that sublethal damage repair is less efficient in tumour cells than in normal cells and in areas of hypoxia or low pH. Proportionately more DNA damage is repairable with smaller radiation doses (fractions). Half-time for sublethal damage repair is in the order of hours with about 95 per cent being complete within 6 hours.

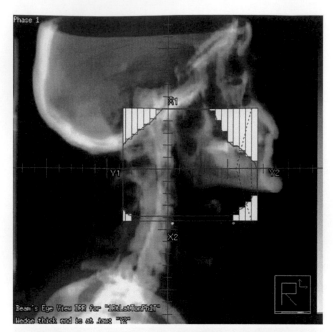

Figure 42.4 Digitally reconstructed radiograph (from CT planning data) showing right lateral field shaped by multileaf collimator used to shield parts of the mouth and skull base in the treatment of a man with a T_4N_2 tongue base carcinoma. A matching field to cover the inferior neck is also used (not shown).

TUMOUR CELL KINETICS AND RESPONSE TO RADIOTHERAPY

Cell proliferation and loss

Rates of cellular proliferation of most tumours exceed that of most normal tissues. The ultimate and measurable increase in tumour size is a result of the balance between proliferation and cell loss from necrosis, desquamation and apoptosis. Potential doubling times (T_{pot}) calculated from incorporation of ^{3}H-thymidine are therefore substantially less than actual doubling times. In a series of head and neck squamous cancers, values of T_{pot} range from 2 to 67 days (median 6.4 days).[4] In a study investigating the effects of treatment delays, actual doubling times ranged from 15 to greater than 234 days (median 99 days).[5] More rapidly proliferating tumours may be those that are less well differentiated or have other adverse histological features. Only the fate of tumour cells with clonogenic potential (between 1 and 10 per cent of all tumour cells) will determine the response to treatment. At any one time, not all cells with clonogenic potential will be actively proliferating – with a lower proportion in hypoxic areas.

As tumour cells proliferate, stromal cells also proliferate in response to growth factors produced by tumour and stromal cells. Proliferation of vascular endothelium, in response to vascular endothelial growth factor (VEGF), is crucial to the continuing growth of tumour cells and the balance between rate of expanse of the tumour and its supporting vascular network will influence the development of hypoxia and necrosis.[6]

Intrinsic radiosensitivity

Accurate prediction of response to radiotherapy would be valuable in advising patients about treatment options. Conventional histological features correlate poorly with response to radiotherapy and assays which measure the fraction of cultured tumour cells surviving a 2 Gy dose of radiotherapy (SF_2) are not routinely available. Such assays may take several weeks and not all attempts to culture tumour cells are successful. Cell cultures effectively exclude the additional problem of hypoxia present *in vivo*. In a study of 84 head and neck tumours treated with radiotherapy, local failure was seen in 9 per cent with an SF_2 less than 0.40 (the median value) and in 26 per cent with an SF_2 greater than 0.40.[7] The ultimate response to a 35-fraction course of radiotherapy is SF_2 to the power of 35 so that even small changes in SF_2 can result in significant differences in outcome. Intrinsic radiosensitivity is likely to account for the largest differences between tumours in response to radiotherapy.

Hypoxia

Thomlinson and Gray[8] were the first to demonstrate that tumour cells greater than 100–150 μm from the nearest capillary suffered increasing hypoxia with necrosis present at greater distances. At that time, it was also demonstrated that anoxic cells were 2.5–3.0 times less sensitive to the effects of radiation.[9]

Substantial areas of hypoxia can be identified by the insertion of oxygen electrodes into primary tumour and neck nodes[10] or by imaging with a ^{18}F-labelled nitroimidazole.[11, 12] Greater degrees of hypoxia are associated with worse outcome following radiotherapy.[12, 13]

Human papillomavirus infection and response to radiotherapy

It has recently been recognized that evidence of past human papillomavirus (HPV) infection, determined by HPV-16 DNA *in situ* hybridization, is more common in patients with oropharyngeal cancers and especially in those who have never smoked.[14] Furthermore, in patients with oropharyngeal cancers treated with radiotherapy (with or without chemotherapy), the outcome is significantly better in those with evidence of HPV infection compared to those without.[14, 15, 16, 17] The reasons for greater sensitivity to treatment are as yet unknown, but likely to be more than just younger age and the absence of smoking-related comorbidity.

Changes in cell kinetics and oxygenation during a course of radiotherapy

As tumour cells do not die immediately after irradiation, visible consequences are slow to appear. As cells die, oxygen penetrates progressively further into hypoxic areas stimulating hypoxic cells to proliferate. Oxygenation may improve as treatment progresses, as assessed by oxygen electrodes[10] or by imaging with ^{18}F-labelled misonidazole.[11] In normal tissues, resting cells enter the cell cycle, the cell cycle time shortens and the rate of proliferation increases. This accelerated proliferation accounts for the rapid healing of acutely responding normal tissues, such as mucosa and skin, after an initial latent period. Accelerated proliferation within tumours probably starts within the third week of treatment.[18]

Assessing response to radiotherapy

Generally, it takes up to 4–6 weeks after the end of a course of radiotherapy for maximum tumour response to become evident. Assessment prior to this can be misleading, so a minimum of 8 weeks is preferable before reimaging with CT or carrying out further biopsies. Post-treatment magnetic resonance imaging (MRI) is best left until 12 weeks to allow the general increase in signal in the irradiated area to subside. A systematic review of 27 post-treatment fluorodeoxy-glucose-positron emission tomography (PET) studies showed a positive predictive value of 75 per cent and a negative predictive value of 95 per cent with greater sensitivity of scans performed 10 or more weeks after treatment.[19]

TREATMENT MORBIDITY

The extent of acute and late normal tissue morbidity will depend on the area being treated and the dose received. Modern planning systems permit very accurate dose calculations within normal tissues. This aids shielding (where possible) and better prediction of the consequences of treatment.

Acute toxicity: development

Tiredness is a side effect experienced by most patients. This can date from the very start of treatment and may build up as treatment continues. Chemotherapy adds to tiredness generally. Recovery of pretreatment levels of energy following more intensive courses of chemoradiotherapy can take up to six months. The biological basis of tiredness is poorly understood.

Dryness of the mouth (xerostomia) can develop during the first week of treatment – rather earlier than would be expected from direct tumour cell kill. It is likely that selective radiation damage to the plasma membrane of secretory granules is responsible.[20] Parotid and submandibular salivary flow rates fall rapidly to less than 20 per cent of pretreatment values by the end of the second week.[21] As watery and mucous components of saliva are not affected equally, the initial general dryness gives way to increasing thick sticky saliva beyond the fourth week. Certain foods, particularly bread, become more difficult to swallow. Even when the contralateral salivary glands are spared, the sticky saliva from the irradiated side can predominate in the latter part of treatment and the few weeks following. The effects of dryness may be greater in patients who have lost a submandibular gland as part of a neck dissection.

In the past, there has been undue attention to the parotid gland, ignoring the submandibular gland, in standard radiotherapy planning texts. The contribution of the submandibular gland to resting salivary function is now better understood and the need to spare the submandibular glands increasingly emphasized. Dose–response relationships are now established for both. For the parotid gland, the mean dose for 50 per cent loss of salivary excretion at seven months was 22.5 Gy[22] and for 75 per cent loss at six months, 40 Gy.[23] Recovery can be expected up to 12 months after completion of treatment.[23] Doses to the submandibular glands in excess of 39 Gy were not associated with recovery but at doses < 39 Gy, recovery of salivary flow took place at 3 per cent per month up to 24 months.[24] Where possible, beam arrangements should ensure that dose received by the parotid and submandibular glands should be as low as possible.

Loss of taste accompanies most head and neck radiotherapy and is exacerbated by dryness of the mouth. Loss of taste compounds the problems of maintaining an adequate nutritional intake.

Mucositis develops from the third week of treatment onwards and increases in severity according to the volume irradiated and total dose. The visible reaction progresses from erythema to patchy mucositis (characterized by white patches of fibrinous exudate on an erythematous base) to confluent mucositis (where the exudative patches coalesce). In severe cases, contact bleeding may occur. Confluent mucositis, common toxicity criteria (CTC) grade 3,[25] is seen in 40–80 per cent of patients receiving more than 60 Gy (or equivalent), more frequently in those receiving concurrent chemotherapy or accelerated radiotherapy.[26, 27] Painful swallowing increases progressively and is further aggravated by difficulty clearing thick saliva.

Skin erythema also increases from the third week onwards. Progression is from faint erythema to bright erythema to moist desquamation.

Acute toxicity: management

A systematic review of interventions used for the prophylaxis of mucositis in patients receiving radiotherapy for head and neck cancer identified only antibacterial pastilles as having any objective benefit in reducing the incidence of more severe mucositis.[28] However, these are not widely used because of general concerns about antibiotic resistance.

To relieve symptoms of mucositis, a combination of good mouth care, an antiseptic mouthwash and narcotic analgesics is recommended.[29] Alcohol-based mouthwashes should be avoided as these can sting and may have a drying effect in an already dry mouth; a water-based mouthwash (e.g. Biotene) is preferred. Candidal infection is common during radiotherapy, particularly if chemotherapy is also used, so there should be a low threshold for prescribing antifungals. Fluconazole is preferred as this has been shown to be more effective than oral amphotericin or nystatin in the treatment of oral candidiasis[30, 31] and, as it is absorbed systemically, can treat other sites at risk (e.g. gastrostomy site).

Analgesics in increasing strength are essential, moving from soluble aspirin or paracetamol to soluble cocodamol 30/500 to morphine sulphate solution (Oramorph) in increasing doses. Analgesia given 4-hourly 20–30 minutes before meals can relieve the worst of the pain and help maintain nutrition. Patients requiring higher doses of opiates may benefit from

Limitations of altered fractionation

Straightforward comparisons of radiotherapy regimes are no longer as informative as previously because for more advanced cancers of the head and neck, radiotherapy is no longer given in isolation.

Mathematical extrapolations to determine the most effective regime[66] are limited as these do not take into account the potential additive effect of concurrent chemotherapy or biological agents as the benefit of these may also be related to treatment duration.

Radical versus palliative radiotherapy

In situations where the emphasis is on control of symptoms and quality of life rather than long-term control or cure, lower doses of radiotherapy may be sufficient (equivalent to 30–40 Gy in 15–20 fractions over 3–4 weeks). With a lower total dose, there is more flexibility around fractionation so that, in general, it is preferable to give fewer larger fractions. Examples include 20 Gy in five daily fractions over 1 week, 30 Gy in ten daily fractions over 2 weeks or a single fraction of 10–12 Gy. This reduces the number of patient attendances, especially important where performance status or mobility are reduced or where the patient lives some distance from the oncology centre. Where disease is relatively localized and there is a lower potential for acute side effects, slightly higher doses may be given (e.g. 21 Gy in three daily fractions, 25 Gy in five daily fractions over 1 week or 35 Gy in ten daily fractions over 2 weeks, although these doses do exceed spinal cord tolerance).

Radiotherapy techniques differ for palliative radiotherapy. As total dose is lower, and in many cases within spinal cord tolerance, simpler or varied field arrangements may be used. The aim should be to minimize acute side effects, particularly mucositis. An example would be the use of a direct field angled posteriorly to treat a parapharyngeal mass – irradiation of the pharynx is minimized and spinal cord dose is within tolerance (**Figure 42.5**).

In the AIIMS study, 20 Gy given in five daily fractions over 1 week improved symptoms in approximately 50 per cent of patients.[74] Other studies using rather different schemes, the Hypo trial (30 Gy in five fractions given twice weekly over 2.5 weeks) and QUAD SHOT trial (14 Gy in four fractions over 2 days) showed similar degrees of symptomatic benefit.[75, 76]

As durable relief of symptoms can be related to dose sometimes to the point where a radical course of treatment may be considered to provide the best palliation, the option of giving radical treatment with tight margins and a 4-week schedule (rather than longer) should be considered for those with borderline performance status or comorbidity.

FACTORS INFLUENCING THE EFFECTIVENESS OF RADIOTHERAPY

These factors are summarized in **Table 42.4**.

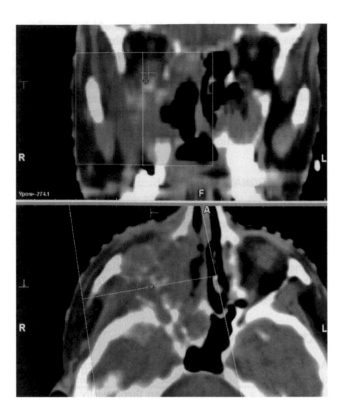

Figure 42.5 Single palliative radiotherapy field directed posteriorly at an oblique angle to treat a recurrent adenoid cystic carcinoma extending from the maxillary antrum into the lower orbit. The oblique angle avoids the contralateral eye and minimises the dose to the nasal cavity which had previously received a course of radical radiotherapy.

Table 42.4 Summary of factors affecting effectiveness of radiotherapy for head and neck cancer.

Factor	% Increase in local control	% Decrease in local control
Concurrent chemotherapy or cetuximab	10%	
70 Gy rather than 66 Gy	5%	
Delays in starting radiotherapy		15% per month
Treatment interruptions		1.4% per extra day
Anaemia		10–15%
Smoking		10–15%

Total dose

A review of the effectiveness of ten different fractionation schedules used in the treatment of T_3N_0 carcinoma of the larynx demonstrates a clear dose–response relationship.[77] On this basis, just increasing the dose from 66 to 70 Gy would be expected to improve local control by 5 per cent. Analysis of the RTOG 9003 trial of accelerated and hyperfractionated regimes indicated an increase in locoregional control of 1 per cent for each 1 Gy increase in effective total dose.[78] The relative merits of different schemes of altered fractionation are considered above and in Chapter 041, Head and neck squamous cell carcinomas: radical radiotherapy, Chapter 42, Postoperative radiotherapy in head and neck cancer and Chapter 043, Chemoradiation in head and neck cancer.

Concurrent treatment with chemotherapy or biological agents

The MACH-NC meta-analysis[79] demonstrated an 8 per cent improvement in local control at five years with concurrent platinum-based chemotherapy. Concurrent treatment with cetuximab produces a benefit of similar magnitude.[80] These strategies are discussed in detail in Chapter 45, Chemoradiation in head and neck cancer and Chapter 46, Biologically targeted agents, but are mentioned here so that their benefits can be considered alongside other factors which impact the effectiveness of radiotherapy.

Delays in starting treatment

Many oncology centres around the world have limited capacity which historically has resulted in significant delays in starting radiotherapy. The current UK standard is that treatment with radical radiotherapy should commence within 4 weeks of the decision to treat and palliative radiotherapy within 2 weeks. Provided there is adequate capacity, this is generally achievable even for patients who require PEG insertion and dental treatment prior to radiotherapy.

A systematic review has shown that delays in commencing radiotherapy significantly reduce locoregional control.[81] This meta-analysis demonstrates a relative risk of locoregional recurrence of 1.15 per month of delay for radiotherapy as primary treatment and 1.28 for postoperative treatment. A similar impact on survival was also seen. Two CT-based studies comparing tumour volumes at diagnosis and at the time of radiotherapy planning showed a mean increase in volume of 46 per cent over a median waiting time of 28 days[5] and a 70 per cent increase over a median interval of 56 days.[82] In the latter study, this equated to an estimated reduction in probability of tumour control of 18 per cent.

Treatment interruptions

Where a course of radiotherapy is prolonged beyond the prescribed duration, local control falls by 1.4 per cent per extra day.[83] Oncology centres routinely move patients between treatment machines to avoid interruptions due to machine servicing, quality assurance or breakdowns. Interruptions due to public holidays, transport failure or intercurrent illness are compensated for by planning a treatment session on a public holiday or at the weekend, by hyperfractionation (treating twice in 1 day with a minimum 6-hour gap) or by refractionation.[84] Refractionation involves adjusting the remaining dose and number of fractions to deliver an equivalent dose in the remaining prescribed time or increasing the total dose (equivalent to 0.9 Gy per day of interruptions) and giving additional fractions. Refractionation is the least preferred option as increases in total dose or dose per fraction may increase the risk of late normal tissue damage.

Anaemia

There is clear evidence that locoregional control and survival are reduced in patients who are anaemic at the time of radiotherapy.[85, 86] From earlier studies it was unclear whether this was related to true radioresistance or due to the milieu in which the tumour had developed or to an interaction between tumour and host. However, in multivariate analysis disease-free survival was more clearly related to the haemoglobin concentration at the end of radiotherapy than to pretreatment haemoglobin.[87] In a study of postoperative radiotherapy, it was the fall in haemoglobin between surgery and radiotherapy, rather than the absolute values, that had the greatest impact on outcome.[88] This detriment with falling haemoglobin is equivalent to a loss of local control of approximately 10–15 per cent for a 2 g/dL fall in haemoglobin.[87, 88] The relationship with haemoglobin at the end of treatment suggests that efforts to maintain haemoglobin to a level ≥ 12.0 g/dL are worthwhile. Blood transfusion is the principal means of maintaining haemoglobin. Erythropoietin analogues cannot at present be recommended for routine use because of concerns that these may stimulate erythropoietin receptors present on some tumour cells.[89] However, in a study using epoetin alpha to counter anaemia during chemoradiation, the detrimental effect of low pretreatment haemoglobin seen in historical controls was abolished by use of epoetin alpha to maintain haemoglobin in the anaemic subgroup.[90] This appears contrary to the results of randomized trials in which epoetin did not improve outcomes in patients treated with radiotherapy alone.[91]

Smoking

Smoking during radiotherapy reduces treatment effectiveness, probably by inhaled carbon monoxide displacing oxygen from haemoglobin. In a study of 973 patients undergoing radiotherapy, local control at five years was significantly worse in active smokers compared to former smokers (80 versus 67 per cent).[92] In two older studies, smoking was a significant adverse factor in univariate but not in multivariate analysis.[93, 94] It would seem prudent, therefore, to encourage patients to stop smoking prior to radiotherapy. Use of a carbon monoxide monitor (of exhaled air) in clinic is a valuable adjunct to other strategies aimed at patients stopping smoking.

NEW DEVELOPMENTS

Intensity-modulated radiotherapy

Although conventional three-dimensional conformal radiotherapy remains a significant step forward compared to

for radiotherapy. *British Journal of Cancer* 1955; **9**: 539–49.

● 9. Gray LH, Conger AD, Ebert M *et al.* The concentration of oxygen dissolved in tissues at the time of irradiation is a factor in radiotherapy. *British Journal of Radiology* 1953; **26**: 638–48.

● 10. Lartigau E, Lusinchi A, Weeger P *et al.* Variations in tumour oxygen tension (pO$_2$) during accelerated radiotherapy of head and neck carcinoma. *European Journal of Cancer* 1998; **34**: 856–61.

● 11. Eschmann SM, Paulsen F, Bedeshem C *et al.* Hypoxia-imaging with 18F-misonidazole and PET: changes of kinetics during radiotherapy of head-and-neck cancer. *Radiotherapy and Oncology* 2007; **83**: 406–10.

● 12. Lehtio K, Eskola O, Viljanen T *et al.* Imaging perfusion and hypoxia with PET to predict radiotherapy response in head-and-neck cancer. *International Journal of Radiation Oncology, Biology, Physics* 2004; **59**: 971–82.

● 13. Thorwarth D, Eschmann SM, Paulsen F, Alber M. A model of reoxygenation dynamics of head-and-neck tumours based on serial 18F-fluoromisonidazole positron emission tomography investigations. *International Journal of Radiation Oncology, Biology, Physics* 2007; **68**: 515–21.

14. Hafkamp HC, Manni JJ, Haesevoets A *et al.* Marked differences in survival rate between smokers and nonsmokers with HPV 16-associated tonsillar carcinomas. *International Journal of Cancer* 2008; **122**: 2656–64.

● 15. Fakhry C, Westra WH, Li S *et al.* Improved survival of patients with human papillomavirus-positive head and neck squamous cell carcinoma in a prospective clinical trial. *Journal of the National Cancer Institute* 2008; **100**: 261–9.

16. Sugiyama M, Bhawal UK, Kawamura M *et al.* Human papillomavirus-16 in oral squamous cell carcinoma: clinical correlates and 5-year survival. *British Journal of Oral and Maxillofacial Surgery* 2007; **45**: 116–22.

17. Worden FP, Kumar B, Lee JS *et al.* Chemoselection as a strategy for organ preservation in advanced oropharynx cancer: response and survival positively associated with HPV16 copy number. *Journal of Clinical Oncology* 2008; **26**: 3138–46.

● 18. Tarnawski R, Fowler J, Skladowski K *et al.* How fast is repopulation of tumour cells during the treatment gap? *International Journal of Radiation Oncology, Biology Physics* 2002; **54**: 229–36.

◆ 19. Isles MG, McKonkey C, Mehanna HM. A systematic review and meta-analysis of the role of positron emission tomography in the follow up of head and neck squamous cell carcinoma following radiotherapy or chemoradiotherapy. *Clinical Otolaryngology* 2008; **33**: 210–22.

● 20. Konings AW, Coppes RP, Vissink A. On the mechanism of salivary gland radiosensitivity. *International Journal of Radiation Oncology, Biology, Physics* 2005; **62**: 1187–94.

● 21. Burlage FR, Coppes RP, Meertens H *et al.* Parotid and submandibular/sublingual salivary flow during high dose radiotherapy. *Radiotherapy and Oncology* 2001; **61**: 271–4.

● 22. Bussels B, Maes A, Flamen P *et al.* Dose-response relationships within the parotid gland after radiotherapy for head and neck cancer. *Radiotherapy and Oncology* 2004; **73**: 297–306.

● 23. Braam PM, Roesink JM, Moerland MA *et al.* Long-term parotid gland function after radiotherapy. *International Journal of Radiation Oncology, Biology, Physics* 2005; **62**: 659–64.

● 24. Murdoch-Kinch CA, Kim HM, Vineberg KA *et al.* Dose-effect relationships for the submandibular salivary glands and implications for their sparing by intensity modulated radiotherapy. *International Journal of Radiation Oncology, Biology, Physics* 2008; **72**: 373–82.

✳ 25. National Cancer Institute. Common terminology criteria for adverse events (CTCAE) and common toxicity criteria (CTC) v3.0. Last updated September 8, 2010. Available from: http://ctep.info.nih.gov/reporting/ctc.html.

● 26. Adelstein DJ, Li Y, Adams GL *et al.* An Intergroup phase III comparison of standard radiation therapy and two schedules of concurrent chemoradiotherapy in patients with unresectable squamous cell head and neck cancer. *Journal of Clinical Oncology* 2003; **21**: 92–8.

● 27. Dische S, Saunders M, Barrett A *et al.* A randomised multicentre trial of CHART versus conventional radiotherapy in head and neck cancer. *Radiotherapy and Oncology* 1997; **44**: 123–36.

◆ 28. Sutherland SE, Browman GP. Prophylaxis of oral mucositis in irradiated head and neck cancer patients: a proposed classification scheme of interventions and meta-analysis of randomised controlled trials. *International Journal of Radiation Oncology, Biology, Physics* 2001; **49**: 917–30.

◆ 29. Scully C, Epstein J, Sonis S. Oral mucositis; a challenging complication of radiotherapy, chemotherapy, and radiochemotherapy. Part 2, diagnosis and management of mucositis. *Head and Neck* 2004; **26**: 77–84.

● 30. Finlay PM, Richardson MD, Robertson AG. A comparative study of the efficacy of fluconazole and amphotericin B in the treatment of oropharyngeal candidosis in patients undergoing radiotherapy for head and neck tumours. *British Journal of Oral and Maxillofacial Surgery* 1996; **34**: 23–5.

● 31. Pons V, Greenspan D, Lozada-Nur F *et al.* Oropharyngeal candidiasis in patients with AIDS: randomized comparison of fluconazole versus nystatin oral suspensions. *Clinical Infectious Diseases* 1997; **24**: 1204–7.

● 32. Salas S, Baumstarck-Barrau K, Alfonsi M *et al.* Impact of the prophylactic gastrostomy for unresectable squamous cell head and neck carcinomas treated with radio-chemotherapy on quality of life: prospective randomised trial. *Radiotherapy and Oncology* 2009; **93**: 503–9.

● 33. Lin LC, Que J, Lin LK, Lin FC. Zinc supplementation to improve mucositis and dermatitis in patients after radiotherapy for head-and-neck cancers: a double-blind, randomized study. *International Journal of Radiation Oncology, Biology, Physics* 2006; **65**: 745–50.

34. Burlage FR, Roesink JM, Kampigna HH *et al*. Protection of salivary function by concomitant pilocarpine during radiotherapy: a double-blind, randomized, placebo-controlled study. *International Journal of Radiation Oncology, Biology, Physics* 2008; **70**: 14–22.

35. Scarantino C, LeVeque F, Swann RS *et al*. Effect of pilocarpine during radiation therapy: results of RTOG 97-09, a phase III randomized study in head and neck cancer patients. *Journal of Supportive Oncology* 2006; **4**: 252–8.

36. Seikaly H, Jha N, Harris JR *et al*. Long-term outcomes of submandibular gland transfer for prevention of postradiation xerostomia. *Archives of Otolaryngology – Head and Neck Surgery* 2004; **130**: 956–61.

37. Brizel DM, Wasserman TH, Henke M *et al*. Phase III randomized trial of amifostine as a radioprotector in head and neck cancer. *Journal of Clinical Oncology* 2000; **18**: 3339–45.

38. Bardet E, Martin L, Calais G *et al*. Subcutaneous compared with intravenous administration of amifostine in patients with head and neck cancer receiving radiotherapy: final results of the GORTEC 2002–02 phase III randomized trial. *Journal of Clinical Oncology* 2011; **29**: 127–33.

39. Sasse AD, Clark LG, Sasse EC, Clark OA. Amifostine reduces side effects and improves complete response rate during radiotherapy: results of a meta-analysis. *International Journal of Radiation Oncology, Biology, Physics* 2006; **64**: 784–91.

40. Buentzel J, Micke O, Adamietz IA *et al*. Intravenous amifostine during chemoradiotherapy for head-and-neck cancer: a randomized placebo-controlled phase III study. *International Journal of Radiation Oncology, Biology, Physics* 2006; **64**: 684–91.

41. Dirix P, Abbeel S, Vanstraelen B *et al*. Dysphagia after chemoradiotherapy for head-and-neck squamous cell carcinoma: dose-effect relationships for the swallowing structures. *International Journal of Radiation Oncology, Biology, Physics* 2009; **75**: 385–92.

42. van der Voet JC, Keus RB, Hart AA *et al*. The impact of treatment time and smoking on local control and complications in T1 glottic cancer. *International Journal of Radiation Oncology, Biology, Physics* 1998; **42**: 247–55.

43. Lee IJ, Koom WS, Lee CG *et al*. Risk factors and dose-effect relationship for mandibular osteoradionecrosis in oral and oropharyngeal cancer patients. *International Journal of Radiation Oncology, Biology, Physics* 2009; **75**: 1084–91.

44. Mendenhall WM. Mandibular osteoradionecrosis. *Journal of Clinical Oncology* 2004; **22**: 4867–8.

45. Wahl MJ. Osteoradionecrosis prevention myths. *International Journal of Radiation Oncology, Biology, Physics* 2006; **64**: 661–9.

46. Springer IN, Niehoff P, Warnke PH *et al*. Radiation caries – radiogenic destruction of dental collagen. *Oral Oncology* 2005; **41**: 723–8.

47. Dijkstra PU, Kalk WW, Roodenburg JL. Trismus in head and neck oncology: a systematic review. *Oral Oncology* 2004; **40**: 879–89.

48. Teguh DN, Levendag PC, Voet P *et al*. Trismus in patients with oropharyngeal cancer: relationship with dose in structures of mastication apparatus. *Head and Neck* 2008; **30**: 622–30.

49. Gowda RV, Henk JM, Mais KL *et al*. Three weeks radiotherapy for T1 glottic cancer: the Christie and Royal Marsden Hospital experience. *Radiotherapy and Oncology* 2003; **68**: 105–11.

50. Silva JJ, Tsang RW, Panzarella T *et al*. Results of radiotherapy for epithelial skin cancer of the pinna: the Princess Margaret Hospital experience, 1982–1993. *International Journal of Radiation Oncology, Biology, Physics* 2000; **47**: 451–9.

51. Hayter CR, Lee KH, Groome PA, Brundage MD. Necrosis following radiotherapy for carcinoma of the pinna. *International Journal of Radiation Oncology, Biology, Physics* 1996; **36**: 1033–7.

52. Schultheiss TE. The radiation dose-response of the human spinal cord. *International Journal of Radiation Oncology, Biology, Physics* 2008; **71**: 1455–9.

53. Jones A. Transient radiation myelopathy (with reference to Lhermitte's sign of electrical paraesthesia). *British Journal of Radiology* 1964; **37**: 727–44.

54. Bhandare N, Monroe AT, Morris CG *et al*. Does altered fractionation influence the risk of radiation-induced optic neuropathy? *International Journal of Radiation Oncology, Biology Physics* 2005; **62**: 1070–7.

55. Parsons JT, Bova FJ, Fitzgerald CR *et al*. Radiation optic neuropathy after megavoltage external beam irradiation: analysis of time-dose factors. *International Journal of Radiation Oncology, Biology, Physics* 1994; **30**: 755–63.

56. Monroe AT, Bhandare N, Morris CG, Mendenhall WM. Preventing radiation retinopathy with hyperfractionation. *International Journal of Radiation Oncology, Biology, Physics* 2005; **61**: 856–64.

57. Ferrufino-Ponce ZK, Henderson BA. Radiotherapy and cataract formation. *Seminars in Ophthalmology* 2006; **21**: 171–80.

58. Jereczek-Fossa BA, Zarowski A, Orecchia R. Radiotherapy-induced ear toxicity. *Cancer Treatment Reviews* 2003; **29**: 417–30.

59. Bhandare N, Antonelli PJ, Morris CG *et al*. Ototoxicity after radiotherapy for head and neck tumours. *International Journal of Radiation Oncology, Biology, Physics* 2007; **67**: 469–9.

60. Dorresteijn LDA, Kappelle AC, Boogerd W *et al*. Increased risk of ischaemic stroke after radiotherapy on the neck in patients younger than 60 years. *Journal of Clinical Oncology* 2002; **20**: 282–8.

61. Haynes JC, Machtay M, Weber RS *et al.* Relative risk of stroke in head and neck carcinoma patients treated with external cervical irradiation. *Laryngoscope* 2002; **112**: 1883–7.

62. Lam WW, Yuen HY, Wong KS *et al.* Clinically underdetected asymptomatic and symptomatic carotid stenosis as a late complication of radiotherapy in Chinese nasopharyngeal carcinoma patients. *Head and Neck* 2001; **23**: 780–4.

63. Alterio D, Jereczek-Fossa BA, Franchi B *et al.* Thyroid disorders in patients treated with radiotherapy for head-and-neck cancer: a retrospective analysis of seventy-three patients. *International Journal of Radiation Oncology, Biology, Physics* 2007; **67**: 144–50.

64. Bhandare N, Kennedy L, Malyapa RS *et al.* Primary and central hypothyroidism after radiotherapy for head-and-neck tumours. *International Journal of Radiation Oncology, Biology, Physics* 2007; **68**: 1131–9.

65. Cheng SW, Wu LL, Ting AC *et al.* Irradiation-induced extracranial carotid stenosis in patients with head and neck malignancies. *American Journal of Surgery* 1999; **178**: 323–8.

66. Fowler JF. Is there an optimum overall time for head and neck radiotherapy? A review, with new modelling. *Clinical Oncology (Royal College of Radiologists (Great Britain))* 2007; **19**: 8–22.

67. Fu KK, Pajak TF, Trotti A *et al.* A Radiation Therapy Oncology Group (RTOG) phase III randomised study to compare hyperfractionation and two variants of accelerated fractionation to standard fractionation radiotherapy for head and neck squamous cell carcinomas: first report of RTOG 9003. *International Journal of Radiation Oncology, Biology, Physics* 2000; **48**: 7–16.

68. Saunders MI, Dische S, Hong A *et al.* Continuous hyperfractionated accelerated radiotherapy in locally advanced carcinoma of the head and neck region. *International Journal of Radiation Oncology, Biology, Physics* 1989; **17**: 1287–93.

69. Bourhis J, Overgaard J, Audry H *et al.* Hyperfractionated or accelerated radiotherapy in head and neck cancer: a meta-analysis. *Lancet* 2006; **368**: 843–85.

70. Overgaard J, Hansen HS, Specht L *et al.* Five compared with six fractions per week of conventional radiotherapy of squamous-cell carcinoma of head and neck: DAHANCA 6&7 randomised controlled trial. *Lancet* 2003; **362**: 933–40.

71. Skladowski K, Maciejewski B, Golen M *et al.* Continuous accelerated 7-days-a-week radiotherapy for head-and-neck cancer: long-term results of phase III clinical trial. *International Journal of Radiation Oncology, Biology, Physics* 2006; **66**: 706–13.

72. Turner SL, Slevin NJ, Gupta NK *et al.* Radical external beam radiotherapy for 333 squamous carcinomas of the oral cavity – evaluation of late morbidity and a watch policy for the clinically negative neck. *Radiotherapy and Oncology* 1996; **41**: 21–9.

73. Bentzen SM, Saunders MI, Dische S, Bond SJ. Radiotherapy-related early morbidity in head and neck cancer: quantitative clinical radiobiology as deduced from the CHART trial. *Radiotherapy and Oncology* 2001; **60**: 123–35.

74. Mohanti BK, Umapathy H, Bahadur S *et al.* Short course palliative radiotherapy of 20 Gy in 5 fractions for advanced and incurable head and neck cancer: AIIMS study. *Radiotherapy and Oncology* 2004; **71**: 275–80.

75. Corry J, Peters LJ, D'Costa I *et al.* The 'QUAD SHOT' – a phase II study of palliative radiotherapy for incurable head and neck cancer. *Radiotherapy and Oncology* 2005; **77**: 137–42.

76. Porceddu SV, Rosser B, Burmeister BH *et al.* Hypofractionated radiotherapy for the palliation of advanced head and neck cancer in patients unsuitable for curative treatment – 'Hypo Trial'. *Radiotherapy and Oncology* 2007; **85**: 456–62.

77. Jackson SM, Hay JH, Flores AD. Local control of T3N0 glottic carcinoma by 60 Gy given over five weeks in 2.4 Gy daily fractions. One more point on the biological effective dose (BED) curve. *Radiotherapy and Oncology* 2001; **59**: 219–20.

78. Withers HR, Peters LJ. Transmutability of dose and time. Commentary on the first report of RTOG 9003. *International Journal of Radiation Oncology, Biology, Physics* 2000; **48**: 1–2.

79. Pignon JP, Maitre A, Bourhis J *et al.* Meta-analyses of chemotherapy in head and neck cancer (MACH-NC): an update. *International Journal of Radiation Oncology, Biology, Physics* 2007; **69**(Suppl. 2): S112–S114.

80. Bonner JA, Harari PM, Giralt J *et al.* Radiotherapy plus cetuximab for squamous-cell carcinoma of head and neck. *New England Journal of Medicine* 2006; **354**: 567–78.

81. Chen Z, King W, Pearcey R *et al.* The relationship between waiting time for radiotherapy and clinical outcomes: a systematic review of the literature. *Radiotherapy and Oncology* 2008; **87**: 3–16.

82. Waaijers A, Terhaard CHJ, Dehnad H *et al.* Waiting times for radiotherapy: consequences of volume increase for the TCP in oropharyngeal carcinoma. *Radiotherapy and Oncology* 2003; **66**: 271–6.

83. Bese NS, Hendry J, Jeremic B. Effects of prolongation of overall treatment time due to unplanned interruptions during radiotherapy of different tumour sites and practical methods for compensation. *International Journal of Radiation Oncology, Biology, Physics* 2007; **68**: 654–61.

84. Royal College of Radiologists. The timely delivery of radical radiotherapy: standards and guidelines for the management of unscheduled treatment interruptions, 3rd edn. London: Royal College of Radiologists, 2008.

85. Cho EI, Sasaki CT, Haffty BG. Prognostic significance of pretreatment haemoglobin for local control and overall survival in T1–2N0 larynx cancer treated with external beam radiotherapy. *International Journal of Radiation Oncology, Biology, Physics* 2004; **58**: 1135–40.

86. Fortin A, Wang CS, Vigneault E. Effect of pretreatment anaemia on treatment outcome of concurrent radiochemotherapy in patients with head and neck cancer. *International Journal of Radiation Oncology, Biology, Physics* 2008; **72**: 255–60.

87. van Acht MJ, Hermans J, Boks DE, Leer JW. The prognostic value of haemoglobin and a decrease in haemoglobin during radiotherapy in laryngeal carcinoma. *Radiotherapy and Oncology* 1992; **23**: 229–35.

88. van de Pol SM, Doornaert PA, de Bree R et al. The significance of anaemia in squamous cell head and neck cancer treated with surgery and postoperative radiotherapy. *Oral Oncology* 2006; **42**: 131–8.

89. Henke M, Mattern D, Pepe M et al. Do erythropoietin receptors on cancer cells explain unexpected clinical findings? *Journal of Clinical Oncology* 2006; **24**: 4708–13.

90. Glaser CM, Millesi W, Kornek GV et al. Impact of haemoglobin level and use of recombinant erythropoetin on efficacy of preoperative chemoradiation therapy for squamous cell carcinoma of the oral cavity and oropharynx. *International Journal of Radiation Oncology, Biology, Physics* 2001; **50**: 705–15.

91. Henke M, Laszig R, Rübe C et al. Erythropoietin to treat head and neck cancer patients with anaemia undergoing radiotherapy: randomised, double-blind, placebo-controlled trial. *Lancet* 2003; **362**: 1255–60.

92. Fortin A, Wang CS, Vigneault E. Influence of smoking and alcohol drinking behaviours on treatment outcomes of patients with squamous cell carcinomas of the head and neck. *International Journal of Radiation Oncology, Biology, Physics* 2009; **74**: 1062–9.

93. Browman GP, Wong G, Hodson I et al. Influence of cigarette smoking on the efficacy of radiation therapy in head and neck cancer. *New England Journal of Medicine* 1993; **328**: 159–63.

94. Marshak G, Brenner B, Shvero J et al. Prognostic factors for local control of early glottic cancer: the Rabin Medical Centre retrospective study of 207 patients. *International Journal of Radiation Oncology, Biology, Physics* 1999; **43**: 1009–13.

95. Kam MK, Leung SF, Zee B et al. Prospective randomised study of intensity-modulated radiotherapy on salivary gland function in early-stage nasopharyngeal carcinoma patients. *Journal of Clinical Oncology* 2007; **25**: 4873–9.

96. Nutting CM, Morden JP, Harrington KJ et al. Parotid-sparing intensity modulated versus conventional radiotherapy in head and neck cancer (PARSPORT): a phase 3 multicentre randomized controlled trial. *Lancet Oncology* 2010; **12**: 127–36.

97. Saarilahti K, Kouri M, Collan J et al. Sparing of the submandibular glands by intensity modulated radiotherapy in the treatment of head and neck cancer. *Radiotherapy and Oncology* 2006; **78**: 270–5.

98. Cannon DM, Lee NY. Recurrence in region of spared parotid gland after definitive intensity-modulated radiotherapy for head and neck cancer. *International Journal of Radiation Oncology, Biology, Physics* 2008; **70**: 660–5.

99. Sanguineti G, Gunn GB, Endres EJ et al. Patterns of locoregional failure after exclusive IMRT for oropharyngeal carcinoma. *International Journal of Radiation Oncology, Biology, Physics* 2008; **72**: 737–46.

100. O'Daniel JC, Garden AS, Schwartz DL et al. Parotid gland dose in intensity-modulated radiotherapy for head and neck cancer: is what you plan what you get? *International Journal of Radiation Oncology, Biology, Physics* 2007; **69**: 1290–6.

101. Shirato H, Shimizu S, Kitamura K, Onimaru R. Organ motion in image-guided radiotherapy: lessons from real-time tumour-tracking radiotherapy. *International Journal of Clinical Oncology* 2007; **12**: 8–16.

102. Lee NY, Mechalakos JG, Nehmeh S et al. Fluorine-18-labelled fluoromisonidazole positron emission and computed tomography-guided intensity-modulated radiotherapy for head and neck cancer: a feasibility study. *International Journal of Radiation Oncology, Biology, Physics* 2008; **70**: 2–13.

103. MacDougall RH, Orr JA, Kerr GR, Duncan W. Fast neutron treatment for squamous cell carcinoma of the head and neck: final report of the Edinburgh randomised trial. *British Medical Journal* 1990; **301**: 1241–2.

104. Maor MH, Errington RD, Caplan RJ et al. Fast-neutron therapy in advanced head and neck cancer: a collaborative international randomised trial. *International Journal of Radiation Oncology, Biology, Physics* 1995; **32**: 599–604.

105. Chan AW, Liebsch NJ. Proton radiation therapy for head and neck cancer. *Journal of Surgical Oncology* 2008; **97**: 687–700.

106. Lodge M, Pijls-Johannesma M, Stirk L et al. A systematic literature review of the clinical and cost-effectiveness of hadron therapy in cancer. *Radiotherapy and Oncology* 2007; **83**: 110–22.

107. Creak AL, Harrington K, Nutting C. Treatment of recurrent head and neck cancer: re-irradiation or chemotherapy? *Clinical Oncology (Royal College of Radiologists (Great Britain))* 2005; **17**: 138–47.

108. Kasperts N, Slotman B, Leemans CR, Langendijk JA. A review on re-irradiation for recurrent and second primary head and neck cancer. *Oral Oncology* 2005; **41**: 225–43.

109. Salama JK, Vokes EE, Chmura SJ et al. Long-term outcome of concurrent chemotherapy and reirradiation for recurrent and second primary head-and-neck squamous cell carcinoma. *International Journal of Radiation Oncology, Biology, Physics* 2005; **64**: 382–91.

43

Head and neck squamous cell carcinomas: radical radiotherapy

PETRA J JANKOWSKA AND CHRIS M NUTTING

Who controls the past controls the future. Who controls the present controls the past.

George Orwell, *Nineteen Eighty-Four*, 1949

INTRODUCTION

For many early-stage head and neck squamous cell carcinomas (HNSCC) surgical excision or radiotherapy (RT) alone have similar cure rates, but have different adverse effect profiles. Radical radiation alone is indicated in the treatment of several early-stage tumours, particularly when organ preservation and/or cosmesis are important. Patient preference should also be taken into account when decisions between surgery and radiation are taken.

RT is frequently employed in the treatment of early cancers of the larynx, oropharynx and hypopharynx, so that natural speech and swallowing, respectively, may be preserved. Equally, radiation may preserve cosmesis and function in patients with cancers of the nasal cavity, columella, paranasal sinuses and ear.

Early oral cancer including superficial (<5 mm thickness), T1 and T2 lesions should be considered for brachytherapy.

Many patients with more locally advanced disease will be treated with a combination of surgery plus postoperative radiotherapy (PORT) or chemoradiotherapy. However, a significant proportion will be unsuitable for radical surgery or combined chemoradiation due to comorbid conditions and this cohort may be offered radical radiotherapy in order to maximize local control, even though long-term cure is only achieved in 30–40 per cent of patients. In the small proportion of patients presenting with metastatic disease, moderate-dose short-course RT may be used to ameliorate local symptoms.

GENERAL PRINCIPLES OF TREATMENT VOLUME AND DEFINITION

Patients with head and neck cancer should be seen in a multidisciplinary setting by a team comprising specialist surgeons, oncologists, pathologists, radiologists and palliative care doctors, together with dietitians, speech and language therapists and clinical nurse specialists. At the initial visit, a full history and examination, including nasendoscopy if relevant, will be carried out. Further pretreatment assessment should include examination under anaesthesia (EUA) and tumour biopsy, imaging in the form of computed tomography (CT) and/or magnetic resonance imaging (MRI) of the head and neck, chest x-ray or CT thorax, full blood count, urea and electrolytes, liver function tests, dietitian assessment, and assessment by a speech and language therapist. In particular, patients with poor dietary intake and a low body mass index should be identified and considered for elective percutaneous gastrostomy or nasogastric feeding.[1] Dental assessment is also essential for any patient in whom the radiation field is likely to include either mandibular or maxillary alveolus, since dental extraction subsequent to a radical dose incurs a greater risk of chronic non-healing ulceration or osteoradionecrosis.[2] Written informed consent, detailing both the acute and late toxicities of radiation, should be obtained prior to embarking on a course of radical treatment. Smoking cessation should be advised since smoking is known to both increase radiation-induced toxicity and reduce cure rates.[3, 4] Alcohol cessation should also be advised at least for the duration of the radiation since, again, toxicity is likely to be increased.

Most patients with early tumours will usually be treated in a single-phase radiation plan, although the field arrangements will vary for each site.

However, tumour sites such as tongue base and hypopharynx, which are associated with a higher risk of occult nodal micrometastasis, are more likely to receive their radiation in two phases. Phase 1 is typically a larger volume encompassing the primary tumour, involved lymph nodes and potential areas of microscopic nodal spread while in phase 2, a smaller volume including the primary tumour and involved lymph nodes alone is treated. Elective irradiation of lymph nodes is indicated when the risk of microscopic lymphatic spread exceeds 15–20 per cent. **Table 43.1**, categorizes the risk of occult micrometastases to lymph nodes, which have been documented from surgicopathological series.[5, 6, 7] Lymph node levels are defined as: level Ia, submental; level Ib, submandibular; level II, upper deep cervical; level III, mid-deep cervical; level IV, lower deep cervical; level V, posterior triangle (**Figure 43.1**). Recommendations for specific node groups to be included in the field of treatment are meant as a guide (**Table 43.2**). The responsible clinician must make the final decision based on the details of the individual case.

A similar two-phase technique is employed if proceeding with total mucosal irradiation and in patients being treated for locally advanced inoperable disease.

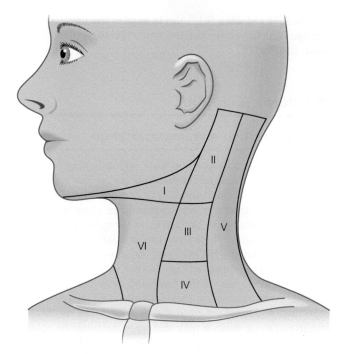

Figure 43.1 The lymph node levels in the neck: I, submental and submandibular; II, upper deep cervical; III, middle deep cervical; IV, lower deep cervical; V, posterior triangle.

Table 43.2 Recommendations for elective lymph node irradiation in patients undergoing definitive radiotherapy for head and neck cancer.

Larynx

T1/T2 N0 glottic	No elective nodal irradiation
T3/T4 N0 glottic	Levels Ib to IV bilaterally
T1/T2 N0 supraglottic	Levels Ib to III bilaterally
All other stages	Levels Ib to V bilaterally

Oropharynx

T1 N0 tonsil	Levels Ib, II ipsilateral
T2 N0 tonsil (lateralized)	Levels Ib to IV ipsilateral
T1/T2 N1 tonsil (lateralized)	Levels Ib to V ipsilateral
T2 N0 tonsil (approaching midline)+other sites	Levels Ib to V bilaterally
All other stages and subsites	Levels Ib to V bilaterally

Hypopharynx

All stages and subsites	Levels Ib to V bilaterally

Nasal cavity

Any T, N0	No elective nodal irradiation
Any T, N+	Levels Ib to V bilaterally

Paranasal sinuses

Any T, N0	Lateral pharyngeal/
Any T, N+	retropharyngeal lymph node

Oral cavity

T1/T2 N0 (lateralized primary)	Levels I, II ipsilateral
T2 N1 (lateralized primary)	Levels I to V ipsilateral
T2 N0 (primary approaching midline)	Levels I to IV bilateral
All other stages	Levels I to V bilateral

Table 43.1 The risk of nodal metastases based on tumour site and location.

High risk (>60%)	Nasopharynx Oropharynx Hypopharynx Supraglottis
Moderate risk (20–60%)	Oral cavity Advanced larynx Salivary gland (parotid, submandibular, etc.)
Low risk (<20%)	Early glottic Nasal cavity Paranasal sinuses Skin
Predominantly unilateral risk	Early tonsil Well-lateralized oral cavity Parotid
Bilateral risk	Tongue base Hypopharynx (pyriform sinus) Advanced larynx Nasopharynx

Palliative radiation fields aim to employ the simplest beam arrangement to cover macroscopic disease while limiting acute toxicity.

PLANNING TECHNIQUE

Patient position and immobilization

The anatomy of the head and neck region is very complex, with bony structures, soft tissues and air cavities all present within a relatively small volume. In addition to the tumour, many critical structures are frequently in close proximity, such as the spinal cord, brainstem, optic apparatus, mucosa and salivary glands. These structures are defined as organs at risk (OAR). Although OAR may lie close to the tumour volume, internal organ motion is relatively limited. Therefore, immobilization of the head and neck region using a custom-made cabulite or thermoplastic shell should ensure reproducible patient set up to within 3 mm.[8] The mechanical stability of these shells is such that large areas may be cut out to maximize skin sparing during treatment. Thermoplastic shells are more convenient but have been associated with less stability in the past, and so were reserved for the palliative setting. However, the repositioning accuracy of the newer thermoplastic shells is comparable to that of cabulite, particularly when more locating points are used.[9, 10, 11, 12] The addition of a tattoo on the body may also help with this. The main disadvantage of the cabulite shells, apart from the time factor, is that by virtue of their method of attachment to the treatment couch, necessary limitations are imposed on the radiation beam directionality. This has implications for the delivery of intensity-modulated radiotherapy (IMRT). In contrast, newer carbon fibre head and neck boards are available for use with the thermoplastic shells, and are likely to become standard in the future. In the meantime, before adopting any changes, it is recommended that departments assess their own system, comparing it to any new proposed system, because of differences in attachment to bed, number of locating points used and head rest used.[13] This enables the estimation of both set-up systematic and random errors that one might expect, prior to the introduction of new systems.

Prior to the manufacture of an immobilization shell, the head and neck position, shell extent, requirements for mouth bite and full planning details should be specified.

For most sites, patients are immobilized in the head neutral position with the spinal cord straight. This enables matching between photon and electron fields along a straight line in front of the spinal cord, if necessary, during the second phase of treatment. However, patients being treated with IMRT are likely to be immobilized in the neck extended position in order to limit the volume of oral cavity irradiated.

Any patient with palpable lymphadenopathy should have this marked with wire and a simulator image taken to facilitate planning at subsequent visits. This step may be omitted, however, if virtual simulation using a CT scan is planned, where tumour definition is more easily apparent.

Mouth bites are used primarily in tumours of the oral cavity, nasal cavity and maxillary sinus. The action of the mouth bite is to open the jaw and depress the tongue. Thus it may be possible to exclude either the upper or lower half of the mouth from the treatment field, thereby reducing the acute toxicity of the treatment. Caution is required in the immobilization of patients with early tongue tumours with a mouth bite, however, since the mouth bite may push the mobile tongue posteriorly and superiorly out of the radiation field.

Volume definition

The International Commission on Radiation Units and Measurements (ICRU) Reports 50 and 62 contain recommendations on how to report a treatment in external beam radiotherapy.[14, 15] In particular, they specify the concepts of the volumes needing to be treated. The gross tumour volume (GTV) and clinical target volume (CTV) are pure oncological concepts. The GTV is defined as the macroscopically identifiable tumour, while the CTV allows a margin around the GTV to account for the potential spread of subclinical disease. The margin used for CTV requires knowledge of the natural history of the tumour as well as any relevant risk factors in a given patient. The planning target volume (PTV), a concept which was refined in the ICRU 62 report, takes into account two components of movement. The internal margin (IM) takes into account variations in size, shape and position of the CTV in relation to anatomical reference points, while the set-up margin (SM) accounts for uncertainties in patient–beam positioning and relates to technical factors such as accuracy of set up and immobilization of the patient.

Delivery of dose to the PTV depends on the tumour type, the need for radical as opposed to elective radiation, and the nearby organs at risk. OAR (e.g. spinal cord, parotid gland) have defined tolerance doses which have been summarized in **Table 43.3**.[16]

With regard to the elective irradiation of a nodal target volume, consensus guidelines were recently published in order to define a reproducible standard applicable internationally.[17, 18]

Volume localization

Conventional radiotherapy planning employs the use of a radiotherapy simulator to define the fields and has been

Table 43.3   Tolerance doses of specific organs at risk.

Organ	Normal tissue tolerance (2 Gy/fraction)
Lens	6 Gy
Cornea	40 Gy
Retina	50 Gy
Optic nerve	50 Gy
Optic chiasm	50–55 Gy
Spinal cord	44–48 Gy
Brainstem	48–54 Gy
Parotid gland	30 Gy
Lacrimal gland	30 Gy

standard practice in most treatment centres for many years. Typically, field borders are defined in relation to standard bony anatomical landmarks which represent the extent of a given tumour subsite. These field borders may then be modified in individual patients. This planning method does not use the GTV, CTV and PTV definitions outlined in the ICRU 50 and 62 reports. Instead, the field borders represent the PTV plus a physical margin for penumbra.[19] Most commonly, lateral parallel opposed fields are used to treat the target volume. For more complex plans, such as a wedged pair beam arrangement, the PTV is marked on a patient outline taken through an appropriate level, often the central slice, with the PTV then being manually reconstructed from orthogonal simulator films. The clinical results, as well as the toxicities, from such treatments are well described and expected.

Computed tomography planning is, however, increasingly used for head and neck cancer patients. The ICRU 50 and 62 recommendations should be followed and the responsible clinician should define the GTV, CTV, PTV and OAR. The outlining of these structures should be done with the aid of diagnostic imaging, including CT and MRI, as well as clinical examination, flexible nasendoscopy, and notes from all EUA and relevant operations.[20] This enables accurate definition of both the GTV for the primary as well as the nodal GTV and CTV.

A planning CT scan with intravenous contrast is recommended, since this gives better definition of the primary and nodal GTV.[21, 22] CT planning also results in more accurate dosimetry, as well as being essential for inverse planning and IMRT.[23]

Early tumours of the head and neck are frequently best assessed clinically or endoscopically, since cross-sectional imaging such as CT or MRI may not easily identify small lesions of the larynx, oral cavity and oropharynx. However, CT and MRI are useful in the assessment of tumours where the signal intensity of the tumour compared to the adjacent normal tissue is more contrasting, such as nasal cavity or paranasal sinus tumours.

CTV definition for radical radiotherapy is controversial. The magnitude of the margin required to 'grow' the GTV to the CTV is taken to be between 1 and 2 cm, and accounts for the estimated subclinical spread of disease.[24, 25] It therefore necessitates sound knowledge of the natural history of the disease and patterns of local tumour extension. However, where a tumour is known to exhibit significant submucosal spread, e.g. pyriform sinus cancer, this margin may be increased. Equally, where there is an anatomical barrier to spread, e.g. bone and air cavities, this margin may be reduced.

The recent publication of consensus guidelines for both the elective irradiation of lymph nodes and nodal irradiation in the involved or postoperative setting has been a valuable contribution for nodal CTV localization.[17, 18] The carotid arteries are important structures in the definition of the deep cervical lymph nodes. Therefore, as previously stated, the use of intravenous contrast with CT scan is recommended. Where lymph node metastases are present in addition to the primary tumour, they each require localization as a separate GTV, with a 1–2 cm margin added for CTV as for the primary. Again, this margin may be reduced where there is an anatomical barrier to spread.

A final margin accounting for both internal organ motion and set-up error is added to the CTV to derive the final PTV. In the head and neck region, most internal organ motion is minimal and therefore the magnitude of this margin is largely dependent on the immobilization technique and accuracy of set up.[8, 26] A margin of 3–5 mm, based on the accuracy of immobilization, is sufficient for most primary sites, although for tumours of the hypopharynx and larynx, where movement occurs on swallowing and breathing, a margin of at least 5 mm may be preferable.

Outlining of OAR is essential in CT planning, since these are usually the dose-limiting structures. The OAR relevant to head and neck tumour outlining include the brain, brainstem, spinal cord, optic apparatus (lens, eye, retinae, optic nerves and chiasm), parotid glands, mandible and thyroid gland. Their tolerance doses have previously been summarized (**Table 43.3**).[16] All OAR in close proximity to the PTV, or falling within the likely path of one of the radiation fields, should be outlined in their entirety. This enables accurate cumulative dose–volume histograms (DVHs) to be derived. Such DVHs can be derived for both photon and electron fields, and give a mathematical estimation of the maximum point dose to an OAR, as well as the mean and minimum dose to other volumes, such as the PTV. An example of a DVH for PTV, spinal cord and brainstem is demonstrated in **Figure 43.2**.

IMRT is a new technology in three-dimensional conformal radiotherapy (3D CRT), where by virtue of the beam intensity varying across the treatment field, radiation can be delivered to the PTV with greater sparing of the surrounding normal tissues.[27, 28, 29] While 3D CRT uses radiation beams of uniform intensity, in IMRT, the tumour is treated with multiple small beams of variable intensity, which are achieved by use of a static or dynamic multileaf collimator. Highly conformal dose distributions can therefore be produced, including concave shapes, such as that seen where a tumour is wrapped around an OAR, e.g. parotid gland or spinal cord. IMRT is currently being used both in protocols for the reduction of treatment-related toxicity and also in dose escalation trials, in order to improve local tumour control.[30, 31, 32] IMRT planning is dependent on the inverse planning algorithm. In addition to outlining the target volume and OAR, the clinician must generate constraints in the form of dose volume points. The computer algorithm, using the 'inverse method' is then capable of generating significant dose gradients between the target volume and the adjacent structures. For the target volume, the constraints are usually the prescription dose ± 5 per cent, and for OAR the tolerance dose to a small volume of that organ.[33, 34]

Online real-time image guidance (IG) protocols for tumour volume localization are also currently under assessment, including for patients with head and neck cancer.[35] This requires the implementation of kilovoltage cone-beam CT on board a linear accelerator and will become increasingly available in the clinical, as well as the research, setting. Preliminary studies have shown that residual set-up errors reduce with increasing frequency of IG during the course of external beam radiotherapy for head and neck cancer patients. Tomotherapy is a helical system of RT delivery which offers both IMRT and IGRT advances for HNSCC patients.[36]

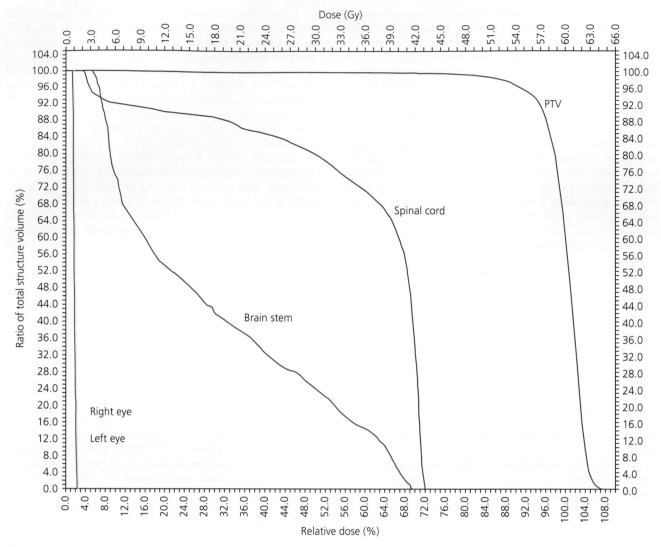

Figure 43.2 Cumulative DVH for PTV, spinal cord and brainstem.

Dose prescription

Every dose prescription should specify the total dose, the number of fractions or treatments, the schedule of treatment delivery (daily, twice daily, etc.), the prescription point and the photon or electron beam energy. Plans should be normalized to the ICRU reference point. The plan should subsequently be checked to ensure adequate PTV coverage, dose homogeneity, and also that the doses to OAR are within tolerance. Cumulative DVHs are helpful for this purpose.

For radical treatment courses for squamous cancers of the head and neck, tumour tissue and OAR will usually be treated close to tolerance, in order to optimize the probability of local control and cure. Conventional radiotherapy involves daily radiation, Monday to Friday, with a dose of 1.8–2 Gy per fraction to a total dose of 66–70 Gy.[37, 38, 39] Some centres, however, use a hypofractionated regime, delivering 55 Gy in 20 fractions daily, Monday to Friday over 4 weeks (2.75 Gy per fraction).[40, 41, 42, 43]

In T1/T2 N0 tumours of the head and neck, where the area to be irradiated does not exceed a field size of 42 cm^2,

this 4-week hypofractionated schedule may be adopted, on the basis that smaller volumes will tolerate the larger doses per fraction better. Nevertheless, most US centres do not give doses of greater than 1.8–2 Gy per fraction.

For large volume disease, where surgery has been deemed inappropriate or not possible, there will usually be a target volume for macroscopic disease, which includes the primary tumour and involved lymph nodes, as well as an elective target volume. In this setting, the former, high-dose volume is frequently overlying the spinal cord, in the lateral projection of the field. This necessitates the use of a two-phase technique in order to maintain the dose to the spinal cord within tolerance. Macroscopic disease should receive 66–70 Gy in 1.8–2 Gy per fraction. Microscopic disease in the elective target volume should receive 44–50 Gy in 1.8–2 Gy per fraction.

Conventionally, 50 Gy is the dose considered to be required to sterilize microscopic disease. Data from both the CHART (continuous hyperfractionated accelerated radiotherapy) trials and Europe demonstrated no significant excess of level 5 neck recurrences with elective doses of 44–46 Gy.[25, 39] However,

Table 43.4 An outcome-based comparison of various fractionation schedules.

Fractionation	Tumour growth rate indication	Radiobiological principles	Data for tumour response	Data on complications
Conventional	Average	Standard		
Accelerated fractionation	Rapid	Reduced overall treatment time prevents tumour cell repopulation		
DAHANCA 6 & 7 trial (pure acceleration)			5-year LRC, 66 vs 57% ($p = 0.01$); 5-year DFS, 72 vs 65% ($p = 0.04$); no difference OS	More acute mucositis, no difference in late complication rate
CHART (accelerated # with total dose reduction)			No difference in LRC, DFS or OS	More acute mucositis, reduced late effects
GORTEC 94-02 (accelerated # with total dose reduction)			2-year LRC, 58 vs 34% ($p < 0.01$); no difference in OS	More acute mucositis ($p < 0.01$), similar late toxicity
RTOG 90-03 (accelerated # with concomitant boost)			Greater LRC ($p = 0.05$); trend to improved DFS ($p = 0.054$); no difference in OS	More acute mucositis, no difference in late toxicity
Hyperfractionation	Slow	Greater number of fractions, usually of smaller dose per fraction, allows reoxygenation, allows stem cell repopulation and spares late damage		
RTOG 90-03 (Hyperfractionation with higher overall dose)			Higher LRC ($p = 0.045$); trend to improved DFS ($p = 0.067$); no difference in OS	More acute mucositis, no difference in late effects
EORTC trial (Hyperfractionation with higher total dose)			5-year LRC, 59% vs 40% ($p = 0.02$); particular benefit in T3 tumours	More acute mucositis, no difference in late toxicity

DFS, disease-free survival; LRC, locoregional control; OS, overall survival.

this is a comparatively low-risk site for recurrence in most cases.

For locally advanced disease, the outcome with radical radiation may be improved by using altered fractionation regimes (**Table 43.4**)[37, 38, 44, 45] or through the addition of concomitant platinum-based chemotherapy (see Chapter 45, Chemoradiation in head and neck cancer).[46] There are also data to suggest that unplanned prolongation of the overall time of treatment detrimentally affects local control rates, and, thereby, tumour cure rates.[47] This is important to consider at the outset of a patient's treatment, since there are many predictable and unpredictable interruptions possible.

For radical radiation, the prescription point is defined as the ICRU reference point, or intersection point. However, for IMRT plans, where the isocentre of each treatment segment may not be located within the target, the dose is specified to the median.

Field arrangement and beam modification

Lateral parallel opposed fields and a wedged pair field arrangement are the most commonly employed, although more complex beam arrangements are sometimes necessary. These are discussed below under Site-specific treatment planning.

The most common methods of beam modification used in radical radiotherapy are the use of wedges and shielding.

A radiation beam may be modified by the introduction of a wedge which alters the dose distribution, due to greater absorption of radiation through the thicker end of the wedge (**Figure 43.3**). In head and neck radiation, wedges are used primarily to improve dose homogeneity of unilateral wedged pair fields (**Figure 43.4**), although they may also be employed to compensate for the natural curvature of skin surfaces, or for a sloping target volume.

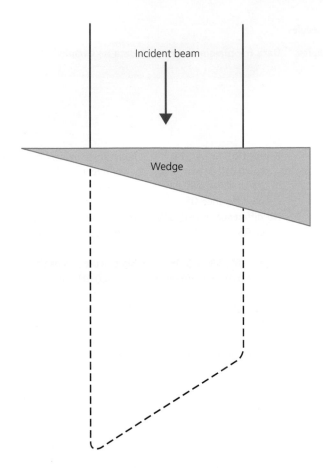

Figure 43.3 Radiation beam modified by introduction of wedge, showing greater attenuation of the beam through the thicker end of the wedge.

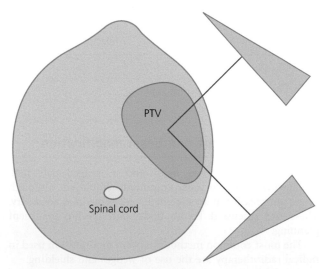

Figure 43.4 Unilateral wedged pair: dose homogeneity improved through the use of wedged radiation fields.

Shielding is the method of shaping the radiation beam for conformal treatments. Most centres achieve this through the use of multileaf collimators.[48] Typically there are 20–80 leaves arranged in opposing pairs which can be positioned under computer control to create an irregular field which conforms to the tumour shape. However, some still use customized alloy blocks which must manually be placed on a template prior to irradiation.

Implementation of treatment

Radiographers, who are responsible for the day-to-day implementation of treatments, must check for shell loosening during the course of therapy. This is particularly relevant in patients who experience significant weight loss. Here, the effect of shell loosening results in inaccuracies of target volume, and importantly, OAR localization, and it is advisable to make a new shell, and replan the volume.[49]

For most treatments, the shell can be cut out, to reduce dose to skin, unless the tumour extends close to the skin, such as laryngeal cancer involving the anterior commissure.

Verification

Prior to treatment, the treatment isocentre, radiation fields and beam shaping are verified against the treatment plan. This may be achieved either using fluoroscopy in a simulator or immediately prior to treatment using electronic portal imaging (EPI). Tolerance of ± 3 mm is usually acceptable (unless critical OAR are very close to the PTV when tolerance levels may be more stringent). During the initial 3 days of radiotherapy, EPI should be used to verify RT field position and confirm set-up reproducibility which continues to be monitored throughout the remainder of the treatment course.[50]

Toxicity of radiation and care during treatment

Patients will have given written informed consent prior to commencement of treatment. Toxicity of RT may be categorized as acute and late. Acute effects occur during the RT, and would usually be expected to have largely resolved within 4–6 weeks of a radical treatment course. By contrast, late effects begin to occur from months after treatment, and some may not develop until years afterwards.

Expected acute toxicities vary according to the primary site irradiated.[51, 52] Skin erythema and tenderness may occur. For doses exceeding 60 Gy, or for larger fraction sizes, skin breakdown or desquamation may occur, which may either be dry or moist. A mucositis commonly occurs from the second to third week.[53] This may be accompanied by dysphagia, odynophagia and ulceration. A dry mouth secondary to salivary, particularly parotid gland irradiation, is usual from the third week onwards. Hoarseness is usual with irradiation of the larynx, and patients should be monitored closely for the development of stridor, particularly in the setting of T3/T4 tumours or subglottic disease at diagnosis. Hair loss in the irradiated areas is expected, but is usually reversible, depending on the fraction size. Irradiation of the mucous membranes of the nasal cavity also results in dryness and crusting, as well as transient bleeding. If the entrance of the nasolacrimal duct is in the radiation field, patients may experience epiphoria.

The late effects of radiation depend on the area treated and the dose per fraction, as well as total dose, delivered during treatment. Salivary gland irradiation in excess of 26–30 Gy will usually result in permanent xerostomia.[54] This, in combination with the severe mucositis often seen in treatments to the oral cavity and oropharynx, may result in long-term swallowing difficulties and percutaneous endoscopic gastrostomy dependence, and appears to be related to the radiation dose, the concomitant use of chemotherapy, advancing age, and the presence of neck disease at diagnosis.[55] Irradiation of the mandibular or maxillary alveolus put the patient at risk of osteoradionecrosis in the event of future dental work required.[2] Irradiation of the pterygoid muscles may result in trismus, which is ideally identified before interference with nutrition.[56] The risk of second malignancy resulting from conventional irradiation is reported to be approximately 1 per cent per ten years following RT, although this figure may increase with the widespread adoption of IMRT, where a greater volume of normal tissue is exposed to lower doses of radiation.[57] In contrast, the background risk of developing a second smoking- or alcohol-related malignancy is about 20 per cent.

It is therefore good practice for all head and neck patients undergoing a course of radical radiotherapy to be seen in a weekly review clinic by a clinical oncologist, a head and neck clinical nurse specialist (CNS), a dietician, and a speech and language therapist (SALT).[58] Following completion of treatment, and as part of ongoing follow up in a joint head and neck clinic, continued review by a dietician, SALT and head and neck CNS may be advisable.

SITE-SPECIFIC TREATMENT PLANNING

Larynx

The larynx is divided into three regions: the supraglottis (laryngeal epiglottis, false vocal cords, ventricles, aryepiglottic folds and arytenoids), the glottis (true vocal cords, anterior and posterior commissures) and the subglottis (10 mm below the free edge of the vocal cords to the inferior border of the cricoid cartilage). Each has its own natural history and pattern of spread, which dictates treatment recommendations.

Immobilization for all larynx cancer patients should be in the supine position with the cervical spine straight.

GLOTTIC TUMOURS

Most stage T1/T2, N0 glottic tumours are treated with radical radiotherapy, with surgery reserved for salvage after radiotherapy failure.[59] The local control rate with definitive radiotherapy for T1 lesions is approximately 90 per cent and for T2 lesions, 70–80 per cent. Controversy remains about which modality gives the best voice quality, though irradiation is generally preferred as it preserves natural voice and avoids a tracheostomy.[60]

Typically, a lateral parallel opposed field arrangement is used, with 5 cm (T1) or 6 cm (T2) square fields centred on the vocal cord (1 cm below thyroid promontory and anterior to the lower border of C5 cervical vertebra).

For T1 lesions, the radiotherapy portal extends from the lower border of the hyoid bone superiorly, to the lower border of the cricoid cartilage inferiorly. Anteriorly, the field border should be in air at the field centre, and posteriorly through the anterior part of the vertebral body (**Figure 43.5**). Usually, 10–20° wedges are used as missing tissue compensators. There is no requirement to give elective nodal irradiation, due to the extremely low incidence of cervical nodal metastases from early glottic tumours, although part of the mid-cervical lymph nodes (level III) is within the volume.

For T2 tumours, the field size is extended based on the supraglottic and/or subglottic disease extension. In cases of extensive subglottic extension, it is recommended that the paraoesophageal and paratracheal lymph nodes are included.

Where glottic tumours extend to the anterior commissure, tumour underdosage is a risk due to the skin-sparing effects of the megavoltage beam. In such cases, the immobilization shell should not be cut out, and it may even be necessary to increase the dose to the skin by the addition of bolus to the shell anteriorly. If the calculated dose is still low, a further improvement in the dose may be seen by reducing or removing the wedge from each lateral field.

In some patients, it will not be possible to deliver lateral fields to the larynx due to high shoulder position or short neck. In this situation, an anterior oblique wedged pair field arrangement is more appropriate (**Figure 43.6**). For conventional planning, this requires an outline to be taken through the field centre, or alternatively, a PTV can be localized by CT planning.

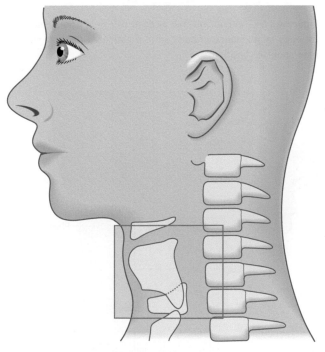

Figure 43.5 Radiotherapy for a T1/T2 N0 carcinoma of the glottis.

Dose prescription

The dose prescription, dependent on field size, is as follows:

- $< 36 \, cm^2$, 50 Gy in 16 fractions treating daily, five fractions a week;
- $36-42 \, cm^2$, 55 Gy in 20 fractions treating daily, five fractions a week;[61]
- $> 42 \, cm^2$, 64–66 Gy in 2 Gy per fraction, treating daily, five fractions a week.

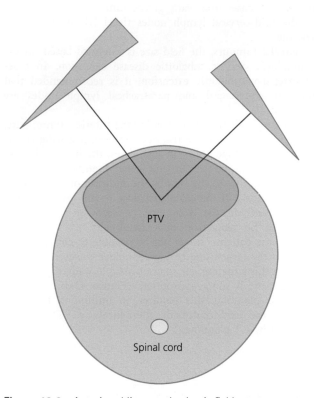

Figure 43.6 Anterior oblique wedged pair field arrangement for early larynx cancer irradiation in a patient with short neck or high shoulder position.

SUPRAGLOTTIC TUMOURS

Radical radiation is indicated for most early (T1/T2, N0) supraglottic tumours. However, in contrast to glottic disease, the supraglottic region has richer lymphatics and, consequently, a higher incidence of occult lymph node metastases in levels II and III. All patients, therefore, require elective nodal irradiation of these levels. This is achieved through the use of a two-phase technique (**Figure 43.7**). Phase I includes the primary tumour, the whole larynx, the pre-epiglottic space and the cervical lymph nodes bilaterally in levels Ib, II and III anterior to the spinal cord. Phase II includes the primary tumour and larynx only. Parallel opposed wedged fields are used for both phases.

Dose prescription

The total dose is 66–70 Gy in 2 Gy per fraction, treating daily, five fractions a week, to macroscopic disease and 44–50 Gy in 2 Gy per fraction, treating daily, five fractions a week, to microscopic disease; for example, phase I: 50 Gy/25#/5 weeks; phase II: 20 Gy/10#/2 weeks.

SUBGLOTTIC TUMOURS

Subglottic tumours are rare, and usually present with locally advanced disease requiring surgery followed by adjuvant radiotherapy. However, for patients with early-stage disease, definitive radiation is a recognized larynx preservation approach. Although the incidence of cervical lymph node metastases is rare, the involvement of paratracheal nodes is estimated at 50 per cent, and therefore these nodes should be treated electively. The radiation portal should extend from the top of the thyroid cartilage superiorly to the mid-trachea inferiorly. This requires the use of either an anterior oblique beam arrangement or a coronal technique (**Figure 43.8**), in order that good coverage of the inferior-most area is achieved.

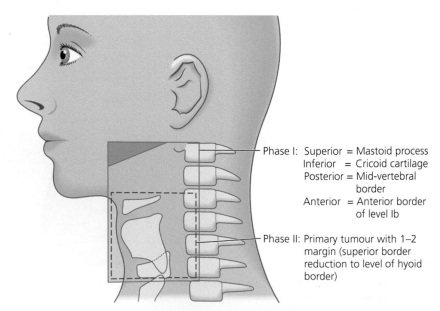

Phase I: Superior = Mastoid process
Inferior = Cricoid cartilage
Posterior = Mid-vertebral border
Anterior = Anterior border of level Ib

Phase II: Primary tumour with 1–2 margin (superior border reduction to level of hyoid border)

Figure 43.7 Radiotherapy technique for node negative supraglottic carcinoma.

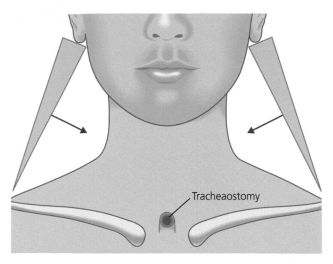

Figure 43.8 Coronal technique for treatment of laryngeal bed and tracheostomy site.

Dose prescription

Dose prescription is 66–70 Gy in 2 Gy per fraction, treating daily, five fractions a week.

LOCALLY ADVANCED DISEASE OF THE LARYNX

Increasingly, stage III/IV tumours of the glottis, supraglottis and subglottis are treated with primary chemoradiation as an alternative to surgery and PORT.[62] This maximizes organ preservation rates, maintaining natural speech and swallowing.[63] However, where patients are not fit for surgery or chemoradiation due to pre-existing comorbid conditions, they may also be considered for radical radiotherapy, as an option to optimize local control, ahead of first-line palliation.

The target volume will include the larynx, pre-epiglottic space, involved lymph nodes and all lymph node areas at risk of involvement with occult metastases, namely, levels Ib, II, III, IV and V in all patients bilaterally. This is achieved with a two- or three-phase technique, depending on the anatomical site(s) of involved lymph nodes, and a combination of megavoltage photon fields and matched electron fields. Phase I will include the primary tumour, the entire larynx, pre-epiglottic space and bilateral cervical lymph node levels Ib–V with radiation delivered using a combination of lateral opposed photon beams and a matched lower anterior neck photon field. This neck field is matched below the level of the cricoid cartilage and therefore allows midline shielding of the spinal cord. Laterally, some shielding of the lungs below the clavicles is also possible (**Figure 43.9**). In phase II, the posterior border of the lateral portals is brought anterior to the spinal cord, and matched electron fields, used because their rapid dose reduction at depth limits the dose to this critical OAR, are applied bilaterally to the posterior level II and level V lymph nodes. In cases where the involved lymph nodes are at or below the level of the larynx, a further superior field border reduction is possible in phase III. One should note that where IMRT has been introduced into routine practice, there is no need for electron fields.

Dose prescription

The total dose is 66–70 Gy in 2 Gy per fraction, treating daily, five fractions a week, to macroscopic disease and 44–50 Gy in 2 Gy per fraction, treating daily, five fractions a week, to microscopic disease; for example, phase I: 50 Gy/25#/5 weeks; phase II: 20 Gy/10#/2 weeks.

Oropharynx

The oropharynx is divided into four main subsites: the tonsil, tongue base, soft palate and posterior pharyngeal wall. Treatment recommendations are guided by natural history as well as the laterality of the tumour, with the long-term outcome for patients treated with radical RT being equivalent to primary surgery.[64, 65] All lesions of the oropharynx have a relatively high risk of nodal metastasis. Where a lesion is well lateralized, e.g. tumour confined to tonsillar fossa, the risk of contralateral nodal metastasis is low (15 per cent) and a unilateral irradiation technique may be employed.[66] This results in sparing of the contralateral normal tissues, especially the contralateral parotid gland. By contrast, midline tumours, such as tongue base and soft palate, may metastasize to either side of the neck, necessitating bilateral neck irradiation, which inevitably causes xerostomia. Conventional beam arrangement with irradiation of both parotid glands results in xerostomia in >75 per cent of cases. IMRT should therefore be considered wherever possible for such patients otherwise planned for parallel opposed radiation portals.[67]

TONSIL

Small (T1/T2, N0) well-lateralized tumours of the tonsil are amenable to treatment with irradiation alone. Immobilization is in the supine position with the cervical spine straight. The target volume for the macroscopic dose includes the tonsillar fossa while the ipsilateral cervical lymph nodes, levels Ib–IV, are treated to a microscopic dose. This is achieved by using a wedged pair field technique to treat the tonsil, with anterior and posterior oblique radiation portals (see **Figure 43.4**), extending from the hard palate superiorly to the lower border of the hyoid bone inferiorly. A modest wedge of approximately 30–45° is required for each of the fields to improve dose homogeneity. This field arrangement encompasses the upper cervical lymph nodes levels Ib–II. At the level of the hyoid bone, a matched ipsilateral anterior neck radiation portal is used to treat the cervical lymph node levels II–IV.

Dose prescription

The total dose is 66–70 Gy in 2 Gy per fraction, treating daily, five fractions a week, to macroscopic disease and 44–50 Gy in 2 Gy per fraction, treating daily, five fractions a week, to microscopic disease; for example, phase I: 50 Gy/25#/5 weeks; phase II: 20 Gy/10#/2 weeks.

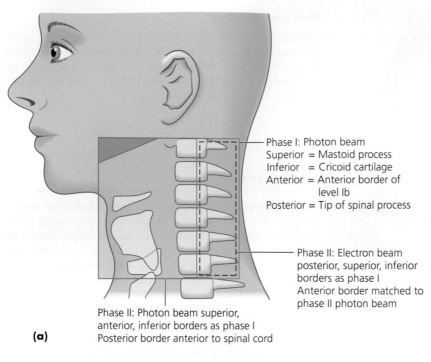

Phase I: Photon beam
Superior = Mastoid process
Inferior = Cricoid cartilage
Anterior = Anterior border of
level Ib
Posterior = Tip of spinal process

Phase II: Electron beam
posterior, superior, inferior
borders as phase I
Anterior border matched to
phase II photon beam

Phase II: Photon beam superior,
anterior, inferior borders as phase I
Posterior border anterior to spinal cord

(a)

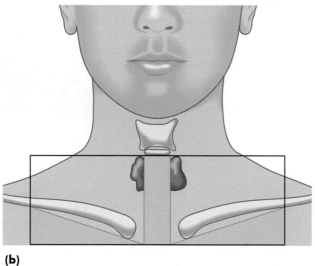

(b)

Figure 43.9 (a) Radiotherapy technique for locally advanced laryngeal carcinoma. Field borders for phase I and II will be coincident and are depicted as smaller for illustrative purposes only. (b) Radiotherapy technique for anterior neck field matching at cricoid level, with midline spinal cord and infraclavicular shielding.

TONGUE BASE

Most tongue base tumours present with locally advanced and/or node positive disease, which are best treated with radical chemoradiation, since resection is usually associated with poor swallow and speech function.[68, 69] However, small tongue base tumours (T1/T2) presenting early (N0), particularly exophytic tumours without fixity, may be offered radical radiotherapy, with locoregional control rates of approximately 70 per cent.[70] However, either side of the neck may harbour occult lymph node metastases, so bilateral neck irradiation to levels Ib–V is mandatory.

Immobilization is in the supine position with the cervical spine straight. The radiation technique employs the use of lateral parallel opposed fields to the primary tumour and upper echelon lymph nodes, with the field extending from the hard palate superiorly to the lower border of the hyoid bone inferiorly. Anteriorly, the CTV extends to include the

level Ib lymph nodes or 1 cm anterior to the tumour, whichever is the more anterior. Posteriorly, the CTV includes the posterior level II and level V lymph nodes. After 40–44 Gy, the posterior border is reduced to come off the spinal cord and the primary tumour continues to the radical dose. The posterior upper neck is treated with applied electron fields to complete the dose for microscopic disease (**Figure 43.10**). The lymph nodes below the level of the hyoid bone are treated with a bilateral anterior neck field with midline shielding as described above under Larynx, but with matching at the level of the hyoid bone.

Dose prescription

The total dose is 66–70 Gy in 2 Gy per fraction, treating daily, five fractions a week, to macroscopic disease and 44–50 Gy in 2 Gy per fraction, treating daily, five fractions a week, to

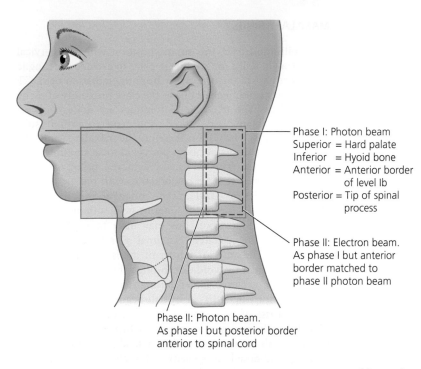

Phase I: Photon beam
Superior = Hard palate
Inferior = Hyoid bone
Anterior = Anterior border
              of level Ib
Posterior = Tip of spinal
               process

Phase II: Electron beam.
As phase I but anterior
border matched to
phase II photon beam

Phase II: Photon beam.
As phase I but posterior border
anterior to spinal cord

Figure 43.10 Radiotherapy technique for oropharyngeal tumours using parallel opposed fields. Field borders for phase I and II will be coincident and are depicted as smaller for illustrative purposes only.

microscopic disease; for example, phase I: 50 Gy/25#/5 weeks; phase II: 20 Gy/10#/2 weeks.

SOFT PALATE

Immobilization is in the supine position with the cervical spine straight.

For early (T1/T2) node-negative tumours, elective nodal irradiation is not necessary.[71] The target volume is therefore the GTV with a 2 cm margin, and can be irradiated with small lateral opposed radiation portals to the radical dose.

Dose prescription

The total dose is 66–70 Gy in 2 Gy per fraction, treating daily, five fractions a week.

LOCALLY ADVANCED OROPHARYNGEAL CARCINOMA

Patients with locally advanced or node positive disease who are not fit for chemoradiotherapy or for consideration of surgery and adjuvant radiation, may be considered for definitive radiation alone, to maximize their chances of long-term palliation. The radiation technique is similar to that for tongue base tumours, where bilateral neck irradiation is undertaken. However, it is important to note that all involved lymph node areas must receive a *macroscopic* tumour dose, including those in the posterior neck, which may be treated with electrons in the second phase of treatment.

Dose prescription

The total dose is 66–70 Gy in 2 Gy per fraction, treating daily, five fractions a week, to macroscopic disease and 44–50 Gy in 2 Gy per fraction, treating daily, five fractions a week, to microscopic disease; for example, phase I: 50 Gy/25#/5 weeks; phase II: 20 Gy/10#/2 weeks.

Hypopharynx

The hypopharynx has three recognized subsites: the pyriform fossa, the postcricoid region and the posterior pharyngeal wall. All are characterized by a high incidence of nodal metastases as well as submucosal spread. Therefore, even in the case of early primary tumours, elective nodal irradiation is necessary. As tumours of the hypopharynx have a tendency to present with locally advanced disease, the majority will be treated with radical chemoradiation, if an organ preservation approach is desired.[72] Dose escalation approaches, such as with IMRT, should also be considered where possible.[73] Nevertheless, for patients unable to tolerate concomitant platinum-based chemotherapy, and for whom surgery is not feasible, radical radiation is an option.[74]

PYRIFORM FOSSA

Immobilization is in the supine position with the cervical spine straight. The target volume includes the primary tumour and levels Ib–V lymph nodes bilaterally. The radiation technique usually involves the use of lateral opposed beams to treat the primary disease, involved nodes and upper cervical lymph nodes in phase I, with a small matched lower anterior split neck field to treat the lower echelon lymph nodes. The lateral radiation portals extend superiorly from the skull base to the lower border of the cricoid cartilage inferiorly. Then, as for treatment of the tongue base, the posterior border is reduced to come off the spinal cord at 40–44 Gy with the phase II lateral photon fields, while the posterior cervical nodes are boosted to the appropriate dose using matched electron fields. Where patients have a short neck or high shoulder position, sometimes it may not be possible to achieve adequate coverage of the most inferior aspects of the disease, and the coronal technique may be necessary (see **Figure 43.8**). Since it is technically difficult to match an electron field posteriorly to an anterior coronal field, in such cases, the phase I coronal plan, encompassing the posterior lymph nodes, should receive 44 Gy in 22 fractions, before coming off spinal cord for phase II of the plan. This ensures that the posterior lymph nodes are treated to the highest possible elective dose.

Dose prescription

The total dose is 66–70 Gy in 2 Gy per fraction, treating daily, five fractions a week, to macroscopic disease and 44–50 Gy in 2 Gy per fraction, treating daily, five fractions a week, to microscopic disease; for example, phase I: 50 Gy/25#/5 weeks; phase II: 20 Gy/10#/2 weeks.

POSTERIOR PHARYNGEAL WALL AND POSTCRICOID REGION

Immobilization is in the supine position with the cervical spine and upper thoracic spine as straight as possible. This may require imaging in the simulator to define the optimal patient position prior to making the shell. For both posterior pharyngeal wall and postcricoid tumours, an inherent radiation planning difficulty is the ability to adequately cover the inferior-most extent of disease once a margin has been added for CTV and PTV. The CTV includes the primary tumour with a 2 cm (posterior pharyngeal wall) or 5 cm (post-cricoid) margin craniocaudally and levels Ib–V lymph nodes bilaterally. It is therefore usually necessary to use the coronal technique described above, although even this may not achieve an adequate dose distribution in the superior mediastinum. In this instance, a low-weighted anterior field with a superior to inferior wedge may increase the dose in this region, although often at the expense of spinal cord dose. Where there are overt lymph node metastases at presentation, radiation may have to be palliative, as the full dose cannot be delivered to all the PTV without compromising the OAR, in particular the spinal cord.

Dose prescription

The total dose is 66–70 Gy in 2 Gy per fraction, treating daily, five fractions a week, to macroscopic disease and 44–50 Gy in 2 Gy per fraction, treating daily, five fractions a week, to potential microscopic disease.

Nasal cavity and paranasal sinuses

The main sites are the maxillary sinus, ethmoid sinus and nasal cavity. Most patients are best treated with a combination of surgery with radiation and/or chemotherapy, since most lesions present when they are locally advanced, frequently invade several adjacent sinuses, may invade the orbit and not infrequently invade the anterior and/or middle cranial fossa.[75] Definitive radiation is possible, however, for the occasional early tumour.[76] It may also be offered for advanced unresectable disease, although five-year survival rates for the latter do not usually exceed 10 per cent. In the case of advanced lesions where chemotherapy is not possible, one should consider optimizing the results of radical radiation by using an altered fractionation regime.[38]

MAXILLARY SINUS

Immobilization is in the supine position with the cervical spine straight and a mouth bite in place to exclude the tongue and lower part of the oral cavity from the radiation field. CT planning is recommended due to the close proximity of many critical OAR. The majority of tumours are node negative, even if locally quite advanced, and tend to exhibit submucosal spread. The CTV is therefore the maxillary sinus, the ethmoid sinus, the nasal cavity, pterygoid fossa and the lateral pharyngeal node. This is usually achieved using a heavily weighted anterior field in combination with one or two lateral fields (**Figure 43.11**). The ipsilateral eye should be shielded if possible from the anterior field, although in cases of frank orbital invasion this may have to be limited to shielding of the ipsilateral lacrimal gland, to avoid xerophthalmia. The anterior border of the lateral fields should be non-divergent to avoid exit through the contralateral lens. This may be achieved either through angling of the lateral field posteriorly by 5–10° or by half-beam blocking. The area at greatest risk of underdose is the posteromedial part of the PTV. It may be necessary to consider a further 'in-field' IMRT boost to this area ('field within a field') to improve PTV coverage and dose homogeneity, although care must be taken with the dose to the optic chiasm and brainstem. It may be necessary to introduce shielding to these structures thus compromising PTV coverage, if their tolerance is exceeded. Under these circumstances, patients must be clear that radiation is unlikely to effect long-term cure, rather high-dose palliation of symptoms.

Dose prescription

The total dose is 66–70 Gy in 2 Gy per fraction, treating daily, five fractions a week.

ETHMOID SINUS

Immobilization is again in the supine position with the cervical spine straight and a mouth bite in place, with CT planning recommended due to the close proximity of the optic apparatus. Where available, a planning MRI scan may be performed, and co-registered with the planning CT, as this further aids identification of the OAR and helps with target volume definition. The CTV should include both ethmoid sinuses, the nasal cavity, the medial half of the maxilla on the ipsilateral side and the pterygoid fossa. A three-field plan, using a heavily weighted anterior field and two lateral fields, similar to the arrangement in maxillary sinus tumours, usually achieves the best dose homogeneity. Again, lymph node metastases are rare, so there is no need for elective lymph node irradiation to be undertaken. Occasionally, patients present with very small (T1) tumours, such that the radiation portals can be confined to covering the ethmoid sinuses and nasal cavity alone using superior and inferior anterior oblique fields (**Figure 43.12**).

Dose prescription

The total dose is 66–70 Gy in 2 Gy per fraction, treating daily, five fractions a week.

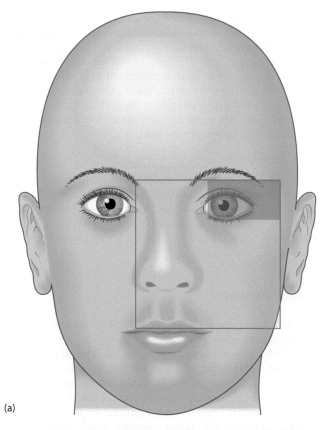

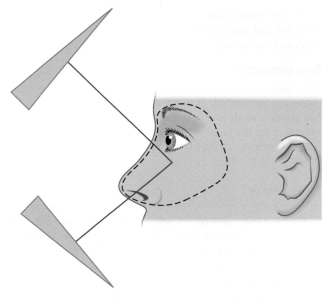

Figure 43.12   Radiotherapy technique for small ethmoid sinus tumours, using superior and inferior anterior oblique fields. Laterally, shielding of the lenses and lacrimal glands is possible.

the primary lesion and a 1 cm margin. The field arrangement may be either an anterior wedged pair of photon fields, or in more advanced disease, a three-field technique similar to maxilla/ethmoid sinus plans, where the entire nasal cavity is included in the CTV.

Dose prescription

The total dose is 66–70 Gy in 2 Gy per fraction, treating daily, five fractions a week.

NASAL COLUMELLA/VESTIBULE

Radiation is often undertaken in the first instance to avoid deformity. Patient immobilization is undertaken as previously. The natural history of nasal columella tumours is such that tumours with seemingly localized presentation may infiltrate quite deeply submucosally along the nasal septum. By contrast, vestibule tumours tend to be more locally confined. The local control rate for vestibule tumours treated with radiation is in the order of 80–90 per cent at five years.[77] Vestibule tumours and small lesions of the nasal columella, without evidence of extension up the nasal cavity and/or septum, may be treated with appositional electrons, with the CTV including the primary tumour with a 2 cm margin. In order to produce a homogeneous tissue density for deposition of dose, the nose may be 'built up' using a wax block externally and wax nostril plugs internally. This is usually a relatively small volume, and may therefore be treated with the hypofractionated regime given below.

With more locally advanced lesions, CT planning is recommended, with the CTV including the primary tumour with a 1 cm margin and the entire nasal septum. An anterior oblique wedged pair field arrangement usually achieves good dose homogeneity, although occasionally a three-field technique as for nasal cavity irradiation may be necessary. In cases where tumour is in the build-up region of the radiation

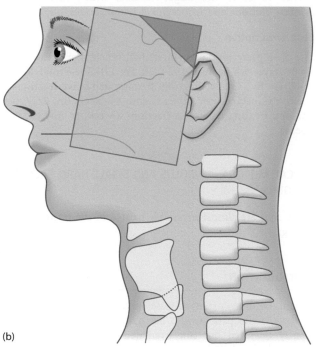

Figure 43.11   (a) Anterior field for a left maxillary antrum tumour; (b) lateral field for a left maxillary antrum tumour.

NASAL CAVITY

For tumours of the nasal cavity being treated with radical radiation, rather than surgery, immobilization and CT planning are recommended. Again, the probability of lymph node metastases is extremely low, such that the CTV includes

beam, the immobilization shell should not be cut out over this area, and the additional application of wax bolus may be necessary to increase the dose to the PTV at the skin surface.

Dose prescription

The dose prescription for small lesions confined to the columella or vestibule is 55 Gy in 20 fractions, treating daily, five times a week and that for more advanced lesions, with extension up the nasal septum/cavity is 66–70 Gy in 2 Gy per fraction, treating daily, five times a week.

Oral cavity

The oral cavity is divided into several subsites: the oral tongue, floor of mouth, buccal mucosa, alveolus and hard palate. Published data suggest that most oral cavity tumours are best treated with surgery, followed by adjuvant radiation with or without chemotherapy, depending on the presence of intermediate or high risk pathological features.[78, 79, 80] However, small (T1/T2), superficial (<5 mm thickness) lesions of the oral tongue and floor of mouth should be considered for interstitial brachytherapy.[81, 82] It is also possible to offer definitive radiation to patients with early lesions when surgery is not possible for comorbid reasons.

In lesions being considered for interstitial brachytherapy (brachy = Greek, short distance), an anaesthetic assessment is required in addition to the other preparatory measures for radiation described previously. Interstitial brachytherapy consists of surgically implanting small radioactive sources directly into the target tissues. It is therefore helpful to conduct this procedure with the assistance of the surgical oncologist. Most head and neck brachytherapy treatments use low dose rate (LDR) temporary iridium-192, with an activity of approximately 50 cGy per hour, or 10 Gy per day. All interstitial implants rely on classic systems which define rules governing the distribution of the radioactive sources, the dose specification and also to aid dose calculation. These systems enable advance planning of interstitial implants and the one most frequently used in head and neck brachytherapy is the Paris system.[83, 84] The Paris system is a simple system, founded on empirical clinical practice and mathematical calculations, and is adaptable to many clinical situations, since it is applicable to both single- and multi-plane implants. Paris rules specify that implants should be parallel, uncrossed and straight. Wire spacing should be equidistant from 5 to 20 mm, with wire separation determined by target volume thickness and wire length being approximately 1.5 times the target volume length. These are the features which the clinician must aim for when implanting the volume, and which the physicist will use to determine the precise duration of implantation in order to deliver the prescribed dose.

ORAL TONGUE

Small superficial lesions may be treated with interstitial brachytherapy. Usually two to three iridium-192 hairpins are required to implant the target volume. The CTV includes the primary lesion with a 1 cm margin.

For patients unsuitable for brachytherapy, but also not suitable for surgery, definitive external beam radiation (EBRT) may be offered. Immobilization is in the supine position with the cervical spine straight, and a mouth bite may be considered. The CTV includes the primary tumour with a 2 cm margin, which if well lateralized, may be achieved with a wedged pair field arrangement (see above under Oropharynx). However, for tumours that either are more deeply infiltrating or approaching the midline, lateral parallel opposed beams are required, since the CTV is then expanded to include irradiation of the neck.

Dose prescription

The dose prescription for interstitial brachytherapy is 60 Gy over 6 days with iridium-192 LDR. For EBRT, the total dose is 66–70 Gy in 2 Gy per fraction, treating daily, five fractions a week, to macroscopic disease and 44–50 Gy in 2 Gy per fraction, treating daily, five fractions a week, to microscopic disease.

FLOOR OF MOUTH

Again, small, superficial lesions may be treated with interstitial brachytherapy as above.

If EBRT is considered, the mouth should be held open during immobilization with a mouth bite, to limit the dose to the upper oral cavity, in particular the hard palate. Tumours of the floor of mouth are frequently in the midline, such that EBRT requires the use of lateral parallel opposed radiation portals to cover the target volume, which includes the primary tumour and locoregional lymph nodes.

Dose prescription

The dose prescription for interstitial brachytherapy is 60 Gy over 6 days with iridium-192 LDR. For EBRT the total dose is 66–70 Gy in 2 Gy per fraction, treating daily, five fractions a week, to macroscopic disease and 44–50 Gy in 2 Gy per fraction, treating daily, five fractions a week, to microscopic disease.

BUCCAL MUCOSA, ALVEOLUS AND SMALL HARD PALATE TUMOURS

These sites are almost invariably treated in the postoperative setting.

Reirradiation

Patients with recurrent disease largely fall into four categories: (1) the patient who has disease recurring in a previously operated but not irradiated site; (2) disease in a previously irradiated site and amenable to surgical salvage; (3) disease in a previously irradiated site, not amenable to further surgery where reirradiation may be considered; (4) recurrent disease associated with other distant metastases, or other comorbidities, such that a further radical dose of radiation would be inappropriate. Within these broad categories, the cause of recurrence can be attributed to radiation resistance, geographical miss, or the development of a second primary HNSCC (for review, see Creak et al.[85]). Tumours occurring due to geographical miss, and arising in the penumbra region of the previous RT field, or in the low-dose region, and second primary tumours, often occurring after a tumour-free interval of several years, should be considered for reirradiation.

RATIONALE FOR REIRRADIATION

Only one-third of HNSCC recurrences are amenable to salvage surgery, with a median survival of approximately nine months.[86] Palliative chemotherapy with a cisplatin-based regimen, while associated with response rates of 20–40 per cent and median survival of between five and nine months, is often associated with significant morbidity, and is only usually recommended for patients with WHO performance status 0–1.[87]

As a comparison, for carefully selected patients the locoregional control (LRC) rate with reirradiation ranges from 20 to 60 per cent, with a recognized cohort of patients surviving beyond five years (five-year survival, 10–93 per cent).[88, 89]

The clinical judgement lies between proceeding with palliative chemotherapy or whether to risk irradiation to a site where there will inevitably be overlap of past and current fields. The clinician must be guided by features such as the time elapsed since previous irradiation, the total dose previously received as well as the dose fractionation, the critical structures previously in proximity to the target volume and whether they were irradiated short of tolerance, as well as the patient's performance status and personal wishes. It should be possible to determine the maximum dose to OAR given previously, and factor in a degree of 'recovery' depending on time elapsed since treatment.[90, 91] Nevertheless, the reirradiation dose is almost always limited by the dose to OAR. The risks of normal tissue toxicity are greater, so the patient must take an informed decision. However, there may be more durable palliation and disease control with this modality than with chemotherapy.

The planning technique is as above, with cautious consideration of CTV definition, based on CT planning scans performed with intravenous contrast.

Table 43.5 details the patient and treatment factors to be considered when planning reirradiation.

REIRRADIATION WITH BRACHYTHERAPY

For T1/T2 locally recurrent disease of the oropharynx or nasopharynx, without evidence of regional lymph node metastasis, LDR iridium-192 implant brachytherapy may be considered, employing the afterloading technique. When a mean dose of 60 Gy is achieved, five-year local control rates as high as 80 per cent for rT1 and 67 per cent for rT2 may be seen, although the overall survival at five years is lower at 30 per cent, due to the high incidence of other alcohol- and smoking-related comorbid disease.[92, 93, 94]

REIRRADIATION WITH EXTERNAL BEAM RADIOTHERAPY ALONE

This approach has been most successful in rT1/rT2 disease of the larynx. Again, the optimum dose is 60 Gy or greater, with either conventional or altered fractionation, giving five-year actuarial local control and survival rates of approximately 60 and 90 per cent. Notably, the majority of local failures went on to have salvage total laryngectomy.[88]

REIRRADIATION WITH CONCOMITANT CHEMOTHERAPY

The addition of concomitant chemotherapy to reirradiation is associated with considerable toxicity. However, for carefully selected patients, where optimal debulking has been possible, with only microscopic residual disease, this is an approach again associated with some long-term survivors.[95]

REIRRADIATION WITH IMRT

Some patients develop recurrence within, or at the periphery of a previous radiation portal, but at a site not suited to surgical salvage, such as the skull base or infratemporal fossa.

Table 43.5 Patient and treatment factors to consider for reirradiation.

	Anatomical site	Nasopharynx and larynx recurrence associated with a more favourable outcome than other sites
Patient factors	Category of disease	Second primary tumours usually more responsive to reirradiation than recurrent disease, as less likely to be radioresistant
		Life expectancy at least 6 months
	Treatment-free interval	Reirradiation 3 years or more since first irradiation associated with improved 1-year survival compared with reirradiation within 3 years
		If RT given >2 years ago, at no more than 2 Gy/#, possibly up to 60% recovery for late-responding tissues with α/β ratio of 2
	Late toxicity	Better outcomes seen where there is absence of late toxicity from first irradiation
Treatment factors	Surgery	Debulking surgery to be carried out where feasible as this confers better outcomes than no surgical debulk
	Radiation dose	Reirradiation to be delivered with a therapeutic dose of at least 50 Gy

RT, radiotherapy.

Reirradiation with IMRT is an attractive option in this setting since this technique affords the advantage over conventional RT of a greater normal tissue-sparing effect while delivering highly conformal RT to the tumour.[96] In series reported to date, the LRC has been excellent, with acceptable acute toxicity. Longer follow up is needed to evaluate late toxicity and overall survival.[97, 98]

- Ongoing developments in radiation technology include the introduction of IMRT and IGRT into mainstream clinical practice.

KEY EVIDENCE

- Radiotherapy is a key modality in the treatment of head and neck cancer, providing high rates of tumour control and organ preservation in early stage tumours.
- For patients with advanced stage tumours, radiotherapy is usually combined either with chemotherapy or used in the postoperative setting.
- Appropriate use of advanced radiotherapy technologies can reduce side effects and improve outcomes for head and neck patients.

KEY LEARNING POINTS

- An important consideration in radiotherapy planning is patient positioning and immobilization to ensure reproducibility of treatments.
- ICRU Reports 50 and 62, as well as the consensus guidelines, should dictate the delineation of GTV, CTV, PTV, nodal target volume and the organs at risk.
- Early tumours, particularly those with low risk of lymph node disease, are often treated in a single phase, with conventionally planned volumes and simple radiation fields.
- Some early, superficial tumours, particularly those sited in the oral cavity, may be suitable for treatment with interstitial brachytherapy.
- More locally advanced tumours, and those with a higher risk of lymph node disease, are often treated in two or more phases, using CT-planned volumes and more complex radiation fields.
- For conventionally fractionated treatments (1.8–2 Gy per fraction) the dose needed to adequately treat macroscopic disease is 66–70 Gy, while 44–50 Gy is needed to sterilize microscopic disease.
- For locally advanced disease, the results of definitive radiation may be improved by using an altered fractionation regime or by the addition of chemotherapy.
- Recurrent disease should be carefully considered for optimal surgical debulking and reirradiation.

REFERENCES

1. Mangar S, Slevin N, Mais K, Sykes A. Evaluating predictive factors for determining enteral nutrition in patients receiving radical radiotherapy for head and neck cancer: A retrospective review. *Radiotherapy and Oncology* 2006; **78**: 152–8.
2. Jereczek-Fossa BA, Orecchia R. Radiotherapy-induced mandibular bone complications. *Cancer Treatment Reviews* 2002; **28**: 65–74.
3. Browman GP, Wong G, Hodson I *et al.* Influence of cigarette smoking on the efficacy of radiation therapy in head and neck cancer. *New England Journal of Medicine* 1993; **328**: 159–63.
4. Terhaard CH, Snippe K, Ravasz LA *et al.* Radiotherapy in T1 laryngeal cancer: prognostic factors for locoregional control and survival, uni- and multivariate analysis. *International Journal of Radiation Oncology, Biology, Physics* 1991; **21**: 1179–86.
5. Candela FC, Kothari K, Shah JP. Patterns of cervical node metastases from squamous carcinoma of the oropharynx and hypopharynx. *Head and Neck* 1990; **12**: 197–203.
6. Lindberg R. Distribution of cervical lymph node metastases from squamous cell carcinoma of the upper respiratory and digestive tracts. *Cancer* 1972; **29**: 1446–9.
7. Shah JP, Candela FC, Poddar AK. The patterns of cervical lymph node metastases from squamous carcinoma of the oral cavity. *Cancer* 1990; **66**: 109–13.
8. Humphreys M, Guerrero Urbano MT, Mubata C *et al.* Assessment of a customised immobilisation system for head and neck IMRT using electronic portal imaging. *Radiotherapy and Oncology* 2005; **77**: 39–44.
9. Sharp L, Lewin F, Johansson H *et al.* Randomized trial on two types of thermoplastic masks for patient immobilization during radiation therapy for head-and-neck cancer. *International Journal of Radiation Oncology, Biology, Physics* 2005; **61**: 250–6.
10. Gilbeau L, Octave-Prignot M, Loncol T *et al.* Comparison of setup accuracy of three different thermoplastic masks for the treatment of brain and head and neck tumors. *Radiotherapy and Oncology* 2001; **58**: 155–62.
11. Fuss M, Salter BJ, Cheek D *et al.* Repositioning accuracy of a commercially available thermoplastic mask system. *Radiotherapy and Oncology* 2004; **71**: 339–45.
12. Boda-Heggemann J, Walter C, Rahn A *et al.* Repositioning accuracy of two different mask systems – 3D revisited: comparison using true 3D/3D matching with cone-beam CT. *International Journal of Radiation Oncology, Biology, Physics* 2006; **66**: 1568–75.

13. Roques T, Dagless M, Tomes J. Randomized trial on two types of thermoplastic masks for patient immobilization during radiation therapy for head-and-neck cancer: in regard to Sharp *et al.* (*International Journal of Radiation Oncology, Biology,* Physics 2005; 61: 250–6). *International Journal of Radiation Oncology, Biology, Physics* 2005; 62: 942; author reply 943.

* 14. The International Commission on Radiation Units and Measurements (ICRU). *ICRU Report 50, Prescribing and reporting photon beam therapy.* Bethesda, MD: ICRU, 1993.

* 15. The International Commission on Radiation Units and Measurements (ICRU). ICRU Report 62, Prescribing, recording and reporting photon beam therapy (Supplement to ICRU Report 50), ICRU: Bethesda, MD, 1999.

16. Emami B, Lyman J, Brown A *et al.* Tolerance of normal tissue to therapeutic irradiation. *International Journal of Radiation Oncology, Biology, Physics* 1991; 21: 109–22.

* 17. Gregoire V, Eisbruch A, Hamoir M, Levendag P. Proposal for the delineation of the nodal CTV in the node-positive and the post-operative neck. *Radiotherapy and Oncology* 2006; 79: 15–20.

* 18. Gregoire V, Levendag P, Ang KK *et al.* CT-based delineation of lymph node levels and related CTVs in the node-negative neck: DAHANCA, EORTC, GORTEC, NCIC, RTOG consensus guidelines. *Radiotherapy and Oncology* 2003; 69: 227–36.

19. Dobbs JBA, Ash D. *Practical radiotherapy planning.* London: Arnold, 1999.

20. Nutting CBM, Harrington KJ, Henk JM. *Geometric uncertainties in radiotherapy: head and neck cancer.* London: British Institute of Radiology, 2003.

♦ 21. Newbold K, Partridge M, Cook G *et al.* Advanced imaging applied to radiotherapy planning in head and neck cancer: a clinical review. *British Journal of Radiology* 2006; 79: 554–61.

22. Geets X, Daisne JF, Tomsej M *et al.* Impact of the type of imaging modality on target volumes delineation and dose distribution in pharyngo-laryngeal squamous cell carcinoma: comparison between pre- and per-treatment studies. *Radiotherapy and Oncology* 2006; 78: 291–7.

23. Liauw SL, Amdur RJ, Mendenhall WM *et al.* The effect of intravenous contrast on intensity-modulated radiation therapy dose calculations for head and neck cancer. *American Journal of Clinical Oncology* 2005; 28: 456–9.

24. Wijers OB, Levendag PC, Tan T *et al.* A simplified CT-based definition of the lymph node levels in the node negative neck. *Radiotherapy and Oncology* 1999; 52: 35–42.

25. Levendag P, Braaksma M, Coche E *et al.* Rotterdam and Brussels CT-based neck nodal delineation compared with the surgical levels as defined by the American Academy of Otolaryngology-Head and Neck Surgery. *International Journal of Radiation Oncology, Biology, Physics* 2004; 58: 113–23.

26. Astreinidou E, Bel A, Raaijmakers CP *et al.* Adequate margins for random setup uncertainties in head-and-neck IMRT. *International Journal of Radiation Oncology, Biology, Physics* 2005; 61: 938–44.

27. Nutting C. Intensity-modulated radiotherapy (IMRT): the most important advance in radiotherapy since the linear accelerator? *British Journal of Radiology* 2003; 76: 673.

♦ 28. Guerrero, Urbano MT, Nutting CM. Clinical use of intensity-modulated radiotherapy: part I. *British Journal of Radiology* 2004; 77: 88–96.

♦ 29. Guerrero, Urbano MT, Nutting CM. Clinical use of intensity-modulated radiotherapy, part II. *British Journal of Radiology* 2004; 77: 177–82.

30. Clark CH, Miles EA, Urbano TG *et al.* Quality assurance for an IMRT trial: pre-trial exercises for PARSPORT. *Clinical Oncology (Royal College of Radiologists (Great Britain))* 2007; 19: S6.

31. Kwong DL, Sham JS, Leung LH *et al.* Preliminary results of radiation dose escalation for locally advanced nasopharyngeal carcinoma. *International Journal of Radiation Oncology, Biology, Physics* 2006; 64: 374–81.

● 32. Clark CH, Bidmead AM, Mubata CD *et al.* Intensity-modulated radiotherapy improves target coverage, spinal cord sparing and allows dose escalation in patients with locally advanced cancer of the larynx. *Radiotherapy and Oncology* 2004; 70: 189–98.

♦ 33. Verhey LJ. Comparison of three-dimensional conformal radiation therapy and intensity-modulated radiation therapy systems. *Seminars in Radiation Oncology* 1999; 9: 78–98.

34. Verhey LJ. Issues in optimization for planning of intensity-modulated radiation therapy. *Seminars in Radiation Oncology* 2002; 12: 210–18.

35. Zeidan OA, Langen KM, Meeks SL *et al.* Evaluation of image-guidance protocols in the treatment of head-and-neck cancers. *International Journal of Radiation Oncology, Biology, Physics* 2007; 67: 670–7.

36. van Vulpen M, Field C, Raaijmakers CP *et al.* Comparing step-and-shoot IMRT with dynamic helical tomotherapy IMRT plans for head-and-neck cancer. *International Journal of Radiation Oncology, Biology, Physics* 2005; 62: 1535–9.

● 37. Horiot JC, Bontemps P, van den Bogaert W *et al.* Accelerated fractionation (AF) compared to conventional fractionation (CF) improves loco-regional control in the radiotherapy of advanced head and neck cancers: results of the EORTC 22851 randomized trial. *Radiotherapy and Oncology* 1997; 44: 111–21.

● 38. Fu KK, Pajak TF, Trotti A *et al.* A radiation therapy oncology group (RTOG) phase III randomized study to compare hyperfractionation and two variants of accelerated fractionation to standard fractionation radiotherapy for head and neck squamous cell carcinomas: first report of RTOG 9003. *International Journal of Radiation Oncology, Biology, Physics* 2000; 48: 7–16.

● 39. Dische S, Saunders M, Barrett A et al. A randomised multicentre trial of CHART versus conventional radiotherapy in head and neck cancer. *Radiotherapy and Oncology* 1997; **44**: 123–36.

40. Short S, Krawitz H, Macann A et al. TN/TN glottic carcinoma: a comparison of two fractionation schedules. *Australasian Radiology* 2006; **50**: 152–7.

41. Sanghera P, McConkey C, Ho KF et al. Hypofractionated accelerated radiotherapy with concurrent chemotherapy for locally advanced squamous cell carcinoma of the head and neck. *International Journal of Radiation Oncology, Biology, Physics* 2007; **67**: 1342–51.

42. Madhava K, Hartley A, Wake M et al. Carboplatin and hypofractionated accelerated radiotherapy: a dose escalation study of an outpatient chemoradiation schedule for squamous cell carcinoma of the head and neck. *Clinical Oncology (Royal College of Radiologists (Great Britain))* 2006; **18**: 77–81.

◆ 43. Fowler JF. Biological factors influencing optimum fractionation in radiation therapy. *Acta Oncologica* 2001; **40**: 712–17.

◆ 44. Overgaard J, Hansen HS, Specht L et al. Five compared with six fractions per week of conventional radiotherapy of squamous-cell carcinoma of head and neck: DAHANCA 6 and 7 randomised controlled trial. *Lancet* 2003; **362**: 933–40.

◆ 45. Bourhis J, Etessami A, Wilbault P et al. Altered fractionated radiotherapy in the management of head and neck carcinomas: advantages and limitations. *Current Opinion in Oncology* 2004; **16**: 215–19.

● 46. Pignon JP, Bourhis J, Domenge C, Designe L. Chemotherapy added to locoregional treatment for head and neck squamous-cell carcinoma: three meta-analyses of updated individual data. MACH-NC Collaborative Group. Meta-analysis of chemotherapy on head and neck cancer. *Lancet* 2000; **355**: 949–55.

◆ 47. Van den Bogaert W, Van der Leest A, Rijnders A et al. Does tumor control decrease by prolonging overall treatment time or interrupting treatment in laryngeal cancer? *Radiotherapy and Oncology* 1995; **36**: 177–82.

48. Cheung KY, Choi PH, Chau RM et al. The roles of multileaf collimators and micro-multileaf collimators in conformal and conventional nasopharyngeal carcinoma radiotherapy treatments. *Medical Physics* 1999; **26**: 2077–85.

49. Senkus-Konefka E, Naczk E, Borowska I et al. Changes in lateral dimensions of irradiated volume and their impact on the accuracy of dose delivery during radiotherapy for head and neck cancer. *Radiotherapy and Oncology* 2006; **79**: 304–9.

50. de Boer JC, Heijmen BJ. A new approach to off-line setup corrections: combining safety with minimum workload. *Medical Physics* 2002; **29**: 1998–2012.

51. Mendes RL, Nutting CM, Harrington KJ. Managing side effects of radiotherapy in head and neck cancer. *Hospital Medicine* 2002; **63**: 712–17.

52. Vissink A, Jansma J, Spijkervet FK et al. Oral sequelae of head and neck radiotherapy. *Critical Reviews in Oral Biology and Medicine* 2003; **14**: 199–212.

53. Scully C, Epstein J, Sonis S. Oral mucositis: a challenging complication of radiotherapy, chemotherapy, and radiochemotherapy, part 1, pathogenesis and prophylaxis of mucositis. *Head and Neck* 2003; **25**: 1057–70.

54. Jellema AP, Slotman BJ, Doornaert P et al. Unilateral versus bilateral irradiation in squamous cell head and neck cancer in relation to patient-rated xerostomia and sticky saliva. *Radiotherapy and Oncology* 2007; **85**: 83–9.

55. Al-Othman MO, Amdur RJ, Morris CG et al. Does feeding tube placement predict for long-term swallowing disability after radiotherapy for head and neck cancer? *Head and Neck* 2003; **25**: 741–7.

56. Vissink A, Burlage FR, Spijkervet FK et al. Prevention and treatment of the consequences of head and neck radiotherapy. *Critical Reviews in Oral Biology and Medicine* 2003; **14**: 213–25.

57. Hall EJ. The inaugural Frank Ellis Lecture – Iatrogenic Cancer: the impact of intensity-modulated radiotherapy. *Clinical Oncology (Royal College of Radiologists (Great Britain))* 2006; **18**: 277–82.

58. Machin J, Shaw C. A multidisciplinary approach to head and neck cancer. *European Journal of Cancer Care (England)* 1998; **7**: 93–6.

59. Mendenhall WM, Parsons JT, Stringer SP et al. T1-T2 vocal cord carcinoma: a basis for comparing the results of radiotherapy and surgery. *Head and Neck Surgery* 1988; **10**: 373–7.

● 60. Spaulding MB, Fischer SG, Wolf GT. Tumor response, toxicity, and survival after neoadjuvant organ-preserving chemotherapy for advanced laryngeal carcinoma. The Department of Veterans Affairs Cooperative Laryngeal Cancer Study Group. *Journal of Clinical Oncology* 1994; **12**: 1592–9.

● 61. Wiernik G, Alcock CJ, Bates TD et al. Final report on the Second British Institute of Radiology Fractionation Study: short versus long overall treatment times for radiotherapy of carcinoma of the laryngo-pharynx. *British Journal of Radiology* 1991; **64**: 232–41.

62. Mantz CA, Vokes EE, Kies MS et al. Sequential induction chemotherapy and concomitant chemoradiotherapy in the management of locoregionally advanced laryngeal cancer. *Annals of Oncology* 2001; **12**: 343–7.

63. Fung K, Lyden TH, Lee J et al. Voice and swallowing outcomes of an organ-preservation trial for advanced laryngeal cancer. *International Journal of Radiation Oncology, Biology, Physics* 2005; **63**: 1395–9.

64. Mendenhall WM, Stringer SP, Amdur RJ et al. Is radiation therapy a preferred alternative to surgery for squamous cell carcinoma of the base of tongue? *Journal of Clinical Oncology* 2000; **18**: 35–42.

65. Mendenhall WM, Amdur RJ, Stringer SP et al. Radiation therapy for squamous cell carcinoma of the tonsillar

region: a preferred alternative to surgery? *Journal of Clinical Oncology* 2000; **18**: 2219–25.

66. O'Sullivan B, Warde P, Grice B *et al*. The benefits and pitfalls of ipsilateral radiotherapy in carcinoma of the tonsillar region. *International Journal of Radiation Oncology, Biology, Physics* 2001; **51**: 332–43.

67. Pacholke HD, Amdur RJ, Morris CG *et al*. Late xerostomia after intensity-modulated radiation therapy versus conventional radiotherapy. *American Journal of Clinical Oncology* 2005; **28**: 351–8.

68. Harrison LB, Zelefsky MJ, Armstrong JG *et al*. Performance status after treatment for squamous cell cancer of the base of tongue – a comparison of primary radiation therapy versus primary surgery. *International Journal of Radiation Oncology, Biology, Physics* 1994; **30**: 953–7.

69. Allal AS, Nicoucar K, Mach N, Dulguerov P. Quality of life in patients with oropharynx carcinomas: assessment after accelerated radiotherapy with or without chemotherapy versus radical surgery and postoperative radiotherapy. *Head and Neck* 2003; **25**: 833–9discussion 839–40.

70. Wang CC, Montgomery W, Efird J. Local control of oropharyngeal carcinoma by irradiation alone. *Laryngoscope* 1995; **105**: 529–33.

71. Selek U, Garden AS, Morrison WH *et al*. Radiation therapy for early-stage carcinoma of the oropharynx. *International Journal of Radiation Oncology, Biology, Physics* 2004; **59**: 743–51.

● 72. Lefebvre JL, Chevalier D, Luboinski B *et al*. Larynx preservation in pyriform sinus cancer: preliminary results of a European Organization for Research and Treatment of Cancer Phase III trial. EORTC Head and Neck Cancer Cooperative Group. *Journal of the National Cancer Institute* 1996; **88**: 890–9.

73. Johansson J, Blomquist E, Montelius A *et al*. Potential outcomes of modalities and techniques in radiotherapy for patients with hypopharyngeal carcinoma. *Radiotherapy and Oncology* 2004; **72**: 129–38.

74. Nakamura K, Shioyama Y, Kawashima M *et al*. Multi-institutional analysis of early squamous cell carcinoma of the hypopharynx treated with radical radiotherapy. *International Journal of Radiation Oncology, Biology, Physics* 2006; **65**: 1045–50.

75. Hoppe BS, Stegman LD, Zelefsky MJ *et al*. Treatment of nasal cavity and paranasal sinus cancer with modern radiotherapy techniques in the postoperative setting – the MSKCC experience. *International Journal of Radiation Oncology, Biology, Physics* 2007; **67**: 691–702.

76. Katz TS, Mendenhall WM, Morris CG *et al*. Malignant tumors of the nasal cavity and paranasal sinuses. *Head and Neck* 2002; **24**: 821–9.

77. Langendijk JA, Poorter R, Leemans CR *et al*. Radiotherapy of squamous cell carcinoma of the nasal vestibule. *International Journal of Radiation Oncology, Biology, Physics* 2004; **59**: 1319–25.

78. Edwards DM, Johnson NW. Treatment of upper aerodigestive tract cancers in England and its effect on survival. *British Journal of Cancer* 1999; **81**: 323–9.

● 79. Cooper JS, Pajak TF, Forastiere AA *et al*. Postoperative concurrent radiotherapy and chemotherapy for high-risk squamous-cell carcinoma of the head and neck. *New England Journal of Medicine* 2004; **350**: 1937–44.

● 80. Bernier J, Domenge C, Ozsahin M *et al*. Postoperative irradiation with or without concomitant chemotherapy for locally advanced head and neck cancer. *New England Journal of Medicine* 2004; **350**: 1945–52.

81. Marsiglia H, Haie-Meder C, Sasso G *et al*. Brachytherapy for T1-T2 floor-of-the-mouth cancers: the Gustave-Roussy Institute experience. *International Journal of Radiation Oncology, Biology, Physics* 2002; **52**: 1257–63.

82. Leung TW, Wong VY, Kwan KH *et al*. High dose rate brachytherapy for early stage oral tongue cancer. *Head and Neck* 2002; **24**: 274–81.

◆ 83. Gillin MT, Kline RW, Wilson JF, Cox JD. Single and double plane implants: a comparison of the Manchester system with the Paris system. *International Journal of Radiation Oncology, Biology, Physics* 1984; **10**: 921–5.

84. Marinello G, Wilson JF, Pierquin B *et al*. The guide gutter or loop techniques of interstitial implantation and the Paris system of dosimetry. *Radiotherapy and Oncology* 1985; **4**: 265–73.

◆ 85. Creak AL, Harrington K, Nutting C. Treatment of recurrent head and neck cancer: re-irradiation or chemotherapy? *Clinical Oncology (Royal College of Radiologists (Great Britain))* 2005; **17**: 138–47.

86. Mabanta SR, Mendenhall WM, Stringer SP, Cassisi NJ. Salvage treatment for neck recurrence after irradiation alone for head and neck squamous cell carcinoma with clinically positive neck nodes. *Head and Neck* 1999; **21**: 591–4.

● 87. Forastiere AA, Metch B, Schuller DE *et al*. Randomized comparison of cisplatin plus fluorouracil and carboplatin plus fluorouracil versus methotrexate in advanced squamous-cell carcinoma of the head and neck: a Southwest Oncology Group study. *Journal of Clinical Oncology* 1992; **10**: 1245–51.

88. Wang CC, McIntyre J. Re-irradiation of laryngeal carcinoma – techniques and results. *International Journal of Radiation Oncology, Biology, Physics* 1993; **26**: 783–5.

89. Stevens KR Jr, Britsch A, Moss WT. High-dose reirradiation of head and neck cancer with curative intent. *International Journal of Radiation Oncology, Biology, Physics* 1994; **29**: 687–98.

● 90. Nieder C, Milas L, Ang KK. Tissue tolerance to reirradiation. *Seminars in Radiation Oncology* 2000; **10**: 200–9.

91. Ang KK, Jiang GL, Feng Y *et al*. Extent and kinetics of recovery of occult spinal cord injury. *International Journal of Radiation Oncology, Biology, Physics* 2001; **50**: 1013–20.

92. Peiffert D, Pernot M, Malissard L *et al.* Salvage irradiation by brachytherapy of velotonsillar squamous cell carcinoma in a previously irradiated field: results in 73 cases. *International Journal of Radiation Oncology, Biology, Physics* 1994; **29**: 681–6.

93. Mazeron JJ, Langlois D, Glaubiger D *et al.* Salvage irradiation of oropharyngeal cancers using iridium 192 wire implants: 5-year results of 70 cases. *International Journal of Radiation Oncology, Biology, Physics* 1987; **13**: 957–62.

94. Hall CE, Harris R, A'Hern R *et al.* Le Fort I osteotomy and low-dose rate Ir192 brachytherapy for treatment of recurrent nasopharyngeal tumours. *Radiotherapy and Oncology* 2003; **66**: 41–8.

95. Haraf DJ, Weichselbaum RR, Vokes EE. Re-irradiation with concomitant chemotherapy of unresectable recurrent head and neck cancer: a potentially curable disease. *Annals of Oncology* 1996; **7**: 913–18.

♦ 96. Nutting C, Dearnaley DP, Webb S. Intensity modulated radiation therapy: a clinical review. *British Journal of Radiology* 2000; **73**: 459–69.

97. Lu TX, Mai WY, Teh BS *et al.* Initial experience using intensity-modulated radiotherapy for recurrent nasopharyngeal carcinoma. *International Journal of Radiation Oncology, Biology, Physics* 2004; **58**: 682–7.

98. Chen YJ, Kuo JV, Ramsinghani NS, Al-Ghazi MS. Intensity-modulated radiotherapy for previously irradiated, recurrent head-and-neck cancer. *Medical Dosimetry* 2002; **27**: 171–6.

44

Postoperative radiotherapy in head and neck cancer

ANDREW HARTLEY AND NELLIE CHEAH

The difficulty in life is the choice.

George Moore

INTRODUCTION

The role of postoperative radiotherapy is important in the treatment of head and neck cancer. The delivery involves close collaboration between head and neck surgeons and oncologists. Patient selection, dosage of postoperative radiotherapy and optimum treatment starting and completion time have yet to be fully determined. This chapter will briefly cover some historical aspects of the development of postoperative radiotherapy in head and neck cancer and the current usual practice.

EVIDENCE FOR THE USE OF POSTOPERATIVE RADIOTHERAPY IN SQUAMOUS CELL CARCINOMA

Any consideration of the role of postoperative radiotherapy in squamous cell carcinoma of the head and neck is hindered by a lack of prospective randomized trials. This dearth of quality data has resulted from difficulties in performing studies which randomize patients to no radiotherapy when the results from surgery alone for advanced clinical stages have historically been poor. For example, in a series of 71 patients with either extracapsular lymph nodal extension

and/or positive resection margins the three-year local control rate for patients with both these factors was 0 per cent.[1]

It is therefore difficult to estimate the benefit of postoperative radiotherapy in a given stage and site of tumour let alone assess the therapeutic ratio of tumour control over side effects in a patient with their individual comorbidity and performance status. Retrospective data or other studies with methodological flaws have to be relied upon to give clinicians some idea of the likely benefit of such treatment. In one series, 140 patients with stage 3 and stage 4 buccal mucosal cancer were 'randomized' to surgery or surgery followed by 58–65 Gy postoperative radiotherapy. Disease-free survival at three years was 38 per cent in the surgery alone arm and 68 per cent in the postoperative radiotherapy arm ($p < 0.005$). The preference of surgeons in the study to assign patients to the postoperative radiotherapy group if they were node positive regardless of the randomization resulted in an excess of node positive patients in this arm (70 versus 6 per cent, $p = 0.05$). This imbalance together with the heterogeneity of the radiotherapy dose and small sample size allow few conclusions on the precise effect of postoperative radiotherapy to be drawn. However, it is reasonable to conclude some likelihood of a beneficial effect given the superior disease-free survival despite higher nodal stage.[2]

In a small study, 51 patients with completely resected head and neck cancer were randomized to no further treatment or 50 Gy in 25 fractions postoperatively. Again, despite randomization, there was an excess of histologically node positive disease in the postoperative radiotherapy arm (63 versus 84 per cent). There was also a non-significant decrease in all recurrences (distant and local considered together) (56 versus 37 per cent). This difference was felt to be largely due to relapse in the non-operated contralateral neck (15 per cent), and the authors concluded no significant benefit from postoperative radiotherapy as such relapses may often be surgically salvaged.[3]

In a non-randomized series ($n = 125$) prior to the advent of single multidisciplinary teams within major hospitals, patients with head and neck cancer seen by general surgeons were not routinely sent for postoperative radiotherapy whereas those cases seen by specialist head and neck surgeons were considered. The three-year local control rate for patients with extracapsular spread was higher with postoperative radiotherapy (31 versus 66 per cent; $p = 0.03$) than it was for patients irradiated with positive margins (41 versus 49 per cent; $p = 0.04$), with the most significant difference in local control occurring in patients with both these factors (0 versus 68 per cent; $p = 0.001$). Disease-free survival was also increased with postoperative radiotherapy in this series (25 versus 45 per cent; $p = 0.0001$).[1]

While none of these studies reaches currently acceptable standards of evidence, it is reasonable to assume some effect of postoperative radiotherapy on reducing recurrence. However, given the likely hypoxic environment in the postoperative surgical bed might radiotherapy given preoperatively be more efficacious? Two randomized prospective studies have examined this question. Forty-nine patients with hypopharyngeal cancer were randomized to 50 Gy completed 2 weeks prior to a laryngopharyngectomy and neck dissection, or the same surgery followed within 4 weeks by 55 Gy. The preoperative arm fared generally worse than the postoperative with more carotid haemorrhage (5 versus 1), less patients undergoing surgery (17/25 versus 24/24), more cancer deaths (11 versus 6) and five-year survival was 20 versus 56 per cent.[4] In a larger study of 277 patients, there was significantly higher locoregional control (LRC) with postoperative radiotherapy of 60 Gy when compared with 50 Gy preoperative radiotherapy ($p = 0.04$). There was no difference in overall survival due to distant metastases and second primary tumours in the postoperative arm.[5] These studies suggest that if combined modality treatment is to be employed in resectable head and neck cancer radiotherapy should be employed postoperatively.

INDICATIONS FOR POSTOPERATIVE RADIOTHERAPY

Several groups have identified pathological factors based on the available literature which enable classification of patients postoperatively into high, medium and low risk disease. As above, the presence of nodal disease with extracapsular spread is considered in all systems as a marker of high risk disease where postoperative radiotherapy is mandatory.[1, 6, 7] In addition, the CHARTWEL group at Mount Vernon randomizing patients to conventional or accelerated postoperative radiotherapy considered as high risk the presence of an involved surgical margin or four of the following factors: excision margins less than 5 mm, stage T3/T4, perineural or vascular invasion, poor differentiation, oral cavity primary, multicentre primary, more than four nodes positive, soft tissue invasion and dysplasia or carcinoma *in situ* at the resection margin.[6] Patients with two of these

factors were assessed at intermediate risk with all other patients judged at low risk and not considered for postoperative radiotherapy.

The MD Anderson group considered patients with either extracapsular spread or two of the following factors at high risk: oral cavity primary, involved surgical margins, perineural invasion, more than one node involved, more than one nodal group involved, largest node greater than 3 cm, and an interval between surgery and radiotherapy greater than 6 weeks.[7, 8] Patients with one of these factors were considered at intermediate risk. These classifications have been used to assign patients to varying dose levels and fractionation schedules in the prospective trials described below.

Following laryngectomy in addition to the factors described above, the presence of transglottic disease, a preoperative tracheostomy and lymph node involvement in level 6 are additional risk factors.

EVIDENCE FOR DOSE ESCALATION AND ACCELERATION OF POSTOPERATIVE RADIOTHERAPY

The main body of evidence with regard to the appropriate postoperative dose of radiotherapy for a given risk disease is derived from a study of 302 patients performed at the MD Anderson Cancer Center between 1983 and 1991.[7] Using a point system dependent on adverse pathological variables, patients were assigned to a low risk or high risk group. The low, medium and high risk groups described above were subsequently formulated based on the results from this study. Patients assigned as low risk were initially randomized to postoperative doses of either 52–54 Gy in 29–30 fractions or 63 Gy in 35 fractions. An interim analysis after only two years showed a higher rate of recurrence in the lower dose arm and so for the rest of the study the dose in this arm was increased to 57.6 Gy in 32 fractions. In the high risk group, patients were randomized between 63 Gy in 35 fractions and 68.4 Gy in 38 fractions. After the initial dose adjustment in the low risk arm, and in the high risk arm throughout the whole study, there was no significant advantage in the use of a higher dose of radiotherapy when analysing the study as originally planned. However, the primary tumour local control for patients receiving 63 Gy in 35 fractions was identical at 89 per cent for patients in both the low and high risk groups suggesting that the initial pathological scoring system was flawed, prompting the subsequent analysis of pathological features leading to the system described above. Subgroup analysis of patients with extracapsular nodal extension identified a significant increase in local control between the 57.6 and 63 Gy arms (52 versus 74 per cent; $p = 0.03$).

The conclusions from this study are that a dose less than 57.6 Gy in 32 fractions is suboptimal for postoperative radiotherapy and that patients with extracapsular spread should receive at least 63 Gy in 35 fractions. The lack of a dose response above 57.6 Gy in all patients led the same group to examine the possibility that accelerated repopulation might nullify any additional dose due to prolongation of overall treatment time.

In a second study at MD Anderson between 1991 and 1995, 213 patients were assigned to the low, medium and high risk groups as per the system derived from the above study.[8] Low risk patients without any adverse risk factors did not receive radiotherapy and had similar five-year local control to patients with one risk factor (other than extracapsular spread) who received 57.6 Gy in 32 fractions (90 versus 94 per cent). There were similar rates of distant metastases between these two groups (3 versus 4 per cent) and a non-significant difference in five-year survival (83 versus 66 per cent). The high risk group with either extracapsular extension alone or two risk factors had a significantly lower rate of local control and overall survival (68 per cent, $p = 0.003$ and 42 per cent, $p = 0.0001$) together with a higher rate of distant metastases (33 per cent). This group of 151 patients was randomized to 63 Gy in 35 fractions delivered in 1.8 Gy fractions either once daily over 7 weeks or once daily for the first 3 weeks and then twice a day with a 6-hour interval for the last 2 weeks with an overall treatment time of 5 weeks. This accelerated arm resulted in a trend towards improved local control ($p = 0.11$) and a trend towards improved overall survival ($p = 0.08$).

EFFECT OF DELAY BETWEEN SURGERY AND POSTOPERATIVE RADIOTHERAPY

The optimal timing of postoperative radiotherapy has yet to be determined although overall treatment time (OTT) is a known important factor in treatment of head and neck cancer treated with radiotherapy alone. The potential doubling time of squamous cell carcinomas in head and neck cancers can be as few as 5 days, hence higher total dose may be required to maintain tumour control if treatment duration is prolonged. Relapsed tumours were found to have shorter doubling time than those that did not as found in a flow cytometry study of 70 patients although it did not reach statistical significance (5.3 versus 6.1 days, $p = $ NS).[9]

Another radiobiology factor is the concept of accelerated repopulation whereby the tumours grow even more quickly after surgery and may be related to increase in tumour growth factors and inflammatory response in the areas of wound healing.[10]

With combined modality of treatment of surgery and postoperative radiotherapy, radiobiological considerations of potential doubling time and accelerated repopulation suggest that delays in commencing postoperative radiotherapy may be detrimental to the outcomes. However, no randomized control trial has addressed the optimal timing of postoperative radiotherapy specifically.

A series from Memorial Sloan-Kettering Cancer Center with more than 100 patients with stages 3 and 4 squamous cell carcinoma of head and neck had a higher incidence of regional failure when radiotherapy was delayed by more than 6 weeks after surgery.[11] However, the results could be confounded by suboptimal radiation doses as the majority of patients who failed received less than 56 Gy. When patients who had treatment delays of more than 6 weeks were analysed into groups of patients receiving less than 56 Gy versus at least 60 Gy, the latter had better LRC suggesting a compensatory effect by a higher radiotherapy dose. Moreover, the relapse incidence of the latter group was similar to another group receiving at least 60 Gy and who started treatment within the first 6 weeks after surgery. The authors concluded that a delay in postoperative radiotherapy may not have a negative impact provided the radiation dose is more than 60 Gy.

A retrospective study in France of 420 patients did not find delays in starting postoperative radiotherapy to be a statistically significant factor for locoregional relapse or survival.[12] The patients were treated with doses of 45–55 Gy if margins were > 5 mm or node negative, 56–65 Gy if margins were < 5 mm or node positive, and 66–74 Gy if margins were microscopically positive or if there was extracapsular nodal spread. The patients were divided into starting treatment ≤ 30 or > 30 days. Of the patients, 19.5 per cent had radiotherapy starting > 50 days after surgery.

The authors offered several explanations for the negative results. First, the rate of locoregional relapse at 18.3 per cent was possibly too low to be influenced by the delays in radiotherapy. They postulated the low incidence of relapse was affected by the increased incidence of metastasis, second primaries and unrelated deaths. Second, the inclusion criterion of complete macroscopic resection might mean the impact of radiotherapy delays was limited as residual cancer cells might be minimal. Third, tissue hypoxia following surgery might make residual cancer cells more resistant to the effects of radiotherapy. Therefore, they concluded that delay in starting postoperative radiotherapy might not be such an important factor as suggested by radiobiological considerations.

Amdur et al.[13] reported an older series of 134 patients of whom 96 per cent were stage 3 and 4, who achieved macroscopic clearance following surgery and who were treated with continuous course radiotherapy. They did not find the interval between surgery and starting radiotherapy (ranging from 1 to 10 weeks) was a significant factor based on multivariate analysis.

However, a few studies found the delay in starting postoperative radiotherapy and the OTT of combined modality treatment might influence outcomes.[8, 14, 15, 16, 17]

An MD Anderson prospective randomized trial of 213 patients addressed the issue of postoperative radiotherapy or no further treatment after surgery. They found that high risk patients who received conventional fractionated radiotherapy over 7 weeks had a lower LRC ($p = 0.03$) and lower survival rates ($p = 0.01$) if there was > 6 weeks delay between surgery and radiotherapy.[8] There was no significant effect in high risk patients who received accelerated radiotherapy over 5 weeks, even if there was a delay in starting postoperative radiotherapy.

When they looked into OTT, which takes into account the time of surgery until the time of completing radiotherapy, the LRC and survival were lower in the groups who had prolonged OTT. The five-year actuarial LRC for OTT < 11 weeks was 76 per cent compared with 62 per cent for 11–13 weeks and 38 per cent for > 13 weeks ($p = 0.002$); and the corresponding survival rates were 48, 27 and 25 per cent ($p = 0.03$). Hence, the authors suggested that OTT should be taken into account and the treatment of surgery and postoperative radiotherapy should be considered as a package that needs to be delivered in a coordinated fashion. However,

While there is a lack of phase III randomized trials comparing concurrent chemoradiation as a sole treatment modality versus surgery,[41] several randomized trials have investigated concurrent chemoradiation versus radiotherapy alone in the treatment of locally advanced squamous cell carcinoma of the head and neck cancer, as well as in nasopharyngeal carcinoma. A summary of these seminal trials is presented in **Table 45.4**.[42, 43, 44, 45, 46, 47, 48, 49] While associated with increased acute toxicity, concurrent chemoradiation has been demonstrated in these trials to be superior to radiotherapy alone or to induction chemotherapy followed by radiotherapy in terms of improving local control rates. However, not all the trials have shown a survival benefit in favour of concurrent chemoradiation over the alternative approaches. Nonetheless, on the basis of these seminal studies, concurrent chemoradiation remains the standard of care for the management of patients with locally advanced, non-metastatic head and neck cancer. Alternative methods of delivering chemotherapy, for example using a weekly schedule of cisplatin chemotherapy instead of the 3-weekly schedule used currently, have been investigated to alleviate the acute toxicity associated with concurrent platinum-based chemoradiation. Amifostine is a cytoprotective agent which has been investigated in randomized trials to reduce

mucositis and xerostomia commonly associated with concurrent chemoradiation.[50, 51]

Altered fractionation and concurrent chemotherapy

As discussed above, altered fractionation radiotherapy has been shown to be superior to standard fractionation radiotherapy in a meta-analysis of 15 trials.[16] Results of this meta-analysis in concert with the positive results in favour of concurrent chemoradiation over radiotherapy alone led to the development of several randomized trials investigating altered fractionation schedules with concurrent chemotherapy to further improve local control and overall survival. Brizel et al. randomized 116 patients with locally advanced head and neck cancer to hyperfractionated radiotherapy alone (75 Gy in 1.25 Gy twice daily fractions) or the same schedule with two cycles of concurrent cisplatin-based chemotherapy.[45] Patients treated with concurrent chemotherapy had a statistically significant improvement in local control and overall survival. Budach et al. randomized 384 patients with locally advanced head and neck cancer to altered

Table 45.4 Randomized phase III trials of definitive chemoradiation versus radiation in advanced head and neck cancer.

Trial	Patient population	Trial arms	Local control rates	Overall survival rates
Adelstein et al.[42]	Unresectable HNC (n = 271)	RT (arm A) vs CRT (arm B) vs split-course CRT (arm C)	NR	3-year projected: 23% (arm A) vs 37% (arm B) (p = 0.014) vs 27% (arm C) (NS)
Forastiere et al.[43]	Stage III/IV laryngeal carcinoma (n = 518)	RT (arm A) vs CRT (arm B) vs C-RT (arm C)	5-year rates: 51% (arm A) vs 68.8% (arm B) vs 54.9% (arm C) (p = 0.002 A vs) (p = 0.001 B vs C) (p = NS B vs C)	5-year rates: 55% in all three arms (NS)
Denis et al.[44]	Stage III/IV oropharynx carcinoma (n = 226)	RT (arm A) vs CRT (arm B)	5-year rates: 24.7% (arm A) vs 47.6% (arm B) (p = 0.002)	5.5-year rates: 15.8% (arm A) vs 22.4% (arm B) (p = 0.05)
Brizel et al.[45]	Advanced HNC (n = 116)	RT (arm A) vs CRT (arm B)	3-year rates: 44% (arm A) vs 70% (arm B) (p = 0.01)	3-year rates: 34% (arm A) vs 55% (arm B) (p = 0.07)
Budach et al.[46]	Advanced HNC (n = 384)	RT (arm A) vs CRT (arm B)	5-year rates: 37.4% (arm A) vs 49.9% (arm B) (p = 0.001)	5-year rates: 23.7% (arm A) vs 28.6% (arm B) (p = 0.023)
Al-Sarraf et al.[47]	NPC (n = 147)	RT (arm A) vs CRT (arm B)	Crude rates: 74% (arm A) vs 90% (arm B)	3-year rates: 47% (arm A) vs 78% (arm B) (p = 0.005)
Wee et al.[48]	NPC (n = 221)	RT (arm A) vs CRT (arm B)	Crude rates: 91% (arm A) vs 92% (arm B)	3-year rates: 65% (arm A) vs 80% (arm B) (p = 0.006)
Chan et al.[49]	NPC (n = 350)	RT (arm A) vs CRT (arm B)	4-year rates: 68% (arm A) vs 80% (arm B) (p = 0.051)	5-year rates: 58.6% (arm A) vs 70.3% (arm B) (p = 0.049)

CRT, chemoradiation; C-RT, induction chemotherapy followed by radiotherapy; HNC, head and neck cancer; NPC, nasopharyngeal carcinoma; NR, not reported; NS, not significant; RT, radiotherapy alone.

fractionation radiotherapy alone versus altered fractionation radiotherapy with concurrent mitomycin C-based chemotherapy.[46] Patients randomized to the radiotherapy alone arm in this study received a total radiation dose of 77.6 Gy compared to 70.6 Gy for patients randomized to the concurrent chemotherapy arm. Nonetheless, patients randomized to the concurrent chemotherapy arm also had a statistically significant improvement in local control and progression-free survival. Several other randomized trials have also reported positive results in favour of concurrent altered fractionation chemoradiation[52, 53, 54] with the exception being a study by Staar et al.[55] in which patients underwent a second randomization to either receive or not receive granulocyte colony-stimulating factor (G-CSF). G-CSF was given to reduce the risk of treatment-related mucositis, and it has been hypothesized that administration of G-CSF may have inadvertently led to stimulation of tumour clonogens. A meta-analysis of 32 trials of altered fractionation radiotherapy with or without concurrent chemotherapy concluded that concurrent chemotherapy was associated with a significant improvement in overall survival regardless of the radiation fractionation schedule used.[56]

The question as to whether concurrent modified fractionation chemoradiation is superior to conventional fractionation concurrent chemoradiation remains unanswered.[57] This key issue is being addressed in two large randomized controlled trials in Europe and the United States, the results of which are awaited with great anticipation. The US RTOG 01-29 study is comparing standard fractionation concurrent chemoradiation versus altered fractionation concurrent chemoradiation and the European-based GORTEC study is a three-arm study comparing concurrent altered fractionation chemoradiation versus 'very accelerated' radiotherapy alone versus standard chemoradiation.

Adjuvant concurrent chemoradiation for head and neck cancer

Following surgery for head and neck cancer, the presence of inadequate resection margins, multiple lymph node involvement or extranodal spread predicts for a high risk of local recurrence. Adjuvant radiotherapy has been shown to reduce the risk of local recurrence compared to preoperative radiotherapy.[58] Results of previously published randomized trials demonstrated superiority of concurrent chemoradiation over radiotherapy alone in the adjuvant setting.[59, 60] Results of these smaller trials have been confirmed by two landmark trials published simultaneously in 2004. The European-based EORTC trial by Bernier et al. randomized 334 patients to adjuvant radiotherapy or cisplatin-based concurrent chemoradiation.[61] The addition of chemotherapy to radiotherapy resulted in a statistically significant improvement in local control rates, progression-free survival and overall survival. In the US-based RTOG trial reported by Cooper et al. the addition of cisplatin chemotherapy to adjuvant radiotherapy significantly improved local control rates and disease-free survival but not overall survival when compared to radiotherapy alone.[62] An 'entente cordiale' pooling of their results published in 2005 demonstrated a significant survival benefit for adjuvant concurrent chemoradiation in patients with positive margins or lymph node involvement with

extracapsular spread.[63] There was a trend in favour of chemoradiation in patients with stage III–IV disease, presence of perineural infiltration, and lymphovascular invasion.

Meta-analysis of concurrent chemoradiation in head and neck cancer

A large number of randomized trials designed to investigate chemotherapy given as neoadjuvant (induction), concurrent (concomitant, synchronous, simultaneous) and, less frequently, adjuvant (following definitive treatment) have now been reported with many of the earlier studies drawing conflicting conclusions, possibly because of small sample sizes and because of the use of less effective chemotherapy agents. Meta-analyses have greatly improved our understanding of the benefit and limitations of these techniques. Results of neoadjuvant and adjuvant chemotherapy are discussed below under Neoadjuvant chemotherapy in head and neck cancer.

The first meta-analysis reported by Stell and Rawson was based upon a review of 23 randomized trials of adjuvant chemotherapy in squamous carcinoma of the head and neck,[64] none of which were individually large enough to detect the anticipated survival improvement of the order of 5 per cent. Only synchronous and or maintenance trials appeared to confer benefit. Perhaps unexpectedly, cisplatin containing regimens offered no benefit and patients treated with the commonly used vinblastine, bleomycin and methotrexate regimen fared worse. While the incidence of locoregional recurrence was reduced in the chemotherapy arms, the distant metastasis rate was unchanged. Toxicity was poorly reported in these trials; however, the average mortality rate in nine series was an alarming 6.5 per cent, an unacceptable figure by current standards. A larger meta-analysis of 54 randomized trials published by Munro reiterated Stell's findings with cisplatin containing regimens once again failing to confer a survival advantage.[65] However, single agent simultaneous chemotherapy increased survival by 12.1 per cent with a corresponding confidence interval of 5–19 per cent.

Over the last 15 years, many more trials have reached maturity. In 2000 the Meta-analysis of Chemotherapy on Head and Neck Cancer (MACH-NC) collaborative published its first meta-analysis based upon individual patient data, which included almost 11 000 patients from 63 randomized trials.[66] The same group published, in 2009, an updated meta-analysis involving 17 346 patients from 93 randomized trials.[67] The addition of chemotherapy to radiotherapy was shown to give an absolute benefit of 4.5 per cent at five years in improving overall survival from head and neck cancer. The same group have performed a meta-analysis of 11 randomized trials in nasopharyngeal carcinoma, and concluded that chemotherapy confers an absolute benefit of 6 per cent at five years in improving survival from nasopharyngeal carcinoma.[68]

Concomitant epidermal growth factor receptor inhibition and radical radiotherapy in head and neck cancer

The epidermal growth factor receptor (EGFR) is a member of the ErbB/HER family of receptor tyrosine kinases.

It possesses an extracellular N-terminal ligand-binding domain, a transmembrane region and a C-terminal intracellular domain which includes the kinase domain and multiple phosphorylation sites.[69] The great majority of squamous cell carcinomas of the head and neck express EGFR.[70] Activation of EGFR activates intracellular signal transduction pathways which are potent oncogenic regulators of tumour cell growth, invasion, angiogenesis and metastasis.[69] High EGFR levels in tumours are associated with adverse outcome and exposure of tumour cells to ionizing radiation increases the level of EGFR expression, the blockade of which increases cell sensitivity to radiation.[71, 72]

Cetuximab is a human–murine chimeric immunoglobulin-G monoclonal antibody that competitively binds to the extracellular domain of EGFR. Phase I and II studies indicated safety and efficacy in head and neck squamous carcinoma and were shown to reverse platinum resistance.[73] Bonner *et al.* undertook a multicentre, randomized controlled trial in which 424 patients with advanced head and neck squamous cell carcinoma were randomized to radiotherapy alone versus radiotherapy with concomitant cetuximab.[74] Cetuximab was given initially as a loading dose of $400 \, mg/m^2$ a week prior to commencing radiotherapy then weekly throughout at a dose of $250 \, mg/m^2$. Radiotherapy was defined as high dose although the schedules varied according to the trial centre. Daily fractionation to the US of 70 Gy in 35 fractions over 7 weeks was commonly employed as was hyperfractionated and concomitant boost accelerated irradiation. There was a statistically significant overall survival benefit in favour of the cetuximab treatment arm (36.4 versus 45.6 per cent, $p = 0.018$).[75] Patients receiving cetuximab experienced more infusion reactions and acneiform skin reactions; patients experiencing at least a grade 2 acneiform skin reaction had a statistically better survival compared to those experiencing a grade 1 reaction. A major criticism of this study remains that the standard arm in the trial was not concurrent chemoradiation which is now accepted as the standard of care in locally advanced head and neck cancer, hence despite clear benefits the use of cetuximab concomitant with radiotherapy cannot be accepted as the new standard of care. It seems unlikely that such a trial will be performed in the future. In practice, cetuximab concomitant with radiotherapy is often reserved for patients with locally advanced head and neck cancer considered not to be fit enough to withstand the rigors of platinum-based concurrent chemoradiation. The RTOG 0522 randomized trial comparing the addition of cetuximab to cisplatin-based concurrent accelerated chemoradiation may provide further useful data for the role of cetuximab in locally advanced head and neck cancer.

Neoadjuvant chemotherapy in head and neck cancer

The rationale for chemotherapy in head and neck cancer was founded upon high response rates observed with a variety of chemotherapy agents including methotrexate, vinblastine, bleomycin, 5-fluorouracil, cisplatin, carboplatin and the taxanes, either alone or in combination. In early studies, chemotherapy was mostly used in an attempt to downstage disease prior to definitive local therapies and to reduce the incidence of distant metastases. These neoadjuvant chemotherapy schedules were initially investigated in non-randomized trials using historical or case-matched controls, which suggested a major advance in overall survival. However, such encouraging results were not subsequently borne out by randomized controlled trials, at least, not until very recently. The issue of using neoadjuvant chemotherapy for 'organ preservation' is worthy of note, an approach which was driven by the objective of avoiding ablative surgery in advanced disease. The Veterans Affairs study randomized patients between induction chemotherapy followed by radiotherapy versus surgery followed by postoperative radiotherapy. Those receiving chemotherapy underwent surgery and radiotherapy if a partial response was not achieved. Two-thirds of the patients treated in the conservation arm retained their larynx, although overall survival was the same.[76] This trial was heavily criticized for the absence of a radiotherapy alone arm. Consequently, the Intergroup trial R91-11 was initiated, comparing induction chemotherapy and radiotherapy versus concurrent chemoradiation versus radiotherapy alone;[43] the addition of chemotherapy reduced the incidence of distant metastases and improved disease-free survival compared to radiotherapy alone; however, there was no difference in overall survival rates between the three arms. Concurrent chemoradiation was significantly superior to induction chemotherapy for organ preservation and local recurrence rates. Similar criticism as for the Veterans Affairs trial can also be levelled at the EORTC trial reported by Lefebvre, which investigated pyriform sinus cancer using a similar strategy resulting in a comparable conclusion albeit with a lower, 35 per cent, rate of pharyngeal preservation.[77] These trials are frequently quoted as offering standards of care, but their conclusions should now be reconsidered in the context of the high quality meta-analyses exploring the role of chemotherapy in head and neck cancer.

The latest meta-analysis by the MACH-NC collaborative examined 31 trials of induction chemotherapy involving 5311 patients and a median follow up of 6.1 years.[67] Neoadjuvant chemotherapy offers a statistically non-significant absolute benefit of 2.4 per cent at five years ($p = 0.18$). Furthermore, the authors conclude concurrent chemoradiation offers a significantly greater benefit than induction chemotherapy. These results reflect the findings of earlier meta-analyses discussed previously in this chapter.

Reasons for the failure of neoadjuvant chemotherapy in increasing survival from head and neck cancer remain unclear and several hypotheses have been suggested. The concept that tumours treated with chemotherapy may become more aggressive despite apparent down-staging was supported by a study of tumour cell kinetics using flow cytometry in 97 patients with oropharyngeal cancer which demonstrated significantly increased mean labelling indices and shorter potential doubling times following induction chemotherapy compared to pretreatment measurements, particularly in poorly responding tumours.[78] Alternatively, the possible benefits of neoadjuvant chemotherapy for responding patients may be offset by the adverse effect of delaying surgery or radiotherapy in non-responding patients. A potential survival advantage may also be eroded by excess mortality associated with the high incidence of intercurrent disease, mainly second tumours and vascular disease, in this group of patients, which may be further offset by toxic-related deaths resulting from chemotherapy, which was all too common in the 1980s. Finally, the chemotherapy schedules used in earlier studies were often devoid of a platinum agent.

As treatment for patients with locally advanced head and neck cancer has improved local control rates, there has been increasing interest in attempts to reduce the rates of distant metastases as a strategy for improving survival from head and neck cancer. While cisplatin with or without 5-fluorouracil has been the mainstay of chemotherapy in head and neck cancer for nearly two decades, the development of newer chemotherapy agents, in particular the taxanes, has offered new scope in the treatment of head and neck squamous carcinoma. This class of chemotherapy agents enhances microtubule formation, thereby suppressing microtubule dynamics required for mitotic function, effectively blocking cell cycle progression resulting in cellular apoptosis.[79] Phase II studies demonstrated greater activity when docetaxel was added to cisplatin and 5-fluorouracil in advanced disease compared to cisplatin plus 5-fluorouracil alone.[80]

Based on the results of these phase II trials, the TAX 323 and TAX 324 randomized trials investigated the addition of docetaxel to cisplatin and 5-fluorouracil chemotherapy as neoadjuvant treatment in unresectable head and neck cancer. TAX 323 was a European-based trial which randomized 358 patients with stage III–IV squamous cell carcinoma of the head and neck to receive up to four cycles of neoadjuvant chemotherapy with docetaxel, cisplatin, 5-fluorouracil (TPF) (docetaxel ($75 \, mg/m^2$, day 1), cisplatin ($750 \, mg/m^2$, day 1) and 5-fluorouracil ($750 \, mg/m^2$, days 1–5)) or cisplatin, 5-fluorouracil (PF) (cisplatin ($100 \, mg/m^2$, day 1) and 5-fluorouracil ($1000 \, mg/m^2$, days 1–5)).[81] Patients with stable or responsive disease then underwent radical radiotherapy. At a median of 51 months, the addition of docetaxel was associated with a statistically significant improvement in response rates to chemotherapy, progression-free survival and overall survival. Surprisingly, quality of life was better in the TPF arm and although there was a higher incidence of grade 3 and 4 neutropenia, thrombocytopenia was less frequent compared to the PF arm.

The TAX 324 was a US-based study and randomized 501 patients to receive up to three cycles of neoadjuvant TPF or PF chemotherapy.[82] While the dose of docetaxel was the same as in TAX 323, patients in TAX 324 received $100 \, mg/m^2$ of cisplatin and $1000 \, mg/m^2$ of 5-fluorouracil in both arms. Following chemotherapy, patients received carboplatin-based concurrent chemoradiation. Once again, the addition of docetaxel resulted in a statistically significant improvement in progression-free and overall survival.

The same combinations of chemotherapy have also been compared in a randomized trial investigating an organ preservation strategy in 213 patients with locoregionally advanced laryngeal and hypopharyngeal cancer.[83] After three cycles, non-responders underwent surgery followed by post-operative radiotherapy while responders underwent radiotherapy. The overall response rates were higher for those treated with TPF, with corresponding laryngeal preservation rates at three years of 70.3 and 57.5 per cent ($p = 0.03$), respectively, in favour of docetaxel-based chemotherapy.

Hitt et al. reported a randomized phase III trial of 382 patients with locoregionally advanced squamous cancer of the head and neck, randomized to neoadjuvant chemotherapy with cisplatin and 5-fluorouracil or the same

regimen with paclitaxel.[84] Following three cycles, patients responding to chemotherapy were treated with cisplatin-based concurrent chemoradiation. The addition of paclitaxel significantly improved response rates and progression-free survival, with a trend towards overall survival.

Results of these trials indicate that both neoadjuvant docetaxel and paclitaxel improve locoregional control and overall survival in patients with locally advanced head and neck cancer. Nevertheless, several unanswered questions remain; how does induction TPF chemotherapy followed by platinum-based concurrent chemoradiation compare to platinum-based concurrent chemoradiation alone? Can taxanes be used safely and effectively concomitant with radiotherapy? What is the optimum management of patients who fail to respond to neoadjuvant TPF chemotherapy? Is there a role for EGFR inhibition in the context of taxane-based neoadjuvant chemotherapy?

Palliative chemotherapy in locally advanced/metastatic head and neck cancer

Up to two-thirds of patients with head and neck cancer present with locally advanced disease, half of whom relapse within two years of definitive treatment. Ten per cent of patients have de novo metastatic disease. The prognosis for these patients remains dismal with a median survival of seven to eight months.[1] Although the survival benefit of palliative chemotherapy over best supportive care has not been demonstrated in an adequately powered randomized trial,[85] palliative chemotherapy with cisplatin and 5-fluorouracil remains the generally accepted standard of care based on results of several randomized trials.[86, 87, 88, 89, 90] As discussed earlier, there is increasing interest in the role of EGFR inhibition in the treatment of head and neck cancers. While a randomized phase III placebo-controlled trial of 117 patients failed to demonstrate a survival benefit for the addition of cetuximab to cisplatin chemotherapy,[91] a second trial involving 442 patients demonstrated a statistically significant survival benefit for the addition of cetuximab to platinum-based palliative chemotherapy.[92]

ADVANCES IN RADIATION DELIVERY IN HEAD AND NECK CANCERS

From two-dimensional planning through conformal radiotherapy to intensity modulated radiotherapy

The aim of radiotherapy planning is to deliver a homogenous dose to the primary tumour and potential areas of micrometastatic disease while minimizing the dose to the organs at risk. Accurate tumour localization is central to radiotherapy planning and it is important to have the following information to hand: findings of clinical examination including examination under anaesthesia; operation notes and intraoperative findings; relevant histopathology report; results of any radiological investigations including computed tomography (CT), magnetic resonance imaging (MRI) and [18]FDG-positron emission tomography (PET) scans.

For more than two decades conventional two-dimensional (2D) planning has utilized standard orthogonal x-ray films taken by a simulator, a diagnostic x-ray machine connected to a television screen which is geometrically identical to the linear accelerator (see **Figure 45.1**) or cobalt-60 treatment unit. Cross wires mounted in the light beam from the simulator define the size of the area to be treated. As diagnostic x-rays have poor soft tissue resolution the radiotherapist defines the area to be treated on the simulator films using bony landmarks together with clinical and radiological knowledge of the position and extent of the tumour. Resultant volumes are therefore relatively crudely derived from 2D x-ray films with, at best, assumed knowledge of the position of critical soft tissue structures, tumour and organs at risk.

Fast computers introduced in the 1990s permitted the use of CT scanning and other axial slice imaging modalities to allow the radiotherapist to define the tumour and organ at risk using software which permits a three-dimensional (3D) reconstruction of these volumes. The radiation beams should 'conform' as closely as possible to the shape of the tumour, which are by no means simple cuboidal, cylindrical or even spheroidal structures. This is even more exemplified when associated tumour masses coexist in close proximity, for example a primary tumour with locally involved nodes surrounded by normal tissues. The 3D software allows the radiation beams to be shaped by the linear accelerator to achieve this objective hence the term 'conformal radiotherapy' (see **Figure 45.2**). The software also calculates the dose of radiation delivered to specific volumes of both the tumour bearing target and normal tissue 'organs at risk' and displays these by dose–volume histograms (see **Figure 45.3**) thus providing the radiotherapist with a tool for determining precise dosimetric information for accuracy of treatment and of risk of damage to normal tissues. While long established in the US and northern Europe, 3D conformal radiotherapy has only recently become available in many UK centres.

3D conformal radiotherapy has undoubtedly been a major step forward. Nevertheless, the radiation beam arrangements are relatively simple and do not permit complex coverage of convex shapes, for example when a high radiation dose curves around an organ at risk such as the spinal cord, brain stem or major salivary glands, as is frequently required in nasopharyngeal irradiation.

The development of intensity modulated radiotherapy (IMRT) is a potential leap ahead. Multiple beams of varying intensities allow the creation of irregular shapes, if necessary with concave contours[93, 94] (**Figure 45.4**). Most of the data supporting the use of IMRT come from single institution phase II trials; preliminary results have been most encouraging in both squamous cell head and neck cancer[95, 96, 97, 98] and nasopharyngeal carcinoma.[99, 100, 101] The ability to reduce toxicity by avoidance of critical organs at risk, specifically the parotid glands, without compromising tumour coverage and control has been clearly demonstrated. Quality

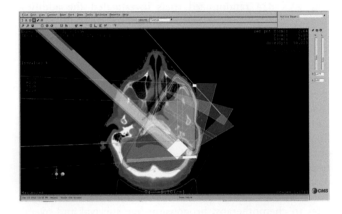

Figure 45.2 Conformal radiotherapy plan to treat carcinoma of the left parotid gland.

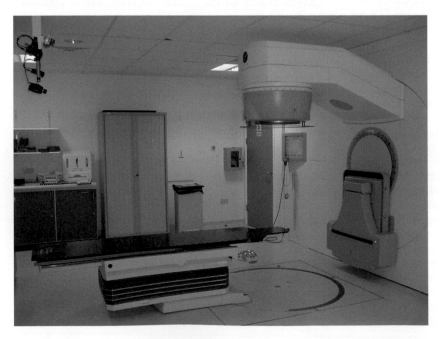

Figure 45.1 A 6MV Elekta linear accelerator.

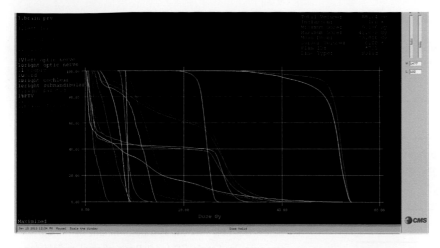

Figure 45.3 Dose–volume histogram for the plan shown in **Figure 45.2**, demonstrating dose to the target volume and also to the organs at risk.

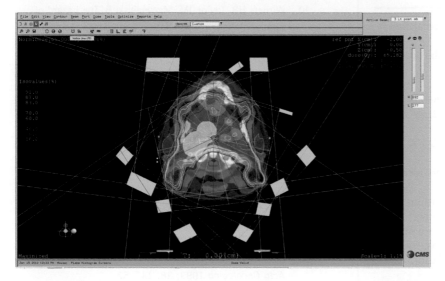

Figure 45.4 A radiotherapy plan demonstrating intensity modulated radiotherapy (IMRT) to treat nasopharyngeal carcinoma in a young patient.

of life has been shown to be improved when comparing IMRT to 3D conformal radiotherapy by a recent French matched pair analysis cohort study[102] and is the subject of the UK PARSPORT trial. The technology is rapidly gaining a prime position in the treatment of head and neck cancer in the Western world, although disappointingly the UK is once more lagging behind the US and northern Europe. No single imaging modality is entirely accurate and image fusion technology, particularly the use of PET with CT, may improve the ability to define the tumour volume during the process of radiotherapy planning.[103, 104]

Nevertheless, there is a potential downside to IMRT. Since multiple beams are used, often seven or more as compared to two or three with 2D or 3D conformal radiotherapy, a larger volume of normal tissue receives low dose radiation with concerns being raised about the potential of an increased risk of second malignancies.[105]

IMRT is unquestionably a new gold standard, although we must proceed with vigilance. It will undoubtedly be included in future fractionation and combined modality studies with the ultimate aim of achieving even greater enhancement of the therapeutic ratio between tumour destruction and normal tissue tolerance.[106]

AREAS FOR FUTURE RESEARCH

Areas for future research are as follows:

- The late effects of recent developments in therapy must be continually monitored and researched.
- Gross tumour target definition requires further investigation and validation of imaging methodologies if we are to use new techniques of more closely targeted radiotherapy (IMRT) safely.
- The efficacy and safety of the combinations and permutations of these new technologies is yet to be confirmed by the following studies:
  - synchronous chemoradiotherapy – 3D conformal radiotherapy versus IMRT (GORTEC 2004-01 trial);
  - synchronous chemoradiotherapy – modified versus conventional fractionation (GORTEC 99-02 and RTOG H029 trials);
  - IMRT or 3D conformal (non-randomized) accelerated radiotherapy+synchronous chemotherapy ± cetuximab (RTOG 0522 trial);
  - role of taxane induction chemotherapy followed by concomitant chemoradiotherapy compared to

concomitant chemoradiotherapy alone (DeCIDE, PARADIGM and GORTEC trials).

- Is there a role for combining EGFR inhibitors such as cetuximab with taxanes and in what sequence?

KEY EVIDENCE

The evidence base for most recent developments in non-surgical management of head and neck cancer is of high quality, primarily level I.

KEY LEARNING POINTS

- Multidisciplinary team working is essential for ensuring optimum care.
- Commence treatment as soon as possible after diagnosis and staging.
- Avoid treatment interruption.
- Use alimentation support, i.e. percutaneous endoscopic gastrostomy feeding when large areas of mucosa are being irradiated.
- 3D conformal radiotherapy should be a UK standard.
- Modified radiation fractionation confers local control and survival advantage.
- Platinum-based concurrent chemoradiation confers local control and survival advantage.
- Consider use of cetuximab synchronous with radiotherapy in those patients unsuitable for platinum-based concurrent chemoradiation.

REFERENCES

◆ 1. Arigis A, Karamouzis MV, Raben D, Ferris RL. Head and neck cancer. *Lancet* 2008; **371**: 1695–1709.

◆ 2. Burri RJ, Lee NY. Concurrent chemotherapy and radiotherapy for head and neck cancer. *Expert Review of Anticancer Therapy* 2009; **9**: 293–302.

◆ 3. Bucci MK, Bevan A, Roach M III. Advances in radiation therapy: conventional to 3D, to IMRT, to 4D, and beyond. *CA A Cancer Journal for Clinicians* 2005; **55**: 117–34.

4. Radiotherapy dose-fractionation. BFCO(06)1. The Royal College of Radiologists Board of Faculty of Clinical Oncology 2006. Last acessed March 2, 2009. Available from: https://www.rcr.ac.uk/publications.aspx?pageID = 149&publications = 229.

5. Williams MV, James ND, Summers ET *et al*. National survey of radiotherapy fractionation practice in 2003. *Clinical Oncology (Royal College of Radiologists (Great Britain))* 2006; **18**: 3–14.

6. Hendry JH, Roberts SA, Slevin NJ *et al*. Influence of radiotherapy treatment time on control of laryngeal cancer: comparison between centres in Manchester, UK and Toronto, Canada. *Radiotherapy and Oncology* 1994; **31**: 14–22.

7. Gowda RV, Henk JM, Mais KL *et al*. Three weeks radiotherapy for T1 glottic cancer: the Christie and Royal Marsden Hospital experience. *Radiotherapy and Oncology* 2003; **68**: 105–11.

8. Fowler JF. Is there an optimum overall time for head and neck radiotherapy? A review, with new modelling. *Clinical Oncology (Royal College of Radiologists (Great Britain))* 2007; **19**: 8–22.

9. Steele GG. Cell survival as a determinant of tumour response. In: Steele GG (ed.). *Basic clinical radiobiology*, 3rd edn. London: Arnold, 2002.

10. Withers HR, Taylor JM, Maclejewski B. The hazard of tumour clonogen repopulation during radiotherapy. *Acta Oncologica* 1988; **27**: 131–46.

11. Hoffstetter S, Marchal C, Peiffert D *et al*. Treatment duration as a prognostic factor for local control and survival in epidermoid carcinomas of the tonsillar region treated by combined external beam irradiation and brachytherapy. *Radiotherapy and Oncology* 1997; **45**: 141–8.

12. Robertson C, Robertson AG, Hendry JH *et al*. Similar decreases in local tumour control are calculated for treatment protraction and for interruptions in the radiotherapy of carcinomas of the larynx in four centres. *International Journal of Radiation Oncology, Biology, Physics* 1998; **40**: 319–29.

13. Disch S, Saunders MI. The CHART regimen and morbidity. *Acta Oncologica* 1999; **38**: 147–52.

14. Cox JD, Pajak TF, Marcial VF *et al*. ASTRO plenary: interfraction interval is a major determinant of late effects, with hyperfractionated radiation therapy of carcinomas of upper respiratory and digestive tracts: results from Radiation Therapy Oncology Group protocol 8313. *International Journal of Radiation Oncology, Biology, Physics* 1991; **20**: 1191–5.

● 15. Horiot JC, Le Fur R, N'Guyen T *et al*. Hyperfractionation versus conventional fractionation in oropharyngeal carcinoma: final analysis of a randomized trial of the EORTC cooperative group of radiotherapy. *Radiotherapy and Oncology* 1992; **25**: 231–41.

● 16. Bourhis J, Overgaard J, Audry H *et al*. Hyperfractionated or accelerated radiotherapy in head and neck cancer: a meta-analysis. *Lancet* 2006; **368**: 843–54.

17. Jackson SM, Weir LM, Hay JH *et al*. A randomised trial of accelerated versus conventional radiotherapy in head and neck cancer. *Radiotherapy and Oncology* 1997; **43**: 39–46.

18. Poulsen MG, Denham JW, Peters LJ *et al*. A randomised trial of accelerated and conventional radiotherapy for stage III and IV squamous carcinoma of the head and

neck: a Trans-Tasman Radiation Oncology Group Study. *Radiotherapy and Oncology* 2001; **60**: 113–22.

19. Overgaard J, Hansen HS, Specht L *et al.* Five compared with six fractions per week of conventional radiotherapy of squamous-cell carcinoma of head and neck: DAHANCA 6&7 randomised controlled trial. *Lancet* 2003; **362**: 933–40.

20. Hliniak A, Gwiazdowska B, Szutkowski Z *et al.* A multicentre randomized/controlled trial of a conventional versus modestly accelerated radiotherapy in the laryngeal cancer: influence of a 1 week shortening overall time. *Radiotherapy and Oncology* 2002; **62**: 1–10.

21. Skladowski K, Macieejewski B, Golen M *et al.* Continuous accelerated 7-days-a-week radiotherapy for head-and-neck cancer: long-term results of a phase III clinical trial. *International Journal of Radiation Oncology, Biology, Physics* 2006; **66**: 706–13.

22. Fu KK, Pajak TF, Trotti A *et al.* A Radiation Therapy Oncology Group (RTOG) phase III randomized study to compare hyperfractionation and two variants of accelerated fractionation to standard fractionation radiotherapy for head and neck squamous cell carcinomas: first report of RTOG 9003. *International Journal of Radiation Oncology, Biology, Physics* 2000; **48**: 7–16.

23. Horiot JC, Bontemps P, van den Bogaert W *et al.* Accelerated fractionation (AF) compared to conventional fractionation (CF) improves loco-regional control in the radiotherapy of advanced head and neck cancers: results of the EORTC 22851 randomized trial. *Radiotherapy and Oncology* 1997; **44**: 111–21.

24. Dische S, Saunders M, Barrett A *et al.* A randomised multicentre trial of CHART versus conventional radiotherapy in head and neck cancer. *Radiotherapy and Oncology* 1997; **44**: 123–36.

25. Saunders M, Rojas AM, Dische S. CHART revisited: a conservative approach for advanced head and neck cancer. *Clinical Oncology* 2008; **20**: 127–33.

26. Awwad HK, Lotayef M, Shouman T *et al.* Accelerated hyperfractionation (AF) compared to conventional fractionation (CF) in the postoperative radiotherapy of locally advanced head and neck cancer: influence of proliferation. *British Journal of Cancer* 2002; **86**: 517–23.

27. Sanghera P, McConkey C, Ho K-F *et al.* Hypofractionated accelerated radiotherapy with concurrent chemotherapy for locally advanced squamous cell carcinoma of the head and neck. *International Journal of Radiation Oncology, Biology, Physics* 2007; **67**: 1342–51.

28. Janssen HL, Haustermans KM, Balm AJ, Begg AC. Hypoxia in head and neck cancer: how much, how important? *Head and Neck* 2005; **27**: 622–38.

29. Fazekas J, Pajak TF, Wasserman T *et al.* Failure of misonidazole-sensitized radiotherapy to impact upon outcome among stage III–IV squamous cell carcinoma of the head and neck. *International Journal of Radiation Oncology, Biology, Physics* 1987; **13**: 1155–60.

30. Overgaard J, Hansen HS, Andersen AP *et al.* Misonidazole combined with split-course radiotherapy in the treatment of invasive carcinoma of larynx and pharynx: report from the DAHANCA 2 study. *International Journal of Radiation Oncology, Biology, Physics* 1989; **16**: 1065–8.

31. Van den Bogaert W, van den Schueren E, Horiot JC *et al.* The EORTC randomized trial on three fractions per day and misonidazole (trial no. 22811) in advanced head and neck cancer: long-term results and side effects. *Radiotherapy and Oncology* 1995; **35**: 91–9.

32. Lee DJ, Cosmatos D, Marcial VA *et al.* Results of an RTOG phase III trial (RTOG 85-27) comparing radiotherapy plus etanidazole with radiotherapy for locally advanced head and neck carcinomas. *International Journal of Radiation Oncology, Biology, Physics* 1995; **15**: 567–76.

33. Eschwège F, Sancho-Garnier H, Chassagne D *et al.* Results of a European randomized trial of Etanidazole combined with radiotherapy in head and neck carcinomas. *International Journal of Radiation Oncology, Biology, Physics* 1997; **39**: 275–81.

34. Overgaard J, Hansen HS, Overgaard M *et al.* A randomised double-blind phase III study of nimorazole as a hypoxic radiosensitizer of primary radiotherapy in supraglottic larynx and pharynx carcinoma. Results of the Danish Head and Neck Cancer Study (DAHANCA) Protocol 5-85. *Radiotherapy and Oncology* 1998; **46**: 135–46.

35. Gandara DR, Lara PN Jr, Goldberg Z *et al.* Tirapazamine: prototype for a novel class of therapeutic agents targeting tumour hypoxia. *Seminars in Oncology* 2002; **29**: 102–9.

36. Kaanders JH, Pop LA, Marres HA *et al.* Accelerated radiotherapy with carbogen and nicotinamide (ARCON) for laryngeal cancer. *Radiotherapy and Oncology* 1998; **48**: 115–22.

37. Harrison LB, Chadha M, Hill RJ *et al.* Impact of tumour hypoxia and anaemia on radiation therapy outcomes. *Oncologist* 2002; **7**: 492–508.

38. Lee WR, Berkey B, Marcial V *et al.* Anaemia is associated with decreased survival and increased locoregional failure in patients with locally advanced head and neck carcinoma: a secondary analysis of RTOG 85-27. *International Journal of Radiation Oncology, Biology, Physics* 1998; **42**: 1069–75.

39. Prosnitz RG, Yao B, Farrell CL *et al.* Pretreatment anaemia is correlated with the reduced effectiveness of radiation and concurrent chemotherapy in advanced head and neck cancer. *International Journal of Radiation Oncology, Biology, Physics* 2005; **61**: 1087–95.

40. Lutterbach J, Guttenberger R. Anaemia is associated with decreased local control of surgically treated squamous cell carcinomas of the glottis larynx. *International Journal of Radiation Oncology, Biology, Physics* 2000; **48**: 1345–50.

41. Soo KC, Tan EH, Wee J *et al.* Surgery and adjuvant radiotherapy vs concurrent chemoradiotherapy in stage III/IV nonmetastatic squamous cell carcinoma head and

neck cancer: a randomised comparison. *British Journal of Cancer* 2005; **93**: 279–86.

42. Adelstein DJ, Li Y, Adams GL *et al.* An Intergroup phase III comparison of standard radiation therapy and two schedules of concurrent chemoradiotherapy in patients with unresectable squamous cell head and neck cancer. *Journal of Clinical Oncology* 2003; **21**: 92–8.

43. Forastiere AA, Goepfert H, Maor M *et al.* Concurrent chemotherapy and radiotherapy for organ preservation in advanced laryngeal cancer. *New England Journal of Medicine* 2003; **349**: 2091–8.

44. Denis F, Garaud P, Bardet E *et al.* Final results of the 94-01 French Head and Neck Oncology and Radiotherapy Group randomized trial comparing radiotherapy alone with concomitant radiochemotherapy in advanced-stage oropharynx carcinoma. *Journal of Clinical Oncology* 2004; **22**: 69–76.

45. Brizel DM, Albers ME, Fisher SR *et al.* Hyperfractionated irradiation with or without concurrent chemotherapy for locally advanced head and neck cancer. *New England Journal of Medicine* 1998; **338**: 1798–804.

46. Budach V, Stuschke M, Budach W *et al.* Hyperfractionated accelerated chemoradiation with concurrent fluorouracil-mitomycin is more effective than dose-escalated hyperfractionated accelerated radiation therapy alone in locally advanced head and neck cancer: final results of the Radiotherapy Cooperative Clinical Trials Group of the German Cancer Society 95-06 prospective randomized trial. *Journal of Clinical Oncology* 2005; **23**: 1125–35.

47. Al-Sarraf M, LeBlanc M, Giri SPG *et al.* Chemoradiotherapy versus radiotherapy in patients with advanced nasopharyngeal cancer: phase III randomized Intergroup Study 0099. *Journal of Clinical Oncology* 1998; **16**: 1310–17.

48. Wee J, Tan EH, Tai BC *et al.* Randomized trial of radiotherapy versus concurrent chemoradiotherapy followed by adjuvant chemotherapy in patients with American Joint Committee on Cancer/International Union Against Cancer stage III and IV nasopharyngeal cancer of the endemic variety. *Journal of Clinical Oncology* 2005; **23**: 6730–8.

49. Chan ATC, Leung SF, Ngan RKC *et al.* Overall survival after concurrent cisplatin-radiotherapy compared with radiotherapy alone in locoregionally advanced nasopharyngeal carcinoma. *Journal of the National Cancer Institute* 2005; **97**: 536–9.

50. Buentzel J, Micke O, Adamietz IA *et al.* Intravenous amifostine during chemoradiotherapy for head-and-neck cancer: a randomised placebo-controlled phase III study. *International Journal of Radiation Oncology, Biology, Physics* 2006; **64**: 684–91.

51. Hensley ML, Hagerty KL, Kewalramani T *et al.* American Society of Clinical Oncology 2008 clinical practice guideline update: use of chemotherapy and radiation therapy protectants. *Journal of Clinical Oncology* 2009; **27**: 127–45.

52. Jeremic B, Shibamoto Y, Milicic B *et al.* Hyperfractionated radiation therapy with or without concurrent low-dose daily cisplatin in locally advanced squamous cell carcinoma of the head and neck: a prospective randomized trial. *Journal of Clinical Oncology* 2000; **18**: 1458–64.

53. Dobrowsky W, Naudé J. Continuous hyperfractionated accelerated radiotherapy with/without mitomycin C in head and neck cancers. *Radiotherapy and Oncology* 2000; **57**: 119–24.

54. Bensadoun RJ, Bénézery K, Dasssonville O *et al.* French multicentre phase III randomised study testing concurrent twice-a-day radiotherapy and cisplatin/5-fluorouracil chemotherapy (BiRCF) in unresectable pharyngeal carcinoma: results at 2 years (FNCLCC-GORTEC). *International Journal of Radiation Oncology, Biology, Physics* 2006; **64**: 983–94.

55. Staar S, Rudat V, Stuetzer H *et al.* Intensified hyperfractionated accelerated radiotherapy limits the additional benefit of simultaneous chemotherapy – results of a multicentric randomized German trial in advanced head-and-neck cancer. *International Journal of Radiation Oncology, Biology, Physics* 2001; **50**: 1161–71.

56. Budach W, Hehr T, Budach V *et al.* A meta-analysis of hyperfractionated and accelerated radiotherapy and combined chemotherapy and radiotherapy regimens in unresected locally advanced squamous cell carcinoma of the head and neck. *BMC Cancer* 2006; **6**: 28; accessed January 7, 2010. Available from: www.biomedcentral.com/content/pdf/1471-2407-6-28.pdf.

57. Jeremic B, Milicic B, Dagovic A *et al.* Radiation therapy with or without concurrent low-dose daily chemotherapy in locally advanced, nonmetastatic squamous cell carcinoma of the head and neck. *Journal of Clinical Oncology* 2004; **22**: 3540–8.

58. Tupchong L, Scott CB, Blitzer PH *et al.* Randomized study of preoperative versus postoperative radiation therapy in advanced head and neck carcinoma: long-term follow-up of RTOG study 73-03. *International Journal of Radiation Oncology, Biology, Physics* 1991; **20**: 21–8.

59. Haffty BG, Son YH, Sasaki CT *et al.* Mitomycin C as an adjunct to postoperative radiation therapy in squamous cell carcinoma of the head and neck: results from two randomized clinical trials. *International Journal of Radiation Oncology, Biology, Physics* 1993; **27**: 241–50.

60. Bachaud JM, David JM, Boussin G, Daly N. Combined postoperative radiotherapy and weekly cisplatin infusion for locally advanced squamous cell carcinoma of the head and neck: preliminary report of a randomised trial. *International Journal of Radiation Oncology, Biology, Physics* 1991; **20**: 243–6.

61. Bernier J, Domenge C, Ozsahin M *et al.* Postoperative irradiation with or without concomitant chemotherapy for locally advanced head and neck cancer. *New England Journal of Medicine* 2004; **350**: 1945–52.

62. Cooper JS, Pajak TF, Forastiere AA *et al.* Postoperative concurrent radiotherapy and chemotherapy for high-risk squamous-cell carcinoma of the head and neck. *New England Journal of Medicine* 2004; **350**: 1937–44.

63. Bernier J, Cooper JS, Pajak TF *et al.* Defining risk levels in locally advanced head and neck cancers: a comparative analysis of concurrent postoperative radiation plus chemotherapy trials of the EORTC (#22931) and RTOG (#9501). *Head and Neck* 2005; **27**: 843–50.

64. Stell PM, Rawson NS. Adjuvant chemotherapy in head and neck cancer. *British Journal of Cancer* 1990; **61**: 779–87.

65. Munro AJ. An overview of randomised controlled trials of adjuvant chemotherapy in head and neck. *British Journal of Cancer* 1995; **71**: 83–91.

66. Pignon JP, Bourhis J, Domenge C *et al.* Chemotherapy added to locoregional treatment for head and neck squamous cell carcinoma: three meta-analyses of updated individual data. *Lancet* 2000; **355**: 949–55.

67. Pignon JP, le Maître A, Maillard E *et al.* Meta-analysis of chemotherapy in head and neck cancer (MACH-NC): an update on 93 randomised trials and 17,346 patients. *Radiotherapy and Oncology* 2009; **92**: 4–14.

68. Baujat B, Audry H, Bourhis J *et al.* Chemotherapy in locally advanced nasopharyngeal carcinoma: an individual-patient data meta-analysis of eight randomised trials and 1753 patients. *International Journal of Radiation Oncology, Biology, Physics* 2006; **64**: 47–56.

69. Kalyankrishna S, Grandis JR. Epidermal growth factor receptor biology in head and neck cancer. *Journal of Clinical Oncology* 2006; **24**: 2666–72.

70. Cohen EEW. Role of epidermal growth factor receptor pathway-targeted therapy in patients with recurrent and/or metastatic squamous cell carcinoma of the head and neck. *Journal of Clinical Oncology* 2006; **24**: 2659–65.

71. Ang KK, Berkey BA, Tu X *et al.* Impact of epidermal growth factor receptor expression on survival and pattern of relapse with advanced head and neck carcinoma. *Cancer Research* 2002; **62**: 7350–6.

72. Bonner JA, Maihle NJ, Folven BR *et al.* The interaction of epidermal growth factor and radiation in human head and neck squamous cell carcinoma cell lines with vastly different radiosensitivities. *International Journal of Radiation Oncology, Biology, Physics* 1994; **29**: 243–7.

73. Baselga J, Trigo JM, Bourhis J *et al.* Phase II multicenter study of the antiepidermal growth factor receptor monoclonal antibody cetuximab in combination with platinum-based chemotherapy in patients with platinum-refractory metastatic and/or recurrent squamous cell carcinoma of the head and neck. *Journal of Clinical Oncology* 2005; **23**: 5568–77.

74. Bonner JA, Harari PM, Giralt J *et al.* Radiotherapy plus cetuximab for squamous cell carcinoma of the head and neck. *New England Journal of Medicine* 2006; **354**: 567–78.

75. Bonner JA, Harari PM, Giralt J *et al.* Radiotherapy plus cetuximab for locally advanced head and neck cancer: 5-year survival data from a phase 3 randomised trial, and relation between cetuximab-induced rash and survival. *Lancet Oncology* 2010; **11**: 21–8.

76. Spaulding MB, Fischer SG, Wolf GT. Tumour response, toxicity, and survival after neoadjuvant organ-preserving chemotherapy for advanced laryngeal carcinoma. The Department of Veterans Affairs Cooperative Laryngeal Cancer Study Group. *Journal of Clinical Oncology* 1994; **12**: 1592–9.

77. Lefebvre JL, Chevalier D, Luboinski B *et al.* Larynx preservation in pyriform sinus cancer: preliminary results of a European Organisation for Research and Treatment of Cancer phase III trial. EORTC Head and Neck Cancer Cooperative Group. *Journal of the National Cancer Institute* 1996; **88**: 890–9.

78. Bourhis J, Wilson G, Wibault P *et al.* Rapid tumour cell proliferation after induction chemotherapy in oropharyngeal cancer. *Laryngoscope* 1994; **104**: 468–72.

79. Perez EA. Microtubule inhibitors: differentiating tubulin-inhibiting agents based on mechanisms of action, clinical activity and resistance. *Molecular Cancer Therapeutics* 2009; **8**: 2086–95.

80. Pignon JP, Syz N, Posner M *et al.* Adjusting for patient selection suggests the addition of Docetaxel to 5-fluorouracil-cisplatin therapy may offer survival benefit in squamous cell cancer of the head and neck. *Anticancer Drugs* 2004; **15**: 331–40.

81. Vermoken JB, Remenar E, van Herpen C *et al.* Cisplatin, fluorouracil, and docetaxel in unresectable head and neck cancer. *New England Journal of Medicine* 2007; **357**: 1695–704.

82. Posner MR, Hershock DM, Blajman CR *et al.* Cisplatin and fluorouracil alone or with docetaxel in head and neck cancer. *New England Journal of Medicine* 2007; **357**: 1705–15.

83. Pointreau Y, Garaud P, Chapet S *et al.* Randomized trial of induction chemotherapy with cisplatin and 5-fluorouracil with or without docetaxel for larynx preservation. *Journal of the National Cancer Institute* 2009; **101**: 498–506.

84. Hitt R, López-Pousa A, Martínez-Trufero J *et al.* Phase III study comparing cisplatin plus fluorouracil to paclitaxel, cisplatin, and fluorouracil induction chemotherapy followed by chemoradiotherapy in locally advanced head and neck cancer. *Journal of Clinical Oncology* 2005; **23**: 8636–45.

85. Colevas DA. Chemotherapy options for patients with metastatic or recurrent squamous cell carcinoma of the head and neck. *Journal of Clinical Oncology* 2006; **24**: 2644–52.

86. Forastiere AA, Metch B, Schuller DE *et al.* Randomized comparison of cisplatin plus fluorouracil and carboplatin plus fluorouracil versus methotrexate in advanced squamous-cell carcinoma of the head and neck: a

Southwest Oncology Group study. *Journal of Clinical Oncology* 1992; **10**: 1245–51.

87. Jacobs C, Lyman G, Velez-Garcia E *et al.* A phase III randomized study comparing cisplatin and fluorouracil as single agents and in combination for advanced squamous cell carcinoma of the head and neck. *Journal of Clinical Oncology* 1992; **10**: 257–63.

88. Clavel M, Vermorken JB, Cognetti F *et al.* Randomized comparison of cisplatin, methotrexate, bleomycin and vincristine (CABO) versus cisplatin and 5-fluorouracil (CF) versus cisplatin (C) in recurrent or metastatic squamous cell carcinoma of the head and neck. A phase III study of the EORTC Head and Neck Cooperative Group. *Annals of Oncology* 1994; **5**: 521–6.

89. Gibson MK, Li Y, Murphy B *et al.* Randomized phase III evaluation of cisplatin plus fluorouracil versus cisplatin plus paclitaxel in advanced head and neck cancer (E1395): an intergroup trial of the Eastern Cooperative Oncology Group. *Journal of Clinical Oncology* 2005; **23**: 3562–7.

90. Forastiere AA, Leong T, Rowinsky E *et al.* Phase III comparison of high-dose paclitaxel + cisplatin + granulocyte colony-stimulating factor versus low-dose paclitaxel + cisplatin in advanced head and neck cancer. Eastern Cooperative Oncology Group Study E1393. *Journal of Clinical Oncology* 2001; **19**: 1088–95.

91. Burtness B, Goldwasser MA, Flood W *et al.* Eastern Cooperative Oncology Group. Phase III randomized trial of cisplatin plus placebo compared with cisplatin plus cetuximab in metastatic/recurrent head and neck cancer: an Eastern Cooperative Oncology Group study. *Journal of Clinical Oncology* 2005; **23**: 8646–54.

● 92. Vermorken JB, Mesia R, Rivera F *et al.* Platinum-based chemotherapy plus cetuximab in head and neck cancer. *New England Journal of Medicine* 2008; **359**: 1116–27.

93. Xia P, Fu KK, Wong GW *et al.* Comparison of treatment plans involving intensity-modulated radiotherapy for nasopharyngeal carcinoma. *International Journal of Radiation Oncology, Biology, Physics* 2000; **48**: 329–37.

◆ 94. Gregoire V, Maingon P. Intensity modulated radiation therapy in head and neck squamous cell carcinoma: state of the art and future challenges. *Cancer Radiothérapie* 2005; **9**: 42–50.

95. Chao KS, Ozyigit G, Tran BN *et al.* Patterns of failure in patients receiving definitive and postoperative IMRT for head-and-neck cancer. *International Journal of Radiation Oncology, Biology, Physics* 2003; **55**: 312–21.

96. Chao KS, Ozyigit G, Blanco AI *et al.* Intensity-modulated radiation therapy for oropharyngeal carcinoma: impact of

tumour volume. *International Journal of Radiation Oncology, Biology, Physics* 2004; **59**: 43–50.

97. Eisbruch A, Ten Haken RK, Kim HM *et al.* Dose, volume, and function relationships in parotid salivary glands following conformal and intensity-modulated irradiation of head and neck cancer. *International Journal of Radiation Oncology, Biology, Physics* 1999; **45**: 577–87.

98. Dawson LA, Anzai Y, Marsh L *et al.* Patterns of local-regional recurrence following parotid sparing conformal and segmental intensity-modulated radiotherapy for head and neck cancer. *International Journal of Radiation Oncology, Biology, Physics* 2000; **46**: 1117–26.

99. Lee N, Xia P, Quivey JM *et al.* Intensity-modulated radiotherapy in the treatment of nasopharyngeal carcinoma: an update of the UCSF experience. *International Journal of Radiation Oncology, Biology, Physics* 2002; **53**: 12–22.

100. Kwong DL, Pow EH, Sham JS *et al.* Intensity-modulated radiotherapy for early-stage nasopharyngeal carcinoma: a prospective study on disease control and preservation of salivary function. *Cancer* 2004; **101**: 1584–93.

101. Wolden SL, Chen WC, Pfister DG *et al.* Intensity-modulated radiation therapy (IMRT) for nasopharynx cancer: update of the Memorial Sloan-Kettering experience. *International Journal of Radiation Oncology, Biology, Physics* 2006; **64**: 57–62.

102. Graff P, Lapeyre M, Desandes E *et al.* Impact of intensity-modulated radiotherapy on health-related quality of life for head and neck cancer patients: matched pair comparison with conventional radiotherapy. *International Journal of Radiation Oncology, Biology, Physics* 2007; **67**: 1309–17.

103. Paulino AC, Koshy M, Howell R *et al.* Comparison of CT- and FDG-PET-defined gross tumour volume in intensity-modulated radiotherapy for head-and-neck cancer. *International Journal of Radiation Oncology, Biology, Physics* 2005; **61**: 1385–92.

104. Schwartz DL, Ford EC, Rajendran J *et al.* FDG-PET/CT-guided intensity modulated head and neck cancer radiotherapy: a pilot investigation. *Head and Neck* 2005; **27**: 478–87.

105. Kry SF, Salehpour M, Followill DS *et al.* The calculated risk of fatal secondary malignancies from intensity-modulated radiation therapy. *International Journal of Radiation Oncology, Biology, Physics* 2005; **62**: 1195–203.

◆ 106. Mendenhall WM, Amdur RJ, Palta JR. Intensity-modulated radiotherapy in the standard management of head and neck cancer: promises and pitfalls. *Journal of Clinical Oncology* 2006; **24**: 2618–23.

46

Biologically targeted agents

KEVIN J HARRINGTON

The odds of hitting your target go up dramatically when you aim at it

Mal Pancoast

INTRODUCTION

The non-surgical management of head and neck cancer has undergone a number of significant changes in the last decade. These include: (1) the application of technological advances in radiation delivery as a means of reducing normal tissue toxicity and potentially increasing dose to tumour tissue;[1, 2, 3, 4, 5] (2) the clear demonstration of the superiority of concomitant chemoradiotherapy over radiotherapy alone in both definitive[6] and adjuvant settings;[7, 8] and (3) the identification of some of the molecular biological processes that drive the disease and the development of new therapies that target specifically them.[9]

Improved understanding of the molecular biology of cancer has fundamentally changed the search for new therapies for malignant disease. Central to this change has been the realization that cancer is a genetic disease that occurs when the information contained in cellular (DNA) is corrupted or decoded aberrantly. These changes are manifest as altered patterns of gene expression which are detected in cancer cells in terms of derangement of normal protein function. In simple terms, the genetic changes that result in the development of cancers can be considered to mediate two general effects: (1) enhancement of the activity of genes that stimulate cell growth, survival and spread and (2) reduction of the actions of genes that repress these processes. As a consequence of these changes, cancer cells acquire the properties that allow them to grow in an uncontrolled fashion, invade adjacent normal tissues, recruit a dedicated blood supply, spread to distant metastatic sites and develop resistance to anticancer therapies.

In this chapter, the key normal cellular processes that are altered in head and neck cancer cells will be described. This essential background information will form the basis of a discussion of the new therapeutic opportunities that are now being assessed in clinical trials and will facilitate an attempt to predict important new targeted treatment combinations for head and neck cancer.

MOLECULAR BIOLOGY OF HEAD AND NECK CANCER

The genetic code

The genetic code is contained in DNA molecules that are packaged in chromosomes in the nucleus of the cell. DNA molecules consist of a sugar-phosphate backbone (deoxyribose sugars joined by phosphate linkages) with each sugar bearing one of four nucleotide bases (the purines adenine (A) and guanine (G) and the pyrimidines thymine (T) and cytosine (C)). Two DNA strands twist around one another to form a double helix with the bases forming hydrogen bonds with specific partners in the opposite strand: A is only able to form pairs with T; C is only able to form pairs with G (**Figure 46.1**). The helix is wound around nucleosomes, consisting of histone proteins, and is further condensed to form chromatin. The entire genetic code consists of approximately 3.2×10^9 bases and contains approximately 30 000 genes, which account for only about 1 per cent of the genome. The DNA sequence within a gene comprises so-called exons and introns. The exons represent the protein-coding regions that

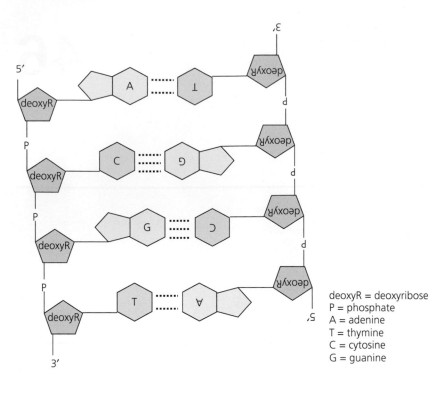

deoxyR = deoxyribose
P = phosphate
A = adenine
T = thymine
C = cytosine
G = guanine

Figure 46.1 The structure of DNA. DNA consists of a double helix composed of a deoxyribose sugar-phosphate backbone and four bases (adenine, guanine, thymine and cytosine). The four bases form hydrogen bonds with specific bases on the opposite strand. A binds with T and C binds with G.

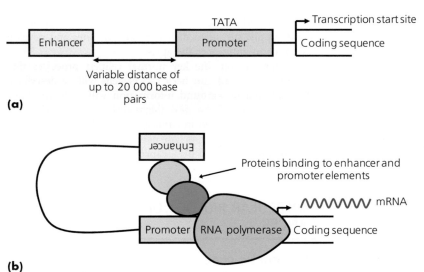

Figure 46.2 Schematic representation of transcriptional control elements involved in the regulation of gene expression. (a) The coding sequence of a gene is controlled by a proximal upstream promoter element (Promoter) and a distal enhancer. The promoter contains a TATA-box sequence which acts as a binding site for the TATA factor. (b) Binding of regulatory proteins to enhancer and promoter regions regulates their interaction and the assembly of the transcriptional machinery and subsequent mRNA synthesis.

are translated at the ribosome, whereas the introns are non-encoding and are edited (spliced) out before translation can occur.

The function of genes is to make proteins and this process occurs in two steps. First, because the DNA code is confined to the nucleus, its information must be carried to the site of protein production by a messenger ribonucleic acid (mRNA) molecule. This process of making a copy of the information in the DNA code is called transcription (**Figure 46.2**). RNA differs from DNA in two ways: (1) the sugar backbone contains ribose (not deoxyribose) and (2) thymine is replaced by uracil (U). The process by which genetic information is transcribed into mRNA, transported to the ribosome and translated into a cellular protein is complex and subject to multiple levels of control. Regulation of transcription is the key initiating event in the process and is mediated by the

interaction between enhancer/promoter elements in the DNA and specific proteins (>100 individual subunits) that bind to them. At the transcription start site, a DNA-dependent RNA polymerase II is recruited and begins to synthesize an mRNA molecule that is said to be complementary to the coding strand of DNA. This means that the DNA sequence that is being transcribed serves as a template for the production of a specific mRNA molecule, e.g. the DNA sequence CGTATACG becomes GCAUAUGC in the mRNA (note the substitution of U for T in RNA). This mRNA molecule is then subjected to a number of so-called post-transcriptional modifications that include splicing out of introns and processing the ends of the molecule to make it ready for export from the nucleus to the cytoplasm. Many human genes (approximately 60 per cent) can undergo alternate splicing of the mRNA transcripts which means that one gene can give rise to the production of a number of different protein molecules. Once the mRNA is in the cytoplasm it may be degraded by cellular small interfering RNA molecules (siRNA) before translation occurs. If the mRNA reaches the ribosome, it is decoded into a specific protein molecule through the process of translation, which is based on the fact that groups of three nucleotides represent specific amino acids (e.g. the sequence AUG encodes methionine). It is the protein products of genes that mediate the functional (phenotypic) changes that we recognize as cancer.

Cancer genes

The functions of two classes of genes (oncogenes and tumour suppressor genes) lie at the heart of any understanding of the biology of cancer (reviewed in Ref. 10).

Oncogenes are derived from mutated versions of normal cellular genes (called proto-oncogenes) that encode proteins that control cell proliferation, survival and spread. In normal cells, the expression of proto-oncogenes is very tightly regulated to avoid uncontrolled cell growth. In cancer, abnormalities of proto-oncogenes are responsible for uncontrolled cell division, enhanced survival (even in the face of anticancer treatment) and dissemination. Oncogenes are phenotypically dominant – i.e. a single mutated copy of a proto-oncogene is sufficient to promote cancer – and are almost never responsible for inherited cancer syndromes, with the exception of Ret in hereditary endocrine tumours. Oncogenes can be activated in three ways to cause cancers (see **Figure 46.3**): (1) gene mutation involves the acquisition of a specific defect in the sequence of a gene such that the gene has enhanced function (e.g. Ras in pancreatic and colorectal cancers); (2) gene amplification occurs when a gene retains its normal sequence – but the gene is multiply repeated in the chromosome (e.g. N-myc in neuroblastoma); (3) gene translocation involves the gene being moved from its normal chromosomal position (locus) to a new position (usually on a different chromosome) where it comes under the influence of a new, more active promoter element (e.g. c-myc in Burkitt lymphoma) or forms

a novel fusion protein (e.g. bcr-abl in chronic myeloid leukaemia).

Tumour suppressor genes (TSG) are normal cellular genes whose function involves inhibition of cell proliferation and survival. They are frequently involved in controlling cell cycle progression and apoptosis. TSG are phenotypically recessive – i.e. the function of both copies must be lost in order to promote cancer – and are responsible for inherited cancer syndromes. In familial cancer syndromes, individuals inherit a germ line mutation in one copy (allele) of a TSG such that every cell in the body is affected. It is, therefore, highly likely that at least one cell in the body will suffer complete loss of TSG function because only one copy has to be mutated (so-called loss of heterozygosity). As a result, hereditary cancer syndromes often give rise to multiple cancers at an early age.

The hallmarks of cancer

Hanahan and Weinberg[11] described six key changes that occur in cancers and which are largely responsible for driving their malignant behaviour (**Box 46.1**).

This schema provides a useful way of thinking about the different ways in which cancer can be targeted. However, for individual tumour types, it is becoming clear that some of these processes may represent better targets than others. In the following sections, the individual hallmarks of cancer will

---

Box 46.1   The hallmarks of cancer

- Growth factor independence or self-sufficiency
- Ability to recruit a dedicated blood supply
- Avoidance of programmed cell death (apoptosis)
- Insensitivity to anti-growth signals
- Immortalization by reactivation of telomerase
- Ability to invade adjacent normal tissues and metastasize to distant sites

---

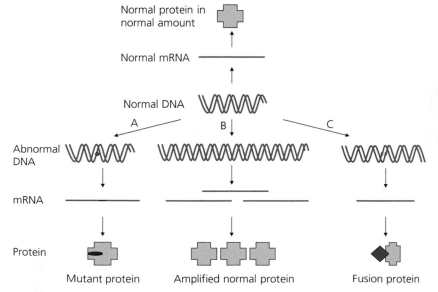

Figure 46.3 Oncogenic activation can occur via three pathways. Normal gene expression leads to formation of normal mRNA and expression of a normal protein in normal amounts. A. Specific mutations in the sequence of the DNA code lead to alterations in the amino acid sequence of the protein, giving it enhanced activity. B. Increased numbers of normal copies of the gene (amplification) result in the formation of increased amounts of normal protein. C. Translocation of part of DNA from one chromosomal location to another can result in the generation of a fusion protein with enhanced biological activity.

be discussed and their potential as targets for therapeutic intervention in head and neck cancer will be reviewed.

TARGETING GROWTH FACTOR INDEPENDENCE

A general scheme for the function of growth factor receptors and their ligands in promoting head and neck cancer cell growth (and other effects) is shown in **Figure 46.4**. In this case, binding of the cognate ligand to the specific ligand-binding domain on the extracellular component of the growth factor receptor (GFR) leads to a change in the shape of the protein that allows it to form a dimer (two protein molecules) with another identical GFR (homodimer) or with other members of the same receptor family (heterodimer). This dimerization process results in the intracytoplasmic domains of the adjacent receptors each adding phosphate groups to tyrosine residues on the other. For this reason, these receptors are known as tyrosine kinase receptors. Phosphorylation of tyrosine residues in the tails of the receptors leads to a cascade of signals via so-called secondary messengers such that the binding of a protein on the cell surface is able to influence the behaviour of the cell. Under normal circumstances, activation of growth factor receptors is very tightly controlled – as is the synthesis and release of the ligands that bind to them. The signalling pathway is normally responsible for regulating physiological cellular processes, such as epithelial tissue development and response to injury.

c–erbB receptor family

One extremely important family of GFR is represented by the c–erbB receptors of the transmembrane type I receptor tyrosine kinase family. This family comprises four members: the epidermal growth factor receptor (EGFR) or c-erbB-1, c-erbB-2/neu/HER-2, c-erbB-3/HER-3 and c-erbB-4/HER-4.[12, 13] They consist of a large glycosylated extracellular ligand-binding domain, a hydrophobic transmembrane component and an intracellular domain with tyrosine kinase activity.

Head and neck cancer cells very frequently (>90 per cent) usurp normal EGFR-mediated signalling pathways.[12] By doing so, they are able to gain a growth and survival advantage over neighbouring normal cells. Cancer cells exploit three main strategies for achieving self-sufficiency in growth factors: (1) they manufacture and release growth factors which stimulate their own receptors (autocrine signalling) and those of their immediate neighbours (paracrine signalling); (2) they alter the number, structure or function of the growth factor receptors on their surface such that they are more likely to send a growth signal to the nucleus (even in the absence of the cognate ligand); (3) they deregulate the signalling pathway downstream of the growth factor receptor so that it is permanently turned on (constitutively active).

Squamous cell cancer of the head and neck is probably the most clearly described example of EGFR-driven oncogenesis because this is the dominant signalling pathway responsible for the malignant features of the disease and overexpression has been shown to correlate with poor survival.[14, 15] Currently, 12 major ligands with a shared EGF-like motif and affinity for the family of c-erbB receptors are known. The consequences of receptor dimerization and activation and subsequent intracellular signalling provide mechanistic explanations for many of the features that characterize head and neck cancers.[16] EGFR is a 170 kDa protein and the founding member of the receptor family.[17] In contrast to certain tumour types where EGFR gene amplification or mutation is implicated, overexpression of the receptor, without gene amplification, appears to be the dominant process in squamous cell cancer of the head and neck (SCCHN). Elevated levels of EGFR mRNA and protein and of the ligand transforming growth factor-alpha (TGFα) are present in normal mucosa several centimetres from a malignant lesion. TGFα upregulation is also detectable in pre-invasive lesions and mild dysplasia, consistent with the theory of 'field cancerization' due to exposure to environmental chemical carcinogens.[18, 19, 20] Upregulation of EGFR is a significant early event in the progression from pre-invasive mucosal dysplasia to invasive head and neck cancer and is most marked in lesions displaying greater dysplasia.[20]

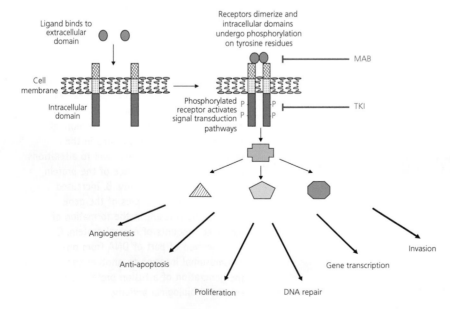

Figure 46.4 Growth factor independence can lead to sustained signalling in pathways that control essential biological functions, such as growth, apoptosis, angiogenesis, invasion and DNA damage repair. Signal transduction can be blocked by monoclonal antibodies (MAB) that target the extracellular domain of the receptor or by small molecule tyrosine kinase inhibitors (TKI) that interact with enzymatic activity in the intracellular part of the receptor.

Several studies have shown links between EGFR over-expression and head and neck cancer oncogenesis and progression.[21, 22, 23] In an experimental xenograft model where highly metastatic sublines were isolated by *in vivo* selection from nodal metastases, EGFR was one of only 33 differentially expressed genes, showing a two-fold upregulation.[24] A mutated version of EGFR (EGFRvIII) is the most common of seven known variants of EGFR. Deletion of exons 2–7 of the EGFR gene results in a truncated extracellular domain and constitutive activation of the intracellular tyrosine kinase, which continuously triggers multiple downstream phosphorylation cascades. EGFRvIII can associate with and activate wild-type EGFR in the absence of ligand. This particular mutation is common in tumour types such as glioblastoma multiforme and non-small cell lung cancer, and has recently been reported to be present in 42 per cent of head and neck cancers.[25]

The c-erbB-2 receptor is a 185 kDa receptor-like phosphoglycoprotein with no known exogenous ligand. When highly overexpressed it may spontaneously dimerize and autoactivate, but it is more frequently activated by heterodimerization with other erbB receptors. The contribution of c-erbB-2 expression to the pathogenesis of head and neck cancer is less well defined than in other tumour types such as breast and ovarian cancer. However, c-erbB-2:c-erbB-3 heterodimers are potent inducers of the PI3-kinase anti-apoptotic pathway[26] as c-erbB-3 can bind directly to the PI3-kinase p85 subunit. Increasing expression of c-erbB-2 has been shown in parallel with acquisition of a more malignant phenotype in a series of oral carcinomas, which may imply a role in progression.[23, 27] The distribution of c-erbB-3 protein in tissues is different from that of EGFR and c-erbB-2. It does not have intrinsic tyrosine kinase activity but it can be transphosphorylated by both EGFR and c-erbB2. Its overexpression (but not amplification) has been found in head and neck cancer cell lines and in some cases it has been related to malignant potential. There has been comparatively little investigation of erbB-3 and erbB-4 in clinical samples from head and neck cancers, probably due to the low detection (~10 per cent) in immunohistochemical surveys of clinical specimens.[28] Xia *et al.* have indicated that expression of all four receptors is associated with shortened survival in patients with oral squamous cell carcinoma, with the combination of EGFR, erbB-2 and erbB-3 (but not erbB-4) giving the greatest prognostic information.[29]

c-erbB receptor family as a therapeutic target

c-erbB receptors represent an extremely attractive molecular target in head and neck cancers, because their overexpression in tumour cells offers the prospect of antitumour selectivity (see **Figure 46.5**). Two classes of drugs have entered clinical trials: (1) monoclonal antibodies (MAB) directed against the extracellular domain of the receptor and (2) small molecules inhibiting receptor tyrosine kinase (TK) activity (so-called TKi). The relative advantages and disadvantages of EGFR blocking agents are detailed in **Table 46.1**.

Anti-EGFR monoclonal antibodies

A number of MAB have been developed for clinical evaluation. They differ from one another in terms of their species of origin (murine, chimeric or fully humanized) and the specific part (epitope) of the target protein that they recognize. Cetuximab (C225, Erbitux®) is a human–murine chimeric monoclonal antibody against EGFR which has undergone extensive preclinical and clinical evaluation. *In vitro* studies have demonstrated antitumour activity against several tumour cell lines through a range of mechanisms including an antiproliferative effect, direct cytotoxicity and the potentiation of the cytotoxic effects of chemotherapy or radiotherapy.[30, 31, 32, 33] In addition, *in vivo* experiments have demonstrated anti-angiogenic actions.[34] This agent has been evaluated in early stage clinical trials with favourable indications of efficacy in combination with chemotherapy or radiotherapy.[35, 36, 37, 38, 39]

The most significant trial to date reporting on the impact of EGFR inhibition in combination with radiotherapy was conducted using cetuximab in patients with head and neck

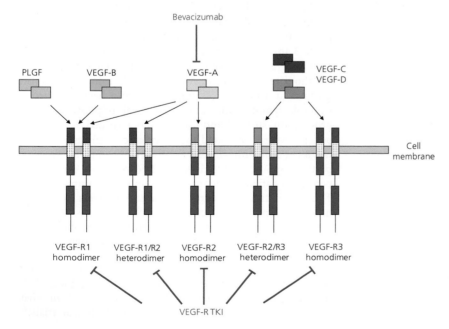

Figure 46.5 Vascular endothelial growth factor (VEGF) receptor signalling. VEGF-R can form homo- or heterodimeric complexes that are capable of binding different activating ligands. VEGF-A is the dominant ligand involved in signalling through VEGF-R2 to mediate new blood vessel formation in tumours. Activation of this receptor can be inhibited by binding of the ligand by an anti-VEGF-A antibody (bevacizumab) or by small molecule VEGF-receptor tyrosine kinase inhibitors (VEGF-R TKI).

Table 46.1 Advantages and disadvantages of epidermal growth factor receptor blockade as a therapeutic strategy.

Advantages	Disadvantages
Prevent accelerated repopulation	Stasis in resistant phase of cell cycle
Enhance apoptotic signalling	Promote tumour hypoxia
Reduce invasion	Enhance normal tissue toxicity
Inhibit pro-angiogenic signalling	Off-target systemic toxicity
Inhibit DNA repair	

cancer.[40] Four hundred and twenty-four patients with locally advanced head and neck cancer were randomly allocated to treatment with either radical radiotherapy alone or in combination with weekly cetuximab. The combination treatment arm had significantly improved locoregional control (24.4 months versus 14.9 months; hazard ratio 0.68, $p = 0.005$), improved progression-free survival (hazard ratio 0.70, $p = 0.006$) and improved overall survival (hazard ratio 0.74, $p = 0.03$). Other than a higher incidence of rash and infusion reactions, the grade 3 and greater toxic effects did not differ significantly between the two groups. Further studies are in progress addressing the use of cetuximab in combination with radical chemoradiotherapy in patients with locally advanced head and neck cancer.

Cetuximab has also recently been shown to improve the outcome of palliative chemotherapy in a large randomized phase III study.[41] This is the first new agent to demonstrate an improvement in survival in the setting of relapsed/metastatic head and neck cancer. In this study in 442 eligible patients with untreated recurrent or metastatic SCCHN, cisplatin ($100 \, mg/m^2$) or carboplatin (area under the curve of $5 \, mg/mL/min$) plus 5-fluorouracil ($1 \, g/m^2$ per day for 4 days) was administered every 3 weeks for a maximum of six cycles. Two hundred and twenty-two patients received the same chemotherapy plus cetuximab ($400 \, mg/m^2$ initially, then $250 \, mg/m^2$ per week) for a maximum of six cycles. Patients with stable disease who received chemotherapy plus cetuximab continued with cetuximab until disease progression or unacceptable toxicity. Adding cetuximab to platinum-based chemotherapy with fluorouracil significantly prolonged the median overall survival from 7.4 months in the chemotherapy alone group to 10.1 months in the group that received chemotherapy plus cetuximab (hazard ratio for death, 0.80; 95 per cent confidence interval, 0.64–0.99; $p = 0.04$). The median progression-free survival time was prolonged from 3.3 to 5.6 months (hazard ratio for progression, 0.54; $p < 0.001$) and the response rate increased from 20 to 36 per cent ($p < 0.001$).

A number of other monoclonal antibodies have entered clinical trials. They include agents such as zalutumumab and panitumumab.[42, 43, 44] These agents differ from cetuximab, which is a chimeric human–murine antibody, in terms of their degree of humanization. Randomized evaluations of these agents in settings that are similar to those in which cetuximab has proven activity are ongoing and are likely to yield interesting and important data in the near future.

Small molecule tyrosine kinase inhibitors

Gefitinib (ZD1839, Iressa®) is a low-molecular weight tyrosine kinase inhibitor (TKI) that is highly specific for EGFR. By competing with adenosine triphosphate (ATP) on the intracellular domain of EGFR it has been shown to prevent receptor autophosphorylation, with resultant antiproliferative effects observed in a variety of human xenograft models. Furthermore, combining gefitinib with cytotoxic chemotherapy increases growth inhibition and apoptotic cell death.[45, 46, 47]

Four phase I studies have evaluated gefitinib in more than 250 patients, of whom 28 had head and neck cancer.[48, 49, 50, 51] Gefitinib was well-tolerated at doses from 150 to $800 \, mg/m^2$, the most frequent grade 1 or 2 toxicities being diarrhoea (47–55 per cent), asthenia (44 per cent) and an acneiform follicular rash (46–64 per cent). Antitumour activity, including both partial responses and cases of prolonged stable disease, was observed at all doses. Clinically meaningful stable disease was achieved in 50 per cent of patients with head and neck cancer, and quality of life ratings also remained stable during treatment, except in one study where they improved significantly over time.[52]

A phase II study has evaluated oral gefitinib ($500 \, mg/day$) as first- or second-line monotherapy in 52 patients with recurrent or metastatic head and neck cancer, most of whom had previously received combination chemotherapy or radiotherapy.[53, 54] Of these, 47 patients were evaluable for tumour response and an objective partial response rate of 10.6 per cent (one complete response) was demonstrated. Disease control, defined as objective tumour response plus stable disease, was achieved in 53 per cent of patients and was sustained for more than six months in 13 per cent of patients. The response rates and survival times of patients who received gefitinib as first-line therapy were not significantly different to those of patients who had received prior chemotherapy. Overall, the median times to progression and death were 3.4 months and 8.1 months, respectively, with an estimated one-year survival of 29 per cent. These results are more favourable than those achieved with chemotherapy in this setting, but with the additional benefit of reduced treatment-related toxicity. There was only a single case of grade 4 toxicity (hypercalcaemia), a 4–6 per cent incidence of grade 3 toxicity (anorexia, diarrhoea, nausea and hypercalcaemia), grade 1 or 2 skin rash in 48 per cent and grade 1 or 2 diarrhoea in 50 per cent. A second study using single-agent gefitinib at a dose of $500 \, mg/day$ has also been reported.[55] Clinical, symptomatic and radiological response, time to progression, survival and toxicity were recorded. Forty-seven patients were treated and the observed clinical response rate was 8 per cent with a disease control rate (complete response, partial response, stable disease) of 36 per cent. Thirty-four percent of patients experienced a symptomatic improvement. The median time to progression and survival were 2.6 and 4.3 months, respectively. Acneiform folliculitis was the most frequent toxicity observed (76 per cent), but the majority of cases were grade 1 or 2. Only four patients experienced grade 3 toxicity of any type (all cases of folliculitis).

Lapatinib is an oral dual TK inhibitor with action against both EGFR (c-erbB1, HER-1) and c-erbB2 (HER-2).[56, 57] It has demonstrated activity both *in vitro* and *in vivo*, as well as showing tolerability in phase I clinical trials.[57]

A placebo-controlled randomized phase 0 biomarker study has been performed with this agent in patients with advanced head and neck cancer. A single agent response rate of 17 per cent was reported, with biomarker evidence of significantly reduced proliferation and receptor phosphorylation in the lapatinib-treated group.[58] A phase I dose escalation study of lapatinib administered during radical chemoradiotherapy has been completed in patients with stage III and IV head and neck cancer.[59] Patients were enrolled in cohorts of escalating lapatinib dose: 500 mg, 1000 mg and 1500 mg/day. Patients received 1 week of lapatinib alone followed by 6.5–7 weeks of the same dose of lapatinib plus radiotherapy 66–70 Gy and cisplatin 100 mg/m^2 on days 1, 22 and 43 of radiotherapy. End points included safety/tolerability and clinical activity. Thirty-one patients were enrolled (seven in each of the 500 mg and 1000 mg cohorts, 17 in the 1500 mg cohort (14 in a safety cohort)). Dose-limiting toxicities (DLT) observed were perforated ulcer in one patient in the 500 mg cohort, and transient elevation of liver enzymes in one patient in the 1000 mg cohort. No DLTs were observed in the 1500 mg cohort. The recommended phase II dose was therefore defined as lapatinib 1500 mg/day with chemoradiation. The most common grade 3–4 adverse events were radiation mucositis, radiation dermatitis, lymphopenia and neutropenia. No patients experienced drug-related symptomatic cardiotoxicity, and no interstitial pneumonitis was reported. The overall response rate was 81 per cent (65 per cent at the recommended phase II dose). The recommended phase II dose is lapatinib 1500 mg/day with chemoradiation in patients with locally advanced SCCHN, and is associated with an acceptable tolerability profile. Based on these findings, randomized phase II and III studies of lapatinib plus chemoradiation have been initiated. The results of these studies are awaited with interest.

TARGETING SUSTAINED ANGIOGENESIS

In normal tissues, the growth of new blood vessels (angiogenesis) is held very tightly in check by a balance between positive (pro-angiogenic) and negative (anti-angiogenic) signals (see **Box 46.2**).

The growth of cancer deposits is intimately related to their ability to secure a blood supply. A small cluster of cancer cells can grow to 60–100 μm by deriving a supply of oxygen and nutrients by direct diffusion, but beyond this size the fledgling tumour must acquire a dedicated blood supply. Cancers acquire their new blood supply by subverting the balance between pro- and anti-angiogenic factors.[60, 61] Essentially, cancers switch to an 'angiogenic phenotype' by upregulating production of pro-angiogenic proteins such as vascular endothelial growth factor (VEGF), basic fibroblast growth factor (bFGF) and platelet-derived growth factor (PDGF) and/or by downregulating production of anti-angiogenic proteins such as thrombospondin-1, angiostatin and endostatin. Cancer-associated endothelial cells have receptors for both growth promoting and inhibitory factors (**Figure 46.5**). Binding of cognate ligand to a VEGF receptor on the endothelial cell causes receptor tyrosine kinase activation and downstream signalling to stimulate endothelial cell proliferation, vessel permeability and migration. The net result is formation of new blood vessels. VEGF production in tumour

---

Box 46.2   Pro- and anti-angiogenic factors

Pro-angiogenic

- Vascular endothelial growth factor (VEGF)
- Basic fibroblast growth factor (bFGF)
- Acidic fibroblast growth factor (aFGF)
- Transforming growth factors-alpha and -beta (TGF-α, TGF-β)
- Platelet-derived growth factor (PDGF)
- Tumour necrosis factor-alpha (TNF-α)

Anti-angiogenic

- Angiostatin
- Endostatin
- Thrombospondin-1 and -2 (TSP-1, TSP-2)
- Interleukins (IL-1β, IL-12, IL-18)
- Antithrombin III

---

cells is frequently under the control of hypoxia inducible factor (HIF)-1α, which is a transcription factor that is activated by low cellular oxygen tension.

Drugs that target angiogenesis can be classified into two main groups: (1) vascular disrupting agents and (2) anti-angiogenic agents.[62] Vascular disrupting agents cause rapid and selective dysfunction of existing tumour vasculature leading to tumour death. Tubulin-destabilizing agents like combretastatin A4 phosphate and ZD6126 are two such agents.[62, 63, 64] The attraction of these agents is their potential ability to deprive large areas of tumour of a blood supply, with resulting widespread tumour cell death. As such, they are likely to lead to tumour regressions. However, their ability to cause vascular shutdown may also theoretically increase the presence of tumour hypoxia – a factor that is known to be correlated with resistance to standard therapeutics. Anti-angiogenic agents work in a completely different fashion by inhibiting new blood vessel formation, without having an effect on established tumour vasculature. This is achieved by either binding VEGF or inhibiting VEGF-R activation.[61] Bevacizumab (Avastin™) is a humanized monoclonal antibody to the VEGFR ligand VEGF-A. VEGF-R tyrosine TKIs also have anti-angiogenic properties through their ability to inhibit phosphorylation of the tyrosine residues in the cytoplasmic domain of the receptor. A number of small molecule TKIs (SU6668, SU5416 (semaxanib), SU11248 (sunitinib), SU11657, PTK787/ZK222584 (vatalanib) and ZD6474) have shown promise in tumour types other than head and neck cancer.[61] It is highly likely that these agents will be assessed in head and neck cancer in combination with chemotherapy and/or radiotherapy.

As regards the combination of vascular disrupting or anti-angiogenic agents with standard therapeutic agents (radiotherapy, chemotherapy), there are a number of theoretical considerations that might suggest that this approach could be detrimental. For example, depriving a tumour of its blood supply (either acutely by vascular disruption or chronically by reducing angiogenesis) is likely to increase tumour hypoxia – a factor that is known to mediate treatment resistance. However, for the anti-angiogenic agents, Jain and colleagues have suggested that treatment can lead to normalization of the tumour vasculature – if the dose and duration of treatment lies within certain parameters.[65, 66] The existence of this so-called 'vascular normalization window' is supported by experimental data, but not yet by clinical trial findings. In addition, for the vascular disrupting drugs, it is possible that they can be used to trap radiosensitizing compounds or cytotoxic drugs within tumour tissue by collapsing the vascular networks that will serve to wash the drug out of the tissue. In view of both of these rationalizations, there is enormous interest in combining anti-VEGF monoclonal antibodies, VEGF-R TKIs and vascular disrupting agents with radiation and/or chemotherapy.

TARGETING THE APOPTOTIC PATHWAY

Normal cells continually audit their viability by assessing the balance of survival (anti-apoptotic) and death (pro-apoptotic) signals that they receive. In normal cells, DNA damage leads to a block in proliferation (cell cycle arrest) while the potential for repair is assessed. If the level of damage exceeds the capacity for repair, the balance of anti- and pro-apoptotic signals tips and the cell undergoes programmed cell death (apoptosis). This prevents maintenance of DNA damage and avoids the risk that mutations will be passed to the progeny of cell division. As such, this mechanism represents a very powerful barrier to the development of cancer.

Loss of normal apoptotic pathway signalling is an extremely common event in cancer. Indeed, two of the best known cancer-associated genes (p53 (TSG) and bcl-2 (oncogene)) are intimately involved in apoptosis. The two main mechanisms of apoptotic signalling (intrinsic and extrinsic pathways) are illustrated in a simplified form in **Figure 46.6**. Cancer cells are able to evade apoptosis through an ability to ignore signals sent through the extrinsic pathway or by resetting the balance of intracellular pro- and anti-apoptotic molecules in favour of inhibition of apoptosis. By circumventing apoptosis, cancer cells can sustain DNA damage without it causing cell death (unless the damage is to a gene that is absolutely

necessary for cell survival). Therefore, cancer cells that have switched off their apoptotic pathway are more likely to be intrinsically resistant to anticancer treatments. In fact, the use of these treatments may promote the accumulation of other mutations that may have a negative influence on the biology of the disease.

Therefore, targeting the apoptotic machinery represents a potentially attractive new therapeutic option in a range of cancers, including head and neck cancer. In general terms, there are two specific strategies that are under investigation: enhancing pro-apoptotic signalling by stimulating the extrinsic pathway and blocking the anti-apoptotic regulators of the intrinsic pathway (**Figure 46.6**).

The first of these approaches has been assessed preclinically and in early phase clinical trials using both recombinant pro-apoptotic receptor ligands (recombinant human apoptotic ligand 2/tumour necrosis factor-related apoptosis inducing ligand (rhApo2L/TRAIL))[67] and monoclonal antibodies that can stimulate the DR4 and DR5 death receptors.[68] Agonistic humanized or human monoclonal antibodies against DR4 and DR5 have been tested in phase I and II trials in patients with advanced cancer (other than head and neck cancer).[68] These trials have shown that these antibodies are well tolerated and are capable of producing prolonged stable disease. Clinical studies in which TRAIL-receptor antibodies are being investigated in combination treatment regimens in patients with advanced cancer are ongoing. It is anticipated that the results from a broad spectrum of cancer therapy clinical trials will identify the activity and toxicity profiles of TRAIL death-receptor antibodies as single agents, or in combination with chemotherapy agents or radiotherapy. Studies in patients with head and neck cancer are ongoing and will be reported in the near future.

The second approach to enhancing apoptosis is targeted blockade of anti-apoptotic signalling pathways. This strategy has largely relied on the approach of using antisense oligo-nucleotides to reduce the expression of proteins such as Bcl-2 in cancer cells. *In vitro* and *in vivo* studies in murine models have suggested that targeted reduction of Bcl-2 expression can enhance the therapeutic efficacy of chemotherapy or radiotherapy in head and neck models.[69, 70]

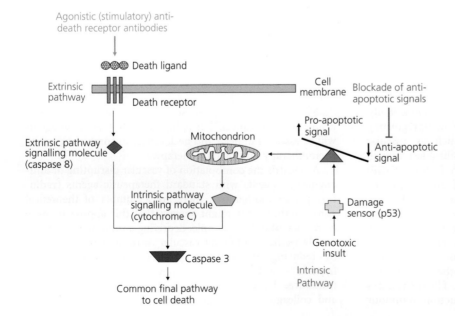

Figure 46.6 Normal apoptotic signalling pathways. Cells can undergo programmed cell death in response to activation of either the intrinsic or extrinsic apoptotic pathway. Cancers frequently subvert these pathways to allow them to survive signals that would lead to the death of normal cells. The extrinsic pathway can be activated by agonistic monoclonal antibodies that can stimulate the DR4 and DR5 death receptors. Alternatively, the intrinsic pathway can be activated by inhibiting anti-apoptotic signalling (e.g. blockade of Bcl-2 or XIAP).

However, this has not yet been tested in patients with head and neck cancer in the clinic. In recent years, another means of blocking anti-apoptotic regulators of the intrinsic pathway has received considerable research attention. This approach is based on blocking the actions of inhibitor of apoptosis proteins[71] A prime example of this group of proteins is provided by the X-linked inhibitor of apoptosis protein (XIAP) which is a component of the final common pathway that inhibits caspases and suppresses apoptosis. XIAP is overexpressed in many cancer cell lines and cancer tissues and its expression has been correlated with resistance to chemotherapy and radiotherapy and to poor clinical outcome. Inhibition of XIAP can be achieved with either antisense oligonucleotides or small molecule inhibitors. *In vitro*, XIAP antagonists produce XIAP knockdown and apoptosis which is associated with sensitization of tumour cells to radiotherapy and cytotoxic drugs.[71] *In vivo*, XIAP antagonists have antitumour effects and sensitize tumours to the effects of chemotherapy. This group of agents is currently undergoing phase I evaluation and may have potential in solid cancers such as head and neck cancer.

TARGETING INSENSITIVITY TO ANTI-GROWTH SIGNALS

There are a number of normal anti-growth signals that counteract the positively acting growth signals described above. Anti-growth signals work either by forcing cells into quiescence (G0 stage of the cell cycle) or by inducing their terminal differentiation such that they are permanently unable to re-enter the cell cycle. Anti-growth signalling is mediated by ligands (e.g. transforming growth factor-beta, TGF-β) that act on cellular receptors (e.g. TGF-β receptor) and send signals to the nucleus via second messengers. These pathways are mainly involved in controlling the cell cycle clock and mediate their effects through proteins that include retinoblastoma protein (Rb), cyclins, cyclin-dependent kinases (CDK) and their inhibitors (CDKi). Abnormalities in anti-growth signalling pathways are extremely common in cancer and play a role in helping cancer cells to progress through the cell cycle. Therefore, loss of Rb and members of the CDKi family and overexpression of certain cyclins and CDK have been shown to occur in a large number of tumour types.

Clinical attempts to target proliferation through cell cycle control are in their very early stages. The cyclin-dependent kinase inhibitor, seliciclib (CYC202; *R*-roscovitine), has been shown to enhance apoptosis in head and neck cancer cells in preclinical studies.[72] It is the first selective, orally bioavailable inhibitor of cyclin-dependent kinases 1, 2, 7 and 9 to enter the clinic and in a phase I trial in 21 patients at doses of 100, 200 and 800 mg twice daily, it caused dose-limiting toxicities at the 800 mg dose.[73] No objective tumour responses were noted, but disease stabilization was recorded in eight patients. Other similar agents are in development and will enter clinical trials in patients with a range of malignancies, including head and neck cancer, in the coming years.

TARGETING CELLULAR IMMORTALIZATION

Normal somatic cells can only undergo a finite number of cell divisions (Hayflick limit) before they enter a period of permanent growth arrest known as replicative senescence. This process occurs as a result of the cells' inability to replicate the ends of their chromosomes (the telomeres) fully at each division. Therefore, over time the telomeres get progressively shorter, effectively acting as molecular clocks that count down the cells' lifespan. In contrast, stem cells and malignant cells have acquired immortality by maintaining the length of their telomeres. In most tumours, this occurs through upregulation of the enzyme telomerase, but in 10–15 per cent of cases a different mechanism, called alternative lengthening of the telomeres, is responsible. Telomerase enzymatic activity involves a large number of proteins, but its two main components are an RNA template (hTR) and a reverse transcriptase enzyme (hTERT): the reverse transcriptase uses the hTR RNA template as a guide in the resynthesis of the DNA sequence of the telomere. Therefore, tumours that have reactivated the expression of telomerase are able to rebuild the parts of their telomeres that they lose with each round of cell division and, so, are able to avoid being sidelined into replicative senescence.

At present, efforts to target the immortalized, stem cell compartment within tumours remains in its infancy. Nonetheless, recognition of the importance of these cells to the overall behaviour of the tumour – in terms of its ability to self-propagate, spread and resist therapeutic intervention – means that active efforts will be made to devise specific targeted therapies against this compartment. Such developments are likely to result in novel approaches to the treatment of a range of tumour types, including head and neck cancer.

TARGETING INVASION AND METASTASIS

Distant metastases cause 90 per cent of cancer deaths. Invasion and metastasis involves careful orchestration of a series of complex biological processes: (1) detachment from immediate neighbours and stroma at the local site; (2) enzymatic digestion of the extracellular matrix followed by specific directional motility; (3) penetration (intravasation) of blood or lymphatic vessels and tumour embolization; (4) survival in the circulation until arrival at the metastatic site that may be chosen on the basis of provision of a favourable supply of appropriate growth factors; (5) it adheres to the endothelium of blood vessels at its destination and extravasates from the vessel; and (6) it begins to proliferate and invade its new location and sets about recruiting a new blood supply.

The development of metastatic disease in locoregional cervical lymph nodes is a hallmark of SCCHN. Such is the predilection of this disease for lymphatic metastasis that patients may present with pathologically involved cervical nodes at any time during the natural history of the disease.[74] The phenomenon of cervical nodal metastasis from an occult primary mucosal site in the head and neck is well recognized.[75] In addition, involved cervical nodes can present synchronously with the primary tumour or metachronously as the first sign of disease relapse. The presence or absence of lymphatic metastasis is the most important prognostic factor for patients with SCCHN.[76] On the basis of this fact, most patients who are diagnosed as having SCCHN will have radiological investigations such as computed tomography (CT) or magnetic resonance imaging (MRI) in an attempt to identify nodal metastases. Even if these tests suggest that the neck is not involved (clinically node negative or cN0 disease), patients frequently undergo prophylactic treatment of the neck, either by elective neck dissection or radiotherapy, in an attempt to ablate occult micrometastases. Such additional treatment carries a significant morbidity for the patient. For those patients who present with N+ disease, there is a greater risk of systemic metastasis which increases with increasing N stage and involvement of nodes lower in the neck (e.g. level IV compared with level I). Identification of a panel of biomarkers that could predict the likelihood of nodal metastases would represent a useful tool for patient selection for elective or adjuvant treatment of the neck. Alternatively, novel therapies that could reduce the risk of local or systemic metastasis would represent a very significant advance in the treatment of head and neck cancer.

There is evolving evidence that the patterns of metastasis of different cancers to specific organs (e.g. head and neck cancer to cervical lymph nodes; breast cancer to liver, bone and brain; lung cancer to brain and adrenal gland) are not random, but appear to be driven by expression of chemokine receptors by tumour cells that allow them to 'seek' a suitable environment in which to establish a colony. Chemokines are small, secreted proteins with characteristic cysteine motifs in their amino acid sequences.[77] Most members of the chemokine superfamily have four cysteines and on this basis they have been classified into four groups (CXC or α, CC or β, C or γ and CXC3 or δ) according to the motif displayed by the first two cysteines. Chemokines interact with their cognate receptors which are G-protein coupled, seven-transmembrane receptors.[78] Chemokines were initially shown to be involved in controlling the targeted migration of haematopoietic cells, but more recently they have been implicated in a diverse range of physiological and pathological functions including wound healing, the control of angiogenesis and the development of tumour metastases. Indeed, there has been an evolving interest in the role of chemokines and their receptors in the process of tumour metastasis in recent years. A landmark study clearly demonstrated that breast cancer cells that expressed the chemokine receptors CXCR4 and CCR7 were capable of preferentially homing to particular tissues.[79]

CCR7 is known to be the functional receptor for SLC (secondary lymphoid organ chemokine). It acts by influencing the migration of activated dendritic cells to regional lymph nodes. In a recent study, a strong association was reported between CCR7 expression and synchronous nodal metastasis in patients with tonsillar cancer.[80] Only 1 of 11 (9.1 per cent) patients with negative CCR7 immunohistochemistry had nodal involvement at presentation, in contrast to 8 of 13 (61.5 per cent) patients with '+' staining, 24 of 27 (88.9 per cent) patients with '++' staining and 29 of 33 (87.8 per cent) patients with '+++' staining. Similarly, the degree of CCR7 immunopositivity was directly correlated with the extent of nodal metastasis at diagnosis, such that 43 of 44 (97.7 per cent) patients with N2 or N3 disease had '++' or '+++' immunostaining at diagnosis. CCR7 staining in the primary tumour was also shown to be associated with disease relapse, systemic metastasis and disease-specific and overall survival.

Blockade of CCR7 signalling has been shown to increase the therapeutic efficacy of cisplatin and anti-EGFR therapy in

murine models of head and neck cancer.[81] Similar effects in a breast cancer model have been reported with blockade of another chemokine receptor (CXCR4).[82] Clearly, this is an interesting area for future clinical development, although there have not yet been any clinical trials of targeted anti-chemokine therapeutics.

CONCLUSIONS

Despite significant improvements in treatment outcome in patients with SCCHN that have resulted from technological advances in radiation delivery and the use of cytotoxic chemotherapy, there is still a pressing need for novel therapies. In the last two decades, the molecular biology revolution has provided us with a new framework for developing specific targeted therapies. The first major success of this approach was the development of the anti-EGFR monoclonal antibody cetuximab which has been shown to increase control rates in newly diagnosed disease (in combination with radiotherapy) and to prolong survival in relapsed disease (in combination with chemotherapy). This agent is likely to be the frontrunner of a series of new agents that will target specific molecular defects in head and neck cancer. It is likely that the next wave of developments will include active small molecule inhibitors of EGFR (and other members of the c-erbB family of receptors), anti-angiogenic agents and drugs that can increase pro-apoptotic signalling in cancer cells. As with cetuximab, it is most likely that these new agents will first find a niche in the context of combination regimens with standard anticancer therapeutics.

KEY EVIDENCE

- The addition of drug treatment (cytotoxic chemotherapy) to radiation therapy has resulted in significant improvements in progression-free and overall survival rates.[6,7,8] These data point to the potential benefits of more targeted drugs that can interact with specific hallmarks of cancer to achieve patient benefit.
- Proof-of-principle data for the use of targeted drugs in combination with standard anticancer therapies have been provided by the randomized phase III trial of cetuximab plus radiotherapy.[40] Further studies of agents capable of targeting the hallmarks of cancer are under way.

KEY LEARNING POINTS

- The hallmarks of cancer have been described and provide a rational basis for developing novel targeted biological agents for use against head and neck cancers.
- Targeted agents are unlikely to exert significant single-agent activity against head and neck

cancer, but may be active as part of combination regimens with standard anticancer therapies, such as radiation and chemotherapy.

- Studies in which EGFR has been targeted with specific monoclonal antibodies have provided a strong rationale for developing this approach in combination with radiotherapy in patients with locally advanced disease.
- Anti-angiogenic treatments represent attractive potential therapeutics, but their integration alongside standard therapies will require careful evaluation of treatment scheduling in order to avoid the risks of antagonistic interactions.
- Drugs which have the capacity to enhance apoptosis, insensitivity to anti-growth signals and telomerase reactivation all have the potential to increase the activity of radiotherapy and/or chemotherapy.
- Specific drugs capable of targeting the metastatic process are desperately needed as a means of reducing the number of patients who experience systemic disease relapse following successful locoregional treatment.

REFERENCES

1. Nutting C. Intensity-modulated radiotherapy (IMRT): the most important advance in radiotherapy since the linear accelerator? *British Journal of Radiology* 2003; **76**: 673.
2. Lee NY, Le QT. New developments in radiation therapy for head and neck cancer: intensity-modulated radiation therapy and hypoxia targeting. *Seminars in Oncology* 2008; **35**: 236–50.
3. Guerrero Urbano T, Clark CH, Hansen VN *et al.* A phase I study of dose-escalated chemoradiation with accelerated intensity modulated radiotherapy in locally advanced head and neck cancer. *Radiotherapy and Oncology* 2007; **85**: 36–41.
4. Bhide S, Clark C, Harrington K. Nutting CM. Intensity modulated radiotherapy improves target coverage and parotid gland sparing when delivering total mucosal irradiation in patients with squamous cell carcinoma of head and neck of unknown primary site. *Medical Dosimetry* 2007; **32**: 188–95.
5. Miles EA, Clark CH, Urbano MT *et al.* The impact of introducing intensity modulated radiotherapy into routine clinical practice. *Radiotherapy and Oncology* 2005; **77**: 241–6.
* 6. Pignon JP, Bourhis J, Domenge C, Designe L. Chemotherapy added to locoregional treatment for head and neck squamous-cell carcinoma: three meta-analyses of updated individual data. MACH-NC Collaborative Group. Meta-analysis of chemotherapy on head and neck cancer. *Lancet* 2000; **355**: 949–55.
● 7. Bernier J, Domenge C, Ozsahin M *et al.* European Organization for Research and Treatment of Cancer Trial 22931. Postoperative irradiation with or without concomitant chemotherapy for locally advanced head and neck cancer. *New England Journal of Medicine* 2004; **350**: 1945–52.
● 8. Cooper JS, Pajak TF, Forastiere AA *et al.* Radiation Therapy Oncology Group 9501/Intergroup. Postoperative concurrent radiotherapy and chemotherapy for high-risk squamous-cell carcinoma of the head and neck. *New England Journal of Medicine* 2004; **350**: 1937–44.
9. Singh B. Molecular pathogenesis of head and neck cancers. *Journal of Surgical Oncology* 2008; **97**: 634–9.
10. Harrington KJ. Biology of cancer. *Medicine* 2008; **36**: 1–5.
◆ 11. Hanahan D, Weinberg RA. The hallmarks of cancer. *Cell* 2000; **100**: 57–70.
◆ 12. Rogers SJ, Harrington KJ, Rhys Evans P *et al.* Biological significance of c-erbB family oncogenes in head and neck cancer. *Cancer and Metastasis Reviews* 2005; **24**: 47–69.
13. Khademi B, Shirazi FM, Vasei M *et al.* The expression of p53, c-erbB-1 and c-erbB-2 molecules and their correlation with prognostic markers in patients with head and neck tumors. *Cancer Letters* 2002; **184**: 223–230.
14. Dassonville O, Formento JL, Francoual M *et al.* Expression of epidermal growth factor receptor and survival in upper aerodigestive tract cancer. *Journal of Clinical Oncology* 1993; **11**: 1873–8.
15. Kusukawa J, Harada H, Shima I *et al.* The significance of epidermal growth factor receptor and matrix metalloproteinase 3 in squamous cell carcinoma of the oral cavity. *Oral Oncology* 1996; **32B**: 217–21.
16. O-charoenrat P, Rhys-Evans P, Modjtahedi H, Eccles SA. The role of cerbB receptors and ligands in head and neck squamous cell carcinoma. *Oral Oncology* 2002; **38**: 627–50.
● 17. Downward J, Yarden Y, Mayes E *et al.* Close similarity of epidermal growth factor receptor and v-erb-B oncogene protein sequences. *Nature* 1984; **307**: 521–7.
18. Grandis JR, Tweardy DJ. Elevated levels of transforming growth factor alpha and epidermal growth factor receptor messenger RNA are early markers of carcinogenesis in head and neck cancer. *Cancer Research* 1993; **53**: 3579–84.
19. Shin DM, Ro JY, Hong WK, Hittelman WN. Dysregulation of epidermal growth factor receptor expression in premalignant lesions during head and neck tumorigenesis. *Cancer Research* 1994; **54**: 3153–9.
20. Grandis JR, Tweardy DJ, Melhem MF. Asynchronous modulation of transforming growth factor alpha and epidermal growth factor receptor protein expression in progression of premalignant lesions to head and neck squamous cell carcinoma. *Clinical Cancer Research* 1998; **4**: 13–20.
21. Ibrahim SO, Vasstrand EN, Liavaag PG *et al.* Expression of c-erbB proto-oncogene family members in squamous cell carcinoma of the head and neck. *Anticancer Research* 1997; **17**: 4539–46.

22. Werkmeister R, Brandt B, Joos U. Clinical relevance of erbB-1 and -2 oncogenes in oral carcinomas. *Oral Oncology* 2000; **36**: 100–5.

23. Wilkman TS, Heitanen JH, Malstrom MJ, Kontiinen YT. Immunohistochemical analysis of the oncoprotein c-erbB-2 expression in oral benign and malignant lesions. *International Journal of Oral and Maxillofacial Surgery* 1998; **27**: 209–12.

24. Chen Z, Zhang K, Zhang X et al. Comparison of gene expression between metastatic derivatives and their poorly metastatic parental cells implicates crucial tumor–environment interaction in metastasis of head and neck squamous cell carcinoma. *Clinical and Experimental Metastasis* 2003; **20**: 335–42.

● 25. Sok JC, Coppelli FM, Thomas SM et al. Mutant epidermal growth factor receptor (EGFRvIII) contributes to head and neck cancer growth and resistance to EGFR targeting. *Clinical Cancer Research* 2006; **12**: 5064–73.

26. Hellyer NJ, Kim MS, Koland JG. Heregulin-dependent activation of phosphoinositide 3-kinase and Akt via the ErbB2/ErbB3 co-receptor. *Journal of Biological Chemistry* 2001; **276**: 42153–61.

27. Hou L, Shi D, Tu SM et al. Oral cancer progression and c-erbB-2/neu proto-oncogene expression. *Cancer Letters* 1992; **65**: 215–20.

28. Bei R, Pompa G, Vitolo D et al. Co-localization of multiple ErbB receptors in stratified epithelium of oral squamous cell carcinoma. *Journal of Pathology* 2001; **195**: 343–8.

29. Xia W, Lau Y-K, Zhang H-Z et al. Combination of EGFR, HER-2/neu and -3 is a stronger predictor for the outcome of oral squamous cell carcinoma than any individual family members. *Clinical Cancer Research* 1999; **5**: 4164–74.

30. Barnes CJ, Kumar R. Epidermal growth factor receptor family tyrosine kinases as signal integrators and therapeutic targets. *Cancer and Metastasis Reviews* 2003; **22**: 301–7.

● 31. Huang SM, Harari PM. Modulation of radiation response after epidermal growth factor receptor blockade in squamous cell carcinomas: inhibition of damage repair, cell cycle kinetics, and tumor angiogenesis. *Clinical Cancer Research* 2000; **6**: 2166–74.

32. Harari PM, Huang SM. Head and neck cancer as a clinical model for molecular targeting of therapy: combining EGFR blockade with radiation. *International Journal of Radiation Oncology, Biology, Physics* 2001; **49**: 427–33.

33. Herbst RS, Kim ES, Harari PM. IMC-C225, an anti-epidermal growth factor receptor monoclonal antibody, for treatment of head and neck cancer. *Expert Opinion on Biological Therapy* 2001; **1**: 719–32.

34. Huang SM, Li J, Harari PM. Molecular inhibition of angiogenesis and metastatic potential in human squamous cell carcinomas after epidermal growth factor receptor blockade. *Molecular Cancer Therapeutics* 2002; **1**: 507–14.

35. Baselga J, Pfister D, Cooper MR et al. Phase I studies of anti-epidermal growth factor receptor chimeric antibody C225 alone and in combination with cisplatin. *Journal of Clinical Oncology* 2000; **18**: 904–14.

36. Shin DM, Donato NJ, Perez-Soler R et al. Epidermal growth factor receptor-targeted therapy with C225 and cisplatin in patients with head and neck cancer. *Clinical Cancer Research* 2001; **7**: 1204–13.

● 37. Robert F, Ezekiel MP, Spencer SA et al. Phase I study of anti-epidermal growth factor receptor antibody cetuximab in combination with radiation therapy in patients with advanced head and neck cancer. *Journal of Clinical Oncology* 2001; **19**: 3234–43.

38. Herbst RS, Arquette M, Shin DM et al. Phase II multicenter study of the epidermal growth factor receptor antibody cetuximab and cisplatin for recurrent and refractory squamous cell carcinoma of the head and neck. *Journal of Clinical Oncology* 2005; **23**: 5578–87.

39. Baselga J, Trigo JM, Bourhis J et al. Phase II multicenter study of the antiepidermal growth factor receptor monoclonal antibody cetuximab in combination with platinum-based chemotherapy in patients with platinum-refractory metastatic and/or recurrent squamous cell carcinoma of the head and neck. *Journal of Clinical Oncology* 2005; **23**: 5568–77.

● 40. Bonner JA, Harari PM, Giralt J et al. Radiotherapy plus cetuximab for squamous-cell carcinoma of the head and neck. *New England Journal of Medicine* 2006; **354**: 567–78.

● 41. Vermorken JB, Mesia R, Rivera F et al. Platinum-based chemotherapy plus cetuximab in head and neck cancer. *New England Journal of Medicine* 2008; **359**: 1116–27.

42. Heymach JV, Nilsson M, Blumenschein G et al. Epidermal growth factor receptor inhibitors in development for the treatment of non-small cell lung cancer. *Clinical Cancer Research* 2006; **12**: 4441s–5s.

43. Wu M, Rivkin A, Pham T. Panitumumab: human monoclonal antibody against epidermal growth factor receptors for the treatment of metastatic colorectal cancer. *Clinical Therapeutics* 2008; **30**: 14–30.

44. Kruser TJ, Armstrong EA, Ghia AJ et al. Augmentation of radiation response by panitumumab in models of upper aerodigestive tract cancer. *International Journal of Radiation Oncology, Biology, Physics* 2008; **72**: 534–42.

45. Baselga J, Averbuch SD. ZD1839 ('Iressa') as an anticancer agent. *Drugs* 2000; **60**(Suppl. 1): 33–40.

46. Sirotnak FM, Zakowski MF, Miller VA et al. Efficacy of cytotoxic agents against human tumor xenografts is markedly enhanced by coadministration of ZD1839 (Iressa), an inhibitor of EGFR tyrosine kinase. *Clinical Cancer Research* 2000; **6**: 4885–92.

47. Norman P. ZD-1839 (AstraZeneca). *Current Opinion in Investigational Drugs* 2001; **2**: 428–34.

48. Baselga J, Rischin D, Ranson M et al. Phase I safety, pharmacokinetic, and pharmacodynamic trial of ZD1839, a selective oral epidermal growth factor receptor tyrosine kinase inhibitor, in patients with five selected solid tumor types. *Journal of Clinical Oncology* 2002; **20**: 4292–302.

49. Ranson M, Hammond LA, Ferry D et al. ZD1839, a selective oral epidermal growth factor receptor-tyrosine kinase inhibitor, is well tolerated and active in patients with solid, malignant tumors: results of a phase I trial. *Journal of Clinical Oncology* 2002; **20**: 2240–50.

50. Herbst RS, Maddox AM, Rothenberg ML et al. Selective oral epidermal growth factor receptor tyrosine kinase inhibitor ZD1839 is generally well-tolerated and has activity in non-small-cell lung cancer and other solid tumors: results of a phase I trial. *Journal of Clinical Oncology* 2002; **20**: 3815–25.

51. Nakagawa K, Tamura T, Negoro S et al. Phase I pharmacokinetic trial of the selective oral epidermal growth factor receptor tyrosine kinase inhibitor gefitinib ('Iressa', ZD1839) in Japanese patients with solid malignant tumors. *Annals of Oncology* 2003; **14**: 922–30.

52. LoRusso PM, Herbst RS, Rischin D et al. Improvements in quality of life and disease-related symptoms in phase I trials of the selective oral epidermal growth factor receptor tyrosine kinase inhibitor ZD1839 in non-small cell lung cancer and other solid tumors. *Clinical Cancer Research* 2003; **9**: 2040–8.

● 53. Cohen EE, Rosen F, Stadler WM et al. Phase II trial of ZD1839 in recurrent or metastatic squamous cell carcinoma of the head and neck. *Journal of Clinical Oncology* 2003; **21**: 1980–7.

54. Cohen EE, Kane MA, List MA et al. Phase II trial of gefitinib 250 mg daily in patients with recurrent and/or metastatic squamous cell carcinoma of the head and neck. *Clinical Cancer Research* 2005; **11**: 8418–24.

55. Kirby AM, A'Hern RP, D'Ambrosio C et al. Gefitinib (ZD1839, Iressa) as palliative treatment in recurrent or metastatic head and neck cancer. *British Journal of Cancer* 2006; **94**: 631–6.

56. Xia W, Mullin RJ, Keith BR et al. Anti-tumor activity of GW572016: a dual tyrosine kinase inhibitor blocks EGF activation of EGFR/erbB2 and downstream Erk1/2 and AKT pathways. *Oncogene* 2002; **21**: 6255–63.

57. Burris HA III, Hurwitz HI, Dees EC et al. Phase I safety, pharmacokinetics, and clinical activity study of lapatinib (GW572016), a reversible dual inhibitor of epidermal growth factor receptor tyrosine kinases, in heavily pretreated patients with metastatic carcinomas. *Journal of Clinical Oncology* 2005; **23**: 5305–13.

58. Del Campo JM, Sebastian P, Hitt R et al. Effect of lapatinib on apoptosis and proliferation: results of a phase II randomised study in patients with locally advanced squamous cell carcinoma of the head and neck (SCCHN). *Annals of Oncology* 2008; **19** (Suppl. 8); viii217 (Abstr. 6880).

● 59. Harrington KJ, El-Hariry IA, Holford CS et al. Phase I study of lapatinib in combination with chemoradiation in patients with locally advanced squamous cell carcinoma of the head and neck. *Journal of Clinical Oncology* 2009; **27**: 1100–7.

◆ 60. Folkman J. Angiogenesis. *Annual Review of Medicine* 2006; **57**: 1–18.

◆ 61. Seiwert TY, Cohen EE. Targeting angiogenesis in head and neck cancer. *Seminars in Oncology* 2008; **35**: 274–85.

62. Lippert JW 3rd. Vascular disrupting agents. *Bioorganic and Medicinal Chemistry* 2007; **15**: 605–15.

63. el-Zayat AA, Degen D, Drabek S et al. *In vitro* evaluation of the antineoplastic activity of combretastatin A-4, a natural product from *Combretum caffrum* (arid shrub). *Anticancer Drugs* 1993; **4**: 19–25.

64. Chaplin DJ, Pettit GR, Parkins CS, Hill SA. Antivascular approaches to solid tumour therapy: evaluation of tubulin binding agents. *British Journal of Cancer Supplement* 1996; **27**: S86–8.

◆ 65. Jain RK. Normalization of tumor vasculature: an emerging concept in antiangiogenic therapy. *Science* 2005; **307**: 58–62.

66. Fukumura D, Jain RK. Tumor microvasculature and microenvironment: targets for anti-angiogenesis and normalization. *Microvascular Research* 2007; **74**: 72–84.

67. Ashkenazi A, Holland P, Eckhardt SG. Ligand-based targeting of apoptosis in cancer: the potential of recombinant human apoptosis ligand 2/tumor necrosis factor-related apoptosis-inducing ligand (rhApo2L/TRAIL). *Journal of Clinical Oncology* 2008; **26**: 3621–30.

68. Buchsbaum DJ, Forero-Torres A, LoBuglio AF. TRAIL-receptor antibodies as a potential cancer treatment. *Future Oncology* 2007; **3**: 405–9.

69. Yip KW, Mocanu JD, Au PY et al. Combination bcl-2 antisense and radiation therapy for nasopharyngeal cancer. *Clinical Cancer Research* 2005; **11**: 8131–44.

70. Lacy J, Loomis R, Grill S et al. Systemic Bcl-2 antisense oligodeoxynucleotide in combination with cisplatin cures EBV+ nasopharyngeal carcinoma xenografts in SCID mice. *International Journal of Cancer* 2006; **119**: 309–16.

71. Danson S, Dean E, Dive C, Ranson M. IAPs as a target for anticancer therapy. *Current Cancer Drug Targets* 2007; **7**: 785–94.

72. Mihara M, Shintani S, Kiyota A et al. Cyclin-dependent kinase inhibitor (roscovitine) suppresses growth and induces apoptosis by regulating Bcl-x in head and neck squamous cell carcinoma cells. *International Journal of Oncology* 2002; **21**: 95–101.

73. Benson C, White J, De Bono J et al. A phase I trial of the selective oral cyclin-dependent kinase inhibitor seliciclib (CYC202; R-Roscovitine), administered twice daily for 7

days every 21 days. *British Journal of Cancer* 2007; **96**: 29–37.

74. Munro AJ, MacDougall RH, Stafford ND. Head and neck chapter. In: Price P, Sikora K (eds). *Treatment of cancer.* London: Chapman and Hall Medical, 2002: 313–90.

75. De Braud F, al-Sarraf M. Diagnosis and management of squamous cell carcinoma of unknown primary tumor site of the neck. *Seminars in Oncology* 1993; **20**: 273–8.

76. Layland MK, Sessions DG, Lenox J. The influence of lymph node metastasis in the treatment of squamous cell carcinoma of the oral cavity, oropharynx, larynx and hypopharynx: N0 versus N+. *Laryngoscope* 2005; **115**: 629–39.

◆ 77. Rossi D, Zlotnik A. The biology of chemokines and their receptors. *Annual Review of Immunology* 2000; **18**: 217–42.

78. Gerard C, Rollins BJ. Chemokines and disease. *Nature Immunology* 2001; **2**: 108–15.

79. Muller A, Homey B, Soto H *et al.* Involvement of chemokine receptors in breast cancer metastasis. *Nature* 2001; **410**: 50–6.

80. Pitkin L, Corbishley C, Dalton P *et al.* Expression of CC chemokine receptor 7 in tonsillar cancer predicts cervical nodal metastasis, systemic relapse and survival. *British Journal of Cancer* 2007; **97**: 670–7.

81. Wang J, Seethala RR, Zhang Q *et al.* Autocrine and paracrine chemokine receptor 7 activation in head and neck cancer: implications for therapy. *Journal of the National Cancer Institute* 2008; **100**: 502–12.

82. Liang Z, Wu T, Lou H *et al.* Inhibition of breast cancer metastasis by selective synthetic polypeptide against CXCR4. *Cancer Research* 2004; **64**: 4302–8.

47

Multidisciplinary team working

ANDREW DAVIES, IÑIGO TOLOSA, ZOË NEARY, DES McGUIRE, DEBRA FITZGERALD, KATE REID AND RICHARD WIGHT

> to cure sometimes, to relieve often, to comfort always
>
> Anonymous (fifteenth century)

INTRODUCTION

Head and neck cancer (HNC) has been portrayed as one of the most devastating cancers. The decision to treat HNC is confounded by the balance of eradicating disease against the cost to the patient's contentment with the consequences of the treatment. Chapter 10, Quality of life, describes the impact of malignancy and the detrimental effects that treatment has on a patient's quality of life. With the commitment to improve survival outcomes for HNC patients, and by aiming to address both the physical and psychosocial concerns following treatment, multidisciplinary team (MDT) working has been the standard for HNC care. MDT working should be an integral part of a health professional's routine in cancer care, and MDT meetings are an essential step for making decisions in the planning of treatment and rehabilitation for HNC patients. Due to this, it is worthwhile familiarizing oneself with the structure, objectives, management and collaboration of the MDT. This chapter focuses on the 'team' required for treating HNC, providing an overview of the benefits of MDT working and how the MDT can help reduce patients' distress using good communication skills. The chapter also expands on the roles of key individuals involved during the different stages of the patient's journey

and, finally, highlights the importance of data collection to provide outcomes which will help future patients.

In the United Kingdom, the Calman–Hine report[1] recommended site-specific MDTs meet regularly to discuss patients and agree on treatment decisions. Multidisciplinary team working ensures the patient receives the benefits and expertise of a range of specialists for their diagnosis and treatment, and that care is given according to recognized guidelines (**Box 47.1**). Due to HNC being a heterogeneous group of diseases with multifaceted health-related issues, it is recognized that patients may require the involvement of a large team of health professionals from different disciplines (**Box 47.2**). The MDT gives optimal care for HNC patients by contributing to the decision-making process and addressing a variety of post-treatment issues. Although not all members will be initially involved with the patient and different interventions involving different disciplines may come at different stages during the patient's pathway, it vital that each member can provide time and expertise for the quality and the continuity of patient care.

For MDT working to be effective, it is important for each member to understand the role of the individuals within the team.[2] This comprehension of the responsibility each member has helps with the cooperation between professionals and ensures that patients receive optimal and timely care. Clarity of the strengths and limitations of the MDT facilitates the communication between specialities and helps create a supportive working environment for the MDT meetings. It can be a difficult balance between working as an independent practitioner and working as a team member with other autonomous professionals. The goal of providing a cure for

Box 47.1 Benefits of multidisciplinary team working

- Provides structure to the patient's pathway
- Formulates consensus about treatment plans
- TMN staging
- Brings together extensive health professional experience
- Improves team communication, coordination and consistency
- Ensures all information and investigations have been completed
- Opportunities for a learning environment
- Reciprocated team support
- Captures data and audits for service improvement
- Highlights research prospect and recruitment to clinical trials

Box 47.2 Members of the head and neck multidisciplinary team (MDT)

- Head and neck consultants
- Consultant oncologists
- Consultant thyroid surgeon
- Radiologist
- Histopathologist
- Clinical nurse specialist
- Palliative care specialist
- Speech and language therapists
- Dietictian
- MDT coordinator
- Mental health specialist
- Hospital social worker
- Prosthetic specialist
- Restorative dentist
- Outpatient and ward nursing staff
- Research nurse
- Complementary therapy

any individual patient may be the common aim of the MDT meeting, but the views on the best way of achieving this may differ. The very nature of HNC means that disagreements about what is in the patient's best interest will exist between MDT members. Conflicts of judgement should not be seen as negative, since such discussions improve patient care and may highlight the need for further research in a particular area. Teams do not automatically function because a group of professionals have come together. The role of the clinical MDT lead ensures discussion is focused on the patient's best interest in a composed and respectful atmosphere.[3] The clinical lead needs to ensure that that the MDT provides appropriate input to reach a consensus of opinion. Members of the MDT also have a duty to voice their concerns, but ultimately to uphold the outcome of the meeting.

There is no universal model of how the meetings should run. They may be based on national, regional and local policies and guidelines. Some surgery, for instance that involving the thyroid gland, may have a well-established treatment pathway but the meeting should not simply be a 'rubber stamp' exercise. The size of the tumour or the patient's prognosis does not necessarily determine the level of distress a patient may experience and each case needs to be assessed individually. Sometimes not all the patient's information is available for the MDT meeting. Logistical problems may occur when obtaining information from satellite centres. Initial investigations may have been inadequate to confirm the stage of the cancer. A decision to treat may be delayed because of concerns about the patient's capacity to consent for treatment or the ability to cope with the effects of treatment. Further assessment of comorbidities may be necessary before a decision can be reached. Some decisions within the MDT may show that either surgery or radiotherapy may be equally appropriate to offer the patient, and the decision then comes down to informed consent and patient choice. Sometimes the patient may disagree with the MDT's decision and occasionally ask for a second opinion.

CORE CLINICAL COMMUNICATION SKILLS

The way in which MDT members communicate with the patient can have a direct effect on quality of life. Complicated cases do not always require complex solutions, and the distress experienced by the patient can be managed with good clinical communication skills. Good communication is about the clinician's and MDT's adaptable approach to patient care, pre-planning consultation and reflecting on the patient's and personal experience of the case. Having good communication skills is not something you can read from a script. It can be likened to performing surgery, theoretical knowledge is vital but there is no substitute for practical experience.

Over 30 years of research has shown a key hindrance to a successful consultation is not time, but lack of effective training. Following training focused on eliciting patient concerns, clinicians improve their ability to gather clinical and relevant patient experience data: this leads to more accurate diagnosis, greater doctor–patient concordance, much reduced complaints and an increased likelihood of the patient understanding and following clinical and lifestyle suggestions. In the United Kingdom, 3-day advanced communication skills training workshops approved by the National Cancer Action Team Workshops are open and compulsory to core members of the cancer MDTs. Participants are expected to improve their confidence and skills in advanced communication skills, but also in providing others with constructive and specific feedback on their own communication skills. Good internal communication skills help to achieve a cooperative and effective MDT. Consultations can then be proactively and openly managed.

Patients may not remember all the details about their diagnosis, but they will remember the manner in which the information was conveyed. If the patient feels the consultation is hectic then it may leave an unhelpful and possibly incorrect impression of how their treatment may be. The key is to encourage a therapeutic working relationship with the patient and their loved ones from the first meeting. The aim is to encourage an open, honest and trustworthy rapport between you and the patient, giving them confidence to share their concerns and feel they have been understood. The purpose of clinical communication is to elicit our patients' thoughts and feelings and to respond to both with integrity and empathy, providing them with our clinical and human understanding. The goals are to obtain and attend to the patient's concerns; to agree on their priorities; to tailor our information to their concerns and communication preferences; and to agree with the MDT a joint plan of action. In the process, we can learn how our patients prefer to discuss their condition and try to understand the impact it has on them.

Before the consultation

Before the consultation it is necessary to:

- Prepare what information might need to be conveyed or obtained, but remember you will be holding back until the patient's agenda, expectations and concerns are fully elicited.
- Provide a quiet, private space with minimal or preferably no interruptions (no staff coming in halfway through the consultation, no bleeps, mobiles or other calls). A chaotic consultation space will make it impossible for either clinicians or patients to focus on the task in hand. If you are interrupted or the management of your clinic means that intrusion is unavoidable, warn the patient of this before you start. Disruption may tell the patient that you are too busy to listen. This can prevent them raising their concerns. Discuss how you will manage the disruption and when you will continue the consultation.
- Help yourself and your patients by training them to attend your consultations well prepared. Invite them to bring their key issues in writing, as well as a trusted relative or friend, and offer written information about your team and service. Be prepared to reiterate this information in the consultation when necessary.
- Use tools that elicit a wide range of concerns and help them prioritize those for you, such as quality of life measures (see Chapter 10, Quality of life) or the NCCN distress thermometer. Choosing a tool that would be useful to your MDT allows both patients and clinicians to bypass social taboos or blocks, and leads to a more focused discussion of the patient's key concerns in areas such as family, practical, emotional, spiritual and physical problems.
- Prepare a physical space where you can sit next to the patient, with additional chairs for relatives. Avoid obstacles such as desks. Have writing materials to hand, position them so that both you and the patient can see what you write and use them as a joint planner and record of the consultation. The patient will then be able to see that their concerns are being documented.
- Remember that patients will bring up most of their key concerns in the first 90 seconds of the consultation (the patient monologue), but that we tend to interrupt them after only 17 seconds! Once we have interrupted, we are less likely to elicit their concerns, even if we ask

appropriate questions; by then, we have already programmed them not to tell us.

During the consultation

During the consultation, it is necessary to:

- Welcome your patient and companions in a culturally appropriate manner, inviting them to come in and get comfortable.
- Introduce yourself: name, title, position in the team.
- Find out how they would like to be addressed and who they would like present at the consultation.
- Establish the amount of time available today for your consultation.
- Establish the purpose of the consultation from the patient perspective; clarify the patient's desired outcome.
- Draw out their concerns and needs prior to the consultation, actively listen to cues about concerns and distress, then explore them tentatively and respectfully: 'You say you've had "terrible pain". I understand pain itself is very distressing and we will discuss its treatment in a moment. Can I also ask you whether you have concerns about this pain?' It might be that the pain is made worse by an undisclosed fear of malignancy or recurrences. If that was the case, both the pain and the concern can be addressed.
- Most doctors believe that patients will bring up difficult issues as appropriate, whereas most patients believe they should not bring them up until the doctor has expressed an interest. This leads to most concerns not being discussed. The solution is for the clinician to ask open directive questions that elicit the concerns.
- Once a full history has been taken and the patient's needs ascertained, summarize your understanding and check it with the patient.
- Align your knowledge to systematically address both their concerns and their information needs.
- Find your balance: patient-centred and respectful but clear and precise as appropriate. Keep your sentences short and clear, your questions even more so.
- Allow pauses for questions, and to check the patient's and companion's understanding.
- Timing is everything: as the consultation progresses, new patient concerns will arise; elicit these and the impact on patient and family. Acknowledge them and explore them further as appropriate.
- Signal key transitions in the consultation: i.e. from your information gathering to your delivering, from physical symptoms to key concerns, from impact on the person to that on the family.
- Show your interest in the patient's understanding by requesting their summary of the discussion so far.
- Find ways of expressing support, or of reinforcing patient coping skills that seem to work for them.
- At appropriate times, check with the patient and family how the communication is going. If it is a difficult consultation, you can acknowledge this and still ask 'I realize we are talking about a very difficult situation, would it be OK to check how we are progressing?', 'Is

there something I am doing that makes this more difficult?'
- Maintain a culturally appropriate body language throughout.

Closing the consultation

When closing the consultation, the following details should be observed:

- Calmly explore further areas: 'What issues are important to you that we have not addressed fully?', then later: 'What have we not discussed yet?' Tone and body language can convey the difference between genuine interest, or a rush to finish the consultation.
- It is best to avoid cursory closing questions like: 'Any other questions?', since the negative wording ('any') and the positioning at the end of the consultation are actually interpreted as cues to end the conversation, even when we mean to give an opportunity to bring up further issues.
- Summarize key points, including both clinical and other worries and concerns. Research using quality of life measures shows that, if clinicians move beyond the physical symptoms and discuss patients' concerns and quality of life in the consultation, the patients report being less distressed by their symptoms six months later (and the consultation lasts the same amount of time).
- List the action points that have been jointly agreed in the consultation. Identify members of the MDT who may need to be involved.
- State any actions which are to be taken by you. Identify any issues you are referring on to colleagues. Also clarify any action you have agreed the patient or family will take.
- Set a time to review progress in a future consultation.
- Provide a record of the consultation: written, audio recording, etc.
- Show your appreciation for your patient's effort to let you know about their concerns, whether these are physical or not.
- If there is no more time but some issues are still pending, negotiate how they are going to be addressed, i.e. at a later appointment, with a colleague or other service.

After the consultation

After the consultation, the following details should be attended to:

- When the patient leaves the room, reflect on the consultation and make a note of issues that were brought up but not fully addressed so that they can be attended to next time.
- Get feedback on your strengths and weaknesses from patients: use questionnaires and patient interviews at regular intervals.
- Get regular feedback on your strengths and weaknesses from colleagues, especially after complex consultations: discuss possible improvements and put them into

practice during your next consultation with that specific patient, whenever possible.
- Review your own practice by studying video or audio recordings of successful and unsuccessful consultations.
- Get specialist feedback from professional trainers: this can be live or through analysis of audio/video recordings. You can learn which consultations are most difficult for you and focus on improving them.
- Clinicians need not find the answers to all the patient's concerns: most patients will benefit from voicing them and thinking them through with their clinician. Even though we are trained to solve problems, it is important to value the support we can offer our patients to think through their key concerns. This is likely to lead to an improved doctor–patient relationship and often guides the patient to find their own answers.

There are power imbalances in the relationship between the patient and the MDT that need to be addressed. The patient is at a disadvantage through the fear and uncertainty that HNC can create, reducing their confidence, especially at a time when they are particularly psychologically vulnerable. It is therefore important that MDT includes a health professional trained in dealing with the wide range of the mental health issues.

The presence of the clinical nurse specialist at diagnosis is fundamental to help address the possible disparity between the information being given by the clinician and the level of understanding the patient has at this time. The diagnosis and plan of treatment may need to be discussed at a slow pace, often with many repetitions, to allow the patient to come to terms with the situation and give informed consent. The patient should leave the consultation feeling the discussion was both compassionate and constructive.

THE ROLE OF THE CLINICAL NURSE SPECIALIST

The clinical nurse specialist (CNS) takes a leading role in the coordination of care for patients coping with a diagnosis of HNC, any subsequent treatment and supportive care. Many health professionals are involved in the assessment of each patient's clinical, nutritional and psychological state in order to inform treatment planning and management. The CNS liaises with them all and also assesses non-medical needs.

At the time of diagnosis and presentation of treatment options, patients and carers are given a great deal of information which needs to be presented in an appropriate and timely way to meet individual needs. This involves informed discussion between patients and health professionals involved in their treatment and rehabilitation. The involvement of a CNS promotes a holistic and organized approach to assessment and problem solving prior to treatment commencing. The aim is to help patients and carers gain a realistic understanding of the treatment involved and the rehabilitation required to achieve an acceptable outcome.

Support and information giving

It has been suggested[4] that all patients should be offered the opportunity to see a CNS before final decisions are made about their disease and its treatment. Many patients are given their diagnosis in the outpatient department. They should be encouraged to bring a relative or friend with them.[5, 6] Best practice suggests that a CNS should be present at the time of giving a diagnosis of HNC to offer support and take notes on the treatment options presented by the medical staff. This method of practice ensures accurate recording of the treatment plan proposed. Often the patient and carer are unable to retain all the information presented at the time of diagnosis. This can be repeated in a timely fashion on the patient's request either over the telephone or during further MDT pretreatment consultations. A written record of the diagnosis in medical and layman's terms plus the proposed treatment options should be offered to the patient before leaving the department. In addition, contact details of the health professionals involved in the treatment programme should be provided for the patient and carers. It is important that the patient understands that help and support is available if needed and that further opportunities to clarify information and ask questions will be provided.[7]

It is well recognized that patients retain very little of the verbal information given in a consultation. This is even more problematic when a diagnosis of cancer is also given.[8] Time and privacy should be provided in a safe supportive way following the medical consultation. Most patients appreciate having the opportunity to go to a quiet, private room where they can have time to take in and clarify the information they have been given, express emotions and compose themselves before returning home.

Information needs

Recent research suggests that unmet information needs may contribute significantly to psychological distress.[9, 10] Information should be readily available and be provided by specialist professionals who have good communication skills. The value of good quality written information should not be underestimated. Nurses have an important role in developing and providing this information leading to the potential of improving quality of life.[11] In the early stages, around the time of diagnosis and treatment planning, information is required about the disease, as well as surgery, radiotherapy or chemotherapy. When treatment has been completed, there is a greater need for more supportive information, such as access to practical help and psychological support.

The King's Fund report on HNC care[12] makes clear recommendations regarding information provision as follows:

- People want access to information and advice at all stages of the patient journey: during initial investigations, subsequent diagnosis, throughout treatment and follow up.
- Information should be presented in a timely fashion, with open access a few days after diagnosis in order to have questions answered once the diagnosis has had time to sink in. This illustrates the importance of providing contact details of the specialist support team and arranging a pretreatment appointment for assessment and information giving.
- Information on the impact and side effects of treatment on their lives.
- Information on support services and support groups.

- What to look out for if they suspect a recurrence of their cancer and who to contact.

The CNS assists in many ways during the provision of patient information,[13] from translating medical words and terms into an understandable form to timing the delivery of appropriate written information and suggesting appropriate websites. The CNS will also introduce patient visitors who will talk about their experiences to newly diagnosed patients, and also coordinate patient rehabilitation programmes and support groups.

Pretreatment assessment

In order to provide information about treatment planning, there needs to be an assessment of each patient's clinical, nutritional and psychological state (**Box 47.3**).[4] These aspects of care can be considered by the appropriate health professionals in pretreatment assessment clinics. Information gathered can then inform the rest of the MDT when final decisions on treatment planning are made. Key health professionals involved in pretreatment assessment should include a clinical nurse specialist, dietitian, speech and language therapist, specialist/restorative dentist, anaesthetist and an assessment from a mental health specialist.

Following diagnosis, the CNS has a role in coordinating these appointments according to individual needs before the first treatment. A series of meetings is often required to provide timely information and achieve informed consent. When appropriate information is elicited it becomes obvious that many issues require attention and intervention prior to treatment.

Box 47.3   Areas of assessment

- Presenting symptoms/symptom control requirements
- Comorbidity
- Performance status
- Emotional state
- Psychological state/previous experience
- Existing anxiety and depression
- Alcohol dependence
- Nicotine dependence
- Dentition
- Nutritional status
- Social support network
- Relationships
- Coping skills ability
- Literacy skills
- Financial status/work and professional issues
- Likely equipment requirements
- Previous experience of cancer
- Previous experience of hospitals and treatment
- Anaesthetic assessment

Referral

Pretreatment assessment includes communication and liaison with other health professionals both within the hospital and community care setting. This is especially important for patients who will have communication difficulties post-operatively.[14] This may involve the patient being referred on to community nursing teams, substance misuse services, smoking cessation services and social and benefit advisors. Social services can be initiated at the pretreatment stage in relation to family care issues or financial problems. Another area of consideration is the provision of medical equipment, such as suction and nebulizer units and communication aids.

Pretreatment education

Patients can be helped to cope with a cancer diagnosis and treatment by careful 'coaching' from the CNS.[6] The aims of education are to:

- fully inform about all potential treatment options and their anticipated effects;
- facilitate a positive secondary appraisal of a previously perceived threatening situation;
- facilitate pretreatment preparation with information on timing of events and likely outcomes;
- guide the patient and family towards suitable coping strategies.

Coping ability

Nursing care should be aimed at developing a therapeutic relationship with the patient and family in order to facilitate the development of coping strategies.[6] Continual contacts with the medical team is necessary to enhance the patient's feeling of personal control. However, this may be difficult to achieve.[9]

The CNS can act as the front-line point of contact either via the telephone or in the outpatient department to elicit concerns and advise on appropriate interventions, referring on to the medical team if necessary. Essentially, the CNS navigates the patient and family through the system and also assists the patients to cope with the diagnosis, providing quality, individually tailored information to promote understanding of the proposed treatment. Achieving informed consent contributes to long-term coping ability. This process cannot be achieved by a single health professional and requires input from many MDT members.

Post-treatment considerations

If patients have been well informed pretreatment, they are likely to recover more quickly. Encouraging self-care promotes a reduction in anxiety. This means that the patient's perception of control increases and dependence decreases.[15] Research has illustrated that psychosocial problems of head and neck cancer patients change with time following their diagnosis.[16] Medical problems improve with time but psychological problems including anxiety and anger can get worse. Decreased quality of life may reflect patient burnout.[9, 16] This phenomenon may be decreased, if adequate coping skills are acquired.

Patients can also suffer late side effects to treatment which causes further psychological distress.[17] This illustrates the importance of the continued availability of the specialist support team to the patient and carers, so that appropriate interventions can be initiated. It is the role of the CNS to establish a network of health professionals and resources to meet the patient's needs and requirements at different stages of their disease, treatment and supportive care. Regular outpatient follow up by health professionals, known to the patient, will promote continuity and accurate assessment of changing symptoms.

Pain is a significant problem following surgery for HNC[18] and those who have had both surgery and radiotherapy are more likely to have pain than those treated with radiotherapy alone. On direct questioning, it is evident that a significant number of patients do not use regular pain control medication. With appropriate assessment and advice, nurses can assist patients to manage their pain effectively. Specialist pain teams both within the hospital and community settings should be available if initial pain management interventions have been ineffective.

Supportive interventions

After survival itself, patients rate emotional and physical well-being very highly.[19] The use of complementary therapies has grown over recent years, and in many cancer centres forms part of an integrated programme of psychosocial care and support at all stages of the disease.

As previously discussed, for the patient negotiating the stages of investigation, diagnosis and treatment can be an anxious and frustrating time. Once side effects of treatment are subsiding, the threat of recurrence is ever present. The years following cancer treatment can be complicated with physical and psychological difficulties and general well-being can deteriorate. HNC patients find that physical problems can cause significant psychological distress.[16] Indeed, the after-effects, such as dry mouth, taste changes, swallowing difficulties and altered body image have been described as so bad that patients regret ever having had treatment.[19]

The CNS has a role in developing supportive interventions aimed at improving the emotional well-being of the patient, aiming to relieve some of the distress, anxiety, pain and side effects from diagnosis and treatment. If delivered well by appropriately trained and supervised staff complementary therapies, such as reflexology, aromatherapy, acupuncture and massage can be effective in relieving some of the symptoms experienced. It is appropriate to add that complementary therapies provided in a hospital setting are offered to complement medical treatment and not as an alternative.

THE ROLE OF SPEECH AND LANGUAGE THERAPY

Introduction

Swallowing and communication are two activities that as humans we take for granted. These behaviours are far from perfunctory; they are also both highly coordinated and pleasurable. They are ways of being able to express and share enjoyment. For any patient who is limited in their ability to communicate and swallow, social events and, in particular, celebrations have to be coped with in novel and frequently significantly adapted ways. An outsider, or even those familiar with the patient do not easily identify many of the symptoms or feelings associated with the changes that the HNC patient has to tolerate. The patient, in their social environments, should they still choose to try and still be a part of them, may well have to suppress emotions of loss and frustration as family and friends tell them how well they look and how well they are coping.

The assessment and prediction of swallowing and communication abilities for an individual patient is complex. It is part of the team's responsibility to describe and translate in terms that the patient and their family will understand the current and future effects of the cancer or treatment on the patient's ability to carry on with their life. Specifically because the anatomical areas that may be most threatened are so involved with swallowing and communication there is a need as part of clinical trials for these functions to be evaluated. Clinicians find it difficult to answer accurately patients' enquiries as to how they are likely to be affected by the recommended treatment long term.

Members of the MDT are aware how differently HNC patients present with their symptoms. Two patients who may clinically have a similar site and size of tumour can react emotionally and behaviourally very differently to the diagnosis and management of their disease. The results of any assessment may also not truly reflect the patient's function within their daily life. A patient with little impairment may have poor function and vice versa. Patients' illness perceptions when diagnosed can explain some of the variance of the quality of life data that are collected.[20] While swallowing and speech are a part of the domains that are measured, there is also an awareness that patients adjust and change with their attitudes over the course of time,[21] so that despite similar function reported by the patient there is a decrease in the perceived difficulty in swallowing a year after treatment.

As members of the team, it is important to remain receptive to these changes and support the patient as they try to maintain what in their terms is an acceptable level of quality of life. The use of disease-specific quality of life assessments has been reviewed.[22] They allow patients at an individual level to score their specific symptoms which must then be acted upon at a clinical level.[23] Such information can help inform and shape the goals of the speech and language therapist (SLT).

Inevitably, as a result of the site and effect of the diagnosed tumours SLTs working with HNC patients are likely to have the opportunity to assess and help patients with their dysphagia and communication needs. The Improving Outcomes Guidelines (2004) produced by the National Institute for Clinical Excellence[4] recommended that as part of the MDT, SLTs should meet and assess patients pretreatment. At whatever stage, the therapist first meets the patient, is important that they are able to assess the communication and swallowing symptoms accurately and have an opinion as to whether there is a way of improving the status of the patient with reference to two fundamental areas of life and function.

What the research says

As clinicians looking for information with specific reference to swallowing and communication, it soon becomes apparent that there are only a small number of papers that make reference to these functions. Where clinical trials have been conducted and swallowing measured they have been described as crude and non-standardized.[24] The randomized control trial methodology – cause and effect – is difficult to apply to this population. The more complex the topic, the less amenable it is to systematic review because of the multiple comparisons, range of treatments and outcomes that are studied.[25] The heterogeneous nature of the patients and the interaction of some of the effects have been reported.[20, 26] One needs to be mindful that much of the early data did not report on baseline pretreatment information, which means it is difficult to distil what may be a disease effect as opposed to a treatment effect. What is encouraging to note is that the measuring of quality of life and function are being seen as publishable end points alongside mortality statistics.[27, 28, 29, 30, 31] For clinicians the reality is that, as a result of so much variability, informing patients on the likely outcome of their speech and swallow needs to be carried out at an individual level.

The normal swallow

Swallowing is complex and involves cranial nerves, and the muscles that are innervated by them, transporting a liquid or solid bolus from the oral cavity through the pharynx into the oesophagus to the stomach. The normal process is quick, coordinated, automatic and safe. Tasting and chewing are controlled for the most part by the tongue and the lips, with the oral tongue moving the bolus in a controlled manner around the mouth until it has been manipulated well enough to allow a swallow into the pharynx.[32] There is a need for the build up of pressure in order to move the bolus, and while this is achieved in part by the tongue, the closure of the soft palate, the elevation of the larynx and the adduction of the vocal cords ensure that the bolus whether it is liquid or solid passes, without pooling, or escape into the oesophagus via the cricopharyngeus. Elevation and anterior movement of the laryngeal complex allows the cricopharyngeal muscle to open,[33] which explains why there can be limited success in performing a cricopharyngeal myotomy on the HNC patient.[34] Efficient movement of bolus relies on more than just muscle relaxation.

If one is reminded of the dynamic, precise and strong muscle pattern that is required to swallow safely, and relates the effects of the tumour or the treatment to the process, it is possible to build up predictions as to how the swallow or speech may be affected in general terms which will guide the team in their further assessment.

The assessment of swallowing

Liaison with members of the nutritional team will allow the MDT to judge whether the patient will be able to maintain adequate calorific intake during their treatment or whether they should be advised to have alternative methods of feeding. Close liaison with dietetic colleagues allows for the full dysphagic history to be gathered and acted upon.

Assessments fall into two categories:

- Subjective based on observation including bedside assessment[35] and by discussion/case history taking with the patient and their family.
- Objective (flexible endoscopic evaluation of swallowing (FEES)[36] and video fluoroscopy swallowing study (VFSS)[19]) both of which can define the pathophysiology of the swallow and help establish a rehabilitation programme with identifiable goals for the patient.[37, 38]

While **Table 47.1**, is by no means extensive, from a clinical point of view it highlights the main issues that one will consider when deciding upon which objective measure is best suited to the assessment. The ideal is that both investigations are available and depend on the information which is being sought.

Swallowing pretreatment

At pretreatment, HNC patients demonstrate a less efficient swallow.[39] Of the 352 patients assessed using VFSS in this study 59 per cent complained of difficulty swallowing, with those who had oral tumours and smaller tumours less likely to complain of dysphagia. Swallow function was worse for patients with oral and pharyngeal lesions than laryngeal lesions and with increased tumour stage. The conclusions of the study were that the patients, despite their symptoms, had highly functional swallows. In a study that investigated the swallowing function of stage III and IV HNC patients pretreatment, patients with laryngeal and hypopharyngeal

tumours had the most severe dysfunction.[40] This study did not find that swallowing function was correlated with tumour site or overall stage, which would add evidence to the adaption of patients to their dysfunction. In another study of pretreatment speech and swallowing by the use of regression techniques, in a number of patients with tumours of oral tongue and anterior floor of mouth, articulation was significantly reduced. In addition, the percentage of those with oral tongue and tongue base tumours that were also affected also significantly related to swallowing efficiency.[41] While the research does not allow for precise predictions to be made, it underlines the diverse nature of the symptoms and findings that can be identified in patients.

Of course, there is more to swallowing than solely the biomechanical process. Mood (depression, anxiety), change in taste, fatigue, pain on swallowing (odynophagia) and lifestyle will all influence appetite and may mean that a patient is not maintaining their normal weight. It is important for the MDT to bear in mind the different causes of reduced oral intake and to understand these changes within the context of the patient's normal lifestyle, which may or may not include high consumption of alcohol and tobacco.[42] The pretreatment stage is a valuable opportunity in which there is time to build an informed assessment of a patient's symptoms and how they might have already adapted to some of the changes caused by the disease process.

Swallowing disorders after surgery

If the therapist has seen the patient presurgery, judgements can be made as to how the surgery has impacted upon the patient. The SLT needs to assess the effect of the surgery on the patient's speech and swallow before the patient starts to

Table 47.1   Description of flexible endoscopic evaluation of swallow (FEES) and video fluoroscopy swallowing study (VFSS)

Assessment	FEES	VFSS
Description	View via nasendoscopy swallowing a range of bolus consistencies both liquid and solid	Radiographically image and record swallow of various bolus consistencies mixed with radio opaque material
Visualize	Dynamic view from velum to larynx in colour	Dynamic view of all oral tract structures in black and white from lips through to top of oesophagus. Laterally and anterior/posterior not simultaneously
Stage of swallow assessed	Pharyngeal	Pre-oral, oral, pharyngeal and oesophageal
Advantages	Good view of anatomical structures	Able to study temporal nature of swallow
	Able to check sensation with scope	Good for viewing effect of therapy techniques, repercussions on other stages of swallow
	Assess pooling of secretions	Silent aspiration evident
	Good assessment of velopharyngeal wall competence	Objective tool for research
	Able to view effect of recommended therapy techniques, e.g. good vocal cord closure	No part of the swallow is obscured during the process
	Repeatable at regular intervals	Well-developed descriptors of swallow
	Portable	
Disadvantages	Cannot view oral and oesophageal phase	Cannot be taken to the patient
	If swallow is complete, laryngeal elevation cannot visualize swallow at height of laryngeal elevation 'white out'	Unable to view swallow for long periods, has to be snapshot radiation exposure

trial oral intake. While in the acute stages of recuperation the need to heal will preclude eating and drinking. The SLT is still able to informally assess the patient's oral movements and their ability to deal with their saliva. This may include giving the patient an opportunity to try and communicate and give feedback on how they feel about any changes in their communication abilities. It is worth noting that research reports that a tracheostomy tube does not increase the likelihood of aspiration, and that neither the presence of the tube nor decannulation causes a deterioration or improvement in swallowing function. The presence of comorbidities predispose the patient to dysphagia and aspiration rather than the tracheostomy tube per se.[43]

As a general guide, the larger the resection and the more dynamic the structure resected the more one may expect the speech and swallow to be affected. A study on oral/oral pharyngeal resected patients concluded that the total volume of tongue resected, and percentage of tongue base resected had an impact on postoperative swallowing function.[44] In further studies investigating the effect of flaps, patients with comparable site of resection and percentage of oral tongue or tongue base resection had the same or better function if primary closure could be achieved in comparison to those who had a flap reconstruction.[45, 46]

At a laryngeal level, patients requiring a supracricoid laryngectomy are at risk of aspiration, and need the input of SLTs to identify and carry out swallowing and voice rehabilitation in order to prevent repeated aspiration, and to facilitate a return to oral intake and functional voice. Patients need to be carefully selected for the procedure in the knowledge that they are likely to have a period of aspiration after the surgery.[47] For patients who undergo a laryngectomy, the presumed outcome has been that they cannot aspirate and therefore have minimal dysphagic symptoms. The incidence of dysphagia for this patient population has been underreported.[48] The removal of the larynx results in an increased level of resistance of a bolus to flow through the pharynx into the upper oesophagus. To compensate for this, the patient has to increase the pressure from the tongue to overcome the altered pharynx.[49] If there is reduced tongue base pressure, there is prolonged bolus transit times and poor clearance of residue. The effects on the patient's quality of life and any reduced function are varied, and reduced function does not always lead to reduced quality of life.[50] If the disease process is such that there is a need to use a graft or stomach transposition, there may be subsequent dysphagia symptoms for the patient to adjust to.

Swallowing disorders after surgery and radiotherapy

Patients recommended as a result of their pathology to have radiotherapy will experience effects from treatment which may include neuromuscular damage and fibrosis of the irradiated tissues.[51] The implications of the treatment are that the oral and pharyngeal stages of swallowing are affected. In a small study of patients who had either had surgery and radiotherapy or surgery, only the latter group were reported to have slower oral transit times, due to xerostomia, greater pharyngeal residue and reduced cricopharyngeal opening due

to what is termed a reduction in the pharyngeal bolus driving pressure.[52] The same authors further explained the reduction in the pharyngeal bolus driving pressure as a consequence of radiation-induced fibrosis on the soft tissues, and that specifically the affect resulted in reduced tongue base retraction, a decreased bulging of the posterior pharyngeal wall, and a reduced duration of contact of the tongue base to the posterior pharyngeal wall.[53]

Swallowing disorders from chemotherapy and radiotherapy

Current research now indicates that radiotherapy and chemotherapy can affect the function of patients' swallow and quality of life issues. The term 'organ preservation' seems to have been used because there is not a specific date on which the tumour has been excised. There is plenty of evidence showing both short- and long-term radiotherapy and chemoradiotherapy have an effect on the patient's ability to return to normal diet.[54, 55, 56] Based on retrospective analysis of patient data, aspiration is a silent morbidity following chemoradiotherapy, and it is underreported because of the silent nature of the symptom in HNC patients.[57] While cure has got to be seen as the main objective of the treatment, it is important for clinicians to discuss with patients that there are going to be some changes in their swallowing abilities. The research remains sparse with information in terms of post one-year treatment, and much of the difficulty in trying to compare the expected effects is that the disease and treatments have many variables. When analysing saliva production post-chemoradiotherapy at 12 months post-treatment, saliva production was found to be significantly decreased which then impacted on the patients' perceptions of their swallowing ability and therefore their dietary choices.[58] In a study that investigated 170 patients who had been treated using both objective and subjective measures, it was the patients three months post-treatment who often had reduced oral intake and had a delayed pharyngeal swallow, incomplete laryngeal vestibule closure, reduced laryngeal elevation and a rating of a non-functional swallow, i.e. demonstrated aspiration, residue within the pharynx and prolonged transit times. Over time at 6 and 12 months, reduced laryngeal elevation and a rating of non-functional swallow remained significant to reduced oral intake, with poor cricopharyngeal opening appearing as a new relationship.[59] It is beyond the remit of this chapter to review these data in detail, but the precise nature of the symptoms described would allow a hypothesisn-driven treatment plan to remediate or at least minimize some of the symptoms that are being described. In the clinical situation SLTs are moving from merely describing the symptoms to what rehabilitation and compensatory techniques can be used to try and improve the oral intake and communication of the patient.

Speech and language interventions

In a review of swallowing dysfunction and rehabilitation strategies for HNC patients, the behavioural and therapeutic procedures used by SLTs to eliminate aspiration and increase the volume of oral intake are described.[60] The

from the United Kingdom reported that 53 per cent patients were hospitalized during the last month of life: the reasons for admission included bleeding episodes (17 per cent), pain problems (9 per cent), breathing difficulties (9 per cent), swallowing difficulties (9 per cent), inability to cope (6 per cent) and a fracture (3 per cent).[13]

In most cases, the terminal phase is relatively straight-forward in patients with HNC.[79] Thus, it is feasible to consider the option of a home death, particularly as the literature suggests that most cancer patients would prefer to die at home. In such circumstances, it is important that the patient and their families are provided with not only appropriate medical support, but also with adequate practical support (e.g. social services, physical aids). Nevertheless, it appears that most head and neck cancer patients die in hospital, rather than at home or in other care settings.[80, 81, 82] A recent study from the United Kingdom reported that 62 per cent of patients died in a hospital, 19 per cent died in a hospice, 16 per cent died at home and 3 per cent died in a nursing home.[80] There are numerous explanations (but little supportive information) to explain the high rate of hospital deaths (and the low rate of home deaths).[83] Nevertheless, a study from Israel reported that patients who died at home tended to be younger and had better symptom control than those who died in a hospital.[84]

In most instances, head and neck cancer patients die as a result of gradual deterioration in their condition[79, 80, 81] Furthermore, as discussed above, the majority of patients have a relatively uneventful terminal phase (i.e. from the health professional viewpoint).[79] Nevertheless, in some instances, HNC patients die as a result of an acute complication of their disease (e.g. airway obstruction, haemorrhage), or an acute event not directly related to the disease (e.g. myocardial infarction, pulmonary embolism). **Table 47.3** demonstrates the reported cause of death among a cohort of HNC patients admitted to a hospice in the United Kingdom.[79]

An MDT approach is as valid in the terminal phase of the illness as in the earlier phases of the disease process. This means that while specialist palliative care professionals are experienced in dealing with problems relating to symptom control, they are often less able, for example, to deal with problems relating to tracheostomy tubes or enteral feeding tubes. In addition, the transition from 'active treatment' to 'palliative care' may be made easier by the ongoing support of familiar healthcare professionals (e.g. CNS in head and neck oncology).

Finally, although the focus of end-of-life care is on the patient, it is important that the needs of the family are not overlooked. Family members often require psychological support during the terminal phase of the illness, but they may also require more practical assistance at this time (e.g. advice on legal matters/financial issues). Furthermore, it is important that ongoing/future problems are identified and that strategies are put in place to combat them. For example, it is possible to identify a person at increased risk of an abnormal bereavement reaction and to arrange appropriate support for such a person following the patient's death.[85]

QUALITY OF DEATH

Increasingly, the concept of quality of death has been highlighted in the literature. Quality of death, like quality of life, is a subjective phenomenon, which encompasses physical, psychological, spiritual and social domains. Not surprisingly, the concept of a 'good death' varies from individual to individual, and may vary within an individual over a period of time. It is influenced by a number of factors including personal circumstances, religion and culture.[86] Importantly, there are certain discrepancies between what healthcare professionals and patients and their families consider being a good death;[87, 88, 89] these discrepancies need to be acknowledged, since they could have implications for the provision of end-of-life care. Steinhauser et al.[90] identified factors important for a good death from four groups of people: seriously ill patients, recently bereaved families, doctors and other professionals (e.g. nurses, social workers). The factors that were common to all the groups are shown in **Box 47.5**. However, a number of other factors were highlighted by the group of seriously ill patients, including being mentally alert, not being a burden, planning funeral arrangements and coming to peace with God.

Provision of palliative care

In the United Kingdom, the provision of specialist palliative care is relatively comprehensive, although there are significant geographical variations in the type of services available.[91] Specialist palliative care services are found in both the primary care setting and also the secondary care setting. For example, in 2006 there were 221 hospice inpatient units, 257 hospice daycare centres, 356 home care teams and 114 'hospice at home' teams in the UK.[91] Similarly in 2006, there were 305 hospital support teams.[91] It should be noted that the constitution of these services are extremely variable, and the roles adopted by these services are also extremely variable. For example, some hospice inpatient units will provide respite care, while others will only provide admission for symptom control or terminal care.

Table 47.3 Causes of death in head and neck patients receiving palliative care.[14]

Cause of death	Number of patients ($n = 36$)
Progressive disease[a]	17 (47%)
Bronchopneumonia	9 (25%)
Massive haemorrhage	3 (8%)
Airway obstruction	2 (6%)
Myocardial infarction	2 (6%)
Cardiac failure	2 (6%)
Other	1 (2%)

[a]Condition gradually deteriorated.

Box 47.5   Common factors for a 'good death'

- Adequate pain/symptom control
- Clear decisions about management
- Being treated as a 'whole person'
- Making preparations for death
- Achieving a sense of completion

The specialty of palliative care developed as a result of deficiencies in the care of dying cancer patients. The general consensus is that specialist palliative care has improved the end-of-life care of cancer patients, and there is increasing research evidence to back up this impression.[92] However, a significant proportion of cancer patients do not receive specialist palliative care at the end of life. In an attempt to address the latter issue, a number of end-of-life initiatives have been introduced in various countries. In the UK, the Department of Health's End of Life Initiative (www.endoflifecare.nhs.uk) includes support for the Gold Standards Framework in primary care (www.goldstandardsframework.nhs.uk),[93] the Liverpool Care Pathway in secondary care (www.lcp-mariecurie.org.uk)[94] and Preferred Place of Care tools. It should be noted that similar end-of-life strategies have been developed in other countries.

THE ROLE OF DATA COLLECTION

Introduction

The 1995 Calman–Hine Report (a policy framework for commissioning cancer services),[1] identified significant variability in cancer services and care provision in the United Kingdom. These variable outcomes helped shape the National NHS Cancer Plan,[69] and the subsequent National Institute for Health and Clinical Excellence (NICE) report on improving outcomes in head and neck cancers (2004)[4] and more recently 'Improving outcomes: a strategy for cancer'.[95] Recommendations in these documents for improving quality of service provision highlight the importance of clinical data collection and subsequent clinical audit. Audit allows variations in management and outcome to be assessed and helps identify possible contributory factors to these variations, such as inconsistency in standards of clinical practice, variability in resource or differing levels of comorbidity or disease extent. For all head and neck cancer units to be able to contribute to national prospective audit and long-term population-based studies requires the use of a standardized minimum data set.

Evolution of a minimum data set

In April 1999, the British Association of Head and Neck Oncologists (BAHNO)[96] published a National Minimum Data Set to collect the minimum data required utilizing national coding systems, e.g. OPCS4, ICD10 and TNM staging, to allow cross-comparison of care and incorporated the Royal College of Pathologists' 1998 histopathology minimum data set.[97]

NATIONAL CANCER DATASET

BAHNO[98] actively contributed with other specialist societies to work led by the then NHS Information Authority (now the NHS Information Centre for Health and Social Care (NHSIC)) to deliver the National Cancer Dataset (NCDS).

The NCDS was designed to meet the requirements for:

- cancer registration;
- clinical governance (national risk-adjusted clinical audit data are a key component);
- local data (research and publication, capacity/demand);
- NHS performance management (ensures national waiting times' targets are met).

Version 1,[99] published in 2000, included generic data fields applicable to all cancers and this was accompanied by a data manual defining all items and codes. The dataset was designed to incorporate events during a patient's journey, i.e. referral to follow up or death, incorporating diagnostic imaging and procedures, staging and care plan (MDT); surgical and oncology treatments; resective pathology and included site-specific items relevant to head and neck cancer. A series of updates to the NCDS has been published with a revised version the National Clinical Outcomes dataset to be released in late 2012.

DEVELOPMENT OF NATIONAL CANCER AUDIT

The National Clinical Audit Support Programme (NCASP) originally commissioned by the Healthcare Commission (formerly CHI) was initiated in 2001 to deliver national comparative audit based upon the NCDS subset for head and neck cancer. NCASP also supported professional bodies working in lung cancer (LUCADA), bowel cancer (NBO-CAP), oesophagogastric cancer (NOGCA) and mastectomy and reconstruction (NMBRA).

NCASP AND BAHNO

In 2002, agreement was reached for BAHNO together with a multiprofessional Head and Neck Clinical Reference Group to work with NCASP to develop a collaborative approach to national audit, and in 2004 a head and neck national database, DAHNO (Data for Head and Neck Oncology), was deployed in England. Data were received from Wales for the first time in 2006, collected via transfer from the Cancer Network Information System Cymru (CaNISC). The DAHNO project aims for secure centralized data collection, rapid comparative reporting, mortality and data quality tracking, and works towards providing the public and commissioners with access to risk-adjusted comparative clinical audit data, as well as assurance of multiprofessional care provision.

The first phase of DAHNO included all patients with a new diagnosis of squamous cell carcinoma of the oral cavity or larynx. Phase II extended the anatomic sites to include pharynx (naso-, oro- and hypo-) and major salivary gland, and additional data fields relating to specialist nursing, nutrition, swallowing and surgical voice restoration.

The fledgling first annual report published by DAHNO in 2006 showed 1038 cases which compares to 25 per cent of the expected total in England.[100] Subsequent annual reports have shown steady improvements in case ascertainment, and included Welsh data.[101] The sixth (2011) report[102] includes 95 per cent of the expected total for England and Wales, some 6400 cases, with submission from all but two trusts delivering head and neck cancer care. The main findings of the sixth annual report are: improved assurance of delivery of multiprofessional care, increased levels of T and N pretreatment staging and risk factor recording, and improvements were seen in the length of time patients waited for key aspects of care. Delays to radiotherapy remained a challenge.

Key case-mix factors considered in DAHNO are:

- age and sex (patient demographics);
- deprivation (derived from area of residence at time of diagnosis);
- comorbidity using the ACE-27 comorbidity index (presence and level of decompensation from other illnesses);
- performance status using ECOG (ability to perform tasks of daily living);
- stage at presentation using UICC TNM staging at time of treatment decision (to include presenting site, histological type and anatomic extent of disease).

The initial DAHNO reports concentrated on timeliness and delivery of pathway processes and provision of multi-disciplinary assessment, but in the sixth report variation in the delivery of care pathways (e.g early larynx treatment) have been examined. Future reporting will move to look at case-mix adjusted outcomes in order to clearly identify areas of good and poor practice with a view to improving overall patient care. To be able to accurately draw comparative conclusions, it is very important for contributors to include case-mix factors so that 'like' can be compared with 'like'.

THYROID CANCER AND NATIONAL AUDIT

While a National Cancer Dataset has been derived for thyroid cancer, this has not as yet been translated into a national comparative audit. In thyroid cancer, there are significant differences in clinical pathways compared with those of other sites within the head and neck. Thyroid cancer is a much rarer cancer with a better prognosis and, usually, a longer diagnostic pathway and follow-up period. In most cases, the first definitive and curative treatment for thyroid cancer is a diagnostic hemi-thyroidectomy which inevitably means the data have to be collected retrospectively and the patient will not be discussed at MDT until after the first treatment. The British Association of Endocrine and Thyroid Surgeons (BAETS) has maintained a national clinical audit database covering thyroid, parathyroid, adrenal and pancreatic surgery which also encompasses benign thyroid cases. BAETS membership is not mandatory for surgeons who perform endocrine surgery and therefore analysis may not provide a reliable picture of national practice. However, if a surgeon is a member of BAETS, then it is compulsory to participate in the national audit. The third national audit report was published in 2009.[103] Clinical data are entered via a secure web browser-based database and the annually updated data set is informed by current evidence-based clinical practice. The database facilitates anonymised analysis on clinical outcomes and practice, as well as a demographic analysis of disease incidence. The National Cancer Intelligence Network (NCIN) (www.ncin.org.uk) is currently actively engaging clinical groups who manage thyroid cancer to facilitate a process to enable audit in thyroid cancer.

CLINICAL AUDIT AND PEER REVIEW

The National Cancer Peer Review Programme seeks to support quality assurance and enables improvement of services in head and neck cancer. A group of peer reviewers performs assessment of compliance by cancer networks and individual units against a set of detailed measures (standards of service). The outcomes of the peer review programme aim to identify shortcomings in the quality of cancer services where they occur, so that rectification and improvements can be made and confirm that services are of approved quality. The 2011 peer review round has, for the first time, included Clinical Lines of Enquiry (www.cquins.nhs.uk), which take findings from DAHNO, as well as identifying additional local areas for audit. These aim to provide a greater focus within peer review on clinical issues, and to span different professional contributions along the patient pathway.

Cancer waiting times' targets, December 2005

As from the first quarter of 2006, it became mandatory for all trusts to report waiting times for all their newly diagnosed cancer patients. This was for government monitoring of targets from referral to first definitive treatment for patients with suspected cancer referred urgently by their general practitioner (62 days) and from decision to treat to first definitive treatment for all sources of referral (31 days) (**Figure 47.2**). This required patient pathways to be streamlined resulting in reduced waiting times for diagnostic tests and changes in the way hospitals work together. An additional benefit is greater focus on cancer data collection, as the only way for hospitals to monitor where patients are on their pathway and how long they have before the targets are breached, is to collect data on each patient.

The continuation of cancer wait times monitoring was affirmed in 'Improving outcomes: A strategy for cancer' (2011).[95]

Key principles of data collection

BEST PRACTICE

Currently, units use combinations of data collection methods including paper proformas and expansion of current outpatient notation forms; direct data entry to DAHNO or commercial databases; uploads to DAHNO from a third-party patient clinical information system or custom-made Microsoft Access databases or spreadsheets, and creation of automatic links to existing electronic hospital information systems. Best practice workshops have confirmed that the most successful will be led by one committed individual whose role is to promote and oversee collection, collation,

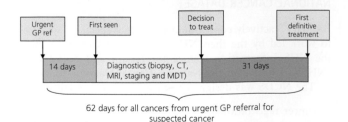

Figure 47.2   Cancer waiting times' targets.

quality control and analysis of head and neck data. This individual can be a clinician or an administrative data manager, an MDT coordinator or medical secretary. Certainly, multidisciplinary team support and direct involvement of members is crucial as clinical data include everyone involved in the patient's journey. The dilemma is not only about where and how to collect the data, but who is going to input the data, as every member of the multidisciplinary team will inevitably have a busy workload. Often the person who leads the data process is one who has an avid interest in technology, and has a keen desire to see and act on the results of cancer information and strives to attain the highest standards of patient care by the team.

TRUST-WIDE STRATEGY

In an ideal situation, a trust-wide strategy should be developed to use the same software for data collection which will inevitably prevent repetition, inconsistency and misinterpretation of core data. In this way, data can be shared and used for different purposes, such as cancer waiting times' data measuring and monitoring the 14-, 31- and 62-day waiting times' targets; national audits; local clinicians' use for research, audit and management; and audits of local demand and activity, etc. IT departments should be involved in linking the database to existing hospital electronic information systems, such as patient information systems, radiology and pathology systems, oncology tracking systems, etc.

MULTIDISCIPLINARY TEAM MEETING

The multidisciplinary team meeting to discuss a patient's care plan is the central focal point for decision and planning, at which time all professionals involved with each patient should be present. Data on diagnosis, morphology, tumour site and clinical pretreatment staging, comorbidity, performance status, social history and risk factors should be available. This is the ideal time to raise, capture and identify any missing data while the appropriate personnel are all together and any ambiguous data items can be discussed. An individual team member should be responsible for recording and this can be a data manager, MDT coordinator, secretary or clinician. The lead clinician should ensure that all the data required and the care plan are made clear and that there are no missing data at this point, before proceeding to the following patient.

It is imperative to use the NHS number wherever possible as it is this identifier which will be used in national audit. To encourage individuals to input data to a database, rewards in the form of automatically generated correspondence such as discharge letters, GP letters, monitoring reports, MDT meeting lists and minutes, monitoring and tracking reports should be incorporated. Wherever possible, prospective data collection at source should be the ultimate goal, since retrospective data gleaned from hospital notes is time-consuming, may lead to misinterpretation and will be of lesser quality to data collected prospectively. It is essential that any database is networked across the hospital so that any number of individuals can contribute to the database at any time by adding their contribution to the patient record. This will also mean data are secure and backed up.

The clinician should be able to trust the data being collected and this can only be gained by clinical ownership and direct involvement in the process. In reality, not every single item needs to be checked (signed off), but each consultant should be satisfied that the patient record makes clinical sense and the diagnosis, pretreatment staging, clinical status and care plan information are correct, and that subsequent audit submissions are valid. Collection of clinical data must not be viewed solely as an administrative exercise, but as an integral part of the clinician's role, and for national comparative audit to be successful, clinical audit contribution should be an aspect included within everyone's appraisal and personal development.

KEY EVIDENCE

The role of speech and language therapy

- The gold standard of research methodology – the randomized control trial design – is not well suited to the study of HNC patients' swallowing and communication difficulties. Disease, patient and treatment variables[25] impinge upon the cause and effect paradigm.
- As members of the MDT, SLTs are well placed to assess and review the impact of the disease and treatments on patients both in terms of changes to the oral tract[60] and the impact on quality of life.[20, 26]
- While it is wholly appropriate to review the literature with reference to the impact of disease and treatment on patients' function,[24, 45, 53, 59] it is also essential that clinical judgement at an individual level is maintained in order to explore the interaction of the patient's adaptive practices to the symptoms that they present with.[26]

The role of data collection

- National comparative head and neck cancer audit is established across the NHS in England and Wales.[102]
- The future agenda in cancer audit has been set out in 'Improving outcomes: A strategy for cancer' (2011).[95] Recommendations for improving quality of service provision highlight the importance of clinical data collection and subsequent clinical audit.

KEY LEARNING POINTS

The role of the clinical nurse specialist

- The clinical nurse specialist (CNS) is a core member of the multidisciplinary team.
- The CNS is key to the coordination of care for the patient and a point of contact for them, the family and carers.

- Information needs to be presented to meet individual needs in a timely way.
- Involvement of a CNS promotes holistic needs assessment and care.

The role of speech and language therapy

- Swallowing and communication may be affected by either the disease, the treatment directly or the patient's reaction to the changes that are enforced.
- Swallowing is timed and coordinated, and patients show adaptive behaviours prior to treatment. SLTs work as integral members of the MDT and relate closely with many members of the team on a daily basis.
- SLTs are well placed to offer ongoing assessment, management and support to the HNC patient which is so much more easily achieved if they are able to meet the patient at the pretreatment stage.
- Research needs to be seen in the context of the individual patient because each patient will present with a unique set of variables that the team have to work with.
- The larger the resection required and the more dynamic the structure affected, the more dysphagic or communication difficulties are predicted.
- Radiotherapy and chemoradiotherapy may impact on the coordination of swallowing and speech in the short or long term as a result of the fibrosing of soft tissues.
- Objective and subjective assessments will help devise strategies which include postures, changed consistencies, swallowing manoeuvres and exercises to start or safely maintain oral intake and communication.

The role of palliative care

- Palliative care involves the management of the physical, psychological, spiritual and social complications of cancer.
- Palliative care is not synonymous with terminal care.
- Palliative care may be applicable to patients with early disease.

The role of data collection

- Clinician confidence in the data being collected, can only be gained by clinical ownership and direct involvement in the process, and should be seen as an integral part of the clinician's role.
- The multidisciplinary team meeting to discuss a patient's care plan is the central focal point for decision and planning and is an ideal point at which data can be collected at which time all professionals involved with each patient should be present.
- The NHS number should be recorded for all patients as it is the key linkage in assimilating information from different sources.

- A trust-wide strategy for cancer information is the preferred route to allow use of the same software for data collection which will inevitably prevent repetition, inconsistency and misinterpretation of core data.
- The recent introduction of Clinical Lines of Enquiry aims to provide a greater focus within peer review on clinical issues, and to span different professional contributions along the patient pathway. The national lines of enquiry use information from DAHNO.

REFERENCES

1. Department of Health. A policy framework for commissioning cancer services: a report by the Expert Advisory Group on Cancer to the Chief Medical Officers of England and Wales. London: HMSO, 1995.
2. Fleissig A, Jenkins V, Catt S, Fallowfield L. Multidisciplinary teams in cancer care: are they effective in the UK? *Lancet Oncology* 2006; **7**: 935–43.
3. Ruhstaller T, Roe H, Thurlimann B, Nicoll JJ. The multidisciplinary meeting: an indispensable aid to communication between different specialities. *European Journal of Cancer* 2006; **42**: 2459–63.
4. National Institute for Clinical Excellence. Guidance on cancer services – improving outcomes in head and neck cancers. The manual. London: NICE, 2004.
5. British Thyroid Association. Guidelines for the management of thyroid cancer in adults. Informing the patient. London: BTA, 2002: 6.
6. Feber T. *Head and neck oncology nursing*. London: Whurr Publishers, 2000.
7. Dear S. Breaking bad news: caring for the family. *Nursing Standard* 1995; **10**: 31–3.
8. Buckman R. *How to break bad news. A guide for health professionals*. London: Pan Books, 1994.
9. Ziegler L, Newell R, Stafford N, Lewin R. A literature review of head and neck cancer patients information needs, experiences and views regarding decision-making. *European Journal of Cancer Care* 2004; **13**: 119–26.
10. Edwards D. Head and neck cancer services: views of patients, their families and professionals. *British Journal of Oral and Maxillofacial Surgery* 1998; **36**: 99–102.
11. Semple C, McGowan B. Need for appropriate written information for patients, with particular reference to head and neck cancer. *Journal of Clinical Nursing* 2002; **11**: 585–93.
12. Edwards D. *Face to face: patient, family and professional perspectives of head and neck cancer care*. London: King's Fund, 1997.
13. Owen-Hafiz C. The role of the specialist nurse. In: Mazzaferri EL, Harmer C, Mallick UK, Kendall-Taylor P

(eds.). *Practical management of thyroid cancer.* London: Springer, 2006: 59–63.

14. Dobbins M, Gunson J, Bale S *et al.* Improving patient care and quality of life after laryngectomy/glossectomy. *British Journal of Nursing* 2005; **14**: 634–40.

15. Dropkin M. Body image and quality of life after head and neck surgery. *Cancer Practice* 1999; **7**: 309–13.

16. Rapoport Y, Kreitler S, Chaitchik S *et al.* Psychosocial problems in head and neck cancer patients and their change with time since diagnosis. *Annals of Oncology* 1993; **4**: 69–73.

17. Bjordal K, Kassa S. Psychological distress in head and neck cancer patients 7–11 years after curative treatment. *British Journal of Cancer* 1995; **71**: 592–7.

18. Whale Z, Lyne PA, Papanikolaou P. Pain experience following radical treatment for head and neck cancer. *European Journal of Oncology Nursing* 2001; **5**: 112–20.

19. Young J, Howells N. Providing complementary therapies in a cancer hospital. In: Barraclough J (ed.). *Integrated cancer care. Holistic, complementary and creative approaches.* Oxford: Oxford University Press, 2001.

20. Scharloo M, Baatenburg de Jong R, Langeveld Ton PM *et al.* Quality of life and illness perceptions in patients with recently diagnosed head and neck cancer. *Head and Neck* 2005; **27**: 857–63.

21. Morton RP. Studies in the quality of life of head and neck cancer patients: a result of a two year longitudinal study and a comparative cross-sectional cross-cultural survey. *Laryngoscope* 2003; **113**: 1091–110.

◆ 22. Ringash J, Bezjak A. A structured review of Quality of life instruments for head and neck cancer patients. *Head and Neck* 2001; **23**: 201–13.

23. Funk GF, Karnell LH, Smith RB, Christensen AJ. Clinical significance of health status assessment measures in head and neck cancer: what do quality-of-life scores mean? *Archives of Otolaryngology – Head and Neck Surgery* 2004; **130**: 825–9.

◆ 24. Frowen JJ, Perry AR. Swallowing outcomes after radiotherapy for head and neck cancer: a systematic review. *Head and Neck* 2006; **28**: 932–44.

25. Hicks C. Concepts and theories II: operationalism and its legacy. In: Brown B, Crawford P, Hicks C (eds). *Evidence-based research: dilemmas and debates in health care.* Buckingham: Open University Press, 2003.

26. Llewellyn CD, McGurk M, Weinman J. Head and neck cancer: to what extent can psychological factors explain differences between health-related quality of life and individual quality of life? *British Journal of Oral and Maxillofacial Surgery* 2006; **44**: 351–7.

27. Lovell S, Wong H, Loh K *et al.* Impact of dysphagia on quality-of-life in nasopharyngeal carcinoma. *Head and Neck* 2005; **27**: 864–72.

28. List MA, Mumby P, Haraf D *et al.* Performance and quality of life outcome in patients completing concomitant chemoradiotherapy protocols for head and neck cancer. *Quality of Life Research* 1997; **6**: 274–84.

29. Nordgren M, Jannert M, Boysen M *et al.* Health-related quality of life in patients with pharyngeal carcinoma: a five-year follow-up. *Head and Neck* 2006; **28**: 339–49.

30. Rogers SN, Lowe D, Fisher SE *et al.* Health-related quality of life and clinical function after primary surgery for oral cancer. *British Journal of Oral and Maxillofacial Surgery* 2002; **40**: 11–18.

31. Schliephake H, Jamil MU. Prospective evaluation of quality of life after oncologic surgery for oral cancer. *International Journal of Oral and Maxillofacial Surgery* 2002; **31**: 427–33.

32. Kahrilas PJ, Logemann JA, Lin S, Ergun GA. Pharyngeal clearance during swallowing: a combined manometric and videofluoroscopic study. *Gastroenterology* 1992; **103**: 128–36.

33. Jacob P, Kahrilas PJ, Logemann JA *et al.* Upper esophageal sphincter opening and modulation during swallowing. *Gastroenterology* 1989; **97**: 1469–78.

34. Jacobs JR, Logemann J, Pajak TF *et al.* Failure of cricopharyngeal myotomy to improve dysphagia following head and neck cancer surgery. *Archives of Otolaryngology – Head and Neck Surgery* 1999; **125**: 942–6.

● 35. Logemann JA. *Evaluation and treatment of swallowing disorders.* Austin, TX: Pro-Ed, 1998.

36. Langmore SE. Role of flexible laryngoscopy for evaluating aspiration. *Annals of Otology, Rhinology and Laryngology* 1998; **107**: 446.

● 37. Logemann J. *Manual for video fluoroscopic study of swallowing,* 2nd edn. Austin, TX: Pro-Ed, 1993.

38. Simental AA Jr, Carrau RL. Assessment of swallowing function in patients with head and neck cancer. *Current Oncology Reports* 2004; **6**: 162–5.

39. Pauloski BR, Rademaker AW, Logemann JA *et al.* Pretreatment swallowing function in patients with head and neck cancer. *Head and Neck* 2000; **22**: 474–82.

40. Stenson KM, MacCracken E, List M *et al.* Swallowing function in patients with head and neck cancer prior to treatment. *Archives of Otolaryngology – Head and Neck Surgery* 2000; **126**: 371–7.

41. Colangelo LA, Logemann JA, Rademaker AW. Tumor size and pretreatment speech and swallowing in patients with resectable tumors. *Otolaryngology – Head and Neck Surgery* 2000; **122**: 653–61.

◆ 42. Blot WJ, McLaughlin JK, Winn DM *et al.* Smoking and drinking in relation to oral and pharyngeal cancer. *Cancer Research* 1988; **48**: 3282–7.

43. Leder SB, Joe JK, Ross DA *et al.* Presence of a tracheotomy tube and aspiration status in early, post surgical head and neck cancer patients. *Head and Neck* 2005; **27**: 757–61.

44. Pauloski BR, Rademaker AW, Logemann JA *et al.* Surgical variables affecting swallowing in patients treated for oral/oropharyngeal cancer. *Head and Neck* 2004; **26**: 625–36.

45. McConnel FM, Pauloski BR, Logemann JA. Functional results of primary closure vs flaps in oropharyngeal reconstruction. A prospective study of speech and

swallowing. *Archives of Otolaryngology – Head and Neck Surgery* 1998; **124**: 625–30.

46. Zuydam AC, Lowe D, Brown JS *et al.* Predictors of speech and swallowing function following primary surgery for oral and oropharyngeal cancer. *Clinical Otolaryngology* 2005; **30**: 428–37.

47. Farrag TY, Koch WM, Cummings CW *et al.* Supracricoid laryngectomy outcomes: the Johns Hopkins experience. *Laryngoscope* 2007; **117**: 129–32.

48. Ward EC, Bishop B, Frisby J, Stevens M. Swallowing outcomes following laryngectomy and pharyngolaryngectomy. *Archives of Otolaryngology – Head and Neck Surgery* 2002; **128**: 181–6.&dopt=Abstract">PMID: 12574769

49. McConnel FM, Cerenko D, Mendolsohn MS. Dysphagia after total laryngectomy. *Otolaryngologic Clinics of North America* 1988; **21**: 721–6.

50. Deleyiannis FW, Weymuller EA Jr, Coltrera MD, Futran N. Quality of life after laryngectomy: are functional disabilities important? *Head and Neck* 1999; **21**: 319–24.

51. Pauloski BR, Rademaker AW, Logemann JA *et al.* Relationship between swallow motility disorders on videofluorography and oral intake in patients treated for head and neck cancer with radiotherapy with or without chemotherapy. *Head and Neck* 2006; **28**: 1069–76.

52. Pauloski BR, Rademaker AW, Logemann JA, Colangelo LA. Speech and swallowing in irradiated and non irradiated post surgical oral cancer patients. *Otolaryngology – Head and Neck Surgery* 1998; **118**: 616–24.

53. Pauloski BR, Logemann JA. Impact of tongue and posterior pharyngeal wall biomechanics on pharyngeal clearance in irradiated postsurgical oral and oropharyngeal cancer patients. *Head and Neck* 2000; **22**: 120–31.

54. Kotz T, Abraham S, Beitler JJ *et al.* Pharyngeal transport dysfunction consequent to an organ-sparing protocol. *Archives of Otolaryngology – Head and Neck Surgery* 1999; **125**: 410–13.

55. Lazarus CL, Logemann JA, Pauloski BR *et al.* Swallowing disorders in head and neck cancer patients treated with radiotherapy and adjuvant chemotherapy. *Laryngoscope* 1996; **106**: 1157–66.

56. Smith RV, Kotz T, Beitler JJ, Wadler S. Long-term swallowing problems after organ preservation therapy with concomitant radiation therapy and intravenous hydroxyurea: initial results. *Archives of Otolaryngology – Head and Neck Surgery* 2000; **126**: 384–9.

57. Nguyen NP, Frank C, Moltz CC *et al.* Aspiration rate following chemoradiation for head and neck cancer: an underreported occurrence. *Radiotherapy and Oncology* 2006; **80**: 302–6.

58. Logemann JA, Smith CH, Pauloski BR. Effects of xerostomia on perception and performance of swallow function. *Head and Neck* 2001; **23**: 317–21.

59. Pauloski BR, Rademaker AW, Logemann JA *et al.* Relationship between swallow motility disorders on videofluorography and oral intake in patients treated for head and neck cancer with radiotherapy with or without chemotherapy. *Head and Neck* 2006; **28**: 1069–76.

♦ 60. Mittal BB, Pauloski BR, Haraf DJ *et al.* Swallowing dysfunction – preventative and rehabilitation strategies in patients with head and neck cancer treated with surgery, radiotherapy and chemotherapy: a critical review. *International Journal of Radiation Oncology, Biology, Physics* 2003; **57**: 1219–30.

61. Logemann JA, Rademaker AW, Pauloski BR, Kahrilas PJ. Effects of postural change on aspiration in head and neck surgical patients. *Otolaryngology – Head and Neck Surgery* 1994; **110**: 222–7.

62. Veis S, Logemann JA, Colangelo L. Effects of three techniques on maximum posterior movement of the tongue base. *Dysphagia* 2000; **15**: 142–5.

63. Lazarus C, Logemann JA, Song CW *et al.* Effects of voluntary maneuvers on tongue base function for swallowing. *Folia Phoniatrica et Logopaedica* 2002; **54**: 171–6.

64. Logemann JA, Pauloski BR, Rademaker AW, Colangelo LA. Super-supraglottic swallow in irradiated head and neck cancer patients. *Head and Neck* 1997; **19**: 535–40.

65. Lazarus C, Logemann JA, Gibbons P. Effects of manoeuvres on swallowing function in a dysphagic oral cancer patient. *Head and Neck* 1993; **15**: 419–24.

66. Kahrilas PJ, Logemann JA, Krugler C, Flanagan E. Volitional augmentation of upper esophageal sphincter opening during swallowing. *American Journal of Physiology* 1991; **260**: G450–6.

67. Lazarus CL. Effects of radiation therapy and voluntary manoeuvres on swallow functioning in head and neck cancer patients. *Clinics in Communication Disorders* 1993; **3**: 11–20.

68. World Health Organization. National Cancer Control Programmes. *Policies and managerial guidelines*, 2nd edn. Geneva: WHO, 2002.

∗ 69. Department of Health. The NHS cancer plan. London: DOH, 2000.

∗ 70. National Institute for Clinical Excellence. Improving supportive and palliative care for adults with cancer. The manual. London: NICE, 2004.

71. Booth S, Davies A (eds). *Palliative care consultations in head and neck cancer*. Oxford: Oxford University Press, 2006.

72. Davies A. Oral problems. In: Booth S, Davies A (eds). *Palliative care consultations in head and neck cancer*. Oxford: Oxford University Press, 2006: 77–89.

♦ 73. Berger AM, Portenoy RK, Weissman DE (eds). *Principles and practice of palliative care and supportive oncology*, 2nd edn. Philadelphia: Lippincott Williams & Wilkins, 2002.

74. Doyle D, Hanks G, Cherny NI, Calman K (eds). *Oxford textbook of palliative medicine*, 3rd edn. Oxford: Oxford University Press, 2004.

75. Kaasa S, Loge JH. Quality of life in palliative medicine – principles and practice. In: Doyle D, Hanks G, Cherny NI, Calman K (eds). *Oxford textbook of palliative medicine*, 3rd edn. Oxford: Oxford University Press, 2004: 196–210.

76. Calman KC. Quality of life in cancer patients – an hypothesis. *Journal of Medical Ethics* 1984; **10**: 124–7.

77. Fardy M. Oro-facial cancer – is there more to treatment than surgery and radiotherapy? *Palliative Care Today* 1997; **6**: 20–1.

78. Rhys Evans PH, Patel SG. Introduction. In: Rhys Evans PH, Montgomery PQ, Gullane PJ (eds). *Principles and practice of head and neck oncology*. London: Martin Dunitz, 2003: 3–13.

● 79. Forbes K. Palliative care in patients with cancer of the head and neck. *Clinical Otolaryngology and Allied Sciences* 1997; **22**: 117–22.

● 80. Ethunandan M, Rennie A, Hoffman G et al. Quality of dying in head and neck cancer patients: a retrospective analysis of potential indicators of care. *Oral Surgery, Oral Medicine, Oral Pathology, Oral Radiology, and Endodontics* 2005; **100**: 147–52.

81. Shedd DP, Carl A, Shedd C. Problems of terminal head and neck cancer patients. *Head and Neck Surgery* 1980; **2**: 476–82.

82. Leitner C, Rogers SN, Lowe D, Magennis P. Death certification in patients whose primary treatment for oral and oropharyngeal carcinoma was operation: 1992–1997. *British Journal of Oral and Maxillofacial Surgery* 2001; **39**: 204–9.

83. Gomes B, Higginson IJ. Factors influencing death at home in terminally ill patients with cancer: systematic review. *British Medical Journal* 2006; **332**: 515–21.

84. Talmi YP, Bercovici M, Waller A et al. Home and inpatient hospice care of terminal head and neck cancer patients. *Journal of Palliative Care* 1997; **13**: 9–14.

85. Kissane DW. Bereavement. In: Doyle D, Hanks G, Cherny NI, Calman K (eds). *Oxford textbook of palliative medicine*, 3rd edn. Oxford: Oxford University Press, 2004: 1137–51.

86. Walter T. Historical and cultural variants on the good death. *British Medical Journal* 2003; **327**: 218–20.

87. Payne SA, Langley-Evans A, Hillier R. Perceptions of a "good" death: a comparative study of the views of hospice staff and patients. *Palliative Medicine* 1996; **10**: 307–12.

88. Steinhauser KE, Clipp EC, McNeilly M et al. In search of a good death: observations of patients, families and providers. *Annals of Internal Medicine* 2000; **132**: 825–32.

89. Clark J. Freedom from unpleasant symptoms is essential for a good death. *British Medical Journal* 2003; **327**: 180.

90. Steinhauser KE, Christakis NA, Clipp EC et al. Factors considered important at the end of life by patients, family, physicians, and other care providers. *Journal of the American Medical Association* 2000; **284**: 2476–82.

91. Help the Hospices. Hospice and palliative care directory United Kingdom and Ireland 2006. London: Help the Hospices, 2006.

92. Finlay IG, Higginson IJ, Goodwin DM et al. Palliative care in hospital, hospice, at home: results from a systematic review. *Annals of Oncology* 2002; **13** (Suppl. 4): 257–64.

✳ 93. Thomas K. *Caring for the dying at home: companions on the journey*. Abingdon: Radcliffe Medical Press, 2003.

✳ 94. Ellershaw J, Wilkinson S. *Care of the dying: a pathway to excellence*. Oxford: Oxford University Press, 2003.

95. Department of Health. Improving outcomes: a strategy for cancer. London: DoH. Available from: www.dh.gov.uk/en/Publicationsandstatistics/Publications/PublicationsPolicyAndGuidance/DH_123371.

96. British Association of Head and Neck Oncologists. BAHNO national minimum and advisory head and neck cancer data sets version 1. London: British Association of Head and Neck Oncologists, 1999.

97. Royal Collection of Pathologists. Minimum data set for head and neck carcinoma histopathology reports. London: Royal Collection of Pathologists, 1998.

98. British Association of Otorhinolaryngologists – Head and Neck Surgeons. Effective head and neck cancer management. Third consensus document. London: ENT UK, 2002.

99. NHS Information Centre. National cancer dataset version 1. London: NHS Information Centre.

100. NHS Health and Social Care Information Centre. DAHNO First Annual Report: key findings from the National Head and Neck Cancer Audit for the period January 2004 to November 2005. London: The Information Centre, 2006.

101. National Head and Neck Cancer Audit. Available from: www.ic.nhs.uk/services/national-clinical-audit-support-programme-ncasp/audit-reports/head-and-neck-cancer.

102. Data for Head and Neck Oncology (DAHNO). Annual report. Available from: www.ic.nhs.uk/webfiles/Services/NCASP/audits%20and%20reports/Head_and_Neck_Cancer_Audit_2010/NHS_Head_Neck_Cancer_Audit_ERRATA.pdf.

103. British Association of Endocrine and Thyroid Surgeons (BAETS). Third National Audit Report. 2009. Available from: www.baets.org.uk/Pages/BAETS%203rd%20National%20Audit.pdf.

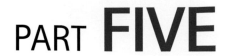

PART **FIVE**

RECONSTRUCTION

Section editors: Ralph W Gilbert and David Soutar

48

Basic principles of head and neck plastic surgery

TAIMUR SHOAIB

Every act of creation is first an act of destruction.

Pablo Picasso

INTRODUCTION

In head and neck surgery, there are several reconstructive principles. We should aim to replace like with like, there should be movement where movement is needed, we should use thin pliable tissue when mobility is important and bulk where filling is required. Static supports may be needed when tissue ptosis is likely to be predicted and colour matching with excellent tissue handling skills are required to achieve cosmesis, epithelial cover should be robust and we should consider the need for potential future surgery to ensure we keep our options available and not 'burn any bridges'. Lastly, and perhaps most importantly in the twenty-first century, it behoves the contemporary plastic surgeon to be mindful of the need to keep at the forefront of his mind the need to minimize donor site morbidity. Head and neck reconstruction encompasses plastic surgery of the oral cavity, the oropharynx, the pharynx, the midface and bones, complex aesthetic structures, the head and neck skin and facial reanimation.

HISTORY OF HEAD AND NECK RECONSTRUCTION

Historically, the cheek flap and the forehead flap were probably the first flaps described for head and neck reconstruction. The cheek flap was first described for nasal reconstruction by Sushruta in 600–800BC, and so plastic surgery as a specialty was born over 2000 years ago in India, as was the specialty of head and neck reconstruction. In his book, the Sushruta Samhita (roughly translated as Sushruta's Compendium), Sushruta wrote detailed notes on nasal reconstruction. In India at that time, the nose was seen as a symbol of dignity and respect. Prisoners, adulterers and other criminals would have their nose amputated as punishment. Sushruta described the use of a template made from a leaf which was then placed on the cheek from where the flap was raised. The cheek rhinoplasty flap of Sushruta was later modified by using a forehead flap, based probably on the supratrochlear vessels or midline forehead vessels and became known as the traditional method of Indian rhinoplasty. It was when British surgeons working in India saw the results of Indian rhinoplasty on a man called Cowasjee that the procedure was described in the *Madras Gazette* and the October 1794 issue of the *Gentleman's Magazine of London*. The first reported case of an Indian rhinoplasty in the Western world was performed by Joseph Constantine Carpue in 1815 and the procedure gained popularity subsequently within Europe and the USA. Nasal reconstruction also formed the basis of the pedicled medial arm flap, described by Gasparo Tagliacozzi who lived between 1546 and 1599 in Bologna in Italy. He described the procedure in his manuscript *De Curtorum Chirurgia Per Insitionem*, noting that the skin of the medial arm was thin and had few hairs. He described a multistage technique in which skin of the medial arm was raised as a bipedicled flap, the donor site was left to heal, the flap was then attached to the defect in the nose or lip, with the arm immobilized and the flap pedicle was divided some time later.

Although the median forehead flap, based on the supratrochlear vessels, was first described for nasal reconstruction, the other type of forehead flap based on the superficial temporal artery was used by McGregor[1] in 1963 for intraoral reconstruction. This workhorse flap in head and neck reconstruction was followed by descriptions of the deltopectoral flap by Bakamjian[2] in 1965 and the pectoralis major flap in 1979 by Ariyan.[3] In 1983, after the advent of the operating microscope for microvascular reconstruction, the free radial forearm flap was popularized by Soutar[4] for oral cancer and has remained a popular workhorse flap since. Now, with the rapid recent advancements in perforator flap knowledge, we can use almost any area of skin and soft tissue and thin the area harvested to create a well-contoured, size-matched flap while simultaneously minimizing donor site morbidity,[5] and perforator flaps are increasingly being used and described for head and neck reconstruction.

MUCOSAL RECONSTRUCTION

In mucosal head and neck cancer, the priorities in the reconstructive principles differ for reconstruction at different sites in the upper aerodigestive tract. For example, reconstruction of the floor of mouth has different principles to reconstruction of the posterior pharynx, and so on. It is also becoming increasingly clear that functional outcomes are more dependent on the size of the excision and the structures involved in the excision, rather than the type of reconstruction used though, clearly, reconstruction using robust and reliable techniques with careful attention to the principles of reconstruction in these areas plays an important role in the ultimate final outcome.

The principles of reconstruction in the oral cavity following oral cancer excision remain to maximize functional results. Functions of the oral cavity include the articulation component of speech, tongue mobility to propel food and clear the oral cavity of food debris, and mobility of the tongue tip to prevent pooling of saliva in the sump areas of the anterior and lateral floor of mouth. The oral cavity consists of the lips, alveolus, buccal mucosa, hard palate, anterior two-thirds of the tongue (the mobile tongue), the floor of mouth and the retromolar trigone. The main priorities of reconstruction are maintenance of tongue mobility, maintenance of a lingual sulcus, maintenance of mouth opening, avoidance of bulk where native tissue is thin and avoidance of convexities at sites of concavity. Tongue mobility allows a sweeping movement to clear food debris, to allow food to be propelled to the appropriate regions of the mouth for chewing and for food to be passed into the oropharynx for further processing. The tongue also shapes much of the air that is vibrated to produce intelligible speech. To create speech, we must have air flowing into the mouth; that air needs to be vibrated to create a sound, and that air needs to be shaped to create consonants and vowels. The tongue plays an important role, along with the lips, teeth and oropharynx in shaping air that is already vibrating and also in creating the vibrations for the sibilant subset of the fricative sounds (such as sh-, ch- and j-).

Much of the muscle of the tongue can be removed and function maintained; however, a tongue that is tethered will not be mobile. Without a mobile tongue, the speech, swallowing and chewing functions of the tongue will be difficult to maintain. Notably, even a small amount of the oral tongue may be removed and tethered laterally or anteriorly and this will lead to poor tongue function in view of the lack of mobility of the tongue. For example, if a small mobile lateral tongue tumour is excised and directly closed, if the tongue defect is sutured to the lateral floor of the mouth, tongue mobility will be unnecessarily restricted. Similarly, an anterior ventral tongue defect sutured to the anterior floor of mouth will lead to restriction in tongue protrusion and elevation, again leading to unnecessarily reduced tongue function. Direct closure of lateral tongue defects should be considered with a vertically orientated scar to prevent lateral tethering, and closure of the ventral and tongue tip should be considered with a longitudinally orientated scar.

Oral sensation is of great importance in maintaining oral function and many reconstructions are reasonably sensate when a sensory nerve is used to reinnervate the reconstruction. When free flaps are used for oral reconstruction, an appropriate cutaneous nerve may be harvested and a neurorrhaphy performed with a nearby sensory cranial nerve. Although there are reports of improved function and sensation following such a nerve repair, the results are in limited groups of patients studied. Nevertheless, an attempt should be made to offset some of the sensory changes after ablative surgery by performing a sensate reconstruction. For total glossectomy defects, some authors have suggested using reinnervated muscle flaps for both tongue muscle power and sensation. However, it is difficult to imagine how a reinnervated large muscle would perform the delicate and fine movements of an organ as sophisticated as the tongue.

The oropharynx consists of the tonsils, the soft palate, part of the posterior pharyngeal wall, the tonsolingual angle and the posterior one-third of the tongue (the base of the tongue). Reconstruction of the oropharynx is designed to prevent nasal escape and hypernasality, thereby maintaining velopharyngeal competence. Nasal escape occurs when fluid or food material inadvertently passes from the oropharynx to the nasopharynx, usually during swallowing. Hypernasality occurs when air passes inadvertently from the oropharynx to the naspharynx, usually during plosive consonant production.

The velopharyngeal musculature consists of palatoglossus, palatopharyngeus, levator veli palatini, tensor veli palatini and the musculus uvalae muscles. These are innervated by the trigeminal nerve and vagus nerves and interact during swallowing and speech to maintain normal function. Following ablative surgery to the posterior oral cavity or oropharynx, some or all of these muscles will no longer function normally and the unreconstructed defect will be left with velopharyngeal incompetence. Maintaining velopharyngeal competence therefore forms one of the main reconstructive principles in oropharyngeal reconstruction and there are several ways of performing this including providing bulk, performing a pharygoplasty and dynamizing the reconstruction.

If the reconstruction is a bulky flap, the normal concavity of the soft palate is converted to a convexity. This means that the normal working and moving muscles do have to move such a long distance to provide closure of the velopharyngeal aperture. Bulky flaps include most myocutaneous flaps and some fascicutaneous flaps, such as the anterolateral thigh flap in people of European origin. Paradoxically, some reconstructive plastic surgeons feel a thin flap in such situations is a better option, as some of the flap is then able to move to assist with closure of the velopharyngeal aperture. Based on this principle, it is also possible to dynamize a thin flap. For example, the radial forearm flap may be taken with a distal strip of palmaris longus tendon as it heads toward the palm. This strip of tendon may be hitched to the normal working muscles on the contralateral side of the velum to the ablative surgery. Although the tendon of palmaris longus does not directly attach to the skin of the forearm, from where the flap has been raised, there is dynamic movement of the flap following such a procedure in the long term, and this can be seen on flexible nasendoscopy of the soft palate post-operatively when the patient is asked to make a plosive consonant. Lastly, a pharyngoplasty performed at the same time as the reconstruction also serves to narrow the velopharyngeal aperture. The pharyngoplasty used is usually a superiorly based flap, but varies according to the extent of ablative surgery. All these methods serve to improve the functional outcome of what can potentially be destructive surgery with noticeable functional impairment. By using one or a combination of these principles very effective rehabilitation can be achieved to allow the patient to speak, swallow and chew well.

In summary, reconstruction of the mucosal surfaces of the upper aerodigestive tract follows some important and fundamental principles. The reconstructive surgeon needs to be aware of the structures excised and the shape of the defect both at rest and during functional activity. By being mindful of these principles, we can make an attempt to maximize functional outcomes.

SKIN RECONSTRUCTION

In external skin and soft tissue reconstruction, the principles of reconstruction differ from those of mucosal reconstruction. The main principles in skin reconstruction are to orientate scar lines in the lines of election, to consider reconstruction of aesthetic subunits, to replace like with like, to be aware of the colour differences in the head and neck skin compared to skin elsewhere and to mimic the contours of the head and neck with the reconstruction used, avoiding bulk where thinness is needed and vice versa. Finally, with large reconstructions on tissues that are likely to drag with time and gravity, the reconstructive surgeon should elevate the tissues and hitch mobile structures to immobile structures. The skin of the head and neck can be considered in terms of the anatomic site, and so reconstructive principles differ at the scalp, the forehead, the upper face, the midface, the lower face, the central face, the lateral face and the neck. All these areas have their own unique characteristics and qualities with differences in reconstruction priorities.

The scalp is where many people have hair-bearing skin that benefits from being replaced following excision. Where hair replacement is required, then the scalp can be reconstructed using a number of options including scalp rotation flaps, scalp interdigitating flaps or rhomboid flaps. By using skin graft on hair-bearing skin, the patient is left with a patch of alopecia; however, this does not seem to concern a large number of our patients who have skin cancers of the scalp. The scalp skin has limited elasticity but can be expanded using tissue expansion. In this two-stage technique, an expandable saline-filled implant with a silicone outer shell is positioned into the layer between the galea and the periosteum under the skin requiring growth. Expansion occurs over a period of several weeks until the desired skin size increase has taken place, and a second-stage procedure is performed to remove the expander and reposition the newly formed skin over the defect requiring coverage. In most patients with cancers, the time delay between expander insertion and completion of the expansion process is too long for safe oncologic practice, and for scalp defects this is usually a delayed reconstruction procedure.

The forehead skin is similarly limited in its elasticity, and in those places within the forehead where there is movement it is occasionally undesirable to use this movement for reconstructive local flaps. Tissue expansion can be used in the forehead. For example, around the eyebrow region there is considerable movement but this is needed for facial expression and abnormally positioning a brow is to be avoided. Forehead reconstruction is often possible with skin grafts and local flaps. When a forehead flap is used as a donor flap, then some authors argue for letting part of the donor site heal by secondary intention. There is little wound contracture because of the bony base of the defect and much wound healing takes place by epithelial growth as opposed to wound contraction. Although wound healing by secondary intention at the forehead takes place over a protracted period, the ultimate aesthetic result is often better than if resurfaced with a split skin graft.

The midface consists of the area between the lower eyelids and angle of the mouth and has central and lateral components. The midface is a very prominent part of the facial anatomy and is highly visible. Light usually falls from above onto the midface and the human eye and brain is used to seeing contour differences and contrast differences. Accordingly, central midface reconstruction should ensure that contours are maintained, a suitable colour match is achieved and scars are placed in lines of election and run as close to possible as parallel to these. Useful local flaps for midface reconstruction include V–Y flaps, W-plasties or Z-plasties for cheek scar revisions, cheek rotation flaps, cervicofacial flaps and MACS (minimal access cranial suspension) facelift-type reconstructions with excision of Burrow's triangles in the postauricular region for reconstruction of defects anterior to the root of the helix in the sideburn region. Local flaps such as rhomboid flaps on the cheek can sometimes lead to prominent scars that run perpendicular to lines of election and are often a second choice for reconstruction. Regional flaps for reconstruction of the cheek, such as the deltopectoral flap and the forehead flap based on the superficial temporal vessels, often provide excellent colour-matched results, but have the disadvantage of being two-stage procedures and the donor site often needs a skin graft in places. When reconstructing the midface, it is important to avoid tension on the lower eyelid at the end of the procedure. Additionally, because of gravity and inflammatory oedema, tissue ptosis takes place over the course of time and can lead to late development eyelid malposition or ectropion. Tension on the lower eyelid at the end of the procedure, pulling the lid down, should not be the case and never improves with watchful waiting. To avoid tissue ptosis in the midface, one or two carefully placed deep sutures are occasionally needed to hitch the mobile structures of the midface to immobile structures. The most immobile structure in the midface is the facial skeleton and the use of anchors or bony tunnels occasionally helps in securing the mobile to immobile sutures to prevent cheek ptosis dragging down the lower eyelid. Although the lower eyelid does form part of the midface, reconstruction of the lower eyelid itself is included below under Eyelid reconstruction.

The lower face is far more forgiving, but reconstruction here must prevent lateral ptosis of the angle of the mouth. A ptotic angle of mouth leads to oral incompetence and dental show at rest, both of which are undesirable outcomes following lower facial reconstruction. Oral competence is also an integral part of lip reconstruction which is discussed below under Lip reconstruction. Neck skin reconstruction involving large areas often requires local or free flaps. The radial forearm flap was first used as a means of neck reconstruction in head and neck surgery following burn contractures, and the qualities of the flap reflect the principles of reconstruction. The neck skin needs to be thin, pliable, needs to permit movement in many vectors and there should be a good colour and contour match with the surrounding skin. Examples of local flaps used for neck reconstruction include deltopectoral flaps, pectoralis major muscle flaps with skin grafts, supraclavicular artery perforator flaps and local neck skin random pattern flaps. Whenever neck skin is incised for use as a local flap, the incisions must be placed in a manner which will permit subsequent incisions for a neck dissection without compromising skin flap vascularity.

Clearly, the larger the skin defect in any area of the head and neck, the more likely the need for free flap reconstruction. The choices for free flaps are many, and include muscle flaps with overlying skin grafts (which seem to give excellent colour and contour matching to the surrounding skin, in the author's experience), fasciocutaneous flaps, cutaneous flaps and musculocutaneous flaps.

BONY RECONSTRUCTION

The bones commonly requiring reconstruction in the head and neck are the mandible and the maxilla. The history of head and neck bony reconstruction dates back to ancient Egypt and China with prosthetics. Towards the end of the nineteenth century, bone grafts were first performed, and microsurgical reconstruction was described from the late 1970s onwards.[6] Nowadays, our principles of reconstruction are to provide cosmesis, speech, swallowing, chewing and dental occlusion and restoration, either with dentures or with dental implants. Our decision-making in bony reconstruction of the mid and lower face depends on the extent of the defect, the need for postoperative radiotherapy, the presence of radionecrosis, the state of the potential donor vessels in the region, the fitness of the patient, the height of the native mandible requiring reconstruction, the presence of teeth and the availability of donor sites.

Mandibular reconstruction

Mandibular reconstruction may be performed with no reconstruction, plate reconstruction, bone graft reconstruction, and vascularized bone either on a pedicled or free flap. When no reconstruction is performed of an anterior mandible defect, the patient is left with a so-called 'Andy Gump deformity'. Andy Gump was a cartoon character in an American comic book between 1917 and 1959 who had no chin whatsoever. No reconstruction of an excised mandible will lead to severe retrognathia with loss of anterior tongue support, oral incompetence with severe difficulties of speech, swallowing and chewing. The soft tissues collapse around the dead space created by the loss of anterior mandible leading to the deformity. This type of defect is rarely seen nowadays and even in the most unfit of patients we have an option of using a plate-only reconstruction. Mandibular reconstruction plates nowadays are usually malleable locking 2.0 or 2.4 mm plates. Commonly used are the low profile plates with threaded plate holes for screws with threaded heads, providing an internal or external fixation device for increased bony stability. These titanium plates are one of the means of maintaining dental occlusion prior to mandibular excision, and they can be resterilized following tumour excision. Additionally, the plates can be prebent using stereolithographic models for greater accuracy. At least three screws should be used in the native mandible at either end of the reconstruction plate for stability.

In addition to using a plate-only reconstruction, a plate can be used as a template for bony reconstruction which can be vascularized or non-vascularized. Vascularized bone is preferred in mandibular reconstruction because of the large forces generated by normal jaw movements and vascularized bone is more robust. Of all the vascularized bone flaps that are available the commonly used ones for the mandible are the fibular flap, the vascularized iliac crest flap (more commonly referred to as the deep circumflex iliac artery flap or DCIA flap), the scapular flap and the radial forearm osteocutaneous flap. There are advantages and disadvantages to each flap.

The fibular flap provides a long straight segment of vascularized bone, based on the peroneal artery. The flap can contain skin and muscle depending on how it is raised. Harvesting the flap is performed under tourniquet control and allows a two-team approach in the operating theatre – one team can perform the head and neck surgery and the other team can perform the flap surgery. The flap is raised and subsequent osteotomies are performed on the harvested bone, and these can be either closing wedge osteotomies where a triangular wedge-shaped portion of bone is removed and the two remaining bony segments are plated. Alternatively, open wedge osteotomies may be performed in which the bone is fractured and fixed to a reconstruction plate which forms a framework for the bony shape required. The peroneal artery is a good size match for many of the branches of the external carotid artery and the peroneal veins tend to be large, thin-walled vessels with multiple valves. The fibula can provide enough length to reconstruct a mandible from angle to angle, but neomandibular height is limited with this reconstruction.

The deep circumflex iliac artery provides vascularized bone from the iliac crest. The flap may incorporate the internal oblique muscle, supplied by the ascending branch of the deep circumflex iliac artery, and skin overlying the iliac crest, supplied by perforating branches of the artery, for a composite flap for reconstruction of all the layers of the lower face. The iliac crest can be taken for a considerable height allowing for adequate neomandibular height reconstruction. Use of the internal oblique muscle provides excellent lining tissue after it mucosalizes and recreates the normal situation of a tightly bound mucosa to the underlying mandible. Long-term orthopantomograms of patients at our institution have shown neomandibular remodelling almost indistinguishable from the native mandible. Donor site morbidity is a significant consideration for this flap and has been reduced by utilizing only the inner plate of the iliac crest.

The scapular provides a robust segment of bone when incorporated in the scapular flap. The flap is based on the cutaneous branch of the circumflex scapular artery and the vascular pedicle passes through the triangular space above teres major, the long head of triceps and the subscapularis. A segment of the lateral border of the scapula may be harvested along with a cuff of surrounding muscle and significant muscle dissection is required to harvest the bony segment. The patient needs to be turned during the procedure so that the reconstructive surgeon may gain access to the flap following the head and neck surgery.

The radial forearm flap provides up to 10 cm of bone when raised as an osteocutaneous free flap. The vessels supplying the bone pierce through flexor pollicis longus, arising on the deep aspect of the radial artery, and a cuff of this muscle is harvested when raising the flap as an osteocutaneous flap. Bone between the attachments of pronator teres and brachioradialis may be raised and in an average adult this provides approximately 10 cm of bone. A boat-shaped segment of bone taking less than one-third of the circumference of the radius should be taken, to avoid weakening radius, reducing the risk of subsequent fracture. Only one osteotomy may be made in the bone thereby reducing the length to 5 cm of a double segment of bone. Osseointegration cannot be performed in the reconstructed mandible and donor site morbidity is potentially considerable. The radius is weakened, and options to increase the strength of the radius after harvesting the flap include the use of a 2.4 mm straight fixation plate between the two ends of the bone and the use of cancellous bone graft from the iliac crest to replace the bone removed. An above elbow cast is used for 6 weeks postoperatively when a plate is not used for radial reconstruction.

In summary, mandibular reconstruction may be performed using a variety of techniques, and the choice of the surgeon depends on mandibular height (which is particularly relevant in dentate patients), the length of bone needed, the number of osteotomies planned, future osseointegration, flap familiarity (though it could be argued that the reconstructive surgeon should be familiar with most flaps), donor site availability and morbidity, the position of donor vessels and flap composition.

Maxillary reconstruction

Maxillectomy defects are most commonly created following excision of carcinomas, but other bony and sinus diseases can lead to the need for maxillary reconstruction. In general, narrow and superficial defects are more likely to need obturators. The wider and taller the defect, the greater the need to use vascularized tissue. When reconstructing a maxillectomy defect, consideration needs to be given to oronasal closure, velopharyngeal competence, the position of the globe of the eye, the height of the cheeks, dental rehabilitation with either implants or dentures. These are the principles of maxillary reconstruction.

Obturator reconstruction is a very effective and surgically simple method of oronasal closure. However, in larger and wider defects, vascularized reconstruction is generally used. Options include the DCIA flap and non-vascularized iliac crest supported by vascularized muscle. Since the maxilla has less force acting on it than the mandible, the latter option is mechanically sound. There are advantages and disadvantages to each method of reconstruction.

Obturator closure is a relatively simple procedure for the patient to tolerate (and for the surgeon to perform). Usually, at the end of the procedure, the defect is filled with a malleable material which subsequently hardens. This allows an obturator to be made by the prosthetician which the patient can insert and remove as required. An obturator is ideal for smaller defects.

Ideally, larger defects require flap reconstruction. The two options that seem to have found favour among reconstructive surgeons are the DCIA flap and vascularized muscle with non-vascularized bone graft. The DCIA flap provides well-vascularized composite tissue in the form of bone, muscle and skin if required and fills the maxillectomy defect very effectively. The main disadvantages of the procedure are donor site morbidity and the pedicle length which necessitates either anastomosing the flap vessels to the facial vessels in the face or to vessels in the neck but with the additional use of vein grafts. However, there is only one donor site and harvesting can be performed at the same time as resection. Muscle flaps with bone grafts include the rectus muscle or lattisimus dorsi muscle, which have long pedicles and muscles that can be tailored in their size and shape to match the defect. The bone graft from the iliac crest is inset with miniplates and the muscle is sutured into the defect. Some surgeons use skin grafts to reline the nasal passageways with a naspharyngeal tube left *in situ* for a few weeks to prevent blockage of the nasal airway. A dental plate is usually secured with small screws to help compress the muscle into the correct shape for the first couple of weeks in the postoperative period.

RECONSTRUCTION OF COMPLEX AESTHETIC UNITS

The face is a complex structure and defects often involve complex aesthetic units either in the central face or in the lateral face. The central face complex units include lips, nose, eyebrows and eyelids. The lateral complex units include the external ear.

Lip reconstruction

The principles of lip reconstruction are to maintain oral competence, to maintain labial sensation, to maintain a lower sulcus and to maintain aperture size. Oral competence is maintained with correct alignment of the orbicularis oris muscle, along with careful suturing of full-thickness defects in multiple layers. Aperture size is maximized using tissue

49

Local flaps

NICHOLAS WHITE, LOK HUEI YAP AND JOHN C WATKINSON

Replace like with like.

Sir Harold Gillies

INTRODUCTION

This chapter discusses wound closure in the head and neck using grafts and local flaps; these are most commonly used to deal with defects following skin cancer excision, but can also be applied to various other defects around the face and to facilitate wound closure following resections in the aerodigestive tract. Primary closure is always the first option to be considered when closing surgical wounds, however if this cannot be achieved then the use of skin grafts and local flaps are of use. A graft is a piece of tissue that has no blood supply of its own and is dependent upon the blood supply of the recipient site to survive, whereas a flap is a piece of tissue with its own blood supply and its survival is not dependent upon the recipient site. The basic principles of wound closure, skin grafts and local flaps are discussed and their use in reconstruction of different regions of the head and neck are then illustrated.

WOUND CLOSURE

Following ablative cancer surgery in the head and neck many defects can be directly closed if they are small and enough tissue is available locally. For larger defects, closure of the wound can only be achieved through the use of grafts, local flaps, pedicled flaps, free flaps or a combination of these techniques. Areas of the face, head and neck facilitate direct closure because of the availability of lax skin; this is particularly true in the elderly as the skin loses its elasticity with

age. The concept of relaxed skin tension lines are useful when considering where to place skin incisions (**Figure 49.1**).[1] These lines are parallel to the natural skin wrinkles and tend to be perpendicular to the underlying muscle fibres. Ideally, surgical incisions should be placed parallel to these lines and,

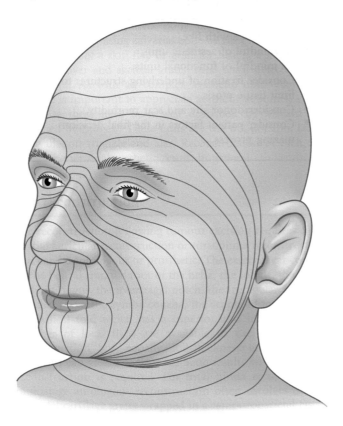

Figure 49.1 Relaxed skin tension lines.

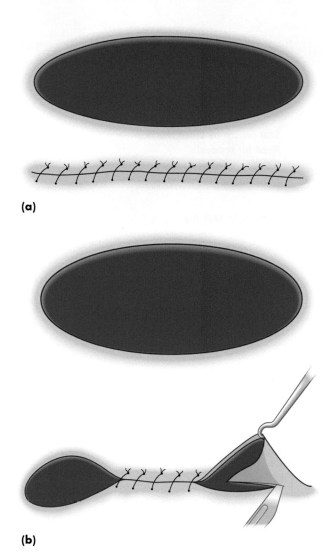

(a)

(b)

Figure 49.2 (a) An elliptical excision with a length three times the width. (b) An ellipse which is too short leading to dog ears at the ends of the closed wounds.

in particular, the scar from a direct closure of a defect should be in a relaxed skin tension line. This is because it will be under the least tension as skin contraction is at its greatest when a scar is perpendicular to the relaxed skin tension lines.

Elliptical excision

Classically, a defect is designed as an ellipse three times as long as it is wide. This is the best dimension to take account of skin stretch and elasticity to approximate the wound edges with the least tension. If an ellipse is too short then excess skin (dog ears) can form an unsightly appearance (**Figure 49.2**). If there is uncertainty about the direction of the relaxed skin tension line then the lesion can be excised as a circle with the correct margins to obtain clearance. The skin edges of the wound can then be pulled together in various directions to assess in which axis there is the least tension. The circle can then be extended as an ellipse perpendicular to this axis and then closed.

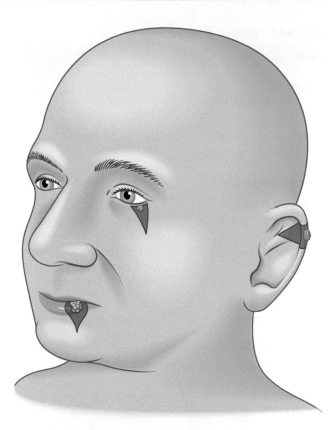

Figure 49.3 Wedge excision technique in the lip, eyelid and ear.

Wedge excision

An alternative to excising lesions as an ellipse is to excise them as a wedge. Lesions located at the free edge of tissue such as the eyelid, lips of helical rim of the ear can be excised in this fashion and then closed directly (**Figure 49.3**). It should be remembered that these free edges are not just skin but composite tissue and should be closed in layers to obtain optimal function and appearance. In the case of lips these layers are mucosa, orbicularis oris and skin; in the ear, cartilage and skin on both the anterior and posterior surface; and in eyelids, conjunctiva, tarsal plate, orbicularis oculi and skin.

Suture materials

Many suture materials and techniques have been used to primarily close defects in the head and neck. These can be permanent or absorbable sutures which can be placed through the skin or buried within it; recently, skin adhesives and tapes have been developed which can be used instead of sutures. Each has their own advantages and disadvantages and these are summarized in **Table 49.1**. There are no correct or incorrect techniques and due consideration should be given to the method of wound closure on a case by case basis.

SKIN GRAFTS

Grafting of skin originated in India over 3000 years ago,[2] where surgeons from the tile-making caste took skin grafts

Table 49.1   Methods of wound closure.

Material	Advantages	Disadvantages
Sutures		
Non-absorbable cutaneous	Simple and effective	Wound dehiscence if removed too early
		Scarring if left too long
Absorbable cutaneous	No need for removal	Scar caused by stitch marks
Non-absorbable subcuticular	Minimal scar	Need for removal
		Risk of wound dehiscence
Absorbable subcuticular	No need for removal	Retention of foreign body
Fasteners		
Skin tapes	Can effectively approximate wound edges	Need to be kept dry
	Easy to apply and remove	
Skin staples	Fast wound closure in long incisions	Need removal which can be painful
	Evert wound edges well	
Skin adhesives	Simple and fast to apply	May need deeper sutures to prevent wound dehiscence
Alternatives		
Secondary intention	Useful for small superficial wounds	May take some time until fully healed
		Risk of an unsightly scar

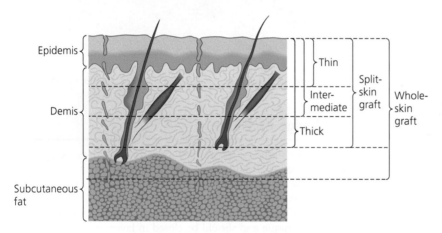

Figure 49.4   Differing depths of skin grafts.

from the gluteal region to repair traumatic defects of the face. The first report in the English language was in 1817 when Sir Astley Cooper grafted a full-thickness piece of skin from a man's amputated thumb onto the stump for coverage. Lawson[3] reported successful elective full-thickness skin grafting in 1871, which was followed by Ollier,[4] a French surgeon, describing a split-thickness skin graft in 1872. Thiersch,[5] from Germany, was the first to recognize the importance of recipient site for graft survival, and in 1875 Wolfe used a full-thickness skin graft taken from the patient's forearm to treat a traumatic ectropion of the lower lid following a gunpowder explosion. Full-thickness skin grafting of the eyelids is now a procedure with which Wolfe's name has become synonymous.[6]

In 1929 Brown and Blair[7] differentiated between full-thickness and split-thickness skin grafts; they identified the advantages and disadvantages of each and using their techniques consistent, acceptable results were achieved. Medawar[8] studied the underlying biology of healing skin grafts in the 1940s. His work described the cellular changes in both the epidermis and dermis giving the technique of skin grafting a scientific basis and laying the foundation of modern transplant immunology.[9]

Skin grafts can be split-thickness, full-thickness or composite. Split-thickness skin grafts (STSG) contain epidermis and a variable amount of dermis whereas full-thickness skin grafts (FTSG) contain epidermis and all of the dermis. In practice, there is a spectrum of depth of skin grafts from thin to thick as shown in **Figure 49.4**. Composite grafts consist of two different tissue types, such as skin and cartilage or septal mucosa and cartilage.[10] The part of the body from which the skin is taken is the donor site and the area onto which the skin is transplanted is the recipient site or bed. An autograft is a graft taken from one part of an individual's body and transferred to a different part of that same individual. An isograft is a graft between genetically identical individuals, such as identical twins. An allograft is taken from another individual of the same species. A xenograft is when the donor is of a different species to the recipient. The terminology used in skin grafting is summarized in **Table 49.2**.

Table 49.2 Skin graft terminology.

Composition	
Split-thickness	Part of the dermis
Full-thickness	All of the dermis
Composite	Skin and another tissue
Graft origin	
Autograft	Same person
Isograft	Identical twin
Allograft	Same species
Xenograft	Different species
Alloplastic	Synthetic

Graft survival

Once a skin graft has been harvested, it has been detached from its blood supply and is, temporarily, not viable. In order to survive permanently, it has to become reattached and obtain a new blood supply from its recipient site; this process is known as 'take'. Successful take of a skin graft is dependent upon the extent and speed at which vascular perfusion is returned to the graft. This is determined by the characteristics of the graft itself, the characteristics of the bed on which the graft is laid and the conditions under which the graft is applied to the bed.

Under comparable conditions, two properties of a graft determine its take. These are the blood supply of the skin from which the graft was harvested, as a graft taken from a highly vascular donor area will heal better than a graft from a poorly perfused area, and the metabolic activity of the skin graft at the time of its application to the recipient bed. This metabolic activity will direct how the graft responds to the period of ischaemia before it undergoes successful revascularization.

The recipient wound bed must have an adequate blood supply to support the skin graft. Muscle and fascia act readily as recipient beds whereas fat is less suitable. Bone covered with periosteum will take a graft but exposed bone will not, however burring bone and allowing it to granulate (such as the outer table of the skull) will facilitate graft take. Healthy granulation tissue covering a pre-existing wound on the head and neck will also take a graft but any necrotic tissue has to be debrided first.

To obtain successful graft take, the conditions have to be optimized. These conditions can be either specific to graft location or systemic. The graft has to be immobile and in direct contact with the bed. Numerous methods of attachment of grafts, such as tie-over dressings, have been described and shearing forces which make the graft move from side to side have to be avoided. The most frequent cause of graft loss is the presence of a haematoma which separates a graft from its bed. Scrupulous haemostasis and either meshing or fenestrating the graft may help to prevent this. Infection is another common cause of graft loss and if suspected should be treated with systemic and/or topical antibiotic agents. Common pathogens include *Streptococcus pyogenes*, *Pseudomonas aeruginosa* and methicillin-resistant *Staphlococcus aureus* which can all destroy fibrin and prevent graft adherence.[11] In addition to these local conditions, systemic conditions of the patient can also influence skin graft take.

These include diabetes mellitus, smoking, previous radiotherapy and chemotherapy, as well as nutritional status.

Graft adhesion and revascularization

Two processes allow the skin graft to adhere to the recipient site. The first is fibrin adherence which takes place in the first 2–3 days; during this time the graft is held to the recipient bed by a thin layer of fibrin from both the wound bed and undersurface of the graft.[12] Within 48 hours, this fibrin starts to break down and adhesion to the bed is maintained by the proliferation of fibroblasts and the deposition of collagen.[13]

Once the graft is adherent, two separate processes keep the skin graft alive. The first of these is called serum imbition.[14] Immediately after a graft is inset it absorbs plasma that is leaking from the recipient bed. This provides temporary nourishment for the graft and is demonstrated by the graft gaining weight and swelling. The process keeps the graft alive for the first 48 hours, after which vascular flow through the graft begins to be re-established. The second process is collectively known as graft revascularization. This is a combination of cut vessels from the host bed lining up with the cut ends of the vessels of the graft to form anastomoses[15] (inosculation) and the ingrowth of new capillary buds from the host into the graft. Ingrowth of vessels into the graft produces new vascular channels[16] (true revascularization) or, alternatively, by the endothelium of the old vessels degenerating but the basement membrane remaining and this acting as a conduit for the capillary buds to travel down[17] (neovascularization). All these processes restore blood flow and continue for approximately a month until revascularization is complete.

Full-thickness or split-thickness skin graft?

The amount of dermis included with the graft determines both the likelihood of survival and the degree of contraction. STSGs can tolerate less vascularity but have a greater amount of contraction. Full-thickness grafts require a better vascular bed for survival but undergo less contracture. Owing to this, split-thickness skin grafts have the best take and can be used under conditions that may cause the failure of FTSGs. However, STSGs tend to contract, have abnormal pigmentation and are susceptible to trauma once healed. In contrast, FTSGs require a more robust blood supply to be acquired from the recipient bed to survive; however, a healed FTSG does not contract as much, resists trauma better and has a better colour match. Sensory recovery of the full-thickness graft is superior to that of the split-thickness graft due to more sensory organs being retained in the transferred tissue, but the innervation takes longer to recover as there is more tissue for new nerves to grow through. These differences are summarized in **Table 49.3**.

Skin graft donor sites

After a STSG is harvested, the donor site heals by re-epithelialization from adenexal structures, such as hair follicles

Table 49.3 Advantages and disadvantages of split-thickness and full-thickness skin grafts.

Factor	Split-thickness skin graft	Full-thickness skin graft
Depth of dermis harvested	Variable amount of dermis	All of the dermis
Chance of successful graft take	More likely to 'take'	Higher risk of graft loss
Graft contraction	Contracts more	Contracts less
Final graft colour once healed	Pigment abnormal	Better colour match
Robustness of healed graft	Susceptible to trauma once healed	More robust once healed
Return of sensation	Limited sensory recovery	Better sensory recovery
Donor site healing	Slow donor site healing by re-epithelialization	Fast donor site healing by primary intention
Size of skin graft which can be harvested	Potentially large volumes of donor skin	Limited availability of donor skin
Graft characteristics	Can be meshed to increase surface area	Primary contraction decreases surface area

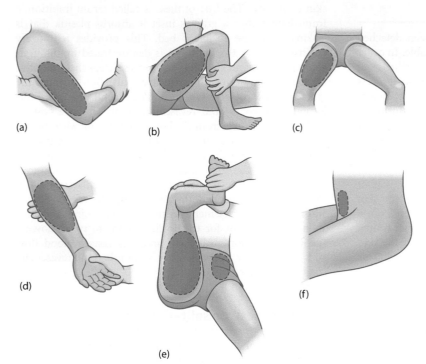

(a)   (b)   (c)

(d)   (e)   (f)

Figure 49.5   Split-thickness skin graft donor sites.

and sweat glands, in the remaining dermis. Resurfacing occurs by the migration of keratinocytes from these structures to cover the wound. As there is no remaining epithelium in full-thickness graft donor sites, the wound needs to be closed directly; this limits the amount of skin that can be harvested and the size of the defect that can be reconstructed using a FTSG. Split-thickness skin grafts can be taken from anywhere on the body.[18] Commonly used areas include the thigh, trunk and buttocks as shown in **Figure 49.5**.

The graft is harvested with either an air or battery powered dermatome or a hand knife such as a Watson knife. The standard thickness which is preset on a dermatome is 0.3–0.4 mm or 10–12/1000 of an inch. The skin can then be either meshed or fenestrated by hand. The donor site is dressed with a non-adherent dressing[19] and left undisturbed for approximately 14 days. Most STSG donor sites are healed by 21 days with minimal scarring but may be discoloured and susceptible to sunburn for two years afterwards.

The thickness and colour of skin varies greatly from different parts of the body and this affects the choice of FTSG donor site. Commonly used sites are pre- and postauricular,

the supraclavicular fossa, the antecubital fossa and the groin as shown in **Figure 49.6**. The FTSG is harvested with a scalpel and is closed directly with sutures to leave a linear scar. The amount of skin that can be taken is limited by the need to obtain a tension-free closure of the donor site. Examples of the use of skin grafts in the head and neck are given in **Figures 49.7** and **49.8**.

PRINCIPLES OF LOCAL FLAPS

Local cutaneous flaps of the head and neck can be classified according to their circulation, composition, contiguity and contour. The circulation of flaps may be random or axial, which means that they are based on an anatomically recognized artery.[20] Flaps can be composed of different tissue types, such as skin, fascia and skin (fasciocutaneous), muscle or muscle and the overlying skin paddle (myocutaneous). The contiguity of a flap means its source. A local flap is composed of tissue adjacent to the defect. A pedicled flap is from a

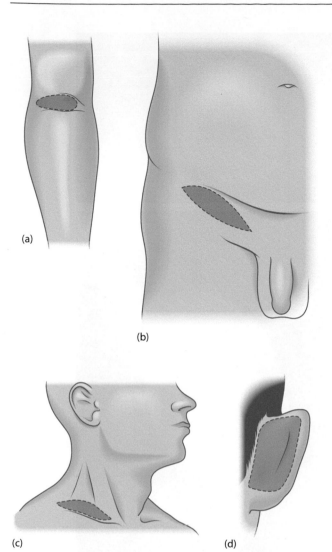

Figure 49.6 Full-thickness skin graft donor sites. (a) Antecubital fossa. (b) Groin. (c) Supraclavicular fossa. (d) Postauricular.

distant part of the body to which it remains attached. A free flap is completely detached from the body and anastomosed to recipient vessels close to the defect. The contour of the flap depends on the method in which it is transferred into the defect. It can either be advanced or moved about a pivot point. A flap is inset into a primary defect. The secondary defect is the site from which the flap is raised. This is usually closed directly but can be grafted or closed by another flap.

When designing a local flap in the head and neck the two most important considerations are appreciation of the cosmetic units and the relaxed skin tension lines. The face can be subdivided into separate units (**Figure 49.9**). It is preferable to use one flap to reconstruct one cosmetic unit and it may be necessary to excise an entire cosmetic unit, beyond the boundary of the original cancer resection, to obtain an optimal result. Conversely, if the resection involves two cosmetic units then two flaps, one for each unit, may be necessary. The donor area from the flap should be from the same cosmetic unit or one adjacent and should not transgress multiple units. Relaxed skin tension lines have already been discussed above under

Wound closure, p. 914. Ideally, the scar from a direct closure of a secondary defect should be in a relaxed skin tension line as it will be under the most tension of any part of the flap.

In order to accurately plan a flap, reverse planning can be used where a template of the primary defect can be reflected onto surrounding skin to help assess where the flap can be raised from to give minimal donor site morbidity. When skin flap is designed randomly, its blood supply is from the base of the flap. Normally the breadth of the base should be no more than the length of the flap to prevent necrosis of the flap (a ratio of 1:1). In the head and neck, the blood supply is good so this can be extended to a ratio of base breadth to flap length of 1:1.5. In an axial flap based on a known artery system, the ratio of base breadth to flap length can be much greater.

Advancement flaps

Advancement flaps may be simple or modified. A simple advancement flap just relies on the skin's elasticity to cover the primary defect. They can also be modified in a number of ways to aid advancement; one example of this is to include Burow triangles at the base of the flap. These are triangles of skin that are excised either side of the base of the flap. This is demonstrated by a Rintalla flap[21] being used to cover a defect of the nasal tip (**Figure 49.10**). A V-Y flap is another modified advancement flap. The flap itself is triangular (or 'V' shaped), the flap is advanced and the secondary defect is closed directly to leave a 'Y'-shaped scar. The nasolabial V-Y advancement flap, shown in **Figure 49.11**, is an axial flap which can be based on either the superior labial artery or the angular artery, both of which are branches of the facial artery. A bipedicled flap receives a blood supply from both ends as it has two bases. It is less prone to necrosis than flaps of similar dimensions which are attached at only one end. An example of this is the Tripier flap[22] for lower eye lid reconstruction (**Figure 49.12**). Skin from the upper lid based on both a medial and a lateral attachment is swung down, like a bucket handle, to provide cover for a defect in the lower lid. To increase the viability of this flap, a strip of the orbicularis oculi muscle can be included making it a musculocutaneous flap.

Pivot flaps

A pivot flap moves about a fixed pivot point and can either be a transposition flap where the flap moves laterally across the pivot point or a rotation flap where the flap is rotated around the pivot point (**Figure 49.13**). When a flap is transposed to cover the primary defect, the secondary defect is normally skin grafted. This secondary defect can be closed directly when a rotation flap is used.

RHOMBOID FLAPS

A rhomboid flap is a type of transposition flap where the donor defect is closed directly.[23] The defect is designed as a rhomboid; each of the limbs of the defect and the flap being raised need to be of equal length and the angles of the

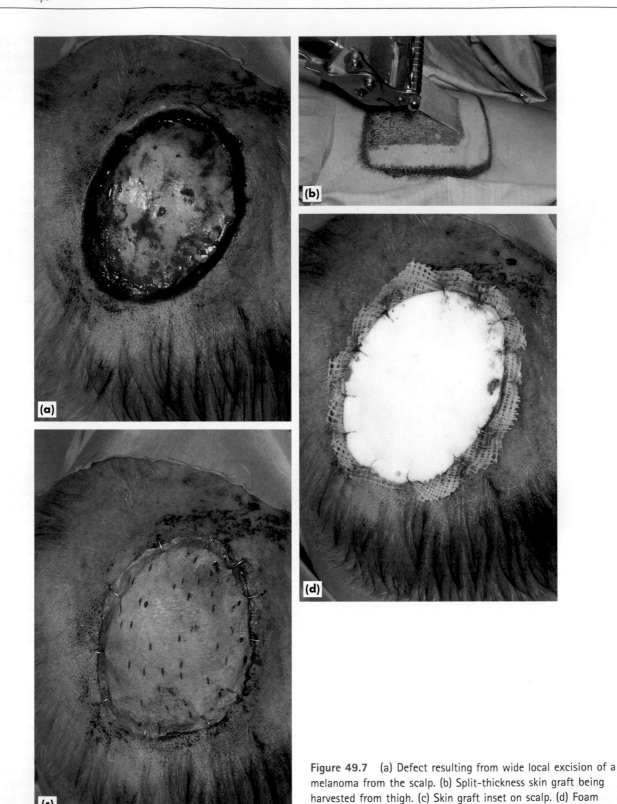

Figure 49.7   (a) Defect resulting from wide local excision of a melanoma from the scalp. (b) Split-thickness skin graft being harvested from thigh. (c) Skin graft inset on scalp. (d) Foam dressing held with surgical clips.

rhomboid need to be 120° and 60°, respectively. The flap needs to be designed so that the scar from the donor site sits parallel to the relaxed skin tension lines. This is demonstrated in **Figure 49.14**. A variation of the rhomboid flap is the Dufourmentel flap,[24] which has equal lengths of the limbs but the angles are 150° and 30°. Other variations of the

geometry of the rhomboid flap have been described.[25] One of these is the 'square peg in the round hole' where the primary defect is circular (as is the case in most clinical situations) and the rhomboid flap is stretched to fill the defect.[26] This reduces the need to excise extra skin in cosmetically sensitive areas such as the face.

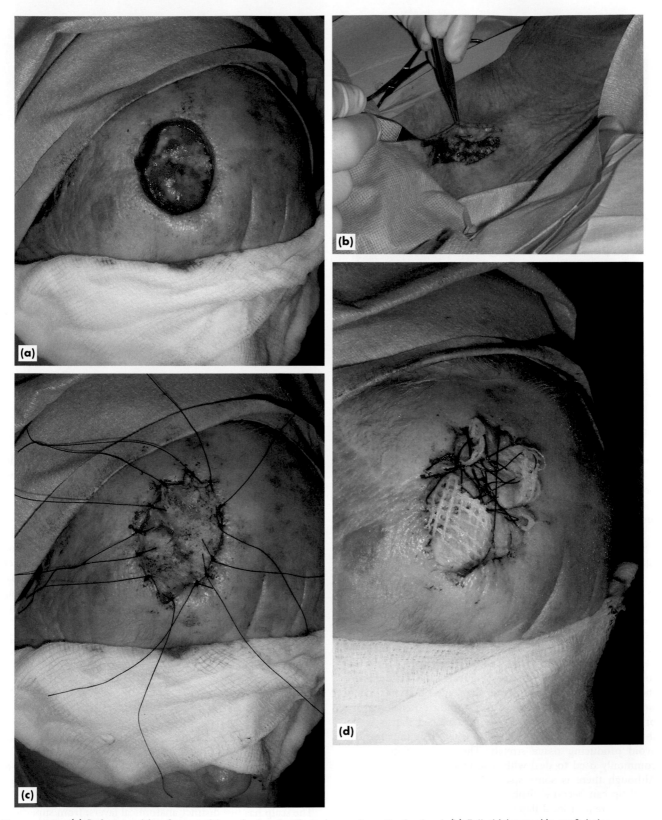

Figure 49.8 (a) Defect resulting from excision of a basal cell carcinoma from the forehead. (b) Full-thickness skin graft being harvested from left supraclavicular fossa. (c) Skin graft inset on forehead. (d) Proflavin wool and paraffin gauze tie-over dressing.

FLAG OR BANNER FLAPS

A number of small transposition flaps can be used around the face and generally the donor site is closed directly. These are termed flag flaps as the piece of tissue moved resembles a flag or banner. These are normally random pattern flaps but can be based on a known artery in some parts of the head or neck. A glabellar flap is an axial transposition 'flag' flap based

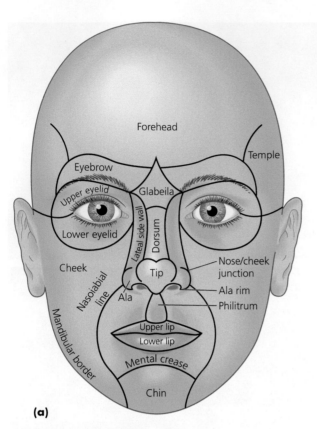

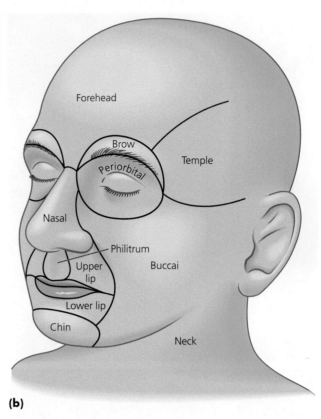

(a)

(b)

Figure 49.9 Cosmetic subunits of the face.

on the supratrochlear artery, a branch of the ophthalmic artery. This allows the flap length to be three times the base breadth and in **Figure 49.15**, is shown covering a defect of the medial canthus. It is transposed to cover the primary defect and the donor site is closed directly.

BILOBED FLAP

A bilobed flap consists of two transposition flaps.[27] The first flap is transposed into the primary defect, the second flap is transposed into the secondary defect (the original site of the first flap) and the tertiary defect (the original site of the second flap) is closed directly. Again, the flap should be designed so that the directly closed tertiary defect is parallel to the relaxed skin tension lines (**Figure 49.16**). Theoretically, the bilobed flap uses less tissue than any other method of wound closure and because of this minimizes tension at the primary defect.[28] The ideal use of a bilobed flap is where there is tissue available locally and where it is important to avoid producing tissue stretch. The bilobed flap is most commonly used to deal with defects at the tip of the nose. Although there is some spare tissue around this area, the nasal tip can become displaced if skin is imported to cover defects here as a local flap.[29]

Rotation flaps

Rotation flaps are large flaps that rotate into the primary defect. The volume of tissue raised in the flap is high when compared to the defect being closed. Normally the flap is a

semicircle and the primary defect is designed as a triangle, like a slice of cake. The flap circumference should be at least eight times the width of the defect. Unlike transposition flaps, where the secondary defect is closed with a skin graft or primarily using skin adjacent to the flap donor site, it is tissue redistribution and skin elasticity of the flap itself that usually permits direct closure of the donor site in the case of rotation flaps. Occasionally, the use of a Burow's triangle or a back cut may be needed. A back cut releases a rotation flap that is too tight by decreasing the tension at the base of the flap and thus the tension of closure at the site of the primary defect. This however does have the risk of devascularizing the flap by decreasing the width of its base. These flaps are useful for dealing with defects of the scalp or cheek (**Figure 49.17**).

RECONSTRUCTION OF SPECIFIC REGIONS OF THE HEAD AND NECK

Scalp

ANATOMY

The scalp has five distinct anatomical layers; from superficial to deep, these are the skin, subcutaneous connective tissue, muscle or aponeurosis (galea), loose areolar tissue and pericranium. The skin of the scalp is the thickest on the human body, ranging from 3 to 8 mm. Beneath the skin, the subcutaneous tissue contains the vessels and nerves supplying the scalp. Deep to this is the muscular-aponeurotic layer consisting of the frontalis muscle anteriorly and the

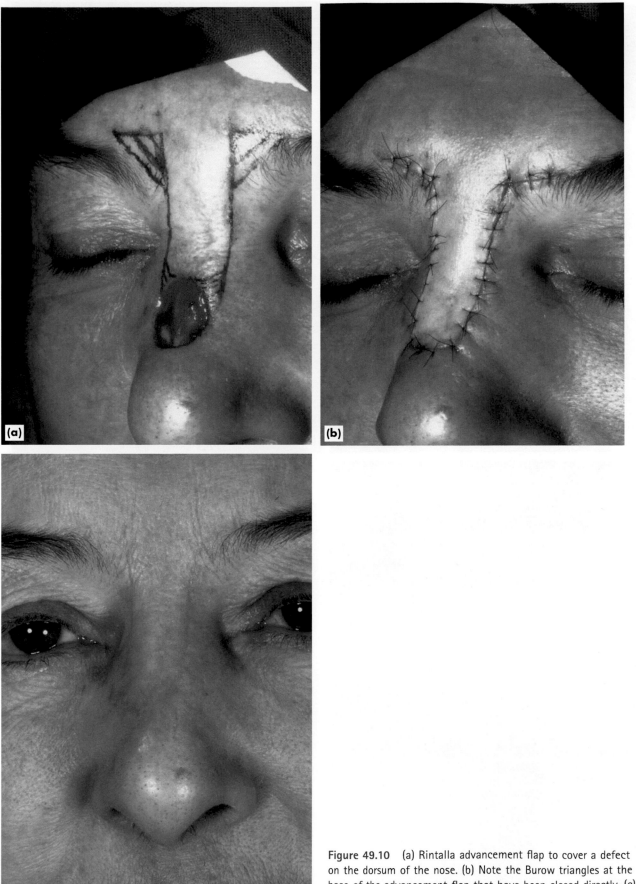

Figure 49.10   (a) Rintalla advancement flap to cover a defect on the dorsum of the nose. (b) Note the Burow triangles at the base of the advancement flap that have been closed directly. (c) The final result.

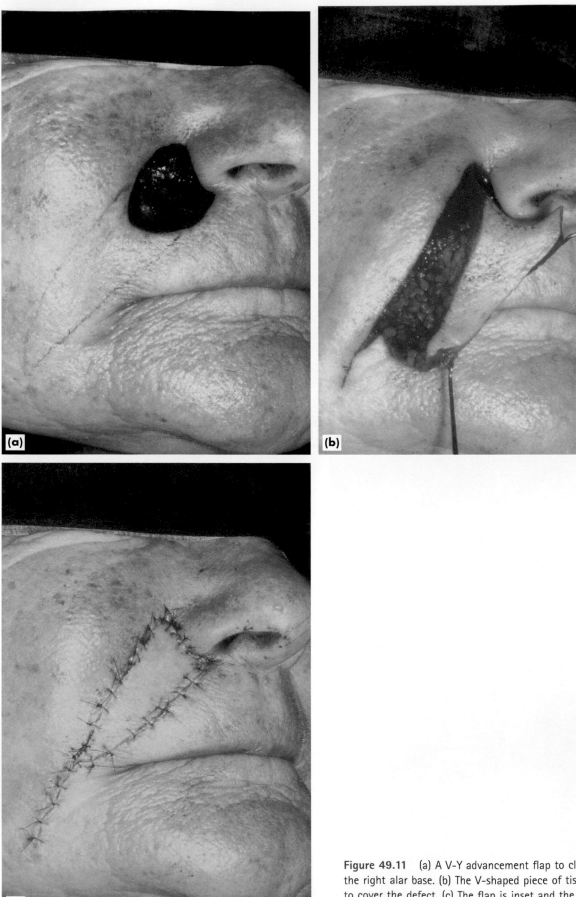

Figure 49.11 (a) A V-Y advancement flap to close a defect on the right alar base. (b) The V-shaped piece of tissue is advanced to cover the defect. (c) The flap is inset and the donor site is closed directly to leave a Y-shaped scar.

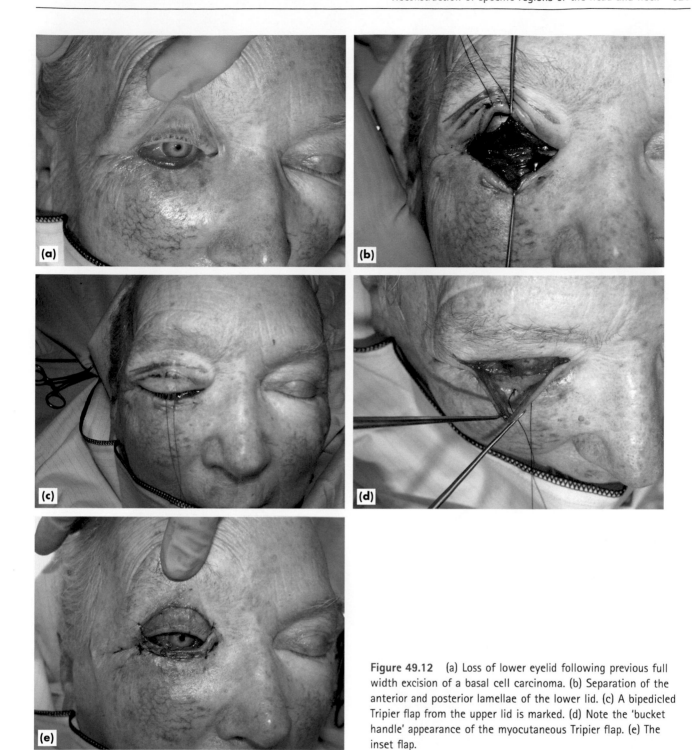

Figure 49.12   (a) Loss of lower eyelid following previous full width excision of a basal cell carcinoma. (b) Separation of the anterior and posterior lamellae of the lower lid. (c) A bipedicled Tripier flap from the upper lid is marked. (d) Note the 'bucket handle' appearance of the myocutaneous Tripier flap. (e) The inset flap.

occipitalis muscle posteriorly. These muscles are connected by an aponeurosis (the galea aponeurotica). Laterally, this aponeurosis is connected to the subcutaneous musculoaponeurotic system (SMAS) of the face. The layer of loose areolar tissue deep to this, also known as the inominate fascia, is an avascular plane. Owing to this, most local flaps of the scalp are raised at this level because it is easy to dissect and relatively bloodless, thus making scalp flaps fasciocutaneous rather than cutaneous. The deepest layer is the pericranium (the periosteum of the skull) which is firmly adherent to the underlying bone. However it can be raised and turned over on itself to form a pericranial flap.[30] This is viable tissue that can cover exposed bone and is capable of taking a skin graft. Laterally, the pericranium is continuous with the deep temporal fascia overlying the temporalis muscle.

BLOOD SUPPLY

The scalp has a rich blood supply from tributaries of both the external and internal carotid arteries (**Figure 49.18**). The paired superficial temporal, posterior auricular and occipital

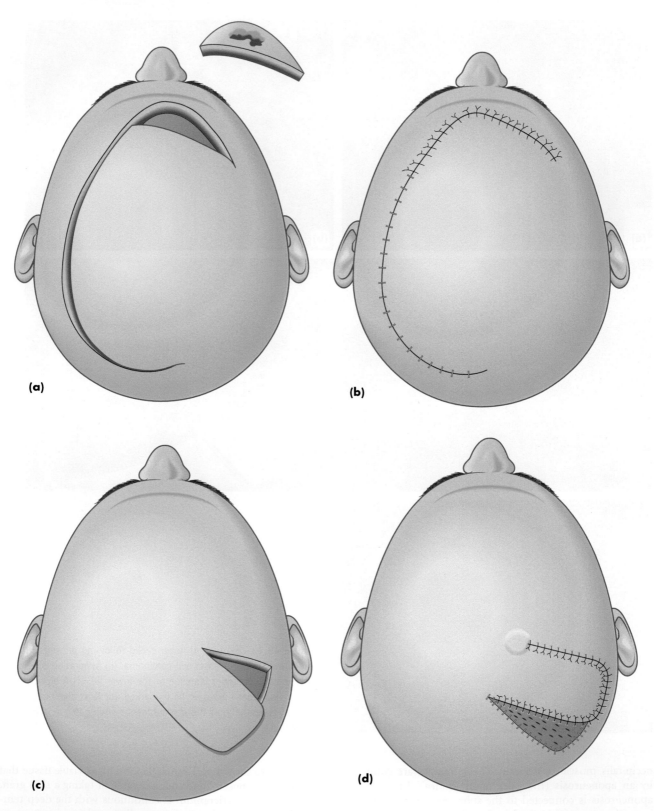

Figure 49.13   (a) A rotation flap is rotated around a pivot point to close a scalp defect. (b) The rotation flap donor site is closed directly. (c) A transposition flap is moved laterally across a pivot point to close a similar scalp defect. (d) The transposition flap donor site is closed with a split-thickness skin graft.

arteries are all branches of the external carotid, whereas the paired supratrochlear and supraorbital arteries are branches of the ophthalmic artery. There are anastomoses between all

these arteries and the entire scalp can survive on any single one of these vessels. However, when planning reconstructions of the scalp using local flaps, it is convenient to think of three

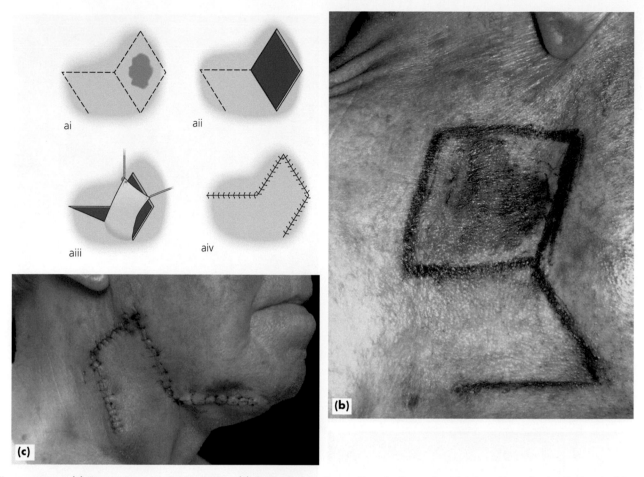

ai

aii

aiii

aiv

(b)

(c)

Figure 49.14 (a) The design of a rhomboid flap. (b) An area of lentigo maligna in the neck which is to be excised and closed with a rhomboid flap. (c) The flap raised and transposed into the defect.

separate axes of blood supply: an anterior axis (supratrochlear and supraorbital), a lateral axis (superficial temporal and posterior auricular) and a posterior axis (occipital). Scalp flaps should contain one of these axes at the base of the flap to provide a reliable vascularity. The venous drainage of the scalp runs parallel to the arterial supply; in addition, venous blood also drains through the diploe of the skull via emissary veins to the dural sinuses.

SCALP FLAPS

Small defects of the scalp can be closed directly. If there is too much skin tension, then the use of a split-thickness skin graft is to be considered. To have a successful take of a skin graft, a healthy recipient bed is needed. This normally means healthy pericranium following the excision of a cutaneous malignancy, most commonly a squamous cell carcinoma. When the excision defect following ablative surgery includes the pericranium and the outer table of the skull is exposed there are two options. The first is burring the outer table to obtain a healthy vascular bed which will take a skin graft or peforming a pericranial turnover flap to provide a graftable bed.[31] However, if adjuvant radiotherapy is to be used, then this may influence the decision to skin graft a scalp defect which is down to bone as there is an increased risk of

breakdown of the recipient site. If this is the case, then a scalp flap should be considered.

Larger defects of the scalp are best treated with a local flap. These can be either rotation or transposition flaps. If a rotation flap is to be used, it has to be designed big enough to cover the primary defect and allow direct closure of the donor site. This normally means that a scalp rotation flap is at least half the area of the patient's scalp. In addition to the size of the scalp flap, back cuts can be useful as well as scoring the undersurface of the flap (the galea) to enable it to stretch adequately. The alternative to a rotation flap is a transposition flap. This does not need to be designed as large as a rotation flap, but the donor defect needs to be covered with a split-thickness skin graft. This leaves a 'bald spot' on the patient's head but, considering the majority of patients are elderly and being treated for a cutaneous malignancy secondary to sun exposure, this is not as cosmetically disfiguring as might be supposed. Other techniques have been described to increase the amount of tissue available for scalp flaps. These include the use of tissue expansion to provide a greater volume of tissue[32] which can be used to provide a larger flap. Alternatively, multiple interdigitating flaps can be used as described by Orticochea.[33, 34] For very large defects, the use of microvascular free tissue transfer needs to be considered,[35] however that is beyond the scope of this chapter.

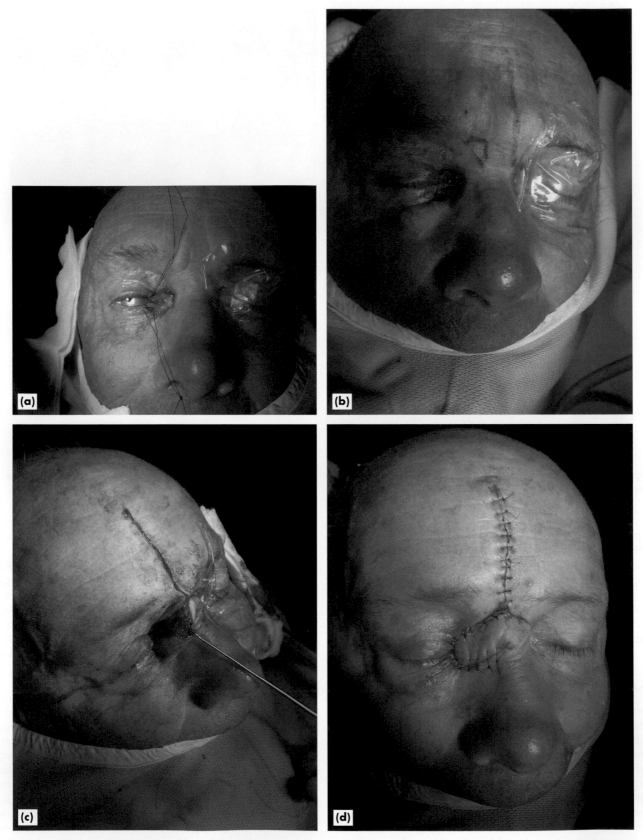

Figure 49.15   (a) A basal cell carcinoma of the right medial canthus. (b) The excision defect and the glabellar transposition flap drawn. (c) The flap transposed with the donor site directly closed. (d) The flap inset into the defect.

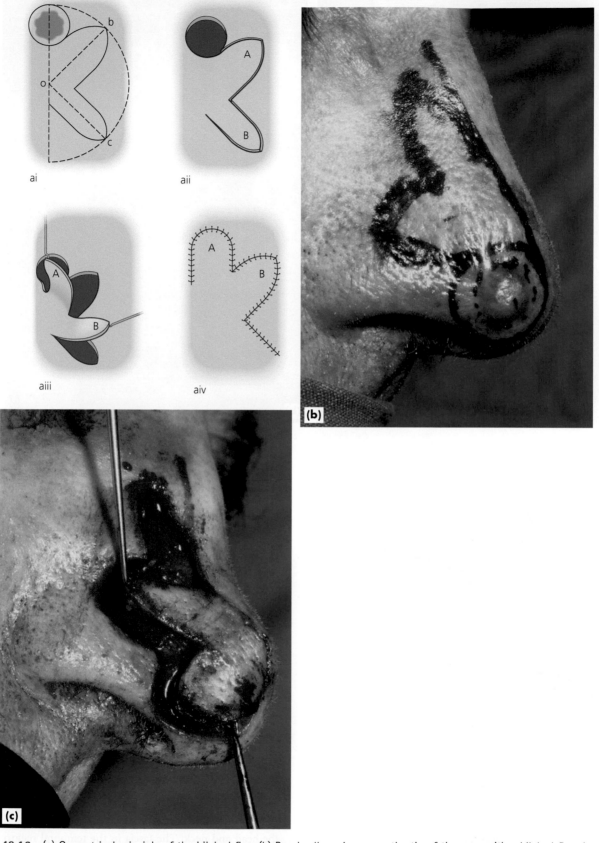

Figure 49.16   (a) Geometrical principle of the bilobed flap. (b) Basal cell carcinoma on the tip of the nose with a bilobed flap drawn. (c) The flap raised and transferred.

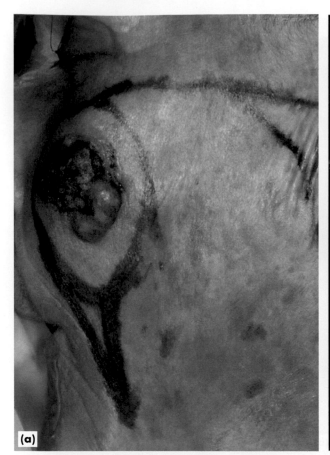

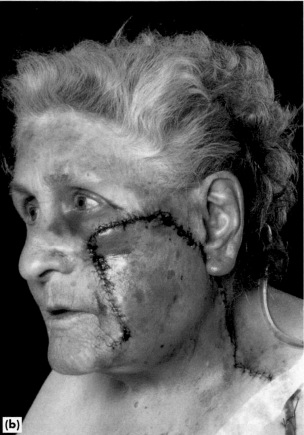

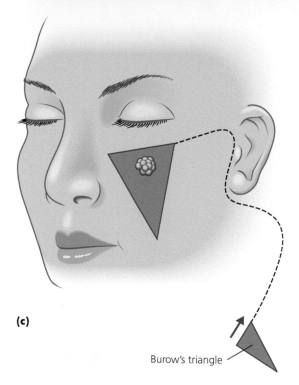

Burow's triangle

Figure 49.17   (a) Squamous cell carcinoma of the cheek with a cheek rotation flap drawn. (b) Closure of the defect with the rotation flap. (c) Diagram of the technique.

TEMPOROPARIETAL FASCIA FLAPS

When discussing scalp flaps it is useful to consider tissue from the scalp that can be used to reconstruct defects around the head and neck. The fascia in the temporal region can be used for this purpose. This fascia has several well-described layers.[36] The superficial temporal fascia (temporoparietal fascia) lies immediately deep to the hair follicles and is in

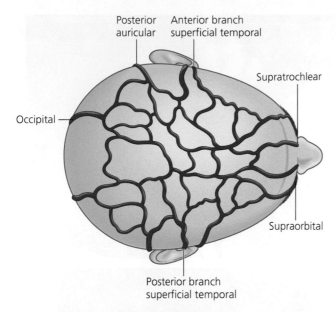

Figure 49.18 The blood supply of the scalp.

continuity with the galea superiorly and the SMAS inferiorly. Deep to this is an avascular layer, known as the innominate fascia, which is in continuity with the loose areolar tissue of the scalp. The deep temporal fascia (or temporalis fascia) is the deepest layer and this is in continuity with the pericranium superiorly. Each of these layers may be used as a local flap to cover defects within their arc of rotation. They are particularly useful in covering exposed bone around the skull base and related structures such as the ear and the orbit.[37] This is shown in **Figure 49.19** where a temporoparietal fascia flap is used to cover the exposed temporal bone following total resection of the external ear and extended neck dissection for a $T_4N_1M_0$ squamous cell carcinoma.

Forehead

The forehead is bounded by the anterior hairline superiorly and the eyebrows inferiorly. The lateral limits are the temporal hairline. Underlying the skin is the frontalis muscle and deep to that the frontal bone. The skin can appear very smooth in younger patients, but in the older population transverse furrows appear, which are more obvious on frowning (contraction of the frontalis muscle). Small defects of the forehead should be directly closed. The forehead is very visible to observers and so care should be taken to place incisions to give minimal scarring. This is done by placing scars horizontally or along the hair line and eyebrow; defects as large as 6 cm can be closed in this way. Distortion of these hair-bearing surfaces can be cosmetically unsightly so for some larger defects where direct closure may cause malposition of the hairline or brow a large full-thickness skin graft would give an adequate result. Larger defects of the forehead can be closed with hatchet flaps which are random rotation flaps with a back cut. They can be single or double and heal with minimal scarring. They are particularly useful for cutaneous malignancies which have been excised with a circular primary defect. Large defects can be closed using this technique and it is possible to preserve the supratrochlear and supraorbital nerves when dissecting the forehead to maintain a sensate forehead.[38] It should be remembered that when using a double hatchet flap the vertical scar should be placed in the centre of the forehead. Other techniques for forehead reconstruction include the use of scalp rotation flaps which can be tissue expanded to produce a larger flap.[39] These however are limited as they import hair-bearing skin into the forehead thus distorting the hairline.

Eyelid

ANATOMY

The anatomy of the periorbital region is complex and without a good understanding of the structure and function of the eyelids periobital excisions and reconstructions should not be undertaken. The upper eyelid and the lower eyelid differ in their roles. The upper eyelid both elevates due to contraction of the levator palpabrae muscle, which is innervated by the oculomotor (3rd cranial) nerve and constricts due to contraction of the orbicularis oculi muscle which is innervated by the facial (7th cranial) nerve. The lower lid is only able to constrict and relax due to the action of orbicularis oculi. This means that the upper lid has a far greater excursion (movement) than the lower lid. Both the upper and lower eyelids are divided into anterior and posterior lamellae. The anterior lamella consists of the skin and the orbicularis oculi muscle, whereas the posterior lamella consists of the conjunctiva and the tarsal plate. The skin of the eyelid is the thinnest in the body (1 mm) and is loosely attached to the orbicularis oculi muscle. This is arranged in a concentric ring around the orbit and upon contracture acts as a sphincter closing the orbital aperture. It can be divided into three parts: an outer orbital part covering bone, and inner preseptal and pretarsal components. Dividing the anterior and posterior lamellae is a septum. This is continuous with the pericranium at the orbital rims and extends to the margin of the eyelid. The tarsal plate forms the skeleton of the eyelid and is a dense sheet of fibrous tissue. The deepest structure of the eyelid is its lining, the conjunctiva, which contains many mucus secreting cells.

EYELID RECONSTRUCTION

Defects in the eyelid can be partial thickness, with either the anterior or posterior lamella having been excised or full thickness. Partial thickness defects of the anterior lamella are best either closed directly if small or covered with a full thickness skin graft. The posterior lamella can be closed with a graft of buccal or hard palate mucosa[40] or a chondromucosal[41] graft from the nasal septum consisting of nasal mucosa and septal cartilage. Full-thickness defects of up to one-quarter of the lid length can be closed directly and this increases to one-third in the elderly population with lax skin. When reconstructing a larger full-thickness defect, it is important to remember that both the anterior and posterior lamellae need to be replaced. This can be done by either using a single flap to reconstruct both layers or by using a flap to reconstruct the anterior lamella and a graft for the posterior lamella. At least one of the two layers must have its own blood supply as a graft placed on another graft will fail.

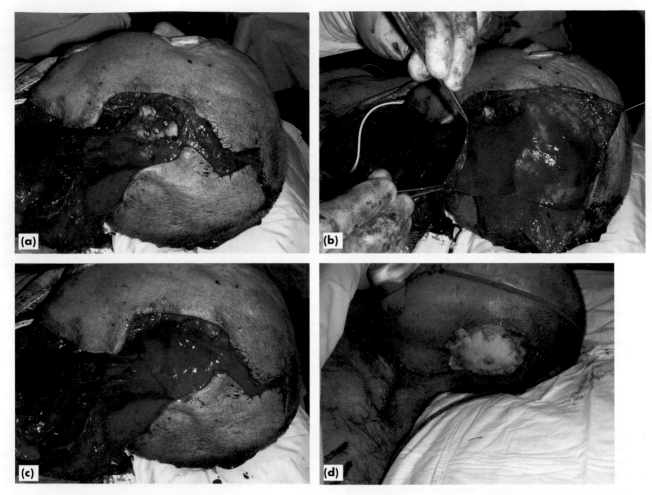

Figure 49.19 (a) Defect following total pinnectomy, parotidectomy and neck dissection for $T_4N_1M_0$ squamous cell carcinoma of the ear. Note the exposed temporal bone with osseointegrated abutments for a prosthetic ear posterior to the external auditory meatus. (b) Temporoparietal fascia flap. (c) The temporoparietal fascia flap inset covering the exposed bone and implants. (d) The temporoparietal fascia flap was then covered with a split-thickness skin graft.

When closing a defect directly, two additional techniques may be used to bring in adjacent lateral tissue to enable a tension-free closure. The first of these is a lateral cantholysis. A horizontal incision is made from the lateral canthus to the orbital rim. The lateral canthal tendon is identified and divided. The lateral part of the lid can then be mobilized medially to close the wound. A second method is to place a z-plasty over the lateral canthus.[42] A z-plasty consists of two interdigitating flaps of equal size and can be used to move tissue from one area to another. To reconstruct larger defects either a rotation or a transposition flap may be used. To reconstruct the lower eyelid a cheek rotation flap may be utilized, whereas a glabellar transposition flap is useful for the upper eyelid (**Figure 49.15**). These can both be combined with a composite graft from the nasal septum to reconstruct both anterior and posterior lamellae separately (**Figure 49.20**).

Nose

It is difficult to close primary defects in the nose directly without distortion, due to a relative lack of skin laxity. The use of full-thickness skin grafts gives very good cosmetic results and these remain the mainstay of nasal reconstruction for superficial defects. The skin grafts will take on recipient beds of subcutaneous tissue or perichondrium. However, if the deep margin has included the perichondrium, the nasal cartilages or is full thickness and has included excision of nasal mucosa then a different approach needs to be used. When constructing a full-thickness defect of the nose, three distinct layers need to be considered and reconstructed: these are nasal lining, nasal support and overlying skin (inside, scaffold and outside). A composite graft taken from the ear is an option when a small nasal rim defect is being reconstructed. This involves taking a full-thickness piece of the ear including both anterior and posterior skin. When the defect is medium sized, then a local flap needs to be used. The undersurface of such a flap can then be skin grafted to replace the nasal lining. Normally this can be a split-thickness skin graft but when support is needed to keep the nasal aperture open then a composite graft from the ear containing just anterior skin and cartilage is used. The cartilage is used as a non-anatomical strut (i.e. not in the normal anatomical position of the alar or lateral cartilages). The local flap options used to cover nasal defects are varied and can include

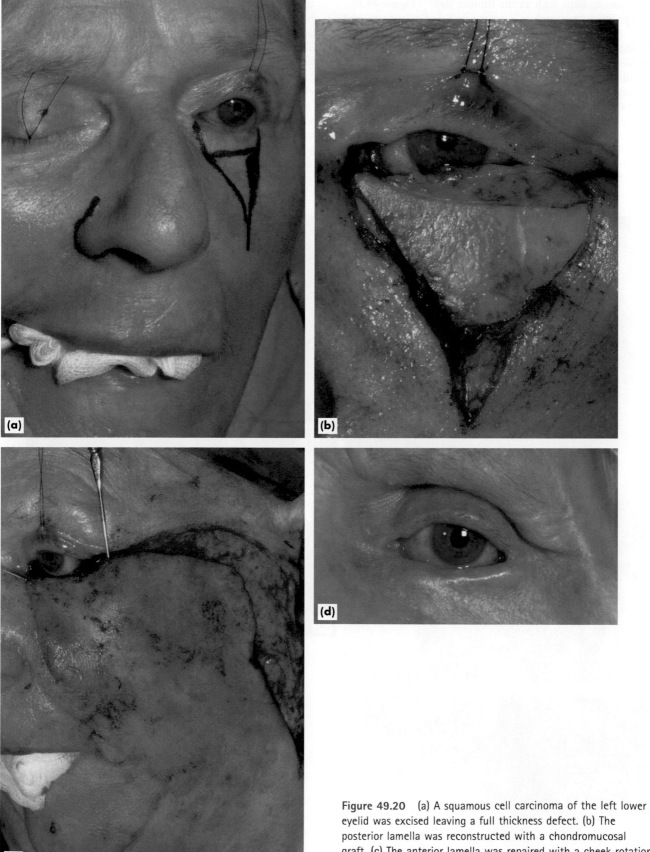

Figure 49.20   (a) A squamous cell carcinoma of the left lower eyelid was excised leaving a full thickness defect. (b) The posterior lamella was reconstructed with a chondromucosal graft. (c) The anterior lamella was repaired with a cheek rotation flap. (d) The final result.

advancement flaps such as the Rintalla flap[21] (**Figure 49.10**), transposition flaps such as a superiorly based axial nasolabial flap (**Figure 49.21**) or a bilobed flap (**Figure 49.16**). In addition to these techniques, microvascular free tissue transfer of a chondrocutaneous flap from the ear has been described.[43]

Larger full-thickness defects of the nose following partial or total rhinectomy are more difficult to manage. A local flap can be used to reconstruct both the lining and skin cover of the nose by folding the flap in two. The most commonly used flaps for this are superiorly based nasolabial flaps. Bilateral flaps can be raised to import a large volume of tissue.[44] An alternative to folding a flap is to use one flap for the lining and another for the cover. The nasolabial flap can be used for the lining as can a random hinge flap where adjacent tissue is raised and flipped over to fill the defect.[45] This technique is more commonly used when the defect has been excised previously and the old wound margins have healed. The flaps used as lining can then be covered with either a skin graft or another flap such as a forehead flap (see below). It has to be remembered that when dealing with a total rhinectomy defect very good results can be obtained using a prosthesis. With the advent of osseointegration a prosthetic nose is both cosmetically acceptable and convenient for the patient.[46] This is a viable alternative to surgical reconstruction.

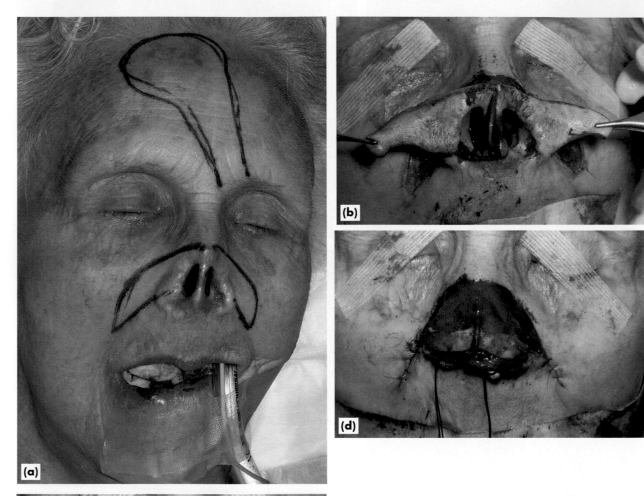

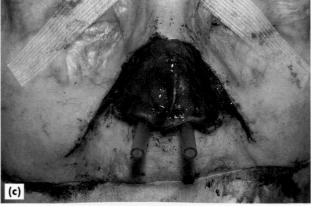

Figure 49.21 (a) Defect following previous excision of large infiltrating squamous cell carcinoma of the nose with bilateral nasolabial and forehead flap marked. (b) Nasolabial flaps raised. (c) Nasolabial flaps inset to provide internal lining of nose. (d) Nasal support provided with auricular cartilage grafts. (e) Forehead flap raised. (f) Forehead flap inset to provide external cover. (g) The final result.

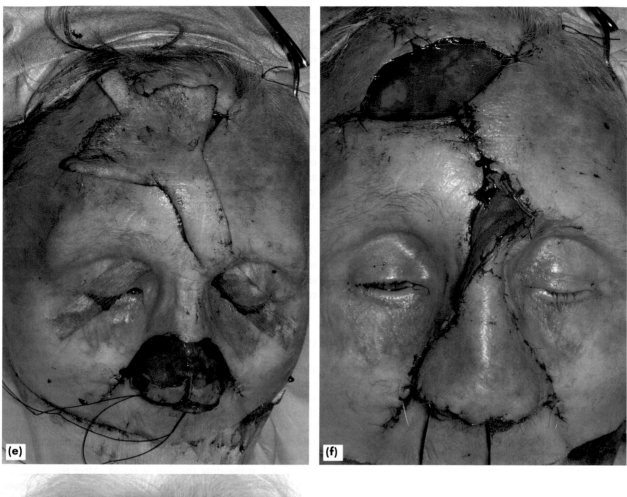

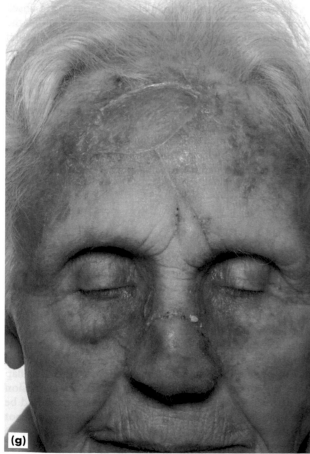

Figure 49.21   Continued

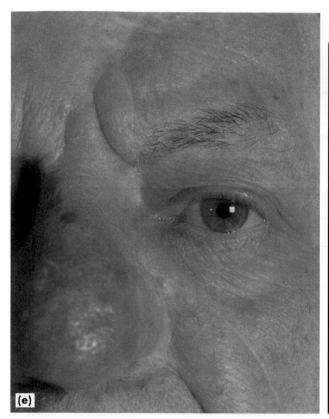

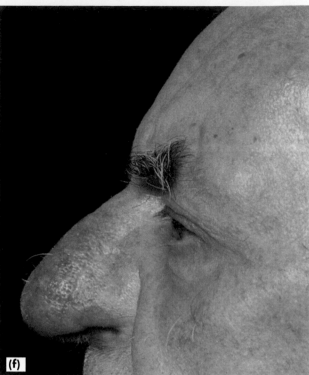

Figure 50.2 Continued.

mucosa and laterally by the external lamina of the muscles of facial expression, the masseter, the buccal fat pad, and the facial artery and vein.

The facial artery, a branch of the external carotid artery, enters the face by curving around the lower border of the mandible at the anterior edge of the masseter muscle. It then follows a tortuous course, passing superiorly and anteriorly to a position just lateral to the commissure of the mouth. At this point it lies deep to the risorius, zygomaticus major muscle and the superficial lamina of the orbicularis oris muscle. It lies superficial to the buccinator muscle and the lateral edge of the deep lamina of the orbicularis oris muscle. At this point in its course it gives off multiple perforating vessels to the cheek and the superior labial artery. It continues superiorly to the angular artery, which reaches the medial canthus. It has communicating branches with the buccal and infraorbital branches.

The FAMM flap is an axial pattern flap based on the facial artery. The flap may be harvested as an inferiorly based flap based on antegrade flow or a superiorly based flap with retrograde flow. The basic harvest technique is to Doppler out the facial artery through the buccal mucosa and map the course of the vessel. For the inferiorly based flap, dissection begins anterosuperiorly to identify the arterial supply to the upper lip with division of the facial artery at this point and then retrograde dissection which includes the mucosa, buccinator, facial artery and the tissue and venous plexus that lies between the artery and the muscle. In the superiorly based flap, the dissection begins inferiorly with visualization and ligation of the facial artery and then a retrograde dissection of the tissues including the buccinator

muscle. A flap of 7–8 cm can be harvested with a thickness of 8–10 mm.

The FAMM flap is ideally suited for reconstruction of small mucosal defects in the oral cavity and, in particular, the mucosa of the lip. The flap can also be rotated across the alveolus to close small defects of the floor of mouth or tongue as well as the palate.

Temporoparietal fascial flap

The temporoparietal flap is a versatile local rotation or free fascial flap for reconstruction of the head and neck or extremities. Golovine first described the flap in the nineteenth century for orbit reconstruction. More recently it has been popularized by Brent and Byrd,[7] and others for microtia repair and auricular reconstruction. Its unique characteristics are a remarkably robust vascular supply with a very thin and pliable flap with minimal donor site morbidity.

The arterial supply of the temporoparietal flap is the superficial temporal artery, a terminal branch of the external carotid artery. The vessel classically has a number of branches above the zygoma with most patients having a prominent frontal branch and dominant branch, which ascends towards the vertex of the skull. The venous drainage is via the superficial temporal vein running with the artery. There is some variation in venous anatomy with a small percentage of patients having venous drainage through the post-auricular vein or occipital veins. The temporoparietal fascia (TPF) lies just under the subcutaneous tissue of the lateral scalp (**Figure 50.5**). The fascia has an inner and an outer layer with the

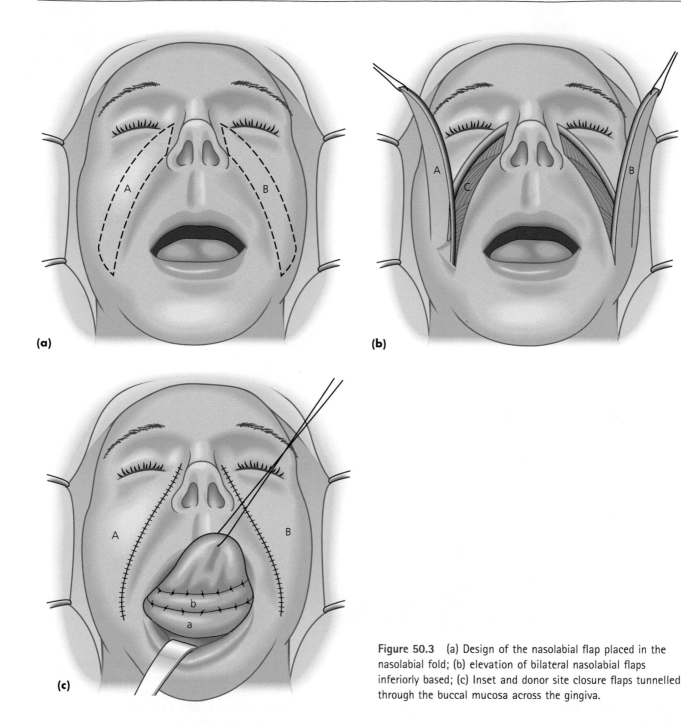

Figure 50.3 (a) Design of the nasolabial flap placed in the nasolabial fold; (b) elevation of bilateral nasolabial flaps inferiorly based; (c) Inset and donor site closure flaps tunnelled through the buccal mucosa across the gingiva.

artery and vein entering between the inner and outer layers and then coursing vertically in the outer layer of the fascia. The outer layer of the TPF extends as the superficial muscular aponeurotic system (SMAS) below the zygoma. A thin muscular layer (the superficial auricular muscle) separates two parts of the outer layer of the fascia below the temporal line. The inner layer of the TPF contains a dense vascular network, which originates from the outer layer. Two nerves have an anatomic relation to the flap. The auriculotemporal nerve, a branch of V3, lies within the superficial layer of the TPF and theoretically could provide for a sensate flap. The frontal branch of the facial nerve traverses over the zygoma in the same plane as the frontal branch of the superficial

temporal artery and can be injured if the dissection is carried too far forward in the plane of this vessel.

For flap harvest, the patient is usually positioned in the supine position, with the drape line along the vertex of the scalp leaving the post-auricular area exposed.

The important landmarks for this flap are the arch of the zygoma, the pinna and the usual landmarks of the facial nerve. The artery usually lies just in front of the pinna and is easily palpated or detected with the Doppler in this location. The artery ascends vertically to the apex with a frontal branch coming off 1–3 cm above the zygomatic arch. The flap is harvested as an elliptical or teardrop shape, above the level of the zygoma. The incision is placed just posterior to the

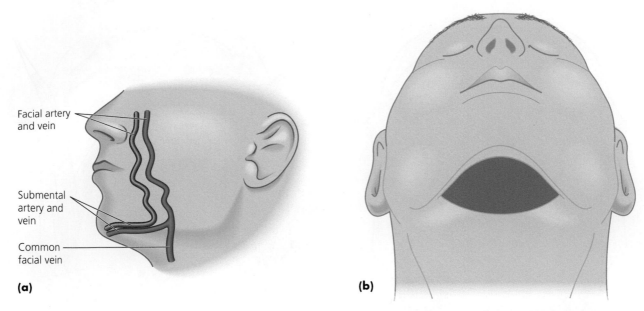

(a)

Facial artery and vein

Submental artery and vein

Common facial vein

(b)

Figure 50.4 (a) Vascular anatomy of the submental island flap; (b) donor site (shaded for the submental island flap).

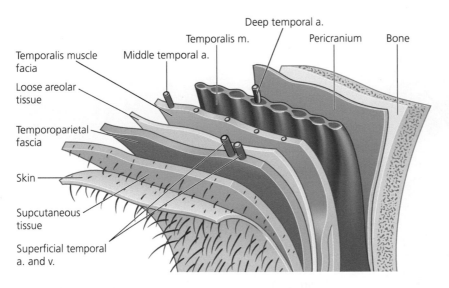

Temporalis muscle facia

Loose areolar tissue

Temporoparietal fascia

Skin

Supcutaneous tissue

Superficial temporal a. and v.

Deep temporal a.

Temporalis m.

Middle temporal a.

Pericranium

Bone

Figure 50.5 The anatomy of the scalp and the blood supply of the temporoparietal fascial flap.

position of the vertical branch and can be either a straight or curvilinear incision into the scalp or can be 'Y' shaped for larger teardrop-shaped flaps. The inferior limit of the incision is usually the tragus, but inferior extensions can be used for extended rotations or if the surgeon wishes to visualize the facial nerve. The initial incision is started just above the zygoma extending into the scalp. The surgeon harvesting this flap for the first time must take great care not to incise too deeply as the pedicle can easily be divided during the incision. The plane of dissection is initiated by defining the level of the superficial temporal fascia just below the subcutaneous fat layer in the scalp. A good landmark is to look for the hair follicles; if they are being transected, the surgeon is elevating the flap too superficially. Once fully mobilized from the overlying skin the flap is incised around its periphery and elevated in the plane just above the temporal fascia. Dissection is carried down to about 2 cm below the arch of the zygoma to ensure an appropriate arc of rotation (**Figure 50.6**).

Clinical applications for this flap include orbital reconstruction including the extenteration cavity, upper and lower eyelids and the eyebrow as a fasciocutaneous hair-bearing flap. The flap has been widely used for auricular reconstruction including microtia and traumatic or oncologic deformities, as well as palate reconstruction and buccal mucosal reconstruction.

DISTANT AXIAL FLAPS

Deltopectoral flap

This flap was described by Bakamjian and Littlewood[8] in 1964 and is an axial pattern flap designed on the anterior chest wall between the line of the clavicle and the level of the anterior axillary fold. Its vascular supply arises from the upper three or four perforating branches of the internal

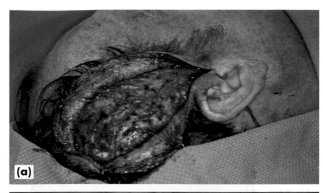

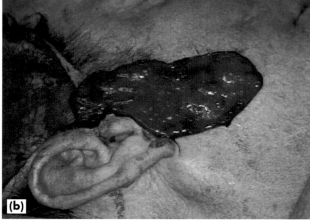

Figure 50.6 (a) Donor site of the temporoparietal flap. (b) Arc of rotation temporoparietal flap.

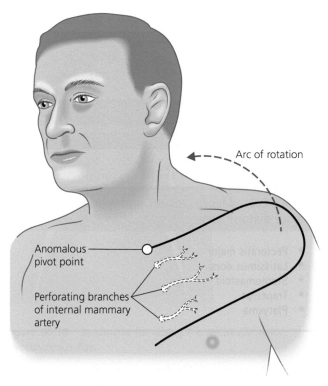

Arc of rotation

Anomalous pivot point

Perforating branches of internal mammary artery

Figure 50.7 Design and planning of the deltopectoral flap. Note the position of the anomalous pivot point at the upper medial end of the flap.

mammary artery, which emerge through the medial end of the intercostal spaces (**Figure 50.7**). Its boundaries are the clavicle superiorly, the acromion laterally and a line running through the anterior axillary fold to above the nipple inferiorly. The flap will extend to any site in the neck and is extremely useful for neck resurfacing. The territory of the perforator vascular system has been shown to extend as far as the groove separating the deltoid from the pectoralis major (deltopectoral groove). Any extension of the flap beyond this should not be regarded as a random component.

The flap is marked out using the landmarks described above and then elevation begins laterally. The pectoral fascia is left on the flap, leaving the muscle fibres below absolutely bare. Any branches of the acromiothoracic axis that are encountered should be ligated.

PLANNING THE TRANSFER

The deltopectoral flap has an anomalous pivot point. There is considerable laxity of the skin on the anterior axillary fold when the arm is abducted. This means that the lower border of the flap is considerably longer than the upper part. The pivot point on the flap is thus at the medial end of the upper limb and not the lower limb. This needs to be taken into account when planning the flap. The donor site is usually covered with a split skin graft.

The uses of a deltopectoral flap are:

* a one-stage reconstruction of the anterior neck skin;

* a two-stage reconstruction as the flap may be passed over existing neck structures to resurface distant sites.

OTHER DISTAL AXIAL CUTANEOUS FLAPS

These include cervical skin flaps and occipitomastoid-based flaps.

Cervical-facial skin flaps of varying shape, size, site and direction may be designed to make good use of lax neck skin for reconstructive purposes. In general, they make use of the side of the neck. They are most frequently used as a primary or salvage procedure for external skin defects of the lower face and cheek. This flap has the unique advantage of providing excellent if not identical colour match for external defects. The nape of neck (Mütter) or posterior scalp flap is a random pattern skin flap, which exploits the neck skin over the trapezius muscle and can be raised on the occipital vessels and extended downwards to the spine of the scapula. It may be swung on its upper pedicle to reconstruct areas in the lower face and submandibular region.

MYOCUTANEOUS AND MUSCLE ONLY AXIAL DISTANT FLAPS

One of the most important discoveries in the last 20 years is that the skin over most parts of the body receives its blood supply from small musculocutaneous arteries (perforating vessels) that enter it from the underlying muscle (**Figure 50.8**). It subsequently became apparent that an obvious way

Box 50.3   Elevating the pectoralis major flap

- Incise the skin down to the underlying muscle.
- Define the inferior and lateral borders of the pectoralis major muscle.
- Mobilize the lateral border of the pectoralis major muscle dissecting the subpectoral plane which is relatively avascular.
- Visualize the pedicle on the deep surface of the muscle running medial to lateral.
- Divide the inferior muscle attachments from the ribs or rectus sheath.
- Mobilize in an upward direction.
- If the skin paddle is thick or excessively mobile place sutures from the dermis of the skin island to the muscle surface to prevent shearing and flap loss.
- Combine mobilization in an upward direction first laterally and then medially.
- Identify the lateral border of the external segment of the muscle.
- Divide the sternal insertion of the muscle at the level of the anterior axillary line and remember to continue in an vertical direction.
- Divide the insertion of the muscle usually with a monopolar cautery to avoid bleeding from the lateral perforators of the pectoral artery.
- The muscle will be now rotated and the vascular pedicle will be clearly identified.

impossible to tube a pectoralis major myocutaneous flap. This should be considered as a salvage technique only as better free tissue transfer techniques are available.

When the above guidelines are followed, there are very few potential pitfalls with this flap. It is highly reliable and even when the skin paddle fails, the underlying muscle will usually survive and can be allowed to granulate and heal by secondary intention, or covered subsequently with a skin graft. It is always worth checking for congenital absence of the pectoralis major, although it is extremely rare with an incidence of 1:11 000. Congenital absence of the sternocostal head is part of Poland's syndrome.

When a conventional flap is used, the skin paddle is designed medial to the nipple, at about the level of the sixth rib. In this area, the skin overlying the muscle is usually relatively thin in males. To achieve similar thickness in females, a design placing the skin island in the inframammary fold oriented transversely or slightly angled superiorly in its medial extent allows for the thinnest flaps. The surgeon considering this flap in females should consider the inframammary incision as the preferred approach.

Latissimus dorsi flap

This flap represents the first myocutaneous flap described in the medical literature.[11] It was repopularized by Olivari[12] in 1976 for the repair of local defects. Further work by Quillen[13]

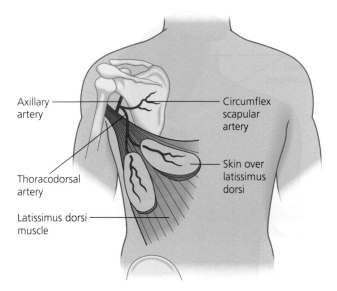

Figure 50.11   Blood supply to the latissimus dorsi flap. The thoracodorsal artery is a continuation of the subscapular artery which comes directly off the axillary artery.

in 1978 described its use for head and neck reconstruction, and it remains a reliable and versatile fundamental component of the surgeon's repertoire.

The muscle is large and triangular in shape and arises from the sacrum and lumbar vertebrae, thoracolumbar fascia, the posterior iliac crest and the lower six thoracic vertebrae. In addition, some slips arise from the lower three ribs and the muscle converges to have a narrow insertion into the intertubercular groove of the humerus. Hence, it forms the posterior wall of the axilla. It is a type V muscle that receives a significant but smaller blood supply from the perforating vessels through the lumbosacral fascia, and a pedicled flap can be based on this to repair defects in the buttock region.

Its major vascular supply arises from the thoracodorsal vessels, which have their origin in the subscapular artery (**Figure 50.11**). This latter artery arises from the axillary artery, gives rise to the circumflex scapular artery about 4 cm from its origin (**Figures 50.12 and 50.13**) and then continues as a thoracodorsal artery to enter the latissimus dorsi about 10 cm from its humeral insertion. Just before its insertion, it gives off a branch, which accompanies branches from the lateral thoracic artery (which also arises from the subscapular artery) and carries on to supply the serratus anterior. Within the latissimus dorsi muscle, the thoracodorsal vessels divide into superior and lateral branches, which allow the muscle to be split into two. Either two flaps can then be taken or just one flap, thereby leaving some muscle behind.

Venous drainage is by the venae comitantes, which accompany the thoracodorsal artery and drain into the axillary vein. The nerve supply is via the thoracodorsal nerve, which is a branch of the posterior cord of the brachial plexus.

Large amounts of tissue are made available using this flap. Flaps measuring 10×8 cm are easily harvested and subsequent primary closure is easily achieved. Even larger amounts of tissue may be taken as a musculocutaneous flap measuring 40×20 cm but this requires skin grafting of the donor defect and may lead to problems with healing on the back.

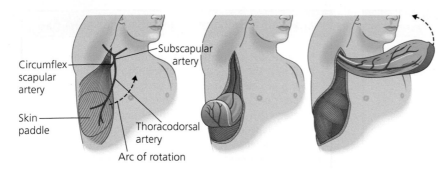

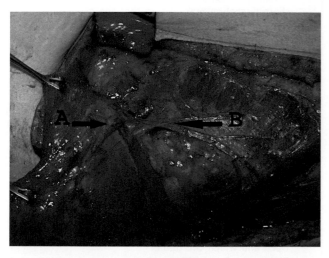

Figure 50.12 Technique of raising the latissimus dorsi flap. When designing for pedicled transfer, an oblique incision is used to allow maximal length to the flap. The dissection begins low down and then the pedicle is identified more proximally as the dissection approaches the axilla.

Figure 50.13 Lateral view of latissimus dorsi pedicle: A, thoracodorsal branch to latissimus dorsi; B, thoracodorsal branch to serratus anterior.

Box 50.4   Advantages of latissimus dorsi flap

- Large amounts of tissue transferred
- Pedicled or free tissue transfer
- Cosmetic advantage, especially females
- Versatile: may be tubed/multiple/osseous components
- When pedicled, can reach the upper face and scalp

Box 50.5   Disadvantages of latissimus dorsi flap

- Very bulky
- Occasional donor site dehiscence
- Reduction in upper limb power
- May require moving of the patient to harvest

A latissimus dorsi flap may not only be raised as a myocutaneous pedicled flap but also used for free tissue transfer. It is reliable, with a long pedicle of > 10 cm, which can be further lengthened by dividing the circumflex scapular artery. The diameter of the subscapular artery at this point is at least 3 mm and the veins are of similar size.

By designing the flap low down on the back, the arc of rotation allows transfer into the head and neck region up to the zygomatic arch and flaps can be made to reach the top of the head (particularly if only muscle is used). The other advantages of this flap are that it does not violate the breast and because it is a large flat muscle, it is possible in extreme circumstances to tube it for total pharyngeal reconstruction. In addition, the subscapular artery offers a variety of flaps, which may be used either singularly or in combination. Therefore, a scapular flap along with a latissimus dorsi flap and serratus anterior flap may all be raised on the same pedicle (**Box 50.4**).

Despite the advantages, it still remains a musculocutaneous flap with thick skin and is therefore more bulky than, for example, a radial free forearm flap. Its use tends to be in resurfacing large defects of the external neck skin and for secondary repair of wound complications such as salivary fistulae. It has an excellent application in reconstructing the total glossectomy defect as the volume of the flap makes it ideal for filling the mucosal defect and the dead space below the resection site. Serious donor site problems are rare but dehiscence and late wound seroma can be a problem.

Congenital absence of the muscle should be checked for prior to surgery, and in athletes and those who do manual work the flap should be raised from the non-dominant side.

Raising the flap usually involves a variable amount of turning of the patient. Some authors advocate the lateral decubitis position that often requires a repositioning manoeuvre following the ablative procedure (see **Box 50.5**). Most surgeons experienced with this flap will harvest it with the patient turned 15 to 30° which obviates the need for the repositioning manoeuvre and allows two team procedures.

RAISING THE FLAP

Small flaps may be raised with the patient supine, but larger flaps require the patient in a rotated position with the arm freely draped so that it may be moved during the flap harvest.

Skin may be raised over the whole area of the muscle, although the vascular supply from the thoracodorsal artery decreases as one approaches the lumbosacral fascia. The posterior axillary fold is marked out and this represents the anterior edge of the muscle. The posterior iliac crest is also marked, together with the tip of the scapula. The skin flap is designed to the appropriate size and shape, with particular

---

Box 50.6 Elevation of latissimus dorsi

- Outline the flap.
- The initial incision exposes the anterior edge of the latissimus dorsi muscle.
- Identify the serratus anterior.
- Do not go **deep** to serratus anterior here: this places the pedicle in jeopardy.
- Identify the branches to serratus and follow them in a retrograde direction to visualize the pedicle to the latissimus dorsi.
- Divide latissimus dorsi inferiorly.
- The muscle flap may be extended beyond the skin island in a lateral to medial and superoinferior direction to provide additional muscle to resurface external defects or provide additional volume to fill defects. Remember at this point that if one is low and on top of the latissimus dorsi, the pedicle is not in jeopardy.
- Elevate the flap in the submuscular plane.
- Identify the pedicle running down the muscle, usually in its central portion. The key to easy identification and protection of the pedicle to latissimus dorsi is to identify the branches to the serratus and follow them superiorly to the take-off from the thoracodorsal. Occasionally, patients will have a separate pedicle to serratus but this is very infrequent. Once the thoracodorsal pedicle is identified divide the vessels to serratus anterior and continue dissecting superiorly.
- Continue the dissection up towards the tip of the scapula.
- The junction of the thoracodorsal vessels with the circumflex scapular vessels to form the subscapular artery can be clearly seen at the upper anterior end of the muscle in the axilla.
- If a longer pedicle is required (as is usual), ligate the circumflex scapular vessels.
- Follow the subscapular vessels into the axilla.

Box 50.7 Delivery of the latissimus dorsi flap

- Ligate the circumflex scapular artery and vein.
- Follow the subscapular vessels into the axilla.
- If a pedicled transfer is to be completed, the flap must be tunnelled into the neck. There are essentially two options, sub- or suprapectoral, with the subpectoral route being the favoured approach. The border of the pectoralis major is identified and dissection deep to the muscle establishes the space between pectoralis major and pectoralis minor. A tunnel may be developed with blunt or sharp dissection making sure that the pedicle to the pectoralis major is kept medially. The surgeon then develops the superior dissection if exposing the clavicle and the clavipectoral fascia has not already performed it. Splitting the pectoralis major then develops a tunnel. The tunnel needs to be wide enough to allow the passage of the muscle without compression, usually the breadth of one's hand.
- Use blunt finger dissection going on top of the pedicle.
- Remember to go 'over pectoralis minor – under pectoralis major'.
- Dissect from above through the clavipectoral fascia, dividing some of the lateral fibres of pectoralis major.
- Open and widen the tunnel.
- Deliver the flap without twisting or rotating the muscle.

---

reference to the length of pedicle. If an arc of rotation is required to facilitate transfer to the head and neck via a pedicled myocutaneous flap, it will usually mean an oblique or vertical design, but if a free flap is required the flap may be harvested in a horizontal direction, which gives a more acceptable scar in young women since it can be hidden behind the bra strap.

Elevation of the latissimus dorsi is shown in **Box 50.6**.

When using the flap as a myocutaneous rotation flap, consideration should be given to not dividing the insertion of the muscle. When the muscle is left intact the insertion prevents twisting of the vascular pedicle and reduces the risk of kinking and venous congestion. If an extended pedicle is required then the tendon must be divided to get additional length.

Delivery of the latissimus dorsi flap is shown in **Box 50.7**.

The donor site is closed primarily in two layers using two large drains, one of which should be left for up to a week to avoid a seroma, which can occur following such a large dissection. This can be avoided by suturing the muscle remnants to the chest wall prior to closure. With a pedicled flap, the muscle should be denervated by dividing the nerve. If a free flap is being used, the thoracodorsal nerve may be preserved and used for reinnervation procedures such as anastomosis to a cross-facial nerve graft for facial reanimation, or following total glossectomy where the maintenance of muscle bulk has been noted following anastomosis to the hypoglossal nerve.

Sternomastoid flap

The sternocleidomastoid muscle, unlike the previously described muscles, does not have a localized vascular hilum. It is supplied segmentally by vessels, which enter the muscle at intervals along its length. There are two principal vessels in its upper half, which consist of two branches of the occipital artery, and in its lower half, a branch from the superior thyroid artery. Further minor arterial branches enter in between. Its use has been described as a myocutaneous flap raised as a composite skin muscle flap, as a myocutaneous skin island flap taking a skin island based over the lower aspect of the muscle (**Figure 50.14**) or as a composite muscle–bone flap used for mandibular reconstruction taking

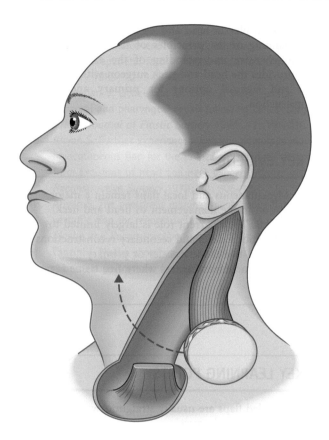

Figure 50.14 Sternomastoid flap.

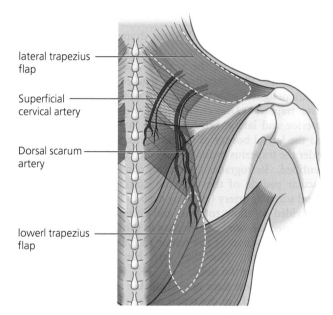

lateral trapezius flap

Superficial cervical artery

Dorsal scarum artery

lowerl trapezius flap

Figure 50.15 The trapezius group of flaps.

a segment of clavicle. Its routine use is not recommended as it has a number of distinct disadvantages (**Box 50.8**).

The sternomastoid flap is therefore rarely used but it may still have a role to play in two situations. First, it can be particularly useful as a muscle-only flap pedicled superiorly to fill small defects in the pharynx and oral cavity, and second, when split along its length and rotated anteriorly, it may be used to cover vessels in the compromised neck.

Trapezius flap

Three basic myocutaneous flaps have been described which make use of trapezius: the upper trapezius, the lateral trapezius and the lower trapezius flaps.[14] These may be pedicled into the head and neck area and, in addition, descriptions of the upper and lateral trapezius flaps to include transfer of the spine of the scapula have been described for mandibular reconstruction. The vascular supply of these flaps is complex and varied depending on the design.

The superiorly based trapezius flap incorporates the upper third of the trapezius muscle and the overlying skin. The flap is supplied predominantly by the occipital artery and its venae comitantes. This flap has a limited used but can be applied for defects of the temporal bone, lateral face or upper neck. The flap is harvested by designing a skin island over the pars descendens of the trapezius muscle with dissection carried out in a retrograde direction along the deep surface of the muscle.

The pars horizontalis (middle) and pars ascendens (lower) of the trapezius muscle form the basis of the lateral and lower

trapezius flaps (**Figure 50.15**). The middle parts of the muscle are supplied mainly by the superficial cervical artery (superficial branch of the transverse cervical artery) and the lower part is supplied by the dorsal scapular artery (deep branch of the transverse scapular artery) and segmental intercostal perforators. The origins of the arteries supplying the trapezius muscle are highly variable and the aforementioned vessels may arise from different trunks.

A recently published anatomic study[15] has demonstrated that the superficial cervical artery always runs lateral to the levator scapulae and rhomboid muscles dividing into a short superior branch and long inferior branch which courses inferiorly with the accessory nerve to the level of the scapular spine. The dorsal scapular artery, the dominant supply to the lower third of the muscle, runs deep to the levator scapulae and minor rhomboid muscles.

The flap with the most utility for head and neck reconstruction is the pedicled lower trapezius myocutaneous flap. This version of the flap has an arc of rotation appropriate for resurfacing of the neck and face, and has great utility as a salvage option when a free tissue transfer has failed or there are no recipient vessels available for anastomosis of a free tissue transfer. The patient is positioned in the lateral

Various muscles (the elevators and depressors of the mandible) are attached to the mandible at a variety of sites. They are responsible for the complex movements required of the mandible in mastication, swallowing and speech.

As the mandible projects anteriorly from its articulation with the skull base, a cantilever system with a fulcrum at the temperomandibular joint is created. This requires the mandible to sustain significant forces particularly in mastication. Tensional forces are created at the upper border and compressional forces at the lower border.

Whatever mode of reconstruction is used, it must be able to withstand these considerable forces.

ANATOMICAL CONSIDERATIONS AND RECONSTRUCTION

The cosmetic deformity and functional loss that occur after mandibular resection depends on the size and location of the segmental defect.

The more anterior the defect, the greater the deformity and loss of function. Posterior defects are much better tolerated but a malocclusion may result in a dentate patient.

CLASSIFICATION OF THE MANDIBULAR DEFECT

Not only the size and location of the mandibular defect should be assessed, but also the associated soft tissue deficit. The size and location of the soft tissue deficiency, the vascularity of the remaining soft tissues, the presence of infection and whether the tissues have been irradiated will determine the best mode of reconstruction. Only a thorough understanding of the defect allows optimal reconstruction.

In 1991, Urken et al.[3] described a classification scheme not only taking into consideration the mandibular defect but also the soft tissue defect.

The mandibular defect can be classified as H, C, L:

H – lateral defects of any length including the condyle
L – as above but the condyle not included
C – entire central segment from lower canine to canine.

The soft tissue defect can be classified as none, skin, mucosal and through and through.[4]

Boyd et al.'s classification[5] uses three upper case and three lower case letters.

For a bony defect, it is similar to the above classification.

A combination of letters is possible, for example a defect from angle to angle of the mandible is LCL.

For a soft tissue defect:

o – neither skin or mucosa affected
s – skin
m – mucosa.

A through and through defect will thus be sm.

The mandibular reconstructive ladder is shown in **Box 51.1**.

> **Box 51.1   Mandibular reconstructive ladder**
>
> - No bony reconstruction
>   - Direct soft tissue closure
>   - Local flaps
>   - Soft tissue interposition
>   - Alloplastic materials
> - Bony reconstruction
>   - Non-vascularized bone with or without soft tissue flap: free bone graft, costochondral graft
>   - Vascularized bone: pedicled flap, free flap
> - Distraction osteogenesis
> - TMJ reconstruction
> - Dental implants

NO BONY RECONSTRUCTION

Advancements in soft tissue reconstruction and thus improving the recipient soft tissue bed has allowed the reconsideration of alloplastic materials to reconstuct the mandible. Improving the soft tissue vascularity around the mandible with free tissue transfer or pedicled flaps reduces previous problems seen with using alloplastic materials in reconstructing the mandible. Kiyokawa et al.[6] reconstructed the oro–mandibular complex using a petoralis major flap with a metal plate in seven patients with no complications.

The ideal alloplastic material must be biocompatible and able to withstand the forces sustained by the mandible in mastication.

Materials that have been used include medical polymers, ceramics and a variety of metals. The initial metal alloys used were vitallium and stainless steel in the form of a plate. However, these were susceptible to screw loosening and fracture. The titanium reconstruction plates and the THORP (titanium hollow osseointegrated reconstruction plate) plate are able to withstand masticatory forces and plate fracture is much rarer. Hoever, plate exposure through the external skin or into the mouth is still a major problem.

Bhathena and Kavarana[7] used a sialastic mandibular implant for mandibular reconstruction in 69 patients. Only 30 per cent of the implants were retained for greater than one year. Chemoradiotherapy was one of the major determinants for extrusion.

Okura et al.[8] in a series of 100 patients reconstructed mandibular defects with bridging plates. The plate survival at five years was 62 per cent. Anterior defects and radiotherapy were major determinants for survival.

Anterior mandibular defects are much more likely to fail than posterior ones.[9] Ninety-two per cent of reconstruction with plates is successful in lateral defects but only 30 per cent with anterior ones. It is also argued that patients who require mandibular reconstruction for advanced cancers will die of their disease within two years and so the use of alloplastic materials is recommended. Shiptzer et al.[10] showed good results of mandibular reconstruction with just plates. There was no plate exposure, extrusion or fracture in 83 per cent of their sample one year and 72 per cent at two years.

As the risk of initial complications with alloplastic reconstructions is less than that with more complex reconstructions, delays in starting adjuvant chemoradiotherapy are less. There is also no evidence that alloplastic metals are responsible for radiation shielding in patients.

Lindquist et al.[11] concluded that functional and aesthetic results were excellent in their series of 34 patients when reconstruction plates were used.

Blackwell et al.[12] in a series of 17 patients abandoned using soft tissue flaps with THORP plates even for lateral defects as the risk of reconstructive failure in their series was as high as 40 per cent.

Kim et al.[13] presented 41 cases reconstructed with AO plates. Twenty-two per cent of patients required plate removal but the incidence varied as to the location of the defect – 52 per cent of anterior, 12 per cent of lateral and 8 per cent of condylar and ramus defects.

Wei et al.[14] looked at 80 patients reconstructed with a reconstruction plate and a soft tissue flap. Thirty-one per cent of surviving patients had required secondary surgery for plate exposure, soft tissue deficiency, intraoral contracture, trismus and lack of gingivolabial sulcus.

Ryu et al.[15] showed that significantly more mandibular plates were lost when the patient had received radiotherapy in the postoperative period.

The patient's quality of life and oral rehabilitation does not appear to be related to the quantity of mandible resected but on the amount of associated tongue resection.

Although some success has been achieved with alloplastic materials, the general consensus among reconstructive surgeons is that the potential problems outweigh any benefits and so this technique is reserved for patients with medical comorbidities.

Technique

The reconstruction plate must be accurately contoured to the shape of the mandible. This can be facilitated by the construction of a three-dimensional model on which the plate is pre-bent. The plate can then be sterilized and placed *in situ* prior to the resection. The cost of the three-dimensional models is countered by improved reconstructive results and a reduction in operative time. It is imperative that the condyles remain in the correct position after reconstruction. If the condylar position is not replicated, the occlusion or mouth opening may be affected. If the tumour has breached the buccal cortex of the mandible (**Figure 51.4**) then it may not be possible to pre-bend a plate intraoperatively. Alternative means of ensuring the condyles remain in their premorbid situation are used. Methods include intermaxillary wire fixation if the patient is dentate or external fixators or the use of three-dimensional models.

In our practice, a 2.0 mm locking plate is used for most cases. This reduces the risk of plate exposure, facilitates placement of dental implants and is easier to bend. In our series of 85 patients over the last five years, we have had no plate fractures. However, if the plate is also carrying a prosthetic mandibular condyle, we use a 2.4 mm locking plate due to the plate being load bearing and increased forces (**Figure 51.5**). The plate must be positioned to allow optimal placement of the bone to ensure good aesthetics and subsequent implant placement.

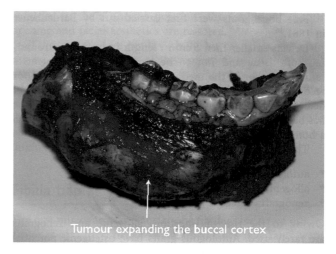

Figure 51.4   Tumour breaching the buccal cortex and so intraoperative plate bending made more complicated.

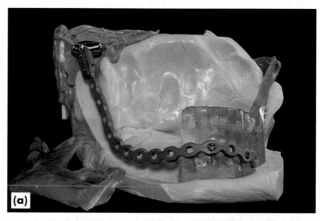

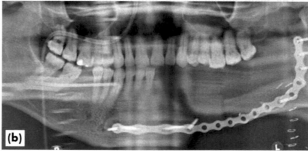

Figure 51.5   A large plate with a prosthetic condyle attached to a plate (a) and a 2.0 mm locking plate (b).

The overlying soft tissue closure must be watertight to reduce the risk of infection and fistula formation.

NON-VASCULARIZED BONE WITH OR WITHOUT SOFT TISSUE FLAP

Free bone grafts

Free bone grafts may be in the form of block grafts or particulate cancellous bone in metallic trays.

mandibular defects. They had no flap failures or fractures of the radius. They concluded that with rigid fixation, fractures of the radius are rare.

Edmonds et al.[47] in cadaveric studies reported that a radial composite flap decreases the strength of the radius by 82 per cent but by plating the radius the strength is increased by 75 per cent.

The main advantages are:

- thin pliable skin
- consistent anatomy
- good pedicle length
- two team operating possible.

The disadvantages are:

- poor bone quality and quantity
- poor healing over tendons may lead to tendon exposure
- poor cosmetic result
- risk of fracture of the residual radius
- altered sensation to the thumb due to injury to superficial branches of the radial nerve
- decreased function of the hand.[48]

PREOPERATIVE ASSESSMENT

The patency of the ulnar artery must be ensured by carrying out the Allen test – both the ulnar and radial arteries are compressed with finger pressure, with the wrist in flexion and the hand closed. The hand is then opened and the wrist returned to neutral and the hand is seen to be pale. The ulnar artery is then released and the time taken for the hand to return to normal colour is noted.

CONSENT

The patient must be warned about the risk of fracture of the residual radius, parasthesia of the thumb and the poor wound healing.

ANATOMY

The brachial artery gives off two main branches, the radial and ulnar arteries. The hand is supplied by a communication between these arteries via the superficial and deep palmar arches (**Figure 51.15**). As long as the arches are intact, the radial artery can be sacrificed without impairing the vascularity of the hand. Venous drainage can be via the deep venous system (the two venae comitantes accompanying the radial artery) or via the superficial system (based around the cephalic vein). Nearly all the flexor aspect of the forearm skin can be taken for the flap.

TECHNIQUE

The arm is exsanguinated and the flap is raised under tourniquet control. The right-sized and -shaped skin paddle is marked over the flexor aspect of the forearm over the radial artery. The more distal that this is positioned, the longer the pedicle. The radial, ulnar and brachial arteries are marked.

The skin is incised at the ulnar aspect of the paddle and the skin is raised laterally in a subfascial plane. Care must be taken not to injure the ulnar vessels and the paratenon must be kept over the flexor tendons. Dissection proceeds laterally until the lateral aspect of the flexor carpi radialis is reached. The distal aspect of the skin paddle is incised and the radial artery and its two accompanying venae comitantes are seen and ligated. The incision is then extended laterally, taking care not to damage the cephalic vein or the radial cutaneous nerve, and the skin is elevated medially until the brachioradialis is reached.

The flexor carpi radialis tendon is retracted medially to expose the flexor pollicis muscle and the tiny perforators that travel to the radius through it. An incision is made through the flexor pollicis at the ulnar aspect. Care must be taken to leave as much flexor pollicis attached to the radius as possible. Unicortical cuts are then made through the flexor aspect of the radius leaving 70 per cent of the radius in situ.

The arm is then rotated and the brachioradialis is retracted laterally. The bone cuts are made through the lateral aspect of the radius, again just unicortically, and leaving 70 per cent of the radius in situ, but join the flexor cuts proximally and distally (**Figure 51.16**).

By this technique only the exact predicted amount of radius is removed reducing the risk of fracture. Only 30 per cent of the radius should be removed.[49]

The risk of fracture is reduced even further by using a locking 2.4 mm plate with bicortical screws to strengthen the residual radius (**Figure 51.17**). The skin of the forearm is replaced with a full-thickness skin graft from the abdomen. The arm is then immobilized in a plaster of Paris back slab.

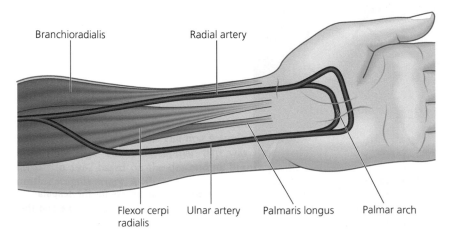

Figure 51.15 Blood supply to the arm. The radial and ulnar arteries terminate to form the superficial and deep palmar arches.

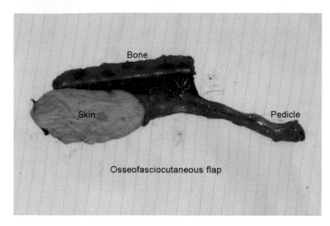

Figure 51.16 Osseocutaneous flap illustrating the small amount of bone, a thin skin paddle and the long vascular pedicle.

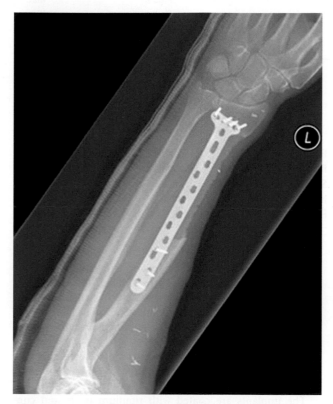

Figure 51.17 The radius plated with a T-shaped plate to reduce the incidence of radial fracture.

COMPLICATIONS

The main morbidity from this flap is the high risk of fracture of the radius. However, this can be reduced by not removing greater than a third of the radius and plating it prophylactically. Healing over the flexor tendons may also be poor. There is a high probability of sensory impairment over the thumb.

The flap is reserved for defects that do not require bicortical bone to re-establish structural integrity and, in particular, where the soft tissue needs are more critical than the bony ones. There are also situations where it may not be possible to raise any other bony flap.

Although early studies advocated using the osteocutaneous radial forearm flap for mandibular reconstruction, other superior donor sites have relegated it to a minor role.

Comparison of bony flaps

When bony flaps are compared, the bone quality and quantity (**Table 51.1**), skin quality (**Table 51.2**) and other factors (**Table 51.3**) must be taken into consideration. The tables are the author's personal preferences for each flap.

Wilson et al.[50] compared patients who had undergone hemimandibulectomy and were either reconstructed with bone or just soft tissue. They concluded that restoration of mandibular continuity led to improved function and a superior quality of life.

Chen et al.[51] concluded that in their experience the absolute indications for free vascularized bone transfer are:

1. osteoradionecrosis of the mandible or an irradiated tissue bed
2. hemimandibular reconstruction with the free end in the glenoid fossa
3. long segmental defects
4. inadequate skin or mucosa to reconstruct soft tissue defects
5. failure of reconstruction by other modes
6. near total mandibular reconstruction.

Success of composite reconstructions are now approaching 95 per cent.[52]

DISTRACTION OSTEOGENESIS

Distraction osteogenesis is the technique of growing new bone by distraction (stretching) of pre-existing bone. Ilizarov[53] applied the principles of distraction osteogenesis to treat thousands of patients with limb defects. There are four main stages:

1. Osteotomy – cuts through the bony cortex.
2. Latency – (time between osteotomy and the start of distraction. It allows formation of a primitive callus).
3. Distraction – The callus is stretched at a rate of 1 mm per day. If the rate is less than 0.5 mm per day, there is a risk of early fusion. If the rate is greater than 1.5 mm per day, there is a risk of fibrous union. The optimum rate of 1.0 mm per day is ideally divided into four movements of 0.25 mm per day.
4. Consolidation – the new bone is stabilized for up to 4 weeks.

The initial bone formed is non-lamellar and gradually gets replaced by lamellar bone.

Kuriakose et al.[54] treated four patients with distraction with defects between 3.5 and 6.5 cm.

Mandibular distraction devices used to be extraoral, but intraoral devices are now available. Extraoral devices leave unsightly facial scars.

The efficacy of distraction in previously irradiated mandible has been shown by Gantous et al.[55] in a canine model.

Table 51.1 Bone quality.

	Good	→	→	Poor
Contour	Iliac	Fibula	Scapula	Radial
Implants	Iliac	Fibula	Scapula	Radial
Bone quality	Iliac	Fibula	Scapula	Radial
Bone length	Fibula	Iliac	Scapula	Radial
Anterior dentate	Iliac	Scapula	Fibula	Radial
Posterior dentate	Iliac	Fibula	Scapula	Radial
Anterior edentulous	Fibula	Iliac	Scapula	Radial
Posterior edentulous	Fibula	Iliac	Scapula	Radial

Table 51.2 Skin quality.

	Good	→	→	Poor
Reliability of skin	Radial	Scapula	Fibula	Iliac
Ease of placement	Scapula	Fibula	Radial	Iliac
Thickness	Radial	Fibula	Scapula	Iliac
Extensive soft tissue resection	Scapula	Fibula	Iliac	Radial

Table 51.3 Other factors.

	Good	→	→	Poor
Ease of harvest	Fibula	Radial	Scapula	Iliac
Pedicle length	Fibula	Radial	Scapula	Iliac
Pedicle size	Fibula	Scapula	Radial	Iliac
Two team operating	Fibula	Iliac	Radial	Scapula
Donor site	Scapula	Fibula	Iliac	Radial

Rubio-Bueno[56] distracted five patients with intraoral distractors for segmental defects of 35–80 mm. They were successful in three of the five patients. In one patient there was intraoral exposure of the distractor and one patient died.

Distraction is likely to be better for dental prosthesis and implants in view of the better bone quality, quantity and the ability to produce normal mucosa. However, it is time-consuming with occlusal disturbance likely as it is difficult to get all the vectors of movement right. Although distraction has been shown to be possible in the irradiated canine model, its use in patients who have received radiotherapy is still in question.

DENTAL IMPLANTS

For the complete rehabilitation of a patient after mandibular resection, mandibular continuity needs to be restored and the dentoalveolar structures reconstructed.

Any patient who has undergone resection of the mandible with or without soft tissue resection has disturbed internal anatomy and altered sensation despite reconstruction. The alveolar bone height is reduced with poor lingual and labial sulci and the tongue anatomy and mobility may also be reduced. Cancer sufferers may also have received radiotherapy and be suffering from a dry mouth. All these factors make conventional dentures difficult to wear.

Osseointegration is the incorporation of metal into living bone. There is no fibrous connective tissue intervening between the implant and bone. The bone is able to remodel under loading of the implant.

The soft tissue around which the implant exits the bone has to be keratinized and attached mucosa otherwise chronic inflammation may result.

The implants are coated with titanium oxide and contamination must be avoided at the time of placement. Care must also be taken to ensure that the bone is not overheated and damaged during placement of the implant.

Although implants may be loaded immediately, integration rates are more predictable if loading is delayed.

The use of hyperbaric oxygen in irradiated patients may increase implant survival rates.

TEMPEROMANDIBULAR RECONSTRUCTION

If at all possible, the mandibular condyle should be preserved but tumour resection should never be compromised. If the condyle is preserved, the new bone must be fixed to it. Every

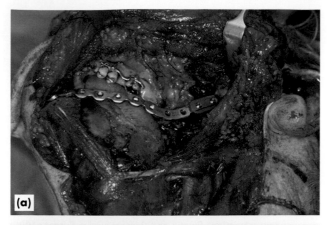

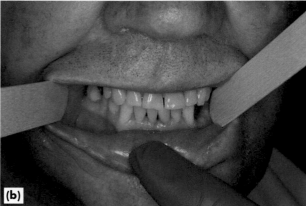

Figure 51.18 (a) A prosthetic condyle on a 2.4 mm plate before the fibula was osteotomized and plated in position. (b) The patient occlusion postoperatively.

effort must be made to position the condyle in the glenoid fossa at its preoperative position.

Where the condylar head needs to be sacrificed for tumour resection, the bony flap can be placed directly into the glenoid fossa. The shape and size of the fibula make it the ideal bony flap for temperomandibular reconstruction.

However, if the patient is dentate, a prosthetic condylar head used within a bony flap provides a more predictable occlusion (**Figure 51.18**).

CONCLUSION

The aims of mandibular reconstruction are to restore form and function, cover any defects causing minimal morbidity, and maximizing quality of life. This requires thorough defect analysis, assessment of all donor sites, knowledge of all the modes of reconstruction and working in a multidisciplinary environment.

It is important that every unit treating patients with mandibular tumours possesses the full repertoire of reconstruction so the most suitable modality is chosen for each patient. Free tissue transfer is now the gold standard in reconstruction of the mandible. It is an extremely reliable method of reconstruction, particularly in a hostile recipient bed. However, it requires specialized teams and significantly longer operating times. Postoperative morbidity and possible

loss of form and function at the donor site are important considerations.

REFERENCES

- 1. Rogers S, Devine J, Lowe D *et al.* Longitudinal quality of life after mandibular reconstruction for oral cancer: a comparison between rim and segmental resection. *Head and Neck* 2004; **26**: 59–62.
- 2. Komisar A. The functional result of mandibular reconstruction. *Laryngoscope* 1990; **100**: 364–74.
- ◆ 3. Urken ML, Weinberg H, Vickery C *et al.* Oromandibular reconstruction using microvascular composite free flaps. Report of 71 cases and a new classification scheme for bony, soft tissue, and neurologic defects. *Archives of Otolaryngology – Head and Neck Surgery* 1991; **117**: 733–44.
- 4. Takushima A, Harii K, Asato H *et al.* Mandibular reconstruction using microvascular free flaps. *Plastic Reconstructive Surgery* 2001; **108**: 1555–63.
- ◆ 5. Boyd JB, Gullane PJ, Rotstein LE. Classification of mandibular defects. *Plastic and Reconstructive Surgery* 1993; **92**: 1266–75.

6. Kiyokawa K, Tai Y, Inove Y. Reliable minimally invasive oro-mandibular reconstruction using metal plate rolled with pectoralis major myocutaneous flap. *Journal of Craniofacial Surgery* 2001; **12**: 326–36.

7. Bhathena HM, Kavarana NM. Primary reconstruction of the mandible in head and neck cancer with sialastic implant – a review of 69 cases. *Acta Chirugiae Plasticae* 1998; **40**: 31–5.

◆ 8. Okura M, Isomura ET, Lida S, Kogo M. Long term outcome and factors influencing bridging plates for mandibular reconstruction. *Oral Oncology* 2005; **41**: 791–8.

9. Schusterman MA, Reece KP, Kroll SS *et al*. Use of the AO plate for mandibular reconstruction in cancer patients. *Plastic and Reconstructive Surgery* 1991; **88**: 588–93.

10. Shiptzer T, Gullane PJ, Neligar PC *et al*. The free vascularised flap and the flap plate options. *Laryngoscope* 2000; **110**: 2056–60.

11. Lindquist C, Sederholm AL, Laine P *et al*. Rigid reconstruction plates for immediate reconstruction following mandibular resection. *Journal of Oral and Maxillofacial Surgery* 1992; **50**: 1158–63.

12. Blackwell KE, Buchbinder D, Urken ML. Lateral mandibular reconstruction using soft tissue free flaps and plates. *Archives of Otolaryngology – Head and Neck Surgery* 1996; **122**: 672–8.

13. Kim NR, Donoff RB. Critical analysis of mandibular reconstruction using AO plates. *Journal of Oral and Maxillofacial Surgery* 1992; **50**: 1152–7.

◆ 14. Wei FC, Celik N, Yang WG *et al*. Complications after reconstruction by plate and soft-tissue free flap in composite mandibular defects and secondary salvage reconstruction with osteocutaneous flap. *Plastic Reconstructive Surgery* 2003; **112**: 37–42.

15. Ryu JK, Stern RL, Robinson MG *et al*. Mandibular reconstruction using a titanium plate: the impact of irradiation. *International Journal of Radiation Oncology, Biology, Physics* 1995; **32**: 627–34.

16. Bardenheuer F. Verhandlung der Deutsch Gesellschaft Zentrabilothek. *Chirugie* 1892; **21**: 68.

17. Foster RD, Anthony JP, Sharma A, Pogrel MA. Vascularised bone flaps versus non vascularised bone grafts for mandibular reconstruction. *Head and Neck* 1999; **21**: 66–71.

18. Millard DR Jr, Maisels DO, Batsone JH. Immediate repair of radical resection of the anterior arch of the lower jaw. *Plastic Reconstructive Surgery* 1967; **39**: 153–61.

19. Lawson W, Loscalzo L, Baek S *et al*. Experience with immediate and delayed mandibular reconstruction. *Laryngoscope* 1982; **92**: 5–10.

20. Wolfe SA. Autogenous bone grafts versus alloplastic materials in maxillofacial surgery. *Clinics in Plastic Surgery* 1982; **9**: 539–40.

21. Netscher D, Alford EL, Wigoda P *et al*. Free composite myo-osseous flap with serratus anterior and rib. *Head and Neck* 1998; **20**: 106–12.

22. Conley J. Use of composite flaps containing bone for major repairs in the head and neck. *Plastic and Reconstructive Surgery* 1972; **49**: 522–6.

23. Cordeiro PG, Disa JJ, Hidalgo DA. Reconstruction of the mandible with osseous flaps. *Plastic and Reconstructive Surgery* 1999; **104**: 1314–20.

24. Taylor GI, Miller DH, Ham FJ. The free vascularised bone graft: a clinical extension of microvascular techniques. *Plastic and Reconstructive Surgery* 1975; **55**: 533–44.

25. Chen Z, Yan W. The study and clinical application of the osteocutaneous flap of fibula. *Microsurgery* 1983; **4**: 11–16.

● 26. Hidalgo DA. Fibula flap: a new method of mandibular reconstruction. *Plastic and Reconstructive Surgery* 1989; **84**: 71–8.

● 27. Hidalgo DA, Rekwo A. A review of 60 consecutive fibula free flap mandibular reconstructions. *Plastic and Reconstructive Surgery* 1995; **96**: 585–96.

28. Schusterman MA, Reece GP, Miller MJ, Harris S. The osteocutaneous free fibula flap: is the skin paddle reliable? *Plastic and Reconstructive Surgery* 1992; **90**: 787–93.

29. Noncini PF, Wangerin K, Albanese M *et al*. Vertical distraction of a vascularised fibula flap. *Journal of Cranio-Maxillo-Facial Surgery* 2000; **28**: 20–4.

30. Coghlan BA, Townsend P. The morbidity of the free vascularised fibula flap. *British Journal of Plastic Surgery* 1993; **46**: 466–9.

31. Yoshimura M, Shimada T, Hosokawa M. The vasculature of the peroneal tissue transfer. *Plastic and Reconstructive Surgery* 1990; **85**: 917–21.

32. Hidalgo DA. Aesthetic improvements in free flap mandibular reconstruction. *Plastic and Reconstructive Surgery* 1991; **88**: 574–85.

33. Wei FC, Seah CS, Tsai YC *et al*. Fibula osteoseptocutaneous flap for reconstruction of composite mandibular defects. *Plastic and Reconstructive Surgery* 1994; **93**: 294–306.

● 34. Taylor GI, Townsend P, Cordell R. Superiority of the deep circumflex iliac vessels as the supply for free groin flaps. *Plastic and Reconstructive Surgery* 1979; **64**: 595–604.

35. Sanders R, Mayou B. A new vascularised bone graft transferred by microvascular anastomosis as a free flap. *British Journal of Surgery* 1979; **66**: 787–8.

36. Ramasastry SS, Tucker JB, Swartz WM *et al*. The internal oblique muscle flap: an anatomical and clinical study. *Plastic and Reconstructive Surgery* 1984; **73**: 721–33.

● 37. Urken ML, Vickery C, Weinberg H *et al*. The internal oblique-iliac crest osseomyocutaneous free flap in oromandibular reconstruction: a report of 20 cases. *Archives of Otolaryngology – Head and Neck Surgery* 1989; **115**: 339–49.

38. Forrest C, Boyd B, Monktelow R *et al*. The free vascularised iliac crest tissue transfer: donor site complications in eighty two cases. *British Journal of Plastic Surgery* 1992; **45**: 89–93.

39. Saijo M. The vascular territories of the dorsal trunk: a reappraisal for potential flap donor sites. *British Journal of Plastic Surgery* 1978; **31**: 200–4.

40. Nassif TM, Vidal L, Bovet JL *et al.* The parascapular flap: a new cutaneous microsurgical free flap. *Plastic and Reconstructive Surgery* 1982; **69**: 591–600.

41. Teot L, Bosse JP, Moufarrage R *et al.* The scapula crest pedicled bone graft. *International Journal of Microsurgery* 1981; **3**: 257–62.

42. Yang G, Chen B, Gao Y *et al.* Forearm free skin flap transplantation. *National Medical Journal of China* 1981; **61**: 139.

43. Soutar DS, McGregor IA. The radial forearm flap for intra oral reconstruction: the experience of 60 consecutive cases. *Plastic and Reconstructive Surgery* 1986; **78**: 1–8.

44. Soutar DS, Widdowson WP. Immediate reconstruction of the mandible using vascularised segment of radius. *Head and Neck Surgery* 1986; **8**: 232–46.

45. Thoma A, Khanderoo R, Grigenas O *et al.* Oromandibular reconstruction with the radial forearm osteocutaneous flap. *Plastic and Reconstructive Surgery* 1999; **104**: 368–78.

46. Villaret DB, Futran N. The indications and outcomes in the use of the osteocutaneous radial forearm free flap. *Head and Neck* 2003; **25**: 475–81.

47. Edmonds JL, Bowers KW, Toby EB *et al.* Torsional strength of the radius after osteofasciocutaneous free flap harvest with or without bone plating. *Otolaryngology – Head and Neck Surgery* 2000; **123**: 400–8.

48. Boorman JG, Brown JA, Sykes PJ. Morbidity in the forearm flap donor arm. *British Journal of Plastic Surgery* 1987; **40**: 207–12.

49. Swanson E, Boyd JB, Mulholland RS. The radial forearm flap: a biomechanical study of the osteotomised radius. *Plastic Reconstructive Surgery* 1990; **85**: 267–72.

50. Wilson KM, Rizk HM, Armstrong S. Effect of hemimandibulectomy on the quality of life. *Laryngoscope* 1998; **108**: 1574–7.

51. Chen YB, Chen HC, Hahn LH. Major mandibular reconstruction with vascularised bone grafts: indications and selection of donor tissue. *Microsurgery* 1994; **15**: 227–37.

52. Urken ML. Composite free flaps in oromandibular reconstruction: a review of the literature. *Archives of Otolaryngology – Head and Neck Surgery* 1991; **117**: 724–32.

53. Ilizarov GA. Clinical application of the tension – stress effect for limb lengthening. *Clinical Orthopaedics and Related Research* 1990; **250**: 8–26.

54. Kuriakose M, Schnayder Y, DeLacure MD. Reconstruction of segmental mandibular defects by distraction osteogenesis for mandibular reconstruction. *Head and Neck* 2003; **25**: 816–24.

55. Gantous A, Phillips JH, Catton P, Holmberg D. Distraction osteogenesis in the irradiated canine mandible. *Plastic and Reconstructive Surgery* 1994; **93**: 164–8.

56. Rubio-Bueno B, Naval L, Rodriguez-Campo F. Internal distraction osteogenesis with a unidirectional device for reconstruction of mandibular segmental defects. *Journal of Oral and Maxillofacial Surgery* 2005; **63**: 598–608.

Defect-based reconstruction: pharynx

JONATHAN CLARK AND RALPH W GILBERT

> Mistakes are a part of being human. Appreciate your mistakes for what they are: precious life lessons that can only be learned the hard way. Unless it's a fatal mistake, which at least others can learn from.
>
> Al Franken

INTRODUCTION

The technical aspects of pharyngeal reconstruction advanced tremendously over the twentieth century and, in particular, over the last three decades. This has enabled important improvements in functional outcomes, reliability, reduced morbidity and length of hospital stay. Despite these steps forward, the basic concepts of pharyngeal reconstruction have not changed significantly. In the majority of pharyngeal defects, the reconstructive surgeon only aims to achieve a patent and well-sealed tube that permits the passive passage of food and air. Reconstructing laryngopharyngeal defects with an intact larynx is a more complex process. Ingenious techniques have permitted laryngeal preservation in select cases, but speech and swallowing remains unpredictable. While the three-dimensional structure of the laryngopharyngeal unit can be closely replicated, the problems of aspiration due to insensate, adynamic tissue highlight the remarkable complexity of combining deglutition with voice production in a single orifice.

This chapter discusses the history of pharyngeal reconstruction, detailing the major technical advances, and then focuses on current reconstructive methods and their relative merits. Pharyngeal defects can be divided into partial and total (circumferential), depending as to whether the full circumference of the larynx and pharynx has been removed.

Partial pharyngeal defects are further subdivided into simple and complex, depending on whether the larynx has been extirpated. Complex defects are those where the larynx is preserved, either in part (partial laryngectomy and pharyngectomy) or in its entirety (pharyngectomy without laryngectomy). These defects are termed 'complex' because reconstructive techniques need to focus not only on creating a patent conduit but on minimizing disabling aspiration and facilitating functional speech.

The morbidity, major and minor, associated with pharyngeal reconstruction is substantial and methods of minimizing this are continually being sought. The repercussions of the present chemoradiation era are now being felt by ablative and reconstructive surgeons alike, particularly in the area of pharyngolaryngectomy. Novel approaches to minimize pharyngocutaneous fistula by the use of highly vascularized free or regional tissue have limited success and the effect of chemoradiation on the residual native tissue impairs coordinated deglutition. As a result, patients may require long-term feeding tubes despite a patent reconstruction. Although organ preservation protocols have enabled functional larynx preservation in many patients with advanced larynx and hypopharyngeal tumours, more sophisticated techniques need to be developed to determine which patients will perform poorly with these protocols.

Functional outcomes are poorly documented in the present literature and objective evidence to support one reconstruction over another is remarkably scant. Putting this aside, one should consider the dramatic improvements in functional outcomes that have been achieved through regional and free flap reconstruction. The common problem of three permanent cervical stomas is, in the majority, now a complication of the past. Despite these advances, survival following total laryngopharyngectomy remains unfavourable and this needs to be considered in the reconstructive algorithm. Minimizing perioperative morbidity is important so that patients can enjoy quality time out of the hospital environment with early and reliable return to functional speech, swallowing and social interaction.

GOALS OF RECONSTRUCTION

The goals of reconstruction of pharyngeal defects, in particular following surgical resection of hypopharyngeal and laryngeal cancers are primarily to restore a patent pharyngeal conduit that permits acceptable speech and swallowing. Secondary goals are to prevent complications, in particular pharyngocutaneous fistula and pharyngeal stricture, but also to minimize systemic and donor site morbidity. The optimal reconstructive technique depends upon a number of factors including the nature of the defect, prior treatment, patient comorbidity, disease-related outcomes (survival) and the reconstructive surgeon's experience. Minimizing operative morbidity for patients with advanced malignancy is particularly important. The reconstruction should facilitate early discharge so that patients can enjoy quality time out of the hospital environment. Prolonged, complex multistage reconstructions may be inappropriate for patients with a limited life expectancy if simple and reliable alternatives are available. **Table 52.1**, summarizes the components of an ideal reconstruction based on those described by Couch.[1] Currently, no method fulfils all of these criteria.

HISTORY OF LARYNGOPHARYNGEAL RECONSTRUCTION

The history and evolution of pharyngo-oesophageal reconstruction illustrates the complex issues regarding functional restoration for patients undergoing circumferential resections. The introduction of free tissue transfer has increased

Table 52.1   Ideal pharyngeal reconstruction.

Surgical
Facilitate resection with adequate surgical margins
Allow two team approach to reduce operative time
Simple technique that is reproducible

Morbidity
Highly reliable flap
Low complication rate, in particular fistula and stricture
Prevention of life-threatening complications, in particular
    vascular rupture and mediastinitis
Low donor site morbidity
Flap vascularity to withstand adjuvant therapy and promote
    neovascularization in radiated tissue

Functional and quality of life
Single-stage procedure with short hospital stay
Short time to swallowing and normal diet
Quality voice with normal intelligibility
Functional tissue, in particular sensation and dynamic
    reconstruction for patients where the larynx is preserved

the complexity but substantially reduced the morbidity of many forms of head and neck reconstruction. Currently, free flap reconstruction is preferred for most cases except where there is significant cervical oesophageal involvement or substantial patient comorbidity. The increasing application of chemoradiation organ preservation protocols has challenged the reliability of standard reconstructive techniques. This has led surgeons to apply new methods to minimize complications, in particular pharyngocutaneous fistula, skin flap necrosis, major vessel rupture and late stricture.

Cervical skin flaps for staged reconstruction

The first methods of laryngopharyngeal reconstruction preceded the anatomical description of axial and regional flap reconstruction and were based on random pattern skin flaps. Czerny[2] reported local skin flap reconstruction as early as 1877, only a few years following the initial description of total laryngectomy by Billroth in 1874.[3] The early literature is dominated by European surgeons such as Mikulicz[4] (1886) and Trotter[5] (1913), who both described similar techniques to Czerny. These early techniques were multistage and highly unreliable and did not gain general acceptance. Modifications by Wookey[6] in 1942 resulted in a more reliable two-stage reconstruction which was more widely applied (**Figure 52.1**). Despite the improved technique there are inherent problems with cervical skin flaps and complications occurred in over 90 per cent of patients.[7] Multiple stages necessitate a prolonged period where the patient endured a separate pharyngostome (oropharynx) and oesophagostome, resulting in aspiration of saliva into the open tracheostome.

Radiotherapy was standard treatment for laryngeal cancer in many parts of the Western world in the early twentieth

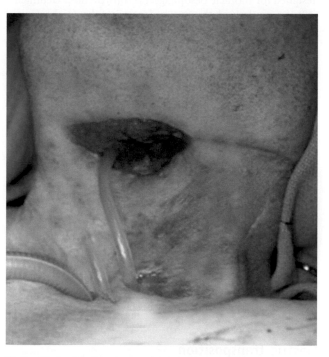

Figure 52.1   Tracheostome, pharyngostome and oesophagostome in a patient being prepared for a Wookey flap reconstruction.

century. Using cervical skin within the radiation field often resulted in partial flap necrosis, wound breakdown and pharyngocutaneous fistula, particularly as radiotherapy was poorly regulated in terms of dose and fields. Life-threatening complications, such as mediastinitis and major vessel rupture, were likely sequelae and long-term complications were also problematic, in particular pharyngeal stricture for 'successful' reconstructions. These techniques were not suitable where a substantial length of oesophagus was resected. The next stage in skin flap reconstruction did not evolve until Bakamjian[8] described the deltopectoral flap more than two decades later. Alternative techniques included skin grafts placed over temporary or permanent synthetic implants, however results were at best unreliable.[9, 10, 11]

Transposed viscera for pharyngo–oesophageal reconstruction

Early descriptions of using pedicled viscera to reconstruct the oesophagus extend back to the turn of the century where Wiillstein (1904) described the use of pedicled jejunum,[12] Kelling (1911) described colonic transfer[13] and Jianu (1912) described the gastric tube.[14] At a similar time Denk (1913) described the technique of blunt oesophagectomy in the animal model and cadaver.[15] However, over a half century transpired before these techniques were to be applied to pharyngo-oesophageal reconstruction.

The gastric tube was well established in Europe following Kirschner's (1920) work.[16] Additional length was achieved through modifications by Mes (1948),[17] who used an isoperistaltic tube based on the right gastroepiploic vessels, and Gavriliu and Georgescu[18] (1955) with an antiperistaltic tube relying on the left gastroepiploic arcade; however, these were designed for thoracic oesophageal reconstruction. Heimlich[19] (1961) popularized the reversed gastric tube in the United States, and further modifications allowed extension of the reconstruction to reach the oropharynx where this was applied to the total laryngopharyngectomy–oesophagectomy defect for cervical oesophageal cancer before 1970.[20] Prior to both of these publications Goligher and Robin[21] (1954) used pedicled colon to reconstruct the pharyngo-oesophagus, utilizing both right and left colon.

Both the reverse gastric tube and pedicled colon continued to be used with relative frequency into the early 1980s, predominantly with extra-anatomic placement of the conduit in a subcutaneous or substernal position. While these reconstructions were prone to the cardiopulmonary complications of thoracoabdominal surgery, generally they were reliable when performed as a two-stage reconstruction. The primary limitation of oesophagocoloplasty is the functional delay of food passage from oropharynx to stomach, which is a marked problem in nearly 50 per cent of patients.[22] This technique still has a role in patients unsuitable for alternative techniques, in particular following gastric necrosis complicating gastric transposition where the oesophagus has already been removed.

Gastric transposition

The introduction of single-stage anatomic reconstruction of the pharynx and oesophagus is generally credited to Ong and Lee who described three cases of gastric transposition in 1960.[23] However, Shefts and Fischer reported a one-stage procedure in 1949 for cervical oesophageal cancer.[24] Ong and Lee argued that laryngopharyngectomy was essentially a palliative procedure and that effective palliation could not be achieved by multistage operations. The initial descriptions involved three body cavities; however, the morbidity of gastric transposition was minimized by performing a closed chest (blunt) transhiatal oesophagectomy and pull-up as reported by LeQuesne and Ranger in 1966.[25] This concept was not original, being based on work by Denk[15] (1913) and Turner[26] (1933) half a century earlier. Gastric transposition effectively replaced reversed gastric tube, oesophagocoloplasty and other techniques for pharyngo-oesophageal reconstruction. Its popularity increased such that some surgeons advocated its use for all patients requiring pharyngolaryngectomy (**Figure 52.2**).[27]

Functional results of gastric 'pull-up', in terms of stricture and swallowing were superior compared to prior techniques. Rapid restoration of swallowing and early discharge from hospital represented a major advance, especially when compared to multistage techniques. Unfortunately, the major morbidity and mortality following gastric transposition has been formidable. Wei et al.[28] reviewed the literature on 978 patients undergoing gastric transposition after pharynolaryngo-oesophagectomy and demonstrated a 16 per cent mortality and 37 per cent major morbidity. Institutions performing this technique regularly have been able to reduce mortality over time. Wei et al. reported that mortality in their institution prior to 1980 was 31 per cent but declined to 9 per cent after 1985. Anastomotic leak similarly decreased from 23 to 9 per cent. Despite this improvement, others have argued that a 10 per cent mortality rate remains excessive and that a body cavity should not be entered unless necessary.[29, 30] Since microvascular reconstruction has become routine, gastric transposition is increasingly reserved for tumours with significant cervical oesophageal extension.[28] While there are no strict limitations on how high the stomach can reach, it is recognized that pedicled enteric flaps become less reliable approaching the skull base. In these cases, it is advisable to 'supercharge' the stomach with a cervical microvascular anastomosis. Recent advances have focused on laparoscopic

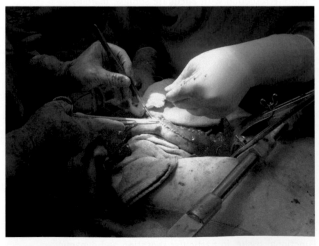

Figure 52.2 Stomach being tubed in preparation for gastric transposition to neck.

and thoracoscopic dissection to further minimize morbidity; however, this technique is in its infancy.[31]

Pedicle and axial flap reconstruction

The deltopectoral flap represented a major advance in non-enteric reconstruction of the pharynx.[8] This was a superior technique compared to local skin flaps because it used tissue outside the irradiated field and had the advantage of an axial blood supply for most of its length. Furthermore, it provides thin and pliable tissue. It has remained an essential part of the head and neck reconstructive surgeon's armamentarium and has recently been revived in the guise of the internal mammary artery perforator (IMAP) flap (**Figure 52.3**).[32, 33] The deltopectoral flap was highly reliable and effectively replaced Wookey-type skin flap reconstructions. However, it represented a two-stage reconstruction with a controlled distal pharyngostome (**Figure 52.4**). Consequences of this were a prolonged time to oral intake, multiple hospital admissions and long-term stricture. Fredrickson et al.[34] demonstrated that the average time to swallowing was 90 days over seven admissions compared to 12 days for gastric transposition. In patients with a limited life expectancy from advanced

hypopharyngeal cancer this represented an unacceptable delay. As a result, the deltopectoral flap's main niche was reconstructing the substantial number of patients not likely to tolerate the significant cardiopulmonary insult imposed by gastric transposition.

Ariyan is best known for his description of the 'workhorse' flap that revolutionized head and neck reconstruction in 1979, the pectoralis major pedicled myocutaneous flap.[35] However, prior to this, he had already used the trapezius and sternomastoid muscle flaps for pharyngeal reconstruction.[36] The pectoralis major flap was used frequently for non-circumferential pharyngeal defects and the first reports of 'tubing' the flap for circumferential reconstruction were by Withers et al.[37] Owing to its bulk many surgeons found this difficult to perform[38, 39] particularly in females. Fabian[40] described partial tubulation of the flap combined with skin graft of the prevertebral fascia as an alternative method for circumferential defects.

Few flaps have been used as extensively as the pectoralis major and total flap failure is very unusual. The technique is excellent for selected patients with non-circumferential defects as shown in **Figure 52.5**. However, problems with partial flap necrosis are not rare, particularly when attempting to thin or fold the flap, place it under tension or use tissue at the limits of its vascular territory. As a result pharyngocutaneous fistula is reported in 13–63 per cent of pharyngeal reconstructions.[29, 40, 41, 42, 43, 44] Inappropriate application of bulky flaps may result in pharyngeal obstruction, poor quality TEP voice[45] and long-term stricture, particularly where adjuvant radiotherapy is used. These restrictions have limited its widespread application for circumferential defects despite its ease of harvest.[1] Other limitations include patients with low oesophageal resections and long or complex defects. The development of reliable microvascular reconstruction has called into question the blanket application of the pectoralis major flap, particularly for reconstruction of the circumferential laryngopharyngeal defect. Despite this, we still consider regional musculocutaneous flaps, such as the pectoralis major and latissimus dorsi, as the first choice for salvaging complicated scenarios in a

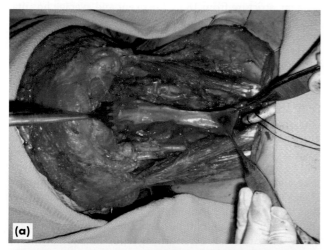

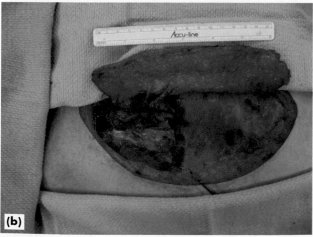

Figure 52.3 Vertical internal mammary perforator (IMAP) flap raised in preparation for inset to partial pharyngectomy defect.

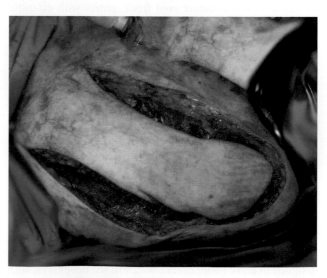

Figure 52.4 Deltopectoral flap.

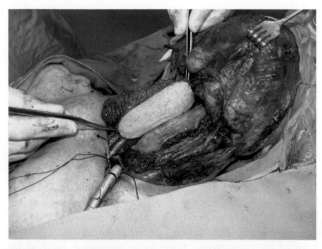

Figure 52.5 Pectoralis major myocutaneous flap being inset to partial laryngopharyngectomy defect.

hostile neck following flap necrosis, pharyngocutaneous fistula and major vessel rupture.[46]

Enteric free flap reconstruction

It is surprising that the first successful free tissue transfer in a human preceded the description of both gastric transposition and the deltopectoral flap. The natural appeal of jejunum to replace the laryngopharynx and oesophagus led Seidenberg[47] to use this for pharyngeal reconstruction in 1959. The availability of the operating microscope, modern instrumentation and suture material has made this commonplace. Series of free jejunal autotransplantation were first reported using the canine model,[48] and following this, human series emerged in the 1970s.

Free jejunal transfer is by far the most widely reported flap for circumferential pharyngeal reconstruction. A literature review[49] of 595 circumferential reconstructions is summarized in **Table 52.2**, alongside the authors' own experience. Accurately determining the complication rate associated with free jejunal transfer is difficult because morbidity varies so widely in the literature even from centres with extensive experience.[49, 50, 51, 52, 53, 54, 55, 56] For example, Triboulet[39] published a single institutional French series comparing free jejunal transfer ($n = 77$) with gastric transposition ($n = 127$). They found a substantially higher fistula rate in the jejunal group (32.5 versus 15.7 per cent), whereas other authors have found the reverse. As expected, cardiopulmonary complications were greater in the gastric transposition group (22.1 versus 6.5 per cent). This supports the concept that institutional experience has considerable bearing on morbidity and other treatment-related outcomes.

The popularity of the free jejunum relates in part to the aesthetic similarity to oesophagus, ease of harvest and that only two mucosal anastomoses are required in the neck, that is, there is no vertical suture line. Jejunum is very versatile and any length can be provided to allow superior extension to the skull base or inferiorly to the abdomen for total oesophageal replacement.[52] It is also amenable to techniques designed to allow better calibre match to the oropharyx, such as 'double barrelling',[1, 50, 57] which also prevent problems

Table 52.2 Circumferential reconstructions.

	Shanghold et al.[49] (%)	Clark et al.[64] (%)
Mortality	4	0
Flap failure	9	7
Abdominal complications	6	10
Fistula	17	20
Stricture	11	20
Oral diet	82	97
TEP speech	14	33

associated with uncoordinated peristalsis.[58] Sarukawa et al.[59] reported a large Japanese series with 269 patients undergoing free jejunal transfer over a 12-year period. They emphasize the importance of standardization to facilitate a replicable technique which minimizes morbidity and improves functional outcomes. One critical aspect is keeping the jejunum under tension, as redundancy has a marked adverse effect on swallowing and vocal rehabilitation. This series also demonstrates that outcomes improve over time in experienced units. Pharyngocutaneous fistula reduced from 18 to 5 per cent, stricture from 18 to 3 per cent and average hospital stay from 32 to 24 days. Flap failure, however, was unchanged at approximately 2 per cent, although early revision surgery decreased from 12 to 4 per cent.

Disa et al.[60] reported a large North American series with 90 consecutive patients undergoing free jejunal transfer. Flap failure was 2 per cent, the fistula rate was 10 per cent, mortality occurred in one patient and late stricture in 8 per cent. One of the major limitations of jejunum is dysphagia due to uncoordinated peristalsis. This is reflected by the fact that while 88 per cent maintained oral nutrition, less than 65 per cent had an unrestricted diet. Peristaltic action decreases with time and is also diminished by postoperative radiotherapy. High rates of tracheo-oesophageal speech (60 per cent) have been reported using jejunum;[61, 62] however, this is unusual and few reports have critically and objectively appraised the quality of that speech. Peristalsis, again, is unhelpful, with the typical 'wet' quality being interrupted by contractions. Radiotherapy also aids tracheo-oesophageal speech by reducing secretions and intrinsic muscle activity.[63]

Free jejunal transfer has been used extensively at our institution, but we now avoid its use for the reasons described above. In addition, many patients are nutritionally deplete with major cardiopulmonary comorbidity. This makes laparotomy a high-risk procedure which should be avoided where there are suitable alternatives. Where laparotomy is indicated, we favour the gastro-omental free flap as the enteric reconstruction of choice.[64] Further advances in free jejunal transfer have been achieved by reducing the donor site morbidity through laparoscopic harvest. Only small series have been published to date,[65, 66, 67] but nonetheless demonstrating that it is a viable option.

Compared to jejunum, the gastro-omental flap has had limited application in pharyngeal reconstruction. Despite this, it is not a newcomer to the reconstructive arena, with free transfer of gastric antrum reported by Hiebert and

Cummings[68] in 1961 and omental transfer in 1972.[69] The combined use of both stomach and omentum to reconstruct the pharynx was subsequently described in 1979 by Baudet.[70] Recently, this flap has undergone revival as a result of the 'organ preservation era' where fistula rates for salvage surgery exceed 30 per cent and wound complications approach 50 per cent in recent post-chemoradiation series.[71, 72]

Genden *et al.*[73] described the suitability of this flap in a series of high-risk patients. Similarly, we have used it almost exclusively for salvage after either high-dose accelerated radiotherapy or concurrent chemoradiation.[74] This composite flap is unique because the omentum can be draped over the pharyngeal anastomoses, exposed vasculature and microvascular anastomosis as demonstrated in **Figures 52.6** and **52.7**. Hence, if a leak occurs it is rapidly walled off, preventing major sequelae such as high volume fistulae, neck sepsis, mediastinitis and vascular rupture. Early experience has documented radiological fistula rates between 0 and 16 per cent in an extremely high-risk group of patients.[63, 73, 74, 75] While the stomach has intrinsic muscular activity, the gastric tube does not develop significant persistalsis and tracheo-oesophageal speech does not have the typical wet character of jejunum despite secretory mucosa. The flap is versatile in terms of length and width, and pedicle length is good and easily harvested. Donor complications are similar to jejunum with a risk of respiratory compromise, bowel obstruction, enteric leak and hernia, and in addition the prepyloric (antrum) region needs to be avoided to prevent pyloric stenosis. Laparoscopic harvest has not been reported, but is likely to be feasible.[1]

Free colon transfer has not become a popular technique for laryngopharyngeal reconstruction but continues to be used for laryngopharyngectomy with oesophagectomy, mainly as a pedicled flap, in certain institutions. The unique anatomy of the ileocaecal valve and appendix has been used by some authors to full advantage.[76, 77] While these innovative techniques hold some promise, there are no comparative data to show whether they are useful in the mainstream. In general, the patulous nature of colon results in poor quality tracheoesophageal speech.[1]

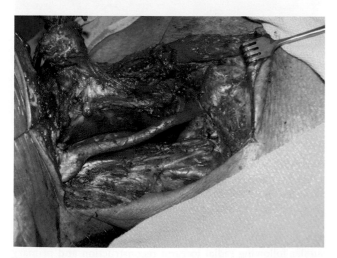

Figure 52.6 Exposed right internal carotid artery and subclavian artery during circumferential pharyngolaryngectomy. This patient is at high risk of a vascular rupture in the event of a salivary fistula.

Fasciocutaneous free flaps reconstruction

The forearm flap was first described in the Chinese literature[78] in the late 1970s and then reported in the English literature by Song *et al.* in 1982.[79] It has become the most common flap for head and neck reconstruction because of its ease of harvest, long pedicle, versatility and reliability. Harii and Ebihara[80] popularized it as a tubed flap for pharyngeal reconstruction in 1985, initially reporting its use in 12 circumferential defects (**Figure 52.8**). At a similar time, Hayden[81] was using the lateral thigh flap as an alternative tubed fasciocutaneous flap after it was first reported in 1983.[82] The lateral thigh flap had the distinct advantage of being able to harvest a large area of tissue with primary closure of the donor site; however, its harvest is relatively complex when compared to the anterolateral thigh flap, which otherwise has similar properties.

Early experience with tubed fasciocutaneous free flap reconstruction of the hypopharynx was plagued by an unacceptably high stricture rate, predominantly at the distal pharyngeal anastomosis. A variety of methods have been reported to overcome this problem. The most popular techniques have been either to break up the suture line using a V- or Z-plasty[83, 84] or by stenting the anastomosis with a salivary bypass tube.[85, 86] Deschler[87] reviewed the English literature and compared 919 free jejunal autografts with 179 fasciocutaneous free flaps (mainly radial forearm). Overall flap failure was higher in the jejunal group (7.5 versus 1.8 per cent), but other complications such as fistula (17 versus 23 per cent) and stricture (9.1 versus 16 per cent) were similar or lower.

Recently, the anterolateral thigh (ALT) flap has all but replaced the lateral thigh flap, mainly because it has all of the advantages of the lateral thigh flap but is comparatively easy to harvest. This flap was described by Song[88] and then popularized by Wei following some large Taiwanese series. It is particularly suited to the Asian population, who generally have minimal subcutaneous fat in the thigh, and in selected centres this is now considered the fasciocutaneous flap of choice.[89, 90] In other ethnic groups, the thigh may be thicker making it difficult to tube,[91] not unlike the pectoralis major flap. The ALT flap can be thinned to provide an 'ultra-thin' flap, however this reduces the vascular territory to approximately 80 per cent of what is usual and may reduce flap reliability either due to trauma to the small perforators or disruption of the subdermal plexus.[92]

We have reported our experience with the ALT for both general head and neck reconstruction[93] and specifically for pharyngeal reconstruction[86] (**Figure 52.9**). Recent data suggest that the ALT is replacing the radial forearm for fasciocutaneous hypopharyngeal reconstruction, mainly due to donor site morbidity, but also the fistula rate may be lower than that of the radial forearm.[64] We perform a subfascial dissection and use the dense layer of fascia lata as a second layer to bolster the pharyngeal anastomoses, and in a series of 14 circumferential reconstructions only one patient developed a radiological leak and there were no clinical fistulas.[86] The stricture rate was 14 per cent where a salivary bypass tube was used to stent the anastomosis compared to 20 per cent for jejunum.[64] The salivary tube is sutured to a feeding tube which is then fixed to the nasal septum to prevent migration and can be removed in the outpatient clinic without sedation.

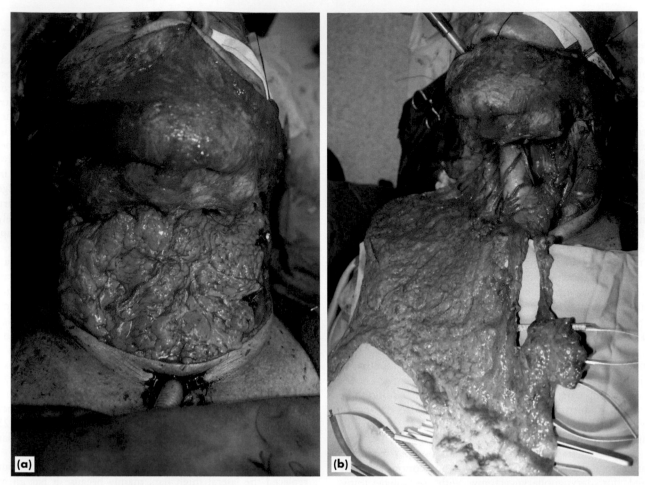

Figure 52.7 Gastro-omental free flap showing inset stomach and omentum wrapped around all tissue to contain any potential salivary leaks.

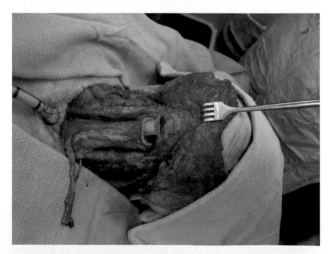

Figure 52.8 Tubed radial forearm free flap used to reconstruct circumferential pharyngeal defect over a salivary bypass tube.

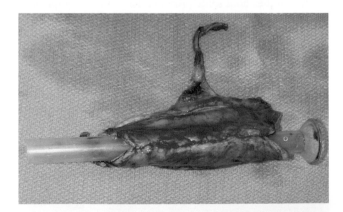

Figure 52.9 Anterolateral thigh (ALT) free flap rolled to create a tube over a salivary bypass tube. The ALT flap can be harvested with the fascia lata of the leg and used as a second layer of closure to prevent fistulas.

There is increasing evidence to suggest that fasciocutaneous flaps are superior to jejunal flaps with regards to tracheo-oesophageal speech and deglutition while avoiding the morbidity of laparotomy. Anthony *et al.*[94] demonstrated that objective parameters of tracheo-oesophageal speech were similar following radial forearm reconstruction and primary mucosal closure after total laryngectomy. More recently, Yu *et al.*[95, 96] compared patients undergoing ALT flap reconstruction with jejunal reconstruction and found that the ALT was superior in terms of achieving a complete oral diet

(95 versus 65 per cent) and fluent speech (89 versus 22 per cent) with no significant difference in fistula or long-term stricture rates.

RECONSTRUCTION OF PARTIAL LARYNGOPHARYNGEAL DEFECTS

Partial defects: simple

Partial defects are those where the full circumference of the laryngopharyngeal complex is not removed. These are subdivided into simple partial defects where the larynx has been removed and complex defects where the larynx is retained, in part or in entirety. Simple defects are termed such because the aim of reconstruction is essentially to provide enough tissue to allow closure of the defect without narrowing or fistula. In fact, classical total laryngectomy presents us with a simple defect where minimal piriform fossa mucosa is resected and the defect can, in fact, be closed primarily. In general, native mucosa is the optimal tissue for reconstruction where possible, although following high-dose radiotherapy or chemoradiation there may be a role for covering this anastomosis with well-vascularized tissue to prevent or minimize the high likelihood of fistulalization.[97]

Several options are available for reconstruction of simple partial defects of the laryngopharynx. Conceptually, these are divided into defects where external skin is required and those where it is not. The authors do not consider that the tissue used is critical to functional outcomes as it does not need to be tubed or folded, which necessitates a thin pliable flap. As a result, most of the issues of flap selection revolve around donor site morbidity, cosmesis and reliability.

PARTIAL DEFECTS: SIMPLE WITH EXTERNAL SKIN

In patients where an external skin defect requires replacement the simplest option is a pectoralis major pedicled flap and skin graft on the muscle. This is a good option where simplicity, time and reliability are crucial. Regional muscle flaps are particularly suitable in the context of active pharyngocutaneous fistula or flap necrosis where the neck is hostile and free flap reconstruction is high risk. The latissimus dorsi flap can act as a substitute for the pectoralis major flap for partial pharyngeal reconstruction, but requires some rotation of the torso for harvest.

Alternatively, an internal mammary-based flap may be used to create external lining. This may be the classical deltopectoral flap or the more recently IMAP flap.[22, 32] The internal mammary flaps are good options for peristomal cover where a skin graft and its dressing can be problematic, and has the advantage of providing thin, pliable material with good colour match, depending on prior therapy, ethnicity and sun exposure (**Figure 52.10**). The IMAP flap has some advantages over the traditional deltopectoral flap. These include the ability to close the donor site primarily, although this is not likely to be possible where a pectoralis major flap has been taken from the same hemi-thorax. The IMAP can also be used to close the mucosal defect without a controlled fistula and two flaps can be used to reconstruct

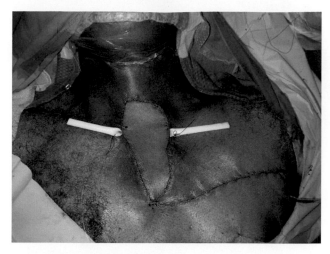

Figure 52.10 Thin, pliable skin of upper chest with good colour match to neck is available with deltopectoral and internal mammary perforator (IMAP) flaps.

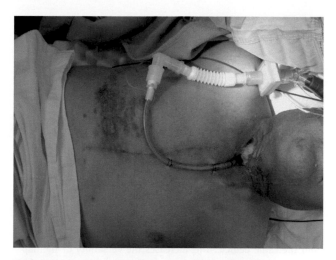

Figure 52.11 Internal mammary perforator (IMAP) flap necrosis causing pharyngocutaneous fistula, further complicated by herpes zoster infection due to immune suppression.

both internal and external lining simultaneously. Unfortunately, being a perforator flap the IMAP flap is less robust and anecdotal experience suggests that it is less reliable than the deltopectoral flap (**Figure 52.11**). While a pectoralis major flap can be used for external lining, its bulk makes it suboptimal around the tracheostomal and not used in our reconstructive algorithm.

The chest donor site is problematic from an aesthetic point of view, particularly in females where the combination of a pectoralis major flap primarily closed and deltopectoral flap skin grafted is a highly disfiguring combination (**Figure 52.12**). There appears to be considerable variance in psychosocial impact based on ethnicity, age, personal preference and donor site. In the current era, where free flap reconstruction is commonplace and highly reliable, we believe that donor sites need to be carefully chosen taking all factors into consideration.

Possibly the most suitable reconstruction of simple partial defects requiring external skin cover is the double paddle

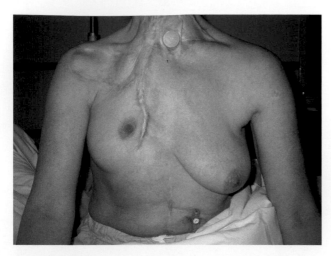

Figure 52.12 Combination of pectoralis major flap and deltopectoral flap for laryngopharyngeal reconstruction in a female patient causing disfigurement.

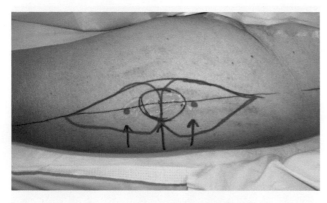

Figure 52.13 The anterolateral thigh flap often has multiple perforators that can be used to supply separate skin paddles from the same pedicle. This increases the versatility of the flap and can be used to reconstruct both pharyngeal and skin defects simultaneously without folding the flap.

anterolateral thigh free flap. The anterolateral thigh flap is unique in that most patients have multiple long perforators arising from the descending branch of the lateral circumflex femoral vessels.[88, 89, 90, 91, 92] This can be assessed preoperatively by Doppler mapping and allows the flap to be divided into separate islands that can be used to reconstruct both the internal and external defects without a de-epithelialized segment (**Figure 52.13**). Colour match is variable depending on sun exposure and ethnicity. Certainly any fasciocutaneous flap can be used with a de-epithelialized segment to create internal and external lining, however orientation becomes critical in this setting and if a leak occurs this segment will re-epithelialize and form a chronic fistula.

PARTIAL DEFECTS: SIMPLE WITH INTACT EXTERNAL SKIN

Reconstruction of these defects is relatively simple. Either regional or free tissue flaps can be used with similar outcomes. The pectoralis major flap has been extensively used

for this purpose and appears to be well suited as long as there is not excessive subcutaneous fat. Other regional flaps are also reasonable options for closing these defects. In centres with microvascular expertise a fasciocutaneous free flap (such as the radial forearm or ALT) avoids the donor site concerns in the chest and is arguably more reliable. Numerous other flaps have been used for these defects, such as jejunum opened on the antimesenteric border, and optimal choice also depends on institutional expertise as much as flap selection.

TRACHEO–OESOPHAGEAL PUNCTURE

The choice of flap does not appear to significantly impact on voice outcomes for these simple partial reconstructions, although there are minimal data to verify this. Bulky flaps may interfere with speech in the short term, however after two to three months atrophy is sufficient to overcome this problem for musculocutaneous flaps. This may not be the case if there is excessive subcutaneous fat. Timing of tracheo-oesophageal puncture is controversial and based on theoretical concerns rather than evidence. Due to the thickness of the pectoralis major flap, early placement of a tracheo-oesophageal puncture valve is difficult if it has to be placed through the flap itself and will need to be resized numerous times. In this situation, secondary puncture is preferred after the muscle has atrophied. Free fasciocutaneous and enteric flaps do not atrophy to the same degree, however all flaps undergo some remodelling and placing a primary puncture though the flap may concern the reconstructive surgeon.

Often enough native mucosa is retained that the puncture passes through the oesophagus rather than the flap. In this case, personal preference and resources will dictate timing of puncture. Our preference is to avoid primary placement outside the setting of a standard total laryngectomy and primary closure because of complexity and the risk of fistula, particularly in the context of chemoradiation. Patient and institutional factors need to be taken into consideration, in particular cognition, motivation, visual acuity and manual dexterity are more important in ultimate tracheo-oesophageal speech success than flap selection. If there is any doubt, we favour secondary puncture since care of the laryngostoma is more difficult with a tracheo-oesophageal fistula in place in the early postoperative period (**Figure 52.14**).

Partial defects: complex

Small defects confined to the lateral pyriform sinus or posterior pharyngeal wall with larynx preservation can be closed primarily while larger defects require reconstruction with a regional or free flap. Preference should be given to thin pliable flaps, such as the forearm or thigh flaps, depending on body habitus. Free jejunum has also been used as a mucosal patch to reconstruct partial defects or bypass postcricoid stricture.[58] Our practice has been to combine flap reconstruction with a silastic salivary stent for 6 weeks when stricture is likely. Most patients require a tracheotomy until swelling subsides and the stent is removed.

Complex pharyngolaryngeal resections are not new concepts, being pioneered in the mid-twentieth century, and represent extensions of partial laryngeal surgery with

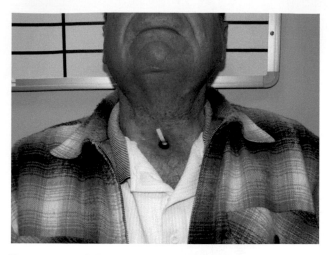

Figure 52.14 Delayed tracheo-oesophageal puncture in a patient who underwent a gastro-omental flap reconstruction of a total laryngopharyngectomy defect for postcricoid squamous cell carcinoma after radiotherapy for glottic cancer ten years earlier. Note the skin telangiectasia and depigmentation from radiotherapy.

important contributions by Alonso, Ogura, Biller, Pearson, Laccourreye, Bocca and others (see **Table 52.3**). The advent of free tissue reconstruction held much promise in allowing patients to undergo increasingly more radical larynx preserving procedures. While numerous techniques have been described, reconstructive surgery has not proved to be the panacea for the triad of dysphonia, dysphagia and aspiration that plagues laryngeal reconstruction. The success of these techniques can be unpredictable and depends on patient, tumour and treatment factors.

Reconstruction of the hypopharynx usually results in some initial aspiration and is more severe if part of the larynx is resected concurrently. Patient compliance and motivation are important factors and elderly patients or those with significant cardiopulmonary disease are unlikely to tolerate this. The chances of successful reconstruction, defined as return to oral nutrition without a gastrostomy tube and functional speech, are further diminished in patients who have previously been treated with radiotherapy or chemoradiation for numerous reasons. Partial laryngeal surgery has demonstrated that the minimal functional apparatus is preservation of a single cricoarytenoid unit. Without this, there are currently no reconstructive techniques that allow speech and swallowing without a tracheostoma. In patients undergoing concurrent hypopharyngectomy, there are multiple factors which may interfere with deglutition, described below.

Prior radiotherapy causes problems related to fibrosis, oedema and xerostomia. Elevation of the laryngeal apparatus is restricted, food is poorly lubricated, sensation is altered and normal coordinated pharyngeal contraction is impaired. When partially replaced with insensate, non-contractile and structurally aberrant tissue such as a free flap the result is laryngeal penetration and without adequate laryngeal reflexes, aspiration follows. The ultimate outcome then depends on severity of aspiration, pulmonary reserve and the individual's ability to compensate through dietary modification, physical manoeuvres and cough.

Numerous methods of resection and reconstruction of complex partial defects have been described. Many are extensions of horizontal or partial laryngectomy and very few have been tested in large series outside of a single institution in the modern era. Examples of the basic defects and references are described in **Table 52.3**. The authors believe that in appropriately selected patients these are reasonable options with the aim of functional organ preservation.

CIRCUMFERENTIAL DEFECTS

Figure 52.15 summarizes the authors' current reconstructive algorithm for circumferential defects of the laryngopharynx. Most patients are reconstructed using free vascularized tissue which has increased the complexity but substantially reduced the morbidity of pharyngeal reconstruction. Free tissue is preferred except in situations where there is significant cervical oesophageal involvement.

Cervical oesophageal involvement

For tumours extending to the cervical oesophagus that require a laryngo-pharyngo-oesophagectomy, we favour gastric transposition. Alternative methods include pedicled or free jejunal flaps and colonic transfer depending on institutional expertise. There is no clearly defined cut-off at which the extent of oesophageal involvement necessitates total oesophagectomy either from an oncologic or reconstructive perspective, although a 2 cm margin on the distal extent of the tumour is preferable. We use free tissue reconstruction for all patients where a hand-sewn anastomosis can be performed to the proximal oesophagus safely. This depends on patient body habitus; however, in general, if the tumour extends below the thoracic inlet (first rib) it will be difficult to inset a free flap and gastric transposition is preferred. Circular stapled anastomoses have been described and facilitate anastomosis in the mid to upper thorax but anastomotic leak in this location is potentially disastrous. Functional problems include regurgitation, dumping syndrome and poor tracheo-oesophageal speech due to the patulous nature of the vibratory segment of stomach wall.[1, 113]

Gastric 'pull-up' has been used widely, however there are multiple technical aspects that necessitate an experienced thoracoabdominal surgeon to deliver the stomach into the neck; in particular, adequate Kocherisation of the duodenum, atraumatic handling of the right gastroepiploic vasculature, tubing to lengthen the stomach, minimal blind dissection of the thoracic oesophagus and, above all, tension-free anastomosis in the neck. Transhiatal thoracoscopy has been used to minimize bind dissection and subsequent haemorrhage. In patients where a high anastomosis is required, supercharging the stomach by microvascular anastomosis of the left gastric or gastroepiploic vessels may decrease distal necrosis and subsequent fistula. Given that gastric necrosis is not infrequently associated with mortality, we suggest that this procedure should only be performed by surgeons with considerable expertise or training in this technique. **Figure 52.16** demonstrates the disastrous complication of gastric necrosis following transposition.

Table 52.3 Complex partial defects.

Procedure	Description	Reconstruction	Reference
Extended supraglottic laryngectomy or supraglottic hemilaryngopharyngectomy	Resection of supraglottis with epilaryngeal or medial piriform sinus	Primary closure, with musculoperichondrial flap	Alonso,[98] Ogura et al.,[99] Bocca et al.,[100] Chevalier et al.,[101] Makeieff et al.[102]
Partial laryngopharyngectomy or extended vertical hemilaryngectomy or supracricoid hemilaryngopharyngectomy or partial laryngopharyngectomy with hemicricoid resection	Resection of tissue above or including cricoid, vocal cord, paraglottic space, laryngeal cartilage, pre-epiglottic space, epiglottis and preservation of one cricoarytenoid unit. Incoporating medial piriform	Primary closure with mucoperichondrial flap or ricohyoidopexy or reconstruction with radial forearm free flap	Ogura et al.,[103] Pearson et al.,[104, 105] Laccourreye et al.,[106] Laccourreye et al.,[107] Chantrain et al.,[108] Urken et al.[109]
Lateral pharyngectomy without laryngectomy	Resection of lateral piriform sinus or posterior pharyngeal wall	Primary closure or radial forearm free flap	Ogura et al.,[110] Delaere et al.,[111] Urken et al.[112]

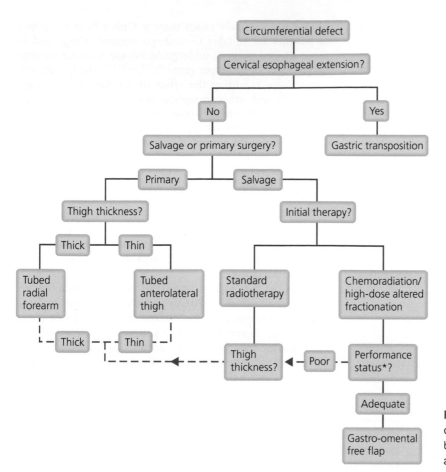

Figure 52.15 Reconstructive algorithm for circumferential laryngopharyngeal defects based on prior treatment, performance status and patient body habitus.

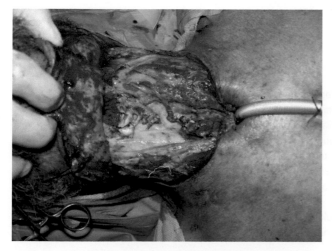

Figure 52.16 Major neck sepsis following necrosis of the stomach after gastric transposition. This complication is frequently followed by catastrophic haemorrhage and is difficult to salvage with any alternative flap since the oesophagus has been removed.

As discussed earlier (see above under Gastric transposition) gastric transposition has been extensively reported in the literature and is associated with a high morbidity and excessive mortality rate in some series. Wei *et al.*[28] reviewed 20 published series between 1966 and 1995 and found that the average major complication and mortality rates were 37 and

Table 52.4 Gastric transposition.

Complication	Goldberg *et al.*[114] (1989)	Clark *et al.*[64] (2005)
Mortality	20%	0%
Major morbidity	46%	66%
Fistula	22%	48%
Stricture	n.a.	29%
Mean length of stay	31 days	34 days

n.a., Not available.

16 per cent, respectively. This was confirmed by reviews at our own institution in 1989 and 2005 as shown in **Table 52.4**.

Primary surgery

Selected patients are not appropriate for organ preservation protocols and while jejunum has been used most widely to reconstruct these defects, there is considerable movement towards tubed fasciocutaneous free flap reconstruction of these defects. There are numerous reasons for this trend including a desire to avoid the inherent risk associated with laparotomy and superior functional outcomes. Jejunal voice tends to have a 'wet' quality and patients often suffer intermittent dysphagia from uncoordinated peristalsis during deglutition.[115, 116, 117]

The forearm and ALT flaps are the most commonly used fasciocutaneous flaps for reconstruction of circumferential defects. The tubed anterolateral thigh flap is ideally suited for reconstruction of these long pharyngeal defects as 8–10 cm width and 15–20 cm length can generally be harvested easily with primary closure of the thigh. The flap is difficult to tube in patients with a 'female distribution' of body fat, particularly in the Western population where obesity is common, even in patients with head and neck cancer. The flap can be thinned, however we prefer to use the fascia lata as an additional layer to bolster the oropharyngeal and oesophageal anastomosis. In patients unsuitable for an ALT flap, we prefer to use a radial forearm free flap, which provides ultra-thin tissue that can readily be tubed. Unfortunately, the donor site after harvest of 15 × 8 cm of forearm skin is particularly noticeable. Stricture has been a problem with all tubed fasciocutaneous flaps and we have adopted the policy of using a silastic salivary bypass tube as a stent in the postoperative period for approximately 6 weeks.[86]

Salvage surgery

Salvage surgery should be considered whenever recurrent disease is resectable, the patient is free of distant metastatic disease and medically fit for surgery. Only a limited number of patients are suitable to undergo surgical salvage and in those selected patients undergoing salvage five-year survival ranges from 18 to 35 per cent.[118, 119, 120, 121] The literature is inconclusive regarding the effect of standard radiotherapy on fistula and other complications following salvage laryngectomy or laryngopharyngectomy. This probably represents variability in dosing, timing and individual tissue response. Since the advent of chemoradiation and high-dose accelerated radiotherapy, the effect on tissue healing and subsequent wound complications has become even more apparent. Grouping patients who received 50–60 Gy of standard fractionated radiotherapy with those receiving ≥70 Gy combined with concurrent cisplatin is inappropriate. Furthermore, timing of salvage surgery may also play a role in the complication rate. Hence our approach has been to select the reconstruction based on prior therapy and individual patient factors.

Where salvage follows standard single daily radiotherapy to a moderate dose (<70 Gy) and the patient has had the usual tissue response to this therapy the risk of fistula is not substantially increased. In these patients, we use a thin fasciocutaneous free flap reconstruction. The preferred flap is the ALT tubed over a size 14 Fr silastic salivary bypass tube. In patients with a thick thigh, tubing and insetting the flap to

Table 52.5 Complications following laryngopharyngectomy and reconstruction.

Immediate	Wound	Haematoma
	Flap	Microvascular occlusion
	Gastric transposition	Tracheal tear
		Pneumothorax
		Thoracic haemorrhage
Early	Wound	Infection
		Dehiscence
		Seroma
	Fistula	Radiological
		Clinical pharyngocutaneous fistula
	Flap	Donor site complications: wound infection/dehiscence; enteric leak; haematoma
		Necrosis: partial; total flap failure
	Vascular	Major vessel rupture
	Cardiopulmonary	Cardiac ischaemia
		Atelectasis/pneumonia
		Pulmonary embolism
		Mediastinitis
	Endocrine/metabolic	Hypoparathyroidism
		Gastric dumping
Late	Donor site	Small bowel construction
		Abdominal hernia
		Limb weakness
		Limb dysaesthesia
	Stricture/stenosis	Pharyngo-oesophageal
		Tracheostomal
	Endocrine	Hypothyroidism
		Hypoparathyroidism
	Functional	Dysphagia
		G-tube dependence
		Poor speech rehabilitation
		Neck and shoulder stiffness/pain

the oesophagus is difficult and in this instance a forearm flap is preferred. Each suture needs to be placed under vision and often this is best achieved by parachuting the flap into position for the posterior wall, passing the salivary tube into the oesophagus and then suturing the anterior wall under vision. The posterior vertical suture line created by tubing the flap is placed against the prevertebral fascia to minimize leak. The salivary bypass tube is sutured to a nasogastric feeding tube and this is sutured to the nasal septum to prevent migration of the stent into the stomach. At 6 weeks postsurgery, the nasal sutures are divided and the nasogastric tube is pulled through the mouth and used to remove the stent without sedation. This has substantially reduced the incidence of long-term stricture that was observed using fasciocutaneous flaps.

In patients who have undergone chemoradiation, high-dose accelerated hyperfractionated radiotherapy, or where a severe tissue response to radiotherapy is observed, the risk of pharyngocutaneous fistula and wound breakdown is increased. Our preference in these patients is to perform a gastro-omental free flap reconstruction (**Figure 52.15**). The primary advantage of this flap is the abundant vascularized omentum which can be draped over the mucosal anastomoses and exposed vasculature. This is very effective in minimizing major complications of pharyngocutaneous fistula and vascular rupture and also has the unexpected advantage of softening the neck skin and subcutaneous tissue which can be a disabling problem. Before planning this reconstruction, an assessment of patient performance status is essential. We believe that in patients with significant cardiopulmonary comorbidity, severe nutritional depletion or prior major abdominal surgery laparotomy is best avoided and these patients should undergo fasciocutaneous free flap reconstruction, as discussed above under Primary surgery. The addition of a regional myogenous flap to cover the anastomosis should be considered at the initial surgery.

COMPLICATIONS

Morbidity following laryngopharyngectomy and reconstruction is difficult to classify because there are many potential complications that may occur. A standard approach is to classify these as immediate, early and late, as shown in **Table 52.5**. Certain sequelae can be directly attributed to the reconstruction or the ablation, however many, such as pharyngocutaneous fistula and stricture, are functions of both. Current data suggest that some form of complication will occur in the majority of patients, especially if minor or anticipated complications, such as hypocalcaemia, are included.[64] **Table 52.6** provides the relative frequencies of early and late morbidity from the University of Toronto. The effect of radiotherapy on fistula and wound complications is inconsistent in the literature. Our experience demonstrated that salvage patients had a 40 per cent radiological pharyngocutaneous fistula rate following radiotherapy compared to 27 per cent in the primary setting. The lack of agreement

Table 52.6 Combined morbidity of all patients undergoing pharyngectomy.

Complications			Frequency	Percentage (%)
Early total			109	71
	Wound		38	25
		Dehiscence	25	16
		Infection	11	7
		Skin necrosis	2	1
	Vascular		14	9
		Haematoma	7	5
		Major vessel rupture	7	5
	Fistula		51	33
	Flap		20	13
		Necrosis	9	6
		Free flap failure	3	4.7[a]
		Donor site	6	4
		Stent migration	4	36[b]
	Cardiopulmonary		21	14
	Hypocalcaemia		69	45
	Other		13	8
Late total			40	26
	Stricture		23	15
	Stomal stenosis		12	8
	Small bowel obstruction		5	9[c]
	Permanent feeding tube		25	16

[a]Percentage of patients undergoing free tissue transfer.
[b]Percentage of patients where salivary stent was used.
[c]Percentage of patients undergoing laparotomy.

regarding effect of radiotherapy reflects the heterogeneity in radiation treatment approaches. In this series, an accelerated hyperfractionated accelerated radiotherapy regimen was routinely used and evidence suggests that high-dose, accelerated and concurrent chemoradiation is certainly a predictor of increased and more severe wound complications. Much effort needs to be invested in minimizing the morbidity associated with these complex procedures.

KEY EVIDENCE

- Common complications after pharyngeal reconstruction are fistula and stricture.
- Hospital length of stay has reduced dramatically with the introduction of gastric transposition and free flap reconstruction of circumferential pharyngeal defects.
- There is little evidence to guide flap selection in pharyngeal reconstruction, however, fasciocutaneous flaps probably provide better quality tracheo-esophageal voice than enteric flaps, but are associated with a higher stricture rate.

KEY LEARNING POINTS

- Pharyngeal defects may be partial or circumferential, simple or complex, depending on whether the larynx has been preserved.
- Common options for pharyngeal reconstruction include pedicled flaps, such as pectoralis major flap or free tissue flaps, which may be fasciocutaneous or enteric.
- The choice of reconstruction depends on patient comorbidity, prior treatment and institutional expertise.

REFERENCES

1. Couch ME. Laryngopharyngectomy with reconstruction. *Otolaryngologic Clinics of North America* 2002; **35**: 1097–114.
2. Czerny F. Neue operationen. *Zentralblatt für Chirurgie* 1877; **4**: 433–4.
3. Gussenbauer C. Uber die erste durch Th. Billroth am Menschen ausgefuhrte Kehlkopf-Extirpation und die Anwendung eines kunstlichen Kehlkopfes. *Langenbecks Archiv für Klinische Chirurgie* 1974; **17**: 343–56.
4. Mikulicz J. Ein Fall von Resection des carcinomatosen Esophagos mit platichem Ersatz des excidirten Stuckes. *Prager Medizinische Wochenschrift* 1886; **11**: 93–7.
5. Trotter W. Operative treatment of diseases of the mouth and pharynx. *Lancet* 1913; **1**: 1075–81.
6. Wookey H. Surgical treatment of carcinoma of the pharynx and upper esophagus. *Surgery, Gynecology and Obstetrics* 1942; **75**: 499–500.
7. Surkin MI, Lawson W, Biller HF. Analysis of the methods of pharyngoesophageal reconstruction. *Head and Neck Surgery* 1984; **6**: 953–70.
8. Bakamjian VY. A two stage method for pharyngoesophageal reconstruction with primary pectoral skin flap. *Plastic and Reconstructive Surgery* 1965; **36**: 173–84.
9. Rob CG, Bateman GH. Reconstruction of the trachea and cervical esophagus: preliminary report. *British Journal of Surgery* 1949; **37**: 202–5.
10. Negus VE. Reconstruction of pharynx after pharyngoesophagolaryngectomy. *British Journal of Plastic Surgery* 1953; **6**: 99–101.
11. Conley JJ. One-stage radical resection of cervical esophagus, larynx, pharynx and lateral neck with immediate reconstruction. *Archives of Otolaryngology* 1953; **58**: 645–54.
12. Wiillstein L. Uber antethorakale oesophago-jejunostomie und operationen nach gleichem prinzipo. *Deutsche Medizinische Wochenschrift* 1904; **31**: 734.
13. Kelling G. Oesophagoplastik mit Hilfe des Querkolon. *Zentralblatt für Chirurgie* 1911; **38**: 1209.
14. Jianu A. Gastronomie und oesophagoplastik. *Deutsche Zeitschrift für Chirurgie* 1912; **118**: 383.
15. Denk W. Zur Radikaloperation des Oesophaguskarzinoms. *Zentralblatt für Chirurgie* 1913; **40**: 1065–8.
16. Kirschner M. Eine neues Verfahren der oesophagoplastik. *Langenbecks Archiv Klinische für Chirurgie* 1920; **114**: 606.
17. Mes G. A new method of oesophagoplasty. *Journal of the International College of Surgeons* 1948; **11**: 270.
18. Gavriliu D, Georgescu L. Esophagoplastic direction a material gastric. *Revista Stiintelor Medicale (Bucharest)* 1955; **3**: 33.
19. Heimlich H. Reconstruction of the entire esophagus with restoration of swallowing with reverse gastric tube. *New York State Journal of Medicine* 1961; **61**: 2478–82.
20. Heimlich HJ. Carcinoma of the cervical esophagus. *Journal of Thoracic and Cardiovascular Surgery* 1970; **59**: 309–18.
21. Goligher J, Robin I. Use of left colon for reconstruction of the pharynx and oesophagus after pharyngectomy. *British Journal of Surgery* 1954; **42**: 283–90.
22. Carlson G, Schusterman M, Guillamonegui O. Total reconstruction of the hypopharynx and cervical esophagus: a 20 year experience. *Annals of Plastic Surgery* 1992; **29**: 408–12.
23. Ong G, Lee T. Pharyngogastric anastomosis after oesophagopharyngectomy for carcinoma of the hypopharynx and cervical oesophagus. *British Journal of Surgery* 1960; **48**: 193–200.
24. Shefts LM, Fischer A. Carcinoma of the cervical esophagus with a one stage total esophageal resection and pharyngogasterostomy. *Surgery* 1949; **25**: 849.

25. LeQuesne L, Ranger D. Pharyngolaryngectomy with immediate pharyngogastric anastomosis. *British Journal of Surgery* 1966; **53**: 105–9.

26. Turner G. Excision of the thoracic esophagus for carcinoma with reconstruction of the extrathoracic gullet. *Lancet* 1933; **2**: 1315.

27. Harrison DFN. Rehabilitation problems after pharyngogastric anastomosis. *Archives of Otolaryngology* 1978; **104**: 244–6.

28. Wei WI, Lam LK, Yuen PW, Wong J. Current status of pharyngolaryngo-esophagectomy and pharyngogastric anastomosis. *Head and Neck* 1998; **20**: 240–4.

29. Spriano G. Pectoralis major myocutaneous flap for hypopharyngeal reconstruction. *Plastic and Reconstructive Surgery* 2002; **110**: 1408–13.

30. Schuller DE, Mountain RE, Nicholson RE et al. One-stage reconstruction of partial laryngopharyngeal defects. *Laryngoscope* 1997; **107**: 247–53.

31. DePaula AL, Macedo ALV, Cernea CR et al. Reconstruction of upper digestive tact: reducing morbidity by laparoscopic pull-up. *Otolaryngology – Head and Neck Surgery* 2006; **135**: 710–13.

32. Vesely MJ, Murray DJ, Novak CB et al. The internal mammary artery perforator flap: an anatomical study and a case report. *Annals of Plastic Surgery* 2007; **58**: 156–61.

33. Yu P, Roblin P, Chevray P. Internal mammary artery perforator (IMAP) flap for tracheostoma reconstruction. *Head and Neck* 2006; **28**: 723–9.

34. Fredrickson J. Gastric pull up vs deltopectoral flap for reconstruction of the cervical oesophagus. *Archives of Otolaryngology* 1981; **107**: 613–16.

35. Ariyan S. One-stage repair of a cervical esophagostome with two myocutaneous flaps from the neck and shoulder. *Plastic and Reconstructive Surgery* 1979; **63**: 426–9.

36. Ariyan S. The pectoralis major myocutaneous flap. A versatile flap for reconstruction in the head and neck. *Plastic and Reconstructive Surgery* 1979; **63**: 73–81.

37. Withers E. Pectoralis major musculocutaneous flap: a new flap in head and neck reconstruction. *American Journal of Surgery* 1979; **138**: 537–43.

38. Genden EM, Kaufman MR, Katz B et al. Tubed gastro-omental free flap for pharyngoesophageal reconstruction. *Archives of Otolaryngology – Head and Neck Surgery* 2001; **127**: 847–53.

39. Triboulet JP. Surgical management of carcinoma of the hypopharynx and cervical esophagus: analysis of 209 cases. *Archives of Surgery* 2001; **136**: 1164–70.

40. Fabian RL. Reconstruction of the laryngopharynx and cervical esophagus. *Laryngoscope* 1984; **93**: 1334–50.

41. Coleman JJ. Reconstruction of the pharynx after resection for cancer. A comparison of methods. *Annals of Surgery* 1989; **209**: 554–60.

42. Stell PM. Some topics in head and neck surgery. Musculocutaneous flap. *Acta Oto-Rhino-Laryngologica Belgica* 1983; **37**: 399–417.

43. Nozaki M, Huang TT, Hayashi M et al. Reconstruction of the pharyngoesophagus following pharyngoesophagectomy and irradiation therapy. *Plastic and Reconstructive Surgery* 1985; **76**: 386–94.

44. Neifeld JP, Merritt WA, Theograj SD et al. Tubed pectoralis major musculocutaneous flaps for cervical esophageal replacement. *Annals of Plastic Surgery* 1983; **11**: 24–30.

45. Deschler DG, Doherty ET, Reed CG, Singer MI. Quantitative and qualitative analysis of tracheoesophageal voice after pectoralis major flap reconstruction of the neopharynx. *Otolaryngology – Head and Neck Surgery* 1998; **118**: 771–6.

46. Watson JS, Lendrum J. One stage reconstruction using a compound latissimus dorsi island flap. *British Journal of Plastic Surgery* 1981; **34**: 87–90.

47. Seidenberg B. Immediate reconstruction of the cervical esophagus by a revascularised jejunal segment. *Annals of Surgery* 1959; **149**: 162–71.

48. Green C, Som M. Free grafting and revascularization of the intestine. I. Replacement of the cervical esophagus. *Surgery* 1966; **60**: 1012–16.

49. Shangold L, Urken M. Jejunal transplantation for pharyngoesophageal reconstruction. *Otolaryngologic Clinics of North America* 1991; **24**: 1321–42.

50. Jones AS, Gati I. Free revascularized jejunal loop repair following total pharyngolaryngectomy for carcinoma of the hypopharynx: report of 90 patients. *British Journal of Surgery* 1996; **83**: 1279–83.

51. Coleman JJ III, Tan KC, Searles JM et al. Jejunal free autograft: analysis of complications and their resolution. *Plastic and Reconstructive Surgery* 1989; **84**: 589–95.

52. Chen HC, Tang YB. Microsurgical reconstruction of the esophagus. *Seminars in Surgical Oncology* 2000; **19**: 235–45.

53. Uchiyama K, Kimata Y, Ebihara S et al. Evaluating the donor site after harvest of free jejunum grafts. *Head and Neck* 2002; **24**: 451–5.

54. Eckardt A, Fokas K. Microsurgical reconstruction in the head and neck region: an 18-year experience with 500 consecutive cases. *Journal of Cranio-Maxillofacial Surgery* 2003; **31**: 197–201.

55. Disa J, Cordeiro P. Microvascular reconstruction of the hypopharynx: defect classification, treatment algorithm, and functional outcomes based on 165 consecutive cases. *Plastic and Reconstructive Surgery* 2003; **111**: 652–60.

56. Schusterman MA, Shestak K, de Vries EJ et al. Reconstruction of the cervical esophagus: free jejunal transfer versus gastric pullup. *Plastic and Reconstructive Surgery* 1990; **85**: 16–21.

57. Benazzo M, Bertino G, Gatti P et al. Atypical reconstructions with free jejunum flap after circumferential pharyngolaryngectomy. *Microsurgery* 2007; **27**: 17–20.

58. Delaere P, Hierner R, Goeleven A, D'Hoore A. Reconstruction for postcricoid pharyngeal stenosis after organ preservation protocols. *Laryngoscope* 2006; **116**: 502–4.

ANATOMIC CONSIDERATIONS AND RECONSTRUCTION

Although the midface skeletal structure is complex in shape, the need to faithfully reconstruct these bones is often not necessary. The region of the paranasal sinuses with the exception of the medial orbital wall does not require reconstruction or obturation as long as there is no oronasal fistula. Resecting the maxilla, however, may result in the loss of support for the orbit, the facial skin and the dentition, and it is in these areas that adequate obturation or reconstruction are essential to avoid facial collapse, ectropion and/or enopthalmos, and the loss of the dentition. It is also essential to reconstruct the nasal bones to avoid nasal collapse although they are generally spared following maxillectomy.

CLASSIFICATION

There have been many attempts to provide a simple and descriptive classification of the maxillectomy defect, which can relate to the method of treatment.[1, 2, 3, 4] The classification proposed by the author[1] is the first to attempt to combine both the surgical (**Box 53.1**) and dental (**Box 53.2**) factors related to maxillectomy and so predict the effect of the defect on the quality of life of the patient as well as the likely requirement in terms of reconstruction.

In simple terms, there is a vertical or surgical defect, which relates to the extent of the resection in the vertical plane from the dentition to the skull base. This defect results in a mainly aesthetic defect as there is initially loss of support of the cheek, then support for the orbit and then loss of the orbit itself. As a result, patients who wear an obturator or undergo reconstruction still have at least half of the functioning dentition, and although they lose binocular vision with the loss of the eye, the vision is still maintained through the orbit that is left. A letter (a, b or c) is added depending on how much of the upper alveolus is removed which is considered as the horizontal or dental component of the defect (see **Figure 53.1**).

Box 53.1   Surgical component (vertical)

- Class 1: The removal of alveolar bone not resulting in an oronasal or oroantral fistula. Resections of the ethmoid and frontal sinus cavity defects, or removal of the lateral nasal wall would fit into this part of the classification. Included in this group is the removal of only palatal bone, which will inevitably result in an oronasal fistula, but leaves the dental bearing part of the maxilla intact.
- Class 2: Partial maxillectomy including the alveolus and antral walls, but not including the orbital rim or the maxillary buttress.
- Class 3: Partial maxillectomy including the floor of the orbit with or without periorbital ± skull base resection.
- Class 4: Partial maxillectomy with orbital exenteration ± anterior skull base resection.

Box 53.2   Dental component (horizontal)

- a: Unilateral alveolar maxilla and hard palate resected. Less than or equal to half the alveolar and hard palate resection not involving the nasal septum or crossing the midline.
- b: Bilateral alveolar maxilla and hard palate resected. Includes a smaller resection that crosses the midline of the alveolar bone including the nasal septum.
- c: The removal of the entire alveolar maxilla and hard palate.

The principle of this classification is that it is simple to remember and relates to the likely need for reconstruction of the higher class of defect, such as class 3 and 4. There was clear evidence that this was the case with the experience in the unit in Liverpool (**Table 53.1**). There was also a correlation with the quality of life outcome, which was less likely to be favourable as the defect became larger whatever the method of facial and oral rehabilitation.[1]

A MULTIDISCIPLINARY APPROACH TO REHABILITATION OF THE MAXILLECTOMY PATIENT

In the management of the maxillary defect, it is not only the method of treatment for the disease that requires the rigours of a multidisciplinary decision-making process but also the method of rehabilitation. At present, there is very little information on patient outcomes in terms of survival and quality of life treated with either prosthetic rehabilitation alone or reconstruction with subsequent dental and facial prostheses. As with many aspects of head and neck cancer management, the evidence base is weak because of the small number of cases, the variety of the pathology, and the publication of case series that represent a single method of management with no comparative analysis. In the Regional Maxillofacial Unit in Liverpool, we have now prospectively entered more than 1600 patients onto the database. There are 153 (**Table 53.1**) patients with the site of the tumour in the palate, maxillary alveolus or paranasal sinuses who have undergone a maxillectomy and 38 have been rehabilitated with obturation and 115 reconstructed with a variety of techniques. Even though there are now between 350 and 400 new patients discussed at the multidisciplinary team meeting (MDT), relatively few of them have tumours requiring maxillectomy.

There are very few data on the comparison of obturation and reconstruction in terms of function and quality of life. A group from Japan found little difference in speech intelligibility between reconstructed (rectus abdominis) and non-reconstructed cases but there were only four patients in each group.[5] We compared a group of 28 patients who underwent either obturation or reconstruction, and completed a series of questionnaires that examined their denture satisfaction as well as their function and quality of life.[6] **Table 53.2** represents the results of the study, which indicate that overall the patients who underwent reconstruction probably fared

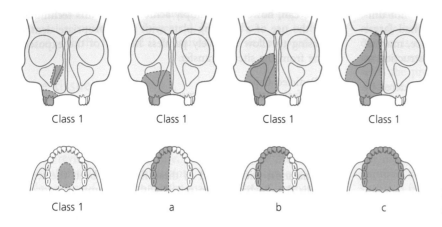

Figure 53.1 Classification of the maxillectomy defect.

Class 1 | Class 1 | Class 1 | Class 1

Class 1 | a | b | c

Table 53.1   Midface rehabilitation and reconstruction in Liverpool (1992–2006).

Method of rehabilitation/reconstruction	Class 1	Class 2	Class 3	Class 4
Obturate	6	28	4	–
Radial (fasciocutaneous)	8	29	–	–
Radial (osteocutaneous)	–	14	4	4
Iliac crest with internal oblique	–	19	14	17
Scapula (thoracodorsal)	–	–	–	2
Fibula (osteocutaneous)	–	2	–	–
Latissimus dorsi	–	–	–	2
Rectus abdominis	–	–	–	1

Table 53.2   Comparison of obturation and reconstruction.

	Obturation	Reconstruction	*p* value
Classification			
1	1	1	
2a	7	6	
2b	1	5	
3a/b	1	2	
4a/b	–	3	
Not available		1	
Radiotherapy	10% (1/10)	19% (3/18)	
University of Washington Questionnaire (cumulative score)			
Cumulative score	74	75	0.68
EORTC head and neck (35% with problem during the last week)			
Pain in your mouth	60	22	0.04
Soreness in your mouth	80	33	0.05
Problems opening mouth wide	30	39	0.98
Gained weight	20	61	0.06
Oral symptom check list (% item present)			
Aware upper teeth	90	40	0.06
Self-conscious	50	9	0.06
Denture satisfaction % satisfied (NB. 8 patients in reconstructed group)			
Satisfied with upper denture	50	100	0.07
Satisfied with function	40	100	0.03

In such a situation it may be necessary to use a radial forearm flap (**Figure 53.1**) for the larger defects but a local palatal flap, buccal fat pad or greater palatine island flap may close the fistula successfully. Ostectomies that involve the lateral nasal wall typically following the excision of an inverted papilloma do not need reconstruction and can be left to epithelialize with no functional or aesthetic deficit.

CLASS 2 (a–c)

This is the classic hemimaxillectomy defect in which the orbital floor is left intact although a varying height of the maxillary buttress and anterior wall may be removed. The letters a, b or c represent: a, less than half the upper alveolus; b, more than half the upper alveolus; and c, the whole of the functioning upper alveolus. The success of obturation will decrease as more of the upper alveolus is removed. Not only will there be no chance of retaining any upper teeth in a class c, but it becomes more difficult to supply a functioning prosthesis the more of the palate and upper alveolus is removed.

Class 2a

By definition a class 2a involves only half of the upper alveolus and, as such, only a unilateral tuberosity resection is required leaving support of the nose with an intact nasal septum. In this situation there is no chance of nasal collapse and the collapse of the lateral face is unlikely with the retention of the malar arch.

It is not necessary to reconstruct the maxilla posterior to the first molar tooth. It is often necessary to include a resection of the posterior unilateral maxilla for retromolar tumours encroaching on the region of the maxillary tuberosity. In this situation, it is better to carry out a formal posterior maxillectomy including the pterygoid plates in order to obtain a clear margin of resection. These defects will require a flap to reconstruct the cheek, posterior tongue and in some cases the mandible, in which case the choice of reconstruction is decided by the soft tissue or mandibular defect. The soft tissue portion of the flap is all that is required to close the posterior maxillary defect.

For class 2a defects that involve the anterior maxilla, bone will be required if the patient is to be restored to normal dental function. This is an essential part of the planning for the reconstruction considering that an obturator can provide a dental restoration as well as restoration of the facial contour. This is especially true for class 2a defects in which there is a residual functioning alveolus and often sufficient bone to reliably support a prosthesis. The additional advantage of being able to screen the defect by removing the obturator and the simplicity of the surgery may make it difficult to justify a complex reconstruction.

Reconstructive options

This defect is too large for local flaps unless used in conjunction with a free tissue transfer or a pedicled flap. The temporalis flap has been used extensively for this defect but the harvest of split calvarial bone is very difficult in the temporal region. Techniques have been described using this flap in combination with titanium mesh and autogenous iliac crest (non-vascularized)[21] or a titanium implant fashioned

from a stereolithographic model.[17] The problem with both techniques is the risk of flap dehiscence, and postoperative radiotherapy introduces a high risk of failure.

All of the composite free tissue transfer options have been described (**Table 53.3**) and, in my opinion, the best option is probably the fibula flap, mainly on account of the adequate bone for a low maxillectomy and the longer pedicle (**Figure 53.2**). The tendency for the soft tissue component of this flap to fibrose to the bone is an advantage in the maxilla as it prevents the redundant skin from falling down into the mouth. This makes the pre-implant surgery less difficult and allows a better implant to bone interface. The disadvantage of using skin to line the oral part of the reconstruction is the

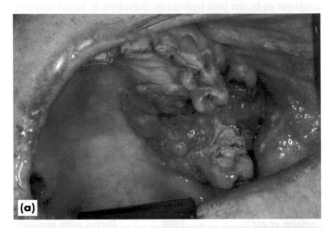

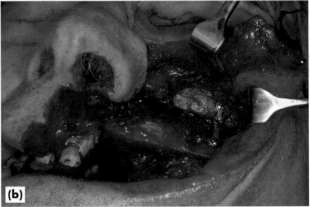

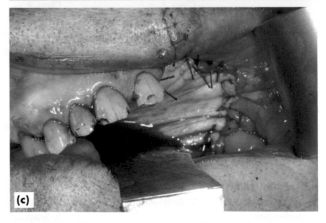

Figure 53.2 Class 2a reconstructed with fibula flap. The height and width of the bone is adequate for facial and lip support, as well as for dental implants if required.

need for palatal or mucosal grafting techniques to provide an adequate bone to implant interface. Although the iliac crest with internal oblique provides an ideal implant to bone relationship, the shorter pedicle makes the anastomotic surgery more difficult, which can result in the need for vein grafts and a subsequent higher failure rate. As the fibula can achieve equivalent results, even though the pre-implant surgery will require grafting, the use of the iliac crest and internal oblique, although providing an excellent result, may be considered an overcomplicated solution.

The scapula can also be used for this type of defect, but the skin to bone relationship is less favourable. Although there is much more versatility in the placement of the skin island compared to the fibula, the skin is thicker, complicating the graft preparation site if implants are to be placed. On the other hand, the flap has been described as being raised with the teres major muscle although this is limited in its placement in the oral cavity compared to internal oblique, which is a flatter and longer muscle harvest. It is possible to lengthen the artery of this flap by harvesting the thoracodorsal artery and using that as the anastomoses to the recipient artery. To achieve this, the subscapular artery is tied off and the dissection continued from the circumflex scapula artery in a retrograde manner to the branching of this artery into the latissimus dorsi muscle. Another option is to use the latissimus dorsi muscle and the tip of the scapula on the thoracodorsal angular artery (TDAA).[27] This will provide an excellent soft tissue reconstruction and reasonable bone base for implants. The main disadvantage of using the subscapular system is the need to turn the patient or the difficulty of a two team approach when this site is so close to the head and neck.

The composite radial forearm flap has also been advocated for this defect but the bone is of very poor quality to accept implants essential for a full dental rehabilitation and there are concerns over the donor site, although the use of a bone plate to protect the forearm for postoperative fractures has proved successful.[29]

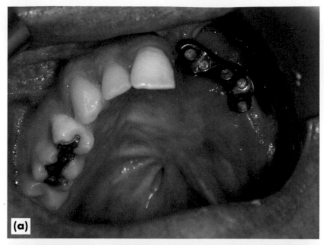
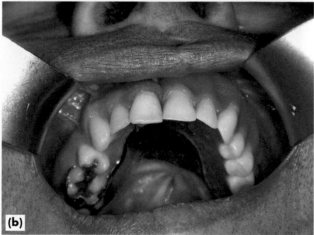

Figure 53.3   (a, b) Class 2b (crossing the midline palate) reconstructed with iliac crest and internal oblique with an implant-retained bar system for denture retention and support. Note the excellent healing properties of the epithelialized muscle base, which facilitate the pre-implant surgery.

Class 2b and c

This defect crosses the midline and can involve bone up to the height of the orbit which can include the perinasal bone that supports the alar base, as well as providing the central upper alveolus. If the maxillectomy is low and only involving the height of the alveolus and not including the maxillary buttresses that support the alar base then the fibula flap can provide sufficient height of bone. This flap may be less reliable if the defect includes the anterior maxillary buttresses, in which case some form of midfacial collapse may occur, especially if a large part of the nasal septum has also been resected. This problem has been highlighted in the literature using a horizontally orientated iliac crest with internal oblique which was compared with a similar defect treated with the vertical orientation of the same flap (**Figure 53.3**).[19] The cases were reported to demonstrate the problem of the loss of central midfacial support in the vertical component, which would be very difficult to restore with a fibula flap that has not been folded over (double-barrelled).

CLASS 3a

This is the most complex of all the midfacial defects because the orbit is retained, but the whole of the anterior maxilla is lost including the upper alveolus. In cases of orbital exenteration, there is a need for an orbital prosthesis, which can disguise some of the failures in restoring the orbital rim or facial contour. If the eye is retained, then the reconstructive aims include avoiding enophthalmos, ectropion, epiphora, hypoglobus and scleral show, while at the same time restoring the orbital floor and medial wall, as well as the anterior maxilla and the upper alveolus so vital to a full dental rehabilitation.

The anatomy of the maxillary bones and relations has been outlined but it is worth emphasizing the nature of this defect in terms of what has been removed before considering the reconstructive options. The maxilla is a bone which is lined by oral mucoperiosteum which is fixed and immobile in the oral cavity. In the nasal region, the bone is also covered with mucoperiosteum and the sinuses include a ciliated epithelium. In simple terms, this is a large bone covered by mucoperiosteum, which has relatively little vital function apart from the support of the teeth, the facial tissues and the orbit. The most important loss of function is not related to nasal breathing or the sense of smell but the use of the teeth, with its resultant effect on the ability to chew normally and maintain a reasonable appearance. In reconstructive terms, the task is to restore a fixed bone in the midface, which if done with accuracy can completely restore all the potentially lost functions as well as achieve an excellent long-term aesthetic result. The failure to use bone as the main element in the reconstructive option will result in a reasonable short-term result but a poor long-term outcome without a satisfactory oral rehabilitation.

Reconstructive options

In the management of the class 3 defect, the surgical and dental rehabilitation team must decide on the complete reconstruction of the defect which includes the orbital floor, facial contour and dental alveolus, or the support of the orbit and obturation of the facial contour and dental alveolus. Obturation alone with a non-vascularized support for the orbital floor will have a high risk of enophthalmos and ectropion with poor function and aesthetics. In basic terms, there are seven main options that have been described in the literature, which can fulfil the necessary requirements:

1. The use of the temporalis flap with either full-thickness cranial bone or the coronoid process to

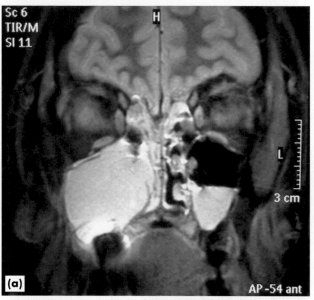

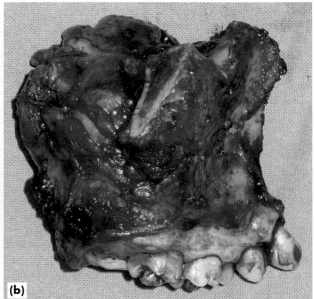

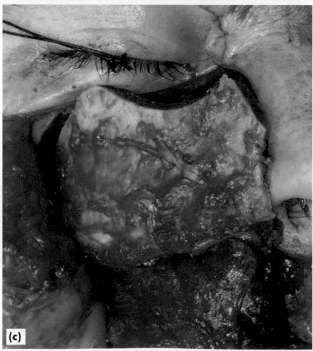

Figure 53.4 Class 3a reconstructed with iliac crest and internal oblique. (a) Magnetic resonance image scan showing an extensive ameloblastoma involving the floor and medial wall of the orbit. (b) The surgical specimen emphasizes the point that the resulting defect is a loss of bone and mucoperiosteum, which can be replaced by bone and muscle. (c) The iliac crest can be fashioned to fit with the nasal bones, the anterior alveolus and the zygomatic buttress to ensure a stable graft in the long term. (d) In this case we have used titanium mesh to reconstruct the floor and medial wall of the orbit. Alternatives include bone from the iliac crest or the calvarium. (e) The overall facial result shows the avoidance of enopthalmos and ectropion six months following the completion of the surgery. We plan an implant-retained dental prosthesis and minimal revision of the anterior part of the graft.

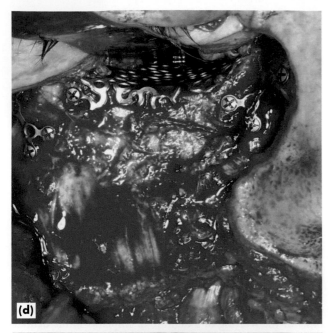

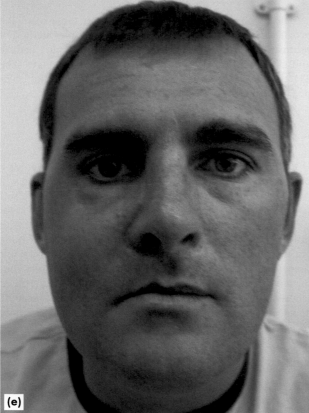

Figure 53.4 Continued.

reconstruct the orbital floor with supporting obturation.

2. The use of a temporoparietal flap with split-thickness calvarial bone to reconstruct the orbital floor with supporting obturation.

3. Reconstruction of the orbital floor with non-vascularized bone or titanium mesh and a soft tissue free flap and obturation.

4. Reconstruction of the orbital floor with non-vascularized bone or titanium mesh and closure of the fistula with a soft tissue vascularized flap.

5. Reconstruction of the orbital floor, facial contour and dental alveolus with non-vascularized bone or titanium mesh and a soft tissue vascularized flap.

6. Reconstruction of the orbital floor and facial contour and closure of the fistula with an osteocutaneous free flap.

7. Complete reconstruction of the orbital floor, facial contour and the dental alveolus with an osteocutaneous free flap followed by dental rehabilitation with either tissue-borne or implant-retained dental prosthesis (**Figure 53.4**).

The use of a vascularized pedicle flap, such as the temporalis or the temperoparietal flap in conjunction with obturation, is a good option if the decision is to use obturation as the main support of the facial contour and the provision of a dental appliance. In this situation, the orbital floor is adequately supported and there is sufficient space for the prosthodontist to find undercuts to retain a reasonable functioning obturator. The use of obturation without orbital support risks poor orbital function and appearance due to contraction and fibrosis involving the orbital floor and adnexae. This option allows a simple reconstruction, which can be performed quickly and thus keeps the morbidity of the necessary surgery to a minimum.

I question the use of free tissue transfer when the dental rehabilitation is an obturator.[23] This means that there will be skin lining the orbital floor and the side of the nose, which will hinder the retention of the obturator. This option also commits the patient to a prolonged procedure involving microvascular techniques. If the patient is motivated and fit enough to undergo free tissue transfer as part of the reconstructive option then it seems sensible to use an osteocutaneous flap and obviate the need for obturation.

The most important part of the reconstruction is the orbital floor and rim if that has also been resected. If a soft tissue free flap is chosen, then this bone requires reconstruction from one of the main donor sites, which is often split-thickness cranial bone. Cordeiro et al.[21] have used the iliac crest as a non-vascularized bone graft for orbital floor and maxillary reconstruction in conjunction with a rectus abdominis flap. This technique requires two donor sites and risks inadequate vascularization of the bony reconstruction. It does fulfil the principle, however, that the bone graft is sealed from the nasal cavity and the air and covered with vascularized tissue on all sides. There is little doubt that non-vascularized bone which is open to the nasal or oral cavity has a high risk of infection and failure.

If the option is to use one of the osteocutaneous flaps then the most important area for bone restoration is the orbital rim and floor to retain the orbit in the correct horizontal plane and avoid ectropion. In this situation, it is difficult to arrange the bone for the fibula or the scapula to fulfil the requirements of orbital and facial support and the provision of adequate bone in the dental alveolus for an implant-retained prosthesis. The fibula will require two osteotomies to provide bone along the orbital rim, vertically down the side of the nose and horizontally along the dental alveolus. The orientation of the skin paddle becomes very difficult in such a situation and the pedicle length is shortened considerably as at least 12 cm of bone is required for this approach. The method still leaves some poor support of the facial skin in the area where no bone has been placed. The scapula bone at least has the necessary height to span the width between the orbital rim and the dental alveolus providing support for the facial skin, but the bone is very thin in the region of the orbit if the lateral rim is used for the alveolus limiting the reconstructive options.

Mark Urken[30] popularized the use of the internal oblique with the iliac crest raised on the deep circumflex iliac artery and vein. The bulk of the bone harvested allowed immediate mandibular reconstruction with the placement of implants at the same time to reduce the rehabilitation period.[31] This flap relies on the healing of the internal oblique muscle in the oral cavity as a mucosal reconstruction and, although there is some inevitable contraction, the appearance and feel of this tissue is the most natural reconstruction available. In the maxilla, the contraction, of the tissue is an advantage, both as part of the reconstructed nasal lining and the hard palate. Both these structures are immobile and lined by mucoperiosteum, and the internal oblique becomes epithelialized and forms a structure, which reflects the tissue that has been removed. The anterior iliac crest is the best site for a bone graft except for the posterior crest for which a vascularized option is not available. The combination of an excellent source of bone, both in height and depth as well as the muscle, which can be used to obturate the defect, is the ideal option in the reconstruction of the class 3 defect.

The main alternative to this option is the use of the angle of the scapula raised on the angular artery, which is a branch of the thoracodorsal artery and so allows either latissimus dorsi, teres major or serratus anterior, and/or skin to be raised on the same pedicle (TDAA).[27] The principle advantage of this option is the long pedicle, which allows easier anastomoses from the larger vessels in the neck. The main problem is the small amount of fairly thin bone from the angle of the mandible, which may not be sufficient to provide both a functioning alveolus and adequate reconstruction of the orbital rim and floor. The patient usually requires turning or at best the access to the site is limited during the necessary head and neck surgery carried out as part of the tumour ablation. The advantage of using muscle as the replacement for the oral and nasal mucosa is maintained with this option.

Box 53.3 demonstrates a class 3 reconstruction.

CLASS 3b and c

When the defect crosses the midline, then the iliac crest is the only donor site providing sufficient bone that can cross the midface to the opposite canine or premolar region and provide height to support the orbit. The flap is capable of supporting both orbits and spanning the dental alveolus reconstructing the lost bone between the zygomatic buttresses.

CLASS 4a

Although this is a larger defect with a greater potential for intracranial extension the problems of reconstruction are considerably reduced because the orbit is removed usually by exenteration rather than enucleation. In this situation, some of the facial collapse can be compensated for by the orbital prosthesis if a soft tissue reconstruction is preferred. The loss of the nasal bones will add to the reconstructive problem and often a non-vascularized graft is required supported by vascularized muscle in much the same way that the orbital floor and medial wall is reconstructed for class 3a–c defects.

The advantage of the iliac crest with internal oblique is the use of the muscle to line the nasal and oral cavity and provide a vascularized base for the safe healing of the eye socket. If vascularized tissue is not placed to support the dead space lost by the orbit then the eyelid skin remaining may dehisce and form a nasocutaneous fistula. Although this can be covered by an orbital prosthesis there will be the problem of encrustation and low-grade inflammation. The iliac crest will restore the orbital rim but there is no need to reconstruct the orbital floor, as the normal contracture of the eye socket will result in sufficient space for the placement of the orbital prosthesis. The reconstructed maxilla will supply sufficient bone to fully support the facial tissues and provide a natural base for the wearing of a denture or implants in the dentate case.

There is a reasonable argument that in these cases the prognosis is generally poor and therefore a simpler method of reconstruction using a soft tissue flap with a longer pedicle and sufficient bulk to obturate the defect is adequate. The TDAA with latissimus dorsi provides a longer and safer pedicle and is an option we have used successfully.

CLASS 4b and c

If the resection crosses the midline of the dental alveolus a bony reconstruction of the alveolar ridge and alar region will result in a much better result than a compromise with a soft tissue flap alone. There will be inevitable facial and nasal collapse, which cannot be adequately obturated and with little chance of any dental rehabilitation. The use of bone grafts such as non-vascularized iliac crest supported by a soft tissue free flap has been reported with good results, but bilateral defects require a larger graft and a higher risk of failure. In this situation, the iliac crest is ideal, but the scapula angle with latissimus dorsi can be useful and may be more reliable in terms of flap perfusion and survival.

AVOIDING COMPLICATIONS IN MIDFACE RECONSTRUCTION WITH FREE FLAPS

The reconstruction of the midface is the most complex reconstructive problem facing the surgeon even after the development of free tissue transfer techniques. The main reason for this is the increased distance from the reconstructive site to the recipient vessels in the neck. The temptation in such a situation is to choose a flap with a long pedicle, which works well as long as the flap is able to restore form and function. It has occurred to me that the unpopularity of the iliac crest and internal oblique muscle in midface reconstruction is related to the morbidity of the donor site and the

---

Box 53.3   Case presentation of class 3 reconstruction with iliac crest and internal oblique

A 32-year-old man presented with a swelling of the right cheek, which had been increasing in size over the last two months. An oral biopsy was reported as an ameloblastoma. Magnetic resonance imaging (MRI) and computed tomography (CT) showed an extensive tumour filling and perforating the right maxillary sinus and extending to involve the floor of the orbit and the right nasoethmoid sinus.

The planned surgical procedure was a maxillectomy extending to the right ethmoid sinus and including the rim, floor and medial orbital wall. The defect would result in a classical class 3a defect with preservation of the nasal septum and the nasal bones. In this situation, the prognosis is excellent and the patient is looking forward to a normal lifespan with an optimum functional and aesthetic result.

The options of a reconstruction or a prosthetic solution were discussed in detail with the patient and his partner and a decision made to reconstruct the defect. It was decided to place any implants as a secondary procedure.

In this situation, the iliac crest with internal oblique can offer an ideal reconstruction, which faithfully restores the lost bone and mucoperiosteum. In such a situation, there is no need to compromise the patient's fitness or the length or complexity of the reconstructive surgery.

The ablation was carried out through a Weber-Ferguson incision and an en bloc resection was possible. During the ablative surgery it was possible to raise the iliac crest with internal oblique in a standard manner according to Urken's description.[30] In this technique, the pedicle is approached from the abdominal side and the inguinal ligament and other attachments to the anterior superior iliac spine can be maintained. Additional pedicle length can be achieved by starting the most proximal bone cut 3–4 cm posterior to the anterior superior iliac spine. A template can be obtained of the maxillary defect, which can help in the modelling process during insetting of the flap.

In order to use the facial artery and vein as end-to-end anastomoses, the submandibular gland is removed to allow easier access to these vessels. If the pedicle is too short to reach the neck, which is often the case, a vertical incision can be made to allow easier access while protecting the mandibular branch of the facial nerve. The flap is inset into the bone, and in this case a titanium mesh sheet was used to reconstruct the floor of the orbit and the medial wall. This was well supported on the iliac crest, which was more than 1 cm thick in this area. The bone is orientated as described previously, with the muscle obturating the oroantral fistula and lining the lateral nasal wall. The muscle also fills the dead space and reduces the risk of infection.

Postoperatively there were no complications that required intervention and the overall result is reasonable. Some points about this case are worth looking at in more detail. One of the problems in this case has been the slight ptosis of the facial skin around the right eye, even with bone in place. This could be avoided or at least improved upon by hitching up the orbital tissue with sutures passed through small burr holes in the grafted bone. In such a case, the accuracy of the reconstruction of the orbital floor could be improved by making a mirror image template of the left orbital floor following the construction of a stereolithographic model. We have decided to make no orbital correction as the minimal epiphora is acceptable and the patient is pleased with the result. Further surgery is planned to place implants into the graft and, at the same time, some reduction of the graft on the facial side will be carried out.

---

short length of the pedicle. While accepting that the pedicle length is short compared to the fibula flap, the osteocutaneous scapula flap also has a short pedicle unless retrograde dissection along the thoracodorsal artery is carried out. This will still leave a relatively short vein, as retrograde flow is not possible due to multiple valves in the thoracodorsal vein.

The evidence for an increased morbidity relating to the iliac crest has not been supported in the literature. In Liverpool, we carried out a study to compare the fibula and iliac crest donor sites and found that the morbidity was equivalent.[32] Similarly, retrospective non-comparative reports have shown a related morbidity, which has been acceptable. In the one main study from Toronto in which the outcome using iliac crest and fibula was compared for mandibular reconstruction, the failure rate was higher for the fibula series.[33] Similarly, Urken et al.[34] has published 137 consecutive iliac crest flaps with and without internal oblique with a failure rate of 4 per cent, which included 27 scapula, 46 fibula and 30 cases with double free flaps. There was no comment relating to a higher failure rate for any particular donor site. He also reported on the morbidity of the donor sites with major complications occurring in one fibula case that required a free latissimus dorsi or tissue loss and poor healing, and one iliac crest donor site that underwent the

repair of an abdominal wall hernia. He reported early gait problems in all patients with either a fibula or iliac crest donor site, but only two patients required assisted ambulation with a cane (donor site not specified).

The standard approach in Liverpool for patients requiring a midface reconstruction with a free flap in which the pedicle length may be insufficient to reach the larger vessels in the neck is as follows:

1. The submandibular gland may be removed with preservation of the facial vessels in continuity. If there is a need for a selective neck dissection then, if possible, the facial artery and vein are dissected out and kept in continuity. For modified radical neck dissections a planned vein graft is required but the facial artery may still be useable.
2. The submandibular incision can be extended vertically with dissection and preservation of the mandibular branch of the facial nerve to improve access to carry out the anastomoses.
3. In some cases, an arterial and venous vein graft can be prepared to allow the pedicle to be passed into the neck and in proximity to the larger arteries and veins in the neck. This can also be done with a temporary

shunt using the saphenous vein from the artery to the venous system, which can then be divided, and the anastomoses carried out knowing that at least two of the four anastomoses are working.

4. The methods of lengthening the pedicle for the iliac crest and the scapula have been mentioned, but this is especially useful in the scapula flap where the dissection can follow the thoracodorsal artery rather than into the subscapular system. The thoracodorsal artery is then anastomosed to the recipient artery and the blood flows in a retrograde manner into the circumflex arterial system. Using the angular branch of the thoracodorsal system to the angle of the scapula also lengthens the pedicle, but the bone stock is much less for the larger defects although the latissimus dorsi muscle offers the advantage of a natural looking epithelialized muscle base.

In our experience the main problem has been the poor run-off in the arterial system. In only one case have we required to provide a vein graft in the venous system as a result of the honeycombed septae that were present in the preferred recipient site of the anastomoses. Sometimes it is possible to use the retromandibular vein if sufficient length can be dissected out.

Box 53.4 illustrates the actions to be taken in the event of an arterial anastomoses that will not perfuse the flap.

Box 53.4

- If the run-off from the facial artery looks reasonable, then consider redoing the anastomoses and using a bolus of intravenous heparin (50–80 units/kg) prior to the release of the clamps.
- If the run-off from the facial artery is poor, then you can consider the following options:
  - fashion either an arterial (radial donor site) or venous (saphenous or cephalic site) graft and use that to run from the external carotid system once the run-off is adequate (usually the facial artery);
  - dissect out the external carotid artery up to its bifurcation to the maxillary and superficial temporal arteries and bring that forward for an end-to-end anastomoses to the deep circumflex iliac artery.

NB. Intravenous heparin must be used with caution in maxillectomy cases due to the increased risk of bleeding, and in my practice this is limited to a single i.v. bolus (50–80 units/kg), as well as routine deep-vein thrombosis prophylaxis.

It is routine in our practice to leave other parts of the closure so that the anastomoses and the flap can be finally checked at least 45 minutes after the completion of the microsurgery. We would also advise the use of the Cook-Swartz[35] continuous Doppler readout of the arterial or venous flow when using a muscle flap as these are often difficult to monitor from clinical observation alone.

KEY EVIDENCE

The level of evidence is either a case series (level 4) or expert opinion without explicit critical appraisal based on first principles. The attempts to classifiy the defects by the author and Cordeiro represent good reviews,[1, 2] and although attempts have been made to compare reconstruction to prosthetic rehabilitation[6] the evidence is also weak.

KEY LEARNING POINTS

- A multidisciplinary approach between ablative and reconstructive surgeons and the expert in oral and facial rehabilitation is essential.
- Muscle provides the best reconstruction of the lateral nasal walls and the oral cavity, which can be supplied by the iliac crest with internal oblique or the thoracodorsal angular artery flap with teres major, latissimus dorsi or serratus anterior.
- It is essential to reconstruct the orbital floor if the eye is retained in high maxillectomies (class 3), for which the iliac crest with internal oblique is probably the best option.
- There is no evidence that midface reconstruction as opposed to obturation compromises the oncological outcome.
- The careful preparation and preservation of the recipient vessels in continuity into the maxillary region will result in better reconstructive options, less need for vein grafting and thus a higher flap success rate.

REFERENCES

1. Brown JS, Rogers SN, McNally DN, Boyle M. A modified classification for the maxillectomy defect. *Head and Neck* 2000; 22: 17–26.
2. Cordeiro PG, Santamaria E. A classification system and algorithm for reconstruction of maxillectomy and midfacial defects. *Plastic and Reconstructive Surgery* 2000; 105: 2331–46.
3. Larson DL. A classification system and algorithm for reconstruction of maxillectomy and midfacial defects. *Plastic and Reconstructive Surgery* 2000; 105: 2347–8.
4. Cordeiro PG, Bacilious N, Schantz S, Spiro R. The radial forearm osteocutaneous "sandwich" free flap for reconstruction of the bilateral subtotal maxillectomy defect. *Annals of Plastic Surgery* 1998; 40: 397–402.

5. Matsui Y, Ohno K, Shirota T et al. Speech function following maxillectomy reconstructed by rectus abdominis myocutaneous flap. *Journal of Cranio-Maxillo-Facial Surgery* 1995; **23**: 160–4.

● 6. Rogers SN, Lowe D, McNally D et al. Health-related quality of life after maxillectomy: a comparison between prosthetic obturation and free flap. *Journal of Oral and Maxillofacial Surgery* 2003; **61**: 174–81.

7. Bradley P, Brockbank J. The temporalis muscle flap in oral reconstruction. A cadaveric, animal and clinical study. *Journal of Maxillofacial Surgery* 1981; **9**: 139–45.

8. Tideman H, Samman N, Cheung LK et al. Immediate reconstruction following maxillectomy: a new method. *International Journal of Oral and Maxillofacial Surgery* 1993; **22**: 221–5.

9. Curioni C, Toscano P, Fioretti C, Salerno G. Reconstruction of the orbital floor with the muscle-bone flap (temporal muscle with coronoid process). *Journal of Maxillofacial Surgery* 1983; **11**: 263–8.

10. Choung PH, Nam IW, Kim KS. Vascularized cranial bone grafts for mandibular and maxillary reconstruction. The parietal osteofascial flap. *Journal of Cranio-Maxillo-Facial Surgery* 1991; **19**: 235–42.

11. Genden EM, Buchbinder D, Urken ML. The submental island flap for palatal reconstruction: a novel technique. *Journal of Oral and Maxillofacial Surgery* 2004; **62**: 387–90.

12. Kim JT, Kim SK, Koshima I et al. An anatomic study and clinical applications of the reversed submental perforator-based island flap. *Plastic and Reconstructive Surgery* 2002; **109**: 2204–10.

13. Cheung LK, Samman N, Tideman H. Reconstructive options for maxillary defects. *Annals of the Royal Australasian College of Dental Surgeons* 1994; **12**: 244–51.

14. Hai HK. Repair of palatal defects with unlined buccal fat pad grafts. *Oral Surgery, Oral Medicine, Oral Pathology* 1988; **65**: 523–5.

15. Hashikawa K, Tahara S, Ishida H et al. Simple reconstruction with titanium mesh and radial forearm flap after globe-sparing total maxillectomy: a 5-year follow-up study. *Plastic and Reconstructive Surgery* 2006; **117**: 963–7.

16. Guelfucci B, Bizeau A, Gras R et al. Reconstruction of the palatal vault by free forearm cutaneosu flap in oncology. *Annales d'Oto-laryngologie et de Chirurgie Cervico Faciale* 2001; **118**: 233–7.

17. Nakayama B, Hasegawa Y, Hyodo I et al. Reconstructing a three dimensional orbitozygomatic skeletal model of titanium mesh plate and soft tissue free flap transfer following total maxillectomy. *Plastic and Reconstructive Surgery* 2004; **114**: 631–9.

18. Kim JH, Rosenthal EL, Ellis T, Wax MK. Radial forearm osteocutaneous free flap in maxillofacial oromandibular reconstruction. *Laryngoscope* 2005; **115**: 1697–701.

● 19. Brown JS, Jones DC, Summerwill A et al. Vascularized iliac crest with internal oblique muscle for immediate reconstruction after maxillectomy. *British Journal of Oral and Maxillofacial Surgery* 2002; **40**: 183–90.

20. Kelly CP, Moreira-Gonzalez A, Ali MA et al. Vascular iliac crest with inner table of the ilium as an option in maxillary reconstruction. *Journal of Craniofacial Surgery* 2004; **15**: 23–8.

21. Cordeiro PG, Santamaria E, Kraus DH et al. Reconstruction of total maxillectomy defects with preservation of the orbital contents. *Plastic and Reconstructive Surgery* 1998; **102**: 1874–84.

22. Davison SP, Boehmier JH, Ganz JC, Davidson B. Vascularized rib for facial reconstruction. *Plastic and Reconstructive Surgery* 2004; **114**: 15–20.

23. Sakuraba M, Kimata Y, Ota Y et al. Simple maxillary reconstruction using free tissue transfer and prostheses. *Plastic and Reconstructive Surgery* 2003; **111**: 594–8.

● 24. Peng X, Mao C, Yu GY et al. Maxillary reconstruction with the free fibula flap. *Plastic and Reconstructive Surgery* 2005; **115**: 1562–9.

25. Yazar S, Cheng MH, Wei FC et al. Osteomyocutaneous peroneal artery perforator flap for reconstruction of composite maxillary defects. *Head and Neck* 2006; **28**: 297–304.

26. Granick MS, Ramasastry SS, Newton ED et al. Reconstruction of complex maxillectomy defects with the scapular-free flap. *Head and Neck* 1990; **12**: 377–85.

● 27. Uglesic V, Virag M, Verga S et al. Reconstruction following radical maxillectomy with flaps supplied by the subscapular artery. *Journal of Cranio-Maxillo-Facial Surgery* 2000; **28**: 153–60.

28. Yamamoto K, Takagi N, Miyashita Y et al. Facial reconstruction with latissimus dorsi myocutaneous island flap following total maxillectomy. *Journal of Cranio-Maxillo-Facial Surgery* 1987; **15**: 288–90.

29. Villaret DB, Futran NA. The indications and outcomes in the use of the osteocutaneous radial forearm free flap. *Head and Neck* 2003; **25**: 475–81.

● 30. Urken ML, Vickery C, Weinberg H et al. The internal oblique-iliac crest osseomyocutaneous microvascular free flap in head and neck reconstruction. *Journal of Reconstructive Microsurgery* 1989; **5**: 203–14.

31. Urken ML, Buchbinder D, Weinberg H et al. Primary placement of osseointegrated implants in microvascular mandibular reconstruction. *Otolaryngology – Head and Neck Surgery* 1989; **101**: 56–73.

32. Rogers SN, Lakshmiah SR, Narayan B et al. A comparison of the long-term morbidity following deep circumflex iliac and fibula free flaps for reconstruction following head and neck surgery. *Plastic and Reconstructive Surgery* 2003; **112**: 1517–25.

33. Shpitzer T, Neligan PC, Gullane PJ et al. The free iliac crest and fibula flaps in vascularized oromandibular reconstruction: comparison and long-term evaluation. *Head and Neck* 1999; **21**: 639–47.

34. Urken ML, Weinberg H, Buchbinder D *et al*. Microvascular free flaps in head and neck reconstruction. Report of 200 cases and review of complications. *Archives of Otolaryngology – Head and Neck Surgery* 1994; **120**: 633–40.

35. Oliver DW, Whitaker IS, Giele H *et al*. The Cook-Swartz venous Doppler probe for the post-operative monitoring of free tissue transfers in the United Kingdom: a preliminary report. *British Journal of Plastic Surgery* 2005; **58**: 366–70.

Defect-based reconstruction: skull base

RALPH W GILBERT AND MARC COHEN

The only source of knowledge is experience.

Albert Einstein

INTRODUCTION

Since the introduction of craniofacial resection by Smith and Ketcham in the 1950s and 1960s, the treatment of skull base neoplasm has changed dramatically.[1,2] The treatment of an expanded number of lesions, with significantly decreased morbidity, is indicative of a number of critical advances. The evolution of multidisciplinary teams that specialize in the management of patients with cranial base tumours has been instrumental in the improvement of outcomes. These teams include a head and neck surgeon, neurosurgeon, reconstructive surgeon, as well as nonsurgical specialists, such as radiologists and pathologists. Advances in imaging have provided heightened understanding of anatomy and routes of tumour spread. In the past two decades, devices such as angled endoscopes, image guidance and specialized instrumentation have led to a paradigm shift with respect to the viability of an endoscopic approach to select lesions of the anterior skull base. Perhaps even more integral to the decreased morbidity of skull base surgery have been advances in reconstruction. Adequate and effective reconstruction of the skull base is important because of the location of the defect and the potential morbidity associated with reconstructive failure. Reconstruction after skull base surgery is a broad topic, for which a multitude of specific considerations need to be evaluated before a decision is made regarding the most appropriate intervention (**Table 54.1**).

As in other areas of the head and neck, the critical issues are maintenance of structure, function and aesthetics (**Table 54.2**). Inadequate separation of intracranial contents and the skin or mucosal surfaces leads to extremely high risk of central nervous system complications, including cerebrospinal fluid leak, meningitis and pneumocephalus. Of paramount importance in skull base reconstruction is a watertight dural closure. Furthermore, it is imperative that the reconstruction supports the brain and maintains a safe barrier between the central nervous system and the extracranial cavity. This barrier must eliminate dead space and cover vital structures including the central nervous tissue, as well as the carotid artery. In large resections, soft tissue bulk is required to maintain structure, function and aesthetics. Although not always required, significant resections of the anterior fossa involving the orbital rims or maxilla may

Table 54.1 Specific factors influencing reconstruction.

Location of skull base defect	Anterior skull base
	Middle or central skull base
	Posterior skull base
Size of Skull Base Defect	
Components of Defect	Bone
	Dura
	Brain
History of surgery altering reconstructive option	Prior use of local flap options
Factors hindering healing	History of radiation or chemoradiation
	Anticipated adjuvant treatment
	Diabetes or other systemic factors
	Contamination or infection

Table 54.2 Critical factors in skull base reconstruction.

Isolation of central nervous system	Watertight dural closure
	Soft tissue barrier external to dura
	Protection of critical vessels
	Obliteration of dead space
Maintenance of appropriate structure and facial form	Well-vascularized soft tissue that obliterates dead space
Oronasal separation	Bone grafts or flaps where appropriate
Reconstruction of orbitomaxillary complex	
Opportunity for prosthetic rehabilitation	Support for orbital prosthesis
	Adequate environment for dental implants
	Appropriate local tissue for auricular prosthesis

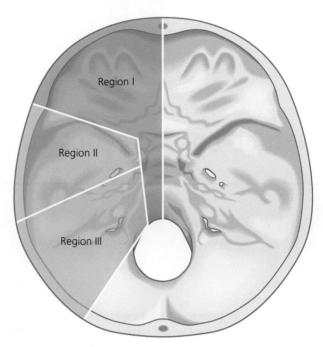

Figure 54.1 Illustration of classification of skull base defects. Region I, anterior skull base; region II, middle central skull base; region III, lateral skull base.

require bone reconstruction. Finally, skull base reconstruction may be necessary to provide a framework for the placement of orbital, dental or auricular prostheses.

SKULL BASE ANATOMY

The cranial base forms the floor on which the intracranial contents rest. It may be divided into three regions internally: the anterior, middle and posterior fossae. The extracranial skull base forms the roof of the paranasal sinuses and orbit, nasopharynx and infratemporal fossa (**Figure 54.1**). The anterior fossa extends from the anterior wall of the frontal sinus to the lesser wings of the sphenoid bone. The anterior fossa includes the cribriform plate of the ethmoid, roof of the ethmoid, crista galli and planum sphenoidale. The lateral aspect of the floor of the anterior cranial fossa provides the roof of the orbit. The middle fossa extends anteriorly from the lesser wings of the sphenoid to the anterior aspect of the petrous bone posteriorly. This encompasses the greater wing and body of the sphenoid sinus, as well as the anterior surface of the temporal pyramid. The extracranial aspect of the middle fossa corresponds with the infratemporal fossa. The posterior fossa involves the clivus, temporal bone pyramid and the entire occipital bone.

As benign and malignant processes can affect multiple regions of the skull base, a number of groups have classified regions based on the surgical approach. Jackson and Hide[3] divided the region into anterior and posterior regions based on the pattern of tumour spread. Jones et al.[4] labelled their surgical regions in concordance with the specific fossa and divided the skull into anterior, middle and posterior regions. Irish et al.[5] divided the skull base into three regions based on the anatomic and tumour correlates. Region I tumours extend from the anterior fossa to the clivus and foramen magnum posteriorly. Region II includes the middle fossa, as well as the infratemporal and pterygopalatine fossa. Region III is composed of the posterior fossa with possible tumour extension to the posterior aspect of the middle fossa. Nomenclature such as 'anterior skull base' generally refers to

lesions in region I and 'lateral skull base' refers to lesions of both regions II and III. Lesions of region I arise from the sinuses or orbit and are accessed via traditional open anterior craniofacial resection or endoscopic techniques. Region II lesions are most frequently accessed through an infratemporal approach with a hemicoronal incision, which may be combined with a mandibulotomy or transtemporal approach as needed. Region III lesions are lesions of the ear and temporal bone and are approached with a transtemporal approach.

SPECIFIC OPTIONS FOR RECONSTRUCTION OF THE SKULL BASE

As reconstruction of the cranial vault can involve a number of different grafts and flaps, the most commonly used options will be described first, followed by discussion of the specific considerations of the unique areas of the skull base (**Table 54.3**).

Grafts

Free grafts are nonvascularized tissues that heal initially via imbibition from surrounding tissues until inosculation and angiogenesis commences. Skin grafts were used routinely in the early stages of skull base surgery. These grafts, placed as dural patches or as overlay grafts, have extremely high rates of necrosis with subsequent cerebrospinal fluid (CSF) leak. Ketcham et al.[6] reported a nearly 50 per cent CSF leak rate in the early patient population undergoing craniofacial resection with skin graft reconstruction. While there is no role for primary skin grafting in modern skull base reconstruction,

Table 54.3   Specific options for reconstruction of the skull base.

Free grafts	Skin graft
	Fat
	Muscle
	Fascia lata
Local	Pericranial
	Galeal
	Temporalis
	Paramedian forehead/glabellar
	Scalp
	Nasoseptal
Regional	Pectoralis major
	Latissimus dorsi
	Trapezius flap
Free tissue	Rectus abdominis
	Radial forearm
	Anterolateral thigh
	Scapular system
	Iliac crest
	Gastro-omental
Allografts	Acellular dermis
	Bone
	Lyophilized dura
	Fibrin
Alloplasts	Titanium plates
	Hydroxyapatite
	Polyethylene

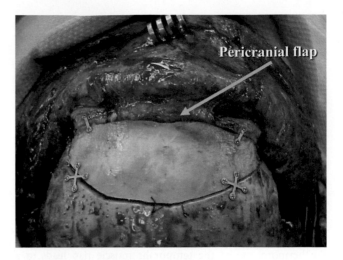

Figure 54.2   Illustration of a pericranial flap inset below the bone flap to reconstruct the anterior skull base.

there is a role for other free grafts. Fascia lata of the lateral thigh, or more locally available tissue such as temporalis fascia, provide material to overlay for dura or to obliterate small, well-contained spaces. Furthermore, fat, most often taken from the periumbilical area, can be used to obliterate dead space, most frequently used in the lateral skull base in the setting of primary interventions for benign disease. Disadvantages of free fat include the inability to heal when infected and the significant reduction of volume with time. Most surgeons would not use grafts if the resection site is in continuity with mucosal surfaces or in the setting of previous radiation impacting on the ability of the graft to heal. Furthermore, anticipation of adjuvant therapy would provide a relative contraindication to the use of free grafts. Free bone grafts, when necessary, can be obtained via split calvarial bone or a portion of a craniectomy. When this is inadequate bone stock, iliac crest bone may be harvested. However, most bony defects of the skull base need not be repaired, with the exception of the orbitomaxillary unit.

Local flaps

The use of local flaps in the field of skull base reconstruction was a significant advance in the early era of skull base surgery. Local tissue is mobilized and rotated or advanced, with critical emphasis on maintenance of the vascular supply. The use of local flaps is logical, as these tissues are relatively easy to harvest and have minimal donor site morbidity, usually located within the field of the ablation. Disadvantages of local

flaps include the availability of a limited stock of tissue precluding these as an option for large defects. Furthermore, the local tissues of revision cases or cases following radiation often have inadequate vascularity to be used for reliable reconstruction.

The most common local flap used in anterior skull base reconstruction is the galeal/pericranial flap. The pericranial flap, first described by Johns et al. in 1981,[7] is based on the bilateral supratrochlear and supraorbital arteries. The pericranial flap is dissected in a subgaleal plane to the supraorbital rims and then the pericranium is incised and carefully dissected anteriorly, preserving the blood supply. The advantages of this flap include its relative ease of harvest and the fact that the blood supply has been shown to be hearty, even when assessed by Doppler techniques.[8] This flap can provide a layer of separation between the central nervous structures and the paranasal sinuses for anterior skull base defects greater than 3.0×4.0 cm.[9] The galeal-pericranial flap includes the pericranium, as well as the galea and frontalis muscle, for a more hearty, well-vascularized option. In addition, a pericranial flap can be used in conjunction with a free bone graft ± titanium mesh with success in the appropriately selected patient.[10] Disadvantages of pericranial flaps include the inability to obliterate dead space and tenuous blood supply in the setting of prior surgery or radiation (**Figure 54.2**).

The scalp and forehead flaps have been used as a local flap for skull base reconstruction.[11, 12, 13] Unfortunately, these options for reconstruction are restricted by the limited tissue available for extension to the posterior aspect of the anterior cranial base. The forehead flap is supplied by the supratrochlear artery and can only be considered in the use of extremely small central defects in the anterior skull base. Furthermore, this flap is difficult to pass through the area of the defect and leaves an aesthetic donor site morbidity. Therefore, these flaps are infrequently used in the modern era of skull base reconstruction.

The temporal flap system is the most common local flap system used for the lateral skull base. The temporal flap system includes the temporoparietal fascia, the deep temporal fascia and the temporalis muscle. The temporoparietal fascia is based on the superficial temporal artery and can extend to and be used for reconstruction of the posterior fossa, as well as the middle fossa or infratemporal fossa. This local flap can provide an adequate separation of intracranial and extracranial contents without the ability to obliterate a large amount of dead space. Furthermore, temporoparietal fascia can be used as reconstruction after orbital exenteration. The temporalis muscle blood supply arises from the deep temporal artery via the maxillary artery and the middle temporal artery from the superficial temporal artery. Despite publications illustrating the utility of the temporalis muscle flap in anterior cranial fossa reconstruction, the temporalis local flap has limited applications to most clinicians, mainly limited to lateral soft tissue reconstruction.[14, 15] The disadvantages of this flap include limited mobility and compromise of vascularity with access to the skull base. Furthermore, use of the temporalis muscle flap leads to a hollowing out of the temporal fossa. Alloplastic implants are available to obviate this secondary deformity, however should be used cautiously in patients who are undergoing adjuvant therapy.

Regional flaps

Regional flaps are frequently used in head and neck reconstruction. In general, these axial flaps have the advantages of reliable blood supply, ease of harvest and significant amount of soft tissue available. Over the past decade, the limitations of regional flaps for skull base reconstruction have become evident, as these flaps are often limited in their reach into various defects. In addition, the distal aspect of these flaps, the area most critical for safe reconstruction, is the most sensitive to ischaemia. Therefore, in current practice, the use of regional flaps is limited, mainly to moderate-sized defects of the lateral skull base.

The pectoralis major flap is a pedicled myocutaneous flap based on the pectoral branch of the thoracoacromial artery that has been used in anterior and lateral skull base reconstruction.[16] This flap is tunnelled under the neck skin, over the clavicle, to the recipient site. This flap has limited reach to the paranasal sinuses and cannot extend superior to the inferior orbital rim; lateral extension of the pectoralis major flap is limited approximately to the area of the ear. As in other regional flaps, the distal tip of the pectoralis major flap is susceptible to necrosis. Furthermore, there can be unacceptable aesthetic ramifications of the pectoralis major flap harvest, especially in female patients.

The latissimus dorsi pedicled flap is a myocutaneous flap based on the thoracodorsal artery which branches off the subscapular vessels. The latissimus dorsi muscle can be elevated with or without the overlying skin. This flap has a large arc of rotation across the axilla. While the pedicled latissimus dorsi flap can reach most skull base defects when dissected fully, it is most useful in lateral skull base defects with large soft tissue components. The lower trapezius flap has also been used for skull base reconstruction. The inferiorly based trapezius flap, with blood supply from the dorsal scapular artery, has a long arc of rotation. The skin paddle may be fashioned to cover large areas of the lateral skull base. Care must be taken to preserve the blood supply

to this flap if a neck dissection is being performed at the same time.

Free tissue transfer

Over the past 20 years, free tissue transfer has been used to provide vascularized tissue for the most complex skull base defects. Because free flaps are not limited by a pedicle arc and there are multiple viable donor sites, there are numerous flap options. Furthermore, free tissue transfer provides the ability to recruit multiple tissue types and a variety of bulk depending on the defect characteristics. Increased complexity, leading to greater operative time is tempered by the ability to engage two teams. Most high volume centres have flap transfer success greater than 95 per cent, justifying the use of free tissue transfer in the reconstruction of skull base defects.[17, 18, 19, 20] The utility of free tissue transfer has been supported by the work of numerous authors at high volume centres. Neligan et al.[21] demonstrated significantly decreased morbidity with free flap reconstruction in comparison with patients undergoing a pedicled regional flap reconstruction. In this series from Princess Margaret Hospital, pedicled reconstructions had a complication rate of 75 per cent, compared with 34 per cent in the free flap cohort. Interestingly, the complication rate in the locally reconstructed group was similar to that of the free flap cohort, suggesting that regional flaps are less appropriate for reconstruction of the skull base, regardless of the defect. Furthermore, in a series from Memorial Sloan Kettering Cancer Center, Califano et al.[17] showed that major complication rates for patients undergoing free tissue transfer were comparable with those undergoing local or regional reconstruction (31 versus 35 per cent), despite a significant increase in complexity and extent of defect. Heth et al.[18] confirmed these data showing comparable levels of wound complications following local or free flap reconstructions of the skull base. Data from MD Anderson Cancer Center revealed an acceptable level of complications (30–36 per cent) with free tissue transfer for reconstruction of skull base defects.[19, 20]

A majority of publications describe microvascular reconstruction of the anterior and middle cranial base with a selected group of flaps; these include the radial forearm free flap, rectus abdominis and latissimus dorsi.[21, 22, 23] Lateral skull base reconstruction is most commonly performed with anterolateral thigh or scapular system of free flap. The following is a description of the most commonly used free flaps for skull base reconstruction.

RECTUS ABDOMINUS FLAP

The rectus abdominis free flap is based on the deep inferior epigastric artery and is either a myogenous or myocutaneous flap. The rectus abdominis was the initial workhorse flap in skull base reconstruction because of the amount of soft tissue that can be used for obliteration of a large defect.[24, 25] In a study of 35 patients, of whom most underwent reconstruction with a rectus abdominis free flap after skull base surgery, Teknos et al.[26] cited an acceptable cerebrospinal fluid leak rate of 8.6 per cent, with the incidence of meningitis less than 3 per cent. The specific advantages to this flap include long vascular pedicle, relative ease of harvest and large amount of soft tissue. In addition for cranial procedures, the flap can be harvested with a two team approach and does not require repositioning. The disadvantages of this reconstruction include a flap that can be too bulky for the purposes of skull base reconstruction. Furthermore, the rectus abdominis has the propensity to undergo significant atrophy which can be both an advantage and a disadvantage. The deep inferior epigastric perforator (DIEP) flap can also be used incorporating a smaller island of muscle and fascia with a reduction in donor site morbidity (**Figure 54.3**).

FREE FOREARM FLAP

The radial forearm free flap is a versatile flap that is based on the radial artery. This fasciocutaneous flap has the advantage of a relative ease of dissection and a long vascular pedicle. This flap provides the appropriate bulk for dural coverage and is thus optimal for anterior skull base defects lacking a large dead space.[27, 28] However, this flap lacks adequate soft tissue for use with larger defects and almost all lateral skull base defects. Chepeha *et al.* have shown acceptable risk of morbidity (35 per cent), in those patients undergoing salvage

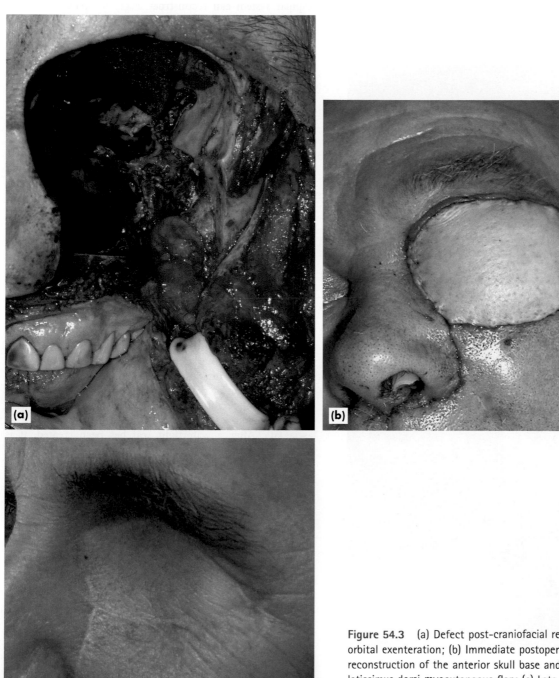

Figure 54.3   (a) Defect post-craniofacial resection including orbital exenteration; (b) Immediate postoperative result with reconstruction of the anterior skull base and dural defect with latissimus dorsi myocutaneous flap; (c) Late postoperative result latissimus dorsi flap, note muscular atrophy and suitability for ocular prosthetic.

anterior skull base resections who are reconstructed with forearm free flaps (**Figure 54.4**).[29]

ANTEROLATERAL THIGH FLAP

The anterolateral thigh free flap is a fasciocutaneous flap based on the perforators of the descending branch of the lateral circumflex femoral artery. The main advantage of this free flap is the ability to reconstruct larger defects, optimal for use in lateral skull base reconstruction. The pedicle is shorter than that of the radial forearm free flap. Hanasono et al.[30] have shown the anterolateral thigh free flap to be useful in skull base surgery (mainly lateral defects) with an overall complication rate of 29 per cent.

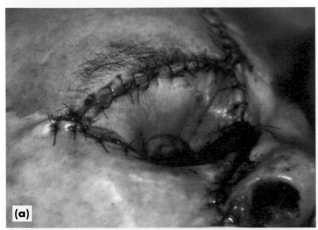

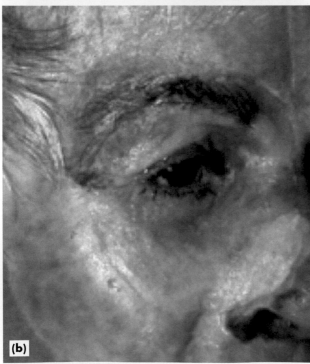

Figure 54.4 (a) Anterior skull base and exenteration reconstructed with a free forearm flap to create orbital depth for prosthetic reconstruction. (b) Prosthetic result with osseointegrated prosthesis.

SCAPULAR SYSTEM OF FLAPS

The scapular/parascapular system of free flaps include the parascapular, scapular, as well as latissimus dorsi flaps based on the circumflex scapular and thoracodorsal arteries. The circumflex scapular artery provides nutrient blood supply to the lateral border of the scapula. In addition, the angular artery, most commonly from the thoracodorsal artery, supplies the scapular tip and a distinct osseous flap may be harvested based on this vasculature. This system of flaps can by harvested as cutaneous, myocutaneous or osteomyocutaneous in consistency. The advantages of this system of flaps are the versatility of defects for which it can be utilized. The scapular system can reconstruct large, complex, composite defects of the skull base and orbitomaxillary complex. The bulk of tissue available makes using the latissimus dorsi flap an ideal soft tissue option for large lateral skull base defects. Furthermore, the bony scapula flaps are particularly suited for orbitomaxillary reconstruction; the vascularized bone provides a contour approximating either the palate or the anterior maxillary sinus wall. In addition, free bone obtained from the scapula can be used to the orbital floor. The disadvantages of the scapular system of flaps include the complexity of harvest, unique positioning, as well as a relatively short pedicle when using the circumflex scapular nutrient arteries to the lateral aspect of the scapula. When the angular branch is used for harvest of the scapula tip, there is sufficient pedicle length for skull base reconstruction without the need for vein grafts (**Figure 54.5**).

Specific sites of reconstruction

ANTERIOR SKULL BASE

Resection of anterior cranial base tumours often places central nervous system structures in continuity with adjacent mucosa of the nasopharynx or paranasal sinuses. After resection of tumours of the anterior skull base with or without resection of brain parenchyma, the initial most critical aspect of reconstruction is dural closure, with either primary techniques or use of autologous tissues, such as fascia lata. After a watertight seal has been created, it is

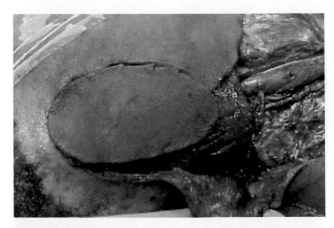

Figure 54.5 Rectus abdominus flap for reconstruction of lateral temporal bone defect (note volume matching).

imperative to place a vascularized soft tissue barrier, such as a pericranial flap, to protect and support the dural reconstruction. In dural defects that are unable to be closed, a large soft tissue barrier may be used to primarily seal and protect the intracranial contents. In addition, in patients who have undergone or will be undergoing radiation therapy, vascularized tissue coverage is critical to prevent wound breakdown and complication.

For most defects, the pericranial flap is the workhorse in the anterior cranial base, as it can provide dural coverage as far posteriorly as the clivus. Furthermore, this layer can be easily tacked to surrounding tissue providing the necessary barrier. In patients with large dural defects including orbital exenteration, our preference is to use a free flap combined with local flaps.[21] Situations favouring free flap reconstruction include tumour factors, patient factors and others. In patients who have had prior pericranial flaps or who have had prior irradiation or will be undergoing radiation, we favour free tissue reconstruction. Interestingly, some authors have shown that patients who receive preoperative radiotherapy have significantly higher rates of complication using the pericranial flaps than those receiving postoperative radiotherapy.[31] In the largest single institution report on skull base reconstruction, Hanasono et al.[20] advocate the use of free tissue transfer for skull base reconstruction in patients who have received preoperative radiation, chemotherapy or who have had previous surgery. Furthermore, surgeons should consider microvascular reconstruction in patients undergoing secondary reconstruction in an infected field with questionable local tissues. In addition, ablations that leave significant adjacent tissue defects require free flap reconstruction. These include resections involving the orbitomaxillary buttresses, orbit, maxilla and nose. Appropriate reconstruction of these areas, which have critical functional and aesthetic ramifications, cannot be understated.

Special consideration should be made for reconstructions that require bone. Defects of the midline anterior skull base do not need to be reconstructed. However, defects of the frontal sinus, orbital rims, maxillae or larger defects of the skull require bony reconstruction. Bone substitutes and different types of mesh are frequently used for repair of flat bones of the skull, however these are inappropriate if the space is in continuity with the paranasal sinuses or in the setting of preoperative radiation or planned adjuvant therapy. Reconstruction of the orbital floor can be performed with autologous bone.

The complexity of the orbit has led Chepeha et al.[32] to advocate for a subgrouping of defects in this region. They divided orbital defects into three groups, the first being orbital exenteration cavity alone, the second being the exenteration cavity with less than 30 per cent of the orbital rim excised, and the third being orbital exenteration cavity with resection of overlying skin, as well as the malar eminence or other bony areas. This group advocated for reconstruction of group 1 defects with a radial forearm free flap, group 2 defects with osseocutaneous forearm free flaps, and group 3 defects with osseocutaneous scapula free flaps. In a retrospective evaluation of reconstruction of anterior and middle cranial base defects of the orbitomaxillary complex at Memorial Sloan Kettering Cancer Center, Chiu et al.[23] described their approach, which entailed the use of the rectus abdominis in 97 per cent of patients, with the placement of nonvascularized bone in 11 per cent of patients. The incidence of complications was low, with a 0 per cent incidence of flap loss and a 7 per cent incidence of postoperative CSF leak. Interestingly, in patients undergoing maxillectomy with preservation of orbital contents, 52 per cent of these patients had eyelid complications or orbital position anomaly, highlighting the challenges related to adequate orbitomaxillary reconstruction. In all patients undergoing surgery of the orbitomaxillary unit with breach of the lacrimal apparatus, a dacryocystorhinostomy is to be performed to prevent epiphora or the need for a secondary procedure.

Our group favours use of the scapular tip bone flap for complex skull base reconstruction with orbitomaxillary involvement. As stated prior, this vascularized bone flap provides the advantages of similar shape to the palate or anterior maxillary sinus wall with local bone stock appropriate for reconstruction of the inferior orbital rim. The presence of a long pedicle and minimal donor site morbidity make this an optimal option for select anterior skull base defects. We have published on the successful use of this flap in our first 29 patients.[33, 34] There were no flap failures and eight patients (28 per cent) had orbital complications (five patients had ectropion and three had epiphora). All eight patients were treated successfully with minor secondary procedures.

For skull base defects that are small (usually less than 2 cm), created via an endoscopic approach, nasoseptal flaps are appropriate. The Hadad-Bassagasteguy flap, first described in 2006, provides adequate local tissue for local reconstruction of defects created using minimally invasive skull base surgery.[35] The nasoseptal flap is currently the standard of endoscopic reconstructive techniques as it is reliable, available bilaterally, and is easy to harvest in those trained in endoscopic techniques. As with other local flaps, nasoseptal flaps may be taken down and reused for revision cases.[36] In patients without viable tissue for a nasoseptal flap, the inferior turbinate pedicle flap is also an option for small skull base defects. For even larger defects of the skull base after extended endoscopic skull base resections, authors have recently published on novel techniques, such as bilateral nasoseptal flaps, as well as endoscopically harvested pericranial flaps.[37, 38] However, the limitation in endoscopic skull base surgery is inadequate reconstructive techniques for large defects or defects with high flow cerebrospinal fluid leaks.

Middle and central skull base

As in treatment of the anterior cranial base, critical to reconstruction of skull base defects of the middle skull base is watertight closure of the dura with soft tissue separation of the central nervous system and extracranial contents. In contrast to anterior defects, watertight closure of middle fossa defects is difficult, especially in the parasellar area. Therefore, an overlay of vascularized tissue in this area is critical. As in defects of the anterior vault, small defects of the bony skull base without dural disruption can be obliterated with a variety of tissue. Following endoscopic skull base surgery involving the sellar area, free fat or fascia lata can be used to obliterate dead space and create a barrier. However, larger defects are not adequately treated with this option. Certain cases of large dural defects without history of radiation can be repaired with a pericranial flap. In patients with large defects or with history of radiation, a free tissue transfer is indicated for reconstruction. Free tissue transfer options for the central skull base include myogenous flaps (such as the latissimus dorsi or the rectus abdominis), fasciocutaneous options (such as the radial forearm free flap) or enteric options (such as the gastro-omental flap, which provides a large amount of well-vascularized tissue that is able to fill soft tissue defects). Small bony defects of the middle skull base do not require reconstruction. If the defect extends to involve the orbital rims, zygoma, mandible, maxilla or temporal region, consideration must be given to bony reconstruction.

Lateral skull base reconstruction

Following transtemporal approaches, there is often a lateral skull base defect in which it is not feasible to perform a watertight dural closure. These defects are often as a result of surgical ablation of benign disease and adjuvant therapy is infrequently warranted. In this case, reconstruction involves placement of a soft tissue barrier alone. Some authors have shown good results using synthetic material, such as hydroxyapatite for reconstruction of the selected lateral skull base defect.[39] Care must be exercised on the use of alloplastic materials as they have a risk of extrusion, especially in those undergoing radiation treatment or where there is potential communication with the paranasal sinuses or mastoid cavity.

When vascularized tissue is desired, either a temporoparietal fascia pedicled flap or a temporalis muscle flap may be used. Some authors advocate the use of pectoralis major or trapezius regional flaps for reconstruction of composite lateral skull base defects.[40, 41, 42] When the patient has undergone preoperative radiation or postoperative radiation is anticipated, a free tissue transfer must be considered. The most commonly used options for free flaps in the lateral skull base include the anterolateral thigh, rectus abdominis and scapular system of flaps. In an evaluation of reconstruction after temporal bone resection, Dean et al.[43] cited an acceptable 15 per cent overall complication rate, in their series of 65 patients undergoing a variety of reconstruction (greater than 80 per cent free flaps). Moukarbel et al.[44] demonstrated a low rate of complications, with a 5 per cent flap complication rate using scapular flaps for 60 patients undergoing lateral skull base reconstruction. O'Connell et al.,[45] in a study evaluating 65 patients undergoing free flap reconstruction for lateral skull base and scalp reconstruction (68 per cent latissimus dorsi), demonstrated 100 per cent flap success with one patient requiring a re-exploration for venous thrombosis. Using data from two tertiary centres, Rosenthal et al.[46] proposed an algorithm for reconstruction of periauricular and lateral skull base defects; for patients with periauricular defects with preservation of the external auditory canal, the group suggested reconstruction with a radial forearm free flap. For patients with lateral temporal bone resection with auricular preservation, the anterolateral thigh free flap is the preferred reconstruction. Finally, patients undergoing lateral temporal bone resection with total auriculectomy require either the anterolateral thigh free flap or the rectus abdominis flap (**Figure 54.6**). Bony defects rarely require reconstruction in this area, unless the defect extends anterior to the

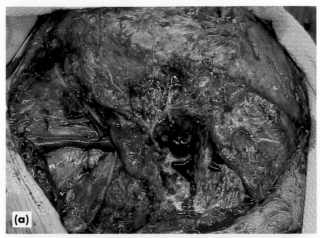

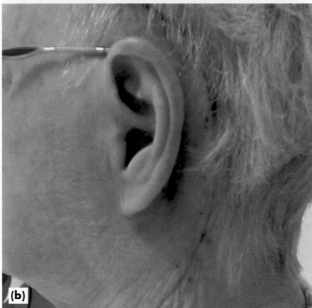

Figure 54.6 (a) Defect post-lateral temporal bone resection with ear and facial nerve preservation. (b) Postoperative result defect reconstructed with de-epithelialized anterolateral thigh flap for reconstruction of volume (note natural ear position).

mandible, orbit or other functionally or aesthetically critical area. Our philosophy is to use the appropriate flap for the defect size, staying focused on matching the volume of the reconstruction and the principles of skull base reconstruction.

Special consideration should be given to the patient undergoing facial nerve sacrifice. If clear margins can be obtained, facial nerve repair should be offered to all patients. As with trauma, if the nerve can be coapted without tension, then primary anastomosis may be performed. In the case that tension is present, primary repair should not be attempted and a nerve graft should be performed. Cable nerve grafts are usually performed using sural nerve, medial antebrachial cutaneous nerve or greater auricular nerve. Hanasono et al.[20] demonstrated evidence of reinnervation at 12 months in 75 per cent of patients undergoing facial nerve repair. Falcioni et al.[47] demonstrated 46 per cent of 56 patients undergoing facial nerve grafting recovered to a grade III on the House–Brackmann scale. The most important predictor of long-term function was repair prior to 12 months of injury. If a nerve stump cannot be identified proximally, consideration should be made to a hypoglossal nerve or a trigeminal nerve (motor nerve to masseter) to facial nerve graft. Without a viable distal nerve stump, muscle transposition of the masseter or temporalis should be considered. In the delayed setting, there are multiple options for facial nerve rehabilitation in the setting of proximal nerve stump absence: these include cross-facial nerve grafting with or without free muscle transfer or free muscle transfer innervated by the trigeminal nerve (nerve to masseter). When innervated options are not an option, a static sling can provide symmetry at rest. An important concern is the safety of the cornea. In patients with anticipated facial paralysis, a gold weight should be inserted in the upper lid. In the case of anticipated temporary paresis, the clinician should provide aggressive corneal care, including artificial tears, lubrication, and in some cases, tarsorrhaphy to prevent corneal injury.

Patients undergoing auriculectomy during skull base surgery are typically unable to undergo surgical reconstruction of the ear. Local tissue loss and scarring in the setting of treatment for malignant disease requiring adjuvant therapy, render autogenous reconstruction very challenging. Prosthetic reconstruction of the ear can be invaluable and provides outstanding aesthetic results. Auricular prosthesis may be retained with an osseointegrated framework or may be attached to the soft tissue reconstruction with tissue adhesive daily.

COMPLICATIONS OF SKULL BASE RECONSTRUCTION

Relating to the proximity of the skull base to critical structures, complications following reconstruction of this area can be devastating. The reported range of complications after skull base reconstruction is wide, ranging from approximately 10 to 60 per cent, with an international collaborative study citing a rate of 36 per cent.[22, 48, 49, 50, 51] Postoperative mortality was shown to be approximately 5 per cent. The incidence of postoperative complications is likely decreasing secondary to the increased expertise of multidisciplinary teams, improved reconstruction and better postoperative management. A decrease in complication rate may be tempered by expanded indications for surgical intervention, as well as intensification of neoadjuvant and adjuvant treatments.

The most feared complications of skull base reconstruction are those that arise from persistent contiguity of the central nervous system and the extracranial region. This leads to early complications, including unresolving cerebrospinal fluid leaks, predisposing to central nervous system (CNS) infection, such as meningitis, skull base osteomyelitis and abscess. Furthermore, persistent communication may progress to life-threatening tension pneumocephalus. As in all complex reconstruction, there is a risk of wound complication. As stated previously, the use of a regional pedicled flap places patients at higher risk for wound complication, likely related to marginal flap necrosis. Local flaps have a greater risk of wound complication in the patient who has

undergone radiation treatment or has comorbidity such as diabetes mellitus. The risk of free tissue transfer failure is relatively low, with most authors publishing approximately 95 per cent success rates with a range of 86–100 per cent.[19, 21, 24, 52, 53] Late complications of skull base reconstruction include facial deformity and inappropriate globe position, causing diplopia, malocclusion and trismus. Contributing factors that may lead to these outcomes include lack of bony support in the reconstruction, tissue atrophy or postoperative radiation fibrosis. Secondary procedures are often required to correct late complications of skull base surgery.

CONCLUSION

The ability to reconstruct the skull base following open and minimally invasive procedures is the most important predictor of operative success in oncologic procedures of the skull base. The formation of multidisciplinary skull base teams, advances in imaging and postoperative management, as well as the evolution of ablative and reconstructive techniques have dramatically reduced the morbidity of skull base surgery. Specific patient and tumour factors, including histology, location and size, as well as previous treatment, drive the selection of the appropriate skull base reconstruction. Adhering to the principles of reconstruction including providing a watertight dural seal, obliteration of dead space and maintaining the separation between the intracranial structures and the external skin and mucosal surfaces of the paranasal sinuses will provide the patient with greatest opportunity for a complication-free recovery.

KEY EVIDENCE

- The use of local flaps for small defects and free tissue transfer for large defects have been shown to have a significantly decreased complication rate compared to regional flaps.[21]
- The use of free tissue transfer limits morbidity in patients who have undergone preoperative chemotherapy, radiation or surgery.[20]

KEY LEARNING POINTS

- Management of patients with skull base lesions requires multidisciplinary teams of clinicians experienced in diagnosis, ablation and reconstruction of tumours in this critical area.
- Every patient should have treatment individualized to the specific tumour and patient factors, including previous treatment and plans for adjuvant therapy.
- Critical to skull base reconstruction is the creation of a watertight dural seal, obliteration

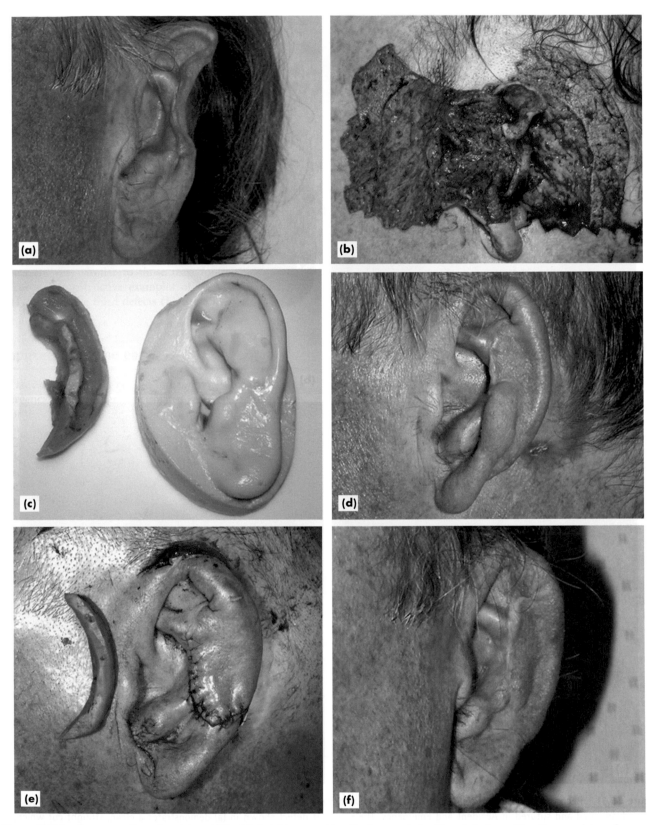

Figure 55.12 Reconstruction of auricle, middle third. A 63-year-old patient presented with a defect resulting from excision of a squamous cell carcinoma of the middle third of the pinna (a). Open dissection demonstrates the combined cartilage and soft tissue defects (b). A bespoke cartilage segment was carved from costal cartilage. In this patient, the costal cartilage was wide and thick enough to allow fabrication of the helical rim, antihelical segment and the base plate in one piece (c, left). A prosthetic model of the proportions of the normal ear was prepared preoperatively and used as a guide (c, right). Part of the lobular tissue was preserved with the skin envelope to maintain blood supply to the envelope at the conclusion of the first stage (d). This was trimmed and inset at the second stage, six months later (e, right). A C-shaped block of cartilage was further harvested and inset to maintain projection (e, left) which was then resurfaced with a superficial temporal artery flap with a scalp skin graft overlay. The final result (f) shows an improved contour, well-defined rim and satisfactory definition of the antihelix, albeit with a small residual scar.

Keloids of the ear

Keloids of the ear[18] typically occur in the ear lobes following piercing. They are much more common in the Asian and Afro-Carribean population and are a difficult problem to treat. The treatment options include intralesional injection of steroids (triamcinolone/prednisolone), which may be used in sequence or in conjunction with the use of localized pressure (ear clips) or surgery (intralesional excision). Patients should be cautioned that treatment does not yield uniform results and that recurrence is frequent. In patients with repeated recurrences, surgical options may be restricted.

THE FUTURE OF EAR RECONSTRUCTION

The aim of ear reconstruction is to create an anatomically accurate biological unit of living tissue which is matched to the patient. One of the stated disadvantages of using costal cartilage is that it has to be harvested as a separate procedure, and the full frame construct assembled from constituent cartilages. This results in longer operative times. There is potential pain, discomfort and healing problems with the chest wall harvest site, although with updated methods of nerve blocks and accurate closure these are much reduced compared to previously.[19] A prefabricated, histocompatible tissue-engineered frame would save both surgical and postoperative healing time.[20] Various materials have been trialled to provide the endoskeletons on which cultured chondroblastic and chondrocytic elements can be implanted, but these have so far only reached the cellular viability stage. Although cartilage can be successfully cultured in the laboratory, cultured cartilage is soft and lacks the rigidity and projectile strength of costal cartilage.

Costal cartilage-based auricular framework fabrication with well-vascularized local/regional tissue is the current gold standard for autologous reconstruction, and looks likely to remain so for the immediate future.

KEY EVIDENCE

- A retrospective analysis of 62 patients[21] following ear reconstruction showed that both children and adults reported improvement in social and leisure activities, postoperatively. There were similar improvements for patients undergoing both autologous and alloplastic reconstructions. Patients rated the appearances higher than the surgeons.
- A panel review of the outcomes of 51 microtia reconstructions[22] showed gradual improvement in results over time, and that the learning curve for microtia surgery is a long one.
- A prospective assessment of the psychosocial changes after autologous ear reconstruction in 21 patients,[23] compared to 23 patients who decided not to undergo surgical procedures, demonstrated significant improvements after surgery. More than 80 per cent of the patients would repeat their reconstructions if faced with the same surgical decision again, while 66 per cent reported good integration of the reconstructed ear with their body image.

KEY LEARNING POINTS

Anatomy

- The pinna is centred on the Frankfort horizontal plane (line drawn from the infraorbital foramen to the upper aspect of the external auditory meatus).
- The upper border of the pinna is level with the lateral aspect of the eyebrow.
- The lower border of the pinna is level with the alar base.
- The pinna is located one ear-length backwards from the lateral canthus.

Multidisciplinary management of ear reconstruction

Ear reconstruction is a multidisciplinary enterprise and should include input from the following specialties:

- otolaryngology
- plastic surgery
- clinical prosthetics
- craniofacial surgery
- audiology
- speech and language therapy
- clinical genetics

General reconstructive options

- A strong cartilage frame is required to resist the forces of secondary scar contracture.
- The height of the reconstruction can be matched to that of the opposite side in unilateral cases.
- A properly constructed autologous reconstruction is permanent, resistant to infection and requires no maintenance.
- If the patient is a child, they should be of an age where they are able to participate in the decisions regarding surgery.

Summary

- Beware of incorporating scar tissue into a repair.
- The liberal use of vascularized tissue is recommended.
- There is as yet no ideal alloplastic implant.
- Scalp skin grafts provide the best texture and colour match.
- Costal cartilage provides the best tissue for framework reconstruction.

REFERENCES

- 1. Tanzer RC. Total reconstruction of the external ear. *Plastic and Reconstructive Surgery* 1959; **23**: 1–15.
  2. Tanzer RC. Deformities of the auricle. In: Converse JM (ed). *Reconstructive plastic surgery*, 2nd edn. Philadelphia: WB Saunders, 1977: 1675–6.
  3. Brent B. The acquired auricular deformity: a systematic approach to its analysis and reconstruction. *Plastic and Reconstructive Surgery* 1977; **59**: 475–85.
- 4. Nagata S. A new method of total reconstruction of the auricle for microtia. *Plastic and Reconstructive Surgery* 1993; **92**: 187–201.
- 5. Nakajima H, Imanishi N, Minabe T. The arterial anatomy of the temporal region and the vascular basis of various temporal flaps. *British Journal of Plastic Surgery* 1995; **48**: 439–50.
  6. Da Vinci LVII. On the proportions and on the movements of the human figure. In: Richter JP (ed). *The literary works of Leonardo Da Vinci*. Plate VII. London: Sampson Low, Marston, Searle and Rivington, 1883; I: 310.
- 7. Tolleth H. Artistic anatomy, dimensions, and proportions of the external ear. *Clinics in Plastic Surgery* 1978; **5**: 337–45.
  8. Brent B. The correction of microtia with autogenous cartilage grafts: I. The classic deformity. *Plastic and Reconstructive Surgery* 1980; **66**: 1–12.
  9. Brent B. The correction of microtia with autogenous cartilage grafts, II. Atypical and complex deformities. *Plastic and Reconstructive Surgery* 1980; **66**: 13–21.
- 10. Brent B. Technical advances in ear reconstruction with autogenous rib cartilage grafts: personal experience with 1200 cases. *Plastic and Reconstructive Surgery* 1999; **104**: 319–34.
  11. Nagata S. Modification of the stages in total reconstruction of the auricle: Part IV. Ear elevation for the constructed auricle. *Plastic and Reconstructive Surgery* 1994; **93**: 254–66; discussion 267–8.

  12. Tan ST, Abramson DL, MacDonald DM, Mulliken JB. Molding therapy for infants with deformational auricular anomalies. *Annals of Plastic Surgery* 1997; **38**: 263–8.
- 13. Antia NH, Buch V. Chondrocutaneous advancement flap for the marginal defect of the ear. *Plastic and Reconstructive Surgery* 1967; **39**: 472–7.
  14. Dieffenbach JF. *Die Operative Chirurgie*. Leipzig: PA Brockhas, 1845.
  15. Salyapongse A, Maun LP, Suthunyarat P. Successful replantation of a totally severed ear. *Plastic and Reconstructive Surgery* 1979; **64**: 706–7.
  16. Pribaz JJ, Crespo LD, Orgill DP *et al*. Ear replantation without microsurgery. *Plastic and Reconstructive Surgery* 1997; **99**: 1868–72.
  17. Lin SC, Chiu HY, Yu JC, Lee JW. Replantation of part of an ear as an open fan composite graft. *British Journal of Plastic Surgery* 1997; **50**: 135–8.
  18. Cheng LH. Keloids of the ear lobe. *Laryngoscope* 1972; **82**: 673–81.
- 19. Kawanabe Y, Nagata S. A new method of costal cartilage harvest for total auricular reconstruction: part I. Avoidance and prevention of intraoperative and postoperative complications and problems. *Plastic and Reconstructive Surgery* 2006; **117**: 2011–18.
  20. Xu JW, Johnson TS, Motarjem PM *et al*. Tissue-engineered flexible ear-shaped cartilage. *Plastic and Reconstructive Surgery* 2005; **115**: 1633–41.
- 21. Horlock N, Vögelin E, Bradbury ET *et al*. Psychosocial outcome of patients after ear reconstruction: a retrospective study of 62 patients. *Annals of Plastic Surgery* 2005; **54**: 517–24.
- 22. Suutarla S, Rautio J, Klockars T. The learning curve in microtia surgery. *Facial Plastic Surgery* 2009; **25**: 164–8.
- 23. Steffen A, Wollenberg B, König IR, Frenzel H. A prospective evaluation of psychosocial outcomes following ear reconstruction with rib cartilage in microtia. *Journal of Plastic, Reconstructive and Aesthetic Surgery* 2010; **63**: 1466–73.

The management of the paralysed face

PATRICK ADDISON AND PETER C NELIGAN

What sunshine is to flowers, smiles are to humanity. These are but trifles, to be sure; but, scattered along life's pathway, the good they do is inconceivable.

Joseph Addison (1672–1719)

INTRODUCTION

Facial nerve paralysis is a distressing and disfiguring condition because of the loss of facial symmetry and expression both at rest and during voluntary movement. Resting tone and coordinated movement of the muscles of facial expression not only convey the aesthetics of the face but facilitate verbal and non-verbal communication. Consequently, these patients have a tendency to avoid social interactions and may retreat from society altogether. In congenital or early-onset facial paralysis the child's psychosocial development may be severely compromised. In addition, the loss of normal ocular and oral function can result in corneal exposure keratitis, epiphora and difficulty with speech and alimentation. Collapse of the internal nasal valve may create respiratory difficulties and the specialized functions of taste, hearing and lacrimal gland secretion may also be impaired. Facial paralysis therefore results in a combination of functional and aesthetic concerns often associated with profound psychosocial difficulties.

Although there are many aetiologies underlying congenital and acquired facial paralysis, the reconstructive techniques currently practised are relatively few and the management of the patient depends more upon the duration and extent of paralysis than its cause. The management plan is therefore based upon a thorough assessment of the patient's individual requirements and motivation, their general health and their suitability for operative intervention. The involvement of a multidisciplinary team variably comprising plastic surgeons, neurosurgeons, neurologists, oncologists, otolaryngologists, ophthalmologists, psychologists and physiotherapists helps ensure a favourable outcome.

For clarity, the word 'paralysis' refers to complete loss of muscle movement, whereas 'paresis' is a partial loss or weakness. 'Palsy' incorporates both paralysis and paresis. The terms are used interchangeably in this chapter.

HISTORY OF SURGERY FOR FACIAL PALSY

The Scottish surgeon Sir Charles Bell first identified the facial nerve as the motor supply to the muscles of facial expression in 1829. Fifty years later, Drobnick performed the first facial nerve repair by coaptation of the facial and spinal accessory nerves and in 1927, Bunnell attempted the first intratemporal repair of the facial nerve.[1]

For cases where facial nerve repair was not possible, other reconstructive techniques were sought. In 1971, Thompson reported the first series of non-vascularized muscle transplants for facial paralysis using the palmaris longus and extensor digitorum brevis muscles. He subsequently advocated microneural coaptation to the contralateral facial nerve.[2, 3] With the development of refined microsurgical technique and equipment in the 1970s, Scaramella pioneered the use of cross-facial nerve grafting as a technique for the reinnervation of unilateral facial paralysis, heralding the modern era of reanimation surgery.[4]

Harii *et al.* described the first successful use of vascularized free muscle transfer for facial reanimation, using the gracilis muscle to reproduce a smile in 1976.[5] Initially, the gracilis transfer was innervated by the motor branch to the temporalis muscle, but later, the cross-facial nerve graft was used, allowing more spontaneous rehabilitation.[6] Today, free tissue transfer remains the gold standard of facial reanimation surgery, yielding excellent and reproducible results.[7, 8, 9] In 1982, Terzis and Manktelow described the dual innervated pectoralis minor transfer making use of two separate cross-facial nerve grafts to improve independent motor control for eyelid closure and lip elevation[10] although the technique has proved less useful than first anticipated. Manktelow also described the 'minitransfer' of a thinned segment of the gracilis as a means of reducing bulk in the cheek without compromising muscle power or excursion.[11]

Free muscle transfer with cross-facial nerve grafting is normally a two-stage procedure with at least six months between operations. Recently, interest has again focused on single-stage procedures, making use of a variety of donor muscles with long nerves that obviate the need for cross-facial nerve grafting.[12, 13, 14, 15, 16]

Although reconstruction of the smile remains one of the greatest challenges in facial paralysis surgery, its other manifestations must also be addressed. A number of adjunctive techniques have been developed to correct brow ptosis and eyelid closure, and a variety of static procedures are designed to achieve facial symmetry at rest for those patients unable or unwilling to undergo free muscle transfer.

FUNCTIONS OF THE FACIAL NERVE

The frontalis, orbicularis oris and oculi, zygomaticus major, levator labii superioris and depressor labii inferioris are functionally the most important muscles innervated by the facial nerve. In the upper face, paralysis of the frontalis results in ptosis of the forehead and brow that worsens over time with gravity and the loss of skin elasticity associated with ageing. As a result, the patient may appear to be angry, depressed or unduly serious, the upper visual field may be obstructed and some loss of facial expression is inevitable. Impaired orbicularis oculi contraction prevents normal eyelid closure and may compromise the ability to blink. Globe exposure is further exacerbated by retraction of the upper eyelid due to the unopposed action of the levator palpebrae muscle. Elevation of the upper lid is a function of the occulomotor nerve (CN III) and the sympathetic nervous system and is therefore preserved in pure facial nerve paralysis. Loss of tone in the lower lid due to paralysis of the orbicularis and the effects of gravity, results in ectropion and loss of contact between the globe and the canalicular system, precluding normal tear drainage. These factors, combined with lacrimal gland dysfunction, result in desiccation of

the globe, exposure keratitis and epiphora, as well as an expressionless, staring eye.

It is important to appreciate that congenital or neonatal facial palsy rarely produces the same severity of ocular symptoms. The eye appears to tolerate exposure relatively well and the soft tissue elasticity is better. However, as the child grows into adulthood, the same problems may arise.

In the mid and lower face, there are other significant functional and aesthetic consequences of facial paralysis. The perioral retractor muscles normally lift the upper lip, depress the lower lip and move the oral commissures outward while the orbicularis oris allows pursing and protrusion of the lips and assists with labial speech production. Buccinator helps control the food bolus when chewing and prevents food accumulation in the buccal sulcus. Poor oral continence, drooling, cheek biting and poor speech are troublesome symptoms for many patients, and for some the collapse of the nasal valve due to the loss of cheek muscle tone may cause difficulties with nasal breathing. Loss of these functions has predictable results, but the inability to produce a spontaneous and symmetrical smile is perhaps the most devastating of all because patients may be perceived to be emotionally and mentally abnormal on account of their physical appearance.

Each of these symptoms and signs of facial paralysis may be uni- or bilateral, partial or complete. Although unilateral facial paralysis is far more common, the bilateral condition is functionally more severe and leaves the patient totally devoid of facial movement and expression even though the face is relatively symmetrical at rest.

FACIAL NERVE ANATOMY

The facial nerve is composed of approximately 10 000 neurons, 70 per cent of which supply the muscles of facial expression together with the stylohyoid, posterior belly of the digastric and the stapedius muscles. The remainder comprises the 'nervus intermedius', which carries somatosensory fibres from the anterior two-thirds of the tongue and parasympathetic secretomotor fibres to the parotid, submandibular, sublingual and lacrimal glands. The facial nerve also contains a few general somatic afferent fibres, which join the auricular branch of the vagus nerve to supply sensation to the external auditory meatus, and visceral afferents, which innervate the mucous membranes of the nose, palate and pharynx via the greater palatine nerve. It is an embryological derivative of the second branchial arch.

The anatomy of the facial nerve is described as having a central, intratemporal and extratemporal course (**Figure 56.1**).[17, 18]

Central course

Motor and sensory neurons originate at the pre- and post-central gyri of the cerebral cortex, passing through the internal capsule and upper midbrain to the pons, where they synapse in the facial nerve nucleus. The tracts supplying the upper face cross back and forth in the pons, whereas those to the lower face cross only once. As a result, the facial

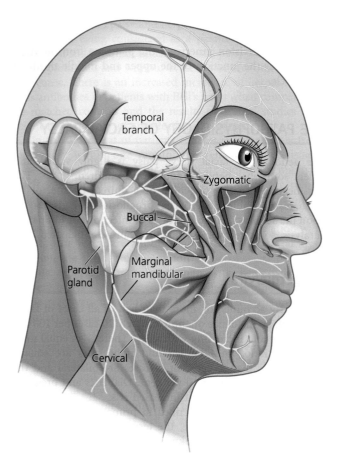

Figure 56.1 Facial nerve anatomy. The extratemporal facial nerve.

nerve nucleus receives bilateral cortical projections destined for the upper facial muscles, and unilateral projections innervating the lower facial muscles. Clinically, an injury proximal to this level will spare function in the orbicularis oculi and frontalis muscles allowing for eyelid closure and forehead elevation.

The facial nerve nuclei receive afferent input from both the trigeminal nerve and acoustic nuclei, respectively forming a component of the corneal and stapedial reflexes.

Neurons exiting the facial nerve nucleus pass around the abducens nucleus as they emerge from the brainstem. A lesion near the fourth ventricle may therefore involve both these nerves and the superior salivatory nucleus resulting in a dry eye, as well as cranial nerve (CN) VI and VII dysfunction.

The facial nerve's parasympathetic fibres originate in the superior salivatory nucleus and travel with the trigeminal nerve (CN V). The lacrimal nerve travels with V1, the ptery-gopalatine nerve with V2 and the lingual nerve/chorda tympani with V3.

The facial nerve emerges from the brainstem accompanied by the nervus intermedius, which lies between the facial nerve superiorly and the vestibulocochlear nerve inferiorly. The nervus intermedius conveys taste fibres from the anterior two-thirds of the tongue via the chorda tympani and from the soft palate via the palatine and greater petrosal nerves. In addition, preganglionic parasympathetic innervation of the submandibular, sublingual and lacrimal glands are carried with the nervus intermedius, as is a small sensory component from the skin of the auricle and postauricular area.

The facial nerve, the nervus intermedius and the vestibulocochlear nerve are in close proximity at the cerebellopontine angle and in the internal auditory canal. Consequently, lesions at these levels can result in disturbances of lacrimal function, taste, salivary flow, hearing, balance and facial movement.

Approximately 2 cm after leaving the brainstem, the nerves enter the internal auditory canal.

Intratemporal course

The facial nerve travels through the narrow petrous temporal bone for a distance of 2.5–3 cm, occupying up to 50 per cent of the canal's volume. Here, it is vulnerable to inflammatory processes and to traumatic injuries of the bone, such as basal skull fractures. The canal is divided into three segments.

After traversing the short and narrow labyrinthine segment, the facial nerve changes direction at the geniculate ganglion to enter the tympanic segment of the bony canal. Here, the nervus intermedius and the facial nerve form a common trunk. The geniculate ganglion is joined by afferent fibres from the chorda tympani. Three nerves branch from the ganglion: the greater superficial petrosal nerve carrying secretomotor fibres to the lacrimal gland; the lesser petrosal nerve carrying secretory fibres to the parotid gland; and the external petrosal nerve, an inconstant branch carrying sympathetic fibres to the middle meningeal artery.

The distal portion of the facial nerve emerges from the middle ear between the posterior wall of the external auditory canal and the horizontal semicircular canal. Here, the facial nerve reaches the beginning of the mastoid segment. Three branches exit from this segment of the facial nerve: the nerve to the stapedius muscle; the chorda tympani; and the nerve from the auricular branch of the vagus. The facial nerve continues vertically down the anterior wall of the mastoid process to the stylomastoid foramen. At this point, the nerve contains only sensory and motor fibres. A branch exits the nerve just below the stylomastoid foramen and innervates the posterior wall of the external auditory canal and a portion of the tympanic membrane.

Extracranial course

Immediately after exiting the stylomastoid foramen, the facial nerve gives off a posterior auricular branch, which innervates the superior and posterior auricular and the occipitalis muscles, as well as providing sensation to an area behind the earlobe. Two separate small branches innervate the stylohyoid muscle and posterior belly of the digastric.

As the facial nerve passes from the stylomastoid foramen to the posterior border of the parotid, it passes anterior to the posterior belly of the digastric, lateral to the styloid process and external carotid artery then posterior to the facial vein. Surgical landmarks to the facial nerve include the tragal pointer and the posterior belly of the digastric. In children, the facial nerve will be found more superficially because of incomplete development of the parotid gland and pneumatization of the mastoid.

Table 56.2 Effects of facial nerve injury by region.

Site of Injury	Effect	Signs and symptoms	Investigations
Extracranial facial nerve injury	Muscles of facial expression	Brow ptosis Inability to close eyes Lower lid laxity Facial asymmetry	Facial movement
Tympanomastoid	Taste fibres Salivary glands Stapedius muscle	Loss of taste Dry mouth Hyperacousis	Taste test Salivary test Stapedial reflex
Geniculate ganglion	Lacrimal gland Mucosal glands	Dry eye Dry nose	Schirmer's test
Internal acoustic canal	Cranial nerve VIII	Loss of hearing and balance	Audiology
CNS		Sparing of frontalis and orbicularis function	CNS examination

CNS, central nervous system.

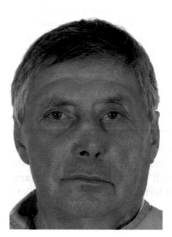
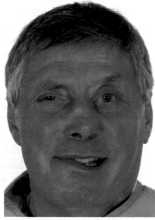

Figure 56.2 Synkinesis. Note closure of the eye when the patient attempts to smile.

discomfort and oral competence. In terms of reconstructive options, some patients are concerned primarily with facial symmetry at rest, while others will seek facial reanimation in order to be able to smile.

The initial evaluation of facial movement and expression can be made during the history taking. Subsequently, the examiner should specifically and systematically identify the functioning muscles and grade their power. Asking the patient to raise their brow, close their eyes, smile, show their teeth and pucker their lips will reveal most deficiencies. Synkinesis, seen most commonly as eye closure with smiling, should be noted (**Figure 56.2**). The degree of voluntary movement of the facial muscles can be graded or classified, and monitored by systems such as those of House and Brackmann (**Table 56.3**).[28, 29] Digital photography and video can help document the condition and assess future response to treatment.

The head and neck examination should include the ears, eyes, parotid glands and neck as well as a thorough evaluation of the function of all the cranial nerves. Formal audiological and ophthalmologic examination may be appropriate, and radiological, electrophysiological and other special tests arranged.

On examination of the eye, visual acuity and corneal sensation should be assessed. The height of the palpebral aperture should be recorded bilaterally. The palpebral fissure

normally narrows with smiling and failure to do so can result in an unsatisfactory aesthetic. The presence of a Bell's reflex should be sought, as this will affect the degree of corneal exposure when the patient attempts to close the eye. Finally, lower eyelid position and tone should also be recorded and compared with the normal side (**Figure 56.3**).

The lower face should be observed at rest and with animation. Asymmetry of the nose and mouth are noted and can be measured using a hand-held transparent ruler (**Figure 56.4**) which is convenient and reproducible, although more sophisticated computer imaging techniques are available.[19] The position of the vermilion border at the base of the nose, mid upper lip and oral commissure can be measured with respect to the dental midline and horizontal plane both at rest and during maximal smile. The strength and direction of pull while smiling on the normal side are documented and act as a guide to reconstruction.[19] With a unilateral paralysis, there is often weakening of the nasolabial fold, deviation of the philtrum and entire oral sphincter toward the normal side and depression of the commissure at rest.

In children, the physical examination and subsequent radiological and neurophysiological testing are similar to adults but subject to some limitations of cooperation. Physical examination may reveal other cranial nerve palsies or

Table 56.3 The House–Brackmann classification of facial nerve function.

Grade	Description	Characteristics
I	Normal	Normal facial function in all areas
II	Mild dysfunction	Slight weakness or synkinesis
III	Moderate dysfunction	Obvious asymmetry, but not disfiguring, synkinesis, contracture, or hemifacial spasm; complete eye closure with effort
IV	Moderately severe dysfunction	Obvious weakness or disfiguring asymmetry; normal symmetry and tone at rest; incomplete eye closure
V	Severe dysfunction	Only barely perceptible motion; asymmetry at rest
VI	Total paralysis	No movement

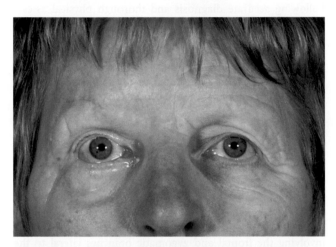

Figure 56.3 The upper and lower eyelids in facial paralysis. Note upper lid retraction and scleral show on the patient's right side. The frontal rhytids are absent on the right.

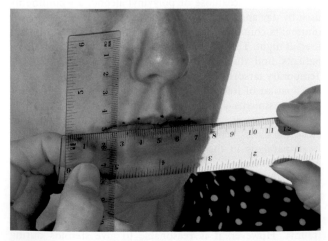

Figure 56.4 Ruler measurement of lip and commissure excursion.

other congenital anomalies. These should be investigated and managed appropriately.

Thoughtful consideration and assessment of potential nerve and muscle donor sites for reanimation procedures should also be made.

INVESTIGATIONS FOR FACIAL PALSY

Blood tests

Routine preoperative blood tests may be ordered according to the patient's general health and the proposed operation. Supplementary special investigations may also be necessary to determine the aetiology of facial palsy based upon the history and physical examination. These may include fluorescence *in situ* hybridization for velocardiofacial syndrome, toxoplasmosis, rubella, cytomegalovirus and herpes simplex screening. When syndromic cases are suspected, chromosomal analysis may be indicated.

Imaging studies

Computed tomography (CT) and magnetic resonance imaging (MRI) are useful in the diagnosis of injury to, or tumour around, the intratemporal or intracranial portions of the facial nerve. The path of the facial nerve can be seen, and swelling or disruption noted.[30] Associated abnormalities of the ear, skull base and mandible suggest a developmental aetiology of the paralysis. MRI provides the best definition of the nerve and the surrounding soft tissue and gadolinium can be used to enhance soft tissue resolution. Aplasia or hypoplasia of the nerve strongly suggests a developmental aetiology whereas haematoma and soft tissue swelling point to a traumatic origin.

Electrophysiology

Electrophysiological testing can help to determine the site and extent of injury, the potential for recovery and progression. The following tests are performed by percutaneous stimulation of the facial nerve. They are, however, of little value in patients with incomplete paralysis.

The nerve excitability test (NET) is low-cost and practicable, but subjective.[31] A stimulating electrode is placed over the stylomastoid foramen, and the threshold current required to produce a twitch on the paralysed side of the face is compared with the contralateral side. A difference of greater than 3.5 mA indicates a poor prognosis for return of facial function.

The maximum stimulation test (MST) is a modified version of the NET. The difference between the stimulus required to depolarize all facial nerve branches on the paralysed and contralateral sides is compared and graded. An equal or slightly decreased response on the involved side favours complete recovery. An absent or markedly decreased response carries a poor prognosis. Sequential testing allows for assessment of recovery.

Electroneuronography (ENoG) is an objective, qualitative measurement of neural degeneration. Following facial nerve stimulation, muscle response is recorded. The peak-to-peak amplitude of the evoked compound action potential is proportional to the number of intact axons. The normal and paralysed sides of the face are compared. A reduction in amplitude on the involved side to 10 per cent or less of the normal side indicates a poor prognosis, whereas reduction of less than 90 per cent within 3 weeks of injury suggests a very high likelihood of spontaneous recovery. ENoG studies are useful in determining the timing and the need for surgical intervention.[32]

The NET, MST and ENoG are useful in the degenerative phase but will give normal results during the first 72 hours after injury until nerve degeneration reaches the site of the test stimulus. Furthermore, these tests rely on comparison with a normal contralateral facial nerve, and so, are of no use in bilateral paralysis.

Fibrillation potentials indicating axonal degeneration do not appear until 10–14 days post-onset of facial paralysis. After this time, however, electromyography (EMG) can be used to assess the potential for muscle recovery. Needle electrodes are placed into the muscle and action potentials generated by voluntary and involuntary activity are recorded. Fibrillation potentials indicate degeneration and polyphasic potentials indicate reinnervation. The latter appear between 6 and 12 weeks before clinical return of function is noted.

Newborns who present with a complete facial nerve paralysis should undergo electrophysiological testing within the first 3 days to differentiate congenital and traumatic aetiologies. In traumatic cases, the nerve can be stimulated for up to 5 days post-injury and fibrillation potentials will be seen on EMG at 10–14 days. In congenital cases, neither usually occurs.

Topographical testing

Specific tests can be used to localize the site of injury to the facial nerve and therefore assist in diagnosis and management. If the lesion is distal to a particular branch of the nerve, the function of that branch will be spared. Moving distally from the brainstem, these tests include the stapedial reflex test (stapedial branch), taste testing (chorda tympani), salivary flow rates and pH (chorda tympani):

- Schirmer's test evaluates lacrimation, a function of the greater superficial petrosal nerve. A strip of filter paper is placed in the lower conjunctival fornix bilaterally. After 3–5 minutes, the length of the strip that is moist is compared to the normal side. A reduction of 25 per cent or a total of less than 25 mm in 5 minutes is abnormal and indicates injury to the greater superficial petrosal nerve or to the facial nerve proximal to the geniculate ganglion. When local anaesthetic is used to avoid reflex tearing, the test is called Schirmer's 2.
- Stapedial reflex testing evaluates the stapedius branch of the facial nerve. A loud tone is presented to either ear evoking a reflex movement of the stapedius muscle and a change in the tension of the tympanic membrane. This can be recorded and compared with the normal side. In Bell's palsy, absence of the stapedial reflex during the

first 2 weeks is common and is usually of no prognostic significance.
- Taste sensation to the anterior two-thirds of the tongue is carried by the chorda tympani and can be assessed by placing salt, sugar or lemon juice on the tongue. The test is, however, extremely subjective. Tongue biopsy may reveal the absence of taste papillae within 10 days of symptom onset.
- Salivary flow rates can be assessed to evaluate the integrity of the chorda tympani by cannulation of Wharton's duct, but the test is difficult to perform. A 25 per cent reduction in flow from the involved side is considered abnormal, as is a salivary pH of less than 6.1.

In practical terms, these tests are rarely carried out because interpretation is difficult; a careful history and examination supplemented with CT and MRI provide the most useful information.

THE TREATMENT OF FACIAL PALSY

Following accurate diagnosis and thorough physical assessment (see **Figure 56.5**), the probability of spontaneous recovery of nerve function must be estimated and supplemented by appropriate use of electrophysiological testing. Time should be allowed for such recovery to occur spontaneously, and intervention should be limited to conservative therapies or temporary surgical procedures to protect the eye from exposure keratitis.

Further treatment of facial paralysis can be medical or surgical.

Medical therapy

The most urgent consideration in facial palsy is protection of the eye. Exposure keratitis is prevalent in facial nerve injury involving the frontal and zygomatic branches lateral to the outer canthus.

Conservative measures aimed at protecting the eye include the use of artificial tears during the daytime and ointment at night. Drops containing hydroxypropyl cellulose, hydroxypropyl methylcellulose or polyvinyl alcohol are commonly used by day and may reduce excessive reflex tearing. Thicker ointments containing petrolatum, mineral oil or lanolin are used at night. The eye may be taped closed at night but many patients find this process awkward and prone to failure. Temporary tarsorrhaphy may be required to protect the eye in anticipation of functional recovery and regular ophthalmologic assessments should be arranged.

In some cases, medication may speed the resolution of facial paralysis. Harris et al. recommended that traumatic facial paralysis in the newborn be managed conservatively with corticosteroids.[33] A recent randomized control trial of steroid and antiviral use in patients over 16 years old supports the use of the former only.[34] No prospective randomized studies are available that evaluate the efficacy of steroid use in the newborn with facial paralysis caused by birth trauma. However, it is reasonable to give steroids during the 5-week observation period before decompression or exploration of the nerve is undertaken. This approach is

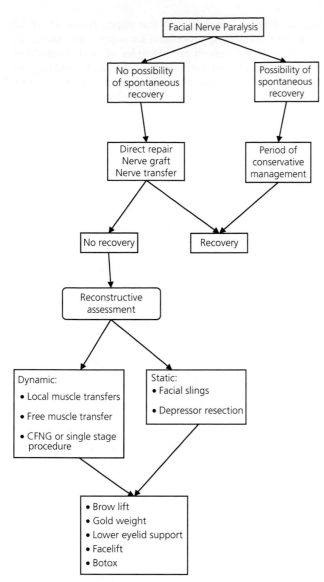

Figure 56.5   An algorithm for the management of facial paralysis.

similar to treatment of adult acute idiopathic facial paralysis. A combination of steroids and antiviral agents may be used in the treatment of Bell's palsy and Ramsay Hunt syndrome.[35],[36] Surgery to decompress the nerve is rarely required.

Other medical treatments for facial palsy include the use of botulinum toxin in the management of synkinesis, hyperkinesis and facial asymmetry. Although the effects wear off after only three to four months, the technique yields good results in the control of these sequelae, particularly following facial reinnervation procedures. Botox or local anaesthetic can also be used prior to definitive resection of the depressor anguli oris muscle to address lower lip asymmetry, allowing patients to assess the benefits of surgery without committing to it. In cases of upper eyelid retraction with corneal exposure keratitis where spontaneous motor recovery is anticipated, Botox can be used to paralyse the levator palpebrae muscle.

Neuromuscular therapy may be employed in patients with partial facial nerve palsy and makes use of specific exercises and biofeedback. In addition, the input of speech therapists and psychologists may be useful.

Surgical therapy

GENERAL PRINCIPLES

A variety of surgical options are available for the treatment of facial palsy and new techniques are frequently described. It is important to select procedures that will most likely address the needs and expectations of the patient and which fall within the capabilities of the operating surgeon.

A distinction must be made between an acute facial nerve injury in which the function of the paralysed muscles may be restored by timely intervention and a chronic state where depletion of the motor end plates and muscle atrophy preclude successful reinnervation. The cut-off is generally between 12 and 18 months following the onset of paralysis. Beyond this time period, denervated muscle exhibits irreversible degeneration and patients become dependent upon static procedures to improve facial function and symmetry, or upon the transfer of functioning muscle to the face for dynamic reconstruction.

In contrast to developmental cases, early exploration and nerve repair should be considered in all traumatic facial palsies. If a temporal bone fracture is present on CT scanning, surgical exploration of the facial nerve should be undertaken as soon as possible. The nerve must be fully exposed and decompressed and any haematoma within the nerve sheath must be evacuated.

When possible, direct coaptation of the divided nerve produces optimal results. Intraoperative nerve stimulation can be very helpful to assist in locating the distal branches of the nerve only in the first 2 or 3 days following the injury. In cases where the facial nerve is injured medial to the lateral canthus of the eye, the rich anastomotic network may obviate the need for exploration and repair.

Nerve repair should be tension free. Sharp penetrating trauma including inadvertent iatrogenic injury is most amenable to direct repair. Crushing injuries such as those caused by neonatal forceps delivery, result in scarring of longer segments of the facial nerve. This, and resection of the nerve on oncological grounds, necessitates the use of interpositional nerve grafts. Cable grafts may be required, particularly in proximal deficiencies, if the donor nerve is of insufficient calibre. Donor nerves include the sural nerve, which is remote from the zone of injury and, less commonly, the great auricular nerve, which is readily accessible. Sacrifice of these nerves results in reduced sensation to the lateral border of the foot or the lower half of the ear, respectively. Rarely, the hypoglossal nerve, supraclavicular nerve and the medial cutaneous antebrachial nerve are used as graft donors.

Recovery following direct nerve repair or grafting can be satisfactory even though a comparatively small number of axons are regenerated. Muscle tone and movement usually return at around six months postoperatively. Even following technically perfect nerve repairs however, synkinesis, facial spasm and mass movement are frequent complications, particularly in proximal repairs.

Direct coaptation or nerve grafting may be either impossible or inappropriate. This scenario commonly arises when the facial nerve lesion is within the central nervous system or the temporal bone and no proximal facial nerve stump is available for repair. In long-standing palsies, the motor end plates to the mimetic muscles are permanently lost and nerve repair serves no purpose.

When the proximal facial nerve stump is not available for repair, but the distal branches and motor end plates are still intact, alternative donor nerves may be used. A cross-facial nerve graft (VII to VII) can be used and has the theoretical advantage of providing natural, spontaneous facial muscle control although there is significant loss of axons through the graft, resulting in weak function. Consequently, the cross-facial nerve graft is better suited to powering free muscle transfers and alternative donor nerves are sought to innervate the innate facial muscles when appropriate. These include the glossopharyngeal, spinal accessory, phrenic, trigeminal (masseter) and hypoglossal nerves. Control of facial muscles reinnervated in this way can be unnatural, uncoordinated and prone to synkinesis. The hypoglossal nerve is most commonly used and has been effective in cases of bilateral facial palsy associated with Möbius syndrome.[37] In Möbius syndrome, there is bilateral facial and abducens nerve paralysis often associated with a broad range of other conditions. The absence of the facial nerve on either side compels the use of alternative donor nerves for reanimation procedures. The masseter nerve is proving to be a popular and well tolerated alternative.[38] Tongue atrophy and associated difficulty with mastication, speech and swallowing are known complications of hypoglossal nerve transfer.[39, 40, 41] The masseter nerve is gaining in popularity as the first choice of donor nerve in this scenario as donor morbidity is minimal and some patients seem to regain spontaneous muscle movement.[42, 43]

Nerve transfers can be used as a temporary measure to 'babysit' the facial muscles and maintain their motor end plates until a cross-facial nerve graft can be brought over from the normal side.[44] The hypoglossal nerve is most commonly used for this purpose and can be coapted end-to-end with the facial nerve stump with loss of hemitongue function,[45] or, to preserve some of this function, the nerve can be partially divided and coapted end to side to the facial nerve stump with a nerve graft.[46]

Finally, direct neurotization of denervated muscle has been reported with variable results. This involves burying a donor nerve directly into the muscle. However, such a technique is only suitable for isolated partial muscle paralysis.[47]

CHRONIC FACIAL PALSY

The management of stable, long-standing facial paralysis is governed by the assumption that there will be no further recovery in facial movement and the anticipation of a worsening of facial symmetry as the patient ages. Static procedures are designed to alter the facial posture and symmetry at rest and may improve oral continence and nasal valve collapse. They do not provide voluntary facial movement, but may reduce the distortion produced by muscle activity in the normal half of the face. Brow lifts, blepharoplasties, weighting of the upper eyelid, lower lid canthopexies and sling procedures for support and symmetry of the cheek and mouth are examples of static procedures. They are generally less demanding of the patient and surgeon alike and may therefore be more appropriate in the older, comorbid or less-motivated patient who wants a relatively quick fix and accepts the limitations of these procedures. Although resting facial symmetry is improved, asymmetry is again apparent during animation of the normal contralateral face.

Dynamic procedures, on the other hand, aim to reproduce movement in the paralysed face, improving symmetry both at rest and in motion. Such procedures are appropriate for younger or well-motivated patients as the procedures and rehabilitation are both long and complex. Many patients will require a combination of static and dynamic procedures to address different areas of the face.

The specific procedures available for facial reanimation will be considered by region.

The brow

Normally, brow ptosis can be compensated in the non-paralysed face by contraction of the frontalis muscle, raising the brow and upper eyelid. In lower motor neuron facial palsies affecting the temporal branch, brow ptosis may eventually contribute to the obstruction of the visual axis, especially in older patients with long-standing paralysis. A ptosis of 3–4 mm is apparent to most people. Loss of forehead movement per se is otherwise not a major concern for most patients but may contribute to the cosmetic deformity.

Static procedures are most appropriate to address brow ptosis. A suprabrow excision of redundant forehead skin and subcutaneous tissue, made along the line of the hair follicles, is often sufficient and the resultant scar is subtle, although some parasthesiae in the supraorbital nerve area may result (**Figure 56.6**). The outcome can be made more durable if the brow is secured to the periosteum of the frontal bone. Alternatively, conventional or endoscopic brow lifts may be undertaken. The contralateral brow may also need to be addressed.

The upper and lower eyelids

Inability to close the eye fully and loss of the blink reflex due to orbicularis muscle paralysis renders the cornea prone to injury, which can be painful and cause blindness. The ectropic lower eyelid exacerbates the problem by interfering with tear transport, resulting in epiphora. An early ophthalmologic assessment and accurate measurements of the degree of ptosis should be made. As with the brow, static procedures are currently more successful in addressing the upper and lower lid deficiencies. The most common corrective procedure involves the placement of a shaped gold weight in the upper eyelid, anterior to and secured to the tarsal plate with permanent sutures.[48] The ideal weight can be estimated preoperatively by taping trial weights to the eyelid skin in clinic. The lightest weight required to bring the lids to within 1–2 mm of closure is preferred; this is generally around 1 g. The operation can be carried out under local or

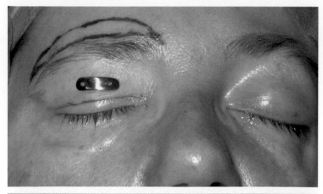

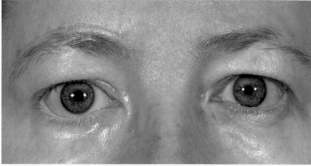

Figure 56.6   Suprabrow excision. Note preoperative asymmetry.

general anaesthetic, when combined with other procedures (**Figure 56.7**). Complications include under or over-correction, a visible bulge, infection and extrusion of the implant. Securing the weight with sutures may reduce the exposure rate. Overall though, gold weights permit complete eye closure in 82 per cent of patients.[49]

Spring devices are available for lid closure but placement and adjustment of tension can be difficult and complications are more common. Permanent tarsorraphy may be required to aid eye closure when there is little expectation of recovery, but the visual field is compromised and the appearance of the eye can be unsatisfactory.

For dynamic eyelid closure, transfer of a strip of temporalis muscle has been described. A thin strip of this muscle, based inferiorly, is extended with two strips of fascia or tendon, passed through the upper and lower eyelid, and fastened to the medial canthal ligament (**Figure 56.8**).[50] Because the upper eyelid is responsible for most movement, a static sling may be placed in the lower lid and a temporalis transfer in the upper lid only. Undesirable side effects include a slit-like palpebral aperture with lateral movement and skin wrinkling of the lateral lid region on closure. Frequently there is an obvious muscle bulge over the lateral orbital margin and there will be some synkinetic eyelid movement when chewing, which may assist irrigation of the globe. The procedure can however provide forceful and complete eyelid closure.

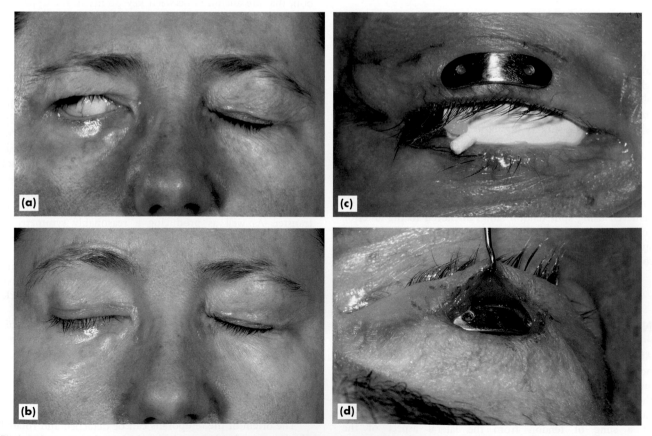

Figure 56.7   Gold weight insertion to upper eyelid. Note incomplete eye closure preoperatively on paralysed side and a normal Bell's reflex. Postoperatively, there is near complete eyelid closure. The patient has also had a direct brow lift.

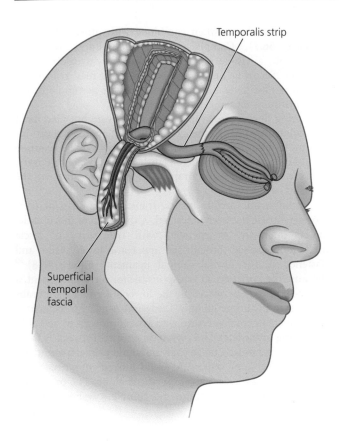

Temporalis strip

Superficial temporal fascia

Figure 56.8   Dynamic eyelid procedure.

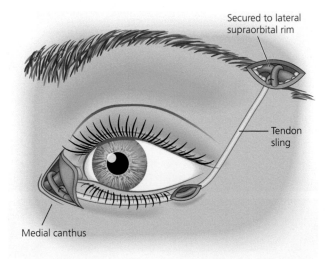

Secured to lateral supraorbital rim

Tendon sling

Medial canthus

Figure 56.9   Lower eyelid tendon sling for ectropion.

Free platysma transfer has also been described for dynamic ocular reanimation.[51] Innervation of this muscle transfer requires a separate cross-facial nerve transfer to which the cervical branch of the facial nerve contained in the platysma transfer is coapted. The vascular pedicle of this transfer is very small, usually about 0.5 mm in diameter which makes the surgery highly technically demanding. The frontal branch of the superficial temporal system is used to revascularize the platysma.

For lower lid ectropion, wedge excision of the lateral lower eyelid and lateral canthopexy can be performed, but are prone to relapse. More definitive lower lid support can be achieved using split tendon slings anchored to the anterior component of the medial canthal ligament and threaded subcutaneously along the subciliary margin of the lower lid to the superolateral orbital margin (**Figure 56.9**).

Nasal airway

Airway obstruction on the side of the paralysis may occur. The normal side of the face pulls the lower portion of the nose away from the paralysed side and gravity causes drooping of the nasal base on the same side. Correction of airway collapse can be obtained using an intranasal spreader graft or by means of a sling of tendon from the lateral aspect of the alar base up to the orbital margin.[52] However, correction of the lower face and lips will often ease the nasal obstruction.

The smile

The mid-third of the face is the most important area involved in the generation of a smile and is the most challenging region in facial paralysis surgery. In the elderly patient, those in poor health or unwilling to undergo more major surgery, static procedures to improve facial symmetry utilize slings of plantaris, palmaris or second or third toe extensor tendon, fascia lata or, less commonly, Gore-tex® or Endotine® ribbon, that are anchored between key points in the upper lip and modiolus, and the fascia overlying the zygoma or temporalis (**Figure 56.10**). 'Thread lifting' has also been successfully employed in some cases to improve facial symmetry with relatively little risk. Careful preoperative measurements of lip position at rest and during attempted smiling improve the accuracy of postoperative symmetry. Overcorrection is frequently required in anticipation of some stretching of the sling and relaxation of the facial tissues postoperatively. Facelift procedures can be combined with static slings to elevate ptotic cheek tissue and excise redundant skin. Children have good facial tone at rest, and generally do not benefit from static procedures.

Dynamic reanimation of the smile is appropriate for well-motivated patients with no contraindications to free muscle transfer. As well as producing a reasonably symmetrical, dynamic smile, the soft tissue defect that may result from prior parotidectomy or facial atrophy may be improved. If the distal facial nerve stump, motor end plates and muscle are still viable, an attempt can be made to bring in alternative nerve supply to power the muscle. If not, local muscle transposition or free muscle transfer will be necessary.

Muscle transposition makes use of local muscle to reanimate the face. Such procedures obviate the need for microneurovascular procedures, but the results are often less satisfactory and the donor site morbidity more significant. The temporalis or masseter muscles can be used for this transposition technique, but the latter can result in impediment to mastication and speech.[11]

The origin of the temporalis can be detached and rotated distally towards the nasolabial fold and anchored to the orbicularis oris muscle by means of periosteal extensions (the

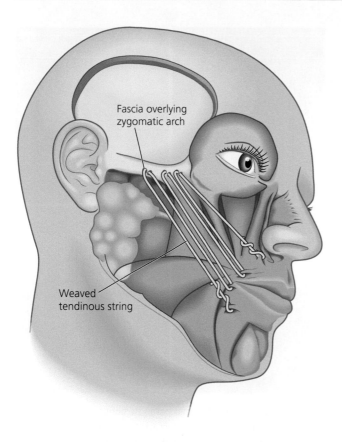

Figure 56.10 Static sling to cheek.

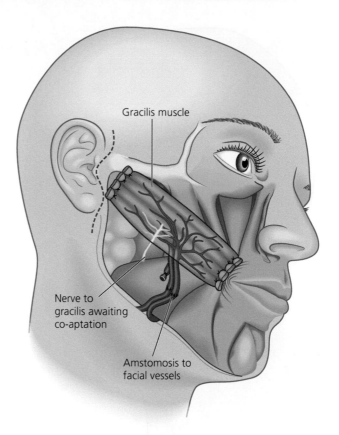

Figure 56.11 Gracilis transfer. The muscle is secured and anastomosed to the facial vessels.

Rubin transfer), but this technique leaves a temporal hollow and a bulge over the zygoma.[53] Alternatively, the temporalis can be disinserted from the mandible by osteotomy of the coronoid process, which is then secured to the nasolabial fold and the upper lip using tendon or fascia lata graft (the McGlaughlin procedure).[54]

Significantly better results are usually obtained using free muscle transfer.[55] In contrast to muscle transposition, free muscle transfers can be freely positioned to achieve optimum results. Various donor muscles have been described including the gracilis, pectoralis minor, rectus abdominis, latissimus dorsi, extensor carpi radialis brevis, serratus anterior, tensor fascia lata and abductor hallucis. The gracilis muscle is a popular donor, having appropriate excursion and a good neurovascular pedicle length. The muscle can be harvested simultaneously with the exposure in the face and thinned *in situ* to avoid excessive bulk. The anterior division of the obturator nerve supplies the muscle, and its length can allow for coaptation to a cross-facial nerve graft at the upper lip. Another common donor muscle for free transfer is the pectoralis minor raised on the medial and lateral pectoral nerves.[56] This muscle has the advantage of a strong tendinous insertion, which allows secure anchoring in the face. Donor site morbidity is minimal and, in theory at least, the dual nerve supply allows for single-stage smile and eye closure restoration by splitting of the flap. The muscle transfer is then secured to the area of the insertion of zygomaticus major and levator labii on the upper lip, and to the fascia overlying the zygomatic arch (**Figure 56.11**). Each muscle has its advocates and the appropriate choice probably depends as much upon surgeon experience as anticipated activity and donor site morbidity.

Of course, muscle transfers require innervation. In the absence of a useable ipsilateral facial nerve, the most desirable donor motor supply for facial reanimation would seem to be the contralateral facial nerve. The obvious advantage of using this nerve is that rehabilitation of facial function will be relatively spontaneous and straightforward. Interconnections between buccal branches of the facial nerve permit the sacrifice of one or two of these branches for facial reanimation without causing significant motor loss at the donor side. Only branches that produce a smile on stimulation should be used and these are identified through intraoperative nerve stimulation. A cross-facial nerve graft is often required to reach the paralysed cheek as part of a two-stage procedure. The sural nerve is the most common donor, providing ample length and appropriate diameter. Partial sensory loss along the lateral border of the foot results following nerve harvest but this is rarely problematic for the patient. Following coaptation to the donor nerve and tunnelling of the graft across the upper lip, axonal regeneration proceeds at a rate of approximately 1–3 mm/day. Clinically, an advancing Tinel's sign is elucidated but may take several months to reach its destination, during which time the facial muscles may lose their ability to be reinnervated (**Figure 56.12**).[57] Alternatively, a simpler, single-stage procedure has made effective use of the latissimus dorsi muscle with the thoracodorsal nerve which can be more than 15 cm long.[12] Other single-stage procedures using gracilis,[15] rectus femoris[14] and abductor hallucis[13] have been described, although these may be less effective.

As described above, the hypoglossal nerve can be used as an alternative motor supply to the distal facial nerve stump,

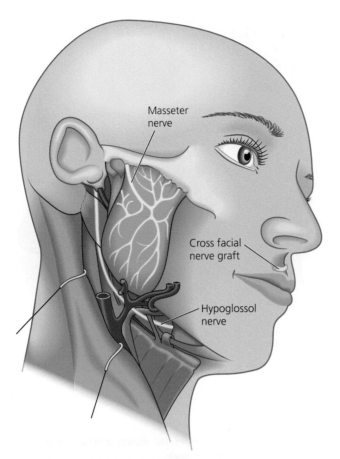

Figure 56.12 Donor nerves for facial reanimation. Note the masseter and hypoglossal nerves and the cross-facial nerve graft.

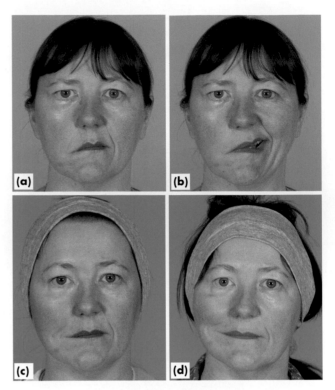

Figure 56.13 Unilateral facial paralysis before and after reanimation with free gracilis to Masseter nerve. (a) At rest preoperatively; (b) attempted smile preoperatively; (c) at rest postoperatively; (d) smiling postoperatively.

although the patient may experience swallowing and speech difficulties as well as synkinesis. For this reason, the use of the hypoglossal nerve is discouraged in young children whose speech is yet to develop and may be contraindicated in patients with pre-existing difficulties with swallowing. Some studies have shown that these complications can be minimized by transposition of a portion of the hypoglossal nerve only. Alternatively, the hypoglossal nerve can be used to innervate the facial nerve temporarily (babysitting), until a cross-facial graft is prepared.

The motor nerve to the masseter muscle is increasingly used as a donor for free muscle transfer. It has the advantage of proximity to the operative site and so reconstruction can be carried out in a single stage with little donor site morbidity (**Figure 56.13**). Use of the masseter nerve also appears to result in better excursion of the lip postoperatively relative to the cross-facial nerve graft.[58] For this reason, its use may be indicated in patients whose predisposition or occupation requires them to smile frequently, those with a heavy face, and older patients in whom a cross-facial nerve graft is known to be less successful. Initial concern that the masseter nerve would not allow production of a spontaneous smile has not proved true. In a recent study, 80 per cent of patients were able to smile without biting and 60 per cent were able to smile spontaneously with the aid of therapy and biofeedback.[7] A dual innervation approach has recently been described where the

latissimus dorsi muscle is innervated from both the contralateral facial nerve and the ipsilateral masseter in the hope of gaining the benefits of both.[59]

The facial or superficial temporal vessels are normally used for microvascular anastomoses to the flap pedicle.

The lower lip

The lower lip is animated by the orbicularis, the depressors anguli oris and labii inferioris, mentalis and the platysma. Marginal mandibular nerve palsy causes elevation of the ipsilateral lower lip and drooling. It also affects the symmetry of the smile. Direct neurotization of the depressors can be attempted by cross-facial nerve grafting, but this is infrequently used. Static slings between the lateral orbicularis oris muscle and the zygomatic arch have been used to improve resting posture.[60] Alternatively, improved lower lip symmetry can be achieved by resection of the depressor anguli oris muscle on the normal side of the lip, while sparing the branches of the mental nerve.[61] A similar effect can be achieved temporarily using Botox, or very briefly with local anaesthetic. This can allow the patient to assess the effect before committing to a more permanent procedure (**Figure 56.14**).[62] Transfer of the anterior belly of the digastric or platysma has also been used successfully but is infrequently undertaken.[63, 64] On occasion, a wedge excision of the flaccid lower lip is required.

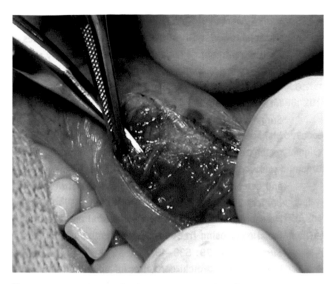

Figure 56.14 Lower lip depressor resection. Branches of the mental nerve are seen and spared.

FOLLOW-UP CARE AND REHABILITATION

In the early postoperative period, free muscle transfers must be closely monitored by clinical assessment of colour and capillary refill if a skin paddle is used. More commonly, however, the muscle flap is entirely buried and flap viability can only be assessed with the help of Doppler, and occasionally, implantable thermocouple devices.

After facial reanimation, return of function takes many months but physical therapy including biofeedback and facial expression exercises making use of a mirror should begin early to achieve optimal results. When a cross-facial nerve graft is used for reanimation, muscle activity may take four to six months to appear but rehabilitation is relatively straightforward. With the masseter nerve as a donor, rein-nervation of the muscle takes only two to three months but the rehabilitation is, naturally, more demanding for the patient. Donor site morbidity, including parasthesiae, tongue atrophy in patients with facial nerve–hypoglossal nerve transposition, and difficulty with mastication in patients with masseter or temporalis transfer, should be evaluated. If a nerve other than the contralateral facial has been used as the motor supply, synkinesis and difficulty in controlling the smile can be expected. With the masseter nerve, the patient must at first learn to control the smile by clenching of the teeth. The strength of the smile will be proportionate to the strength of the bite, which the patient can learn to control. In time, the majority of patients can learn to smile without biting and, in some cases, without conscious thought.

COMPLICATIONS

Facial reanimation and static procedures are subject to the same general complications as any surgery including infection, haematoma (3 per cent) and delayed wound healing. In addition, there is a risk of flap failure either in terms of arterial (5 per cent) or venous thrombosis (3 per cent), muscle necrosis (1 per cent) or motor function (3 per cent). Occasional loss of function at the donor site occurs and this may include partial tongue atrophy or contralateral facial weakness. With infants and young children, growth and development should be carefully monitored. The facial nerve is involved with the control of oral competence in the oral phase of swallowing and the ability to suck. Feeding may therefore be impaired. Speech development may also be hampered and therapy is an important adjunct to surgical therapy.

OUTCOME AND PROGNOSIS

More than 90 per cent of adults with Bell's palsy and children with facial nerve paralysis caused by blunt trauma will recover spontaneously. In other cases, including congenital paralysis, the optimal outcome of facial symmetry at rest, during voluntary movement, and spontaneous emotive movement, is rarely fully achieved without surgical intervention. Bilateral cases, which are most often congenital, suffer from asymmetry even after surgical reanimation, because of the difficulties of obtaining identical muscle placement, innervation and excursion on each side. Under comparable circumstances, however, children often fare better than adults following reanimation procedures.

In adults, an overall improvement can be anticipated in the vast majority of patients following microvascular free tissue transfer. Women and younger patients appear to do better in terms of muscle function and speed of recovery compared with men. Patients with a developmental cause of facial nerve paralysis also appear to do better than those with post-traumatic facial nerve paralysis. This may be because free muscle transfer in developmental palsies generates facial movement where there was none, whereas reanimation of traumatic facial palsies will never achieve preoperative function: patient satisfaction is correspondingly diminished. In terms of donor muscle selection, patients with pectoralis minor muscle transfer may regain function earlier than with gracilis. The best results are obtained by surgeons who commonly manage facial paralysis patients using techniques with which they are highly experienced.

SUMMARY

Facial paralysis engenders many distinct aesthetic and functional problems. A careful individual assessment and management plan are prerequisites for a successful and satisfactory outcome. Paralysis with the prospect of spontaneous resolution must be given time to occur, but interim treatment may be required to protect the exposed cornea and maximize the viability of the motor end plates. In long-standing cases, facial asymmetry and the inability to smile are often the primary indications for reconstruction, but other functional and aesthetic defects are also of great importance. A variety of static and dynamic procedures is available and should be chosen and tailored to the individual needs of the patient. While reconstructive techniques continue to improve, current therapy has its limitations and aims to provide good ocular and oral function, and an acceptable

probably the first to recommend transplantation of actual teeth around 1100AD. This was the established standard of care for many centuries until the high failure rate and risks of disease transmission came to be recognized.

Between the sixteenth and twentieth centuries, attempts at replacing the dentition with homologous teeth, gold-wire baskets, iron posts and china pegs were reported, although the results invariably were not. More recently, various implant designs have been developed, all based on an increasing understanding of biocompatibility, tissue healing and functional requirements.

Osseointegration is now well established, and the biological basis for success in both oral and facial rehabilitation is better understood. The number of implants placed increases year on year. Within the dental community it is now considered essential to discuss implants with suitable patients and to offer them as a viable treatment option. Equally, patients with congenital or acquired deformities of the head and neck should have access to multidisciplinary teams with skills that include osseointegrated implants and prostheses, to allow them to benefit from a comprehensive approach to reconstruction.

IMPLANT DESIGNS

Subperiosteal implants

Subperiosteal implants were devised 70 years ago. They are designed to rest on the bone and under the periosteum, distributing masticatory forces over a wide area. Until recently, these implants required a two-stage surgical approach. At the first operation, the subperiosteal flaps were reflected, and an impression taken of the underlying bone. The implant was produced on the model, cast from this impression and placed into the mouth at a second operation. With computed tomography (CT), and computer-aided design, computer-aided manufacture (CADCAM), the creation of an accurate model of the jaw is now possible. The implant can be produced from this computer-generated model and inserted in a single surgical procedure.

Subperiosteal implants are connected to the bone by fibrous tissue, although some exhibit direct bony contact in places. The transmucosal abutment posts that emerge through the gum and are used to retain a denture are an integral part of the implant.

The facility to coat the implants with hydroxyapatite, as an aid to integration, the refinement of the substructure design and the development of accurate CADCAM-derived models have resulted in renewed interest in this implant type in recent years. Subperiosteal implants remain of value in selected edentulous cases where narrow ridges or deep undercuts and severe angulations preclude endosteal implants.[5] They can be produced quickly and can be specifically designed to avoid anatomical structures or localized defects. Loading is possible immediately after soft tissue healing. The denture is extremely stable as the implant spreads the masticatory load over a wide area of bone. The patient can remove the denture to maintain oral hygiene.

Subperiosteal implants are not appropriate in the very atrophic jaw or in the post-resection patient as the area of available bone on which the implant frame can lie is reduced. Consequently, the load transmitted to the bone during function is increased, causing resorption of bone.

Endosteal implants

Endosteal implants are surgically placed into bone (**Figure 57.1**). This type of implant had been tried for centuries with limited success due to inadequate osseointegration. A variety of materials has been used including platinum-iridium, vitallium, stainless steel, aluminium hydroxide, chrome cobalt and titanium and titanium alloys.

Until recently, few designs had been based on thorough research and development. Swedish and Swiss groups working in the 1950s and 1960s provided the foundation for the current explosion of interest in dental endosseous implants. These implants broadly fall into two groups as detailed in the following subsections.

ROOT FORM IMPLANTS

Root form implants are the most commonly used, and many companies produce a number of differing designs. The designs are beginning to converge towards an accepted norm as the benefits of certain features are recognized and developed with successive generations of implants. Most implants are threaded and screw inserted. The threads mechanically lock the implant into the bone and achieve primary stability, i.e. stability at the time of insertion rather than due to later osseointegration.

Early implant designs had surfaces that were machined and relatively smooth. The bone to surface contact achieved by these implants was relatively low, and consequently they were long and relied on bicortical engagement of the jaws to achieve the stability that was required for successful osseointegration. These smooth surface implants tend to be longer (up to 20 mm or so in length).

Virtually all systems now rely on roughened surfaces. Some implants have chemically treated surfaces, to improve bone healing. The implants rely on surface roughness and an implant diameter slightly larger than that of the drilled hole to achieve primary stability. The roughened surface enlarges the surface area and promotes increased bone to implant surface contact once integrated. Due to the increased surface area for osseointegration, these implants can be produced in smaller lengths (typically 6–12 mm), and do not require bicortical engagement of the jaws for reliable fixation during healing and subsequent prosthetic reconstruction.

Some implants are coated with hydroxyapatite. In theory, this surface should allow the formation of ionic bonds with the bone and provide a greater bone to implant contact. The implants have been advocated for use in the cancellous bone of the maxilla. Some concerns have been expressed over the durability of the coating.

A recent development is that of very long implants (up to 55 mm in length) (**Figure 57.2**), which can engage areas of good quality bone remote from the defect or area to be reconstructed. These 'Zygomaticus' (Nobel Biocare Management, Zurich, Switzerland) implants were originally designed for reconstruction of the edentulous atrophic maxilla,

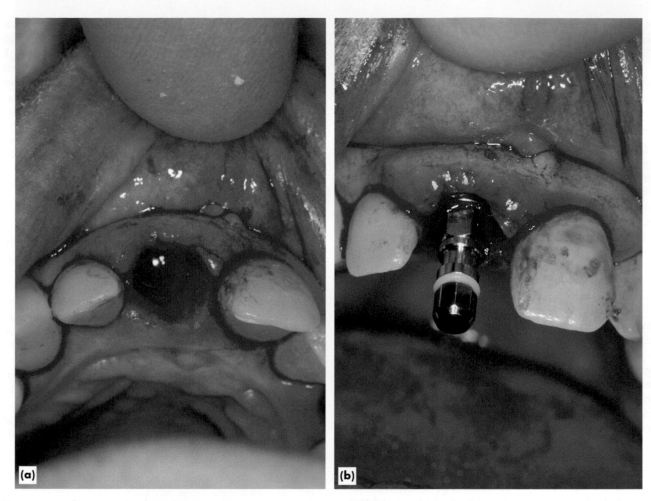

Figure 57.1   Straumann implant placed into the bone of an extraction socket.

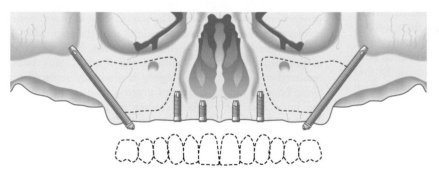

Figure 57.2   Diagram of Zygomaticus® implants used in an edentulous maxilla.

(**Figure 57.2**) but they are useful in the management of complex composite defects of the face and jaws.

All implants come pre-packaged and pre-sterilized. This avoids potential contamination prior to implant placement, either by metal contamination from non-titanium instruments or organic contamination from tissue contact. These factors have been reported as interfering with success.[6]

Recent innovations have been aimed at increasing the surface area of the implants; e.g. at the micro level, by experimenting with different textures, and chemically treating the surface to increase the attractiveness of the surface to bone progenitor cells, and at the macro level, by increasing the diameter of the implants.

Wide implants are available in shorter lengths and are primarily designed for use in areas of reduced bone height and where the greater surface area improves their load-carrying abilities, such as the posterior mandible. The shorter implants can be placed to avoid the inferior dental (ID) nerve or the maxillary sinus. They may also be used where primary stability of the normal diameter implants cannot be achieved and there is a need to engage more cortical bone between the buccal and lingual cortices. This can improve primary stability and osseointegration.

Wide diameter implants may have a role in orbital reconstructions where the frontal sinus encroaches on the supraorbital rim, and in auricular reconstructions and BAHA placement where the mastoid air cells limit bone depth in the temporal bone.

METAL SELECTION, SURFACE CHARACTERISTICS AND THE PROCESS OF OSSEOINTEGRATION

Metals, either as single element materials or alloys, have favourable characteristics for use as implants. They are strong, and easy to machine and manufacture. Metals are often reactive (except for the noble metals such as gold and silver). Most pure metals on contact with air become covered in an oxide layer and it is this oxide layer that is in contact with the host issues.

Leventhal[7] introduced titanium as a suitable biocompatible metal for orthopaedic surgery in 1951. Commercially pure titanium and titanium alloys are the basis for the majority of osseointegrated implants in current use. Millions of titanium implants have been placed over the past 40 years and there are no series reporting allergic reactions or carcinogenicity.

Early investigations into osseointegration established predictable techniques for tooth replacement. A specialized periodontal ligament surrounds a tooth but not an implant. Implants are in contact with either fibrous tissue (fibrous encapsulation) or bone (osseointegration). The latter are more successful and root form, cylindrical implants are now produced with the aim of achieving this.

The concept of osseointegration is based on work undertaken by Dr Per-Ingvar Brånemark in the 1950s and early 1960s. Optical chambers made out of titanium were implanted into rabbit tibias to study *in vivo* bone and marrow function. Once healed, these chambers could not be removed because the bone had grown directly against the titanium frames. Animal models were developed to investigate the potential of these findings.[8] From these results, titanium implants were developed to replace the dentition. Success rates in terms of implant survival and marginal bone loss now exceed those of the original Branemark fixtures which, nevertheless, remain the gold standard against which other systems are compared.

Predictable osseointegration requires the gentle and minimally traumatic placement of a biocompatible implant into bone. The implant should not be mobile at the time of insertion; it should exhibit primary stability. A period of undisturbed healing should follow prior to loading with a prosthesis. Implants can be loaded immediately in certain situations;[9] however, preliminary results suggest that this approach may be associated with a higher failure rate and less predictable soft tissue responses.[10]

THE IMPLANT AND TISSUE INTERFACE

The precise mechanism of osseointegration remains under investigation, although the physiology of bone healing, with which it is intimately associated, is well documented.[10] Osseointegration is not restricted to titanium or titanium alloys. Aluminium oxide ceramics, tantalum, stainless steel and cobalt- and nickel-based alloys have all been shown to osseointegrate. Titanium remains the material of choice. It can be easily machined into shapes that are small enough to be placed in the jaws and facial bones and yet strong enough to withstand masticatory loads of up to 500 N. Recent developments with zirconium/titanium alloys have shown that implants made from these alloys are stronger than titanium alone and can be machined as smaller units for easier placement where bone volume is limited.

A thin oxide layer covers the surface of pure titanium after contact with air. This titanium oxide is inert, practically insoluble and very resistant to body fluids. More extensive oxide growth occurs on titanium implants subjected to biological tissues.[11] Macrophages in particular, may contribute to development of the oxide layer by excreting proteolytic enzymes, cytokines, superoxide and hydrogen peroxide.[12] It is hypothesized that the actual interface between the titanium implant and living tissue is a hydrated titanium peroxy matrix.

The formation of such a matrix is unique to titanium. Of fundamental importance is that bone predictably grows on the surface of a titanium implant. Contaminated titanium surfaces have been shown to impede the colonization of human osteoblast cells which only adhere to and cover the surface of clean implants.

Implant placement causes bleeding and an acute inflammatory response in the bone immediately adjacent to the implant. The implant surface becomes coated with the products of acute inflammation. Macrophages remove bone and metallic debris. Undifferentiated mesenchymal cells migrate into the area and produce an extracellular matrix. Within 1 week of implant placement, these cells develop into osteoblasts and produce osteoid. The osteoid gradually organizes into an increasingly dense procallus, with further mesenchymal cells differentiating into osteoblasts and fibroblasts. The osteoblasts produce fibres that have the potential to calcify. The fibrocartilagenous callus that develops matures into woven bone by the 3rd week. The remodelling of woven bone involves the recruitment of osteoclasts into the area. After 7 weeks, lamellar bone is being laid down. This is more mineralized and further stabilizes the implant. Any bone rendered non-vital by the surgery is gradually replaced by living bone. A very thin layer of proteoglycan exists between the bone and the implant surface of all osseointegrated implants. This layer is up to 500 nm thick. In effect, the body fails to recognize the implant as a foreign body and it becomes incorporated into bone as part of the wound healing process.

The final stages of healing involve maturation of the bone at the implant interface. There is an increase in bone hardness and density that is associated with loading and functional use, and which is ongoing even a year after implant placement. This correlates with Wolff's law, which states that bone tends to develop the structure best suited to resist forces prevailing upon it.

The soft tissue interface between the skin or mucosa and the implant is equally important. It consists of both epithelium and connective tissue. A rough implant surface has been demonstrated to promote connective tissue attachment. However, as maintenance of good hygiene and the avoidance of plaque accumulation within the mouth, and organic debris from the surrounding skin, is impossible on this roughened surface, endosseous implants are designed to have smooth components in contact with the soft tissues. This facilitates mechanical cleaning.

The connective tissue fibres run parallel to the implant surface in this situation, forming a tight cuff rather than a direct attachment. A peri-implant sulcus is formed and lined with non-keratinized epithelium during soft tissue healing. The epithelial cells are in direct contact with the implant. This is analogous to the junctional tissue of the normal oral periodontium that surrounds tooth roots. As in all clinical situations, epithelium does not contact bone, and a layer of connective tissue exists between the marginal bone and the epithelium. Where submerged, two-stage implants are used, the placement of the abutment results in epithelium growing down to the implant abutment junction. If this is at or below the bone level, some resorption occurs as connective tissue always separates the epithelium from the bone. In practice, this apparent shortcoming does not compromise long-term success.

Inflammation and excessive loading can cause bone resorption.[13] Where peri-implant disease develops, the sulcal epithelium desquamates, exposing the underlying connective tissue, which becomes inflamed. This inflammation induces osteoclast activity and chemical mediator release from cells adjacent to the implant surface. As this tissue is less well differentiated than that around teeth where a protective periodontal membrane exists, progressive bone loss can be more rapid. Within the bone, premature loading or overload (as can occur through occlusal trauma, or the non-passive fit of a bar linking implants) causes areas of pressure concentration, osteoclastic activity and angular bone loss at the implant site. This is particularly damaging during the healing phase when osseointegration has not fully developed and the immature bone resorbs easily. Overloading, even after several years, can cause microfractures in the bone that may heal with scar tissue and cause implant mobility to develop.

The combination of inflammation and overload is particularly harmful, but separately or together, the end is the same as osseointegration is progressively lost and the implant fails.

ANATOMICAL CONSIDERATIONS

Bone density varies within the jaws, at different sites in the face, and between individuals. The greater the proportion of cortical bone to cancellous bone, the better the long-term osseointegration results, hence mandibular implants have higher success rates than maxillary implants. Within the facial skeleton, implants at the nasal bridge should be long enough to engage the frontal bone, and those around the orbit are best placed in the upper outer quadrant where bone density is greatest, avoiding the frontal sinus. However, care is required in the preparation of dense bone where the risk of overheating during drilling is greatest.

The presence of adequate bone volume is a prerequisite for the successful placement and subsequent osseointegration of an implant. Patients who most need implants often have the least volume of bone. Congenital deformities, such as severe hemifacial microsomia or Treacher Collins syndrome, are associated with underdevelopment of the temporal bone, limiting sites for implant placement and subsequent BAHA

and auricular prostheses. Tooth loss results in acquired patterns of bone resorption which compromise implant placement and have been classified.[14] Specific features of the various facial anatomical sites used for implant placement are considered below.

Maxilla

Maxillary bone is less dense, and the proximity of the nasal floor, maxillary sinuses and the incisive foramen can all have an impact on implant placement. The loss of part of the upper jaw, either due to trauma or after resection, further exacerbates the difficulties.

Tooth loss and subsequent bone resorption concentrates bone stock between the lateral nasal wall and the maxillary sinus. This canine buttress, running up towards the pyriform rim, is the most predictable site for implant placement in the upper jaw. The maxillary tuberosity can also be used. It consists of low density cancellous bone which may compromise osseointegration and is often too posterior for easy use. The perpendicular plate of the palatine bone and the pterygoid plates of the sphenoid bone lie posterior and medial to the tuberosity. Implants can be placed in this region via the tuberosity. However, access can be limited, and the angulation of insertion required to engage the plates can cause difficulties with the prosthetic reconstruction, particularly if trismus exists due to previous surgery or radiotherapy. Implant placement from the maxilla into the zygomatic body via the maxillary sinus is now a well-recognized procedure, and can avoid the need for bone gradting.

Following tooth loss, buccal and vertical bone resorption narrows the maxillary arch width and increases the interarch distance between the jaws. If the dental arches are to occupy the original form, the implants have to be angled away from the sagittal plane, resulting in greater lateral load on the implants. The greater the intermaxillary distance, the larger the prosthesis that is required to restore normal jaw relationships and the greater the load carried by each implant. These factors have to be taken into account when planning the number and size of implants to be used in the reconstruction.

In the atrophic upper jaw, maxillary ridge width and height are reduced. Additional bone augmentation techniques may be required, such as ridge expansion, guided tissue regeneration using membranes and bone grafting of the ridge, sinus floor and nasal floor.

Mandible

Mandibular bone is predominantly cortical around a central cancellous core. The genial undercut should be taken into consideration when assessing the depth of bone available near the mandibular symphysis. The true depth is frequently less than the apparent depth. A lateral cephalogram x-ray will demonstrate this feature and allow accurate measurement of the available bone. Cone beam CT scanning is now readily available. The anatomy of the jaws is easy to appreciate as implant placement can now be predetermined using planning software.

The genial tubercles can lie above the level of the ridge in the very atrophic mandible where they can compromise implant placement. Surgical removal of the prominence may be required.

The mylohyoid ridge creates a lingual undercut in the molar regions. Avoidance of lingual perforation through the cortical plate during implant placement is important as haemorrhage into the floor of the mouth can have life-threatening consequences.[15] In practice, this may preclude using the full height of bone available above the inferior dental nerve. Clinical assessment at the time of patient evaluation can be supplemented with tomograms or coronal CT scans to demonstrate the relevant anatomy.

The ID nerve runs a variable course from the lingula to the mental foramen and influences implant placement.[16] Bicortical engagement is only possible proximal to the mental foramen, unless the implants are inserted either buccal or lingual to the nerve or the nerve itself is transposed laterally at the time of implant placement. A safer alternative is to use short, wide implants and place them above the nerve.

Prior to emergence from the mental foramen, the nerve loops anteriorly to a variable extent. This is often apparent on a panoral tomogram. Care is required when placing an implant immediately in front of the mental foramen, so that this anterior loop is undamaged and lip sensation preserved.

In the very atrophic mandible, the mental foramen may lie on or lingual to the alveolar ridge. To protect the nerve, careful dissection in this area is required during the reflection of a buccal subperiosteal flap.

Extraoral implant sites

TEMPORAL BONE

The anatomy of the temporal bone is complex and becomes unpredictable in patients with congenital deformity, such as Treacher Collins and hemifacial/craniofacial microsomia. Where practical, the external auditory meatus (EAM) is the landmark for correct implant placement, as the auricular prosthesis will be fitted around this. If the meatus or ear remnants are in the wrong position, then assessment against the other side (if normal) or using anthropometric landmarks, such as the Frankfort plane and alar tragal line, may be required to correctly site implants (**Figure 57.3**).

The outer table of the temporal bone is usually dense cortex into which implants can be placed easily. The implants should be placed in the posterior, upper quadrant, 18–22 mm from the centre of the EAM, ideally 15 mm apart, and two or three in number.[17] Although the mastoid air cells may underlie the cortex, the cells become progressively smaller away from the mastoid apex and in the normal temporal bone they rarely prevent implant placement. The position of the posterior cranial fossa and the sigmoid and superior petrosal sinus may vary, but it is usually in children that these structures are encountered or in congenital deformity where the temporal bone is very atrophic or underdeveloped. The shallow depth of bone available mandates the use of short, extraoral implants. If encountered, the dura can be pushed away from the implant during insertion. Should the vascular sinuses be encountered, then the rapid insertion of the

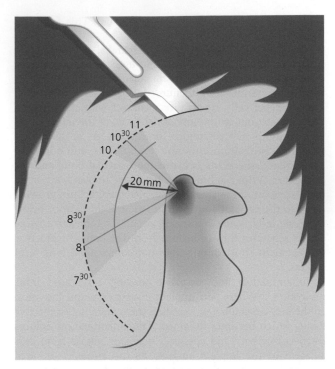

Figure 57.3   Diagram showing implant sites for a right ear prosthesis.

implant quickly plugs the hole and haemorrhage is arrested. Cerebrospinal fluid (CSF) leaks are rare.

Implants are generally avoided in children, as osseointegration can impair normal growth of adjacent bone. However, the benefit of a BAHA on hearing, and therefore speech and language development, and the fact that 80 per cent of skull growth has been achieved by the age of two years, means that early implant placement confers significant advantages to this select group of young patients.

ORBIT

Orbital prostheses present special problems. The normal eye moves constantly, whereas a prosthesis is static and the eyelids do not move. Careful implant placement is crucial if the prosthesis is to compare well with the normal side. It should sit deep enough within the socket such that symmetry in all three planes is maintained when compared to the normal eye. The proximity of the frontal, ethmoid and maxillary sinuses, and the thin cortical edge to the orbital rim, limits the areas where implants can successfully be placed (**Figure 57.4**).

In practice, most orbital implants are placed in the upper, outer orbital rim (lateral to the frontal sinus) and into the body of the zygoma. The bone of the medial orbital wall is too thin for implant anchorage. A posteroanterior x-ray or CT scan will show the anatomical landmarks that influence and limit implant placement and, in contrast to auricular implants, imaging is essential when planning orbital implant placement.

Narrow orbital rims should be drilled back until 5 mm width is achieved. Conventional oral implants can be placed directed up into the frontal bone and down into the zygoma. The flange on extraoral implants often ulcerates through the

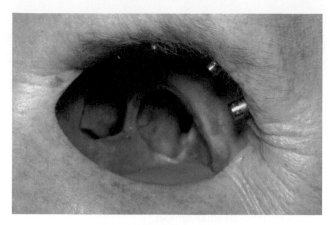

Figure 57.4   Ideal implant sites in the left orbit.

overlying skin with time and these fixtures are best avoided wherever possible at this site. Correct angulation of the implant ensures that the emergence profile of the implant abutment is within the orbital cavity. In practice, this limits the length of implant that can be used because the hand piece and the implant have to be positioned within the orbit at the time of placement if the correct line of insertion is to be achieved. A surgical template showing the proposed position of the prosthesis in the orbit is a useful guide to correct implant position in all three planes.

NOSE

The prosthetic nose is best produced as a single aesthetic unit. It is therefore sometimes better to undertake excision of the whole nose if an autogenous reconstruction is not going to be attempted. The alae, columella, anterior nasal septum and nasal bone need to be removed so that implants can be placed without interference from surrounding tissues. The best support and retention for the prosthesis relies on placing implants as far apart as possible around the nasal rim. In practice, this confines placement to the pyriform rim inferiorly and the nasal bridge superiorly. Flood and Russell[18] describe placing the implants upside down into the nasal floor, so that they emerge under the nostril. However, atrophy of the anterior maxilla in edentulous patients can limit the length of implant that can be placed at this site. Greater bone is available laterally, in the region of the canine buttress, so that oral implants can be angled downwards and backwards into the strut of bone that separates the medial aspect of the maxillary sinus from the lateral nose. The depth available is limited by the height of the palate. In the nasal bridge region, the nasal bones are very thin and frequently fracture or split along the midline suture if an implant is placed at this level. Consequently, resecting the nasal bone back to the nasion allows implant placement in the wider, denser bone of the frontal bone, and again, oral implants can be used to good effect at this site. It is important that the implant is angled so that the emergence profile is behind the line of the nasal bridge (**Figure 57.5**).

The recent development of the zygomaticus implants has given greater flexibility to nasal reconstruction as these implants can be placed horizontally from the middle of the nasal defect through the maxillary sinus under the eye and

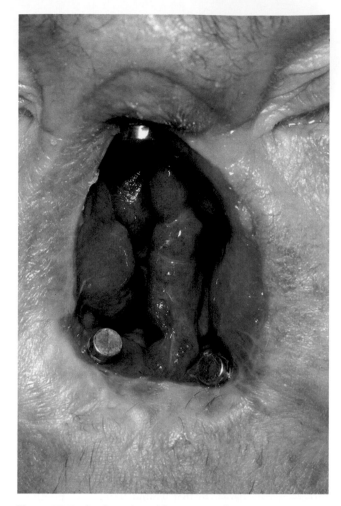

Figure 57.5   Implants in a rhinectomy patient.

engage the cortical bone of the zygoma. They are particularly useful where the anterior maxilla has been lost and pyriform rim implants are not possible (**Figure 57.6**).

PATIENT ASSESSMENT AND PLANNING

Many implant failures can be traced back to poor preoperative assessment. The suitability of a patient for implants is based on general and local factors. The following factors should be considered:

- General factors: impaired immune system, smoking, previous radiotherapy; psychological factors: body image/psychiatric disorders, attitudes to complex dentistry, hygiene and aftercare.
- Local factors: available bone, quality of bone, quality of soft tissue, peri-implant infections.

Medical factors

Absolute contraindications to implant treatment are rare, but can include immunosuppression (either by disease or drug therapy) and psychiatric disorders, including those associated with abnormal perceptions of body image. Susceptibility to

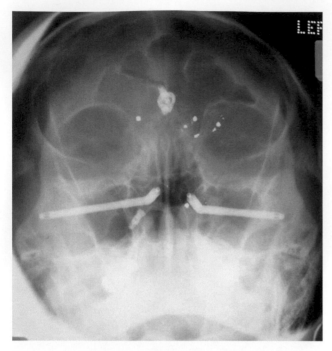

Figure 57.6 Zygomaticus implants used where lateral nateral nasal bone is missing.

infective endocarditis, and patients with prosthetic joint replacements, need consideration, although the risks of implant-related infections are probably very low. In view of the x-rays needed, it is prudent to avoid implant placement during pregnancy.

Diabetes should be well controlled before any elective surgery is considered, so that wound healing is optimized. Osteoporosis, in our experience, is not a problem, although longer healing times with careful loading of the implants is appropriate.

Smoking

Smoking has a detrimental effect on implant osseointegration and long-term survival.[19] Patients should be warned of this during the preoperative assessment. Where it is decided to undertake treatment, consideration should be given to over-engineering the reconstruction, so that an increased risk of failure is built into the treatment plan and sufficient implants will remain to support any superstructure.

Previous radiotherapy

Radiotherapy to the head and neck does not preclude implant placement, but failure rates approaching 50 per cent have been reported.[20]

Hyperbaric oxygen (HBO) both before and after implant placement may minimize the onset of osteoradionecrosis and subsequent late implant loss. Twenty dives before and ten dives after surgery, at two atmospheres pressure, are recommended. Failure rates may then be reduced to less than 10 per cent.[21] Trials are ongoing to substantiate this benefit and also the incidence of osteoradionecrosis.

Not all patients are suitable for HBO and it is not universally available. Absolute contraindications include untreated pneumothorax, optic neuritis, existing neoplasia and active infections. Caution is needed in those patients with middle ear disease who will require grommets before HBO. Those with chronic obstructive pulmonary disease whose respiratory drive may be compromised in an oxygen-rich environment and who are more susceptible to a pneumothorax also need careful assessment.

HBO is thought to act by a number of mechanisms:

- Hyperoxygenation of poorly perfused tissues.
- Vasoconstriction, without compromising oxygen availability to the tissues.
- It is bactericidal to anaerobes.
- Peroxidase activity in macrophages is promoted, rendering them more effective in killing bacteria.[22]
- Promotes vascular ingrowth to a hypoxic area.
- Bone matrix production and bone mineralization is increased.[23]
- Promotes osteoclast activity and enhances necrotic bone removal.
- Enhances erythrocyte deformation to improve oxygen delivery to damaged tissues.

Local factors

Local factors include poor hygiene, ongoing cutaneous or periodontal disease, and dental neglect. Any physical or mental disability that may prevent meticulous cleaning of the fixtures should give rise to concern over the patient's suitability for implants. The presence of active epithelial or connective tissue disease, such as erosive lichen planus, pemphigus and pemphigoid, is a contraindication. In these conditions, poor wound healing and loss of soft tissue integrity around the implant is likely to compromise the overall outcome.

Counselling

Once a patient has been screened for contraindications to implant placement, it is important to establish that the patient's expectations are realistic at the outset and are balanced against those which are clinically achievable and appropriate. Where more than one clinician is involved in the treatment, it is particularly important that all parties have a clear understanding of each other's role, and a common purpose developed. Many problems (and subsequent litigation) relating to implant cases can be traced back to errors of communication and misunderstandings during the preoperative assessment.

Diagnostic wax-up/models

A diagnostic 'wax-up' is essential for most intraoral and extraoral implant cases. It can be used as a guide for the correct emergence profile of the implants (**Figure 57.7**). The clinician can use the wax model of the proposed prosthesis to determine the reconstructive options (fixed bridge or

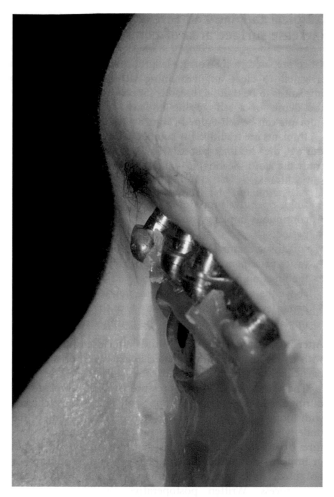

Figure 57.7 Unfavourable implant angulation for a left orbital prosthesis.

removable denture/obturator, surface area to be covered by the ear, nose, etc.) and the ideal sites for implant placement. The patient can also assess the set up for appearance. Where practical, all parties should agree on this diagnostic stage before continuing with treatment. Skeletal and occlusal influences on intraoral prostheses are dealt with in standard prosthodontic texts.

Once approved, the set up should be retained and duplicated in clear acrylic. Should problems later arise with the construction and appearance of the superstructure then the original set up is still available to refer back to. The clear acrylic set up can be used as an accurate template or stent from which the implant sites and angles of insertion can be transferred from the study casts, directly to the patient's mouth during the operation.

CADCAM models/CT-3D imaging

Software programs are now available, such as SimPlant8 (Materialise/Columbia Scientific, Leuven, Belgium), which allow CT data to be manipulated so that ideal implant sites can be identified, in terms of the height, width and depth of available bone. Once the appropriate implant sites, angles of insertion and lengths have been determined, the data can be

used to produce customized surgical templates. These templates fit directly onto the proposed operative site and guarantee correct implant position and angulation. The correct implant length can be preselected.

Within the mouth, it is much easier and less expensive to achieve acceptable aesthetics with an implant-supported denture than with a fixed prosthesis (bridge). If a fixed prosthesis is used, the teeth are often very long to compensate for the increased interarch distance that occurs in the edentulous jaw. Long teeth can be disguised with pink porcelain or acrylic to mimic a more normal gum margin.

The site of implant placement is determined according to superstructure design, patient factors and radiographic findings. All patients should have a panoral tomogram and periapical x-rays of existing teeth as a minimum if oral implants are planned. Posteroanterior facial views are useful for orbital implants (to show the extent of the frontal and maxillary sinus) and fine cut CT with the facility for 3D reformatting for other sites in the face.

Where a patient has an original denture, it can often be modified or remade to allow for implant placement. It can be converted or copied into an obturator if a maxillectomy is to be undertaken. Acrylic dentures are easily adjusted during the healing phase to avoid loading implants and the operative sites and causing unnecessary pain and implant loss through overload.

Meticulous records should be kept throughout treatment and thereafter to form the basis for prospective studies, audit, appraisal of success or failure, and as defence against litigation. Patients should be well aware of the implications of implant treatment in terms of hygiene and recall appointments. Anything less than meticulous cleaning and regular attendance for review can jeopardise the long-term success of the case. The treatment plan, alternatives, possible complications and cost (where appropriate) should be documented and signed by the patient as part of the consent process before commencing any implant treatment.

Setting up an implant programme needs careful consideration of the workload and costs, including maintenance of the prostheses, for the life of the patient. As the patient cohort increases, so does the cost of replacing prostheses, bars, abutments and the occasional lost implant.

SURGICAL TECHNIQUES

Anaesthesia

Surgery can be undertaken under local anaesthetic, with or without sedation, or general anaesthetic. Local anaesthetic alone can be advantageous, particularly when placing implants for oral reconstruction. During implant placement, even using a template, difficult interarch and opposing tooth relationships need continuous intraoperative assessment. This is best achieved by maintaining full patient cooperation.

Prophylactic antibiotics

Antibiotics are recommended during the surgical phase. A single, 3-g dose of amoxycillin given orally 1 hour

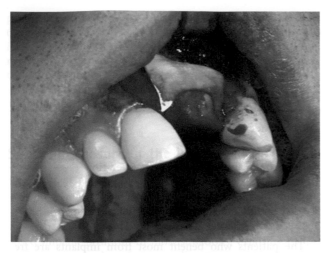

Figure 57.9 Resorbable barrier membrane over a bone graft in the anterior maxilla.

Dahlin demonstrated that isolating a bony defect from fibrous tissue invasion using ePTFE allowed bony healing within the defect.[34] Those defects not isolated were filled with fibrous tissue with very little bony ingrowth.

Membranes can be used to optimize a site for implant placement, or to encourage bone ingrowth to an area of deficiency around an existing implant. This can be either at the time of implant placement or after osseointegration, if evidence of bone loss becomes apparent. The membranes are most effective when protecting a bone graft or bone substitute during the healing period.

The membrane should be larger than the defect to be augmented. It should be kept clear of adjacent structures as flap dehiscence can occur, with detrimental effects on healing.[35]

Tension-free, soft tissue closure over the implanted membrane is essential if premature exposure of the membrane is to be avoided. Infection can result with loss of any regeneration gained. The membrane should be removed if there is any clinical evidence of inflammation present during the healing phase. Wherever possible, the membrane is left in place for at least six months. This allows adequate time for bony regeneration and maturation. Removal earlier than this leaves an augmented site with soft immature tissue that tends to resorb. Resorbable membranes do not need to be removed, unless infected. Successful long-term osseointegration in membrane-regenerated bone is well established.

Where significant bony deficiencies exist, then the use of barrier techniques alone are not appropriate and bone grafts are needed. The local supply of this is most deficient in those patients who need it most. To overcome this deficiency other sites may be used, such as the iliac crest, tibia or cranium. An alternative is to use bone graft substitutes. Autogenous bone is the material against which other materials are compared.

Various bone graft substitutes have been advocated. The substitutes can be divided into osteoconductive or osteoinductive materials. Osteoconduction implies bone apposition onto and into a framework and occurs from existing bone or bone progenitor cells. Osteoinductive materials convert undifferentiated cells into osteoblast or chondroblasts. Autogenous bone is capable of both of the above as well as osteogenesis, the production of bone in the absence of undifferentiated cells.

Most osteoconductive materials are synthetic alloplasts, usually ceramics. The two main groups of ceramics used in conjunction with implants are tricalcium phosphate (TCP) and hydroxyapatite (HA) derived from a variety of sources. They are biocompatible substances that bond strongly to bone.

TCP is more soluble than HA and is partially resorbable. This occurs at a rate equivalent to the ingrowth of normal bone and is related to the manufacturing process of the TCP.[36]

Hydroxyapatite is the major inorganic component of bone. It has good compressive but poor tensile strength. The porous type of particulate HA is most frequently used with osseointegrated implants. Pore sizes of 150 μm facilitate ingrowth of mineralized bone.[37]

Osseoinductive materials are mainly allografts derived from screened human donors, such as demineralized freeze-dried bone. The manufacturing process activates bone morphogenic proteins (BMP) that are present in the bone collagen matrix. These have been purified and isolated as a number of different osseoinductive substances and are predominantly present in cortical bone. The use of synthetically produced BMP in the future may overcome increasing reticence to the use of human-derived bone by both patients and clinicians.[38]

These materials have applications in the management of localized bony defects, frontal and maxillary sinus augmentation and the treatment of peri-implant deficiencies, either at the time of placement or later during salvage surgery.

ADJUNCTIVE IMPLANT TECHNIQUES

Where local factors adversely affect conventional implant placement, a number of procedures have been developed to modify the local anatomy and aid implant placement.

Upper jaw

In the atrophic upper jaw, implant placement may require:

- prior or simultaneous sinus grafting
- placement of implants in the tuberosity or pterygoid plates
- ridge expansion
- nasal floor grafting
- onlay grafting.

There has been a gradual evolution in sinus grafting procedures with current techniques offering predictable success rates. Implant placement into augmented sinuses is associated with at least 80 per cent long-term osseointegration in most series. Where sufficient bone exists to provide primary stability for the implant, the sinus lining can be elevated either with osteotomes or the implant itself, resulting in predictable osseointegration.[29]

Tatum[39] developed a modified Caldwell-Luc procedure, placing bone grafts or a variety of osseoinductive and osseoconductive materials under the elevated sinus mucosa, to good effect (**Figure 57.10**).

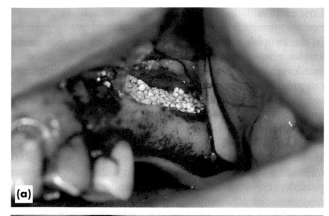

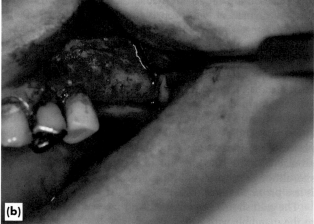

Figure 57.10   (a) Intraoperative view of a left maxillary sinus floor augmentation with hydroxyapatite; (b) healing at six months.

The area to be grafted can be approached via an appropriately reflected soft tissue flap. The lateral antral wall can be carefully drilled and intruded on the sinus lining, or the window removed completely. Elevation of the intact antral lining in the subperiosteal plane requires careful dissection through the antrostomy. Septa within the antrum can be seen on preoperative x-rays or scans and avoided or included in the dissection as appropriate. The cavity to be grafted is bounded by the antral lining and bony window above, the medial and lateral sinus walls and the floor of the sinus. Care should be taken not to obstruct the osteum of the sinus with overzealous grafting. While autogenous bone is the ideal, in practice, the volume that can be collected intraorally is limited. The volume can be supplemented with a bone substitute. Good results have been achieved with hydroxyapatite, demineralized freeze-dried bone, glass derivatives and tricalcium phosphate.[36, 37] In the author's experience, with informed consent, patients prefer to avoid human-derived bone if possible.

The bony window is replaced or a collagen sheet used to cover the antrostomy and the flaps closed without tension. Antibiotics are continued for 5 days. Nasal decongestants are not routinely used.

Enlarged frontal sinuses can be similarly grafted prior to orbital implant placement. Grafting is usually undertaken prior to implant placement with a healing period of at least six months.

In the atrophic premaxillary region, the nasal floor can be elevated, and grafts placed to allow anterior implant placement.

Where there is considerable maxillary deficiency, onlay grafts can be used to widen and vertically augment the alveolar ridge. Bone can be harvested from the external oblique ridge of the mandible (ramus graft) or from the iliac crest or calvarium if more volume is required (**Figure 57.11**).

An example is shown (**Figure 57.12**) where implant placement through onlay grafts was undertaken with osseointegration and subsequent reconstruction of all implants. In this case, the bone grafts were retained with 2 mm miniscrews, and the implants lag screwed through the buccal onlay grafts into the residual bone of the maxilla.

Where the maxilla is very atrophic, the deficiency can be corrected with a Le Fort I osteotomy, advancing the maxilla downwards and forwards, and interpositional bone grafts. However, the Le Fort fragment is fragile and often resorbs. The procedure in many cases has been superseded by conventional grafting.

Distraction osteogenesis techniques and distractors have been adapted for augmentation of the alveolus and closure of defects by bone transport. In selected cases, the techniques

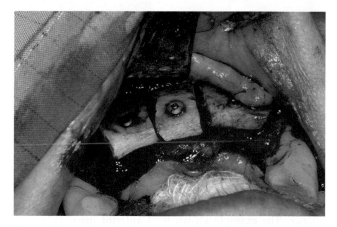

Figure 57.11   Mandibular ramus graft used to increase height and width of anterior maxilla.

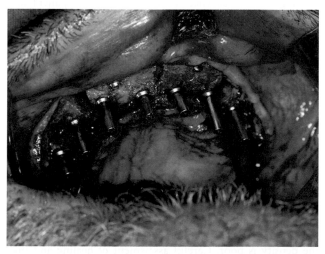

Figure 57.12   Simultaneous implants with iliac crest bone grafting.

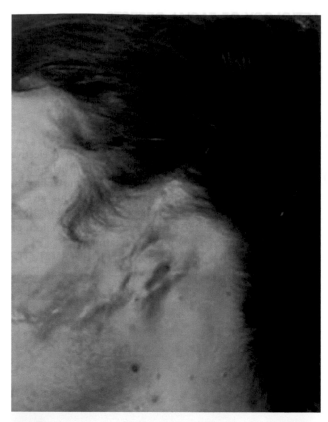

Figure 58.2 Traumatic injury.

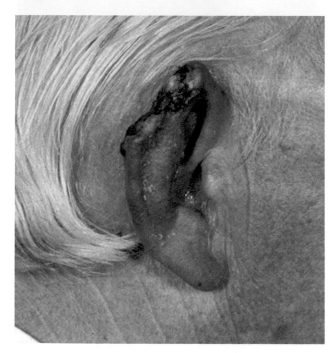

Figure 58.3 Infiltrating tumour.

the loss of vital structures and create potential impairment of function, such as sight, hearing, swallowing, speech, taste and smell. Loss of self-esteem and self-confidence are very real issues for these patients.

Every effort should be made to use the patient's own tissue and, if necessary, surgical procedures are undertaken in stages until the optimal result is obtained. If surgery is not possible (or will involve multiple procedures with an unpredictable result), then prostheses can be considered.

For patients with tumours, the defect size is determined by the amount of tissue that has to be removed during ablative resection. How the defect is left is of paramount importance if a prosthesis is to be used as it will determine the final aesthetic result. Ideally, thin skin cover is always preferable as this allows for an optimum interface between defect and prosthesis. Bulky flaps are to be avoided as they restrict contouring and positioning of prostheses and will not allow mirror imaging of existing symmetrical structures, such as eyes.

Defect reconstruction

The reconstruction of hard and soft tissues is a combination of art and science. Major defects in the craniofacial region have challenged the skills of the reconstructive surgeon. The use of microvascular free-flap transfer of hard and soft tissue to the mandible, maxilla, cranial and midface regions has greatly improved the outcome for patients. Surgical techniques have advanced using autogenous tissues to replace aesthetically difficult areas, such as the nose and ear. The results of these reconstructions, however, can be highly variable with consistent results difficult to achieve without a very high level of specialization.

It may be that the decision is not to reconstruct immediately as there may be a need to look for evidence of recurrent disease at the defect site, prior to any secondary reconstruction. Alternatively, the defect may be obliterated with a large bulky flap to close a large surgical cavity and perhaps bury residual disease prior to radiotherapy. This can have the advantage of closing communication between oral and nasal components but with limited or unacceptable aesthetics and function.

Craniofacial defects should be reconstructed as soon as the patient's condition allows. This is an important factor for all patients, including those with a poor prognosis. With the standard of autogenous or prosthetic techniques available it is not acceptable for patients with facial deformity to be precluded from leading as normal a life as possible.

Small soft tissue defects are reconstructed by covering with skin grafts, deeper defects by the use of local flaps (**Figure 58.4**). Large defects usually require coverage by a free flap. Bony defects may be reconstructed by a non-vascularized bone graft, provided that there is sufficient soft tissue coverage with non-irradiated tissue. For defects of both hard and soft tissue, a composite free flap containing bone and skin is preferred. Skeletal fixation is obtained using internal fixation with plates and screws. Sites of composite free flaps include iliac crest, fibula, scapula and radius. Radial forearm flaps have a large surface area of skin to volume; this makes them thin and suitable for both intraoral and extraoral mucosal or skin defects. However, limited bone volume can be harvested with this flap from the radius. The use of bulky flaps can compromise aesthetics and make prosthetic options impracticable. Smaller, thinner flaps and skin grafting may give coverage without compromising prosthetic possibilities. The two options are compared in **Table 58.1**.

Table 58.1 Comparison of surgical and prosthetic reconstruction.

Surgical		Prosthetic	
Advantages	**Disadvantages**	**Advantages**	**Disadvantages**
Uses patient's own tissue	May prevent inspection of defect site (for tumour patients)	Immediate temporary reconstruction	Non-mobile tissue
Reconstruction at same time as resection may be possible	May require multiple procedures	Inspection of defect (tumour patients)	Requires skilled prosthetist
More acceptable to patient	Variable aesthetic result: depends on quality of donor and recipient site	Predictable results	Long-term follow up required
Does not require prosthetic maintenance/replacements	Separate donor site often required	Easily modifiable	Replacement prosthesis required
		Does not preclude future surgical reconstruction	

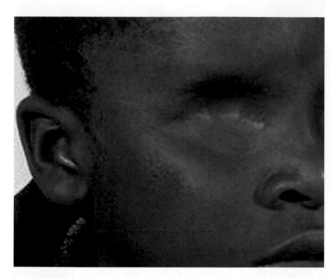

Figure 58.4 Orbital defect following exteneration.

Defect sites

AURICULAR DEFECTS

The incidence of malformation of the external ear occurs in 1 in 10 000 live births.[3] Auricular defects frequently appear in combination with those of the external auditory canal and middle ear. Unilateral microtia may be associated with facial malformations involving the first and second branchial arch. Unilateral or bilateral microtia can be part of a bilateral condition, such as Treacher Collins syndrome.

Children born with congenital defects can invoke feelings of anxiety and guilt, causing the parents to seek an immediate solution. This should be resisted and reassurance should be given to parents with an explanation of potential treatments available. Delay in treatment will allow sufficient growth to occur for an optimum aesthetic result to be achieved and for the child to understand and be involved in the process.[4] The introduction of families to parents with children of the same condition is very useful in allaying fears that their child is alone in suffering this condition.

Patients are best assessed by a multidisciplinary team, which should include ENT, maxillofacial, prosthetists and plastic surgery colleagues. Depending on the severity of the condition, a variety of treatment options may need to be considered.

The importance of hearing to development should never be overlooked or considered less important than aesthetics and should be a priority. If necessary, a bone anchored hearing aid (BAHA) should precede ear reconstruction.

A realistic age for successful prosthetics in children is 10–12 years and onwards. Our experience is that before this age children are not sufficiently developed physically or psychologically to commit to a long-term treatment regime.

Many patients referred for prosthetics have had disappointing autogenous reconstructions. This should not be used as a reason to preclude further consideration of this, as cooperation between prosthetics and autogenous reconstruction is vital to achieve a balanced and appropriate treatment for the varied range of patients with auricular defects.[5] There have been great improvements in autogenous reconstructive techniques with major contributions by Brent[6] and Nagata.[7] With improved techniques, more consistent aesthetic results can be achieved, but specialization is as important as technique to achieve these standards. The decision to opt for the prosthetic option is easer when an autogenous reconstruction is totally impractical, such as the presence of compromised skin or following tumour resection.

Indications for auricular prostheses include:

- lack of autogenous tissue;
- irradiated area;
- failed autogenous reconstruction;
- cancer resection;
- absence of lower half of pinna;
- microtia;
- patient preference;
- craniofacial anomaly;
- traumatic defect.

Microtia cases can predictably be reconstructed with a prosthesis, but have the disadvantage of long-term follow up. Treatment can compromise any future autogenous reconstruction by removal of ear remnants or compromise available soft tissue. The amount of ear left (particularly the lower third) or the position and shape of remnants can make autogenous reconstruction a more viable option. There is a role for both autogenous and prosthetic options in auricular reconstruction and both options, working to complement each other, can only benefit patient treatment regimes.

Once treatment is decided upon, careful planning is required to determine the stages and timing of treatment. The prosthetist should be involved in all stages of treatment if prosthetics is the chosen option.

NASAL DEFECTS

Nasal defects are predominantly a result of tumour surgery or traumatic loss; congenital absence is an extremely rare entity. The goal of reconstruction is to construct an aesthetically pleasing and 'functional' nose. Autogenous reconstruction must address the underlining bone and cartilage support, skin coverage, and reconstruction of the nasal lining.

Acquired defects produce a variety of midface deformities dependent on the extent of traumatic injury or ablative resection. Smaller defects are easier to reconstruct using autogenous methods. The cosmetic anatomy of the nose is classified in five aesthetic units: dorsum, lateral tip, tip, alar lobule and soft tissue triangle, as described by Burget and Menick.[8] The majority of acquired defects are confined to skin. Skin grafts from the postauricular or preauricular area are ideal because of colour and texture match in the proximal two-thirds of the nose. The distal tip requires 'thicker' coverage and is usually best reconstructed with a composite flap.

The decision to reconstruct is dependent on the health of the patient, the quality and availability of donor tissue, the presence of any residual disease and patient choice. The defect may also involve orbital and maxillectomy components and this should be considered in treatment planning.

If the lip is to be sacrificed, it is essential to reconstruct the competent boundaries if possible. This can be achieved by using local, regional or free flaps.[9] Prosthetic reconstruction is difficult in these cases because of the mobility of the surrounding tissue and the functional seal required for lip competence. Large prostheses can be difficult to stabilize and retain.

The use of osseointegration in the midface region can dramatically improve anchorage and enable complex and dynamic junctions to be accommodated within the prosthesis.[10]

Placing fixtures at the time of ablative surgery gives great advantages. It significantly reduces the time before prosthetic rehabilitation can commence. In some cases, immediate reconstruction can be started. Fixtures are best placed in bone prior to any radiotherapy, thereby increasing implant osseointegration and survival rate. Implants are ideally placed around the circumference of the defect, in the nasal rim and into the nasal bridge. It is often necessary to trim back thin bone to allow placement into wider bone. Intraoral fixtures should always be used to take advantage of as much depth of bone in the premaxilla and nasal bridge sites as possible. It can be advantageous to utilize zygomatic implants which use good quality bone at distant sites[11] while providing stability for prostheses at the defect site. It is important to involve the

prosthetist as early as possible so that impressions can be taken of the facial structures prior to ablative surgery. This enables a template to be constructed for use as a starting point in reconstructive planning of the lost tissues (**Figure 58.5**).

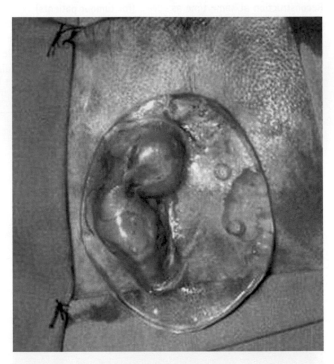

Figure 58.5   Implant template for congenital ear defect.

ORBITAL DEFECTS

Any defect that is confined only to the globe is treated with an 'indwelling prosthesis', which sits behind the lids. These prostheses, which are self-retaining, are often historically referred to as 'glass eyes', although they are now, at least in the UK, made in acrylic. Defects including the loss of orbital contents and the lids are more extensive and an orbital prosthesis will often be the treatment of choice.

The majority of patients requiring orbital prostheses have acquired defects as a result of tumour surgery. These can also include defects extending into the maxilla and or nasal area. The type of surgery for which prosthetics is required is shown in **Table 58.2**.

Reconstruction in this area is complicated by the presence of neighbouring sinuses. Any extension into the sinuses may produce a chronic discharge. In these cases, the opening can be obliterated or closed over with skin cover or a flap. Where

Table 58.2   Orbital surgery requiring prostheses.

Term	Tissue lost	Solution
Evisceration	Cornea	Cosmetic shell
Enuculation	Eye	Artificial eye
Exenteration	Eye and orbital contents	Orbital prosthesis

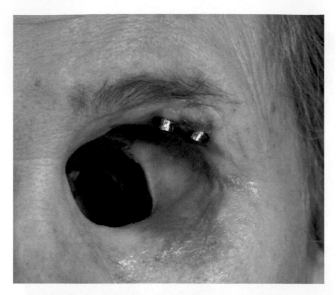

Figure 58.6 Orbital defect with implants.

there is a congenital deformity, any rudimentary eye, conjunctiva or eyelids and lashes should be removed. This should result in a deep orbital socket and a skin boundary with restricted movement to enhance prosthetic stability.

For patients who are to receive orbital prostheses, it is important that there is sufficient depth within the defect to position the eye unit and achieve symmetry with the normal side. Bulky flaps often preclude this and it is essential that consideration be given to this or further reversionary surgery will be required (**Figure 58.6**).

Extraoral implant placement can be carried out at the same time as ablative surgery or as a planned secondary procedure.

ORAL CAVITY

Intraoral prosthetics are well documented in technical and dental literature. This section will only cover prosthetics in relation to ablative surgery.

The surgical management of oral cancer requires understanding and skills in assessment, access, ablative and reconstruction surgery. Prosthetic input may be required in dealing with complex and difficult defects. Removal of soft and hard tissue has a dramatic effect on function; small defects can be closed by local flaps with free tissue transfer available for larger defects. While surgical reconstruction has improved and it is the treatment of choice, there are occasions where prosthetics is a suitable option, or it can be used if a surgical reconstruction has failed.

The objective of prosthetic rehabilitation in patients with defects of the orofacial region is the restoration of form, function and appearance. In patients with orofacial cancer, a decision should be made as to whether immediate or staged surgical reconstruction is advocated. If possible, a one-stage procedure should be used. Surgery involving the oral cavity will require preoperative dental checks and any necessary treatment should be undertaken prior to surgery. When a maxillary resection requires an intermediate obturator,

impressions are required preoperatively to enable design and construction of the plate.

The design needs to consider how the plate is to be retained, the approximate extent of the resection and whether any teeth are to be lost or utilized for retention. The type of dressing/pack is important as the type of pack can affect the design of the plate.

In the maxilla, the bony margins and alveolus should be trimmed such that primary closure of the surrounding tissues can be achieved. The hard palate pterygoid plates and nasal septum should be examined and cut back to provide a smooth, non-sharp surface and, where possible, covered with local mucosa.

Following a maxillectomy, it is important to remove the coronoid process of the mandible as it can dislodge and break the seal of a definitive prosthesis. Retaining the coronoid contributes to postoperative trismus due to temporalis shortening; trismus is further exacerbated by postoperative radiotherapy.

The surgical plate is essential to immediately restore speech and mastication and to provide support for soft tissue. Any prosthesis must be able to be modified at the time of surgery to accommodate any surgical variations that may be necessary.

The obturator is retained by using skeletal wiring, bone screws through the acrylic plate or by clasping to existing teeth. It is possible to use fast setting, expandable, silastic foam as both a dressing medium and to provide retention by a mechanical attachment to the plate.[12] This technique requires the dental plate to be held in place and the foam is poured or syringed into the defect. The foam will expand to fill the defect and sets around the retentive posts that are incorporated into the underside of the plate. The foam can easily be trimmed with scissors to give a flexible and very accurate fitting 'bung' which obturates the defect and provides support and retention to the plate.

Technical requirements for surgical splint construction include:

- dental impressions;
- approximate extent of resection;
- method of retaining plate;
- type of dressing/pack (**Figure 58.7a**).

Recent surgical developments and the use of digital technology has changed how these patients are managed. With the use of computer-generated models, it is now possible to plan the surgical resection and construct prebent plates that will fit exactly the remaining anatomy and be used as both a template and provide fixation for the free tissue bony flap. When carefully planned, these custom plates can be used for both maxillary and mandibular reconstructions and improve patient outcomes and greatly reduce surgical time.

From a prosthetic perspective, this means that a dental plate is no longer required for the ablative surgical stage as the defect is reconstructed from the patient's own tissue. Technical input is still required but in the form of planning and in the custom construction of the plates.

Patients can then go forward for conventional or implant-retained prosthetics to restore the dentition (**Figure 58.7b–e**).

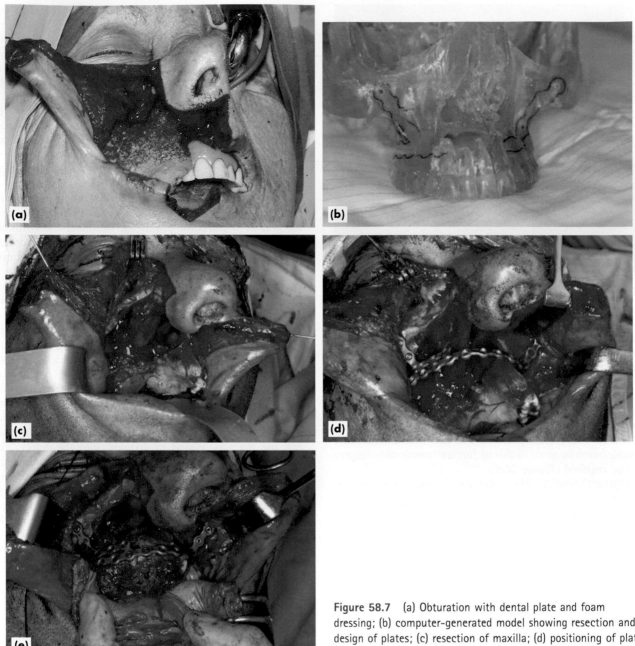

Figure 58.7   (a) Obturation with dental plate and foam dressing; (b) computer-generated model showing resection and design of plates; (c) resection of maxilla; (d) positioning of plate; (e) fixation of bony flap.[13]

Extraoral prosthesis construction

Once a decision has been taken to provide a patient with a facial prosthesis, a series of technical/clinical procedures is commenced. The retention options for the prosthesis are discussed with the patient. Clinical assessment should be carried out to establish the size and extent of the planned prosthesis and where the prosthetic margins will be finished. Soft tissue examination will help identify any mobile areas that could compromise marginal integrity of the prosthesis. Computed tomography (CT)/magnetic resonance imaging (MRI) and plain x-rays will assess the skeletal structure for potential implant sites. Impressions are taken to provide a working cast of the defect.

If the prosthesis is retained using conventional methods, unless any preprosthetic surgery is required, prosthetic construction can be commenced immediately. In patients selected for implants, it is essential to plan the optimum position for retention without compromising aesthetics. A template is constructed and used during the surgical treatment to identify implant sites for the surgeon.[13]

It is helpful to use x-ray images to determine bone depth and quality. The use of 3D computer-generated models and implant software programs can be invaluable in complex cases. Surgical guides can be made directly from the CT scan data either resting on the soft tissue or directly onto the underlying bone. However, in many cases, such as the mastoid bone, these are of less value as even in children with thin bone, as encountered in early BAHA placement, it is unlikely to change the outcome.[14] If air cells or poor quality bone are encountered in the planned positions, it is only necessary to move from the planned position until sound bone is encountered. The template will keep implant placement within acceptable limits.

In patients having ablative surgery, recent experience has shown that there is a great benefit in placing the fixtures at the time of resection.[15] It is particularly helpful in those who are to receive postoperative radiotherapy, as the osseointegration process is established before the bone is irradiated with improved survival rate compared to fixtures inserted into compromised bone. This also reduces the number of surgical procedures and the time between surgery and the fitting of the prosthesis.

The decision on fixture placement has to be made following tumour clearance and is ideally made by the surgeon and prosthetist based on the availability of bone and the usability of potential sites.

STAGES IN PROSTHETIC CONSTRUCTION

Various technical stages are involved in the fabrication of prostheses (**Figure 58.8a**):

- impression (**Figure 58.8b**)
- pattern
- mould
- processing
- fitting.

An impression is taken of the defect to create a master cast on which a wax pattern is sculptured. This can be adjusted and aligned on the patient to achieve the desired contour and orientation.

When completed, a two- or three-part mould is constructed and, using the lost-wax technique, a void is created which is then replaced by the prosthetic material. The materials of choice are silicone elastomers, which are individually coloured to match patient skin shades (**Figure 58.8c**).

FACIAL PROSTHESIS RETENTION METHODS

The success of facial prostheses depends not just on aesthetics but on the retentive qualities. The prosthesis must be comfortable and give confidence to the wearer. Methods of retention can be categorized as follows:

- adhesive
- anatomical/mechanical
- implant.

With some prosthetic devices, retention can be retained by virtue of the anatomical location, for example an artificial eye held in place by the eyelids. This also disguises any margins. Facial prostheses do not always have this convenient camouflaging; therefore, the design must take this into account to minimize any compromise of margin integrity.

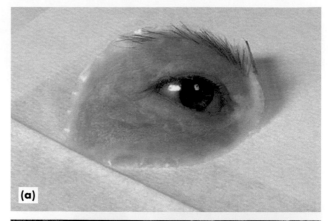

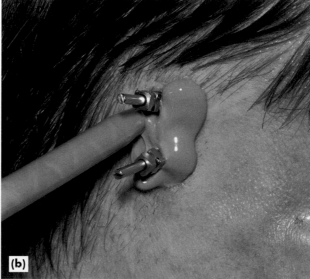

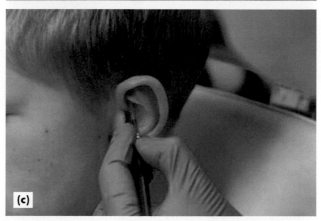

Figure 58.8 (a) Orbital prostheses; (b) impression of auricular defect incorporating implants; (c) extrinsically tinting prostheses.

Adhesive

Until the advent of implants, adhesives were often the method of choice for extraoral prostheses, providing good aesthetics if used carefully by a compliant patient. The adhesives used are waterproof and, if correctly applied, the prosthesis will remain in position for many hours (**Figure 58.9**). Most problems are encountered by the continual

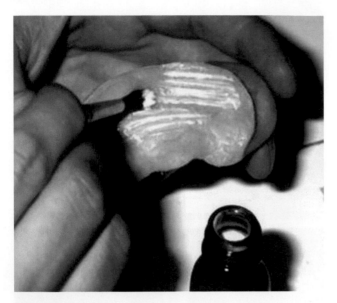

Figure 58.9   Applying adhesive to prostheses.

fitting and removal of the prosthesis. This can have a detrimental effect, particularly on the fine edges of the prosthesis. Patients will need a certain amount of dexterity to be able to locate and position the prosthesis. The type and quality of the skin can influence the choice of adhesive and the suitability of this technique. Patients with broken or compromised skin are best treated with other retentive methods. Allergic reactions to the adhesive are well recognized.

Mechanical/anatomical

Mechanical retention of facial prostheses is the oldest form of retention. Early retention included spring bands and straps. Spectacle frames are the mainstay of mechanical retention for facial prostheses. Mechanical retention can be incorporated into interlocking intra- and extraoral prosthetic combinations, such as an obturator linked to an orbital prosthesis. Spectacle-retained prostheses are still useful in cases where simplicity and ease of location is of paramount importance. They have a particular application in the elderly and patients who have dexterity problems. The prosthesis is attached to the spectacle frame which means that the patient is not able to remove their glasses without revealing the defect. The adjustment of the glasses is important as it will have a direct bearing on the location and fit of the prosthesis.

Anatomical retention is possible in patients who have favourable undercuts. These are the result of soft tissue contracture, such as in a maxillectomy defect where a soft tissue band contracts to give a ledge over which an obturator rim can be rotated, or in areas where soft silicone flanges may be expanded to create retention via gentle, local, expansive pressure.

Obtaining the correct amount of retentive pressure is difficult and care must be exercised not to ulcerate the tissue as a result of overload. This technique is more suited to intraoral defects. Obturator-retained extraoral prostheses are more likely to be affected by facial movements and can cause the loss of marginal integrity.

Implant retained

Implants provide a stable and secure method of retention. The margins of any implant-retained prosthesis can be very thin as they are much less likely to tear than those around adhesive-retained prostheses. Thin margins offer the best possible aesthetics.

Implants were first used in extraoral sites in Sweden in 1977. This is now an established technique that provides predictable results for patients with various craniofacial defects.[16] Implants allow prostheses to be extremely stable and secure. The prosthesis is generally retained in place by a rigid bar with clips or by magnets incorporated into the prosthesis and connecting to magnetic caps on the implant.[17]

The number of implants required for retention of any prosthesis is determined by the size and shape of the defect. Auricular defects that involve only the pinna will usually only require two implants for adequate retention. This is achieved by a bar and clip arrangement. In cases where bone quality is poor or when the tissue has been irradiated, it is advisable to overengineer the reconstruction and place further fixtures as 'sleepers' in case of future failures.

Following fixture placement, the size of the abutment that attaches to the implant and which emerges through the skin is determined by the thickness of the tissue and the aesthetic requirements. It may be advisable to initially place healing abutments and then the prosthetist can select the optimal abutment type and size following the healing phase. These healing abutments can also be used in selected circumstances when the implants are placed in a transcutaneous fashion rather than submerged. The abutments are, in turn, fitted with the appropriate prosthetic components, depending on the retentive elements selected for prosthesis attachment. If necessary, angled abutments can be used to overcome problems with implant placement and to aid prosthesis location. In certain cases, prosthetic components can be connected directly to the fixture.

The bar and clip arrangement has the advantage that the clips are adjustable and the bar design can be modified to keep the retention components low proile and within the margins of the prosthesis. The bar is connected by gold screws into the abutments (**Figure 58.10**).

Magnets have a role with some patients in auricular cases and retention can be further enhanced by using lip magnets which have increased resistance to lateral dislodgement. Magnets are particularly useful in orbital and midface cases where bar construction is difficult or complex and location of the prosthesis could be difficult for the patient. They also have a role in patients with limited manual dexterity or impaired vision as they are easier to clean and maintain. Ball attachments can also be utilized but are not favoured by the authors. They have been superseded by locator-type attachments which have a greater surface area and are more tolerant of divergent angulations.

The advantages and disadvantages of implant-retained extraoral prostheses are summarized in **Table 58.3**.

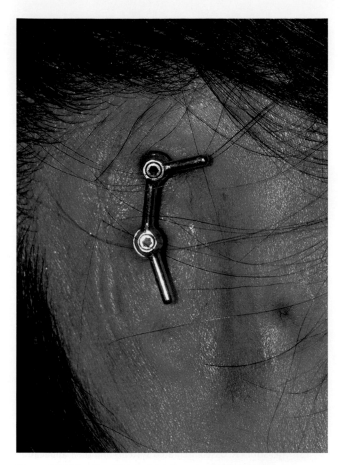

Figure 58.10 Bar attachment for prosthetic retention.

Table 58.3 Implant-retained extraoral prostheses.

Advantages	Disadvantages
Secure retention	Two-stage surgery usually
Fine margins of prosthesis	required
Positive location	Planning required for implant
Prosthesis or patient not	positioning and defect site
affected by adhesive	Expensive components
Spectacles can be removed	Patient must maintain hygiene
independently of prosthesis	Possible skin reaction around the
	abutments
	Success rates compromised
	postradiotherapy

PATIENT FOLLOW-UP MANAGEMENT

The choice of a prosthetic reconstruction results in an ongoing commitment for the prosthetic team and the patient. The patient needs to maintain a significant level of hygiene, particularly if there are skin-penetrating abutments. They have to exercise care in seating and cleaning the prosthesis and commit to long-term follow up.

The success of the reconstruction reflects the ability of the prosthetist to design a functional and well-fitting prosthesis. The prosthetist should give instructions on how to position, apply and remove the prosthesis with details of any instructions regarding wearing. It is important that the prosthesis does not restrict the patient's activities and lifestyle. Implant-borne prostheses give the most predictable results, but should not be considered the only option.

Dealing with patients with facial disfigurement is very demanding and requires an understanding of patient expectations, tempered with a realization of what is practical or possible.[18] Patient reactions to facial disfigurement vary greatly. Time spent with patients in consultation is important in building a relationship to enable sensible and practical options to be considered.

Quality of life outcomes are now a welcome and vital issue to be considered in patient management.[19] Patients require lifelong follow up for maintenance and adjustment of prostheses, examination of any implants, abutments and the local skin.[20] The commitment to long-term management must be discussed with the patient.

CURRENT DEFICIENCIES AND FUTURE DEVELOPMENTS

There have been many developments in materials used for the production of prostheses. The advent of the percutaneous osseointegrated implant has dramatically improved the potential for retention of any prosthesis. However, many of the construction methods and mould-making techniques have changed little and remain highly skilled and time-consuming. Each prosthesis is individually produced and the use of high technology has been difficult to adapt or, to date, is not cost-effective.

With advances in computer software using CT data, there are programs available that allow 3D simulation of facial reconstructive methods including osteotomy and distraction procedures. Data from medical scanners (CT, MRI) can be used to reproduce physical models of human anatomy via rapid prototyping (RP). Several RP techniques exist, the most common being stereolithography. The basic principle of creating a 3D structure is to build layers using the CT data and an optical scanning system that draws a shape one layer at a time onto the surface of the liquid photosensitive resin until the desired model is completed.

It is possible to have individual implant templates for either soft tissue or direct bone contact to allow exact implant placement. Precise anatomical models (3D) made by RP enable surgeons to view and evaluate their treatment plans. On this physical model, osteotomy lines or drilling holes can be indicated and trial surgery can be undertaken. These models can be used, if necessary, to pre-bend plates ready for surgical procedures. The applications of these models can be advantageous in both facial reconstruction and in the production of obturator prostheses for maxillary defects and designing and planning cranioplasties for skull defects.

Improvements in surgical techniques and the advent of specialization have enabled more accurate and aesthetic reconstructions to be performed. While prosthetic materials continue to be improved and refined, these surgical improvements may render prostheses to be necessary in a more limited format. The necessity of treating tumours by ablative surgery in the future may be reduced by other treatment regimes and therefore the necessity to surgically or prosthetically reconstruct these defects could be reduced.

The use of current technology and digital imaging in processing complex shapes and patterns is now achievable and readily available. In certain circumstances, it can produce moulds and patterns that are difficult to duplicate by conventional methods. It remains to be seen whether the use of this technology is cost-effective in individual cases, or is just another method of obtaining the same result. As with most new techniques, there is a tendency to overuse. Careful evaluation of each individual case should be a balance between the need to obtain the optimal result and the cost-effectiveness of the process. These technological advances are an essential and welcome addition to reconstructive surgical and prosthetic practice.

KEY LEARNING POINTS

- Have realistic expectations.
- Follow reconstructive ladder.
- Be able to offer all options to the same standard.
- Keep prosthetics simple and user friendly.
- Spend time with patients to establish a full understanding of procedures.
- Make sure patients have an expected time frame.

ACKNOWLEDGEMENTS

The role and practice of medical and surgical disciplines has become increasingly specialized with patients treated in centres with a high concentration of complex cases. These centres with their multidisciplinary teams and expertise can help to provide the comprehensive care necessary to deal with the demands required to deliver a head and neck service. To meet patient prosthetic expectations can be technically, clinically and emotionally challenging, and we would like to acknowledge the work of our colleague Peter Jeynes (MIMPT) for his expertise and support in the prosthetic management of these patients.

REFERENCES

1. Conroy B. The history of facial prostheses. *Clinics in Plastic Surgery* 1983; **10**: 689–707.
2. Manigula AJ, Stucker FJ, Stepnick DW (eds). *Surgical reconstruction of the face and anterior skull base*. Philadelphia: WB Saunders, 1999: 3.
3. Proops DW. Bone anchored hearing aids and prostheses. *Journal of Laryngology and Otology* 1993; **107**: 99–100.
4. Waterfield LJ, Worrollo SJ, Wake MJC, Proops DW. The position of BAHA in relation to a bone anchored auricular prostheses. *Journal of Maxillofacial Prosthetics and Technology* 1997; **1**: 1–9.
5. Wilkes G, Wolfaardt J. Auricular defects: treatment options. In: Branemark P-I, Tolman DE (eds). *Osseointegration in craniofacial construction*. Carol Stream, IL: Quintessence, 1998: 141–53.
6. Brent B. The correction of microtia with autogenous cartilage. *Plastic and Reconstructive Surgery* 1980; **66**: 13–21.
7. Nagta S. A new method of total reconstruction of the auricle for microtia. *Plastic and Reconstructive Surgery* 1993; **92**: 187–201.
8. Burget GC, Menick FJ. The subunit principle in nasal reconstruction. *Plastic and Reconstructive Surgery* 1985; **76**: 239–47.
9. Jackson I. Chapter 12, Management of soft tissue. In: Branemark P-I, Tolman DE (eds). *Osseointegration in craniofacial construction*. Carol Stream, IL: Quintessence, 1998: 127–39.
10. Beumer J III, Roumanas E, Nishimura R. Advances in osseointegrated implants for dental and facial rehabilitation following major head and neck surgery. *Seminars in Surgical Oncology* 1995; **11**: 200–7.
11. Weicher T, Schetter D, Nohor C. Titanium implants in the zygoma as retaining elements after hemimaxillectomy. *International Journal of Oral and Maxillofacial Implants* 1997; **12**: 211–14.
12. Buckle JP. Adaptation and application of silicone foams. *Journal of Maxillofacial Prosthetics and Technology* 1998; **2**: 27–9.
13. Tjellstrom A. Osseointegrated systems and their application in head and neck surgery. *Advances in Otolaryngology – Head and Neck Surgery* 1989; **3**: 39–70.
14. Proops DW. The Birmingham bone anchored hearing aid progamme: surgical methods and complications. *Journal of Larynology and Otology* 1996; **21**: 7–12.
15. Dover MS, Worrollo SJ. Prosthetic rehabilitation of the facial area. *Current Opinion in Otolaryngology and Head and Neck Surgery* 2002; **10**: 129–33.
16. Tjellström A, Portmann D. Osseointegrated implants in facial prosthesis and hearing aids. *Revue de Laryngologie, Otologie, Rhinologie* 1992; **113**: 439–45.
17. Johnson F, Cannavina G, Brook I, Watson J. Facial prosthetics: techniques used in the retention of prostheses following ablative cancer surgery or trauma and for congenital defects. *European Journal of Prosthodontics and Restorative Dentistry* 2000; **8**: 5–9.
18. Newton T, Fiske J, Foote O *et al*. Preliminary study of the impact of loss of part of the face and its prosthetic reconstruction. *Journal of Prosthetic Dentistry* 1999; **82**: 585–90.
19. Sloan JA, Tolman DE, Anderson JD. Patients with reconstruction of craniofacial or intra oral defects; development of instruments to measure quality of life. *International Journal of Oral and Maxillofacial Implants* 2001; **16**: 225–45.
20. Habakuk SW. Care of the facial prostheses. In: McKinstry RE (ed.). *Fundamentals of facial prostheses*. Arlington, VA: ABI Professional Publications, 1995: 193–9.

APPENDIX: CASE REPORTS

Case report A

This female patient underwent a total rhinectomy for a squamous cell carcinoma of the nose. This was followed by a course of radical radiotherapy of 55 Gy in 20 fractions. Her initial management was with an adhesive-retained nasal prosthesis, but this had limitations in terms of stability and aesthetics. She was then transferred to our unit for her prosthetic management and consideration for extraoral implants to retain her nasal prosthesis. Given her radiotherapy exposure, hyperbaric oxygen therapy was undertaken for 20 sessions pre- and 10 sessions post-implant placement at a pressure of 2.2 ATA with oxygen breathing for 90 minutes. Three implants were placed in the base of the nose 13, 10 and 15 mm in length. The implants were allowed to heal undisturbed for six months before exposure, following which a new prosthesis was made, retained by a bar and clip giving very secure anchorage (**Figure 58.11**).

As a general rule, we no longer use extraoral implants for the retention of facial prostheses, with the exception of ears. In almost all cases, conventional implants such as those used for intraoral reconstruction are suitable. There are clear advantages to using longer implants in terms of long-term survival and load-carrying ability.

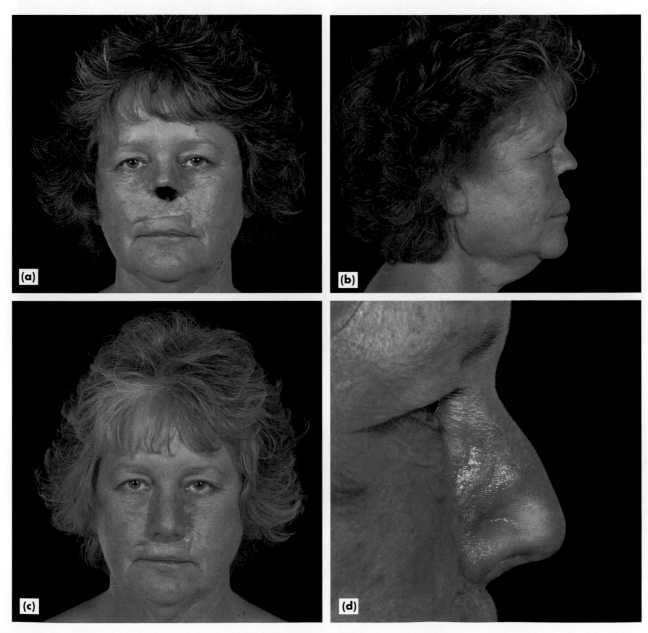

Figure 58.11   Case A, Rinectomy: (a,b) Nasal defect; (c,d) with prostheses.

Case report B

In 1990, a female patient underwent a total rhinectomy and right neck dissection for a squamous cell carcinoma of the nose. Her initial management was with a spectacle-retained nasal prosthesis, but this had limitations in terms of stability and aesthetics. In 1997, she was referred to us and under a general anesthetic had three standard Brånemark fixtures placed, one 10 mm implant in the nasal bridge, extending up into the anterior wall of the fontal sinus and two 13 mm implants placed obliquely downwards into the pyriform rim of the nasal sill (**Figure 58.12a**). The implants were allowed to heal undisturbed for six months before exposure. Magnets have been used to retain the nasal prosthesis (**Figure 58.12b**). The patient is now freed from using spectacles and has much greater confidence in the prosthesis, particularly when playing with her grandchildren (**Figure 58.12c** and **58.12d**).

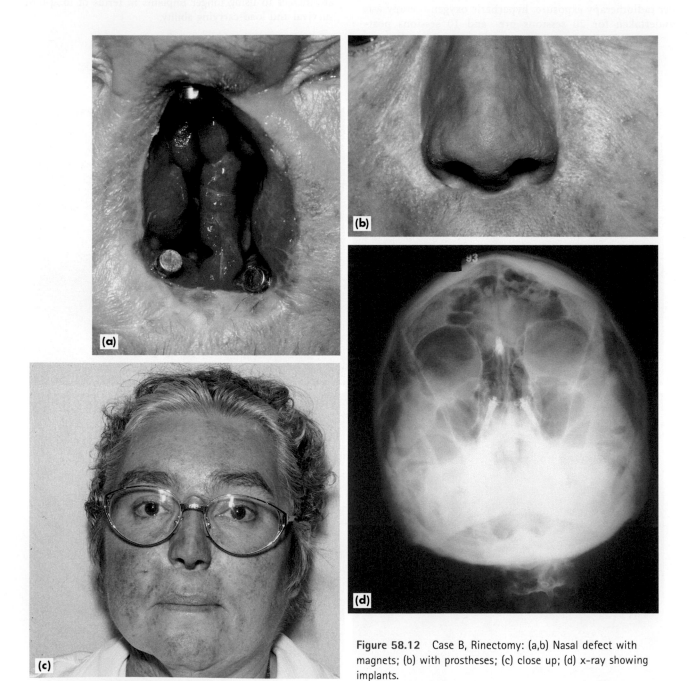

Figure 58.12   Case B, Rinectomy: (a,b) Nasal defect with magnets; (b) with prostheses; (c) close up; (d) x-ray showing implants.

Case report C

This female patient had a craniofacial resection for an adenoidcystic carcinoma resulting in a right orbital exteneration. Extraoral implants were placed for retention for an orbital prosthesis. Initially four implants were placed and three were utilized using magnets for retention; the remaining implant was left as a 'sleeper' to be used if required in the future. This patent has now had implants for over 20 years, during which time one was removed because of inherit pain and one lost. Two further implants have been placed and retention is now via a bar and clip arrangement. The patient has consistently used the prosthesis on a daily basis only removing it at night (**Figure 58.13**).

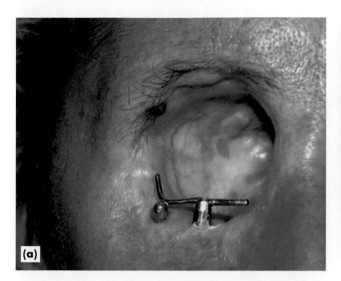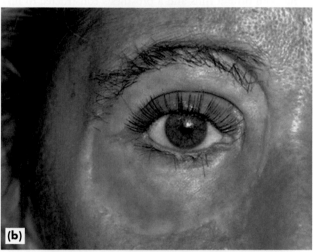

Figure 58.13   Case C, Orbital exteneration: (a) Orbital defect; (b) with prostheses.

Case report D

At the age of 19, this male sustained a gunshot injury to his midface that rendered him blind (**Figure 58.14**). His mother cared him for until his mid-40s when he was referred to our unit. A large mucocele of the frontal sinus was present and surgically removed, together with debridement of the frontal sinus and bone grafting of the anterior skull base. Once all residual infection had been treated, implants were placed around both orbital rims and a prosthesis constructed to fill the orbital and nasal defects (**Figure 58.14b** and **58.14c**). Although blind, the psychological benefit to this patient and that of his mother can best be expressed by the letter she wrote to the department on completion of treatment.

> As a mother and on behalf of my son, I wish to convey to you all my most sincere thanks and admiration for your skills, your care, your unique approach and above all your commitment and professionalism to your work. He has been transformed both visually and spiritually. He enjoys company and has the confidence to meet and make new friends. He wakes in the morning looking forward to another day at last feeling equal and acceptable to everyone. I cannot explain to you how grateful we both are to you all.

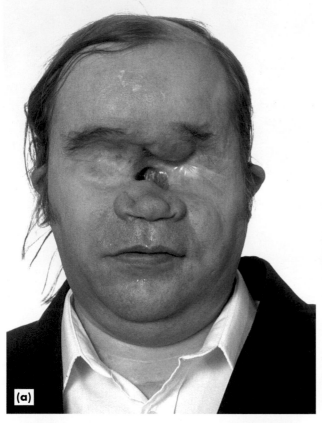

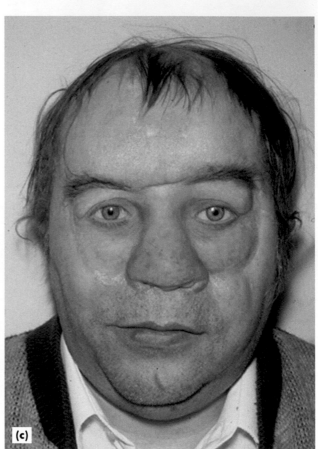

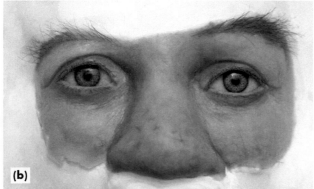

Figure 58.14   Case D, Traumatic midface defect: (a) Facial defect; (b) prostheses; (c) prostheses *in situ*.

Case report E

This young girl presented with a lesion on the left ear which was diagnosed as nodular melanoma.

Treatment was a pinnectomy with insertion of two 4 mm extraoral implants for an immediate prosthetic reconstruction. The external abutments were also placed during this procedure. The prosthesis was fitted within three months of the ablative surgery when the skin had fully healed and osseointegration of implants had occurred. Retention was by using a bar and clips method which gives very secure fixation.

Autogenous reconstruction was not considered an option at this stage because of the pathology. Close observation of the defect was considered essential in the initial and intermediate stages. The prosthesis will not prevent any autogenous reconstruction should that be considered in the future (**Figure 58.15**).

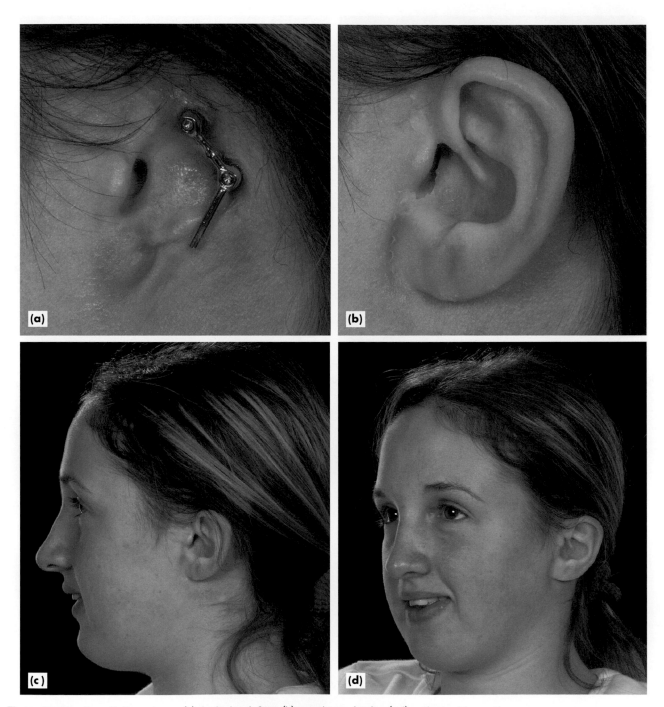

Figure 58.15 Case E, Pinnectomy: (a) Auricular defect; (b) prostheses *in situ*; (c,d) patient with prostheses.

Case report F

This patient had an infiltrating basal cell carcinoma left pinna extending into the external auditory meatus. Treatment was pinnectomy, coverage with split skin graft and osseointegrated implants.

Two 4 mm fixtures were placed with abutments as a one stage procedure.

Fabrication of the prostheses was commenced following healing of the defect area and integration of the implants. The prosthesis was retained using a bar framework. Patients are given full instruction on the care and fitting of the prostheses.

It is also important to involve them in the process during construction in terms of projection and form, etc. This helps with building confidence and having input to the final appearance (**Figure 58.16**).

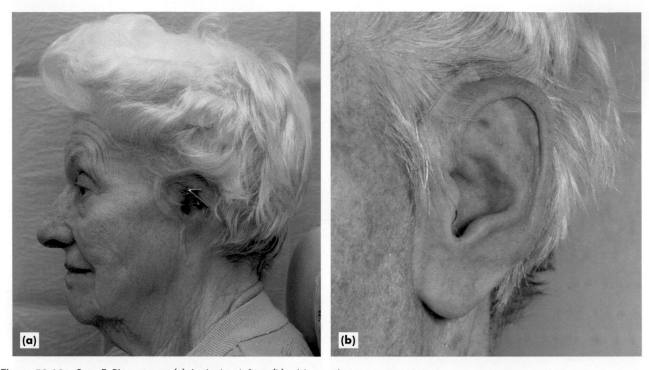

Figure 58.16   Case F, Pinnectomy: (a) Auricular defect; (b) with prostheses.

59

Voice restoration

REHAN KAZI, PETER RHYS-EVANS AND PETER CLARKE

Nothing that I can do will change the structure of the universe. But maybe, by raising my voice I can help the greatest of all causes – goodwill among men and peace on earth.

Albert Einstein

INTRODUCTION

Despite advances in conservative laryngeal surgery and radiotherapy, laryngectomy still remains the procedure of choice for advanced-stage laryngeal carcinoma and relapse after radiotherapy. However, the procedure results in a life-long stoma, loss of normal voice, loss of nasal function and lung function changes. Increased cough and mucus and reduced swallowing efficiency are also common.[1]

Functional rehabilitation of patients has improved in the last two decades as increasing emphasis on primary voice restoration and quality of life have become as important as cure and survival. Concern about loss of natural voice is very often traumatic for the laryngectomee, but with preoperative counselling from speech and language therapists and modern surgical voice restoration, good quality voice results should be the norm.

TYPES OF ALARYNGEAL SPEECH

For normal speech production, a moving column of air from the lungs is exhaled through the adducted vocal cord producing a tone which is modified by the articulators into speech. Following laryngectomy, not only is the vibratory source removed, but the air supply (lungs) is disconnected from the articulators. Attempts to develop voice after laryngectomy have utilized an external sound source (e.g. electrolarynx and Cooper Rand®), or used the pharyngeal mucosa as a vibratory sound source, utilizing the oesophagus rather than the lungs as an air supply (oesophageal speech) or reconnecting the lungs to the pharynx with a surgical shunt (e.g. Staffieri®, Amatsu®) or with a valved prosthesis in a fistula (e.g. Blom Singer®, Groningen®, Provox®).[1, 2] In the future, possible laryngeal transplantation or artificial laryngeal implantation can be foreseen.

Electrolarynx

There are two types of electrolarynges, an external type that is placed against the neck (the most common) and an oral type (intraoral placement device). The neck placement type is placed flush to the skin on the side of the neck, under the chin or on the cheek. The sound vibration is transmitted through a metal or plastic head on the device and transmitted through the tissues in the pharynx, hypopharynx and the oral cavity and then articulated normally.[1] Most neck placement devices can also be converted into an intraoral device by using an adapter. A small tube is placed in the oral cavity and the generated sound is then articulated. The intraoral feature may be useful in the postoperative period when tenderness can prevent the adequate placement of an electrolarynx on the neck (**Figure 59.1**).

The main advantages of the electrolarynx are its relatively short learning time, the ability to use it immediately postoperatively, its relative low cost and its minimal maintenance. The main disadvantages include the mechanical, monotonous and robot-like sound quality, the necessity to use a hand to operate the controls and dependence on batteries.[2, 3, 4, 5]

Oesophageal speech

Oesophageal speech was the mainstay of alaryngeal communication until the early 1980s and had been used as a method of voice restoration for over 100 years. It entails trapping air in the mouth or pharynx and propelling it into the oesophagus.[3, 4, 5, 6, 7, 8] The patient can then reflux the air up through the oesophagus, vibrating the pharyngeal mucosa or 'pharyngo-oesophageal (PE) segment'. This produces a belch-like sound that can be articulated by the tongue, lips and teeth. The vibratory segment is located in

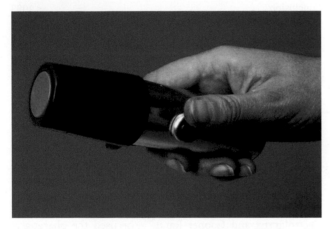

Figure 59.1   Image of a classic representative electrolarynx.

the lower cervical region, corresponding to C5 to C7. The cricopharyngeus and thyropharyngeus contribute to the formation of the vibratory segment (**Figure 59.2**).

The advantages of oesophageal speech are that it requires no batteries and no apparatus need be purchased or maintained, it does not sound mechanical and it does not require additional surgery, and it provides hands-free speech. The major disadvantage of it is that very few laryngectomees are successful users. Success rates for intelligible post-laryngectomy oesophageal speech varies from 14 to 75 per cent and to acquire oesophageal speech requires 30–50 hours of intense speech therapy.[4, 5, 6, 7, 8, 9, 10, 11]

Tracheoesophageal voice using voice prosthesis

Since the introduction of the first useful, reliable voice prosthesis by Singer and Blom in 1980, the success rate of vocal rehabilitation after total laryngectomy has improved considerably.[1, 2, 3, 4] Prosthetic voice restoration is presently the method of choice for most medical professionals treating laryngectomized patients, and has transformed the expectation and quality of voice production after total laryngectomy over the past 25 years. The technique involves creating a simple tracheo-oesophageal puncture between the posterior wall of the tracheostome and the upper oesophagus into which a one-way silicone valve is inserted. Occlusion of the stoma allows air during exhalation to be shunted into the pharynx. Sound is then produced by vibrating the mucosa of the pharyngo-oesophageal segment.[1, 2] Speech is then produced by articulation of this sound in the oral cavity. The one-way valve prevents salivary and liquid soiling the airway (**Figure 59.3**).

Initially, the puncture technique was used as a secondary procedure in patients with previous laryngectomy who failed to achieve oesophageal speech, but the consistently good results and superior quality of voice prompted

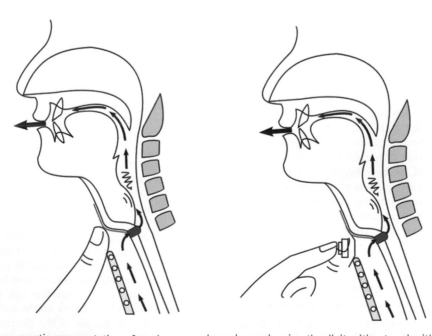

Figure 59.2   Line diagrammatic representation of trachea-oesophageal speech using the digit without and with a HME.

Hamaker *et al.* in 1985 to incorporate the tracheo-oesophageal puncture at the time of laryngectomy as a primary procedure.[12, 13, 14, 15]

The advantages of tracheo-oesophageal voice over oesophageal voice are many. It is more quickly and easily attained, it is more intelligible, natural sounding, and has improved intensity and duration of speech, achieving more words with one breath when compared to oesophageal speakers. Although the vibrating PE segment, the resonating vocal tract and the articulators are the same, the major difference between fistula and oesophageal speech is in the volume and capacity of the air reservoir leading to louder and more sustained voice.

Since its air supply is pulmonary, tracheo-oesophageal speech is closer to laryngeal speech than oesophageal speech on a range of voice parameters, such as fundamental frequency, jitter, shimmer, words per minute and maximum phonation time (**Table 59.1**).[10, 11, 12, 13, 14]

For patients undergoing laryngectomy, the gold standard for voice rehabilitation is the rapid restoration of near-normal speech within 2–3 weeks of operation with primary tracheo-oesophageal puncture and voice prosthesis. The contraindications to doing this routinely are few, but careful selection of patients will help to reduce disappointment and failure. In established laryngectomees, careful investigation and selection is more critical for secondary voice restoration in order to achieve success.[1] In all cases, there are a number of anatomical, physiological, psychological and social factors that need to be considered.

SELECTION CRITERIA FOR PRIMARY SPEECH RESTORATION

Primary voice restoration

Primary voice restoration is now standard practice and patients undergoing laryngectomy should feel confident that they will be able to talk shortly after their operation. There are few contraindications to primary puncture at the time of laryngectomy.[1, 15, 16, 17, 18] Even if there are concerns about dexterity or a patient's ability to manage their prothesis, most should be offered this as many will cope well and if there are continuing concerns it is easily reversible by removing the prosthesis. However, if the upper oesophagus is resected and replaced with jejunum or stomach, it is preferable to delay voice restoration for some weeks. Equally, if the trachea is separated from the upper oesophagus, consideration should be given to delaying the formation of the puncture. If circumferential resection and reconstruction is limited to the pharynx, it is quite reasonable to undertake a primary voice restoration provided that the lower anastomosis is well above the proposed puncture site (**Table 59.2**).[19, 20, 21, 22, 23, 24, 25]

Surgical technique of primary voice restoration

Certain fundamental principles and modifications have been incorporated into the laryngectomy technique to ensure good predictable voice results with minimal risk of complications.

SURGICAL TECHNIQUE

Of prime importance is the need to resect all diseased tissue to provide good oncological results. There are, however, a number of fundamental steps that improve the voice and swallowing results and these should be undertaken if they do not compromise the oncological resection.[1, 3, 15, 16, 17, 18, 26]

The laryngectomy is carried out in the usual fashion conserving as much pharyngeal mucosa as possible, particularly over the postcricoid region, the piriform fossae and the vallecullae, provided safe clearance from the tumour is obtained. The thyropharyngeus and cricopharyngeaus muscles should be dissected off the thyroid laminae on both sides preserving as much muscle as possible. For hypopharyngeal tumours, the mucosa of the uninvolved piriform fossa is carefully preserved to minimize the need for flap reconstruction. Ideally, a transverse mucosal width of at least 6 cm is necessary to enable adequate swallowing and effortless tracheo-oesophageal speech. Augmentation of the pharynx

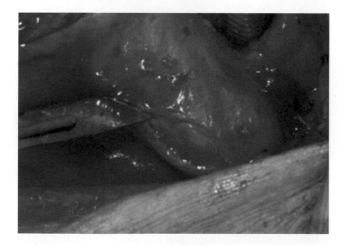

Figure 59.3 Myotomy through full thickness of upper oesophageal muscles.

Table 59.1 Comparison between laryngeal, oesophageal and tracheo-oesophageal speech.

Physical requirements	Laryngeal speech	Oesophageal speech	Tracheo-oesophageal speech
Initiator	Lungs 500 mL	Oesophageal air 40–70 mL	Lungs 500 mL
Vibrator	Vocal cords	Pharyngo-oesophageal segment	Pharyngo-oesophageal segment
Articulators	Tongue, teeth, lips, soft palate	Tongue, teeth, lips, soft palate	Tongue, teeth, lips, soft palate

Adapted from Rhys-Evans *et al.*[1]

Table 59.2 Primary versus secondary puncture.

Timing of insertion	Advantages	Disadvantages
Primary	One operation No nasogastric tube Rapid return of voice Lung powered speech Minimal time off work Oesophageal voice useable	Initial sensitive stoma Postoperative radiotherapy may delay speech
Delayed	Healing stabilized May have developed oesophageal speech	Two operations Considerable time off work Aphonic for much longer Fear of second operation Myotomy may be necessary Greater voice failure rate

Adapted from Rhys-Evans et al.[1]

with a flap is preferable if the residual mucosal strip is under 6 cm, otherwise stenosis is likely with significant functional impairment.

Cricopharyngeal myotomy

Once the larynx is removed, a myotomy of the upper oesophageal sphincter is carried out. This is important to avoid hypertonicity and spasm of these muscles during attempted phonation and to allow expansion of the upper oesophagus providing an air 'reservoir' below the PE segment. Hypertonicity or spasm will interrupt the flow of air to a varying degree, restricting or completely stopping voice production. This spasm appears to be caused by reflex contraction of cricopharyngeal and constrictor muscles when the upper oesophagus is distended with air. It seems to be a cause of tracheo-oesophageal puncture speech failure in 10–12 per cent of patients (**Figure 59.3**).[1, 3, 27]

A short posterior midline myotomy is carried out with a scalpel over a distance of 4–5 cm from just below the level of the tracheo-oesophageal puncture site into the fibres of thyropharyngeus. This divides the circular muscle fibres in the upper oesophagus and the cricopharyngeus. It is important that all muscle fibres are cut. It is unclear whether assessment of the upper oesophageal sphincter with a finger can predict the development of spasm and there seems little contraindication to doing a myotomy on all patients, indeed it may also improve swallow. One of the conclusions of the European multicentre audit of speech and swallowing results after laryngectomy was that myotomy improved voice outcomes.

A unilateral pharyngeal plexus neurectomy has been advocated in the past as an alternative method of constrictor relaxation. Three to five branches of the plexus entering the lateral wall of the pharynx are exposed and tested with a nerve stimulator before cautery and division. This is not in widespread use however.

Tracheo-oesophageal puncture

The puncture is positioned in the midline about 10–15 mm below the cut end of the posterior tracheal wall. The tip of a pair of curved artery forceps is inserted through the pharyngeal defect and advanced into the upper oesophagus just as far as the puncture site, tenting up the mucosa. A scalpel

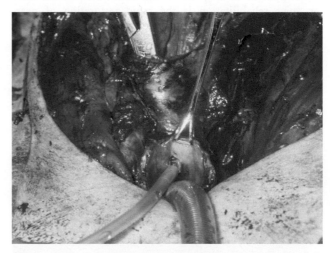

Figure 59.4 Primary puncture and insertion of stomagastric tube. A prosthesis may also be inserted primarily.

is used to incise minimally and horizontally through the mucosa and muscle on to the tip of the forceps, which are then advanced into the tracheal lumen and opened to grasp the tip of a 14NG tube or Foley catheter (**Figure 59.4**).[1]

The forceps and the catheter are then withdrawn through the fistula tract and the tip of the catheter is passed distally down the oesophagus. The catheter is anchored to the skin above the stoma at the end of the procedure. Absorbable sutures between the oesophageal wall and the posterior aspect of the trachealis on either side of the proposed position of the puncture secure the party wall and avoids inadvertent separation.

Pharyngeal closure

A horizontal closure of the pharyngeal defect is preferred using an interrupted or continuous absorbable mucosal suture and then an interrupted muscle layer. This produces a wider pharynx above the PE segment which has been shown to improve resonance for speech. A 'T' closure results in a three-point junction which probably increases the risk of leak and fistula. Significant resection of the hypopharynx will necessitate a flap reconstruction. The thyropharyngeus

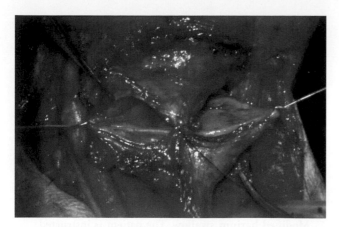

Figure 59.5   Horizontal closure of pharyngeal defect.

constrictor muscle is then brought together anteriorly with mattress sutures. The purpose is to try to create a suitable, 'tonic' PE segment at the optimal site in the pharynx with a good air reservoir below it and a wide resonating pharyngeal segment above (**Figure 59.5**).

While the upper oesophagus needs to be relaxed so that it does not respond to air being injected through the valve by going into spasm, the neopharynx or PE segment needs to provide an area where the mucosa is in apposition to allow it to vibrate efficiently and produce strong voice. Repairing the thyropharyngeus provides this vibratory segment. Conversely, if the muscles or PE segment wall are hypotonic (e.g. after total pharyngolaryngectomy and reconstruction, or if the thyropharyngeus is not repaired) the voice will be weak because there is minimal or absent muscle in the wall to create a PE segment.

Repair of the suprahyoid muscles

Following repair of the thyropharyngeus, it is important to suture the suprahyoid muscles down to the thyropharyngeus. This strengthens the mucosa above the repair thus avoiding a pseudoepiglottis and anterior pouch which can significantly affect swallow and also reattaches the middle constrictor and other suprahyoid muscles which are important in the swallow reflex (**Figure 59.6**).

Reinnervation of the pharynx

The cut ends of the superior laryngeal nerves and the recurrent laryngeal nerves may be reimplanted into the muscular wall of the reconstructed pharynx and upper oesophagus respectively in the hope that this may restore some sensory and motor reinnervation.[1] It is felt that this can only have a potentially beneficial effect on neuromuscular coordination of the reconstructed 'neolarynx', although obviously it is difficult to measure any effect objectively.

Stoma reconstruction

The size, shape and contour of the stoma and surrounding skin are important to aid digital occlusion of the stoma and help ensure optimal adhesion of the tracheostoma valve housing. In order to avoid unnecessary tracheal retraction, at laryngectomy the trachea should not be transected too low and the margins of the trachea can be sutured to the medial margins of the sternomastoid muscles to secure it near the

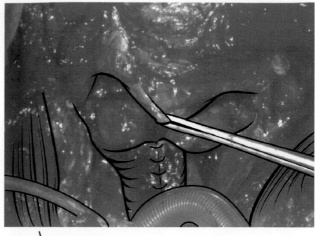

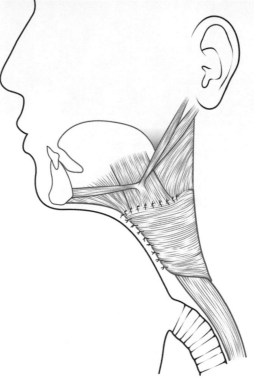

Figure 59.6   Repair of the suprahyoid muscles after repair of thyropharyngeus/cricopharyngeus.

skin. If the tendons of the sternomastoid muscle are prominent, they could be safely divided to ensure a smooth and circular stomal appearance (**Figure 59.7**).

SECONDARY VOICE RESTORATION

The technique of tracheo-oesophageal puncture with prosthetic voice restoration was originally developed for those patients who had failed to achieve adequate oesophageal speech. A preliminary videofluoroscopy will determine whether it is necessary to carry out a constrictor myotomy at the same operation and other procedures, such as stoma revision, may also be indicated at the same time. The selection of suitable patients has previously been discussed.

Assessment

Post-laryngectomy, the patient needs a tonic pharyngo-oesophageal segment to provide a satisfactory vibratory source for tracheo-oesophageal (TO) speech.[1] The first step in assessing patients who present for secondary voice restoration after laryngectomy, when they have failed oesophageal speech acquisition, should be an assessment of PE segment tonicity (**Tables 59.3** and **59.4**).

TONICITY

This is best assessed with videofluoroscopy. Therapeutic options for pharyngo-oesophageal spasm include pharyngeal

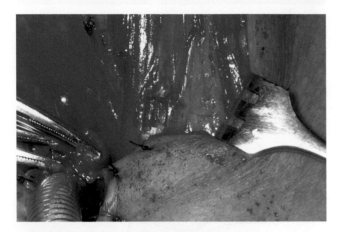

Figure 59.7 Division of the sternomastoid tendon to help flatten the peristomal skin for easier adhesion of heat and moisture exchanger.

constrictor myotomy, unilateral pharyngeal plexus neurectomy, and more recently, chemical denervation of the pharyngo-oesophageal segment through the use of *Clostridium botulinum* toxin. Botulinum toxin is a potent neurotoxin, producing neuromuscular blockade by restricting the release of acetylcholine.

Videofluoroscopy

The most reliable and accurate way of assessing PE segment physiology after a laryngectomy is with videofluoroscopy.[27, 28, 29, 30, 31, 32, 33] This has three important components: a modified barium swallow, an oesophageal insufflation test and attempted phonation (**Figure 59.8**).

1. **Modified barium swallow.** The patient is instructed to swallow barium liquid while the pharynx is screened, initially from the front and then in a lateral position. The flow of barium is followed through the pharynx and the PE segment into the oesophagus and any hold up or delay due to spasm or stricture is noted, as well as any fistula or diverticulum.
2. **Oesophageal insufflation test.** This procedure also called the taub test simulates airflow to the oesophagus at the level of a tracheo-oesophageal puncture. A soft rubber catheter with eyelets at its proximal end is inserted transnasally to the upper oesophagus below the level of the PE segment. Air is passed from an air cylinder through the tube at a slow flow rate (i.e. 0.5 L/min) and the patient is asked to pantomime counting one to ten and/or prolonging a vowel sound. This is simultaneously recorded audiovisually.

Table 59.3 Videofluoroscopy assessment of pharyngeal constrictor tone.

Pharyngo-oesophageal segment	Ba swallow	Phonation	Assisted phonation (Taub test)	
Tonic	Passes easily	Good voice	Stronger sustained voice	
Hypotonic	Passes easily	Weak voice	More sustained, stronger with digital pressure	
Hypertonic	Normal or slower passage	Intermittent tight voice	Intermittent tight voice	Gastric distension
Spasm	Some hold up and residue above pharyngo-oesophageal segment	No voice, no air goes into oesophagus	Minimal voice, explosive segment release as pressure increases	Gastric distension
Stricture	Permanent hold up	No voice	No voice	

Table 59.4 Management strategy for voice restoration.

Pharyngo-oesophageal tonicity	Management
Hypotonic	Tracheo-oesophageal valve with digital pressure
Tonic	Tracheo-oesophageal valve
Hypertonic	Tracheo-oesophageal valve + pharyngeal constrictor myotomy (± botulinum neurotoxin injection)
Spasm	Tracheo-oesophageal valve + pharyngeal constrictor myotomy (± botulinum neurotoxin injection)
Stricture	Tracheo-oesophageal valve + pharyngeal flap augmentation

3. **Attempted phonation.** An alternative method of oesophageal insufflation was described by Blom et al.[28, 29, 30, 31, 32, 33] A catheter is inserted transnasally a distance of approximately 25 cm from the nares and connected to an adapter attached with adhesive to the peristomal skin. The patient occludes the adapter and diverts pulmonary air to the oesophagus as he or she attempts to produce sustained voicing (**Figure 59.8**). Passing is based on the ability to sustain uninterrupted phonation of a vowel for 8 seconds and to count continuously from 1 to 15.

Selection criteria for secondary voice restoration have been summarized in the **Table 59.5**.

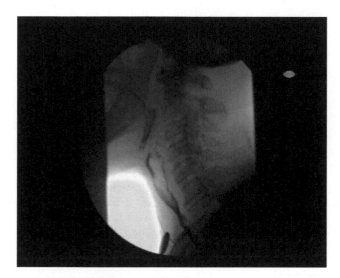

Figure 59.8 Videofluoroscopic image of a good trachea-oesophageal speaker.

Table 59.5 Selection criteria for secondary voice restoration.

Selection criteria
1. Patient must be motivated
2. Patient should be mentally stable
3. Patient must have adequate understanding of post-surgical anatomy and of the tracheo-oesophageal puncture voice prosthesis
4   Patient should not have an alcohol or other substance dependency
5. Patient must demonstrate adequate manual dexterity and ability to manage prosthesis
6. Visual acuity must be sufficient for purposes of managing tracheostoma and prosthesis
7. Patient should demonstrate positive tonicity results following oesophageal air insufflation test
8. Patient should not have significant pharyngeal stenosis or stricture
9. Patient must have adequate pulmonary support for prosthesis use
10. Patient should have stoma of adequate depth and diameter for prosthesis to avoid airway occlusion
11. Patient should have an intact tracheo-oesophageal party wall

PATIENT CRITERIA FOR TRACHEO-OESOPHAGEAL PUNCTURE PROCEDURE

Surgical technique

The method described by Singer and Blom in 1980 has provided a reliable technique for restoration of good quality lung-powered speech, but significant problems associated with the rigid endoscopic technique have been described, particularly concerning access down to the stoma level. Similar problems with access using the rigid endoscope prompted the first author to develop an alternative method using a modified pair of curved Lloyd-Davies forceps, which has been used successfully in a series of 94 secondary voice punctures since 1984, with no failed or abandoned procedures.

The forceps are inserted alongside a pharyngeal speculum into the oesophageal opening under direct vision and advanced down to the level of the tracheostome where the tip can be seen and palpated as it tents up the posterior tracheal wall in a similar way to the primary puncture technique.[2] An incision is made through the posterior wall of the stoma in the midline on to the tips of the forceps, which are advanced into the trachea. The end of a 14FG catheter is then introduced into the opened tips of the forceps and withdrawn into the pharynx, passed caudally and released. The catheter is sutured to the skin above the tracheostome and, if a Foley catheter is used, the balloon is inflated with 1.5 mL of saline to prevent dislodgement (**Figure 59.9**).

A normal diet is resumed after the procedure and the stenting catheter remains in place for a period of 2–7 days depending on whether a myotomy has been carried out simultaneously. It is then removed and, after measuring the length of the tract, a suitable Blom-Singer prosthesis is inserted.

Botulinum toxin injection

Botulinum toxin is used to provide a chemical neurectomy and is the treatment of choice for failed tracheo-oesophageal

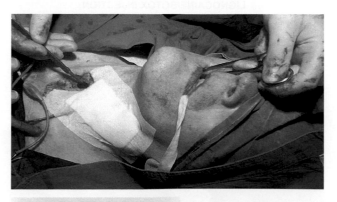
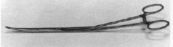

Figure 59.9 Secondary voice restoration using a long curved artery forceps as used by Mr Rhys-Evans.

speech when caused by spasm or hypertonicity. Myotomy is reserved for circumstances where botulinum is ineffective or is required repeatedly (**Figure 59.10**).[33, 34, 35, 36, 37]

TYPES OF VOICE PROSTHESES

Two basic types of valve are available from the InHealth Group (High Wycombe, UK): the 'standard' valves, including the original 'duckbill' valve and the modified 'low-pressure' or 'low-profile' valves (**Figure 59.11**).[1] The second type is the 'indwelling' valve. Each has particular features that may be more appropriate for some patients than others. The 'duckbill' valve incorporates a slit aperture over its tip that has a higher airway resistance than the low-pressure valve. The duckbill voice prosthesis is a first-generation device that is economical and durable. Its slit valve design is slightly higher in resistance to airflow through it than the hinged flap valve of the low-pressure style.

The low-pressure style of voice prosthesis is easily and atraumatically inserted using the gel cap insertion system.

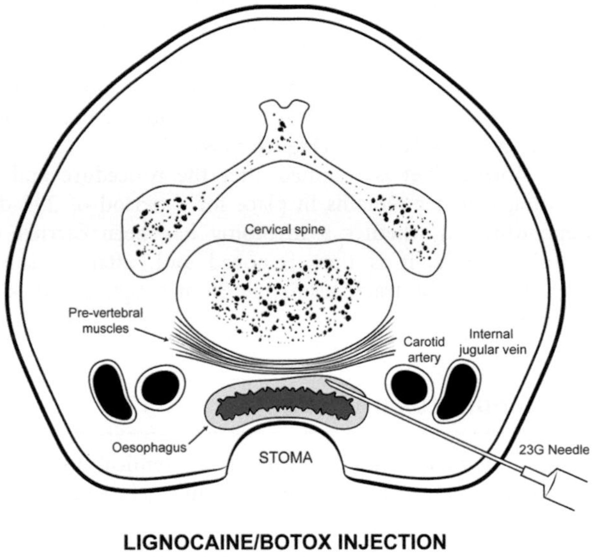

![Diagram of cervical spine cross-section showing lignocaine/botox injection technique with labels: Cervical spine, Pre-vertebral muscles, Carotid artery, Internal jugular vein, Oesophagus, STOMA, 23G Needle]

LIGNOCAINE/BOTOX INJECTION

Figure 59.10 Technique for injecting botulinum toxin into the upper oesphageal sphincter muscles.

The 16Fr diameter is routinely used unless a reduction in effort to produce voice is required and can be demonstrated with the larger 20Fr diameter. A simple test for this is to have the user momentarily produce voice through an open puncture. This simulates the effect of a larger opening because there is no prosthesis occupying space. If voice is significantly easier to produce, the larger 20Fr diameter low-pressure prosthesis is indicated.

The indwelling style of low-pressure voice prosthesis has enhanced-retention collar dimensions (i.e. larger and thicker), which secure it without the need for a neck strap and tape. It is ideal for patients who are unable or unwilling to routinely remove, clean and reinsert a regular-style voice prosthesis.

The indwelling voice prosthesis is cleaned *in situ* without removal and is replaced by a qualified speech-language pathologist or otolaryngologist, usually twice a year. The Provox 2 voice prosthesis is an indwelling style recessed hinged valve supported by a radiopaque, fluoroplastic ring, which is fastened in the shaft of the prosthesis.

Selecting a prosthesis

Careful selection of patients is important for achieving optimal results, but the variety of valves now available has widened the potential population of patients suitable for the prosthesis.[1] Several sizes and styles of tracheo-oesophageal prostheses are available and this issue has been considered in detail below under Troubleshooting tracheo-oesophageal punctures: problems and solution. Selecting a valve should be a conscientious decision and five main issues should be considered:

1. **Candidate dexterity**. If the patient and his or her spouse appear able and willing to participate in prosthesis management, a valve with no restrictions on placement procedures should be considered. Indwelling devices, although touted for their advanced design, must be inserted by a trained professional. This stipulation creates a situation of patient dependency on the health-care professional. Autonomy offered by devices that can be changed without restriction is appealing to many patients. Conversely, if the patient is unable or unwilling to

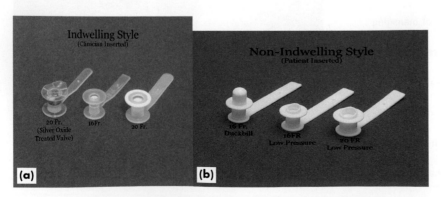

Figure 59.11 Current (a) indwelling and (b) non-indwelling Blom-Singer valves.

change the valve independently, an indwelling style device offers more security from dislodgement.

2. **Phonatory effort**. Before any prosthesis is inserted, phonation should be sampled with a patent puncture tract. The perceptual quality and effort of that sample guides decision-making. For example, if the voice quality is effortless, loud and consistent, then the patient may do well with a higher-resistance device with increased durability. If the voice quality is strained and effortful, a lower-resistance device of greater diameter (20F) may be appropriate. The duckbill valve may be used initially to start prosthetic voice rehabilitation since this is easier to fit and change, as well as being more economical. Once the healing process has stabilized, a more permanent choice of valve can be made. It is also the device of choice for a person who experiences a problem with 'inhaling' air through a low-pressure prosthesis during quiet inhalation, resulting in excessive stomach gas.

3. **Thickness of the party wall**. The length of the TO fistula varies from person to person and should be accurately estimated using the measuring device to determine the length of the prosthesis to be used. Every effort must be paid to obtain a snug fit. A too long prosthesis will cause a 'pistoning effect' and consequently leakage around the prosthesis, while a too short prosthesis may result in aphonia.

4. **Durability**. Occasionally, the device that provides the least phonatory effort also has a patient-specific tendency to malfunction rapidly. If the device recurrently leaks in less than a couple of months with no treatable cause (e.g. candida infection), a device with higher resistance and durability should be considered.

5. **Cost**. Prices for valves vary widely and cost issues should be considered when devices are comparable in style and performance. Certain health insurance policies do not cover prosthetic supplies. Patients without prosthesis coverage should be provided cost options when selecting a device.

General steps for fitting a prosthesis

Correct fitting of and appropriate training with the voice prosthesis are critical to success with this method of alaryngeal speech. With both primary and secondary tracheo-oesophageal voice restoration procedures, the surgeon punctures the tracheo-oesophageal party wall and places a 16Fr catheter to maintain the hole. About a week after the primary voice restoration procedure, a barium swallow is performed to confirm a patent neopharynx without a leak and the patient can be begun on oral diet. At this time, the catheter is removed and an appropriately sized Blom-Singer voice prosthesis placed. As the amount of neopharyngeal healing necessary to withstand the pressures generated during speech production is greater than that needed for the passage of a good bolus, we generally wait a few more days before voice rehabilitation is begun in non-irradiated patients or about a week in irradiated patients. Following secondary puncture, the prosthesis may be fitted after 2–3 days unless a myotomy has been carried out, in which case fitting is best delayed for a week (**Figures 59.12, 59.13, 59.14, 59.15, 59.16, 59.17** and **59.18**).

The clinician's task involves removing the catheter, measuring the tracheo-oesophageal puncture tract length,

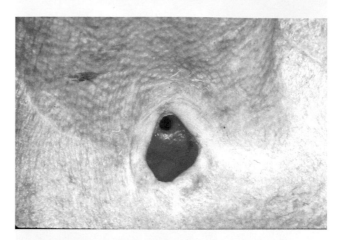

Figure 59.12 Image showing the TE puncture with the catheter removed (image courtesy Dr Eric Blom).

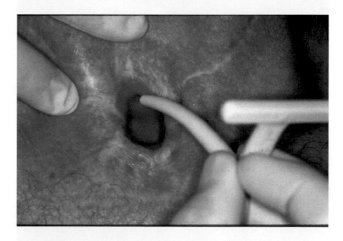

Figure 59.13 Image showing the dilator being gently advanced into the TE puncture (image courtesy Dr Eric Blom).

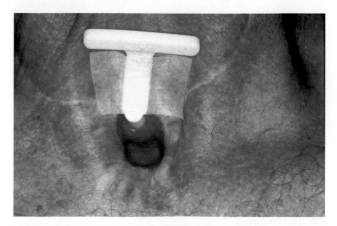

Figure 59.14 Image showing the dilator securely fastened in the TE puncture (image courtesy Dr Eric Blom).

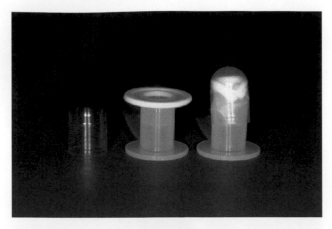

Figure 59.15 Image showing a gelcap mounted on the indwelling valve (image courtesy Dr Eric Blom).

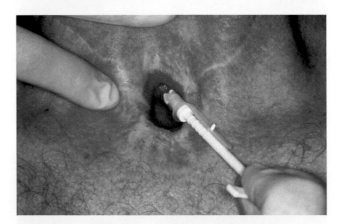

Figure 59.16 Gelcap-mounted valve loaded on the insertor being gently advanced into the TE puncture (image courtesy Dr Eric Blom).

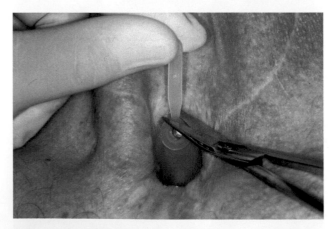

Figure 59.17 With the valve securely confirmed in place, the strap is cut (only for indwelling) (image courtesy Dr Eric Blom).

determining the type, length and diameter of prosthesis to use, dilating the tract to accept easily either a 16Fr or a 20Fr device, inserting the voice prosthesis, and, finally, confirming safe placement.

A speech–language pathologist is the professional usually responsible for initial and ongoing prosthesis fitting, teaching

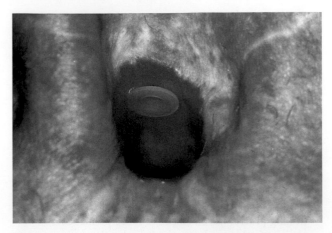

Figure 59.18 An indwelling valve sitting securely in place (image courtesy Dr Eric Blom).

removal and reinsertion, care and maintenance, and tracheo-oesophageal voice restoration rehabilitation. Once the voice prosthesis has been fitted, three equally important tasks must be taught. The first involves facilitating production of the best possible tracheo-oesophageal speech. The second deals with safe and correct voice prosthesis changing, unless an indwelling prosthesis has been selected. The third concerns hygiene of the voice prosthesis and stoma area.

1. Evaluate phonation with a patent puncture tract called 'open tract' voice and stoma occlusion to rule out technique/valve problems.
2. Measure the length of the puncture tract.
3. Select and prepare prosthesis.
4. Dilate the puncture tract to slightly wider than the prosthesis.
5. Align the prosthesis with the puncture tract for insertion; alignment is more important than pressure.
6. Ask the patient to drink liquid and watch for any leak through or around the prosthesis.
7. Assess patient phonation with stoma occlusion.

TROUBLESHOOTING TRACHEO-OESOPHAGEAL PUNCTURES: PROBLEMS AND SOLUTION

At first glance, the tracheo-oesophageal puncture technique appears to be a straightforward method of alaryngeal voice restoration requiring nothing more than 'making a hole and sticking in a valve'. However, nothing could be further from the truth, as any experienced clinician can verify. Surgeons and clinicians should recognize that, as with any surgical technique, success is dependent on sufficient knowledge, training and accrued clinical experience. The tracheo-oeso-phageal puncture technique and the application of its asso-ciated prosthetic valves are not always problem free. Although problems and complications occur related to the best efforts for voice restoration for the laryngectomized patient, they are manageable when they are recognized early and a methodical treatment plan is formulated.

Problems related to tracheo-oesophageal punctures and prosthetic devices are mentioned, along with typical causes and corresponding solutions.[38, 39, 40, 41, 42, 43]

Leakage problems

Leakage at the puncture site into the trachea can occur and is usually first noted with fluids, which cause immediate coughing on swallowing. It is important to determine on close examination with good light whether leakage is through or around the valve since the causes and management are quite different.

LEAKAGE THROUGH THE PROSTHESIS

Leakage through the prosthesis may be due to a number of reasons. A faulty or defective valve is usually evident immediately; valve distortion may occur due to excessive compression of the middle part of the prosthesis, for example when the tract has just been dilated up from 16Fr to accommodate a 20Fr valve, which may result in a slightly gaping flap. It is advisable to dilate established tracts slowly by keeping an intermediate-sized catheter in for several hours or preferably overnight before inserting the larger diameter valve. Leakage may also occur if small pieces of debris or undissolved gelatin from the gel cap hold the valve open. The prosthesis should be removed for inspection to make sure it closes completely and then reinserted and checked with a further drink of liquid. Leakage through the prosthesis may be due simply to the natural lifespan of the valve, but this can vary enormously from a few weeks to over a year. Careful cleaning of the delicate valve mechanism either with the prosthesis removed or *in situ* will prolong its usage. Some patients prefer to remove the prosthesis regularly, perhaps once or twice a week, and replace it with another, alternating the two valves for some considerable time. The spare prosthesis is kept in hydrogen peroxide or other cleaning fluid to prevent accumulation of debris or infecting organisms.

Microbial colonization of the prosthesis, predominantly with *Candida albicans* is the most common cause of leakage through the valve due to distortion of the valve mechanism.[38, 39, 40, 41] Much effort has been devoted to trying to find a prophylactic method of protecting the silicone prosthesis from microbial colonization, but so far without success. Routine use of nystatin suspension (500 000 units twice daily swished around the mouth for 4 minutes) is effective in reducing colonization and almost doubling the lifespan of a valve, but full compliance is often difficult (**Figure 59.19**).

Distortion and leakage through the duckbill prosthesis may be due to compression of the protruding valve against the posterior oesophageal wall. This is often relieved by changing to a low profile valve.

LEAKAGE AROUND THE VALVE

A satisfactory seal around the tracheo-oesophageal prosthesis depends on the natural elasticity of the surrounding party wall tissues to provide a 'snug' fit around the shaft of the valve. It is also important to have a correct measured length of prosthesis so that the retention collar on the anterior wall of the oesophagus is closely applied to the mucosa to provide a good circumferential seal and to prevent movement or dislodgement. Leakage of liquid around the prosthesis is a

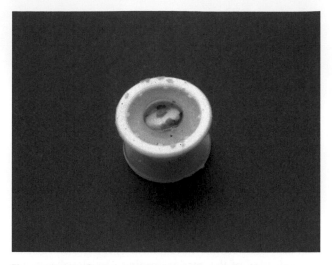

Figure 59.19 Fungal colonization over an indwelling valve (image courtesy Dr Eric Blom).

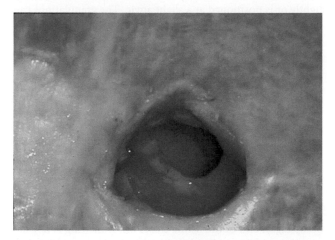

Figure 59.20 Image of a widely dilated TEP that will naturally cause leakage around the valve (image courtesy Dr Eric Blom).

difficult problem and may be due to a number of reasons. A prosthesis that is too long acts as a piston and dilates the tracheo-oesophageal tract as the prosthesis moves in and out. It is essential that the length of the tract is correctly measured and the appropriate length prosthesis is selected, particularly during the first six months as the postoperative oedema settles and the thickness of the party wall decreases (**Figure 59.20**).[38, 39, 40, 41, 42, 43]

Another important reason is a 'troubled' or 'compromised' party wall. It is defined as a thin, dilated mobile party wall that is or is in danger of leaking around the prosthesis. This is often seen in cachetic, thin individuals who have received radiotherapy in the past, is less than 6–8 mm in length and wider than 22–24Fr. Attempts at putting in a larger prosthesis may only result in enlargement of the tract and greater leakage. A troubled party wall should be managed with minimal interventional trauma, down-sizing to allow shrinkage and use of a silicon antileakage ring. If this fails, surgical intervention in the form of a submucosal purse-string suture or tissue augmentation with bioplastique may be attempted. An effective long-term solution for a chronic thin leaking compromised party wall is closure of the puncture site and reconstruction with a decent layer of muscle, preferably non-irradiated tissue. In some cases, an inferiorly based pedicled sternomastoid muscle flap can be sandwiched between the trachea and the oesophagus using a three-layer closure, with successful repuncture of the tract about three months later. In some instances where there is significant loss of surface mucosa, a pedicled myocutaneous flap may be required to achieve satisfactory closure.

Granulations

Some of the early valves had an inferiorly placed portal that frequently became blocked with granulation tissue and which eventually occluded the valve lumen. This has been resolved by elimination of the inferior opening. Occasionally, granulations arise around the prosthesis on the posterior wall of the trachea due to irritation if the edge of the valve is digging into the mucosa. This may occur if the prosthesis fits too tightly or is positioned at a slight angle. The granulations can be removed easily and cauterized and the position of the valve corrected.[1]

Fibrous ring

When the prosthesis has been used for some period of time, it may gradually become surrounded by an increasingly thick ring of fibrous tissue that forms a 'doughnut' around the tracheal end of the valve.[1] This has the effect of gradually lengthening the tract so that the posterior end of the prosthesis is gradually drawn forwards into the tract. If not recognized, the patient's voice will slowly deteriorate requiring increasing effort and eventually fail completely as the oesophageal end of the fistula closes off. If the ring is not too prominent, the tract can be resized and a longer valve fitted. Otherwise, excision of the fibrous ring is recommended (**Figure 59.21**).

Valve extrusion

The prosthesis may become dislodged during cleaning or coughing, or for other reasons, and if not replaced immediately the tract will close down.[1] A catheter or dilator can be used instead to keep the tract open until the prosthesis can be replaced. Unless the fistula has closed down completely, it is usually possible to dilate it up successfully, and for this purpose a serial set of soft urethral catheters is useful. Alternatively, progressive dilatation of a stenosed puncture tract may be possible with a set of curved metal male urethral dilators, but these should only be used by experienced clinicians. Occasionally, valves may need to be retrieved with bronchoscopy if inhaled.

Aphonia

Aphonia following secondary voice restoration (SVR) using a valve may have a number of reasons. Often this is due to a

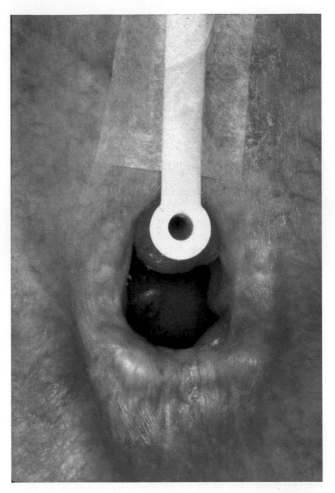

Figure 59.21 Non-indwelling valve surrounded by a classic fibrous ring (image courtesy Dr Eric Blom).

clogged device either by food debris or undissolved gelatin from the gel cap at the time of insertion. The prosthesis should be removed for inspection to make sure the valve is functional. Another reason could be a duckbill prosthesis that is compressed against the posterior oesophageal wall. This is often relieved by changing to a low profile valve. Other reasons include incomplete insertion that requires resizing and finally repuncture for a puncture closure.

Hypertonicity/spasm

Failure to carry out a myotomy at the time of laryngectomy may lead to voice failure because of hypertonicity or spasm of the pharyngeal constrictors. This can be demonstrated on videofluoroscopy as described earlier in the chapter and corrected with botulinum neurotoxin injection or a long myotomy (**Figure 59.22**).[29, 30, 31, 32, 33]

Pseudovallecula

This invariably occurs if the pharynx has been sewn up with a vertical closure at laryngectomy. The anterior pouch at the tongue base and the coronal fibrous web behind it may cause

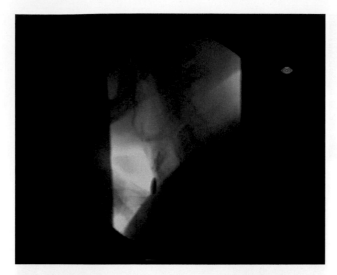

Figure 59.22   Videofluoroscopic image of a hypertonic PE segment during voicing.

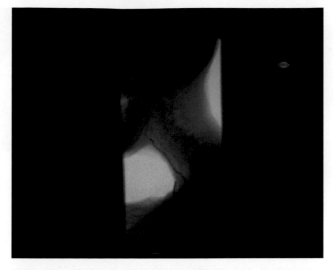

Figure 59.23   Videofluoroscopic image of a hypotonic PE segment during voicing.

dysphagia with the patient having to make several swallowing attempts to get food down through the narrowed opening into the hypopharynx. This shows up well on videofluoroscopy. Correction is easily achieved by endoscopic division of the web using a similar technique to excision of the cricopharyngeal bar in the pharyngeal pouch.

Stenosis

This may occur if insufficient mucosa/skin has been used for reconstruction of the hypopharynx or at the anastomotic site following total pharyngolaryngectomy. It may also develop slowly after jejunum transposition due to ischaemic contracture if the mesenteric blood supply is compromised. Dilatation may be sufficient if the narrowing is not severe, but reconstruction of the pharynx may be necessary.

Hypotonic voice

A reconstructed hypopharynx typically produces a hypotonic voice due to loss or absence of muscular tone, which can be shown on videofluoroscopy. Voice quality may be improved using digital pressure or by wearing an elastic band over the pharynx on the anterior neck.[30, 31, 32]

Excessive flatulence

Excessive collection of air in the stomach is a disturbing and sometimes painful problem in tracheo-oesophageal voice users and may be due to several different causes. During normal respiration, oesophageal pressure is negative during inspiration; this may cause slight opening of the valve and small amounts of air may be sucked into the oesophagus and swallowed into the stomach. Replacement of the prosthesis with a higher resistance duckbill valve may provide a solution. In a similar way, if the PE segment is hypotonic (**Figure 59.23**), excessive air ingestion may occur from the mouth

during normal inspiration due to the negative oesophageal pressure. In patients with a hypertonic PE segment or stricture, excessive expiratory effort is needed to force air through the vocal tract and some air may be driven in a reverse direction down into the stomach. Problems with tonicity is managed as outlined above under Tonicity.

Macrostomia

Occasionally, the tracheostoma opening is too large for the patient to achieve airtight finger or thumb occlusion during speech. Use of a silicone laryngectomy tube may help or the patient may find that a tracheostoma valve housing attached to the peristomal skin will allow better occlusion or preferably use of the hands-free stoma valve. Surgical reduction of the stoma is rarely needed.

Microstomia

Until the peristomal scar tissue has stabilized after a few months following laryngectomy, it has a natural tendency to contract and most patients will need to wear a laryngectomy tube or button to prevent stenosis. They may also feel more comfortable and 'safer' wearing something, particularly at night. If the stoma size reduces to less than 2 cm, it becomes difficult to manage a prosthesis and under 1 cm breathing becomes difficult. The stoma can usually be dilated with buttons or laryngectomy tubes, but if the stenosis is well established it may be necessary to carry out a stomaplasty.[1] The preferred technique is bilateral Y–V advancements with excision of scar tissue as necessary.

Excessive stomal mucus

During the first six months or so following laryngectomy, excessive mucus discharge and coughing can be a problem. Most cases settle with the use of a heat and moisture exchanger system.

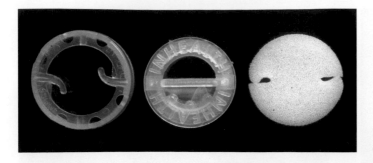

Figure 59.24 Different parts of a classic heat and moisture exchanger (image courtesy Dr Eric Blom).

HEAT AND MOISTURE EXCHANGE SYSTEMS

Heat and moisture exchange systems (HME systems) have been used for years during anaesthesia and in medical intensive care units (ICU). The working mechanism of a passive heat and moisture exchanger is simple but quite effective. The head and moisture exchanger is placed over the tracheostoma so that all the respired air passed through the device. During expiration, the air passes through the heat and moisture exchanger, where the air loses some of its heat. Because the water vapour content of the air is directly related to the air temperature, water vapour condenses as soon as the temperature and moisture exchanger, which retains water and heat at the same time, is used. The air leaving the heat and moisture exchanger contains less heat and moisture than when no heat and moisture exchange is in use. During inspiration, cool and dry ambient air passes through the heat and moisture exchanger and pains some of the heat and moisture preserved in the device. A heat and moisture exchanger effectively protects the trachea and the lower airway from drying and cooling and considerably reduces the burden of air-conditioning on the lower respiratory tract (**Figures 59.24** and **59.25**).[44, 45, 46, 47, 48]

Another function of head and moisture exchangers is the resistance to airflow. Raising airway resistance has a positive effect on tissue oxygen saturation in the laryngectomized patient. Presumably by preventing alveolar collapse, the optimum lung ventilation : perfusion ratio is maintained. The last function of heat and moisture exchanger filters is that they have some particle filtering capability, although the efficiency is not known. Patients should use the HME system for at least two weeks to assess its potential benefit. In addition, all heat and moisture exchanger filters need to be replaced at least every 24 hours. This avoids the risk of heat and moisture preservation decrease, and more importantly, it limits the microbial overgrowth of the filter and the associated risks of airway contamination.

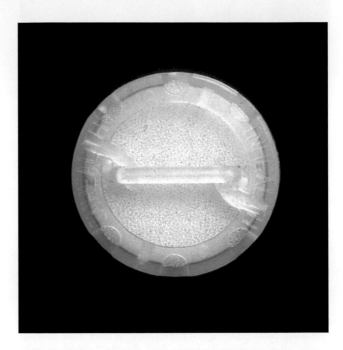

Figure 59.25 Classic representative head and moisture exchanger (image courtesy Dr Eric Blom).

HANDS–FREE TRACHEOSTOMA VALVES

Tracheostoma valves provide two primary functions: hands-free speech and housing for heat and moisture filters. The tracheostoma breathing valve device consists of two parts: an external housing and an adjustable valve. The valve remains open during quiet respiration and automatically closes in

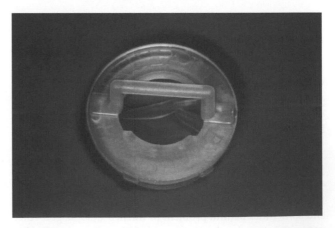

Figure 59.26 Classic representative hands-free device (image courtesy Dr Eric Blom).

response to an increase in expiratory flow to allow speech production (**Figures 59.26**, **59.27** and **59.28**).

There are two types of housing: the first is the standard peristomal housing which is attached to the peristomal skin

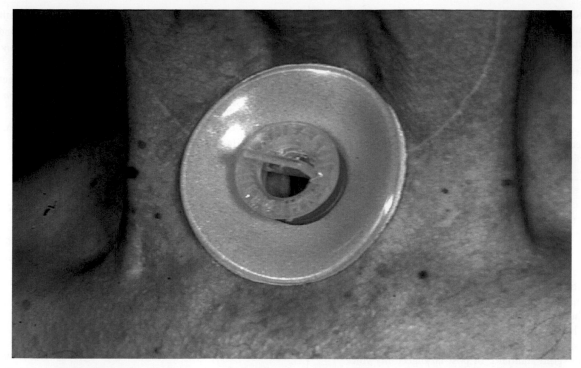

Figure 59.27 Image showing the open valve to facilitate breathing in a hands-free device (image courtesy Dr Eric Blom).

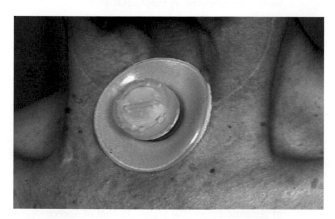

Figure 59.28 Image showing the valve closed to enable voicing in a hands-free device (image courtesy Dr Eric Blom).

with an adhesive disc and a layer of liquid adhesive. The second type of housing is the Barton button, developed by Barton and Associates in 1988, which uses intraluminal rather than peristomal attachment. It is composed of soft, silicone rubber which conforms to the patient's stoma. An adequate adhesive seal is essential to generate hands-free speech. Without a tight external seal, stomal air escape reduces the amount of airflow available for speech.

CONCLUSION

The great advance of this time is that laryngeal cancer is treatable with voice preservation or restoration, and that patients are no longer condemned to silence while they await the results of their cancer treatments. They can face the challenge of cure of laryngeal cancer with the knowledge that normal quality of life is possible.

Successful voice restoration for alaryngeal speakers can be attained with any of the three speech options. Although, no single method is considered best for every patient, the tracheo-oesophageal puncture has become the preferred method in the past decade. Since the first description of a tracheo-oesophageal voice prosthesis in 1980, many new devices have been developed, and several of the original devices have been modified. In many centres now, voice prostheses have replaced oesophageal speech as the gold standard for voice rehabilitation.

Despite the potential facility of voice production with the tracheo-oesophageal puncture, careful attention must be directed to PE segment integrity, valve selection and troubleshooting. Despite new device designs in recent years, candidal infestation of the prostheses and leakage continues to remain a problem. Successful tracheo-oesophageal voice restoration in laryngectomy patients can be very rewarding, but the cost and other problems associated with maintaining prostheses are often prohibitive, especially in Third World countries.

Finally, remember voice restoration is a process, not a prosthesis!

KEY EVIDENCE

- The advantages of voice prosthesis are numerous and include immediate voice production, relatively low complication rates, reversibility to other forms of rehabilitation and possibility of sustained speech. The speech is more fluent which is closer to laryngeal speech than oesophageal speech on a range of voice parameters, such as fundamental frequency, jitter, shimmer, words per minute and maximum phonation time.[1, 2]

- Problems related to tracheo-oesophageal punctures and prosthetic devices, such as leakage through and around the prosthesis reducing the valve life continue to challenge clinicians around the world.[38, 39, 40, 41, 42, 43]

KEY LEARNING POINTS

- Total laryngectomy results in a permanent stoma, change in voice, olfactory and gustatory changes which affect the overall quality of life of the patient.[1, 2, 3]
- The advantages of surgical voice restoration using voice prosthesis has made this modality the 'gold standard' of post-laryngectomy voice rehabilitation.[1, 2, 7]
- The last three decades has seen tremendous technical improvements in the valve design, methods of insertion with the introduction of hands-free, low pressure, indwelling and fungal-resistant valves.[1]
- Despite new device designs in recent years, candidal infestation of the prostheses and leakage continues to remain a problem. Successful tracheo-oesophageal voice restoration in laryngectomy patients can be very rewarding, but the cost and other problems associated with maintaining prostheses can be prohibitive, especially in Third World countries.[1, 2]
- Although the end result of acquiring adequate voice rehabilitation is the desired choice, the process of acquiring this requires focused efforts and commitment both from the patient, as well as the clinician.[1, 3]

REFERENCES

1. Rhys-Evans P, Montgomery PQ, Gullane PJ. *Principles and practice of head and neck oncology*. London: Martin Dunitz, 2003.
2. Kazi R, Singh A, De-Cordova J *et al.* A New self-administered questionnaire to determine patient experience with Blom-Singer Voice Prostheses. *Journal of Postgraduate Medicine* 2005; **51**: 253–9.
3. Blom ED. Evolution of tracheoesophageal voice prostheses. In: Blom ED, Singer MI, Hamaker RC (eds). *Tracheoesophageal voice restoration following total laryngectomy*. San Diego: Singular, 1998: 1–8.
4. Gussenbauer C. Ueber cie Erste Durch Th. Billroth Am Menschen Ausgefuhrte Kehlkopf-Exstirpation Und die Anwendung Eines Kunstlichen Kehlkopfes. *Archiv fur Klinische Chirurgie* 1874; **17**: 334–56.
5. Taub S, Spiro RH. Vocal rehabilitation of laryngectomees: preliminary report of a new technique. *American Journal of Surgery* 1972; **124**: 87–90.
6. Edels Y. Pseudo voice, its theory and practice. In: Edels Y (ed.). *Laryngectomy: diagnosis to rehabilitation*. Beckenham: Croom-Helm, 1983: 107–42.
7. Kazi R, Kanagalingam J, Venkitaraman R *et al.* Electroglottographic and perceptual evaluation of tracheoesophageal speech. *Voice* 2009; **23**: 247–54.
8. van As CJ, Hilgers FJ, Verdonck-de Leeuw IM, Koopmansvan Beinum F. Acoustical analysis and perceptual evaluation of tracheoesophageal prosthetic voice. *Journal of Voice* 1998; **12**: 239–48.
9. Pindzola RH, Cain BH. Acceptability ratings of tracheoesophageal speech. *Laryngoscope* 1988; **98**: 394–7.
10. Robbins J. Acoustic differentiation of laryngeal, esophageal and tracheoesophageal speech. *Journal of Speech and Hearing Research* 1984; **27**: 577–85.
11. Qi Y, Weinberg B. Characteristics of voicing source waveforms produced by esophageal and tracheoesophageal speakers. *Journal of Speech and Hearing Research* 1995; **38**: 536–48.
12. Blood GW. Fundamental frequency and intensity measurements in laryngeal and alaryngeal speakers. *Journal of Communication Disorders* 1984; **17**: 319–24.
13. Moon JB, Weinberg B. Aerodynamic and myoelastic contributions to tracheoesophageal voice production. *Journal of Speech and Hearing Research* 1987; **30**: 387–95.
14. van As CJ, Koopmans-van Beinum FJ, Pols LC, Hilgers FJ. Pols LCW. Perceptual evaluation of tracheoesophageal speech by naive and experienced judges through the use of semantic differential scales. *Journal of Speech, Language, and Hearing Research* 2003; **46**: 947–59.
15. Kazi R, Kiverniti E, Prasad V *et al.* Multidimensional assessment of female tracheoesophageal prosthetic speech. *Clinical Otolaryngology* 2006; **31**: 511–17.
16. Singer MI, Blom ED. An endoscopic technique for restoration of voice after laryngectomy. *Annals of Otology, Rhinology, and Laryngology* 1980; **89**: 529–33.
17. Singer MI, Blom ED, Hamaker RC. Further experience with voice restoration after total laryngectomy. *Annals of Otology, Rhinology, and Laryngology* 1981; **90**: 498–502.
18. Hamaker RC, Singer MI, Blom ED, Daniels HA. Primary voice restoration at laryngectomy. *Archives of Otolaryngology* 1985; **111**: 182–6.
19. Rhys-Evans PH. Tracheo-oesophageal puncture without tears: the forceps technique. *Journal of Laryngology and Otology* 1991; **105**: 748–9.
20. Salamoun W, Swartz WM, Johnson JT *et al.* Free jejunal transfer for reconstruction of the laryngopharynx.

Otolaryngology – Head and Neck Surgery 1987; **96**: 149–50.

21. Wilson PS, Bruce-Lockhart FJ, Johnson AP, Rhys Evans PH. Speech restoration following total pharyngolaryngectomy with free jejunal repair. *Clinical Otolaryngology* 1994; **19**: 145–8.

22. Ong GB, Lee TC. Pharyngogastric anastomosis after oesophagopharyngectomy for carcinoma of the hypopharynx and cervical oesophagus. *British Journal of Surgery* 1960; **48**: 193–200.

23. Huntley TC, Borrowdale RW. Tracheoesophageal voice restoration following laryngopharyngectomy and laryngopharyngoesophagectomy In: Blom ED, Singer MI, Hamaker RC (eds). *Tracheoesophageal voice restoration following total laryngectomy.* San Diego: Singular, 1998.

24. Shangold LM, Urken ML, Lawson W. Jejunal transplantation for pharyngoesophageal reconstruction. *Otolaryngologic Clinics of North America* 1991; **24**: 1321–42.

25. Anthony JP, Singer MI, Mathes SJ. Pharyngoesophageal reconstruction using the tubed radial forearm flap. *Clinics in Plastic Surgery* 1994; **21**: 137–47.

26. Freeman SB, Hamaker RC. Tracheoesophageal voice restoration at time of laryngectomy In: Blom ED, Singer MI, Hamaker RC (eds). *Tracheoesophageal voice restoration following total laryngectomy.* San Diego: Singular, 1998p.19–25.

27. Blom ED, Singer MI, Hamaker RC. An improved esophageal insufflation test. *Archives of Otolaryngology* 1985; **111**: 211–12.

28. Perry A, Edels Y. Recent advances in the assessment of failed oesophageal speakers. *British Journal of Disorders of Communication* 1985; **20**: 229–36.

29. Kazi R, Singh A, Mullen G et al. Can objective parameters derived from the videofluoroscopic assessment of post-laryngectomy valved speech replace the current subjective measures? An e-tool based analysis. *Clinical Otolaryngology* 2006; **31**: 518–24.

30. Perry A. Preoperative tracheoesophageal voice restoration assessment and selection criteria. In: Blom ED, Singer MI, Hamaker RC (eds). *Tracheoesophageal voice restoration following total laryngectomy.* San Diego: Singular, 1998: 9–18.

31. Cheesman AD, Knight J, McIvor J, Perry A. Tracheooesophageal 'puncture speech': an assessment technique for failed oesophageal speakers. *Journal of Laryngology and Otology* 1986; **100**: 191–9.

32. McIvor J, Evans PF, Perry A, Cheesman AD. Radiological assessment of post-laryngectomy speech. *Clinical Radiology* 1990; **41**: 312–16.

33. Simpson IC, Smith JC, Gordon MT. Laryngectomy: the influence of muscle reconstruction on the mechanism of oesophageal voice production. *Journal of Laryngology and Otology* 1972; **86**: 961–90.

34. Trudeau MD, Schuller DE, Hall DA. The effects of radiation on tracheo-oesophageal puncture. *Archives of Otolaryngology* 1989; **115**: 1116–17.

35. Singer MI, Blom ED, Hamaker RC. Pharyngeal plexus neurectomy for alaryngeal speech rehabilitation. *Laryngoscope* 1986; **96**: 50–4.

36. Hamaker RC, Cheesman AD. Surgical management of pharyngeal constrictor muscle hypertonicity. In: Blom ED, Singer MI, Hamaker RC (eds). *Tracheoesophageal voice restoration following total laryngectomy.* San Diego: Singular, 1998.

37. Hoffman HT, Fischer H, Vandemark D et al. Botulinum neurotoxin injection after total laryngectomy. *Head and Neck* 1997; **19**: 92–7.

38. Blom ED. Tracheoesophageal valves: problems, solutions and directions for the future. *Head and Neck Surgery* 1988; **2**(Suppl.): S142–5.

39. Silver FM, Gluckman JL, Donegan JO. Operative complications of tracheo-oesophageal puncture. *Laryngoscope* 1985; **95**: 1360–2.

40. Garth RJN, McRae A, Rhys Evans PH. Tracheooesophageal puncture: a review of problems and complications. *Journal of Laryngology and Otology* 1991; **105**: 750–4.

41. Ward PH, Andrews JC, Mickel RA et al. Complications of medical and surgical approaches to voice restoration after total laryngectomy. *Head and Neck Surgery* 1988; **10**: 124–8.

42. Wei WK, Lam KH, Choi S, Wong J. Late problems after pharyngogastric anastomosis for cancer of the larynx and hypopharynx. *American Journal of Surgery* 1984; **148**: 509–12.

43. Blom ED, Singer MI, Hamaker RC. Tracheostoma valve for post laryngectomy voice rehabilitation. *Annals of Otology, Rhinology, and Laryngology* 1982; **91**: 576–8.

44. Jay S, Ruddy J, Cullen RJ. Laryngectomy: the patient's view. *Journal of Laryngology and Otology* 1991; **105**: 934–8.

45. Kazi R, Kanagalingam J, Prasad V et al. Quality of life outcome measures following total laryngectomy: assessment using the UW-QOL scale. *ORL* 2006; **69**: 100–6.

46. Kazi R, Singh A, De-Cordova J et al. Voice-related quality of life in laryngectomees: assessment using the VHI and V-RQOL symptom scales. *Journal of Voice* 2007; **21**: 728–34.

47. Ackerstaff AH, Hilgers FJ, Aaronson NK et al. Improvements in respiratory and psychosocial functioning following total laryngectomy by use of heat and moisture exchanger. *Annals of Otology, Rhinology, and Laryngology* 1993; **102**: 878–83.

48. Hilgers FJM, Aaronson NK, Ackerstaff AH et al. The influence of a heat and moisture exchanger (HME) on the respiratory symptoms after total laryngectomy. *Clinical Otolaryngology* 1991; **16**: 152–6.

DIRECTIONS FOR FUTURE RESEARCH AND DEVELOPMENTS IN HEAD AND NECK CANCER SURGERY

PART SIX

DIRECTIONS FOR FUTURE RESEARCH AND
DEVELOPMENTS IN HEAD AND NECK
CANCER SURGERY

60

Robotics, laryngeal transplantation, gene therapy, growth factors and facial transplantation

DAVID G GRANT, MICHAEL L HINNI AND MARTIN A BIRCHALL

> The future is already here – it's just not evenly distributed.
>
> William Gibson

INTRODUCTION

Some predictions are better than others (**Figure 60.1**). We were taught at medical school that 'half the treatments we employ are useless; it is just that we don't know which half'. Thus, we entirely expect that much of the vision laid out below will return to haunt us just as much as titles containing 'modern', 'new' and 'future' haunt all authors as the pages yellow with time. Nonetheless, taken with a side portion of healthy scepticism, here is our take on some of the more exciting developments of today and a vision of a possible future for our specialty.

THE FUTURE OF HEAD AND NECK CANCER

Ninety per cent of the head and neck cancer we see and treat today is smoking-related squamous cell disease. Although Sir Richard Doll in Oxford pointed out the clear associations between smoking and cancer in the 1950s,[1] governments have only started to embrace the challenge of stopping people smoking in very recent years. World Bank predictions show a depressing picture of escalating tobacco deaths for most of the twenty-first century, due to increased consumption by developing countries and the cohort effect (**Figure 60.2**).

Meanwhile, life expectancy in Western countries continues to grow (**Figure 60.3**).[2] Since increasing age is the next biggest risk factor for head and neck cancer after smoking, the combined effect is a steady increase in the demand for head and neck cancer treatment for many decades to come. Our generation will not be short of people to treat.

TECHNOLOGY LEADING OR LED?

The past 50 years has seen little change in survival from head and neck cancer: technical changes in reconstruction and rehabilitation have improved the quality of survivorship. The limited, but much vaunted, gains of combined medical therapy have in reality still left ablative surgery at the core of care for over two-thirds of patients.[3] Technology, however, is driving change. Like cardiac surgery before us (**Figure 60.4**), one vision sees head and neck surgery replaced by interventional physicians and technicians and rendered irrelevant by effective molecular therapies. A rump may live on, the slave of technocrats and health ministers.

Alternatively, head and neck surgeons can develop a vision; become the beacon for scientists, physicians and engineers to follow towards a new future, where people who have had head and neck cancer look, talk, eat and drink, and laugh just like everyone else. In this vision, the future head and neck surgeon plays two roles:

1. The pilot of one-stop head and neck offices, where diagnosis, prognosis and treatment selection are all performed in one sitting, using internal and external techniques.

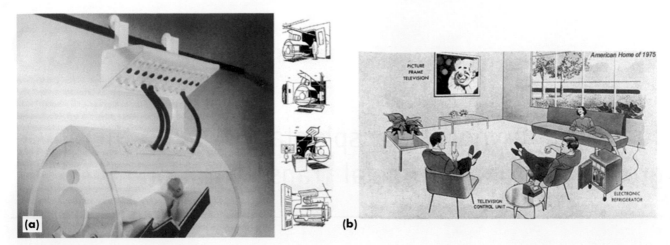

Figure 60.1 Making predictions is notoriously hazardous. (a) 1970s architects predicted hospitals in which patients would be ferried around in their own capsules, not even leaving to undergo surgery. (b) A better stab was made by 'The Technician' accurately predicting flat-screen TV, remote control and small refrigerators.

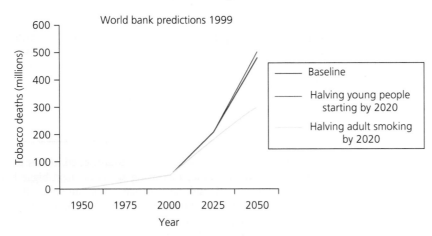

Figure 60.2 World Bank predictions of tobacco-related deaths. Strategies to halve the numbers of young people smoking by 2020 will have a negligible effect on mortality, while halving adult smoking will still lead to a doubling in deaths by 2050. A plateau is not expected until beyond the middle of this century.

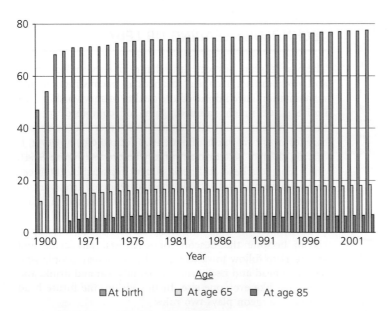

Figure 60.3 US Center for Population Health and Statistics. The average life expectancy of Western populations continues to grow steadily.

2. The restorer of normal human interactions, with stem cells, nanotechnology, robotics and transplantation at his or her disposal to restore appearance and function.

Contemplating this vision briefly may allow us to prepare adequately for the future. Whether or not it becomes reality, ploughing the same furrow we have followed for the last 20 years or more might court extinction or relegation. We

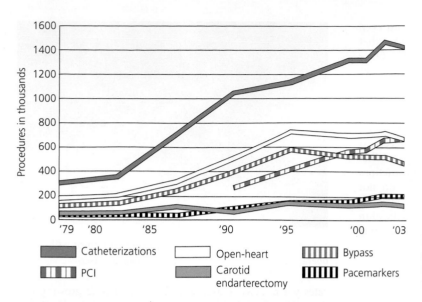

Figure 60.4   Centers for Disease Control data showing the fall off in cardiac surgery as interventional techniques expanded in recent years. Is the same happening to head and neck surgery?

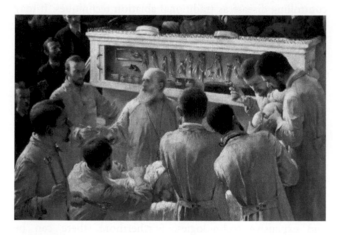

Figure 60.5   Theodor Billroth trains future surgeons on his programme in Vienna, circa 1882. Billroth embedded research and scholarship in the training of all his pupils.

propose that head and neck surgeons should engage with the world's best scientists right now. As the second part of this prescription, we need to embed sufficient scholarship in surgical training to permit the next generation to lead and not be led. Present trends in surgical education should not, therefore, exclude scholarship in the drive to produce pure (and by definition inflexible and soon-to-be-extinct) artisans. In this way, we can future-proof our craft and the central position held by head and neck surgeons in head and neck cancer care for generations to come.

SCHOLARSHIP AND TRAINING

Theodor Billroth (**Figure 60.5**) had many seminal achievements. His operations, many of them 'firsts', such as laryngectomy and gastrectomy, developed in the middle of the nineteenth century are still performed (with modifications) today. Arguably, one of the keys to the longevity of his innovations was the establishment of the world's first formal surgical training programme. Integral to this programme was

scholarship, including research. The drive to streamline surgical training in many countries has tended to lead to a simplified view of what a surgeon is. As surgical curricula developed, it has been difficult to persuade politically driven mandarins to allow time for reflection and research. If we neglect this, however, we will be signing up to a view of surgeons as technicians, taking their place on 'treatment centre' assembly lines.

Training in research skills in a world of dizzyingly accelerating technological change can no longer be regarded as optional, however. Only someone who has learnt how to interpret new research (and the best way to learn is by doing) will be able to appraise and assimilate new technologies appropriately and in a timely manner. Furthermore, scientists need people who can place their new work in the context of real human cancer. For all their skills, oncologists do not have the same intimate relationship with and understanding of head and neck cancer and its functional sequelae as head and neck surgeons. Therefore, we need to place future surgeons closer to the science–patient interface than has previously been envisaged.

THE REPLACEMENT OF ABLATIVE SURGERY

We are certainly living in something of an evidence-free zone compared to most other surgical oncology specialties. Randomized controlled trials are very rare indeed, and while there are many barriers and difficulties, oncologists will always hold the whip hand in deciding the direction of services unless surgeons are able to provide level 1 evidence for what they expound. In fact, if we did nothing more than apply all our present knowledge in a thorough, evidence-based way in every country, we would almost certainly make major inroads into morbidity and mortality, even without the development of anything novel.

However, this is to ignore that technology is now the heartbeat of our societies and economies. The company which rests on its laurels and does not embrace technological change rapidly goes out of business. As architects have found, for example, when building a structure designed to last even 25 years, 'future-proofing' it for all possible technologies that the incumbents may wish to use is already impossible. Once again, the best defence against the future, for the surgeon, as well as the architect, is scholarship, with which comes the flexibility to meet the future head on.

So, let us assume that the promises of gene therapy, antiangiogenesis drugs, immunotherapy and all the other drugs in phase 1 and 2 trials will bear fruit. With injections and tablets, the tumours shrink away before our eyes. What will we be left to do surgically? The answer is reconstruction, regeneration and repair. Even if the magic bullets do not come along, advances in these areas of biomedicine make us beholden to investigate the full potential of their application in postoperative patients. The aim is normal-appearing, normal-talking and normal-swallowing patients throughout.

Here, we present some of the best of today and a little of tomorrow, to set the stage on which our trainees must ultimately walk.

MINIMALLY INVASIVE SURGERY, LASERS AND ROBOTICS

Minimally invasive surgery (MIS) represents an emerging philosophy in head and neck cancer whereby the surgeon gains access to the tumour through the body's natural orifices, or through small incisions with the assistance of video endoscopy. Indeed, in some cases, the surgeon may no longer directly see or touch the structures that they are operating on. Surgical damage to uninvolved tissues and structures can be avoided as the patient is not disassembled from the outside to gain access to a tumour. Proponents of minimally invasive techniques maintain that patients experience less pain and fewer complications and recover faster, with greater preservation of anatomical and physiological function than compared to open surgery. Numerous authors have described transnasal endoscopic approaches to the anterior cranial base and clivus.[4, 5] Salivary tumours and thyroid cancers are now routinely being removed through incisions as small as 2 cm with the use of specialized instruments and endoscopes.

For head and neck squamous cell carcinomas, MIS has evolved with removal of tumours of the pharynx and larynx through the natural orifice of the mouth using specialized endoscopic instruments, microscopes and lasers leaving wounds to heal by secondary intention.[6, 7] No definitive taxonomy has been decided for such procedures but terms such as natural orifice transluminal endoscopic surgery (NOTES), endoscopic laser surgery (ELS) and transoral laser microsurgery (TLM) have all gained in popularity.[8, 9, 10] Of special mention is TLM. In TLM, the tumour is removed often in a piecemeal fashion, generally using carbon dioxide laser, under an operating microscope (**Figure 60.6**). This approach, it is argued, permits a more 'logical' tumour resection where the tumour is divided and its depth mapped using frozen section. This preserves as much normal tissue as possible and with the smallest volume of normal tissue removed, assures a complete margin in all dimensions. TLM, therefore, has a diagnostic element as it confirms tumour extent and 'following' the tumour can prevent under-treatment. Advocates point to the acceptable local control

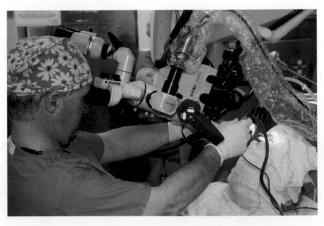

Figure 60.6 Transoral laser microsurgery performed with an operating microscope-mounted carbon dioxide laser.

rates when TLM is used and, indeed, there is growing evidence that for select tumours this method is as effective in controlling disease as traditional ablation techniques. It may be that in preserving local microcirculation, TLM can also provide optimal conditions for the effects of adjuvant radiotherapy.[11, 12, 13, 14, 15]

Advantages of MIS and the techniques mentioned above are that patients suffer less morbidity, fewer tracheostomies and reconstructions, shorter hospital stays, and can return to health faster and with improved function compared with traditional surgical and non-surgical techniques. Furthermore, the use of MIS does not preclude any further treatment strategy should the patient experience recurrent or second primary disease. The disadvantages of minimally invasive surgical methods include the abandonment of traditional bias, start-up costs including instrumentation and training, as well as those associated with maintaining both evolving and expensive technologies. Furthermore, there can be technical drawbacks of occasional discomforts associated with limited access and poor line-of-sight visualization.

Lasers

Critical to the development of MIS are new technologies that permit precise tissue instrumentation and visibility through the limiting natural orifices or small incisions. Line-of-sight visibility may at times be impossible, as can be line-of-sight delivery of cutting instruments including lasers. The carbon dioxide laser with its power and absorption characteristics remains the current optimum instrument for use in the aerodigestive tract. The long wavelength (10 600 nm) and physical properties of this laser have, until recently, mandated deploying the beam in a direct path from a mounted mirror manipulator to the end organ. This adds risk to the procedure and limits the workspace of the laser within the patient which can prove particularly problematic as tumour size increases or patient anatomy does not permit line-of-sight delivery. The Omni Guide System (Omni Guide, Cambridge, MA, USA), has been developed to deliver a CO_2 laser via a flexible hollow core fibre. This system allows enhanced delivery of the laser to areas of the head and neck in which the direct visualization required for conventional linear CO_2

laser systems cannot be acquired.[16, 17] Thus, for the first time, CO_2 energy can be delivered non-line-of-sight and has been surgically used in middle ear surgery, particularly on the stapes footplate, in the nose, sinus and anterior cranial fossa floor, as well as in the upper aerodigestive tract, including the pleural cavity, pleural pharynx, hypopharynx and larynx. This fibre has even been utilized to release gastro-esophageal strictures following minimally invasive bariatric surgery.

Other fibre-based laser technologies are emerging and beginning to find application in the treatment of head and neck cancer. Thulium ion-based continuous wave lasers have similar properties to CO_2 lasers and have demonstrated promise for benign laryngeal and tracheal disease, as well as for cancer.[18, 19] As the wavelength of this laser is only 2013 nm, it can be delivered by a glass fibreoptic fibre, yet retains water as a chromophore. This laser offers smooth vaporization associated with excellent haemostasis similar to that realized with the potassium titanyl phosphate (KTP) laser, but with less risk of deep tissue penetration as it has an absorption length of only 0.180 nm.[20] Arteries 2 mm in size and smaller are reliably sealed with this laser, thus, bleeding during surgery is significantly less than that encountered with CO_2. In addition, the authors have recently utilized the holmium laser. Similar to the thulium, this fibre-delivered laser energy has excellent tissue interaction properties, less bleeding than CO_2 and less associated margin necrosis than that observed with the thulium-based laser. KTP, Nd YAG and argon may also have utilization in MIS, particularly in treating vascular tumours and malformations. In the future, these wavelengths, as well as other light therapies, will likely become more prevalent in the treatment of both benign and malignant diseases of the head and neck through MIS in both the operating theatre setting, as well as the outpatient setting. As interest, experience and instrumentation for MIS evolve, patients will be able to experience the benefits of MIS for increasingly unfavourable anatomic or tumour characteristics. Furthermore, in conjunction with advances in surgical robotics, the continued progress of light technology will be an integral part of the future ability of minimally invasive surgery.

Robotics

Nothing quite seems to capture the imagination more than the possibility of a robot performing surgery on a human being. For many years now, the subject of robotic surgery is one that has fascinated both the public and medical profession alike. Over the last half century, the medical robot has maintained a continuous presence in the literature and media of science fiction writers and perhaps no other aspect of future science receives such enthusiastic prediction than machines taking over the role of doctors.

While the potential benefits of medical robots cannot be denied, what of the wider philosophical questions that arise from the transfer of that most trusted and intimate of relationships from man to machine? Can the surgeon be replaced by a collection of computer chips, sensors and actuators? In this section, we will explore the history and development of contemporary surgical robotics, existing robotic technology, and likely near-term future developments.

Asimov's three laws of robotics

1. A robot may not injure a human being, or, through inaction, allow a human being to come to harm.

2. A robot must obey the orders given to it by human beings, except where such orders would conflict with the First Law.

3. A robot must protect its own existence, as long as such protection does not conflict with the First or Second Law.

Figure 60.7 Asimov's three laws of robotics.

The originator of the term 'robot' was Czech painter, poet, and writer Josef Čapek. Josef introduced the term to his brother Karel Čapek, a fellow writer, who used the expression to describe several characters in his stage play 'R.U.R. (Rossum's Universal Robots)' which had its premiere in 1920. Prophetically, the play examines the moral and ethical dilemmas created by the use of 'artificial people', called robots, as slave or factory labour. The etymological origins of the word 'robot' can be found in the Czech *robota* meaning 'compulsory labour' derived from the Old Church Slavonic *rabota* or 'servitude'.[21] More widely known perhaps is the term 'robotics' and the famous 'three laws' penned by the science-fiction writer Isaac Asimov (**Figure 60.7**). Despite enthusiasm for the creation of the 'three laws', they were in reality a narrative device employed by Asimov in his fiction writing and were never actually meant to function in real life. Apart from the fact that the laws require the robot to have some form of human-like intelligence, which robots still lack, the laws themselves do not actually work very well. Indeed, Asimov repeatedly showed them to be false in his robot novels, showing time and again how these seemingly watertight rules could produce unintended consequences.[22]

While the literary aspects of robotics are easily dealt with, the precise technical definition of what a robot is remains more of a challenge. The International Organization for Standardization (ISO) defines a robot under ISO 8373. A robot is, 'an automatically controlled, reprogrammable, multipurpose manipulator programmable in three or more axes, which may be either fixed in place or mobile for use in industrial automation applications'.[23] Some find this definition too simplistic, i.e. a microwave oven could be considered a robot by this standard. Others would say that for a machine to be a robot, it should appear to have intent or agency. 'Mental' agency is considered the ability of a robot to make choices, while 'physical' agency is a belief that whatever the controlling device of the machine, the robot should possess limbs or limb-like components. In November 2007, the Society of American Gastrointestinal and Endoscopic Surgeons (SAGES) and the Minimally Invasive Robotic Association (MIRA) produced a consensus document on robotic surgery. The document examined four areas of robotic surgery: training, clinical applications, risks of surgery/cost–benefit analysis and future research. The authors defined 'robotic surgery' as 'a surgical procedure or technology that adds a computer technology-enhanced device to the interaction between a surgeon and a patient during a surgical operation and assumes some degree of control heretofore completely reserved for the surgeon.[24]

The ability of the current generation of surgical robotics is perhaps less alluring than the science fiction. Most readers will now be familiar with the popular da Vinci surgical robotics system (Intuitive Surgical, Sunnyvale, CA, USA). The da Vinci surgical robots are in fact telemanipulators and are controlled by a surgeon sitting at a remote console. The surgeon is provided with a stereoscopic visual display that is collocated with control handles that direct movements of the instruments inside the patient's body (**Figure 60.8a**). As the surgeon directly controls the motion of instruments in the surgical field, the level of autonomy and mental 'agency' in the da Vinci robot is very low. The da Vinci system has been used for a number of types of minimally invasive surgery, including cardiac, abdominal and urology, and, more recently, in head and neck surgery where some authors have reported success in the removal of select tumours through the mouth (**Figure 60.8b–d**).[25, 26, 27] Cadaver experience is also emerging in select centres with the use of robotic transmaxillary approaches to the anterior cranial face.[5] Proponents of robotic surgery point to minimal invasiveness, decreased pain, faster recovery and lower morbidity when compared to equivalent open surgical procedures. Furthermore, motion scaling increases precision and reduces the larger hand movements required by humans while eliminating tremor. Finally, as one author puts it, the robot

surgeon 'suffers no fatigue, does not lose interest or require praise'.[28]

In contrast to using two hands and perhaps a foot pedal, the robotic surgeon seated at a console with the current S-series da Vinci robot can control four arms. One of these arms holds the three-dimensional video camera, a second when used typically holds a retractor, while the remaining two arms are used to interact with the tissue. These latter two working arms generally include a grasping instrument and a cutting instrument. If a surgeon wishes to change instruments, it is necessary that an assistant remove the robotic arm from the patient or operative field, change the instrument and reinsert it into the surgeon's line of sight. Seated at the console, the surgeon can then resume the operation with the new or different instrument. The image of the operative field to the surgeon is truly a three-dimensional one. While the surgeon typically controls the working robotic tool on the right of the visual field with the right hand and the tool on the left of the visual field with the left hand, this control can be easily reversed such that the instrument in the surgeon's right visual field could be controlled by the left hand and vice versa. If one considers that degrees of freedom are measured by the number of joints in the human hand (wrist, metacarpophalangeal and phalangeal), approximately three or four degrees of freedom of motion can be realized. All surgeons have experienced difficulties sewing at one time or another in a cramped operative field. Current robotic tools have a minimum of six degrees of freedom within an inch of the tool's tip with no radioulnar rotational limitations as

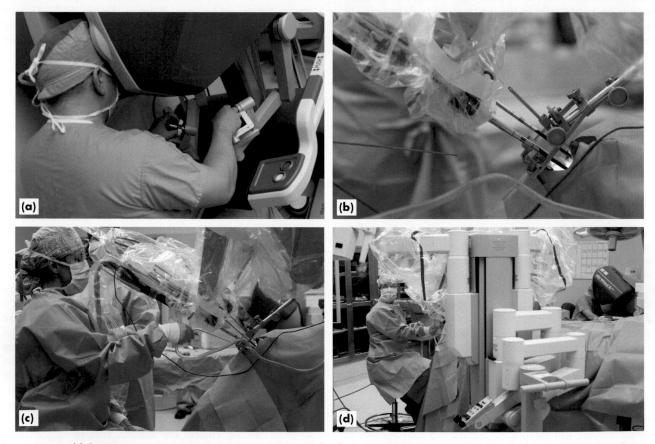

Figure 60.8 (a) Surgeon console for the da Vinci surgical robot. (b–d) Three robotic arms of the da Vinci are inserted through the patient's mouth for transoral robotic surgery.

found in the human forearm. These additional degrees of freedom provide vastly superior freedom of movement than that found with traditional open surgery using human hands or laparoscopic instrumentation. While expensive, the enhanced optical visualization with ability to zoom, the enhanced degrees of freedom, the absolute precision with no tremor, and the optical ability to see around corners, afford current robotic surgeons distinct advantages that should not be dismissed out of hand.

The current generation of robots is expensive, bulky and somewhat unwieldy, and may present particular difficulties in the head and neck arena at present. In addition to the current exorbitant expense, some detractors point to the learning curve, the need for better head and neck instrumentations (for example, transoral retractors) and the lack of tactile or haptic feedback from the robot as the system currently exists. While there may be some debate about the place of robotics in the future of head and neck surgery, it is essential that head and neck surgeons be familiar with certain key characteristics and terminology which will be of use in the design and development of the next generation of surgical robots (**Table 60.1**).

Advancements we can expect to see in robotic surgery in the near future will be in scale and in integration of robotics with fusion of technologies, such as image guidance and computer control. Developments in the area of force feedback will be vital to maintain safety and accuracy as will the development of robotic simulators and patient rehearsal systems. With increasing image and computer control, operators will be able to define 'no go' areas or 'virtual restraints' which will protect surrounding structures or even facilitate head-up graphic representations.[29] It is already possible for surgeons using a patient's computed tomography (CT) scans and magnetic resonance imaging (MRI) to practise an operation in advance of the actual one. Such 'immersion environments' will represent a total fusion of robotics, imaging and allied technologies, permitting a fully interactive graphic visual and oral environment for the surgeon to work in. Advancements in the technologies of haptics currently permit tools on the International Space Station to sense and detect, and distinguish, different types of metal. Preliminary experiments using sensors to detect on contact benign and malignant diseases are underway and exciting.[30]

The most critical near-term issue for the head and neck surgeons concerns the entire existing robotic platform. The arms are designed to rotate around an axis of 15 cm. While ideally suited for the abdominal and thoracic cavities, we have noted it can be quite cumbersome when all of these instruments are placed through the mouth. Space can be quite tight and the instruments are often thumping against teeth or the three-dimensional telescope. Not only is there a great need for better and smaller instrumentations, but the existing design needs to be significantly miniaturized for use in the upper aerodigestive tract. An essential next step for robotics within the aerodigestive tract will be single port access, where endoscope and manipulators are delivered via a single arm or port access. There is some way to go before robots will be autonomously operating on human beings. Artificial intelligence research continues to evolve with exciting new developments occurring in numerous areas, including genetic algorithms and evolutionary

Table 60.1 Important characteristics of robot design and technology.[78]

Characteristic	
Degrees of freedom	Defines the number of independent motions of which a robot is capable, i.e. the number of 'knobs' one can turn to control the tool tip
Resolution workspace	The smallest incremental movement the robot can make or measure
Inertia	All of the area the end effector can reach, the robots workspace is limited by the length of its links, joint limits and collisions with itself and obstructing anatomy
Stiffness	The inertia of a robot is related to its size and material. Higher inertia leads to sluggish movement and a gain in kinetic energy with motion
Force dynamic range	The stiffer the robot is and the less spring-like give it has, the easier it will be to maintain control and accuracy
Force feedback	The ratio between the highest and lowest forces that the robot can exert is known as the 'force dynamic range'
Bandwith of motion	Force feedback control allows the operator of a robot to feel the forces that the robot is exerting on its environment. Sometimes referred to as 'haptics'. As the surgeon's hand moves quickly, the robot's bandwith must be higher than the frequency with which the surgeon is moving or it will fall behind the command

intelligence. New evolving robotic technology will bring significant ethical and legal implications for robotic surgeries.

REPLACEMENT AND REPAIR

Tissue engineering

Regenerative medicine and tissue engineering require two complementary ingredients: cells to replace those lost or damaged, and an ideal milieu in which they can thrive. Great strides are being made in both these areas.

Cells may be obtained as primary cultures from existing, adult, differentiated cells. The big advantage of such an approach over transplantation is that, provided the source of the cells is the recipient patient, there are no questions over rejection and immunosuppression. Primary cells have been used to populate trachea[31] and organ scaffolds as disparate as the bladder and heart.[32, 33] Alternatively, it is possible to use adult mesenchymal stem cells (obtained from bone marrow, fat or other sources) and use culture conditions and growth factors to persuade them to develop into the cell type required.[34, 35] Thus, for example, we have taken adult fat-derived stem cells and used them to generate Schwann cells with the aim of supporting cranial nerve regeneration. In practice, bioengineers are already growing up all the requisite building blocks of head and neck organs in most of our major universities: cartilage, nerve, bone, epithelium and even muscle.

Traditional culture methods are two-dimensional. In order to develop new head and neck tissues, differentiating or differentiated cells need to be grown in three-dimensional matrices in order to truly mimic the cell–cell contact and nutrient environments they will encounter when they are implanted. One approach is to use allogeneic, cadaveric human tissues and decellularize them. However, although these form anatomically contoured supports, questions remain over their true allogenicity. Synthetic polymers have been tried.[36] However, these tend to excite a local immune response, and have high porosity with micrometre-sized fibres, when nanometer dimensions are necessary to truly nest a human cell.[37] An ideal biological scaffold will be: (1) derived from biological sources; (2) made of basic units which can be 'designed' to fit purpose; (3) biodegraded at a controlled rate; (4) non-toxic; (5) supportive of all-round cell–cell interactions; (6) non-inflammatory; (7) cost-effective to produce; (8) transportable; (9) compatible with physiological conditions in man; (10) compatible with other biomaterials. This is a tall order, and one certainly not met by the few matrices presently available,[38] which are, to be fair, aimed primarily at laboratory work and are really little advance on two-dimensional culture on a simple substrate. However, a number of new approaches have arisen from chemistry with self-assembling peptides at the fore.[39] These can incorporate the active regions of guidance or growth molecules as well, such as adhesion molecules, to provide a tailored and 'intelligent' scaffold for replacement tissue growth.

Tissue engineering, stem cell technology and nanotechnology (see below under Nanotechnology) all offer the possibility of creating 'off-the-shelf' tissues and organs. We have already successfully used tissue-engineered patches to reconstruct trachea and bronchus in the clinic,[40] and have used fat-derived stem cells to generate nerve and Schwann cells for reinnervation, while others have 'grown' tissues such as muscle, and 'organs' from stem cells.[41] Combined with implantable, and increasingly small and biocompatible, pacemakers, it is theoretically possible to construct all the component parts of a larynx and make them function as such. However, experience to date with late twentieth century tissue transfer techniques and laryngeal prostheses suggests caution in such predictions.[42] Success in generating phonation and airway protection usually demands a permanent tracheostomy,[43] while success in achieving an adequate airway may lead to problems with phonation and aspiration of food.[44] The human larynx is a unique, three-tiered sphincter supplied by more fine motor control fibres than any other part of the body. It successfully juggles the quite opposing requirements of phonation, deglutition and respiration with ease. Furthermore, it may have an important role in mediating tolerance to inhaled and ingested antigens.[45] We believe that research into tissue engineering for laryngeal, tracheal and other head and neck organ replacement is absolutely justified.

We believe that tissue engineering techniques will offer a better way for long segment replacement of the tracheal airway than transplantation. Tissue engineering applies the principles of engineering, material science and biology towards the development of biological substitutes that restore, maintain or improve tissue function.[46] This process of fabricating new, physiologic, functioning tissues may be obtained by (1) guided tissue regeneration with engineered matrices alone, (2) injection of allogenic or xenogenic cells alone or (3) use of cells seeded on or within matrices (cell matrix construct), with the latter two approaches the most common. The use of isolated cell or cell substitutes avoids potential surgical complications and allows cell manipulation before injection, but has the drawback of possible rejection or loss of function.[41] The use of seeded matrices, the most common method in tissue engineering, is particularly relevant in the present context because these structures are biocompatible, bioabsorbable, non-immunogenic, supportive of cell attachment and growth, and inductive of angiogenesis. They may be created either by isolating the cells from the host's body with a permeable membrane allowing exchange of nutrients (closed system) or by culturing *in vitro* the isolated cells and seeding them on to a scaffold, either synthetic or natural, that is implanted into the host after a given cultivation time (open system).[47] Available evidence suggests that single tissue constructs are unlikely to suffice, and that only a composite (mucosa, connective tissue, cartilage) tissue-engineered graft may substitute functionally for the native airway. We are presently working towards this goal.

Transplantation

Laryngotracheal transplantation has been explored experimentally since almost the dawn of organ transplantation itself.[48, 49] Laryngectomy for irreversible laryngeal disease, usually cancer, is a nineteenth century invention, and leaves recipients with impairment of many of the functions that allow us to interact as human beings. Combined with the recognition that a century of effort has failed to provide autologous or synthetic solutions that can replicate the complex functions of the larynx, the impetus to provide total replacement has been compelling. Despite this need and 40 years of research, however, there has only been one properly documented human total laryngeal transplant.[50] Replacement of the trachea is theoretically less problematic as it does not perform complex neuromuscular actions, unlike the larynx. Nonetheless, the multiplicity of surgical and prosthetic options, augmented by the promise of tissue engineering as above, makes it unlikely that transplantation has anything to offer for static organs.

The arguments against transplantation are persuasive. They are costly and difficult procedures, with unquantified morbidity and mortality.[51] They are presently suitable for only a tiny number of patients. As long as we cannot functionally reinnervate, their outcomes will be no better than those having conventional supportive treatments, such as tracheostomy, laser treatment, sleeve resection and reconstruction.[52] The major target population for transplantation has cancer, and immunosuppression of this group is at best hazardous and at worst unethical.[53] In due course, scientific advances will cure such cancers anyway, and tissue engineering and stem cell technology will provide much better forms of reconstruction.[46] Besides, most people with a laryngectomy have a perfectly acceptable quality of life, so there is no real need for transplantation. These are all cogent arguments which mean that the otolaryngological and thoracic surgical communities are, at best, divided on the future of laryngotracheal transplantation.

There is little doubt that retrieval and implantation of a larynx or trachea represents a major challenge. However, major head and neck cancer operations often take more than 6 hours, and involve a similar number of individual, if different, steps to those required for a transplant, so time alone is not a major consideration. Tracheostomy and gastrostomy are already routine. In our large animal (pig) model, implantation takes a median of 5.5 hours (range, 2.3–9.0).[54] In the National Health Service (NHS), an all-day head and neck cancer operation, preceded by all the necessary preparation and followed by 3 weeks as an inpatient and associated drug costs currently (2010) comes to around £37 000 (US$74 000: Guy's Hospital, London tariff). Our estimates suggest an identical figure for laryngeal and tracheal transplantation for the first six months. However, the continuing costs of immunosuppression give an additional monthly cost of between £350 and £500 (US$700–1000) thereafter (extrapolated from human lung transplant modelling).[55] Our work on tracheal transplantation, also in pigs, suggests a shorter operating time, but similar long-term costs.[56, 57] We argue that these excess costs, for laryngeal transplantation at least, may not be excessive given the potential returns in quality of life.

A failed historical attempt to graft an unmatched, unvascularized mucosal patch into the skeleton of a larynx from which a cancer had been resected has given rise to much pessimism regarding the potential of airway transplantation.[51] However, the qualified success of the first complete, revascularized laryngeal transplant has changed the picture considerably. The recipient, whose larynx had been damaged by trauma, has only had two possible acute rejection episodes in the first few months, and subsequently has regained normal swallowing and speech.[50, 58] On the downside, he retains a tracheostomy and is still on low-dose immunosuppression. Nonetheless, he is essentially well and working as a professional speaker some ten years later (Strome, personal communication). The tolerability of the procedure receives further support from the quality of life rapidly attained by porcine recipients in our own series.

The ideal pool of patients for the first trials would also be those who have irreversible damage due to trauma, as was the case for the 1998 laryngeal transplant. Such patients can generally be managed satisfactorily by conventional techniques,[52] so the pool of potential recipients for early trials at least is small, perhaps between one and 200 in the United Kingdom. Nonetheless, for the reasons stated above, it is both sensible and ethical to transplant this group before embarking on the major challenge of cancer patients. The argument that was used for the first heart transplants, for example, that there is nothing to lose by trials does not apply to either group as death is far from inevitable, even from advanced laryngeal cancer. The operation is targeted at restoration of quality of life and not quantity.

There are approximately 1000 laryngectomies carried out per annum in the UK for cancer.[59] While many of these patients have poor performance status and/or are elderly,

there is a subpopulation of younger, fitter patients with disease limited within the laryngeal skeleton that would be good potential recipients of a transplant. Immunosuppressed patients are, of course, more likely to develop cancers. However, correcting for premorbid smoking and drinking habits, there is little concrete evidence for an increase in head and neck cancer in transplant recipients.[53] Furthermore, increasing numbers of liver transplants are being carried out for patients with hepatic cancer, with good overall results. Although some patients might argue otherwise, it is counterintuitive to immunosuppress someone in order to provide a short-term quality of life gain, only for them to die much sooner from recurrent disease. This is not only what happened to the 1969 patient,[51] but also to the world's first tongue transplant recipient, who also had advanced squamous cancer, in 2004.[60] When we asked laryngectomees this very question, they also flagged this as a major concern.[61]

Part of the problem here lies in our limited understanding of laryngeal and tracheal immunology, although, as with other areas of transplant research, detailed scientific study has led to as many questions as answers to date.[62] For example, there is an unexplained, but possibly significant, difference in graft dendritic cell responses to transplantation between subsites of the same organ, which may lead to differential rates of rejection (**Figure 60.3**). The present documented human laryngeal transplant is maintained on tacrolimus, which may raise the potential for recurrence if applied to patients who have had a cancer laryngectomy. A major breakthrough may have been reached, however, by the startling discovery that rapamycin, and its derivative everolimus, is not only an effective immunosuppressant, but also inhibits the growth of squamous cell cancer *in vitro* and in a rat model.[63] Although the potential effects on wound healing may mitigate against using rapamycin as part of a starting regimen,[64] its early introduction thereafter is almost certainly indicated. This may bring clinical trials in the main, and increasingly a large, target population much closer than we previously thought.

Almost certainly, however, the key issue in determining the viability of laryngeal transplantation is the establishment of functional reinnervation. It has long been known that direct repair of the recurrent laryngeal (main motor) nerve in man does not lead to functional recovery, but rather to a functionless synkinesis where adductor and abductor nerve fibres do not return to their appropriate target muscles.[65] This conundrum has led to nerve and muscle transfer techniques, which 'rob Peter to pay Paul' with mixed evidence of clinical effectiveness to date,[36, 66, 67, 68] although improvements are possible with careful selective intralaryngeal reinnervation.[69] We and others have hypothesized that part of the failure of these techniques lies in the slow rate of progression of reinnervation (1 mm/day), which allows aberrant intralaryngeal sprouting to occur.[70] Thus, we have applied neurotrophins *in vitro* and in nerve transfer experiments in pigs with the aim of improving the speed and accuracy of reinnervation with encouraging results.[71] These methods are now undergoing clinical trials in equine patients with recurrent nerve paralysis and favourable outcomes here should pave the way for similar trials in man. Meanwhile, progress is being made in the development of laryngeal pacemakers, triggered to stimulate abductor (opening) muscles on inspiration. Such devices offer the prospect of immediate return of appropriate respiratory function to a transplanted larynx and might be useful either on a long-term basis, or as a 'babysitter', preserving muscle fibre morphology and type-distribution until reinnervation occurs as a result of selective or transfer techniques, with or without neurotrophin support.

As alternatives to transplantation for patients where conventional reconstruction techniques will not suffice, several experimental and clinical lines of research have been evaluated for tracheal replacement: synthetic substitutes, modified to avoid tissue reaction; implantation of nonviable tissues, including fixed trachea; adaptation and transfer of autogenous tissues, with or without scaffolding of foreign materials as patches or tubes; and tissue engineering as above. All but the latter, which is still developing, have ultimately failed to reproduce a predictable or dependable tracheal substitute, the Achilles heels being the unique vascular supply of the cervical and intrathoracic trachea and biological issues.

The five-year survival of patients undergoing laryngectomy is around 40 per cent. Thus, many people live for years without a larynx. Although there is a very active minority who make the most of things and a few who actually return to work thereafter, the impact on quality of life is profound. A functioning larynx is necessary for normal speech, swallowing, lifting, coughing, straining, sniffing, smelling, tasting and even kissing. These are the very functions that allow us to function in human society, and the impact of their loss should not be underestimated. Many patients become reclusive and depressed, despite putting a brave face on when presenting for follow up in clinic.[72] The loss of a long segment of trachea is, of course, incompatible with life. Our survey of the views of laryngectomees on the acceptability of laryngeal transplantation demonstrated widespread support for the idea, provided the questions of reinnervation and immunosuppression were satisfactorily addressed.[61] Thus, while for some people laryngectomy represents a challenge to be fought and overcome, for many it represents withdrawal from society and most would accept the risks of a transplant if it meant a return to normal functioning and to normal human society.

The arguments against laryngeal transplantation are strong, but may be balanced, individually, by counterarguments. We propose that a twin track of research into airway transplantation, alongside research into tissue-engineering strategies, is essential if we are to be confident that we may ultimately offer functional alternatives to the dehumanizing effects of a mutilating operation (laryngectomy) which has changed little in 150 years.[73]

NANOTECHNOLOGY

Another exciting development that promises much for the future is nanotechnology or nanomedicine. The term 'nanotechnology', derived from the Greek *nanos* or 'dwarf', generally refers to engineering and manufacturing at the molecular or nanometre length scale. One nanometre (nm) is 1 billionth, or 10^{-9} of a metre. To put that scale in context, the comparative size of a nanometre to a metre is the same as that of a marble to the size of the earth. Or put another way, a nanometre is the amount a man's beard grows in the time it takes him to raise the razor to his face. Nanoscale devices are

smaller than human cells (10 000–20 000 nm in diameter) and organelles and similar in size to large biological macromolecules, such as enzymes and receptors. Haemoglobin, for example, is approximately 5 nm in diameter, while the lipid bilayer surrounding cells is 6 nm thick. Nanoscale devices smaller than 50 nm could easily enter most cells, while those

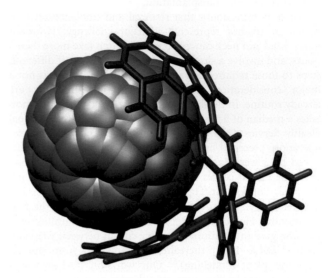

Figure 60.9   A double concave hydrocarbon buckycatcher, a crystal structure of molecular tweezers composed of two corannulene pincers clasping a C60 fullerene. (Copyright of M Stone).

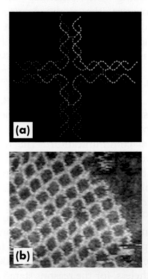

Figure 60.10   Self-assembled DNA nanostructures. (a) DNA 'tile' structure consisting of four branched junctions oriented at 90° intervals. These tiles serve as the primary 'building block' for the assembly of the DNA nanogrids shown in (b). Each tile consists of nine DNA oligonucleotides as shown. (b) An atomic force microscope image of a self-assembled DNA nanogrid. Individual DNA tiles self-assemble into a highly ordered periodic two-dimensional DNA nanogrid. (Copyright Wikimedia (http://upload.wikimedia.org/wikipedia/commons/5/55/DNA_nanostructures.png)).

smaller than 20 nm could transit in and out of blood vessels. As a result, nanoscale devices can readily interact with biomolecules on both the cell surface and within the cell, in ways that do not alter the behaviour and biochemical properties of those molecules.

Constructing nanoscale machines involves two main concepts.[74] In the first, called the 'bottom-up' approach, materials and devices are built from molecular components which assemble themselves chemically by principles of molecular recognition. A variety of molecular machines have been synthesized in this way, including molecular motors switches, sensors and tweezers (**Figure 60.9**). In addition, DNA nanotechnology is an interesting area of current research that uses the bottom-up, self-assembly approach for nanotechnological goals. In DNA nanotechnology, the unique molecular recognition properties of DNA and other nucleic acids is utilized to create self-assembling branched DNA molecules with useful properties. In this application, DNA is used as a structural material rather than as a carrier of biological information to construct three-dimensional structures, such as lattices or tiles (**Figure 60.10**).

In the second, 'top-down' approach, nano-objects are constructed from larger entities without atomic-level control.

These methods create smaller devices by using larger ones to direct their assembly. Microelectromechanical systems (MEMS) is the technology of the very small, and merges at the nanoscale into nanoelectromechanical systems (NEMS) and nanotechnology. NEMS have become practical as they are constructed using modified semiconductor fabrication technologies, normally used to make electronics. These include moulding and plating, wet and dry etching and electro discharge machining, and other technologies capable of manufacturing very small devices. Examples of such nanomachines are shown in **Figure 60.11**.

n the United States, the current potential applications for molecular and NEMS nanoscale technology are being targeted as an important part of the future portfolio of both the National Institute of Health (NIH) and National Institute of Cancer (NIC).[75] Examples of future nanotechnology include 'Trojan Horse' photoactive tumoricidal nanoparticles delivered via monocytes to facilitating cancer therapies in hypoxic areas of tumours.[76] Researchers are also developing nanodevices that can deliver therapeutic doses of radiotherapy within tumours (nanobrachytherapy) with reduced side effects to the surrounding tissues.[77] Gold-coated nanoparticles preferentially accumulate in tumours and research is

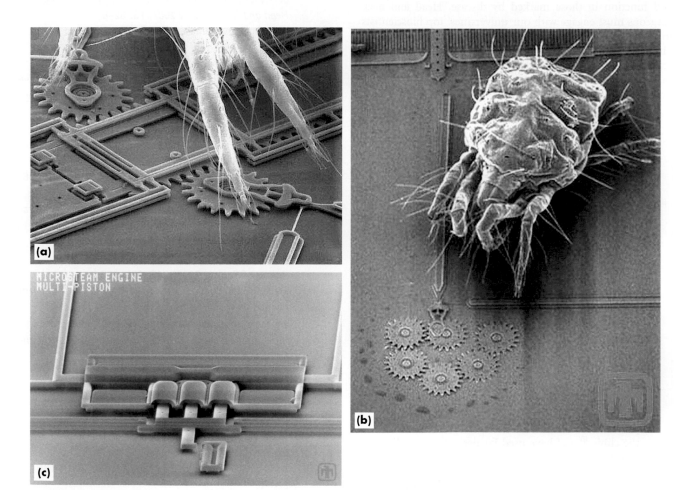

Figure 60.11 Nanoelectomechanical systems (NEMS). (a) Spider mite with legs on a mirror drive assembly; (b) a gear chain with a mite approaching; (c) triple-piston microsteam engine. Water inside three compression cylinders is heated by electric current and vaporizes, pushing the piston out. Capillary forces then retract the piston once the current is removed. (Courtesy of Sandia National Laboratories, SUMMiT™ Technologies, www.memes.sandia.gov).

underway using associated or combined laser technology to selectively thermocoagulate malignant tissue. The Apple Corporation recently announced progress on the development of a 'smart pill' allowing patients, with the use of their Apple computer, to program the specific timed release of their medication based on their individual needs. In the future, we may possibly see multifunctional nanoscale devices called 'nanoclinics' that will have the capability to make *in vivo* diagnosis with molecular nanosensors, treat tumours with a variety of tumoricidal nanodevices and report back their findings while monitoring response to therapy and recurrence.

CONCLUSIONS

It is not possible in a chapter of this size, as the saying goes, to cover the full exciting vista of biotechnology now and in the future. We believe that whether or not complete medical 'cures' for squamous cell carcinoma of the head and neck are developed, the head and neck surgeon of the future will have twin roles as 'pilot' of high-tech outpatient and operating room procedures, and as restorer of normal structure and function in those marked by disease. Head and neck surgeons must engage with our universities' top bioscientists to keep treatment of our patients at the forefront of advance. Finally, we must equip our future specialists with the scholarship to walk alongside the scientists and to adapt to whatever future, this or a completely different one, is presented to them.

KEY LEARNING POINTS

- Minimally invasive surgery (MIS) represents an emerging philosophy in head and neck cancer. Advantages include less morbidity, fewer tracheostomies and reconstructions, shorter hospital stays and improved function compared with traditional surgical and non-surgical techniques.[12, 13, 14, 15]
- In the near future, advancements we can expect to see in robotic surgery will be in scale and in integration of robotics with fusion technologies, such as image guidance and computer control.
- Tissue engineering, stem cell technology and nanotechnology all offer the possibility of creating 'off-the-shelf' tissues and organs. We have already successfully used tissue-engineered patches to reconstruct trachea and bronchus in the clinic,[40] and have used fat-derived stem cells to generate nerve and Schwann cells for reinnervation, while others have 'grown' tissues such as muscle, and 'organs' from stem cells.[41] Tissue engineering will offer a better way for long segment replacement of the tracheal airway than transplantation.

REFERENCES

1. Doll R, Hill AB. Smoking and carcinoma of the lung; preliminary report. *British Medical Journal* 1950; **2**: 739–48.
2. Office of Statistics. Population estimates 2007: Available from: www.statistics.gov.uk/CCI/nugget.asp?ID = 6.
3. Birchall M, Bailey D, King P. Effect of process standards on survival of patients with head and neck cancer in the south and west of England. *British Journal of Cancer* 2004; **91**: 1477–81.
4. Kassam AB, Gardner P, Snyderman C et al. Expanded endonasal approach: fully endoscopic, completely transnasal approach to the middle third of the clivus, petrous bone, middle cranial fossa, and infratemporal fossa. *Neurosurgical Focus* 2005; **19**: E6.
5. Hanna EY, Holsinger C, DeMonte F, Kupferman M. Robotic endoscopic surgery of the skull base: a novel surgical approach. *Archives of Otolaryngology – Head and Neck Surgery* 2007; **133**: 1209–14.
6. Ambrosch P. The role of laser microsurgery in the treatment of laryngeal cancer. *Current Opinion in Otolaryngology and Head and Neck Surgery* 2007; **15**: 82–8.
7. Hartl D. [Transoral laser resection for head and neck cancers]. *Bulletin du Cancer* 2007; **94**: 1081–6.
8. Davis RK, Kriskovich MD, Galloway EB 3rd et al. Endoscopic supraglottic laryngectomy with postoperative irradiation. *Annals of Otology, Rhinology and Laryngology* 2004; **113**: 132–8.
9. Grant DG, Salassa JR, Hinni ML et al. Carcinoma of the tongue base treated by transoral laser microsurgery. Part one: Untreated tumors, a prospective analysis of oncologic and functional outcomes. *Laryngoscope* 2006; **116**: 2150–5.
10. Flora ED, Wilson TG, Martin IJ et al. A review of natural orifice translumenal endoscopic surgery (NOTES) for intra-abdominal surgery: experimental models, techniques, and applicability to the clinical setting. *Annals of Surgery* 2008; **247**: 583–602.
11. Pradier O, Christiansen H, Schmidberger H et al. Adjuvant radiotherapy after transoral laser microsurgery for advanced squamous carcinoma of the head and neck. *International Journal of Radiation Oncology, Biology and Physics* 2005; **63**: 1368–77.
12. Grant DG, Salassa JR, Hinni ML et al. Transoral laser microsurgery for untreated glottic carcinoma. *Otolaryngology – Head and Neck Surgery* 2007; **137**: 482–6.
13. Grant DG, Salassa JR, Hinni ML et al. Transoral laser microsurgery for carcinoma of the supraglottic larynx. *Otolaryngology – Head and Neck Surgery* 2007; **136**: 900–6.
14. Hinni ML, Salassa JR, Grant DG et al. Transoral laser microsurgery for advanced laryngeal cancer. *Archives of Otolaryngology, Head and Neck Surgery* 2007; **133**: 1198–204.

15. Martin A, Jackel MC, Christiansen H et al. Organ preserving transoral laser microsurgery for cancer of the hypopharynx. Laryngoscope 2008; **118**: 398–402.

16. Holsinger FC, Prichard CN, Shapira G et al. Use of the photonic band gap fiber assembly CO_2 laser system in head and neck surgical oncology. Laryngoscope 2006; **116**: 1288–90.

17. Jacobson AS, Woo P, Shapshay SM. Emerging technology: flexible CO_2 laser WaveGuide. Otolaryngology – Head and Neck Surgery 2006; **135**: 469–70.

18. Ayari-Khalfallah S, Fuchsmann C, Froehlich P. Thulium laser in airway diseases in children. Current Opinion in Otolaryngology and Head and Neck Surgery 2008; **16**: 55–9.

19. Koufman JA, Rees CJ, Frazier WD et al. Office-based laryngeal laser surgery: a review of 443 cases using three wavelengths. Otolaryngology – Head and Neck Surgery 2007; **137**: 146–51.

20. Teichmann HO, Herrmann TR, Bach T. Technical aspects of lasers in urology. World Journal of Urology 2007; **25**: 221–5.

21. 'Robot'. Merriam Webster Online Dictionary. 2008. Accessed April 5, 2008. Available from: www.merriam-webster.com/dictionary/robot.

22. Asimov I. The robots of dawn. New York: Bantham Books, 1994.

23. International Organization for Standardization. ISO8373, 1996. Available from: www.iso.org/iso/iso_catalogue/catalogue_ics/catalogue_detail_ics.htm?csnumber=26798&ICS1=25&ICS2=40&ICS3=30.

24. Herron DM, Marohn M. A consensus document on robotic surgery. Surgical Endoscopy 2008; **22**: 313–25; discussion 1–2.

25. Solares CA, Strome M. Transoral robot-assisted CO_2 laser supraglottic laryngectomy: experimental and clinical data. Laryngoscope 2007; **117**: 817–20.

26. Weinstein GS, O'Malley BW Jr, Snyder W, Hockstein NG. Transoral robotic surgery: supraglottic partial laryngectomy. Annals of Otology, Rhinology, and Laryngology 2007; **116**: 19–23.

27. Genden EM, Desai S, Sung CK. Transoral robotic surgery for the management of head and neck cancer: a preliminary experience. Head and Neck 2009; **31**: 283–9.

28. Gerhardus D. Robot-assisted surgery: the future is here. Journal of Healthcare Management 2003; **48**: 242.

29. Satava RM. Emerging technologies for surgery in the 21st century. Archives of Surgery 1999; **134**: 1197–202.

30. Andrews RJ, Mah RW. The NASA Smart Probe Project for real-time multiple microsensor tissue recognition. Stereotactic and Functional Neurosurgery 2003; **80**: 114–19.

31. Genden EM, Mackinnon SE, Yu S et al. Pretreatment with portal venous ultraviolet B-irradiated donor alloantigen promotes donor-specific tolerance to rat nerve allografts. Laryngoscope 2001; **111**: 439–47.

32. Atala A, Bauer SB, Soker S et al. Tissue-engineered autologous bladders for patients needing cystoplasty. Lancet 2006; **367**: 1241–6.

33. Mirensky TL, Breuer CK. The development of tissue-engineered grafts for reconstructive cardiothoracic surgical applications. Pediatric Research 2008; **63**: 559–68.

34. Kafienah W, Mistry S, Perry MJ et al. Pharmacological regulation of adult stem cells: chondrogenesis can be induced using a synthetic inhibitor of the retinoic acid receptor. Stem Cells 2007; **25**: 2460–8.

35. Suzuki T, Kobayashi K, Tada Y et al. Regeneration of the trachea using a bioengineered scaffold with adipose-derived stem cells. Annals of Otology, Rhinology, and Laryngology 2008; **117**: 453–63.

36. Birchall M, Idowu B, Murison P et al. Laryngeal abductor muscle reinnervation in a pig model. Acta Otolaryngologica 2004; **124**: 839–46.

37. Gelain F, Horii A, Zhang S. Designer self-assembling peptide scaffolds for 3-d tissue cell cultures and regenerative medicine. Macromolecular Bioscience 2007; **7**: 544–51.

38. Kleinman HK, McGarvey ML, Hassell JR et al. Basement membrane complexes with biological activity. Biochemistry 1986; **25**: 312–18.

39. Bromley EH, Channon K, Moutevelis E, Woolfson DN. Peptide and protein building blocks for synthetic biology: from programming biomolecules to self-organized biomolecular systems. ACS Chemical Biology 2008; **3**: 38–50.

40. Macchiarini P, Walles T, Biancosino C, Mertsching H. First human transplantation of a bioengineered airway tissue. Journal of Thoracic and Cardiovascular Surgery 2004; **128**: 638–41.

41. Vacanti JP, Langer R. Tissue engineering: the design and fabrication of living replacement devices for surgical reconstruction and transplantation. Lancet 1999; **354**(Suppl. 1): S132–4.

42. Tack JW, Rakhorst G, van der Houwen EB et al. In vitro evaluation of a double-membrane-based voice-producing element for laryngectomized patients. Head and Neck 2007; **29**: 665–74.

43. Pearson BW. Subtotal laryngectomy. Laryngoscope 1981; **91**: 1904–12.

44. Sesterhenn AM, Dunne AA, Werner JA. Complications after CO_2 laser surgery of laryngeal cancer in the elderly. Acta Otolaryngologica 2006; **126**: 530–5.

45. Barker E, Haverson K, Stokes CR et al. The larynx as an immunological organ: immunological architecture in the pig as a large animal model. Clinical and Experimental Immunology 2006; **143**: 6–14.

46. Langer R, Vacanti JP. Tissue engineering. Science 1993; **260**: 920–6.

47. Fuchs JR, Nasseri BA, Vacanti JP. Tissue engineering: a 21st century solution to surgical reconstruction. Annals of Thoracic Surgery 2001; **72**: 577–91.

48. Work WP, Boles R. Larynx: replantation in the dog. *Archives of Otolaryngology* 1965; **82**: 401–2.

49. Ogura JH, Harvey JE, Mogi G *et al.* Further experimental observations of transplantation of canine larynx. *Laryngoscope* 1970; **80**: 1231–43.

50. Strome M, Stein J, Esclamado R *et al.* Laryngeal transplantation and 40-month follow-up. *New England Journal of Medicine* 2001; **344**: 1676–9.

51. Kluyskens P, Ringoir S. Follow-up of a human larynx transplantation. *Laryngoscope* 1970; **80**: 1244–50.

52. Grillo HC. Tracheal replacement: a critical review. *Annals of Thoracic Surgery* 2002; **73**: 1995–2004.

53. Birkeland SA, Lokkegaard H, Storm HH. Cancer risk in patients on dialysis and after renal transplantation. *Lancet* 2000; **355**: 1886–7.

54. Birchall MA, Bailey M, Barker EV *et al.* Model for experimental revascularized laryngeal allotransplantation. *British Journal of Surgery* 2002; **89**: 1470–5.

55. Sharples LD, Taylor GJ, Karnon J *et al.* A model for analyzing the cost of the main clinical events after lung transplantation. *Journal of Heart and Lung Transplantation* 2001; **20**: 474–82.

56. Macchiarini P. Trachea-guided generation: déjà vu all over again? *Journal of Thoracic and Cardiovascular Surgery* 2004; **128**: 14–16.

57. Macchiarini P, Mazmanian GM, de Montpreville VT *et al.* Experimental tracheal and tracheoesophageal allotransplantation. Paris-Sud University Lung Transplantation Group. *Journal of Thoracic and Cardiovascular Surgery* 1995; **110**: 1037–46.

58. Lorenz RR, Hicks DM, Shields RW Jr *et al.* Laryngeal nerve function after total laryngeal transplantation. *Otolaryngology – Head and Neck Surgery* 2004; **131**: 1016–18.

59. Wight RG, Puttnam G. *Database for head and neck oncology.* First annual report. London: NHS Executive, 2006.

60. Birchall MA. Tongue transplantation. *Lancet* 2004; **363**: 1663.

61. Potter CP, Birchall MA. Laryngectomees' views on laryngeal transplantation. *Transplant International* 1998; **11**: 433–8.

62. Rees LE, Jones PH, Ayoub O *et al.* Smoking influences the immunological architecture of the human larynx. *Clinical Immunology* 2006; **118**: 342–7.

63. Knott PD, Tamai H, Strome M *et al.* RAD inhibition of sarcoma growth: implications for laryngeal transplantation. *American Journal of Otolaryngology* 2007; **28**: 375–8.

64. Knight RJ, Villa M, Laskey R *et al.* Risk factors for impaired wound healing in sirolimus-treated renal transplant recipients. *Clinical Transplantation* 2007; **21**: 460–5.

65. Crumley RL. Laryngeal synkinesis revisited. *Annals of Otology, Rhinology, and Laryngology* 2000; **109**: 365–71.

66. Fex S. Functioning remobilization of vocal cords in cats with permanent recurrent laryngeal nerve paresis. *Acta Otolaryngologica* 1970; **69**: 294–301.

67. Crumley RL. Phrenic nerve graft for bilateral vocal cord paralysis. *Laryngoscope* 1983; **93**: 425–8.

68. Marie JP, Dehesdin D, Ducastelle T, Senant J. Selective reinnervation of the abductor and adductor muscles of the canine larynx after recurrent nerve paralysis. *Annals of Otology, Rhinology, and Laryngology* 1989; **98**: 530–6.

69. Damrose EJ, Huang RY, Ye M *et al.* Surgical anatomy of the recurrent laryngeal nerve: implications for laryngeal reinnervation. *Annals of Otology, Rhinology, and Laryngology* 2003; **112**: 434–8.

70. Lewis WS, Crumley RL, Blanks RH, Pitcock JK. Does intralaryngeal motor nerve sprouting occur following unilateral recurrent laryngeal nerve paralysis? *Laryngoscope* 1991; **101**: 1259–63.

71. Kingham PJ, Hughes A, Mitchard L *et al.* Effect of neurotrophin-3 on reinnervation of the larynx using the phrenic nerve transfer technique. *European Journal of Neuroscience* 2007; **25**: 331–40.

72. Devins GM, Stam HJ, Koopmans JP. Psychosocial impact of laryngectomy mediated by perceived stigma and illness intrusiveness. *Canadian Journal of Psychiatry* 1994; **39**: 608–16.

73. Stell PM. The first laryngectomy. *Journal of Laryngology and Otology* 1975; **89**: 353–8.

74. Silva GA. Introduction to nanotechnology and its applications to medicine. *Surgical Neurology* 2004; **61**: 216–20.

75. US Department of Health and Human Services, National Institutes of Health. Cancer nanotechnology plan. A strategic initiative to transform clinical oncology and basic research through the directed application of nanotechnology. Available from: http://nano.cancer.gov/objects/pdfs/Cancer_Nanotechnology_Plan-508.pdf. National Cancer Institute, July 2004.

76. Choi MR, Stanton-Maxey KJ, Stanley JK *et al.* A cellular Trojan Horse for delivery of therapeutic nanoparticles into tumors. *Nano Letters* 2007; **7**: 3759–65.

77. Khan MK, Minc LD, Nigavekar SS *et al.* Fabrication of {198AuO} radioactive composite nanodevices and their use for nanobrachytherapy. *Nanomedicine* 2008; **4**: 57–69.

78. Camarillo DB, Krummel TM, Salisbury JK Jr. Robotic technology in surgery: past, present, and future. *American Journal of Surgery* 2004; **188**(Suppl.): 2S–15S.

Index

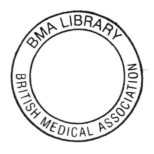